HOW TO USE

The Pearson Nurse's Drug Guide 2023

CLASSIFICATIONS AND PROTOTYPE DRUGS

The classifications used in this book are based on the system used by the American Hospital Formulary Service (AHFS). This book further classifies drugs by therapeutic uses, enabling the nurse to identify drugs in the same class that have similar indications for use. Thus, the book provides a framework for understanding how drugs in a given class are used in clinical practice. The pharmacologic classification appears immediately after the **Classification** heading, followed by the **Therapeutic** classification. In general, drugs in a class will have similar actions, uses, adverse effects, and nursing implications. Therefore, we have selected certain drugs that are representative of a classification or its subclassification—**prototype drugs**—to aid the nurse in understanding the classification of drugs. Prototype drug monographs are identified with a small icon. **Pr** The user can refer to the prototype drug to develop a better understanding of drugs that belong within the same classification or subclassification. When a drug belongs to a classification that has a designated prototype drug, that prototype is identified directly below the therapeutic classification. Medications that are designated by the Institute for Safe Medication Practices (ISMP) as **high alert** medications **A** have an icon indicating this. All prototype drugs are highlighted in **bold** type in the index for quick identification. Some drugs have a unique mechanism of action or therapeutic effect. In these cases, there is no prototype drug to be identified.

AMIODARONE HYDROCHLORIDE Pr

(a-mee'oh-da-rone)

Cordarone, Nexterone, Pacerone

Classification: ANTIARRHYTHMIC, CLASS III

Therapeutic: CLASS III ANTIARRHYTHMIC; ANTIANGINAL

PREGNANCY CATEGORY

In December 2014, the FDA released a final rule replacing the historic "letter categories" with new detailed subsections describing the risk of medication exposure in the real-world context of caring for pregnant patients. Refer to Appendix C, *FDA Pregnancy Information*, for additional details.

CONTROLLED SUBSTANCES

In the United States, **Controlled Substances** are classified as belonging to one of five schedules (I to V) according to abuse potential. Schedule I has the highest and Schedule V has the lowest potential for abuse. When a drug is a controlled substance, information about the schedule of the drug is found at the bottom of the yellow box. Refer to Appendix B, *U.S. Schedules of Controlled Substances*, for a complete description of each schedule.

AVAILABILITY

Because drugs come in a variety of dosages and forms, the authors include a section devoted to **Availability** in each monograph. This section identifies the available dosage forms (e.g., tablets, capsules).

> **AVAILABILITY** Tablet; injection

ACTION & *THERAPEUTIC EFFECT*

Each monograph describes the **Action** by which the specific drug produces physiologic and biochemic changes at the cellular, tissue, and organ levels. This information helps the user understand how the drug works in the body and makes it easier to learn its adverse reactions, and cautious uses. The ***Therapeutic Effect,*** which is set in italics for clarity and ease of use is the reason why a drug is prescribed. Therapeutic effectiveness of the drug can be determined by monitoring improvement in the condition for which the drug is prescribed.

> **ACTION & *THERAPEUTIC EFFECT*** Acts directly on all cardiac tissues by prolonging duration of action potential and refractory period. Slows conduction time through the AV node and can interrupt the reentry pathways through the AV node. *Effective in prevention or suppression of cardiac arrhythmias.*

USES AND UNLABELED USES

The therapeutic applications of each drug are described in terms of approved (i.e., FDA-labeled) **Uses** and **Unlabeled Uses.** An unlabeled use is one that does not appear on the drug label or in the manufacturer's literature but is supported by medical literature or expert consensus.

> **USES** Prophylaxis and treatment of life-threatening ventricular arrhythmias and supraventricular arrhythmias, particularly with atrial fibrillation.
>
> **UNLABELED USES** Treatment of nonexertional angina, conversion of atrial fibrillation to normal sinus rhythm, paroxysmal supraventricular tachycardia, ventricular rate control due to accessory pathway conduction in pre-excited atrial arrhythmia, after defibrillation and epinephrine in cardiac arrest, AV nodal reentry tachycardia.

CONTRAINDICATIONS AND CAUTIOUS USE

Many drugs have **Contraindications** and therefore should not be used in specific conditions, such as during pregnancy or pathologic disorders. In other cases, the drug requires **Cautious Use** because of a greater than average risk of untoward effects.

> **CONTRAINDICATIONS** Hypersensitivity to amiodarone, iodine, or benzyl alcohol; cardiogenic shock, severe sinus bradycardia, second- or third-degree AV block unless a pacemaker is available, severe sinus-node dysfunction or sick sinus syndrome, bradycardia causing syncope (except in patients with functioning

pacemaker); congenital or acquired QR prolongation syndromes, or history of torsades de pointes; pregnancy (category D); lactation.

CAUTIOUS USE Severe hepatic disease, cirrhosis; Hashimoto's thyroiditis, goiter, thyrotoxicosis, or history of other thyroid dysfunction; severe hepatic impairment; HF, older adults; Fabry disease especially with visual disturbances; electrolyte imbalance, hypokalemia, hypomagnesemia, hypovolemia; preexisting lung disease, COPD; open heart surgery.

ROUTE & DOSAGE

The **Routes and Dosages** are highlighted in a blue box for easy access. Route of administration is specified as subcutaneous, IM, IV, PO, PR, nasal, ophthalmic, vaginal, topical, aural, intradermal, or intrathecal. Dosages are listed according to indication or FDA-approved labeled use(s). The guide includes adult, adolescent, geriatric, and pediatric dosages, as well as dosages for neonates and infants whenever applicable. This section also indicates dosage adjustments for renal impairment (based on creatinine clearance), hepatic impairment, patients undergoing hemodialysis, and obese patients (based on ideal body weight), as well as chemotherapeutic dosage adjustments based on toxicity adjustments. Additionally, information about the need for dosage adjustments based on pharmacogenetic variables [e.g., cytochrome (CYP) system of enzymes] is provided as available.

ROUTE & DOSAGE

Arrhythmias

Adult: **PO Loading Dose** 800–1600 mg/day in 1–2 doses for 1–3 wk **PO Maintenance Dose** 400–600 mg/day in 1–2 doses; **IV Loading Dose** 150 mg over 10 min followed by 360 mg over next 6 h; **IV Maintenance Dose** 540 mg over 18 h (0.5 mg/min), may continue at 0.5 mg/min; **Convert IV to PO** Duration of infusion less than 1 wk use 800–1600 mg; **PO,** 1–3 wk use 600–800 mg; **PO,** greater than 3 wk use 400 mg

Child: **IV** 5 mg/kg then repeat (max: 300 mg total)

Hepatic Impairment Dosage Adjustment

Adjustment only suggested in severe hepatic impairment

ADMINISTRATION

Drug administration is an important primary role for the nurse. Organized by different routes, the **Administration** section lists comprehensive instructions for administering, handling, and storing medications.

ADMINISTRATION

- Note: Correct hypokalemia and hypomagnesemia prior to initiation of therapy.

Oral

- Give consistently with respect to meals. Avoid grapefruit juice.
- Note: Only a prescriber experienced with the drug and treatment of life-threatening

- arrhythmias should give loading doses.
- Note: GI symptoms commonly occur during high-dose therapy, especially with loading doses. Symptoms usually respond to dose reduction or divided dose given with food, including milk.

INTRAVENOUS DRUG ADMINISTRATION

Within the **Administration** section of appropriate monographs, the authors highlight intravenous drugs, indicated by a vertical color bar. This section provides users with comprehensive instructions on how to **Prepare** and **Administer** direct, intermittent, and continuous intravenous medications. When different from adults, intravenous administration and preparation for pediatric patients is provided. It also includes **Solution/Additive** and **Y-Site** incompatibility for every monograph, where appropriate, to indicate which drugs and solutions should not be mixed with the intravenous drug. This is crucial information for drug administration. A chart for **Y-Site Compatibility** for common intravenous drugs is located inside the back cover of this drug guide. These enhancements eliminate the need for additional resources for intravenous administration.

Intravenous

PREPARE: **IV Infusion: First rapid loading dose infusion:** Add 150 mg (3 mL) amiodarone to 100 mL D5W to yield 1.5 mg/mL. **Second infusion during first 24 h (slow loading dose and maintenance infusion):** Add 900 mg (18 mL) amiodarone to 500 mL D5W to yield 1.8 mg/mL. **Maintenance infusions after the first 24 h:** Prepare concentrations of 1–6 mg/mL amiodarone. Note: Use central line to give concentrations greater than 2 mg/mL.

ADMINISTER: **IV Infusion:** Initial infusion rate should not exceed 30 mg/min. Loading dose is usually given over 10 min in adults and 20–60 min in children. Note: See manufacturer's guidelines for **Nexterone** administration.

INCOMPATIBILITIES: **Solution/additive: Aminophylline, amoxicillin/clavulanic acid, cefazolin, floxacillin, furosemide. Y-site: Acyclovir, allopurinol, amifostine, aminocaproic acid, aminophylline, amoxicillin, ampicillin, ampicillin / sulbactam, argatroban, atenolol, bivalirudin, cefamandole, cefazolin, cefotaxime, cefotetan, ceftazidime, ceftopribole, chloramphenicol, cytarabine, dantrolene, dexamethasone, diazepam, digoxin, doxorubicin, ertapenem, fludarabine, fluorouracil, foscarnet, fosphenytoin, ganciclovir, gemtuzumab, heparin, hydrocortisone, imipenem/cilastatin, ketorolac, leucovorin, levofloxacin, magnesium sulfate, mechlorethamine, melphalan, meropenem, methotrexate, micafungin, mitomycin, paclitaxel, pentobarbital, phenytoin, piperacillin, piperacillin/tazobactam, potassium acetate, potassium phosphate, sodium bicarbonate, sodium phosphate, SMZ/TMP, thiopental, thiotepa, tigecycline, verapamil.**

ADVERSE EFFECTS

Virtually all drugs have **Adverse Effects** that may be bothersome to some individuals but not to others. Adverse effects with an incidence of ≥5% are listed by body system or organs. The most common adverse effects (those with reported incidence over 25%) appear in *italic* type, whereas those that are life-threatening are underlined. Users of the drug guide will find a key at the bottom of every page as a quick reminder. Events are organized following a head to toe patient assessment model.

> **ADVERSE EFFECTS** **CV:** Bradycardia, *hypotension* (IV), sinus arrest, cardiogenic shock, CHF, arrhythmias; AV block. **Respiratory:** (Pulmonary toxicity) Alveolitis, pneumonitis (fever, dry cough, dyspnea), interstitial pulmonary fibrosis, *fatal gasping syndrome* with IV in children. **CNS:** Peripheral neuropathy (*muscle weakness,* wasting numbness, tingling), *fatigue,* abnormal gait, dyskinesias, *dizziness,* paresthesia, headache. **HEENT:** *Corneal microdeposits,* blurred vision, optic neuritis, optic neuropathy, permanent blindness, corneal degeneration, macular degeneration, photosensitivity. **Endocrine:** Hyperthyroidism or hypothyroidism; may cause neonatal hypo- or hyperthyroidism if taken during pregnancy. **Skin:** Slate-blue pigmentation, *photosensitivity,* rash. **GI:** *Anorexia, nausea, vomiting, constipation,* hepatotoxicity. **Other:** With chronic use, angioedema.

DIAGNOSTIC TEST INTERFERENCE

Diagnostic Test Interference describes the effect of the drug on various tests and alerts the nurse to possible misinterpretations of test results when applicable. Also listed are lab tests that may have inaccurate results due to effects of the drug. The name of the specific test altered is highlighted in ***bold italic*** type.

> **DIAGNOSTIC TEST INTERFERENCE** Affects ***thyroid function tests***, causing an increase in serum T_4 and serum reverse T_3 levels, and a decline in serum T_3 levels.

INTERACTIONS

When applicable, this section lists individual drugs, drug classes, foods, and herbs that have relevant interactions with the drug discussed in the monograph. Drugs may interact to inhibit or enhance one another. Thus, drug interactions may improve the therapeutic response, lead to therapeutic failure, or produce specific adverse reactions. Only drugs that have been shown to cause clinically significant and documented interactions with the drug discussed in the monograph are identified. Note that generic drugs appear in **bold** type, and drug classes appear in SMALL CAPS.

> **INTERACTIONS** **Drug:** Significantly increases **digoxin** levels; enhances pharmacologic effects and toxicities of **disopyramide, procainamide, quinidine, flecainide, lidocaine, lovastatin, simvastatin;** anticoagulant effects

of ORAL ANTICOAGULANTS enhanced; **verapamil, diltiazem,** BETA-ADRENERGIC BLOCKING AGENTS may potentiate sinus bradycardia, sinus arrest, or AV block; may increase **phenytoin** levels 2- to 3-fold; **cholestyramine** may decrease amiodarone levels; **fentanyl** may cause bradycardia, hypotension, or decreased output; may increase **cyclosporine** levels and toxicity; **cimetidine** may increase amiodarone levels; **ritonavir** may increase risk of amiodarone toxicity, including cardiotoxicity; **simvastatin** doses over 20 mg increase risk of rhabdomyolysis; **loratadine** use may increase risk of QT prolongation. **Food: Grapefruit juice** may increase amiodarone concentrations. **Herbal: Echinacea** may increase hepatotoxicity, **St. John's wort** may decrease efficacy.

PHARMACOKINETICS

This section identifies how the drug moves throughout the body. **Pharmacokinetics** lists the mechanisms of absorption, distribution, metabolism, elimination, and half-life when known. It also provides information about onset, peak, and duration of the drug action. Where appropriate, information appears for protein-binding and CYP450 impact.

PHARMACOKINETICS Absorption: 22–86% absorbed. **Onset (PO):** 2–3 days to 1–3 wk. **Peak:** 3–7 h. **Distribution:** Concentrates in adipose tissue, lungs, kidneys, spleen; crosses placenta; 96% protein bound. **Metabolism:** Extensively in liver; undergoes some enterohepatic cycling; via CYP2C8 and 3A4. **Elimination:** Excreted chiefly in bile and feces; also in breast milk. **Half-Life:** Biphasic, initial 2.5–10 days, terminal 40–55 days.

NURSING IMPLICATIONS

Under the headings **Black Box Warning, Assessment & Drug Effects,** and **Patient & Family Education,** the nurse can quickly and easily identify needed information and incorporate it into the appropriate steps of the nursing process. Before administering a drug, the nurse should read **Nursing Implications** to determine the assessments that should be made before and after administration of the drug, the indicators of drug effectiveness, laboratory tests recommended for individual drugs, and the essential patient and/or family education related to the drug.

BLACK BOX WARNING

The U.S. Food and Drug Administration (FDA) can require a pharmaceutical manufacturer to place a warning in the literature describing potentially serious or life-threatening risks associated with a prescription drug. This type of warning is commonly referred to as a "black box warning" because it appears in the manufacturer's literature printed as a box outlined in black. If a drug has a black box warning, the warning will appear in each monograph directly under the **Nursing Implication** heading.

NURSING IMPLICATIONS

Black Box Warning

Amiodarone has been associated with pulmonary toxicity (sometimes severe and potentially fatal), liver injury (ranging from mild to severe), and development of arrhythmias (heart block or sinus bradycardia).

Assessment & Drug Effects

- Monitor BP carefully during infusion and slow the infusion if significant hypotension occurs; bradycardia should be treated by slowing the infusion or discontinuing if necessary. Monitor heart rate and rhythm and BP until drug response has stabilized; report promptly symptomatic bradycardia. Sustained monitoring is essential because drug has an unusually long half-life.
- Monitor for S&S of: Adverse effects, particularly conduction disturbances and exacerbation of arrhythmias, in patients receiving other antiarrhythmic drugs; drug-induced hypothyroidism or hyperthyroidism (see Appendix F), especially during early treatment period; pulmonary toxicity (progressive dyspnea, fatigue, cough, pleuritic pain, fever) throughout therapy.
- Monitor for elevations of AST and ALT. If elevations persist or if they are 2–3 times above normal baseline readings, reduce dosage or withdraw drug promptly to prevent hepatotoxicity and liver damage.
- Auscultate chest periodically or when patient complains of respiratory symptoms. Check for diminished breath sounds, rales, pleuritic friction rub; observe breathing pattern. Drug-induced pulmonary function problems **must be** distinguished from CHF or pneumonia. Keep prescriber informed.
- Anticipate possible CNS symptoms within a week after amiodarone therapy begins. Proximal muscle weakness, a common side effect, intensified by tremors presents a great hazard to the ambulating patient. Assess severity of symptoms. Supervision of ambulation may be indicated.
- Monitor lab tests: Baseline and periodic serum electrolytes (i.e., potassium and magnesium); baseline and semiannual LFTs; baseline and periodic thyroid functions.

Patient & Family Education

- Check pulse daily once stabilized, or as prescribed. Report a pulse less than 60.
- Take oral drug consistently with respect to meals. Do not drink grapefruit juice while taking this drug.
- Become familiar with potential adverse reactions and report those that are bothersome to the prescriber.
- Use dark glasses to ease photophobia; some patients may not be able to go outdoors in the daytime even with such protection.
- Follow recommendation for regular ophthalmic exams, including funduscopy and slit-lamp exam.
- Wear protective clothing and a barrier-type sunscreen that physically blocks penetration of skin by ultraviolet light to prevent a photosensitivity reaction (erythema, pruritus); avoid exposure to sun and sunlamps.

THERAPEUTIC EFFECTIVENESS

Therapeutic effectiveness of a drug can be determined by monitoring improvement in the condition for which the drug is prescribed, and by using the **Assessment & Drug Effects** section. Drugs have multiple uses or indications. Therefore, it is important to know why a drug is being prescribed for a specific patient (**Uses** and **Unlabeled Uses**). In the italicized sentences at the end of the **Action &** ***Therapeutic Effect*** section in all monographs, specific indicators of the effectiveness of the drug are provided. Additionally, in the **Route & Dosage** table for each drug, the dosages are listed according to the indications for FDA-labeled use(s) of the drug. Furthermore, the **Therapeutic** classifications listed within the tan box at the beginning of the monograph provide the nurse with further assistance in determining and evaluating the therapeutic effectiveness of the drug.

PEARSON NURSE'S DRUG GUIDE 2023

Kelly M. Shields, PharmD
Associate Dean and Professor of Pharmacy Practice
Raabe College of Pharmacy
Ohio Northern University
Ada, Ohio

Kami L. Fox, DNP, RN, APRN, CPNP-PC
Director/Chair and Associate Professor of Nursing
Ohio Northern University
Ada, Ohio

Christina Liebrecht, DNP, RN, CNE
Associate Professor of Nursing
Ohio Northern University
Ada, Ohio

Pearson

Content Management: Kevin Wilson
Content Production: Michael Giacobbe
Product Management: SPi Global
Product Marketing: Brian Hoel
Rights and Permissions: SPi Global

Please contact https://support.pearson.com/getsupport/s/ with any queries on this content

Notice: The authors and the publisher of this volume have taken care to make certain that the doses of drugs and schedules of treatment are correct and compatible with the standards generally accepted at the time of publication. Nevertheless, as new information becomes available, changes in treatment and in the use of drugs become necessary.

The reader is advised to carefully consult the instruction and information material included in the package insert of each drug or therapeutic agent before administration. This advice is especially important when using, administering, or recommending new and infrequently used drugs. The authors and publisher disclaim all responsibility for any liability, loss, injury, or damage incurred as a consequence, directly or indirectly, of the use and application of any of the contents of this volume.

Cover Image by kavione/Shutterstock

CIP available at the Library of Congress.

4 2022

Pearson

ISBN-10: 0-13-767668-9
ISBN-13: 978-0-13-767668-2

CONTENTS

To

Rick, Kris, Leah, and Katelyn for their willing sacrifice of time and their patience.

♦

To

Frostie, the first nurse that loved and cared for me. My parents Karron, Marion, and my family: Ken, Amelia, Nolan, and Sophia for their unconditional love, support, and guiding light that allow me to provide safe and compassionate care to others.

♦

My family—Amanda, Rachel, and Brie—Thank you for all of your love, encouragement, laughter, and support and in loving memory of my husband, Jay. And, my students, who soak up learning and inspire me.

♦

And a special thank you to Billie Ann Wilson and Margaret T. Shannon;

without whom this work would not have been possible

ABOUT THE AUTHORS

Kelly M. Shields is currently Associate Dean and Professor of Pharmacy Practice at Ohio Northern University's RaabeCollege of Pharmacy. She holds a Doctor of Pharmacy from Butler University and completed a fellowship in Natural Product Information and Research at University of Missouri-Kansas City. She has practiced pharmacy in retail, community, and academic settings and has worked as a freelance medical writer.

Kami L. Fox is the Director of Nursing and the School of Health and Behavioral Sciences. She is an Associate Professor of Nursing at Ohio Northern University. She holds a BS and MS in Nursing from Wright StateUniversity in Dayton, Ohio, and a DNP from the University of Toledo. She is a certified pediatric nurse practitioner in primary care.

Christina M. Liebrecht is Associate Professor of Nursing at Ohio Northern University. She holds a BS in Nursing from University of Toledo, an MS in Nursing from Walden University, and Doctorate in Nursing Practice from the University of Toledo. She has a focus on medical surgical nursing, fundamentals of nursing, and nursing education as well as the use of simulation to support student learning and safe practice. She continues to practice as a medical surgical nurse in the acute care setting.

PHARMACY CONSULTANT

A special acknowledgment to **Zachary Woods, PharmD, RPh,** who is a tremendous addition to the author team as a contributor for the monographs of the new drugs in this edition. We are grateful for his expertise and for his valued input.

EDITORIAL REVIEW PANEL

We wish to thank the following individuals for conducting thorough reviews of the drug information in this book for its accuracy, currency, relevance, presentation, accessibility, and use. Their feedback guided us in developing a better book for nurses.

Nile Barnes, Pharm.D.
The University of Texas at Austin
Austin, TX

Karen Bastianelli, Pharm.D.
University of Minnesota
Duluth, MN

Kalin M. Clifford, Pharm.D.
Texas Tech University Health Center
Dallas, TX

Vinh N. Kieu, Pharm.D
George Mason University
Fairfax, VA

PREFACE

Pearson Nurse's Drug Guide 2023 is a current and reliable reference designed to provide comprehensive information needed to make appropriate decisions regarding drug administration. This new edition includes 15 new monographs for drugs recently approved by the Food and Drug Administration (FDA), and over 220 updates to drug indications, available dosage forms, adverse effects, dosages, and more.

Each drug monograph provides the necessary information for safe and effective drug administration. The user should read all the information provided. Occasionally, the user will be referred to Appendix E, *Glossary of Key Terms, Clinical Conditions, and Associated Signs and Symptoms*. This unique glossary provides valuable information regarding common assessment findings related to therapeutic effectiveness or ineffectiveness of specific drugs.

The authors recognize that the decision-making process related to drug administration is a cyclical one. For example, assessments are made both prior to and after drug administration. Thus, nursing diagnoses and interventions may change as a result of an *achieved therapeutic effect, therapeutic failure, manifestation of an adverse effect,* or *demonstration of a learning need*. The authors believe that the users of this drug reference will find that the clear and logical design of the drug monographs facilitates decision making and supports the nursing process.

Since physicians, advanced practice nurses, and other health professionals have prescriptive privileges, the term *prescriber* is used throughout this book.

ORGANIZATION

The ***Pearson Nurse's Drug Guide 2023*** is user friendly. To help readers better understand how to use the drug guide, the authors illustrate and describe all the components of a drug monograph in the ***How to Use the Pearson Nurse's Drug Guide 2023,*** immediately after the front cover of the book.

In this drug guide, all drugs are listed alphabetically according to their generic names. Pharmacologic classifications are paired with therapeutic classifications for every drug monograph for ease of use by nurse clinicians and students alike. Each drug is indexed by both its generic and trade names in the back of the guide to make it easier for the user to locate individual drug monographs. Trade names followed by a maple leaf indicate that brand of the drug is available in Canada.

If a drug is not listed in the alphabetical section, it may be a combination drug, which is a drug made up of more than one generic component. Common combination drugs are listed under their trade names in the index and in Appendix D, *Prescription Combination Drugs*. The appendix identifies the generic components and the amount of each active ingredient contained in the combination. Users of this drug guide will find the page numbers for monographs of the component drugs in this appendix to make access to this information easier and faster.

Medications that are designated by the Institute for Safe Medication Practices (ISMP) are designated as "hight alert" medications and have an icon indicating this.

APPENDICES

Several helpful tables and charts in this drug guide include: Appendix A, *Ocular Medications, Low Molecular Weight Heparins, Inhaled Corticosteroids, Topical Corticosteroids*, and *Topical Antifungal Agents*; Appendix B, *U.S. Schedules of Controlled Substances*; Appendix C, *FDA Pregnancy Information*; Appendix D, *Prescription Combination Drugs*; Appendix E, *Glossary of Key Terms, Clinical Conditions, and Associated Signs and Symptoms*; Appendix F, *Abbreviations*; Appendix G, *Herbal and Dietary Supplement Table*; Appendix H, *Vaccines*, which highlights vaccines commonly seen/administered in practice.

INDEX

The index in the ***Pearson Nurse's Drug Guide 2023*** is perhaps the most often-used section in the entire book. All generic, trade, and combination drugs are listed in this index. Whenever a trade name is listed, the generic drug monograph is listed in parentheses. Additionally, classifications are listed and identified in SMALL CAPS, whereas all prototype drugs are highlighted in **bold** type. Drugs belonging to various classifications and subclassifications, including therapeutic classes, are also cross-referenced in this index. As a special feature, the index includes entries for combination drugs with index references to component drugs as well as the combination drug reference to Appendix D.

Medications listed in Appendix A (*Ocular Medications, Low Molecular Weight Heparins, Inhaled Corticosteroids, Topical Corticosteroid, and Topical Antifungal Agents*) or Appendix H (*Vaccines*) are also cross-referenced in the index.

ACKNOWLEDGMENTS

We wish to express our appreciation to our past and present students who have provided the inspiration for this work. It is for these individuals and all who strive for excellence in patient care that this work was undertaken.

Kelly M. Shields, PharmD
Kami L. Fox, DNP, RN, APRN, CPNP-PC
Christina Liebrecht, DNP, RN, CNE

ABACAVIR SULFATE

(a-ba′ca-vir)

Ziagen

Classification: ANTIRETROVIRAL; NUCLEOSIDE REVERSE TRANSCRIPTASE INHIBITOR (NRTI)

Therapeutic: ANTIRETROVIRAL (NRTI)

Prototype: Lamivudine

AVAILABILITY Tablet; oral solution

ACTION & *THERAPEUTIC EFFECT* Abacavir inhibits the activity of viral reverse transcriptase (RT) by competing with natural DNA nucleoside and by incorporation into viral DNA. Abacavir prevents viral DNA replication. Results in inhibited viral replication.

USES Treatment of HIV-1 infection in combination with other antiretroviral agents.

CONTRAINDICATIONS Hypersensitivity to abacavir; serious and sometimes fatal hypersensitivity to abacavir have been reported; lactic acidosis; creatinine clearance of less than 50 mL/min; severe hepatomegaly with severe steatosis; moderate to severe hepatic impairment; lactation.

CAUTIOUS USE Patients with HLA-B*5701 allele (high risk for hypersensitivity reaction); prior resistance to another nucleoside reverse transcriptase inhibitor (NRTI); history of cardiac disease; hypertension, hyperlipidemia, DM, smoking; older adults; pregnancy (high level of transfer across the human placenta). Safe use in children younger than 3 mo has not been established.

ROUTE & DOSAGE

HIV Infection

Adult: **PO** 300 mg bid or 600 mg once daily

Child (3 mo–16 yr): **PO** 8 mg/kg bid (max: 300 mg bid) OR *Patients weighing 14 to less than 20 kg:* **PO** 150 mg twice bid; *21 to less than 25 kg:* **PO** 150 mg in morning and 300 mg in the evening; *greater than 25 kg:* **PO** 300 mg twice daily

Hepatic Impairment Dosage Adjustment

Mild (Child-Pugh class A): 200 mg bid

ADMINISTRATION

Oral

- May be administered with or without food.
- Store tablets and liquid at 20°–25°C (68°–77°F). Liquid may be refrigerated.

ADVERSE EFFECTS **CNS:** Insomnia, abnormal dreams, *headache, fever*, dizziness, depression, anxiety **Skin:** *Rash*. **GI:** Increased liver function tests. **Other:** Hypersensitivity reactions (including fever, skin rash, fatigue, nausea, vomiting, diarrhea, abdominal pain); malaise; lethargy; myalgia; arthralgia.

INTERACTIONS **Drug: Alcohol** may increase abacavir blood levels Can decrease effect of **cladribine.**

PHARMACOKINETICS **Absorption:** Rapidly absorbed. **Distribution:** Distributes into extravascular space and erythrocytes; 50% protein bound. **Metabolism:** Metabolized by alcohol dehydrogenase and glucuronyl transferase to inactive metabolites. **Elimination:** 84% in urine, primarily as inactive metabolites; 16% in feces. **Half-Life:** 1.5 h.

NURSING IMPLICATIONS

Black Box Warning

*Abacavir has been associated with serious and sometimes fatal hypersensitivity reactions, especially in those with the HLA-B*5701 allele, and with lactic acidosis and severe hepatomegaly, sometimes fatal.*

Assessment & Drug Effects

- Monitor for S&S of hypersensitivity: Fever, skin rash, fatigue, GI distress (nausea, vomiting, diarrhea, abdominal pain). Withhold drug and immediately notify prescriber if hypersensitivity develops.
- Monitor for S&S of lactic acidosis [e.g., hyperventilation, lethargy, plasma pH less than 7.35 and lactate greater than 5–6 mol/L (mEq/L)], hepatomegaly, and renal insufficiency. Withhold drug and immediately notify prescriber for S&S of acidosis or hepatotoxicity.
- Monitor lab tests: Baseline screening for HLA-B*5701; periodic LFTs, BUN and creatinine, CBC with differential, triglyceride levels, and blood glucose (especially in diabetics).

Patient & Family Education

- Take drug exactly as prescribed at indicated times. Missed dose: Take immediately, then resume dosing schedule. Do not double a dose.
- Withhold drug immediately and notify prescriber at first sign of hypersensitivity or liver damage (see Assessment & Drug Effects).
- Carry Warning Card provided with drug at all times.

ABALOPARATIDE

(a-bal′oh-par′a-tide)

Tymlos

Classification: PARATHYROID AGENTS

Therapeutic: PARATHYROID HORMONE ANALOG

AVAILABILITY Subcutaneous injection, multiuse pen

ACTION & *THERAPEUTIC EFFECT* Analog of human parathyroid hormone related peptide, which acts as an agonist at the PTH1 receptor. *Results in stimulation of osteoblast function and increased bone mass.*

USES Osteoporosis in postmenopausal women, at high risk of fracture, who have failed or cannot tolerate other therapies.

CAUTIOUS USE Urolithiasis; pregnancy; lactation. Safety and efficacy in children not established.

ROUTE & DOSAGE

Osteoporosis

Adult: **Subcutaneous** 80 mcg daily

ADMINISTRATION

Subcutaneous

- Inject subcutaneously into the periumbilical region of the abdomen.
- Rotate sites each day and administer at approximately the same time each day.

ADVERSE EFFECTS **CNS:** *Dizziness, headache,* fatigue. **Endocrine:** *Increased uric acid,* hypercalcemia. **Skin:** *Erythema at injection site, swelling at injection site,* pain at injection site. **GI:** *Nausea,* upper abdominal pain. **Urinary:** *Hypercalciuria.* **Cardiac:** Palpitations, orthostatic hypotension, tachycardia.

PHARMACOKINETICS **Absorption:** 36% bioavailability. **Distribution:** 70% protein bound. **Metabolism:** Proteolytic degradation into small peptide groups. **Elimination:** Urine. **Half-Life:** 1.7 h.

NURSING IMPLICATIONS

Black Box Warning

Abaloparatide was associated with an increased risk of osteosarcoma in animal studies; avoid use in patients with increased risk for osteosarcoma at baseline.

Assessment & Drug Effects

- Monitor for and report orthostatic hypotension.
- Monitor serum calcium; bone mineral density (BMD) should be evaluated 1–2 yr after initiating therapy and every 2 yr thereafter.

Patient & Family Education

- Notify prescriber immediately if you experience bone pain, pain anywhere that does not go away, a lump, or swelling under the skin that is tender.
- Notify prescriber if you have signs of high calcium levels such as weakness, confusion, feeling tired, headache, upset stomach, vomiting, constipation, or bone pain.
- Notify prescriber if you experience signs or symptoms of allergic reaction such as rash, hives, itching, shortness of breath, wheezing, cough, swelling of the face, lips, tongue, or throat; or any other signs.
- To lower the chance of feeling dizzy, change positions and sit and stand slowly. Be careful going up and down stairs.

ABAMETAPIR

(a-ba-MET-a-pir)

Xeglyze

Classifications: ANTIPARASITIC AGENT; PEDICULOCIDE

Therapeutic: PEDICULOCIDE

AVAILABILITY Topical suspension

ACTION & *THERAPEUTIC EFFECT* A metalloproteinase inhibitor impacting the physiological processes critical to egg development and survival of lice. *Used to stop the development and survival of head lice.*

USES Treatment of head lice infestation.

CONTRAINDICATIONS There are no contraindications per manufacturer labeling.

CAUTIOUS USE Use with caution with pediatric patients; in neonates, may be associated with "gasping syndrome"; pregnancy (adverse effects not observed in animal reproduction studies); lactation.

ROUTE & DOSAGE

Head lice treatment

Adult/Adolescent/Children (6 month old or greater):
Topical Apply contents of one bottle (210 mL) to hair and scalp

ADMINISTRATION

Topical

- Not for oral, opthalmic, or intravaginal use.
- Shake bottle well before use; apply to dry hair and massage into scalp and throughout hair. Avoid contact with eyes; rinse with warm water for 10 minutes. Wash hands after application. Hair may be shampooed at any time after treatment.

- Use in conjunction with overall lice management program (wash or dry-clean all recently worn clothing, hats, used bedding, and towels; wash personal care items such as combs, brushes, and hair clips in hot water; and use a fine-tooth comb or special nit comb to remove dead lice and nits.
- Store at 20°-25° C (68°-77°F).

ADVERSE EFFECTS **HEENT:** Eye irritation **Skin:** Erythema, burning, rash **Other:** Hair color changes

INTERACTIONS **Drug:** Avoid combination with, or use of, CYP1A2 (e.g., **duloxetine**, **theophylline**), CYP2B6 (e.g., **bupropion**, **efavirenz**), or CYP3A4 (e.g., **midazolam**, **simvastatin**, **tacrolimus**) substrates within 2 weeks of application, as abametapir will increase concentration of these medications.

PHARMACOKINETICS **Peak:** 0.5–1.5 h **Distribution:** 91–92% protein-bound **Metabolism:** Extensively metabolized by CYP1A2 **Half-Life:** 21 h

NURSING IMPLICATIONS

Assessment & Drug Effects

- Assess head, hair, and skin surfaces for presence of lice and nits. Teach patient appropriate application.

Patient & Family Education

- Seek medical help immediately if you have any of the following signs or symptoms of an allergic reaction such as rash; hives; itching; red, swollen, blistered, or peeling skin with or without fever; wheezing; tightness in the chest or throat; trouble breathing, swallowing, or talking; unusual hoarseness; or swelling of the mouth, face, lips, tongue, or throat.

ABATACEPT

(a-ba-ta'sept)

Orencia

Classification: BIOLOGIC AND IMMUNOLOGICAL; IMMUNOMODULATOR; DISEASE-MODIFYING ANTIRHEUMATIC DRUG (DMARD)

Therapeutic: ANTIRHEUMATIC (DMARD); ANTI-INFLAMMATORY

AVAILABILITY Lyophilized powder for injection; solution for injection

ACTION & *THERAPEUTIC EFFECT* Inhibits T-cell (T-lymphocyte) activation by binding to CD80 and CD86, thereby blocking full activation of T-lymphocytes. Activated T-lymphocytes are found in the synovium of patients with RA. *It relieves RA symptoms, slows progression of structural damage, and improves RA physical function in adults with active RA who have had an inadequate response to other drugs.*

USES Treatment of moderate to severe rheumatoid arthritis, psoriatic arthritis or treatment of polyarticular juvenile idiopathic arthritis.

CONTRAINDICATIONS Known hypersensitivity to abatacept, live vaccines; active infections; coadministration with anakinra, TNF antagonists, other biologic RA therapy; lactation.

CAUTIOUS USE COPD; malignancies; pregnancy (category C); children younger than 6 yr.

ROUTE & DOSAGE

Rheumatoid Arthritis/Active Psoriatic Arthritis

Adult (weight less than 60 kg): **IV** Initial dose: 500 mg every 2 wk × 3 doses; *weight 60–100 kg:*

750 mg every 2 wk × 3 doses; *weight greater than 100 kg:* 1000 mg every 2 wk × 3 doses; then every 4 wk; **Subcutaneous** 125 mg weekly

Juvenile Idiopathic Arthritis

Child (6 yr or older, weight less than 75 kg): **IV** 10 mg/kg, repeat at wk 2 and 4, then monthly (max: 1000 mg); *weight 75–100 kg:* 750 mg at wk 2 and 4, then monthly; *weight at least 100 kg:* 1000 mg at wk 2 and 4, then monthly
Child (2 yr or older, weight 50 kg or more): **Subcutaneous** 125 mg once weekly; *weight 25–50:* 87.5 mg once weekly; *weight 10–25 kg:* 50 mg once weekly

ADMINISTRATION

Subcutaneous

- Abatacept for subcutaneous injection is supplied in a 125-mg/mL prefilled syringe.
- Do not remove the small bubble of air in the syringe and do not pull back on the plunger head before injection.
- Ensure that the full contents of the syringe are injected. Rotate injection sites.
- Prefilled syringes must be stored at 2°–8°C (36°–46°F). Do not freeze.
- Allow prefilled syringe and autoinjector to warm to room temperature for 30–60 min prior to administration.

Intravenous

- Note: The prefilled syringe is for subcutaneous injection only. Do not use for IV infusion.

PREPARE: **IV Infusion:** Use the supplied silicone-free disposable syringe with an 18–21-gauge needle to reconstitute the vial. ▪ Add 10 mL sterile water to each 250 mL to yield 25 mg/mL. ▪ To avoid foaming, gently swirl until completely dissolved. Do not shake or vigorously agitate. ▪ After dissolving, vent the vial with a needle to dissipate any foam. ▪ The reconstituted solution **must be** further diluted to a total of 100 mL as follows: From a 100-mL NS IV bag, remove a volume equal to the total volume of abatacept in the reconstituted vials (e.g., for two vials, remove 20 mL). Using the supplied silicone-free syringe, slowly add the reconstituted abatacept to the IV bag and gently mix. ▪ Discard any unused abatacept.

ADMINISTER: **IV Infusion:** Use a 0.2–1.2-micron low-protein-binding filter. Infuse over 30 min.

INCOMPATIBILITIES: **Solution/additive:** Should not be infused in the same intravenous line with other agents. **Y-site:** Should not be infused in the same intravenous line with other agents.

- Store at 2°–8°C (36°–46°F). Protect from light.

ADVERSE EFFECTS **CV:** Hypertension. **Respiratory:** *Nasopharyngitis,* upper respiratory infection, cough. **CNS:** *Headache,* dizziness. **GI:** *Nausea,* dyspepsia. **GU:** Urinary tract infection. **Musculoskeletal:** Back pain. **Other:** *Infection,* antibody development.

INTERACTIONS **Drug:** TNF ANTAGONISTS increase the risk of serious infections. Avoid use of LIVE VACCINES. Avoid use of **anakinra.**

PHARMACOKINETICS Half-Life: 13.1 days (IV); 14.3 days (subcutaneous). Time to onset approximately 2 wk.

NURSING IMPLICATIONS

Assessment & Drug Effects

- Prior to initiating treatment with abatacept, screen for latent TB infection with a TB skin test.
- Prior to initiating treatment with abatacept, screen for hepatitis.
- Monitor for S&S of hypersensitivity (e.g., hypotension, urticaria, and dyspnea); discontinue infusion and notify prescriber if any of these occur.
- Monitor for S&S of infection. Withhold drug and notify prescriber if patient develops a serious infection.

Patient & Family Education

- Report any of the following to a healthcare provider: Any type of infection, a positive TB skin test, a recent vaccination, a persistent cough, unexplained weight loss, fever, sore throat, or night sweats.
- Report S&S of an allergic reaction that may develop within 24 h of receiving abatacept (e.g., hives, swollen face, eyelids, lips, tongue, throat, or trouble breathing).
- Do not accept immunizations with live vaccines while taking or within 3 mo of discontinuing abatacept.

ABEMACICLIB

(uh-beh'muh-sy'klib)

Verzenio

Classification: ANTINEOPLASTIC AGENT; CYCLIN-DEPENDENT KINASE INHIBITOR

Therapeutic: ANTINEOPLASTIC

AVAILABILITY Tablet

ACTION & *THERAPEUTIC EFFECT* Potent small molecule cyclin-dependent kinase inhibitor that blocks retinoblastoma tumor suppressor protein phosphorylation and prevents progression through cell cycle resulting in arrest of the G1 phase. *Results in decreased tumor size.*

USES Monotherapy in HR-positive, HER2-negative advanced or metastatic breast cancer in patients with disease progression following endocrine therapy and prior chemotherapy in metastatic setting. Used in combination with fulvestrant for treatment of HR-positive, HER2-negative advanced or metastatic breast cancer in women with disease progression following endocrine therapy.

CAUTIOUS USE Hepatic impairment; pregnancy; lactation. Safety and efficacy in children not established.

ROUTE & DOSAGE

Breast Cancer

Adult: **PO Monotherapy** 200 mg bid until disease progression or unacceptable toxicity; **PO Combination therapy** 150 mg bid (in combination with fulvestrant and potential gonadotropin releasing hormone agonist) until disease progression or unacceptable toxicity

Toxicity Dosage Adjustment

See package insert

ADMINISTRATION

Oral

- Administer at approximately the same times each day.

- May be administered with or without food. Swallow whole, do not crush, chew, or split tablets.

ADVERSE EFFECTS **Respiratory:** *Cough.* **CNS:** *Dizziness, headache, fatigue.* **Endocrine:** *Increased serum creatinine*; dehydration. **Skin:** *Alopecia.* **Hepatic:** *Increased serum ALT/AST.* **GI:** *Weight loss, nausea, decreased appetite, abdominal pain, vomiting, constipation, stomatitis, xerostomia, dysgeusia.* **Musculoskeletal:** *Arthralgia.* **Hematologic:** *Anemia, decreased lymphocyte count, neutropenia,* thrombocytopenia, leukopenia. **Other:** *Infection, fever,* venous thromboembolism.

INTERACTIONS **Drug:** Abemaciclib is a substrate of CYP3A4 (major); avoid combination with strong inducers (e.g., carbamazepine, phenytoin, rifampin). **Herbal:** St. John's wort.

PHARMACOKINETICS **Absorption:** 45% bioavailability (after single 200-mg oral dose). **Distribution:** 96% protein bound. **Metabolism:** Hepatic, CYP3A4, forms active metabolites. **Elimination:** 81% in feces, 3% in urine. **Half-Life:** 18.3 h; up to 55 h in patients with severe hepatic impairment.

NURSING IMPLICATIONS

Assessment & Drug Effects

- Monitor for and report S&S of severe diarrhea, dehydration, or infection.
- Use effective form of birth control; notify doctor immediately if you become pregnant.
- Perform pregnancy testing prior to initiating treatment.
- Monitor lab tests: CBC with differential, platelet count, and LFTs at baseline, every 2 wk for the first 2 mo, then monthly for 2 mo.

Patient & Family Education

- Notify prescriber if you experience signs or symptoms of allergic reaction such as rash; hives; itching; shortness of breath; wheezing; cough; swelling of the face, lips, tongue, or throat; or any other signs.
- Bleeding may occur with this medication. Be careful to avoid injury. Use a soft toothbrush and an electric razor.
- Notify prescriber right away if you have signs of a blood clot such as chest pain or pressure; coughing up blood; shortness of breath; swelling, warmth, numbness, change of color, or pain in the leg or arm; or trouble speaking or swallowing.
- Use effective form of birth control while on this medication and for 3 wk after your last dose. Notify prescriber immediately if you become pregnant.

ABIRATERONE ACETATE

(a'bir-a'ter-one as'e-tate)

Yonsa, Zytiga

Classification: ANTINEOPLASTIC; ANTIANDROGEN; ANDROGEN BIOSYNTHESIS INHIBITOR

Therapeutic: ANTIANDROGEN

AVAILABILITY Tablet

ACTION & *THERAPEUTIC EFFECT* Inhibits the enzyme required for androgen biosynthesis in testicular, adrenal, and prostatic tumor tissues. *Decreased levels of serum testosterone and other androgens slow the growth of androgen-sensitive carcinomas.*

USES Metastatic castration-resistant prostate cancer.

CONTRAINDICATIONS Severe hepatic impairment (Child-Pugh

class C); pregnancy (may cause fetal harm or loss).

CAUTIOUS USE History of CV disease (e.g., heart failure, hypertension, recent MI, ventricular arrhythmias); hypokalemia; fluid retention; concurrent steroid therapy, especially during dosage adjustment or with concurrent infection or stress; moderate hepatic impairment (Child-Pugh class B). Abiraterone is not indicated for use in children.

ROUTE & DOSAGE

Metastatic Prostate Cancer

Adult: **PO** (Zytiga) 1000 mg once daily in combination with **PO** prednisone 5 mg bid; (Yonsa) **PO** 500 mg daily in combination with PO methylprednisolone 4 mg bid

Hepatic Impairment Dosage Adjustment

Moderate impairment (Child-Pugh class B): **PO** 250 mg once daily (Zytiga) or 125 mg once daily (Yonsa)
Severe impairment (Child-Pugh class C score): Do not use

ADMINISTRATION

Oral

- Give on an empty stomach 1 h before or 2 h after food.
- Tablets should be swallowed whole with water. Do not crush or chew tablet.
- Women who are or may be pregnant must use gloves to handle abiraterone.
- Store at 15°–30°C (59°–86°F).

ADVERSE EFFECTS **CV:** *Arrhythmia,* cardiac failure, chest pain or discomfort, *hypertension,* edema. **Respiratory:** *Cough,* upper respiratory tract infection, dyspnea, nasopharyngitis. **CNS:** Fatigue, insomnia, headache. **Endocrine:** Elevated triglycerides, hyperglycemia, hypernatremia, hypokalemia, hypophosphatemia, hot flash. **Dermatologic:** Skin rash. **Hepatic:** Elevated ALT and AST, elevated total bilirubin. **GI:** *Diarrhea,* dyspepsia, constipation. **GU:** Nocturia, *urinary frequency, urinary tract infection,* hematuria. **Musculoskeletal:** *Joint discomfort and swelling, muscle discomfort,* bone fracture. **Hematologic:** Lymphocytopenia, bruising. **Other:** Fever.

INTERACTIONS **Drug:** Abiraterone can increase concentration of drugs requiring CYP2D6 (e.g., **dextromethorphan, thioridazine**). Strong inhibitors of CYP3A4 (e.g., **ketoconazole, itraconazole, clarithromycin, atazanavir, nefazodone, saquinavir, telithromycin, ritonavir, indinavir, nelfinavir, voriconazole**) increase abiraterone; while inducers of CYP3A4 (e.g., **phenytoin, carbamazepine, rifampin, rifabutin, rifapentine, phenobarbital**) decrease levels of abiraterone. **Herbal: St. John's wort** may decrease abiraterone concentration. **Food:** Must be taken on an empty stomach.

PHARMACOKINETICS **Distribution:** Over 99% plasma protein bound. **Metabolism:** In the liver to an active metabolite via CYP3A4. **Elimination:** Fecal (88%) and renal (5%). **Half-Life:** 14–17 h.

NURSING IMPLICATIONS

Assessment & Drug Effects

- Monitor BP and cardiac function especially with a history of CV disease.

- Monitor for and report signs of fluid retention (e.g., sudden weight gain, peripheral edema).
- Monitor for and report S&S of hypokalemia or hepatotoxicity (see Appendix F). Withhold drug and notify prescriber if AST/ALT is above 5 × ULN or bilirubin above 3 × ULN.
- Monitor lab tests: Baseline LFTs, then q2wk for first 3 mo, then monthly thereafter; periodic serum electrolytes (especially potassium).

Patient & Family Education

- Do not take this drug within 2 h before or 1 h after consuming food.
- A condom should be used during sexual intercourse with a woman who is or could become pregnant.
- Report any of the following to a healthcare provider: Sudden weight gain, swelling of feet or legs, palpitations, unusual weakness, muscle pain, S&S of a urinary tract infection.

ACAMPROSATE CALCIUM

(a-cam-pro′sate)

Campral

Classification: SUBSTANCE ABUSE DETERRENT

Therapeutic: SUBSTANCE ABUSE INHIBITOR

AVAILABILITY Delayed release tablet

ACTION & *THERAPEUTIC EFFECT* Thought to interact with CNS glutamate and GABA neurotransmitter systems and help restore normal balance between neuronal excitation and inhibition. *Reduces craving for alcohol intake due to chronic use, but does not cause alcohol aversion or a disulfiram-like reaction as a result of ethanol ingestion.*

USES Maintenance of abstinence from alcohol in patients with alcoholism.

CONTRAINDICATIONS Hypersensitivity to acamprosate calcium or any of its components; suicidal ideation; severe renal impairment (CrCl less than 30 mL/min).

CAUTIOUS USE Moderate renal impairment; depression; pregnancy (category C); lactation. Safety and efficacy of acamprosate not established in adolescents or children younger than 18 yr.

ROUTE & DOSAGE

Maintenance of Alcohol Abstinence

Adult: **PO** Two 333-mg tablets tid

Renal Impairment Dosage Adjustment

CrCl 30–50 mL/min: 333 mg tid; *less than 30 mL/min:* Do not use

ADMINISTRATION

Oral

- Ensure that the drug is not chewed or crushed. It **must be** swallowed whole.
- Store at 15°–30°C (59°–86°F).

ADVERSE EFFECTS **CV:** Palpitation, syncope. **Respiratory:** Rhinitis, cough, dyspnea, pharyngitis, bronchitis. **CNS:** Depression, anxiety, insomnia, asthenia, dizziness, paresthesia, headache, somnolence, decreased libido, amnesia, abnormal thinking, tremor. **HEENT:** Abnormal vision, taste perversion. **Endocrine:** Peripheral edema, weight gain. **Skin:** Pruritus, diaphoresis, rash. **GI:** *Diarrhea,* nausea, vomiting, anorexia, flatulence, dry mouth, abdominal pain, dyspepsia, constipation, increased appetite.

GU: Impotence. **Musculoskeletal:** Musculoskeletal pain. **Other:** Flu syndrome, chills.

PHARMACOKINETICS Absorption: 11% bioavailability. **Metabolism:** Not metabolized. **Elimination:** Renal. **Half-Life:** 20–33 h.

NURSING IMPLICATIONS

Assessment & Drug Effects

- Monitor for S&S of depression or suicidal thinking.
- Monitor for: Impaired judgment or thinking; dizziness or impaired motor skills. Take appropriate protective measures.

Patient & Family Education

- Report any alcohol consumption while taking acamprosate.
- Report promptly any of the following: Unusual anxiousness or nervousness; depression or suicidal thoughts; burning or tingling sensations in arms, legs, hands, or feet; chest pains or palpitations; difficulty urinating.
- Do not drive or engage in other hazardous activities until reaction to the drug is known.

ACARBOSE (Pr)

(a-car′bose)

Precose

Classification: ANTIDIABETIC; ALPHA-GLUCOSIDASE INHIBITOR

Therapeutic: ANTIDIABETIC

AVAILABILITY Tablet

ACTION & *THERAPEUTIC EFFECT* Delays digestion of carbohydrates by inhibition of pancreatic amylase and intestinal enzymes, resulting in slowed absorption of glucose molecules into the bloodstream and inhibits metabolism of sucrose to glucose and fructose. *Reduces postprandial serum insulin and glucose peaks.*

USES In conjunction with diet and exercise for type 2 diabetes.

UNLABELED USES Adjunctive treatment of type 1 diabetes.

CONTRAINDICATIONS Inflammatory bowel disease, diabetic ketoacidosis, cirrhosis, colon ulcers, partial bowel obstruction, predisposition for obstruction; lactation.

CAUTIOUS USE GI distress or liver disorders, pregnancy (category B); children younger than 18 yr.

ROUTE & DOSAGE

Type 2 Diabetes Mellitus

Adult: **PO** Start with 25 mg daily to tid with meals, titrate to individual response (max: 150 mg/day for 60 kg or less, 300 mg/day for greater than 60 kg)

ADMINISTRATION

Oral

- Remove drug from foil wrapper immediately before administration.
- Give drug with first bite at each of the three main meals.
- Do not store above 25°C (77°F). Keep tightly closed and protect from moisture.

ADVERSE EFFECTS GI: *Flatulence, diarrhea, abdominal pain.*

INTERACTIONS Drug: SULFONYLUREAS may increase hypoglycemic effects. Drugs that induce hyperglycemia (e.g., THIAZIDES, CORTICOSTEROIDS, PHENOTHIAZINES, ESTROGENS, **phenytoin, isoniazid**) may decrease effectiveness of acarbose. Carefully monitor if using **chloroquine** as hypoglycemia may result. May decrease the effect of **digoxin. Herbal: Ginseng** may increase hypoglycemic effects.

PHARMACOKINETICS Absorption: 0.5–2% is absorbed intact from GI tract. **Peak:** Peak blood glucose reduction approximately 70 min after dose. **Metabolism:** In GI tract by intestinal bacteria and digestive enzymes. **Elimination:** 35% in urine, 51% in feces. **Half-Life:** 2 h.

NURSING IMPLICATIONS

Assessment & Drug Effects

- Treat hypoglycemia with dextrose; not with sucrose (table sugar).
- Monitor lab tests: Frequent blood glucose and periodic HbA1C; periodic serum creatinine levels; serum transaminase levels every 3 mo during first year of treatment then periodically.

Patient & Family Education

- Note: Acarbose prevents the breakdown of table sugar. Have a source of dextrose, such as dextrose paste, available to treat low blood sugar.
- Monitor closely blood glucose, especially following dosage changes.
- Report abdominal distress; dietary adjustment or dosage reduction may be warranted.
- Monitor weight and report significant changes.

ACEBUTOLOL HYDROCHLORIDE

(a-se-byoo-toe′lole)

Classification: BETA-ADRENERGIC ANTAGONIST; ANTIHYPERTENSIVE; CLASS II ANTIARRHYTHMIC

Therapeutic: ANTIHYPERTENSIVE; CLASS II ANTIARRHYTHMIC

Prototype: Propranolol

AVAILABILITY Capsule

ACTION & *THERAPEUTIC EFFECT* Beta$_1$–selective adrenergic blocking agent with mild sympathomimetic activity. *Decreases both systolic and diastolic BP at rest and during exercise. Exhibits antiarrhythmic activity (class II antiarrhythmic agent).*

USES Treatment of hypertension. Management of ventricular premature beats.

UNLABELED USES Thyrotoxicosis.

CONTRAINDICATIONS Overt CHF, second- or third-degree AV block, severe bradycardia, cardiogenic shock; acute bronchospasm, pulmonary edema; lactation.

CAUTIOUS USE Impaired cardiac function, well-compensated CHF, mesenteric or peripheral vascular disease; cerebrovascular disease; patients undergoing major surgery involving general anesthesia; renal or hepatic impairment; labile diabetes mellitus; hyperthyroidism; bronchospastic disease (asthma, emphysema); avoid abrupt withdrawal; pregnancy (category B); children younger than 12 yr.

ROUTE & DOSAGE

Hypertension

Adult: **PO** 200–400 mg/day in 1–2 divided doses (max: 1200 mg/day)

Ventricular Arrhythmias

Adult: **PO** 200–400 mg/day in 1–2 divided doses; may be increased to 1200 mg/day

Renal Impairment Dosage Adjustment

CrCl less than 50 mL/min: Reduce dose by 50%; *less than 25 mL/min:* Reduce dose by 75%; *intermittent hemodialysis:* Reduce dose by 75%

ADMINISTRATION

Oral

- Check BP and apical pulse before administration. If heart rate is less than 60 bpm or other ordered parameter, consult prescriber.
- May be administered with or without food.
- Drug is usually discontinued gradually over a period of 2 wk.
- Store at 15°–30°C (59°–86°F).

ADVERSE EFFECTS **CNS:** Fatigue, dizziness, headache.

DIAGNOSTIC TEST INTERFERENCE False-negative test results possible (see **propranolol**).

INTERACTIONS **Drug:** Other HYPOTENSIVE AGENTS, DIURETICS increase hypotensive effect; NSAIDS blunt hypotensive effect; decreases hypoglycemic effect of **glyburide;** increases bradycardia and sinus arrest with **amiodarone.** Do not use with **rivastigmine** as it may enhance bradycardia.

PHARMACOKINETICS **Absorption:** Average bioavailability of 40%. (In geriatric patients, bioavailability increases twofold.) **Onset of Action:** 1–2 h. **Peak:** 3 h. **Distribution:** Minimally into CSF; crosses placenta; is excreted in breast milk. **Metabolism:** In liver. **Elimination:** In urine, feces. **Half-Life:** 3–4 h.

NURSING IMPLICATIONS

Assessment & Drug Effects

- Monitor BP and cardiac status throughout therapy. Observe for and report marked bradycardia or hypotension.
- Monitor I&O ratio and pattern and report changes to prescriber (e.g., dysuria, nocturia, oliguria, weight change).
- Monitor for S&S of CHF, especially peripheral edema, dyspnea, activity intolerance.
- Monitor lab tests: Periodic tests for drug-induced positive ANA titer during long-term therapy, especially in women and older adults; periodic CBC with long-term therapy.

Patient & Family Education

- Know parameters for withholding drug (e.g., pulse less than 60).
- Do not breastfeed while taking this drug without consulting prescriber.
- Note: Common adverse effects include insomnia, drowsiness, and confusion.
- Do not drive or engage in potentially hazardous activities until response to drug is known.
- Do not increase, decrease, omit, or discontinue drug regimen without advice from the prescriber. Abrupt withdrawal may worsen angina or precipitate MI in patient with heart disease.
- Contact prescriber promptly at the first signs or symptoms of CHF (see Appendix F).

- Monitor for loss of glycemic control if diabetic.
- Note: Drug may mask symptoms of hypoglycemia and potentiate insulin-induced hypoglycemia in diabetics.
- Avoid use of OTC oral cold preparations and topical nasal decongestants unless approved by the prescriber.

ACETAMINOPHEN, (PARACETAMOL) Pr

(a-seat-a-mee'noe-fen)

Abenol ♣, A'Cenol, Acephen, Anacin-3, Anuphen, APAP, Atasol ♣, Campain ♣, Dolanex, Exdol ♣, Halenol, Liquiprin, Ofirmev, Panadol, Pedric, Robigesic ♣, Rounox ♣, Tapar, Tempra, Tylenol, Tylenol Arthritis, Valadol

Classification: NONNARCOTIC ANALGESIC, ANTIPYRETIC

Therapeutic: NONNARCOTIC ANALGESIC; ANTIPYRETIC

AVAILABILITY Suppository; tablet/caplet; extended release tablet/capsule; liquid; injection

ACTION & *THERAPEUTIC EFFECT* Produces analgesia by elevation of the pain threshold. Reduces fever by inhibiting the action of endogenous pyrogens on the heat-regulating centers in the brain by blocking the formation and release of prostaglandins in the CNS. *It provides temporary analgesia for mild to moderate pain. In addition, acetaminophen lowers body temperature in individuals with a fever.*

USES Fever reduction. Temporary relief of mild to moderate pain. Generally as substitute for aspirin when the latter is not tolerated or is contraindicated.

CONTRAINDICATIONS Hypersensitivity to acetaminophen or phenacetin. Acute liver failure has been associated with doses that exceed 4000 mg per day.

CAUTIOUS USE Repeated administration to patients with anemia, G6PD deficiency, renal or hepatic disease; arthritic or rheumatoid conditions affecting children younger than 12 yr; alcoholism; malnutrition; thrombocytopenia; bone marrow depression, immunosuppression; pregnancy (category C).

ROUTE & DOSAGE

Mild to Moderate Pain, Fever

Adult: **PO** 325–650 mg q4–6h (max: 4 g/day); **PR** 650 mg q4–6h (max: 4 g/day); **IV** 1000 mg q6h or 650 q4h prn
Child: **PO** 10–15 mg/kg q4–6h **PR** *2–5 yr:* 120 mg q4–6h (max: 720 mg/day); *6–12 yr:* 325 mg q4–6h (max: 2.6 g/day)
Child (2 yr or older): **IV** 15 mg/kg/dose q6h or 12.5 mg/kg/dose q4h prn
Neonate: **PO** 10–15 mg/kg q6–8h

ADMINISTRATION

Oral

- Ensure that extended release tablets are not crushed or chewed. These must be swallowed whole.
- Chewable tablets should be thoroughly chewed and wetted before they are swallowed.
- Do not coadminister with a high carbohydrate meal; absorption rate may be significantly retarded.
- Store in light-resistant containers at room temperature, preferably at 15°–30°C (59°–86°F).

Rectal

- Insert suppositories beyond the rectal sphincter.

Intravenous

PREPARE: **Intermittent:** For adults and adolescents weighing 50 kg (110 lb) or more, give without dilution by attaching a vented IV set directly to the 100-mL (1000-mg) vial. For patients weighing less than 50 kg (110 lb), withdraw the needed dose from a sealed 1000-mg vial and place in an empty sterile container (e.g., plastic IV bag, syringe) for infusion.

ADMINISTER: **Intermittent:** Infuse over 15 min. For small-volume pediatric doses up to 60 mL, use a syringe pump to administer over 15 min. Store at controlled temperature and use within 6 h after opening.

ADVERSE EFFECTS **Other:** Negligible with recommended dosage; rash; anorexia, nausea, vomiting, dizziness, lethargy, diaphoresis, chills, epigastric or abdominal pain, diarrhea; onset of hepatotoxicity: elevation of serum transaminases (ALT, AST) and bilirubin; hypoglycemia, hepatic coma, acute renal failure (rare); neutropenia, pancytopenia, leukopenia, thrombocytopenic purpura, hepatotoxicity in alcoholics, renal damage.

DIAGNOSTIC TEST INTERFERENCE False increases in ***urinary 5-HIAA*** (5-hydroxyindoleacetic acid) by-product of serotonin; false decreases in ***blood glucose*** (by ***glucose oxidase–peroxidase procedure***); false increases in urinary glucose (with certain instruments in glucose analyses); and false increases in ***serum uric acid*** (with ***phosphotungstate method***). High-dose or long-term therapy: ***Hepatic, renal, and hematopoietic function*** (periodically).

INTERACTIONS **Drug: Cholestyramine** may decrease acetaminophen absorption. With chronic coadministration, BARBITURATES, **carbamazepine, phenytoin,** and **rifampin** may increase potential for chronic hepatotoxicity. Chronic, excessive ingestion of **alcohol** will increase risk of hepatotoxicity.

PHARMACOKINETICS **Absorption:** Rapid and almost complete absorption (PO); less complete absorption from rectal suppository. **Peak:** 0.5–2 h. **Duration:** 3–4 h. **Distribution:** In all body fluids; crosses placenta. **Metabolism:** Extensively in liver. **Elimination:** 90–100% of drug excreted as metabolites in urine; excreted in breast milk. **Half-Life:** 1–3 h.

NURSING IMPLICATIONS

Black Box Warning

Doses in excess of 4000 mg/day have been associated with acute liver failure.

Assessment & Drug Effects

- Monitor for S&S of: Hepatotoxicity, even with moderate acetaminophen doses, especially in individuals with poor nutrition or who have ingested alcohol (3 or more alcoholic drinks daily) over prolonged periods; poisoning, usually from accidental ingestion or suicide attempts; potential abuse from psychological dependence (withdrawal has been associated with restless and excited responses).

Patient & Family Education

- Do not take other medications (e.g., cold preparations) containing acetaminophen without medical advice; overdosing and chronic use can cause liver damage and other toxic effects.

- Do not self-medicate adults for pain more than 10 days (5 days in children) without consulting a prescriber.
- Do not use this medication without medical direction for: Fever persisting longer than 3 days, fever over 39.5°C (103°F), or recurrent fever.
- Do not give children more than 5 doses in 24 h unless prescribed by prescriber.

ACETAZOLAMIDE

(a-set-a-zole′a-mide)

Apo-Acetazolamide ♣

Classification: CARBONIC ANHYDRASE INHIBITOR

Therapeutic: DIURETIC; ANTICONVULSANT; ANTIGLAUCOMA

AVAILABILITY Tablet; sustained release capsule; powder for injection

ACTION & *THERAPEUTIC EFFECT* A potent carbonic anhydrase inhibitor that decreases the secretion of aqueous humor in the eye, retards excessive abnormal discharges from CNS neurons, and increases renal loss of bicarbonate ions, which carry out sodium, water, and potassium thus lowering intraocular pressure. *Reduces seizure activity and intraocular pressure. Additionally, it has a diuretic effect.*

USES Reduction of intraocular pressure in open-angle glaucoma and secondary glaucoma; preoperative treatment of acute closed-angle glaucoma; acute mountain sickness/high-altitude cerebral edema.

UNLABELED USES Metabolic alkalosis, urinary alkalinization; idiopathic intracranial hypertension.

CONTRAINDICATIONS Hypersensitivity to acetazolamide, sulfonamides, or any component of the formulation; marked renal and hepatic disease; Addison disease or other types of adrenocortical insufficiency; hyponatremia, hypokalemia, hyperchloremic acidosis; prolonged administration to patients with hyphema; chronic noncongestive angle-closure glaucoma.

CAUTIOUS USE Hypersensitivity to sulfonamides and derivatives (e.g., thiazides), history of hypercalciuria; DM, renal impairment; gout, patients receiving digitalis, obstructive pulmonary disease, older adults; respiratory acidosis; pregnancy (limited data available related to use during pregnancy).

ROUTE & DOSAGE

Close Angle Glaucoma

Adult: **PO/IV** 500 mg once

Altitude Sickness Prevention

Adult: **PO** 1250 mg q12h before climb and continued until at same elevation for 2 days

Renal Impairment Dosage Adjustment

CrCl 10–50 mL/min: Extend interval to q12h; *less than 10 mL/min:* Use not recommended

Hemodialysis Dosage Adjustment

Administer postdialysis

ADMINISTRATION

Oral

- Administer diuretic dose in the morning to avoid interrupted sleep.

- Give with food or meals to minimize GI upset.
- Note: If tablet(s) cannot be swallowed, soften tablet(s) (not sustained release form) in 2 tsp of hot water and add 2 tsp of honey/syrup to disguise bitter taste; avoid syrups containing alcohol or glycerin, or crush tablet(s) and suspend in syrup (250–500 mg/5 mL syrup). Prepare just before administration. Drug does not dissolve in fruit juices.
- Store oral preparations at controlled room temperature.

Intravenous

PREPARE: **Direct:** Reconstitute each 500-mg vial with at least 5 mL of sterile water for injection to yield approximately 100 mg/mL. ▪ May be used as prepared or further diluted. **IV Infusion:** Dilute reconstituted solution with D5W or NS. Use within 24 h of reconstitution.

ADMINISTER: **Direct:** Give at a rate of 500 mg or fraction thereof over 3 min. **IV Infusion:** Give as a continuous infusion over 4–8 h.

INCOMPATIBILITIES: **Solution/additive:** **multivitamin** **Y-site:** **Diltiazem, tacrolimus, TPN**.

ADVERSE EFFECTS

CV: Flushing. **CNS:** Paresthesias, malaise, disorientation, depression, ataxia, convulsions, dizziness, excitement, headache, fatigue, flaccid paralysis. **HEENT:** Auditory disturbance, tinnitus. **Endocrine:** Increased excretion of calcium, potassium, magnesium, and sodium, growth retardation, hyperglycemia, hyperuricemia. **Skin:** Allergic skin reaction, skin photosensitivity, toxic epidermal necrolysis, urticaria. **GI/Hepatic:** Anorexia, nausea, vomiting, dysgeusia, melena, diarrhea, hepatic insufficiency. **GU:** Glycosuria, hematuria, polyuria, renal failure, crystalluria. **Hematologic:** Bone marrow depression with agranulocytosis, hemolytic anemia, aplastic anemia, leukopenia, thrombocytopenia, purpura. **Other:** Exacerbation of gout, Stevens-Johnson syndrome, anaphylaxis, fever.

DIAGNOSTIC TEST INTERFERENCE

Monitor for false-positive ***urinary protein*** determinations. Interfers with serum uric acid levels, may lead to false-negative aldosteron/renin ration.

INTERACTIONS

Drug: Renal excretion of AMPHETAMINES, **ephedrine, flecainide, quinidine, procainamide,** TRICYCLIC ANTIDEPRESSANTS may be decreased, thereby enhancing or prolonging their effects. Renal excretion of **lithium** may be increased. **Amphotericin B** and CORTICOSTEROIDS may accelerate **potassium** loss. Puts patients on high doses of SALICYLATES at high risk for SALICYLATE toxicity. May increase adverse effects of CARBONIC ANHYDRASE INHIBITORS.

PHARMACOKINETICS

Absorption: Well absorbed from GI tract. **Onset:** 1 h regular release; 2 h sustained release; 2 min IV. **Peak:** 2–4 h reg; 8–18 h sustained; 15 min IV. **Duration:** 8–12 h reg; 18–24 h sustained; 4–5 h IV. **Distribution:** Distributed throughout body; crosses placenta. **Elimination:** In urine. **Half-Life:** 2.4–5.8 h.

NURSING IMPLICATIONS

Assessment & Drug Effects

- Establish baseline weight before initial therapy and weigh daily thereafter when used to treat edema.
- Monitor for S&S of: Mild to severe metabolic acidosis; potassium loss,

which is greatest early in therapy (see hypokalemia in Appendix F).
- Monitor I&O especially when used with other diuretics.
- Monitor lab tests: Baseline serum electrolytes, periodic CBC with differential; monitor growth in pediatric patients; monitor intraocular pressure 30 to 60 minutes after administration.

Patient & Family Education

- Maintain adequate fluid intake (1.5–2.5 L/24 h; 1 liter is approximately equal to 1 quart) to reduce risk of kidney stones.
- Do not breastfeed while taking this drug without consulting prescriber.
- Report any of the following: Numbness, tingling, burning, drowsiness, and visual problems, sore throat or mouth, unusual bleeding, fever, skin or renal problems.
- Eat potassium-rich diet and take potassium supplement when taking this drug in high doses or for prolonged periods.
- Use caution when engaging in hazardous activities until reaction to drug is known.

ACETYLCYSTEINE Pr

(a-se-til-sis'tay-een)

Acetadote, N-Acetylcysteine, Mucomyst, Parvolex ♣

Classification: MUCOLYTIC; ANTIDOTE

Therapeutic: MUCOLYTIC; ANTIDOTE

AVAILABILITY Solution for inhalation; solution for injection

ACTION & *THERAPEUTIC EFFECT* Probably acts by disrupting disulfide linkages of mucoproteins in purulent and nonpurulent bronchial secretions. In acetaminophen overdose, it helps to prevent hepatotoxicity by serving as a substrate for the toxic metabolites of acetaminophen. *Lowers viscosity and facilitates the removal of secretions. Removes the toxic metabolites of acetaminophen.*

USES Adjuvant therapy in patients with abnormal mucous secretions in acute and chronic bronchopulmonary diseases, and in pulmonary complications of cystic fibrosis and surgery, tracheostomy, and atelectasis. Also used in diagnostic bronchial studies and as an antidote for acute acetaminophen poisoning.

UNLABELED USES Meconium ileus; prevention of radiocontrast-induced renal dysfunction.

CONTRAINDICATIONS Hypersensitivity to acetylcysteine; patients at risk of gastric hemorrhage.

CAUTIOUS USE Patients with asthma, severe hepatic disease, esophageal varices, peptic ulcer disease; debilitated patients with severe respiratory insufficiency; older adults; pregnancy (category B); lactation.

ROUTE & DOSAGE

Mucolytic

Adult: **Inhalation** 1–10 mL of 20% solution q4–6h or 2–20 mL of 10% solution q4–6h; **Direct Instillation** 1–2 mL of 10–20% solution q1–4h

Child: **Inhalation** 3–5 mL of 20% solution or 6–10 mL of 10% solution 3–4 × day

Infant: **Inhalation** 1–2 mL 20% solution or 2–4 mL of 10% solution 3–4 × day

Acetaminophen Toxicity

Adult/Child: **PO** 140 mg/kg followed by 70 mg/kg q4h for 17 doses (use a 5% solution)
Adult/Adolescent/Child: **IV** 150 mg/kg infused over 60 min, followed by 50 mg/kg over 4 h, then 100 mg/kg over 16 h; total dose 300 mg/kg over 21 h

ADMINISTRATION

Inhalation and Instillation

- Prepare dilution within 1 h of use; drug does not contain an antimicrobial agent. A light purple discoloration does not significantly impair drug's effectiveness.
- Dilute the 20% solution with NS or water for injection. The 10% solution may be used undiluted.
- Give by direct instillation into tracheostomy (1–2 mL of 10–20% solution).
- Instruct patient to clear airway, if possible, coughing productively prior to aerosol administration to ensure maximum effect.
- Store opened vial in refrigerator to retard oxidation; use within 96 h.
- Store unopened vial at 15°–30°C (59°–86°F), unless otherwise directed.

Oral

- Dilute the 20% solution 1:3 with cola, orange juice, or other soft drink to make a 5% solution. If administered via a gastric tube, water may be used as the diluent.
- Freshly prepare all diluted solutions and use within 1 h of preparation.

Intravenous

PREPARE: **IV Infusion:** Acetylcysteine reacts with certain metals and rubber; use IV equipment made of plastic or glass. ▪ Dilute all required doses in D5W as follows: For loading dose, add a dose equal to 150 mg/kg to 200 mL; for second dose, add a dose equal to 50 mg/kg to 500 mL; for third dose, add a dose equal to 100 mg/kg to 1000 mL. ▪ Note: The total IV volume should be reduced for patients less than 40 kg and for those with fluid restriction. In small children, individualize the total IV volume to avoid water intoxication and hyponatremia.
ADMINISTER: **IV Infusion:** Give loading dose over 60 min, second dose 1 over 4 h, third dose 2 over 16 h. Complete all infusions over 21 h.
INCOMPATIBILITIES: **Y-site: Ceftazidime.**

- Store reconstituted solution for up to 24 h at 15°–30°C (59°–86°F).

ADVERSE EFFECTS

Respiratory: Bronchospasm, rhinorrhea, burning sensation in upper respiratory passages, epistaxis. **CNS:** Dizziness, drowsiness. **GI:** Nausea, *vomiting*, stomatitis, hepatotoxicity (urticaria).

PHARMACOKINETICS

Onset: 1 min. **Peak:** 5–10 min. **Metabolism:** Deacetylated in liver to cysteine.

NURSING IMPLICATIONS

Assessment & Drug Effects

- During IV infusion, carefully monitor for fluid overload and signs of hyponatremia (i.e., changes in mental status).

- Monitor for S&S of aspiration of excess secretions, and for bronchospasm (unpredictable); withhold drug and notify prescriber immediately if either occurs.
- Have suction apparatus immediately available. Increased volume of respiratory tract fluid may be liberated; suction or endotracheal aspiration may be necessary to establish and maintain an open airway. Older adults and debilitated patients are particularly at risk.
- Nausea and vomiting may occur, particularly when face mask is used, due to unpleasant odor of drug and excess volume of liquefied bronchial secretions.
- Monitor lab tests: ABGs, pulmonary functions, and pulse oximetry as indicated; baseline serum acetaminophen level (for toxicity), LFTs, bilirubin, serum electrolytes, BUN, and plasma glucose.

Patient & Family Education

- Report difficulty with clearing the airway or any other respiratory distress.
- Report nausea, as an antiemetic may be indicated.
- Note: Unpleasant odor of inhaled drug becomes less noticeable with continued use.

ACITRETIN

(a-ci-tree'tin)

Soriatane

Classification: RETINOID
Therapeutic: ANTIPSORIATIC
Prototype: Isotretinoin

AVAILABILITY Capsule

ACTION & *THERAPEUTIC EFFECT* Binds to the retinoic acid receptors in the skin, thus modifying gene expression, epithelial cell growth, and cell differentiation. *Resulting actions are anti-inflammatory and antiproliferative with keratinocyte differentiation normalized within the epithelium.*

USES Treatment of severe psoriasis in adults.

UNLABELED USES Eczema.

CONTRAINDICATIONS Hypersensitivity to acitretin or sensitivity to parabens; hepatoxicity; hepatitis; severe renal impairment or renal failure, development of psychiatric symptoms (depression, etc.); pregnancy (known teratogen and contraindicated in females who are or may become pregnant) for at least 3 yr after use; lactation.

CAUTIOUS USE Patients with impaired hepatic function, history of mental illness; DM; obesity, history of pancreatitis, hypertriglyceridemia, hypercholesterolemia, coronary artery disease, retinal disease, degenerative joint disease.

ROUTE & DOSAGE

Psoriasis

Adult: **PO 25–50 mg daily with main meal**

ADMINISTRATION

Oral

- Administer as single dose with main meal to enhance absorption.
- Store at 15°–25°C (59°–77°F) and protect from light. After opening, avoid exposure to high temperatures and humidity.

ADVERSE EFFECTS **CV:** Flushing, edema. **Respiratory:** Sinusitis. **CNS:** Headache, depression, aggressive feelings and thoughts of self-harm, insomnia, somnolence.

HEENT: Blurred vision, blepharitis, conjunctivitis, decreased night vision/night blindness, eye pain, photophobia; earache, tinnitus; taste perversion. **Skin:** *Alopecia, skin peeling, dry skin, nail disorders, pruritus, rash, cheilitis, skin atrophy, paronychia,* abnormal skin odor and hair texture, cold/clammy skin, increased sweating, purpura, seborrhea, skin ulceration, sunburn. **GI:** *Dry mouth, increased liver function tests, increased triglycerides and cholesterol,* hepatitis, gingival bleeding, gingivitis, increased saliva, stomatitis, thirst, ulcerative stomatitis, abdominal pain, diarrhea, nausea, tongue disorder. **Other:** *Hyperesthesia, paresthesias, arthralgia, progression of existing spinal hyperostosis, rigors,* back pain, hypertonia, myalgia, fatigue, hot flashes, increased appetite; *Rhinitis, epistaxis, xerophthalmia.*

INTERACTIONS **Drug:** Use with **ethanol** increases teratogenic risk; interferes with the contraceptive efficacy of **progestin**-only ORAL CONTRACEPTIVES. Do not use with **methotrexate** or TETRACYCLINES. May increase photosensitizing effect of **aminolevulinic acid**. **Food:** Avoid supplemental **vitamin A** or vitamins containing **vitamin A.**

PHARMACOKINETICS **Absorption:** Rapidly from GI tract, optimal absorption when taken with food. **Peak:** 2–5 h. **Distribution:** Crosses placenta, distributed into breast milk, 99% protein bound. **Metabolism:** Active metabolite, *cis*-acitretin. **Elimination:** In both urine and feces. **Half-Life:** 49 h acitretin, 63 h *cis*-acitretin.

NURSING IMPLICATIONS

Black Box Warning

Severe birth defects and/or fetal death have occurred when either parent is/was treated with acitretin. Hepatotoxicity has occurred infrequently.

Assessment & Drug Effects

- Monitor for S&S of pancreatitis or loss of glycemic control in diabetics. Report either condition immediately to prescriber.
- Monitor lab tests: Baseline and q1–2wk (until response to drug is known) lipid profile and LFTs; periodic blood glucose and HbA1C.

Patient & Family Education

- If either parent has been treated with acitretin, use two forms of effective contraception for 1 mo before and at least 3 yr following therapy because of the serious risk of fetal deformities that could result from exposure to this medication.
- Do not breastfeed while taking this drug.
- Note: Transient worsening of psoriasis may occur during early therapy.
- Review common adverse effects of drug; lag time of 2–3 mo may be necessary before drug effect is evident.
- Discontinue drug and report immediately to prescriber if visual problems develop.
- Note: Dry eyes with decreased tolerance for contact lenses may occur.
- Do not drink alcohol while taking this drug; it increases risk of

hepatotoxicity and hypertriglyceridemia; females should avoid alcohol during and for 2 mo following therapy.
- Avoid excessive amounts of vitamin A (consult prescriber).
- Do not donate blood for 3 yr following therapy.
- Avoid excessive exposure to sunlight or UV light.

ACLIDINIUM BROMIDE

(a-cli-di'ni-um bro'mide)

Tudorza Pressair

Classification: ANTICHOLINERGIC; ANTIMUSCARINIC; ANTISPASMODIC; BRONCHODILATOR

Therapeutic: BRONCHODILATOR

Prototype: Atropine

AVAILABILITY Powder for inhalation

ACTION & *THERAPEUTIC EFFECT* A long-acting antimuscarinic, anticholinergic agent that inhibits the action of acetylcholine at muscarinic receptors in bronchial smooth muscles. *Promotes bronchodilation and relieves bronchospasms associated with COPD.*

USES Treatment of bronchospasm associated with chronic obstructive pulmonary disease (COPD).

CONTRAINDICATIONS Hypersensitivity to aclidinium; hypersensitivity to milk proteins; acute or paradoxical episodes of bronchospasm.

CAUTIOUS USE Narrow-angle glaucoma; urinary retention; hypersensitivity to milk proteins; pregnancy (category C); lactation. Safety and efficacy in children younger than 18 yr not established.

ROUTE & DOSAGE

Chronic Obstructive Pulmonary Disorder

Adult: **Oral Inhalation** 400 mcg bid

ADMINISTRATION

Inhalation

- Open pouch immediately before first use.
- Prior to each use, remove protective cap from inhaler and prepare inhaler by pressing and releasing the green button causing the control window to change from red to green.
- Instruct the patient to keep inhaling until a "click" is heard to ensure that the full dose has been given.
- Store inhaler inside the sealed pouch at 15°–30°C (59°–86°F).

ADVERSE EFFECTS **Respiratory:** Nasopharyngitis. **CNS:** Headache.

INTERACTIONS **Drug:** Additive anticholinergic effects if used in combination with another ANTICHOLINERGIC AGENT.

PHARMACOKINETICS **Absorption:** 6% bioavailability. **Onset:** 30 min. **Metabolism:** Broken down to inactive metabolites. **Elimination:** Renal (54–65%) and fecal (20–33%). **Half-Life:** 5–8 h.

NURSING IMPLICATIONS

Assessment & Drug Effects

- Monitor peak flow or pulmonary function studies.

- Monitor closely anyone with a history of hypersensitivity to atropine.
- Monitor I&O and assess for urinary retention.
- Monitor for and report promptly S&S of narrow-angle glaucoma (e.g., severe eye pain, eye edema and redness, often accompanied by nausea and vomiting).

Patient & Family Education

- Do not use as a rescue medication.
- Stop using aclidinium and report to prescriber if paradoxical bronchospasms occur.
- Report to prescriber if you experience painful urination or have difficulty passing urine (e.g., frequent urination, urination in weak stream or drips).
- Report promptly any of the following signs of acute narrow-angle glaucoma: Eye pain or discomfort, blurred vision, visual halos, colored images, or red eyes.

ACYCLOVIR, ACYCLOVIR SODIUM

(ay-sye'kloe-ver)

Zovirax

Classification: ANTIVIRAL

Therapeutic: ANTIVIRAL; ANTI-HERPES

AVAILABILITY Capsule; tablet; oral suspension; injection; ointment, cream

ACTION & *THERAPEUTIC EFFECT* It preferentially interferes with DNA synthesis of herpes simplex virus types 1 and 2 (HSV-1 and HSV-2) and varicella-zoster virus, thereby inhibiting viral replication. *Acyclovir reduces viral shedding and formation of new lesions and speeds healing time. It demonstrates antiviral activity against herpes virus simiae (B virus), Epstein-Barr (infectious mononucleosis), varicella-zoster, and cytomegalovirus, but does not eradicate the latent herpes virus.*

USES Parenterally for treatment of viral encephalitis, treatment of herpes simplex, and treatment of varicella-zoster virus (shingles/chickenpox). Used orally for herpes simplex treatment, and prophylaxis and treatment of varicella-zoster virus (shingles/chickenpox). Used topically for herpes labialis (cold sores), initial episodes of herpes genitalis and in non-life-threatening mucocutaneous herpes simplex virus infections in immunocompromised patients.

UNLABELED USES Treatment of eczema herpeticum caused by HSV localized and disseminated herpes zoster, CMV prophylaxis, pharyngitis, stomatitis, varicella prophylaxis, new onset Bell palsy, cytomegalovirus prevention.

CONTRAINDICATIONS Hypersensitivity to acyclovir and valacyclovir.

CAUTIOUS USE Renal insufficiency, dehydration, seizure disorders, or neurologic disease; immunocompromised individuals; older adults; pregnancy (if there is a clinical need, it is considered safe to use).

ROUTE & DOSAGE

Cold Sores

Adult/Adolescents (12 yr or older): **Topical** Apply 5 × day for 4 days

Genital Herpes Simplex (Initial episode)

Adult: **PO** 400 mg tid or 200 mg five times per day for 7–10-day

cycle; **IV** 5–10 mg/kg q8h × 2–7 days **Topical** Apply q3h 6 × day × 7 days
Child: **PO** 40 to 80 mg/kg/d divided in 3–4 doses × 7–10 days

Herpes Simplex in Immunocompromised Patient

Adult: **PO** 400 mg tid × 5–10 days **IV** 5–10 mg/kg q8h × 2–7 days
Child: **PO** 20 mg/kg tid × 7–10 days **IV** 5 mg/kg q8h × 5–7 days

HSV genital infection suppression

Adult/Adolescent: **PO** 400 mg bid

Herpes Zoster

Adult/Adolescent: **PO** 800 mg q4h × 7 days
Child: **PO** 80 mg/kg/day in 5 divided doses

Herpes Zoster (in immunocompromised patients)

Adult/Adolescent: **IV** 10–15 mg/kg q8h × 7 days
Child (less than 12 yr): **IV** 10 mg/kg q8h × 7–10 days

HSV central nervous system infection (encephalitis)

Adult: **IV** 10 mg/kg q8h × 10 days
Child (3 mo to less than 12 yr): **IV** 10–15 mg/kg q8h × 14–21 days

Varicella Zoster Treatment

Adult: **IV** 10 mg/kg q8h × 7 days PO 800 mg 5 times per day × 5–7 days
Child/Adolescent: **PO** 20 mg/kg (max: 800 mg) qid × 5 days initiated within 24 h of onset of rash

Obesity Dosage Adjustment

Patient dose should be calculated using IBW.

Renal Impairment Dosage Adjustment

IV administration: CrCl 25–50 mL/min: Standard dose q12h; *10–25 mL/min:* Standard dose q24h; *less than 10 mL/min:* Give half normal dose q24h (see package insert for neonatal renal impairment adjustment)
PO administration: 10–25 mL/min: if usual dose is 800 mg 5 times/day administer 800 mg q8h; *less than 10 mL/min:* if usual dose is 800 mg 5 times/day administer 200 mg q12h

ADMINISTRATION

Oral

- Shake suspension well prior to use.
- Administer with or without food.
- Store capsules in tight, light-resistant containers at 15°–30°C (59°–86°F) unless otherwise directed.

Topical

- Wash hands thoroughly before and after treatment of lesions and after handling and disposition of secretions.
- Apply approximately ½ inch of cream or ointment ribbon for each 4 square inches of surface area. Use sufficient ointment or cream to completely cover lesions.
- Apply topical preparation with finger cot or surgical glove.
- Store at 15°–25°C (59°–78°F) unless otherwise directed.

Intravenous

PREPARE: **Intermittent:** Reconstitute by adding 10 mL sterile water for injection to 500-mg vial to yield 50 mg/mL. Note: Do not use bacteriostatic water for injection containing benzyl alcohol. Shake well. ▪ Further dilute to 7 mg/mL or less to reduce risk of renal injury and phlebitis. Example: Add 1 mL of reconstituted solution to 9 mL of diluent to yield 5 mg/mL. ▪ Use standard electrolyte and glucose solutions (e.g., NS, LR, D5W) for dilution.

ADMINISTER: **Intermittent:** Administer by constant infusion over at least 1 h to prevent renal tubular damage. Rapid or bolus IV administration **must be** avoided. ▪ Monitor IV flow rate carefully; infusion pump or microdrip infusion set preferred. ▪ Avoid extravasation.

INCOMPATIBILITIES: **Solution/additive:** **Dobutamine, dopamine, tramadol.** **Y-site:** **Amifostine, aminocaproic acid, amphotericin B, ampicillin/sulbactam, amsacrine, aztreonam, capreomycin, cefepime, chlorpromazine, ciprofloxacin, codeine, dacarbazine, daptomycin, daunorubicin, dexrazoxane, diazepam, dobutamine, dolasetron, dopamine, doxorubicin, epinephrine, epirubicin, eptifibatide, esmolol, fenoldopam, foscarnet, garenoxacin, gemcitabine, gemtuzumab, haloperidol, hydralazine, hydroxyzine, idarubicin, irinotecan, ketamine, ketorolac, labetalol, levofloxacin, lidocaine, mesna, methadone, midazolam, mitomycin, mycophenolate, nicardipine, nitroprusside, ondansetron, palonosetron, pentamidine, phenylephrine, phenytoin, piperacillin/tazobactam, potassium phosphate, procainamide, prochlorperazine, promethazine, quinupristin/dalfopristin, sargramostim, sodium phosphate, streptozocin, ticarcillin/clavulanate, topotecan, TPN, vecuronium, verapamil, vinorelbine.**

▪ Refrigerated reconstituted solution may precipitate; however, crystals will redissolve at room temperature. ▪ Store acyclovir powder and reconstituted solutions at controlled room temperature, preferably at 15°–30°C (59°–86°F) unless otherwise directed by manufacturer. ▪ Use reconstituted solution within 12 h. Use diluted solution within 24 h.

ADVERSE EFFECTS **CNS:** Malaise, lethargy, fatigue. **GI:** *Nausea, vomiting*. **GU:** Increased BUN and serum creatinine. **Other:** Inflammation or phlebitis at IV injection site, sloughing (with extravasation), thrombocytopenic purpura.

INTERACTIONS **Drug:** Do not use with **cladribine, foscarnet, tizanidine**; **zidovudine** may cause increased drowsiness and lethargy. Do not use with LIVE VACCINES.

PHARMACOKINETICS **Absorption:** Oral dose is 15–30% absorbed. **Peak:** 1.5–2 h after oral dose. **Distribution:** Into most tissues with lower levels in the CNS; crosses placenta. **Metabolism:** Drug is primarily excreted unchanged. **Elimination:** Renally eliminated; also excreted in breast milk. **Half-Life:** 2.5–5 h.

NURSING IMPLICATIONS

Assessment & Drug Effects

- Observe infusion site during infusion and for a few days following infusion for signs of tissue damage.

- Monitor I&O and hydration status. Keep patient adequately hydrated during first 2 h after infusion to maintain sufficient urinary flow and prevent formation of renal stones. Consult physician about amount and length of time oral fluids need to be pushed after IV drug treatment.
- Monitor for S&S of: Reinfection in pregnant patients; acyclovir-induced neurologic symptoms in patients with history of neurologic problems; drug resistance in immunocompromised patients receiving prolonged or repeated therapy; acute renal failure with concomitant use of other nephrotoxic drugs or preexisting renal disease.
- Monitor for adverse effects and viral resistance with long-term prophylactic use of the oral drug.
- Monitor lab tests: Baseline and periodic renal function tests, particularly with IV administration.

Patient & Family Education

- Start therapy as soon as possible after onset of S&S for best results.
- Maintain a good fluid intake while receiving this drug.
- Do not exceed recommended dosage, frequency of drug administration, or specified duration of therapy. Contact prescriber if relief is not obtained or adverse effects appear.
- Cleanse affected areas with soap and water 3–4 × daily prior to topical application; dry well before application. With application to genitals, wear loose-fitting clothes over affected areas.
- Refrain from sexual intercourse while herpes lesions are present; neither topical nor systemic drug prevents transmission to other individuals.
- Avoid topical drug contact in or around eyes. Report unexplained eye symptoms to prescriber immediately (e.g., redness, pain); untreated infection can lead to corneal keratitis and blindness.

ADALIMUMAB

(a-da-lim′u-mab)

Humira

Classification: BIOLOGICAL RESPONSE MODIFIER; IMMUNOMODULATOR; TUMOR NECROSIS FACTOR (TNF) MODIFIER; DISEASE-MODIFYING ANTIRHEUMATIC DRUG (DMARD)

Therapeutic: ANTIRHEUMATIC; DMARD; ANTI-INFLAMMATORY

Prototype: Etanercept

AVAILABILITY Solution for injection

ACTION & *THERAPEUTIC EFFECT*

A recombinant monoclonal antibody that neutralizes the effects of tumor necrosis factor (TNF)-alpha by blocking its interaction with cell surface TNF receptors. This mechanism blocks the normal inflammatory and immune responses controlled by TNF-alpha. *Reduces the levels of acute phase inflammatory reactants (C-reactive protein, ESR, interleukin-6), thus decreasing overall joint inflammation; also reduces levels of enzymes that produce tissue remodeling responsible for cartilage destruction. In RA, it reduces the overproduction of TNF-alpha (principally by macrophages) in rheumatoid joints. Reduces epidermal thickness and inflammatory cell infiltration in plaque psoriasis.*

USES Treatment of moderate to severe rheumatoid arthritis or psoriatic arthritis, polyarticular juvenile arthritis, ankylosing spondylitis, plaque psoriasis, treatment of Crohn disease, ulcerative colitis, uveitis.

UNLABELED USES Management of Crohn disease after surgical resection.

CONTRAINDICATIONS Hypersensitivity to adalimumab or mannitol; live vaccines; development of lupus-like syndrome while using adalimumab; neoplastic disease.

CAUTIOUS USE History of recurrent infection or conditions predisposing to infection; recurrent history of sensitivity to monoclonal antibodies; CHF; neurologic disease; patients residing in areas with endemic TB or histoplasmosis; latent TB infection prior to therapy; history of or carriers of Hepatitis B; demyelinating disorders; Crohn disease; ulcerative colitis; surgery; older adults; pregnancy (use with caution during pregnancy); lactation. Safe use in children younger than 4 yr has not been established.

ROUTE & DOSAGE

Rheumatoid Arthritis/Ankylosing Spondylitis/Psoriatic arthritis

Adult: **Subcutaneous** 40 mg every other wk

Polyarticular Juvenile Arthritis

Adolescent/Child (2 yr or older and 30 kg or more): **Subcutaneous** 40 mg every other wk
Adolescent/Child (2 yr or older and 15–30 kg): **Subcutaneous** 20 mg every other wk *Child (2 yr or older and 10–15 kg):* **Subcutaneous** 10 mg every other wk

Crohn Disease/Moderate Ulcerative Colitis

Adult/Adolescent/Child (5 yr or older and over 40 kg): **Subcutaneous** Initial dose of 160 mg on day 1 or split over 2 consecutive days then 80 mg at wk 2, followed by 40 mg every other wk beginning at wk 4
Child/Adolescent (5 yr or older and 20–40 kg): **Humira only Subcutaneous** 80 mg then 40 mg 2 wk later, followed by 20 mg every other wk starting at wk 4

Plaque Psoriasis

Adult: **Subcutaneous** 80 mg then after 1 wk 40 mg every other wk

Noninfectious Uveitis

Adult: **Subcutaneous** 30 mg, then 40 mg every other wk
Children 2 yr and older, weight 30 kg or greater: **Subcutaneous** 40 mg every other wk; *weight 15 kg to less than 30 kg:* 20 mg every other wk; *weight 10 kg to less than 15 kg:* 10 mg every other wk

ADMINISTRATION

Subcutaneous

- Leave at room temperature for 15 to 30 min prior to use.
- Inspect prefilled syringe for particulate matter and discoloration prior to subcutaneous injection.
- Rotate injection sites and do not inject into skin that is red, bruised, tender, or hard. After injecting the drug, do not rub the site. Inject in thigh or lower abdomen sites.
- Discard any remaining solution in prefilled syringe, as it contains no preservatives.
- Store in original carton at 2°–8°C (38°–46°F). Protect from light. Do not use beyond the expiration date.

ADVERSE EFFECTS **CV:** Hypertension, hyperlipidemia, hypercholesterolemia. **Respiratory:** Sinusitis, flu-like symptoms. **CNS:** Headache. **Hepatic:** Increased serum alkaline phosphatase. **GI:** Nausea, abdominal pain. **GU:** Urinary tract infection, hematuria. **Musculoskeletal:** Increased creatine phosphokinase, back pain. **Hematologic:** Positive ANA titer. **Integumentary:** Skin rash. **Other:** *Infection*, antibody development, injection site reaction, hypersensitivity reaction, accidental injury.

INTERACTIONS **Drug:** Do not give LIVE VIRUS VACCINES to patient on adalimumab; not recommended for use with other TNF BLOCKERS (**etanercept, infliximab, rilonacept, anakinra**). Do not use with **abatacept, tofacitinib**, or **rituximab**. Do not use with IMMUNOSUPPRESSANTS.

PHARMACOKINETICS **Absorption:** 64% absorbed from subcutaneous injection site. **Peak:** 131 h. **Distribution:** Minimal beyond vascular/synovial space. **Elimination:** Higher clearance in presence of anti-adalimumab antibodies, lower clearance with increasing age. **Half-Life:** 10–20 days.

NURSING IMPLICATIONS

Black Box Warning

Adalimumab has been associated with increased risk of severe, potentially fatal, infections. Children and adolescents are at risk for development of malignancies.

Assessment & Drug Effects

- Monitor for latent TB prior to initiating therapy.
- Monitor for and report lupus-like syndrome (e.g., joint pain, rash on cheeks or arms that is sensitive to sun).
- Monitor for and report promptly S&S of infection, including TB. Monitor known HBV carriers for signs of active HBV infection during therapy and for several months after therapy is discontinued.
- Monitor for signs and symptoms of worsening heart failure.
- Monitor neurologic status closely. Report any change in status such as blurred vision or paresthesia.
- Monitor lab tests: CBC with differential.

Patient & Family Education

- Live vaccines should not be accepted by persons taking this drug.
- Report promptly any of the following to the prescriber: Unexplained joint pain, rash on cheeks or arms, fever, sore throat or other signs of infection, changes in vision, numbness or tingling in extremities.
- Severe and sometimes deadly infections have happened in patients who take this drug. Caution should be taken to minimize exposure to infectious agents.

ADAPALENE

(a-da′pa-leen)

Differin

Classification: ANTIACNE; RETINOID

Therapeutic: ANTIACNE

Prototype: Isotretinoin

AVAILABILITY Gel; cream; lotion

ACTION & *THERAPEUTIC EFFECT*

A topical retinoid-like compound that modulates cellular differentiation, keratinization, and inflammatory processes related to the pathology of acne vulgaris. Topical adapalene may normalize the differentiation of epithelial follicular cells. *Adapalene decreases the inflammatory process and acne formation.*

USES Treatment of acne vulgaris.

UNLABELED USES Rosacea.

CONTRAINDICATIONS Hypersensitivity to adapalene or any of the components of the gel, irritating topical products, and sunburn; skin abrasion, eczema, seborrheic dermatitis.

CAUTIOUS USE Pregnancy (category C); lactation. Safety and efficacy in children younger than 12 yr not established.

ROUTE & DOSAGE

Acne
Adult/Adolescent: Apply once daily to affected areas in evening

ADMINISTRATION

Topical

- Apply a thin film to clean skin, avoiding eyes, lips, mucous membranes, cuts, abrasions, eczematous or sunburned skin.
- Do not apply to skin recently treated with preparations containing sulfur, resorcinol, or salicylic acid.
- Store at 20°–25°C (68°–77°F).

ADVERSE EFFECTS **Skin:** *Erythema, scaling, dryness, pruritus, burning,* skin irritation, stinging, acne flares, sunburn.

PHARMACOKINETICS **Absorption:** Minimal through intact skin. **Elimination:** Primarily in bile.

NURSING IMPLICATIONS

Assessment & Drug Effects

- Monitor therapeutic effectiveness, which is indicated by improvement after 8–12 wk of treatment; early therapy may be marked by apparent worsening of acne.
- Note: Cutaneous reactions (e.g., erythema, scaling, pruritus) are common and normally diminish after first month of therapy.

Patient & Family Education

- Apply only as directed; excessive application will not result in faster healing but will cause marked redness, peeling, and discomfort.
- Minimize exposure to sunlight and sunlamps, and use sunscreen and protective clothing as needed.

ADEFOVIR DIPIVOXIL

(a-de′fo-vir)

Hepsera

Classification: ANTIVIRAL; NUCLEOTIDE ANALOG

Therapeutic: ANTIVIRAL

AVAILABILITY Tablet

ACTION & *THERAPEUTIC EFFECT* Inhibits human hepatitis virus (HBV) DNA polymerase (reverse transcriptase) by competing with its DNA and by causing DNA chain termination after its incorporation into viral DNA. *Resulting in inhibition of HBV DNA replication.*

USES Treatment of chronic hepatitis B.

CONTRAINDICATIONS Hypersensitivity to adefovir; untreated or unknown human immunodeficiency virus (HIV); exacerbations of hepatitis B, especially in patients who have discontinued anti-hepatitis B therapy; lactation.

CAUTIOUS USE Decreased cardiac function due to concomitant disease or other drug therapy; concomitant use of highly nephrotoxic drugs; renal dysfunction; coadministration with drugs that reduce renal function or compete for active tubular secretion; older adults; pregnancy (limited information related to use in pregnancy; use of other agents during pregnancy is recommended); children younger than 2 yr. Appropriate infant immunizations should be used to prevent neonatal acquisition of the hepatitis B virus.

ROUTE & DOSAGE

Hepatitis B

Adult: **PO** 10 mg daily (duration varies based on HBeAg status, duration of HBV suppression, presence of cirrhosis)

Renal Impairment Dosage Adjustment

CrCl 20–49 mL/min: 10 mg q48h; *10–19 mL/min:* 10 mg q72h

Hemodialysis Dosage Adjustment

10 mg q7days following dialysis

ADMINISTRATION

Oral

- May be given without regard to food.
- Store in original container at 15°–30°C (59°–86°F).

ADVERSE EFFECTS **Respiratory:** Cough. **CNS:** Headache. **Endocrine:** *Increased ALT, AST,* increased creatine kinase, amylase, lactic acidosis. **Hepatic/GI:** Abdominal pain, flatulence, diarrhea, dyspepsia, exacerbation of hepatitis after discontinuation of therapy, hepatomegaly. **GU:** *Hematuria,* nephrotoxicity. **Musculoskeletal:** Weakness, back pain.

INTERACTIONS **Drug:** **Tenofovir** may increase concentration of adefovir; avoid use with **tolvaptan, cladribine**.

PHARMACOKINETICS **Absorption:** Adefovir dipivoxil is a prodrug. **Peak:** 1–4 h. **Distribution:** Minimal protein binding. **Metabolism:** Adefovir dipivoxil is rapidly converted to active adefovir. **Elimination:** Primarily in urine. **Half-Life:** 7.5 h.

NURSING IMPLICATIONS

Black Box Warning

Adefovir has been associated with severe, acute exacerbations of hepatitis, nephrotoxicity, HIV resistance, lactic acidosis, and severe hepatomegaly with steatosis.

Assessment & Drug Effects

- Withhold drug and notify prescriber if lactic acidosis is suspected [e.g., hyperventilation, lethargy, plasma pH less than 7.35, and lactate greater than 5–6 mol/L (mEq/L)].
- Monitor for and promptly report S&S of hepatomegaly with steatosis, or other signs of liver injury.
- Monitor lab tests: Baseline and periodic renal function tests (monitor more often with preexisting impairment or other risk factors for renal impairment); periodic LFTs, creatinine kinase, serum amylase, and routine blood chemistries including serum electrolytes.

Patient & Family Education

- Report any of the following to prescriber: Blood in urine, unexplained weakness, or exacerbation of S&S of hepatitis.
- Patients who discontinue adefovir should be monitored at repeated intervals over a period of time for hepatic function.

ADENOSINE

(a-den'o-sin)

Adenocard, Adenoscan

Classification: ANTIARRHYTHMIC

Therapeutic: ANTIARRHYTHMIC

AVAILABILITY Injection

ACTION & *THERAPEUTIC EFFECT* Slows conduction through the atrioventricular (AV) and sinoatrial (SA) nodes. Can interrupt the reentry pathways through the AV node. *Restores normal sinus rhythm in patients with paroxysmal supraventricular tachycardia.*

USES Conversion to sinus rhythm of paroxysmal supraventricular tachycardia (PSVT) including PSVT associated with accessory bypass tracts (Wolff-Parkinson-White syndrome). "Chemical" thallium stress test.

UNLABELED USES Afterload-reducing agent in low-output states; to prevent graft occlusion following aortocoronary bypass surgery; to produce controlled hypotension during cerebral aneurysm surgery.

CONTRAINDICATIONS AV block, preexisting second- and third-degree heart block or sick sinus rhythm without pacemaker because a heart block may result.

CAUTIOUS USE Asthmatics, unstable angina, stenotic valvular disease, hypovolemia; hepatic and renal failure; pregnancy (category C).

ROUTE & DOSAGE

Supraventricular Tachycardia

Adult/Adolescent (weight 50 kg or more): **IV** 6-mg bolus initially; after 1–2 min may give two additional 12-mg bolus doses for a total of 3 doses.
Do not exceed 12 mg in any one dose.
Neonate/Infant/Child: **IV** 0.05–1-mg/kg bolus; additional doses may be increased by 0.05–1 mg/kg q2min (max: 12 mg/dose)

Stress Thallium Test

Adult: **IV** 140 mcg/kg/min × 6 min (max: 0.84 mg/kg total dose)

ADMINISTRATION

Intravenous

Make sure solution is clear at time of use.
- Discard unused portion (contains no preservatives).

PREPARE: **Direct:** No dilution is required.
ADMINISTER: **Direct:** *Supraventricular Tachycardia:* Give rapid bolus over 1–2 sec. *Thallium Stress Test:* Give bolus over 6 min.
- If given by IV line, administer as proximally as possible, and follow with a rapid saline flush.

- Store at room temperature 15°–30°C (59°–86°F). Do not refrigerate, as crystallization may occur. If crystals do form, dissolve by warming to room temperature.

ADVERSE EFFECTS CV: *Transient facial flushing,* sweating, palpitations, chest pain, atrial fibrillation or flutter. **Respiratory:** Shortness of breath, transient *dyspnea,* chest pressure. **CNS:** Headache, lightheadedness, dizziness, tingling in arms (from IV infusion), apprehension, blurred vision, burning sensation (from IV infusion). **GI:** Nausea, metallic taste, tightness in throat. **Other:** Irritability in children.

INTERACTIONS Drug: Dipyridamole can potentiate the effects of adenosine; **theophylline** will block the electrophysiologic effects of adenosine; **carbamazepine** may increase risk of heart block.

PHARMACOKINETICS Absorption: Rapid uptake by erythrocytes and vascular endothelial cells after IV administration. **Onset:** 20–30 sec. **Metabolism:** Rapid uptake into cells; degraded by deamination to inosine, hypoxanthine, and adenosine monophosphate. **Elimination:** Route unknown. **Half-Life:** 10 sec.

NURSING IMPLICATIONS

Assessment & Drug Effects

- Monitor for S&S of bronchospasm in asthma patients. Notify prescriber immediately.
- Use a hemodynamic monitoring system during administration; monitor BP and heart rate and rhythm continuously for several minutes after administration.
- Note: Adverse effects are generally self-limiting due to short half-life (10 sec).
- Note: At the time of conversion to normal sinus rhythm, PVCs, PACs, sinus bradycardia, and sinus tachycardia, as well as various degrees of AV block, are seen on the ECG. These usually last only a few seconds and resolve without intervention.

Patient & Family Education

- Note: Flushing may occur along with a feeling of warmth as drug is injected.

ADO-TRASTUZUMAB EMTANSINE

(A-doh-tras-too'zoo-mab em-tan'seen)

Kadcyla

Classification: IMMUNOMODULATOR; MONOCLONAL ANTIBODY; ANTINEOPLASTIC; ANTI-HUMAN EPIDERMAL GROWTH FACTOR RECEPTOR (ANTI-HER)

Therapeutic: ANTINEOPLASTIC; IMMUNOMODULATOR; ANTI-HER

Prototype: Trastuzumab

AVAILABILITY Powder for injection

ACTION & *THERAPEUTIC EFFECT* Binds to the HER2 receptors on the cell surface and is then brought into the cell, where it is degraded into catabolites that disrupt the microtubule networks in the cell, resulting in cell cycle arrest and apoptotic cell death. *Causes death of HER2-positive breast cancer cells.*

USES Treatment of patients with HER2-positive, metastatic breast cancer who previously received trastuzumab and a taxane, separately or in combination.

CONTRAINDICATIONS Pregnancy (category D).

CAUTIOUS USE Interstitial lung disease or pneumonitis; hypersensitivity; thrombocytopenia; lactation.

ROUTE & DOSAGE

HER2-Positive, Metastatic Breast Cancer

Adult: **IV** 3.6 mg/kg q 3wk

Hepatic Impairment Dosage Adjustment

AST/ALT greater than 5 to less than or equal to 20 × ULN: Withhold therapy; resume with dosage reduction when AST/ALT is less than or equal to 5 × ULN

Total bilirubin greater than 3 to less than or equal to 10 × ULN: Withhold therapy; resume with dosage reduction when total bilirubin less than or equal to 1.5 × ULN

Permanently discontinue use if AST/ALT is greater than 3 × ULN and total bilirubin is greater than 2 × ULN

Thrombocytopenia

Platelet count 25,000/mm³ to less than 50,000 mm³: Withhold therapy; resume at same dose when platelet count is greater than or equal to 75,500 m³
Platelet count less than 25,000/mm³: Withhold treat; resume with dosage reduction when platelet count is greater than or equal to 75,500 m³

Recommended Dosage Reduction Schedule for Adverse Events

First reduction: 3 mg/kg
Second reduction: 2.4 mg/kg
Discontinue if further reduction is required

ADMINISTRATION

Intravenous

Give antipyretics prior to infusion. **Do not** substitute ado-trastuzumab emtansine (Kadcyla) for or with trastuzumab (Herceptin).

PREPARE: **IV Infusion:** Slowly inject 5 mL SW for injection or 8 mL SW for injection into the 100-mg or 160-mg vial, respectively, to yield 20 mg/mL. Swirl gently until dissolved but **do not shake.** Reconstituted solution will be clear to slightly opalescent. Should be used immediately.
From the 20-mg/mL reconstituted vial, withdraw the needed dose and add to 250 mL NS. Gently invert bag to dissolve. **Do not shake.**

ADMINISTER: **IV Infusion:** Infuse through a 0.22-micron in-line, non–protein filter. Give first infusion over 90 min; give subsequent infusions over 30 min if prior infusions well tolerated.

INCOMPATIBILITIES: **Solution/additive:** Do not mix with dextrose. **Y-site:** Do not mix or administer as an infusion with other medications.

- Store at 2°–8°C (36°–46°F) if not used immediately. Discard after 4 h.

ADVERSE EFFECTS **CV:** Hypertension, left ventricular dysfunction. **Respiratory:** Cough, dyspnea, epistaxis, pneumonitis. **CNS:** Dizziness, *headache*, insomnia. **HEENT:** Blurred vision, conjunctivitis, dry eye, lacrimation. **Endocrine:** *AST/ALT increase*, bilirubin increase, blood alkaline phosphatase increase, hemoglobin decrease, hypokalemia. **Skin:** Pruritus, rash. **GI:** Abdominal pain, *constipation*, diarrhea, dry mouth, dyspepsia, *nausea*, stomatitis, vomiting. **GU:** Urinary tract infection. **Musculoskeletal:** Arthralgia, *musculoskeletal pain*, myalgia. **Hematological:** Anemia, neutropenia, *thrombocytopenia*. **Other:** Asthenia, chills, *fatigue*, hypersensitivity reactions, infusion-related reaction, peripheral edema, peripheral neuropathy, pyrexia.

INTERACTIONS **Drug:** Strong CYP3A4 inhibitors (e.g., **ketoconazole, itraconazole, clarithromycin, atazanavir, indinavir, nefazodone, nelfinavir, ritonavir, saquinavir, telithromycin, voriconazole**) may increase the levels of ado-trastuzumab.

PHARMACOKINETICS **Distribution:** 93% plasma protein bound. **Metabolism:** In liver to active and inactive compounds. **Half-Life:** 4 d.

NURSING IMPLICATIONS

Black Box Warning

Ado-trastuzumab emtansine has been associated with severe, potentially fatal, hepatotoxicity, and reduction in left ventricular ejection fraction. It can cause fetal harm and fetal death.

Assessment & Drug Effects

- Monitor for S&S of a hypersensitivity reaction during and for at least 90 min after IV infusion. Slow or stop infusion if a significant infusion-related or hypersensitivity reaction occurs.
- Monitor vital signs frequently during and after IV infusion.
- Monitor for S&S of neurotoxicity. Withhold dose and report to prescriber if Grade 3 or 4 neuropathy develops.
- Monitor for and report promptly S&S of acute hepatitis and/or CHF.
- Monitor pulmonary status and report S&S of pulmonary toxicity (e.g., dyspnea, cough, fatigue, and pulmonary infiltrates).
- Monitor lab tests: Initial HERS2 testing to determine eligibility; prior to each dose, LFTs and platelet count.

Patient & Family Education

- Do not breastfeed while being treated with this drug.
- Use effective means of contraception during and for 6 mo after the last dose of this drug.
- Notify prescriber immediately if you suspect you are pregnant.
- Notify prescriber immediately if you experience S&S of liver damage (e.g., nausea, vomiting, right upper abdominal pain, jaundice, dark urine, generalized itching, anorexia), shortness of breath, cough, swelling of the ankles/legs, palpitations, weight gain of more than 5 lb in 24 h, dizziness, or loss of consciousness.

AFATINIB

(a-fa'ti-nib)

Gilotrif

Classification: ANTINEOPLASTIC; KINASE INHIBITOR

Therapeutic: ANTINEOPLASTIC

Prototype: Erlotinib

AVAILABILITY Tablet

ACTION & *THERAPEUTIC EFFECT*

Epidermal growth factor receptors (EGFR) are expressed or overexpressed in many cancers. EGFR expression is associated with poor prognosis (i.e., development of metastasis and resistance to chemotherapy, hormonal therapy, and radiation therapy). *Inhibits up-regulation or overexpression of EGRF in cancer cells, thus diminishing their capacity for cell proliferation, cell survival, and decreasing their invasive capacity and metastases.*

USES First-line treatment of patients with metastatic non-small cell lung cancer (NSCLC) whose tumors have epidermal growth factor receptor (EGFR) exon 19 deletions or exon 21 (L858R) substitution mutations as detected by an FDA-approved test.

CONTRAINDICATIONS Life-threatening bullous, blistering, or exfoliative skin lesions; confirmed interstitial lung disease (ILD); severe drug-induced hepatic impairment; persistent ulcerative keratitis; symptomatic left ventricular dysfunction; severe or intolerable adverse reaction occurring at a dose of 20 mg per day; pregnancy (category D); lactation.

CAUTIOUS USE Diarrhea, bullous and exfoliative skin disorders, keratitis; mild to moderate interstitial lung disease; metastatic breast cancer; mild to moderate hepatic impairment; patients with HER2-positive metastatic breast cancer. Safety and efficacy in children not established.

ROUTE & DOSAGE

Non-Small Cell Lung Cancer (NSCLC)

Adult: **PO** 40 once daily

Toxicity Dosage Adjustment

Hold therapy for any of the following:
National Cancer Institute Common Terminology Criteria for Adverse Effects (NCI CTCAE) Grade 3 or higher

Diarrhea greater than or equal to Grade 2 persisting for 2 or more consecutive days while on antidiarrheal medication

Grade 2 cutaneous reactions that are prolonged (greater than or equal to 7 days) or intolerable

Hepatotoxicity Dosage Adjustment

Grade 2 or higher renal toxicity

When toxicity resolves, resume therapy at 10 mg/d less than dose that caused toxicity. Permanently discontinue if toxicity occurs at dose of 20 mg/day.

Dosage Adjustment with Concomitant Use of P-gp Inhibitors or Inducers

P-gp inhibitor: Reduce dose to 30 mg/day if not tolerated. If P-gp inhibitor is discontinued, resume previous dose.
P-gp inducer: Increase dose to 50 mg/day as tolerated. If P-gp inducer is discontinued, wait 2–3 wk and resume previous dose.

ADMINISTRATION

Oral

- Give on an empty stomach at least 1 h before or 2 h after a meal.
- Store at 20°–25°C (68°–77°F).

ADVERSE EFFECTS **Respiratory:** Epistaxis, rhinorrhea. **HEENT:** Conjunctivitis. **Endocrine:** ALT/AST increased, increased serum bilirubin, decreased appetite, decreased weight, *hypokalemia*. **Skin:** *Dermatitis acneiform, dry skin,* pruritus, *rash*. **GI:** Cheilitis, *diarrhea, stomatitis,* nausea, vomiting, decreased appetite. **Other:** Cystitis, *paronychia*, pyrexia.

INTERACTIONS **Drug:** Inhibitors of P-gp (e.g., **amiodarone, azithromycin, cyclosporine A, diltiazem, erythromycin, itraconazole, ketoconazole, nelfinavir, quinidine, ritonavir, saquinavir, tacrolimus, verapamil**) can increase the levels of afatinib. Inducers of P-gp (e.g., **carbamazepine, phenobarbital, phenytoin, rifampin**) can decrease the levels of afatinib. **Herbal: St. John's wort** can decrease the levels of afatinib.

PHARMACOKINETICS **Absorption:** 92% bioavailable. **Peak:** 2–5 h. **Distribution:** 95% plasma protein bound. **Metabolism:** Minimal metabolism in liver. **Elimination:** Primarily fecal (85%). **Half-Life:** 37 h.

NURSING IMPLICATIONS

Assessment & Drug Effects

- Monitor vital signs throughout the course of therapy.
- Monitor for diarrhea; withhold drug and notify prescriber if diarrhea lasts more than 48 h or if patient shows S&S of dehydration.
- Monitor for and report skin lesions (e.g., rash, erythema). Withhold drug and notify prescriber if blistering occurs.

- Monitor for and report eye inflammation, excessive lacrimation, light sensitivity, blurred vision, and eye pain.
- Monitor lab tests: Baseline and periodic LFTs; periodic serum electrolytes.

Patient & Family Education

- Women should use highly effective means of birth control during and for at least 2 wk after termination of therapy. Notify prescriber immediately if a pregnancy occurs or is suspected.
- Promptly report if diarrhea develops; seek medical attention promptly for severe or persistent diarrhea.
- Minimize sun exposure with protective clothing and use of sunscreen.
- Report promptly new or worsening symptoms of adverse effects on the heart or lungs (e.g., trouble breathing, shortness of breath, cough, fever, exercise intolerance, fatigue, swelling of the ankles/legs, palpitations, or sudden weight gain).
- Report symptoms of liver damage (e.g., yellow skin or eyes, dark urine, right-sided abdominal pain, lethargy, easy bleeding or bruising).
- Report immediately eye pain, swelling, redness, blurred vision, or other vision changes.

ALBENDAZOLE

(al-ben′da-zole)

Albenza

Classification: ANTHELMINTIC
Therapeutic: ANTHELMINTIC
Prototype: Praziquantel

AVAILABILITY Tablet; chewable tablet

ACTION & THERAPEUTIC EFFECT A broad-spectrum oral anthelmintic agent that causes selective degeneration of cytoplasmic microtubules in intestinal helminths and larvae. *Causes decreased ATP production in the helminths, resulting in energy depletion, which kills the worms.*

USES Treatment of neurocysticercosis caused by pork tapeworm (*Taenia solium*), hydatid disease caused by the larval form of dog tapeworm (*Echinococcus granulosus*).

UNLABELED USES Giardiasis, pinworm infection, hookworm infection, microsporidiosis.

CONTRAINDICATIONS Hypersensitivity to the benzimidazole class of compounds or any components of albendazole.

CAUTIOUS USE Hepatic dysfunction; bone marrow suppression; pregnancy (category C); lactation; children younger than 6 yr.

ROUTE & DOSAGE

Neurocysticercosis

Adult/Adolescent/Child: (6 yr or older, weight less than 60 kg): **PO** 15 mg/kg/day divided bid for 8–30-day cycle (max: 800 mg/day); *weight 60 kg or more:* 400 mg bid for 8–30 days

Hydatid Disease

Adult/Child: (6 yr or older, weight less than 60 kg) 15 mg/kg/day divided bid × 28 days, then 14 days drug free and repeat for 2 more cycles (max: 800 mg/day); *weight 60 kg or more:* 400 mg bid for 28-day cycle (then 14 days without drug and repeat regimen for 3 cycles)

ADMINISTRATION

Oral

- In young children, tablets should be crushed or chewed and swallowed with water.
- Administer with a high-fat meal to increase absorption.
- Do not exceed maximum total daily dose of 800 mg.
- Store at 20°–25°C (68°–77°F).

ADVERSE EFFECTS CNS: Headache. **Hepatic:** Increased liver enzymes. **GI:** Abdominal pain, nausea, vomiting.

INTERACTIONS Drug: Carbamazepine, phenytoin and **phenobarbital** may decrease serum concentrations. **Food:** Avoid **grapefruit juice;** it may increase serum concentration of drug.

PHARMACOKINETICS Absorption: Poorly absorbed, absorption enhanced with a fatty meal. **Peak:** 2–5 h. **Distribution:** 70% protein bound; widely distributed, including cyst fluid and CSF; secreted into animal breast milk. **Metabolism:** In liver to active metabolite. **Elimination:** In bile. **Half-Life:** 8–12 h.

NURSING IMPLICATIONS

Assessment & Drug Effects

- Withhold drug and notify prescriber if WBC count falls below normal or liver enzymes are elevated.
- Obtain baseline ophthalmic exam for retinal lesions.
- Assess pregnancy status and ensure proper use of birth control prior to therapy.
- Monitor lab tests: Prior to each 28-day cycle and q2wk during cycle, WBC count, absolute neutrophil count, and LFTs.

Patient & Family Education

- Take with meals (see ADMINISTRATION), but avoid grapefruit juice while taking this drug.
- Do not become pregnant during or for at least 1 mo after therapy.

ALBIGLUTIDE

(al-bi-glu′tide)

Classification: ANTIDIABETIC; GLUCAGON-LIKE PEPTIDE-1 RECEPTOR AGONIST; INCRETIN MIMETIC

Therapeutic: ANTIDIABETIC

Prototype: Exenatide

AVAILABILITY Lyophilized powder for reconstitution

ACTION & *THERAPEUTIC EFFECT* An agonist of glucagon-like peptide-1 (GLP-1). Enhances glucose-dependent insulin secretion by the pancreas, suppresses glucagon secretion, and slows gastric emptying, thereby decreasing glucagon stimulation of hepatic glucose output and insulin demand. *Improves glycemic control by reducing fasting and postprandial glucose concentrations in patients with type 2 diabetes.*

USES Type 2 diabetes mellitus in combination with diet and exercise.

CONTRAINDICATIONS Hypersensitivity to albiglutide; Type 1 diabetes; personal or family history of medullary thyroid carcinoma; history of Multiple Endocrine Neoplasia Syndrome type 2 (MEN2); pancreatitis; lactation.

CAUTIOUS USE History of pancreatitis; concurrent insulin secretagogues (e.g., sulfonylureas) or insulin; hypoglycemia; renal impairment; pregnancy (use with caution). Safety and efficacy in children younger than 18 yr not established.

ROUTE & DOSAGE

Type 2 Diabetes Mellitus

Adult: **Subcutaneous** 30 mg wk; may increase to 50 mg wk

ADMINISTRATION

Subcutaneous

- Reconstitute powder with the diluent contained in the pen device. Refer to manufacturer's product labeling for full reconstitution instructions. Administer within 8 h of reconstitution.
- Inject into the upper arm, thigh, or abdomen; use a different injection site each wk.
- Administer on the same day each wk, without regard to meals or time of day. The day may be changed, as long as the last dose was at least 4 days before.
- Administer as separate injections if using with insulin (do not mix).
- Store unused pens at 2°–8°C (36°–46°F); may be stored at room temperature (up to 30°C [86°F]) for up to 4 wk prior to use.

ADVERSE EFFECTS **Respiratory:** Cough, *upper respiratory tract infection*. **Endocrine:** *Hypoglycemia*. **Skin:** Rash, erythema, itching at injection site. **GI:** *Diarrhea, nausea*. **Musculoskeletal:** Arthralgia, back pain.

INTERACTIONS **Drug:** Albiglutide causes a delay of gastric emptying and may alter the absorption of concomitantly administered oral medications. May increase risk of hypoglycemia with **insulin detemir, pasireotide,** or sulfonylureas. May decrease the effectiveness of **sincalide**.

PHARMACOKINETICS **Onset:** 3–5 days. **Metabolism:** Degradation to small peptides. **Half-Life:** 5 days.

NURSING IMPLICATIONS

Black Box Warning

Albiglutide belongs to a class of drugs that has been associated with thyroid-C cell tumors.

Assessment & Drug Effects

- Monitor for S&S of pancreatitis (acute abdominal pain with/without vomiting). If pancreatitis is suspected, withhold drug and notify prescriber immediately.
- Monitor lab tests: Periodic HbA1C and renal function tests.

Patient & Family Education

- Teach patient and caregivers proper preparation and administration of subcutaneous injection.
- If a dose is missed, inject as soon as possible within 3 days after the missed dose; then resume on the usual day.
- If more than 3 days have passed since the dose was missed, omit the missed dose and resume at the next regularly scheduled weekly dose. Report promptly symptoms of thyroid tumors (e.g., mass in the neck, difficulty swallowing or breathing, persistent hoarseness).
- Report promptly any of the following: Abdominal pain, severe dizziness, fainting, problems with urination, or signs of hypoglycemia.
- Women of childbearing age should consider stopping albiglutide at [illegible] planned pr[illegible]
- Do not bre[illegible] sulting pres[illegible]

ALBUTEROL

(al-byoo'ter-ole)

Pro-Air HFA, Proventil HFA, Ventolin HFA

Classification: BRONCHODILATOR (RESPIRATORY SMOOTH MUSCLE

RELAXANT); BETA-ADRENERGIC AGONIST
Therapeutic: BRONCHODILATOR

AVAILABILITY Tablet; syrup; capsule for inhalation; solution for inhalation; actuation; breath-activated aerosol powder.

ACTION & THERAPEUTIC EFFECT Moderately selective $beta_2$-adrenergic agonist that acts prominently on smooth muscles of trachea, bronchi, uterus, and vascular supply to skeletal muscles. Produces bronchodilation by relaxing smooth muscles of bronchial tree. *Bronchodilation decreases airway resistance, facilitates mucous drainage, and increases vital capacity.*

USES To relieve bronchospasm associated with reversible obstructive airway diseases. Prevention of exercise-induced bronchospasm.

CONTRAINDICATIONS Hypersensitivity to albuterol or any component of the formulation; severe hypersensitivity to milk proteins; congenital long QT syndrome. Use of oral syrup in children younger than 2 yr. Use of inhalator in children younger than 4 yr.

CAUTIOUS USE Cardiovascular disease, renal impairment, hypertension, hyperthyroidism, diabetes mellitus, older adults; history of seizures; hypersensitivity to sympathomimetic amines or to fluorocarbon propellant used in inhalation aerosols; pregnancy (category C).

ROUTE & DOSAGE

Bronchospasm

Adult: **PO** 2–4 mg 3–4 × day, 4–8 mg sustained release q12h; **Inhaled** 1–2 inhalations q4–6h; **Nebulized** 2.5 mg 3–4 × daily PRN
Child (2 to younger than 6 yr): **PO** 0.1–0.2 mg/kg tid (max: 4 mg/dose); *6 to younger than 12 yr:* 2 mg 3–4 × day; *Child (6–11 yr):* **Inhaled** 1 inhalations q4–6h;
Child (4 yr and younger): **Nebulized** 0.63 to 2.5 mg q4-6h

Prevention of Exercise-Induced Bronchospasm

Adult: **Inhaled** 2 inhalations 5 min prior to exercise
Child (4 yr or older): **Inhaled** 1–2 inhalations 5 min prior to exercise

ADMINISTRATION

Oral

- Do not crush extended release tablets.
- Store tablets and syrup at 2°–25°C (36°–77°F) in tight, light-resistant container.

Inhalation

- ProAir Respiclick inhaler device is breath-actuated and does not require priming. Do not use spacer.
- Metered-dose inhaler should be shaken well before use. Prime prior to first use. Use of spacer is recommended.
- Administer albuterol inhalation aerosol canister only with the actuator provided.
- Store canisters at 15°–30°C (59°–86°F) away from heat and direct sunlight.

ADVERSE EFFECTS **CV:** Tachycardia. **Respiratory:** Upper respiratory tract infection, rhinitis, bronchospasm, nasopharyngitis, exacerbation of asthma, throat irritation. **CNS:** Excitement, nervousness, tremor, shakiness, headache, dizziness. **Hepatic:** Increased serum ALT. **GI:** Nausea, vomiting. **Musculoskeletal:** Muscle cramps, musculoskeletal pain. **Hematologic:** Decreased hematocrit and hemoglobin. **Other:** Increased serum glucose, fever.

DIAGNOSTIC TEST INTERFERENCE

Small increases in ***aldosterone*** may occur.

INTERACTIONS

Drug: With **epinephrine,** other SYMPATHOMIMETIC BRONCHODILATORS, possible additive effects; TRICYCLIC ANTIDEPRESSANTS potentiate action on vascular system; BETA-ADRENERGIC BLOCKERS may decrease bronchodilation, may enhance the QTc-prolonging effect of QTc-Prolonging Agents.

PHARMACOKINETICS

Onset: Inhaled: 10–25 min; PO: 30 min. **Peak:** Inhaled: 0.5–2 h; PO: 2.5 h. **Duration:** Inhaled: 3–6 h; PO: 4–6 h (8–12 h with sustained release). **Metabolism:** In liver by CYP3A4; may cross the placenta. **Elimination:** 76% of dose eliminated in urine in 3 days. **Half-Life:** 3–5 h.

NURSING IMPLICATIONS

Assessment & Drug Effects

- Monitor therapeutic effectiveness, which is indicated by significant subjective improvement in pulmonary function within 60–90 min after drug administration.
- Monitor for: S&S of fine tremor in fingers, which may interfere with precision handwork; CNS stimulation, particularly in children 2–6 yr (hyperactivity, excitement, nervousness, insomnia), tachycardia, GI symptoms. Report promptly to prescriber.
- Consult prescriber about giving last albuterol dose several hours before bedtime, if drug-induced insomnia is a problem.
- Monitor lab tests: Periodic ABGs, pulmonary functions, and pulse oximetry.

Patient & Family Education

- Review directions for correct use of medication and inhaler (see ADMINISTRATION).
- Do not increase number or frequency of inhalations without advice of prescriber.
- Notify prescriber if albuterol fails to provide relief because this can signify worsening of pulmonary function, and a reevaluation of condition/therapy may be indicated.
- Note: Albuterol can cause dizziness or vertigo; take necessary precautions.
- Do not use OTC drugs without prescriber approval. Many medications (e.g., cold remedies) contain drugs that may intensify albuterol action.

ALCLOMETASONE DIPROPIONATE

(al-clo-met′a-sone)

See Appendix A-4.

ALENDRONATE SODIUM

(a-len′dro-nate)

Binosto, Fosamax

Classification: BISPHOSPHONATE; BONE METABOLISM REGULATOR

Therapeutic: BONE METABOLISM REGULATOR

Prototype: Etidronate

AVAILABILITY

Tablet; effervescent tablet; oral solution

ACTION & *THERAPEUTIC EFFECT*

Inhibits osteoclast-mediated bone resorption leading to an indirect increase in bone mineral density.

Decreases bone resorption, thus minimizing loss of bone density.

USES Prevention and treatment of osteoporosis; Paget disease. Treatment of glucocorticoid-induced osteoporosis.

CONTRAINDICATIONS Hypersensitivity to alendronate or other bisphosphonates; achalasia, esophageal stricture, severe renal impairment (CrCl less than 35 mL/min); hypocalcemia; inability to stand or sit upright for at least 30 min.

CAUTIOUS USE Renal impairment, CHF, restricted sodium intake; hyperphosphatemia, liver disease, fever or infection, active upper GI problems; osteonecrosis of the jaw; pregnancy (category C); lactation.

ROUTE & DOSAGE

Treatment of Osteoporosis

Adult: **PO** 10 mg once/day (max: 40 mg/day) or 70 mg qwk

Prevention of Osteoporosis

Adult: **PO** 5 mg daily or 35 mg qwk

Treatment of Steroid-Induced Osteoporosis

Adult: **PO** 5 mg daily or 10 mg daily in postmenopausal females who are not receiving estrogen

Treatment of Paget Disease

Adult: **PO** 40 mg once/day for 6 mo

ADMINISTRATION

Oral

- Correct hypocalcemia before administering alendronate.
- Administer in the morning at least 30 min before the first food, beverage, or medication. Do not administer within 2 h of calcium-containing foods, beverages, or medications. At least 30 min should elapse after alendronate dose before taking any other drugs.
- *Tablet:* Give with 8 oz of plain water.
- *Effervescent tablet:* Dissolve in 4 oz of plain water at room temp. Wait at least 5 min after effervescence stops. Stir the solution for approximately 10 seconds just before administration.
- *Oral solution:* Give with at least 2 oz of water.
- Keep patient sitting up or ambulating for 30 min after taking drug and until the first food of the day is eaten.
- Store according to manufacturer's directions.

ADVERSE EFFECTS **Endocrine:** Decreased serum calcium, decreased serum phosphatase. **GI:** Abdominal pain, acid regurgitation. **Musculoskeletal:** Musculoskeletal pain.

INTERACTIONS **Drug: Calcium/Iron/Magnesium** decrease concentration of alendronate **Aspirin** increases risk of GI bleed. *Food:* **Calcium** and food (especially dairy products) reduce alendronate absorption.

PHARMACOKINETICS **Absorption:** 0.5–1% from GI tract (absorption significantly decreased by calcium and food). **Onset:** 3–6 wk. **Duration:** 12 wk after discontinuation. **Distribution:** Rapid skeletal uptake. **Metabolism:** Not metabolized. **Elimination:** Up to 50% excreted unchanged in urine. **Half-Life:** Up to 10 yr.

NURSING IMPLICATIONS

Assessment & Drug Effects

- Diagnostic test: Bone density scan evaluated 1–2 yr after initiating therapy and every 1–2 yr thereafter.

- Discontinue drug if the CrCl less than 35 mL/min.
- Monitor lab tests: Baseline and periodic albumin-adjusted serum calcium, serum phosphate, serum alkaline phosphatase; periodic renal function tests and LFTs.

Patient & Family Education

- Review directions for taking drug correctly (see ADMINISTRATION).
- Report fever, especially when accompanied by arthralgia and myalgia.
- Need for good oral hygiene and regular dental exams.

ALFENTANIL HYDROCHLORIDE

(al-fen′ta-nill)

Alfenta

Classification: NARCOTIC OPIATE AGONIST ANALGESIC; GENERAL ANESTHETIC

Therapeutic: NARCOTIC ANALGESIC; GENERAL ANESTHETIC

Prototype: Morphine

Controlled Substance: Schedule II

AVAILABILITY Injection

ACTION & THERAPEUTIC EFFECT A narcotic agonist analgesic with CNS effects that appear to be related to interaction of drug with opiate receptors. *Analgesia is mediated through changes in the perception of pain at the spinal cord and at higher levels in the CNS.*

USES General anesthesia induction and maintenance, and sedation maintenance.

UNLABELED USES Severe pain.

CONTRAINDICATIONS Coagulation disorders, bacteremia, infection at injection site; lactation.

CAUTIOUS USE Older adults, history of pulmonary disease; pregnancy (category C). Safety in children younger than 12 yr is not established.

ROUTE & DOSAGE

Anesthesia

Adult: **IV** induction 130–245 mcg/kg; maintenance 0.5–1.5 mcg/kg/min

Conscious Sedation

Adult: **IV** 3–8 mcg/kg then 3–5 mcg/kg q5–20 min or continuous infusion of 0.25–1 mcg/kg/min (total 3–40 mcg/kg)

Obesity Dosage Adjustment

Dose based on IBW

Hepatic Impairment Dosage Adjustment

Maintenance dosage adjustment recommended

ADMINISTRATION

Intravenous

PREPARE: **Direct or Continuous:** Alfentanil is available in a concentration of 500 mcg/mL. Small volumes may be given direct IV undiluted or diluted in 5 mL of NS. ▪ For IV infusion, add 20 mL of alfentanil to 230 mL of compatible IV solution to yield 40 mcg/mL. Compatible IV solutions include NS, D5/NS, D5W, and LR. ▪ Note: Alfentanil may be diluted to concentrations of 25–80 mcg/mL.

ADMINISTER: **Direct:** Administer over at least 3 min. Do not administer more rapidly. **Continuous:** Administer at a rate of 0.25–1 mcg/kg/min. Note: Dose may be individualized.

INCOMPATIBILITIES: **Y-site:** **Amphotericin B, amphotericin B**

(lipid), dantrolene, diazepam, diazoxide, lansoprazole, pantoprazole, phenytoin, sulfamethoxazole/trimethoprim.

- Store at 15°–30°C (59°–86°F). Avoid freezing.

ADVERSE EFFECTS **CV:** Hypotension, hypertension, tachycardia, bradycardia. **Respiratory:** Apnea, respiratory depression, dyspnea. **CNS:** Dizziness, euphoria, drowsiness. **GI:** *Nausea,* vomiting, anorexia, constipation, cramps. **Other:** Thoracic muscle rigidity, flushing, diaphoresis; extremities feel heavy and warm.

INTERACTIONS **Drug:** BETA-ADRENERGIC BLOCKERS increase incidence of bradycardia; CNS DEPRESSANTS such as BARBITURATES, TRANQUILIZERS, NEUROMUSCULAR BLOCKING AGENTS, OPIATES, and INHALATION GENERAL ANESTHETICS may enhance the cardiovascular and CNS effects of alfentanil in both magnitude and duration; enhancement or prolongation of postoperative respiratory depression also may result from concomitant administration of any of these agents with alfentanil.

PHARMACOKINETICS **Onset:** 2 min. **Duration:** Injection 30 min; continuous infusion 45 min. **Distribution:** Crosses placenta. **Metabolism:** In liver by CYP3A4. **Elimination:** Excreted in breast milk. **Half-Life:** 46–111 min.

NURSING IMPLICATIONS

Assessment & Drug Effects

- Monitor for S&S of increased sympathetic stimulation (arrhythmias) and evidence of depressed postoperative analgesia (tachycardia, pain, pupillary dilation, spontaneous muscle movement) if a narcotic antagonist has been administered to overcome residual effects of alfentanil.
- Evaluate adequacy of spontaneous ventilation carefully during postoperative period.
- Monitor vital signs carefully during postoperative period; check for bradycardia, especially if patient is also taking a beta blocker.
- Note: Dizziness, sedation, nausea, and vomiting are common when drug is used as a postoperative analgesic.

Patient & Family Education

- Report unpleasant adverse effects when drug is used for patient-controlled analgesia.

ALFUZOSIN

(al-fuz′o-sin)

UroXatral, Xatral ♣

Classification: ALPHA-ADRENERGIC ANTAGONIST

Therapeutic: GENITOURINARY SMOOTH MUSCLE RELAXER

Prototype: Tamsulosin

AVAILABILITY Tablet

ACTION & THERAPEUTIC EFFECT A short-acting, selective antagonist at alpha-1 receptors with a low incidence of hypotension and sexual dysfunction. Alpha-1 receptors cause contraction of smooth muscle in the prostate, prostatic capsule, prostatic urethra, bladder base, and bladder neck. *Blockade of alpha-1 receptors by alfuzosin causes smooth muscles in the bladder neck and prostate to relax, thereby reducing pressure on the urethra and improving urine flow rate. This results in a reduction in BPH symptoms.*

USES Treatment of symptomatic benign prostatic hypertrophy (BPH).

UNLABELED USES Facilitate expulsion of ureteral stones

CONTRAINDICATIONS Hypersensitivity to alfuzosin; moderate or severe hepatic insufficiency; angina; QT prolongation; carcinoma of the prostate.

CAUTIOUS USE Coronary artery disease, cardiac arrhythmias; mild hepatic disease; severe renal impairment; dizziness, light-headedness, orthostatic hypotension; pregnancy (considered safe for use during pregnancy).

ROUTE & DOSAGE

Benign Prostatic Hypertrophy

Adult: **PO** 10 mg daily

ADMINISTRATION

Oral

- Give immediately after same meal each day.
- Ensure that extended release tablet is not crushed or chewed. It **must be** swallowed whole.
- Store at 15°–30°C (59°–86°F). Protect from light and moisture.

ADVERSE EFFECTS **CV:** Orthostatic hypotension. **CNS:** Dizziness.

INTERACTIONS **Drug:** Increased risk of hypotension with other ANTIHYPERTENSIVE AGENTS or PDE5 INHIBITORS, PROTEASE INHIBITORS may increase alfuzosin levels and toxicity. Contraindicated with ANTIRETROVIRAL PROTEASE INHIBITORS or potent CYP3A4 inhibitors.

PHARMACOKINETICS **Absorption:** 80% protein bound **Peak:** 8 h. **Metabolism:** In liver by CYP3A4. **Elimination:** 69% in feces, 24% in urine. **Half-Life:** 10 h.

NURSING IMPLICATIONS

Assessment & Drug Effects

- Monitor CV status and BP, especially with concurrent antihypertensive drugs or inhibitors of CYP3A4. See INTERACTIONS.
- Check postural vital signs for orthostatic hypotension within a few hours following administration.
- Withhold drug and report new or worsening angina to prescriber.
- Monitor urine flow.
- Monitor lab tests: PSA.

Patient & Family Education

- Inform prescriber about all other prescription, nonprescription, or herbal drugs being taken.
- Make position changes slowly to minimize dizziness.
- Do not drive or engage in other hazardous activities until reaction to drug is known.

ALIROCUMAB

(a-lir-o-cu′mab)

Praluent

Classification: MONOCLONAL ANTIBODY; PROPROTEIN CONVERTASE SUBTILISIN KEXIN TYPE 9 (PCSK9) INHIBITOR; ANTILIPIDEMIC; LIPID LOWERING

Therapeutic: ANTILIPIDEMIC

AVAILABILITY Prefilled pens and solutions for injection

ACTION & *THERAPEUTIC EFFECT* Inhibits the binding of an enzyme (proprotein convertase subtilisin kexin type 9 [PCSK9]) to LDL-C receptors in the liver, thus releasing the receptors to attach to LDL-C and clear LDL-C from the bloodstream. *Lowers the level of LDL-C in the bloodstream reducing the risk of CV disease.*

USES Adjunct treatment for adults with heterozygous familial hypercholesterolemia; primary hyperlipidemia; secondary prevention of cardiovascular events.

CONTRAINDICATIONS Serious hypersensitivity to alirocumab or any component of the formulation.

CAUTIOUS USE Pregnancy; lactation. Safety and efficacy in children younger than 18 yr not established.

ROUTE & DOSAGE

Heterozygous Familial Hypercholesterolemia

Adult: **Subcutaneous** 75 mg q2wk; may increase to 150 mg q2wk

Primary Hyperlipidemia

Adult: **Subcutaneous** 75 mg q2wk or 300 mg q4wk; may increase to max of 150 mg q2wk

ADMINISTRATION

Subcutaneous

- Warm prefilled pen or syringe to room temperature for 30–40 min. Do not shake.
- Inject into the thigh, abdomen, or upper arm; rotate injection site with each injection. Do not coadminister with any other injectable drug.
- Store at 2°–8°C (36°–46°F) and protect from light. Do not leave unrefrigerated at 25°C (77°F) for more than 24 h.

ADVERSE EFFECTS **Respiratory:** Cough. **Endocrine:** Elevated liver enzymes. **GI:** Diarrhea. **Other:** Hypersensitivity reactions, influenza, injection site reactions, antibody development.

PHARMACOKINETICS **Peak:** 3–7 days. **Metabolism:** Peptide degradation. **Half-Life:** 17–20 days.

NURSING IMPLICATIONS

Assessment & Drug Effects

- Monitor for hypersensitivity reactions. Withhold drug and notify prescriber if hypersensitivity develops (e.g., hypersensitivity vasculitis, pruritus, rash, and urticaria).
- Monitor lab tests: Baseline lipid profile then periodically thereafter; periodic LFTs.

Patient & Family Education

- Discontinue the drug and seek prompt medical attention if any signs or symptoms of serious allergic reactions occur (e.g., skin rash, itching, burning, pain).
- Prefilled syringes should not be reused.

ALISKIREN

(a-lis′ki-ren)

Tekturna

Classification: RENIN ANGIOTENSIN SYSTEM ANTAGONIST; ANTIHYPERTENSIVE

Therapeutic: DIRECT RENIN INHIBITOR; ANTIHYPERTENSIVE

AVAILABILITY Tablet

ACTION & *THERAPEUTIC EFFECT* A direct renin inhibitor that reduces plasma renin activity and inhibits the conversion of angiotensinogen to angiotensin I (ANG I) and subsequent production of angiotensin II (ANG II). *Lowers blood pressure by decreasing vasoconstriction and aldosterone production, thus reducing sodium reabsorption and fluid retention.*

USES Treatment of hypertension.

CONTRAINDICATIONS Hypersensitivity to aliskiren; hyperkalemia; hypercalcemia; diabetics who are receiving ARBs or ACE inhibitors; dehydration, hypovolemia or salt depletion; pregnancy (category D second and third trimester); lactation; hypotension.

CAUTIOUS USE Patients with CrCl less than 30 mL/min; history of angioedema; respiratory disorders; history of airway surgery; DM; moderate renal impairment; renal stenosis, severe heart failure, post-MI; older adults; pregnancy (category C first trimester); children younger than 18 yr.

ROUTE & DOSAGE

Hypertension

Adult: **PO** 150 mg once daily (can increase to 300 mg once daily)

ADMINISTRATION

Oral

- Give consistently at same time daily with or without meals.
- Store at 15°–30°C (59°–86°F) and protect from light.

ADVERSE EFFECTS CNS: *Headache, dizziness.* **Endocrine:** Hyperkalemia. **Skin:** Angioedema, rash. **GI:** *Diarrhea.* **Neuromuscular and Skeletal:** Increased creatine phosphokinase. **Renal:** Increased blood urea nitrogen, increased serum creatinine.

INTERACTIONS Drug: Enhances effects of other ANTIHYPERTENSIVE AGENTS. DIURETIC effect may be reduced. **Ketoconazole** increases the plasma level of aliskiren, while **irbesartan** decreases its plasma level.

PHARMACOKINETICS Absorption: 2.5%. **Peak:** 1–3 h; clinical effect seen in 2 wk. **Metabolism:** Less than 10% via liver. **Elimination:** Primarily in stool. **Half-Life:** 24 h.

NURSING IMPLICATIONS

Black Box Warning

Aliskiren has been associated with fetal injury and/or death.

Assessment & Drug Effects

- Monitor for hypotension at the initiation of therapy, following dosage change, and on a regular basis throughout.
- Monitor for angioedema, which may occur any time during treatment. Withhold drug and immediately report to prescriber.
- Monitor lab tests: Periodic serum electrolytes, especially with concurrent ACE inhibitor.
- Evaluate renal status prior to beginning therapy. Assess BUN, serum potassium, and serum creatinine.

Patient & Family Education

- Discontinue drug and notify healthcare provider immediately if pregnancy occurs.
- Full therapeutic effect is usually obtained by 2 wk of therapy.
- Report immediately any of the following: Swelling about the face, lips, tongue; difficulty breathing or swallowing; swelling of hands or feet.
- High-fat meals interfere with the absorption of this drug. Do not take drug following a high-fat meal.
- Do not use salt substitutes or potassium supplements without consulting prescriber.
- Monitor lab tests: Periodic serum potassium.

ALITRETINOIN (9-*cis*-RETINOIC ACID)

(a-li-tre′ti-noyne)

Panretin

Classification: ANTIACNE (RETINOID)

Therapeutic: ANTIACNE

Prototype: Isotretinoin

AVAILABILITY Gel

ACTION & *THERAPEUTIC EFFECT* Naturally occurring retinoid that binds to and activates all known retinoid receptors in cells, which regulate cellular differentiation and proliferation in both healthy and neoplastic cells. *Inhibits the growth of Kaposi sarcoma (KS) in HIV patients. It does not prevent the development of new KS lesions.*

USES Treatment of cutaneous lesions of AIDS-related Kaposi sarcoma.

UNLABELED USES Cutaneous T-cell lymphomas.

CONTRAINDICATIONS Hypersensitivity to alitretinoin or other retinoids including vitamin A; when systemic anti-KS therapy is required; pregnancy (category D); lactation.

CAUTIOUS USE Cutaneous T-cell lymphoma. Safety and efficacy in children younger than 18 yr, or adults 65 yr or older, are unknown.

ROUTE & DOSAGE

Cutaneous Kaposi Sarcoma

Adult: **Topical** Apply sufficient gel to cover lesions bid, may increase application to 3–4 × daily if tolerated

ADMINISTRATION

Topical

- Apply gel liberally over lesions; avoid unaffected skin and mucous membranes.
- Dry 3–5 min before covering with clothes. Do not cover with occlusive dressing.
- Store at 15°–30°C (59°–86°F).

ADVERSE EFFECTS **Skin:** Erythema, edema, vesiculation, *rash, burning pain,* pruritus, exfoliative dermatitis, excoriation, paresthesia.

INTERACTIONS **Drug:** Increased toxicity with insect repellents containing DEET.

PHARMACOKINETICS **Absorption:** Minimal.

NURSING IMPLICATIONS

Assessment & Drug Effects

- Monitor for S&S of dermal toxicity (e.g., erythema, edema, vesiculation).

Patient & Family Education

- Allow up to 14 wk for therapeutic response.
- Discontinue drug immediately if pregnancy occurs.
- Avoid exposure of medicated skin to sunlight or sun lamps.
- Contact prescriber if inflammation, swelling, or blisters appear on medicated areas.

ALLOPURINOL

(al-oh-pure′i-nole)

Aloprim, Apo-allopurinol-A ♣, Zyloprim

Classification: ANTIGOUT

Therapeutic: ANTIGOUT

AVAILABILITY Tablet; powder for injection

ACTION & *THERAPEUTIC EFFECT* Reduces endogenous uric acid by selectively inhibiting action of xanthine oxidase, the enzyme responsible for converting hypoxanthine to xanthine and xanthine to uric acid (end product of purine catabolism). *Urate pool is decreased by the lowering of both serum and urinary uric acid levels, and hyperuricemia is prevented.*

USES To control hyperuricemia, gout, nephrolithiasis, renal calculus, uric acid nephropathy.

CONTRAINDICATIONS Hypersensitivity to allopurinol; as initial treatment for acute gouty attacks; idiopathic hemochromatosis (or those with family history); HLA-B*5801 genotype (strongly associated with allopurinol-induced severe cutaneous reactions).

CAUTIOUS USE Impaired hepatic or renal function, bone marrow suppression, pregnancy (category C). Use with caution when performing tasks that require mental alertness due to CNS effects.

ROUTE & DOSAGE

Treatment of Hyperuricemia

Adult /Adolescent/Child (10 yr and older): **PO** 600–800 mg/day (in divided doses); **IV** 200–400 mg/m²/day (max: 600 mg/day) in 1–4 divided doses

Child (younger than 10 yr): **PO** 300 mg/day; *(younger than 6 yr):* **PO** 150 mg/day; **IV** 200 mg/m²/day in 1–4 divided doses

Treatment of Recurrent Renal Calculi

Adult: **PO** 200–300 daily (may divide dose)

Gout

Adult: **PO** 100 mg daily increase as needed for patient response (max: 800 mg/day)

Renal Impairment Dosage Adjustment

CrCl 10–20 mL/min: **PO** 200 mg/day; **IV** 100 mg; *3–9 mL/min:* 100 mg daily; *less than 3 mL/min:* 100 mg with extended interval between doses (24 h or more)

Hemodialysis Dosage Adjustment

See package insert

ADMINISTRATION

Oral

- Give after meals.
- Administer fluids for sufficient urine output.
- Store at 15°–30°C (59°–86°F) in a tightly closed container.

Intravenous

PREPARE: **Intermittent:** Reconstitute a single dose vial (500 mg) with 25 mL of sterile water for injection to yield 20 mg/mL. ▪ **Must be** further diluted with NS or D5W to a concentration of 6 mg/mL or less. ▪ Note: Adding 2.3 mL of diluent yields 6 mg/mL.

ADMINISTER: **Intermittent:** Usually administered over 30 min.

INCOMPATIBILITIES: **Solution/additive:** **Amikacin, amphotericin B, carmustine, cefotaxime, chlorpromazine, cimetidine, clindamycin, cytarabine, dacarbazine, daptomycin, daunorubicin, diltiazem, diphenhydramine, doxorubicin, doxycycline, droperidol, epirubicin, ertapenem, etoposide, floxuridine, gentamicin, haloperidol, hydroxyzine, idarubicin, imipenem-cilastatin, irinotecan, mechlorethamine, meperidine, methylprednisolone, metoclopramide, metoprolol, minocycline, mycophenolate, nalbuphine, netilmicin, ondansetron, palonosetron, pancuronium, potassium acetate, prochlorperazine, promethazine, sodium bicarbonate, streptozocin, tacrolimus, tobramycin, vecuronium, vinorelbine.**

ADVERSE EFFECTS **CNS:** Drowsiness, headache. **Skin:** Urticaria or pruritus, rash, pruritic maculopapular rash, toxic. **GI:** Nausea, vomiting, diarrhea, abdominal discomfort. **Hematologic:** (Rare) Agranulocytosis, aplastic anemia, bone marrow depression, thrombocytopenia. **Other:** Hepatotoxicity, increased liver enzymes, increased serum alkaline phosphatase, acute gout.

DIAGNOSTIC TEST INTERFERENCE

Possibility of elevated blood levels of ***alkaline phosphatase*** and ***serum transaminases (AST, ALT),*** and decreased blood Hct, Hgb, leukocytes.

INTERACTIONS

Drug: Alcohol may inhibit renal excretion of uric acid; **ampicillin, amoxicillin** increase risk of skin rash; enhances anticoagulant effect of **warfarin;** toxicity from **azathioprine, mercaptopurine, cyclophosphamide, cyclosporin** increased; increases hypoglycemic effects of **chlorpropamide;** THIAZIDES increase risk of allopurinol toxicity and hypersensitivity (especially with impaired renal function); ACE INHIBITORS increase risk of hypersensitivity; high-dose **vitamin C** increases risk of kidney stone formation. Do not use with **didanosine** or **pegloticase.**

PHARMACOKINETICS

Absorption: 80–90% from GI tract. **Onset:** 24–48 h. **Peak:** 2–6 h. **Metabolism:** 75–80% to the active metabolite oxypurinol. **Elimination:** Slowly excreted in urine; excreted in breast milk. **Half-Life:** 1–3 h; oxypurinol, 18–30 h.

NURSING IMPLICATIONS

Assessment & Drug Effects

- Monitor for therapeutic effectiveness, which is indicated by normal serum and urinary uric acid levels usually by 1–3 wk, gradual decrease in size of tophi, absence of new tophaceous deposits (after approximately 6 mo), with consequent relief of joint pain and increased joint mobility.
- Monitor for S&S of an acute gouty attack, which is most likely to occur during first 6 wk of therapy.
- Monitor patients with renal disorders more often; they tend to have a higher incidence of renal stones and drug toxicity problems.
- Report onset of rash or fever immediately to prescriber; withhold drug. Life-threatening toxicity syndrome can occur 2–4 wk after initiation of therapy (more common with impaired renal function) and is generally accompanied by malaise, fever, and aching, a diffuse erythematous, desquamating rash, hepatic dysfunction, eosinophilia, and worsening of renal function.
- Monitor lab tests: Baseline then monthly CBC, LFTs, and kidney function tests; serum uric acid q1–2wk; periodic urine pH.

Patient & Family Education

- Drink enough fluid to produce urinary output of at least 2000 mL/day (fluid intake of at least 3000 mL/day). (Note that 1000 mL is approximately equal to 1 quart.) Report diminishing urinary output, cloudy urine, unusual color or odor to urine, pain or discomfort on urination.
- Report promptly the onset of itching or rash. Stop drug if a skin rash appears, and report to prescriber.
- Do not drive or engage in potentially hazardous activities until response to drug is known.

ALMOTRIPTAN

(al-mo-trip′tan)

Axert

Classification: SEROTONIN 5-HT_1 RECEPTOR AGONIST

Therapeutic: ANTIMIGRAINE

Prototype: Sumatriptan

AVAILABILITY Tablet

ACTION & *THERAPEUTIC EFFECT*

Selective agonist that binds with serotonin receptors within cranial arteries. Causes vasoconstriction and decreases inflammation and neurotransmission. *This results in constriction of cranial vessels that become dilated during a migraine attack and reduces signal transmission in the pain pathways.*

USES Treatment of migraine headache with or without aura.

CONTRAINDICATIONS Hypersensitivity to almotriptan malate; significant cardiovascular disease such as ischemic heart disease, coronary artery vasospasms, MI, angina, arteriosclerosis, cardiac arrhythmias, history of cerebrovascular events, or uncontrolled hypertension; stroke, Wolff-Parkinson-White syndrome, within 24 h of receiving another 5–HT_1 agonist or an ergotamine-containing or ergot-type drug; basilar or hemiplegic migraine.

CAUTIOUS USE Significant risk factors for coronary artery disease unless a cardiac evaluation has been done; hypertension; risk factors for cerebrovascular accident; diabetes; colitis; smoking; obesity; peripheral vascular disease, impaired liver or kidney function, Raynaud disease, older adults; pregnancy (category C); lactation; children.

ROUTE & DOSAGE

Migraine Headache

Adult: **PO** 6.25–12.5 mg; if headache returns, may repeat after at least 2 h (max: 25 mg/day)

Renal Impairment Dosage Adjustment

CrCl less than 30 mL/min: 6.25 mg (max: 12.5 mg/day)

Hepatic Impairment Dosage Adjustment

6.25 mg (max: 12.5 mg/day)

ADMINISTRATION

Oral

- Do not give within 24 h of an ergot-containing drug.
- Administer any time after symptoms of migraine appear.
- Do not administer a second dose without consulting the prescriber for any attack during which the FIRST dose did **not** work.
- Give a second dose if headache was relieved by first dose but symptoms return; however, wait at least 2 h after the first dose before giving a second dose.
- Do not give more than two doses in 24 h.
- Store at 15°–30°C (59°–86°F).

ADVERSE EFFECTS **CNS:** Drowsiness.

INTERACTIONS **Drug: Dihydroergotamine, methysergide,** other 5-HT_1 AGONISTS may cause prolonged vasospastic reactions; SSRIS, could cause serotonin syndrome; MAOIS should not be used with 5-HT_1 AGONISTS. Strong CYP3A4 inhibitors may increase concentration of almotriptan.

PHARMACOKINETICS Absorption: Well absorbed, 70% reaches systemic circulation. **Peak:** 1–3 h. **Distribution:** 35% protein bound. **Metabolism:** 27% metabolized by monoamine oxidase. **Elimination:** 75% renally, 13% in feces. **Half-Life:** 3–4 h.

NURSING IMPLICATIONS

Assessment & Drug Effects

- Monitor cardiovascular status carefully following first dose in patients at relatively high risk for coronary artery disease (e.g., postmenopausal women, men over 40 yr, persons with known CAD risk factors) or who have coronary artery vasospasms.
- Report to prescriber immediately chest pain or tightness in chest or throat that is severe or does not quickly resolve following a dose of almotriptan.
- Pain relief usually begins within 10 min of ingestion, with complete relief in approximately 65% of all patients within 2 h.
- Monitor BP, especially in those being treated for hypertension.

Patient & Family Education

- Notify prescriber immediately if symptoms of severe angina (e.g., severe or persistent pain or tightness in chest, back, neck, or throat) or hypersensitivity (e.g., wheezing, facial swelling, skin rash, or hives) occur.
- Do not take any other serotonin receptor agonist (e.g., Imitrex, Maxalt, Zomig, Amerge) within 24 h of taking almotriptan.
- Advise prescriber of any drugs taken within 1 wk of beginning almotriptan.
- Check with prescriber regarding drug interactions before taking any new OTC or prescription drugs.
- Report any other adverse effects (e.g., tingling, flushing, dizziness) at next prescriber visit.

ALOGLIPTIN

(a-loh-glip'tin)

Nesina

Classification: ANTIDIABETIC; INCRETIN MODIFIER; DIPEPTIDYL PEPTIDASE-4 (DPP-4) INHIBITOR

Therapeutic: ANTIDIABETIC; HORMONE MODIFIER; DPP-4 INHIBITOR

Prototype: Sitagliptin

AVAILABILITY Tablet

ACTION & *THERAPEUTIC EFFECT* Slows inactivation of incretin hormones that are released by the intestine. As plasma glucose rises following food intake, incretin hormones stimulate release of insulin from the pancreas and lower glucagon secretion, resulting in reduced hepatic glucose production. *Lowers both fasting and postprandial plasma glucose levels.*

USES Adjunct treatment of type 2 diabetes mellitus.

CONTRAINDICATIONS History of a serious hypersensitivity reaction (e.g., anaphylaxis, angioedema, or severe cutaneous reactions) to alogliptin-containing products; acute pancreatitis.

CAUTIOUS USE Hepatic dysfunction; concurrent use of insulin secretagogue (e.g., sulfonylurea) or insulin; renal impairment; older adults; heart failure; renal dysfunction; pregnancy (category B); lactation. Safety and efficacy in children not established.

ROUTE & DOSAGE

Type 2 Diabetes Mellitus

Adult: **PO** 25 mg once daily

Renal Impairment Dosage Adjustment

CrCl greater than or equal to 30 mL/min to 59 mL/min: 12.5 mg once daily
CrCl less than 30 mL/min: 6.25 mg once daily

ADMINISTRATION

Oral

- May be given without regard to meals.
- Note that dosage adjustment is recommended for moderate to severe renal impairment.
- Store at 20°–25°C (68°–77°F).

ADVERSE EFFECTS **Respiratory:** Nasopharyngitis, upper respiratory tract infection. **GU:** Decreased estimated GFR, impaired renal function.

INTERACTIONS May increase effect of SULFONYLUREA or **insulin**. May cause hypoglycemia with FLUOROQUINOLONES.

PHARMACOKINETICS **Absorption:** 100% bioavailable. **Peak:** 1–2 h. **Distribution:** 20% protein bound. **Metabolism:** In liver. **Elimination:** Renal (76%) and fecal (13%). **Half-Life:** 21 h.

NURSING IMPLICATIONS

Assessment & Drug Effects

- Monitor for and report S&S of significant GI distress, including nausea, vomiting, and diarrhea.
- Monitor for S&S of hypoglycemia when used in combination with a sulfonylurea drug or insulin.
- Monitor lab tests: Baseline and periodic CrCl; baseline LFTs; periodic fasting and postprandial plasma glucose and HbA1C.

Patient & Family Education

- Stop taking this drug and notify prescriber immediately if you have an allergic reaction (e.g., swelling of your face, lips, throat; difficulty swallowing or breathing; raised, red areas on your skin (hives); skin rash, itching, flaking, or peeling.
- Contact prescriber if you experience unexplained symptoms of liver problems (e.g., nausea or vomiting, abdominal pain, unusual tiredness, loss of appetite, dark urine, yellowing of your skin or the whites of your eyes).
- Taking this drug with another drug that can lower your blood sugar, increasing your risk of hypoglycemia.

ALOSETRON

(a-lo′se-tron)

Lotronex

Classification: SEROTONIN 5-HT_3 RECEPTOR ANTAGONIST
Therapeutic: GI

AVAILABILITY Tablet

ACTION & *THERAPEUTIC EFFECT* Potent and selective serotonin (5-HT_3) receptor antagonist. Serotonin 5-HT_3 receptors are extensively located on enteric neurons of the GI tract. Activation of these receptors affects amount of visceral pain experienced, transit time in the colon, and GI secretions. *Alosetron significantly controls GI pain, and severe diarrhea related to irritable bowel syndrome.*

USES Treatment of severe chronic irritable bowel syndrome (IBS) in women whose predominant symptom is diarrhea and whose symptoms have lasted longer than 6 mo and have failed to respond to conventional therapy.

CONTRAINDICATIONS Constipation, ischemic colitis, development of ischemic bowel symptoms such as sudden onset of rectal bleeding, bloody diarrhea, new or sudden worsening of abdominal pain; history of chronic or severe constipation, intestinal obstruction, toxic megacolon, GI adhesions, GI perforation, active diverticulitis, history of, or current Crohn disease or ulcerative colitis; hypersensitivity to alosetron; thrombophlebitis, hypercoagulable state, inability to comply with Patient–Prescriber Agreement; severe hepatic impairment; lactation.

CAUTIOUS USE Hepatic insufficiency, renal impairment; older adults; pregnancy (category B). Safety and efficacy in children not established.

ROUTE & DOSAGE

Irritable Bowel Syndrome

Adult: **PO** Start with 0.5 mg bid for 4 wk, may increase to 1 mg bid if tolerated

ADMINISTRATION

Oral

- Ensure that the patient has signed the Patient–Prescriber Agreement prior to administering alosetron.
- Do not give this drug if the patient has constipation.
- Review the contraindications for this drug, and ensure that the patient has none of the conditions for which the drug is contraindicated.
- Store at 25°C (77°F).

ADVERSE EFFECTS **CV:** Tachyarrhythmias. **CNS:** Anxiety. **Skin:** Sweating, urticaria. **GI:** *Constipation*, abdominal pain, nausea, distention, reflux, hemorrhoids, hyposalivation, dyspepsia, ischemic colitis. **GU:** Urinary frequency. **Other:** Malaise, fatigue, cramps, pain.

INTERACTIONS **Drug: Fluvoxamine** increases alosetron serum level.

PHARMACOKINETICS **Absorption:** Rapidly absorbed, average bioavailability of 50–60%. **Peak:** 1 h. **Distribution:** 82% protein bound. **Metabolism:** Extensively in liver by CYP2C9. **Elimination:** 73% in urine, 24% in feces. **Half-Life:** 1.5 h.

NURSING IMPLICATIONS

Black Box Warning

Alosetron has been associated with infrequent, but serious and potentially fatal, GI adverse effects, including ischemic colitis and serious complications of constipation.

Assessment & Drug Effects

- Monitor for and report immediately signs of ischemic colitis such as new or worsening abdominal pain, bloody diarrhea, or blood in the stool.
- Withhold drug and notify prescriber if patient has not had adequate control of IBS symptoms after 4 wk of treatment with 1 mg twice a day.
- Monitor carefully patients who have decreased GI motility (e.g., older adults, persons receiving other drugs that may decrease GI motility) as they may be at greater risk of serious complications of constipation.
- Monitor carefully patients with any degree of hepatic insufficiency, as they may be more susceptible to adverse drug effects.

- Monitor periodically for cardiac arrhythmias, especially with preexisting cardiovascular disease.

Patient & Family Education

- Read the Medication Guide before starting alosetron and each time you refill your prescription.
- Do not start taking alosetron if you are constipated.
- Discontinue alosetron immediately and contact your prescriber if you experience any of the following: Constipation, new or worsening abdominal pain, bloody diarrhea, or blood in the stool.
- Contact your prescriber immediately if constipation does not resolve after discontinuation of alosetron. Resume alosetron again only if constipation has resolved and your prescriber directs you to begin taking the medication again.
- Stop taking alosetron and contact your prescriber if IBS symptoms are not adequately controlled after 4 wk of taking 1 tablet twice a day.

ALPRAZOLAM

(al-pray′zoe-lam)

Xanax, Xanax XR

Classification: ANXIOLYTIC; SEDATIVE-HYPNOTIC; BENZODIAZEPINE

Therapeutic: ANTIANXIETY; SEDATIVE-HYPNOTIC

Prototype: Lorazepam

Controlled Substance: Schedule IV

AVAILABILITY Tablet; extended release tab; oral concentrate; orally disintegrating tablet

ACTION & *THERAPEUTIC EFFECT* A CNS depressant that appears to act at the limbic, thalamic, and hypothalamic levels of the CNS. *Has antianxiety and sedative effects with addictive potential.*

USES Management of anxiety disorders or for short-term relief of anxiety symptoms. Also used as adjunct in management of anxiety associated with depression and agitation, and for panic disorders, such as agoraphobia.

UNLABELED USES Acute vertigo.

CONTRAINDICATIONS Sensitivity to benzodiazepines; acute narrow-angle glaucoma; pulmonary disease; use alone in primary depression or psychotic disorders, bipolar disorders, organic brain disorders; myasthenia gravis; pregnancy (potential to cause harm to fetus); lactation.

CAUTIOUS USE Impaired hepatic function; history of alcoholism; renal impairment, hepatic disease; geriatric and debilitated patients; children younger than 18 yr. Effectiveness for long-term treatment (greater than 4 mo) not established.

ROUTE & DOSAGE

Anxiety Disorders

Adult: **PO** Immediate release: 0.25 mg tid (max: 10 mg/day) Extended release: 0.5–1 mg daily, may increase at 3 day intervals (max: 10 mg/day)

Geriatric: **PO** Immediate release: 0.25 mg bid to tid; Extended release: 0.5 mg daily

Hepatic Impairment Dosage Adjustment

Advanced liver disease immediate release forms 0.25 mg bid-tid; extended release forms 0.5 mg daily.

ADMINISTRATION

Oral

- Reduce drug gradually when discontinuing drug.
- Store in light-resistant containers at 20°–25°C (68°–77°F), unless otherwise directed.

ADVERSE EFFECTS **CV:** Tachycardia, hypotension, ECG changes. **Respiratory:** Dyspnea. **CNS:** *Drowsiness, sedation,* dizziness, depression, confusion, fatigue, clumsiness, unsteadiness, rigidity, tremor, restlessness, ataxia, memory loss, irritability, cognitive dysfunction, confusion. **HEENT:** Blurred vision. **Endocrine:** Weight gain, weight loss, change in libido, menstrual disease. **Skin:** Skin rash. **GI:** Change in appetite, constipation, xerostomia, nausea. **GU:** Difficulty in micturition.

INTERACTIONS **Drug: Alcohol** and other CNS DEPRESSANTS, ANTICONVULSANTS, ANTIHISTAMINES, BARBITURATES, NARCOTIC ANALGESICS, BENZODIAZEPINES, **thalidomide** compound CNS depressant effects; CYP 3A4 inhibitors (ex **itraconazole, ketoconazole, clairthromycin,** etc.) **cimetidine,** TRICYCLIC ANTIDEPRESSANTS increase alprazolam levels (decreased metabolism); ORAL CONTRACEPTIVES may increase or decrease alprazolam effects. **Herbal: Kava, valerian** may potentiate sedation; **St. John's wort** decreases serum level of alprazolam.

PHARMACOKINETICS **Absorption:** Rapidly absorbed. **Peak:** 1–2 h. **Distribution:** Crosses placenta. **Metabolism:** Oxidized in liver to inactive metabolites by CYP3A4. **Elimination:** Renal elimination. **Half-Life:** 12–15 h.

NURSING IMPLICATIONS

Assessment & Drug Effects

- Monitor for S&S of drowsiness and sedation, especially in older adults or the debilitated; they may require supervised ambulation and/or fall precautions.
- Monitor respiratory and cardiovascular status.
- Assess risk for abuse, misuse, and addiction.

Patient & Family Education

- Make position changes slowly and in stages to prevent dizziness.
- Do not use alcohol, other CNS depressants, or OTC medications containing antihistamines (e.g., sleep aids, cold, hay fever, or allergy remedies) without consulting prescriber.
- Do not drive or engage in potentially hazardous activities until response to drug is known.
- Taper dosage following continuous use; abrupt discontinuation of drug may cause withdrawal symptoms: Nausea, vomiting, abdominal and muscle cramps, sweating, confusion, tremors, convulsions.

ALPROSTADIL (PGE_1)

(al-pross′ta-dil)

Caverject, Edex, Muse, Prostin VR Pediatric

Classification: PROSTAGLANDIN
Therapeutic: PROSTAGLANDIN
Prototype: Epoprostenol

AVAILABILITY Injection; powder for injection; urethral suppository

ACTION & *THERAPEUTIC EFFECT* Preserves ductal patency by relaxing smooth muscle of ductus arteriosus. Alprostadil induces penile erection by relaxing the smooth muscles of the corpus cavernosum and dilating the cavernosal arteries

Common adverse effects in *italic*; life-threatening effects underlined; generic names in **bold**; classifications in SMALL CAPS; ♣ Canadian drug name; ⊙ Prototype drug; ⚠ Alert

and their penile arterioles. *Preserves ductal patency by relaxing smooth muscle of ductus arteriosus. It induces penile rigidity and erection by penile blood engorgement.*

USES Temporary measure to maintain patency of ductus arteriosus in infants with ductal-dependent congenital heart defects until corrective surgery can be performed. Also used in erectile dysfunction.

CONTRAINDICATIONS Ductus arteriosus respiratory distress syndrome (hyaline membrane disease); neonates with respiratory distress syndrome; hypersensitivity to alprostadil; patients with penile implants. **Muse, Edex:** Women, children, and newborns; lactation. **Muse:** Patients with urethral stricture, inflammation/infection of glans penis, severe hypospadias, acute or chronic urethritis; sickle cell disease or trait, thrombocytopenia, thrombocytosis; polycythemia, multiple myeloma.

CAUTIOUS USE Ductus arteriosus; bleeding tendencies; cardiovascular disease; erectile dysfunction; hypersensitivity to alprostadil; leukemia; penile anatomic deformations; patients on anticoagulants, vasoactive or antihypertensive drugs; pregnancy (category C).

ROUTE & DOSAGE

To Maintain Patency of Ductus Arteriosus

Neonate: **IV** 0.05–0.1 mcg/kg/min, may increase gradually (max: 0.4 mcg/kg/min)

Erectile Dysfunction of Vasculogenic, Psychogenic, or Mixed Etiology

Adult: **Intracavernosal** Initiate with 2.5 mcg; if inadequate response, increase dose by 2.5 mcg. May then increase dose in 5 mcg increments until a suitable erection occurs, not exceeding 1 h in duration (max: 60 mcg).
Adult: **Intraurethral (Muse)** 125 mcg or 250 mcg; dose adjusted to patient satisfaction (max: 2 ×/24 h)

Erectile Dysfunction of Pure Neurogenic Etiology

Adult: **Intracavernosal** Initiate with 1.25 mcg; if inadequate response, increase dose by 1.25 mcg, then increase by 2.5 mcg, may then increase dose in 5 mcg increments until a suitable erection occurs, not exceeding 1 h in duration; wait 24 h between doses (max: 60 mcg)

ADMINISTRATION

Intracavernosal Injection

- Administer only after proper training in the penile injection technique. Refer to information on administration provided to the patient by the manufacturer.
- Use reconstituted solutions immediately.
- Store dry powder at or below 25°C (77°F) for up to 3 mo. Do not freeze.

Transurethral Insertion

- Refer to information on insertion of urethral suppository into the urethra provided to the patient by the manufacturer.

Intravenous

PREPARE: **Continuous:** Dilute 500 mcg alprostadil with NS or D5W to volume appropriate for pump delivery system. ▪ Prepare fresh solution q24h. Discard unused portions. ▪ A 500-mcg ampule diluted in 250 mL yields a concentration of 2 mcg/mL.

ADMINISTER: **Continuous:** Infuse at rate of 0.05–0.1 mcg/kg/min up to a maximum of 0.4 mcg/kg/min. ▪ Reduce infusion rate immediately if arterial pressure drops significantly or if fever occurs. ▪ Discontinue promptly, if apnea or bradycardia occurs.

▪ Store at 2°–8°C (36°–46°F) unless otherwise directed by manufacturer. Protect from freezing.

ADVERSE EFFECTS **CV:** *Flushing,* bradycardia, hypotension, syncope, tachycardia; CHF, ventricular fibrillation, shock. **Respiratory:** Apnea. **CNS:** *Fever,* seizures, lethargy. **Skin:** Rash on face and arms, alopecia. **GI:** Diarrhea, gastric regurgitation. **GU:** Oliguria, anuria, *penile pain,* prolonged erection, priapism, penile fibrosis, injection site hematoma/ecchymosis, penile rash and edema, prostatitis, perineal pain. **Hematologic:** Disseminated intravascular coagulation (DIC), thrombocytopenia. **Other:** Leg pain.

INTERACTIONS **Drug:** May increase anticoagulant properties of **warfarin;** ANTIHYPERTENSIVE AGENTS increase risk of hypotension.

PHARMACOKINETICS **Onset:** 15 min to 3 h. **Metabolism:** Rapidly in lungs. **Elimination:** Through kidneys. **Half-Life:** 5–10 min.

NURSING IMPLICATIONS

Black Box Warning

Alprostadil has been associated with apnea in neonates.

Assessment & Drug Effects

Ductus Arteriosus

- Monitor for apnea especially during the first hour of infusion.
- Monitor therapeutic effectiveness, which is indicated by increased blood oxygenation (Po_2), usually evident within 30 min, in infants with cyanotic heart disease; increased pH in those with acidosis, increased systemic BP and urinary output, return of palpable pulses, and decreased ratio of pulmonary artery to aortic pressure in infants with restricted systemic blood flow.
- Monitor arterial pressure, ECG, heart rate, BP, respiratory rate, and temperature, throughout the infusion.
- Monitor lab tests: Arterial blood gases and blood pH throughout the infusion.

Patient & Family Education

Erectile Dysfunction

- Follow carefully directions for penile injection provided by the manufacturer.
- Do not change dose without consulting the prescriber.
- Do not use intracavernosal injection more often than 3 × wk; allow at least 24 h between uses.
- Do not use more than 2 urethral suppository systems in a 24 h period.
- Report promptly any of the following: Nodules or hard tissue in penis; penile pain, redness, swelling, tenderness; or curvature of the erect penis.
- Seek immediate medical attention if an erection persists longer than 6 h.

ALTEPLASE RECOMBINANT

(al'te-plase)

Activase, Cathflo Activase

Classification: THROMBOLYTIC, TISSUE PLASMINOGEN ACTIVATOR

Therapeutic: THROMBOLYTIC ENZYME

Common adverse effects in *italic;* life-threatening effects underlined; generic names in **bold;** classifications in SMALL CAPS; ♣ Canadian drug name; ⊙ Prototype drug; ⚠ Alert

AVAILABILITY Injection

ACTION & *THERAPEUTIC EFFECT* A recombinant DNA-derived form of human tissue-type plasminogen activator that promotes thrombolysis by forming the active proteolytic enzyme, plasmin. *Plasmin is capable of degrading fibrin, fibrinogen, and factors V, VIII, and XII.*

USES Acute MI management; acute ischemic stroke management; lysis of pulmonary embolism; reestablishing patency of occluded IV catheter.

UNLABELED USES Lysis of arterial occlusions in peripheral and bypass vessels; DVT, intravascular catheter occlusion, parapneumonic pleural effusions.

CONTRAINDICATIONS Hypersensitivity to alteplase; active internal bleeding, history of cerebrovascular accident (within 3 mo), aneurysm, recent (within 3 mo) intracranial or interspinal surgery or trauma, intracranial neoplasm, increased intracranial pressure; arteriovenous malformation, severe uncontrolled hypertension, likelihood of left heart thrombus, acute pericarditis, bacterial endocarditis, severe liver or renal dysfunction, septic thrombophlebitis; neurological deficit.

CAUTIOUS USE Recent major surgery (within 10 days), cerebral vascular disease, recent GI or GU bleeding, recent trauma, renal impairment, hypertension, hemorrhagic ophthalmic conditions; age greater than 75 yr; children; pregnancy (category C); lactation.

ROUTE & DOSAGE

Acute MI

Adult: **IV** 60 mg over first hour, 20 mg/h over second hour, and 20 mg over third hour (for a total of 100 mg over 3 h). *Accelerated schedule with heparin and aspirin (weight greater than 67 kg):* 15 mg bolus, then 50 mg over next 30 min, then 35 mg over next 60 min. *Accelerated schedule with heparin and aspirin (weight 67 kg or less):* 15 mg bolus, then 0.75 mg/kg (not to exceed 50 mg) over next 30 min, then 0.5 mg/kg (not to exceed 35 mg) over next 60 min

Acute Ischemic Stroke/Thrombotic Stroke

Adult: **IV** 0.9 mg/kg over 60 min with 10% of dose as an initial bolus over 1 min (max: 90 mg)

Pulmonary Embolism (Activase only)

Adult: **IV** 100 mg infused over 2 h

Reopen Occluded IV Catheter (Cathflo Activase only)

Adult/Child (greater than 30 kg): **IV** Instill 2 mg/2 mL into dysfunctional catheter for 2 h. May repeat once if needed. *Child (weight 10–29 kg):* **IV** Instill 110% of internal lumen volume (max: 2 mg in 2 mL). May repeat if function not restored within 2 h.

ADMINISTRATION

Intravenous

PREPARE: **IV Infusion:** Reconstitute the *50 mg vial* as follows: Do not use if vacuum in vial has been broken. Use a large-bore needle (e.g., 18 gauge) and do not prime needle with air. ▪ Dilute contents of vial with sterile water for injection supplied by manufacturer. ▪ Direct stream of sterile water into the lyophilized cake. Slight foaming is usual. Allow to stand until bubbles dissipate. Resulting concentration is 1 mg/mL. ▪ Reconstitute the *100-mg vial* using supplied transfer device for reconstitution. Follow manufacturer's directions.

ADMINISTER: **IV Infusion:** ▪ Start IV infusion as soon as possible after the thrombolytic event, preferably within 6 h. ▪ Administer drug as reconstituted (1 mg/mL) or further diluted with an equal volume of NS or D5W to yield 0.5 mg/mL. **Acute MI:** 3-h infusion: Administer 60% of total dose in the first hour for acute MI, with 6–10% given as a bolus dose over 1–2 min and remainder of first dose infused over hour 1. Follow with second dose (20% of total) over hour 2, and third dose (20% of total) over hour 3. ▪ For patients weighing less than 65 kg calculate dose using 1.25 mg/kg over 3 h. See accelerated schedule under Route & Dosage. **Pulmonary embolism:** Administer entire dose over a 2-h period. **Acute ischemic stroke:** Give 0.9 mg/kg (not to exceed 90-mg total dose) over 60 min with 10% of the total dose administered as an initial IV bolus over 1 min. ▪ Do not exceed a total dose of 100 mg. Higher doses have been associated with intracranial bleeding. ▪ Follow infusion of drug by flushing IV tubing with 30–50 mL of NS or D5W.

▪ Reconstituted drug is stable for 8 h in above solutions at room temperature (2°–30°C; 36°–86°F). Because there are no preservatives, discard any unused solution after that time.

INCOMPATIBILITIES: **Solution/additive:** **Dobutamine, dopamine, heparin.** **Y-site:** **Bivalirudin, dobutamine, dopamine, heparin, nitroglycerin.**

▪ Store above reconstituted solutions at room temperature 2°–30°C (36°–86°F) for no longer than 8 h. Discard any unused solution after that time.

ADVERSE EFFECTS **Hematologic:** Internal and superficial bleeding (cerebral, retroperitoneal, GU, GI), stroke.

PHARMACOKINETICS **Peak:** 5–10 min after infusion completed. **Duration:** Baseline values restored in 3 h. **Metabolism:** In liver. **Elimination:** In urine. **Half-Life:** 26.5 min.

NURSING IMPLICATIONS

Assessment & Drug Effects

- Monitor for S&S of excess bleeding q15min for the first hour of therapy, q30min for second to eighth hour, then q8h.
- Monitor neurologic checks throughout drug infusion q30min and qh for the first 8 h after infusion.
- Protect patient from invasive procedures because spontaneous bleeding occurs twice as often with alteplase as with heparin. IM injections are contraindicated. Minimize physical manipulation of patient during thrombolytic therapy to prevent bruising.
- Check vital signs frequently. Be alert to changes in cardiac rhythm.
- Report signs of bleeding: Gum bleeding, epistaxis, hematoma, spontaneous ecchymoses, oozing at catheter site, increased pain from internal bleeding. Stop the infusion, then resume when bleeding stops.
- Use the radial artery to draw ABGs. Pressure to puncture sites, if necessary, should be maintained for up to 30 min.
- Continue monitoring vital signs until laboratory reports confirm

anticoagulant control; patient is at risk for postthrombolytic bleeding for 2–4 days after intracoronary alteplase treatment.
- Monitor lab tests: Baseline CBC, aPTT, PT, INR; Hct and Hgb, and platelet count as needed.

Patient & Family Education
- Report promptly any of the following: Sudden severe headache, blood in urine, bloody or tarry stool, any sign of bleeding or oozing from injection/insertion sites.
- Remain quiet and on bedrest while receiving this medicine.

ALTRETAMINE
(al-tre′ta-meen)

Classification: ANTINEOPLASTIC; ALKYLATING
Therapeutic: ANTINEOPLASTIC
Prototype: Cyclophosphamide

AVAILABILITY Capsule

ACTION & *THERAPEUTIC EFFECT*
A synthetic cytotoxic antineoplastic drug with an unknown mechanism of action. Its metabolites have cytotoxic properties. *Altretamine has demonstrated neoplastic activity in patients resistant to alkylating agents.*

USES Ovarian cancer.

CONTRAINDICATIONS Hypersensitivity to altretamine, severe bone marrow depression, neurologic toxicity, neurologic disease; pregnancy (may cause fetal harm if administered during pregnancy); lactation.

CAUTIOUS USE Concerns related to bone marrow suppression, gastrointestinal toxicity, and neurotoxicity. Safety and efficacy in children not established.

ROUTE & DOSAGE

Ovarian Cancer

Adult: **PO** 260 mg/m²/day for 14 or 21 consecutive days in a 28-day cycle

ADMINISTRATION

Oral
- Give only under supervision of a qualified prescriber experienced in the use of antineoplastics.
- Give in 4 divided doses after meals and at bedtime.
- Hazardous agent; use appropriate precautions for handling and disposal.
- Altretamine is usually discontinued for 14 days or longer and restarted at 200 mg/m²/day if any of the following occur: Platelet count less than 0.075 mL; severe GI intolerance; WBC count less than 2000/mm³, granulocyte count less than 1000/mm³; or progressive neurotoxicity.
- Store at room temperature, 15°–30°C (59°–86°F).

ADVERSE EFFECTS **CNS:** *Paresthesias, peripheral numbness, ataxia.* **GI:** *Nausea, vomiting,* anorexia. **GU:** Increased blood urea nitrogen, increased serum creatinine. **Hematologic:** <u>Leukopenia, anemia, thrombocytopenia.</u> **Hepatic:** Increased serum alkaline phosphatase.

INTERACTIONS **Drug:** Concomitant administration of TRICYCLIC ANTIDEPRESSANTS (**imipramine, amitriptyline**), MONOAMINE OXIDASE INHIBITORS, or **selegiline** result in orthostatic hypotension. Use with other IMMUNOSUPPRESSANTS will increase immune suppression. Use with MYELOSUPPRESSIVE AGENTS close monitoring is required.

Do not administer LIVE VACCINES, consider delaying administration of INACTIVATED VACCINES. Avoid use with **sargramostim, filgrastim**. **Palifermin** increases duration of oral mucositis. **Herbal:** Echinacea may reduce efficacy. **Food: Vitamin B_6** supplementation may decrease effect.

PHARMACOKINETICS **Absorption:** Rapidly from GI tract. Approximately 25% reaches systemic circulation. **Metabolism:** Rapidly demethylated in the liver. **Elimination:** 62% of the dose is excreted in the urine in 24 h. **Half-Life:** 4.7–10 h.

NURSING IMPLICATIONS

Black Box Warning

Altretamine has been associated with severe neurotoxicity and bone marrow suppression.

Assessment & Drug Effects

- Perform a neurologic examination regularly; assess for the presence of paresthesias, peripheral numbness, ataxia, decreased sensations, and alterations in mood or consciousness.
- Withhold medication if neurologic symptoms fail to resolve with dose reduction. Notify prescriber.
- Monitor for nausea and vomiting, which are related to the cumulative dose of altretamine. After several weeks some patients develop tolerance to the GI effects. Antiemetics may be required to control GI distress.
- Use with caution in patients previously treated with **myelosuppressive** drugs or with preexisting neurotoxicity.
- Monitor lab tests: Prior to each course of therapy and monthly, CBC with differential.

Patient & Family Education

- Taking altretamine after meals or with food or milk may decrease nausea.
- Report symptoms indicative of neurotoxicity to prescriber (paresthesias, peripheral numbness, ataxia, decreased sensations, and alterations in mood or consciousness).

ALUMINUM HYDROXIDE (Pr)

(a-lu′mi-num)

ALternaGEL, Alu-Cap, Alugel, Alu-Tab, Amphojel, Dialume

ALUMINUM CARBONATE, BASIC

Basaljel

ALUMINUM PHOSPHATE

Phosphaljel

Classification: ANTACID; ADSORBENT

Therapeutic: ANTACID

AVAILABILITY **Aluminum Hydroxide:** Tablet; capsule; suspension; **Aluminum Carbonate, Basic:** Tablet; capsule; suspension; **Aluminum Phosphate:** Tablet; capsule; suspension

ACTION & *THERAPEUTIC EFFECT* Nonsystemic antacid with moderate neutralizing action. Reduces acid concentration and pepsin activity by raising pH of gastric and intraesophageal secretions. *Reduces gastric acidity by neutralizing the stomach acid content. Aluminum carbonate lowers serum phosphate by binding dietary phosphate to form insoluble aluminum phosphate, which is excreted in feces.*

USES Symptomatic relief of gastric hyperacidity associated with gastritis, esophageal reflux, and hiatal hernia; adjunct in treatment of gastric and duodenal ulcer. More commonly used in combination with other antacids. Aluminum carbonate is used primarily in conjunction with a low phosphate diet to reduce hyperphosphatemia in patients with renal insufficiency and for prophylaxis and treatment of phosphatic renal calculi.

CONTRAINDICATIONS Prolonged use of high doses in presence of low serum phosphate.

CAUTIOUS USE Renal impairment; gastric outlet obstruction; older adults; decreased bowel activity (e.g., patients receiving anticholinergic, antidiarrheal, or antispasmodic agents); patients who are dehydrated or on fluid restriction; pregnancy (category C).

ROUTE & DOSAGE

Antacid (Hydroxide and Phosphate)

Adult: **PO** 600 mg tid or qid

Antacid (Carbonate)

Adult: **PO** 10–30 mL of regular suspension or 5–15 mL of extra strength suspension or 2 capsules or tablets q2h

Phosphate Lowering (Carbonate)

Adult: **PO** 10–30 mL of regular suspension or 5–15 mL of extra strength suspension or 2–6 capsules or tablets 1 h p.c. and at bedtime

ADMINISTRATION

Oral

- Tablet **must be** chewed until it is thoroughly wetted before swallowing.
- Note for antacid use: Follow well-chewed tablet with one-half glass of water or milk; follow liquid preparation (suspension) with water to ensure passage into stomach. For phosphate lowering: Follow tablet, capsule, or suspension with full glass of water or fruit juice.
- Store at 15°–30°C (59°–86°F) in tightly closed container.

ADVERSE EFFECTS **CNS:** Dialysis dementia (thought to be due to aluminum intoxication). **Endocrine:** Hypophosphatemia, hypomagnesemia. **GI:** *Constipation*, fecal impaction, intestinal obstruction.

INTERACTIONS **Drug:** Aluminum will decrease absorption of **chloroquine, cimetidine, ciprofloxacin, digoxin, isoniazid,** IRON SALTS, NSAIDS, **norfloxacin, ofloxacin, phenytoin, phenothiazines, tetracycline, thyroxine. Sodium polystyrene sulfonate** may cause systemic alkalosis.

PHARMACOKINETICS **Absorption:** Minimal absorption. **Peak:** Slow onset. **Duration:** 2 h when taken with food; 3 h when taken 1 h after food. **Elimination:** In feces as insoluble phosphates.

NURSING IMPLICATIONS

Assessment & Drug Effects

- Note number and consistency of stools. Constipation is common and dose related. Intestinal obstruction from fecal concretions has been reported.
- Monitor lab tests: Periodic serum calcium and phosphorus levels with prolonged high-dose therapy or impaired renal function.

Patient & Family Education

- Increase phosphorus in diet when taking large doses of these antacids for prolonged periods; hypophosphatemia can develop within 2 wk of continuous use of these antacids. The older adult in a poor nutritional state is at high risk.

- Antacid may cause stools to appear speckled or whitish.
- Report epigastric or abdominal pain; it is a clinical guide for adjusting dosage. Keep prescriber informed. Pain that persists beyond 72 h may signify serious complications.
- Seek medical help if indigestion is accompanied by shortness of breath, sweating, or chest pain, if stools are dark or tarry, or if symptoms are recurrent when taking this medication.
- Seek medical advice and supervision if self-prescribed antacid use exceeds 2 wk.

ALVIMOPAN

(al-vi-mo′pan)

Entereg

Classification: PERIPHERAL OPIOID RECEPTOR ANTAGONIST; GI MOTILITY STIMULANT

Therapeutic: GI MOTILITY STIMULANT

AVAILABILITY Capsule

ACTION & *THERAPEUTIC EFFECT* Morphine and other postop analgesics are mu-opioid receptor agonists known to inhibit GI motility and prolong the duration of postoperative ileus. Alvimopan is a selective antagonist of mu-opioid receptors. *It competitively antagonizes the effect of morphine on contractility, shortening the duration of postop ileus.*

USES To accelerate the time to upper and lower gastrointestinal recovery after partial large- or small-bowel resection surgery with primary anastomosis.

UNLABELED USES Constipation, opioid-induced constipation.

CONTRAINDICATIONS Therapeutic doses of opioids for greater than 7 consecutive days immediately preoperative; end-stage renal disease; severe hepatic impairment (Child-Pugh class C).

CAUTIOUS USE Recent exposure to opioids; surgery for complete bowel obstruction; history of CAD or MI; pregnancy (category B); lactation. Safety and efficacy in children not established.

ROUTE & DOSAGE

Acceleration of Postoperative GI Recovery

Adult: **PO** 12 mg 0.5–5 h preoperative; then 12 mg bid up to 7 days

ADMINISTRATION

Oral

- Give preop dose 30 min–5 h before surgery.
- Do not exceed 15 doses (maximum allowed).
- Store at 15°–30°C (59°–86°F).
- Note: Hospitals **must be** registered in and have met all of the requirements for the **Entereg** Access Support and Education (E.A.S.E.) program in order to use alvimopan.

ADVERSE EFFECTS **Endocrine:** Hypokalemia. **GI:** Constipation, dyspepsia, flatulence. **GU:** Urinary retention. **Musculoskeletal:** Back pain. **Hematologic:** Anemia.

INTERACTIONS **Food:** Decreased extent and rate of absorption if taken with a high-fat meal.

PHARMACOKINETICS **Absorption:** Bioavailability 6%. **Peak:** 2 h. **Distribution:** 90–94% plasma protein bound. **Metabolism:** By intestinal flora. **Elimination:** Fecal (primary) and renal (35%). **Half-Life:** 10–18 h.

NURSING IMPLICATIONS

Assessment & Drug Effects

- Monitor frequently for return of bowel sounds and ability to pass flatus.
- Monitor closely patients with impaired renal function for adverse effects.
- Report to prescriber increasing abdominal pain, diarrhea, nausea and vomiting.
- Monitor lab tests: Serum potassium in those predisposed to hypokalemia.

Patient & Family Education

- Report promptly increasing abdominal pain and nausea.

AMANTADINE HYDROCHLORIDE

(a-man'ta-deen)

Gocovri, Osmolex ER

Classification: ANTIVIRAL; CENTRAL-ACTING DOPAMINE AGONIST; ANTIPARKINSON

Therapeutic: ANTIVIRAL; ANTIPARKINSON

AVAILABILITY Capsule; tablet; oral syrup; extended release capsule, extended release tablet

ACTION & *THERAPEUTIC EFFECT* Mechanism of action related to antiviral activity is poorly understood but may be due to prevention of release of infectious viral nucleic acid into the host cell. Mechanism of action in parkinsonism may be related to release of dopamine from neuronal storage sites. *Active against several strains of influenza A virus. Effective in management of symptoms of parkinsonism when used in conjunction with other antiparkinson agents.*

USES Treatment of Parkinson disease; drug-induced extrapyramidal symptoms.

UNLABELED USES Tardive dyskinesia, multiple sclerosis-related fatigue, traumatic brain injury.

CONTRAINDICATIONS Hypersensitivity to amantadine or rimantadine, closed-angle glaucoma; suicidal ideation; lactation.

CAUTIOUS USE History of epilepsy or other types of seizures; CHF, peripheral edema, orthostatic hypotension; recurrent eczematoid dermatitis; psychoses, severe psychoneuroses; hepatic disease; renal impairment; older adults, cerebral arteriosclerosis; pregnancy (use with caution during pregnancy). Safety in children younger than 1 yr for Influenza A is not established.

ROUTE & DOSAGE

Parkinson Disease

Adult: **PO** (immediate release) 100 mg bid, may increase based on response to 300 mg/day **PO** (extended release) 137 mg capsule daily then after 1 week increase to 274 mg daily OR 129 tablet daily then after 1 week increase to 322 mg daily.

Drug-Induced Parkinsonism

Adult: **PO** 100 mg bid (max: 300 mg/day in divided doses if needed) **PO** (Extended release tablet) 129 mg daily

Renal Impairment Dosage Adjustment

Varies based on dosage form; consult package insert

ADMINISTRATION

Oral

- Do not crush, chew, or divide capsules. If needed, sprinkle entire contents on a small amount of soft food and administer immediately without chewing.
- Give with water, milk, or food.
- Use supplied calibrated device for measuring syrup formulation.
- Schedule medication in the morning or, with q12h dosing, schedule 2nd dose several hours before bedtime. If insomnia is a problem, suggest patient limit number of daytime naps.
- Store in tightly closed container preferably at 20°–25°C (68°–77°F) unless otherwise directed by manufacturer. Avoid freezing.

ADVERSE EFFECTS **CV:** Orthostatic hypotension, peripheral edema, syncope. **CNS:** *Dizziness, light-headedness,* headache, ataxia, irritability, anxiety, *nervousness, difficulty in concentrating,* mood or other mental changes, confusion, visual and auditory hallucinations, *insomnia,* nightmares, depression, paranoia, falling. **GI:** Anorexia, *nausea,* dry mouth, decreased appetite, constipation. **GU:** UTI, BPH. **Hematologic:** Bruising.

INTERACTIONS **Drug: Alcohol** enhances CNS effects; may potentiate effects of ANTICHOLINERGICS. Use with **bupropion** can increase restlessness/agitation Do not use with **alizapride, amisulpride,** ANTIPSYCHOTICS, **metoclopramide, sulipride, live influenza vaccine**.

PHARMACOKINETICS **Absorption:** Almost completely absorbed from GI tract. **Onset:** Within 48 h. **Peak:** 1–4 h. **Distribution:** Through body fluids. **Metabolism:** Not metabolized. **Elimination:** 90% unchanged in urine. **Half-Life:** 10–22 h (prolonged in renal insufficiency).

NURSING IMPLICATIONS

Assessment & Drug Effects

- Monitor effectiveness. Note that with parkinsonism, maximum response occurs within 2 wk–3 mo. Effectiveness may wane after 6–8 wk of treatment; report change to prescriber.
- Monitor and report: Mental status changes; nervousness, difficulty concentrating, or insomnia; loss of seizure control; S&S of toxicity, especially with doses above 200 mg/day.
- Monitor for and report promptly suicidal ideation, especially in those with a history of psychiatric disorders.
- Establish a baseline profile of the patient's disabilities to accurately differentiate disease symptoms and drug-induced neuropsychiatric adverse reactions.
- Monitor vital signs for at least 3 or 4 days after increases in dosage; also monitor urinary output.
- Monitor for and report reduced salivation, increased akinesia or rigidity, and psychological disturbances that may develop within 4–48 h after initiation of therapy and after dosage increases with parkinsonism.
- Monitor lab tests: Renal function (baseline and as clinically indicated).

Patient & Family Education

- Make all position changes slowly, particularly from recumbent to upright position, in order to minimize dizziness.
- Report any of the following to prescriber: Shortness of breath, peripheral edema, significant weight gain, dizziness or light-headedness, inability to

concentrate, and other changes in mental status, suicidal ideation, difficulty urinating, and visual impairment.

- Do not drive, and exercise caution with potentially hazardous activities until response to the drug is known.
- Note: People with Parkinson disease should not discontinue therapy abruptly; doing so may precipitate a parkinsonian crisis with severe akinesia, rigidity, tremor, and psychic disturbances. Adhere to established dosage regimen.

AMCINONIDE

(am-sin'oh-nide)

See Appendix A-4.

AMIFOSTINE

(am-i-fos'teen)

Ethyol

Classification: CYTOPROTECTIVE

Therapeutic: CYTOPROTECTIVE

AVAILABILITY Solution for injection

ACTION & THERAPEUTIC EFFECT Amifostine reduces cytotoxic damage induced by radiation or antineoplastic agents; this protective effect appears to be mediated by the formation of a metabolite of amifostine that removes free radicals from normal cells exposed to cisplatin. *Amifostine is cytoprotective in the kidney, bone marrow, and GI mucosa, but not in the brain or spinal cord. The cytoprotection results in decreased myelosuppression and peripheral neuropathy.*

USES Reduction of the cumulative renal toxicity associated with cisplatin, xerostomia.

UNLABELED USES Reduction of paclitaxel toxicity, bone marrow suppression prophylaxis.

CONTRAINDICATIONS Sensitivity to aminothiol compounds or mannitol, patients with potentially curable malignancies, hypotensive patients or those who are dehydrated, exfoliated dermatitis; lactation.

CAUTIOUS USE Patients at risk for hypocalcemia, cardiovascular disease (i.e., arrhythmias, CHF, TIA, CVA); radiation therapy; renal disease; pregnancy (category C).

ROUTE & DOSAGE

Renal Protection

Adult: **IV** 910 mg/m² once daily prior to chemotherapy

Reduction of Xerostomia

Adult: **IV** 200 mg/m² prior to radiation therapy

ADMINISTRATION

Intravenous

Give antiemetics, adequately hydrate, and defer antihypertensives for 24 h prior to administration. Do not administer if patient is hypotensive or dehydrated. Consult prescriber.

PREPARE: **IV Infusion:** Reconstitute by adding 9.7 mL of NS injection to a single-dose vial to yield 50 mg/mL. ▪ May be further diluted with NS to a concentration as low as 5 mg/mL.

ADMINISTER: **IV Infusion:** Infuse over no more than 15 min, beginning 30 min before chemotherapy; place patient in supine position prior to and during infusion. ▪ For xerostomia, infuse over 3 min; begin 15–30 min before radiation.

INCOMPATIBILITIES: **Solution/additive:** Do not mix with any solutions other than NS. **Y-site: Acyclovir, amphotericin B, amphotericin B lipid, cefoperazone, chlorpromazine, cisplatin, ganciclovir, hydroxyzine, minocycline, mycophenolate, prochlorperazine, quinupristin-dalfopristin.**

- Store reconstituted solution at 15°–30°C (59°–86°F) for 5 h or refrigerate up to 24 h.

ADVERSE EFFECTS CV: *Transient reduction in blood pressure.* **GI:** *Nausea, vomiting.* **Other:** Infusion reactions (flushing, feeling of warmth or coldness, chills, dizziness, somnolence, hiccups, sneezing), hypocalcemia, hypersensitivity reactions.

INTERACTIONS Drug: ANTIHYPERTENSIVES could cause or potentiate hypotension.

PHARMACOKINETICS Onset: 5–8 min. **Metabolism:** In liver to active free thiol metabolite. **Elimination:** Renally excreted. **Half-Life:** 8 min.

NURSING IMPLICATIONS

Assessment & Drug Effects

- Monitor for S&S of hypocalcemia and fluid balance if vomiting is significant.
- Monitor BP every 5 min during infusion. Stop infusion if systolic BP drops significantly from baseline (e.g., 20% drop in systolic BP), and place patient flat with legs raised. Restart infusion if BP returns to normal in 5 min.

Patient & Family Education

- Know and understand adverse effects.

AMIKACIN SULFATE

(am-i-kay′sin)

Amikin

Classification: AMINOGLYCOSIDE ANTIBIOTIC

Therapeutic: ANTIBIOTIC

Prototype: Gentamicin

AVAILABILITY Solution for injection

ACTION & *THERAPEUTIC EFFECT* Appears to inhibit protein synthesis in bacterial cells and is usually bactericidal. *Effective against a wide range of gram-negative bacteria, including many strains resistant to other aminoglycosides. Also effective against penicillinase- and non-penicillinase-producing Staphylococcus.*

USES Primarily for short-term treatment of serious infections of respiratory tract, bones, joints, skin, and soft tissue, CNS (including meningitis), peritonitis burns, recurrent urinary tract infections (UTIs).

UNLABELED USES Intrathecal or intraventricular administration, in conjunction with IM or IV dosage.

CONTRAINDICATIONS History of hypersensitivity or toxic reaction with an aminoglycoside antibiotic; lactation.

CAUTIOUS USE Impaired renal function; eighth cranial (auditory) nerve impairment; preexisting vertigo or dizziness, tinnitus, or dehydration; fever; myasthenia gravis; parkinsonism; hypocalcemia; older adults, premature infants, neonates and infants; pregnancy (category C).

ROUTE & DOSAGE

Moderate to Severe Infections

Adult: **IV/IM** 5–7.5 mg/kg loading dose, then 7.5 mg/kg q12h (max: 15 mg/kg/day) for 7–10 days
Child: **IV/IM** 5–7.5 mg/kg loading dose, then 5 mg/kg q8h or 7.5 mg/kg q12h for 7–10 days (max: 1.5 g/day)
Neonate: **IV/IM** 10 mg/kg loading dose, then 7.5 mg/kg q12h for 7–10 days

Uncomplicated UTI

Adult: **IV/IM** 250 mg q12h

Obesity Dosage Adjustment

Calculate dose based on IBW

Renal Impairment Dosage Adjustment

CrCl greater than 60 mL/min: Normal dose q8h; *40–60 mL/min:* Normal dose q12h; *20–39 mL/min:* Half dose q24h; *less than 20 mL/min:* Administer loading dose then monitor closely

Hemodialysis Dosage Adjustment

Administer dose postdialysis or give ⅔ dose as supplemental dose

ADMINISTRATION

Intramuscular

- Use the 250 mg/mL vials for IM injection. Calculate the required dose, and withdraw the equivalent number of mLs from the vial.
- Give deep IM into a large muscle.

Intravenous

Verify correct IV concentration and rate of infusion with prescriber for neonates, infants, and children.

PREPARE: **Intermittent:** Add contents of 500-mg vial to 100 or 200 mL D5W, NS injection, or other diluent recommended by manufacturer. ▪ For pediatric patients, volume of diluent depends on patient's fluid tolerance. ▪ Note: Color of solution may vary from colorless to light straw color or very pale yellow. Discard solutions that appear discolored or that contain particulate matter.

ADMINISTER: **Intermittent:** Give a single dose (including loading dose) over at least 30–60 min by IV infusion. ▪ Increase infusion time to 1–2 h for infants. ▪ Monitor infusion rate carefully. A rapid rise in serum amikacin level can cause respiratory depression (neuromuscular blockade) and other signs of toxicity.

INCOMPATIBILITIES: **Solution/additive:** **Aminophylline, amphotericin B, ampicillin,** CEPHALOSPORINS, **chlorothiazide, heparin,** PENICILLINS, **phenytoin, vitamin B complex with C.** **Y-site:** **Allopurinol, amphotericin B, azithromycin, hetastarch, propofol.**

- Store at 15°–30°C (59°–86°F) unless otherwise directed.

ADVERSE EFFECTS **CNS:** Neurotoxicity: Drowsiness, unsteady gait, weakness, clumsiness, paresthesias, tremors, convulsions, peripheral neuritis. **HEENT:** *Auditory–ototoxicity,* high-frequency hearing loss, complete hearing loss (occasionally permanent); tinnitus; ringing or buzzing in ears; *Vestibular:* Dizziness, ataxia. **Endocrine:**

Hypokalemia, hypomagnesemia. **Skin:** Skin rash, urticaria, pruritus, redness. **GI:** Nausea, vomiting, hepatotoxicity. **GU:** Oliguria, urinary frequency, hematuria, tubular necrosis, azotemia. **Other:** Superinfections.

INTERACTIONS **Drug:** ANESTHETICS, SKELETAL MUSCLE RELAXANTS have additive neuromuscular blocking effects; **acyclovir, amphotericin B, bacitracin, capreomycin, cephalosporins, colistin, cisplatin, carboplatin, methoxyflurane, polymyxin B, vancomycin, furosemide, ethacrynic acid** increase risk of ototoxicity and nephrotoxicity.

PHARMACOKINETICS **Peak:** 30 min IV; 45 min to 2 h IM. **Distribution:** Does not cross blood–brain barrier; crosses placenta; accumulates in renal cortex. **Elimination:** 94–98% renally in 24 h, remainder in 10–30 days. **Half-Life:** 2–3 h in adults, 4–8 h in neonates.

NURSING IMPLICATIONS

Black Box Warning

Nephrotoxicity and ototoxicity (both vestibular and auditory) can occur, especially with preexisting renal damage and/or high doses. Neuromuscular blockade and respiratory paralysis have been reported especially in those treated with anesthetics or neuromuscular blocking agents.

Assessment & Drug Effects

- Baseline tests: Before initial dose, C&S; renal function and vestibulocochlear nerve function (and at regular intervals during therapy; closely monitor in the older adult, patients with documented ear problems, renal impairment, or during high-dose or prolonged therapy).
- Monitor peak and trough amikacin blood levels: Draw blood 1 h after IM or immediately after completion of IV infusion; draw trough levels immediately before the next IM or IV dose.
- Monitor for and promptly report S&S of: Ototoxicity [primarily involves the cochlear (auditory) branch; high-frequency deafness usually appears first and can be detected only by audiometer]; indicators of declining renal function; respiratory tract infections and other symptoms indicative of superinfections.
- Monitor for and report auditory symptoms (tinnitus, roaring noises, sensation of fullness in ears, hearing loss) and vestibular disturbances (dizziness or vertigo, nystagmus, ataxia).
- Monitor and report any changes in I&O, oliguria, hematuria, or cloudy urine. Keeping patient well hydrated reduces risk of nephrotoxicity; consult prescriber regarding optimum fluid intake.
- Monitor respiratory status especially in those who have received anesthetics, neuromuscular blocking agents or multiple transfusions of citrated blood.
- Monitor lab tests: Baseline and frequent serum creatinine and BUN, complete urinalysis.

Patient & Family Education

- Report immediately any changes in hearing or unexplained ringing/roaring noises or dizziness, and problems with balance or coordination.

AMILORIDE HYDROCHLORIDE

(a-mill′oh-ride)

Classification: DIURETIC, POTASSIUM-SPARING

Therapeutic: DIURETIC, POTASSIUM-SPARING; ANTIHYPERTENSIVE

Prototype: Spironolactone

AVAILABILITY Tablet

ACTION & *THERAPEUTIC EFFECT* Induces urinary excretion of sodium and reduces excretion of potassium, calcium, magnesium, and hydrogen ions by direct action on distal renal tubules. *Lowers blood pressure by excretion of sodium ion and water from the kidney while sparing potassium excretion.*

USES Adjunctive treatment of heart failure, hypertension.

UNLABELED USES Ascites, hypokalemia, edema.

CONTRAINDICATIONS Hypersensitivity to amiloride; elevated serum potassium (greater than 5.5 mEq/L) anuria, acute or chronic renal insufficiency; evidence of diabetic nephropathy; type 1 diabetes mellitus; metabolic or respiratory acidosis.

CAUTIOUS USE Debilitated patients; diet-controlled or uncontrolled diabetes mellitus; COPD; severe hepatic disease; older adult; pregnancy (category B); lactation. Safe use in children not established.

ROUTE & DOSAGE

HTN, HF, Hypokalemia

Adult: **PO** 5–10 mg/day, may increase up to 20 mg/day

ADMINISTRATION

Oral

- Give once/day dose in the morning and schedule the second bid dose early to avoid interrupting sleep.
- Give with food to reduce possibility of gastric distress.
- Store at 15°–30°C (59°–86°F) in a tightly closed container unless otherwise directed.

ADVERSE EFFECTS **Respiratory:** Cough, dyspnea. **CNS:** Dizziness, fatigue, headache. **Endocrine:** Hyperkalemia. **GI:** Abdominal pain, change in appetite, constipation, diarrhea, nausea, vomiting. **GU:** Impotence. **Musculoskeletal:** Muscle cramps, weakness.

DIAGNOSTIC TEST INTERFERENCE May lead to false-negative aldosterone/renin ratio (ARR).

INTERACTIONS **Drug:** Use with **triamterene** or **eplerenone** may cause hyperkalemia. **Sotalol** may cause cardiotoxicity. ACE INHIBITORS (e.g., **captopril**), **spironolactone,** POTASSIUM SUPPLEMENTS may cause hyperkalemia with cardiac arrhythmias; possibility of increased **lithium** toxicity (decreased renal elimination); possibility of altered **digoxin** response; NSAIDS may attenuate antihypertensive effects. Concurrent use of **bupropion** may decrease renal clearance. **Food:** POTASSIUM-CONTAINING SALT SUBSTITUTES or foods high in **potassium** increase risk of hyperkalemia.

PHARMACOKINETICS **Absorption:** 50% from GI tract. **Onset:** 2 h. **Peak:** 3–4 h. **Duration:** 24 h. **Elimination:** 20–50% unchanged in urine, 40% in feces. **Half-Life:** 6–9 h.

NURSING IMPLICATIONS

Black Box Warning

Amiloride has been associated with severe, potentially fatal hyperkalemia especially in the elderly and those with renal impairment or diabetes.

Assessment & Drug Effects

- Monitor for S&S of hyperkalemia and hyponatremia. Hyperkalemia occurs in about 10% of patients receiving amiloride, and serum potassium can rise suddenly and without warning. It is more common in older adults and patients with diabetes or renal disease.

- Monitor ECG as warranted.
- Monitor lab tests: Serum potassium levels, particularly when therapy is initiated, whenever dosage adjustments are made, and during any illness that may affect kidney function; periodic BUN, creatinine, for patients with renal or hepatic dysfunction, diabetes mellitus, older adults, or the debilitated.
- Monitor blood pressure, I&O, daily weights.

Patient & Family Education

- Learn S&S of hyperkalemia and hyponatremia and report to prescriber immediately.
- Do not take potassium supplements, salt substitutes, high intake of dietary potassium unless prescribed by prescriber.
- Do not drive or engage in potentially hazardous activities until response to drug is known.

AVAILABILITY Solution for injection; tablet; syrup

AMINOCAPROIC ACID

(a-mee-noe-ka-proe′ik)

Amicar

Classification: COAGULATOR; SYSTEMIC HEMOSTATIC

Therapeutic: ANTIHEMORRHAGIC; ANTIFIBRINOLYTIC

ACTION & *THERAPEUTIC EFFECT* Synthetic hemostatic agent with specific antifibrinolysis action. Inhibits plasminogen activator substance, and to a lesser degree plasmin (fibrinolysin), which is concerned with destruction of clots. *Acts as an inhibitor of fibrinolytic bleeding.*

USES To control excessive bleeding resulting from systemic hyperfibrinolysis; also used in urinary fibrinolysis associated with severe trauma, anoxia, shock, urologic surgery, and neoplastic diseases of GU tract.

UNLABELED USES To prevent hemorrhage in hemophiliacs undergoing dental extraction; as a specific antidote for streptokinase or urokinase toxicity; to prevent recurrence of subarachnoid hemorrhage, especially when surgery is delayed; for management of amegakaryocytic thrombocytopenia; and to prevent or abort hereditary angioedema episodes.

CONTRAINDICATIONS Severe renal impairment; active disseminated intravascular clotting (DIC); upper urinary tract bleeding (hematuria); hemophilia; benzyl alcohol hypersensitivity, especially in neonates; paraben hypersensitivity; lactation.

CAUTIOUS USE Cardiac, renal, or hepatic disease; renal impairment; history of pulmonary embolus or other thrombotic diseases; hypovolemia; pregnancy (category C).

ROUTE & DOSAGE

Hemostatic

Adult: **PO/IV** 4–5 g during first hour, then 1–1.25 g qh for 8 h or until bleeding is controlled (max: 30 g/24h)
Child: **PO/IV** 100 mg/kg or 3 g/m^2 during first hour, then 33.3 mg^2/kg qh qh (max: 18 g/m^2/24 h)

Renal Impairment Dosage Adjustment

Reduce dose to 15–25% of normal dose

 Common adverse effects in *italic;* life-threatening effects underlined; generic names in **bold;** classifications in SMALL CAPS; ♣ Canadian drug name; Ⓟ Prototype drug; ⚠ Alert

ADMINISTRATION

Oral

- Note: May need to give patient as many as 10 tablets or 4 tsp for a 5 g dose during the first hour of treatment.

Intravenous

PREPARE: **IV Infusion:** Dilute parenteral aminocaproic acid before use. ▪ Each 4 mL (1 g) is diluted with 50 mL of NS, D5W, or LR.
ADMINISTER: **IV Infusion:** Prescriber orders specific IV flow rate. ▪ Usual rate is 5 g or a fraction thereof over first hour (5 g/250 mL). ▪ Give each additional gram over 1 h. Avoid rapid infusion to prevent hypotension, faintness, and bradycardia or other arrhythmias.
INCOMPATIBILITIES: **Solution/additive:** **Fructose solution.**

- Store in tightly closed containers at 15°–30°C (59°–86°F) unless otherwise directed. Avoid freezing.

ADVERSE EFFECTS **CV:** Faintness, orthostatic hypotension; dysrhythmias; thrombophlebitis, thromboses. **CNS:** Dizziness, malaise, headache, seizures. **HEENT:** Tinnitus, nasal congestion. Conjunctival erythema. **Skin:** Rash. **GI:** Nausea, vomiting, cramps, diarrhea, anorexia. **GU:** Diuresis, dysuria, urinary frequency, oliguria, reddish-brown urine (myoglobinuria), acute renal failure. Prolonged menstruation with cramping.

DIAGNOSTIC TEST INTERFERENCE ***Serum potassium*** may be elevated (especially in patients with impaired renal function).

INTERACTIONS **Drug:** ESTROGENS, ORAL CONTRACEPTIVES may cause hypercoagulation.

PHARMACOKINETICS **Absorption:** Rapidly from GI tract. **Peak:** 2 h. **Distribution:** Readily penetrates RBCs and other body cells. **Elimination:** 80% as unmetabolized drug in 12 h.

NURSING IMPLICATIONS

Assessment & Drug Effects

- Check IV site at frequent intervals for extravasation.
- Observe for signs of thrombophlebitis. Change site immediately if extravasation or thrombophlebitis occurs (see Appendix F).
- Monitor and report S&S of myopathy: Muscle weakness, myalgia, diaphoresis, fever, reddish-brown urine (myoglobinuria), oliguria, as well as thrombotic complications: Arm or leg pain, tenderness or swelling, Homans' sign, prominence of superficial veins, chest pain, breathlessness, dyspnea. Drug should be discontinued promptly.
- Monitor vital signs and urine output.
- Monitor lab tests: With prolonged therapy, periodic creatine phosphokinase and urinalyses for early detection of myopathy.

Patient & Family Education

- Report difficulty urinating or reddish-brown urine.
- Report arm or leg pain, chest pain, or difficulty breathing.

AMINOPHYLLINE (THEOPHYLLINE ETHYLENEDIAMIDE)

(am-in-off'i-lin)

Classification: BRONCHODILATOR; RESPIRATORY SMOOTH MUSCLE RELAXANT; XANTHINE
Therapeutic: BRONCHODILATOR
Prototype: Theophylline

AVAILABILITY Solution for injection

ACTION & THERAPEUTIC EFFECT A xanthine derivative that relaxes smooth muscle in the airways of the lungs and suppresses the response of the airways to stimuli that constrict them. *It is a respiratory smooth muscle relaxant that results in bronchodilation.*

USES Treatment of acute exacerbations of symptoms and reversible airflow obstruction due to asthma or other chronic lung diseases.

UNLABELED USES Reversal of adenosine-, dipyridamole-, or regadenoson-induced adverse reactions during nuclear cardiac stress testing.

CONTRAINDICATIONS Hypersensitivity to xanthine derivatives or to ethylenediamine component; cardiac arrhythmias.

CAUTIOUS USE Severe hypertension, cardiac disease, arrhythmias; impaired hepatic function; diabetes mellitus; hyperthyroidism; glaucoma; prostatic hypertrophy; fibrocystic breast disease; history of peptic ulcer; neonates and young children, older adults; COPD, acute influenza or patients receiving influenza immunization; pregnancy (category C); lactation.

ROUTE & DOSAGE

Bronchospasm

Adult: **IV Loading Dose** 6 mg/kg over 30 min; **IV Maintenance Dose** *Nonsmoker:* 0.5 mg/kg/h; *smoker:* 0.8 mg/kg/h; *CHF or cirrhosis:* 0.1–0.2 mg/kg/h

Child: **IV Loading Dose** 6 mg/kg IV over 30 min; **IV Maintenance Dose** *1–9 yr:* 1 mg/kg/h; *9 yr or older:* 0.8 mg/kg/h; **IV** *6–11 mo:* 0.7 g/kg/h; *2 to less than 6 mo:* 0.5 mg/kg/h

Neonatal Apnea

Neonate: See package insert

Obesity Dosage Adjustment

Calculate dose based on IBW

ADMINISTRATION

Intravenous

Verify correct IV concentration and rate of infusion with prescriber for neonates, infants, and children.

PREPARE: **IV Infusion:** Dilute loading dose in 100–200 mL NS, D5W, D5/NS, or LR. For continuous or intermittent infusion dilute in 500–1000 mL. ▪ Do not use aminophylline solutions if discolored or if crystals are present.

ADMINISTER: **IV Infusion:** Infuse at the ordered rate (mg/kg/h).

INCOMPATIBILITIES: **Solution/additive:** **Amikacin, atracurium, bleomycin, cefepime, cefoperazone, ceftazidime, ceftriaxone, chlorpromazine, ciprofloxacin, clindamycin, corticotropin, dimenhydrinate, dobutamine, doxorubicin, epinephrine, hydralazine, hydroxyzine, insulin, isoproterenol, levorphanol, meperidine, methylprednisolone, midazolam, minocycline, morphine, nafcillin, norepinephrine, papaverine, penicillin G, pentazocine, procaine, prochlorperazine, promazine, promethazine, trimecaine, verapamil, vitamin B complex with C, zinc.** **Y-site:** **Amiodarone, ampicillin, ascorbic acid, atracurium,**

azathioprine, buprenorphine, chlorpromazine, ciprofloxacin, clarithromycin, dantrolene, daunorubicin, dexrazoxane, diazepam, diazoxide, dimenhydrinate, diphenhydramine, dobutamine, dolasetron, doxorubicin, epinephrine, epirubicin, fenoldopam, ganciclovir, garenoxacin, gemtuzumab, haloperidol, hydralazine, hydroxyzine, idarubicin, isoproterenol, lansoprazole, magnesium, midazolam, minocycline, mitomycin, moxifloxacin, mycophenolate, norepinephrine, ondansetron, oritavancin, papaverine, pefloxacin, pentamidine, pentazocine, phenytoin, prochlorperazine, promazine, quinupristin/dalfopristin, SMZ/TMP, thiamine, topotecan, TPN, vancomycin, verapamil, vinorelbine, warfarin.

- Store at 15°–30°C (59°–86°F) in tightly closed containers unless otherwise directed.

ADVERSE EFFECTS **CNS:** Headache, insomnia, irritability, restlessness, seizure. **GI:** Diarrhea, nausea, vomiting. **GU:** Transient diuresis. **Musculoskeletal:** Tremor. **Integumentary:** Allergic skin reaction, exfoliative dermatitis.

INTERACTIONS **Drug:** Increases **lithium** excretion, lowering **lithium** levels; **cimetidine,** high-dose **allopurinol** (600 mg/day), **ciprofloxacin, fluvoxamine, erythromycin, troleandomycin** can significantly increase **theophylline** levels. **Herbal: St. John's wort** may decrease effect.

DIAGNOSTIC TEST INTERFERENCE: Plasma glucose, uric acid, free fatty acids, total cholesterol, HDL, HDL/LDL ratio, and urinary free cortisol excretion may be increased. Theophylline may decrease triiodothyronine.

PHARMACOKINETICS **Absorption:** Most products are 100% absorbed from GI tract. **Peak:** IV 30 min; uncoated tablet 1 h; sustained release 4–6 h. **Duration:** 4–8 h; varies with age, smoking, and liver function. **Distribution:** 40% protein bound, crosses placenta. **Metabolism:** Extensively in liver; by CYP1A2. **Elimination:** Parent drug and metabolites excreted by kidneys; excreted in breast milk. **Half-Life:** 3.7 h (child); 7.7 h (adult).

NURSING IMPLICATIONS

Assessment & Drug Effects

- Monitor for S&S of toxicity (generally related to theophylline serum levels over 20 mcg/mL). Observe patients receiving parenteral drug closely for signs of hypotension, arrhythmias, and convulsions until serum theophylline stabilizes within the therapeutic range.
- Monitor and record vital signs and I&O. A sudden, sharp, unexplained rise in heart rate may indicate toxicity.
- Note: Older adults, acutely ill, and patients with severe respiratory problems, liver dysfunction, or pulmonary edema are at greater risk of toxicity due to reduced drug clearance.
- Note: Children appear more susceptible to CNS stimulating effects of xanthines (nervousness, restlessness, insomnia, hyperactive reflexes, twitching, convulsions). Dosage reduction may be indicated.
- Monitor lab tests: Periodic serum theophylline levels.

Patient & Family Education

- Note: Use of tobacco tends to increase elimination of this drug (shortens half-life), necessitating higher dosage or shorter intervals than in nonsmokers.
- Report excessive nervousness or insomnia. Dosage reduction may be indicated.
- Note: Dizziness is a relatively common side effect, particularly in older adults; take necessary safety precautions.
- Do not take OTC remedies for treatment of asthma or cough unless approved by prescriber.

AMINOSALICYLIC ACID

(a-mee-noe-sal-i-sil′ik)

Paser

Classification: ANTITUBERCULOSIS
Therapeutic: ANTITUBERCULOSIS
Prototype: Isoniazid

AVAILABILITY Granule packets

ACTION & *THERAPEUTIC EFFECT* Suppresses growth and multiplication of *Mycobacterium tuberculosis* by preventing folic acid synthesis. Aminosalicylates reportedly have potent hypolipemic action. *Aminosalicylates are an effective anti-infective alone or in combined therapy and reduce serum cholesterol and triglycerides by lowering LDL and VLDL.*

USES Treat tuberculosis along with other medications.

CONTRAINDICATIONS Hypersensitivity to aminosalicylates, salicylates, or to compounds containing *para*-aminophenyl groups (e.g., sulfonamides, certain hair dyes); G6PD deficiency, use of the sodium salt in patients on sodium restriction or CHF; lactation.

CAUTIOUS USE Impaired renal and hepatic function; blood dyscrasias; goiter; gastric ulcer; pregnancy (teratogenic effects have been reported in animal reproduction studies).

ROUTE & DOSAGE

Tuberculosis

Adult/Adolescent/Child: **PO** 4 g 2–3 × day (max: 12 g)

ADMINISTRATION

Oral

- Mix granules in applesauce or yogurt, or suspend in an acidic drink such as fruit juice or tomato juice. Do not administer granules that have lost their tan color.
- Give with or immediately following meals to reduce irritative gastric effects.
- Store in tight, light-resistant containers in a cool, dry place, preferably at 15°–30°C (59°–86°F), unless otherwise directed.

ADVERSE EFFECTS **CNS:** Psychotic reactions. **Hepatic/GI:** *Anorexia, nausea, vomiting, abdominal distress, diarrhea,* acute hepatitis. **GU:** Renal (irritation), crystalluria. **Hematologic:** Leukopenia, agranulocytosis, thrombocytopenia, hemolytic anemia. **Other:** Fever. With long-term administration, goiter.

DIAGNOSTIC TEST INTERFERENCE Aminosalicylates may interfere with urine ***urobilinogen*** determinations (using ***Ehrlich's reagent***) and may cause false-positive ***urinary protein*** and ***VMA*** determinations (with ***diazo reagent***); false-positive ***urine glucose*** may result with ***cupric sulfate tests*** (e.g., ***Benedict's solution***), but reportedly not with ***glucose oxidase reagents*** (e.g., ***TesTape***,

Clinistix). Reduces ***serum cholesterol,*** and possibly ***serum potassium, serum PBI,*** and 24-h ***I-131 thyroidal uptake*** (effect may last almost 14 days).

INTERACTIONS **Drug:** Increases hypoprothrombinemic effects of ORAL ANTICOAGULANTS; decreased intestinal absorption of **cyanocobalamin, folic acid, digoxin;** may decrease concentration of **sulfinpyrazone**. Concurrent use increases risk of toxic effects of NSAIDS. Increased risk of Reye syndrome with **varicella** or **influenza** vaccinations.

PHARMACOKINETICS **Absorption:** Almost completely from GI tract; sodium form more rapidly absorbed than the acid. **Peak:** 1.5–2 h. **Duration:** 4 h. **Distribution:** Well distributed to tissue and body fluids except CSF unless meninges are inflamed. **Metabolism:** In liver. **Elimination:** Greater than 80% in urine in 7–10 h. **Half-Life:** 1 h.

NURSING IMPLICATIONS

Assessment & Drug Effects

- Monitor for abrupt onset of fever, particularly during the early weeks of therapy, and clinical picture resembling that of infectious mononucleosis (malaise, fatigue, generalized lymphadenopathy, splenomegaly, sore throat), as well as minor complaints of pruritus, joint pains, and headache, which strongly suggest hypersensitivity; report these symptoms promptly.
- Monitor I&O and encourage fluids. High concentrations of drug are excreted in urine, and this can cause crystalluria and hematuria.
- Monitor lab tests: Liver function, thyroid function.

Patient & Family Education

- Note: Hypersensitivity reactions may occur after a few days, but most commonly in the fourth or fifth week; report promptly.
- Notify prescriber if sore throat or mouth, malaise, unusual fatigue, bleeding or bruising occurs.
- Note: Therapy generally lasts about 2 yr. Adhere to the established drug regimen, and remain under close medical supervision to detect possible adverse drug effects during the treatment period. Resistant TB strains develop more rapidly when drug regimen is interrupted or is sporadic.
- Do not take aspirin or other OTC drugs without prescriber's approval.
- Discard drug if it discolors (brownish or purplish); this signifies decomposition.

AMIODARONE HYDROCHLORIDE (Pr)

(a-mee′oh-da-rone)

Cordarone, Nexterone, Pacerone

Classification: ANTIARRHYTHMIC, CLASS III

- **Therapeutic:** CLASS III ANTIARRHYTHMIC; ANTIANGINAL

AVAILABILITY Tablet; injection

ACTION & *THERAPEUTIC EFFECT* Acts directly on all cardiac tissues by prolonging duration of action potential and refractory period. Slows conduction time through the AV node and can interrupt the reentry pathways through the AV node. *Effective in prevention or suppression of cardiac arrhythmias.*

USES Prophylaxis and treatment of life-threatening ventricular arrhythmias and supraventricular arrhythmias, particularly with atrial fibrillation.

UNLABELED USES Treatment of nonexertional angina, conversion of atrial fibrillation to normal sinus rhythm, paroxysmal supraventricular tachycardia, ventricular rate control due to accessory pathway conduction in preexcited atrial arrhythmia, after defibrillation and epinephrine in cardiac arrest, AV nodal reentry tachycardia.

CONTRAINDICATIONS Hypersensitivity to amiodarone, iodine, or benzyl alcohol; cardiogenic shock, severe sinus bradycardia, second- or third-degree AV block unless a pacemaker is available, severe sinus-node dysfunction or sick sinus syndrome, bradycardia causing syncope (except in patients with functioning pacemaker); congenital or acquired QR prolongation syndromes, or history of torsades de pointes; pregnancy (category D); lactation.

CAUTIOUS USE Severe hepatic disease, cirrhosis; Hashimoto thyroiditis, goiter, thyrotoxicosis, or history of other thyroid dysfunction; severe hepatic impairment; CHF, older adults; Fabry disease especially with visual disturbances; electrolyte imbalance, hypokalemia, hypomagnesemia, hypovolemia; preexisting lung disease, COPD; open heart surgery.

ROUTE & DOSAGE

Arrhythmias

Adult: **PO Loading Dose** 800–1600 mg/day in 1–2 doses for 1–3 wk; **PO Maintenance Dose** 400–600 mg/day in 1–2 doses; **IV Loading Dose** 150 mg over 10 min followed by 360 mg over next 6 h; **IV Maintenance Dose** 540 mg over 18 h (0.5 mg/min), may continue at 0.5 mg/min; **Convert IV to PO** Duration of infusion less than 1 wk use 800–1600 mg; **PO;** 1–3 wk use 600–800 mg; **PO;** greater than 3 wk use 400 mg

Child: **IV** 5 mg/kg then repeat (max: 300 mg total)

Hepatic Impairment Dosage Adjustment

Adjustment only suggested in severe hepatic impairment

ADMINISTRATION

- Note: Correct hypokalemia and hypomagnesemia prior to initiation of therapy.

Oral

- Give consistently with respect to meals. Avoid grapefruit juice.
- Note: Only a prescriber experienced with the drug and treatment of life-threatening arrhythmias should give loading doses.
- Note: GI symptoms commonly occur during high-dose therapy, especially with loading doses. Symptoms usually respond to dose reduction or divided dose given with food, including milk.

Intravenous

PREPARE: **IV Infusion: First rapid loading dose infusion:** Add 150 mg (3 mL) amiodarone to 100 mL D5W to yield 1.5 mg/mL. **Second infusion during first 24 h (slow loading dose and maintenance infusion):** Add 900 mg (18 mL) amiodarone to 500 mL D5W to yield 1.8 mg/mL. **Maintenance infusions after the first 24 h:** Prepare concentrations of 1–6 mg/mL amiodarone. Note: Use central line to give concentrations greater than 2 mg/mL.

ADMINISTER: **IV Infusion:** Initial infusion rate should not exceed 30 mg/min. Loading dose is usually given over 10 min in adults and 20–60 min in children. Note: See manufacturer's guidelines for **Nexterone** administration.

INCOMPATIBILITIES: **Solution/additive:** **Aminophylline, amoxicillin/clavulanic acid, cefazolin, floxacillin, furosemide.** **Y-site:** **Acyclovir, allopurinol, amifostine, aminocaproic acid, aminophylline, amoxicillin, ampicillin, ampicillin/sulbactam, argatroban, atenolol, bivalirudin, cefamandole, cefazolin, cefotaxime, cefotetan, ceftazidime, ceftobiprole, chloramphenicol, cytarabine, dantrolene, dexamethasone, diazepam, digoxin, doxorubicin, ertapenem, fludarabine, fluorouracil, foscarnet, fosphenytoin, ganciclovir, gemtuzumab, heparin, hydrocortisone, imipenem/cilastatin, ketorolac, leucovorin, levofloxacin, magnesium sulfate, mechlorethamine, melphalan, meropenem, methotrexate, micafungin, mitomycin, paclitaxel, pentobarbital, phenytoin, piperacillin, piperacillin/tazobactam, potassium acetate, potassium phosphate, sodium bicarbonate, sodium phosphate, SMZ/TMP, thiopental, thiotepa, tigecycline, verapamil.**

- Store at 15°–30°C (59°–86°F) protected from light, unless otherwise directed.

ADVERSE EFFECTS

CV: Bradycardia, *hypotension* (IV), sinus arrest, cardiogenic shock, CHF, arrhythmias; AV block. **Respiratory:** (Pulmonary toxicity) Alveolitis, pneumonitis (fever, dry cough, dyspnea), interstitial pulmonary fibrosis, *fatal gasping syndrome* with IV in children. **CNS:** Peripheral neuropathy (*muscle weakness,* wasting numbness, tingling), *fatigue,* abnormal gait, dyskinesias, *dizziness,* paresthesia, headache. **HEENT:** *Corneal microdeposits,* blurred vision, optic neuritis, optic neuropathy, permanent blindness, corneal degeneration, macular degeneration, photosensitivity. **Endocrine:** Hyperthyroidism or hypothyroidism; may cause neonatal hypo- or hyperthyroidism if taken during pregnancy. **Skin:** Slate-blue pigmentation, *photosensitivity,* rash. **GI:** *Anorexia, nausea, vomiting, constipation,* hepatotoxicity. **Other:** With chronic use, angioedema.

DIAGNOSTIC TEST INTERFERENCE

Affects thyroid function tests, causing an increase in serum T_4 and serum reverse T_3 levels, and a decline in serum T_3 levels.

INTERACTIONS

Drug: Significantly increases **digoxin** levels; enhances pharmacologic effects and toxicities of **disopyramide, procainamide, quinidine, flecainide, lidocaine, lovastatin, simvastatin;** anticoagulant effects of ORAL ANTICOAGULANTS enhanced; **verapamil, diltiazem,** BETA-ADRENERGIC BLOCKING AGENTS may potentiate sinus bradycardia, sinus arrest, or AV block; may increase **phenytoin** levels 2- to 3-fold; **cholestyramine** may decrease amiodarone levels; **fentanyl** may cause bradycardia, hypotension, or decreased output; may increase **cyclosporine** levels and toxicity; **cimetidine** may increase amiodarone levels; **ritonavir** may increase risk of amiodarone toxicity, including cardiotoxicity; **simvastatin** doses over 20 mg increase risk of rhabdomyolysis; **loratadine** use may increase risk of QT prolongation. **Food: Grapefruit juice** may increase amiodarone concentrations. **Herbal: Echinacea** may increase hepatotoxicity, **St. John's wort** may decrease efficacy.

PHARMACOKINETICS **Absorption:** 22–86% absorbed. **Onset (PO):** 2–3 days to 1–3 wk. **Peak:** 3–7 h. **Distribution:** Concentrates in adipose tissue, lungs, kidneys, spleen; crosses placenta; 96% protein bound. **Metabolism:** Extensively in liver; undergoes some enterohepatic cycling; via CYP2C8 and 3A4. **Elimination:** Excreted chiefly in bile and feces; also in breast milk. **Half-Life:** Biphasic, initial 2.5–10 days, terminal 40–55 days.

NURSING IMPLICATIONS

Black Box Warning

Amiodarone has been associated with pulmonary toxicity (sometimes severe and potentially fatal), liver injury (ranging from mild to severe), and development of arrhythmias (heart block or sinus bradycardia).

Assessment & Drug Effects

- Monitor BP carefully during infusion and slow the infusion if significant hypotension occurs; bradycardia should be treated by slowing the infusion or discontinuing if necessary. Monitor heart rate and rhythm and BP until drug response has stabilized; report promptly symptomatic bradycardia. Sustained monitoring is essential because drug has an unusually long half-life.
- Monitor for S&S of: Adverse effects, particularly conduction disturbances and exacerbation of arrhythmias, in patients receiving other antiarrhythmic drugs; drug-induced hypothyroidism or hyperthyroidism (see Appendix F), especially during early treatment period; pulmonary toxicity (progressive dyspnea, fatigue, cough, pleuritic pain, fever) throughout therapy.
- Monitor for elevations of AST and ALT. If elevations persist or if they are 2–3 times above normal baseline readings, reduce dosage or withdraw drug promptly to prevent hepatotoxicity and liver damage.
- Auscultate chest periodically or when patient complains of respiratory symptoms. Check for diminished breath sounds, rales, pleuritic friction rub; observe breathing pattern. Drug-induced pulmonary function problems **must be** distinguished from CHF or pneumonia. Keep prescriber informed.
- Anticipate possible CNS symptoms within a week after amiodarone therapy begins. Proximal muscle weakness, a common side effect, intensified by tremors presents a great hazard to the ambulating patient. Assess severity of symptoms. Supervision of ambulation may be indicated.
- Monitor lab tests: Baseline and periodic serum electrolytes (i.e., potassium and magnesium); baseline and semiannual LFTs; baseline and periodic thyroid functions.

Patient & Family Education

- Check pulse daily once stabilized, or as prescribed. Report a pulse less than 60.
- Take oral drug consistently with respect to meals. Do not drink grapefruit juice while taking this drug.
- Become familiar with potential adverse reactions, and report those that are bothersome to the prescriber.
- Use dark glasses to ease photophobia; some patients may not be able to go outdoors in the daytime even with such protection.
- Follow recommendation for regular ophthalmic exams, including funduscopy and slit-lamp exam.
- Wear protective clothing and a barrier-type sunscreen that physically blocks penetration of skin by ultraviolet light to prevent a photosensitivity reaction (erythema, pruritus); avoid exposure to sun and sunlamps.

AMISULPRIDE

(am-ee-sul-pride)

Barhemsys

Classifications: DOPAMINE AGONIST

Therapeutic: ANTIEMETIC

AVAILABILITY Solution for injection

ACTION & *THERAPEUTIC EFFECT* Selective dopamine-2 (D_2) and dopamine-3 (D_3) receptor antagonist. Interferes with subsequent activations of CTZ and the relay of stimuli to the vomiting center. Helpful to prevent or decrease postoperative nausea and vomiting.

USES To prevent or treat nausea/vomiting association with surgery/diagnostic procedures.

CONTRAINDICATIONS Known hypersensitivity to amisulpride, patients with congenital long QT syndrome.

CAUTIOUS USE Patients with preexisting arrhythmias/cardiac conduction disorders, hypokalemia, hypomagnesemia, congestive heart failure, and patients taking medications or who have other medical conditions known to prolong the QT interval.

ROUTE & DOSAGE

Prevention of Postoperative Nausea and Vomiting

Adult: **IV** 5 mg

Treatment of Postoperative Nausea and Vomiting

Adult: **IV** 10 mg

ADMINISTRATION

Intravenous

PREPARE: **Direct:** Dilution is not required prior to administration Visually inspect and discard if any particulate matter or discoloration is noted

ADMINISTER: **Direct:** Administer within 12 hours of vial removal from protective carton. Infuse over 1–2 minutes as a single dose. May flush line with D5W or NS

INCOMPATIBILITIES: None reported

- Store vial in protective carton at a controlled room temperature between 20° and 25°C (68° and 77°F). Protect from light.

ADVERSE EFFECTS (> 5%) **CV:** Dose and concentration dependent prolongation of the QT interval **CNS:** Light-headedness, dizziness, fainting, and new onset of seizures may indicate prolonged QT interval **Endocrine:** Increased prolactic levels **Skin:** Injection site pain

INTERACTIONS **Drugs:** may decrease effect of anti parkinson agents (**levodopa**); closely monitor other drugs affecting QT interval

PHARMACOKINETICS **Onset:** **Peak:** End of infusion **Distribution:** 127–144L; 25–30% protein bound **Elimination:** 74% excreted unchanged in urine; 23% in feces **Half-Life:** 4–5 h

NURSING IMPLICATIONS

Assessment & Drug Effects

- Absence or decreased nausea and vomiting
- Monitor ECG in patients with preexisting cardiac conduction disorders, electrolyte disorders, congestive heart failure or patients taking medication that causes a prolonged QT interval
- Monitor lab tests: electrolytes

Patient & Family Education

- Notify prescriber for lightheadedness, dizziness, fainting, or seizures

AMITRIPTYLINE HYDROCHLORIDE

(a-mee-trip'ti-leen)

Apo-Amitriptyline ♣, Levate ♣

Classification: TRICYCLIC ANTIDEPRESSANT

Therapeutic: ANTIDEPRESSANT

Prototype: Imipramine

AVAILABILITY Tablet

ACTION & *THERAPEUTIC EFFECT* Inhibits the reuptake of serotonin (5-HT) and norepinephrine from the synaptic gap; also inhibits norepinephrine reuptake to a moderate degree. Restoration of the levels of these neurotransmitters is a proposed mechanism of its antidepressant action. *Interference with the reuptake of serotonin and norepinephrine results in the antidepressant activity of amitriptyline.*

USES Major depressive disorder.

UNLABELED USES Chronic fatigue syndrome, fibromyalgia, functional dyspepsia, prophylaxis of chronic tension headache, insterstitial cystitis, irritable bowel syndrome, migraine prophylaxis, neuropathic pain, postherpetic neuralgia, sialorrhea.

CONTRAINDICATIONS TCA hypersensitivity; acute recovery period after MI, cardiac arrhythmias, AV block, long-QT prolongation; suicidal ideation; history of seizure disorders; lactation, children younger than 12 yr.

CAUTIOUS USE Prostatic hypertrophy, history of urinary retention or obstruction; angle-closure glaucoma; diabetes mellitus; history of hematologic disorders; history of alcoholism; GERD, BPH; hyperthyroidism; patient with cardiovascular, hepatic, or renal dysfunction; patient with suicidal tendency, bipolar disorder; paranoid patients: ultrarapid, intermediate, and poor CPY2D6 metabolizers; electroshock therapy; elective surgery; schizophrenia; respiratory disorders; Parkinson disease; seizure disorders; older adults, adolescents. Fetal and infant risk cannot be ruled out.

ROUTE & DOSAGE

Depression

Adult: **PO** 75 mg/day in divided doses, may gradually increase to 150–300 mg/day
Geriatric: **PO** 10–25 mg daily at bedtime
Child 9–12 years: **PO** 1 mg/kg/day in 3 divided doses

Pharmacogenetic Dosage Adjustment

CYP2D6 poor metabolizers: Dose at 60–75% of normal dose

ADMINISTRATION

Oral

- Give with or immediately after food to reduce possibility of GI irritation. Tablet may be crushed if patient is unable to take it whole; administer with food or fluid.
- Give increased doses preferably in late afternoon or at bedtime due to sedative action that precedes antidepressant effect.
- Note that dose is usually tapered over 2 wk at discontinuation to prevent withdrawal symptoms (headache, nausea, malaise, musculoskeletal pain, panic attack, weakness).
- Store at controlled room temperature 20–25°C (68–77°F), in a well-closed container, protected from light.

ADVERSE EFFECTS **CV:** *Orthostatic hypotension*, sudden cardiac death, myocardial infarction, tachycardia, palpitation, ECG changes. **CNS:** *Drowsiness, sedation, dizziness*, nervousness, restlessness, fatigue, *headache*, insomnia, abnormal movements (extrapyramidal symptoms), seizures. **HEENT:** *Blurred vision*, mydriasis. **Skin:** Alopecia, urticaria. **GI:** *Dry mouth*, increased appetite especially for sweets, *constipation*, weight gain, sour or metallic taste, nausea, vomiting. **GU:** *Urinary retention*. **Other:** Worsening depression.

INTERACTIONS **Drug:** Avoid drugs affecting QT interval. CNS DEPRESSANTS, **alcohol,** HYPNOTICS, barbiturates, SEDATIVES potentiate CNS depression; ANTICOAGULANTS, ORAL, may increase hypoprothrombinemic effect; **levodopa,** SYMPATHOMIMETICS (e.g., **epinephrine, norepinephrine**), possibility of sympathetic hyperactivity with hypertension and hyperpyrexia; MAO INHIBITORS, possibility of severe reactions, toxic psychosis, cardiovascular instability; **methylphenidate** increases plasma TCA levels; THYROID DRUGS may increase possibility of arrhythmias; **cimetidine** may increase plasma TCA levels. **Herbal: St. John's wort** may cause serotonin syndrome.

PHARMACOKINETICS **Absorption:** Rapidly from GI tract. **Peak:** 2–12 h. **Distribution:** Crosses placenta. **Metabolism:** In liver (CYP2D6). **Elimination:** Primarily in urine; enters breast milk. **Half-Life:** 10–50 h.

NURSING IMPLICATIONS

Black Box Warning

Amitriptyline has been associated with increased risk of suicidal thinking and behavior in children and adolescents, especially during the first few months of treatment.

Assessment & Drug Effects

- Monitor for S&S of drowsiness and dizziness (initial stages of therapy); institute measures to prevent falling. Monitor for overdose or suicide ideation especially in children and adolescents and in patients who use excessive amounts of alcohol.

- Eye examinations (including glaucoma testing) are recommended particularly for older adults, adolescents, and patients receiving high doses/prolonged therapy.
- Monitor BP and pulse rate in patients with preexisting cardiovascular disease. Assess for orthostatic hypotension especially in older adults. Withhold drug if there is a rise or fall in systolic BP (by 10–20 mmHg), or a sudden increase or a significant change in pulse rate or rhythm. Notify prescriber.
- Monitor I&O, including bowel elimination pattern.
- Monitor lab tests: Baseline and periodic amitriptyline level (level greater than 300 mg/mL associated with increased adverse effects); periodic blood glucose.

Patient & Family Education

- Monitor weight; drug may increase appetite or a craving for sweets.
- Understand that tolerance/adaptation to anticholinergic actions (see Appendix F) usually develops with maintenance regimen. Keep prescriber informed.
- Symptom improvement may not be noted for a few weeks.
- Do not suddenly discontinue the drug without consulting a health-care provider.
- Avoid alcohol.
- Relieve dry mouth by taking frequent sips of water and increasing total fluid intake.
- Make position change slowly and in stages to prevent dizziness.
- Do not drive or engage in potentially hazardous activities until response to drug is known.
- Do not use OTC drugs without consulting prescriber while on TCA therapy; many preparations contain sympathomimetic amines.
- Note: Amitriptyline may turn urine blue-green.

AMLODIPINE

(am-lo′di-peen)

Norvasc

Classification: CALCIUM CHANNEL BLOCKER; ANTIHYPERTENSIVE

Therapeutic: ANTIHYPERTENSIVE; ANTIANGINAL

Prototype: Nifedipine

AVAILABILITY Tablet

ACTION & *THERAPEUTIC EFFECT*

A calcium channel blocking agent that selectively blocks calcium influx across cell membranes of cardiac and vascular smooth muscle without changing serum calcium concentrations. It reduces coronary vascular resistance, increases coronary blood flow, decreases peripheral vascular resistance, increases oxygen delivery to myocardial tissue, and increases cardiac output. *Amlodipine reduces systolic, diastolic, and mean arterial blood pressure. It also decreases pain due to angina.*

USES Treatment of mild to moderate hypertension and stable/variant angina.

CONTRAINDICATIONS Hypersensitivity to amlodipine; hypotension; severe obstructive coronary artery disease; severe aortic stenosis; lactation.

CAUTIOUS USE Hepatic impairment; concomitant use with

hypotension; CHF, severe obstructive CAD, ventricular dysfunction; older adults; GERD; hepatic disease; pregnancy (category C); children younger than 6 yr.

ROUTE & DOSAGE

Hypertension

Adult: **PO** 5–10 mg once daily
Geriatric: Start with 2.5 mg, adjust dose at intervals of not less than 2 wk
Adolescent/Child (6 yr or older): **PO** 2.5–5 mg daily (max: 10 mg)

Stable/Vasospastic Angina

Adult: **PO** 5–10 mg daily (usually 10 mg)

Hepatic Impairment Dosage Adjustment

Start with 2.5 mg, adjust dose at intervals of not less than 2 wk

ADMINISTRATION

Oral

- Give drug without regard to meals.
- Note: Doses are usually titrated upward over a period of 14 days or more rapidly if warranted.
- Store at 15°–30°C (59°–86°F).

ADVERSE EFFECTS **CV:** Palpitations, flushing tachycardia, *peripheral or facial edema*, bradycardia, chest pain, syncope, postural hypotension. **Respiratory:** Dyspnea. **CNS:** Light-headedness, fatigue, *headache*. **Skin:** Flushing, rash. **GI:** Abdominal pain, nausea, anorexia, constipation, dyspepsia, dysphagia, diarrhea, flatulence, vomiting. **GU:** Sexual dysfunction, frequency, nocturia. **Other:** Arthralgia, cramps, myalgia.

INTERACTIONS **Drug: Adenosine** may increase the risk of bradycardia; **bosentan** may decrease efficacy of amlodipine; additive hypotensive effects with other ANTIHYPERTENSIVE AGENTS; AZOLE ANTIFUNGALS (e.g., **fluconazole, itraconazole**) may inhibit metabolism of amlodipine; **itraconazole** may increase edema. Use caution with **ezetimibe** or **simvastatin** due to increased risk of myopathy. CYP3A4 inducers (**rifampin, rifabutin, carbamazepine, phenytoin**) may increase needed amlodipine dose. **Food: Grapefruit juice** may increase amlodipine levels. **Herbal: Ephedra, ma huang, melatonin** may antagonize antihypertensive effects. **St. John's wort** may reduce clinical efficacy.

PHARMACOKINETICS **Absorption:** Greater than 90% absorbed from GI tract. **Peak:** 6–9 h. **Duration:** 24 h. **Distribution:** Greater than 95% protein bound. **Metabolism:** In liver (CYP3A4) to inactive metabolites. **Elimination:** In urine (less than 5–10% excreted unchanged), 20–25% in feces. **Half-Life:** Less than 45 yr: 28–69 h; greater than 60 yr: 40–120 h.

NURSING IMPLICATIONS

Black Box Warning

Amlodipine has been associated with fetal injury and death.

Assessment & Drug Effects

- Monitor BP for therapeutic effectiveness. BP reduction is greatest after peak levels of amlodipine are achieved 6–9 h following oral doses.
- Monitor for S&S of dose-related peripheral or facial edema that may not be accompanied by weight gain; rarely, severe edema

may cause discontinuation of drug.

- Monitor BP with postural changes. Report postural hypotension. Monitor more frequently when additional antihypertensives or diuretics are added.
- Monitor heart rate; dose-related palpitations (more common in women) may occur.

Patient & Family Education

- Discontinue drug immediately and report to prescriber if pregnancy is suspected.
- Do not breastfeed while taking this drug.
- Report significant swelling of face or extremities.
- Exercise caution when standing and walking due to possible dose-related light-headedness/dizziness.
- Report shortness of breath, palpitations, irregular heartbeat, nausea, or constipation to prescriber.

AMOXICILLIN

(a-mox-i-sill'in)

Amoxil, Apo-Amoxi ♣

Classification: ANTIBIOTIC; AMINOPENICILLIN

Therapeutic: ANTIBIOTIC

Prototype: Ampicillin

AVAILABILITY Tablet; capsule; powder for suspension; extended release tablet; chewable tablet

ACTION & *THERAPEUTIC EFFECT* Broad-spectrum semisynthetic aminopenicillin and analog of ampicillin. Like other penicillins, amoxicillin inhibits the final stage of bacterial cell wall synthesis. It results in bacterial cell lysis and death. *Active against both aerobic gram-positive and aerobic gram-negative bacteria.*

USES Infections of ear, nose, throat, lower respiratory tract, GU tract, skin, and soft tissue caused by susceptible bacteria.

UNLABELED USES Treatment of anthrax, prophylaxis against infective endocarditis, treatment of Lyme disease, prosthetic joint infection.

CONTRAINDICATIONS Hypersensitivity to penicillins and cephalosporins; infectious mononucleosis.

CAUTIOUS USE History of or suspected atopy or allergy (hives, eczema, hay fever, asthma); history of cephalosporin or carbapenem hypersensitivity; colitis, dialysis, diarrhea, GI disease; viral infection, syphilis, severe hepatic impairment; renal impairment or failure, diabetes mellitus, leukemia, pregnancy (category B); lactation—infant risk cannot be ruled out.

ROUTE & DOSAGE

Mild to Moderate Infections

Adult: **PO Immediate release** 500 mg –1 g q8–12 h
Child/Infant (3 mo or older): **PO** 25–50 mg/kg/day (max: 60–80 mg/kg/day) divided q8h
Neonate/Infant (younger than 3 mo): **PO** 20–30 mg/kg/day divided q12h (max dose 500 mg)

Severe Infections

Adult: **PO** 875mg q12h or 500 mg q8h
Child/Infant: **PO** 80–100 mg/kg/day divided q8h (max dose 500 mg)

Pharyngitis

Adult/Adolescent: **PO Extended release** 775 mg daily × 10d;

Immediate release 500 mg bid or 1 g daily x 10 days

Lower Respiratory Tract Infection

Adult: **PO** 1 g 3 times daily
Adolescent/Child/Infant (over 3 months): **PO** 90 mg/kg/day divided q12h (max dose 4000 mg/day)

Rhinosinusitis

Adult: **PO** 500 mg q8h **or** 875 mg q12h x 5–7 days
Adolescent/Child (over 2 yr): **PO** 45 mg/kg/day divided q12 h

Skin/Soft Tissue Infection

Adult: **PO** 500 mg TID x 5 days

Otitis Media

Child/Infant (over 2 mo): **PO** 80–90 mg/kg/day divided q12h

ADMINISTRATION

Oral

- Ensure that chewable tablets are chewed or crushed before being swallowed with a liquid.
- Do not crush or chew extended release tablets.
- May be taken with or without food.
- Shake suspension or pediatric drops.
- Place reconstituted pediatric drops directly on child's tongue or add to formula, milk, fruit juice, water, ginger ale, or other soft drink. Have child drink all the prepared dose promptly.
- Refrigeration is preferred but not required. Store capsules 125-mg and 250-mg unconstituted powder in tightly covered containers at 20°C (68°F) unless otherwise directed. Store 200-mg, 400-mg chewable tablets, 500-mg and 750-mg tablets, 200-mg and 400-mg unreconstituted powder at 25°C (77°F). Reconstituted oral suspensions are stable for 14 days at room temperature.

ADVERSE EFFECTS (<u>> 5%</u>) **CNS:** Headache. **GI:** Diarrhea.

DIAGNOSTIC TEST INTERFERENCE False-positive reactions may occur with **Clinitest, Benedict's solution,** or **Fehling's solution.**

INTERACTIONS **Probenecid** prolongs the activity of amoxicillin. ORAL CONTRACEPTIVE efficacy may be reduced. Levels of **methotrexate** may be increased. Increase monitoring in patients taking ANTICOAGULANTS. Avoid LIVE VACCINES.

PHARMACOKINETICS **Absorption:** Nearly complete absorption. **Peak:** 1–2 h (immediate release); 3 h (extended release). **Distribution:** Diffuses into most tissues and body fluids, except synovial fluid and CSF (unless meninges are inflamed); crosses placenta; distributed into breast milk in small amounts. **Metabolism:** In liver. **Elimination:** 60% in urine. **Half-Life:** 1–1.3 h.

NURSING IMPLICATIONS

Assessment & Drug Effects

- Determine previous hypersensitivity reactions to penicillins, cephalosporins, and other allergens prior to therapy.
- Monitor for S&S of an urticarial rash (usually occurring within a few days after start of drug) suggestive of a hypersensitivity reaction. If it occurs, look for other signs of hypersensitivity (fever, wheezing, generalized itching, dyspnea), and report to prescriber immediately.

- Report onset of generalized, erythematous, maculopapular rash (ampicillin rash) to prescriber. Ampicillin rash is not due to hypersensitivity; however, hypersensitivity should be ruled out.
- Monitor for and report diarrhea, which may indicate pseudomembranous colitis.
- Monitor lab tests: Baseline C&S prior to initiation of therapy, CBC, periodic renal, hepatic, and hematologic functions with prolonged therapy.

Patient & Family Education

- Take drug around the clock, do not miss a dose, and continue therapy until all medication is taken, unless otherwise directed by prescriber.
- Drug may decrease the effectiveness of oral contraceptives with concurrent use. Use alternative methods of birth control.
- Report to prescriber onset of diarrhea, vomiting, rash, and other possible symptoms of superinfection (see Appendix F).

AMOXICILLIN AND CLAVULANATE POTASSIUM

(a-mox-i-sill'in)

Augmentin, Augmentin-ES600, Clavulin ♣

Classification: BETA-LACTAM ANTIBIOTIC; AMINOPENICILLIN

Therapeutic: ANTIBIOTIC

Prototype: Ampicillin

AVAILABILITY Chewable tablet; tablet; oral suspension; sustained release tablet

ACTION & *THERAPEUTIC EFFECT* As a beta-lactam antibiotic, amoxicillin is bactericidal. It inhibits the final stage of bacterial cell wall synthesis. *Effectiveness of ampicillin is synergistic in combination with clavulanic acid. Clavulanic acid in combination with ampicillin inhibits enzyme (beta-lactamase) degradation of amoxicillin and by synergism extends both spectrum of activity and bactericidal effect of amoxicillin against many gram-positive and gram-negative strains of beta-lactamase-producing bacteria resistant to amoxicillin alone.*

USES Lower respiratory tract infections, acute bacterial rhinosinusitis, community-acquired pneumonia, otitis media, skin and skin structure infections, and UTI.

UNLABELED USES Diabetic foot infection, COPD exacerbation, intra-abdominal infection

CONTRAINDICATIONS Hypersensitivity to penicillins; infectious mononucleosis; patient with previous history of drug-induced cholestasis, jaundice, or other hepatic dysfunction; severe renal impairment.

CAUTIOUS USE Allergic disorders; cephalosporin hypersensitivity; GI disorders; colitis; hepatic or renal impairment; older adults; pregnancy (category B); lactation—infant risk is minimal.

ROUTE & DOSAGE

Mild to Moderate Infections

Adult: **PO Immediate release** 500 mg q8–12h **or** 875 mg q12h; **Extended release** 2 g q 12h

Otitis Media

Adult: **PO Immediate release** 875 mg BID or 500 mg q8h × 5–7 days

Child/Infant (over 3 months): **PO** 90 mg amoxicillin/kg/day divided q12h × 10 days

Rhinosinusitis

Adult: **PO Immediate Release** 500 mg q8h or 875 mg q12h × 5–7days

Pneumonia, community-acquired

Adolescent/Child/Infant (over 3 mo): **PO** 90 mg amoxicillin/kg/day divided q12h (max dose 4000 mg/day)

ADMINISTRATION

Oral

- Give at the start of a meal to minimize GI upset and enhance absorption.
- Reconstitute oral suspension by adding amount of water specified on container to provide a 5-mL suspension. Tap bottle before adding water to loosen powder, then add water in 2 portions, shaking suspension well before each addition.
- Shake suspension well just before administration of each dose.
- Give dialysis patient an additional 2 doses on the day of dialysis; one dose during and another dose after dialysis.
- Store dry powder and tablets in tight containers at or below 25° C (77°F). Reconstituted oral suspension should be refrigerated at 2°–8°C (36°–46°F), then discarded after 10 days.

ADVERSE EFFECTS (≥ 5%) Skin: Diaper rash, rash. **GI:** Diarrhea, loose stool.

DIAGNOSTIC TEST INTERFERENCE May interfere with ***urinary glucose*** determinations using ***cupric sulfate, Benedict's solution, Clinitest.***

INTERACTIONS Drug: Probenecid prolongs the activity of amoxicillin. ORAL CONTRACEPTIVE efficacy may be reduced. Levels of **methotrexate** may be increased. Increase monitoring in patients taking anticoagulants. Do not administer LIVE VACCINES.

PHARMACOKINETICS Absorption: Nearly complete absorption. **Peak:** 1–2 h. **Distribution:** Diffuses into most tissues and body fluids, except synovial fluid and CSF (unless meninges are inflamed); crosses placenta; distributed into breast milk in very small amounts. **Metabolism:** In liver. **Elimination:** 50–73% of the amoxicillin and 25–45% of the clavulanate dose excreted in urine in 2 h. **Half-Life:** Amoxicillin 1–1.3 h, clavulanate 0.78–1.2 h.

NURSING IMPLICATIONS

Assessment & Drug Effects

- Determine previous hypersensitivity reactions to penicillins, cephalosporins, and other allergens prior to therapy.
- Monitor for S&S of an urticarial rash (usually occurring within a few days after start of drug) suggestive of a hypersensitivity reaction. If it occurs, look for other signs of hypersensitivity (fever, wheezing, generalized itching, dyspnea), and report to prescriber immediately.
- Monitor for and report diarrhea, which may indicate pseudomembranous colitis.
- Monitor for improvement of bacterial infection.
- Monitor lab tests: Baseline C&S prior to initiation of therapy and as needed during treatment, CBC. In prolonged therapy, monitor LFTs and renal function tests.

Patient & Family Education

- Female patients should report onset of symptoms of *Candidal vaginitis* (e.g., moderate amount of white, cheesy, nonodorous vaginal discharge; vaginal inflammation and itching; vulvar excoriation, inflammation, burning, itching). Therapy may have to be discontinued.
- Drug may decrease effectiveness of oral contraceptives. Other forms of birth control should be used.
- Report onset of diarrhea and other possible symptoms of superinfection to prescriber (see Appendix F).

AMPHETAMINE SULFATE

(am-fet'a-meen)

Adderall, Adderall XR

Classification: CEREBRAL STIMULANT; ANOREXIANT

Therapeutic: CEREBRAL STIMULANT

Controlled Substance: Schedule II

AVAILABILITY Tablet; sustained release capsules

ACTION & THERAPEUTIC EFFECT Marked stimulant effect on CNS thought to be due to action on cerebral cortex and possibly the reticular activating system. Acts indirectly on adrenergic receptors by increasing synaptic release of norepinephrine in the brain and by blocking reuptake of norepinephrine at presynaptic membranes. *CNS stimulation results in increased motor activity, diminished sense of fatigue, alertness, wakefulness, and mood elevation. Anorexigenic effect thought to result from direct inhibition of hypothalamic appetite center as well as mood elevation.*

USES Narcolepsy, attention-deficit/hyperactivity disorder in children and adults (hyperkinetic behavioral syndrome, minimal brain dysfunction). Use as short-term adjunct to control exogenous obesity not generally recommended because of its potential for abuse.

CONTRAINDICATIONS Hypersensitivity to sympathomimetic amines; history of drug abuse; severe agitation; hyperthyroidism; diabetes mellitus; moderate to severe hypertension, advanced arteriosclerosis, angina pectoris or other cardiovascular disorders; Gilles de la Tourette disorder; glaucoma; during or within 14 days after treatment with MAOIs; lactation.

CAUTIOUS USE Mild hypertension; pregnancy (category C); children younger than 3 yr.

ROUTE & DOSAGE

Narcolepsy

Adult: **PO** 5–60 mg/day divided q4–6h in 2–3 doses
Child (12 yr or older): **PO** 10 mg/day, may increase by 10 mg at weekly intervals; *6–12 yr:* 5 mg/day, may increase by 5 mg at weekly intervals

Attention-Deficit/Hyperactivity Disorder

Adult/Adolescent: **PO Extended release** 10 mg once daily in a.m.; may increase by 5–10 mg at weekly intervals if needed (max: 30 mg/day)
Child (6 yr): **PO** 5 mg 1–2 × day, may increase by 5 mg at weekly intervals (max: 40 mg/day); *3–5 yr:* 2.5 mg 1–2 × day, may increase by 2.5 mg at weekly intervals; **Extended release** 10 mg once daily in a.m.; may increase by 5–10 mg at weekly intervals if needed (max: 30 mg/day)

Obesity Dosage Adjustment

Adult: **PO** 5–10 mg 1 h before meals

ADMINISTRATION

Oral

- Give first dose on awakening or early in a.m. when prescribed for narcolepsy.
- Give last dose no later than 6 h before patient retires to avoid insomnia.
- Ensure that sustained release capsules are not crushed or chewed.
- Store at 15°–30°C (59°–86°F) unless otherwise directed.

ADVERSE EFFECTS **CV:** *Palpitation,* elevated BP; tachycardia, vasculitis. **CNS:** *Irritability,* psychosis, *restlessness,* nervousness, headache, *insomnia,* weakness, *euphoria,* dysphoria, drowsiness, trembling, hyperactive reflexes. **GI:** Dry mouth, anorexia, unusual weight loss, nausea, vomiting, diarrhea, or constipation. **GU:** Impotence and change in libido with high doses. **Other:** Allergy, urticaria, sudden death (reported in children with structural cardiac abnormalities).

DIAGNOSTIC TEST INTERFERENCE Elevations in ***serum thyroxine (T_4)*** levels with high amphetamine doses.

INTERACTIONS **Drug: Acetazolamide, sodium bicarbonate** decrease amphetamine elimination; **ascorbic acid** increases amphetamine elimination; effects of both amphetamine and BARBITURATES may be antagonized if given together; **furazolidone** may increase BP effects of amphetamines, and interaction may persist for several weeks after **furazolidone** is discontinued; **guanethidine** antagonizes antihypertensive effects; because MAO INHIBITORS, **selegiline** can precipitate hypertensive crisis (fatalities reported), do not administer amphetamines during or within 14 days of these drugs; PHENOTHIAZINES may inhibit mood elevating effects of amphetamines; TRICYCLIC ANTIDEPRESSANTS enhance amphetamine effects through increased **norepinephrine** release; BETA AGONISTS increase cardiovascular adverse effects.

PHARMACOKINETICS **Absorption:** Rapid. **Peak effect:** 1–5 h. **Duration:** Up to 10 h. **Distribution:** All tissues, especially CNS. **Metabolism:** In liver. **Elimination:** Renal; excreted into breast milk. **Half-Life:** 10–30 h.

NURSING IMPLICATIONS

Black Box Warning

Amphetamine has high abuse potential, and misuse can cause severe cardiovascular adverse effects as well as sudden death.

Assessment & Drug Effects

- Monitor drug use and be alert for signs of misuse.
- Monitor for S&S of toxicity in children. Response to this drug is more variable in children than adults; acute toxicity has occurred over a wide dosage range.
- Monitor for S&S of insomnia or anorexia. Report complaints to prescriber. Dosage reduction may be required.
- Monitor BP and HR, especially in those with hypertension.
- Monitor diabetics closely for loss of glycemic control.

- Monitor growth in children; drug may be discontinued periodically to allow for normal growth.
- Note: Drug's excitatory and euphoric effects are associated with a high abuse potential.

Patient & Family Education

- Keep prescriber informed of clinical response and persistent or bothersome adverse effects. This drug exerts a stimulating effect that masks fatigue; after exhilaration disappears, fatigue and depression are usually greater than before, and a longer period of rest is needed.
- Report insomnia or undesired weight loss.
- Do not drive or engage in potentially hazardous tasks until response to drug is known.
- Rinse mouth frequently with clear water, especially after eating, to relieve mouth dryness; increase fluid intake, if allowed; chew sugarless gum or sourballs.
- Note: Meticulous oral hygiene is required because decreased saliva encourages demineralization of tooth surfaces and mucosal erosion.
- Avoid caffeine-containing beverages because caffeine increases amphetamine effects.
- Note that drug is usually tapered gradually following prolonged administration of high doses. Abrupt withdrawal may result in lethargy, profound depression, or other psychotic manifestations that may persist for several weeks.

AMPHOTERICIN B (Pr)

(am-foe-ter'i-sin)

Fungizone

Classification: ANTIFUNGAL

Therapeutic: ANTIFUNGAL

AVAILABILITY Powder for injection

ACTION & THERAPEUTIC EFFECT Antifungal agent that binds to the cell membrane and causes a leakage of intracellular components. *It can be fungistatic or fungicidal at higher concentrations, depending on sensitivity of fungus.*

USES Used intravenously for a wide spectrum of potentially fatal systemic fungal (mycotic) infections. Alternative treatment for patients with New World mucocutaneous leishmaniasis.

UNLABELED USES Treatment of candidiasis, talaromycosis.

CONTRAINDICATIONS Hypersensitivity to amphotericin; lactation—infant risk cannot be ruled out.

CAUTIOUS USE Severe bone marrow depression; renal function impairment; anemia; pregnancy (category B).

ROUTE & DOSAGE

Systemic Infections

Adult: **IV Test Dose** 1 mg dissolved in 20 mL of D5W by slow infusion (over 20–30 min); **IV Maintenance Dose** 0.3 to 1.5 mg/kg/day infused over 4–6 h
Child: **IV Test Dose** 0.1 mg/kg up to 1 mg dissolved in 20 mL of D5W by slow infusion (over 20–60 min); **IV Maintenance Dose** 0.25 to 0.5 mg/kg/dose once daily infused over 4–6 h, may increase by 0.25 mg/kg/day as needed (max: 1.5 mg/kg)

Renal Impairment Dosage Adjustment

The dose can be reduced or interval extended

ADMINISTRATION

Intravenous

PREPARE: Typically prepared by pharmacy service due to complex technique required for IV solution preparation. Reconstitute 50-mg vial with 10 mL sterile water only for an injection concentration of 5 mg/mL. Further dilute in D5W only. Max concentration for peripheral infusion, 0.1 mg/mL.

ADMINISTER: **Intermittent:** May use a 1-micron filter. ▪ Infuse total daily dose over 2–6 h. Use longer infusion time for better tolerance. ▪ **Alert:** Rapid infusion of any amphotericin can cause cardiovascular collapse. If hypotension or arrhythmias develop stop infusion and notify prescriber. ▪ Protect IV solution from light during administration. ▪ Note incompatibilities. When given through an existing IV line, flush before and after with D5W. ▪ Initiate therapy using the most distal vein possible and alternate sites with each dose if possible to reduce the risk of thrombophlebitis. ▪ Check IV site frequently for patency.

INCOMPATIBILITIES: **Solution/additive:** Any **saline**-containing solution (precipitate will form), PARENTERAL NUTRITION SOLUTIONS, **amikacin, calcium chloride, calcium gluconate, chlorpromazine, cimetidine, ciprofloxacin, diphenhydramine, dopamine, edetate calcium disodium, gentamicin, kanamycin, magnesium sulfate, meropenem, metaraminol, penicillin G, polymyxin, potassium chloride, prochlorperazine, streptomycin, verapamil.** **Y-site:** **Acyclovir, alemtuzumab, alfentanil, allopurinol, amifostine, amikacin, ampicillin, amsacrine, anidulafungin, atenolol, atracurium, atropine, azithromycin, aztreonam, benztropine, bivalirudin, bleomycin, bretylium, bumetanide, butorphanol, calcium chloride, cangrelor, capreomycin, carboplatin, caspofungin, cefamandole, cefepime, cefotetan, cefpirome, ceftaroline, ceftizoxime, ceftobiprole, Ceftolozane/tazobactam, chloramphenicol. Chlorpromazine, cimetidine, cisplatin, clindamycin, codeine, cyanocobalamin, cyclophosphamide, cytarabine, dacarbazine, dantrolene, daptomycin, daunorubicin, dexamethasone, dexmedetomidine, dexrazoxane, diazepam, digoxin, diphenhydramine, dobutamine, docetaxel, dolasetron, dopamine, doxorubicin, doxorubicin liposome, edetate, enalaprilat, ephedrine, epinephrine, epirubicin, epoetin alfa, eptifibatide, ertapenem, esmolol, etoposide, famotidine, fenoldopam, filgrastim, fluconazole, fludarabine, foscarnet, fosfomycin, ganciclovir, garenoxacin, gemcitabine, gemtuzumab, glycopyrrolate, granisetron, haloperidol, hydralazine, hydrocortisone, hydroxyzine, idarubicin, irinotecan, isoproterenol, ketorolac, labetalol, lansoprazole, leucovorin, levofloxacin, lidocaine, linezolid, mechlorethamine, melphalan, meperidine, meropenem, mesna, methadone, methotrexate, methylprednisolone, metoclopramide, metoprolol, metronidazole, midazolam, minocycline, mitomycin, mitoxantrone, mivacurium, morphine, mycophenolate, nafcillin, nalbuphine, netilmicin, nicardipine, nitroprusside, norepinephrine, ondansetron, oritavancin,**

oxacillin, paclitaxel, palonosetron, pamidronate, pancuronium, pantoprazole, papaverine, pemetrexed, penicillin, pentamidine pentazocine, phentolamine, phenylephrine, phenytoin, piperacillin, piperacillin/tazobactam, plazomicin, polymyxin B, potassium chloride, prochlorperazine, promethazine, propofol, propranolol, protamine, pyridoxine, quinupristin/dalfopristin, rituximab, rocuronium, sodium bicarbonate, streptomycin, succinylcholine, sulfamethoxazole/trimethoprim, telavancin, thiamine, tigecycline, tirofiban, tobramycin, tolazoline, topotecan, trastuzumab, vancomycin, vasopressin, vecuronium, verapamil, vinblastine, vincristine, vinorelbine, voriconazole.

- Store according to manufacturer's recommendations for reconstituted and unopened vials.

ADVERSE EFFECTS (No percentages of occurrence reported) **CV:** Hypotension, cardiac arrest. **CNS:** Headache, sedation, muscle pain, arthralgia, weakness. **HEENT:** Ototoxicity with tinnitus, vertigo, loss of hearing. **Endocrine:** *Hypokalemia, hypomagnesemia*. **Skin:** Dry, erythema, pruritus, burning sensation; allergic contact dermatitis, exacerbation of lesions. **GI:** Nausea, vomiting, diarrhea, epigastric cramps, anorexia, weight loss. **GU:** Nephrotoxicity, urine with low specific gravity. **Hematologic:** Anemia, thrombocytopenia. **Other:** Hypersensitivity (pruritus, urticaria, skin rashes, fever, dyspnea, anaphylaxis); *fever, chills*. Pain; arthralgias, thrombophlebitis (IV site), superinfections.

INTERACTIONS **Drug:** AMINOGLYCOSIDES, **capreomycin, cisplatin, carboplatin, colistin, cyclosporine, foscarnet, mechlorethamine, methoxyflurane, furosemide, vancomycin** increase the possibility of nephrotoxicity; CORTICOSTEROIDS potentiate hypokalemia; with DIGITALIS GLYCOSIDES, hypokalemia increases the risk of **digitalis** toxicity. Increased risk of hypotension with **amifostine, bromperidol, or obinutuzumab**.

PHARMACOKINETICS **Peak:** 1–2 h after IV infusion. **Duration:** 20 h. **Distribution:** Minimal amounts enter CNS, eye, bile, pleural, pericardial, synovial, or amniotic fluids; similar plasma and urine concentrations. **Elimination:** Excreted renally; can be detected in blood up to 4 wk and in urine for 4–8 wk after discontinuing therapy. **Half-Life:** 15–48 h.

NURSING IMPLICATIONS

Black Box Warning

Amphotericin should be reserved for progressive and potentially fatal fungal infections.

Assessment & Drug Effects

- Monitor for S&S of local inflammatory reaction or thrombosis at injection site, particularly if extravasation occurs.
- Monitor cardiovascular and respiratory status and observe patient closely for adverse effects during initial IV therapy. If a test dose (1 mg over 20–30 min) is given, monitor vital signs every 30 min for 2–4 h. Febrile reactions (fever, chills, headache, nausea) occur in 20–90% of patients, usually 1–2 h after beginning infusion, and subside within 4 h after drug is discontinued. The severity of this reaction usually decreases with continued therapy. Keep prescriber informed.

- Monitor I&O and weight. Report immediately: Oliguria, any change in I&O ratio and pattern, or appearance of urine [e.g., sediment, pink or cloudy urine (hematuria)], abnormal renal function tests, unusual weight gain or loss. Generally, renal damage is reversible if drug is discontinued when first signs of renal dysfunction appear.
- Report to prescriber and withhold drug if BUN exceeds 40 mg/dL or serum creatinine rises above 3 mg/dL. Dosage should be reduced or drug discontinued until renal function improves.
- Consult prescriber for guidelines on adequate hydration and adjustment of daily dose as a possible means of avoiding or minimizing nephrotoxicity.
- Report promptly any evidence of hearing loss or complaints of tinnitus, vertigo, or unsteady gait. Tinnitus may not be a complaint in older adults or the very young. Other signs of ototoxicity (i.e., vertigo or hearing loss) are more reliable indicators of ototoxicity in these age groups.
- Baseline C&S prior to initiation of therapy; baseline and periodic BUN, serum creatinine, creatinine clearance; periodic CBC, serum electrolytes (especially K^+, Mg^{++}, Na^+, Ca^{++}), and LFTs. Pulmonary function tests for patients with recent or concomitant leukocyte transfusion.

Patient & Family Education

- Maintain a high fluid intake of 2–3 L (approximately 2–3 qts) of fluid daily if not directed otherwise.
- May cause skin discoloration
- Report promptly chills, fever, unusual weakness, lightheadedness, loss of appetite, weight loss, diarrhea, nausea, vomiting, blurred or double vision, racing pulse, swelling in the legs, shortness of breath, confusion, bruising, pink-colored urine, bleeding without injury in nose or gums.

AMPHOTERICIN B LIPID-BASED

Abelcet, AmBisome

Classification: ANTIFUNGAL

Therapeutic: ANTIFUNGAL

Prototype: AMPHOTERICIN B

AVAILABILITY **Abelcet:** Suspension for injection; **AmBisome:** Powder for injection

ACTION & *THERAPEUTIC EFFECT* Antifungal that selectively binds to sterols in fungus cell membranes, which leads to a leakage of cellular contents and fungal cell death. *Fungicidal at higher concentrations, depending on sensitivity of fungus.*

USES Used intravenously for a wide spectrum of systemic fungal (mycotic) infections; cryptococcal meningitis in patients with HIV.

UNLABELED USES Treatment of candiduria, fungal endocarditis, meningitis, septicemia; fungal infections of urinary bladder and urinary tract; visceral leishmaniasis.

CONTRAINDICATIONS Hypersensitivity to amphotericin or any of its components; lactation—infant risk cannot be ruled out.

CAUTIOUS USE Severe bone marrow depression; renal function impairment; anemia; pregnancy (category B).

ROUTE & DOSAGE

Systemic Infections (Abelcet)

Adult/Adolescent/Child: **IV** 5 mg/kg/day

(AmBisome)

Adult/Child: **IV** 3–6 mg/kg/day

Cryptococcal Meningitis in HIV *(AmBisome)*

Adult: **IV** 3–4 mg/kg/day

Leishmaniasis *(AmBisome)*

Adult (Immunocompetent): **IV** 3 mg/kg/day on days 1–5, 14, and 21; may repeat if necessary. *Immunocompromised:* 4 mg/kg/day on days 1–5, 10, 17, 24, 31, and 38

ADMINISTRATION

Intravenous

PREPARE: Each brand of amphotericin is prepared differently according to manufacturer's directions. ▪ Refer to specific manufacturer's guidelines for preparation of IV solutions.

ADMINISTER: **IV Infusion:** Flush existing line with D5W before infusion. Do not use normal saline; it may cause a precipitate. Invert infusion bag several times before administering and every 2 hours if infusion exceeds 2 hours. Give at a rate of 2.5 mg/kg/h. Do not use an in-line filter.

ALERT: Rapid infusion of any amphotericin can cause cardiovascular collapse. If hypotension or arrhythmias develop, interrupt infusion and notify prescriber. ▪ Protect IV solution from light during administration. ▪ Note incompatibilities. When given through an existing IV line, flush before and after with D5W. ▪ Initiate therapy using the most distal vein possible and alternate sites with each dose if possible, to reduce the risk of thrombophlebitis. ▪ Check IV site frequently for patency.

INCOMPATIBILITIES (Abelcet): **Solution/additive:** Any **saline**-containing solution (precipitate will form), PARENTERAL NUTRITION SOLUTIONS. **Y-site: alatrofloxacin, alemtuzumab, alfentanil, amikacin, ampicillin, ampicillin/sulbactam, aztreonam, bleomycin, calcium salts, capreomycin, caspofungin, cefepime, cefoperazone, cefotaxime, cefotetan, ceftazidime, ceftolozane/tazobactam, chlorpromazine, ciprofloxacin, cisplatin, cyclosporine, dacarbazine, daunorubicin, dexrazoxane, diazepam, digoxin, diltiazem, dobutamine, doxorubicin, doxorubicin liposome, doxycycline, droperidol, epirubicin, erythromycin, etoposide, fosfomycin, gallium, garenoxacin, gatifloxacin, gemcitabine, gemtuzumab, gentamicin, hydroxyzine, idarubicin, imipenem/cilastatin, inamrinone, irinotecan, labetalol, letermovir, leucovorin, levofloxacin, lorazepam, magnesium sulfate, mannitol, mechlorethamine, meperidine, meropenem, metoclopramide, metronidazole, midazolam, minocycline, mitoxantrone, morphine, mycophenolate, nalbuphine, nicardipine, ofloxacin, ondansetron, paclitaxel, pentamidine, phenytoin, potassium phosphate, prochlorperazine, promethazine, propranolol, , quinupristin/dalfopristin, sodium bicarbonate, sodium phosphate, telavancin, teniposide, tobramycin, vancomycin, vecuronium, verapamil, vinblastine, vinorelbine.**

INCOMPATIBILITIES (AmBisome): **Solution/additive:** Any

saline-containing solution (precipitate will form). **Y-site: alemtuzumab, alfentanil, amikacin, ampicillin, ampicillin/sulbactam, atenolol, bivalirudin, bleomycin, calcium salts, capreomycin, cisplatin, dacarbazine, dantrolene, daptomycin, daunorubicin, dexmedetomidine, dexrazoxane, diazepam, diltiazem, dobutamine, dolasetron, dopamine, doxorubicin, doxycycline, epirubicin, erythromycin, esmolol, etoposide, fenoldopam, fluconazole, foscarnet, fosfomycin, gallium, gemcitabine, gemtuzumab, gentamicin, glycopyrrolate, haloperidol, hydralazine, hydroxyzine, idarubicin, imipenem/cilastatin, irinotecan, isavuconazonium, isoproterenol, labetalol, leucovorin, levofloxacin, magnesium sulfate, mechlorethamine, meropenem, mesna, metaraminol, metoprolol, metronidazole, midazolam, milrinone, minocycline, mitoxantrone, morphine, mycophenolate, nalbuphine, naloxone, nicardipine, norepinephrine, ondansetron, pancuronium, pentamidine, phenylephrine, phenytoin, polymyxin B,** POTASSIUM SALTS, **prochlorperazine, promethazine, propranolol, quinupristin/dalfopristin, remifentanil, sodium bicarbonate, sodium acetate, sodium phosphate, sulfamethoxazole/trimethoprim, tirofiban, tobramycin, topotecan, vancomycin, vasopressin, vecuronium, vinorelbine, voriconazole.**

- Do not mix **Abelcet** with any other drugs.
- Store according to manufacturer's recommendations for reconstituted and unopened vials.

ADVERSE EFFECTS (≥ 5%) CV: Hypotension, cardiac arrest. **Other:** Fever, shivering, multiple organ failure.

INTERACTIONS Drug: AMINOGLYCOSIDES, **capreomycin, cisplatin, carboplatin, colistin, cyclosporine, mechlorethamine, furosemide, vancomycin** increase the possibility of nephrotoxicity; CORTICOSTEROIDS potentiate hypokalemia; with DIGITALIS GLYCOSIDES, hypokalemia increases the risk of **digitalis** toxicity.

PHARMACOKINETICS Peak: 1–2 h after IV infusion. **Duration:** 20 h. **Distribution:** Minimal amounts enter CNS, eye, bile, pleural, pericardial, synovial, or amniotic fluids; similar plasma and urine concentrations. **Elimination:** Excreted renally; can be detected in blood up to 4 wk and in urine for 4–8 wk after discontinuing therapy. **Half-Life:** 24–48 h.

NURSING IMPLICATIONS

Assessment & Drug Effects

- Monitor for S&S of local inflammatory reaction or thrombosis at injection site, particularly if extravasation occurs.
- Monitor cardiovascular and respiratory status and observe patient closely for adverse effects during initial IV therapy. If a test dose (1 mg over 20–30 min) is given, monitor vital signs every 30 min for at least 4 h. Febrile reactions (fever, chills, headache, nausea) occur in 20–90% of patients, usually 1–2 h after beginning infusion, and subside within 4 h after drug is discontinued. The severity of this reaction usually decreases with continued therapy. Keep prescriber informed.
- Monitor I&O and weight. Report immediately oliguria, any change in I&O ratio and pattern, or appearance of urine

[e.g., sediment, pink or cloudy urine (hematuria)], abnormal renal function tests, unusual weight gain or loss. Generally, renal damage is reversible if drug is discontinued when first signs of renal dysfunction appear.

- Report to prescriber and withhold drug if BUN exceeds 40 mg/dL or serum creatinine rises above 3 mg/dL. Dosage should be reduced or drug discontinued until renal function improves.
- Consult prescriber for guidelines on adequate hydration and adjustment of daily dose as a possible means of avoiding or minimizing nephrotoxicity.
- Report promptly any evidence of hearing loss or complaints of tinnitus, vertigo, or unsteady gait. Tinnitus may not be a complaint in older adults or the very young. Other signs of ototoxicity (i.e., vertigo or hearing loss) are more reliable indicators of ototoxicity in these age groups.
- Monitor lab tests: Baseline C&S prior to initiation of therapy; baseline and periodic renal function tests; periodic CBC, serum electrolytes (especially K^+, Mg^{++}, Na^+, Ca^{++}), PT/PTT, and LFTs.

Patient & Family Education

- Maintain a high fluid intake of 2–3 L (approximately 2–3 qts) of fluid daily if not directed otherwise.
- Report promptly chills, fever, vomiting, diarrhea, shortness of breath, dizziness, or unusual weakness.

AMPICILLIN (Pr)

(am-pi-sill'in)

Novo-Ampicillin ♣

Classification: ANTIBIOTIC; AMINOPENICILLIN

Therapeutic: ANTIBIOTIC

AVAILABILITY Capsule; injection

ACTION & THERAPEUTIC EFFECT A broad-spectrum, semisynthetic aminopenicillin that is bactericidal but is inactivated by penicillinase (beta-lactamase). Like other penicillins, ampicillin inhibits the final stage of bacterial cell wall synthesis by binding to specific penicillin-binding proteins (PBPs) located inside the bacterial cell wall resulting in lysis and death of bacteria. *Effective against gram-positive bacteria as well as some gram-negative bacteria.*

USES Infections of GU, respiratory, and GI tracts and skin and soft tissues; also bacterial meningitis, respiratory tract infections, bloodstream infection; bacterial endocarditis.

UNLABLED USES: Endocarditis prophylaxis, prosthetic joint infection, osteomyelitis.

CONTRAINDICATIONS Hypersensitivity to ampicillin or other penicillins; infections caused by penicillinase-producing organisms; infectious mononucleosis.

CAUTIOUS USE History of hypersensitivity to cephalosporins; GI disorders; renal disease or impairment; pregnancy—fetal risk cannot be ruled out; lactation—infant risk is minimal.

ROUTE & DOSAGE

Bloodstream Infection

Adult: **IV** 2g q4h

Endocarditis treatment

Adult: **IV** 2 g q4h

Adolescent/Child: **IV** 200–300 mg/kg/day divided q4–6 h (max 12 g/day)

Meningitis

Adult: **IV** 2g q4h × 7–21 days
Child/Infant: **IV** 300–400 mg/kg/day divided q4–6h (max dose 12 g/day)

Mild to moderate infection

Child: **PO** 50–100 mg/kg/day divided q6h (max dose 2000 mg/day); **IV** 50–200 mg/kg/day divided q6h (max dose 8 g/day)

Renal Impairment Dosage Adjustment

CrC; over 50 mL/min: give q6h
CrCl 10–50 mL/min: Give q6–12h; *less than 10 mL/min:* Give q12–24h

ADMINISTRATION

Oral

- Give with a full glass of water on an empty stomach (at least 1 h before or 2 h after meals) for maximum absorption. Food hampers rate and extent of oral absorption.
- Shake a suspension well before measuring the dose.

Intramuscular

- Reconstitute each vial by adding the indicated amount of sterile water for injection or bacteriostatic water for injection (125-mg vial add 1.2 mL to have 125 mg/mL final concentration; 250-mg vial add 1 mL to have 250 mg/mL final concentration; 500-mg vial add 1.8 mL to have 250-mg/mL final concentration; 1 g vial add 3.5 mL to have 250-mg/mL final concentration; 2 g vial add 6.8 mL to have 250 mg/mL. Administer within 1 h of preparation. The 1-g and 2-g vials are intended for IV use, but may be used for an IM administration if the 250-mg and 500-mg vials are not available.
- Withdraw the ordered dose and inject deep IM into a large muscle.

Intravenous

Verify correct IV concentration and rate of infusion with prescriber for administration to neonates, infants, and children.

PREPARE: **Direct/Intermittent:** Reconstitute as follows with sterile water for injection: Add 5 mL to 500-mg vial or fraction thereof; add 7.4 mL to 1-g vial; add 14.8 mL to 2-g vial. Final concentration **must be** 30 mg/mL or less; may be given direct IV as prepared or further diluted in 50 mL or more of NS, D5W, D5/NS, D5W/0.45NaCl, or LR. ▪ Stability of solution varies with diluent and concentration of solution. Solutions in NS are stable for up to 8 h at room temperature; other solutions should be infused within 2–4 h of preparation. Give direct IV within 1 h of preparation. ▪ Wear disposable gloves when handling drug repeatedly; contact dermatitis occurs frequently in sensitized individuals.

ADMINISTER: **Direct/Intermittent:** Infuse 500 mg or less slowly over 3–5 min. Give 1–2 g over at least 15 min. ▪ With solutions of 100 mL or more, set rate according to amount of solution, but no faster than direct IV rate. ▪ Convulsions may be induced by too rapid administration.

- Store dry powder vials of ampicillin sodium at controlled room temperature between 20 and 25°C (68 and 77°F); excursions permitted to 15–30°C (59–86°F).

INCOMPATIBILITIES: **Solution/additive: Amikacin, chlorpromazine, dopamine, etamsylate, gentamicin,**

hydralazine, isoproterenol, prochlorperazine, salbutamol, sodium bicarbonate, tranexamic acid. Y-site: **Aminophylline, amiodarone, amphotericin B, amphotericin B lipid complex, buprenorphine, caspofungin, chlorpromazine, codeine, dacarbazine, dantrolene, daunorubicin, diazepam, diazoxide, diphenhydramine, dobutamine, dolasetron, doxorubicin, doxycycline, epirubicin, fenoldopam, fluconazole, ganciclovir, garenoxacin, hydroxyzine, idarubicin, inamrinone, ketamine, lansoprazole, lorazepam, midazolam, minocycline, mitoxantrone, mycophenolate, nesiritide, nicardipine, ondansetron, pentamidine, pentazocine, phenytoin, prochlorperazine, protamine, quinupristin/dalfopristin, sargramostim, sulfamethoxazole/trimethoprim, topotecan, tranexamic, verapamil, vinorelbine.**

- Store capsules and unopened vials at 15°–30°C (59°–86°F) unless otherwise directed. Keep oral preparations tightly covered.

ADVERSE EFFECTS

(No specific percentage of occurrence reported) **CNS:** Convulsive seizures with high doses. **Skin:** *Rash*. **GI:** *Diarrhea*, nausea, vomiting, pseudomembranous colitis. **Hematologic:** Agranulocytosis, thrombocytopenia. **Other:** Similar to those for penicillin G. Hypersensitivity (pruritus, urticaria, eosinophilia, hemolytic anemia, interstitial nephritis, anaphylactoid reaction); superinfections. Severe pain (following IM); phlebitis (following IV).

DIAGNOSTIC TEST INTERFERENCE

Urine glucose: High urine drug concentrations can result in false-positive test results with ***Clinitest*** or ***Benedict's*** [enzymatic ***glucose oxidase methods*** (e.g., ***Clinistix, Diastix, TesTape***) are not affected].

INTERACTIONS

Drug: Tetracycline may reduce bactericidal effects of ampicillin. Ampicillin may interfere with the contraceptive action of oral contraceptives (**estrogens**). Do not use with LIVE VACCINES. **Food:** Food may decrease absorption of ampicillin, so it should be taken 1 h before or 2 h after meals.

PHARMACOKINETICS

Absorption: Oral dose is 50% absorbed. Peak effect: 5 min IV, 1 h IM, 2 h PO. **Distribution:** Most body tissues; high CNS concentrations only with inflamed meninges; crosses the placenta. **Metabolism:** Minimal hepatic metabolism. **Elimination:** 90% in urine; excreted into breast milk.

NURSING IMPLICATIONS

Assessment & Drug Effects

- Determine previous hypersensitivity reactions to penicillins, cephalosporins, and other allergens prior to therapy. Monitor closely for signs of hypersensitivity during first 30 min after administration.
- Note: Sodium content of IV drug should be considered in patients on sodium restriction.
- Inspect skin daily, and instruct patient to do the same. The appearance of a rash should be carefully evaluated to differentiate a nonallergenic ampicillin rash from a hypersensitivity reaction. Report rash promptly to prescriber.
- Monitor for and report diarrhea, which may indicate pseudomembranous colitis.

- Monitor for improved signs and symptoms of infection
- Monitor lab tests: Baseline C&S prior to initiation of therapy; CBC, baseline and periodic renal, hepatic, and hematologic function tests, particularly during prolonged or high-dose therapy.

Patient & Family Education

- Report diarrhea to prescriber; do not self-medicate. Give a detailed report to the prescriber regarding onset, duration, character of stools, associated symptoms, temperature, and weight loss to help rule out the possibility of drug-induced, potentially fatal pseudomembranous colitis (see Appendix F).
- May decrease the effectiveness of oral contraceptives. Recommend alternate forms of birth control.
- Report S&S of superinfection (onset of black, hairy tongue; oral lesions or soreness; rectal or vaginal itching; vaginal discharge; loose, foul-smelling stools; or unusual odor to urine).
- Report development of a late skin rash, which can be all over the body, itch, and maculopapular.
- Notify prescriber if no improvement is noted within a few days after therapy is started.
- Take medication around the clock with 8 oz of water; continue taking medication until it is all gone (usually 10 days) unless otherwise directed by prescriber or pharmacist.

AMPICILLIN SODIUM AND SULBACTAM SODIUM

(am-pi-sill′in/sul-bak′tam)

Unasyn

Classification: ANTIBIOTIC; AMINOPENICILLIN

Therapeutic: ANTIBIOTIC

Prototype: Ampicillin

AVAILABILITY Injection

ACTION & *THERAPEUTIC EFFECT* Ampicillin inhibits the final stage of bacterial cell wall synthesis by binding to specific penicillin-binding proteins (PBPs) located inside the bacterial cell wall, thus destroying the cell wall. Sulbactam inhibits beta-lactamases, most frequently responsible for transferred drug resistance. Thus, the spectrum of drugs affected by the combination of the two is increased. *Effective against both gram-positive and gram-negative bacteria, including those that produce beta-lactamase and non-beta-lactamase producers. Ampicillin without sulbactam is not effective against beta-lactamase-producing strains.*

USES Treatment of infections due to susceptible organisms in skin and skin structures, intra-abdominal infections, and gynecologic infections.

UNLABELED USE Bite wound infection, treatment of endocarditis, community-acquired pneumonia, surgical site infection.

CONTRAINDICATIONS Hypersensitivity to ampicillin or other penicillins; mononucleosis; infections caused by penicillinase-producing organisms.

CAUTIOUS USE Hypersensitivity to cephalosporins; GI disorders; renal or hepatic disease or impairment; pregnancy (category B) or lactation.

ROUTE & DOSAGE

Usual dosing range

Adult/Adolescent/Child (weight greater than 40 kg): **IV** 1.5–3 g q6h (max: 12g/day)

Child (1 yr or older, less than 40 kg): **IV** 100–300 mg/kg/day divided q6h (max dose: 2000 mg ampicillin/dose)

Diabetic Foot Infection

Adult: **IV** 3g q6h x 2–4 wk

Renal Impairment Dosage Adjustment

CrCl 15–29 mL/min: Give q12h; *5–14 mL/min:* Give q24h

ADMINISTRATION

Intramuscular

- Reconstitute solution with sterile water for injection by adding 3.2 mL diluent to a 1.5-mg vial or add 6.4 mL diluent to a 3-g vial. Each mL contains 250 mg ampicillin and 125 mg sulbactam. Administer within 1 hour of reconstitution.
- Give deep IM into a large muscle. Rotate injection sites.

Intravenous

PREPARE: **Direct/Intermittent:** Reconstitute each 1.5-g vial with 3.2 mL of sterile water for injection to yield 375 mg/mL (250 mg ampicillin/125 mg sulbactam); must further dilute with NS, D5W, D5/NS, D5W/0.45NS, or LR to a final concentration within the range of 3–45 mg/mL.

ADMINISTER: **Direct:** Give slowly over at least 10–15 min. **Intermittent:** Infuse solutions of less than 50 mL over 10–15 min and solutions of 50–100 mL over 15–30 min. With solutions of 100 mL or more, set rate according to amount of solution but no faster than direct IV rate (e.g., 100 mL over 30 min). ▪ Convulsions may be induced by too rapid administration. ▪ Use only freshly prepared solution; administer within 1 h after preparation.

▪ Store unopened vials of powder at or below 30°C (86°F). Temperatures and use within times vary for IV preparations based on diluent.

INCOMPATIBILITIES: **Solution/additive: Ciprofloxacin, tranexamic acid. Y-site: Acyclovir, amiodarone, amphotericin B, amphotericin B lipid complex, azathioprine, caspofungin, chlorpromazine, ciprofloxacin, dacarbazine, dantrolene, daunorubicin, diazepam, diazoxide, dobutamine, dolasetron, doxorubicin, doxycycline, epirubicin, ganciclovir, garenoxacin, hydralazine, hydrocortisone, hydroxyzine, idarubicin, lansoprazole, lorazepam, mechlorethamine, methylprednisolone, midazolam, minocycline, mitoxantrone, mycophenolate, nicardipine, ondansetron, papaverine, pentamidine, pentazocine, phenytoin, prochlorperazine, promethazine, protamine, quinupristin/dalfopristin, sargramostim, SMZ/TMP, topotecan, tranexamic acid, verapamil, vinorelbine.**

- Store powder for injection at 15°–30°C (59°–86°F) before reconstitution. Storage times and temperatures vary for different concentrations of reconstituted solutions; consult manufacturer's directions.

ADVERSE EFFECTS (≥ 5%) Other:

Hypersensitivity (rash, itching, anaphylactoid reaction). Local pain at injection site; thrombophlebitis.

DIAGNOSTIC TEST INTERFERENCE

Urine glucose: High urine drug

concentrations can result in false-positive test results with ***Clinitest*** or ***Benedict's*** [enzymatic ***glucose oxidase methods*** (e.g., ***Clinistix, Diastix, TesTape***) are not affected].

INTERACTIONS **Drug: Tetracycline** may reduce bactericidal effects of ampicillin. Ampicillin may interfere with the contraceptive action of oral contraceptives (**estrogens**).

PHARMACOKINETICS **Peak:** Immediate after IV. **Duration:** 6–8 h. **Distribution:** Most body tissues; high CNS concentrations only with inflamed meninges; crosses placenta; appears in breast milk. **Metabolism:** Minimal hepatic metabolism. **Elimination:** In urine. **Half-Life:** 1 h.

NURSING IMPLICATIONS

Assessment & Drug Effects

- Determine previous hypersensitivity reactions to penicillins, cephalosporins, and other allergens prior to therapy.
- Report promptly unexplained bleeding (e.g., epistaxis, purpura, ecchymoses).
- Monitor patient carefully during the first 30 min after initiation of IV therapy for signs of hypersensitivity and anaphylactoid reaction (see Appendix F). Serious anaphylactoid reactions require immediate use of emergency drugs and airway management.
- Monitor for and report diarrhea, which may indicate pseudomembranous colitis. Observe for and report other S&S of superinfection.
- Monitor I&O ratio and pattern. Report dysuria, urine retention, and hematuria.
- Monitor lab tests: Baseline C&S prior to initiation of therapy; CBC, baseline and periodic renal, hepatic, and hematologic function tests, particularly during prolonged or high-dose therapy.

Patient & Family Education

- Report chills, wheezing, pruritus (itching), respiratory distress, or palpitations to prescriber immediately.
- Report diarrhea to prescriber; do not self-medicate.
- Report development of a skin rash.

ANAGRELIDE HYDROCHLORIDE

(a-na′gre-lyde)

Agrylin

Classification: ANTIPLATELET

Therapeutic: ANTIPLATELET; REDUCER OF PLATELET COUNT

AVAILABILITY Capsule

ACTION & *THERAPEUTIC EFFECT* Causes dose-related reduction in platelet production. It inhibits platelet aggregation by affecting several aggregating agents (e.g., thrombin and arachidonic acid, ADP, and collagen). *Anagrelide is associated with significant decreases in platelet counts and is thought to prevent early changes in shape of platelets.*

USES Essential thrombocythemia.

UNLABELED USES Polycythemia vera, chronic myelogenous leukemia.

CONTRAINDICATIONS Severe hepatic impairment; congenital QT prolongation; a history of acquired QT prolongation; those receiving concomitant QT-prolonging medications; hypokalemia; lactation.

CAUTIOUS USE Cardiovascular disease, mild and moderate hepatic impairment, renal impairment; pulmonary disease; jaundice; patients taking anticoagulants, NSAIDs, antiplatelet agents, other phosphodiesterase 3 (PDE) inhibitors, or serotonin reuptake inhibitors; pregnancy (category C); children.

ROUTE & DOSAGE

Essential Thrombocythemia

Adult (16 yr or older): **PO** Start with 0.5 mg qid or 1 mg bid × 1 wk, may increase by 0.5 mg/day qwk until platelet count is less than 600,000/mcL (max: 10 mg/day)

Hepatic Impairment Dosage Adjustment

0.5 mg daily for 1 wk

ADMINISTRATION

Oral

- Make sure a single dose does not exceed 2.5 mg and dosage increments do not exceed 0.5 mg/day in any 1 wk.
- Maximum daily dose is 10 mg.
- May be administered with or without regard to food.
- Store at 15°–30°C (59°–86°F) in a light-resistant container.

ADVERSE EFFECTS **CV:** Chest pain, peripheral edema, general edema, *palpitations*, peripheral edema, tachycardia. Incidence unknown: Atrial fibrillation, cardiomegaly, cardiomyopathy, heart block, MI, pericardial effusion. **Respiratory:** Cough, dyspnea. **CNS:** *Headache*, dizziness, malaise, paresthesia. **Skin:** Rash, pruritus. **GI:** *Diarrhea*, nausea, abdominal pain, flatulence, vomiting, indigestion. **Musculoskeletal:** *Weakness*, back pain. **Other:** Fever, pain.

INTERACTIONS **Drugs** May have additive effect with agents that affect QT prolongation (e.g., **ziprasidone, bepridil,** etc.) Do not use with **cilostazol. Herbal:** Alfalfa and bilberry may increase bleeding risk.

PHARMACOKINETICS **Absorption:** 70% from GI tract. Food reduces bioavailability. **Onset:** 7–14 days. **Duration:** Increased platelet counts were observed 4 days after discontinuing drug. **Metabolism:** Extensively metabolized (CYP1A2). **Elimination:** Primarily in urine as metabolites. **Half-Life:** 1.3–1.8 h.

NURSING IMPLICATIONS

Assessment & Drug Effects

- Monitor for therapeutic effectiveness, which is indicated by reduction of platelets for at least 4 wk to 600,000/mcL or less or 50% from baseline.
- Monitor for bleeding or thrombosis.
- Monitor for S&S of CHF or myocardial ischemia and compare to baseline ECG.
- Monitor for S&S of renal toxicity in patients with renal insufficiency (creatinine 2 mg/dL or more).
- Monitor for S&S of hepatic toxicity in patients with liver functions greater than 1.5 times upper limit of normal.
- Monitor lab tests: Platelet count q2days for first wk, weekly thereafter until maintenance dose reached; frequent Hgb, WBC count, LFTs, BUN, creatinine, and serum electrolytes while platelet count is being lowered.

Patient & Family Education

- Contact prescriber if palpitations, swelling, breathing difficulty, symptoms of bleeding (vomiting bright red blood or if it looks coffee grounds, black tarry or red stools, bleeding gums, abnormal vaginal bleeding, bruises without reason) or any other distressful symptoms develop.

ANAKINRA

(an-a-kin'ra)

Kineret

Classification: DISEASE-MODIFYING ANTIRHEUMATIC DRUG (DMARD)
Therapeutic: ANTIRHEUMATIC; DMARD

AVAILABILITY Solution for injection

ACTION & *THERAPEUTIC EFFECT* An interleukin-1 (IL-1) receptor antagonist that inhibits IL-1 binding to interleukin receptors present in both bone and cartilage (as well as other tissues). IL-1 is produced in response to inflammation and mediates various responses of tissues, including inflammatory and immunologic responses. *Anakinra competes with interleukin-1 (IL-1) by inhibiting it from binding to its receptor sites in tissues.*

USES Treatment of rheumatoid arthritis; neonatal-onset multisystem inflammatory disease (NOMID).

UNLABELED USES Acute gout flares, recurrent pericarditis.

CONTRAINDICATIONS Hypersensitivity to anakinra, *E. coli*–derived proteins, active infections; live vaccines, pregnancy and lactation.

CAUTIOUS USE Neutropenia, immunosuppressed patients, or patients with frequent, serious infections; asthmatics; patients with latent tuberculosis, older adults; renal impairment; children.

ROUTE & DOSAGE

Rheumatoid Arthritis

Adult: **Subcutaneous** 100 mg daily

NOMID

Adult /Adolescent/Child: **Subcutaneous** 1–2 mg/kg daily, may taper up to usual maintenance dose 3–4 mg/kg/day (max dose: 8 mg/kg/day)

ADMINISTRATION

Subcutaneous Only

- Do not give anakinra if the patient has an active infection.
- Note that anakinra should not ordinarily be given with tumor necrosis factor (TNF) blocking agents.
- Do not shake the syringe.
- Discard any unused portions as the drug contains no preservative.
- Check expiration date and do not use if expired, discolored, or if an excessive number of translucent particles appears in the syringe.
- To decrease injection site reactions, apply a cold compress before/after injection and warm solution to room temperature 30 min before injection.
- Store in the refrigerator at 2°–8°C (36°–46°F). **Do not freeze or shake.** Protect from light.

ADVERSE EFFECTS **CV:** Cardiopulmonary arrest. **Respiratory:** Nasopharyngitis. **CNS:** Headache. **Endocrine:** (not defined) hypercholesterolemia. **Skin:** Bacterial cellulitis. **GI:** Vomiting, nausea, diarrhea. **Musculoskeletal:** Joint pain. **Hematologic:** Eosinophilia, decreased WBCs. **Other:** Fever.

INTERACTIONS **Drug:** Increased risk of infection with live virus vaccine, TUMOR NECROSIS FACTOR MODIFIERS. Increased risk of neutropenia as well as infection with **etanercept, abatacept**, and **infliximab.**

PHARMACOKINETICS Absorption: 95% absorbed subcutaneous site. **Peak:** 3–7 h. **Elimination:** In urine. **Half-Life:** 4–6 h.

NURSING IMPLICATIONS

Assessment & Drug Effects

- Monitor for S&S of infection (e.g., pneumonia or other URI, cellulitis). Stop drug and notify prescriber if these appear.
- Monitor closely patients with impaired renal function for S&S of adverse drug reactions.
- Assess for injection site reactions manifested by erythema, bruising, inflammation, and pain.
- Monitor lab tests: Absolute TB baseline test, complete blood count (CBC), serum creatinine, absolute neutrophil count (ANC) prior to initiating anakinra, monthly for 3 mo, and q3mo thereafter for 1 yr, erythrocyte sedimentation rate (ESR), C-reactive protein, rheumatoid factor levels during long-term therapy.

Patient & Family Education

- Review carefully the "Information for Patients and Caregivers" leaflet for detailed instructions on handling and injecting anakinra.
- Give the injection at approximately the same time every day.
- Leave syringe at room temperature for 30 min, and administer only 1 dose (the entire contents of 1 prefilled glass syringe) per day. Discard any unused portions as the drug contains no preservative. Do not save unused drug.
- Do not permit vaccination with live vaccines while taking anakinra.
- Stop drug and notify prescriber for S&S of upper respiratory, skin, or other infection(s).

ANASTROZOLE

(a-nas'tro-zole)

Arimidex

Classification: ANTINEOPLASTIC; NONSTEROIDAL AROMATASE INHIBITOR

Therapeutic: ANTINEOPLASTIC

AVAILABILITY Tablet

ACTION & *THERAPEUTIC EFFECT*
Anastrozole is a potent and selective nonsteroidal aromatase inhibitor that converts estrone to estradiol. It lowers serum estrogen levels in postmenopausal women without interfering with adrenal steroid synthesis. *Inhibiting the biosynthesis of estrogens is one way to deprive tumors of estrogens and thus restrict tumor growth.*

USES Early and advanced breast cancer with hormone receptor positive or hormone status unknown in postmenopausal women.

CONTRAINDICATIONS Premenopausal women, postmenopausal hormone replacement therapy; severe hepatic disease, pregnancy (category X); lactation.

CAUTIOUS USE Mild to moderate hepatic disease; patients with osteopenia, hypercholesterolemia, or ischemic cardiac disease.

ROUTE & DOSAGE

Breast Cancer

Adult: **PO** 1 mg once daily

ADMINISTRATION

Oral

- The National Institute for Occupational Safety & Health (NIOSH) recommends use of single gloves if intact tablets are handled. If cutting, crushing, or manipulating or handling uncoated tablets, double gloves and protective gown. Prepare in ventilated control device.
- Wear single gloves and eye/face protection when administering if the formulation is hard for the patient to swallow or if the patient may resist, vomit, or spit up.
- Give with or without food.
- Store at 20°–25°C (68°–77°F).

ADVERSE EFFECTS **CV:** Chest pain, hypertension, peripheral edema, *vasodilation*. **Respiratory:** Dyspnea, increased frequency of cough, pharyngitis. **CNS:** Fatigue, mood disorder, anxiety, headache, weakness, insomnia, pain and depression. **HEENT:** Cataracts. **GI:** *Disorder of the gastrointestinal tract*, constipation, diarrhea, abdominal pain, anorexia, indigestion, dry mouth. **GU:** Breast pain, UTI, pelvic pain, vulvovaginitis, breast cancer. **Musculoskeletal:** Bone fracture, muscle and joint pain, osteoporosis. **Hematological:** Lymphedema. **Other:** Accidental injury, pain, cyst.

INTERACTIONS **Drug:** Use with **tamoxifen** may reduce anastrozole plasma levels.

PHARMACOKINETICS **Absorption:** Rapidly absorbed from GI tract. 80% bioavailable. **Distribution:** 40% protein bound. **Metabolism:** 85% metabolized in liver to inactive metabolites. **Elimination:** Mostly in feces. **Half-Life:** 50 h.

NURSING IMPLICATIONS

Assessment & Drug Effects

- Assess for hypotension, complications of edema, thrombotic events, bone pain or fracture, and signs of liver toxicity.
- Monitor bone mineral density at baseline. Mammograms and clinical breast exam at baseline and at least every 2 yr.
- Monitor lab tests: Periodic total cholesterol and lipid profile.

Patient & Family Education

- Recognize common adverse effects and seek information on measures to control discomfort.
- Seek medical attention if you experience signs of depression, suicidal ideation, anxiety, emotional instability, or confusion, chest pain, calf pain, or shortness of breath; unexplained loss of appetite or nausea; jaundice, swelling of arms or legs, severe headache, fatigue, dizzy, vaginal bleeding or vaginitis.

ANGIOTENSIN II

(an-jee-oh-ten′ sin-too)

Giapreza

Classification: VASOACTIVE AGENT

Therapeutic: VASOACTIVE AGENT

AVAILABILITY Solution for injection; single-dose vial

ACTION & *THERAPEUTIC EFFECT* Angiotensin works by increasing vasoconstriction through G-protein-coupled receptors on vascular smooth muscle and increased aldosterone release. *Causes a net increase in blood pressure.*

USES Used to increase blood pressure in patients with septic or other distributive shock.

CAUTIOUS USE A higher incidence of thrombosis has been

reported with angiotensin II use; patients are advised to use VTE prophylaxis.

ROUTE & DOSAGE

Shock

Adult: **IV** Initial: 10–20 ng/kg/min; titrate dose to response every 5 min in increments of up to 15 ng/kg/min as needed; down-titration found in package insert (max maintenance dose: 40 ng/kg/min)

ADMINISTRATION

Intravenous

PREPARE: **IV infusion:** Giapreza should be diluted in 0.9% NS prior to infusion. Specific infusion instructions are in the package insert. Final concentrations will be 5000 ng/mL or 10,000 ng/mL.
- Prepared IV solutions should be used within 24 h.

ADMINISTER: IV Infusion: Administer via continuous intravenous infusion; use of a central line is recommended. Blood pressure should be monitored for response and dose titrated to achieve/maintain goal.

- Store in refrigerator at 2°–8°C (36°–46°F).

ADVERSE EFFECTS **CV:** Thrombosis, thrombocytopenia, tachycardia, peripheral ischemia. **CNS:** Delirium. **Endocrine:** Acidosis, hyperglycemia. **Other:** Fungal infection.

INTERACTIONS **Drug:** Concomitant use of ACE-INHIBITORS (e.g., lisinopril) or ARB-INHIBITORS (e.g., losartan) may increase overall response to angiotensin II.

PHARMACOKINETICS **Absorption:** 100% bioavailability from infusion. **Peak:** 5 min. **Metabolism:** Angiotensin is metabolized through aminopeptidase A and angiotensin converting enzyme 2 (ACE-2) found in plasma, erythrocytes, and other organs. **Half-Life:** Less than 1 min.

NURSING IMPLICATIONS

Assessment & Drug Effects

- Monitor blood pressure.
- Monitor for signs of DVT or thromboembolic event (one-sided swelling, redness, leg pain or cramp, shortness of breath or pain when breathing, chest pain, cough, back pain).

Patient & Family Education

- Report signs of deep vein thrombosis or other clotting: rapid heartbeat, one-sided swelling, redness, leg pain or cramp, shortness of breath or pain when breathing, chest pain, cough, back pain.

ANIDULAFUNGIN

(a-ni-dul'a-fun-gin)

Eraxis

Classification: ECHINOCANDIN ANTIFUNGAL

Therapeutic: ANTIFUNGAL

Prototype: Caspofungin

AVAILABILITY Powder for injection

ACTION & *THERAPEUTIC EFFECT*

Anidulafungin is a semisynthetic echinocandin that inhibits glucan synthase, an enzyme present in fungal cells. Glucan is an essential component of the fungal cell wall; therefore, anidulafungin causes fungal cell death. *Interferes with reproduction and growth of susceptible fungi.*

Common adverse effects in *italic;* life-threatening effects underlined; generic names in **bold;** classifications in SMALL CAPS; ♣ Canadian drug name; ⊕ Prototype drug; ⚠ Alert

USES Treatment of candidemia, esophageal candidiasis, and other *Candida* infections.

UNLABELED USES Candidal endocarditis, oropharyngeal candidiasis, disseminated chronic candidiasis.

CONTRAINDICATIONS Hypersensitivity to anidulafungin or another echinocandin antifungal; lactation.

CAUTIOUS USE Hepatic impairment; fetal risk in pregnancy and infant risk for lactation cannot be ruled out. Safety and efficacy in children not established.

ROUTE & DOSAGE

Candidemia and Other *Candida* Infections

Adult: **IV** 200-mg loading dose on day 1, then 100-mg IV daily for at least 14 days after last positive culture

Esophageal Candidiasis

Adult: **IV** 100-mg loading dose on day 1, then 50-mg IV daily for at least 14 days (and for at least 7 days after resolution of symptoms)

ADMINISTRATION

Intravenous

PREPARE: **IV Infusion:** Reconstitute with sterile water only. The reconstituted solution must be further diluted in NS or D5W to a final concentration of 0.77 mg/mL as follows: Dilute a 50-mg dose in 50 mL IV fluid; dilute a 100-mg dose in 100 mL IV fluid; dilute a 200-mg dose in 200 mL IV fluid.

ADMINISTER: **IV Infusion:** Give at a rate **no greater** than 1.1 mg/min. **Do not** give a bolus dose.

INCOMPATIBILITIES: **Y-site: Amphotericin B conventional, dantrolene sodium, dantrolene, diazepam, ertapenem, gemtuzumab, magnesium, nalbuphine, pemetrexed, phenytoin, potassium, magnesium sulfate, nalbuphine hydrochloride, pemetrexed disodium, phenytoin, sodium bicarbonate, sodium phosphates.**

- Store intact vials at 2°–8°C (36°–46°F); excursions at 25°C (77°F) are permitted for 96 h, and the vial may be returned to storage. Do not freeze. Reconstituted solution can be stored up to 24 h at temperatures up to 25°C (77°F) prior to dilution into the infusion solution (D5W or NS). The infusion solution may be stored for up to 48 h at temperatures up to 25°C (77°F) or stored in the freezer for at least 72 h prior to administration.

ADVERSE EFFECTS **CV:** Hypotension, hypertension, peripheral edema, DVT, chest pain. **Respiratory:** Dyspnea, pleural effusion, cough, pneumonia, respiratory distress. **CNS:** Insomnia, confusion, headache, depression. **Endocrine:** Hypoglycemia, hypomagnesemia, dehydration, hyperglycemia, hyperkalemia. **Skin:** Decubitus ulcer. **Hepatic:** Increased serum alkaline phosphatase. **GI:** Nausea, diarrhea, vomiting, constipation, indigestion, abdominal pain, oral candidiasis. **GU:** UTI, increased serum creatinine. **Musculoskeletal:** Back pain. **Hematologic:** Anemia, leukocytosis, thrombocythemia. **Other:** Fever.

INTERACTIONS **Drug: Cyclosporin** increases overall systemic exposure.

PHARMACOKINETICS **Distribution:** 99% protein bound. **Metabolism:** Nonhepatic degradation to inactive metabolites. **Elimination:** Fecal. **Half-Life:** 26 h.

NURSING IMPLICATIONS

Assessment & Drug Effects

- Prior to initiating therapy with anidulafungin, obtain specimen for fungal culture.
- Monitor for and report S&S of hypersensitivity (e.g., dyspnea, flushing, hypotension, swelling about the face, pruritus, rash, and urticaria), abnormal LFTs, or liver dysfunction (e.g., jaundice, clay-colored stools).
- Discontinue infusion if signs of hypersensitivity appear.
- Monitor cardiac status especially with a preexisting history of dysrhythmias.
- Monitor for S&S hypokalemia and hepatic toxicity (see Appendix F).
- Monitor diabetics for loss of glycemic control.
- Monitor lab tests: Baseline and periodic LFTs.

Patient & Family Education

- Report any of the following immediately if experienced during or shortly after infusion: Difficulty breathing, swelling about the face, itching, rash.
- Report S&S of jaundice to the prescriber: Clay-colored stool, dark urine, yellow skin or sclera, unexplained abdominal pain, or fatigue.

APIXABAN

(a-pix'a-ban)

Eliquis

Classification: ANTICOAGULANT; ANTITHROMBOTIC; SELECTIVE FACTOR XA INHIBITOR

Therapeutic: ANTICOAGULANT; ANTITHROMBOTIC

Prototype: Rivaroxaban

AVAILABILITY Tablet

ACTION & *THERAPEUTIC EFFECT*

A reversible, selective active site inhibitor of factor Xa that does not require antithrombin III for antithrombotic activity; indirectly inhibits platelet aggregation induced by thrombin. *By inhibiting FXa, apixaban decreases thrombin generation and clot development.*

USES Reduction of the risk of stroke and systemic embolism in patients with nonvalvular atrial fibrillation, DVT prophylaxis, treatment of PE.

UNLABELED USE Heparin-induced thrombocytopenia, prevention of stroke/TIA.

CONTRAINDICATIONS Severe hypersensitivity to apixaban; active pathological bleeding; 48 h before surgery; severe hepatic impairment; CrCl less than 25 mL/min; prosthetic heart valves or significant rheumatic heart disease; pregnancy—fetal risk cannot be ruled out; lactation—infant risk cannot be ruled out.

CAUTIOUS USE Moderate hepatic or renal impairment; older adults; patients with postoperative indwelling catheters. Safety and efficacy in children not established.

ROUTE & DOSAGE

Reduction of Stroke and Systemic Embolism

Adult: **PO** 5 mg bid

Adult (with at least 2 of the following: 80 yr or older, weight 60 kg or less, or serum creatinine 1.5 mg/dL or more): **PO** 2.5 mg bid

DVT Prophylaxis

Adult: **PO** 2.5 mg bid × 12 d (after knee replacement) or × 35 d (after hip replacement)

DVT/PE Treatment

Adult: **PO** 10 mg bid × 7 d then 5 mg bid

Dosage Adjustment if Coadministered with Dual CYP3A4 and P-gp Inhibitors

Decrease dose to 2.5 mg bid

Renal Impairment Dosage Adjustment (for patients with Nonvalvular Atrial Fibrillation)

Adult (80 yr or older and/or weighs 60 kg or less with serum creatinine 1.5 mg/dL or more): **PO** 2.5 mg twice daily

ADMINISTRATION

Oral

- May be given without regard to food.
- For patients that have difficulty swallowing, apixaban can be crushed and suspended in apple juice or applesauce for prompt administration. Alternatively, tablets can be crushed and suspended in 60 mL of water and promptly delivered through nasogastric tube.
- Store at 20°–25°C (68°–77°F), with excursions permitted between 15° and 30°C (59° and 86°F).

ADVERSE EFFECTS **Hematological:** *Increased bleeding risk, anemia.*

INTERACTIONS **Drug:** Inhibitors of CYP3A4 and P-gp (e.g., **ketoconazole, itraconazole, ritonavir, clarithromycin**) may increase apixaban levels. Inducers of CYP3A4 and P-gp (e.g., **rifampin, carbamazepine, phenytoin, primidone**) may decrease apixaban levels. Use with POTASSIUM-SPARING DIURETICS may increase serum potassium. NSAIDS may increase bleeding risk. Avoid use with other ANTICOAGULANT or ANTIPLATELET agents. **Vitamin E** increases anticoagulation effect. **Herbal: St. John's wort** may decrease apixaban levels.

PHARMACOKINETICS **Absorption:** 50% bioavailable. **Peak:** 3–4 h. **Distribution:** 87% plasma protein bound. **Metabolism:** In liver (25%). **Elimination:** Renal (27%) and fecal (73%). **Half-Life:** 12 h.

NURSING IMPLICATIONS

Black Box Warning

Discontinuing apixaban without replacement with another anticoagulant increases the risk of thrombotic events.

Assessment & Drug Effects

- Report promptly suspected or overt bleeding. Patients are at higher risk for bleeding with concomitant use of drugs such as aspirin, antiplatelet agents or anticoagulants agents, thrombolytic agents, SSRIs, SNRIs, or NSAIDs.
- Note: There is no established way to reverse anticoagulant effect of apixaban, which can persist for about 24 h after last dose.
- Monitor lab tests: CBC during initiation and at regular intervals (at least yearly), LFTs at initiation and periodically during treatment, renal function tests at initiation and periodically during treatment.

Patient & Family Education

- Do not stop taking this drug without consulting your prescriber.
- If you miss a dose, take it as soon as you remember, but do not take more than one dose at the same time to make up for a missed dose.

- Do not take aspirin or other OTC pain relievers, such as NSAIDs, that could increase the risk of bleeding.
- Warn that small bumps to skin may result in obvious bruising.
- Report promptly to prescriber if you experience any of the following: Unexpected, prolonged, or severe bleeding; red, pink, or brown urine; red or black tarry stools; coughing up blood; vomiting blood or your vomit looks like coffee grounds; unexpected pain, swelling, or joint pain; headaches, feeling dizzy or weak, bowel or bladder dysfunction.
- Be sure to report taking medications to healthcare providers if planning an elective surgery or invasive procedure.
- Do not plan pregnancy or breastfeed while taking this drug. Contact physician if becoming pregnant.

APOMORPHINE HYDROCHLORIDE

(a-po-mor'feen)

Apokyn, Kynmobi

Classification: ANTIPARKINSON; NON-ERGOT DERIVATIVE DOPAMINE RECEPTOR AGONIST

Therapeutic: ANTIPARKINSON

AVAILABILITY Injection; sublingual film

ACTION & *THERAPEUTIC EFFECT* A central dopamine receptor agonist that is thought to stimulate centrally located postsynaptic dopamine D_2-type receptors. *Diminishes hypomobility associated with "off" episodes ("end-of-dose wearing off" and unpredictable "on/off" episodes) in persons with advanced Parkinson disease.*

USES Treatment of "off" episodes associated with advanced Parkinson disease.

CONTRAINDICATIONS Hypersensitivity to the drug or its ingredients (i.e., sodium metabisulfite), benzyl alcohol hypersensitivity; renal failure; QT prolongation; heart failure, or shock; depression, suicidal ideation; decreased alertness, seizures, seizure disorder, unconscious state or coma, decreased alertness; pregnancy—fetal risk cannot be ruled out. Lactation—infant risk cannot be ruled out.

CAUTIOUS USE Hypersensitivity to sulfites; cardiovascular, cerebrovascular, respiratory, renal, or hepatic disease; CNS depression, history of (chronic) depression or suicidal ideation; hypotension; vomiting; bradycardia; hypokalemia and hypomagnesemia; older adult.

ROUTE & DOSAGE

"Off" Episodes of Parkinson Disease

Adult: **Sublingual** 10 mg PRN at intervals ≥ 2 h for "off episodes" (max of 5 doses/day); may increase dose in 5-mg increments q3 days (max single dose 30 mg) at intervals ≥ 2 h **Subcutaneous** Start with a test dose where BP can be closely monitored. Escalate test dose no sooner than 2 h after last dose until dose is not tolerated or patient has response. *See package insert for dosing based on response to test dose*

ADMINISTRATION

Sublingual

- Must be administered whole; do not cut, chew, or swallow. Film disintegrates is about 3 minutes.

- Make sure to separate doses by at least 2 hours.

Subcutaneous

- Aspirate to avoid intravascular injection and ensure the injection is subcutaneous and not intradermal.
- Rotate subcutaneous sites to reduce skin reactions.
- If the patient has not received apomorphine in more than 1 wk, reinstitute it by starting with the initial test dose and titrating to the desired dose.
- Apomorphine causes nausea and vomiting; thus the recommendation is to give 300 mg of trimethobenzamide PO tid, starting 3 days before the first injection and continued for at least the first 2 mo of treatment.
- Store sublingual film at controlled room temperature between 20° and 25°C (68° and 77°F) with excursions permitted between 15° and 30°C (59° and 86°F). Keep in foil pouch until ready to use.
- Store subcutaneous medication at controlled room temperature of 25°C (77°F) with excursions permitted between 15° and 30°C (59° and 86°F).

ADVERSE EFFECTS (≥ 5%) CV: Acute circulatory failure, *peripheral edema, angina,* bradycardia, hypertension, *orthostatic hypotension,* QT prolongation, vasovagal response, syncope. **Respiratory:** *Rhinitis.* **CNS:** CNS depression, *dizziness, drowsiness,* headache, light-headed, euphoria, restlessness, tremor, depression, *dyskinesias, hallucinations.* **Endocrine:** Peripheral edema. **Skin:** Contact dermatitis, *bruising,* granuloma, pruritus, sweating. **GI:** *Nausea, vomiting,* hypersalivation, taste perversions, *swelling of oral cavity structures.* **Other:** Weakness, yawning, tiredness.

INTERACTIONS Drug: Alosetron, dolasetron, granisetron, ondansetron, palonosetron, ANTIHYPERTENSIVES may cause severe hypotension and unconsciousness; **alfuzosin, bepridil, chloroquine, clozapine, cyclobenzaprine, droperidol, flecainide, halofantrine, halothane, levomethadyl,** LOCAL ANESTHETICS, MACROLIDES **(clarithromycin, erythromycin, troleandomycin), maprotiline, mefloquine, methadone, pentamidine,** PHENOTHIAZINES, **probucol, gatifloxacin, gemifloxacin, grepafloxacin, levofloxacin, moxifloxacin, sparfloxacin, tacrolimus,** TRICYCLIC ANTIDEPRESSANTS, **amiodarone, clozapine, disopyramide, dofetilide, dolasetron, haloperidol, ibutilide, mesoridazine, palonosetron, pimozide, procainamide, quinidine, thioridazine, sotalol, ziprasidone** may exacerbate QT_C prolongation; may increase CNS depression with other CNS depressants, including TRICYCLIC ANTIDEPRESSANTS, ANXIOLYTICS, SEDATIVES, HYPNOTICS, **dronabinol,** GENERAL ANESTHETICS, **mirtazapine, nefazodone,** OPIATE AGONISTS, **pramipexole, ropinirole,** SKELETAL MUSCLE RELAXANTS, **tramadol, trazodone.** Do not use with **alizapride, amisulpride, bromperidol**.

PHARMACOKINETICS Absorption: Subcutaneous: Rapid **Onset:** 7–14 min. **Peak:** 10–60 min (subcutaneous); 0.5–1 hr sublingual. **Duration:** Up to 2 h. **Distribution:** 85–90% protein bound. **Metabolism:** Metabolized by glucuronidation, sulfation, and N-demethylation. **Elimination:** Excreted by kidneys. **Half-Life:** 30–60 min (subcutaneous) 1.7 h (sublingual)

NURSING IMPLICATIONS

Assessment & Drug Effects

- Periodic ECG, especially in those with known CV disease.
- Withhold drug and notify prescriber for S&S of torsades de pointes (i.e., palpitations and syncope), especially in those with bradycardia or suspected hypokalemia or hypomagnesemia.
- Monitor closely for orthostatic hypotension, especially when doses are increased, and in patients taking antihypertensive medications and vasodilators (especially nitrates).
- Monitor orthostatic vital signs. Institute fall precautions, especially if orthostatic hypotension occurs.
- Monitor impulsive behaviors that are new or worsened like gambling urges, sexual urges, and uncontrolled spending.
- Monitor for drowsiness and somnolence that could lead to falls.

Patient & Family Education

- Avoid the use of alcohol while taking this drug.
- Report promptly any of the following: Irregular or fast, pounding heartbeat, or palpitations; dizziness, light-headedness, or fainting; unexplained weakness, tiredness, or sleepiness; confusion, hallucinations, or depression; unusual body movements; vomiting; mouth dryness, oral sores, swollen tongue, oral pain, lip ulceration, or prolonged painful erections.
- Encourage slow change in positions from lying to standing.
- Report behaviors that are new or worsened like gambling urges, sexual urges, and uncontrolled spending.
- Do not suddenly stop taking this medication.
- Do not engage in potentially hazardous activities that require mental alertness until reaction to drug is known.
- Doses should be separated by at least 2 hours, and patient should not take more than 5 doses per day.

APRACLONIDINE

(a-pra-clo′ni-deen)

IOPIDINE **See Appendix A-1.**

APREMILAST

(a-prem′i-last)

Otezla

Classification: ANTIARTHRITIC; PHOSPHODIESTERASE 4 INHIBITOR

Therapeutic: ANTIARTHRITIC

AVAILABILITY Tablet

ACTION & *THERAPEUTIC EFFECT* Inhibits the enzyme, phosphodiesterase 4 (PDE4), specific for cAMP, which results in increased intracellular cAMP levels and regulation of numerous inflammatory mediators (e.g., decreased expression of nitric oxide synthase, TNF-alpha, and IL 23). *Decrease pain and inflammation in affected joint and other tissues.*

USES Treatment of adult patients with active psoriatic arthritis.

CONTRAINDICATIONS Known hypersensitivity to apremilast or any components in the formulation; suicidal ideation; unexplained or clinically significant weight loss.

CAUTIOUS USE History of depression and/or suicidal thoughts; weight loss; severe renal impairment; pregnancy (category C); lactation. Safety and efficacy in children younger than 18 yr not established.

ROUTE & DOSAGE

Psoriatic Arthritis

Adult: **PO** 30 mg bid following a 5-day titration: *Day 1:* 10 mg in a.m.; *Day 2:* 10 mg bid; *Day 3:* 10 mg a.m., 20 mg p.m.; *Day 4:* 20 mg bid; *Day 5:* 20 mg a.m., 30 mg p.m.

Renal Impairment Dosage Adjustment

CrCl less than 30 mL/min: 30 mg once daily

ADMINISTRATION

Oral

- Administer without regard to food.
- Tablet **must not be** crushed, chewed, or divided.
- Store below 30°C (86°F).

ADVERSE EFFECTS Respiratory: Bronchitis, nasopharyngitis, upper respiratory tract infection. **CNS:** Depression, *headache,* insomnia, sinus headache, tooth abscess. **Endocrine:** Decreased appetite, decreased weight. **GI:** *Diarrhea,* dyspepsia, *nausea,* vomiting. **Musculoskeletal:** Abdominal pain upper, back pain. **Other:** Fatigue, folliculitis.

INTERACTIONS Drug: Strong CYP450 inducers (i.e., **rifampin**) decrease the levels of apremilast. **Herbal: St. John's wort** may decrease the levels of apremilast.

PHARMACOKINETICS Absorption: 73% bioavailable. **Peak:** 2.5 h. **Distribution:** 68% plasma protein bound. **Metabolism:** Hepatic oxidation and conjugation. **Elimination:** Renal (58%) and fecal (39%). **Half-Life:** 6–9 h.

NURSING IMPLICATIONS

Assessment & Drug Effects

- Monitor weight regularly during therapy. Report significant weight loss.
- Monitor for and report promptly signs or symptoms of depression, suicidal thoughts, or other significant mood changes.
- Monitor lab tests: Periodic renal function test.

Patient & Family Education

- Report promptly to prescriber if you experience any of the following: Excessive weight loss, suicidal thoughts, depression, anxiety, restlessness, irritability, panic attacks, or mood changes.

APREPITANT (Pr)

(a-pre′pi-tant)

Cinvanti, Emend

FOSAPREPITANT

(fos-a-pre′pi-tant)

Emend

Classification: CENTRAL ACTING MISCELLANEOUS; ANTIEMETIC; SUBSTANCE P/NEUROKININ 1 (NK_1) RECEPTOR ANTAGONIST

Therapeutic: ANTIEMETIC

AVAILABILITY Capsule; powder for injection; oral suspension

ACTION & *THERAPEUTIC EFFECT* Aprepitant is a selective substance P/neurokinin 1 (NK_1) receptor antagonist. Substance P and the NK-1 receptors are present in areas in the brain that control the emetic reflex. Aprepitant crosses the blood–brain barrier and occupies brain NK_1 receptors. Peripheral blockade by NK_1 receptor antagonists at receptors located in the GI is an additional hypothesized mechanism of action. *Aprepitant augments the antiemetic activity of the 5-HT_3-receptor antagonist, ondansetron, and inhibits both the acute and delayed phases of emesis induced by chemotherapy agents.*

USES Chemotherapy-induced nausea/vomiting, postoperative nausea/vomiting.

CONTRAINDICATIONS Hypersensitivity to aprepitant; pregnancy—fetal risk cannot be ruled out; lactation—infant risk cannot be ruled out.

CAUTIOUS USE Chemotherapeutic agents metabolized through CYP3A4; severe hepatic impairment; severe renal impairment without dialysis; children younger than 18 yr.

ROUTE & DOSAGE

Chemotherapy-Induced Nausea and Vomiting

Adult: **PO** 125 mg 1 h prior to chemotherapy, then 80 mg q a.m. for the next 2 days in conjunction with other antiemetics or 3 mg/kg (max: 125 mg/dose) 1 h prior to chemotherapy then 2 mg/kg (max: 80 mg/dose) daily for the next 2 days in conjunction with other antiemetics; **IV** (Emend IV) 150 mg on day 1; (Cinvanti IV) 130 mg 20 min prior to chemotherapy

Postoperative Nausea/Vomiting

Adult: **PO** 40 mg within 3 h of anesthesia induction

ADMINISTRATION

Oral

- Ensure that capsule is swallowed whole with a full glass of water. Do not crush or sprinkle the contents of the capsule.
- Can be given without regard to food.
- Swirl suspension when mixing. Do not shake.
- Give 1 h before start of chemotherapy.
- Store suspension in the refrigerator (36°–46°F or 2°–8°C) for up to 72 h. Suspension mixture may be kept at room temperature at 20°–25°C (68°–77°F) for up to 3 h before administration. Keep the desiccant in the original bottle.
- Store capsules at a controlled room temperature between 20° and 25°C (68° and 77°F).

Intravenous (Fosaprepitant)

PREPARE: **Infusion:** Inject 5 mL NS onto the inside of the 150 mg vial to prevent foaming. Swirl gently to dissolve. Withdraw contents of the vial and add to 145 mL NS.
ADMINISTER: **Infusion:** Infuse over 20–30 min. Longer infusion times may be used if patient complains of burning.

- Store vials refrigerated between 2° and 8°C (36° and 46°F). Vials can be stored at room temperature for up to 60 days. Do not freeze. At ambient room temperature, diluted solution is stable for up to 6 h in 0.9% sodium chloride and for up to 12 h in 5% dextrose. Under refrigeration, diluted solution is stable for up to 72 h in 0.9% sodium chloride or 5% dextrose.

ADVERSE EFFECTS (≥ 5%) **CV:** Hypotension. **Respiratory:** Cough, hiccoughs. **CNS:** Dizziness, headache. **Hepatic:** Increased AST and ALT. **GI**: *Constipation, diarrhea, nausea, abdominal pain.* **Hematologic:** Neutropenia, anemia. **Other:** Serious hypersensitivity reactions, serious infusion-related reactions including anaphylaxis and anaphylactic shock, *fatigue*, dehydration.

INTERACTIONS Drug: Increased risk of cardiovascular toxicity with **dofetilide, pimozide;** may decrease **warfarin** concentrations and INR; may decrease levels and effectiveness of ORAL CONTRACEPTIVES; **carbamazepine, griseofulvin, modafinil, rifabutin, rifapentine, phenobarbital, primidone** may decrease antiemetic efficacy; may increase levels of **dexamethasone.** Because aprepitant is a substrate of CYP3A4, many additional drug interactions are possible. Do not use with **eliglustat, flibanserin, lemborexant, lomitapide. Food: Grapefruit juice** may decrease effectiveness of aprepitant. **Herbal: St. John's wort** may decrease effectiveness of aprepitant.

PHARMACOKINETICS Absorption: 60–65% of oral dose reaches systemic circulation. **Peak:** 4 h. **Duration:** 95% protein bound; readily crosses the blood–brain barrier. **Metabolism:** In liver by CYP3A4. **Elimination:** Not renally excreted. **Half-Life:** 9–12 h.

NURSING IMPLICATIONS

Assessment & Drug Effects

- Monitor cardiac status especially with preexisting CV disease or concurrent use of any CYP3A4 substrate drug (e.g., ketoconazole, itraconazole, nefazodone, troleandomycin, clarithromycin).
- Monitor lab tests: PT/INR 7–10 days after 3-day regimen with concurrent warfarin use; phenytoin level with concurrent use; serum electrolytes, UA, and CBC.

Patient & Family Education

- Report immediately to prescriber any of the following: Skin rash; difficulty breathing or shortness of breath; rapid, slow, or irregular heartbeat; changes in BP; dizziness or confusion; unexplained sharp or severe pain in leg or stomach; rectal bleeding. Inform prescriber of all other drugs or herbal products you are using. Do not take new drugs (prescription, OTC, herbal) without first consulting prescriber.
- Use barrier contraception in addition to oral contraceptives while taking drug and one month after discontinuation of the drug.

ARGATROBAN (Prototype)

(ar-ga′tro-ban)

Classification: ANTICOAGULANT; DIRECT THROMBIN INHIBITOR
Therapeutic: ANTITHROMBOTIC; DIRECT THROMBIN INHIBITOR

AVAILABILITY Injection

ACTION & THERAPEUTIC EFFECT
A direct thrombin inhibitor capable of inhibiting the action of both free and clot-bound thrombin. *Reversibly binds to the thrombin active site, thereby blocking clot-forming activity of thrombin.*

USES Prophylaxis or treatment of thrombosis in patients with heparin-induced thrombocytopenia (HIT); prophylaxis or treatment of coronary artery thrombosis during percutaneous coronary interventions (PCI) in patients at risk for HIT.

CONTRAINDICATIONS

Hypersensitivity to argatroban. Any bleeding including intracranial bleeding, GI bleeding, retroperitoneal bleeding; pregnancy—fetal risk cannot be ruled out; lactation—infant risk cannot be ruled out. Safety and efficacy in children less than 18 yr have not been established.

CAUTIOUS USE

Diseased states with increased risk of hemorrhaging; severe hypertension; GI ulcerations, hepatic impairment; spinal anesthesia, stroke, surgery, trauma.

ROUTE & DOSAGE

Heparin-Induced Thrombocytopenia

Adult: **IV** 2 mcg/kg/min, may be adjusted to maintain an aPTT of 1.5–3 × baseline (max: 10 mcg/kg/min)

Hepatic Impairment Dosage Adjustment

0.5 mcg/kg/min, may be adjusted to maintain an aPTT of 1.5–3 × baseline (max: 10 mcg/kg/min)

Prophylaxis or Treatment of Coronary Thrombosis during PCI

Adult: **IV** Initiate at 25 mcg/kg/min, then bolus of 350 mcg/kg administered via a large bore IV line over 3–5 min, then 25 mcg/kg/min by continuous infusion; maintain activated clotting time (ACT) 300–450 sec; *if ACT below 300 sec:* Increase infusion to 30 mcg/kg/min; *if ACT over 450 sec:* Decrease infusion to 15 mcg/kg/min

ADMINISTRATION

Intravenous

Note: Argatroban **must be** diluted to 1 mg/mL prior to infusion.

PREPARE: **Continuous:** Dilute each 2.5 mL vial by mixing with 250 mL of D5W, NS, or LR to yield 1 mg/mL. ▪ Mix by repeated inversion of the diluent bag for 1 min.

ADMINISTER: **Continuous for Heparin-Induced Thrombocytopenia (HIT/HITTS):** Before administration, discontinue heparin and obtain a baseline aPTT. ▪ Give at a rate of 2 mcg/kg/min, or as ordered. Lower initial doses are required with hepatic impairment. ▪ Check aPTT 2 h after initiation of therapy. After the initial dose, adjust dose (not to exceed 10 mcg/kg/min) until the steady-state aPTT is 1.5 to 3 × baseline (not to exceed 100 sec). **Continuous for Percutaneous Coronary Intervention:** Start an infusion at 25 mcg/kg/min, and give a bolus of 350 mcg/kg, via a large bore IV line, over 3–5 min. ▪ Check ACT 5–10 min after the bolus dose. If the ACT is greater than 450 sec, decrease infusion rate to 15 mcg/kg/min. If ACT is less than 300 sec, give an additional bolus of 150 mcg/kg, and increase infusion to 30 mcg/kg/min. ▪ Check ACT q5–10 min to maintain an ACT level 300–450 sec.

▪ Store unopened vials in original carton at room temperature, 25°C (77°F), with excursions permitted between 15° and 30°C (59° and 86°F). Do not freeze. Protect from light. Discard the vial if solution appears cloudy or if insoluble precipitate is observed. ▪ Diluted solutions are stable for 24 h at 25°C (77°F) in ambient indoor light. ▪ Protect from direct

sunlight. Store solutions refrigerated at 2°–8°C (36°–46°F) in the dark. Diluted solutions are chemically stable up to 96 h.
INCOMPATIBILITIES: **Y-site:** **Cefepime, dantrolene, diazepam, phenytoin.**

ADVERSE EFFECTS (≥ 5%)

CV: Hypotension, cardiac arrest, chest pain. **Respiratory:** Dyspnea. **GI:** Diarrhea, nausea, vomiting. **Hematologic:** Major GI bleed, *minor GI bleeding, hematuria, decrease Hgb/Hct*, groin bleed, hemoptysis, brachial bleed. **Other:** Fever, backache, sepsis.

INTERACTIONS

Drug: Heparin results in increased bleeding; may prolong PT with **warfarin;** may increase risk of bleeding with ANTICOAGULANTS, THROMBOLYTICS, NSAIDS, or **vitamin E. Herbal: Feverfew, garlic, ginger, ginkgo** may increase potential for bleeding.

PHARMACOKINETICS

Peak: 1–3 h. **Distribution:** In extracellular fluid; 54% protein bound. **Metabolism:** In liver by CYP3A4/5. **Elimination:** Primarily in bile (78%). **Half-Life:** 39–51 min.

NURSING IMPLICATIONS

Assessment & Drug Effects

- **Heparin-Induced Thrombocytopenia:** Monitor aPTT. Dose adjustment may be needed to reach the target aPTT. Check aPTT 2 h after initiation of therapy. After the initial dose, adjust dose (not to exceed 10 mcg/kg/min), until the steady-state aPTT is 1.5 to 3 × baseline (not to exceed 100 sec).
- Monitor cardiovascular status carefully during therapy.
- Monitor for and report S&S of bleeding: Ecchymosis, epistaxis, GI bleeding, hematuria, hemoptysis.
- Note: Patients with history of GI ulceration, hypertension, recent trauma, or surgery are at increased risk for bleeding.
- Monitor neurologic status and report immediately focal or generalized deficits.
- Monitor lab tests: Baseline and periodic ACT with PCI; baseline and periodic aPTT with heparin-induced thrombocytopenia, platelet count, Hgb and Hct; daily INR when argatroban and warfarin are coadministered.

Patient & Family Education

- Report immediately any of the following to prescriber: Unexplained back or stomach pain; headache; fever; black, tarry stools; blood in urine, coughing up blood; difficulty breathing; dizziness or fainting spells; heavy menstrual bleeding; nosebleeds; unusual bruising or bleeding at any site.
- Monitor blood pressure at home and report low blood pressures to healthcare provider.

ARIPIPRAZOLE

(a-rip′i-pra-zole)

Abilify, Abilify Maintena, Aristada

Classification: ATYPICAL ANTIPSYCHOTIC; DOPAMINE SYSTEM STABILIZER

Therapeutic: ANTIPSYCHOTIC

Prototype: Clozapine

AVAILABILITY

Tablet; disintegrating tablets; oral solution; injection; extended release injection

ACTION & *THERAPEUTIC EFFECT*

Efficacy of aripiprazole may be mediated through a combination of partial agonist activity at D_2 and

5-HT_{1A} receptors and antagonist activity at 5-HT_{2A} receptors. *Partial dopaminergic agonist property of aripiprazole accounts for antipsychotic treatment of schizophrenic and bipolar individuals.*

USES Treatment of schizophrenia, bipolar disorder, treatment resistant major depressive disorder, irritability associated with autism, Tourette syndrome.

UNLABELED USES Agitation associated with psychiatric disorders.

CONTRAINDICATIONS Hypersensitivity to aripiprazole; dementia-related psychosis in elderly due to increased mortality; QT prolongation; suicidal ideation; neuroleptic malignant syndrome (NMS); severe neutropenia; pregnancy—fetal risk cannot be ruled out; lactation—infant risk cannot be ruled out.

CAUTIOUS USE History of seizures or conditions that lower seizure threshold (e.g., Alzheimer dementia); history of suicides; suicidal tendencies, depression; increased risk of suicidality in children, adolescents, and young adults; brain tumor; psychosis related to Alzheimer disease; patients driving or operating heavy machinery; DM; patients with known cardiovascular disease (history of MI or ischemic heart disease, heart failure, or conduction abnormalities), CVA, or conditions that predispose to hypotension (dehydration, hypovolemia, etc.); dysphagia; ethanol intoxication; hyperglycemia; DM; hypothermia; obesity, older adults; adults and children with severe depression; children younger than 10 yr with bipolar mania or schizophrenia, children younger than 6 yr with autistic disorder.

ROUTE & DOSAGE

Schizophrenia

Adult: **PO** 10–15 mg once daily, may increase at 1-wk intervals (max: 30 mg/day); **IM** 400 mg monthly *Adolescent/Child (10 yr or older):* **PO** 2 mg daily, increase to 5mg after 2 days, increase to 10 mg after 2 more days (max 30 mg/day)

Bipolar Disorder

Adult: **PO** 10–15 mg once daily; may increase dose in 5–10 mg/day increments based on response at 1-wk intervals (max 30 mg/day) **IM Abilify Maintena** 400 mg monthly
Adolescent/Child (10 yr or older): **PO** 2 mg daily, increase to 5 mg after 2 days, increase to 10 mg after 2 more days (max 30 mg/day)

Agitation Associated with Schizophrenia/Bipolar

Adult: **IM** 9.75 mg (range: 5.25–15 mg)

Major Depressive Disorder

Adult: **PO** 2–5 mg daily; may increase dose in 5-mg increments at 1-wk intervals (max 15 mg/day)

Irritability Associated with Autism

Adolescent/Child (6 yr or older): **PO** 2 mg daily x 7 days, then 5 mg/day can increase (max: 15 mg/day)

Tourette Syndrome

Child/Adolescent (6 yr or older, weight over 50 kg): **PO** 2 mg daily x 2 days then increase to 5 mg daily, then after 5 days increase to 10 mg daily (max 20 mg/day); *(6 yr or older, weight less than 50 kg):* **PO** *2 mg daily x 2 days then increase to 5 mg/day.*

Pharmacogenetic Dosage Adjustment

Reduced CYP2D6 expression (i.e., poor metabolizers): Reduce to 50% of usual dose

ADMINISTRATION

Oral

- Remove tablet from blister pack immediately before administration. Do not push the tablet through the foil because this could damage the tablet.
- Administer with or without regard to food.
- Orally disintegrating tablet should be given without water; however, if needed, liquid may be given. Do not split orally disintegrating tablet.
- Oral solution can be given up to 6 mo after opening, but should not exceed expiration date.
- Note that dose should be reduced by 50% with concurrent treatment with ketoconazole, quinidine, fluoxetine, or paroxetine.
- Store at 25°C (77°F). Excursions permitted to 15°–30°C (59°–86°F). Use within 6 mo of opening. Protect from light.

Intramuscular

- Inject slowly and deeply into a large muscle.
- Ensure that drug is not injected intravenously or subcutaneously.
- Make sure to rotate between deltoid and gluteal injection sites.
- Store vial at a controlled room temperature of 25°C (77°F), excursions permitted between 15° and 30°C (59° and 86°F). After reconstitution, keep at room temperature.

ADVERSE EFFECTS (≥ 5%) **CNS:** *Anxiety, agitation, insomnia, lightheadedness, somnolence, akathisia, headache,* tremor. **Endocrine:** Weight gain. **GI:** *Nausea, vomiting, constipation.* **Other:** Fever.

INTERACTIONS **Drug:** CYP3A4 inducers (**carbamazepine, phenytoin,** etc.) will decrease aripiprazole levels (may need to double aripiprazole dose); use with CYP2D6 or CYP3A4 inhibitors (**ketoconazole, quinidine, fluoxetine, paroxetine,** etc.) may increase aripiprazole levels (reduce dose by 50%); may cause additive sedation with other SEDATIVES (**alcohol, tramadol,** BARBITURATES, etc.); may enhance effects of ANTIHYPERTENSIVE AGENTS. Do not use with **fluconazole** or **dofetilide** due to risk of QT prolongation. Do not use with **amisulpride,** DOPAMINE AGONISTS, **azelastine.** **Herbal: St. John's wort** may decrease aripiprazole levels. **Food:** High fat meals may delay time to peak plasma levels.

PHARMACOKINETICS **Absorption:** 87% bioavailable. **Distribution:** Extensively protein bound. **Peak:** 3–5 h. **Metabolism:** In liver by CYP3A4 and 2D6. Major metabolite, has some activity. **Elimination:** 55% in feces, 25% in urine. **Half-Life:** 75 h (94 h for metabolite); 146 h (poor metabolizers).

NURSING IMPLICATIONS

Black Box Warning

Aripiprazole has been associated with increased mortality in the elderly with dementia-related psychosis, and suicidal thinking and behavior in children, adolescents, and young adults.

Assessment & Drug Effects

- Monitor for and report immediately worsening depression or suicidal ideation, especially in children, adolescents, and young adults.
- Fall risk assessment: Especially in the elderly patient.
- Monitor cardiovascular status. Assess for and report orthostatic hypotension. Take BP supine then in sitting position. Report systolic drop of greater than 15–20 mmHg. Patients at increased risk are those who are dehydrated, hypovolemic, or receiving concurrent antihypertensive therapy.
- Monitor for S&S of infection especially in elderly patients with dementia.
- Monitor body temperature in situations likely to elevate core temperature (e.g., exercising strenuously, exposure to extreme heat, receiving drugs with anticholinergic activity, or being subject to dehydration).
- Monitor for and report signs of tardive dyskinesia.
- Monitor for and immediately report S&S of neuroleptic malignant syndrome (NMS) (see Appendix F). Withhold drug if NMS is suspected.
- Monitor diabetics for loss of glycemic control.
- Monitor weight BMI, and waist circumference at baseline and at 4, 8, and 12 wk, then quarterly.
- Monitor lab tests: Periodic Hct, Hgb, and blood glucose; periodic CPK and myoglobinuria if NMS is suspected; frequent CBC with differential with history of low WBC or drug-induced low WBC.

Patient & Family Education

- Report promptly deterioration of mental status or behavior (especially suicidal ideation).
- Carefully monitor blood glucose levels if diabetic.
- Do not drive or engage in other potentially hazardous activities until reaction to drug is known.
- Avoid situations where you are likely to become overheated or dehydrated.
- Report any new or increased seizure activity.
- Report any new or increased gambling urges, sexual urges, compulsive eating or buying, or other urges.
- Report any high fevers, racing pulse, muscle rigidity, or altered mental status.
- Report any stiff or jerky movements of the face or body.
- Notify prescriber if you become pregnant or intend to become pregnant while taking this drug.

ASCORBIC ACID (VITAMIN C)

(a-skor'bate)

Ascor, Apo-C ♣, Cecon, Cevalin, CeVi-Sol ♣, Flavorcee, Redoxon ♣, Vita-C

Classification: VITAMIN

Therapeutic: VITAMIN SUPPLEMENT; URINARY ACIDIFIER

AVAILABILITY

Tablet; injection

ACTION & *THERAPEUTIC EFFECT*

Water-soluble vitamin essential for synthesis and maintenance of collagen and intercellular ground substance of body tissue cells, blood vessels, cartilage, bones, teeth, skin, and tendons. Humans are unable to synthesize ascorbic acid in the body therefore, it **must be** consumed daily. *Increases protective mechanism of* *the immune system, thus supporting wound healing and resistance to infection.*

USES Prophylaxis and treatment of scurvy and as a dietary supplement.

UNLABELED USES Methemoglobinemia, severe burns. Widely used as an antioxidant in formulations of parenteral tetracycline and other drugs.

CONTRAINDICATIONS Use of sodium ascorbate in patients on sodium restriction; use of calcium ascorbate in patients receiving digitalis.

CAUTIOUS USE Excessive doses in patients with G6PD deficiency; hemochromatosis, thalassemia, sideroblastic anemia, sickle cell anemia; patients prone to gout or renal calculi; pregnancy—fetal risk cannot be ruled out; lactation-infant risk cannot be ruled out.

ROUTE & DOSAGE

Vitamin C Deficiency
Adult: **PO** 100–300 mg daily; **IV/IM/Subcutaneous** 70–150 mg daily; *Child:* **PO/IV** 100–300 mg/day in divided doses mg/day

ADMINISTRATION

Oral

- Give oral solutions mixed with food.
- Dissolve effervescent tablet in a glass of water immediately before ingestion.

Intravenous

Verify correct IV concentration and rate of infusion for children with prescriber.

PREPARE: **Direct/Continuous/Intermittent:** Give diluted in solutions such as D5W, then add appropriate solutes to create an isotonic solution. ▪ Be aware that parenteral vitamin C is incompatible with many drugs. ▪ Consult pharmacist for compatibility information.

ADMINISTER: **Direct:** Give slowly. Avoid rapid IV injection. **Continuous/Intermittent (preferred):** Give at ordered rate determined by volume of solution to be infused.

INCOMPATIBILITIES: **Solution/additive:** **Bleomycin, nafcillin, sodium bicarbonate, theophylline.** **Y-site:** **Aminophylline, azathioprine, ceftazidime, ceftriaxone, chloramphenicol, dantrolene, diazepam, diazoxide, erythromycin, etomidate, ganciclovir, hydralazine, hydroxocobalamin, inamrinone, midazolam, minocycline, nitroprusside, papaverine, pentamidine, phenobarbital, phenytoin, propofol, sulfamethoxazole/trimethoprim.**

- Store solution in airtight, light-resistant, nonmetallic containers, away from heat and sunlight, preferably at 2–8°C (36–46°F), unless otherwise specified by manufacturer.
- Store oral tablet at room temperature.

ADVERSE EFFECTS **CNS:** Headache (high doses). **GI:** Nausea, vomiting, heartburn, diarrhea, or abdominal cramps (high doses). **GU:** Urethritis, dysuria, crystalluria, hyperoxaluria, or hyperuricemia (high doses). **Hematologic:** Acute hemolytic anemia (patients with deficiency of G6PD); sickle cell crisis. **Other:** Mild soreness at injection site; dizziness and temporary faintness with rapid IV administration.

DIAGNOSTIC TEST INTERFERENCE

High doses of ascorbic acid can produce false-negative results for ***urine glucose*** with ***glucose oxidase*** methods (e.g., ***Clinitest, TesTape, Diastix***); false-positive results with ***copper reduction methods*** (e.g., Benedict's solution, Clinitest). May produce false-negative tests for ***occult blood*** in stools if taken within 48–72 h of test.

INTERACTIONS

Drug: Large doses may attenuate hypoprothrombinemic effects of ORAL ANTICOAGULANTS; SALICYLATES may inhibit ascorbic acid uptake by leukocytes and tissues, Avoid use with **deferoxamine.**

PHARMACOKINETICS

Absorption: Readily absorbed PO; however, absorption may be limited with large doses. **Distribution:** Widely distributed to body tissues; crosses placenta; distributed into breast milk. **Metabolism:** In liver. **Elimination:** Rapidly in urine when plasma level exceeds renal threshold of 1.4 mg/dL.

NURSING IMPLICATIONS

Assessment & Drug Effects

- Monitor for S&S of acute hemolytic anemia, sickle cell crisis.
- Monitor lab tests: Periodic Hct, Hgb, renal function tests and serum electrolytes.

Patient & Family Education

- High doses of vitamin C are not recommended during pregnancy.
- Take large doses of vitamin C in divided amounts because the body uses only what is needed at a particular time and excretes the rest in urine.
- Megadoses can interfere with absorption of vitamin B_{12}.
- Note: Vitamin C increases the absorption of iron when taken at the same time as iron-rich foods.

ASENAPINE

(a-sin′a-peen)

Saphris, Secuado

Classification: ATYPICAL ANTIPSYCHOTIC; SEROTONIN ANTAGONIST;

Therapeutic: ANTIPSYCHOTIC; ANTIMANIC;

Prototype: Clozapine

AVAILABILITY

Sublingual tablet; transdermal patch

ACTION & *THERAPEUTIC EFFECT*

Mechanism of action thought to be related to antagonism of certain CNS dopamine (D_2) and serotonin ($5\text{-}HT_{2A}$) receptors. *Effect on serotonin and dopamine receptors may account for activity of asenapine against the negative symptoms of psychotic disorders.*

USES

Acute treatment of schizophrenia; acute treatment of manic or mixed episodes associated with bipolar disorder (bipolar I disorder).

CONTRAINDICATIONS

Dementia-related psychosis; ketoacidosis; severe neutropenia (ANC less than 1000/mm^3); patients with history of torsades de pointes related to drugs; suicidal ideation; severe hepatic impairment (Child–Pugh class C); pregnancy—fetal risk cannot be ruled out; lactation—infant risk cannot be ruled out.

CAUTIOUS USE

Tardive dyskinesia (especially women), cardiovascular disease (history of MI, ischemic heart disease, HF, conduction abnormalities, bradycardia), cerebrovascular disease, dehydration, hypovolemia, diabetes mellitus; history of seizures; Alzheimer dementia; older adults; history of suicidal tendencies. Use in children younger than 10 yr not established.

ROUTE & DOSAGE

Schizophrenia

Adult: **SL** 5 mg bid; increase up to 10 mg bid as tolerated **Transdermal:** 3.8 mg patch daily may increase to 5.7 mg after 1 wk.

Bipolar Disorder

Adult: **SL** Start at 5–10 mg bid, (max dose 10 mg bid).
Adolescent/Child (10 yr or older): **SL** 2.5 mg bid may increase after 3 days to 5 mg bid then after 3 days increase to 10 mg bid (max 10 mg bid)

ADMINISTRATION

Sublingual

- Tablet must be placed under tongue and allowed to dissolve completely.
- Ensure that tablet is not split, crushed, chewed, or swallowed.
- Eating and drinking should be avoided for 10 min after administration.
- Store at 15°–30°C (59°–86°F).

Transdermal

- Apply to clean, dry and intact skin on upper arm, upper back, abdomen, or hip.
- Rotate application to a different site each time.
- Replace the patch every 24 hours; only wear 1 patch at a time; if patch falls off, apply a new patch.
- Do not cut the patch.
- Showering is permitted, but avoid long exposure to external health sources. Use during swimming, or bathing has not been evaluated.
- Discard the used transdermal patch so that the adhesive sides stick to itself and safely discard.

ADVERSE EFFECTS (≥ 5%)

CNS: Agitation, inner restlessness, *dizziness, extrapyramidal symptoms, somnolence.* **Endocrine:** Hyperglycemia, increased serum cholesterol, triglycerides, increased weight. **GI:** Oral numbness or loss of sensitivity, constipation, dyspepsia, nausea, vomiting.

INTERACTIONS

Drug: Fluvoxamine and **imipramine** can increase asenapine levels. Do not use with medications that cause QT prolongation. Do not use with CNS DEPRESSANTS, DOPAMINE AGONISTS, **amisulpride, azelastine, metoclopramide, paroxetine, sulpiride.**

PHARMACOKINETICS

Absorption: Bioavailability 35%. **Peak:** 0.5–1.5 h. **Distribution:** 95% plasma protein bound. **Metabolism:** In liver via CYP1A2. **Elimination:** 50% renal; 40% fecal. **Half-Life:** 24 h (transdermal); 0.5–1.5 h (sublingual).

NURSING IMPLICATIONS

Black Box Warning

Asenapine has been associated with increased mortality in the elderly with dementia-related psychosis.

Assessment & Drug Effects

- Monitor for suicidal thoughts.
- Monitor BP, HR, and weight. Monitor orthostatic vital signs with concurrent antihypertensive therapy or any condition that predisposes to hypotension (e.g., advanced age, dehydration).
- Monitor for orthostatic hypotension and syncope, especially early in therapy.

- Monitor weight.
- Monitor for S&S of infection especially in elderly patients with dementia.
- Assess fall risk at initiation and recurrently during long-term use.
- Monitor diabetics or those at risk for diabetes for loss of glycemic control.
- Withhold drug and report promptly S&S of neuroleptic malignant syndrome (see Appendix F).
- Monitor lab tests: Baseline and periodic CBC, fasting glucose, lipid profile, LFTs.

Patient & Family Education

- Be alert for and report worsening of condition, including ideas of suicide.
- Make position changes slowly, especially from lying or sitting to a standing position.
- Limit activities and strenuous exercise in extreme heat and stay well hydrated.
- If using the transdermal patch, avoid exposing the patch to heat sources (e.g., Hair dryers, heating pads, electric blankets, heated water beds).
- Each time you place a new patch, remove the old one and place the new one in a different site.
- If diabetic, monitor blood sugar closely for loss of control.
- Monitor weight.
- Stop taking the drug and report immediately any of the following: High fever, muscle rigidity, altered mental status, or palpitations.
- Avoid engaging in hazardous activities until response to drug is known.
- Do not eat or drink for 10 minutes after taking the sublingual tablet.
- Avoid alcohol while taking this drug.

ASPIRIN (ACETYLSALICYLIC ACID) Pr

(as′pe-ren)

A.S.A., Bayer, Bayer Children's, Cosprin, Easprin, Ecotrin, Entrophen ♣, Halfprin, Measurin, Novasen ♣, ZORprin

Classification: NONNARCOTIC ANALGESIC, SALICYLATE; ANTIPYRETIC; ANTIPLATELET

Therapeutic: ANALGESIC; ANTIPYRETIC; ANTIPLATELET

AVAILABILITY Chewable tablet; tablet; enteric-coated tablet; caplet; extended release caplet; sustained release tablet; suppository

ACTION & *THERAPEUTIC EFFECT* Major action is primarily due to inhibiting the formation of prostaglandins involved in the production of inflammation, pain, and fever. **Anti-Inflammatory Action:** Inhibits prostaglandin synthesis. As an anti-inflammatory agent, aspirin appears to be involved in enhancing antigen removal and in reducing the spread of inflammatory substances. **Analgesic Action:** Principally peripheral with limited action in the CNS in the hypothalamus; results in relief of mild to moderate pain. **Antipyretic Action:** Suppress the synthesis of prostaglandin in or near the hypothalamus. Aspirin also lowers body temperature by indirectly causing centrally mediated peripheral vasodilation and sweating. **Antiplatelet Action:** Aspirin powerfully inhibits platelet aggregation. *Reduces inflammation, pain, and fever. Also inhibits platelet aggregation, reducing ability of blood to clot.*

USES To relieve pain of low to moderate intensity. Also for various inflammatory conditions, such as acute rheumatic fever, systemic lupus, rheumatoid arthritis, osteoarthritis, bursitis, and calcific tendonitis, and to reduce fever in selected febrile conditions. Used to reduce recurrence of TIA due to fibrin platelet emboli and risk of stroke in men; to prevent recurrence of MI; as prophylaxis against MI in men with unstable angina.

UNLABELED USES As prophylactic against thromboembolism; to prevent cataract and progression of diabetic retinopathy; and to control symptoms related to gluten sensitivity.

CONTRAINDICATIONS History of hypersensitivity to salicylates including methyl salicylate (oil of wintergreen); patients with "aspirin triad" (aspirin sensitivity, nasal polyps, asthma); chronic rhinitis; acute bronchospasm; nasal polyps, agranulocytosis; head trauma; increased intracranial pressure; intracranial bleeding; history of GI ulceration, bleeding, or other problems; hemophilia, or other bleeding disorders; severe renal or hepatic insufficiency; alcoholism; older adults; pregnancy fetal risk cannot be ruled out; children or teenagers for viral infections, with or without a fever because of association of Reye syndrome; lactation.

CAUTIOUS USE Otic diseases; gout; children with fever accompanied by dehydration; hyperthyroidism; immunosuppressed individuals; asthma; history of GI disease; history of gout; cardiac disease; G6PD deficiency; vitamin K deficiency; preoperatively; Hodgkin disease; alcohol use; hypoprothrombinemia; vitamin K deficiency; prematures, neonates, or children younger than 2 yr, except under advice and supervision of prescriber.

ROUTE & DOSAGE

Mild to Moderate Pain

Adult: **PO** 500–1000 mg q4–6h (max: 4 g/day)

Fever

Adult: **PO/PR** 350–650 mg q4h (max: 4 g/day)
Adolescent: **PO** 325–650 mg q4–6h (max: 4 g/day)

Arthritic Conditions

Adult: **PO** 3 g/day in 4–6 divided doses

Thromboembolic Disorders

Adult: **PO** 81–325 mg daily

TIA Prophylaxis

Adult: **PO** 160–325 mg within 48 h of event

MI Prophylaxis

Adult: **PO** 75–100 mg/day

ADMINISTRATION

Oral

- Give with a full glass of water (240 mL), milk, food, or antacid to minimize gastric irritation.
- Do not give to children or adolescents with chickenpox or flu-like symptoms.
- Enteric-coated tablets should not be crushed or chewed.

Rectal

- Ensure that suppository is inserted beyond the internal sphincter.
- Store at 15°–30°C (59°–86°F) in airtight container and dry environment unless otherwise directed by manufacturer. Store suppositories in a cool place or refrigerate but do not freeze.

ADVERSE EFFECTS **CV:** Cardiac arrhythmia, edema, hypotension, tachycardia. **Respiratory:** Asthma, bronchospasm, dyspnea, hyperventilation, laryngeal edema, noncardiogenic pulmonary edema, respiratory alkalosis, tachypnea. **CNS:** Agitation, cerebral edema, coma, confusion, dizziness, fatigue, headache, hyperthermia, insomnia, lethargy, Reye syndrome. **HEENT:** Hearing loss, tinnitus. **Endocrine:** Acidosis, dehydration, hyperglycemia, hyperkalemia, hypernatremia. **Skin:** Rash, urticaria. **Hepatic:** Hepatitis (reversible), hepatotoxicity. **GI:** Gastrointestinal ulcer, heartburn, nausea, stomach pain, vomiting. **GU:** Postpartum hemorrhage, prolonged gestation, prolonged labor, stillborn infant, increased blood urea nitrogen, increased serum creatinine, renal failure, renal insufficiency. **Musculoskeletal:** Acetabular bone destruction, rhabdomyolysis, weakness, coagulation. **Hematologic:** Anemia, blood disorder, hemolytic anemia, hemorrhage, prolonged prothrombin time, thrombocytopenia.

DIAGNOSTIC TEST INTERFERENCE Bleeding time is prolonged 3–8 days (life of exposed platelets) following a single 325-mg (5 grains) dose of aspirin. Large doses of salicylates equivalent to 5 g or more of aspirin per day may cause prolonged ***prothrombin time*** by decreasing prothrombin production. False-negative results for ***glucose oxidase urinary glucose tests*** (Clinistix); false-positives using the cupric sulfate method (Clinitest); also, interferes with Gerhardt test, VMA determination; 5-HIAA, xylose tolerance test, and T3 and T4; may lead to false-positive aldosterone/renin ratio.

INTERACTIONS **Drug: Aminosalicylic acid** increases risk of SALICYLATE toxicity. Use with **ketorolac** may result in increased GI effects. ACIDIFYING AGENTS decrease renal elimination and increase risk of SALICYLATE toxicity. ANTICOAGULANTS increase risk of bleeding. ORAL HYPOGLYCEMIC AGENTS increase hypoglycemic activity with aspirin doses greater than 2 g/day. CARBONIC ANHYDRASE INHIBITORS enhance SALICYLATE toxicity. CORTICOSTEROIDS add to ulcerogenic effects. **Methotrexate** toxicity is increased. Low doses of SALICYLATES may antagonize uricosuric effects of **probenecid** and **sulfinpyrazone. Herbal: Feverfew, garlic, ginger, ginkgo, evening primrose oil** may increase bleeding potential.

PHARMACOKINETICS **Absorption:** 80–100% absorbed (depending on formulation), primarily in stomach and upper small intestine. **Peak levels:** 15 min to 2 h (depending on form). **Distribution:** Widely distributed in most body tissues; crosses placenta. **Metabolism:** Aspirin is hydrolyzed to salicylate in GI mucosa, plasma, and erythrocytes; salicylate is metabolized in liver. **Elimination:** 50% of dose is eliminated in the urine; excreted into breast milk. **Half-Life:** Aspirin 20–60 min; salicylate 6 h (dose dependent).

NURSING IMPLICATIONS

Assessment & Drug Effects

- Monitor for loss of tolerance to aspirin. Symptoms usually occur 15 min to 3 h after ingestion: Profuse rhinorrhea, erythema, nausea, vomiting, intestinal cramps, diarrhea.
- Monitor closely the diabetic child for need to adjust insulin dose.

Children on high doses of aspirin are particularly prone to hypoglycemia (see Appendix F).

- Monitor for salicylate toxicity. In adults, a sensation of fullness in the ears, tinnitus, and decreased or muffled hearing are the most frequent symptoms.
- Monitor children for S&S of salicylate toxicity manifested by: hyperventilation, agitation, mental confusion, or other behavioral changes, drowsiness, lethargy, sweating, and constipation.

Patient & Family Education

- Use enteric-coated tablets, extended release tablets, buffered aspirin, or aspirin administered with an antacid to reduce GI disturbances.
- Discontinue aspirin use with onset of ringing or buzzing in the ears, impaired hearing, dizziness, GI discomfort or bleeding, and report to prescriber.
- Do not use aspirin for self-medication of pain (adults) beyond 5 days without consulting a prescriber. Do not use aspirin longer than 3 days for fever (adults and children), never for fever over 38.9°C (102°F) in older adults or 39.5°C (103°F) in children and adults under 60 yr or for recurrent fever without medical direction.
- Consult prescriber before using aspirin for any fever accompanied by rash, severe headache, stiff neck, marked irritability, or confusion (all possible symptoms of meningitis).
- Avoid alcohol when taking large doses of aspirin.
- Observe and report signs of bleeding (e.g., petechiae, ecchymoses, bleeding gums, bloody or black stools, cloudy or bloody urine).
- Maintain adequate fluid intake when taking repeated doses of aspirin.

ATAZANAVIR

(a-ta-zan'a-vir)

Reyataz

Classification: ANTIRETROVIRAL; PROTEASE INHIBITOR

Therapeutic: PROTEASE INHIBITOR

Prototype: Saquinavir

AVAILABILITY Capsule; oral powder

ACTION & *THERAPEUTIC EFFECT*

Selectively inhibits protease enzymes need for the replication of HIV and production of mature viruses; reduces the viral load and increases CD4+ cell count. *Protease inhibition renders the virus noninfectious. Because HIV protease inhibitors inhibit the HIV replication cycle midway in the process, they are active in acutely and chronically infected cells.*

USES Treatment of HIV infection in combination with other antiretroviral agents.

CONTRAINDICATIONS Previously demonstrated severe hypersensitivity reaction to atazanavir; severe hepatic insufficiency; ESRD with hemodialysis; Pregnancy: Fetal risk cannot be ruled out. Lactation: Infant risk cannot be ruled out. Not recommended for infants younger than 3 mo.

CAUTIOUS USE Mild to moderate hepatic impairment, hepatitis B or C; elevated bilirubin; severe renal impairment; DM; diabetic ketoacidosis; hemophilia, hepatic disease; hepatitis; jaundice; cholelithiasis, hypercholesterolemia, hypertriglyceridemia; preexisting conduction system disease (e.g., marked first-degree AV block or second- or third-degree AV block); obesity; older adults.

ROUTE & DOSAGE

HIV Infection

Adult/Adolescent/Child (older than 6 yr and weight greater than 40 kg): **PO** 400 mg once/day with a light meal OR 300 mg once/day with 100 mg of ritonavir
Adolescent/Child (6 yr or older and weight at least 25 kg): **PO** 300 mg plus ritonavir (100 mg) once daily
Adolescent/Child (6 yr or older and weight 15–35 kg): **PO** 200 mg plus ritonavir (100 mg) once daily *Child (3 mo or older, weight 15–25 kg):* **PO** 250 mg plus ritonavir (80 mg); *weight 5 kg to less than 10 kg:* **PO** 150 mg plus ritonavir (80 mg) once daily
Infant (3 mo or older, 5 kg to less than 15 kg): **PO** 200 mg (plus 80 mg ritonavir) daily

Hepatic Impairment Dosage Adjustment

Moderate impairment (Child-Pugh class B): Reduce dose to 300 mg once a day. *Severe impairment:* Not recommended for use.

ADMINISTRATION

Oral

- Give with a light meal, not on an empty stomach.
- **Do not** open capsules, they must be given whole.
- May mix oral powder in one tablespoon of food such as applesauce or yogurt. May mix with a minimum of 30 mL of liquid for infants who can drink from a cup. Follow with additional 15 mL to ensure complete dosage is given. For infants less than 6 mo, mix oral powder with infant formula and give using an oral dosing syringe. Draw up an additional 10 mL of infant formula to administer to ensure complete dosage is given. Administration using an infant bottle is not recommended because full dose may not be delivered. Once the powder is mixed, use within 1 h.
- When coadministered with didanosine buffered formulations, give atazanavir (with food) 2 h before or 1 h after didanosine.
- Give 2 h before/1 h after antacids or buffered drugs.
- Store at 15°–30°C (59°–86°F).

ADVERSE EFFECTS CV: Atrioventricular block. **Endocrine:** Hyperglycemia. **Skin:** Rash. **Hepatic:** Hyperbilirubinemia, jaundice, increased serum amylase. **GI:** Nausea. **Hematologic:** Decreased neutrophils.

INTERACTIONS Drug: There are extensive drug interactions reported; check the package insert for complete listing. May increase levels and toxicity of **nevirapine, maraviroc, pibrentasvir, glecaprevir, simvastatin, silodosin, romidepsin, etravirine, voxilaprevir, clarithromycin, fentanyl, cabazitaxel, tipranavir, lurasidone, rifabutin, and rosuvastatin.** Risk of virologic failure may occur with **nevirapine**. Risk of QT prolongation may occur with **mesoridazine, donepezil, hydroxychloroquine, clarithromycin. Atazanavir** levels may be decreased with concurrent **rifampin, famotidine, minocycline, fosamprenavir, tenofovir, efavirenz.** Use with **cyclophosphamide** may increase risk of neutropenia, infection or mucositis. Use with **diltiazem** may increase risk of cardiotoxicity. **Herbal: St. John's**

wort, garlic, red yeast rice may decrease atazanavir levels.

PHARMACOKINETICS Absorption: 68% into systemic circulation; taking with food enhances bioavailability. **Peak:** 2–2.5 h. **Metabolism:** In liver by CYP3A4. **Elimination:** 70% in feces, 13% in urine. **Half-Life:** 7 h.

NURSING IMPLICATIONS

Assessment & Drug Effects

- Monitor CV status and ECG closely, especially with concurrent treatment with other drugs known to prolong the PR interval.
- Monitor for and report promptly S&S of lactic acidosis (see metabolic acidosis, Appendix F).
- Monitor neonates and infants exposed to atazanavir in utero for severe hyperbilirubinemia during the first few days of life.
- Monitor lab tests: Baseline and periodic CD4+ cell count, HIV RNA viral load, and LFTs; total bilirubin if jaundiced; periodic PT/INR with concurrent warfarin therapy; frequent blood glucose, especially if diabetic.

Patient & Family Education

- Do not alter the dose or discontinue therapy without consulting prescriber.
- Inform prescriber of all prescription, nonprescription, or herbal meds being used.
- Report promptly any of the following: Dizziness or light-headedness; muscle pain (especially with concurrent statin therapy); severe nausea, vomiting (especially if red or "coffee-ground" in appearance), stomach pain, black tarry stools; yellowing of skin or whites of eyes; skin rash or itchy skin; sore throat, fever, or other S&S of infection; unexplained tiredness or weakness.
- If taking both sildenafil and atazanavir, promptly report any of the following sildenafil-associated adverse effects: Hypotension, visual changes, or prolonged penile erection.

ATENOLOL

(a-ten′oh-lole)

Tenormin

Classification: BETA-BLOCKER

Therapeutic: ANTIHYPERTENSIVE; ANTIANGINAL

Prototype: Propranolol

AVAILABILITY Tablet

ACTION & *THERAPEUTIC EFFECT*

Atenolol selectively blocks $beta_1$-adrenergic receptors located chiefly in cardiac muscle. Mechanisms for antihypertensive action include central effect leading to decreased sympathetic outflow to periphery, reduction in renin activity with consequent suppression of the renin–angiotensin–aldosterone system, and competitive inhibition of catecholamine binding at beta-adrenergic receptor sites. *Reduces rate and force of cardiac contractions (negative inotropic action); cardiac output is reduced as well as systolic and diastolic BP. Atenolol decreases peripheral vascular resistance both at rest and with exercise.*

USES Management of hypertension, treatment of stable angina pectoris, acute MI. Reduction of cardiovascular mortality and MI prophylaxis.

UNLABELED USES Antiarrhythmic, mitral valve prolapse, tremor, and migraine prophylaxis.

CONTRAINDICATIONS Sinus bradycardia, greater than first-degree heart block, uncompensated heart failure, cardiogenic shock, abrupt discontinuation, untreated pheochromocytoma; pregnancy (category D); lactation.

CAUTIOUS USE Hypertensive patients with CHF controlled by digitalis and diuretics, vasospastic angina (Prinzmetal angina); peripheral vascular disease; bronchospastic disease; asthma, bronchitis, emphysema, and COPD; major depression; diabetes mellitus; impaired renal function, dialysis; myasthenia gravis; pheochromocytoma, hyperthyroidism, thyrotoxicosis; older adults.

ROUTE & DOSAGE

Hypertension

Adult: **PO** 50 mg/day, may increase to 100 mg/day
Child: (1–17 yr): **PO** 0.5–1 mg/kg/day (max: 2 mg/kg/day)

Acute MI

Adult: **PO** 50 mg then 100 mg daily x 6–9 days or until hospital discharge

MI

Adult: **PO** Start 50 mg/day

Angina

Adult: **PO** 50 mg daily may increase to 100 mg daily

Reduction of CV Risk/MI

Adult: **PO** 100 mg/day in 1–2 divided doses

Renal Impairment Dosage Adjustment

CrCl 15–35 mL/min: Max dose: 50 mg/day; *less than 15 mL/min:* Max dose: 25 mg/day

ADMINISTRATION

Oral

- Crush tablets, if necessary, before administration and give with fluid of patient's choice. Administration with orange juice may lower bioavailability more significantly than other foods.
- When drug is discontinued, it should be tapered and not stopped abruptly.
- Store in tightly closed, light-resistant container at 20°–25° C (68°–77°F) unless otherwise directed.

ADVERSE EFFECTS **CV:** Bradyarrhythmia, cold extremities, *hypotension*. **CNS:** dizziness. **Other:** Depression, *fatigue*.

INTERACTIONS **Drug: Atropine** and other ANTICHOLINERGICS may increase atenolol absorption from GI tract; NSAIDS may decrease hypotensive effects; may mask symptoms of a hypoglycemic reaction induced by **insulin,** SULFONYLUREAS. Risk of bradycardia is increased by use of **dronedarone, diltiazem, verapamil, fenoldopam, clonidine, rivastigmine, fingolimod. Prazosin, terazosin** may increase severe hypotensive response to first dose of atenolol. May have additive electrophysiologic effects with **amiodarone.**

DIAGNOSTIC TEST INTERFERENCE Increased glucose; decreased HDL; may lead to false-positive aldosterone/renin ratio (ARR).

PHARMACOKINETICS **Absorption:** 50% of dose absorbed. **Peak:** 2–4 h. **Duration:** 24 h. **Distribution:** Does not readily cross blood–brain barrier. **Metabolism:** No hepatic metabolism. **Elimination:** 40–50% in urine; 50–60% in feces. **Half-Life:** 6–7 h.

NURSING IMPLICATIONS

Black Box Warning

Abruptly stopping atenolol in patients with angina may cause severe exacerbation of angina, MI, and ventricular arrhythmias.

Assessment & Drug Effects

- Measure trough BP (just prior to scheduled dose) to determine efficacy.
- Check apical pulse before administration in patients receiving digitalis (both drugs slow AV conduction). If below 60 bpm (or other ordered parameter), withhold dose and consult prescriber.
- Monitor BP throughout dosage adjustment period. Consult prescriber for acceptable parameters.
- Monitor diabetics for loss of glycemic control.
- Monitor renal function in geriatric patients.

Patient & Family Education

- Do not abruptly discontinue this drug.
- Adhere closely to dose regimen. Sudden discontinuation of drug can exacerbate angina and precipitate tachycardia or MI in patients with coronary artery disease, and thyroid storm in patients with hyperthyroidism.
- Make position changes slowly and in stages, particularly from recumbent to upright posture.
- If diabetic, closely monitor blood glucose values.

ATOMOXETINE

(a-to-mox′e-teen)

Strattera

Classification: MISCELLANEOUS PSYCHOTHERAPEUTIC

Therapeutic: ADHD AGENT

AVAILABILITY Capsule

ACTION & *THERAPEUTIC EFFECT* Selective inhibition of the presynaptic norepinephrine transporter, resulting in norepinephrine reuptake inhibition. *Improved attentiveness, ability to follow through on tasks with less distraction and forgetfulness, and diminished hyperactivity.*

USES Acute and maintenance treatment of attention-deficit/hyperactivity disorder (ADHD) in adults and children.

CONTRAINDICATIONS Hypersensitive to atomoxetine or any of its constituents; concomitant use or use within 2 wk of MAOIs; narrow-angle glaucoma; structural cardiac abnormalities or other serious heart problems; pheochromocytoma or history of pheochromocytoma; jaundice or liver injury; suicidal ideation; major depressive disorder (MDD); lactation.

CAUTIOUS USE Severe liver injury may progress to liver failure or death in a small percentage of patients. History of hypertension, tachycardia, cardiovascular or cerebrovascular disease; any condition that predisposes to hypotension; urinary retention or urinary hesitancy; history of bipolar disorder; history of suicidal tendencies; increased risk of suicidal ideation in children and adolescents; pregnancy (category C).

ROUTE & DOSAGE

ADHD

Adult/Adolescent/Child (older than 6 yr and weight greater than 70 kg): **PO** Start with 40 mg in morning. May increase after 3 days to target dose of 80 mg/day q.a.m. or as divided dose. May increase (max: 100 mg/day if needed)

Child/Adolescent (weight less than 70 kg): **PO** Start with 0.5 mg/kg/day. May increase after 3 days to target dose of 1.2 mg/kg/day. Administer q.a.m. or divided dose (max: 1.4 mg/kg or 100 mg, whichever is less)

Hepatic Impairment Dosage Adjustment

Child–Pugh class B: Initial and target doses should be reduced to 50% of the normal dose

Child–Pugh class C: Initial dose and target doses should be reduced to 25% of normal dose

Pharmacogenetic Dosage Adjustment/Patients Receiving Concurrent CYP2D6 Inhibitors

CYP2D6 poor metabolizers: Children/adolescents (weight less than 70 kg): Start at 0.5 mg/kg, adjust upward only after 4 wk if well tolerated; *adults/adolescents (weight greater than 70 kg):* Start at 40 mg/day, adjust upward only after 4 wk if well tolerated; do not exceed 80 mg

ADMINISTRATION

Oral

- Note that total daily dose in children and adolescents is based on weight. Determine that ordered dose is appropriate for weight prior to administration of drug.
- Note manufacturer recommends dosage adjustments with concomitant administration of strong CYP2D6 inhibitors (e.g., paroxetine, fluoxetine, quinidine). Consult prescriber.
- Store at 15°–30°C (59°–86°F).

ADVERSE EFFECTS **CV:** Increased blood pressure, sinus tachycardia, palpitations. **Respiratory:** *Cough,* rhinorrhea, nasal congestion, sinusitis. **CNS:** Dizziness, *headache,* somnolence, crying, tearfulness, irritability, mood swings, *insomnia,* depression, tremor, early morning awakenings, paresthesias, abnormal dreams, decreased libido, sleep disorder, suicidal ideation. **HEENT:** Mydriasis. **Endocrine:** Hot flushes, sexual dysfunction, weight loss. **Skin:** Dermatitis, pruritus, increased sweating. **Hepatic:** Hepatotoxicity. **GI:** *Upper abdominal pain,* constipation, dyspepsia, *nausea, vomiting, decreased appetite,* anorexia, dry mouth, diarrhea, flatulence, severe liver injury (rare). **GU:** Urinary hesitation/retention, dysmenorrhea, ejaculation dysfunction, impotence, delayed onset of menses, irregular menstruation, prostatitis; priapism, male pelvic pain. **Musculoskeletal:** Arthralgia, myalgia. **Other:** Flu-like syndrome, flushing, fatigue, fever, rigors.

INTERACTIONS **Drug: Albuterol** may potentiate cardiovascular effects of atomoxetine; CYP2D6 inhibitors (**fluoxetine, paroxetine, quinidine**) may increase atomoxetine levels and toxicity; MAOIS may precipitate a hypertensive crisis; may attenuate effects of ANTIHYPERTENSIVE AGENTS.

PHARMACOKINETICS **Absorption:** Well absorbed from GI tract. **Distribution:** 98% protein bound. **Peak:** 1–2 h. **Metabolism:** In liver by CYP2D6. **Elimination:** Primarily in urine. **Half-Life:** 5.2 h.

NURSING IMPLICATIONS

Black Box Warning

Atomoxetine has been associated with increased suicidal thinking and behavior in children and adolescents.

Assessment & Drug Effects

- Evaluate for continuing therapeutic effectiveness especially with long-term use.
- Report increased aggression and irritability, as these may indicate a need to discontinue the drug.
- Monitor children and adolescents for behavior changes that may indicate suicidal ideation, including aggression and anxiety that may be precursors of it.
- Monitor cardiovascular status especially with preexisting hypertension.
- Monitor HR and BP at baseline, following a dose increase, and periodically while on therapy.
- Monitor lab tests: Periodic LFTs.

Patient & Family Education

- Instruct patients on S&S of liver toxicity.
- Report any of the following to the prescriber: Indicators of suicidal ideation in children and adolescents; chest pains or palpitations, urinary retention or difficulty initiating voiding urine, appetite loss and weight loss, or insomnia.
- Make position changes slowly if you experience dizziness with arising from a lying or sitting position.
- Do not drive or engage in potentially hazardous activities until reaction to the drug is known.

ATORVASTATIN CALCIUM

(a-tor-va'sta-tin)

Lipitor

Classification: REDUCTASE INHIBITOR (STATIN)

Therapeutic: ANTILIPEMIC; STATIN
Prototype: Lovastatin

AVAILABILITY Tablet

ACTION & THERAPEUTIC EFFECT

An inhibitor of HMG-CoA, an enzyme essential to hepatic production of cholesterol; increases the number of hepatic LDL receptors, thus increasing LDL uptake and catabolism. *Atorvastatin reduces LDL and total triglyceride (TG) production as well as increases the plasma level of high-density lipids (HDL).*

USES Adjunct to diet for the reduction of LDL cholesterol and triglycerides in patients with primary hypercholesterolemia, hypertriglyceridemia, and mixed dyslipidemia, prevention of cardiovascular disease in patients with multiple risk factors.

CONTRAINDICATIONS Hypersensitivity to atorvastatin, myopathy, active liver disease, unexplained persistent transaminase elevations, hepatic encephalopathy, hepatitis, active hepatic disease; jaundice, rhabdomyolysis; uncontrolled seizure disorders; pregnancy or women who may become pregnant; lactation.

CAUTIOUS USE Hypersensitivity to other HMG-CoA reductase inhibitors, history of liver disease, older adults; uncontrolled hypothyroidism, diabetes mellitus, renal impairment; patients with previous history of stroke; patients with ALS; patients who consume substantial quantities of alcohol; surgery. Safety and efficacy in children younger than 10 yr not established.

ROUTE & DOSAGE

Hypercholesterolemia/Prevention of Cardiovascular Disease

Adult: **PO** Start with 10–40 mg daily, may increase up to 80 mg/day

Child/Adolescent (10 to younger than 17 yr): **PO** Start with 10 mg daily, may increase up to 20 mg/day

ADMINISTRATION

Oral

- May be given at any time of day with or without food.
- Store at 20°–25°C (68°–77°F).

ADVERSE EFFECTS **Respiratory:** Nasopharyngitis. **CNS:** Insomnia. **Endocrine:** Diabetes mellitus. **GI:** Diarrhea, nausea, indigestion. **GU:** UTIs. **Musculoskeletal:** Joint, muscle, and limb pain. **Other:** Pain.

INTERACTIONS **Drug:** Risk of myopathy increases if used with **posaconazole, ritonavir, fosamprenavir, letermovir, pibrentasvir, lopinavir, gemfibrozil, erythromycin, saquinavir.** Atorvastatin concentrations may increase with **nelfinavir, telaprevir, tipranavir, elbasvir, simeprevir.** May increase **digoxin** levels 20%, increases levels of **norethindrone; erythromycin** may increase atorvastatin levels 40%; Concurrent use of **lopinavir** or **ritonavir** requires decrease of dose of **atorvastatin.** **Food: Grapefruit juice** (greater than 1 qt/day) may increase risk of myopathy and rhabdomyolysis. Fiber may decrease effect, separate doses.

PHARMACOKINETICS **Absorption:** Rapidly from GI tract. 30% reaches the systemic circulation. **Onset:** Initial effects with 48 h. **Peak:** Plasma concentration, 1–2 h; effect 2–4 wk. **Distribution:** 98% or greater protein bound. Crosses placenta, distributed into breast milk of animals. **Metabolism:** In the liver by CYP3A4 to active metabolites. **Elimination:** Primarily in bile; **Half-Life:** 14 h; 20–30 h for active metabolites.

NURSING IMPLICATIONS

Assessment & Drug Effects

- Monitor for therapeutic effectiveness, which is indicated by reduction in the level of LDL-C. Monitor diabetics for loss of glycemic control.
- Assess for muscle pain, tenderness, or weakness; and, if present, monitor CPK level (discontinue drug with marked elevations of CPK or if myopathy is suspected).
- Monitor carefully for digoxin toxicity with concurrent digoxin use.
- Monitor prediabetics and diabetics for loss of glycemic control.
- Monitor lab tests: Lipid levels within 2–4 wk after initiation of therapy or upon change in dosage; LFTs at 6 and 12 wk after initiation or elevation of dose, and periodically thereafter; periodic HbgA1c.

Patient & Family Education

- Report promptly any of the following: Unexplained muscle pain, tenderness, or weakness, especially with fever or malaise; yellowing of skin or eyes; stomach pain with nausea, vomiting, or loss of appetite; skin rash or hives.
- Do not take drug during pregnancy because it may cause birth defects. Immediately inform prescriber of a suspected or known pregnancy.

- Inform prescriber regarding concurrent use of any of the following drugs: Erythromycin, niacin, antifungals, or birth control pills.
- Minimize alcohol intake while taking this drug.
- Do not eat large amounts of grapefruit or drink more than 1 L/day of grapefruit juice.

ATOVAQUONE

(a-to′va-quone)

Mepron

Classification: ANTIPROTOZOAL

Therapeutic: ANTIPROTOZOAL

AVAILABILITY Oral suspension

ACTION & *THERAPEUTIC EFFECT* Atovaquone is an antiprotozoal with antipneumocystic activity, including *Pneumocystis carinii* (PCP) and the *Plasmodium* species. The site of action in PCP is linked to inhibition of the electron transport system in the mitochondria. This results in the inhibition of nucleic acid and ATP synthesis. *Effective against* P. carinii *and the* Plasmodium *species, as well as other protozoans.*

USES Mild to moderate *P. jirovecii* pneumonia (PCP) in immunocompromised patients intolerant of co-trimoxazole.

UNLABELED USES May be effective in the treatment of cerebral toxoplasmosis.

CONTRAINDICATIONS History of potential life-threatening allergies to atovaquone, pregnancy—fetal risk cannot be ruled out, lactation—infant risk cannot be ruled out.

CAUTIOUS USE Severe PCP, concurrent pulmonary diseases, older adults, impaired hepatic function; gastric disorders.

ROUTE & DOSAGE

***Pneumocystis Jirovecii* Pneumonia (PJP)**

Adult: **PO** 750 mg bid or 1500 once daily 21 days

ADMINISTRATION

Oral

- Give with meals because food significantly enhances absorption.
- Shake suspension well before each use.
- Store at room temperature 15°–25°C (59°–77°F) unless otherwise directed by the manufacturer. Do not freeze.

ADVERSE EFFECTS (≥ 5%) **Respiratory:** Cough, *rhinitis*, sinusitis. **CNS:** *Headache*, insomnia. **Skin:** Rash, pruritus. **Hepatic:** Increased liver enzymes. **GI:** *Diarrhea, nausea*, vomiting. **Other:** Fever.

DIAGNOSTIC TEST INTERFERENCE May cause increase in **amylase** and other **liver function tests.**

INTERACTIONS **Drug:** Concurrent **ritonavir, efavirenz** or RIFAMYCINS may reduce **atovaquone** serum levels. **Zidovudine** may increase risk of bone marrow toxicity. **Food:** Oral absorption is increased 3- to 4-fold when administered with food, especially with fatty foods.

PHARMACOKINETICS **Absorption:** 47% bioavailable. **Duration:** 6–23 wk after a 3-wk course of therapy. **Distribution:** Penetrates poorly into cerebrospinal fluid; greater than 99.9% protein bound. **Metabolism:** Not metabolized. **Elimination:** Greater than 94% in feces over 21 days (enterohepatically cycled). **Half-Life:** 2–3 days.

NURSING IMPLICATIONS

Assessment & Drug Effects

- Assess for therapeutic failure in patients with GI disorders that may limit absorption of drug.
- Monitor respiratory function, chest films and sputum staining with microscopy.
- Monitor lab tests: Periodic CBC with differential, arterial blood gases, blood glucose, serum sodium, LFTs in patients with known hepatic impairment, creatinine, BUN, and serum amylase.

Patient & Family Education

- Take this drug with meals.
- Note: It is necessary to take this drug exactly as prescribed because it is slowly eliminated from the body.
- Review adverse effects with the patient and or family: Rash, nausea, vomiting diarrhea, headache, cough, runny nose, insomnia, and fever.

ATOVAQUONE/PROGUANIL HYDROCHLORIDE

(a-to′va-quone/pro′gua-nil)

Malarone

Classification: ANTIMALARIAL

Therapeutic: ANTIMALARIAL

Prototype: Chloroquine

AVAILABILITY Tablets

ACTION & *THERAPEUTIC EFFECT* Combination of two antimalarial drugs. Atovaquone inhibits electron transport system in mitochondria of the malaria parasite, thus interfering with nucleic acid and ATP synthesis of the parasite. Proguanil interferes with DNA synthesis of the malaria parasite. *This drug combination has synergistic activity toward malarial treatment because each component has a different mode of action.*

USES Prevention and treatment of malaria due to *P. falciparum,* even in chloroquine-resistant areas.

CONTRAINDICATIONS Known hypersensitivity to atovaquone or proguanil; severe malaria. Pregnancy—fetal risk cannot be ruled out, lactation—infant risk cannot be ruled out.

CAUTIOUS USE Cerebral malaria, complicated malaria, pulmonary edema; renal failure, renal impairment; hepatic disease; lactation; older adults; African Americans, Chinese, Japanese; diarrhea, emesis, GI disease; hepatic disease, infection, sunlight (UV) exposure.

ROUTE & DOSAGE

Prevention of Malaria

Adult: **PO** 250-mg/100-mg tablet daily with food starting 1–2 days before travel to malarial area, through travel and continuing for 7 days after return

Child **PO** Dose varies based on weight; confirm dosing with package insert

Treatment of Malaria

Adult: **PO** 1000-mg/400-mg single daily dose for 3 days

Child **PO** Dose varies based on weight; confirm dosing with package insert

ADMINISTRATION

Oral

- Give at the same time each day with food or a drink containing milk.

- Give a repeat dose if vomiting occurs within 1 h after dosing.

ADVERSE EFFECTS **Respiratory:** Cough. **CNS:** *Headache*, dizziness, weakness and fatigue. **Skin:** Pruritus. **Hepatic:** Increased LFTs. **GI:** *Nausea, abdominal pain, diarrhea*, dyspepsia.

INTERACTIONS **Drug: Rifampin, rifabutin, tetracycline** may decrease serum levels; **metoclopramide** may decrease absorption. Do not use with **dapsone, efavirenz, lumefantrine.**

PHARMACOKINETICS **Absorption: Atovaquone (A),** Poor, absorption improved when taken with a fatty meal; **Proguanil (P),** Extensively absorbed. **Duration: A,** 6–23 wk after a 3-wk course of therapy. **Distribution: A,** Penetrates poorly into cerebrospinal fluid; greater than 99.9% protein bound; **P,** 75% protein bound. **Metabolism: A,** Not metabolized; **P,** Metabolized by CYP2C19 to cycloguanil. **Elimination: A,** Greater than 94% in feces over 21 days (enterohepatically cycled); **P,** Primarily in urine. **Half-Life: A,** 2–3 days; **P,** 12–21 h.

NURSING IMPLICATIONS

Assessment & Drug Effects

- Monitor for S&S of parasitemia in patients receiving tetracycline and in those experiencing diarrhea or vomiting.
- Note: Only use metoclopramide to control vomiting if other antiemetics are not available.
- Monitor lab tests: Periodic LFTs, especially with long-term therapy, parasitemia in patients who are vomiting.

Patient & Family Education

- Take this drug at the same time each day for maximum effectiveness with a milky drink.
- Note: Absorption of this drug may be reduced with diarrhea and vomiting. Consult prescriber if either of these occurs.
  - If vomiting occurs within of 1 hour of taking the drug, take a second dose, and notify provider if vomiting continues.

ATRACURIUM BESYLATE

(a-tra-kyoor'ee-um)

Classification: NONPOLARIZING SKELETAL MUSCLE RELAXANT; NEUROMUSCULAR ANTAGONIST

Therapeutic: SKELETAL MUSCLE RELAXANT

AVAILABILITY Solution for injection

ACTION & *THERAPEUTIC EFFECT* Inhibits neuromuscular transmission by binding competitively with acetylcholine at muscle end plate receptors. *Synthetic skeletal muscle relaxant that produces short duration of neuromuscular blockade, exhibits minimal direct effects on cardiovascular system, and has less histamine-releasing action.*

USES Adjunct for general anesthesia to produce skeletal muscle relaxation during surgery; to facilitate endotracheal intubation. Especially useful for patients with severe renal or hepatic disease, limited cardiac reserve, and in patients with low or atypical pseudocholinesterase levels.

CONTRAINDICATIONS Myasthenia gravis.

CAUTIOUS USE When appreciable histamine release would be hazardous (as in asthma or anaphylactoid reactions, significant cardiovascular disease), neuromuscular disease (e.g., Eaton–Lambert syndrome), carcinomatosis, electrolyte or acid–base imbalances, dehydration, impaired pulmonary function; pregnancy (category C); lactation; children younger than 1 mo.

ROUTE & DOSAGE

Skeletal Muscle Relaxation

Adult/Child (2 yr or older): **IV** 0.4–0.5 mg/kg initial dose, then 0.08–0.1 mg/kg bolus 20–45 min after the first dose and q15–25 min thereafter; reduce doses if used with general anesthetics
Child (1 mo to less than 2 yr): **IV** 0.3–0.4 mg/kg

Mechanical Ventilation

Adult: **IV** 5–9 mcg/kg/min by continuous infusion

ADMINISTRATION

- Verify correct concentration and rate of infusion for infants and children with prescriber.

Intravenous

PREPARE: **Direct:** Give initial bolus dose undiluted. **Continuous:** Maintenance dose **must be** diluted with NS, D5W, or D5/NS. Maximum concentration should be 0.5 mg/mL. Do not mix in same syringe or administer through same needle as used for alkaline solutions [incompatible with alkaline solutions (e.g., barbiturates)].
ADMINISTER: **Direct:** Give as bolus dose over 30–60 sec. **Continuous:** Give infusion at rate required to maintain desired effect.

INCOMPATIBILITIES: **Solution/additive:** **Lactated Ringer's, aminophylline, cefazolin, heparin, nitroprusside, sodium nitroprusside.** **Y-site:** **Aminophylline, amphotericin B, cefonicid, cefoperazone, cefoxitin, ceftazidime, dantrolene, diazepam, diazoxide, furosemide, ganciclovir, indomethacin, pantoprazole, pentobarbital, phenobarbital, phenytoin, propofol, sodium bicarbonate.**

- Store at 2°–8°C (36°–46°F) to preserve potency unless otherwise directed. Avoid freezing.

ADVERSE EFFECTS **CV:** Bradycardia, tachycardia. **Respiratory:** Respiratory depression. **Other:** Increased salivation, anaphylaxis.

INTERACTIONS **Drug:** GENERAL ANESTHETICS increase magnitude and duration of neuromuscular blocking action; AMINOGLYCOSIDES, **bacitracin, polymyxin B, clindamycin, lidocaine, parenteral magnesium, quinidine, quinine, trimethaphan, verapamil** increase neuromuscular blockade; DIURETICS may increase or decrease neuromuscular blockade; **lithium** prolongs duration of neuromuscular blockade; NARCOTIC ANALGESICS present possibility of additive respiratory depression; **succinylcholine** increases onset and depth of neuromuscular blockade; **phenytoin** may cause resistance to or reversal of neuromuscular blockade.

PHARMACOKINETICS **Onset:** 2 min. **Peak:** 3–5 min. **Duration:** 60–70 min. **Distribution:** Well distributed to tissues and extracellular fluids; crosses placenta; distribution into breast milk unknown. **Metabolism:** Rapid nonenzymatic degradation in bloodstream. **Elimination:** 70–90% in urine in 5–7 h. **Half-Life:** 20 min.

NURSING IMPLICATIONS

Assessment & Drug Effects

- Note: Personnel and equipment required for endotracheal intubation, administration of oxygen under positive pressure, artificial respiration, and assisted or controlled ventilation **must be** immediately available.
- Evaluate degree of neuromuscular blockade and muscle paralysis to avoid risk of overdosage by qualified individual using peripheral nerve stimulator.
- Monitor BP, pulse, and respirations, and evaluate patient's recovery from neuromuscular blocking (curare-like) effect as evidenced by ability to breathe naturally or to take deep breaths and cough, keep eyes open, lift head keeping mouth closed, adequacy of hand-grip strength. Notify prescriber if recovery is delayed.
- Note: Recovery from neuromuscular blockade usually begins 35–45 min after drug administration and is almost complete in about 1 h. Recovery time may be delayed in patients with cardiovascular disease, edematous states, and in older adults.
- Monitor lab tests: Baseline serum electrolytes, acid–base balance, and renal function tests.

ATROPINE SULFATE (Pr)

(a'troe-peen)

Atropen, Atropair ♣

Classification: ANTICHOLINERGIC; ANTIMUSCARINIC; ANTIARRHYTHMIC

Therapeutic: ANTISECRETORY; ANTIARRHYTHMIC; BRONCHODILATOR

AVAILABILITY Solution for injection, ophthalmic ointment, ophthalmic drops

ACTION & THERAPEUTIC EFFECT Acts by selectively blocking all muscarinic responses to acetylcholine (ACh). Antisecretory action (vagolytic effect) suppresses sweating, lacrimation, salivation, and secretions from nose, mouth, pharynx, and bronchi. Blocks vagal impulses to heart causing decreased AV conduction time, increased HR and cardiac output, and shortened PR interval. *Potent bronchodilator when bronchoconstriction has been induced by parasympathomimetics, and decreases bronchial secretions. Decreases GI spasm. Produces mydriasis and cycloplegia by blocking responses of iris sphincter muscle and ciliary muscle of lens to cholinergic stimulation. Increases heart rate and cardiac output.*

USES Antidote for anticholinesterase poisoning, treatment of symptomatic sinus bradycardia. **Ophthalmic Use:** To produce mydriasis and cycloplegia before refraction and for treatment of anterior uveitis and iritis. **Preoperative Use:** To suppress salivation, perspiration, and respiratory tract secretions.

CONTRAINDICATIONS Hypersensitivity to belladonna alkaloids; angle-closure glaucoma; parotitis; intestinal atony, paralytic ileus, achalasia, pyloric stenosis, obstructive diseases of GI tract, severe ulcerative colitis, toxic megacolon; tachycardia; acute hemorrhage; myasthenia gravis, pregnancy—fetal risk cannot be ruled out, lactation—infant risk cannot be ruled out.

CAUTIOUS USE Myocardial infarction, hypertension, hypotension;

coronary artery disease, CHF, tachy-arrhythmias; gastric ulcer, hiatal hernia with reflux esophagitis; hyperthyroidism; COPD; autonomic neuropathy; hepatic or renal disease; debilitated patients; Down syndrome; autonomic neuropathy, spastic paralysis, brain damage in children; patients exposed to high environmental temperatures; patients with fever; BPH; older adults; infants.

ROUTE & DOSAGE

Preanesthesia

Adult: **IV/IM/Subcutaneous** 0.4–1 mg 30–60 min before surgery; repeat Q4h PRN (max **total** dose 3 mg)
Child/Infant: **IV/IM/Subcutaneous** 0.02 mg/kg/dose (max dose: 0.5 mg/dose); 30–60 minutes before surgery; repeat q4–6 h PRN; maximum **total** dose: 1 mg/procedure

Bradycardia

Adult: **IV/IM** 0.5 mg q3–5min (max: 3 mg)
Adolescent/Child: **IV/IM** 0.02 mg/kg (max dose 0.5 mg); may repeat once in 5 min

Organophosphate Antidote

Adult: **IV/IM** 1–6 mg repeat q3–5 min PRN; double dose until muscarinic signs and symptoms subside (may need up to 50 mg); **IM** (Atropen) 2 mg as soon as exposure is known; can administer 2 additional doses in rapid succession 10 min after first dose.
Child/Infant: **IV/IM** 0.05 mg/kg q5—10 min until muscarinic signs and symptoms subside; repeat q5–10 min PRN

Cycloplegia

Adult: **Ophthalmic** 1 drop of solution or small amount of ointment in eye 1 h before the procedure
Child: **Ophthalmic** 1 drop in eye 40 min prior to maximum dilation time

ADMINISTATION

Ocular

- Use a gloved finger to compress the lacrimal sac for 2–3 min after instillation to prevent excessive systemic absorption.
- Store ointment between 15° and 30°C (59° and 86°F). Store solution between 15° and 25°C (59° and 77°F).

Subcutaneous/Intramuscular

- Inject undiluted. When using AtroPen, inject into the outer thigh at a 90-degree angle.
- Store auto-injector at controlled room temperature of 25°C (77°F) with excursions between 15° and 30°C (59° and 86°F). Do not freeze. Protect from light.

Intravenous

PREPARE: **Direct:** Give undiluted or diluted in up to 10 mL of sterile water.
ADMINISTER: **Direct:** Give 1 mg or fraction thereof over 1 min directly into a Y-site.
INCOMPATIBILITIES: **Solution/additive: Pantoprazole. Y-site: Amphotericin B (conventional), dantrolene, diazepam, diazoxide, pantoprazole, phenytoin, SMZ/TMP, thiopental.**

- Store at room temperature 20°–25°C (68°–77°F) in protected airtight, light-resistant containers unless otherwise directed by manufacturer.

ADVERSE EFFECTS **CV:** Hypertension or hypotension, ventricular tachycardia, palpitation, paradoxical bradycardia, AV dissociation, atrial or ventricular fibrillation. **Respiratory:** Respiratory depression. **HEENT:** Mydriasis, blurred vision, photophobia, eye dryness, local redness, glaucoma. **GI:** Dry mouth with thirst, constipation. **GU:** Urinary hesitancy and retention.

DIAGNOSTIC TEST INTERFERENCE **Upper GI series:** Findings may require qualification because of anticholinergic effects of atropine (reduced gastric motility and delayed gastric emptying). **PSP excretion test:** Atropine may decrease urinary excretion of PSP (phenolsulfonphthalein).

INTERACTIONS **Drug:** **Amantadine,** ANTIHISTAMINES, ANTICHOLINERGICS, TRICYCLIC ANTIDEPRESSANTS, **quinidine, disopyramide, procainamide** add to anticholinergic effects. **Levodopa** effects decreased. **Methotrimeprazine** may precipitate extrapyramidal effects. Antipsychotic effects of PHENOTHIAZINES are decreased due to decreased absorption. Avoid use with **clozapine, eluxadoline** due to increased risk of constipation. Therapeutic effect of **levosulpiride, macimorelin, secretin, sincalide.** Avoid use with **potassium chloride.**

PHARMACOKINETICS **Absorption:** Well absorbed from all administration sites. Peak effect: 30 min IM, 2–4 min IV, 1–2 h subcutaneous. **Duration:** Inhibition of salivation 4 h. **Distribution:** In most body tissues; crosses blood–brain barrier and placenta. **Metabolism:** In liver. **Elimination:** 77–94% in urine in 24 h. **Half-Life:** adult 2–3 h.

NURSING IMPLICATIONS

Assessment & Drug Effects

- Monitor vital signs. HR is a sensitive indicator of patient's response to atropine. Be alert to changes in quality, rate, and rhythm of HR and respiration and to changes in BP and temperature.
- Initial paradoxical bradycardia following IV atropine usually lasts only 1–2 min; it most likely occurs when IV is administered slowly (more than 1 min) or when small doses (less than 0.5 mg) are used. Postural hypotension occurs when patient ambulates too soon after parenteral administration.
- Note: Frequent and continued use of eye preparations, as well as overdosage, can have systemic effects. Some atropine deaths have resulted from systemic absorption following ocular administration in infants and children.
- Monitor I&O, especially in older adults and patients who have had surgery (drug may contribute to urinary retention).
- Monitor CNS status. Older adults and debilitated patients sometimes manifest drowsiness or CNS stimulation (excitement, agitation, confusion) with usual doses of drug or other belladonna alkaloids. Supervision of ambulation may be indicated.
- Monitor infants, small children, and older adults for "atropine fever" (hyperpyrexia due to suppression of perspiration and heat loss), which increases the risk of heatstroke.
- Patients receiving atropine via inhalation sometimes manifest mild CNS stimulation with doses in excess of 5 mg and mental depression and other mental disturbances with larger doses.

Patient & Family Education

- Follow measures to relieve dry mouth: Adequate hydration; small, frequent mouth rinses with tepid water; meticulous mouth and dental hygiene; gum chewing or sucking sugarless sourballs.
- Note: Drug causes drowsiness, sensitivity to light, blurring of near vision, and temporarily impairs ability to judge distance. Avoid driving and other activities requiring visual acuity and mental alertness.
- Discontinue ophthalmic preparations and notify prescriber if eye pain, conjunctivitis, palpitation, rapid pulse, or dizziness occurs.
- Notify provider if unable to void urine.

AURANOFIN

(au-rane'eh-fin)

Ridaura

Classification: GOLD COMPOUND; IMMUNOLOGIC; ANTI-INFLAMMATORY; ANTIRHEUMATIC

Therapeutic: ANTI-INFLAMMATORY; ANTIRHEUMATIC

AVAILABILITY Capsule

ACTION & *THERAPEUTIC EFFECT* Strongly lipophilic and almost neutral in solution, properties that may facilitate transport across cell membranes. Has immunomodulatory and anti-inflammatory effects, although mechanism of action is not understood. Gold is taken up by macrophages possibly causing inhibition of phagocytosis and lysosomal enzyme release resulting in an anti-inflammatory effect. Gold also causes decreased serum immunoglobulin concentrations and rheumatoid factor titers resulting in immunomodulatory effect. *Auranofin is immunomodulatory and anti-inflammatory.*

USES Management of rheumatoid arthritis.

CONTRAINDICATIONS History of gold-induced necrotizing enterocolitis, renal disease, exfoliative dermatitis or bone marrow aplasia; recent radiation therapy, history of severe toxicity from previous exposure to gold or other heavy metals; uncontrolled CHF; marked hypertension; SLE; pregnancy—fetal risk cannot be ruled out; lactation—infant risk cannot be ruled out.

CAUTIOUS USE Inflammatory bowel disease, rash, liver disease, renal disease; history of bone marrow depression; pulmonary disorders, older adults; DM; CHF.

ROUTE & DOSAGE

Rheumatoid Arthritis

Adult: **PO** 6 mg/day in 1–2 divided doses, may increase to 6–9 mg/day in 3 divided doses after 6 mo (max: 9 mg/day)

ADMINISTRATION

Oral

- Give capsule with food or fluid of patient's choice.
- Store at 15°–30°C (59°–86°F); protect from light and moisture.
- Note: Expiration date is 3 yr after date of manufacture.

ADVERSE EFFECTS (≥ 5%) **HEENT:** *Conjunctivitis* **Skin:** *Rash, pruritus,* dermatitis, urticaria. **GI:** *Diarrhea;* vomiting, anorexia, dysphagia; *stomatitis.* **GU:** Proteinuria.

INTERACTIONS Drug: No significant interactions.

PHARMACOKINETICS Absorption: 25% from small intestine. **Peak:** 2 h. **Distribution:** Highest concentrations in kidneys, spleen, lungs, adrenals, and liver; unknown if crosses placenta; small amounts distributed into breast milk. **Elimination:** 60% of absorbed gold eliminated in urine, remainder in feces. **Half-Life:** 21–31 days.

NURSING IMPLICATIONS

Black Box Warning

Gold toxicity, manifested by bone marrow suppression, proteinuria, hematuria, pruritus, rash, stomatitis, and persistent diarrhea may occur.

Assessment & Drug Effects

- Monitor for therapeutic effectiveness, which develops slowly and is not usually apparent for 3–4 mo.
- Report any of the following S&S promptly: Unexplained bleeding or bruising, metallic taste, sore mouth; pruritus, rash; diarrhea and melena; yellow skin and sclera; unexplained cough or dyspnea.
- Monitor lab tests: Periodic CBC with differential and platelet count; periodic LFTs and renal function tests.

Patient & Family Education

- Report adverse effects of therapy, especially abdominal cramping and pain; discontinuance of therapy may be necessary.
- Report metallic taste persistent diarrhea and pruritus with or without rash. These are among earliest symptoms of impending gold toxicity.
- Do not change dosage (dose or dose interval) by omission, increase, or decrease without first consulting prescriber.
- Use antidiarrheal OTC drug and high-fiber diet for drug-induced diarrhea.
- Avoid exposure to sunlight or to artificial ultraviolet light to prevent photosensitivity reaction.
- Rinse mouth with water frequently for symptomatic treatment of mild stomatitis. Avoid commercial mouth rinses; clean teeth with soft toothbrush and gentle brushing to avoid gingival trauma. Floss at least once daily.
- Notify provider of cough, fever, chills, or rash.

AVANAFIL

(a-van'a-fil)

Stendra

Classification: PHOSPHODIESTERASE (PDE) INHIBITOR; IMPOTENCE AGENT

Therapeutic: IMPOTENCE AGENT

Prototype: Sildenafil

AVAILABILITY Tablet

ACTION & THERAPEUTIC EFFECT

Enhances the effect of nitric oxide (NO) release in the corpus cavernosum during sexual stimulation. NO causes increased levels of cGMP, producing smooth muscle relaxation in the corpus cavernosum and allowing inflow of blood into the penis. NO inhibits PDE5, an enzyme responsible for degrading cGMP in the corpus cavernosum. *Promotes sustained erection only in the presence of sexual stimulation.*

USES Treatment of erectile dysfunction.

CONTRAINDICATIONS

Hypersensitivity to avanafil; severe hepatic impairment (Child–Pugh class C); severe renal impairment (CrCl less than 30 mL/min).

CAUTIOUS USE

Preexisting cardiovascular disease; bleeding disorders; active peptic ulcer disease; mild-to-moderate renal or hepatic impairment; alcohol consumption; concurrent antihypertensive drugs; pregnancy (category C). Safety and efficacy in children younger than 18 yr not established.

ROUTE & DOSAGE

Erectile Dysfunction

Adult: **PO** 50–100 mg 30 min prior to sexual activity (max: 200 mg once daily); *Concurrent moderate CYP34A inhibitor:* Max dose: 50 mg/24 h

ADMINISTRATION

Oral

- May be given without regard to food.
- Should be taken only once daily.
- Store at 20°–30°C (77°–86°F).

ADVERSE EFFECTS

CV: Abnormal electrocardiogram, hypertension. **Respiratory:** Bronchitis, nasal congestion, nasopharyngitis, sinus congestion, sinusitis, upper respiratory tract infection. **CNS:** Dizziness, headache. **GI:** Constipation, diarrhea, dyspepsia, nausea. **Musculoskeletal:** Arthralgia, back pain. **Other:** Back pain, flushing, influenza, rash.

INTERACTIONS

Drug: Coadministration with **alcohol,** ALPHA$_1$ ANTAGONISTS (i.e., **doxazosin, terazosin**), ANTIHYPERTENSIVE AGENTS (i.e., **amlodipine, enalapril**), **sodium nitroprusside** or ORGANIC NITRATES (i.e., **isosorbide mononitrate, nitroglycerin**) may cause an excessive decrease in blood pressure. Strong (i.e., **atazanavir, clarithromycin, indinavir, itraconazole, ketoconazole, nefazodone, nelfinavir, ritonavir, saquinavir, telithromycin**) and moderate (i.e., **aprepitant, diltiazem, erythromycin, fluconazole, fosamprenavir, verapamil**) inhibitors of CYP3A4 can increase the levels of avanafil. **Food: Grapefruit juice** may increase the levels of avanafil.

PHARMACOKINETICS

Onset: 30–45 min. **Distribution:** 99% plasma protein bound. **Metabolism:** Hepatic transformation to active and inactive compounds. **Elimination:** Fecal (62%) and renal (21%). **Half-Life:** 5 h.

NURSING IMPLICATIONS

Assessment & Drug Effects

- Monitor cardiac response to drug, including changes in BP and HR.
- Assess for and report promptly sudden loss of vision, decrease or loss of hearing, or tinnitus.

Patient & Family Education

- Take no more than once daily.
- Ensure that prescriber has a complete list of all other concurrent medications.

- Report promptly painful erections or prolonged erections lasting 4 h or longer.
- Stop taking drug and seek immediate medical attention for any of the following: Sudden decrease or loss of hearing, with or without tinnitus and dizziness; sudden loss of vision.
- Reduce or eliminate alcohol consumption when using this drug.

AXITINIB

(ax-i′ti-nib)

Inlyta

Classification: ANTINEOPLASTIC; TYROSINE KINASE INHIBITOR

Therapeutic: ANTINEOPLASTIC

Prototype: Erlotinib

AVAILABILITY Tablet

ACTION & THERAPEUTIC EFFECT

Inhibits receptor tyrosine kinases, including vascular endothelial growth factor receptors. These receptors are implicated in pathologic angiogenesis and tumor growth. Thought to inhibit renal tumor growth and cancer progression.

USES Treatment of advanced renal cell carcinoma.

CONTRAINDICATIONS Hypertensive crisis; active brain hemorrhage; recent GI bleeding or perforation; within 24 h of elective surgery; reversible posterior leukoencephalopathy syndrome (RPLS); pregnancy; lactation.

CAUTIOUS USE Hypertension; heart failure; hepatic impairment; renal impairment; mild-to-moderate proteinuria; history of CVA, TIA, MI, or retinal artery occlusion; wound healing complications; hypo- and hyperthyroidism; history of grade 3 or 4 venous thrombosis; wound healing complications; hypo- and hyperthyroidism; history of GI bleeding. Safety and efficacy in children younger than 18 yr not established.

ROUTE & DOSAGE

Renal Cell Carcinoma

Adult: **PO** 5 mg bid; can titrate up to 10 mg bid or down to 2 mg bid

Hepatic Impairment Dosage Adjustment

Moderate impairment (Child–Pugh Class B): Reduce starting dose to approximately half

ADMINISTRATION

Oral

- National Institute of Safety and Health (NIOSH) recommends use of single gloves when handling tablets or capsules or administering from a unit-dose package.
- May be given without regard to food.
- Ensure that tablets are swallowed whole with sufficient water.
- Do not re-administer if patient vomits; wait until next scheduled dose.
- Store at 20°–25°C (68°–77°F).

ADVERSE EFFECTS **CV:** *Hypertension.* **Respiratory:** Cough, dyspnea. **CNS:** *Fatigue, voice disorder,* headache. **Endocrine:** *Decreased serum bicarbonate, hypocalcemia, hyperglycemia, weight loss,* hypothyroidism, hypernatremia, hyperkalemia, hypoalbuminemia, hyponatremia, hypophosphatemia, hypoglycemia. **Skin:** *Palmar-plantar erythrodysesthesia,* xeroderma. **Hepatic/GI:** *Increased serum ALP,* increased serum ALT, increased serum AST, *diarrhea, decreased appetite, nausea,* increased serum lipase, *increased serum amylase,* vomiting, constipation, mucosal inflammation, stomatitis, abdominal pain, dyspepsia. **GU:** Proteinuria, *increased serum creatinine.* **Hematologic:** Anemia, *lymphocytopenia,* hemorrhage, thrombocytopenia, leukopenia.

INTERACTIONS **Drug:** Strong CYP3A4/5 inhibitors (i.e., **atazanavir, clarithromycin, indinavir, itraconazole, ketoconazole, nefazodone, nelfinavir, ritonavir, saquinavir, telithromycin**) may increase the levels of axitinib. Strong (i.e., **carbamazepine, dexamethasone, phenobarbital, phenytoin, rifabutin, rifampin, rifapentine**) and moderate (i.e., **bosentan, efavirenz, etravirine, modafinil, nafcillin**) CYP3A4/5 inducers may decrease the levels of axitinib. **Food: Grapefruit** or **grapefruit juice** may increase the levels of axitinib. **Herbal: St. John's wort** may decrease the levels of axitinib.

PHARMACOKINETICS **Absorption:** 58% bioavailability. **Peak:** 2.5–4.1 h. **Distribution:** 99% plasma protein bound. **Metabolism:** Extensive hepatic metabolism (CYP P450 3A4/5 (CYP3A4), CYP2C19, CYP1A2). **Elimination:** Fecal (41%) and renal (23%). **Half-Life:** 2.5–6.1 h.

NURSING IMPLICATIONS

Assessment & Drug Effects

- Monitor BP at baseline and frequently throughout therapy.
- Assess for and report promptly S&S suggestive of thromboembolic events (e.g., DVT, TIA, chest pain).
- Monitor for and report promptly S&S of hemorrhage, GI perforation, or fistula formation.
- Monitor lab tests: Baseline and periodic thyroid function tests, LFTs, CBC with differential, serum electrolytes, serum glucose, and urinalysis for proteinuria.
- Perform pregnancy test prior to therapy in females of reproductive potential.

Patient & Family Education

- Frequent monitoring of BP is recommended throughout therapy.
- Exercise caution with activities that could result in bleeding.
- Report promptly any of the following: Unexplained bleeding episodes; persistent or severe abdominal pain; any neurologic deficit (e.g., seizure, confusion, visual disturbances, frequent or severe headaches).
- Men and women should use effective means of birth control during therapy.
- Contact your prescriber immediately if you or your partner becomes pregnant during treatment.
- Do not breastfeed while receiving this drug.

AZACITIDINE

(a-za-ci'ti-deen)

Vidaza

Classification: ANTINEOPLASTIC; ANTIMETABOLITE (PYRIMIDINE)

Therapeutic: ANTINEOPLASTIC

Prototype: Fluorouracil

AVAILABILITY Powder for injection

ACTION & THERAPEUTIC EFFECT Promotes hypomethylation of DNA, restoring normal gene differentiation and proliferation. Also exerts direct toxicity to abnormal hematopoietic cells in the bone marrow. *Cytotoxic effects of azacitidine cause the death of rapidly dividing cancer cells that are no longer responsive to normal growth control mechanisms.*

USES Treatment of myelodysplastic syndrome, specifically refractory anemia.

UNLABELED USES Acute myelogenous leukemia.

CONTRAINDICATIONS Hypersensitivity to azacitidine or mannitol; advanced malignant hepatic tumors, myelodysplastic syndrome with hepatic impairment; hepatotoxicity; vaccination; active infection; dental work; intramuscular injections, if platelets are less than 50,000 mm^3; pregnancy (category D); lactation.

CAUTIOUS USE Hypoalbuminemia (less than 3 g/dL), hepatic disease; bone marrow depression; dental disease; history of varicella zoster or other herpes infections; renal impairment, renal failure; older adults. Safety and efficacy in children not established.

ROUTE & DOSAGE

Myelodysplastic Syndrome

Adult: **Subcutaneous/IV** 75 mg/m^2 once daily for 7 days repeat every 4 wk; may increase to 100 mg/m^2 if no beneficial response is seen after 2 treatment cycles and no toxicity other than nausea and vomiting has occurred

Myelosuppression Dosage Adjustment

See package insert

ADMINISTRATION

Subcutaneous

- Reconstitute by slowly injecting 4 mL of sterile water for injection into 100-mg vial to yield 25 mg/mL. Invert 2–3 times and gently rotate until a uniform suspension is achieved. The suspension will be cloudy. If not used immediately, see directions for storage.
- Doses greater than 4 mL should be divided equally into 2 syringes and injected into 2 separate sites. Rotate sites for each injection (thigh, abdomen, or upper arm). Give subsequent injections at least 1 in. from an old site and never into areas where the site is tender, bruised, red, or hard.
- Storage: Reconstituted suspension may be kept in the vial or syringe. May refrigerate for up to 8 h. Before use, suspension may be kept at room temperature for up to 30 min. Resuspend by inverting the syringe 2–3 times and gently roll between the palms for 30 sec immediately before administration.

Intravenous

PREPARE: Reconstitute vial with 10 mL SWFI to form a 10-mg/mL solution. Vigorously shake or roll vial until solution is dissolved and clear. Mix in 50–100 mL NS or lactated Ringer's injection for infusion.

ADMINISTER: **Intermittent:** Infuse over 10–40 min; infusion must be completed within 1 h of reconstitution.

INCOMPATIBILITIES: **Solution/Admixture:** **Sodium bicarbonate, D5W, normal saline, Lactated Ringer's, hetastarch.**

ADVERSE EFFECTS **CV:** Peripheral edema, chest pain, heart murmur. **Respiratory:** Cough, dyspnea, pharyngitis, epistaxis, nasopharyngitis, upper respiratory infection, pneumonia, crackles, rhinorrhea. **CNS:** *Fatigue, rigors,* headache, dizziness, anxiety, depression, malaise, pain, insomnia. **HEENT:** Gingival hemorrhage. **Endocrine:** *Fever,* weight loss, hypokalemia. **Skin:** Erythema, pallor, skin lesion, skin rash, pruritus, diaphoresis, injection site reactions. **GI:** *Nausea, vomiting, constipation, diarrhea,* anorexia, abdominal pain, abdominal tenderness. **Musculoskeletal:** *Weakness,* arthralgia, limb pain, back pain, myalgia. **Hematologic:** *Thrombocytopenia, anemia, neutropenia, leukopenia,* lymphadenopathy, bruising, petechia, bone marrow depression.

INTERACTIONS **Drug:** Do not use with LIVE VACCINES. Use of **tacrolimus, pimecrolimus** may increase side effects.

PHARMACOKINETICS **Peak:** 30 min. **Metabolism:** In liver. **Elimination:** By kidneys. **Half-Life:** 4 h.

NURSING IMPLICATIONS

Assessment & Drug Effects

- Monitor for S&S of drug toxicity in those with renal insufficiency.
- Withhold drug and notify prescriber for any of the following: S&S of hepatic or renal insufficiency; lab values that indicate leukopenia, neutropenia, thrombocytopenia, or hepatic or renal insufficiency; or serum bicarbonate levels less than 20 mEq/L.
- Monitor lab tests: Baseline LFTs, electrolytes, and serum BUN and creatinine; baseline and periodic CBC with differential.

Patient & Family Education

- Promptly report S&S of infection or indication of unusual bleeding tendencies (e.g., dark, tarry stools and easy bruising).
- Women should avoid becoming pregnant and men should not father a child while taking this drug.

AZATHIOPRINE

(ay-za-thye′oh-preen)

Azasan, Imuran

Classification: IMMUNOSUPPRESSANT

Therapeutic: IMMUNOSUPPRESSANT; ANTI-INFLAMMATORY

Prototype: Cyclosporine

AVAILABILITY Tablet; powder for injection

ACTION & *THERAPEUTIC EFFECT* Antagonizes purine metabolism and appears to inhibit DNA, RNA, and normal protein synthesis in rapidly growing cells. *Suppresses T cell effects before transplant rejection. Has immunosuppressant and anti-inflammatory properties.*

USES Adjunctive agent to prevent rejection of kidney allografts. Also used in patients with active rheumatoid arthritis.

UNLABELED USES SLE, lupus nephritis, Crohn disease, pemphigus, nephrotic syndrome, hepatitis, immune thrombocytopenia, multiple sclerosis, myasthenia gravis, psoriasis, uveitis and other inflammatory and immunologic diseases.

CONTRAINDICATIONS Hypersensitivity to azathioprine or mercaptopurine; clinically active infection, immunization of patient or close family members with live virus vaccines; anuria; pancreatitis; patients previously treated with alkylating agents (increased risk of neoplasms), concurrent radiation therapy; development of GI toxicity to drug; pregnancy (category D); lactation.

CAUTIOUS USE Impaired kidney and liver function; MG; serious infections. Safety and efficacy in children not established.

ROUTE & DOSAGE

Kidney Transplant Rejection

Adult: **PO** 3–5 mg/kg/day initially, may be able to reduce to 1–3 mg/kg/day; **IV** 3–5 mg/kg/day initially, may be able to reduce to 1–3 mg/kg/day; switch to **PO**

Rheumatoid Arthritis

Adult: **PO** 1 mg/kg/day initially, may be increased by 0.5 mg/kg/day at 6-wk intervals if needed up to 2.5 mg/kg/day; then reduce dose every 4 wk until lowest effective dose is reached

Obesity Dosage Adjustment

Doses calculated on IBW

Renal Impairment Dosage Adjustment

CrCl 10–50 mL/min: Administer 75% of normal dose; *less than 10 mL/minute:* Administer 50% of normal dose

ADMINISTRATION

Oral

- Give oral drug in divided doses (as prescribed) with food or immediately after meals to minimize gastric disturbances.

Intravenous

PREPARE: **Direct/Intermittent:** Reconstitute by adding 10 mL sterile water for injection into vial; swirl until dissolved. May be given as prepared or further diluted with 50 mL NS, D5W, or D5/NS. ▪ Reconstituted solution may be stored at room temperature but **must be** used within 24 h after reconstitution (contains no preservatives).

ADMINISTER: **Direct/Intermittent:** May infuse over 30 min to 8 h. Typical infusion time is 30–60 min or longer. If longer infusion time is ordered, the final volume of the IV solution is increased appropriately. Check with prescriber.

INCOMPATIBILITIES: **Y-site: amikacin, aminophylline, ampicillin/sulbactam, ascorbic acid, aztreonam, bumetanide, buprenorphine, butorphanol, calcium chloride,** CEPHALOSPORINS, **chloramphenicol, chlorpromazine, cimetidine, clindamycin, dantrolene, diazepam, diazoxide, diphenhydramine, dobutamine, dopamine, doxycycline, ephedrine, epinephrine, esmolol, famotidine, ganciclovir, gentamicin, haloperidol, hydralazine, hydrocortisone, hydroxyzine, imipenem/cilastin, isoproterenol, ketorolac, labetalol, lidocaine, magnesium sulfate, meperidine, metaraminol, midazolam, minocycline, morphine, nafcillin, nalbuphine, netilmicin, nitroprusside, norepinephrine, ondansetron, papaverine, pentamidine, pentazocine, phenylephrine,**

phenytoin, piperacillin, procainamide, prochlorperazine, promethazine, pyridoxine, ritodrine, rocuronium, sodium bicarbonate, streptokinase, succinylcholine, sulfamethoxazole/trimethoprim, tacrolimus, theophylline, thiamine, ticarcillin, tobramycin, tolazoline, vancomycin, verapamil.

- Store at 15°–30°C (59°–86°F) in tightly closed, light-resistant containers unless otherwise directed.

ADVERSE EFFECTS **CNS:** Malaise. **Hepatic:** Hepatotoxicity, increased serum alkaline phosphatase, increased serum bilirubin. **GI:** Nausea, vomiting. **Musculoskeletal:** Myalgia. **Hematologic:** *Leukopenia*, neoplasia, thrombocytopenia. **Other:** Fever, increased susceptibility to infection.

DIAGNOSTIC TEST INTERFERENCE Azathioprine may decrease plasma and urinary ***uric acid*** in patients with gout.

INTERACTIONS **Drug: Allopurinol, febuxostat, pimecrolimus, ribavirin** increases effects and toxicity of azathioprine. **Tubocurarine** and other NONDEPOLARIZING SKELETAL MUSCLE RELAXANTS may reverse or inhibit neuromuscular blocking effects. **Cyclosporine** concentrations may be decreased. ACE INHIBITORS may cause anemia or leukopenia.

PHARMACOKINETICS **Absorption:** Readily from GI tract. **Distribution:** Crosses placenta. **Metabolism:** Extensively in liver to active metabolite mercaptopurine. **Elimination:** In urine. **Half-Life:** 3 h.

NURSING IMPLICATIONS

Black Box Warning

Chronic use of azathioprine has been associated with development of lymphoma.

Assessment & Drug Effects

- Monitor therapeutic efficacy, which usually requires 6–8 wk of therapy for patients with rheumatoid arthritis (improvement in morning stiffness and grip strength). If no improvement has occurred after 12-wk trial period, drug is generally discontinued.
- Monitor for toxicity. Drug has a high toxic potential. Because it may have delayed action, dosage should be reduced or drug withdrawn at the first indication of an abnormally large or persistent decrease in leukocyte or platelet count.
- Monitor vital signs. Report signs of infection.
- Monitor I&O ratio; note color, character, and specific gravity of urine. Report an abrupt decrease in urinary output or any change in I&O ratio.
- Monitor for signs of abnormal bleeding [easy bruising, bleeding gums, petechiae, purpura, melena, epistaxis, dark urine (hematuria), hemoptysis, hematemesis]. If thrombocytopenia occurs, invasive procedures should be withheld, if possible.
- Monitor lab tests: Baseline CBC with differential and platelet count, then weekly during 1st mo, and twice during both 2nd and 3rd mo, or more frequently if indicated (e.g., by dosage or therapy changes); periodic LFTs and renal function tests throughout therapy.

Patient & Family Education

- Chronic use of this drug has been associated with development of blood cancers in patients with inflammatory bowel disease.

- Avoid contact with anyone who has a cold or other infection and report signs of impending infection. Exercise scrupulous personal hygiene because infection is a constant hazard of immunosuppressive therapy.
- Practice birth control during therapy and for 4 mo after drug is discontinued. This drug is associated with potential hazards in pregnancy.
- Do not receive/take vaccinations or other immunity-conferring agents during therapy because they may precipitate unusually severe reactions due to the immunosuppressive effects of the drug.

AZELAIC ACID

(a'ze-laic)

Azelex, Finacea

Classification: ANTIACNE

Therapeutic: ANTIACNE

Prototype: Isotretinoin

AVAILABILITY Cream; gel

ACTION & *THERAPEUTIC EFFECT* Azelaic acid is a naturally occurring dicarboxylic acid. Antimicrobial action is attributable to inhibition of microbial cellular protein synthesis. A normalization of keratinization of the follicle occurs, and it reduces the number of acne lesions. *Reduces the number of inflammatory pustules and papules.*

USES Mild to moderate inflammatory acne vulgaris, mild to moderate rosacea.

CONTRAINDICATIONS Hypersensitivity to any component in the drug.

CAUTIOUS USE Dark complexion, pregnancy (category B); lactation. Safety and efficacy in children younger than 12 yr not established.

ROUTE & DOSAGE

Acne Vulgaris, Rosacea

Adult/Child (12 yr and older): **Topical** Apply thin film to clean and dry area bid

ADMINISTRATION

Topical

- Wash and dry skin thoroughly prior to application of drug.
- Apply by thoroughly massaging a thin film of the cream or gel into the affected area. Avoid occlusive dressing.
- Wash hands before and after application of cream or gel.
- Store at 15°–30°C (59°–86°F).

ADVERSE EFFECTS **Skin:** Pruritus, burning, stinging, tingling, erythema, dryness, rash, peeling, irritation, contact dermatitis, vitiligo depigmentation, hypertrichosis. **Other:** Worsening of asthma.

PHARMACOKINETICS **Absorption:** Approximately 4% absorbed through the skin. **Onset:** 4–8 wk. **Distribution:** Into all tissues. **Metabolism:** Partially by beta oxidation in liver. **Elimination:** Primarily in urine. **Half-Life:** 12 h.

NURSING IMPLICATIONS

Assessment & Drug Effects

- Assess for signs of hypopigmentation, and report immediately.
- Monitor for sensitivity or severe irritation, which may warrant drug dosage reduction or discontinuation.

Patient & Family Education

- Learn proper application of cream or gel, and avoid contact with eyes or mucous membranes.
- Wash eyes with copious amounts of water if contact with medication occurs.
- Note: Transient pruritus, burning, and stinging are common; however, severe skin irritation or hypopigmentation should be reported.

AZELASTINE HYDROCHLORIDE

(a-ze-las'teen)

Astelin, Astepro, Optivar

Classification: ANTIHISTAMINE; H_1-RECEPTOR ANTAGONIST; NASAL AND OCULAR ANTIHISTAMINE

Therapeutic: ANTIHISTAMINE

Prototype: Diphenhydramine

AVAILABILITY Nasal spray; ophthalmic solution

ACTION & THERAPEUTIC EFFECT Potent histamine H_1-receptor antagonist and inhibitor of mast cell release of histamine. *Effective in the symptomatic treatment of seasonal allergic rhinitis and as a nasal decongestant.*

USES Allergic conjunctivitis, allergic rhinitis, ocular pruritus, vasomotor rhinitis.

CONTRAINDICATIONS Hypersensitivity to azelastine; pregnancy (category C). Safety and efficacy in children younger than 5 yr nasal spray use not established.

CAUTIOUS USE Hepatic or renal disease; asthmatics; older adults; lactation. **Astepro** nasal spray in children younger than 5 yr.

ROUTE & DOSAGE

Allergic Rhinitis

Adult/Adolescent: **Intranasal** 1–2 sprays/nostril bid

Child (5–11 yr): **Intranasal** 1 spray/nostril bid

Perennial Allergic Rhinitis (Astepro only)

Adult/Adolescent: **Intranasal** 2 sprays/nostril bid

Ocular Pruritus

See Appendix A-1.

ADMINISTRATION

Intranasal

- Prime delivery unit before first use (see manufacturer's instructions).
- Instruct patient to clear nasal passages prior to drug installation; then tilt head forward slightly and sniff gently when drug is sprayed into each nostril.
- Store the bottle upright at room temperature, 15°–30°C (59°–86°F).

ADVERSE EFFECTS **Respiratory:** Pharyngitis, *rhinitis,* paroxysmal sneezing, *cough,* asthma. **CNS:** *Headache, somnolence.* **HEENT:** *Bitter taste,* nasal burning, epistaxis, conjunctivitis. **Endocrine:** Weight gain. **GI:** Dry mouth, nausea. **Other:** Fatigue, dizziness.

INTERACTIONS **Drug: Alcohol** and CNS DEPRESSANTS, sedating ANTIHISTAMINES may cause reduced alertness.

PHARMACOKINETICS **Absorption:** 40% from nasal inhalation. **Peak:** 2–3 h. **Metabolism:** Active metabolites. **Elimination:** Primarily in feces. **Half-Life:** 22 h.

NURSING IMPLICATIONS

Assessment & Drug Effects

- Monitor level of alertness especially in older adults and with concurrent use of other CNS depressants.

Patient & Family Education

- Follow manufacturer's directions for priming the metered dose spray unit before first use and after storage of greater than 3 days.
- Tilt head forward while instilling spray. Avoid getting spray in eyes.
- Do not drive or engage in potentially hazardous activities until response to drug is known.
- Avoid concurrent use of CNS depressants, such as alcohol, while taking this drug.
- Discard spray unit and dispensing package bottle after 3 mo.

AZILSARTAN MEDOXOMIL

(ay′-zil-sar′-tan me-dox′-oh-mil)

Edarbi

Classification: ANGIOTENSIN II RECEPTOR ANTAGONIST; ANTIHYPERTENSIVE

Therapeutic: ANTIHYPERTENSIVE

Prototype: Losartan

AVAILABILITY Tablet

ACTION & *THERAPEUTIC EFFECT* An angiotensin II receptor blocker (ARB) that prevents binding of angiotensin II to AT1 receptors in vascular smooth muscle and other tissues. *Lowers blood pressure thus reducing the risk for fatal and nonfatal cardiovascular events (e.g., stroke and myocardial infarction).*

USES Hypertension, either alone or in combination with other agents.

CONTRAINDICATIONS Concomitant use with aliskiren-containing products with diabetes mellitus. Pregnancy D; lactation.

CAUTIOUS USE Severe CHF, renal artery stenosis, volume depletion, and renal impairment; older adults; women of childbearing age. Safety and efficacy in children younger than 18 yr not established.

ROUTE & DOSAGE

Hypertension

Adult: **PO** 80 mg once daily; consider 40 mg once daily if on high-dose diuretic

ADMINISTRATION

Oral

- May be given without regard to meals.
- Store at 15°–30°C (59°–86°F), and protect from light and moisture.

ADVERSE EFFECTS **CV:** Hypotension, orthostatic hypotension. **Respiratory:** Cough. **CNS:** Dizziness, fatigue. **Endocrine:** Increased serum creatinine. **GI:** Nausea. **Musculoskeletal:** Asthenia, muscle spasm.

INTERACTIONS **Drug:** Concurrent use of azilsartan with NSAIDs may cause deterioration of renal function. Do not use with **aliskiren.** Use with ACE INHIBITORS may increase adverse effects.

PHARMACOKINETICS **Absorption:** 60% bioavailability. **Distribution:** Greater than 99% plasma protein bound. **Metabolism:** In the liver to pharmacologically inactive metabolites via CYP2C9. **Elimination:** Fecal (55%) and renal (42%). **Half-Life:** 11 h.

NURSING IMPLICATIONS

Assessment & Drug Effects

Black Box Warning

*Azilsartan has been associated with fetal injury and fetal death. It must **not be** used by pregnant women.*

- Monitor HR and BP at regular intervals.
- Monitor for and report S&S of orthostatic hypotension, especially with volume depletion or with concurrent diuretic use.
- Monitor lab tests: Renal function tests, serum potassium, and BUN.

Patient & Family Education

- Report to prescriber if you become or plan to become pregnant.
- Stop taking the drug and immediately report to prescriber if you suspect that you are pregnant.
- Make position changes slowly, especially from lying or sitting to standing.
- Report promptly to prescriber if you experience faintness or dizziness or if you develop a rash.

AZITHROMYCIN

(a-zi-thro-mye′sin)

AzaSite, Zithromax

Classification: MACROLIDE ANTIBIOTIC

Therapeutic: ANTIBIOTIC

Prototype: Erythromycin

AVAILABILITY Tablet; oral suspension; solution for injection; ophthalmic drops

ACTION & THERAPEUTIC EFFECT A macrolide antibiotic that reversibly binds to the 50S ribosomal subunit of susceptible organisms and consequently inhibits protein synthesis. *Effective for treatment of mild to moderate infections caused by pyogenic organisms.*

USES Pneumonia, community-acquired, pharyngitis/tonsillitis, COPD exacerbation, chancroid, urethritis due to chlamydia or gonorrhea, skin and skin structure infections due to susceptible organisms, otitis media, *Mycobacterium avium-intracellular* complex infections, acute bacterial sinusitis **AzaSite:** Bacterial conjunctivitis.

UNLABELED USES Bronchitis, Lyme disease, pertussis, traveler's diarrhea, cystic fibrosis, typhoid fever, acne, chlamydia, dental infection.

CONTRAINDICATIONS Hypersensitivity to azithromycin, erythromycin, or any of the macrolide or ketolide antibiotics; history of cholestatic jaundice/hepatic dysfunction associated with prior use of azithromycin; hepatitis.

CAUTIOUS USE Hepatic or renal impairment; GI disease; altered cardiac conduction, ventricular arrhythmias, bradyarrhythmias, QT prolongation; history of torsade de pointes; MG; superinfection; older adults or debilitated persons; GFR less than 10 mL/min; pregnancy (does cross the placenta; however, there is no evidence of risk to humans); lactation; children younger than 6 mo.

ROUTE & DOSAGE

Pneumonia, Community-Acquired

Adult: **PO** 500 mg on day 1, then 250 mg q24h for 4 more days; **IV** 500 mg daily × 3 days

Child (6 mo and older): **PO** extended release 60 mg/kg single dose (max: 2000 mg); *Child (3 mo and older):* **PO** Immediate release 10 mg/kg on day 1, then 5 mg/kg days 2–5 (max: 250 mg/day) **IV** 10 mg/kg daily × 2 days

COPD Exacerbation

Adult: **PO** 500 mg × 1 day then 250 mg daily days 2–5 or 500 mg daily × 3 days

Acute Bacterial Sinusitis

Adult: **PO** 500 mg once daily × 3 days. **Zmax:** Single one-time dose of 2 g
Child (6 mo or older): **PO** 10 mg/kg once daily × 3 days

Babesiosis

Child/Infant: **PO** 10 mg/kg on day 1 (max 500 mg/dose); then 5 mg/kg daily on days 2–10 (max 250 mg/dose)

Syphilis

Adult: **PO** 2 g as a single dose

Chancroid/Cervicitis/Chlamydia

Adult: **PO** 1 g as a single dose
Adolescent/Child (over 45 kg): **PO** 20 mg/kg as single dose (max: 1 g); *Child (45 kg or less):* **PO** 1 g as single dose

Bacterial Conjunctivitis

Adult: **Ophthalmic** 1 drop bid × 2 days then daily × 5 days

ADMINISTRATION

Oral

- Give extended-release oral suspension (Zmax) at least 1 h before or 2 h after a meal. Tablets may be taken without regard to food.
- Suspension should be taken within 12 h of reconstitution.

Intravenous

PREPARE: **Intermittent:** Reconstitute 500-mg vial with 4.8 mL of sterile water for injection and shake until dissolved. ▪ Final concentration is 100 mg/mL. ▪ Solution **must be** further diluted to 1 or 2 mg/mL by adding 5 mL of the 100-mg/mL solution to 500 mL or 250 mL, respectively, of D5W, D5/NS, 0.45NaCl, or other compatible solution.
ADMINISTER: **Intermittent:** Administer 1 mg/mL over 3 h. Infuse 2 mg/mL over 1 h. ▪ Note: Do not give a bolus dose.
INCOMPATIBILITIES: **Solution/additive: Ciprofloxacin. Y-site: Amiodarone, amphotericin B, chlorpromazine, cloxacillin, diazepam, doxorubicin, epirubicin, garenoxacin, gemtuzumab, midazolam, mitoxantrone, mycophenolate, nicardipine, pentamidine, phenytoin, quinupristin/dalfopristin, thiopental.**

- Store drug when diluted as directed for 24 h at or below 30°C (86°F) or for 7 days under 5°C (41°F).

ADVERSE EFFECTS GI: *Nausea, diarrhea,* abdominal pain. **GU:** Elevated BUN and serum creatinine. **Other:** Pain at injection site, local inflammation.

INTERACTIONS Drug: ANTACIDS may decrease peak level of azithromycin; may increase toxicity of **digoxin, cyclosporine, edoxaban, mizolastine. Nelfinavir** may increase side effects of azithromycin. Carefully monitor when used with any other medication that can affect QT interval. Can decreases concentration of medications metabolized by P-glycoprotein (**doxorubicin, pazopanib, etc.**). Effects of **warfarin** may be potentiated. Do not use with LIVE VACCINES. **Food:** suspension (not other forms) has increased absorption when taken with food.

PHARMACOKINETICS **Absorption:** 37% of dose reaches the systemic circulation. **Onset:** 48 h. **Peak:** 2–3 h (immediate release), 3–5 h (extended release). **Distribution:** Extensively into tissues including sputum and vaginal secretions. **Metabolism:** In liver. **Elimination:** 5–12% of dose in urine. **Half-Life:** 60–70 h.

NURSING IMPLICATIONS

Assessment & Drug Effects

- Monitor for and report loose stools or diarrhea, since *C. difficile* **must be** ruled out.
- Report immediately any S&S of hypersensitivity; though rare, these reactions can be serious.
- Assess results of culture and sensitivity tests and allergies prior to beginning therapy.
- Monitor lab tests: Liver function tests, CBC with differential.

Patient & Family Education

- Report onset of loose stools or diarrhea.
- If being used to treat STD, use protection against transmission.

AZTREONAM

(az-tree′oh-nam)

Azactam, Cayston

Classification: ANTIBIOTIC; MONOBACTAM ANTIBIOTIC

Therapeutic: ANTIBIOTIC

Prototype: Imipenem-cilastatin

AVAILABILITY Vial

ACTION & THERAPEUTIC EFFECT Acts by inhibiting synthesis of bacterial cell wall by preferentially binding to specific penicillin-binding proteins (PBP) in the bacterial cell wall. *Highly resistant to beta-lactamases and does not readily induce their formation. Spectrum of activity limited to aerobic, gram-negative bacteria.*

USES Gram-negative infections of urinary tract, lower respiratory tract, skin and skin structures; and for intra-abdominal and gynecologic infections, septicemia, and as adjunctive therapy for surgical infections, community-acquired pneumonia. Inhalation form for cystic fibrosis.

CONTRAINDICATIONS Hypersensitivity to aztreonam; viral infections.

CAUTIOUS USE History of hypersensitivity reaction to penicillin, cephalosporins, or to other drugs; impaired renal or hepatic function, older adults; pregnancy (category B); lactation. For **Cayston** inhalation only: Safety and efficacy not established in pediatric patients younger than 7 yr; patients with FEV_1 less than 25% or greater than 75% predicted, or colonized with *Burkholderia cepacia*.

ROUTE & DOSAGE

Urinary Tract Infection

Adult/Adolescent: **IV/IM** 0.5–1 g q8–12h

Child/Infant (9 mo or older): **IV** 30 mg/kg q6–8h

Moderate to Severe Infections

Adult: **IV/IM** 1–2 g q8–12h (max: 8 g/24 h)
Child: **IV** 30 mg/kg/day q6–8h

Community-Acquired Pneumonia

Adult: **IV** 1–2 g q8–12h or 2 g q6–8h

Cystic Fibrosis Improvement in Respiratory Symptoms

Adult/Adolescent/Child (7 yr or older): **Inhaled** 75 mg tid × 28 days

Renal Impairment Dosage Adjustment

CrCl 10–30 mL/min: Reduce dose 50%; *less than 10 mL/min:* Reduce dose by 75%

Hemodialysis Dosage Adjustment

Reduce dose to 12.5% and give after hemodialysis

ADMINISTRATION

Inhalation

- Administer immediately after reconstitution.
- Administer only via an Altera Nebulizer System after patient has used a bronchodilator. Short-acting bronchodilators can be taken 15 min–4 h before Cayston. Long-acting bronchodilators can be taken 30 min–12 h before Cayston.

Intramuscular

- Reconstitute with at least 3 mL of diluent/gram of drug for IM injection. Immediately and vigorously shake vial to dissolve. Suitable diluents include sterile water for injection; bacteriostatic water for injection (with benzyl alcohol and propyl parabens); NS 0.9% for injection.
- Give IM injections deeply into large muscle mass such as the upper outer quadrant of the gluteus maximus or lateral thigh. Rotate injection sites.

Intravenous

Verify correct IV concentration and rate of infusion/injection with prescriber before giving to neonates, infants, and children.

PREPARE: **Direct** Reconstitute a single dose with 6–10 mL of sterile water for injection. ▪ Immediately shake vial until solution is dissolved. May be given direct IV as prepared or further diluted for IV infusion. ▪ Reconstituted solutions are colorless to light straw yellow and turn slightly pink on standing. **For intermittent infusion:** Each gram of reconstituted aztreonam **must be** further diluted in at least 50 mL of D5W, NS, or other solution approved by manufacturer to yield a concentration not to exceed 20 mg/mL.

ADMINISTER: **Direct:** Give over 3–5 min. **Intermittent:** Give over 20–60 min through Y-site.

INCOMPATIBILITIES: **Solution/additive:** **Ampicillin, metronidazole, nafcillin.** **Y-site:** **Acyclovir, alatrofloxacin, amphotericin B, amphotericin B cholesteryl complex, amsacrine, azathioprine, azithromycin, chlorpromazine, dantrolene, daunorubicin, erythromycin, ganciclovir, milrinone acetate, indomethacin, lansoprazole, lorazepam, metronidazole, mitomycin, mitoxantrone, mycophenolate, oritavancin, pantoprazole, papaverine, pentamidine, pentazocine, pentobarbital, phenytoin, prochlorperazine, streptozocin, trastuzumab.**

B

ADVERSE EFFECTS **CNS:** Headache, dizziness, confusion, paresthesias, insomnia, seizures. **HEENT:** Tinnitus, nasal congestion, sneezing, diplopia. **Skin:** Rash, purpura, erythema multiforme, exfoliative dermatitis, diaphoresis; petechiae, pruritus. **GI:** Nausea, *diarrhea*, vomiting, elevated liver function tests. **Hematologic:** Eosinophilia. **Other:** Hypersensitivity (urticaria, eosinophilia, anaphylaxis). Local reactions (phlebitis, thrombophlebitis (following IV), pain at injection sites), superinfections (gram-positive cocci), vaginal candidiasis.

DIAGNOSTIC TEST INTERFERENCE Aztreonam may cause transient elevations of ***liver function tests,*** increases in ***PT*** and ***PTT,*** minor changes in ***Hgb,*** and positive ***Coombs test.***

INTERACTIONS **Drug:** **Imipenem-cilastatin, cefoxitin** may be antagonistic.

PHARMACOKINETICS **Peak:** 1 h IM. **Distribution:** Widely distributed including synovial and blister fluid, bile, bronchial secretions, prostate, bone, and CSF; crosses placenta; distributed into breast milk in small amounts. **Metabolism:** Not extensively metabolized. **Elimination:** 60–70% in urine within 24 h. **Half-Life:** 1.6–2.1 h.

NURSING IMPLICATIONS

Assessment & Drug Effects

- Inspect IV injection sites daily for signs of inflammation. Pain and phlebitis occur in a significant number of patients.
- Monitor for and report loose stools or diarrhea because pseudomembranous colitis (see Appendix F) **must be** ruled out.
- Monitor for S&S of opportunistic infections (rectal or vaginal itching or discharge, fever, cough) and promptly report onset to prescriber. Overgrowth of nonsusceptible organisms, particularly *Staphylococci, Streptococci,* and fungi, is a threat, especially in patients receiving prolonged or repeated therapy.
- Monitor lab tests: Baseline C&S prior to initiation of therapy. Baseline and periodic renal function tests, particularly in older adults and in those with history of renal impairment.

Patient & Family Education

- Determine previous hypersensitivity reactions to penicillins, cephalosporins, and other allergens prior to therapy.
- Report promptly any of the following: Unexplained diarrhea or loose stools, any sign of allergic reaction, any worsening symptoms.
- Note: IV therapy may cause a change in taste sensation. Report interference with eating.

BACITRACIN

(bass-i-tray′sin)

Classification: ANTIBIOTIC
Therapeutic: ANTIBIOTIC

AVAILABILITY Ophthalmic ointment; topical ointment

ACTION & *THERAPEUTIC EFFECT* Interferes with the bacterial cell membrane by inhibiting cell wall synthesis. *Spectrum of antibacterial activity similar to that of penicillin. Active against many gram-positive organisms. Ineffective against most other gram-negative organisms.*

USES Treatment of superficial infections of skin.

CONTRAINDICATIONS Toxic reaction or renal dysfunction associated with bacitracin; pulmonary disease; atopic individuals.

CAUTIOUS USE Hypersensitivity to neomycin; myasthenia gravis or other neuromuscular disease; renal impairment; pregnancy (category C); lactation.

ROUTE & DOSAGE

Skin Infections

Adult: **Topical** Apply thin layer of ointment bid, tid, as solution of 250–1000 units/mL in wet dressing

ADMINISTRATION

Topical

- Clean affected area prior to application. May be covered with a sterile bandage.
- Store ointments in tightly closed containers at 15°–30°C (59°–86°F) unless otherwise directed.

ADVERSE EFFECTS **HEENT:** Tinnitus. **GI:** Anorexia, nausea, vomiting, diarrhea, rectal itching and burning. **GU:** Nephrotoxicity; dose-related: Increased BUN, uremia, renal tubular and glomerular necrosis (IM route). **Hematologic:** Systemic use: Bone marrow depression, blood dyscrasias; eosinophilia. **Other:** Hypersensitivity (erythema, anaphylaxis). Pain and inflammation at injection site, fever, superinfection, neuromuscular blockade with respiratory depression.

INTERACTIONS **Drug:** With AMINOGLYCOSIDES, possibility of additive nephrotoxic and neuromuscular blocking effects; with **tubocurarine** and other NONDEPOLARIZING SKELETAL MUSCLE RELAXANTS, possibility of additive neuromuscular blocking effects.

PHARMACOKINETICS **Absorption:** Poorly absorbed from intact or denuded skin or mucous membranes. **Duration:** 6–8 h. **Elimination:** Slow renal excretion (10–40% in 24 h).

NURSING IMPLICATIONS

Assessment & Drug Effects

- Prolonged use may result in overgrowth of nonsusceptible organisms, especially *Candida albicans.*

Patient & Family Education

- Report local allergic reactions with topical applications (e.g., itching, burning, redness).
- Apply only as directed by your provider.

BACLOFEN

(bak'loe-fen)

Gablofen, Lioresal, Ozobax

Classification: CENTRAL-ACTING SKELETAL MUSCLE RELAXANT

Therapeutic: SKELETAL MUSCLE RELAXANT

Prototype: Cyclobenzaprine

AVAILABILITY Tablet; oral solution; solution for injection

ACTION & *THERAPEUTIC EFFECT* Centrally acting skeletal muscle relaxant that depresses monosynaptic and polysynaptic afferent reflex activity at spinal cord level. Baclofen stimulates the GABA receptors, which results in decreased excitatory input into alpha-motor neurons. *Reduces skeletal muscle spasm caused by upper motor neuron lesions.*

USES Symptomatic relief of reversible spasticity in multiple sclerosis and in

B

the management of severe spasticity in spinal cord injury or disease.

UNLABELED USES Treatment of alcohol use disorder.

CONTRAINDICATIONS Hypersensitivity to baclofen or any component of the formulation.

CAUTIOUS USE Impaired renal and hepatic function; bipolar disorder, psychosis, schizophrenia, seizure disorders, seizures, stroke, cerebral palsy, depression, DM, dialysis, head trauma, PKU, epilepsy; thrombocytopenia; psychiatric or brain disorders; older adults, lactation, pregnancy (late onset neonatal withdrawal may occur following in utero exposure); children younger than 2 yr.

ROUTE & DOSAGE

Muscle Spasm

Adult: **PO** 5 mg 1–3 times per day, may increase by 5 mg/dose q3days prn (max: 80 mg/day)
Child 8 yr or older: **PO** 5 mg tid, titrate to response(max: 60 mg/day)
Adult: **Intrathecal** Prior to infusion pump implantation, initiate trial dose of 50 mcg/mL bolus administered in intrathecal space over 1 min or less. Observe patient over next 4–8 h for significant decrease in muscle spasm. If response is inadequate, administer second bolus of 75 mcg and observe 4–8 h. May repeat in 24 h with a 100-mcg/2-mL bolus if necessary. *Post-implant titration:* Use screening dose if response lasted longer than 8 h or double screening dose if response lasted less than 8 h and administer over 24 h. After first 24 h, decrease dose by 10–30% q24h until desired response achieved.

Renal Impairment Dosage Adjustment (oral form)

CrCl 51–80 mL/min: Use 5 mg q12h (max 50 mg/day); *CrCl 30–50 mL/min:* Use 2.5 mg q12h (max 40 mg/day); *CrCl less than 30 mL/min:* do not use

ADMINISTRATION

Oral

- Give with food or milk to avoid GI distress.

Intrathecal

- Give by direct intrathecal injection (via lumbar puncture or catheter) over at least 1 min or longer.
- Dilute *only* with sterile, preservative-free NS injection. Baclofen **must be** diluted to a concentration of 50 mcg/mL when preparing test doses.
- Intrathecal infusion pump: Do not abruptly discontinue as serious adverse effects may develop.
- Do not store above 30°C (86°F) in tightly closed container unless otherwise directed.

ADVERSE EFFECTS **CV:** Hypotension. **CNS:** *Transient drowsiness,* confusion, headache, hypotonia, dizziness, paresthesia, insomnia. **GI:** Nausea, constipation, vomiting. **Musculoskeletal:** Asthenia.

INTERACTIONS **Drug: Alcohol,** CNS DEPRESSANTS, MUSCLE RELAXANTS, ANTIHISTAMINES compound CNS depression.

PHARMACOKINETICS **Absorption:** Readily from GI tract. **Distribution:** Minimal amounts cross

B

blood–brain barrier; crosses placenta; distribution into breast milk unknown. **Metabolism:** 15% in liver. **Elimination:** 70–85% in urine within 72 h; some elimination in feces. **Half-Life:** 3–4 h (oral); 1.5 h (intrathecal).

NURSING IMPLICATIONS

Black Box Warning

Abrupt discontinuation of intrathecal baclofen has resulted in severe adverse reactions, including high fever, altered mental status, exaggerated spasticity and muscle rigidity; rarely, rhabdomyolysis, multiple organ-system failure, and death have occurred.

Assessment & Drug Effects

- Supervise ambulation. Initially, the loss of spasticity induced by baclofen may affect patient's ability to stand or walk.
- Monitor for orthostatic hypotension. Fall precautions may be necessary.
- Observe carefully for CNS side effects: Mental confusion, depression, hallucinations. Older adults are especially sensitive to this drug.
- Regular EEG in patients with epilepsy.
- Monitor lab tests: Renal function tests.

Patient & Family Education

- Do not stop this drug unless directed to do so by prescriber. Drug withdrawal needs to be accomplished gradually over a period of 2 wk or more. Abrupt withdrawal following prolonged administration may cause anxiety, agitated behavior, auditory and visual hallucinations, severe tachycardia, acute exacerbation of spasticity, and seizures.
- Note: CNS depressant effects will be additive to other CNS depressants, including alcohol.
- Monitor blood glucose for loss of glycemic control if diabetic.
- Do not drive or engage in other potentially hazardous activities until the response to drug is known.
- Do not self-dose with OTC drugs without prescriber's approval.

BALOXAVIR MARBOXIL

(ba-LOX-A-veer-mar-BOX-el)

Xofluza

Classifications: ANTIVIRAL, ENDONUCLEASE INHIBITOR

Therapeutic: ANITVIRAL

AVAILABILITY Oral tablet

ACTION & *THERAPEUTIC EFFECT*

Inhibits endonuclease activity of a selective polymerase acidic protein, which is required for viral gene transcription resulting in inhibition of influenza virus replication. *Demonstrates antiviral activity against influenza A and B viruses, including strains resistant to standard antiviral agents.*

USES Treatment of uncomplicated acute influenza in patients 12 years of age or older, symptomatic for no more than 2 days.

CONTRAINDICATIONS Hypersensitivity to baloxavir marboxil or any component of the formulation.

CAUTIOUS USE Bacterial infection; pregnancy (adverse events not observed during pregnancy); lactation (unknown if baloxavir marboxil present in breast milk).

B

ROUTE & DOSAGE

Influenza Treatment

Adult/child (12 yr or older and weight 40–80 kg): **PO** 40 mg as single dose; *(weight greater than 80 kg):* **PO** 80 mg as single dose

ADMINISTRATION

Oral

- Initiate within 48 h of influenza symptom onset.
- Administer a single dose with or without food.
- Avoid administration with dairy products, calcium-fortified beverages, polyvalent cation-containing laxatives, or oral supplements (calcium, iron, magnesium, selenium, zinc).
- Store at 20°–25°C (68°–77°F). Store in original blister package.

ADVERSE EFFECTS **Respiratory:** Bronchitis. **GI:** Diarrhea.

INTERACTIONS **Drugs:** Polyvalent cations may decrease serum concentration including **calcium supplements,** CATION-CONTAINING ANTACIDS or LAXATIVES, **iron supplements.** May decrease effectiveness of live attenuated influnza vaccine. **Food:** Avoid coadministration with dairy products.

PHARMACOKINETICS **Absorption:** Readily absorbed from GI tract. **Peak:** 4 h. **Distribution:** 1180 L; 93% protein bound. **Metabolism:** Pro-drug converted primarily by UGT1A3 (major); CYP3A4 (minor). **Elimination:** 14% excreted unchanged in urine; 80% in feces. **Half-Life:** 79 h.

NURSING IMPLICATIONS

Assessment & Drug Effects

- Monitor for potential secondary bacterial infections.

Patient & Family Education

- Notify your doctor or get medical help right away if you have any of the following signs or symptoms of allergic reaction: Rash, hives, itching; red, swollen, blistered, or peeling skin with or without fever; wheezing; tightness in the chest or throat; trouble breathing, swallowing, or talking; unusual hoarseness; swelling of the mouth, face, lips, tongue, or throat; or any dizziness or passing out.

BALSALAZIDE

(bal-sal′a-zide)

Colazal

Classification: MUCOUS MEMBRANE AGENT; ANTI-INFLAMMATORY

Therapeutic: ANTI-INFLAMMATORY

Prototype: Mesalamine (5-ASA)

AVAILABILITY Capsule

ACTION & *THERAPEUTIC EFFECT* A prodrug of mesalamine that remains intact until it reaches the lumen of the colon. Thought to decrease inflammation of the mucous lining of the colon by blocking cyclooxygenase and inhibiting prostaglandin synthesis in the lining of the colon. *An anti-inflammatory agent and a prodrug of 5-ASA.*

USES Treatment of mild to moderately active ulcerative colitis.

CONTRAINDICATIONS Prior hypersensitivity to salicylates, balsalazide.

CAUTIOUS USE Hypersensitivity to mesalamine, sulfasalazine, olsalazine, salicylate. Allergic response to

B

any medications; hepatic or renal impairment; pyloric stenosis; older adults; pregnancy (use with caution during pregnancy); lactation; children younger than 5 yr.

ROUTE & DOSAGE

Ulcerative Colitis

Adult: **PO** 2.25 g capsules tid for 8–12 wk
Adolescent/Child (5 yr or older): 2.25 g (1–3 caps) tid for up to 8 wk or 750 mg tid for up to 8 w

ADMINISTRATION

Oral

- Give in a consistent manner with respect to food intake (i.e., either always with or always without food).
- Capsules may be opened and sprinkled on applesauce for ease of swallowing.
- Maintain adequate hydration during therapy.
- Store at room temperature, preferably at 20°–25°C (68°–77°F).

ADVERSE EFFECTS **Respiratory:** Nasopharyngitis. **CNS:** Headache. **GI:** Abdominal pain, diarrhea, vomiting, exacerbation of ulcerative colitis. **Other:** Fever.

INTERACTIONS Avoid for 6 wk after VARICELLA VACCINE.

PHARMACOKINETICS **Absorption:** Low and variable absorption from the colon. **Distribution:** 99% protein bound. **Metabolism:** Metabolized in colon to release 5-aminosalicylic acid. **Elimination:** Feces.

NURSING IMPLICATIONS

Assessment & Drug Effects

- Monitor for S&S of myelosuppression in patients also receiving azathioprine. Monitor S&S of colitis, including rectal bleeding and frequent stools. Report worsening symptoms.
- Monitor lab tests: Baseline and periodic renal function tests; periodic CBC especially in older adults; hepatic function.

Patient & Family Education

- Report worsening of S&S of colitis to prescriber (e.g., diarrhea, abdominal pain, fever, rectal bleeding).

BARICITINIB

(bar-i sye′ti-nib)

Olumiant

Classification: BIOLOGICAL RESPONSE MODIFIER; JANUS KINASE (JAK) INHIBITOR; DISEASE-MODIFYING ANTIRHEUMATIC DRUG (DMARD)
Therapeutic: JANUS KINASE (JAK) INHIBITOR

AVAILABILITY Tablet

ACTION & *THERAPEUTIC EFFECT* Inhibits janus kinase (JAK) enzymes and interferes with a signaling pathway that transmits extracellular information to the cell nucleus, influencing DNA transcription. *It improves rheumatoid arthritis by inhibiting the production of inflammatory mediators.*

USES Treatment of moderately to severely active rheumatoid arthritis in patients who have had an inadequate response to other therapies. Use with other JAK inhibitors, DMARDS or potent immunosupressants is not recommended.

UNLABELED USES COVID-19 in hospitalized patients.

CONTRAINDICATIONS Serious uncontrolled infection, opportunistic infection or sepsis; live vaccines;

severe hepatic impairment; hepatitis B or C; pregnancy (limited data related to use during pregnancy; consider discontinuation 1 month prior to conception); lactation.

CAUTIOUS USE Active TB or history of herpes virus infection; history of chronic or recurrent infections; history of cardiovascular disease; current or past smokers; history or risk of GI perforation; moderate or severe renal impairment; moderate hepatic impairment; malignancy; older adults; history or active thrombosis; laboratory abnormalities such as neutropenia, anemia, and elevated liver enzymes and lipid levels.

ROUTE & DOSAGE

Rheumatoid Arthritis

Adult: **PO** 2 mg once a day

Renal Impairment Dosage Adjustment

eGFR 30 to 60 mL/minute/1.73 m²: 1 mg once daily. *eGFR <30 mL/minute/1.73 m²:* Use is not recommended.

Hepatic Impairment Dosage Adjustment

Severe impairment: Use is not recommended

Toxicity Dosage Adjustment

Lymphocytes less than 500 cells/m³: Discontinue; ANC less than 1000 cells/mm³: interrupt therapy until ANC greater than 1000 cells/mm³; hemoglobin less than 8 g/dL: interrupt therapy until hemoglobin greater than 8 g/dL

ADMINISTRATION

Oral

- Give with or without food.
- Store at 20°–25°C (68°–77°F); excursions permitted to 15°–30°C (59°–86°F).

ADVERSE EFFECTS **CV:** Thrombosis. **Respiratory:** Upper respiratory tract infections. **Hepatic:** Increased liver enzymes. **GI:** Nausea, Gastrointestinal perforation. **Hematologic:** Anemia, lymphocytopenia. **Other:** Serious infection.

INTERACTIONS **Drug:** Coadministration with strong OAT3 inhibitors (e.g., **probenecid**) may increase baricitinib levels. Coadministration with other potent IMMUNOSUPPRESSIVE DRUGS (e.g., **azathioprine, tacrolimus, cyclosporine,** DMARDS) or MYELOSUPPRESIVE AGENTS increase the risk of added immunosuppression and associated toxic effects. Do not use with LIVE VACCINES; separate inactivated vaccine therapy from baricitinib administration.

PHARMACOKINETICS **Absorption:** 80% bioavailability. **Peak:** 1 h. **Distribution:** 50% protein bound. **Metabolism:** Mainly metabolized through CYP3A4. **Elimination:** Primarily renal elimination: 75% in urine, 20% in feces. **Half-Life:** 12 h.

NURSING IMPLICATIONS

Black Box Warning

Baricitinib has been associated with increased risk of developing serious infections that may lead to hospitalization or death; lymphoma and malignancy have been observed in patients treated with baricitinib; thrombosis, including DVT and PE, and serious cardiovascular-related events

B

(such as heart attack, stroke), sometimes fatal, have occurred in patients treated with baricitinib.

Assessment & Drug Effects

- Assess for improvement of physical function and joint stiffness.
- Assess skin; patients are at increased risk of skin cancer.
- Consider benefits and risks for the individual patient prior to initiating or continuing therapy, particularly in patients who are current or past smokers, those with cardiovascular risk factors, those who develop a malignancy, and those with a known malignancy other than a successfully treated nonmelanoma skin cancer.
- Monitor lab tests: Lymphocyte, neutrophil, platelet count, Hgb, LFTs, lipids; viral hepatitis prior to initiating therapy.

Patient & Family Education

- Notify prescriber of any S&S of infection: fever, redness, swelling, pain, etc. Notify prescriber of any S&S of URI: Congestion, runny nose, cough, sore throat, difficulty breathing.
- Notify prescriber of any S&S of activation of herpes virus or shingles.
- Report signs or symptoms of blood clots such as pain in lower extremities, difficulty or pain with breathing.
- Avoid live vaccines.

BASILIXIMAB

(bas-i-lix'i-mab)

Simulect

Classification: IMMUNOSUPPRESSANT; MONOCLONAL ANTIBODY; INTERLEUKIN-2 RECEPTOR ANTAGONIST

Therapeutic: IMMUNOSUPPRESSANT

AVAILABILITY Powder for injection

ACTION & THERAPEUTIC EFFECT Immunosuppressant agent that is an interleukin-2 (IL-2) receptor monoclonal antibody produced by recombinant DNA technology. Binds to and blocks the interleukin-2R-alpha chain (CD-25 antibodies) on surface of activated T lymphocytes. *Binding to CD-25 antibodies inhibits a critical pathway in the immune response of the lymphocytes involved in allograft rejection.*

USES Prophylaxis of acute renal transplant rejection.

UNLABELED USE Liver transplant rejection prophylaxis.

CONTRAINDICATIONS Hypersensitivity to mannitol or murine protein; serious infection or exposure to viral infections (e.g., chickenpox, herpes zoster); lactation.

CAUTIOUS USE History of untoward reactions to dacliximab or other monoclonal antibodies; pregnancy (category B).

ROUTE & DOSAGE

Transplant Rejection Prophylaxis

Adult/Child (weight greater than 35 kg): **IV** 20 mg within 2 h prior to surgery then 20 mg 4 days posttransplant

Child (weight less than 35 kg, 2–15 yr): **IV** 10 mg within 2 h prior to surgery then 10 mg 4 days posttransplant

ADMINISTRATION

Intravenous

PREPARE: **Direct/IV Infusion:** Add 2.5 mL or 5 mL sterile water for injection to the 10-mg or

B

20-mg vial, respectively. Rock vial gently to dissolve. ▪ May be given as prepared direct IV as a bolus dose or further diluted in an infusion bag to a volume of 50 mL in NS or D5W. The resulting solution has a concentration of 2.5 mg/mL. ▪ Invert IV bag to dissolve but do not shake. ▪ Discard if diluted solution is colored or has particulate matter. ▪ Use IV solution immediately.

ADMINISTER: **Direct:** Give bolus over 20–30 min. **IV Infusion:** Infuse the ordered dose of diluted drug over 20–30 min.

▪ If necessary, the diluted solution may be stored at room temperature for 4 h or at 2°–8°C (36°–46°F) for 24 h. Discard after 24 h. ▪ Store undiluted drug at 2°–8°C (36°–46°F).

ADVERSE EFFECTS **CV:** *Hypertension*, chest pain, hypotension, arrhythmias. **Respiratory:** Dyspnea, URI, cough, rhinitis, pharyngitis, bronchospasm. **CNS:** *Headache*, *tremor*, dizziness, *insomnia*, paresthesias, agitation, depression. **Endocrine:** Hyperkalemia, hypokalemia, hyperglycemia, hyperuricemia, hypophosphatemia, hypocalcemia, increased weight, hypercholesterolemia, acidosis. **Skin:** Poor wound healing, *acne*. **GI:** *Constipation, nausea, diarrhea, abdominal pain*, vomiting, dyspepsia, moniliasis, flatulence, GI hemorrhage, melena, esophagitis, erosive stomatitis. **GU:** Dysuria, UTI, albuminuria, hematuria, oliguria, frequency, renal tubular necrosis, urinary retention, genital edema (male), impotence. **Hematologic:** *Anemia*, thrombocytopenia, thrombosis, polycythemia, hematoma, hemorrhage, hypoproteinemia, leukopenia, purpura. **Neuromuscular:** Tremor. **Other:** Pain, peripheral edema, edema, fever, viral infection, asthenia, arthralgia, acute hypersensitivity reactions with any dose. Cataract, conjunctivitis.

INTERACTIONS **Drug:** Do not use with **alefacept** or LIVE VACCINES. Use with **gefitinib** can increase risk of adverse reactions. **Herbal:** Do not use with **echinacea.**

PHARMACOKINETICS **Distribution:** Binds to interleukin-2R-alpha sites on lymphocytes. **Half-Life:** 7.2 ± 3.2 days in adults, 11.5 ± 6.3 days in children.

NURSING IMPLICATIONS

Assessment & Drug Effects

- Monitor carefully for and immediately report S&S of opportunistic infection or anaphylactic reaction (see Appendix F).
- Monitor CV status with periodic BP measurements.
- Monitor lab tests: Periodic serum electrolytes, lipid profile, and uric acid.

Patient & Family Education

- Report any distressing adverse effects.
- Avoid vaccination for 2 wk following last dose of drug.

BCG (BACILLUS CALMETTE-GUÉRIN)

(ba-cil'lus cal'met-te guer'in)

Tice, TheraCys

Classification: ANTINEOPLASTIC AGENT; IMMUNOMODULATOR

Therapeutic: ANTINEOPLASTIC; IMMUNOMODULATOR

AVAILABILITY Powder for suspension

ACTION & *THERAPEUTIC EFFECT*

BCG vaccine is an attenuated, live bacterial culture of the Bacillus of Calmette and Guérin (BCG) strain of *Mycobacterium bovis* and induces active immunity against *Mycobacterium tuberculosis.* BCG live is thought to cause a local, chronic inflammatory response involving macrophage and leukocyte infiltration of the bladder. This leads to destruction of superficial tumor cells. *BCG vaccine is an immunization agent for tuberculosis (TB). BCG is active immunotherapy that stimulates the immune mechanism to reject the tumor. It enhances the cytotoxicity of macrophages. BCG live is used intravesically as a biological response modifier for bladder cancer in situ.*

USES Carcinoma in situ of the bladder.

CONTRAINDICATIONS Impaired immune responses, immunosuppressive corticosteroid therapy, active TB, concurrent infections; recent TURP, severe hematuria; positive HIV serology; fever; UTI; angioedema; bone marrow suppression; chemotherapy; infection; mycobacterial infection; radiation therapy; tuberculosis; lactation.

CAUTIOUS USE Hypersensitivity to BCG; high risk for HIV; bladder irritation; pregnancy (not recommended for pregnant women).

ROUTE & DOSAGE

Carcinoma of the Bladder

Adult: **Intravesical** 1 vial **TheraCys** into bladder weekly × 6 wk then 1 vial at 3, 6, 12, 18, and 24 mo following the initial dose; 1 vial of **Tice** weekly × 6 wk then monthly × 6–12 mo

ADMINISTRATION

Intravesical Instillation

- **TheraCys:** Dilute 3 vials of **TheraCys** in 50 mL of sterile preservative free NS and instill into bladder slowly by gravity flow via urethral catheter. Patient retains suspension for 2 h and then voids.
- **Important:** Exercise care when handling BCG vaccine to avoid contact with the product. BCG is a biohazardous material.
- Store dry BCG powder, reconstituted vaccine, and diluent refrigerated at 2°–8°C (35°–46°F). Use reconstituted solution within 2 h.

Percutaneous Application

- Apply vaccine with syringe and needle by dropping onto 1- to 2-inch area of horizontally positioned surface of cleansed dry skin in the deltoid region of the arm.
- Pull skin taut and puncture skin with multiple puncture device centered over the vaccine. Apply pressure for 5 seconds.
- Spread vaccine evenly over puncture area.
- Apply loose covering and keep area dry for 24 h.

ADVERSE EFFECTS Respiratory: Flu-like symptoms. **CNS:** Intravesical administration: *Malaise,* chills, fatigue, pain, dizziness. **Skin:** Pustules, skin ulceration at injection site, injection site reaction (itching, tenderness). **GI:** Anorexia, nausea, vomiting, diarrhea, granulomatous hepatitis. **GU:** Intravesical administration: Bladder spasms, clot retention, decreased bladder capacity, decreased urine flow, *dysuria, hematuria,* incontinence, nocturia, UTI, cystitis, hemorrhagic cystitis, penile pain, prostatism, urinary frequency. **Hematologic:** *Anemia,*

B

leukopenia. **Musculoskeletal:** Arthritis, arthralgia, myalgia. **Other:** Infection, fever.

DIAGNOSTIC TEST INTERFERENCE Prior BCG vaccination may result in false-positive ***tuberculin skin test (PPD).*** Following BCG vaccination, tuberculin sensitivity may persist for months to years.

INTERACTIONS Drug: Concurrent antibiotic therapy may diminish therapeutic effect. Avoid IMMUNOSUPPRESSANT and MYELOSUPPRESSIVE agents. Avoid LIVE VACCINES.

NURSING IMPLICATIONS

Black Box Warning

BCG is a biohazardous material. Accidental exposure has resulted in serious, and sometimes fatal, infections.

Assessment & Drug Effects

- Monitor for S&S of systemic BCG infection: Fever, chills, severe malaise, or cough.
- Assess for regional lymph node enlargement and report fistula formation.
- Monitor lab tests: Culture blood and urine if systemic infection is suspected; PPD test prior to vaccination.

Patient & Family Education

- Report promptly S&S of infections including fever, chills, or unexplained fatigue and weakness.
- Retain instillation in bladder for as long as possible (up to 2 h) before voiding.
- Unless instructed otherwise, increase fluid intake to flush bladder after first voiding.
- Disinfect voided urine with bleach for 15 min before flushing.

BECAPLERMIN

(be-cap′ler-min)

Regranex

Classification: PLATELET-DERIVED GROWTH FACTOR (PDGF)

Therapeutic: GROWTH FACTOR

AVAILABILITY Gel

ACTION & THERAPEUTIC EFFECT It induces fibroblast proliferation in new granulation tissue. *It is effective against diabetic neuropathic ulcers that involve subcutaneous or deeper tissue and also have an adequate blood supply. Hence it promotes wound healing of diabetic ulcers.*

USES Lower-extremity diabetic neuropathic ulcers, wound management.

CONTRAINDICATIONS Hypersensitivity to becaplermin; cresol or paraben hypersensitivity; neoplasms at site of application; wounds that close by primary intention; increased risk of death in patients with DM.

CAUTIOUS USE Systemic infection; peripheral vascular disease; ulcer wounds related to arterial or venous insufficiency; thermal, electrical, or radiation burns at wound site; malignancy; older adults; pregnancy (category C); lactation; children younger than 16 yr.

ROUTE & DOSAGE

Diabetic Neuropathic Ulcers

Adult/Adolescent (16 yr or older): **Topical** Calculate the length of gel based on ulcer size and apply once/day until healed; reassess if ulcer not completely healed in 20 wk

ADMINISTRATION

Topical

- Squeeze calculated length of gel onto clean, firm, nonabsorbable surface.
- Apply even layer to ulcer area with clean tongue depressor or cotton swab and cover with saline-moistened dressing. After 12 h, remove dressing, clean ulcer by rinsing with water or saline to remove residual gel, and apply new saline-moistened dressing without becaplermin for next 12 h. Repeat cycle.
- Apply only to ulcers with good blood supply.
- Dosage calculation: Measure greatest length (*L*) and greatest width (*W*) of ulcer in inches or centimeters; using 15-g tube multiply (*L* × *W*) × 0.6 for dose in inches or (*L* × *W*)/4 for dose in cm; using 2-g tube multiply (*L* × *W*) × 1.3 for dose in inches or (*L* × *W*)/2 for dose in cm.
- Store at 2°–8°C (36°–46°F). Do not freeze and do not use beyond expiration date.

ADVERSE EFFECTS **Skin:** Erythematous rash.

PHARMACOKINETICS **Absorption:** Less than 3% absorbed into systemic circulation.

NURSING IMPLICATIONS

Assessment & Drug Effects

- Therapeutic efficacy: 30% decrease in ulcer size after 10 wk or complete healing after 20 wk.
- Monitor for and report appearance of erythematous rash.

Patient & Family Education

- Consult wound care provider who typically recalculates dosage weekly/biweekly.
- Follow directions for application carefully. Gel may be measured out on waxed paper.
- Wash hands prior to application, and do not allow tip of tube to contact ulcer or any surface.
- Report worsening ulceration or development of skin rash.

BECLOMETHASONE DIPROPIONATE

(be-kloe-meth′a-sone)

Beconase AQ, QVAR

See Appendix A-3.

BEDAQUILINE

(bed-ak′wi-leen)

Sirturo

Classification: ANTI-INFECTIVE; ANTITUBERCULOSIS; INHIBITOR OF MYCOBACTERIAL ATP SYNTHETASE

Therapeutic: ANTITUBERCULOSIS

AVAILABILITY Tablet

ACTION & *THERAPEUTIC EFFECT* Bedaquiline inhibits mycobacterial ATP synthase, an enzyme essential for the generation of energy in *Mycobacterium tuberculosis*. *Bedaquiline is bacteriocidal, thus it causes* Mycobacterium tuberculosis *cell death.*

USES Combination therapy in patients with pulmonary multidrug-resistant tuberculosis (MDR-TB) when other effective treatment regimens are not available.

CONTRAINDICATIONS Significant ventricular irregularities; QTcF interval of greater than 500 msec (confirmed by repeat ECG); recent MI; lactation.

CAUTIOUS USE Concurrent use with drugs that prolong the QT segment; severe renal or hepatic impairment; HIV-TB coinfected patients; patients with TB other than in the lungs; older adults; pregnancy (limited information regarding use during pregnancy). Safety and efficacy in children younger than 5 yr not established.

ROUTE & DOSAGE

Treatment of MDR Tuberculosis

Adult/Adolescent/Child over 5 yr and over 30 kg: **PO** 400 mg once daily for 2 wk; reduce to 200 mg 3 times wk with at least 48 h between doses for wk 3–24.

ADMINISTRATION

Oral

- Give with food. Note that bedaquiline should only be used in combination with other drugs to which the patient's TB has been, or is likely to be, susceptible.
- Tablets should be swallowed whole and should not be crushed or chewed.
- Store in a tight, light-resistant container at 15°–30°C (59°–86°F).

ADVERSE EFFECTS **CV:** *Chest pain.* **CNS:** *Headache.* **Respiratory:** Hemoptysis. **Endocrine:** ALT/AST increase, blood amylase increase. **Skin:** Rash. **GI:** *Nausea.* **Musculoskeletal:** *Arthralgia.* **Other:** Anorexia.

INTERACTIONS **Drug:** Inhibitors of CYP3A4 (e.g., **itraconazole, ketoconazole, lopinavir, ritonavir**) may increase the levels of bedaquiline. Coadministration with other QT-prolonging drugs (FLUOROQUINOLONES, MACROLIDES, **amiodarone, clofazimine**) may increase the risk QT prolongation. Alcohol may enhance hepatotoxic effects. Do not administer with LIVE VACCINES. **Herbal: St. John's wort** may decrease bedaquiline levels.

PHARMACOKINETICS **Peak:** 5 h. **Distribution:** Greater than 99.9% plasma protein bound. **Metabolism:** In liver via CYP 3A4. **Elimination:** Primarily feces. **Half-Life:** 5.5 mo (slow release from peripheral tissues).

NURSING IMPLICATIONS

Black Box Warning

Bedaquiline has been associated with an increased risk of death and should be used ONLY when required to provide an effective treatment regimen. QT prolongation can occur with bedaquiline.

Assessment & Drug Effects

- Monitor heart rate and rhythm with periodic ECG. Report promptly rapid rate or irregular beat.
- Monitor for and report promptly S&S of hepatoxicity.
- Monitor lab tests: Baseline and periodic sputum cultures and LFTs.

Patient & Family Education

- During wk 1 and 2, bedaquiline is taken daily.
- During wk 3–24, take no more than 600 mg in a 7-day period (e.g., 200 mg M–W–F).
- Always take bedaquiline with other medicines prescribed for you to treat TB.
- Report promptly to prescriber if you experience any of the following: Irregular or rapid heartbeat; unexplained nausea or vomiting, stomach pain, fever, weakness,

B

itching, unusual tiredness, loss of appetite, light-colored stool, dark urine, yellowing of your skin or the white of your eyes.
- Do not breastfeed while taking this drug.

BELIMUMAB

(be-lim′ue-mab)

Benlysta

Classification: BIOLOGICAL RESPONSE MODIFIER; MONOCLONAL ANTIBODY; IMMUNOLOGIC AGENT

Therapeutic: IMMUNOSUPPRESSANT

Prototype: Basiliximab

AVAILABILITY Powder for injection

ACTION & *THERAPEUTIC EFFECT* A monoclonal antibody that inhibits the survival of B cells, including autoreactive B cells, and reduces the differentiation of B cells into immunoglobulin-producing plasma cells. *Helps control lupus erythematosus by decreasing the level of a specific immunoglobulin G responsible for the damaging effects of lupus.*

USES Treatment of active, autoantibody-positive systemic lupus erythematosus (SLE) in adults who are receiving standard therapy.

CONTRAINDICATIONS Previous hypersensitivity to belimumab; development of progressive multifocal leukoencephalopathy due to belimumab.

CAUTIOUS USE New onset or chronic infection; psychiatric disorders; depression or suicidal behavior; black patients due to low response rate; pregnancy (category C); lactation. Safety and efficacy not established in children.

ROUTE & DOSAGE

Systemic Lupus Erythematosus

Adult: **IV** 10 mg/kg q2wk for 3 doses, then q4wk

ADMINISTRATION

Intravenous

- Use only in a setting capable of managing hypersensitivity reactions.

PREPARE: **IV Infusion:** Place vial at room temperature for 10–15 min. Reconstitute with sterile water for injection by adding 1.5 mL or 4.8 mL to the 120-mg or 400-mg vial, respectively, to yield 80 mg/mL. Minimize foaming by directing stream to side of vial, then swirl gently for 60 sec. Keep at room temperature, swirling for 60 sec q5min until dissolved. Withdraw the required dose of belimumab, then remove from 250 mL of NS a volume equal to the volume of the dose. Add belimumab to the NS and invert to mix.

ADMINISTER: **IV Infusion: Do not** give IV push or bolus. Infuse over 1 h through a dedicated IV line. Do not mix with other solutions or drugs. Monitor closely for S&S of an infusion reaction. Stop infusion, institute supportive measures and notify prescriber if an infusion reaction (or hypersensitivity) is suspected.

INCOMPATIBILITIES: **Solution/additive: Dextrose** solutions.

- May store reconstituted solution for up to 7 h at 2°–8°C (36°–46°F). Protect from light. Total time from reconstitution to completion of infusion should not exceed 8 h.

B

ADVERSE EFFECTS Respiratory: Bronchitis, *nasopharyngitis*, pharyngitis. **CNS:** Depression, insomnia, migraine headache. **GI:** *Diarrhea*, gastroenteritis, *nausea*. **Hematological:** Leukopenia. **Other:** Cystitis, pain in the extremities, *pyrexia*, infection.

PHARMACOKINETICS Half-Life: 19.4 days.

NURSING IMPLICATIONS

Assessment & Drug Effects

- Monitor vital signs often during and after infusion.
- Monitor closely for S&S of infusion reaction or hypersensitivity. Stop the infusion and notify prescriber if any of these occur.
- Monitor closely if a new infection develops.
- Assess for depression, anxiety, or other manifestations of psychiatric problems. Report immediately suicidal ideation.

Patient & Family Education

- Report immediately any of the following: Difficulty breathing, wheezing, rash, itching, swelling of the face or tongue, chest pain, or other discomfort during drug infusion.
- Inform prescriber immediately of new or worsening mental health problems such as anxiety, depression, or thoughts of suicide.
- Live vaccines received within 30 days of beginning or concurrently with belimumab therapy may not be effective. Seek advice of prescriber.
- Do not breastfeed while taking this drug without consulting prescriber.
- Women should use effective means of contraception during and for at least 4 mo following termination of treatment.

BELINOSTAT

(be-lin′o-stat)

Beleodaq

Classification: ANTINEOPLASTIC; HISTONE DEACETYLASE INHIBITOR

Therapeutic: ANTINEOPLASTIC

AVAILABILITY Lyophilized powder for reconstitution

ACTION & THERAPEUTIC EFFECT Inhibits the enzyme, histone de-acetylase, resulting in accumulation of acetyl groups in cells, leading to cell cycle arrest and apoptosis of tumor cells; drug has preferential cytotoxicity toward tumor cells versus normal cells. *Inhibits proliferation of peripheral T-cell lymphoma cells.*

USES Treatment of patients with relapsed or refractory peripheral T-cell lymphoma (PTCL).

CONTRAINDICATIONS Tumor lysis syndrome due to belinostat; pregnancy (category D); lactation.

CAUTIOUS USE Anemia; neutropenia; thrombocytopenia; hepatic impairment; renal impairment. Safety and efficacy in children younger than 18 yr not established.

ROUTE & DOSAGE

Peripheral T-Cell Lymphoma

Adult: **IV** 1000 mg/m^2 on days 1–5 of a 21-day cycle; can repeat every 21 days

Hematologic Toxicity Dosage Adjustment

ANC less than 0.5 × 10^9/L (any platelet count): Reduce dose to 750 mg/m^2

Common adverse effects in *italic*; life-threatening effects underlined; generic names in **bold**; classifications in SMALL CAPS; ♣ Canadian drug name; ⊙ Prototype drug; ⚠ Alert

B

Platelet count less than 25 × 10^9/L (any nadir ANC): Reduce to 750 mg/m^2

Nonhematologic Toxicity Dosage Adjustment

Any CTCAE grade 3 or 4 adverse reaction (except nausea, vomiting, and diarrhea): Reduce to 750 mg/m^2

Recurrence of CTCAE grade 3 or 4 adverse reactions after two dosage reductions: Discontinue therapy

Grade 3 or 4 nausea, vomiting, or diarrhea: Reduce dose only if the duration is greater than 7 days with supportive management

Patients with Reduced UGT1A1 Activity Dosage Adjustment

*Patients homozygous for the UGT1A1*28 allele:* Reduce initial dose to 750 mg/m^2

ADMINISTRATION

Intravenous

This drug is a cytotoxic agent, and caution should be used to prevent any contact with the drug. Follow institutional or standard guidelines for preparation, handling, and disposal of cytotoxic agents.

PREPARE: **IV Infusion:** Reconstitute 500-mg vial with 9 mL SW to yield 50 mg/mL. Swirl vial until dissolved. Further dilute required dose in 250 mL NS.

ADMINISTER: **IV Infusion:** Give over 30 min through a 0.22-micron in-line filter; if infusion site pain occurs, increase infusion time to 45 min.

- Store drug vials at 15°–30°C (59°–86°F). May store reconstituted solution up to 12 h and solutions diluted for infusion up to 36 h (including infusion time) at 15°–30°C (59°–86°F).

ADVERSE EFFECTS

CV: Hypotension, *peripheral edema,* phlebitis, QT prolongation. **Respiratory:** *Cough,* dyspnea, pneumonia. **CNS:** Chills, dizziness, *fatigue,* headache. **Endocrine:** Hypokalemia, increased lactate dehydrogenase, increase serum creatinine. **Skin:** Pruritus, *skin rash.* **GI:** Abdominal pain, constipation, decreased appetite, diarrhea, *nausea, vomiting.* **Hematological:** *Anemia,* thrombocytopenia. **Other:** *Fever,* infection, injection site pain, multiorgan failure.

INTERACTIONS

Drug: Strong inhibitors of UGT1A1 will increase belinostat levels, and concomitant administration is contraindicated.

PHARMACOKINETICS

Distribution: 93–96% plasma protein bound. **Metabolism:** In liver by UGT1A1. **Elimination:** Primarily renal. **Half-Life:** 1.1 h.

NURSING IMPLICATIONS

Assessment & Drug Effects

- Monitor for and report S&S of GI toxicity (e.g., nausea, vomiting, diarrhea), hepatic dysfunction, infection, or tumor lysis syndrome (e.g., weakness or lethargy, edema, cardiac symptoms, shortness of breath, muscle cramp).
- Withhold drug and notify prescriber if an infection is suspected.
- Monitor lab tests: Baseline and weekly CBC with platelets and differential; renal function tests and LFTs at baseline and before each cycle; periodic serum electrolytes.

B

Patient & Family Education

- Report promptly to prescriber if you experience any of the following: Signs of infection, unexplained bleeding, severe dizziness, fainting, irregular heart rate, shortness of breath, or swelling extremities.
- Report promptly signs of liver toxicity such as yellowing of the skin or the white part of eyes (jaundice), dark urine, itching, or pain in the right upper stomach area.
- GI distress is common but report to prescriber significant anorexia, nausea, or diarrhea.
- Women of reproductive age should avoid pregnancy during treatment with this drug.
- Do not breastfeed while taking this drug.

BENAZEPRIL HYDROCHLORIDE

(ben-a′ze-pril)

Lotensin

Classification: ANTIHYPERTENSIVE; RENIN ANGIOTENSIN SYSTEM ANTAGONIST

Therapeutic: ANTIHYPERTENSIVE, ACE INHIBITOR

Prototype: Enalapril

AVAILABILITY Tablet

ACTION & *THERAPEUTIC EFFECT* Lowers blood pressure by specific inhibition of the angiotensin-converting enzyme (ACE) and thus by decreasing angiotensin II (a potent vasoconstrictor) and aldosterone secretion. *Achieves an antihypertensive effect by suppression of the renin–angiotensin–aldosterone system.*

USES Treatment of hypertension.

UNLABELED USES Heart failure, stable CAD, non ST-elevation ACS.

CONTRAINDICATIONS Hypersensitivity to benazepril or another ACE inhibitor; history of angioedema; coadministration with aliskiren in patients with DM; development of jaundice or elevated hepatic enzymes while taking benazepril; pregnancy (crosses the placenta and may be associated with increased risk of fetal malformations); lactation; children with a CrCl less than 30 mL/h.

CAUTIOUS USE Renal impairment, renal-artery stenosis; patients with hypovolemia, receiving diuretics, undergoing dialysis; patients in whom excessive hypotension would present a hazard (e.g., cerebrovascular insufficiency); CHF; hepatic impairment; women of childbearing age; DM; older adults; children younger than 6 yr.

ROUTE & DOSAGE

Hypertension

Adult/Adolescent: **PO** 5–10 mg daily; can titrate up to 40 mg daily

Child (6 yr or older): **PO** 0.2 mg/kg daily as monotherapy (max: 10 mg/day as monotherapy)

Renal Impairment Dosage Adjustment

CrCl less than 30 mL/min: Use 5-mg starting dose.

ADMINISTRATION

Oral

- Consult prescriber about initial dose if patient is also receiving diuretics. Typically an initial dose of 5 mg is used to minimize the risk of hypotension.
- May be administered without regard to food.

- Store at room temperature, but not above 30°C (86°F).

ADVERSE EFFECTS **CV:** Hypotension. **CNS:** *Headache*, dizziness.

DIAGNOSTIC TEST INTERFERENCE May lead to false-negative aldosterone/renin ratio.

INTERACTIONS **Drug:** POTASSIUM-SPARING DIURETICS may increase the risk of hyperkalemia. Benazepril may increase **lithium** toxicity. Use with ANTIHYPERTENSIVES can cause additive effect. Use with **azathioprine** increases risk of myelosuppression. Patients have an increased risk of anaphylactic reaction with **iron dextran.** Contraindicated with **sacubitril/valsartan.** **Herbal:** Do not use with **grass pollen allergen extracts.**

PHARMACOKINETICS **Absorption:** Readily from GI tract; 37% reaches the systemic circulation. **Peak:** 1–2 h. **Duration:** 20–24 h. **Distribution:** Small amounts cross the blood–brain barrier; crosses placenta; small amount excreted in breast milk. **Metabolism:** In liver to active metabolite, benazeprilat. **Elimination:** Benazeprilat is primarily excreted in urine. **Half-Life:** Benazeprilat 10–11 h.

NURSING IMPLICATIONS

Black Box Warning

Benazepril may cause fetal injury and death.

Assessment & Drug Effects

- Assess for hypotension, especially in patients who may be volume depleted (e.g., prolonged diuretic therapy, recent vomiting or diarrhea, salt restriction) or who have CHF.
- Monitor lab tests: Periodic renal function tests during first few weeks of therapy; serum potassium, CBC with differential.

Patient & Family Education

- Discontinue drug and report to prescriber if pregnancy is suspected or detected.
- To minimize dizziness, change positions slowly. Be careful going up and down stairs.
- Do not use salt substitutes unless recommended by prescriber.
- Report swelling of face, eyes, lips, or tongue or difficulty breathing immediately to prescriber.

BENDAMUSTINE

(ben-da-mus′teen)

Belrapzo, Bendeka, Treanda

Classification: ANTINEOPLASTIC; ALKYLATING AGENT

Therapeutic: ANTINEOPLASTIC

Prototype: Cyclophosphamide

AVAILABILITY Solution for injection

ACTION & *THERAPEUTIC EFFECT* Alkylating agent that causes the formation of intrastrand and interstrand crosslinks between DNA molecules, thus resulting in inhibition of DNA replication, repair and transcription. *Active against both dividing and resting neoplastic lymphocytes.*

USES Treatment of chronic lymphocytic leukemia (CLL), indolent B cell non-Hodgkin lymphoma (NHL).

UNLABELED USES Treatment of mantle cell lymphoma.

CONTRAINDICATIONS Known hypersensitivity (e.g., anaphylaxis reaction) to bendamustine or mannitol; infusion reaction; pregnancy (may cause fetal harm); lactation.

CAUTIOUS USE Myelosuppression; mild hepatic or mild-to-moderate renal impairment; grade 3 or 4 infusion reaction; infection; dermatologic toxicity; extravasation; gastrointestinal toxicities; hypokalemia; infection; malignancies; tumor lysis syndrome; children younger than 6 yr.

ROUTE & DOSAGE

Chronic Lymphocytic Leukemia

Adult: **IV** 100 mg/m^2 on days 1 and 2 of a 28-day cycle, up to 6 cycles

Toxicity Dosage Adjustment

Grade 3 or higher hematologic toxicity: Reduce dose to 50 mg/m^2 on days 1 and 2 of each cycle; *if grade 3 or higher toxicity recurs:* Reduce the dose to 25 mg/m^2 on days 1 and 2 of each cycle.
Grade 4 hematologic toxicity: Hold dose until neutrophil above 1000 and platelets above 75,000.

Non-Hodgkin Lymphoma

Adult: **IV** 120 mg/m^2 on days 1 and 2 of a 21-day cycle; up to 8 cycles

Toxicity Dosage Adjustment

Grade 3 or greater nonhematologic toxicity or grade 4 hematologic toxicity: Reduce dose to 90 mg/m^2
Recurrent grade 3 or greater nonhematologic toxicity or recurrent grade 4 hematologic toxicity: Reduce dose to 60 mg/m^2

ADMINISTRATION

Intravenous

Exercise caution in handling and disposal. Avoid contact with skin. Wash immediately with soap and water if contact occurs.

PREPARE: **IV Infusion:** Reconstitute with sterile water for injection; add 5 mL to the 25-mg vial or 20 mL to the 100-mg vial to yield 5 mg/mL; should dissolve completely in 5 min. Withdraw required dose within 30 min of reconstitution and immediately add to 500 mL of NS.

ADMINISTER: **IV Infusion:** Infuse over 30 min for CLL and 60 min for NHL.

ADVERSE EFFECTS **Cardiovascular:** Peripheral edema, tachycardia, chest pain, hypotension. **Respiratory:** Cough, nasopharyngitis. **CNS:** Headache, dizziness, insomnia, chills, fatigue, anxiety, depression. **Endocrine:** Hyperuricemia. **Skin:** Pruritus, rash, night sweats. **Hepatic:** Increased serum bilirubin. **GI:** Diarrhea, *nausea, vomiting,* anorexia, stomatitis, abdominal pain, decreased appetite, dyspepsia, weight loss, constipation, oral candidiasis. **Hematologic:** *Anemia,* leukopenia, lymphocytopenia, bone marrow depression, *neutropenia,* thrombocytopenia, dehydration. **Musculoskeletal:** Back pain, asthenia. **Other:** Hypersensitivity, infection, *pyrexia.*

INTERACTIONS **Drug:** Compounds that inhibit CYP1A2 (**atazanavir, cimetidine, ciprofloxacin, fluvoxamine, omeprazole, zileuton**) will increase levels of bendamustine. Avoid MYELOSUPRESSIVE AGENTS (ex **clozapine, cladribine**) due to additive bone marrow suppression. Do not use with LIVE VACCINES. Do not use with **lenograstim.**

PHARMACOKINETICS Distribution: 95% protein bound. **Metabolism:** Hepatic oxidation by CYP1A2. **Elimination:** Primarily urine (50%). **Half-Life:** 40 min.

NURSING IMPLICATIONS

Assessment & Drug Effects

- Monitor closely for infusion reactions (i.e., chills, fever, pruritus, rash) and signs of anaphylaxis. Reactions are more likely with the second and subsequent cycles. Discontinue infusion immediately, and notify prescriber for severe reactions.
- Maintain adequate hydration status to minimize risk of tumor lysis syndrome.
- Monitor for and report S&S of infection.
- If extravasation occurs, stop infusion immediately and disconnect tubing from IV cannula. Gently aspirate extravasated solution and remove cannula. Apply dry, cold compress for 20 min 4 × daily.
- Monitor lab tests: Baseline and weekly Hgb, CBC with differential, and platelet count; frequent serum potassium and uric acid; frequent renal function tests with preexisting renal impairment; liver function tests.

Patient & Family Education

- Men and women should use reliable contraception to avoid pregnancy during and for 3 mo after bendamustine therapy is completed.
- Do not drive or engage in other dangerous activities until reaction to drug is known.
- Report promptly any of the following: Signs of infection, nausea, vomiting, diarrhea, worsening rash, itching, shortness of breath, cough, or swelling of face, lips, tongue, or throat.

BENZALKONIUM CHLORIDE

(benz-al-koe'nee-um)

Benza, Benzalchlor-50, Germicin, Pharmatex ♣, Sabol, Zephiran

Classification: TOPICAL ANTIBIOTIC

Therapeutic: ANTIBIOTIC

AVAILABILITY Concentrate, solution, tincture/tincture spray

ACTION & *THERAPEUTIC EFFECT* Bactericidal or bacteriostatic action (depending on concentration), probably due to inactivation of bacterial enzyme. *Effective against bacteria, some fungi (including yeasts), and certain protozoa. Generally not effective against spore-forming organisms.*

USES Antisepsis of intact skin, mucous membranes, superficial injuries, and infected wounds; also for irrigations of the eye and body cavities and for vaginal douching. A component of several contact lens wetting and cushioning solutions, and a preservative for ophthalmic solutions.

CONTRAINDICATIONS Casts, occlusive dressings, anal or vaginal packs, lactation.

CAUTIOUS USE Irrigation of body cavities; pregnancy (category C).

ROUTE & DOSAGE

Minor Wounds or Preoperative Disinfection

Adult: **Topical** 1:750 tincture or spray

Preoperative Disinfection of Denuded Skin and Mucous Membranes

Adult: **Topical** 1:10,000–1:2000 solution

B

Wet Dressings

Adult: **Topical** 1:5000 solution

Urinary Bladder Irrigation

Adult: **Topical** 1:20,000–1:5000 solution

Urinary Bladder Instillation

Adult: **Topical** 1:40,000–1:20,000 solution

Irrigation of Deep Infected Wounds

Adult: **Topical** 1:20,000–1:3000 solution

Vaginal Irrigation

Adult: **Topical** 1:5000–1:2000 solution

Sterile Storage of Instruments, Thermometers, Ampules

Adult: **Topical** 1:750 solution

ADMINISTRATION

Topical

- Use sterile water for injection as diluent for aqueous solutions to be instilled in wounds or body cavities. For other uses, fresh sterile distilled water is used.
- Irrigate eyes immediately and repeatedly with water if medication solution stronger than 1:5000 enters eyes; see a prescriber promptly.
- Rinse first with water, then with 70% alcohol, before applying benzalkonium for preoperative skin preparation.
- Consult prescriber about proper dilution of solutions used on denuded skin or inflamed or irritated tissues.
- Store at room temperature, preferably at 15°–30°C (59°–86°F) in airtight container, protected from light.

ADVERSE EFFECTS **Skin:** Erythema, local burning, hypersensitivity reactions. **Other:** Few or no toxic effects in recommended dilutions.

NURSING IMPLICATIONS

Assessment & Drug Effects

- Monitor wounds carefully. Report increasing signs of infection or lack of healing.

BENZOCAINE

(ben'zoe-caine)

Anesthetic Lubricant, Anbesol Cold Sore Therapy, Chigger-Tox, Dermoplast, Foille, Hurricaine, Orajel, Solarcaine, T-Caine

Classification: LOCAL ANESTHETIC (ESTER TYPE); ANTIPRURITIC

Therapeutic: LOCAL ANESTHETIC; ANTIPRURITIC

Prototype: Procaine

AVAILABILITY Aerosol; ointment; lotion; gel; liquid; lozenge

ACTION & THERAPEUTIC EFFECT Produces surface anesthesia by inhibiting conduction of nerve impulses from sensory nerve endings. Almost identical to procaine in chemical structure, but has prolonged duration of anesthetic action. *Temporary relief of pain and discomfort.*

USES Temporary relief of pain and discomfort in pruritic skin problems, minor burns and sunburn, minor wounds, and insect bites. Preparations are also available for toothache, minor sore throat pain, canker sores, hemorrhoids, rectal fissures, pruritus ani or vulvae, and for use as anesthetic-lubricant for passage of catheters and endoscopic tubes.

CONTRAINDICATIONS Hypersensitivity to benzocaine or other PABA derivatives (e.g., sunscreen preparations), or to any of the components in the formulation; use of ear preparation in patients with perforated eardrum or ear discharge; applications to large areas. **Dental Use:** Children younger than 2 yr. **Anesthetic Lubricant:** Infants younger than 1 yr.

CAUTIOUS USE History of drug sensitivity; denuded skin or severely traumatized mucosa; lactation; pregnancy (systemic absorption may occur from mucous membranes or from damaged skin; use on mucous membranes or damaged skin should be avoided during pregnancy).

ROUTE & DOSAGE

Anesthetic

Adult: **Topical** Lowest effective dose (usually 3–4 × per day)
Child: **Topical** Lowest effective dose (usually 3–4 × per day)

ADMINISTRATION

Topical

- Avoid contact of all preparations with eyes, and be careful not to inhale mist when spray form is used.
- Do not use spray near open flame or cautery, and do not expose to high temperatures. Hold can at least 12 inches (30 cm) away from affected area when spraying.
- Avoid contact with eyes or other mucous membranes.
- Store at 15°–30°C (59°–86°F) in tight, light-resistant containers unless otherwise specified.

ADVERSE EFFECTS **Hematologic:** Methemoglobinemia reported in infants. **Dermatologic:** Contact dermatitis, localized erythema, burning, stinging. **Other:** Low toxicity; sensitization in susceptible individuals; allergic reactions, anaphylaxis.

INTERACTIONS **Drug:** Topical **dapsone, prilocaine** may increase methemoglobinemia risk.

PHARMACOKINETICS **Absorption:** Poorly absorbed through intact skin; readily absorbed from mucous membranes. **Peak:** varies based on dosage form. **Duration:** varies based on dosage form. **Metabolism:** By plasma cholinesterases and to a lesser extent by hepatic cholinesterases.

NURSING IMPLICATIONS

Assessment & Drug Effects

- Assess swallowing when used on oral mucosa, as benzocaine may interfere with second (pharyngeal) stage of swallowing; hold food and liquids accordingly.
- Assess for sensitivity. Local anesthetics are potentially sensitizing to susceptible individuals when applied repeatedly or over extensive areas.

Patient & Family Education

- Use specific benzocaine preparation ONLY as prescribed or recommended by manufacturer.
- Discontinue medication if the condition persists, worsens, or if signs of sensitivity, irritation, or infection occur.

BENZONATATE

(ben-zoe′na-tate)

Tessalon Perles, Zonatuss

Classification: ANTITUSSIVE

Therapeutic: COUGH SUPPRESSANT

B

AVAILABILITY Capsule

ACTION & *THERAPEUTIC EFFECT* Nonnarcotic antitussive activity that acts peripherally by anesthetizing the receptors in the respiratory bronchi, lungs, and pleura, thus reducing the cough reflex. *Decreases frequency and intensity of nonproductive cough.*

USES Symptomatic treatment of cough.

UNLABELED USES Hiccups.

CONTRAINDICATIONS Hypersensitivity to benzonatate.

CAUTIOUS USE Pregnancy (category C); lactation; children younger than 10 yr.

ROUTE & DOSAGE

Antitussive
Adult/Child (10 yr or older): **PO** 100 mg tid (max: 600 mg/day)

ADMINISTRATION

Oral

- Ensure that soft capsules called perles are swallowed whole.
- Store in airtight containers protected from light.

ADVERSE EFFECTS **Respiratory:** Hypersensitivity reaction (bronchospasm, laryngospasm, anaphylaxis). **CNS:** Drowsiness, sedation, headache, mild dizziness. **Skin:** Rash, pruritus. **GI:** Constipation, nausea.

INTERACTIONS Use with MAO INHIBITORS may increase risk of hypotension.

PHARMACOKINETICS **Onset:** 15–20 min. **Duration:** 3–8 h.

NURSING IMPLICATIONS

Assessment & Drug Effects

- Auscultate lungs anteriorly and posteriorly at scheduled intervals.
- Observe character and frequency of coughing and volume and quality of sputum. Keep prescriber informed.

Patient & Family Education

- Do not chew or allow perle to dissolve in mouth; swallow whole. If perle dissolves in mouth, the mouth, tongue, and pharynx will be anesthetized. Also, it is unpleasant to taste.
- Use with caution while driving or operating machinery.

BENZPHETAMINE HYDROCHLORIDE

(benz-fet'a-meen)

Regimex

Classification: CEREBRAL STIMULANT; ANOREXIANT

Therapeutic: ANOREXIANT

Prototype: Amphetamine

Controlled Substance: Schedule III

AVAILABILITY Tablet

ACTION & *THERAPEUTIC EFFECT* Indirect-acting sympathomimetic amine with amphetamine-like actions but with fewer side effects than amphetamine. Anorexiant effect thought to be secondary to stimulation of hypothalamus releasing stored catecholamines in the CNS. *Effective as an appetite suppressant.*

USES Short-term management of exogenous obesity.

CONTRAINDICATIONS Known hypersensitivity to sympathomimetic amines; angle-closure glaucoma; advanced arteriosclerosis, angina pectoris, severe cardiovascular disease, moderate to severe hypertension; hyperthyroidism, agitated states; history of drug abuse; lactation; pregnancy (category X).

CAUTIOUS USE Diabetes mellitus; older adults; psychosis; mild hypertension; children younger than 12 yr.

ROUTE & DOSAGE

Obesity

Adult/Adolescent: **PO** 25–50 mg 1–3 × day

ADMINISTRATION

Oral

- Give as a single daily dose, preferably midmorning or midafternoon, according to patient's eating habits.
- Schedule daily dose no later than 6 h before patient retires to avoid insomnia.
- Store in tight, light-resistant containers at 15°–30°C (59°–86°F) unless otherwise directed.

ADVERSE EFFECTS **CV:** *Palpitation,* tachycardia, elevated BP, irregular heartbeat. **CNS:** Euphoria, irritability, hyperactivity, nervousness, *restlessness, insomnia,* tremor, headache, light-headedness, dizziness, depression following stimulant effects. Marked insomnia, irritability, hyperactivity, personality changes, psychosis, dermatoses. **GI:** Xerostomia, nausea, vomiting, diarrhea or constipation, abdominal cramps.

INTERACTIONS **Drug: Acetazolamide, sodium bicarbonate** decrease AMPHETAMINE elimination; **ascorbic acid** increase AMPHETAMINE elimination; BARBITURATES may antagonize the effects of both drugs; **furazolidone** may increase BP effects of AMPHETAMINES, and interaction may persist for several weeks after discontinuation of **furazolidone; guanethidine** antagonizes antihypertensive effects; because MAO INHIBITORS, **selegiline** can cause hypertensive crisis (fatalities reported); do not administer AMPHETAMINES during or within 14 days of these drugs; PHENOTHIAZINES may inhibit mood-elevating effects of AMPHETAMINES; BETA AGONISTS increase AMPHETAMINE'S adverse cardiovascular effects. Do not use with **meperidine.** Do not use with other ANORECTIC AGENTS. **Herbal:** Do not use with **melatonin.**

PHARMACOKINETICS **Absorption:** Readily absorbed from GI tract. **Duration:** 4 h. **Metabolism:** Via CYP3A4. **Elimination:** Renal elimination.

NURSING IMPLICATIONS

Assessment & Drug Effects

- Assess for signs of excessive CNS stimulation: Insomnia, restlessness, tremor, palpitations. These may indicate need for dosage adjustment.
- Monitor vital signs; report elevated BP, tachycardia, and irregular heart rhythm.
- Monitor diabetics for loss of glycemic control.

Patient & Family Education

- Note: Anorexiant effects are temporary, and tolerance may occur; long-term use is not indicated.
- Do not drive or engage in potentially hazardous activities until response to drug is known.
- Do not terminate high-dosage therapy abruptly; GI distress,

stomach cramps, trembling, unusual tiredness, weakness, and mental depression may result.

BENZTROPINE MESYLATE

(benz'troe-peen)

Apo-Benztropine ✦, Cogentin, PMS Benztropine ✦

Classification: CENTRALLY ACTING CHOLINERGIC RECEPTOR ANTAGONIST; ANTIPARKINSON

Therapeutic: ANTIPARKINSON

AVAILABILITY Tablet, injectable solution

ACTION & *THERAPEUTIC EFFECT* Synthetic centrally acting anticholinergic agent that acts by diminishing excess cholinergic effect associated with dopamine deficiency. *Suppresses tremor and rigidity; does not alleviate tardive dyskinesia.*

USES Parkinson disease or parkinsonism, drug-induced extrapyramidal symptoms.

CONTRAINDICATIONS Narrow-angle glaucoma; myasthenia gravis; obstructive diseases of GU and GI tracts; tendency to tachycardia; tardive dyskinesia achalasia, myasthenia gravis; megacolon; children younger than 3 yr.

CAUTIOUS USE Older adults or debilitated patients, patients with poor mental outlook, mental disorders; tachycardia; autonomic neuropathy; enlarged prostate; hypertension; history of renal or hepatic disease; pregnancy (may provide adverse effects in fetus; however, potential benefits may warrant use); lactation; children older than 3 yr.

ROUTE & DOSAGE

Parkinson Disease

Adult: **PO/IM** 0.5–1 mg/day, may gradually increase if needed, usual dose 1–2 mg/day (max 6 mg/day)

Acute Drug-Induced Extrapyramidal Symptoms

Adult: **IV/IM/PO** 1–2 mg daily
Child (3 yr or older): **PO/IM/IV** 0.02–0.05 mg/kg/dose once or twice daily

ADMINISTRATION

Oral

- Give immediately after meals or with food to prevent gastric irritation. Tablet can be crushed and sprinkled on or mixed with food.
- Initiate and withdraw drug therapy gradually; effects are cumulative.
- Store in tightly covered, light-resistant container at 15°–30°C (59°–86°F) unless otherwise directed.

Intramuscular

- Inject undiluted solution deeply into a large muscle.

Intravenous

IV administration to infants and children: Verify correct IV concentration with prescriber.

PREPARE: **Direct:** Give undiluted.

ADMINISTER: **Direct:** Give 1 mg or a fraction thereof over 1 min.

INCOMPATIBILITIES: **Y-site: Amphotericin B, cefoperazone, chloramphenicol, dantrolene, diazepam, diazoxide, furosemide, ganciclovir, indomethacin, pentobarbital, phenytoin, sulfamethoxazole/trimethoprim.**

Common adverse effects in *italic*; life-threatening effects underlined; generic names in **bold**; classifications in SMALL CAPS; ✦ Canadian drug name; Prototype drug; ⚠ Alert

ADVERSE EFFECTS **CV:** Tachycardia. **CNS:** *Sedation*, drowsiness, dizziness, paresthesias; agitation, irritability, restlessness, nervousness, insomnia, hallucinations, delirium, confusion, toxic psychosis, muscular weakness, ataxia, inability to move certain muscle groups. **HEENT:** Blurred vision, mydriasis. **GI:** Nausea, vomiting, *constipation, dry mouth,* distention, <u>paralytic ileus</u>. **GU:** Dysuria, urinary retention. **Other:** Hyperthermia, fever.

INTERACTIONS **Drug: Amantadine,** TRICYCLIC ANTIDEPRESSANTS, MAO INHIBITORS, PHENOTHIAZINES, **procainamide, quinidine** have additive anticholinergic effects and cause confusion, hallucinations, paralytic ileus, monitor closely any agents that have anticholinergic effects. Do not use with **eluxadoline, levosulpiride, potassium salts.**

PHARMACOKINETICS **Onset:** 15 min IM/IV; 1 h PO. **Duration:** 6–10 h.

NURSING IMPLICATIONS

Assessment & Drug Effects

- Monitor I&O ratio and pattern. Advise patient to report difficulty in urination or infrequent voiding. Dosage reduction may be indicated.
- Closely monitor for appearance of S&S of onset of paralytic ileus including intermittent constipation, abdominal pain, diminution of bowel sounds on auscultation, and distention.
- Monitor HR especially in patients with a tendency toward tachycardia.
- Monitor for and report muscle weakness or inability to move certain muscle groups. Dosage reduction may be needed.
- Supervise ambulation and use protective measures as necessary.
- Report immediately S&S of CNS depression or stimulation. These usually require interruption of drug therapy.

Patient & Family Education

- Do not drive or engage in potentially hazardous activities until response to drug is known. Seek help walking as necessary.
- Avoid alcohol and other CNS depressants because they may cause additive drowsiness. Do not take OTC cold, cough, or hay fever remedies unless approved by prescriber.
- Sugarless gum, hard candy, and rinsing mouth with tepid water will help dry mouth.
- Avoid strenuous exercise in hot weather; diminished sweating may require dose adjustments because of possibility of heat stroke.

BETAMETHASONE

(bay-ta-meth'a-sone)

BETAMETHASONE DIPROPIONATE

Diprolene, Sernivo

BETAMETHASONE VALERATE

Luxiq

Classification: ADRENAL CORTICOSTEROID; GLUCOCORTICOID; ANTI-INFLAMMATORY

Therapeutic: ANTI-INFLAMMATORY; ADRENAL CORTICOSTEROID

Prototype: Hydrocortisone

AVAILABILITY **Betamethasone Acetate and Betamethasone Sodium:** 3 mg acetate, 3 mg sodium phosphate/mL suspension; **Betamethasone Benzoate**

B

and Betamethasone Dipropionate: Injection; **Betamethasone Valerate:** Ointment; cream; lotion; foam.

ACTION & *THERAPEUTIC EFFECT*

Synthetic, long-acting glucocorticoid with minor mineralocorticoid properties but strong immunosuppressive, anti-inflammatory, and metabolic actions. *Relieves anti-inflammatory manifestations and is an immunosuppressive agent.*

USES Reduces serum calcium in hypercalcemia, suppresses undesirable inflammatory or immune responses, produces temporary remission in nonadrenal disease, and blocks ACTH production in diagnostic tests. Topical use provides relief of inflammatory manifestations of corticosteroid-responsive dermatoses.

UNLABELED USES Accelerate fetal lung maturation.

CONTRAINDICATIONS Corticosteroid hypersensitivity; idiopathic thrombocytopenic purpura (ITP).

CAUTIOUS USE Fungal infection; acne vulgaris, acne rosacea; Cushing syndrome; vaccination; ocular herpes simplex; osteoporosis; diverticulitis, nonspecific ulcerative colitis, abscess or other pyrogenic infection, peptic ulcer disease; asthmatics; DM; hypertension; renal insufficiency; MG; pregnancy (studies show some association between first trimester systemic corticosteroid use and oral clefts or decreased birth weight; chronic high doses should be avoided); lactation; children.

ROUTE & DOSAGE

Anti-Inflammatory Agent

Adult: **IM** 2.5–9 mg/day depending on severity of disease and patient response as sodium phosphate
Child: **IM** 0.02 to 0.3 mg/kg/day (0.6 to 9 mg/m^2/day) in 3 or 4 divided doses

Topical

See Appendix A-4.

ADMINISTRATION

Intramuscular

- Use Celestone Soluspan for intra-articular, IM, and intralesional injection. The preparation is not intended for IV use. Do not mix with diluents containing preservatives (e.g., parabens, phenol). Shake well prior to use.
- Use 1% or 2% lidocaine hydrochloride if prescribed. Withdraw betamethasone mixture first, then lidocaine; shake syringe briefly.

Intradermal

- Shake well prior to use. Inject a uniform depot, using a 1 mL syringe with 1/2-inch needle. Do not inject subcutaneously.

Intravenous

PREPARE: **Direct/IV Infusion:** Give by direct IV undiluted or further diluted for infusion in D5W or NS.
ADMINISTER: **Direct:** Give over 1 min. **Infusion:** Give at a rate determined by the total amount of IV fluid.

ADVERSE EFFECTS **CV:** Hypertension, syncope, thrombophlebitis, thromboembolism or fat embolism, tachycardia, cardiac arrhythmia, cardiomegaly, circulatory shock, edema. **Respiratory:** Pulmonary edema. **CNS:** Vertigo, headache, increased intracranial pressure with papilledema (usually after discontinuation of medication), mental disturbances, aggravation of preexisting psychiatric conditions, insomnia. **HEENT:** Blindness, blurred vision, cataract, exophthalmos, glaucoma, increased intraocular pressure, papilledema. **Endocrine:** Suppressed linear growth in children, decreased glucose tolerance; hyperglycemia, manifestations of latent diabetes mellitus; hypocorticism; amenorrhea and other menstrual difficulties. Hypocalcemia; *sodium and fluid retention;* hypokalemia and hypokalemic alkalosis; negative nitrogen balance. **Skin:** Skin thinning and atrophy, *acne, impaired wound healing;* ecchymosis, easy bruising; suppression of skin test reaction; hypopigmentation or hyperpigmentation, hirsutism, acneiform eruptions, subcutaneous fat atrophy; allergic dermatitis, urticaria, angioneurotic edema, increased sweating. **GI:** *Nausea,* increased appetite, ulcerative esophagitis, pancreatitis, abdominal distention, peptic ulcer with perforation and hemorrhage. **GU:** Decreased motility and number of sperm; bladder dysfunction. **Musculoskeletal:** Osteoporosis, compression fractures, muscle wasting and weakness, tendon rupture, aseptic necrosis of femoral and humeral heads (all resulting from long-term use). **Hematologic:** Petechia. **With Parenteral Therapy, IV Site:** Pain, irritation, necrosis, atrophy, sterile abscess; Charcot-like arthropathy following intra-articular use; burning and tingling in perineal area (after IV injection). **Other:** Hypersensitivity or anaphylactoid reactions; aggravation or masking of infections; malaise, weight gain, obesity. Most adverse effects are dose and treatment duration dependent.

DIAGNOSTIC TEST INTERFERENCE

May suppress reactions to skin tests.

INTERACTIONS

Drug: BARBITURATES, **phenytoin, rifampin** may reduce pharmacologic effect of betamethasone by increasing its metabolism. Do not use with IMMUNOSUPPRESANTS due to risk of enhanced immunosupressive effects. Do not administer at the same time as vaccines. Use caution with CYP3A4 inducers.

PHARMACOKINETICS

Peak: 1–2 h. **Half-Life:** 6.5 h.

NURSING IMPLICATIONS

Assessment & Drug Effects

- Assess therapeutic efficacy. Response following intra-articular, intralesional, or intrasynovial administration occurs within a few hours and persists for 1–4 wk. Following IM administration response occurs in 2–3 h and persists for 3–7 days.

Patient & Family Education

- Monitor weight at least weekly.
- Discontinue slowly after systemic use of 1 wk or longer. Abrupt withdrawal, especially following high doses or prolonged use, can cause dizziness, nausea, vomiting, fever, muscle and joint pain, weakness.

BETAXOLOL HYDROCHLORIDE

(be-tax'oh-lol)

Betoptic, Betoptic-S

Classification: MIOTIC (ANTIGLAUCOMA); BETA-ADRENERGIC ANTAGONIST; ANTIHYPERTENSIVE

Therapeutic: ANTIGLAUCOMA (MIOTIC); ANTIHYPERTENSIVE

Prototype: Propranolol

B

AVAILABILITY Tablet; ophthalmic solution; ophthalmic suspension

ACTION & *THERAPEUTIC EFFECT* Acts as a $beta_1$-selective adrenergic receptor blocking agent, especially at the cardioselective $beta_1$ receptors. Its antihypertensive effect is thought to be due to: (1) decreasing cardiac output, (2) reducing sympathetic nervous system outflow to the periphery resulting in vasodilatation, and (3) suppression of renin activity in the kidney. It reduces intraocular pressure within the eye by decreasing the production of aqueous humor. *It has antihypertensive and antiglaucoma effects.*

USES Hypertension. Ocular use for intraocular hypertension, chronic open-angle glaucoma (see Appendix A-1).

CONTRAINDICATIONS Hypersensitivity to beta-blockers; sinus bradycardia, AV block greater than first degree, cardiogenic shock, uncompensated cardiac failure; lactation.

CAUTIOUS USE History of CHF, angina; renal impairment, hyperthyroidism or thyroid disease; DM; bronchospastic diseases; evidence of airflow obstruction or reactive airway disease; depression; cardiovascular insufficiency; peripheral vascular disease; older adults; pregnancy (category C); children younger than 18 yr.

ROUTE & DOSAGE

Hypertension

Adult: **PO** 10–20 mg daily (no benefit above 20 mg/day)
Elderly: **PO** Start with 5 mg/day and taper up

Renal Impairment Dosage Adjustment

Initial dose 5 mg daily may increase (max: 20 mg/day)

Chronic Open-Angle Glaucoma/ Ocular Hypertension

See Appendix A-1.

ADMINISTRATION

Oral

- Check pulse before administering betaxolol, oral or ophthalmic. If there are extremes (rate or rhythm), withhold medication and notify prescriber.

Ophthalmic

- Shake ophthalmic suspension before use.
- After instillation of drops, instruct patient to close eyes to distribute medication.
- Apply finger pressure to lacrimal sac for 1–2 min following application.
- Wait 5 min before administering any other ophthalmic drug product.

ADVERSE EFFECTS **CV:** Bradycardia. **CNS:** Fatigue.

INTERACTIONS **Drug:** Use with **dronedarone, diltiazem, verapamil, fenoldopam, disopyramide, fingolimod, clonidine, rivastigmine, crizotinib, amiodarone** may cause additive hypotensive effects or bradycardia.

PHARMACOKINETICS **Absorption:** 90% bioavailable. **Onset:** 0.5–1 h. **Peak:** 3 h. **Duration:** Greater than 12 h. **Metabolism:** In liver. **Elimination:** 80% in urine. **Half-Life:** 12–22 h.

NURSING IMPLICATIONS

Assessment & Drug Effects

- Monitor pulse rate and BP at regular intervals in patients with known heart disease.
- Report promptly onset of bradycardia or signs of CHF.
- Monitor baseline renal function.
- Taper dosage slowly when discontinuing.

Patient & Family Education

- Report unusual pulse rate or significant changes to prescriber according to parameters provided.
- Adhere to regimen EXACTLY as prescribed. Do not stop drug abruptly; angina may be exacerbated; dosage is reduced over a period of 1–2 wk.
- Report difficulty in breathing promptly to prescriber. Drug withdrawal may be indicated.

BETHANECHOL CHLORIDE (Pr)

(be-than'e-kole)

Classification: DIRECT-ACTING CHOLINERGIC

Therapeutic: CHOLINERGIC

AVAILABILITY Tablet

ACTION & *THERAPEUTIC EFFECT* Synthetic choline ester with effects similar to those of acetylcholine (ACh). Acts directly on postsynaptic receptors, and because it is not hydrolyzed by cholinesterase, its actions are more prolonged than those of ACh. Produces muscarinic effects primarily on GI tract and urinary bladder. Increases tone and peristaltic activity of esophagus, stomach, and intestine; contracts detrusor muscle of urinary bladder, usually enough to initiate micturition. *Bethanechol is indicated for the treatment of urinary retention associated with neurogenic bladder.*

USES Acute postoperative and postpartum nonobstructive (functional) urinary retention, and for neurogenic atony of urinary bladder with retention.

UNLABELED USES Anticholinergic syndrome, GERD, ileus.

CONTRAINDICATIONS COPD; latent or active bronchial asthma; hyperthyroidism; recent urinary bladder surgery, cystitis, bacteriuria, urinary bladder neck or intestinal obstruction, peptic ulcer, recent GI surgery, peritonitis; marked vagotonia, pronounced vasomotor instability, AV conduction defects, severe bradycardia, hypotension or hypertension, coronary artery disease, recent MI; epilepsy, parkinsonism; lactation, children younger than 8 yr.

CAUTIOUS USE Urinary retention; bacteriemia; patients at risk for syncope; pregnancy (category C).

ROUTE & DOSAGE

Urinary Retention

Adult: **PO** 5–10 mg hourly until goals attained (max: 50 mg dose), usually 10–50 mg 3–4 × daily

ADMINISTRATION

Oral

- Give on an empty stomach (1 h before or 2 h after meals) to lessen possibility of nausea and vomiting, unless otherwise advised by prescriber.

ADVERSE EFFECTS CV: Hypotension with dizziness, faintness, flushing,

B

orthostatic hypotension (large doses); mild reflex tachycardia, atrial fibrillation (hyperthyroid patients), transient complete heart block. **Respiratory:** Acute asthmatic attack, dyspnea (large doses). **HEENT:** Blurred vision, miosis, lacrimation. **GI:** Nausea, vomiting, abdominal cramps, diarrhea, borborygmi, belching, salivation, fecal incontinence (large doses), urge to defecate (or urinate). **Other:** (Dose-related) Increased sweating, malaise, headache, substernal pain or pressure, hypothermia.

DIAGNOSTIC TEST INTERFERENCE Bethanechol may cause increases in ***serum amylase*** and ***serum lipase,*** by stimulating pancreatic secretions, and may increase ***AST, serum bilirubin,*** and ***BSP retention*** by causing spasms in sphincter of Oddi.

INTERACTIONS Drug: Amoxapine, ANTIMUSCARINICS, **maprotiline,** TRICYCLIC ANTIDEPRESSANTS may decrease the effect of **bethanechol. Neostigmine,** other CHOLINESTERASE INHIBITORS compound cholinergic effects and toxicity; **procainamide, quinidine, atropine, epinephrine** antagonize effects of bethanechol.

PHARMACOKINETICS Absorption: Poorly absorbed. **Onset:** 30 min. **Duration:** 1 h. **Metabolism:** Unknown. **Elimination:** Unknown.

NURSING IMPLICATIONS

Assessment & Drug Effects

- Monitor BP and pulse. Report early signs of overdosage: Salivation, sweating, flushing, abdominal cramps, nausea.
- Monitor I&O. Observe and record patient's response to bethanechol.
- Monitor respiratory status. Promptly report dyspnea or any other indication of respiratory distress.
- Supervise ambulation as indicated by patient response to drug.

Patient & Family Education

- Make position changes slowly and in stages, particularly from lying down to standing.
- Do not stand still for prolonged periods; sit or lie down at first indication of faintness.
- Do not drive or engage in potentially hazardous activities until response to drug is known.
- Note: Drug may cause blurred vision; take appropriate precautions.

BETRIXABAN

(be-trix'a-ban)

Classification: ANTICOAGULANT; ANTITHROMBOTIC; DIRECT ORAL ANTICOAGULANT; FACTOR XA INHIBITOR
Therapeutic: ANTICOAGULANT; ANTITHROMBOTIC

AVAILABILITY Capsule

ACTION & *THERAPEUTIC EFFECT* Inhibits fibrin clot formation via inhibition of factor Xa, which catalyzes the conversion of prothrombin to thrombin. *Reduces venous thromboembolism (VTE) risk.*

USES Venous thromboembolism prophylaxis in hospitalized adults.

CONTRAINDICATIONS Hypersensitivity to betrixaban or components of the capsule; active pathological bleeding.

CAUTIOUS USE Severe hypersensitivity to betrixaban; active pathological bleeding; hepatic impairment; renal impairment; pregnancy; lactation. Safety and efficacy in patients younger than 18 yr not established.

ROUTE & DOSAGE

VTE Prophylaxis

Adult: **PO** 160 mg on day 1, then 80 mg daily for 35–42 days

Renal Impairment Dosage Adjustment

CrCL 15-30 mL/min: 80 mg on day 1, then 40 mg daily for 35–42 days

ADMINISTRATION

Oral

- Give with food at the same time each day.
- Store at 20° to 25°C (68° to77°F).

ADVERSE EFFECTS **CV:** Hypertension. **Respiratory:** Epistaxis. **CNS:** Headache. **Endocrine:** Hypokalemia. **GI:** Nausea. **GU:** UTI, hematuria. **Hematologic:** Hemorrhage.

INTERACTIONS **Drug:** Decrease dose by 50% for patients on P-GLYCOPROTEIN INHIBITORS (e.g., **amiodarone, azithromycin, clarithromycin, ketoconazole, verapamil**). May have additive effects with ANTICOAGULANTS.

PHARMACOKINETICS **Absorption:** 34% bioavailability. **Onset:** Peak effect in 3–4 h. **Metabolism:** Minimal via CYP-independent hydrolysis. **Elimination:** 85% in feces, 11% in urine. **Half-Life:** 19–27 h.

NURSING IMPLICATIONS

Black Box Warning

Betrixaban may be associated with epidural or spinal hematomas in those receiving neuraxial anesthesia or undergoing spinal puncture.

Assessment & Drug Effects

- Monitor for and report S&S of bleeding.
- Renal function prior to initiation and periodically as clinically indicated; Routine monitoring of coagulation tests is not required; anti-FXa assay may be helpful in guiding clinical decisions.

Patient & Family Education

- Notify provider if you use this drug before you have a spinal or epidural procedure.
- Notify prescriber if you experience signs or symptoms of allergic reaction such as rash, hives, itching, shortness of breath, wheezing, cough, swelling of the face, lips, tongue, or throat; or any other signs.
- Notify prescriber immediately if you have signs of bleeding such as throwing up blood or coffee-ground appearing vomit; coughing up blood; blood in the urine; black, red, or tarry stools; bleeding from the gums; vaginal bleeding that is not normal; bruises without a reason or that get bigger; or any bleeding that is very bad or can't be stopped.
- You may bleed more easily. Be careful and avoid injury. Use a soft toothbrush and electric razor.

BEVACIZUMAB

(be-va-ci-zu'mab)

Avastin

Classification: ANTINEOPLASTIC; BIOLOGICAL RESPONSE MODIFIER; MONOCLONAL ANTIBODY

Therapeutic: ANTINEOPLASTIC

AVAILABILITY Injection

ACTION & *THERAPEUTIC EFFECT* Binds to vascular endothelial growth factor (VEGF) and prevents the interaction of VEGF with its

B

receptors on the surface of endothelial cells. This blocks endothelial cell proliferation and new blood vessel formation in tumor cells. *Believed to cause reduction of microvascularization in the tumor inhibiting the progression of metastatic disease.*

USES Metastatic colorectal cancer, non-small cell lung cancer, malignant glioblastoma, metastatic renal cell carcinoma.

UNLABELED USES Age-related macular degeneration.

CONTRAINDICATIONS Nephrotic syndrome; hemorrhage; recent hemoptysis; GI perforation; nephritic syndrome; leucopenia; surgery within 28 days; dental work within 20 days; necrotizing fasciitis; severe arterial thromboembolic event due to drug; hypertensive crisis; pulmonary embolism; posterior reversible encephalopathy syndrome (PRES); nephrotic syndrome due to drug; lactation.

CAUTIOUS USE Hypersensitivity to bevacizumab; renal insufficiency; hypertension, history of arterial thromboembolic, cardiovascular, or cerebrovascular disease; CHF; history of GI bleeding; older adults; pregnancy (category C). Safety and efficacy in children and infants not established.

ROUTE & DOSAGE

Metastatic Colorectal Cancer

Adult: **IV** 5–10 mg/kg q14 days until disease progression; in conjunction with other chemotherapy

Non–Small-Cell Lung Cancer

Adult: **IV** 15 mg/kg q3wk

Glioblastoma/Metastatic Renal Cell Carcinoma

Adult: **IV** 10 mg/kg q14 days in 28-day cycle

ADMINISTRATION

Intravenous

PREPARE: **IV Infusion:** Withdraw the desired dose of 5 mg/kg and dilute in 100 mL of NS injection. ▪ Do not shake and do **not** mix or administer with dextrose solutions. Discard any unused portion.

ADMINISTER: **IV Infusion: Do not** administer IV push or bolus. ▪ Infuse first dose over 90 min; if well tolerated, infuse second dose over 60 min; if well tolerated, infuse all subsequent doses over 30 min.

INCOMPATIBILITIES: **Solution/additive: Dextrose**-containing solutions. **Y-site: Dextrose**-containing solutions.

▪ Store diluted solution at 2°–8°C (36°–46°F) for up to 8 h. Store vials at 2°–8°C (36°–46°F); do not freeze and protect from light.

ADVERSE EFFECTS CV: DVT, *hypertension,* heart failure, hypotension, intra-abdominal thrombosis, cerebrovascular events. **Respiratory:** Upper respiratory infection, epistaxis, dyspnea, hemoptysis. **CNS:** Syncope, *headache,* anxiety, dizziness, confusion, abnormal gait, leukoencephalopathy. **HEENT:** Taste disorder, increased tearing. **Endocrine:** Hypokalemia, hyperbilirubinemia, hyperglycemia, hypoalbuminemia, hypomagnesemia, ovarian failure, weight loss. **Skin:** Exfoliative dermatitis, alopecia. **GI:** *Abdominal pain, diarrhea,* constipation, nausea, vomiting, anorexia, stomatitis, dyspepsia, weight loss, flatulence, dry mouth, colitis, gastrointestinal perforation. **GU:** *Proteinuria*, urinary frequency/urgency. **Musculoskeletal:** Myalgia. **Hematologic:** Leukopenia, *neutropenia*, thrombocytopenia, hemorrhage, *thromboembolism*. **Other:** *Asthenia*, pain, wound dehiscence, tracheoesophageal (TE) fistula formation.

PHARMACOKINETICS Half-Life: 20 days (11–50 days).

NURSING IMPLICATIONS

Black Box Warning

Bevacizumab has been associated with increased risk of potentially fatal GI perforation, wound healing complications, and hemorrhage.

Assessment & Drug Effects

- Monitor for S&S of an infusion reaction (hypersensitivity); infusion should be interrupted in all patients with severe infusion reactions and appropriate therapy instituted.
- Withhold drug and promptly notify prescriber for S&S of CHF, hemorrhage (e.g., epistaxis, hemoptysis, or GI bleeding), or unexplained abdominal pain.
- Monitor BP at least every 2–3 wk; if hypertension develops, monitor more frequently, even after discontinuation of bevacizumab.
- Monitor for dizziness, lightheadedness, or loss of balance. Take appropriate safety measures.
- Monitor lab tests: Urinalysis for proteinuria and 24 h urine if protein 2+ or greater.

Patient & Family Education

- Report any of the following to the prescriber: Bloody or black, tarry stool; changes in patterns of urination; swelling of legs or ankles; increased shortness of breath; severe abdominal pain; change in mental awareness, inability to talk or move one side of the body.

BEXAROTENE

(bex-a-ro′teen)

Targretin

Classification: RETINOID; ANTINEOPLASTIC

Therapeutic: ANTINEOPLASTIC

Prototype: Isotretinoin

AVAILABILITY Capsule; gel

ACTION & THERAPEUTIC EFFECT Selectively binds to retinoid × receptors (RXR). Activation of the RXR pathway leads to cell death by interfering with cellular differentiation and proliferation of cells. *Inhibits the growth of tumor cells of squamous (skin) cell origin inducing tumor regression.*

USES Treatment of cutaneous manifestations of cutaneous T-cell lymphoma, mycosis fungoides.

CONTRAINDICATIONS Hypersensitivity to bexarotene; pregnancy (category X); lactation.

CAUTIOUS USE Hypersensitivity to retinoid agents; CAD; DM; alcoholism, history of pancreatitis, hepatitis; lipid abnormalities; hepatic impairment; thyroid disease; women of childbearing age. Safety and efficacy in children not established.

ROUTE & DOSAGE

T-Cell Lymphoma

Adult: **PO** 300 mg/m^2/day as a single dose if no response after 8 wk, may increase to

B

400 mg/m²/day. Adjust dose downward in 100 mg/m²/day increments if toxicity occurs. **Topical** Apply once every other day × 1 wk increase frequency at weekly intervals to once/day, bid, tid, and qid

ADMINISTRATION

Oral

- Give drug with or immediately following a meal. Ensure that capsules are swallowed whole.
- Do not initiate therapy in a woman of childbearing age until the possibility of pregnancy has been completely ruled out.

Topical

- Apply a generous coating only to skin lesions; avoid normal skin.
- Do not cover with clothing until gel dries.
- Store capsules and gel at 20°–25°C (36°–77°F). Protect from light and avoid high temperatures and humidity after bottle or tube is opened.

ADVERSE EFFECTS **CV:** *Peripheral edema,* hypertension, angina, syncope. **CNS:** Insomnia, depression, agitation. **Endocrine:** *Hyperthyroidism. Hyperlipidemia, hypercholesterolemia,* increased LDH. **Skin:** *Rash, dry skin,* exfoliative dermatitis, alopecia, photosensitivity. **GI:** *Abdominal pain, nausea,* diarrhea, vomiting, anorexia. **Hematologic:** Leukopenia, anemia, hypochromic anemia. **Other:** *Headache, asthenia, infection,* chills, fever, flulike syndrome, back pain, bacterial infection.

PHARMACOKINETICS **Absorption:** Best with a fat-containing meal. **Peak:** 2 h. **Distribution:** Greater than 99% protein bound. **Metabolism:** Metabolized by CYP3A4. **Elimination:** Primarily in bile. **Half-Life:** 7 h.

NURSING IMPLICATIONS

Black Box Warning

The oral form of bexarotene has been associated with serious birth defects.

Assessment & Drug Effects

- Monitor (with oral dose) for S&S of: Hypothyroidism, hypertriglyceridemia, hypercholesterolemia, and pancreatitis.
- Lab tests (with oral dose): Baseline blood lipids, then weekly for 2–4 wk, and every 8 wk thereafter; baseline LFTs then repeat at 1, 2, 4 wk, and every 8 wk thereafter; baseline WBC and thyroid function tests, then repeat periodically thereafter; periodic serum calcium; for females, pregnancy test monthly throughout therapy.
- Withhold oral drug and notify prescriber if triglycerides greater than 400 mg/dL or AST, ALT, or bilirubin greater than 3 × upper limit of normal.

Patient & Family Education

- Use effective methods of contraception (both men and women) while taking/using this drug and for at least 1 mo after the last dose of the drug.
- Do not take this drug if you are or could be pregnant.
- Report immediately any of the following: Swelling in the face, lips, or wheezing; persistent bloating, constipation, diarrhea, vomiting, or stomach pain; persistent headache, severe drowsiness or weakness.
- Report changes in vision to the prescriber. An ophthalmologic evaluation may be needed.
- Limit exposure to sunlight or sun lamps and wear sunscreen.
- Report significant skin irritation.

BEZLOTOXUMAB

(bez-loe-tox′ue-mab)

Zinplava

Classification: ANTITOXIN; MONOCLONAL ANTIBODY

Therapeutic: ANTITOXIN

AVAILABILITY Solution for injection

ACTION & *THERAPEUTIC EFFECT* A human monoclonal antibody that binds to *Clostridium difficile* toxin B and neutralizes it. *Bezlotoxumab binds to a specific epitope on toxin B that is conserved across reported strains of* Clostridium difficile. *It does not have antibacterial activity nor does it bind to* Clostridium difficile *toxin A.*

USES In combination with antibacterial therapy to reduce the recurrence of *Clostridium difficile* infection in patients 18 yr or older who are at high risk for recurrence.

CAUTIOUS USE Heart failure, pregnancy, lactation.

ROUTE & DOSAGE

Clostridium Difficile

Adult: **IV** 10 mg/kg single dose over 60 min

ADMINISTRATION

Intravenous

PREPARE: **IV Infusion:** Do not shake the vial. Withdraw the required volume from the vial and transfer into an intravenous bag of either 0.9% sodium chloride or 5% dextrose to prepare a diluted solution with a final concentration of 1–10 mg/mL. Mix the diluted solution by gentle inversion; do not shake.

ADMINISTER: **IV Infusion:** Infuse over 60 min using a sterile, nonpyrogenic, low-protein binding 0.2–0.5 micron in-line or add-on filter.

- Do not administer IV push.
- Store at room temperature for 16 h or under refrigeration for up to 24 h. If refrigerated, allow solution to come to room temperature before administering.

ADVERSE EFFECTS **CV:** Heart failure, hypertension. **Respiratory:** Dyspnea. **CNS:** Dizziness, headache. **GI:** Nausea. **Other:** Fatigue, *infusion-related reactions*, pyrexia.

INTERACTIONS Due to metabolic catabolism, none are expected.

PHARMACOKINETICS **Metabolism:** Metabolic catabolism. **Half-Life:** 19 days.

NURSING IMPLICATIONS

Assessment & Drug Effects

- Monitor for signs or symptoms of an infusion-related reaction.
- Monitor for elevated BP or signs or symptoms of heart failure.

Patient & Family Education

- This medication is used to lower the chance of a bacterial infection called *Clostridium difficile (C. diff)* from coming back.
- Notify healthcare provider if you are breastfeeding or if you are pregnant or planning to become pregnant.

BICALUTAMIDE

(bi-ca-lu′ta-mide)

Casodex

Classification: ANTINEOPLASTIC; HORMONE

Therapeutic: ANTINEOPLASTIC; NONSTEROIDAL ANTIANDROGEN

Prototype: Flutamide

AVAILABILITY Tablet

B

ACTION & *THERAPEUTIC EFFECT*

Inhibits the pharmacologic effects of androgen by binding to androgen receptors in target tissue. *Prostatic carcinoma is androgen sensitive; it responds to removal of the source of androgen or treatment that counteracts the effects of androgen.*

USES In combination with a luteinizing hormone-releasing hormone (LHRH) analog for stage D2 metastatic prostate cancer.

CONTRAINDICATIONS Hypersensitivity to bicalutamide, pregnancy (contraindicated in women including pregnant women), hepatic failure; lactation.

CAUTIOUS USE Moderate to severe hepatic impairment; glucose intolerance; diabetes mellitus. Safety and efficacy in children not established.

ROUTE & DOSAGE

Advanced Prostate Cancer
Adult: **PO** 50 mg once/day

ADMINISTRATION

Oral

- Give drug at the same time each day.
- May be given without regard to food.
- Start treatment with bicalutamide at the same time as treatment with a luteinizing hormone-releasing hormone (LHRH) analog.
- Store at 15°–30°C (59°–86°F).

ADVERSE EFFECTS **CV:** Hypertension, chest pain, peripheral edema. **Respiratory:** Dyspnea. **CNS:** Dizziness, pain, paresthesia, insomnia, anxiety, headache. **Endocrine:** Hyperglycemia, weight loss, weight gain, gout, hot flash, gynecomastia. **Skin:** Rash, sweating, dry skin, pruritus. **GI:** *Constipation, nausea, diarrhea,* vomiting, increased liver function tests, abdominal pain, orexia, dyspepsia, flatulence. **GU:** Nocturia, hematuria, UTI, impotence, gynecomastia, incontinence, frequency, dysuria, urinary retention, urgency. **Musculoskeletal:** arthritis, back pain, weakness, ostealgia, pain, infection, anemia.

INTERACTIONS **Drug:** May increase effects of ORAL ANTICOAGULANTS. Bicalutamide concentrations may be increased by PROTEASE INHIBITORS, **erythromycin** and other CYP3A4 inhibitors. Efficacy of bicalutamide may be decreased by BARBITURATES and other CYP3A4 inducers. Do not use with PHOTOSENSITIZING AGENTS, **cisapride.**

PHARMACOKINETICS **Absorption:** Readily from GI tract. **Metabolism:** In liver. **Elimination:** In urine and feces. **Half-Life:** 6 days.

NURSING IMPLICATIONS

Assessment & Drug Effects

- Monitor for S&S of disease progression.
- Monitor lab tests: Baseline LFTs, then regularly during first 4 mo of treatment and periodically thereafter; periodic PSA; with concurrent warfarin therapy, frequent PT and INR; periodic CBC, ECG, echocardiogram, serum testosterone, luteinizing hormone. Monitor blood glucose levels in diabetics.

Patient & Family Education

- Report jaundice or any other troubling adverse effects immediately.

BIMATOPROST

(bi-mat'o-prost)
Lumigan
See Appendix A-1.

BISACODYL (Pr)

(bis-a-koe′dill)

Apo-Bisacodyl ✦, Bisacolax, Ducodyl, Dulcolax, Fleet Bisacodyl

Classification: STIMULANT LAXATIVE

Therapeutic: LAXATIVE

AVAILABILITY Delayed release tablet; rectal suppository; enema

ACTION & *THERAPEUTIC EFFECT* Stimulates peristalsis by directly irritating the smooth muscle of the intestine, altering water and electrolyte secretion and leading to intestinal fluid accumulation and laxation. *Induces peristaltic contractions by direct stimulation of sensory nerve endings in the colonic wall.*

USES Temporary relief of acute constipation and for evacuation of colon before GI procedures.

CONTRAINDICATIONS Acute surgical abdomen, nausea, vomiting, abdominal cramps, intestinal obstruction, fecal impaction; use of rectal suppository in presence of anal or rectal fissures, ulcerated hemorrhoids, proctitis, bowel obstruction or perforation, ileus.

CAUTIOUS USE Pregnancy (category C); lactation.

ROUTE & DOSAGE

Laxative

Adult: **PO** 5–15 mg prn (max: 30 mg for special procedures); **PR** 10 mg prn

Bowel Cleansing

Adult: **PR** 10 mg as single dose

ADMINISTRATION

Oral

- Give in the evening or before breakfast because of action time required. Administer with water.
- Ensure that enteric-coated tablets are swallowed whole; they should not be crushed or chewed. Do not give within 1 h of antacids or milk.
- Store tablets in tightly closed containers at temperatures not exceeding 30°C (86°F).

Rectal

- Suppository inserted into rectum pointed end first and retained for 15–20 min.
- **Enema:** Shake well; remove protective shield and insert tip into rectum. Squeeze bottle until nearly all liquid is instilled. Gently remove enema bottle.
- Storage is same as tablets.

ADVERSE EFFECTS Systemic effects not reported. Mild cramping, nausea, diarrhea, fluid and electrolyte disturbances.

INTERACTIONS **Drug:** ANTACIDS will cause early dissolution of enteric-coated tablets, resulting in decreased efficacy. **Herbal:** Use with licorice will increase risk of hypokalemia.

PHARMACOKINETICS **Absorption:** 5–15% from GI tract. **Onset:** 6–12 h PO; 15–60 min PR. **Metabolism:** In liver. **Elimination:** In urine, bile, and breast milk.

NURSING IMPLICATIONS

Assessment & Drug Effects

- Evaluate periodically patient's need for continued use of drug; bisacodyl usually produces 1 or 2 soft-formed stools daily.

B

- Monitor patients receiving concomitant anticoagulants. Indiscriminate use of laxatives results in decreased absorption of vitamin K.

Patient & Family Education

- Add high-fiber foods slowly to regular diet to avoid gas and diarrhea. Adequate fluid intake includes at least 6–8 glasses/day.

BISMUTH SUBSALICYLATE

(bis′muth)

Pepto-Bismol

Classification: ANTIDIARRHEAL; SALICYLATE

Therapeutic: ANTIDIARRHEAL

AVAILABILITY Tablet/capsule; liquid

ACTION & THERAPEUTIC EFFECT Hydrolyzed in GI tract to salicylate, which is believed to inhibit synthesis of prostaglandins responsible for GI hypermotility and inflammation. *It acts as a direct mucosal protective agent. Efficacy as an antidiarrheal appears to be due to direct antimicrobial action and to an antisecretory effect on intestinal secretions exposed to toxins.*

USES Treatment of diarrhea and for temporary relief of dyspepsia.

UNLABELED USES *Helicobacter pylori* associated with peptic ulcer disease, prophylaxis, and treatment of traveler's diarrhea.

CONTRAINDICATIONS Hypersensitivity to aspirin or other salicylates; coagulopathy, severe hepatic impairment; use for more than 2 days in presence of high fever or in children younger than 3 yr unless prescribed by prescriber; chickenpox or flu; dysentery.

CAUTIOUS USE Diabetes and gout; alcoholism; renal impairment; older adults; smoking; pregnancy (use should be avoided in pregnant women); lactation.

ROUTE & DOSAGE

Diarrhea/Dyspepsia

Adult: **PO** 524 mg q30–60 min prn (max: 4200 mg/day)
Child (3 to less than 6 yr): **PO** 87 mg q30–60 min prn (max: 8 doses/day); *6 yr to less than 9 yr:* 175 mg q30–60 min prn (max: 8 doses/day); *9–12 yr:* 262 mg q30–60 min prn (max: 8 doses/day)

ADMINISTRATION

Oral

- Ensure chewable tablets are chewed or crushed before being swallowed and followed with at least 8 oz water or other liquid. Shake liquid well prior to use.
- Store at 15°–30°C (59°–86°F) unless otherwise directed.

ADVERSE EFFECTS CNS: Anxiety, confusion, depression, headache, slurred speech. **HEENT:** Tinnitus, hearing loss. **GI:** Temporary *darkening of stool* and tongue, tongue discoloration. **Musculoskeletal:** Muscle spasm, weakness.

DIAGNOSTIC TEST INTERFERENCE Because bismuth subsalicylate is radiopaque, it may interfere with ***radiographic studies*** of GI tract; increases AST and uric acid.

INTERACTIONS Drug: Bismuth may decrease the absorption of TETRACYCLINES. Do not take with **aspirin, bismuth-containing compounds, dexketoprofen,**

ANTICOAGULANTS, ANTIPLATELTES, **hyaluronidase,** LIVE VACCINES, **methotrexate.**

Herbal: Do not use with ginkgo, or other herbs that may cause bleeding.

PHARMACOKINETICS Absorption: Undergoes chemical dissociation in GI tract to bismuth subcarbonate and sodium salicylate; bismuth is minimally absorbed, but the salicylate is readily absorbed.

NURSING IMPLICATIONS

Assessment & Drug Effects

- Monitor bowel function; note that stools may darken and tongue may appear black. These are temporary effects and will disappear without treatment.

Patient & Family Education

- Note: Bismuth contains salicylate. Use caution when taking aspirin and other salicylates. Many OTC medications for colds, fever, and pain contain salicylates.
- Consult prescriber if diarrhea is accompanied by fever or continues for more than 2 days.
- Note: Temporary grayish black discoloration of tongue and stool may occur.

BISOPROLOL FUMARATE

(bis-o-pro'lol fum'a-rate)

Classification: BETA-ADRENERGIC ANTAGONIST; ANTIHYPERTENSIVE

Therapeutic: ANTIHYPERTENSIVE

Prototype: Propranolol

AVAILABILITY Tablet

ACTION & THERAPEUTIC EFFECT Selective inhibitor of $beta_1$-adrenergic receptors. *Bisoprolol has antianginal properties, especially improving exercise tolerance. It reduces both systolic and diastolic blood pressure at rest and with exercise.*

USES Hypertension.

UNLABELED USES Acute MI, atrial fibrillation, angina, heart failure, migraine prophylaxis, supraventricular arrhythmias.

CONTRAINDICATIONS History of hypersensitivity to bisoprolol, severe sinus bradycardia, second- and third-degree AV block, overt cardiac failure, cardiogenic shock; pulmonary edema; lactation.

CAUTIOUS USE Asthma or COPD bronchospastic disease; PVD; DM; Prinzmetal angina; hyperthyroidism; renal or hepatic insufficiency, CVA; stroke; pregnancy (category C); lactation. Safety and efficacy in children not established.

ROUTE & DOSAGE

Hypertension

Adult: **PO** 5 mg once daily, may increase to 20 mg/day if necessary

Heart Failure

Adult: **PO** 1.25 mg daily, may increase (max: 10 mg daily)

Hepatic Impairment Dosage Adjustment

Start with 2.5 mg daily

Renal Impairment Dosage Adjustment

CrCl less than 40 mL/min: Start with 2.5 mg daily

B

ADMINISTRATION

Oral

- May be administered without regard to meals.
- Note: The half-life of the drug is increased in those with significant liver dysfunction; usual initial dose is 2.5 mg and may be carefully titrated upward if necessary.
- Discontinue drug gradually over a period of 1–2 wk to avoid rebound, withdrawal angina, or hypertension.
- Store at room temperature, 15°–30°C (59°–86°F).

ADVERSE EFFECTS **Respiratory:** Upper respiratory infection. **CNS:** Fatigue.

INTERACTIONS **Drug:** Use with **dronedarone, diltiazem, verapamil, fenoldopam, disopyramide, fingolimod, clonidine, rivastigmine, crizotinib, amiodarone** may increase bradycardia or hypotension.

PHARMACOKINETICS **Absorption:** Readily from GI tract; 82–94% reaches systemic circulation. **Peak:** 2–4 h. **Duration:** 24 h. **Distribution:** Some CNS penetration. **Metabolism:** 50% in liver. **Elimination:** 50–60% unchanged in urine. **Half-Life:** 10–12.4 h.

NURSING IMPLICATIONS

Assessment & Drug Effects

- Monitor BP, HR, ECG, and serum glucose frequently during periods of dose adjustment or drug withdrawal. Monitor postural vital signs for orthostatic hypotension.
- Monitor for activity-induced angina both during therapy and following discontinuation of drug.
- Monitor for and report severe hypotension and bradycardia. Dosage adjustment may be required.
- Monitor diabetics for loss of glycemic control.

Patient & Family Education

- Teach patient to change positions slowly to minimize postural hypotension risk.
- Report orthostatic hypotension and dizziness to prescriber.
- Do not discontinue drug abruptly unless specifically instructed to do so.
- Note: Drug-induced nightmares and unpleasant dreams are possible when taking this drug.
- Monitor blood glucose for loss of glycemic control if diabetic.

BIVALIRUDIN

(bi-val′i-ru-den)

Angiomax

Classification: ANTICOAGULANT; DIRECT THROMBIN INHIBITOR

Therapeutic: ANTITHROMBOTIC

Prototype: Argatroban

AVAILABILITY Solution for injection

ACTION & *THERAPEUTIC EFFECT* Inhibits thrombin by specifically binding to (and thus inhibiting) cell sites required to cleave fibrinogen into fibrin. *Reversibly binds to the thrombin active site, thereby blocking the thrombogenic activity of thrombin.*

USES Used with aspirin as an anticoagulant in patients undergoing percutaneous coronary intervention.

UNLABELED USES Heparin-induced thrombocytopenia complicated by thrombosis.

CONTRAINDICATIONS Hypersensitivity to bivalirudin; cerebral aneurysm, intracranial hemorrhage; patients with increased risk of bleeding (e.g., recent surgery, trauma, CVA, hepatic disease); coagulopathy; lactation.

CAUTIOUS USE Asthma or allergies; blood dyscrasia or thrombocytopenia; GI ulceration, serious hepatic disease; hypertension, renal impairment, pregnancy (may lead to maternal or fetal adverse effects, especially during the third trimester). Safety and efficacy in children not established.

ROUTE & DOSAGE

Ischemic heart disease, PCI

Adult: **IV** 0.75 mg/kg bolus (5 min after the bolus, ACT should be performed and 0.3 mg/kg given if needed) followed by 1.75 mg/kg/h for the duration of the procedure, and up to 4 hours after

Renal Impairment Dosage Adjustment

CrCl less than 30 mL/min: Give maintenance dose of 1 mg/kg/h

Hemodialysis Dosage Adjustment

Give 0.25 mg/kg/h maintenance dose

ADMINISTRATION

Intravenous

PREPARE: **Direct/Continuous:** Direct IV bolus dose and initial 4-h continuous infusion: Reconstitute each 250-mg vial with 5 mL of sterile water for injection; gently swirl until dissolved. ▪ Must further dilute each reconstituted vial in 50 mL of D5W or NS to yield 5 mg/mL. **Continuous:** Subsequent low-dose, continuous infusions: Reconstitute each 250-mg vial as above. ▪ Further dilute each reconstituted vial in 500 mL of D5W or NS to yield 0.50 mg/mL.

ADMINISTER: **Direct:** Give bolus dose over 3–5 sec. **Continuous:** Give 1.75 mg/kg/h for the duration of the PTCA procedure. ▪ Subsequent doses, give 0.2 mg/kg/h for up to 20 h as ordered.

INCOMPATIBILITIES: **Y-site: Alteplase, amiodarone, amphotericin B, amphotericin B (lipid), caspofungin, chlorpromazine, dantrolene, diazepam, lansoprazole, pentamidine, pentazocine, phenytoin, prochlorperazine, quinupristin/dalfopristin, reteplase, streptokinase, vancomycin.**

▪ Store reconstituted vials refrigerated at 2°–8°C (35.6°–46.4°F) for up to 24 h. Store diluted concentrations between 0.5 mg/mL and 5 mg/mL at room temperature, 15°–30°C (59°–86°F), for up to 24 h.

ADVERSE EFFECTS **CV:** *Hypotension,* hypertension, bradycardia. **CNS:** *Headache,* anxiety, insomnia, nervousness. **GI:** *Nausea,* vomiting, dyspepsia, abdominal pain. **GU:** Pelvic pain. **Hematologic:** Bleeding. **Other:** Injection site pain. *Back pain,* pain, fever.

DIAGNOSTIC TEST INTERFERENCE PT/INR levels may become elevated in the absence of warfarin.

INTERACTIONS ANTICOAGULANTS may increase risk of bleeding.

B

Do not use with **mifepristone,** PROGESTINS. **Herbal:** Avoid use with anticoagulant/antiplatelet properties.

PHARMACOKINETICS **Duration:** 1 h. **Distribution:** No protein binding. **Metabolism:** Proteolytic cleavage and renal metabolism. **Elimination:** Renal. **Half-Life:** 25 min.

NURSING IMPLICATIONS

Assessment & Drug Effects

- Monitor cardiovascular status carefully during therapy.
- Monitor for and report S&S of bleeding: Ecchymosis, epistaxis, GI bleeding, hematuria, hemoptysis.
- Patients with history of GI ulceration, hypertension, recent trauma or surgery are at increased risk for bleeding.
- Monitor neurologic status and report immediately: Focal or generalized deficits.
- Monitor lab tests: Baseline and periodic ACT; baseline and periodic BUN and serum creatinine.

Patient & Family Education

- Report any of the following immediately: Unexplained back or stomach pain; black, tarry stools; blood in urine, coughing up blood; difficulty breathing; dizziness or fainting spells; heavy menstrual bleeding; nosebleeds; unusual bruising or bleeding at any site.

BLEOMYCIN SULFATE

(blee-oh-mye′sin)

Classification: ANTINEOPLASTIC; ANTIBIOTIC
Therapeutic: ANTINEOPLASTIC
Prototype: Doxorubicin

AVAILABILITY Powder for injection

ACTION & THERAPEUTIC EFFECT
By unclear mechanism, blocks DNA, RNA, and protein synthesis. A cell cycle-phase nonspecific agent widely used in combination with other chemotherapeutic agents because it lacks significant myelosuppressive activity. *This mixture of cytotoxic antibiotics from a strain of* Streptomyces verticillus *has strong affinity for skin and lung tumor cells, in contrast to its low affinity for cells in hematopoietic tissue.*

USES As single agent or in combination with other agents, as adjunct to surgery and radiation therapy. Squamous cell carcinomas of head, neck, penis, testicles, cervix, and vulva; lymphomas (including reticular cell sarcoma, lymphosarcoma, Hodgkin); malignant pleural effusions.

UNLABELED USES *Mycosis fungoides* and *Verruca vulgaris* (common warts), AIDS-related Kaposi sarcoma.

CONTRAINDICATIONS History of hypersensitivity or idiosyncrasy to bleomycin; pulmonary infection; concurrent radiation therapy; women of childbearing age, pregnancy (category D); lactation.

CAUTIOUS USE Compromised hepatic, renal, or pulmonary function; peripheral vascular disease; history of tobacco use; previous cytotoxic drug or radiation therapy.

ROUTE & DOSAGE

Squamous Cell Carcinoma, Testicular Carcinoma

Adult/Child: **Subcutaneous/IM/IV** 10–20 units/m^2 or 0.25–0.5 units/kg 1–2 × wk (max: 300–400 units)

 Common adverse effects in *italic;* life-threatening effects underlined; generic names in **bold;** classifications in SMALL CAPS; ♣ Canadian drug name; ⊕ Prototype drug; ⚠ Alert

Lymphomas

Adult/Adolescent: **Subcutaneous/IM/ IV** 10–20 units/m^2 1–2 × wk after a 1–2 units test dose × 2 doses

Malignant Pleural Effusion

Adult: **Intrapleural** 60 units single dose

Cervical, Penile, Vulvular, Head-Neck Cancer

Adult: **IV/IM/Subcutaneous** 5–20 units/m^2 (0.25–0.5 units/kg)

Renal Impairment Dosage Adjustment

CrCl 40–50 mL/min: Reduce dose 30%; *CrCl 30–39 mL/min:* Reduce dose 40%; *CrCl 20–29 mL/min:* Reduce dose 45%; *CrCl 10–19 mL/min:* Reduce dose 55%; *CrCl 5–10 mL/min:* Reduce dose 60%

ADMINISTRATION

Note: Due to risk of anaphylactoid reaction, give lymphoma patients 2 units or less for first two doses. If no reaction, follow regular dosage schedule.

Subcutaneous/Intramuscular

- Reconstitute with sterile water, NS, or bacteriostatic water by adding 1–5 mL to the 15-unit vial or 2–10 mL to the 30-unit vial. Amount of diluent is determined by the total volume of solution that will be injected.
- Inject IM deeply into upper outer quadrant of buttock; change sites with each injection.

Intravenous

IV administration to infants and children: Verify correct IV concentration and rate of infusion with prescriber.

PREPARE: **Intermittent:** Dilute each 15 units with at least 5 mL of sterile water or NS. ▪ May be further diluted in 50–100 mL of the chosen diluent. ▪ Do not dilute with any solution containing D5W.

ADMINISTER: **Intermittent:** Give each 15 units or fraction thereof over 10 min through Y-tube of free-flowing IV.

INCOMPATIBILITIES: **Solution/additive: Aminophylline, ascorbic acid, cefazolin, diazepam, hydrocortisone, methotrexate, mitomycin, nafcillin, penicillin G, terbutaline. Y-site: Amphotericin B, dantrolene, diazepam, phenytoin, tigecycline.**

- Store unopened ampules at 15°–30°C (59°–86°F) unless otherwise specified by manufacturer.

ADVERSE EFFECTS **Respiratory:** Pulmonary toxicity (dose and age-related); interstitial pneumonitis, pneumonia, or fibrosis. **CNS:** Headache, mental confusion. **Skin:** Diffuse alopecia (reversible), *hyperpigmentation, pruritic erythema,* vesiculation, acne, thickening of skin and nail beds, *patchy hyperkeratosis,* striae, peeling, bleeding. **GI:** Stomatitis, ulcerations of tongue and lips, anorexia, nausea, vomiting, diarrhea, weight loss. **Hematologic:** Thrombocytopenia, leukopenia, (rare). **Other:** Pain at tumor site; phlebitis; necrosis at injection site, shivering. Hypersensitivity (anaphylactoid reaction); *mild febrile reaction.*

INTERACTIONS **Drug:** Other ANTINEOPLASTIC AGENTS increase bone marrow toxicity; decreases effects of **digoxin, phenytoin,** avoid use with LIVE VACCINES.

B

PHARMACOKINETICS Distribution: Concentrates mainly in skin, lungs, kidneys, lymphocytes, and peritoneum. **Metabolism:** Unknown. **Elimination:** 60–70% recovered in urine as parent compound. **Half-Life:** 2 h.

NURSING IMPLICATIONS

Black Box Warning

Bleomycin has been associated with severe hypersensitivity reactions and severe pulmonary, renal, and hepatic toxicity.

Assessment & Drug Effects

- Monitor closely for an acute reaction (hypotension, hyperpyrexia, chills, confusion, wheezing, cardiopulmonary collapse). Anaphylactoid reaction can be fatal (see Appendix F). It may occur immediately or several hours after first or second dose, especially in lymphoma patients.
- Monitor temperature. Febrile reaction (mild chills and fever) is relatively common and usually occurs within the first few hours after administration of a large single dose and lasts about 4–12 h. Reaction tends to become less frequent with continued drug administration, but can recur at any time.
- Monitor respiratory status and report promptly any of the following: SOB, cough, fatigue, loss of appetite, and weight loss.
- Monitor for and report any of the following: Unexplained bleeding or bruising; evidence of deterioration of renal function (changed I&O ratio and pattern, decreasing creatinine clearance, weight gain, or edema); evidence of pulmonary toxicity (nonproductive cough, chest pain, dyspnea).
- Check weight at regular intervals under standard conditions. Weight loss and anorexia may persist a long time after therapy has been discontinued.
- Report promptly symptoms of skin toxicity (hypoesthesia, urticaria, tender swollen hands) that may develop in second or third week of treatment and after 150–200 units of bleomycin have been administered. Therapy may be discontinued.

Patient & Family Education

- Avoid OTC drugs during antineoplastic treatment period unless approved by prescriber.
- Report skin irritation, which may not develop for several weeks after therapy begins.
- Hyperpigmentation may occur in areas subject to friction and pressure, skinfolds, nail cuticles, scars, and intramuscular sites.

BLINATUMOMAB

(bli-na-tu′mo-mab)

Blincyto

Classification: ANTINEOPLASTIC; IMMUNOMODULATOR; MONOCLONAL ANTIBODY

Therapeutic: ANTINEOPLASTIC

Prototype: Basiliximab

AVAILABILITY Lyophilized powder for reconstitution and injection

ACTION & *THERAPEUTIC EFFECT*

Binds to CD19 on B-cells and CD3 on T-cells. It activates T cells by connecting CD3 on the T-cell with CD19 on B-cells (malignant and benign), thus forming a connection between a cytotoxic T-cell and the cancer target B-cell. It mediates the production of cytolytic proteins, release of inflammatory cytokines, and proliferation of T cells, which result in lysis of CD19-positive cancer cells.

USES Treatment of Philadelphia chromosome-negative relapsed or refractory B-cell precursor acute lymphoblastic leukemia (ALL).

CONTRAINDICATIONS Known hypersensitivity to blinatumomab; cytokine release syndrome (CRS); tumor lysis syndrome; lactation.

CAUTIOUS USE History of hypersensitivity reactions; infection; increased AST, ALT, and GGT; increased bilirubin; neurologic toxicity; neutropenia and febrile neutropenia; pregnancy (category C).

ROUTE & DOSAGE

Acute Lymphocytic Leukemia (ALL)

Adult (45 kg or greater): **IV** Cycle 1: 9 mcg/day on days 1–7 and 28 mcg/day on days 8–28; cycles 2–5: 28 mcg/day on days 1–28

Dosing Adjustments Based on Toxicities

Cytokine Release Syndrome (CRS)

Grade 3: Withhold until resolved, then restart at 9 mcg/day, and increase to 28 mcg/day after 7 days if the toxicity does not recur

Grade 4: Discontinue permanently

Neurological Toxicity

Grade 3: Withhold until grade 1 or less for at least 3 days, then restart at 9 mcg/day, and increase to 28 mcg/day after 7 days; if toxicity reoccurs at 9 mcg/day, or does not resolve in 7 days, discontinue permanently

Grade 4 or if more than one seizure occurs: Discontinue permanently

Other Clinically Relevant Adverse Reactions

Grade 3: Withhold until toxicity level is grade 1 or less, then restart at 9 mcg/day, and increase to 28 mcg/day after 7 days if the toxicity does not recur. If toxicity does not resolve in 14 days, discontinue permanently

Grade 4: Consider discontinuing permanently

ADMINISTRATION

- This drug is a cytotoxic agent, and caution should be used to prevent any contact with the drug. Follow institutional or standard guidelines for preparation, handling, and disposal of cytotoxic agents.
- Premedicate with dexamethasone 20 mg IV 1 h before first dose of each cycle, prior to a step dose (such as cycle 1 day 8), or when restarting infusion after interruption of 4 or more h.

Intravenous

PREPARE: **IV Continuous:** Preparation must be done in a pharmacy in a laminar flow hood.

ADMINISTER: **IV Continuous:** Infuse through a dedicated line with a nonpyrogenic, low protein-binding, 0.2 micron in-line filter at a rate of 10 mL/h for 24 h or 5 mL/h for 48 h. Prime the IV line only with the prepared solution for infusion. Do not prime with NS. Use programmable, lockable, nonelastomeric infusion pump with an alarm to give at a constant flow rate. **Important Note:** Do not flush the infusion line, especially when changing infusion bags.

B

Flushing when changing bags or at completion of infusion can result in excess dosage.

- Store: Solutions for infusion are stable for up to 48 h at 23°–27°C (73°–81°F) or up to 8 days at 2°–8°C (36°–46°F).

ADVERSE EFFECTS **CV:** Alterations in blood pressure, tachycardia. **Respiratory:** *Cough, dyspnea,* pneumonia. **CNS:** Aphasia, cognitive disorder, convulsion, dizziness, encephalopathy, *headache, insomnia,* memory impairment, paresthesia, *tremor.* **Endocrine:** Decreased appetite, decreased immunoglobulins, hyperglycemia, hypoalbuminemia, *hypokalemia,* hypomagnesemia, *hypophosphatemia,* increased ALT/AST, increased blood bilirubin, increased gamma-glutamyl-transferase, increased weight, tumor lysis syndrome. **Skin:** Rash. **GI:** Abdominal pain, *constipation, diarrhea, nausea,* vomiting. **Musculoskeletal:** Arthralgia, back pain, bone pain, pain in extremity. **Hematological:** *Anemia, febrile neutropenia,* leukocytosis, leukopenia, lymphopenia, *neutropenia,* sepsis, thrombocytopenia. **Other:** Chest pain, *chills,* confusion, cytokine release syndrome, disorientation, edema, *fatigue, pathogenic infections, peripheral edema, pyrexia.*

PHARMACOKINETICS **Metabolism:** Protein degradation. **Half-Life:** 2.1 h.

NURSING IMPLICATIONS

Black Box Warning

Blinatumomab has been associated with potentially life-threatening cytokine release syndrome and severe, potentially life-threatening neurological toxicities.

Assessment & Drug Effects

- Monitor for neurotoxicity (e.g., confusion, lack of coordination or balance, speech disorders); if suspected, stop infusion and notify prescriber immediately.
- Monitor for S&S of cytokine release syndrome (e.g., pyrexia, headache, nausea, weakness, hypotension, increased transaminases, and elevated total bilirubin); if suspected, stop infusion and notify prescriber immediately.
- Monitor for S&S of hypokalemia (see Appendix F) or infection, and report if either is suspected.
- Monitor lab tests: Baseline and periodic CBC with differential and LFTs; periodic serum electrolytes.

Patient & Family Education

- Report promptly to prescriber any of the following: Fever, persistent headache, weakness, dizziness, lack of coordination, confusion or disorientation, problems with speech, swelling of extremities.
- Refrain from driving or engaging in hazardous occupations or activities while receiving this drug.
- Women should use reliable means of contraception while receiving this drug.
- Do not breastfeed while receiving this drug.
- If diabetic, monitor for loss of glycemic control.

BORTEZOMIB Pr

(bor-te-zo′mib)

Velcade

Classification: ANTINEOPLASTIC; BIOLOGICAL RESPONSE MODIFIER; PROTEOSOME INHIBITOR

Therapeutic: ANTINEOPLASTIC; SIGNAL TRANSDUCTION INHIBITOR (STI)

B

AVAILABILITY Powder for injection

ACTION & THERAPEUTIC EFFECT An inhibitor of proteasome, which is responsible for regulation of protein expression and degradation of damaged or obsolete proteins within the cell; its activity is critical to activation or suppression of cellular functions, including the cell cycle, oncogene expression, and apoptosis. *Proteasome inhibition may reverse some of the changes that allow proliferation of malignant cells and suppress apoptosis (programmed cell death) in malignant cells.*

USES Treatment of multiple myeloma or mantle cell lymphoma.

UNLABELED USES Follicular lymphoma, antibody-mediated rejection in cardiac transplant.

CONTRAINDICATIONS Hypersensitivity to bortezomib, boron, or mannitol; acute diffuse infiltrative pulmonary disease due to drug; posterior reversible encephalopathy syndrome (PRES); pregnancy (may cause fetal harm if administered during pregnancy); lactation.

CAUTIOUS USE Peripheral neuropathy; history of syncope, dehydration, hypotension; history of allergies, asthma; preexisting electrolyte or acid-base disturbances, especially hypokalemia or hyponatremia; diabetic mellitus; liver disease; myelosuppression, renal impairment; risk factors for cardiac disease; history of peripheral neuropathy or other neurologic disorders; risk factors for pulmonary disorders; GI toxicities. Safety and efficacy in children not established.

ROUTE & DOSAGE

Multiple Myeloma/Mantle Cell Lymphoma (failed previous therapy)

Adult: **IV** Dose varies based on concurrent other medications, see package insert for details. Note doses should be separated by at least 72 hours.

Toxicity Dosage Adjustment

See package insert.

Obesity Dosage Adjustment

Calculate dose based on patient actual body weight

Hepatic Impairment Dosage Adjustment

Moderate/severe impairment (bilirubin above 1.5 × ULN) reduce **initial** dose to 0.7 mg/m^2

ADMINISTRATION

Intravenous

Wear protective gloves and prevent contact with skin.

PREPARE: **Direct:** Reconstitute 3.5-mg vial with 3.5 mL of NS for injection to yield 1 mg/mL. ▪ Discard if not clear and colorless. Label reconstituted drug for IV use. Give within 8 h of reconstitution.

ADMINISTER: **Direct:** Give as a bolus dose over 3–5 sec. Flush before/after with NS.

INCOMPATIBILITIES: **Solution/additive:** Do not recommend mixing or injecting with any other drugs.

Subcutaneous

- Reconstitute 3.5-mg vial with 1.4 mL of NS to yield 2.5 mg/mL. Label reconstituted drug for subcutaneous use.

B

- Inject into thigh or abdomen. Rotate injection sites. New injections sites should be at least one inch from old sites.
- If local site reaction occurs, the less concentrated form (1 mg/mL) for IV bolus injection may be given subcutaneously.
- Store unopened vials at 20°–25°C (68°–77°F). Protect from light.
- Store reconstituted vials at 15°–30°C (59°–86°F). Give within 8 h of reconstitution. May store up to 3 h in a syringe; however, total storage time must not exceed 8 h when exposed to normal indoor lighting.

ADVERSE EFFECTS **CV:** Hypotension. **Respiratory:** *Dyspnea*. **CNS:** Peripheral neuropathy, fatigue, neuralgia, headache, paresthesia, dizziness. **Skin:** *Rash*. **GI:** *Nausea, vomiting, diarrhea, anorexia, abdominal pain, constipation, decreased appetite*. **Musculoskeletal:** *Asthenia*. **Hematologic:** Thrombocytopenia, leukopenia, *neutropenia, anemia*. **Other:** *Fever*.

INTERACTIONS **Drug:** Do not use with CYP3A4 inducers. Hypoglycemia and hyperglycemia have been reported with ANTIDIABETIC AGENTS; ANTIHYPERTENSIVE AGENTS may exacerbate hypotension. Avoid MYLEOSUPPRESSIVE AGENTS. **Food: Grapefruit juice** may increase drug levels.

PHARMACOKINETICS **Distribution:** 85% protein bound. **Metabolism:** In the liver (CYP3A4, CYP2C19, CYP1A2). **Half-Life:** 9–15 h.

NURSING IMPLICATIONS

Assessment & Drug Effects

- Monitor for and report S&S of neuropathy (e.g., hyperesthesia, hypoesthesia, paresthesia, discomfort or neuropathic pain).
- Monitor diabetics for loss of glycemic control.
- Monitor postural vital signs for orthostatic hypotension.
- Monitor for S&S of developing a pulmonary disorder.
- Monitor I&O and assess for S&S of dehydration or electrolyte imbalance if vomiting and/or diarrhea develop.
- Monitor lab tests: CBC with platelet count prior to each dose; baseline and periodic LFTs, renal function; frequent blood glucose in diabetics.

Patient & Family Education

- Report promptly any of the following: Dizziness, light-headedness, or fainting spells; numbness, tingling, or other unusual sensations; signs of infection (e.g., fever, chills, cough, sore throat); bruising, pinpoint red spots on the skin; black, tarry stools, nosebleeds, or any other sign of bleeding.
- Monitor closely blood glucose level if diabetic.
- Report increased S&S of CHF, or acute onset of these S&S.
- Do not drive or engage in other hazardous activities until reaction to drug is known.
- Report any S&S of respiratory difficulty.
- Females should use reliable methods of contraception to avoid pregnancy while on this drug.

BOSUTINIB

(bo-su'ti-nib)

Bosulif

Classification: ANTINEOPLASTIC; KINASE INHIBITOR

Therapeutic: ANTINEOPLASTIC

Prototype: Erlotinib

AVAILABILITY Tablet

ACTION & THERAPEUTIC EFFECT A tyrosine kinase inhibitor that blocks certain enzymes that promote CML. *Slows progression of CML.*

USES Treatment of Philadelphia chromosome-positive chronic myelogenous leukemia (CML) in adults who are resistant or intolerant to prior therapy.

CONTRAINDICATIONS Hypersensitivity to bosutinib; pregnancy (category D); lactation.

CAUTIOUS USE Diarrhea; myelosuppression; renal impairment; hepatic impairment; bone density changes; bone marrow suppression; fluid retention; gastrointestinal toxicity; hemorrhage; pancreatitis; QT prolongation; older adults. Safety and efficacy in children younger than 18 yr not established.

ROUTE & DOSAGE

Chronic Myelogenous Leukemia (CML)

Adult: **PO** 500 mg once daily until disease progression or drug intolerance. May escalate to 600 mg daily if target response levels are not reached and adverse reactions are less than grade 3.

Hepatic Impairment Dosage Adjustment

Child–Pugh A, B, or C: 200 mg daily. *For elevation of ALT/AST levels greater than or equal to 5 × the upper limit of normal (ULN):* Withhold until ALT/AST levels are less than or equal to 2.5 × ULN and reduce dose to 400 mg once daily. *If levels are not less than or equal to 2.5 ULN after 4 wk:* Discontinue bosutinib.

Renal Impairment Dosage Adjustment

CrCl 30–50 mL/min: Reduce initial dose by 100 mg; *less than 30 mL/min:* Reduce initial dose by 200 mg

Treatment-Related Toxicity Dosage Adjustments

Hematologic Toxicity Dosage Adjustment

If ANC is less than 1000 × 10^6/L or platelet count is less than 50,000 × 10^6/L: Hold bosutinib. *If ANC is greater than or equal to 1000 × 10^6/L and platelet count is greater than or equal to 50,000 × 10^6/L within 2 wk:* Resume bosutinib at normal dose. *If recovery takes longer than 2 wks:* Reduce dose by 100 mg/day.

Diarrhea Dosage Adjustment

Grade 3 or 4 diarrhea: Hold bosutinib until recovery to grade 1 toxicity or lower; resume therapy at 400 mg/day

ADMINISTRATION

Oral

- Give with food.
- Tablets should be swallowed whole and not crushed, cut, or chewed.
- Follow proper handling and disposal precautions for anticancer drugs.
- Avoid exposure to crushed or broken tablets.
- Store at 15°–30°C (59°–86°F).

ADVERSE EFFECTS **CV:** Edema, chest pain. **Respiratory:** Respiratory tract infection, cough, dyspnea, nasopharyngitis, pleural effusion, influenza. **CNS:** Fatigue, headache, dizziness. **Endocrine:** *Hypophosphatemia*, hypokalemia, fever. **Skin:** *Skin rash*, pruritus. **Hepatic/GI:** Increased serum ALT and AST, *diarrhea, nausea*, vomiting, *abdominal pain*, increased serum lipase, decreased appetite. **Endocrine/GU:** Renal insufficiency, increased serum creatinine. **Musculoskeletal:** Arthralgia, weakness, back pain. **Hematologic:** *Thrombocytopenia, anemia*, neutropenia, leukopenia.

INTERACTIONS **Drug:** Strong or moderate inhibitors of CYP3A (e.g., **ketoconazole**) and/or P-glycoprotein may increase the levels of bosutinib. Strong or moderate inducers (e.g., **rifampin**) of CYP3A may decrease the levels of bosutinib. PROTON PUMP INHIBITORS (e.g., **lansoprazole, omeprazole**) can decrease the absorption of bosutinib. Do not use with LIVE VACCINES. **Food:** Grapefruit or grapefruit juice may increase the levels of bosutinib. **Herbal:** **St. John's wort** may decrease the levels of bosutinib.

PHARMACOKINETICS **Peak:** 4–6 h. **Distribution:** 94% plasma protein bound. **Metabolism:** Substrate of CYP3A4. **Elimination:** Fecal (91%) and renal (3%). **Half-Life:** 22.5 h.

NURSING IMPLICATIONS

Assessment & Drug Effects

- Monitor closely for GI toxicity.
- Monitor vital signs and assess for fluid retention (e.g., peripheral edema, pleural effusion, pulmonary edema).
- Monitor for S&S of hepatotoxicity.
- Monitor lab tests: CBC with differential weekly for 1 mo and monthly thereafter; monthly LFTs for 3 mo or more often if indicated, then periodically thereafter; renal function; pregnancy test.

Patient & Family Education

- If a dose is missed beyond 12 h, do not take until next scheduled dose.
- Report promptly any of the following: Jaundice; S&S of infection; unusual bruising or bleeding; sudden weight gain or extremity swelling; shortness of breath.
- Women should use effective means of birth control during therapy and for at least 30 days following completion of therapy.
- Contact your prescriber immediately if you become pregnant during treatment.
- Do not breastfeed while receiving this drug.

BRENTUXIMAB

(bren-tuk′see-mab)

Adcetris

Classification: BIOLOGICAL RESPONSE MODIFIER; MONOCLONAL ANTIBODY; CD-30 SPECIFIC ANTIBODY; ANTINEOPLASTIC

Therapeutic: ANTINEOPLASTIC

Prototype: Basiliximab

AVAILABILITY Lyophilized powder for injection

ACTION & *THERAPEUTIC EFFECT* An antibody-drug complex that binds to a protein (CD 30) on the surface of lymphoma cells and is internalized into these cells where it releases a microtubule disrupting agent. *Causes cell cycle arrest and apoptosis of lymphoma cells.*

USES Treatment of Hodgkin lymphoma in patients nonresponsive to autologous stem cell transplant (ASCT) or non-Hodgkin lymphoma.

CONTRAINDICATIONS Development of progressive multifocal leukoencephalopathy (PML) or Stevens–Johnson syndrome; concurrent use with bleomycin; pregnancy (category D); lactation.

CAUTIOUS USE Hypersensitivity to brentuximab due to infusion reaction; bone marrow depression; renal and hepatic impairment; history of peripheral neuropathy; history of pulmonary disease; older adults. Safety and efficacy in children not established.

ROUTE & DOSAGE

Hodgkin Lymphoma or Systemic Anaplastic Large Cell Lymphoma

Adult: **IV** 1.8 mg/kg q3wk for maximum of 16 cycles

Peripheral Neuropathy Dosage Adjustment

Grade 2/3 peripheral neuropathy: Stop treatment until toxicity resolves to grade 1 or better. Reduce dosage to 1.2 mg/kg q3wk; *For grade 4 peripheral neuropathy:* Discontinue treatment

Neutropenia Dosage Adjustment

Grade 3/4 neutropenia: Stop treatment until toxicity resolves to baseline or grade 2 or better. Consider the use of growth factors (CSFs) for subsequent cycles; *grade 4 neutropenia (despite the use of growth factors):* Discontinue treatment or reduce dosage to 1.2 mg/kg IV q3wk

ADMINISTRATION

Intravenous

- Premedication with acetaminophen, an antihistamine, and a corticosteroid are recommended for prior infusion reactions.

PREPARE: **IV Infusion:** Reconstitute each 50-mg vial with 10.5 mL sterile water (SW) for injection to yield 5 mg/mL. Direct the stream of SW onto side of vial and not into powder. Swirl gently to dissolve. Do not shake. Immediately withdraw the required volume of reconstituted solution and add to a minimum of 100 mL of NS, D5W, or LR to produce a final concentration of 0.4–1.8 mg/mL. Invert bag gently to mix.

ADMINISTER: **IV Infusion:** Give over 30 min. Do not give IV push or bolus.

INCOMPATIBILITIES: **Solution/additive:** Do not mix or administer as an IV infusion with any other medicinal products.

- Store refrigerated, if necessary, at 2°–8°C (36°–46°F). Should be used immediately after preparation but no later than 24 h following reconstitution.

ADVERSE EFFECTS **Respiratory:** *Cough*, dyspnea, oropharyngeal pain, *upper respiratory tract infection.* **CNS:** Anxiety, dizziness, headache, insomnia, *peripheral neuropathy.* **Endocrine:** Decreased appetite, weight loss. **Skin:** Alopecia, dry skin, night sweats, pruritus, *rash.* **GI:** *Abdominal pain*, constipation, *diarrhea, nausea, vomiting.* **Musculoskeletal:** Arthralgia, back pain, muscle spasms, myalgia, pain in extremity. **Hematological:** *Anemia*, lymphadenopathy, *neutropenia, thrombocytopenia.* **Other:** Chills, *fatigue*, pain, peripheral edema, *pyrexia.*

B

INTERACTIONS Drug: Monomethyl auristatin E (MMAE), one of the components of brentuximab, is primarily metabolized by CYP3A4. Strong inhibitors of CYP3A4 (e.g., **ketoconazole, delavirdine, indinavir, itraconazole**) may increase the levels of brentuximab. Strong inducers of CYP3A4 (i.e., **phenobarbital, rifampin**) may decrease the levels of brentuximab. **Herbal: St. John's wort** and **Hypericum perforatum** may reduce the levels of brentuximab.

PHARMACOKINETICS Peak: 1–3 d. **Distribution:** 68–82% plasma protein bound. **Metabolism:** Oxidative metabolism. **Elimination:** Primarily fecal. **Half-Life:** 4–6 d.

NURSING IMPLICATIONS

Black Box Warning

Brentuximab has been associated with progressive JC virus infection resulting in progressive multifocal leukoencephalopathy (PML) and death.

Assessment & Drug Effects

- Discontinue infusion immediately and institute supportive measures if hypersensitivity (see Appendix F) is suspected.
- Monitor closely for and report promptly S&S of an infusion reaction (e.g., chills, nausea, dyspnea, pruritus, fever, cough).
- Monitor cardiac status throughout infusion and during the immediate period thereafter.
- Monitor closely for a report of S&S of peripheral neuropathy (e.g., hypo/hyperesthesia, paresthesia, burning sensation, nerve pain, weakness). Withhold drug and notify prescriber for new or worsening grade 2 or 3 neuropathy.
- Monitor lab tests: Baseline and prior to each dose, CBC with differential.

Patient and Family Education

- Report any of the following to prescriber: Chills, rash, or difficulty breathing within 24 h of infusion; numbness or tingling of hands or feet; muscle weakness; fever of 100.5° F or greater; unexplained cough; or pain on urination.
- Women should use effective means of contraception and avoid breastfeeding while being treated with brentuximab.

BREXPIPRAZOLE

(brex-pi-pra′zole)

Rexulti

Classification: ATYPICAL ANTIPSYCHOTIC; ANTIDEPRESSANT

Therapeutic: ANTIPSYCHOTIC; ANTIDEPRESSANT

Prototype: Clozapine

AVAILABILITY Tablets

ACTION & *THERAPEUTIC EFFECT* Exhibits partial agonist activity for 5-HT_{1A} and D_2 receptors and antagonist activity for 5-HT_{2A} receptors. *May improve mood and affect in major depressive disorder, and may improve overall functional capability in schizophrenia.*

USES Adjunctive treatment of major depressive disorder (MDD) and treatment of schizophrenia.

CONTRAINDICATIONS Hypersensitivity to brexpiprazole or any component of the formulation; dementia-related psychosis; suicidal ideation.

CAUTIOUS USE History of suicidal thoughts; extrapyramidal symptoms; hyperglycemia; DM; obesity; orthostatic hypotension; dyslipidemia; seizures; impaired core body temperature regulation; esophageal dysmotility; pregnancy (third trimester); lactation. Safety and efficacy in people younger than 18 yr not established.

ROUTE & DOSAGE

Major Depressive Disorder (MDD)

Adult: **PO** 0.5 to 1 mg once daily; titrate weekly to max of 3 mg

Schizophrenia

Adult: **PO** 1 mg once daily on days 1–4; titrate to 2 mg once daily on days 5–7, then to 4 mg on day 8 (max 4 mg/day)

Pharmacogenetic Dosage Adjustment/Concomitant CYP Inducers or Inhibitors

CYP2D6 poor metabolizers, or taking concomitant strong CYP2D6 or strong CYP3A4 inhibitors: Half of usual dose
CYP2D6 poor metabolizers taking concomitant strong/moderate CYP3A4 inhibitors, or taking concomitant strong/moderate CYP2D6 inhibitors with strong/moderate CYP3A4 inhibitors: One quarter of usual dose
Taking concomitant strong CYP3A4 inducers: Double usual dose over 1–2 wk

ADMINISTRATION

Oral

- May give without regard to food.
- Store at 15°–30°C (59°–86°F).

ADVERSE EFFECTS **Respiratory:** Nasopharyngitis. **CNS:** Akathisia, headache, tremor, drowsiness. **Endocrine:** Increased triglycerides, weight gain. **GI:** Dyspepsia. **Other:** Extra-pyramidal symptoms, fatigue.

INTERACTIONS **Drug:** Concomitant use with strong CYP3A4 inhibitors (e.g., **clarithromycin, itraconazole, ketoconazole**) and/or strong CYP2D6 inhibitors (e.g., **fluoxetine, paroxetine, quinidine**) will increase the blood levels of brexpiprazole. Concomitant use with strong CYP3A4 inducers (e.g., **rifampin**) will decrease the blood levels of brexpiprazole. CNS DEPRESSANTS may enhance side effects. DOPAMINE ANTAGONISTS will diminish therapeutic effect. **Herbal: St. John's wort** will decrease the levels of brexpiprazole.

PHARMACOKINETICS **Absorption:** 95% bioavailable. **Peak:** 4 h. **Distribution:** 99% plasma protein bound. **Metabolism:** Hepatic oxidation. **Elimination:** Renal (25%) and fecal (46%). **Half-Life:** 91 h.

NURSING IMPLICATIONS

Black Box Warning

Brexpiprazole has been associated with increased mortality in elderly patients with dementia-related psychosis, and increased risk of suicidal thoughts and behavior in those 24 yr and younger.

Assessment & Drug Effects

- Monitor mental status; report worsening of clinical S&S and emergence of suicidal thoughts and behaviors.
- Monitor for extrapyramidal symptoms (EPS) such as tardive dyskinesia (see Appendix F). Withhold

B

drug and notify prescriber if EPS develop.

- Monitor BP at baseline, repeat 3 mo after therapy initiated, then yearly thereafter.
- Monitor closely those at risk for aspiration as esophageal dysmotility and dysphagia may occur.
- Monitor weight, BMI, waist circumference at baseline; repeat at 4, 8, and 12 wk or after changing therapy, then q3mo thereafter; report weight gain of 5% or more of initial weight.
- Monitor lab tests: Baseline and periodic CBC with differential, fasting blood glucose, lipid profile, electrolytes, liver function tests.

Patient & Family Education

- Report new or worsening depression symptoms, especially sudden changes in mood, behaviors, thoughts, or feelings.
- Report promptly suicidal thoughts or actions.
- Avoid drinking alcohol while taking this drug.
- Report promptly any of the following: Restlessness; uncontrolled movement on your face, tongue or other body parts; difficulty swallowing; weight gain; excessive urination or thirst; lightheadedness upon arising.
- Avoid becoming overheated and maintain adequate hydration with liquids.
- Women should use effective means of contraception while taking this drug.
- Do not breastfeed while taking this drug without consulting the prescriber.

BRIMONIDINE TARTRATE

(bry-mon′i-deen)

Alphagan P

See Appendix A-1.

BRINZOLAMIDE

(brin-zol′a-mide)

Azopt

See Appendix A-1.

BRIVARACETAM

(briv′a-ra′se-tam)

Brivlera, Briviact ♣

Classification: ANTICONVULSANT

Therapeutic: ANTICONVULSANT

AVAILABILITY Tablet; oral solution; solution for injection

ACTION & *THERAPEUTIC EFFECT* Exact mechanism has not been determined; however, brivaracetam is highly selective for synaptic vesicle protein 2A (SV2A) in the brain. *This is thought to contribute to the anticonvulsant effect.*

USES Adjunctive therapy in the treatment of partial-onset seizures.

CONTRAINDICATIONS Hypersensitivity to brivaracetam.

CAUTIOUS USE Abrupt discontinuation, depression, driving or operating machinery, geriatric, hepatic disease, suicidal ideation, pregnancy (adverse events have been observed in animal reproduction studies), lactation.

ROUTE & DOSAGE

Epilepsy

Adult: **PO/IV** 50 mg bid; may adjust to 25 mg bid or 100 mg bid

Adolescent/Child/Infant (over 1 month) **PO/IV:** weight over

B

50 kg: 25–50 mg bid; *20–49 kg:* 0.5–1 mg/kg/dose bid; *11–20 kg:* 0.5–1.25 mg/kg/dose bid

Hepatic Impairment Dosage Adjustment

Initial dose of 25 mg bid (max dose: 75 mg bid)

ADMINISTRATION

Oral

- May be administered without regard to meals.
- Swallow tablets whole; do not crush or chew tablets.
- Oral solution does not need to be diluted.
- Discard unused oral solution after 5 mo of first opening the bottle.

Intravenous

PREPARE: **IV Infusion:** No need to dilute but can be diluted in 0.9% sodium chloride, LR, or 5% dextrose.

ADMINISTER: **IV Infusion:** May be given intravenously over 2–15 min.

- Store after dilution for no more than 4 h at room temperature.

ADVERSE EFFECTS **CNS:** Ataxia, drowsiness, lethargy, malaise, abnormal gait, dizziness, fatigue, hypersomnia, psychiatric events, sedation. **HEENT:** Nystagmus. **GI:** Nausea, vomiting. **Other:** Asthenia.

INTERACTIONS **Drug: CYP2C19 inducers** (e.g. **rifampin)** increase the levels of brivaracetam. Brivaracetam may increase the levels of **phenytoin** and **carbamazepine**, CNS DEPRESSANTS may have additive adverse effects.

PHARMACOKINETICS **Peak:** 1 h. **Distribution:** Less than 20% plasma protein bound. **Metabolism:** Hepatic to inactive metabolites (via CYP2C19). **Elimination:** Primarily renal (greater than 95%). **Half-Life:** 9 h.

NURSING IMPLICATIONS

Assessment & Drug Effects

- Assess other medications that patient is taking, alternative therapies, or dosage adjustments that might be needed.
- Monitor for signs or symptoms of depression or suicidal ideation.
- Monitor lab tests: Obtain CBC with differential, LFTs, and renal function tests.

Patient & Family Education

- Notify your healthcare provider if you are breastfeeding or if you are pregnant or planning to become pregnant.
- Upon starting this medication, avoid driving or performing other tasks that require you to be alert.
- Call your healthcare provider right away if you feel sad or depressed, nervous, restless, grouchy, panicky; have a change in mood; or have suicidal thoughts.

BRODALUMAB

(broe-dalu′mab)

Siliq

Classification: MONOCLONAL ANTIBODY; ANTIPSORIATIC AGENT; ANTI-INTERLEUKIN-17 RECEPTOR ANTIBODY

Therapeutic: ANTIPSORIATIC

AVAILABILITY Subcutaneous injection, prefilled syringe

ACTION & *THERAPEUTIC EFFECT* Human monoclonal IgG2 antibody that antagonizes the

B

interleukin-17 receptor, a pathway to block cytokine-induced inflammatory response. *Reduces inflammatory response in moderate to severe plaque psoriasis.*

USES Treatment of plaque psoriasis in patients who have not responded, or stopped responding, to other systemic treatments.

CONTRAINDICATIONS Crohn disease.

CAUTIOUS USE Crohn disease; pregnancy; lactation. Safety and efficacy in children not established.

ROUTE & DOSAGE

Psoriasis

Adult: **Subcutaneous** 210 mg once a wk for 3 wk, then 210 mg every 2 wk; discontinue if response not seen after 12–16 wk

ADMINISTRATION

Subcutaneous

- Allow prefilled syringe to reach room temperature for approx 30 min prior to injecting; do not use if solution is not clear, or discolored.
- Administer subcutaneously into the thigh, abdomen more than 2 in from umbilicus, or outer upper arm.
- Do not inject into tissue that is tender, bruised, red, hard, scaly, or affected by psoriasis.

ADVERSE EFFECTS **CNS:** Fatigue. **Hematologic:** Neutropenia, antibody development. **Muscular:** Arthralgia, myalgia. **Other:** *Infection.*

INTERACTIONS Avoid use with live vaccines; unknown influence on CYP450 enzymes. Do not use with **belimumab, cladribine, fingolimod, infliximab, pimecrolimus, tacrolimus, upadacitinib.**

PHARMACOKINETICS **Absorption:** 55% bioavailability. **Distribution:** Follows nonlinear pharmacokinetics. **Onset:** Peak effect in 3 days. **Metabolism:** Similar to endogenous IgG.

NURSING IMPLICATIONS

Black Box Warning

Brodalumab use is associated with an increased risk of suicidal ideation and behavior; advise patients to seek medical attention if symptoms develop while on treatment with brodalumab. Only available through a REMS program.

Assessment & Drug Effects

- Evaluate for tuberculosis infection prior to treatment.
- Monitor for signs of suicidal ideation or behavior.
- Monitor for signs of infection, including active tuberculosis.
- Routine monitoring of coagulation tests is not required; anti-FXa assay may be helpful in guiding clinical decisions.

Patient & Family Education

- Notify prescriber if you have suicidal thoughts or behaviors.
- Notify prescriber if you experience signs or symptoms of allergic reaction such as rash, hives, itching, shortness of breath, wheezing, cough, swelling of the face, lips, tongue, or throat; or any other signs.
- Prior to initiating treatment, notify prescriber if you have been diagnosed with Crohn disease or have active TB.

BROLUCIZUMAB

(BROE-lue-SIZ-ue-mab)

Beovu

Classifications: VASCULAR ENDOTHELIAL GROWTH FACTOR INHIBITOR

Therapeutic: OPHTHALMIC AGENT

AVAILABILITY Solution for intravitreal injection

ACTION & *THERAPEUTIC EFFECT* Inhibits recombinant humanized monoclonal antibody vascular endothelial growth factor. *Suppresses endothelial cell proliferization, neovascularization, and vascular permeability to slow vision loss.*

USES Neovascular age-related macular degeneration

CONTRAINDICATIONS Hypersensitivity to brolucizumab or any component of the formulation; ocular or periocular infections; active intraocular inflammation.

CAUTIOUS USE Endophthalmitis or retinal detachment, increased intraocular pressure, or thromboembolism; pregnancy (may cause fetal harm if administered to a pregnant female); lactation (unknown if present in breast milk).

ROUTE & DOSAGE

Age-Related Macular Degeneration

Adult: **Intravitreal Injection** 6 mg every mo for three doses, followed by 6 mg every 8–12 wk.

ADMINISTRATION

Intravitreal

- For ophthalmic intravitreal injection only.
- Each vial should be used for the treatment of a single eye. If the contralateral eye requires treatment, a new vial and sterile field and supplies should be used.
- Adequate anesthesia and a topical broad-spectrum antimicrobial agent should be administered prior to the procedure.
- Store at 2° to 8°C (36° to 46°F). Protect from light. Unopened vial may be kept at 20° to 25°C (68°F to 77°F)for up to 24 hours prior to use.

ADVERSE EFFECTS **HEENT:** Blurred vision, cataract, conjunctival hemorrhage, intraocular inflammation, eye pain, vitreous opacity. **Other:** Antibody development.

INTERACTIONS **Drug:** No studies have been conducted.

PHARMACOKINETICS **Peak:** 24 h. **Metabolism:** Nonspecific proteolysis. **Elimination:** Passive renal excretion. **Half-Life:** 4 d.

NURSING IMPLICATIONS

Assessment & Drug Effects

- Monitor intraocular pressure (via tonometry) and optic nerve head perfusion immediately following administration.
- Monitor for symptoms of endophthalmitis, retinal detachment, or thromboembolic events.

Patient & Family Education

- Report signs of eye redness, eye pain, changes in vision, or thromboembolic events (stroke, heart attack, or peripheral blood clot) to your provider immediately.

BROMFENAC

(brom'fen-ac)

Xibrom

See Appendix A-1.

B

BROMOCRIPTINE MESYLATE

(broe-moe-krip'teen)

Cycloset, Parlodel

Classification: ERGOT ALKALOID; DOPAMINE RECEPTOR AGONIST

Therapeutic: ERGOT REPLACEMENT; ANTIDYSKINETIC; ANTIPARKINSON; GLYCEMIC CONTROL AGENT

Prototype: Ergotamine

AVAILABILITY Tablet; capsule

ACTION & *THERAPEUTIC EFFECT* Semisynthetic ergot alkaloid derivative and a sympatholytic dopamine D_2 receptor agonist that activates postsynaptic dopamine receptors leading to inhibited pituitary prolactin secretion and enhanced coordinated muscle control. *Restores ovulation and ovarian function in amenorrheic women, thus correcting female infertility secondary to elevated prolactin levels. Activates dopaminergic receptors in CNS resulting in antiparkinsonism effect. Improves glycemic control in Type 2 diabetics.*

USES Acromegaly, hyperprolactinemia, female infertility, Parkinson disease, prolactinoma, pituitary adenoma. As adjunct to diet and exercise in Type 2 diabetes.

UNLABELED USES To prevent postpartum lactation, neuroleptic malignant syndrome.

CONTRAINDICATIONS Hypersensitivity to ergot alkaloids; uncontrolled hypertension; severe ischemic heart disease or peripheral vascular disease; pituitary tumor; lactation. **Cycloset:** Type 1 diabetes mellitus or diabetic ketoacidosis; syncopal migraine due to hypertensive episodes. **Parlodel:** Uncontrolled hypertension; postpartum period in women with history of CAD, or severe cardiovascular conditions; normal prolactin levels, preeclampsia, eclampsia.

CAUTIOUS USE Hepatic and renal dysfunction; history of psychiatric disorder; history of GI bleeding or peptic ulcer; history of MI with residual arrhythmia; pregnancy (category C); children.

ROUTE & DOSAGE

Amenorrhea, Female Infertility

Adult: **PO** 1.25–2.5 mg/day (max: 2.5 mg 2–3 × day)

Parkinson Disease

Adult: **PO** 1.25 day (increase by 2.5 mg q14–28 days)

Acromegaly

Adult: **PO** 1.25–2.5 mg/day for 3 days, then increase by 1.25–2.5 mg q3–7 days until desired effect is achieved, usually 30–60 mg/day in divided doses

Hyperprolactinemia

Adult: **PO** 1.25–2.5 mg/day increase dose by 2.5 mg q2–7 days until response achieved; (usual dose 2.5–15 mg/day)

Adjunct in Type 2 Diabetes (Cycloset)

Adult: **PO** 0.8 mg daily in the a.m., titrate up (normal dose: 1.6–4.8 mg)

ADMINISTRATION

Oral

- Give with meals, milk, or other food to reduce incidence of GI side effects.
- Cycloset: Administer within 2 hr of waking in the morning.

- Store in tightly closed, light-resistant containers, preferably at 15°–30°C (59°–86°F) unless otherwise directed.

ADVERSE EFFECTS **CV:** Orthostatic hypotension. **Respiratory:** Rhinitis. **CNS:** Dizziness, fatigue, headache. **GI:** Constipation, nausea. **Musculoskeletal:** Weakness.

INTERACTIONS **Drug:** Use with TRIPTANS increases risk of vasospastic reactions, use with sulpiride decreases efficacy. ANTIHYPERTENSIVE AGENTS add to hypotensive effects; ORAL CONTRACEPTIVES, **estrogen, progestins** may interfere with effect of bromocriptine by causing amenorrhea and galactorrhea; PHENOTHIAZINES, TRICYCLIC ANTIDEPRESSANTS, **methyldopa, reserpine** can cause an increase in **prolactin,** which may interfere with bromocriptine activity. Do not use with letermovir, isometheptene, amoxapine, or ERGOTS due to increased risk of adverse effects.

PHARMACOKINETICS **Absorption:** 65–95% bioavailable. **Peak:** 1–2 h. **Duration:** 4–8 h. **Metabolism:** In liver by CYP3A4. **Elimination:** 85% in feces in 5 days; 3–6% in urine. **Half-Life:** 6–20 h.

NURSING IMPLICATIONS

Assessment & Drug Effects

- Monitor BP and HR closely during the first few days and periodically throughout therapy.
- Monitor lab tests: Periodic CBC, LFTs, HbA1C, and renal functions with prolonged therapy.

Patient & Family Education

- Make position changes slowly and in stages, especially from lying down to standing, and to dangle legs over bed for a few minutes before walking. Lie down immediately if light-headedness or dizziness occurs.
- Do not drive or engage in other potentially hazardous activities until response to drug is known.
- Avoid exposure to cold, and report the onset of pallor of fingers or toes.
- Note: Use barrier-type contraceptive measures until normal ovulating cycle is restored. Oral contraceptives are contraindicated.

BROMPHENIRAMINE MALEATE

(brome-fen-ir'a-meen)

Veltane

Classification: ANTIHISTAMINE; H_1-RECEPTOR ANTAGONIST

Therapeutic: ANTIHISTAMINE

Prototype: Diphenhydramine

AVAILABILITY Injection; elixir; tablet; ingredient in many oral combination products containing a decongestant, expectorant, and/or analgesic

ACTION & *THERAPEUTIC EFFECT* Antihistamine that competes with histamine for H_1-receptor sites on effector cells in the bronchi and bronchioles, thus blocking histamine-mediated responses. *Effective against upper respiratory symptoms and allergic manifestations.*

USES Symptomatic treatment of allergic manifestations. Also used in various cough mixtures and antihistamine-decongestant cold formulations.

CONTRAINDICATIONS Hypersensitivity to antihistamines; acute asthma; newborns.

CAUTIOUS USE Older adults; prostatic hypertrophy; GI obstruction; asthma; narrow-angle glaucoma; COPD, cardiovascular or

B

renal disease; seizure disorders; hyperthyroidism; pregnancy (category C); lactation.

ROUTE & DOSAGE

Allergy

Adult: **PO** 4–8 mg tid or qid or 8–12 mg of sustained release bid or tid
Geriatric: **PO** 4 mg 1–2 × day
Child (6 yr or older): **PO** 2–4 mg tid or qid or 8–12 mg of sustained release bid (max: 12 mg/24 h); *younger than 6 yr:* 0.5 mg/kg in 3–4 divided doses

ADMINISTRATION

Oral

- Give with meals or a snack to prevent gastric irritation.
- Store in tightly covered container at 15°–30°C (59°–86°F) unless otherwise directed. Elixir should be protected from light. Avoid freezing.

ADVERSE EFFECTS **CNS:** *Sedation,* drowsiness, dizziness, headache, disturbed coordination. **HEENT:** Ringing or buzzing in ears. **Skin:** Rash, photosensitivity. **GI:** Dry mouth, throat, and nose, stomach upset, constipation. **Other:** Hypersensitivity reaction (urticaria, increased sweating, agranulocytosis).

DIAGNOSTIC TEST INTERFERENCE May cause false-negative **allergy skin tests.**

INTERACTIONS **Drug: Alcohol** and other CNS DEPRESSANTS add to sedation.

PHARMACOKINETICS **Peak:** 3–9 h. **Duration:** Up to 48 h. **Distribution:** Crosses placenta. **Elimination:** 40% in urine within 72 h; 2% in feces. **Half-Life:** 12–34 h.

NURSING IMPLICATIONS

Assessment & Drug Effects

- Drowsiness, sweating, transient hypotension, and syncope may follow IV administration; reaction to drug should be evaluated. Keep prescriber informed.
- Note: Older adults tend to be particularly susceptible to drug's sedative effect, dizziness, and hypotension. Most symptoms respond to reduction in dosage.
- Monitor lab tests: Periodic CBC with long-term therapy.

Patient & Family Education

- Acute hypersensitivity reaction can occur within minutes to hours after drug ingestion. Reaction is manifested by high fever, chills, and possible development of ulcerations of mouth and throat, pneumonia, and prostration. Patient should seek medical attention immediately.
- Sugarless gum, lemon drops, or frequent rinses with warm water may relieve dry mouth.
- Do not drive or perform other potentially hazardous activities until response to drug is known.
- Do not take alcoholic beverages or other CNS depressants (e.g., tranquilizers, sedatives, pain or sleeping medicines) without consulting prescriber.

BUDESONIDE

(bu-des′o-nide)

Entocort EC, Pulmicort, Rhinocort Aqua, UCERIS

Classification: ADRENAL CORTICOSTEROID GLUCOCORTICOID; ANTI-INFLAMMATORY
Therapeutic: RESPIRATORY INHALANT; ANTI-INFLAMMATORY; ADRENAL CORTICOSTEROID
Prototype: Hydrocortisone

AVAILABILITY Inhalation powder, nasal spray, nebulizer solution, oral capsule, extended release tablet; rectal foam

ACTION & THERAPEUTIC EFFECT Its anti-inflammatory action on nasal mucosa is thought to be a result of decreased IgE synthesis and decreased arachidonic acid metabolism. *Glucocorticoids have a wide range of inhibitory activities against multiple cell types (e.g., neutrophils, macrophages) and mediators (e.g., histamine, cytokines) involved in allergic and nonallergic/irritant-mediated inflammation.*

USES Treatment of allergic and perennial rhinitis, maintain remission in mild to moderate Crohn disease or ulcerative colitis; prophylaxis for asthma.

UNLABELED USES Autoimmune hepatitis.

CONTRAINDICATIONS Hypersensitivity to budesonide, status asthmaticus, acute bronchospasms; peptic ulcer disease; lactation (**oral**).

CAUTIOUS USE Active or quiescent tuberculosis; infections of respiratory tract; in sun-treated fungal, bacterial, or systemic viral infections or ocular herpes simplex; recent nasal septal ulcers; recurrent epistaxis; nasal surgery or trauma; psychosis; myasthenia gravis; diabetes mellitus; seizure disorders; hepatic impairment. Pregnancy (some studies show an association between first trimester systemic corticosteroid use and oral clefts; may also influence fetal growth; may be used cautiously to treat disease flares in pregnant women); lactation.

ROUTE & DOSAGE

Crohn Disease

Adult: **PO** 9 mg once daily for up to 8 wk, may taper to 6 mg daily for 2 wk prior to discontinuing. May repeat 8-wk course for recurring episodes of active Crohn disease.

Ulcerative Colitis

Adult: **PO** 9 mg daily for up to 8 wk

Asthma Prophylaxis, Rhinitis

See Appendix A-3.

ADMINISTRATION

Oral

- Ensure that capsules and extended release formulations are swallowed whole and not chewed.
- Give only in the morning.
- Avoid grapefruit juice.
- Patients with moderate to severe liver disease should be monitored for increased signs and/or symptoms of hypercorticism. Reducing the dose of Entocort EC capsules should be considered in these patients.
- Store at 25°C (77°F); excursions permitted to 15°–30°C (59°–86°F).

ADVERSE EFFECTS CV: Chest pain, hypertension, palpitations, sinus tachycardia, facial edema. **Respiratory:** Respiratory tract infection, sinusitis, bronchitis. **CNS:** Dizziness, agitation, nervousness, *headache,* agitation, confusion, insomnia, drowsiness. **Endocrine:** Hypokalemia, decreased cortisol, moon face, weight gain. **Skin:** Eczema, pruritus, purpura, rash, alopecia, acne vulgaris, bruising. **GI:** Dyspepsia, oral candidiasis, diarrhea, nausea, vomiting. **GU:** UTI. **Musculoskeletal:** Arthralgia, arthritis, muscle cramps,

B

myalgia, tremor, weakness. **Other:** Arthralgia, fatigue, fever, hyperkinesis, myalgia, asthenia, paresthesia, tremor.

INTERACTIONS **Drug: CYP3A4 inhibitors (e.g. ketoconazole)** may increase oral budesonide concentrations and toxicity; ANTACIDS may decrease the levels of budesonide. **Food: Grapefruit juice** will significantly increase bioavailability of oral budesonide.

PHARMACOKINETICS **Absorption:** 20% (nasal) dose, 6–13% of (orally inhaled) dose, 9% PO dose reaches systemic circulation; PO form is absorbed from duodenum at pH greater than 5.5; oral bioavailability increases 2.5 × in hepatic cirrhosis. **Onset:** 8–12 h inhaled, 2 wk oral. **Peak:** 2 wk inhaled, 8 wk oral delayed by high-fat meal. **Distribution:** 90% protein bound. **Metabolism:** 85% of absorbed dose undergoes first pass metabolism by CYP3A4. **Elimination:** 60% in urine, 40% in feces. **Half-Life:** 2–3.6 h.

NURSING IMPLICATIONS

Assessment & Drug Effects

- Monitor closely for S&S of hypercorticism if concomitant doses of ketoconazole or other CYP3A4 inhibitors (see Drug Interactions) are being given.
- Monitor patients with moderate to severe liver disease for increased S&S of hypercorticism.
- Monitor Bp and weight.
- Monitor lab tests: Periodic serum glucose, electrolytes.

Patient & Family Education

- Notify the prescriber immediately for any of the following: Itching, skin rash, fever, swelling of face and neck, difficulty breathing, or if you develop S&S of infection.
- Do not drink grapefruit juice or eat grapefruit regularly.
- Avoid people with infections, especially those with chickenpox or measles if you have never had these conditions.

BUMETANIDE

(byoo-met′a-nide)

Bumex, Burinex ♣

Classification: LOOP DIURETIC

Therapeutic: DIURETIC; ANTIHYPERTENSIVE

Prototype: Furosemide

AVAILABILITY Tablet; injection

ACTION & *THERAPEUTIC EFFECT* Inhibits sodium and chloride reabsorption by direct action on proximal ascending limb of the loop of Henle leading to increased excretion of water, sodium, chloride, magnesium, phosphate, and calcium. Also appears to inhibit phosphate and bicarbonate reabsorption. *Produces mild hypotensive effects at usual diuretic doses. Controls formation of edema.*

USES Edema, heart failure.

UNLABELED USES Hypertension, nocturia.

CONTRAINDICATIONS Hypersensitivity to bumetanide or to other sulfonamides; anuria, markedly elevated BUN; hepatic coma; ventricular arrhythmias; severe electrolyte deficiency; lactation.

CAUTIOUS USE Hepatic cirrhosis; renal impairment; severe renal disease; history of gout; history of pancreatitis; history of hypersensitivity to furosemide; diabetes mellitus; acute MI; older adults; pregnancy (category C).

ROUTE & DOSAGE

Edema

Adult: **PO** 0.5–2 mg once/day, may repeat at 4–5 h intervals if needed (max: 10 mg/day); **IV/IM** 0.5–1 mg over 1–2 min, repeated q2–3h prn (max: 10 mg/day)

Hypertension

Adult: **PO** 0.5–4 mg/day in divided doses

ADMINISTRATION

Oral

- Give with food or milk to reduce risk of gastrointestinal irritation.
- Administered in the morning as a single dose, either daily or by intermittent schedule.

Intramuscular

- Use undiluted solution for injection.

Intravenous

PREPARE: **Direct/Continuous:** Give direct IV undiluted (typical) or diluted for infusion with D5W, NS, LR.

ADMINISTER: **Direct:** Give IV push at a rate of a single dose over 1–2 min.

INCOMPATIBILITIES: **Solution/additive: Dobutamine. Y-site: Alemtuzumab, amphotericin B, azathioprine, chlorpromazine, dantrolene, diazepam, diazoxide, fenoldopam, ganciclovir, gemtuzumab, haloperidol, midazolam, minocycline, ofloxacin, oritavancin, papaverine, pentamidine, phenytoin, quinupristin/dalfopristin, sulfamethoxazole/trimethoprim, topotecan.**

- Diluted infusion should be used within 24 h after preparation.
- Store in tight, light-resistant container at 15°–30°C (59°–86°F) unless otherwise directed.

ADVERSE EFFECTS **Endocrine:** Hyperuricemia, hypochloremia, hypokalemia, hyponatremia, hyperglycemia. **Renal/GU:** Azotemia, increased serum creatinine.

INTERACTIONS **Drug:** Do not use with **desmopressin** due to increased risk of hyponatremia. AMINOGLYCOSIDES, **cisplatin** increase risk of ototoxicity; bumetanide increases risk of hypokalemia-induced **digoxin** toxicity; NONSTEROIDAL ANTI-INFLAMMATORY DRUGS (NSAIDS) may attenuate diuretic and hypotensive response; may increase risk of lithium toxicity, **probenecid** may antagonize diuretic activity; bumetanide may decrease renal elimination of **lithium; sotalol, dofetilide, droperidol** may increase risk of cardiotoxicity.

DIAGNOSTIC TEST INTERFERENCE May lead to false-negative aldosterone/renin ratio (ARR).

PHARMACOKINETICS **Absorption:** Readily from GI tract. **Onset:** 30–60 min PO; 2–3 min IV. **Peak:** 0.5–2 h PO; 15–30 min IV. **Duration:** 4–6 h PO; 2–3 h IV. **Distribution:** Distributed into breast milk. **Metabolism:** In liver. **Elimination:** 80% in urine in 48 h, 10–20% in feces. **Half-Life:** 60–90 min.

NURSING IMPLICATIONS

Black Box Warning

Bumetanide has been associated with profound diuresis resulting in serious fluid and electrolyte imbalances.

B

Assessment & Drug Effects

- Monitor I&O and report onset of oliguria or other changes in I&O ratio and pattern promptly.
- Monitor weight, BP, and pulse rate. Assess for hypovolemia by taking BP and pulse rate while patient is lying, sitting, and standing. Older adults are particularly at risk for hypovolemia with resulting thrombi and emboli.
- Monitor for S&S of hypomagnesemia and hypokalemia (see Appendix F), especially in those receiving digitalis or who have CHF, hepatic cirrhosis, ascites, diarrhea, or potassium-depleting nephropathy.
- Monitor for hearing difficulty or ear discomfort. Patients at risk of ototoxic effects include those receiving the drug IV, especially at high doses, those with severely impaired renal function, and those receiving other potentially ototoxic or nephrotoxic drugs (see Appendix F).
- Monitor diabetics for loss of glycemic control.
- Monitor lab tests: Baseline and periodic serum electrolytes, blood studies (for dyscrasias), LFTs and kidney function tests, uric acid (particularly patients with history of gout), and blood glucose.

Patient & Family Education

- Report promptly to prescriber symptoms of electrolyte imbalance (e.g., weakness, dizziness, fatigue, faintness, confusion, muscle cramps, headache, paresthesias).
- Eat potassium-rich foods such as fruit juices, potatoes, cereals, skim milk, and bananas while taking bumetanide.
- Report S&S of ototoxicity promptly to prescriber (see Appendix F).
- Monitor blood glucose for loss of glycemic control if diabetic.

BUPRENORPHINE HYDROCHLORIDE

(byoo-pre-nor′feen)

Buprenex, Butrans, Suboxone

Classification: ANALGESIC; NARCOTIC (OPIATE AGONIST–ANTAGONIST)

Therapeutic: NARCOTIC ANALGESIC

Prototype: Pentazocine

Controlled Substance: Schedule III

AVAILABILITY Injection; sublingual tablet; transdermal patch

ACTION & *THERAPEUTIC EFFECT* Opiate agonist–antagonist with agonist activity approximately 30 × that of morphine and antagonist activity equal to or up to 3 × that of naloxone. Respiratory depression occurs infrequently, probably due to drug's opiate antagonist activity. *Dose-related analgesia results from a high affinity of buprenorphine for mu-opioid receptors and as an antagonist at the kappa-opiate receptors in the CNS. Naloxone is an antagonist at the mu-opioid receptor.*

USES *Injectable* used for moderate to severe pain. *Sublingual tablets* used for treatment of opioid dependence.

UNLABELED USES *Injectable* to reverse fentanyl-induced anesthesia. *Sublingual tablets* may be used to ease cocaine withdrawal.

CONTRAINDICATIONS Hypersensitivity to buprenorphine; significant respiratory depression; acute or severe bronchial asthma without resuscitative equipment; paralytic ileus; severe hepatic impairment; lactation.

CAUTIOUS USE Patient with history of opiate use or substance abuse; family or personal history of alcohol dependency or mental illness; unstable cardiac status; personal or family history of QT prolongation; compromised respiratory function [e.g., COPD, cor pulmonale, decreased respiratory reserve, hypoxia, hypercapnia, or preexisting respiratory depression]; hypothyroidism, myxedema, adrenal insufficient including Addison disease; severe renal impairment; mild to moderate hepatic impairment; geriatric or debilitated patients; acute alcoholism, delirium tremens; hypovolemia; cardiovascular disease including acute MI; prostatic hypertrophy, urethral stricture; comatose patient; patients with CNS depression, head injury, or intracranial lesion; history of seizures; biliary tract dysfunction; older or debilitated adults; pregnancy (category C). Safety and efficacy in children not established.

ROUTE & DOSAGE

Postoperative Pain

Adult/Adolescent (13 yr or older): **IV/IM** 0.3 mg q6h up to 0.6 mg q4h or 25–50 mcg/h by IV infusion
Geriatric: **IV/IM** 0.15 mg q6h
Child (2–12 yr): **IV/IM** 2–6 mcg/kg q4–6h prn

Opioid Dependence/Cocaine Withdrawal

Adult/Adolescent: **SL** Initiate with 8 mg daily on day 1 at least 4 h after last opioid dose, 16 mg daily on day 2, then switch to maintenance therapy at the same buprenorphine dose as day 2 (e.g., 16 mg daily). Adjust dose daily until opiate withdrawal effects are suppressed. Maintenance dose range 4–24 mg/day buprenorphine.

Moderate to Severe Pain

Adult: **Topical** One 5 mcg/h patch q7days (titrate at minimum interval of 72 h)

ADMINISTRATION

Sublingual

- Place sublingual tablets under tongue until dissolved. For doses requiring more than two tablets, place all tablets at once under tongue, or if patient cannot accommodate all tablets, place two tablets at a time under tongue.
- Instruct to hold the tablets under tongue until dissolved; advise not to swallow.

Transdermal

- Apply only to intact, hairless or nearly hairless skin. If needed, clip (but do not shave) hair from skin. Prior to application, clean site with clear water and allow to dry completely; do not use soaps, alcohol, oils, or lotions on application site.
- Each system is worn for 7 days. May apply to upper outer arm, upper chest, upper back, or the side of the chest. Tape edges in place if needed.
- Rotate sites. Must wait at least 21 days before reusing a skin site.

Intramuscular

- Give undiluted, deep IM into a large muscle.
- Store at 15°–30°C (59°–86°F); avoid freezing.

Intravenous

PREPARE: **Direct/IV Infusion:** May be given undiluted direct IV or further dilute each 1 mL (0.3 mg) ampule in 50 mL of D5W, NS, D5NS, or LR to yield 6 mcg/mL for infusion. Do not use if discolored or contains particulate matter.

B

ADMINISTER: **Direct:** Give slowly at a rate of 0.3 mg over 2 min to a patient in a recumbent position. **IV Infusion:** Give by slow infusion over 3 min or longer depending on volume of IV solution.

INCOMPATIBILITIES: **Solution/additive: Diltiazem, floxacillin, furosemide, lorazepam. Y-site: Alemtuzumab, aminophylline, amphotericin B cholesteryl sulfate complex, ampicillin, azathioprine, dantrolene, diazepam, diazoxide, doxorubicin liposome, fluorouracil, gemtuzumab, indomethacin, lansoprazole pantoprazole, pentobarbital, phenobarbital, phenytoin, sodium bicarbonate, SMZ/TMP.**

ADVERSE EFFECTS **CV:** Hypotension, vasodilation. **Respiratory:** Respiratory depression, hyperventilation. **CNS:** *Sedation, drowsiness,* dizziness, vertigo, *headache,* amnesia, euphoria, asthenia, *insomnia, pain* (when used for withdrawal), *withdrawal symptoms.* **HEENT:** Miosis. **Skin:** Pruritus, injection site reactions, *sweating.* **GI:** *Nausea,* vomiting, diarrhea, *constipation.*

INTERACTIONS **Drug: Alcohol,** OPIATES, other CNS DEPRESSANTS, BENZODIAZEPINES augment CNS depression; **diazepam** may cause respiratory or cardiovascular collapse; AZOLE ANTIFUNGALS (e.g., **fluconazole**), MACROLIDE ANTIBIOTICS (e.g., **erythromycin**), and PROTEASE INHIBITORS (e.g., **saquinavir**) may increase buprenorphine levels.

PHARMACOKINETICS **Absorption:** Widely variable sublingual absorption. **Onset:** 10–30 min IM/IV. **Peak:** 1 h IM/IV; 2–6 h SL. **Duration:** 6–10 h. **Metabolism:** Extensively in liver by CYP3A4 to active metabolite norbuprenorphine. **Elimination:** 70% in feces, 30% in urine in 7 days. **Half-Life:** 2.2 h IM/IV; 37 h SL.

NURSING IMPLICATIONS

Black Box Warning

Buprenorphine has been associated with severe, potentially fatal respiratory depression; it also has a high potential for abuse. Prolonged use during pregnancy can cause life-threatening neonatal withdrawal syndrome.

Assessment & Drug Effects

- Monitor respiratory status during therapy. Buprenorphine-induced respiratory depression is about equal to that produced by 10 mg morphine, but onset is slower, and if it occurs, it lasts longer.
- Monitor I&O ratio and pattern: Urinary retention is a potential adverse effect.
- Supervise ambulation; drowsiness occurs in 66% of patients taking this drug.
- Monitor lab tests: Baseline LFTs and renal function tests.

Patient & Family Education

- Do not drive or engage in other potentially hazardous activities until response to drug is known.
- Do not use alcohol or other CNS depressing drugs without consulting prescriber. An additive effect exists between buprenorphine hydrochloride and other CNS depressants including alcohol.

B

BUPROPION HYDROCHLORIDE

(byoo-pro′pi-on)

Budeprion XL, Forfivo XL, Wellbutrin, Wellbutrin SR, Wellbutrin XL, Zyban

BUPROPION HYDROBROMIDE

Aplenzin

Classification: ANTIDEPRESSANT
Therapeutic: ANTIDEPRESSANT

AVAILABILITY Tablet; sustained release tablet; extended release tablet; hydrobromide form

ACTION & *THERAPEUTIC EFFECT* The neurochemical mechanism of bupropion is not fully understood. It selectively inhibits the neuronal reuptake of dopamine and norepinephrine, but does not inhibit monoamine oxidase or reuptake serotonin. The primary action is thought to be dopaminergic and/or noradrenergic. *Its antidepressive effect is related to dopaminergic or noradrenergic properties.*

USES Depression, smoking cessation, seasonal affective disorder.

UNLABELED USES Neuropathic pain, ADHD.

CONTRAINDICATIONS Hypersensitivity to bupropion; seizure disorder; current or prior diagnosis of bulimia or anorexia nervosa; suicidal ideation; concurrent 14 days of MAO inhibitor use; head trauma; CNS tumor; recent MI; abrupt discontinuation, lactation.

CAUTIOUS USE Renal or hepatic function impairment; drug abuse or dependence; hypertension, CHF, MI, renal impairment; severe hepatic impairment, hepatic disease, biliary cirrhosis; suicidal tendencies; major depressive disorders (MDD); bipolar disorder, mania, psychosis, schizophrenia; DM; ethanol intoxication, tics, Tourette syndrome; older adults; pregnancy (category C); children younger than 18 yr.

ROUTE & DOSAGE

Depression/Seasonal Affective Disorder

Adult: **PO Immediate release** 100 mg bid then titrate to 100 mg tid; **Sustained release** 150 mg daily then titrate to 150 mg bid (or 300 mg daily Wellbutrin SR); **Aplenzin:** 174 mg daily can increase to 348 mg daily (max: 522 mg/day)
Geriatric: **PO** May require reduced initial dose

Smoking Cessation

Adult: **PO** Start with 150 mg once daily × 3 days, then increase to 150 mg bid (max: 300 mg/day) for 7–12 wk

Hepatic Impairment Dosage Adjustment

Start at lower dose, decrease dose or dosage frequency

ADMINISTRATION

Oral

- Administer as a single dose in the morning. May be given with or without food.
- Immediate release tablets should be given at approximately 6-h intervals, or longer as directed.
- Ensure that extended release and sustained release tablets are not chewed or crushed. They **must be** swallowed whole.
- Store away from heat, direct light, and moisture.

ADVERSE EFFECTS **CV:** Tachycardia. **Respiratory:** Pharyngitis **CNS:** Seizures (the risk of seizure appears to be strongly associated with dose, especially greater than 450 mg/day), *agitation, insomnia, dry mouth, blurred vision, headache, dizziness, tremor.* **Skin:** Rash, diaphoresis. **GI:** *Nausea, vomiting, constipation.* **Other:** Weight loss, weight gain.

INTERACTIONS **Drug:** May increase metabolism of **carbamazepine, cimetidine, phenytoin, phenobarbital**, decreasing their effect; may increase incidence of adverse effects of **levodopa**, contraindicated with MAO INHIBITORS.

PHARMACOKINETICS **Absorption:** Readily from GI tract. **Onset:** 3–4 wk. **Peak:** 1–3 h. **Metabolism:** In liver to active metabolites by CYP2B6; may inhibit CYP2D6. **Elimination:** 80% in urine. **Half-Life:** 8–24 h.

NURSING IMPLICATIONS

Black Box Warning

Bupropion has been associated with increased risk of suicidal thoughts and behavior in children, adolescents, and young adults. Serious neuropsychiatric events have occurred in patients during use and during treatment discontinuation.

Assessment & Drug Effects

- Monitor for therapeutic effectiveness. The full antidepressant effect of drug may not be realized for 4 or more weeks.
- Monitor for and report promptly worsening of depression or suicidal ideation.
- Monitor respiratory status and report promptly S&S of respiratory depression.
- Monitor blood pressure prior to initiation of treatment and periodically.
- Use extreme caution when administering drug to patient with history of seizures, cranial trauma, or other factors predisposing to seizures; during sudden and large increments in dose, seizure potential is increased.
- Report significant restlessness, agitation, anxiety, and insomnia. Symptoms may require treatment or discontinuation of drug.
- Monitor for and report delusions, hallucinations, psychotic episodes, confusion, and paranoia.
- Monitor lab tests: Periodic renal function tests and LFTs.

Patient & Family Education

- Monitor weight at least weekly. Report significant changes in weight (± 5 lb) to prescriber.
- Minimize or avoid alcohol because it increases the risk of seizures.
- Report promptly suicidal thoughts, especially when treated for depression.
- Do not drive or engage in potentially hazardous activities until response to drug is known because judgment or motor and cognitive skills may be impaired.
- Do not abruptly discontinue drug. Gradual dosage reduction may be necessary to prevent adverse effects.
- Do not take any OTC drugs without consulting prescriber.

BUSPIRONE HYDROCHLORIDE

(byoo-spye′rone)

Classification: ANXIOLYTIC

Therapeutic: ANTIANXIETY

AVAILABILITY Tablet

ACTION & *THERAPEUTIC EFFECT*

An anxiolytic with agonist effects on presynaptic dopamine receptors and also a high affinity for serotonin (5-HT_{1A}) receptors. *Antianxiety effect is due to serotonin reuptake inhibition and agonist effects on dopamine receptors of the brain.*

USES Management of generalized anxiety disorder.

UNLABELED USES Augmentation strategy in treatment of unipolar depression.

CONTRAINDICATIONS Hypersensitivity to buspirone; severe renal impairment; severe hepatic impairment; Concomitant use of MAOI therapy; lactation.

CAUTIOUS USE Moderate to severe renal or hepatic impairment, pregnancy—fetal risk cannot be ruled out; lactation—infant risk cannot be ruled out; children less than 18 yr.

ROUTE & DOSAGE

Anxiety

Adult: **PO** 10–15 mg/day in divided doses, may increase by 5 mg/day q2–3days as needed (max: 60 mg/day)
Adolescent/Child (greater than 6 y): **PO** 5mg daily, may increase by 5 mg/day q2–3 days as needed.

Renal Impairment Dosage Adjustment

Do not use in severe impairment.

Hepatic Impairment Dosage Adjustment

Do not use in severe impairment.

ADMINISTRATION

Oral

- Give with food to decrease nausea.
- Store at 15°–30°C (59°–86°F) in tightly closed container unless otherwise directed.

ADVERSE EFFECTS (> 5%) CNS: *dizziness, headache, drowsiness, excitement.* **GI:** *Nausea.*

DIAGNOSTIC TEST INTERFERENCE Buspirone may increase serum concentrations of ***hepatic aminotransferases (ALT, AST)***; may result in a false positive on a ***urinary assay*** for metanephrine/catecholamine.

INTERACTIONS Drug: May cause serotonin syndrome if used with MAO INHIBITORS, **linezold**; increased **haloperidol** serum levels. Strong CYP3A4 inducers (ex **carbamazepine**) or CYP3A4 inhibitors (ex **itraconazole**) may decrease serum concentrations and should be avoided or closely monitored. Use with **erythromycin** may increase risk of adverse effects. **Food: Grapefruit juice** may increase drug levels. **Herbal: St. John's wort** may increase drug levels.

PHARMACOKINETICS Absorption: Readily from GI tract, undergoes first-pass metabolism. **Distribution:** 86% protein bound. **Peak:** 1 h. **Metabolism:** In liver. **Elimination:** 30–63% in urine as metabolites within 24 h. **Half-Life:** 2–4 h.

NURSING IMPLICATIONS

Assessment & Drug Effects

- Monitor for therapeutic effectiveness. Desired response may begin within 7–10 days; however, optimal results take 3–4 wk.

B

Reinforce the importance of continuing treatment to patient.

- Monitor for and report dystonia, motor restlessness, and involuntary repetitious movement of facial or cervical muscle.
- Observe for and report swollen ankles, decreased urinary output, changes in voiding pattern, jaundice, itching, nausea, or vomiting.

Patient & Family Education

- Report any of the following immediately: Involuntary, repetitive movements of face or neck; weakness, nervousness, nightmares, headache, or blurred vision; depression or thoughts of suicide.
- May take with or without food but take consistently.
- Do not use OTC drugs without advice of the prescriber while taking buspirone.
- Do not drive or engage in other potentially hazardous activities until response to drug is known.
- Do not drink alcohol or large amounts of grapefruit juice.

BUSULFAN

(byoo-sul'fan)

Busulfex, Myleran

Classification: ANTINEOPLASTIC; ALKYLATING AGENT

Therapeutic: ANTINEOPLASTIC

Prototype: Cyclophosphamide

AVAILABILITY Tablet; injection

ACTION & *THERAPEUTIC EFFECT* Potent cytotoxic alkylating agent thought to bring about changes in DNA that block replication and cause its cytotoxic effects. *Causes cell death in slowly proliferating stem cells.*

USES Chronic myelogenous leukemia.

UNLABELED USES: Stem cell transplant preparation, resistant essential thrombocytopenia.

CONTRAINDICATIONS *Hypersensitivity to busulfan or components*, Therapy-resistant chronic lymphocytic leukemia; lymphoblastic crisis of chronic myelogenous leukemia; bone marrow depression, immunizations (patient and household members), chickenpox (including recent exposure), herpetic infections; pregnancy—fetal risk cannot be ruled out; lactation—infant risk cannot be ruled out.

CAUTIOUS USE Men and women in childbearing years; hepatic disease; history of gout or urate renal stones; prior irradiation or chemotherapy; history of seizures, history of pulmonary disease, history of cardiac disease.

ROUTE & DOSAGE

Hematopoietic stem cell conditioning

Adult: **IV** 0.8 mg/kg/dose q6h × 4 days

Child: Dose varies based on weight, concurrent medications and institution protocols. See package insert for dosing information

Obesity Dosage Adjustment

In obese patients, use adjusted ideal body weight = IBW + 0.25 × (actual weight − IBW)

ADMINISTRATION

Oral

- Hazardous agent; NIOSH recommends single gloving for administration of intact tablets. If manipulation of tablets is necessary (e.g., to prepare in an oral solution) double glove, wear protective gown, and prepare in controlled device.

- Give at same time each day.
- Give on an empty stomach to minimize nausea and vomiting.
- Store in tightly capped, light-resistant container at 15°–30°C (59°–86°F), unless otherwise specified.

Intravenous

PREPARE: **Intermittent:** Prepare a volume of NS or D5W IV solution that is 10 × the volume of busulfan needed. ▪ Using a 5-micron nylon filter (supplied), withdraw the needed dose of busulfan. Remove needle and filter and use a new, nonfiltered needle to add busulfan to the IV fluid. (Always add busulfan to IV fluid rather than IV fluid to busulfan.) ▪ Mix by inverting the IV bag several times.

ADMINISTER: **Intermittent:** Busulfan is incompatible with polycarbonate; do not use any infusion components (syringes, filter needles, intravenous tubing, etc.) containing polycarbonate. Infuse via a central venous catheter over 2 h with an infusion pump. ▪ Flush line before/after infusion with at least 5 mL D5W or NS.

- Diluted solutions are stable at room temperature at 25°C (77°F) for up to 8 h and at refrigerated temperature between 2° and 8°C (35.6° and 44.6°F) for up to 12 h; this includes infusion time.

ADVERSE EFFECTS (≥ 5%) **Respiratory:** Irreversible pulmonary fibrosis ("busulfan lung"), *cough, shortness of breath*. **Endocrine:** *Hyperglycemia, hypokalemia, hypomagnesemia*. **Skin:** Alopecia, hyperpigmentation, *injection site inflammation, itching, rash*. **Hepatic:** Veno-occlusive disease of the liver. **GI:** *Vomiting, nausea, mucositis, stomatitis, anorexia, abdominal pain*. **GU:** Ovarian failure, acute renal failure. **Hematologic:** Major toxic effects are related to bone marrow failure; agranulocytosis (rare), *pancytopenia*, thrombocytopenia, leukopenia, *anemia*. **Other:** Fever.

INTERACTIONS **Drug: Probenecid, sulfinpyrazone** may increase uric acid levels. Do not administer LIVE VACCINES. Do not use with other agents that can cause immune suppression or hematologic toxicity (**cladribine, deferasirox, deferiprone, dipyrone, fingolimod**, etc.). **Herbal:** Do not use with echinacea.

PHARMACOKINETICS **Absorption:** Readily from GI tract. **Peak:** 1 h. **Metabolism:** In liver by CYP3A4. **Elimination:** 10–50% in urine within 48 h. **Half-life:** 2–3 h.

NURSING IMPLICATIONS

Black Box Warning

Busulfan can cause severe bone marrow hypoplasia. Malignant tumors and acute leukemias have been associated with this drug.

Assessment & Drug Effects

- Withhold drug and notify prescriber immediately at the first sign of abnormal decrease in any of the formed elements of the blood.
- Monitor the following: Vital signs, weight, I&O ratio and pattern. Urge patient to increase fluid intake to 10–12 (8 oz) glasses daily (if allowed) to ensure adequate urinary output.
- Monitor for and report symptoms suggestive of superinfection (see

Appendix F), particularly when patient develops leukopenia.

- Avoid invasive procedures during periods of platelet count depression.
- Monitor lab tests: Baseline and weekly Hgb, Hct, CBC with differential, platelet count; LFTs, kidney function, serum uric acid as needed, serum bilirubin (total and direct).

Patient & Family Education

- Report to prescriber any of the following: Easy bruising or bleeding, cloudy or pink urine, dark or black stools; sore mouth or throat, unusual fatigue, blurred vision, flank or joint pain, swelling of lower legs and feet; yellowing white of eye, dark urine, light-colored stools, abdominal discomfort, or itching (hepatotoxicity).
- Use contraceptive measures during busulfan therapy and for at least 3 mo after drug is withdrawn.
- Report any seizure activity.
- Report signs of cardiac tamponade: Anxiety, restlessness, low blood pressure, light-headedness, dizziness, weakness, fatigue, chest pain, shortness of breath, discomfort that is relieved by sitting or leaning forward.

BUTABARBITAL SODIUM

(byoo-ta-bar′bi-tal)

Butisol Sodium

Classification: BARBITURATE; ANXIOLYTIC; SEDATIVE-HYPNOTIC

Therapeutic: ANTIANXIETY; SEDATIVE-HYPNOTIC

Prototype: Phenobarbital

Controlled Substance: Schedule III

AVAILABILITY Tablet

ACTION & *THERAPEUTIC EFFECT* Intermediate-acting barbiturate that appears to act at thalamus level of the brain, where it interferes with transmission of impulses to the cerebral cortex. *Preoperative sedative agent that also is an effective antianxiety agent.*

USES Sedation induction and maintenance.

CONTRAINDICATIONS Hypersensitivity to barbiturates, history of or latent porphyria; uncontrolled pain; severe respiratory disease; history of addiction; lactation.

CAUTIOUS USE Severe renal or hepatic impairment; acute abdominal conditions; head trauma, history of seizures; history of suicide or depression; history of herpes infection; older adults or debilitated patients; pregnancy (category C).

ROUTE & DOSAGE

Daytime Sedation

Adult: **PO** 15–30 mg tid or qid

Preoperative Sedation

Adult: **PO** 50–100 mg 60–90 min before surgery
Child: **PO** 2–6 mg/kg/dose (max: 100 mg)

ADMINISTRATION

Oral

- Take on an empty stomach (i.e., 1 h before or 2 h after a meal).
- Schedule slow withdrawal following long-term use to avoid precipitating withdrawal symptoms.
- Store at 20°–25°C (68°–77°F).

ADVERSE EFFECTS **CNS:** Drowsiness, ***residual sedation*** ("hangover"), headache.

B

INTERACTIONS Drug: Alcohol and other CNS DEPRESSANTS add to CNS and respiratory depression; butabarbital increases the metabolism of ORAL ANTICOAGULANTS, BETA-BLOCKERS, CORTICOSTEROIDS, **doxycycline, griseofulvin, quinidine**, THEOPHYLLINES, ORAL CONTRACEPTIVES, decreasing their effectiveness. **Herbal: Kava, valerian** may potentiate sedation.

PHARMACOKINETICS Absorption: Readily from GI tract. **Onset:** 40–60 min. **Peak:** 3–4 h. **Duration:** 6–8 h. **Distribution:** Crosses placenta; distributed into breast milk. **Metabolism:** In liver. **Elimination:** In urine primarily as metabolites. **Half-Life:** Average 100 h.

NURSING IMPLICATIONS

Assessment & Drug Effects

- Assess for adverse effects. Older adults and debilitated patients sometimes manifest excitement, confusion, or depression. Children also may react with paradoxical excitement. Side rails may be advisable. Report these reactions to prescriber.

Patient & Family Education

- Do not drive or engage in other potentially hazardous activities until response to drug is known.
- Do not drink alcoholic beverages while taking this drug. Other CNS depressants may produce additive drowsiness; do not take without approval of prescriber.

BUTENAFINE HYDROCHLORIDE

(bu-ten′a-feen)

Lotrimin Ultra, Mentax

Classification: ANTIFUNGAL ANTIBIOTIC

Therapeutic: ANTIFUNGAL

Prototype: Terbinafine

AVAILABILITY Cream

ACTION & THERAPEUTIC EFFECT Exerts antifungal action by inhibiting fungal sterol synthesis that is needed in formation of the fungal cell membrane. *Antifungal effectiveness against interdigital tinea pedis (athlete's foot), tinea corporis (ringworm), and tinea cruris (jock itch).*

USES Treatment of tinea pedis, tinea corporis, and tinea cruris.

CONTRAINDICATIONS Hypersensitivity to butenafine; ophthalmic or vaginal administration.

CAUTIOUS USE Hypersensitivity to naftifine or tolnaftate; pregnancy (category B); lactation; children younger than 12 yr.

ROUTE & DOSAGE

Tinea Pedis

Adult/Child (12 yr or older): **Topical** Apply to affected area and surrounding skin bid × 7 days or daily × 4 wk

Tinea Corporis, Tinea Cruris

Adult/Child (younger than 12 yr): **Topical** Apply to affected area and surrounding skin once daily

ADMINISTRATION

Topical

- Apply sufficient cream to cover affected skin and surrounding areas.
- Do not use occlusive dressing unless specifically directed to do so.
- Store at 5°–30°C (41°–86°F).

ADVERSE EFFECTS Skin: Burning/stinging at application site, contact dermatitis, erythema, irritation, itching.

NURSING IMPLICATIONS

Assessment & Drug Effects

- Note: 2–4 wk of therapy are usually required for effective treatment.

Patient & Family Education

- Discontinue medication and notify prescriber if irritation or sensitivity develops.
- Avoid contact with mucous membranes.
- Wash hands thoroughly before and after application of cream.

BUTOCONAZOLE NITRATE

(byoo-toe-koe'na-zole)

Femstat 3, Gynazole 1

Classification: AZOLE ANTIFUNGAL ANTIBIOTIC

Therapeutic: ANTIFUNGAL

Prototype: Fluconazole

AVAILABILITY Cream

ACTION & *THERAPEUTIC EFFECT* Imidazole derivative with antifungal activity. Alters fungal cell membrane permeability, permitting loss of essential intracellular constituents with consequent loss of ability to replicate. *Has fungicidal effect as well as effectiveness against some gram-positive bacteria.*

USES Local treatment of vulvovaginal candidiasis.

CAUTIOUS USE Hypersensitivity to azole antifungals; HIV patients; diabetes mellitus; pregnancy (category C); lactation; children less than 12 yr.

ROUTE & DOSAGE

Vulvovaginal Candidiasis

Adult: **Topical** 1 applicator full intravaginally at bedtime for 3 days, may be extended another 3 days if needed

Pregnant women: **Topical** 1 applicator full intravaginally at bedtime for 6 days

ADMINISTRATION

Topical Intravaginal

- Continue treatment even during menstruation.
- Store medication at 15°–30°C (59°–86°F); avoid extreme temperature and freezing.

ADVERSE EFFECTS **CNS:** Headache. **Skin:** Itching of fingers. **GU:** Vulvar or vaginal burning, vulvar itching, discharge, soreness, swelling; urinary frequency and burning.

PHARMACOKINETICS **Absorption:** Small amount absorbed systemically from intravaginal administration. **Distribution:** Crosses placenta in animals. **Metabolism:** In liver. **Elimination:** In both urine and feces within 4–7 days. **Half-Life:** 21–24 h.

NURSING IMPLICATIONS

Assessment & Drug Effects

- Monitor for therapeutic effectiveness. Candidiasis in nonpregnant women is usually controlled in 3 days.

Patient & Family Education

- Take medication exactly as prescribed; do not increase or decrease dosage or discontinue or extend treatment period. Contact prescriber if symptoms (vaginal burning, discharge, or itching) persist; drug may be discontinued if acute irritation occurs.
- Patient's sexual partner should wear a condom during intercourse.

BUTORPHANOL TARTRATE

(byoo-tor'fa-nole)

Stadol, Stadol NS

Classification: ANALGESIC; NARCOTIC (OPIATE AGONIST–ANTAGONIST)

 Common adverse effects in *italic;* life-threatening effects underlined; generic names in **bold;** classifications in SMALL CAPS; ♣ Canadian drug name; Prototype drug; Alert

B

Therapeutic: NARCOTIC ANALGESIC
Prototype: PENTAZOCINE
Controlled Substance: Schedule IV

AVAILABILITY Solution for injection; spray

ACTION & *THERAPEUTIC EFFECT* Synthetic, centrally acting analgesic that acts as agonist on one type of opioid receptor and as a competitive antagonist at others. Site of analgesic action believed to be subcortical, possibly in the limbic system of the brain. Respiratory depression does not increase appreciably with higher doses, as it does with morphine, but duration of action increases. *Narcotic analgesic that relieves moderate to severe pain.*

USES Relief of moderate to severe pain, preoperative or preanesthetic sedation and analgesia, obstetric analgesia during labor, cancer pain, renal colic, burns.

UNLABELED USES Musculoskeletal and postepisiotomy pain.

CONTRAINDICATIONS Narcotic-dependent patients; opiate agonist hypersensitivity.

CAUTIOUS USE History of drug abuse or dependence; emotionally unstable individuals; head injury, increased intracranial pressure; acute MI, ventricular dysfunction, coronary insufficiency, hypertension; patients undergoing biliary tract surgery; respiratory depression, bronchial asthma, obstructive respiratory disease; and renal or hepatic dysfunction; prior to labor, pregnancy (category C). Safe use in children under 18 yr not established.

ROUTE & DOSAGE

Pain Relief

Adult: **IM** 1–4 mg q3–4h as needed (max: 4 mg/dose); **IV** 0.5–2 mg q3–4h as needed
Geriatric: **IM/IV** 0.25–1 mg q6–8h; **Intranasal** 1 mg (1 spray) in one nostril, may repeat in 90 sec, then may repeat these 2 doses q3–4h prn

Adjunct to Balanced Anesthesia

Adult: **IV** 2 mg before induction or 0.5–1 mg in increments during anesthesia

Labor

Adult: **IV/IM** 1–2 mg may repeat in 4 h

Renal Impairment Dosage Adjustment

GFR less than 10 mL/min: Use 50% of dose

Hepatic Impairment Dosage Adjustment

Use half normal dose and at least 6 h interval

ADMINISTRATION

Intranasal

- Give 1 spray into one nostril only. One spray provides a 1 mg dose.

Intramuscular

- Give preoperative IM injection 60–90 min before surgery.

Intravenous

PREPARE: **Direct:** Give undiluted.
ADMINISTER: **Direct:** Give at a rate of 2 mg over 3–5 min.
INCOMPATIBILITIES: **Y-site: Amphotericin B cholesteryl, lansoprazole, midazolam.**

C

▪ Store at 15°–30°C (59°–86°F) unless otherwise directed. Protect from light.

ADVERSE EFFECTS **CV:** Palpitation, bradycardia. **CNS:** Drowsiness, *sedation*, headache, vertigo, dizziness, floating feeling, weakness, lethargy, confusion, light-headedness, insomnia, nervousness, respiratory depression. **Skin:** Clammy skin, tingling sensation, flushing and warmth, cyanosis of extremities, diaphoresis, sensitivity to cold, urticaria, pruritus. **GI:** Nausea. **Genitourinary:** Difficulty in urinating, biliary spasm.

INTERACTIONS **Drug: Alcohol** and other CNS DEPRESSANTS augment CNS and respiratory depression.

PHARMACOKINETICS **Onset:** 10–30 min IM; 1 min IV. **Peak:** 0.5–1 h IM; 4–5 min IV. **Duration:** 3–4 h IM; 2–4 h IV. **Distribution:** Crosses placenta; distributed into breast milk. **Metabolism:** In liver in inactive metabolites. **Elimination:** Primarily in urine. **Half-Life:** 3–4 h.

NURSING IMPLICATIONS

Assessment & Drug Effects

- Monitor for respiratory depression. Do not administer drug if respiratory rate is less than 12 breaths/min.
- Monitor vital signs. Report marked changes in BP or bradycardia.
- Note: If used during labor or delivery, observe neonate for signs of respiratory depression.
- Note: Drug can induce acute withdrawal symptoms in opiate-dependent patients.
- Drug is usually withdrawn gradually following chronic administration. Abrupt withdrawal may produce vomiting, loss of appetite, restlessness, abdominal cramps, increase in BP and temperature, mydriasis, faintness. Withdrawal symptoms peak 48 h after discontinuation of drug.

Patient & Family Education

- Lie down to control drug-induced nausea.
- Do not take alcohol or other CNS depressants with this drug without consulting prescriber because of possible additive effects.
- Do not drive or engage in other potentially hazardous activities until response to drug is known.

CABAZITAXEL

(ka-baz'i tax-el)

Jevtana

Classification: ANTINEOPLASTIC; TAXANE

Therapeutic: ANTINEOPLASTIC; ANTIMICROTUBULE

Prototype: Paclitaxel

AVAILABILITY Solution for injection

ACTIONS & THERAPEUTIC EFFECT Cabazitaxel binds to the microtubule network essential for interphase and mitosis of the cell cycle stabilizing the microtubules involved in cell division and preventing their normal functioning. *This antimicrotubular effect results in inhibition of mitosis in cancer cells.*

USES Treatment of prostate cancer.

CONTRAINDICATIONS Neutrophil count of 1500/mm^3 or less; severe hypersensitivity to cabazitaxel or drugs formulated with polysorbate 80; severe hepatic impairment (total bilirubin more than 3 × ULN). Fetal risk has been demonstrated. Infant risk cannot be ruled out.

CAUTIOUS USE Neutropenia; history of hypersensitivity reactions; GI distress (nausea, vomiting, diarrhea); renal or hepatic impairment; patients 65 yr or greater. Patients who receive prior to radiation. Safety and efficacy in children not established.

ROUTE & DOSAGE

Prostate Cancer

Adult: **IV** 20 mg/m^2 over 1 h, repeat q3wk (max: 10 cycles)

Toxicity Dosage Adjustment

Grade 3 or greater neutropenia: Delay treatment until ANC greater than 1500/mm^3. Reduce dose to 20 mg/m^2. Use G-CSF for secondary prophylaxis.
Patients who develop febrile neutropenia: Delay treatment until improvement, and until ANC is greater than 1500/mm^3. Reduce dose to 20 mg/m^2. Use G-CSF for secondary prophylaxis.
Grade 3 or greater diarrhea or persisting diarrhea: Delay treatment until improvement or resolution. Reduce dose or discontinue cabazitaxel if toxicity persists with 15 mg/m^2 dose.

Hepatic Impairment Dosage Adjustment

Total bilirubin 1–1.5 × ULN: Reduce dose to 20 mg/m^2
Total bilirubin 1.5–3 × ULN: Reduce dose to 15 mg/m^2
Total bilirubin more than 3 × ULN: Should not be given to patients

ADMINISTRATION

Intravenous

▪ The National Institute for Occupational Safety and Health (NIOSH) recommends using double gloves and a protective gown when preparing and administering the medication. If there is a chance that the substance may splash or the patient may resist, use eye/face protection.
▪ Premedicate at least 30 min prior to each dose to avoid severe hypersensitivity: Dexamethasone 8 mg (or equivalent), dexchlorpheniramine 5 mg or diphenhydramine 25 mg, and ranitidine 50 mg (or equivalent).
▪ This drug is a cytotoxic agent, and caution should be used to prevent any contact with the drug. Follow institutional or standard guidelines for preparation, handling, and disposal of cytotoxic agents.

PREPARE: **Continuous:** Prepare under aseptic conditions. **Do not** use infusion containers or equipment made with PVC or polyurethane. *First dilution:* Add all of the supplied diluent to the 60-mg vial of cabazitaxel. ▪ Direct flow of diluent onto inside wall of the cabazitaxel vial; inject slowly to limit foaming, then invert vial gently for 45 sec to mix. ▪ Allow vial to stand until foam dissipates then inspect to ensure there are no visible particles. ▪ The resulting solution (10 mg/mL of cabazitaxel) should be further diluted within 30 min. *Second dilution:* Withdraw required dose and dilute in 250 mL or more of NS or D5W to yield a concentration no greater than 0.26 mg/mL. Solution should be clear without precipitate. ▪ Use first dilution immediately.

ADMINISTER: **Continuous:** Infuse over 1 h through a 0.22-micron in-line filter. **Do not** use tubing containing PVC or polyurethane. ▪ Monitor closely during infusion for S&S of hypersensitivity. Stop infusion immediately and institute supportive care should a hypersensitivity reaction occur.
INCOMPATIBILITIES: **Solution/additive:** Unknown. **Y-site:** Unknown.

▪ Store undiluted at 15°–30°C (59°–86°F). First dilution should be used immediately. Second dilution may be stored for 8 h at room temperature (including 1 h infusion time) or for a total of 24 h if refrigerated (including 1 h infusion time).

ADVERSE EFFECTS **CV:** Peripheral edema, cardiac arrhythmia, hypotension. **Respiratory:** Cough, Dyspnea. **CNS:** *Fatigue*, weakness, peripheral neuropathy, dizziness, headache. **Endocrine:** Weight loss, dehydration. **Skin:** Alopecia. **GI:** Abdominal pain, constipation, decreased appetite, *diarrhea*, *nausea*, *vomiting*. **GU:** Hematuria, dysuria, UTI. **Musculoskeletal:** Backache, muscle spasm. **Hematologic:** *Anemia*, febrile neutropenia, *leukopenia*, *thrombocytopenia*. **Other:** Fever, *infection*.

INTERACTIONS **Drug:** Coadministration of CYP3A4 inducers (e.g., **carbamazepine, phenobarbital, phenytoin, rifabutin, rifampin, rifapentine**) can decrease the levels of cabazitaxel. Coadministration of strong CYP3A4 inhibitors (e.g., **atazanavir, clarithromycin, indinavir, itraconazole, ketoconazole, nefazodone, nelfinavir, ritonavir, saquinavir, telithromycin, voriconazole**) can increase the levels of cabazitaxel. Do not use with **febuxostat. Food:** Grapefruit juice can increase the levels of cabazitaxel. **Herbal: St. John's wort** can decrease the levels of cabazitaxel.

PHARMACOKINETICS **Distribution:** 89–92% plasma protein bound. **Metabolism:** Extensively metabolized in the liver (CYP 3A4). **Elimination:** Primarily fecal elimination. **Half-Life:** 95 h.

NURSING IMPLICATIONS

Black Box Warning

Cabazitaxel has been associated with deaths from complications of severe neutropenia. Severe hypersensitivity reactions have also occurred.

Assessment & Drug Effects

- Monitor for hypersensitivity reactions especially during cycles 1 and 2. S&S requiring treatment and discontinuation of the drug include: Hypotension, bronchospasm, and generalized rash/erythema. Discontinue immediately, and manage symptoms aggressively.
- Monitor vital signs frequently, especially during the first hour of infusion. Cardiac monitoring may be indicated for those with conduction abnormalities.
- Monitor for S&S of infection. Withhold drug, and notify prescriber immediately if oral temperature reaches 101°F or is sustained at 100.4°F or higher over a 1-h period.
- Monitor for and report promptly severe or persistent diarrhea as it may cause dehydration and electrolyte imbalances.
- Monitor lab tests: Weekly CBC with differential during cycle 1 and prior to each cycle thereafter;

baseline and periodic LFTs and kidney function tests; periodic serum electrolytes, especially if diarrhea occurs.

Patient & Family Education

- Report immediately to prescriber S&S of hypersensitivity during drug infusion: Rash or itching, skin redness, difficulty breathing, chest pain or throat tightness, swelling of face, or feeling faint.
- Report severe or persistent diarrhea or vomiting as additional medications may be required.
- Avoid aspirin, NSAIDs, or alcohol to minimize GI distress.
- Do not drink grapefruit juice while taking this drug.
- Report unusual bruising or bleeding (e.g., blood in urine, or dark tarry stools).
- Use caution with exposure to potential sources of infection during periods when your blood count is low.

CABERGOLINE

(ka-ber′go-leen)

Dostinex

Classification: ERGOT ALKALOID
Therapeutic: DOPAMINE RECEPTOR AGONIST; ANTIPARKINSON
Prototype: Ergotamine

AVAILABILITY Tablet

ACTION & *THERAPEUTIC EFFECT* Cabergoline is a synthetic ergot derivative, long-acting dopamine receptor agonist with a high affinity for D_2 receptors in the anterior pituitary. It also suppresses prolactin secretion. *Cabergoline inhibits both puerperal lactation and pathologic hyperprolactinemia. Exhibits antiparkinsonism effects due to increased levels of dopamine.*

USES Treatment of hyperprolactinemia.

UNLABELED USES Parkinson disease, restless leg syndrome, Cushing syndrome.

CONTRAINDICATIONS Uncontrolled hypertension and hypersensitivity to ergot derivatives; cardiac valvular disorder (active or history), pulmonary, pericardial or retroperitoneal fibrotic disorders; pregnancy-induced hypertension, preeclampsia, eclampsia, lactation.

CAUTIOUS USE Hepatic function impairment; older adults; psychosis; pregnancy (category B). Safety and efficacy in pediatric patients are unknown.

ROUTE & DOSAGE

Hyperprolactinemia
Adult: **PO** Start with 0.25 mg 2 × wk, may increase by 0.25 mg 2 × wk (max: 1 mg 2 × wk)

ADMINISTRATION

Oral

- The National Institute for Occupational Safety and Health (NIOSH) recommends use of single gloves by anyone handling intact tablets, capsules, or administering from a unit-dose package.
- Give on same days each week.

ADVERSE EFFECTS **CNS:** Dizziness, *headache*. **GI:** Constipation, dyspepsia, *nausea*. **Musculoskeletal:** Weakness. **Other:** Fatigue.

INTERACTIONS **Drug:** Concurrent use with PHENOTHIAZINES, BUTYROPHENONES, THIOXANTHENES, **nitroglycerin**, and **metoclopramide** decreases therapeutic effects of both drugs. Use with

C

isoproterenol or **epinephrine** can result in dangerous hypertension. Avoid use with **frovatriptan, sumatriptan, zolmitriptan, almotriptan, eletriptan, naratriptan**, and **rizatriptan.**

PHARMACOKINETICS Absorption: Rapidly absorbed in GI tract, undergoes first-pass metabolism. **Peak:** 1–3 h. **Distribution:** 40–42% protein bound. Crosses placenta. **Metabolism:** Extensively metabolized. **Elimination:** Approximately 22% in urine, 60% in feces. **Half-Life:** 63–69 h.

NURSING IMPLICATIONS

Assessment & Drug Effects

- Monitor for hypotension, especially when given with other drugs known to lower BP.
- Monitor lab tests: Periodic serum prolactin level, electrolytes, serum creatinine, baseline echocardiogram then every 6–12 mo, chest x-ray baseline then periodically.

Patient & Family Education

- Patient should avoid activities that require mental alertness or coordination until drug effects are realized.
- Discontinue this drug once prescriber advises that serum prolactin level has been maintained for 6 mo.

CABOTEGRAVIR AND RILPIVIRINE

(KA-boe-TEG-ra-vir & RIL-pi-VIR-een)

Cabenuva

Classifications: ANTIRETROVIRAL; INTEGRASE INHIBITOR; NON-NUCLEOSIDE REVERSE TRANSCRIPTASE INHIBITOR (NNRTI)

Therapeutic: ANTIRETROVIRAL

AVAILABILITY Suspension for injection as two drug kit

ACTION & *THERAPEUTIC EFFECT* Cabotegravir inhibits HIV integrase by binding to the integrase active site and blocking the strand transfer step of retroviral DNA integration. Rilpivirine is a nonnucleoside reverse transcriptase inhibitor; activity is mediated by noncompetitive inhibition of HIV-1 reverse transcriptase. *Works to inhibit HIV DNA integration.*

USES For treatment of HIV-1 infection as a complete regimen.

CONTRAINDICATIONS Hypersensitivity to cabotegravir, rilpirivrine, or any component of the formulation; concomittant use with uridine diphosphate-glucuronosyl transferase and/or cytochrome P450 3A enzyme inducers (anticonvulsants such as carbamazepine, oxcarbazepine, phenobarbital, phenytoin), antimycobacterials (such as rifabutin, rifampin, rifapentine), systemic dexamethasone (more than a single dose), St. John's wort.

CAUTIOUS USE Depressive disorders, hepatoxicity, hypersensitivity reactions, immunity disorders, renal impairment, QT prolongation; pregnancy (not recommended for use during pregnancy); lactation.

ROUTE & DOSAGE

HIV-1 Infection

Adult: **IM** Injection should be preceded by oral medication lead-in. Initial injection: 600 mg cabotegravir/900 mg rilpivirine 1 month after oral lead-in; following initial dose 400 mg cabotegravir/600 rilpivirine monthly

Common adverse effects in *italic;* life-threatening effects underlined; generic names in **bold;** classifications in SMALL CAPS; ♣ Canadian drug name; ⊙ Prototype drug; ⚠ Alert

ADMINISTRATION

Intramuscular

- Injections much be administered by a healthcare professional.
- Administer in ventrogluteal muscle only; complete dose requires 2 injections: 1 cabotegravir injection and 1 rilpivirine injection. Administer each injection at a separate injection site.
- Remove from refrigeration > 15 minutes prior to injection in order to give at room temperature.; vials may remain in carton at room temperature for < 6 hours.
- Shake each vial vigorously to ensure uniform suspension prior to drawing into syringes. Once drawn into syringes, administer as soon as possible. May remain in syringes for < 2 hours.
- Store at 2°–8° C (36°–46°F).

ADVERSE EFFECTS **Skin:** Injection site reaction (discomfort, induration, swelling, nodule, pain, pruritis). **Musculoskeletal:** Increased CPK. **Other:** Fever.

INTERACTIONS **Drug:** Coadministration with UGT1A1 and UGT1A9 inducers should be avoided; Coadministration with potent CYP3A4 inhibitors (e.g., **ketoconazole**) or CYP3A4 inducers (e.g., **phenobarbital**, **phenytoin**) may influence levels of rilpivirine. Rilpivirine may similarly influence CYP3A4 substrates; May enhance the effects of QT-prolonging agents.

PHARMACOKINETICS **Peak:** Cabotegravir: 7 days; Rilpivirine: 3–4 days. **Distribution:** Cabotegravir: 99% protein-bound; Rilpivirine: 99% protein-bound **Metabolism:** Cabotegravir: Primarily by UGT1A1 (major) and UGT1A9 (minor); Rilpivirine: Primarily through CYP3A4 **Elimination:** Cabotegravir: 27% excreted in urine, 59% feces; Rilpivirine: 6% excreted in urine, 85% feces **Half-Life:** Cabotegravir: 5.6–11.5 weeks; Rilpivirine: 13–28 weeks

NURSING IMPLICATIONS

Assessment & Drug Effects

- Monitor for signs and symptoms of hypersensitivity and/or skin reactions; injection-related reactions.
- Monitor for mood changes.
- Monitor lab values: Baseline and periodic LFTs.

Patient & Family Education

- Seek medical help immediately if you have any of the following signs or symptoms of an allergic reaction such as rash; hives; itching; red, swollen, blistered, or peeling skin with or without fever; wheezing; tightness in the chest or throat; trouble breathing, swallowing, or talking; unusual hoarseness; or swelling of the mouth, face, lips, tongue, or throat.
- Report signs of liver problems such as dark urine, feeling tired, not hungry, upset stomach, stomach pain, light-colored stools, throwing up, or yellow skin or eyes to your provider.
- Report signs of depression, suicidal thoughts, emotional ups and downs, abnormal thinking, anxiety, or lack of interest in life to your provider.

CABOZANTINIB

(ka'-boe-zan'-ti-nib)

Cometriq

Classification: ANTINEOPLASTIC; TYROSINE KINASE INHIBITOR

Therapeutic: ANTINEOPLASTIC

Prototype: Erlotinib

C

AVAILABILITY Gelatin capsule

ACTION & *THERAPEUTIC EFFECT* Cabozantinib inhibits tyrosine kinases, which are enzymes required for cancer cell formation (oncogenesis), metastasis, tumor angiogenesis, and maintenance of the tumor microenvironment. *Slows development of progressive, metastatic medullary thyroid cancer.*

USES Treatment of patients with progressive, metastatic medullary thyroid cancer (MTC).

CONTRAINDICATIONS GI perforation or fistula; severe hemorrhage; MI, cerebral infarction, serious arterial thromboembolic events; wound dehiscence; hypertensive crisis or uncontrollable hypertension; osteonecrosis of the jaw; nephrotic syndrome; reversible posterior leukoencephalopathy syndrome (RPLS); within 28 days of dental procedures; moderate or severe hepatic impairment. Fetal risk cannot be ruled out. Infant risk cannot be ruled out. Discontinue breastfeeding while taking medication and up to 4 mo following the final dose.

CAUTIOUS USE Hypertension; mild hepatic impairment; coadministration of strong CYP3A4 inducers/inhibitors.

ROUTE & DOSAGE

Metastatic Medullary Thyroid Cancer

Adult: **PO** 140 mg once daily until disease progression or unacceptable toxicity occurs

Hepatic Impairment Dosage Adjustment

Child–Pugh class A or B: Reduce starting dose to 80 mg daily

Toxicity Dosage Adjustment

See package insert for details

Dosage Adjustment If Coadministered with a Strong CYP3A4 Inhibitor or Inducer

Strong CYP3A4 Inhibitor: Decrease dose by 40 mg; resume previous dose 2–3 days after discontinuing the strong inhibitor

Strong CYP3A4 Inducer: Increase dose by 20 mg (max: 180 mg); resume previous dose 2–3 days after discontinuing strong inducer

ADMINISTRATION

Oral

- The National Institute for Occupational Safety and Health (NIOSH) recommends the use of single gloves by anyone handling intact tablets, capsules, or administering from a unit-dose package.
- Give with at least 240 mL (8 oz) of water on an empty stomach (at least 2 h before/1 h after eating).
- Capsules must be swallowed whole. They should not be opened or crushed.
- Do not ingest foods or nutritional supplements known to inhibit cytochrome P450 during therapy.
- Do not take a missed dose within 12 h of the next dose.
- Store at 15°–30°C (59°–86°F).

ADVERSE EFFECTS **CV:** *Hypertension*, hypotension, venous thromboembolism. **Respiratory:** Pulmonary embolism, dyspnea, cough. **CNS:** *Fatigue*, voice disorder, headache, anxiety, paresthesia, peripheral

C

neuropathy, dizziness. **Endocrine:** *Hypocalcemia, hypophosphatemia, increased triglycerides, hyperglycemia, hypoalbuminemia, hypomagnesia, hyponatremia, increased gamma-glutamyl transferase, weight loss,* hypothyroidism, hypokalemia, dehydration. **Skin:** *Hair color change,* rash, alopecia, erythema, palmar and plantar redness, swelling, pain. **Hepatic:** *Increased alkaline phosphatase, increased ALT/SGPT, hyperbilirubinemia.* **GI:** *Abdominal pain, constipation, loss of appetite, dental pain, diarrhea, nausea, stomatitis, altered taste, vomiting,* renal carcinoma, mucosal inflammation, dysphagia, dyspepsia, hemorrhoids. **Musculoskeletal:** Joint pain, limb pain, muscle spasm. **Hematologic:** *Lymphocytopenia, neutropenia, thrombocytopenia, decreased hemoglobin,* anemia.

INTERACTIONS

Drug: Strong inhibitors of CYP3A4 (e.g., **atazanavir, clarithromycin, indinavir, itraconazole, ketoconazole, nefazodone, nelfinavir, ritonavir, saquinavir, telithromycin, voriconazole**) can increase the levels of cabozantinib. Strong inducers of CYP3A4 (e.g., **carbamazepine, dexamethasone, phenobarbital, phenytoin, rifampin, rifabutin, rifapentine**) may decrease the levels of cabozantinib. **Food:** Grapefruit juice may increase drug levels. **Herbal: St. John's wort** may decrease the levels of cabozantinib.

PHARMACOKINETICS

Peak: 2–5 h. **Distribution:** Greater than 99.7% plasma protein bound. **Metabolism:** In liver. **Elimination:** Fecal (54%) and renal (27%). **Half-Life:** 55 h.

NURSING IMPLICATIONS

Black Box Warning

Cabozantinib has been associated with GI perforation and fistula formation, and severe, potentially fatal, hemorrhage

Assessment & Drug Effects

- Monitor BP at baseline and periodically thereafter.
- Monitor for S&S of thrombotic events (e.g., MI, PE).
- Monitor for S&S of GI perforation and fistula formation (e.g., blood in stool, hematemesis, abdominal pain).
- Assess for development of hand–foot syndrome (e.g., redness, swelling, blisters, pain in hands and feet).
- Report immediately to prescriber if patient presents with seizures, headache, visual disturbances, confusion or altered mental function.
- Monitor lab tests: Periodic urinalysis for protein.

Patient & Family Education

- Practice good oral hygiene while taking this drug.
- Contact your prescriber immediately if you experience signs of bleeding (e.g., coughing up blood or blood clots, vomiting blood or vomit looks like coffee-grounds, red or black tarry stools, heavy menstrual bleeding).
- Contact prescriber immediately for any of the following: Progressive rash, painful sores in mouth, significant weight loss, or severe diarrhea.
- Do not consume grapefruit or grapefruit juice while taking this drug.
- Take a missed dose as soon as possible, but if the next dose is less than 12 h, skip the missed dose.

C

- Men and women should use effective contraception during therapy and for at least 4 mo after last dose.
- Do not breastfeed while taking this drug.

CAFFEINE

(kaf-een′)

Caffedrine, Dexitac, NoDoz, Quick Pep, S-250, Tirend, Vivarin

CAFFEINE AND SODIUM BENZOATE

CITRATED CAFFEINE

Cafcit

Classification: RESPIRATORY AND CEREBRAL STIMULANT; XANTHINE

Therapeutic: RESPIRATORY AND CEREBRAL STIMULANT

AVAILABILITY Tablet; capsule; caffeine citrate oral solution; caffeine citrate injection

ACTION & *THERAPEUTIC EFFECT* Caffeine is structurally similar to adenosine and is capable of binding to adenosine receptors on the surface of cells without activating them, thereby acting as a competitive inhibitor. Antagonism of adenosine receptors stimulates: The vagal nucleus, reducing heart rate; the vasomotor center, constricting blood vessels; and the respiratory center, increasing respiratory rate. It also promotes release of the neurotransmitters (i.e., monoamines and acetylcholine), which causes stimulant effects. *Effective in managing neonatal apnea, and as an adjuvant for pain control in headaches and following dural puncture. Relief of headache is perhaps due to mild cerebral vasoconstriction action and increased vascular tone.*

USES Orally as a mild CNS stimulant to aid in staying awake and restoring mental alertness, and as an adjunct in narcotic and nonnarcotic analgesia. Used parenterally as an emergency stimulant in acute circulatory failure, as a diuretic, and for neonatal apnea.

UNLABELED USES Topical treatment of atopic dermatitis; to relieve spinal puncture headache.

CONTRAINDICATIONS Acute MI, symptomatic cardiac arrhythmias, palpitations; peptic ulcer; pulmonary disease; insomnia, panic attacks.

CAUTIOUS USE Diabetes mellitus; hiatal hernia; psychotic disorders; dementia; depressive disorders; hepatic disease; hypertension with heart disease; pregnancy (category C); lactation.

ROUTE & DOSAGE

Mental Stimulant

Adult: **PO** 100–200 mg q3–4h prn

Circulatory Stimulant

Adult: **IM** 200–500 mg prn

Apnea of Prematurity (Caffeine Citrate Only)

Neonate (28–33 wk gestation): **PO/IV** 20 mg/kg (loading dose); then, after 24 h, 5 mg/kg/day

ADMINISTRATION

Oral

- Powdered form may be dissolved in the patient's liquid of choice.

Intramuscular

- Give deep IM into a large muscle.

Intravenous

Note: IV route reserved for emergency situations only.

PREPARE: **IV Infusion:** May be diluted for infusion in D5W.

ADMINISTER: **IV Infusion:** A syringe infusion pump is recommended. ▪ Give loading dose over 30 min and maintenance dose over at least 10 min.

INCOMPATIBILITIES: **Y-site: Acyclovir, furosemide, lorazepam, nitroglycerin, oxacillin, pantoprazole.**

ADVERSE EFFECTS **CV:** Tingling of face, flushing, palpitation, tachycardia, arrhythmia, angina, ventricular ectopic beats. **Respiratory:** Tachypnea. **CNS:** *Nervousness, insomnia*, restlessness, irritability, confusion, agitation, fasciculations, delirium, twitching, tremors, clonic convulsions. **HEENT:** Scintillating scotomas, tinnitus. **GI:** Nausea, vomiting; epigastric discomfort, gastric irritation (oral form), diarrhea, hematemesis, kernicterus (neonates). **GU:** Increased urination, diuresis.

DIAGNOSTIC TEST INTERFERENCE Caffeine reportedly may interfere with diagnosis of pheochromocytoma or neuroblastoma by increasing urinary excretion of ***catecholamines, VMA***, and ***5-HIAA*** and may cause false-positive increases in ***serum urate*** (by ***Bittner method***).

INTERACTIONS **Drug:** Increases effects of **cimetidine**; increases cardiovascular stimulating effects of BETA-ADRENERGIC AGONISTS; possibly increases **theophylline** toxicity.

PHARMACOKINETICS **Absorption:** Rapid. **Peak:** 15–45 min. **Distribution:** Widely throughout body; crosses blood–brain barrier and placenta. **Metabolism:** In liver. **Elimination:** In urine as metabolites; excreted in breast milk in small amounts. **Half-Life:** 3–5 h in adults, 36–144 h in neonates.

NURSING IMPLICATIONS

Assessment & Drug Effects

- Monitor vital signs closely, as large doses may cause intensification rather than reversal of severe drug-induced depressions.
- Observe children closely following administration as they are more susceptible than adults to the CNS effects of caffeine.
- Monitor lab tests: Frequent blood glucose and periodic HbA1C levels in diabetics.

Patient & Family Education

- Caffeine in large amounts may impair glucose tolerance in diabetics.
- Do not consume large amounts of caffeine as headache, dizziness, anxiety, irritability, nervousness, and muscle tension may result from excessive use, as well as from abrupt withdrawal of coffee (or oral caffeine). Withdrawal symptoms usually occur 12–18 h following last coffee intake.

CALCIPOTRIENE

(cal-ci′po-tri-een)

Dovonex, Sorilux

Classification: VITAMIN D ANALOG

Therapeutic: VITAMIN D ANALOG

Prototype: Calcitriol

AVAILABILITY Ointment; foam; cream; scalp solution

ACTION & *THERAPEUTIC EFFECT* Calcipotriene is a synthetic vitamin D_3 analog for the treatment

C

of moderate plaque psoriasis. *Calcipotriene controls psoriasis by inhibiting proliferation of psoriatic skin, reducing the number of polymorphonuclear leukocytes (PMNs) in the skin cells, and decreasing the number of epithelial cells.*

USES Treatment of psoriasis.

CONTRAINDICATIONS Hypersensitivity to calcipotriene, hypercalcemia or vitamin D toxicity, psoriatic eruptions, lactation.

CAUTIOUS USE History of nephrolithiasis; dermatoses other than psoriasis; older adults; pregnancy (category C). Safety and efficacy in children not established.

ROUTE & DOSAGE

Adult: **Topical** Apply a thin layer to affected area once or twice daily

ADMINISTRATION

Topical

- Shake can before use. Apply to scalp when hair is dry.
- A thin layer should be applied to the affected skin and rubbed in gently and completely.
- Calcipotriene should not be applied to the face.
- Wash hands before and after application of medication.
- Storage at 15°–25°C (59°–77°F), do not freeze.
- Foam and solution contents are flammable, keep away from heat and flame. Do not puncture or incinerate.

ADVERSE EFFECTS **Skin:** Dermatitis, burning, stinging, erythema, folliculitis, rash, peeling of skin, mild transient itching.

PHARMACOKINETICS **Absorption:** 6% absorbed systemically. **Onset:** 2 wk. **Peak:** 8 wk. **Metabolism:** Recycled via liver. **Elimination:** In bile.

NURSING IMPLICATIONS

Assessment & Drug Effects

- Observe reductions in scaling, erythema, and lesion thickness indicating a positive therapeutic response.
- Significant reduction in psoriatic lesions usually occurs following 1 wk of treatment. Marked improvement is generally noted by the 8th wk of treatment.
- Monitor lab tests: Periodic serum calcium, phosphate, and calcitriol levels during long-term therapy.

Patient & Family Education

- Wash hands before and after application.
- Avoid excessive exposure of treated areas to natural or artificial sunlight, including sun lamps or tanning booths.
- Avoid fire, flame, or smoking during and immediately after foam or solution application, as these products are flammable.
- Treatment with calcipotriene may be indefinite, as reappearance of psoriatic lesions is common following discontinuation of the drug.
- Adverse effects may include burning and stinging with drug application; these are usually transient.
- Do not mix calcipotriene with any other topical medicine.
- Report appearance of facial dermatitis (redness and scaling around mouth and nose).
- If foam gets on face or near the eye, rinse area thoroughly with water.

CALCITONIN (SALMON)
Fortical, Miacalcin
Classification: BONE METABOLISM REGULATOR
Therapeutic: BONE METABOLISM REGULATOR

AVAILABILITY Solution for injection; spray

ACTION & *THERAPEUTIC EFFECT* Calcitonin opposes the effects of parathyroid hormone on bone and kidneys, reduces serum calcium by binding to a specific receptor site on osteoclast cell membrane, and alters transmembrane passage of calcium and phosphorus. Promotes renal excretion of calcium and phosphorus. *Effective in osteoporosis due to inhibition of bone resorption. Effective in symptomatic hypercalcemia by rapidly lowering serum calcium.*

USES Symptomatic Paget disease of bone (osteitis deformans), postmenopausal osteoporosis. Orphan drug approval (calcitonin human): Short-term adjunctive treatment of severe hypercalcemic emergencies.

UNLABELED USES Diagnosis and management of medullary carcinoma of thyroid; treatment of osteogenesis imperfecta.

CONTRAINDICATIONS Hypersensitivity to fish proteins or to calcitonin; hypocalcemia.

CAUTIOUS USE Renal impairment; osteoporosis; pernicious anemia; Zollinger–Ellison syndrome; older adults; pregnancy (category C); lactation. Safe use in children younger than 12 yr not established.

ROUTE & DOSAGE

Paget Disease

Adult: **Subcutaneous/IM** 100 international units/day, may decrease to 50–100 international units/day or every other day

Hypercalcemia

Adult: **Subcutaneous/IM** 4 international units/kg q12h, may increase to 8 international units/kg q6h if needed

Postmenopausal Osteoporosis

Adult: **Subcutaneous/IM** 100 international units/day; **Intranasal** 1 spray (200 international units) daily, alternate nostrils

ADMINISTRATION

Allergy Test Dose

- An allergy skin test is usually done prior to initiation of therapy. The appearance of more than mild erythema or wheal 15 min after intracutaneous injection indicates that the drug should not be given.

Intranasal

- Activate the pump prior to first use; hold bottle upright and depress white side arms 6 times.
- The nasal spray is administered in one nostril daily; alternate nostrils.

Subcutaneous

- Calcitonin human is administered only by subcutaneous injection; calcitonin salmon may be administered by subcutaneous or IM injection.

Intramuscular

- Use IM route when the volume to be injected is greater than 2 mL.
- Rotate injection sites.
- Store calcitonin (human) at or below 25°C (77°F), protected from light, unless otherwise specified by manufacturer.

C

- Store calcitonin (salmon) in refrigerator, preferably at 2°–8°C (36°–46°F) unless otherwise directed.

ADVERSE EFFECTS **Skin:** Inflammatory reactions at injection site, flushing of face or hands, pruritus of earlobes, edema of feet, skin rashes. **GI:** *Transient nausea*, vomiting, anorexia, unusual taste sensation, abdominal pain, diarrhea. **GU:** Nocturia, diuresis, abnormal urine sediment. **Other:** Headache, eye pain, feverish sensation, hypersensitivity reactions, anaphylaxis, tremor. Reported for Cibacalcin only: Urinary frequency, chills, chest pressure, weakness, paresthesias, tender palms and soles, dizziness, nasal congestion, shortness of breath.

INTERACTIONS **Drug:** May decrease serum **lithium** levels.

PHARMACOKINETICS **Onset:** 15 min. **Peak:** 4 h. **Duration:** 8–24 h. **Distribution:** Does not cross placenta; distribution into breast milk unknown. **Metabolism:** In kidneys. **Elimination:** In urine. **Half-Life:** 1.25 h.

NURSING IMPLICATIONS

Assessment & Drug Effects

- Have readily available parenteral calcium, particularly during early therapy. Hypocalcemic tetany is a theoretical possibility.
- Examine urine specimens periodically for sediment with long-term therapy.
- Examine nasal passages prior to treatment with the nasal spray and anytime nasal irritation occurs.
- Nasal ulceration or heavy bleeding are indications for drug discontinuation.
- Monitor for hypocalcemia (see Signs & Symptoms, Appendix F). Theoretically, calcitonin can lead to hypocalcemic tetany. Latent tetany may be demonstrated by Chvostek or Trousseau signs and by serum calcium values: 7–8 mg/dL (latent tetany); below 7 mg/dL (manifest tetany).
- Monitor lab tests: Baseline and periodic serum calcium.

Patient & Family Education

- Watch for redness, warmth, or swelling at injection site and report to prescriber, as these may indicate an inflammatory reaction. The transient flushing that commonly occurs following injection of calcitonin, particularly during early therapy, may be minimized by administering the drug at bedtime. Consult prescriber.
- Maintain your drug regimen to prevent early relapses even though symptoms have improved.
- Ensure that you feel comfortable using the nasal pump properly. Notify prescriber if significant nasal irritation occurs.
- Consult prescriber before using OTC preparations. Some supervitamins, hematinics, and antacids contain calcium and vitamin D (vitamin may antagonize calcitonin effects).

CALCITRIOL (Pr)

(kal-si-trye′ole)

Rocaltrol, Vectical

Classification: VITAMIN D ANALOG

Therapeutic: VITAMIN D ANALOG

AVAILABILITY Capsule; oral solution; solution for injection; ointment

ACTION & THERAPEUTIC EFFECT Synthetic form of an active metabolite of ergocalciferol (vitamin D_2). In the liver, cholecalciferol (vitamin D_3) and ergocalciferol (vitamin D_2) are enzymatically metabolized to calcifediol, an activated form of vitamin D_3 in the kidney. Patients with nonfunctioning kidneys are unable to synthesize sufficient calcitriol. *By promoting intestinal absorption and renal retention of calcium, calcitriol elevates serum calcium levels, decreases elevated blood levels of phosphate and parathyroid hormone. Thus it decreases subperiosteal bone resorption and mineralization defects.*

USES Management of hypocalcemia in patients undergoing chronic renal dialysis and in patients with hypoparathyroidism or pseudohypoparathyroidism. Patients with hyperparathyroidism in moderate to severe chronic renal failure not on dialysis; psoriasis; renal osteodystrophy.

UNLABELED USES Selected patients with vitamin D–dependent rickets, familial hypophosphatemia; osteopetrosis; osteoporosis.

CONTRAINDICATIONS Hypersensitivity to calcitriol; hypercalcemia or vitamin D toxicity.

CAUTIOUS USE Hyperphosphatemia, renal failure; sarcoidosis; patients receiving digitalis glycosides; older adults; pregnancy (category C).

ROUTE & DOSAGE

Hypocalcemia /Secondary Hyperparathyroidism

Adult: **PO** 0.25 mcg/day, may increase to 0.5 mcg/day based on lab values; **IV** 1–2 mcg 3 × wk at the end of dialysis, may need up to 3 mcg 3 × wk

Child (3 yr or older): **PO** *On hemodialysis:* 0.25 mcg/day; may increase based on lab values
Child (1–3 yr): **PO** 0.01–0.015 mcg/kg/day. Monitor closely and adjust as needed

Plaque Psoriasis

Adult: **Topical** Apply to affected areas bid

ADMINISTRATION

Oral

- Oral dose can be taken either with food or milk or on an empty stomach. Discuss with prescriber.
- When given for hypoparathyroidism, the dose is given in the morning.
- Capsule, injection and solution should be protected from heat, light, and moisture. Store in tightly closed container.
- Store solution and ointment at 15°–30°C (59°–87°F). Store capsules at controlled room temperature, 20°–25°C (68°–77°F). Do not refrigerate.

Intravenous

PREPARE: **Direct:** Give undiluted.
ADMINISTER: **Direct:** Give IV push over 30–60 sec.

ADVERSE EFFECTS **CNS:** Headache. **Endocrine:** Hypercalcemia, polydipsia. **Skin:** rash. **GI:** abdominal pain. **GU:** UTI.

INTERACTIONS **Drug:** THIAZIDE DIURETICS may cause hypercalcemia; calcifediol-induced hypercalcemia may precipitate digitalis arrhythmias in patients receiving DIGITALIS GLYCOSIDES. Do not use with **burosumab.**

PHARMACOKINETICS Absorption: Readily absorbed from GI tract. **Onset:** 2–6 h. **Peak:** 10–12 h. **Duration:** 3–5 days. **Metabolism:** In liver. **Elimination:** Mainly in feces. **Half-Life:** 3–6 h.

NURSING IMPLICATIONS

Assessment & Drug Effects

- Effectiveness of therapy depends on an adequate daily intake of calcium and phosphate. The prescriber may prescribe a calcium supplement on an as-needed basis.
- Monitor for hypercalcemia (see Signs & Symptoms, Appendix F). During dosage adjustment period, monitor serum calcium levels particularly twice weekly to avoid hypercalcemia.
- If hypercalcemia develops, withhold calcitriol and calcium supplements and notify prescriber. Drugs may be reinitiated when serum calcium returns to normal.
- Monitor lab tests: Baseline and periodic serum calcium, phosphorus, magnesium, alkaline phosphatase, creatinine; 24-h urinary calcium and phosphorus levels.

Patient & Family Education

- Oral/IV: Discontinue the drug if experiencing any symptoms of hypercalcemia (see Appendix F), and contact prescriber.
- Oral/IV: Do not use any other source of vitamin D during therapy because calcitriol is the most potent form of vitamin D_3. This will avoid the possibility of hypercalcemia.
- Oral/IV: Consult prescriber before taking an OTC medication. (Many products contain calcium, vitamin D, phosphates, or magnesium, which can increase adverse effects of calcitriol.)
- Oral/IV: Maintain an adequate daily fluid intake unless you have kidney problems, in which case consult your prescriber about fluids.
- Stop using ointment and contact physician if severe irritation occurs.
- Avoid natural or artificial sunlight when using ointment.
- Limit ointment use to no more than 2 tubes/wk.

CALCIUM CARBONATE

Apo-Cal ♣, Bio-Cal, Calcite-500, Calsan ♣, Cal-Sup, Caltrate ♣, Chooz, Dicarbosil, Equilet, Mallamint, Mega-Cal, Nu-Cal, Os-Cal, Oystercal, Titralac, Tums

CALCIUM ACETATE

PhosLo

CALCIUM CITRATE

Citracal

CALCIUM PHOSPHATE TRIBASIC (TRICALCIUM PHOSPHATE)

CALCIUM LACTATE

Cal-Lac

Classification: FLUID AND ELECTROLYTIC REPLACEMENT SOLUTION; ANTACID

Therapeutic: NUTRITIONAL SUPPLEMENT; ANTACID

Prototype: Calcium gluconate

AVAILABILITY Calcium carbonate: Tablet. **Calcium acetate:** Tablet. **Calcium citrate:** Tablet. **Calcium phosphate tribasic:** Tablet

ACTION & *THERAPEUTIC EFFECT*

Calcium carbonate is a rapid-acting antacid with high neutralizing capacity and relatively prolonged duration of action. Decreases gastric acidity, thereby inhibiting proteolytic action of pepsin on gastric mucosa. All forms of calcium salts

C

are used for calcium replacement therapy. *Effectively relieves symptoms of acid indigestion and useful as a calcium supplement.*

USES Relief of transient symptoms of hyperacidity as in acid indigestion, heartburn, peptic esophagitis, and hiatal hernia. Also as calcium supplement in treatment of mild calcium deficiency states. Control of hyperphosphatemia in chronic renal failure (calcium acetate).

UNLABELED USES For treatment of hyperphosphatemia in patients with chronic renal failure and to lower BP in selected patients with hypertension.

CONTRAINDICATIONS Hypercalcemia and hypercalciuria (e.g., hyperparathyroidism, vitamin D overdosage, decalcifying tumors, bone metastases), calcium loss due to immobilization, severe renal failure, renal calculi, GI hemorrhage or obstruction, dehydration, digitalis toxicity; hypochloremic alkalosis, ventricular fibrillation, cardiac disease.

CAUTIOUS USE Decreased bowel motility (e.g., with anticholinergics, antidiarrheals, antispasmodics), older adults; **Calcium acetate:** Pregnancy (category B); children.

ROUTE & DOSAGE

All doses are in terms of *elemental calcium:*

- 1 g calcium carbonate = 400 mg (20 mEq, 40%) elemental calcium
- 1 g calcium acetate = 250 mg (12.6 mEq, 25%) elemental calcium; 1 g calcium citrate = 210 mg (12 mEq, 21%) elemental calcium
- 1 g tricalcium phosphate = 390 mg (19.3 mEq, 39%) elemental calcium; calcium lactate = 130 mg (6.5 mEq, 13%) elemental calcium

Supplement for Osteoporosis

Adult: **PO** 1–2 g bid or tid

Antacid

Adult: **PO** 0.5–2 g 4–6 × day

Hyperphosphatemia

Adult: **PO** Calcium acetate 2–4 tablets with each meal

Supplement for Mild Hypercalcemia

Child: **PO** 500 mg/kg/day in divided doses (lactate)

ADMINISTRATION

Oral

- When used as antacid, give 1 h after meals and at bedtime. When used as calcium supplement, give 1–1½ h after meals, unless otherwise directed by prescriber.
- Chewable tablet should be chewed well before swallowing or allowed to dissolve completely in mouth, followed with water. Powder form may be mixed with water.
- Ensure that sustained release form of drug is not chewed or crushed. It **must be** swallowed whole.

ADVERSE EFFECTS **CNS:** Mood and mental changes. **Endocrine:** Hypercalcemia with alkalosis, metastatic calcinosis, hypercalciuria, hypomagnesemia, hypophosphatemia (when phosphate intake is low). **GI:** *Constipation* or laxative effect, acid rebound, nausea, eructation, *flatulence*, vomiting, fecal concretions. **GU:** Polyuria, renal calculi.

INTERACTIONS **Drug:** May enhance inotropic and toxic effects of **digoxin; magnesium** may compete for GI absorption; decreases absorption of TETRACYCLINES, QUINOLONES **(ciprofloxacin).**

PHARMACOKINETICS **Absorption:** Approximately ⅓ of dose absorbed from small intestine. **Distribution:** Crosses placenta. **Elimination:** Primarily in feces; small amounts in urine, pancreatic juice, saliva, breast milk.

NURSING IMPLICATIONS

Assessment & Drug Effects

- Note number and consistency of stools. If constipation is a problem, prescriber may prescribe alternate or combination therapy with a magnesium antacid or advise patient to take a laxative or stool softener as necessary.
- Record amelioration of symptoms of hypocalcemia (see Signs & Symptoms, Appendix F).
- Observe for S&S of hypercalcemia in patients receiving frequent or high doses, or who have impaired renal function (see Appendix F).
- Monitor lab tests: Weekly serum and urine calcium with prolonged therapy and in those with renal dysfunction.

Patient & Family Education

- Do not continue this medication beyond 1–2 wk because it may cause acid rebound, which generally occurs after repeated use for 1 or 2 wk and leads to chronic use. It is potentially dangerous to self-medicate. Do not take antacids longer than 2 wk without medical supervision.
- Avoid taking calcium carbonate with cereals or other foods high in oxalates. Oxalates combine with calcium carbonate to form insoluble, nonabsorbable compounds.
- Do not use calcium carbonate repeatedly with foods high in vitamin D (such as milk) or sodium bicarbonate, as it may cause milk-alkali syndrome: Hypercalcemia, distaste for food, headache, confusion, nausea, vomiting, abdominal pain, metabolic alkalosis, hypercalciuria, polyuria, soft tissue calcification (calcinosis), hyperphosphatemia, and renal insufficiency. Predisposing factors include renal dysfunction, dehydration, electrolyte imbalance, and hypertension.

CALCIUM CHLORIDE

Classification: FLUID AND ELECTROLYTIC REPLACEMENT SOLUTION

Therapeutic: FLUID AND ELECTROLYTE REPLACEMENT

Prototype: Calcium gluconate

AVAILABILITY Solution for injection

ACTION & *THERAPEUTIC EFFECT* Ionizes readily and provides excess chloride ions that promote acidosis and temporary (1–2 days) diuresis secondary to excretion of sodium. *Rapidly and effectively restores serum calcium levels in acute hypocalcemia of various origins and an effective cardiac stabilizer under conditions of hyperkalemia or resuscitation.*

USES Treatment of cardiac resuscitation when epinephrine fails to improve myocardial contractions; for treatment of acute hypocalcemia (as in tetany due to parathyroid deficiency, vitamin D deficiency, alkalosis, insect bites or stings, and during exchange transfusions), for treatment of hypermagnesemia, and for cardiac disturbances of hyperkalemia.

CONTRAINDICATIONS Ventricular fibrillation, hypercalcemia, digitalis toxicity, injection into myocardium or other tissue.

CAUTIOUS USE Digitalized patients; sarcoidosis, renal insufficiency, history of renal stone formation; cardiac arrhythmias; dehydration; diarrhea; cor pulmonale, respiratory acidosis, respiratory failure; pregnancy (category A; category C in high doses).

ROUTE & DOSAGE

All doses are in terms of *elemental calcium:*

- 1 g calcium chloride = 272 mg (13.6 mEq) elemental calcium

Hypocalcemia

Adult: **IV** 0.5–1 g (7–14 mEq) at 1–3 day intervals as determined by patient response and serum calcium levels
Child: **IV** 2.7–5 mg/kg administered slowly

Hypocalcemic Tetany

Adult: **IV** 4.5–16 mEq prn
Child: **IV** 0.5–0.7 mEq/kg tid or qid
Neonate: **IV** 2.4 mEq/kg/day in divided doses

CPR

Adult: **IV** 2–4 mg/kg, may repeat in 10 min
Child: **IV** 20 mg/kg, may repeat in 10 min

ADMINISTRATION

Intravenous

IV administration to neonates, infants, and children: Verify correct IV concentration and rate of infusion with prescriber.

PREPARE: **Direct:** May be given undiluted or diluted (preferred) with an equal volume of NS for injection. ▪ Solution should be warmed to body temperature before administration.

ADMINISTER: **Direct:** Give at 0.5–1 mL/min or more slowly if irritation develops. Avoid rapid administration. ▪ Use a small-bore needle and inject into a large vein to minimize venous irritation and undesirable reactions. ▪ Do not use scalp veins for injection in children. ▪ Following injection, keep recumbent for a short time.

INCOMPATIBILITIES: **Solution/additive:** **Amphotericin B, chlorpheniramine, dobutamine**, concentration-dependent incompatibility with other ELECTROLYTES. **Y-site:** **Amphotericin B cholesteryl complex, propofol, sodium bicarbonate.**

ADVERSE EFFECTS **CV:** (With rapid infusion) hypotension, bradycardia, cardiac arrhythmias, <u>cardiac arrest</u>. **Skin:** Pain and burning at IV site, severe venous thrombosis, necrosis and sloughing (with extravasation). **Other:** Tingling sensation. With rapid IV, sensations of heat waves (peripheral vasodilation), fainting.

INTERACTIONS **Drug:** May enhance inotropic and toxic effects of **digoxin;** antagonizes the effects of **verapamil** and possibly other CALCIUM CHANNEL BLOCKERS.

C

PHARMACOKINETICS Distribution: Crosses placenta. **Elimination:** Primarily in feces; small amounts in urine, pancreatic juice, saliva, and breast milk.

NURSING IMPLICATIONS

Assessment & Drug Effects

- Monitor ECG and BP and observe patient closely during administration. IV injection may be accompanied by cutaneous burning sensation and peripheral vasodilation, with moderate fall in BP.
- Advise ambulatory patient to remain in bed for 15–30 min or more depending on response following injection.
- Observe digitalized patients closely because an increase in serum calcium increases risk of digitalis toxicity.
- Monitor lab tests: Frequent serum pH and serum calcium.

Patient & Family Education

- Remain in bed for 15–30 min or more following injection and depending on response.
- Symptoms of mild hypercalcemia, such as loss of appetite, nausea, vomiting, or constipation may occur. If hypercalcemia becomes severe, call healthcare provider if feeling confused or extremely excited.
- Do not use other calcium supplements or eat foods high in calcium, such as milk, cheese, yogurt, eggs, meats, and some cereals, during therapy.

CALCIUM GLUCONATE (Pr)

(gloo′koe-nate)

Classification: ELECTROLYTE AND WATER BALANCE
Therapeutic: ELECTROLYTE REPLACEMENT SOLUTION

AVAILABILITY Tablet; intravenous solution; capsule

ACTION & THERAPEUTIC EFFECT Calcium gluconate acts like digitalis on the heart, increasing cardiac muscle tone and force of systolic contractions (positive inotropic effect). *Rapidly and effectively restores serum calcium levels in acute hypocalcemia of various origins; also effective as a cardiac stabilizer under conditions of hyperkalemia or resuscitation.*

USES Treatment of acute symptomatic hypocalcemia. Also as antidote for magnesium sulfate, for acute symptoms of lead colic, to decrease capillary permeability in sensitivity reactions, and to relieve muscle cramps from insect bites or stings. Oral calcium may be used to maintain normal calcium balance and to prevent primary osteoporosis. Also in osteoporosis, osteomalacia, chronic hypoparathyroidism, rickets, and as adjunct in treatment of myasthenia gravis and Eaton–Lambert syndrome.

UNLABELED USES To antagonize aminoglycoside-induced neuromuscular blockage, and as "calcium challenge" to diagnose Zollinger–Ellison syndrome and medullary thyroid carcinoma, management of severe hypermagnesemia.

CONTRAINDICATIONS Ventricular fibrillation, metastatic bone disease, injection into myocardium; renal calculi, hypercalcemia, predisposition to hypercalcemia (hyperparathyroidism, certain malignancies); digitalis toxicity.

CAUTIOUS USE Digitalized patients, renal or cardiac insufficiency, arrhythmias; dehydration; diarrhea; hyperphosphatemia;

sarcoidosis, history of lithiasis, immobilized patients; pregnancy (category C). The amount of calcium in breast milk is homeostatically regulated and not altered by maternal calcium intake. Decision to continue or discontinue lactation during therapy should take into account risk of the infant exposure, the benefits of breastfeeding to the infant, and benefits of treatment for the mother.

ROUTE & DOSAGE

All doses are in terms of *elemental calcium:*

- 1 g calcium gluconate = 90 mg (4.5 mEq, 9.3%) elemental calcium

Supplement for Osteoporosis

Adult: **PO** 1–2 g bid to qid
Child: **PO** 45–65 mg/kg/day in divided doses
Neonate: **PO** 50–130 mg/kg/day (max: 1 g)

Hypocalcemia

Adult: **IV** 1–4 g over 2–4 h then reassess calcium measurement
Child: **IV** 200–500 mg/kg/day (max: 2–3 g/dose)

Hypocalcemic Tetany

Adult: **IV** 2–3 g prn
Child: **IV** 100–500 mg/kg/dose, may repeat q6–8h
Neonate: **IV** 200 mg followed by 500 mg/kg/day infusion

CPR

Adult: **IV** 1.5–3 grams over 2–5 min

Hyperkalemia with Cardiac Toxicity

Adult: **IV** 500–800 mg (max: 3 g)

ADMINISTRATION

Oral

- Ensure that chewable tablets are chewed or crushed before being swallowed with a liquid. Powder, take with food or liquid.
- Give with meals to enhance absorption.

Intravenous

PREPARE: **Direct:** May be given undiluted. **Intermittent/Continuous:** May be diluted in 1000 mL of NS.

ADMINISTER: **Direct/Intermittent/Continuous:** Due to the risk of particulates, American Regent, Inc. recommends the use of a 0.22-micron in-line filter for IV administration (1.2-micron filter if admixture contains lipids). ▪ Give slowly, not to exceed 200 mg/min for adults or 100 mg/min for children. Use a small-bore needle into a large vein to avoid possibility of extravasation and resultant necrosis. ▪ With children, scalp veins should be avoided. Avoid rapid infusion. ▪ High concentrations of calcium suddenly reaching the heart can cause fatal cardiac arrest.

INCOMPATIBILITIES: **Solution/additive:** **Amphotericin B, cefamandole, dobutamine, methyl-prednisolone, metoclopramide**, concentration-dependent incompatibility with other ELECTROLYTES. **Y-site:** **Amphotericin B cholesteryl complex, cangrelor, ceftobiprole medocaril, ceftriaxone sodium, dantrolene sodium, diazepam, diazoxide, fluconazole, foscarnet sodium, fosphenytoin sodium, gemtuzumab ozogamicin, inamrinone lactate, indomethacin, lansoprazole, meropenem pantoprazole,**

C

methylprednisolone sodium succinate, minocycline hydrochloride, mycophenolate mofetil hydrochloride, oxacillin sodium, pemetrexed, phenytoin sodium, potassium phosphates, quinupristin-dalfopristin, sodium bicarbonate, sodium phosphates, sulfamethoxazole-trimethoprim, tedizolid phosphate, topotecan hydrochloride.

▪ Injection should be stopped if patient complains of any discomfort. ▪ If extravasation occurs, stop the infusion, disconnect (leave needle/cannula in place); gently aspirate extravasated solution (**do not** flush the line). ▪ Patient should be advised to remain in bed for 15–30 min or more following injection, depending on response.

▪ Store intact IV vials at 20°–25°C (68°–77°F). Do not freeze. Discard unused portion within 4 h after initial puncture. Store oral at room temperature.

ADVERSE EFFECTS **CV:** (With rapid infusion) hypotension, bradycardia, cardiac arrhythmias, <u>cardiac arrest</u>. **Skin:** Pain and burning at IV site, severe venous thrombosis, necrosis and sloughing (with extravasation). **GI:** PO preparation: Chalky taste, constipation, increased gastric acid secretion. **Other:** Tingling sensation. With rapid IV, sensations of heat waves (peripheral vasodilation), fainting.

DIAGNOSTIC TEST INTERFERENCE IV calcium may cause false decreases in ***serum and urine magnesium*** (by ***Titan yellow method***) and transient elevations of ***plasma 11-OHCS*** levels by ***Glenn–Nelson technique***. Values usually return to control levels after 60 min; ***urinary steroid values (17-OHCS)*** may be decreased.

INTERACTIONS **Drug:** May enhance inotropic and toxic effects of **digoxin; magnesium** may compete for GI absorption; decreases absorption of TETRACYCLINES, QUINOLONES **(ciprofloxacin)**; antagonizes the effects of **verapamil** and possibly other CALCIUM CHANNEL BLOCKERS (IV administration).

PHARMACOKINETICS **Absorption:** 30% from small intestine. **Onset:** Immediately after IV. **Distribution:** Crosses placenta. **Elimination:** Primarily in feces; small amounts in urine, pancreatic juice, saliva, and breast milk.

NURSING IMPLICATIONS

Assessment & Drug Effects

- Assess for cutaneous burning sensations and peripheral vasodilation, with moderate fall in BP, during direct IV injection.
- Monitor ECG during IV administration to detect evidence of hypercalcemia: Decreased QT interval associated with inverted T wave.
- Observe IV site closely. Extravasation may result in tissue irritation and necrosis.
- Monitor for hypocalcemia and hypercalcemia (see Signs & Symptoms, Appendix F).
- Monitor lab tests: Frequent serum calcium, phosphorus, albumin, and magnesium during sustained therapy.

Patient & Family Education

- Report S&S of hypercalcemia (see Appendix F) promptly to your care provider.
- Milk and milk products are the best sources of calcium (and

phosphorus). Other good sources include dark green vegetables, soy beans, tofu, and canned fish with bones.

- Calcium absorption can be inhibited by zinc-rich foods: Nuts, seeds, sprouts, legumes, soy products (tofu).
- Check with prescriber before self-medicating with a calcium supplement.

CALCIUM POLYCARBOPHIL

(pol-ee-kar'boe-fil)

FiberCon

Classification: BULK LAXATIVE; ANTIDIARRHEAL

Therapeutic: BULK LAXATIVE; ANTIDIARRHEAL

Prototype: Psyllium hydrophilic mucilloid

AVAILABILITY Tablet

ACTION & *THERAPEUTIC EFFECT* Hydrophilic, bulk-producing laxative that restores normal moisture level and bulk content of intestinal tract. In constipation, retains free water in intestinal lumen, thereby indirectly opposing dehydrating forces of the bowel; in diarrhea, when intestinal mucosa is incapable of absorbing fluid, drug absorbs fecal fluid to form a gel. *Relieves constipation or diarrhea associated with bowel disorders and acute nonspecific diarrhea.*

USES Treatment and prevention of constipation.

CONTRAINDICATIONS GI obstruction, difficulty swallowing.

CAUTIOUS USE Fetal risk is minimal. Lactation, infant risk is minimal. Younger than 12 yr.

ROUTE & DOSAGE

Constipation

Adult: **PO** 1 g 1–4 × day or as needed (max: 6 g/24 h)
Child (6–12 yr): **PO** 500 mg 1–4 × day (max: 3 g/24 h); *3 to less than 6 yr:* 500 mg 1–2 × day (max: 1.5 g/24 h)

ADMINISTRATION

Oral

- Administer with at least 180–240 mL (6–8 oz) water or other fluid of patient's choice when used as a laxative and with at least 60–90 mL (2–3 oz) of fluid when used as an antidiarrheal. Chewed tablets should not be swallowed dry.
- If diarrhea is severe, dose can be repeated every half hour up to maximum daily dose.

ADVERSE EFFECTS **GI:** *Flatulence*, abdominal fullness, intestinal obstruction; laxative dependence (long-term use).

PHARMACOKINETICS **Absorption:** Not absorbed from the intestine. Bowel movement usually occurs within 12–72 h. **Elimination:** In feces.

NURSING IMPLICATIONS

Assessment & Drug Effects

- Evaluate effectiveness of medication. If it is ineffective as an antidiarrheal, report to prescriber.
- Report promptly rectal bleeding, very dark stools, or abdominal pain.

Patient & Family Education

- You will likely have a bowel movement within 12–72 h.
- This is an OTC product. Take this drug exactly as ordered. Do not

C

increase the dose if response is inadequate. Consult prescriber. Do not use other laxatives while you are taking calcium polycarbophil.

CANAGLIFLOZIN

(kan'a-gli-floe'zin)

Invokana

Classification: ANTIDIABETIC; SODIUM-GLUCOSE COTRANSPORTER 2 (SGLT2) INHIBITOR

Therapeutic: ANTIDIABETIC; SGLT2 INHIBITOR

AVAILABILITY Tablet

ACTION & *THERAPEUTIC EFFECT* Inhibits the sodium-glucose cotransporter 2 (SGLT2) in the proximal renal tubules that is responsible for the majority of the reabsorption of filtered glucose in the kidney. *Canagliflozin inhibits SGLT2 thus allowing more glucose to be removed from the bloodstream and excreted by the kidney.*

USES Adjunct therapy for the treatment of type 2 diabetes mellitus in combination with diet and exercise.

CONTRAINDICATIONS History of serious hypersensitivity reaction to canagliflozin; Type 1 DM; severe renal impairment (eGFR of 30 mL/min/1.73m^2), ESRD, or on dialysis; severe hepatic impairment; lactation.

CAUTIOUS USE Hypotension; cardiovascular disease; diabetic ketoacidosis; renal impairment; low systolic blood pressure; increases in low-density cholesterol; moderate hepatic impairment; renal insufficiency, reduced intravascular volume; history of genital mycotic infections especially in uncircumcised men; older adults; pregnancy (category C). Safety and efficacy in children younger than 18 yr not established.

ROUTE & DOSAGE

Type 2 Diabetes Mellitus

Adult: **PO** 100 mg once daily; can increase up to 300 mg once daily

Hepatic Impairment Dosage Adjustment

Severe Impairment: Not recommended

Renal Impairment Dosage Adjustment

eGFR 45–59 mL/min/1.73m^2: Do not exceed 100 mg daily
eGFR less than 45 mL/min/1.73m^2: Not recommended

ADMINISTRATION

Oral

- Give before the first meal of the day.
- Store at 15°–30°C (59°–86°F).

ADVERSE EFFECTS **Endocrine:** Increased serum potassium. **GU:** Increased fungal infections for females, polyuria.

INTERACTIONS **Drug: Rifampin** and other inducers of UGT enzymes (e.g., **phenobarbital, phenytoin, ritonavir, carbamazepine, efavirenz, fosphenytoin**) can decrease the levels of canagliflozin. Canagliflozin can increase the levels of **digoxin**. LOOP DIURETICS increase risk of hypotension.

PHARMACOKINETICS **Absorption:** 65% bioavailable. **Peak:** 1–2 h. **Distribution:** 99% plasma protein bound. **Metabolism:** Glucuronidation by UGT. **Elimination:** Renal (30%) and fecal (52%). **Half-Life:** 10.6–13.1 h.

NURSING IMPLICATIONS

Black Box Warning

Lower limb amputation. An approximate twofold increased risk of lower limb amputations associated in two large randomized, placebo controlled trials in patients with cardiovascular disease (CVD) or were at risk for CVD. Amputations of the toe and midfoot were most frequent.

Assessment & Drug Effects

- Monitor BP throughout therapy as drug causes intravascular volume depletion.
- Monitor for symptomatic hypotension, especially at the initiation of therapy and in the older adult or those taking other drugs that lower BP.
- Monitor blood glucose.
- Monitor for S&S of genital fungal infections.
- Monitor for lower limb and feet ulcerations, sores, or infections.
- Monitor volume status in elderly and those with renal impairment.
- Monitor lab tests: Baseline and periodic kidney function tests; periodic HbA1C, serum potassium (in those predisposed to hyperkalemia), magnesium, phosphate, and lipid profile.

Patient & Family Education

- Monitor blood sugar as directed by prescriber. Note that this drug will cause sugar to appear in your urine.
- Report to prescriber if you experience S&S of hypoglycemia (see Appendix F).
- Report to prescriber any S&S of an allergic reaction (e.g., rash, hives).
- Maintain adequate fluid intake as drug can cause dehydration. Inform prescriber if you experience dizziness upon standing.
- Yeast infections of the vagina and penis (especially in uncircumcised men) may occur. Report promptly for treatment.
- Report S/S of UTI (e.g., frequent urination, blood in urine, pain during urination).
- Report to prescriber if a pregnancy is suspected.
- Discontinue breastfeeding while taking this drug.

CANDESARTAN CILEXETIL

(can-de-sar′tan ci-lex′e-til)

Atacand

Classification: ANGIOTENSIN II RECEPTOR ANTAGONIST

Therapeutic: ANTIHYPERTENSIVE

Prototype: Losartan

AVAILABILITY

Tablet

ACTION & THERAPEUTIC EFFECT

Angiotensin II receptor (type AT_1) antagonist. Angiotensin II is a potent vasoconstrictor and primary vasoactive hormone of the renin–angiotensin–aldosterone system. Candesartan selectively blocks binding of angiotensin II to the AT_1 receptors found in many tissues (e.g., vascular smooth muscle, adrenal glands). *Results in blocking the vasoconstricting and aldosterone-secreting effects of angiotensin II, resulting in an antihypertensive effect. Effectively lowers BP from hypertensive to normotensive range.*

USES

Hypertension, heart failure.

C

CONTRAINDICATIONS Known sensitivity to candesartan or any other angiotensin II (AT_1) receptor antagonist (e.g., losartan, valsartan); primary hyperaldosteronism; bilateral renal artery stenosis; pregnancy (category D); lactation; children younger than 1 yr for hypertension, or children with GFR less than 30 mL/min/1.73 m^2.

CAUTIOUS USE Unilateral renal artery stenosis; aortic or mitral valve stenosis; hypertrophic cardiomyopathy; CHF; DM; moderate hepatic or renal impairment, significant renal failure; children.

ROUTE & DOSAGE

Hypertension

Adult: **PO** Start at 8 mg daily; titrate as needed (range 8–32 mg daily)
Adolescent/Child (6 yr or older weighing more than 50 kg): **PO** 8–16 mg given in single or divided doses; adjust based on response; *6 yr or older weighing less than 50 kg:* 4–8 mg given in single or divided doses; adjust based on response; *1 to younger than 6 yr:* 0.2 mg/kg/day; adjust based on response

Heart Failure

Adult: **PO** Start at 4–8 mg once daily, double the dose at 2-wk intervals as tolerated by the patient until a dose of 32 mg is reached

ADMINISTRATION

Oral

- May be administered with or without food.
- Volume depletion should be corrected prior to initiation of therapy to prevent hypotension.
- Dose is individualized and may be given once or twice daily. The daily dose may be titrated up to 32 mg; larger doses are not likely to provide additional benefit.
- Store between 15° and 30°C (59° and 86°F).

ADVERSE EFFECTS CV: Hypotension. **Respiratory:** URI. **Endocrine:** Hyperkalemia. **GU:** Abnormal renal function.

INTERACTIONS Drug: May increase risk of **lithium** toxicity.

PHARMACOKINETICS Absorption: 15% reaches systemic circulation. **Peak:** Serum concentration, 3–4 h; therapeutic effect, 2–4 wk. **Duration:** 24 h. **Distribution:** Greater than 99% protein bound; crosses placenta; distributed into breast milk. **Metabolism:** Minimally in liver. **Elimination:** Primarily in bile (67%) and urine (33%). **Half-Life:** 9–12 h.

NURSING IMPLICATIONS

Black Box Warning

Candesartan cilexetil has been associated with fetal injury and death.

Assessment & Drug Effects

- Monitor BP as therapeutic effectiveness is indicated by decreases in systolic and diastolic BP within 2 wk with maximal effect at 4–6 wk.
- Monitor for transient hypotension in volume/salt-depleted patients; if hypotension occurs, place in supine position and notify prescriber.

- Monitor BP periodically; through readings, just prior to the next scheduled dose, should be made when possible.
- Monitor lab tests: Periodic BUN and creatinine, serum potassium, LFTs, and CBC with differential.

Patient & Family Education

- Stop taking this drug and inform your prescriber immediately if you become pregnant.
- You may not notice maximum pressure-lowering effect for 6 wk.
- Report episodes of dizziness especially when making position changes.

CAPECITABINE

(cap-e-si′ta-been)

Xeloda

Classification: PYRIMIDINE ANTIMETABOLITE

Therapeutic: ANTINEOPLASTIC

Prototype: 5-Fluorouracil (5-FU)

AVAILABILITY Tablet

ACTION & THERAPEUTIC EFFECT Pyrimidine antagonist and cell cycle specific antimetabolite. Prodrug of 5-FU. Blocks actions of enzymes essential to normal DNA and RNA synthesis. May become incorporated into RNA molecules of tumor cells, thereby interfering with RNA and protein synthesis. *Reduces or stabilizes tumor size in metastatic breast cancer and colorectal cancer.*

USES Metastatic breast cancer and colorectal cancer.

UNLABELED USES Ovarian cancer.

CONTRAINDICATIONS Hypersensitivity to capecitabine, doxifluridine, 5-FU; myelosuppression; dihydropyrimidine dehydrogenase (DPD) deficiency; females of childbearing age; active infection; jaundice; severe renal failure (CrCl less than 30 mL/min); pregnancy; lactation.

CAUTIOUS USE Mild to moderate renal or hepatic dysfunction; bacterial or viral infection; coronary artery disease, angina, cardiac arrhythmias; history of varicella zoster or other herpes infections; older adults; children younger than 18 yr.

ROUTE & DOSAGE

Breast Cancer, Colorectal Cancer

Adult: **PO** 1250 mg/m^2 bid × 2 wk every 21 days

Renal Impairment Dosage Adjustment

CrCl 30–50 mL/min: Reduce dose by 25%; *less than 30 mL/min:* Do not use

Obesity Dosage Adjustment

Dose based on actual body weight

Toxicity Dosage Adjustment

See package insert

ADMINISTRATION

Oral

- Hazardous agent: NIOSH recommends single gloving for administration of intact tablets. Do not crush or cut tablets.
- Pregnancy test: Prior to initiation in women of childbearing potential.
- Morning and evening doses (about 12 h apart) should be given within 30 min after the meal. Water is the preferred liquid for taking this drug.

- Store tightly closed at controlled room temperature between 15° and 30°C (59° and 86°F).

ADVERSE EFFECTS CV: *Edema*, venous thrombosis **CNS:** *Fatigue, burning or prickling sensation in hands or feet*, dizziness. **HEENT:** Eye irritation. **Endocrine:** Dehydration. **Skin:** *Dermatitis*. **Hepatic:** *Hyperbilirubinemia*. **GI:** *Abdominal pain, loss of appetite, nausea, stomatitis, diarrhea, vomiting*, constipation. **Musculoskeletal:** *Weakness*, back pain, joint pain, limb pain. **Hematologic:** *Anemia, leukopenia, lymphocytopenia, neutropenia, thrombocytopenia*. **Other:** Fever.

INTERACTIONS Drug: Leucovorin increases concentration and toxicity of **5-FU**, altered coagulation and/or bleeding reported with **warfarin** and **NSAIDs.** Avoid or monitor closely with other agents that may cause neutropenia (**deferiprone, clozapine**). **Food:** Food decreases extent of absorption.

PHARMACOKINETICS Absorption: Absorption significantly reduced by food. **Peak:** 1.5–2 h. **Distribution:** Approx 35% protein bound. **Metabolism:** Extensively metabolized to 5-FU. **Elimination:** In urine. **Half-Life:** 45 min.

NURSING IMPLICATIONS

Black Box Warning

When capecitabine is given to patients using oral coumarin-derivative anticoagulants (e.g., warfarin), there is increased risk of bleeding and death from hemorrhage. These adverse effects may occur as late as several months after starting capecitabine or even after stopping capecitabine.

Assessment & Drug Effects

- Monitor carefully for S&S of grade 2 or greater toxicity: Diarrhea greater than 4 BMs/day or at night; vomiting greater than 1 time/24 h; significant loss of appetite or anorexia; stomatitis; hand-and-foot syndrome (pain, swelling, erythema, desquamation, blistering); temperature = 100.5° F; and S&S of infection.
- Withhold drug and immediately report S&S of grade 2 or greater toxicity.
- Withhold drug and notify prescriber if PT and INR are prolonged beyond the normal range in those with concurrent warfarin therapy.
- Monitor for dehydration and replace fluids as needed.
- Monitor carefully patients with coronary artery disease for S&S of cardiotoxicity (e.g., increasing angina).
- Monitor lab tests: Periodic CBC with differential and LFTs. Frequent PT and INR with concurrent warfarin therapy. Serum bilirubin, serum creatinine, and serum alkaline phosphatase.

Patient & Family Education

- Report immediately significant nausea, loss of appetite, diarrhea, soreness of tongue, fever of 100.5° F or more, or signs of infection. Review patient drug package insert carefully for more detail.
- For female patients, it is a necessity to use contraceptive methods. Inform prescriber immediately if you become pregnant.

CAPREOMYCIN

(kap-ree-oh-mye′sin)

Capastat

Classification: ANTIBIOTIC; ANTITUBERCULOSIS

Therapeutic: ANTITUBERCULOSIS

Prototype: Isoniazid

C

AVAILABILITY Powder for injection

ACTION & *THERAPEUTIC EFFECT* Polypeptide antibiotic that is bactericidal against strains of *Mycobacterium tuberculosis.* The exact action is not fully known. Should not be used alone. *Effective second-line antimycobacterial in conjunction with other antitubercular drugs.*

USES Treatment of active tuberculosis when primary agents cannot be tolerated or when causative organism has become resistant.

CONTRAINDICATIONS Hypersensitivity to capreomycin, pregnancy—fetal risk cannot be ruled out, lactation—infant risk cannot be ruled out.

CAUTIOUS USE Renal insufficiency (extreme caution); acoustic nerve impairment; history of allergies (especially to drugs); preexisting liver disease; myasthenia gravis. Safe use in children not established.

ROUTE & DOSAGE

Tuberculosis

Adult: **IM/IV** 15 mg/kg daily or 25 mg/kg 3 times per week.

Renal Impairment Dosage Adjustment

See package insert for adjustments

ADMINISTRATION

Intramuscular

- Reconstitute by adding 2 mL of NS injection or sterile water for injection to each 1 g vial. Allow 2–3 min for drug to dissolve completely.
- Make IM injections deep into large muscle mass. Superficial injections are more painful and are associated with sterile abscess. Rotate injection sites.
- Solution may become pale straw color and darken with time, but this does not indicate loss of potency.
- After reconstitution, solution may be stored under refrigeration for use within 24 h.
- Store vials at controlled room temperature between 20° and 25°C (68° and 77°F). Excursions permitted between 15° and 30°C (59° and 86°F). Discard unused portion.

Intravenous

PREPARE: **IV Infusion:** Reconstitute by adding 2 mL of NS or sterile water to each 1 g to yield 370 mg/mL. ▪ Allow 2–3 min to dissolve, then add required dose to 100 mL of NS.

ADMINISTER: **IV Infusion:** Give over 60 min. Avoid rapid infusion.

ADVERSE EFFECTS **CNS:** Neuromuscular blockage (large doses: Skeletal muscle weakness, respiratory depression or arrest). **HEENT:** *Ototoxicity,* eighth nerve (auditory and vestibular) damage. **Endocrine:** lectrolyte imbalances. **GU:** Nephrotoxicity (long-term therapy), tubular necrosis. **Hematologic:** *Eosinophilia.* **Other:** Impaired hepatic function (decreased BSP excretion); IM site reactions: Pain, induration, excessive bleeding, sterile abscesses.

INTERACTIONS **Drug:** Capreomycin may enhance the neuromuscular-blocking effect of AMINOGLYCOSIDES or NEUROMUSCULAR BLOCKERS. Do not administer with LIVE VACCINES.

PHARMACOKINETICS **Peak:** 1–2 h. **Distribution:** Does not cross blood–brain barrier; crosses placenta.

Elimination: 52% in urine unchanged in 12 h; small amount in bile.

C

NURSING IMPLICATIONS

Black Box Warning

Capreomycin has been associated with VIII cranial nerve impairment and renal injury.

Assessment & Drug Effects

- Observe injection sites for signs of excessive bleeding, pain, and inflammation.
- Dosage of capreomycin is typically reduced in patients with impaired renal function, as it is cumulative. Follow renal function tests closely.
- Monitor closely for vestibular and/or auditory nerve impairment especially in those with preexisting renal insufficiency.
- Monitor I&O rates and pattern: Report immediately any change in output or I&O ratio, any unusual appearance of urine, or elevation of BUN above 30 mg/dL.
- Evaluate hearing and balance by audiometric measurements (twice weekly or weekly) and tests of vestibular function (periodically).
- Monitor lab tests: Baseline C&S prior to therapy; baseline and weekly renal function tests; baseline and frequent serum electrolytes and LFTs; WBC count with differential.

Patient & Family Education

- Report any change in hearing or disturbance of balance. These effects are sometimes reversible if drug is withdrawn promptly when first symptoms appear.
- Report and difficulty urinating or poor urine output.
- Ensure that you know about adverse reactions and what to do about them. Report immediately the appearance of any unusual symptom, regardless of how vague it may seem.

CAPSAICIN

(cap-say'i-sin)

Axsain, Capsaicin, Capsin, Capzasin-P, Dolorac, Qutenza, Trixaicin, Zostrix, Zostrix-HP

Classification: TOPICAL ANALGESIC

Therapeutic: TOPICAL ANALGESIC

AVAILABILITY Lotion cream; gel, topical patch

ACTION & *THERAPEUTIC EFFECT* Capsaicin depletes and prevents reaccumulation of Substance P, the primary chemical mediator of pain impulses from the periphery to the CNS. *Renders skin and joints insensitive to pain; therefore, it serves as an effective peripheral analgesic.*

USES Temporary relief of pain from arthritis, neuralgias, diabetic neuropathy, and herpes zoster.

UNLABELED USES Phantom limb pain, psoriasis, intractable pruritus.

CONTRAINDICATIONS Hypersensitivity to capsaicin or any ingredient in the cream.

CAUTIOUS USE Patients on ACE inhibitors. Safety and efficacy in children younger than 2 yr not established.

ROUTE & DOSAGE

Analgesia

Adult/Child (2 yr or older):

Topical Apply to affected area not more than 3–4 × day

Common adverse effects in *italic*; life-threatening effects underlined; generic names in **bold**; classifications in SMALL CAPS; ♣ Canadian drug name; ⊙ Prototype drug; ⚠ Alert

ADMINISTRATION

Topical

- Apply to affected areas only and avoid contact with eyes or broken or irritated skin.
- If applied with bare hand, wash immediately following application.
- Use only nitrile gloves when handling a capsaicin patch.
- Avoid tight bandages over areas of application of the cream.
- If necessary for adherence, clip hair (do not shave) on skin where patch will be applied.
- Patch may be cut (before removing protective liner) to match size and shape of treatment area.
- Leave patch on for 60 min. To ensure contact, a dressing may be applied.
- Following patch removal, apply cleansing gel to treatment area and leave on for at least 1 min.

ADVERSE EFFECTS **CNS:** Concentration greater than 1%: Neurotoxicity, hyperalgesia. **Skin:** *Burning, stinging, redness*, itching. **Other:** Cough.

INTERACTIONS **Drug:** May increase incidence of cough with ACE INHIBITORS.

PHARMACOKINETICS **Onset:** Postherpetic neuralgia: 2–6 wk.

NURSING IMPLICATIONS

Assessment & Drug Effects

- Monitor for significant pain relief, which may require 4–6 wk of application 3 or 4 × daily.
- Monitor for and report signs of skin breakdown, as these generally indicate need for drug discontinuation.

Patient & Family Education

- Report local discomfort at site of application if discomfort is distressing or persists beyond the first 3–4 days of use.
- Use caution in handling contact lenses following application of cream. Wash hands thoroughly before touching lenses.
- Notify prescriber if symptoms do not improve or condition worsens within 14–28 days.

CAPTOPRIL

(kap'toe-pril)

Classification: RENIN ANGIOTENSIN SYSTEM ANTAGONIST; ANTIHYPERTENSIVE

Therapeutic: ANTIHYPERTENSIVE; ACE INHIBITOR

Prototype: Enalapril

AVAILABILITY Tablet

ACTION & *THERAPEUTIC EFFECT* Lowers blood pressure by specific inhibition of the angiotensin-converting enzyme (ACE) utilized by renin in the formation of angiotensin II, a potent vasoconstrictor. ACE inhibition alters hemodynamics without compensatory changes in cardiac output (except in patients with CHF). Inhibition of ACE also leads to decreased circulating aldosterone. *Effective in management of hypertension, and in congestive heart failure with resulting decreases in dyspnea and improved exercise tolerance.*

USES Hypertension; heart failure, diabetic nephropathy, left ventricular dysfunction post MI; proteinuria.

UNLABELED USES Idiopathic edema; hypertensive emergency, ST-elevation myocardial infarction.

CONTRAINDICATIONS History of angioedema, hypersensitivity to captopril or ACE inhibitors; coadministration with aliskiren in patients with DM; hypotension; jaundice, or marked elevations of hepatic enzymes; pregnancy—fetal risk cannot be ruled out.

CAUTIOUS USE Impaired renal function, patient with solitary kidney; collagen-vascular diseases (scleroderma, SLE); autoimmune disease, bone marrow suppression, coronary or cerebrovascular disease; black patients; surgery; cardiomyopathy, aortic stenosis; severe salt/volume depletion; heart failure, hyperkalemia, older adults, children, lactation—infant risk is minimal.

ROUTE & DOSAGE

Hypertension

Adult/Adolescent: **PO** 12.5–25 mg bid or tid, may increase to 50 mg tid (max: 450 mg/day)
Child: **PO** 0.3–0.5 mg/kg/dose q8h; titrate to max of 6/mg/kg/day in divided doses

Heart Failure

Adult: **PO** 25 mg tid; may increase to 50 mg tid if needed (max: 450 mg/day)

Diabetic Nephropathy

Adult: **PO** 25 mg tid

Left Ventricular Function Post MI

Adult: **PO** 6.25 then increase to 12.5 mg tid; can increase to target dose of 50 mg tid

Renal Insufficiency Dosage Adjustment

CrCl 10–50 mL/min: 75% of dose; *less than 10 mL/min:* 50% of dose

ADMINISTRATION

Oral

- Give captopril 1 h before meals. Food reduces absorption by 30–40%.
- Store in light-resistant containers at no more than 30°C (86°F) unless otherwise directed.

ADVERSE EFFECTS **CV:** Tachycardia, first dose hypotension, dizziness, fainting. **Endocrine:** Hyperkalemia. **Skin:** *Maculopapular rash*, urticaria, pruritus, angioedema, photosensitivity. **GI:** Altered taste sensation (loss of taste perception, persistent salt or metallic taste); intestinal angioedema. **GU:** Impaired renal function, nephrotic syndrome, membranous glomerulonephritis. **Other:** Hypersensitivity reactions, serum sickness-like reaction, arthralgia, skin eruptions.

DIAGNOSTIC TEST INTERFERENCE

May lead to false-negative aldosterone/renin ratio.

INTERACTIONS **Drug:** NITRATES, DIURETICS, and ANTIHYPERTENSIVES, **amifostine**, enhance hypotensive effects. POTASSIUM-SPARING DIURETICS **(spironolactone, amiloride)** increase potassium levels. May increase risk of angioedema when used with **pregabalin;** increased risk of hyperkalemia with **aliskiren.** ANTACIDS may decrease absorption. Use with **digoxin** (though common) requires reduction in digoxin dose. Captopril increases risk of side effects when used with **lithium, sacubitril, sodium phosphate. Food:** Decreases absorption; take 30–60 min before meals.

PHARMACOKINETICS **Absorption:** 60–75% absorbed; food may decrease absorption 25–40%.

C

Onset: 15 min. **Peak:** 1–2 h. **Distribution:** To all tissues except CNS; crosses placenta. **Metabolism:** Some liver metabolism. **Elimination:** Primarily in urine; excreted in breast milk.

NURSING IMPLICATIONS

Black Box Warning

Captopril has been associated with fetal injury and death.

Assessment & Drug Effects

- Monitor BP closely following the first dose. A sudden exaggerated hypotensive response may occur within 1–3 h of first dose, especially in those with high BP or on a diuretic and restricted salt intake.
- Monitor therapeutic effectiveness. At least 2 wk of therapy may be required before full therapeutic effects are achieved.
- Monitor lab tests: Baseline urine protein levels and monthly for the first 8 mo of treatment and then periodically thereafter; WBC and differential before therapy is begun and at approximately 2-wk intervals for the first 3 mo of therapy and then periodically thereafter; fasting blood glucose, renal function tests, electrolytes, ECG at baseline, lipid profile, CBC.

Patient & Family Education

- Report to prescriber without delay the onset of unexplained fever, unusual fatigue, sore mouth or throat, easy bruising or bleeding. Mild skin eruptions are most likely to appear during the first 4 wks of therapy and may be accompanied by fever and eosinophilia.
- Taste impairment occurs in 5–10% of patients and generally reverses in 2–3 mo even with continued therapy.
- Notify provider of any joint pain, flushing, cough, chest pain, or palpitations.
- Notify prescriber if you become or suspect you are pregnant.
- Use OTC medications only with approval of the prescriber.

CARBACHOL INTRAOCULAR

(kar′ba-kole)

Miostat

See Appendix A-1.

CARBAMAZEPINE

(kar-ba-maz′e-peen)

Apo-Carbamazepine ♣, Carbatrol, Epitol, Equetro, Mazepine ♣, Pms-Carbamazepine ♣, Tegretol, Tegretol XR

Classification: ANTICONVULSANT

Therapeutic: ANTICONVULSANT; ANTIMANIA

AVAILABILITY

Tablet; extended release tablet; extended release capsule; oral suspension; chewable tablet

ACTION & THERAPEUTIC EFFECT

Inhibits sustained repetitive impulses and reduces posttetanic synaptic transmission in the spinal cord. It limits the spread of seizure activity. Provides relief in trigeminal neuralgia by reducing synaptic transmission within trigeminal nucleus. Unknown mechanism regarding bipolar disorder. *Effective anticonvulsant for a range of seizure disorders and as an adjuvant reduces depressive signs and symptoms and stabilizes mood. It is effective for pain and other symptoms associated with neurologic disorders.*

USES

Focal (partial) onset seizures, generalized onset seizures, bipolar disorder, neuropathic pain.

C

UNLABELED USES Agitation, bipolar major depression.

CONTRAINDICATIONS Hypersensitivity to carbamazepine and to TCAs or MAOI therapy; history of myelosuppression or hematologic reaction to other drugs; leukopenia; bone marrow depression; within 14 d use of MAOI drugs; increased IOP; SLE; hepatic, or renal failure; hyponatremia; coronary artery disease; hypertension; petit mal (absent) seizures, atonic or myoclonic seizures; suicidal ideation; acute intermediate porphyria; presence of HLA-B*1502 gene increases risk of Stevens–Johnson syndrome or toxic epidermal necrolysis especially common in Asian ancestry; pregnancy—fetal risk has been demonstrated; lactation—infant risk cannot be ruled out.

CAUTIOUS USE The older adult; history of cardiac disease or impairment, alcoholism; history of suicidal thoughts; hepatic disease or impairment; cardiac arrhythmias; mixed seizure disorder including atypical absence seizures; history of increased ocular pressure; renal impairment; children younger than 6 yr.

ROUTE & DOSAGE

Focal (Partial) Onset Seizures

Adult: **PO** 2 to 3 mg/kg/day (100–200 mg/day) or up to 400 mg/day, doses may be increased based on seizure control and serum concentrations
Adolescent: **PO** 200 mg bid (immediate release tablets) titrate up by 200 mg/day at weekly intervals
Child: (younger than 6 yr): **PO** 10–20 mg/kg/day in 2–3 divided doses immediate release (tablet) or 4 divided doses (suspension), titrate weekly (max: 35 mg/kg/day); *6–12 yr:* 100 mg bid (immediate release tablet) or 50 mg four times daily (suspension), titrate by 100 mg/day at weekly intervals (max: 1 g/day)

Neuropathic Pain

Adult: **PO** 200–400 mg/day increase by 200 mg/day if needed; usual dose 600–800 mg/day (max: 1.2 g/day)

Bipolar Disorder

Adult: **PO** 100–400 mg/day, may increase q1–4 days up to 600 mg–1.2 g/day (max 1.6 g/day)

ADMINISTRATION

Oral

- NIOSH guidelines: Use single gloves by anyone handling intact tablets or capsules or administering from a unit-dose package. If crushing, splitting, or manipulating or handling the uncoated tablets, use double gloves and a gown. Use double gloves and protective gown, use respiratory, face, and eye protections when handling oral liquid and administering a tube feeding. Be sure to use eye/face protection if the patient may resist or if there is a potential to vomit or spit up.
- Do not administer within 14 days of patient receiving a MAO inhibitor.
- Give with a meal to increase absorption. Extended release may be taken without meals. Extended release capsules may be sprinkled over food (applesauce).
- Ensure that chewable tablets are chewed or crushed before being swallowed with a liquid.

- Ensure that sustained release form of drug is not chewed or crushed. It **must be** swallowed whole.
- Shake suspension well before using.
- Do not administer carbamazepine suspension simultaneously with other liquid medications: A precipitate may form in the stomach.
- Store tablet at less than 30°C (86°F). Protect from light. Store extended release tablet at 25°C (77°F), with excursions permitted between 15° and 30°C (59° and 86°F). Protect from light and moisture. Store suspension at less than 30°C (86°F). Protect from light.

ADVERSE EFFECTS (≥ 5%) **CV:** Hypotension, syncope. **CNS:** Dizziness, vertigo, weakness, drowsiness, disturbances of coordination, ataxia. **HEENT:** Blurred vision tinnitus. **Endocrine:** Hyponatremia. **Skin:** Skin rashes, urticaria. **GI:** Nausea, vomiting, constipation, dry mouth and pharynx. **Hematologic:** Aplastic anemia, *leukopenia* (transient).

DIAGNOSTIC TEST INTERFERENCE May cause false-positive ***TCA screen***; may interact with pregnancy tests.

INTERACTIONS **Drug:** Extensive number of drug interactions, only some are listed here; consult package insert for complete list. Serum concentrations of other ANTICONVULSANTS, **bictegravir,** or **ranolazine, cyclosporine, doxorubicin, elvitegravir, ezogabine, lopinavir** may decrease because of increased metabolism; CALCIUM CHANNEL BLOCKERS, **clarithromycin, erythromycin, ketoconazole, nefazodone, voriconazole**, may increase carbamazepine levels; decreases hypoprothrombinemic effects of ORAL ANTICOAGULANTS; increases metabolism of ESTROGENS, thus decreasing effectiveness of ORAL CONTRACEPTIVES. Reduces concentration of **delavirdine, etravirine**. Do not use with dabigatran. Drugs metabolized by CYP3A4 will have decreased serum concentrations when used with carbamazepine. Carbamazepine can increase adverse effects of **adenosine, clozapine, deferiprone, lamotrigine. Food: Grapefruit juice** may increase carbamazepine concentration. **Herbal: Ginkgo** may decrease anticonvulsant effectiveness.

PHARMACOKINETICS **Absorption:** Slowly from GI tract. **Peak:** Varies based on dosage form. **Distribution:** Widely distributed; high concentrations in CSF; crosses placenta; distributed into breast milk. **Metabolism:** In liver by CYP3A4; can induce liver microsomal enzymes. **Elimination:** In urine and feces. **Half-Life:** Variable due to autoinduction: 25–65 h

NURSING IMPLICATIONS

Black Box Warning

*Serious and sometime fatal dermatologic reactions have occurred with carbamazepine in those who carry the HLA-B*1502 allele (e.g., persons of Asian ancestry). Carbamazepine has been associated with development of aplastic anemia and agranulocytosis.*

Assessment & Drug Effects

- Monitor for therapeutic effectiveness and loss of seizure control. Some patients develop tolerance to the effects of carbamazepine. Reduction of pain when used in neurological syndromes. Improved symptoms of bipolar disorder.

C

- Monitor for the following reactions, which commonly occur during early therapy: Drowsiness, dizziness, light-headedness, ataxia, gastric upset.
- Monitor for and report promptly skin rash or any other sign of dermatologic toxicity.
- Withhold drug and notify prescriber if the following signs occur: RBC less than 4 million/mm^3, Hct less than 32%, Hgb less than 11 g/dL, WBC less than 4000/mm^3, platelet count less than 100,000/mm^3, reticulocyte count less than 20,000/mm^3, serum iron greater than 150 mg/dL.
- Monitor for toxicity, which can develop when serum concentrations are even slightly above the therapeutic range.
- Monitor for worsening of depression, suicidal thoughts or behavior, or any unusual changes in mood or behavior.
- Monitor I&O ratio and vital signs during period of dosage adjustment. Report oliguria, signs of fluid retention, changes in I&O ratio, and changes in BP or pulse patterns.
- Doses higher than 600 mg/day may precipitate arrhythmias in patients with heart disease.
- Confusion and agitation may be aggravated in the older adult.
- Monitor intraocular pressure (IOP) in those with history of elevated IOP
- Monitor lab tests: Prior to initiation of therapy HLA-B*1502 testing is recommended; carbamazepine blood concentrations, baseline and periodic CBC with differential, platelet count, LFTs, and kidney function tests; electrolytes, periodic lipid profile, and serum calcium. Saliva levels can be used to monitor therapeutic drug levels.

Patient & Family Education

- Take tablets and suspension with food.
- Do not mix solution with other fluids. Do not take with grapefruit juice.
- Discontinue drug and notify prescriber immediately if early signs of toxicity or a possible hematologic problem appear (e.g., skin rash, anorexia, fever, sore throat or mouth, malaise, unusual fatigue, tendency to bruise or bleed, petechiae, ecchymoses, bleeding gums, nosebleeds).
- Avoid hazardous tasks requiring mental alertness and physical coordination until reaction to drug is known because dizziness, drowsiness, and ataxia are common adverse effects.
- Report promptly to prescriber development of an unexplained skin reaction.
- Avoid excessive sunlight, as photosensitivity reactions have been reported. Apply a sunscreen (if allowed) with SPF of 12 or above.
- Report any worsening of depression, suicidal ideation, or unusual changes in behavior.
- Carbamazepine may cause breakthrough bleeding and may also affect the reliability of oral contraceptives.
- Be aware that abrupt withdrawal of any anticonvulsant drug may precipitate seizures or even status epilepticus.

CARBIDOPA-LEVODOPA (Pr)

(kar-bi-doe'pa)

Duopa, Rytary, Sinemet

CARBIDOPA

Lodosyn

Classification: DOPAMINE RECEPTOR AGONIST; ANTIPARKINSON

Therapeutic: ANTIPARKINSON

AVAILABILITY **Carbidopa:** Tablet. **Carbidopa/Levodopa:** Tablet; sustained release tablet; orally disintegrating tablet; oral suspension

ACTION & *THERAPEUTIC EFFECT* Carbidopa prevents peripheral metabolism of levodopa and thereby makes more levodopa available for transport to the brain. Carbidopa does not cross blood–brain barrier and therefore does not affect metabolism of levodopa within the brain. *Effective in management of symptoms of Parkinson disease and parkinsonism of secondary origin while improving life expectancy and quality of life.*

USES Symptomatic treatment of Parkinson disease, postencephalitic parkinsonism, and parkinsonism following carbon dioxide and manganese intoxication. Carbidopa is available for use with levodopa when separate titration of each agent is indicated.

CONTRAINDICATIONS Hypersensitivity to carbidopa or levodopa; narrow-angle glaucoma; history of or suspected melanoma; pregnancy—fetal risk cannot be ruled out; lactation—infant risk cannot be ruled out.

CAUTIOUS USE Cardiovascular, hepatic, pulmonary, or renal disorders; history of MI; urinary retention; history of peptic ulcer; psychiatric states; endocrine disease; chronic wide-angle glaucoma; asthma, seizure disorders; Parkinson disease. Safe use in children younger than 18 yr is not established.

ROUTE & DOSAGE

Parkinson Disease

Adult: **PO** Varies based on dosage form and titrated to patient response. See package insert for initial dose and taper schedule.

ADMINISTRATION

Oral

- Ensure that sustained release form of drug (Sinemet CR) is not chewed or crushed. It may be broken in half but otherwise swallowed whole. Extended release capsules may be sprinkled onto 1–2 tablespoons of applesauce, swallow immediately. Orally disintegrating tablet can be administered with dry hands, gently remove and place tablet on top of tongue, can dissolve and be swallowed with saliva; no fluids are needed.
- Give consistently with respect to food. High-protein meals may interfere with absorption of levodopa.
- When patient has been taking levodopa alone, carbidopa-levodopa is usually initiated with a morning dose after patient has been without levodopa for at least 8 h.
- Store in tight, light- and moisture-resistant containers. Extended release tablet and capsule can be stored at room temperature, 25°C (77°F), with excursions permitted between 15° and 30°C (59° and 86°F). Disintegrating tablets can be stored at controlled room temperature between 20° and 25°C (68° and 77°F), with excursion permitted between 15° and 30°C (59° and 86°F).

ADVERSE EFFECTS (≥ 5%) **CNS:** *Involuntary movements (dyskinetic, dystonic, choreiform)*, ataxia, muscle twitching, increase in hand tremor, peripheral neuropathy. **GI:** Nausea. **Other:** Psychological depression.

DIAGNOSTIC TEST False-negative reaction using glucose-oxidase tests for glucosuria; false-positive reaction for urinary glucose; false-positive urine ketones.

INTERACTIONS Drug: MAO INHIBITORS may precipitate hypertensive crisis; ANTICHOLINERGIC AGENTS may enhance levodopa effects but can exacerbate involuntary movements; ANTIPSYCHOTICS, PHENOTHIAZINES, haloperidol, **phenytoin, papaverine** may interfere with levodopa effects. Avoid use with **alizapride, amisulpride, bromperidol, macimorelin, metoclopramide, sulpiride.**

PHARMACOKINETICS Absorption: 40–70% of carbidopa absorbed; carbidopa may enhance absorption of levodopa. **Distribution: Levodopa** widely distributed in most body tissues except CNS; crosses placenta; excreted in breast milk. **Metabolism:** Via decarboxylation and O-methylation. **Elimination:** In urine. **Half-Life:** 1.5 h.

NURSING IMPLICATIONS

Assessment & Drug Effects

- Make accurate observations and report promptly adverse reactions and therapeutic effects. Rate of dosage increase is determined primarily by patient's tolerance and response to levodopa.
- Monitor vital signs, particularly during period of dosage adjustment. Report alterations in BP, pulse, and respiratory rate and rhythm.
- Monitor all patients closely for behavior changes. Patients in depression should be closely observed for suicidal tendencies.
- Monitor for changes in intraocular pressure in patients with chronic wide-angle glaucoma.
- Monitor patients with diabetes carefully for alterations in diabetes control. Frequent monitoring of blood sugar is advised.
- Report promptly abnormal involuntary movement such as facial grimacing, exaggerated chewing, protrusion of tongue, rhythmic opening and closing of mouth, bobbing of head, jerky arm and leg movements, and exaggerated respiration.
- Assess for "on-off" phenomenon: Sudden, unpredictable loss of drug effectiveness ("off" effect), which lasts 1 min–1 h. This is followed by an equally abrupt return of function ("on" effect). Sometimes symptoms can be controlled by increasing number of doses/day.
- Monitor therapeutic effects. Some patients manifest increase in bradykinesia ("leg freezing" or slow body movement). The patient is unable to start walking and frequently falls. Reduction of dosage may be indicated in these patients.
- Patients who require more frequent drug administration are most likely to manifest gradual return of parkinsonian symptoms toward the end of a dose period.
- Compulsive behaviors either new or worsening (gambling, sex, shopping, eating), continually throughout treatment.
- Monitor lab tests: Periodic blood glucose, LFTs, renal function tests, CBC with differential, Hgb and Hct.

Patient & Family Education

- Follow prescriber's directions regarding continuation or discontinuation of levodopa. Both adverse reactions and therapeutic effects occur more rapidly with carbidopa-levodopa combination than with levodopa alone.

- Advise patient that the medication has a "wearing off" effect that may occur before the next dose is administered.
- Report any depression, suicidal or psychotic behavior, including hallucinations.
- Report any new-onset or intense uncontrollable urges (gambling, shopping, sex, etc.)
- Make positional changes slowly and in stages, particularly from recumbent to upright position, dangle your legs a few minutes before standing, and walk in place before ambulating, as some patients experience weakness, dizziness, and faintness. Tolerance to this effect usually develops within a few months of therapy. Support stockings may help. Consult prescriber.
- Report muscle twitching and spasmodic winking promptly, as these may be early signs of overdosage.
- You may notice elevation of mood and sense of well-being before any objective improvement. Resume activities gradually and observe safety precautions to avoid injury.
- Maintain your prescribed drug regimen. Abrupt withdrawal can lead to parkinsonian crisis with return of marked muscle rigidity, akinesia, tremor, hyperpyrexia, mental changes.
- Avoid driving or other hazardous activities until reaction to drug is determined.
- Levodopa may cause urine to darken on standing and may also cause sweat to be dark-colored. This effect is not clinically significant.
- Wear medical identification. Inform all healthcare providers that you are taking carbidopa-levodopa.

CARBINOXAMINE

(car-bi-nox'a-meen)

Karbinal ER

Classification: ANTIHISTAMINE; H_1-RECEPTOR ANTAGONIST

Therapeutic: ANTIHISTAMINE; SEDATING H_1-ANTAGONIST

Prototype: Diphenhydramine

AVAILABILITY Oral suspension; oral solution; tablet

ACTION & *THERAPEUTIC EFFECT* Carbinoxamine competes for H_1-receptor sites on effector cells thus blocking histamine release. *Has antihistaminic, anticholinergic (drying), antitussive, and sedative properties.*

USES Allergic conjunctivitis, allergic rhinitis, rhinorrhea, pruritus, sneezing, urticaria.

CONTRAINDICATIONS Hypersensitivity to carbinoxamine; lower respiratory tract symptoms (including acute asthma); MAOI therapy, MAOI coadministration; lactation; children younger than 2 yr.

CAUTIOUS USE Hypersensitivity to antihistamines of similar structure; history of asthma; COPD; convulsive disorders; increased IOP; hyperthyroidism; hypertension, cardiovascular disease; hepatic disease; diabetes mellitus, prostatic hyperplasia/urinary obstruction, pyloroduodenal obstruction, older adults; pregnancy (category C); young children.

ROUTE & DOSAGE

Allergic Conjunctivitis, Allergic Rhinitis, Rhinorrhea, Pruritus, Sneezing, Urticaria

Adult/Adolescent: **PO** 4–8 mg q6–8h (max: 32 mg/day)

Child (2 to younger than 6 yr): **PO** 0.2–0.4 mg/kg/day divided into 3–4 doses; *6 yr or older:* 2–4 mg q6–8h

ADMINISTRATION

Oral

- Administer on an empty stomach with water. Shake suspension well before administering.
- Store at 15°–30°C (59°–86°F). Protect from light.

ADVERSE EFFECTS CV: Extrasystoles, headache, hypotension, palpitations, tachycardia, chest tightness. **Respiratory:** Dryness of mouth, nose and throat, nasal stuffiness, thickening of bronchial secretions. **CNS:** Acute labyrinthitis, blurred vision, confusion, convulsions, diplopia, disturbed coordination, dizziness, euphoria, excitation, fatigue, headache, hysteria, insomnia, irritability, nervousness, neuritis, paresthesia, restlessness, *sedation*, tinnitus, tremor, vertigo. **HEENT:** Labyrinthitis, tinnitus **Skin:** Drug rash, photosensitivity, urticaria. **GI:** Anorexia, constipation, diarrhea, epigastric distress, heartburn, nausea, vomiting. **GU:** Difficult urination, increased urinary frequency, urinary retention, early menses. **Hematological:** Agranulocytosis, hemolytic anemia, thrombocytopenia. **Other:** Anaphylactic shock, chills, excessive perspiration, polyuria, photosensitivity, weakness.

INTERACTIONS Drug: MAO INHIBITORS may prolong and intensify the anticholinergic effects of carbinoxamine. Carbinoxamine may enhance the effects of TRICYCLIC ANTIDEPRESSANTS, BARBITURATES, **alcohol**, and other CNS DEPRESSANTS.

PHARMACOKINETICS Onset: 15–30 m. **Peak:** 1 h. **Metabolism:** Extensive hepatic metabolism to inactive compounds. **Elimination:** Primarily renal. **Half-Life:** 10–20 h.

NURSING IMPLICATIONS

Assessment & Drug Effects

- Monitor CV status especially with preexisting cardiovascular disease.
- Monitor for adverse effects especially in young children and older adults.
- Supervise ambulation and institute fall precautions as necessary.

Patient & Family Education

- Do not use alcohol and other CNS depressants because of the possible additive CNS depressant effects.
- Do not drive or engage in other potentially hazardous activities until the response to drug is known.
- Increase fluid intake, if not contraindicated; drug has a drying effect (thickens bronchial secretions) that may make expectoration difficult.

CARBOPLATIN

(car-bo-pla'tin)

Paraplatin

Classification: ANTINEOPLASTIC; ALKYLATING AGENT

Therapeutic: ANTINEOPLASTIC

Prototype: Cyclophosphamide

AVAILABILITY Solution for injection

ACTION & THERAPEUTIC EFFECT

It produces interstrand DNA cross-linkages, thus interfering with DNA, RNA, and protein synthesis.

Common adverse effects in *italic*; life-threatening effects underlined; generic names in **bold**; classifications in SMALL CAPS; ♣ Canadian drug name; ◎ Prototype drug; ⚠ Alert

Carboplatin is cell-cycle nonspecific and induces programmed cell death. *Full or partial activity against a variety of cancers resulting in reduction or stabilization of tumor size. Useful in patients with impaired renal function, patients unable to accommodate high-volume hydration, or patients at high risk for neurotoxicity and/or ototoxicity.*

USES Advanced ovarian cancer.

UNLABELED USES Combination therapy for breast, cervical, colon, endometrial, head and neck, and lung cancer; leukemia, lymphoma, and melanoma.

CONTRAINDICATIONS History of severe reactions to carboplatin or other platinum compounds, severe bone marrow depression; significant bleeding; impaired renal function; pregnancy—known teratogen; lactation—infant risk cannot be ruled out.

CAUTIOUS USE Use with other nephrotoxic drugs; coagulopathy; previous radiation therapy; renal and/or hepatic impairment; elderly.

ROUTE & DOSAGE

Ovarian Cancer

Adult: **IV** 360 mg/m^2 q4wk or 300 mg/m^2 q4wk for 6 cycles. Dose will vary if used in combination with other agents.

Renal Impairment Dosage Adjustment

CrCl 41–59 mL/min: Initiate at 250 mg/m^2; *16–40 mL/min:* Initiate at 200 mg/m^2

Obesity Dosage Adjustment

Use actual body weight

ADMINISTRATION

Intravenous

PREPARE: **IV Infusion:** Do not use needles or IV sets containing aluminum. ▪ Immediately before use, reconstitute with either sterile water for injection or D5W or NS as follows: 50-mg vial plus 5 mL diluent; 150-mg vial plus 15 mL diluent; 450-mg vial plus 45 mL diluent. All dilutions yield 10 mg/mL. ▪ May be further diluted for infusion with D5W or NS to concentrations as low as 0.5 mg/mL.

ADMINISTER: **IV Infusion:** Give IV solution over 15 min or longer, depending on total amount of solution and patient tolerance.

▪ NIOSH recommends use of double gloves, protective gown, eye and respiratory protection if not prepared in a control device.

▪ NIOSH recommends administering through a prepared solution via IV tubing that is already attached and primed. Wear double gloves and protective gown. If there is any chance that the patient may resist, liquid may splash, or administered by a feeding tube, use eye protection.

▪ Wash with soap and water thoroughly if solution comes into contact with skin; flush thoroughly with water if solution comes into contact with mucous membranes.

▪ Lengthening duration of administration may decrease nausea and vomiting.

▪ Premedication with a parenteral antiemetic 30 min before and on a scheduled basis thereafter is normally used. ▪ Do not repeat doses until the neutrophil count is at least 2000/mm^3 and platelet count at least 100,000/mm^3.

C

- Store unopened vials at controlled room temperature, 25°C (77°F), with fluctuations permitted between 15° and 30°C (59° and 86°F). Protect from light. Store reconstituted solutions at room temperature 25°C (77°F). Discard 8 h after dilution. ***INCOMPATIBILITIES:*** **Solution/additive:** **Fluorouracil, mesna, sodium bicarbonate.** **Y-site:** **Amphotericin B conventional, amphotericin B cholesteryl complex, chlorpromazine, diazepam, lansoprazole, leucovorin, phenytoin, procainamide, thiopental.**

- Protect from light. Reconstituted solutions are stable for 8 h at room temperature; discard solutions 8 h after dilution.

ADVERSE EFFECTS (≥ 5%) **Endocrine:** *Mild hyponatremia, hypomagnesemia, hypocalcemia, and hypokalemia.* **Skin:** Alopecia. **Hepatic:** Increased alkaline phosphatase, elevated AST/SGOT. **GI:** *Mild to moderate nausea and vomiting,* diarrhea. **GU:** Nephrotoxicity. **Hematologic:** *Thrombocytopenia, leukopenia, neutropenia, anemia.* **Other:** Pain.

INTERACTIONS **Drug:** Use with IMMUNOSPRESSANTS or MYELOSUPRESSIVE AGENTS increases adverse effects. Do not administer with LIVE VACCINES.

PHARMACOKINETICS **Distribution:** Highest concentration in the liver, lung, kidney, skin, and tumors. Not bound to plasma proteins. **Metabolism:** Hydrolyzed in the serum. **Elimination:** Primarily by the kidneys; 60–80% excreted in urine within 24 h. **Half-Life:** 3–6 h.

NURSING IMPLICATIONS

Black Box Warning

Carboplatin has been associated with bone marrow suppression that can be severe, resulting in infection and/or bleeding. Anaphylactic-type reactions have occurred within minutes of administration.

Assessment & Drug Effects

- Monitor closely during first 15 min of infusion because severe allergic reactions have occurred within minutes of carboplatin administration.
- Monitor results of peripheral blood counts. Leukopenia, neutropenia, and thrombocytopenia are dose related and may produce dose-limiting toxicity.
- Monitor for peripheral neuropathy (e.g., paresthesias), ototoxicity, and visual disturbances.
- Monitor serum electrolyte studies because carboplatin has been associated with decreases in sodium, potassium, calcium, and magnesium. Special precautions may be warranted for patients on diuretic therapy.
- Monitor lab tests: Baseline and periodic CBC with differential, platelet count, Hgb and Hct; baseline kidney function tests and prior to each infusion; periodic serum electrolytes.

Patient & Family Education

- Learn about the range of potential adverse effects. Strategies for nausea prevention should receive special attention.
- Avoid vaccines during therapy.
- During therapy you are at risk for infection and hemorrhagic complications related to bone marrow suppression. Avoid unnecessary exposure to crowds

C

or infected persons during the nadir period.

- Report paresthesias (numbness, tingling), visual disturbances, or symptoms of ototoxicity (hearing loss and/or tinnitus), poor urine output, swelling in lower extremities, nausea, confusion and weakness.
- Notify provider of a missed dose.

CARBOPROST TROMETHAMINE (PT)

(kar′boe-prost)

Hemabate

Classification: PROSTAGLANDIN; OXYTOCIC

Therapeutic: OXYTOCIC

AVAILABILITY Solution for injection

ACTION & *THERAPEUTIC EFFECT* Synthetic analog of naturally occurring prostaglandin F_2 alpha with longer duration of biological activity. Stimulates myometrial contractions of gravid uterus at term labor. Mean time to abortion 16 h; mean dose required 2.6 mL. *Effectively stimulates uterine contraction and is used to induce abortion. Useful in treatment of postpartum hemorrhage due to uterine atony unresponsive to usual measures.*

USES Pregnancy termination. Also for refractory postpartum bleeding.

UNLABELED USES To reduce blood loss secondary to uterine atony; to induce labor in intrauterine fetal death and hydatidiform mole.

CONTRAINDICATIONS Acute pelvic inflammatory disease; active cardiac, pulmonary, renal, or hepatic disease; pregnancy (category D); lactation.

CAUTIOUS USE History of asthma; adrenal disease; anemia; hypotension; hypertension; diabetes mellitus; epilepsy; history of uterine surgery; cervical stenosis; fibroids.

ROUTE & DOSAGE

Abortion, Postpartum Bleeding

Adult: **IM** Initial: 250 mcg (1 mL) repeated at 1.5–3.5-h intervals if indicated by uterine response. Dosage may be increased to 500 mcg (2 mL) if uterine contractility is inadequate after several doses of 250 mcg (1 mL), not to exceed total dose of 12 mg or continuous administration for more than 2 days.

ADMINISTRATION

Intramuscular

- Give deep IM into a large muscle. Aspirate carefully before injecting drug to avoid inadvertent entry into blood vessel, which can result in bronchospasm, tetanic contractions, and shock. Do not use same site for subsequent doses.
- Store drug in refrigerator at 2°–4°C (36°–39°F) unless otherwise specified.

ADVERSE EFFECTS **GI:** *Nausea,* diarrhea, vomiting. **Other:** Fever, flushing, chills, cough, headache, pain (muscles, joints, lower abdomen, eyes), hiccups, breast tenderness.

PHARMACOKINETICS **Peak:** 30–90 min. **Elimination:** Renal within 24 h.

NURSING IMPLICATIONS

Assessment & Drug Effects

- Monitor uterine contractions and observe and report excessive

C

vaginal bleeding and cramping pain. Save all clots and tissue for prescriber inspection and laboratory analysis.

- Check vital signs at regular intervals. Carboprost-induced febrile reaction occurs in more than 10% of patients and **must be** differentiated from endometritis, which occurs around third day after abortion.

Patient & Family Education

- Report promptly onset of bleeding, foul-smelling discharge, abdominal pain, or fever.
- Because ovulation may reoccur as early as 2 wk postabortion, consider appropriate contraception.

CARFILZOMIB

(car-fil-zo′mib)

Kyprolis

Classification: ANTINEOPLASTIC; PROTEOSOME INHIBITOR

Therapeutic: ANTINEOPLASTIC

Prototype: Bortezomib

AVAILABILITY Sterile lyophilized powder

ACTION & *THERAPEUTIC EFFECT* Plays a regulatory role in cell proliferation by destroying proteins that trigger cell-cycle progression and cell survival pathways in certain cancers; produces antiproliferative and proapoptotic effects leading to cell death in solid and hematologic tumor cells. *Delays tumor growth in multiple myeloma and other hematologic tumors and solid tumors.*

USES Relapsed or refractory multiple myeloma.

CONTRAINDICATIONS Pregnancy—fetal risk cannot be ruled out; lactation—infant risk cannot be ruled out.

CAUTIOUS USE Cardiac and pulmonary disease; CHF; MI within 6 mo; thrombocytopenia; hepatic disease; renal failure. Avoid oral contraceptives or other hormonal contraceptives with increased risk of thrombosis. Safety and efficacy in children younger than 18 yr not established.

ROUTE & DOSAGE

Multiple Myeloma

Adult: **IV** 20 mg/m^2 on days 1, 2, 8, 9, 15, 16 of 28-day cycle. Increase to 27 mg/m^2 on subsequent 28-day cycles if tolerated.

Hepatic Impairment Dosage Adjustment (develops during treatment)

Grade 3 or 4 liver toxicity: Hold therapy until resolved or return to baseline; may restart at a reduced level (from 27 to 20 mg/m^2 or from 20 to 15 mg/m^2); doses may be re-escalated if tolerated.

Renal Impairment Dosage Adjustment (develops during treatment)

Serum creatinine greater than or equal to 2 × baseline: Hold therapy until return to grade 1 or baseline; may restart at a reduced level (from 27 to 20 mg/m^2 or from 20 to 15 mg/m^2); doses may be reescalated if tolerated.

Obesity Dosage Adjustment Use actual body weight ***Dose Modifications Due to Other Toxicities***

Grade 3 or 4 toxicities: Hold therapy until resolution or a return to baseline; consider reducing the dose one level (27 to 20 mg/m^2

or 20 to 15 mg/m^2); doses may be reescalated if tolerated. Refer to package insert for specifics.

ADMINISTRATION

Intravenous

- Hazardous agent. Single glove during receiving and unpacking. For administration: double gloving, protective gown. Premedication: Give 4 mg dexamethasone prior to all doses during cycle 1, during the first cycle of dose escalation to 27 mg/m^2, and if infusion reaction symptoms appear during subsequent cycles. ▪ Hydration: Prior to each dose in cycle 1, give 250–500 mL of IV, NS, or other IV fluid. Give an additional 250–500 mL of IV fluids as needed. Continue IV hydration, as needed, in all subsequent cycles.

PREPARE: **IV Infusion:** Hazardous agent: Double glove and follow appropriate precautions for handling and disposal. Remove vial from refrigeration just prior to use. Reconstitute 60 mg vial with 29 mL sterile water for injection to yield 2 mg/mL. Direct stream against side of vial to prevent foaming. Swirl gently for 1 min or until completely dissolved. Do not shake. If foam appears, allow to stand until foam dissipates. Withdraw required dose and dilute in 50 mL or 100 mL D5W.

ADMINISTER: **IV Infusion:** Infuse over 10–30 min. **Do not** give as bolus dose. Flush IV line before/after with D5W.

INCOMPATIBILITIES: **Solution/additive:** Do not mix with other solutions or medications. **Y-site:** Do not mix with other solutions or medications.

- May store reconstituted drug up to 24 h refrigerated and up to 4 h at room temperature. Protect from light.

ADVERSE EFFECTS **CV:** Chest wall pain, cardiac arrest, congestive heart failure, anemia myocardial infarction, *peripheral edema*, cardiomyopathy, venous thrombosis, hypertension. **Respiratory:** Cough, *dyspnea*, pneumonia, upper respiratory tract infection. **CNS:** Dizziness, *fatigue*, headache, hypoesthesia, intercranial hemorrhage, insomnia. **Endocrine:** AST increased, hypercalcemia, hyperglycemia, hypokalemia, hypomagnesemia, hyponatremia, hypophosphatemia. **GI:** Anorexia, constipation, *diarrhea*, abdominal pain, *nausea*, vomiting, gastrointestinal hemorrhage. **GU:** Acute renal failure. **Musculoskeletal:** Arthralgia, *back pain*, muscle spasms, pain in extremity. **Hematological:** *Anemia*, leukopenia, lymphopenia, neutropenia, *thrombocytopenia*. **Other:** Asthenia, *fatigue*, *fever*, chills, pain, peripheral edema, pyrexia, tumor lysis syndrome.

INTERACTIONS Consider increasing ANC monitoring if used with **clozapine**. Do not administer with vaccines or MYLEOSUPPRESIVE AGENTS, may increase adverse effects. HORMONAL CONTRACEPTIVES or **leflunomide** may increase risk of thrombosis. **Herbal:** Do not use with Echinacea.

PHARMACOKINETICS **Distribution:** 97% plasma protein bound. **Metabolism:** Extensive hydrolytic metabolism. **Half-Life:** 1 h.

NURSING IMPLICATIONS

Assessment & Drug Effects

- Check for pregnancy status.
- Maintain adequate fluid volume status throughout treatment; closely monitor for fluid overload.

C

- Monitor cardiac and respiratory status closely during drug administration period.
- Monitor for evidence of tumor lysis syndrome (TLS). Signs of TLS include nausea and vomiting, dyspnea, irregular HR, cloudy urine, lethargy, and/or joint discomfort.
- Immediately stop infusion if dyspnea occurs. Do not resume infusion until symptoms return to baseline. Consult prescriber.
- Monitor for peripheral neuropathy.
- Monitor lab tests: Baseline and frequent CBC with differential and platelet count, serum electrolytes, LFTs, and renal function tests.

Patient & Family Education

- Report promptly any of the following: Chest pain, shortness of breath, chills, cough, fever, or swelling of the feet or legs.
- Maintain adequate hydration, especially when experiencing diarrhea or vomiting. Seek guidance from prescriber if experiencing dizziness, lightheadedness, or fainting.
- Do not drive or engage in other potentially dangerous activities until reaction to drug is known.
- Women should use effective means of birth control during therapy and 6 months after final dose.
- Contact your prescriber immediately if you become pregnant during treatment.
- Do not breastfeed while receiving this drug.

CARIPRAZINE

(car-i-pra′zine)

Vraylar

Classification: ATYPICAL ANTIPSYCHOTIC; MOOD STABILIZER

Therapeutic: ANTIPSYCHOTIC; ANTIMANIC; ANTIDEPRESSANT

Prototype: Clozapine

AVAILABILITY Capsules

ACTION & *THERAPEUTIC EFFECT* The mechanism of action is unknown, but may be mediated by partial agonist activity at central dopamine D_2 and serotonin 5-HT_{1A} receptors and antagonist activity at serotonin 5-HT_{2A} receptors. *Stabilizes mood and improves ability to perform activities of daily living.*

USES Treatment of schizophrenia and acute treatment of manic or mixed episodes associated with bipolar I disease.

UNLABELED USES: Agitation associated with dementia

CONTRAINDICATIONS Known hypersensitivity to cariprazine and any component in the formulation; neuroleptic malignant syndrome (NMS); pregnancy—fetal risk cannot be ruled out; lactation—infant risk cannot be ruled out.

CAUTIOUS USE Commitment use of a strong CYP3A4 inhibitor or inducer; tardive dyskinesia; hyperglycemia and DM; dyslipidemia; weight gain; esophageal motility disorder; orthostatic hypotension, history of seizures, elderly.

ROUTE & DOSAGE

Schizophrenia or Bipolar I Disease

Adult: **PO** Initial dose of 1.5 mg once daily; can increase to 3 mg once daily on day 2, then titrate up to 3–6 mg (max 6 mg)

Hepatic Impairment Dosage Adjustment

Severe Impairment: Not recommended

Renal Impairment Dosage Adjustment

Severe Impairment (CrCL < 30 mL/min): Not recommended

Concomitant CYP3A4 Inhibitors and Inducers Dosage Adjustments

Strong CYP3A4 inhibitor: Reduce usual dose by half
Strong CYP3A4 inducer: Not recommended

ADMINISTRATION

Oral

- May be given without regard to food.
- Store at 20°–25°C (68°–77°F) with excursions permitted between 15° and 30°C (59° and 86°F). Protect from light.

ADVERSE EFFECTS (≥ 5%) GI: Indigestion, *vomiting*. **Other:** Restlessness.

INTERACTIONS Drug: Concomitant use with strong CYP3A4 inhibitors (e.g., **itraconazole, ketoconazole**) increases the levels of cariprazine; concomitant use with strong CYP3A4 inducers (e.g., **rifampin, carbamazepine**) decreases the levels of cariprazine. Use with CNS DEPRESSANTS increases risk of adverse effects. Do not use with ANTIPARKINSON AGENTS, **azelastine, amisulpride, cabergoline, metoclopramide, thalidomide. Herbal: St. John's wort** decreases the levels of cariprazine.

PHARMACOKINETICS Peak: 3–6 h. **Distribution:** 91–97% plasma protein bound. **Metabolism:** Hepatic metabolism to both active and inactive metabolites. **Elimination:** Renal. **Half-Life:** 2–4 days.

NURSING IMPLICATIONS

Black Box Warning

Cariprazine has been associated with increased mortality in elderly patients with dementia-related psychosis.

Assessment & Drug Effects

- Monitor for orthostatic hypotension, especially early in treatment.
- Monitor for clinical worsening and emergence of suicidal thoughts and behaviors, especially in the initial few months.
- Monitor closely those at risk for aspiration as esophageal dysmotility and dysphagia may occur.
- Monitor for a report promptly S&S of tardive dyskinesia and neuroleptic malignant syndrome (see Appendix F).
- Monitor weight and report excessive increases in weight gain, BMI, and waist circumference.
- Monitor diabetics for loss of glycemic control.
- Monitor lab tests: Baseline and periodic CBC with differential, blood glucose, and lipid profile.

C

Patient & Family Education

- Use caution with activities requiring mental alertness until response to drug is known.
- Tell patients and caregivers to report any suicidal thoughts and behaviors.
- Use caution when arising from a supine or sitting position, as dizziness or fainting may occur.
- Report promptly any of the following: Restlessness; uncontrolled movement of the face, tongue, or other body parts; weight gain; excessive urination or thirst; lightheadedness upon arising.
- Avoid overheating, and maintain adequate hydration with liquids.
- Monitor blood glucose closely if diabetic.
- Notify prescriber of any other prescription or nonprescription drugs taken as significant drug interactions may occur and dosage adjustments may be warranted.
- Women should use effective means of birth control while taking this drug. Report promptly to prescriber if a pregnancy is suspected.

CARISOPRODOL

(kar-eye-soe-proe′dole)

Soma

Classification: CENTRALLY ACTING SKELETAL MUSCLE RELAXANT

Therapeutic: SKELETAL MUSCLE RELAXANT

Prototype: Cyclobenzaprine

Controlled Substance: Schedule IV

AVAILABILITY Tablet

ACTION & *THERAPEUTIC EFFECT* Centrally acting skeletal muscle relaxant that appears to cause slight reduction in muscle tone leading to relief of pain and discomfort of muscle spasm. *Effective spasmolytic while reducing pain associated with acute musculoskeletal disorders.*

USES Acute treatment of musculoskeletal pain.

CONTRAINDICATIONS Hypersensitivity to carisoprodol and related compounds (e.g., meprobamate, carbamate); acute intermittent porphyria. **Beers Criteria:** Avoid use in the elderly.

CAUTIOUS USE Impaired liver or kidney function, addiction-prone individuals; seizure disorder; pregnancy—fetal risk cannot be ruled out; lactation—infant risk cannot be ruled out; children younger than 16 yr.

ROUTE & DOSAGE

Muscle Spasm

Adult/Adolescent: **PO** 250–350 mg tid for max of 2–3 weeks

ADMINISTRATION

Oral

- Give with food, as needed, to reduce GI symptoms. Last dose should be taken at bedtime.
- Store tablet at controlled room temperature between 20 and 25°C (68 and 77°F) in tightly closed container.

ADVERSE EFFECTS (> 5%) **CNS:** *Drowsiness, dizziness,* vertigo, ataxia, headache, syncope, seizures. **Other:** Drug abuse, drug dependence.

INTERACTIONS **Drug: Alcohol,** CNS DEPRESSANTS potentiate CNS effects. Do not use with **meprobamate**. May decrease serum concentrations of CYP2C19 substrates.

PHARMACOKINETICS **Onset:** 30 min. **Duration:** 4–6 h. **Distribution:** Crosses placenta. **Metabolism:** In liver by CYP2C19. **Elimination:**

By kidneys; excreted in breast milk (2–4 × the plasma concentrations). **Half-Life:** 8 h.

NURSING IMPLICATIONS

Assessment & Drug Effects

- Monitor for allergic or idiosyncratic reactions that generally occur from the first to the fourth dose in patients taking the drug for the first time. Symptoms usually subside after several hours; they are treated by supportive and symptomatic measures.
- Abuse potential is high. Monitor use.

Patient & Family Education

- Avoid driving and other potentially hazardous activities until response to the drug has been evaluated. Drowsiness is a common side effect and may require reduction in dosage.
- Report to prescriber if symptoms of dizziness and faintness persist. Symptoms may be controlled by making position changes slowly and in stages.
- Do not take alcohol or other CNS depressants (effects may be additive) unless otherwise directed by prescriber.
- Discontinue drug and notify prescriber if skin rash, diplopia, dizziness, or other unusual signs or symptoms appear.
- Take a missed dose if it is less than 1 hour of the regular dosing time. If more than 1 hour late, skip the missed dose.

CARMUSTINE

(kar-mus′teen)

BiCNU, Gliadel

Classification: ANTINEOPLASTIC; ALKYLATING

Therapeutic: ANTINEOPLASTIC

Prototype: Cyclophosphamide

AVAILABILITY Solution for injection; wafer

ACTION & THERAPEUTIC EFFECT Highly lipid-soluble compound with cell cycle nonspecific activity against rapidly proliferating cells. Produces cross-linkage of DNA strands, thereby blocking DNA, RNA, and protein synthesis in tumor cells. *Drug metabolites are thought to be responsible for antineoplastic activities. Full or partial activity against a variety of cancers results in reduction or stabilization of tumor size and increased survival rates.*

USES Relapsed/refractory Hodgkin lymphoma, multiple myeloma, tumors of brain, and non-Hodgkin lymphoma.

UNLABELED USES Stem cell conditioning regimen.

CONTRAINDICATIONS History of pulmonary function impairment; recent illness with or exposure to chickenpox or herpes zoster; infection; severe bone marrow depression, decreased circulating platelets, leukocytes, or erythrocytes; pregnancy—fetal risk cannot be ruled out; lactation—infant risk cannot be ruled out.

CAUTIOUS USE Hepatic and renal insufficiency; Patient with bone marrow suppression, patients with nausea and vomiting, patient with previous cytotoxic medication, or radiation therapy; history of herpes infections.

ROUTE & DOSAGE

Brain Tumors, Hodgkin Lymphoma, Multiple Myeloma

Adult: **IV** 150–200 mg/m^2 q6wk or 75–100 mg/m^2 over 2 days q6wk; adjust for hematologic toxicity

C

Glioblastoma Multiforme (Recurrent)
Adult: **Implantation (wafer)** 8 wafers (7.7 mg each) implanted intracranially into in the resection cavity

ADMINISTRATION

Topical

- Follow application directions provided by prescriber.
- NIOSH Use double gloves and protective gown. Eye/face and respiratory protection may be needed. If there is a chance that the substance could splash or the patient may resist, use eye/face protection. If the drug comes into direct contact with skin or mucous membranes, immediately wash the area thoroughly with soap and water.

Intravenous

PREPARE: **IV Infusion:** Wear disposable gloves and protective gown. Hazardous agent. Contact of drug with skin can cause burning, dermatitis, and hyperpigmentation. ▪ Add supplied diluent to the 100-mg vial. Further dilute with 27 mL of sterile water for injection to yield a concentration of 3.3 mg/mL. ▪ Each dose is then added to 100–500 mL of D5W or NS. ▪ Avoid using PVC IV tubing and bags. ▪ Protect from light. Reconstituted solution is stable for 24 h refrigerated to 2°–8°C (36°–46°F) in a glass container. Must use within 8 h at room temperature if protected from light.
ADMINISTER: **IV Infusion:** Infuse a single dose over at least 2 h. Adequate dilution will reduce pain of administration. ▪ Avoid starting infusion into dorsum of hand, wrist, or the antecubital veins; extravasation in these areas can damage underlying tendons and nerves leading to loss of mobility of entire limb. Frequently check rate of flow and blood return during infusion; monitor injection site for extravasation. ▪ If there is any question about patency, line should be restarted.
INCOMPATIBILITIES: **Solution/additive:** **Dextrose 5%, sodium bicarbonate.** **Y-site:** **Allopurinol, dantrolene, diazepam, dobutamine, epinephrine, metoclopramide, phenobarbital, phentolamine, phenytoin, procainamide, promethazine, thiopental.**

▪ Reconstituted solutions of carmustine are clear and colorless and may be stored at 2°–8°C (36°–46°F) for 8 h protected from light. ▪ Store unopened vials at 2°–8°C (36°–46°F), protected from light, unless otherwise directed by manufacturer. ▪ Signs of decomposition of carmustine in unopened vial: Liquefaction and appearance of oil film at bottom of vial. Discard drug in this condition.

ADVERSE EFFECTS

Respiratory: <u>Pulmonary infiltration or fibrosis</u>. **CNS:** Dizziness, confusion, ataxia, headache, *seizures*. **HEENT:** (With high doses) <u>Eye infarctions</u>, retinal hemorrhage, suffusion of conjunctiva. **Skin:** Skin flushing and burning pain at injection site, hyperpigmentation of skin (from contact), alopecia. **GI:** Stomatitis, constipation, *nausea, vomiting, diarrhea*. **GU:** Renal failure, gynecomastia. **Hematologic:** Delayed myelosuppression (dose-related); thrombocytopenia.

INTERACTIONS Drug: Cimetidine may potentiate neutropenia and thrombocytopenia. Do not use with LIVE VACCINES. Use with IMMUNOSUPPRESSANTS or MYELOSUPRESSANTS increases risk of adverse effects.

PHARMACOKINETICS Distribution: Readily crosses blood–brain barrier; CSF concentrations 15–70% of plasma concentrations. **Metabolism:** Rapidly metabolized. **Elimination:** 60–70% in urine in 96 h; 10% via lungs; excreted in breast milk.

NURSING IMPLICATIONS

Black Box Warning

Carmustine has been associated with severe, delayed bone marrow depression leading to hemorrhage and/or severe infection. Pulmonary toxicity may occur even years after termination of treatment.

Assessment & Drug Effects

- Monitor for nausea and vomiting (dose related), which may occur within 2 h after drug administration and persist for up to 6 h.
- Monitor vital signs throughout infusion.
- Monitor IV site closely.
- Monitor blood pressure closely during high-dose BMT infusion; supine positions (Trendelenburg position may be necessary), fluid support and vasopressor support should be available.
- Monitor any delayed wound healing.
- Report symptoms of lung toxicity (cough, shortness of breath, fever) to the prescriber immediately.
- Be alert to signs of hepatic toxicity (jaundice, dark urine, pruritus, light-colored stools) and renal insufficiency (dysuria, oliguria, hematuria, swelling of lower legs and feet).
- Monitor lab tests: Baseline CBC with differential and platelet count, repeat following infusion at weekly intervals for at least 6 wk; baseline and periodic LFTs, renal function tests, and pulmonary function tests.

Patient & Family Education

- Report burning sensation immediately, as carmustine can cause burning discomfort even in the absence of extravasation. Infusion will be discontinued and restarted in another site. Ice application over the area may decrease the discomfort.
- Intense flushing of skin may occur during IV infusion. This usually disappears in 2–4 h.
- You will be highly susceptible to infection and to hemorrhagic disorders. Be alert to hazardous periods that occur 4–6 wk after a dose of carmustine. If possible, avoid invasive procedures (e.g., IM injections, enemas, rectal temperatures) during this period.
- Report promptly the onset of sore throat, weakness, fever, chills, infection of any kind, or abnormal bleeding (ecchymosis, petechiae, epistaxis, bleeding gums, hematemesis, melena).
- Female patients should avoid pregnancy during therapy and for at least 6 mo after completion of therapy or after implantation. Male patients avoid pregnancy in sexual partner during therapy and at least for 3 months after completion of therapy or implantation.

C

CARTEOLOL HYDROCHLORIDE

(car'tee-oh-lole)

Ocupress

Classification: BETA-ADRENERGIC ANTAGONIST; ANTIHYPERTENSIVE

Therapeutic: ANTIHYPERTENSIVE; BETA-ADRENERGIC BLOCKER

Prototype: Propranolol

AVAILABILITY Solution

ACTION & *THERAPEUTIC EFFECT* Carteolol is a beta-adrenergic blocking agent (antagonist) that competes for available beta receptor sites. It inhibits both $beta_1$ receptors (chiefly in cardiac muscle) and $beta_2$ receptors (chiefly in the bronchial and vascular musculature). *It interferes with production and outflow of aqueous humor.*

USES Chronic open-angle glaucoma.

CONTRAINDICATIONS Sinus bradycardia, severe CHF; greater than first-degree heart block, cardiogenic shock, CHF secondary to tachycardia treatable with beta-blockers, overt cardiac failure, hypersensitivity to beta-blocking agents, persistent severe bradycardia, bronchial asthma or bronchospasm, and severe COPD; pulmonary edema.

CAUTIOUS USE CHF patients treated with digitalis and diuretics, peripheral vascular disease; diabetes, hypoglycemia, thyrotoxicosis; renal disease; CVA; pregnancy (category C); lactation.

ROUTE & DOSAGE

Open-Angle Glaucoma

Adult: **Ophthalmic** 1 drop in affected eye bid

ADMINISTRATION

Conjunctival

- For topical use only. Wash hands before use. To avoid contamination, do not touch dropper tip to eyelids or other surfaces.
- Remove contact lenses prior to administration; wait 15 min before reinserting if using products containing benzalkonium chloride.

ADVERSE EFFECTS **HEENT:** Conjunctival hyperemia, lacrimation, and ocular irritation.

INTERACTIONS **Drug:** DIURETICS and other HYPOTENSIVE AGENTS increase hypotensive effect.

PHARMACOKINETICS **Absorption:** 25% reaches systemic circulation. **Metabolism:** In liver to active metabolite. **Elimination:** Primarily in urine.

NURSING IMPLICATIONS

Assessment & Drug Effects

- Assess conjunctiva and corneal surfaces for any edema or discoloration.
- Contact prescriber with patient complaints of eye pain or any disturbances in vision (blurry, cloudy, double vision, or decreased night vision).

Patient & Family Education

- Make sure that dropper does not touch the eye during administration.
- Report to prescriber any drooping of the eyelid, drainage from the eye, changes in vision (blurry, cloudy, double vision, unable to tolerate light, or decreased night vision).
- Do not discontinue medication abruptly because sudden withdrawal may precipitate or exacerbate angina.
- Report slow pulse rate, confusion or depression, dizziness or

light-headedness, skin rash, fever, sore throat, or unusual bleeding or bruising.

- Be cautious while driving or performing other hazardous activities until response to drug is known.
- Take your pulse before and after taking the medication. If it is much slower than normal rate (or less than 50 bpm), check with your prescriber.

CARVEDILOL

(car-ve-di'lol)

Coreg, Coreg CR ♣

Classification: ALPHA- AND BETA-ADRENERGIC ANTAGONIST; ANTIHYPERTENSIVE

Therapeutic: ANTIHYPERTENSIVE; ADRENERGIC BLOCKER

Prototype: Propranolol HCl

AVAILABILITY Tablet; extended release capsule

ACTION & THERAPEUTIC EFFECT Adrenergic receptor blocking agent that contributes to blood pressure reduction. Peripheral vasodilatation and, therefore, decreased peripheral resistance results from alpha$_1$-blocking activity. *An effective antihypertensive agent reducing BP to normotensive range and useful in managing some angina, dysrhythmias, and CHF by decreasing myocardial oxygen demand and lowering cardiac workload.*

USES Management of hypertension, heart failure with reduced ejection fraction.

UNLABELED USES Angina, atrial fibrillation, MI.

CONTRAINDICATIONS Patients with class IV decompensated cardiac failure, abrupt cessation in CAD patients; hypersensitivity to any component of the formulation, possibility of cross-reactivity with other alpha/beta-adrenergic blocking agents; bronchial asthma, or related bronchospastic conditions (e.g., chronic bronchitis and emphysema), pulmonary edema; second- and third-degree AV block, sick sinus syndrome, cardiogenic shock or severe bradycardia, severe hepatic impairment, sick sinus syndrome, pregnancy—fetal risk cannot be ruled out; lactation—infant risk cannot be ruled out.

CAUTIOUS USE Patients on MAOI agents, DM; hypoglycemia; patients at high risk for anaphylactic reaction, PVD; cerebrovascular insufficiencies, major depression, hepatic or renal impairment; pheochromocytoma, thyrotoxicosis, cataract surgery, older adults; children younger than 18 yr.

ROUTE & DOSAGE

Heart Failure

Adult (weight less than 85 kg): **PO Immediate release** Start with 3.125 mg bid × 2 wk, may double dose q2wk as tolerated up to 25 mg bid; *weight greater than 85 kg: max dose* 50 mg bid; **Extended release** 10 mg qd × 2 wk may increase up to 80 mg

Hypertension

Adult: **PO Immediate release** Start with 6.25 mg bid, may increase by 6.25 mg bid (max: 25 mg bid); **Extended release** 20 mg daily, may increase to 40 mg daily (max 80 mg/day)

C

ADMINISTRATION

Oral

- Take baseline blood pressure and pulse rate prior to and following first dose.
- Give with food to slow absorption and minimize risk of orthostatic hypotension.
- Extended release capsules should not be crushed, chewed or divided. Capsules may be opened and sprinkled on applesauce for immediate use.
- Dose increments should be made at 7- to 14-day intervals.
- Store tablets at less than 30°C (less than 86°F). Protect from light and moisture.

ADVERSE EFFECTS (≥ 5%) **CV:** Bradycardia, *hypotension*, peripheral edema. **CNS:** *Dizziness.* **Endocrine:** Hyperglycemia, weight increase. **GI:** Diarrhea. **Other:** *Fatigue.*

DIAGNOSTIC TEST INTERFERENCE May lead to false-positive aldosterone/renin ratio.

INTERACTIONS **Drug: Carvedilol** inhibits P-glycoprotein so may increase concentration of drugs metabolized by that pathway **(ex afatinib, bilastine, doxorubicin,** etc.**)**. Do not use with BETA AGONISTS, ERGOT DERIVATIVES, **rivastigmine**. **Rifampin** significantly decreases **carvedilol** levels; **amiodarone, clonidine,** MAO INHIBITORS may cause hypotension or bradycardia; **carvedilol** may increase **cyclosporine, digoxin** levels and may enhance hypoglycemic effects of **insulin** and oral HYPOGLYCEMIC AGENTS, may enhance hypotensive or heart rate effects of ANTIHYPERTENSIVES. **Herbal:** Grass pollen extracts have increased adverse effects.

PHARMACOKINETICS **Absorption:** Rapidly from GI tract, 25–35% reaches the systemic circulation. **Peak:** Antihypertensive effect 2–5 h. **Distribution:** Greater than 98% protein bound. **Metabolism:** In the liver by CYP2D6, CYP2C9, CYP3A4, CYP 2C19. **Elimination:** Primarily through feces. **Half-Life:** 7–10 h.

NURSING IMPLICATIONS

Assessment & Drug Effects

- Monitor for therapeutic effectiveness, which is indicated by lessening of S&S of CHF and improved BP control.
- Monitor pulse.
- Monitor for worsening of symptoms in patients with PVD.
- Withhold drug and notify prescriber at the first sign of hepatic toxicity (see Appendix F).
- Monitor digoxin levels with concurrent use; plasma digoxin concentration may increase.
- Monitor lab tests: Periodic LFTs and renal function tests.

Patient & Family Education

- Do not abruptly discontinue taking this drug and take with food.
- Make position changes slowly due to the risk of orthostatic hypotension.
- Do not engage in hazardous activities while experiencing dizziness.
- If you have diabetes, the drug may increase effects of hypoglycemic drugs and mask S&S of hypoglycemia.
- Notify provider if develop diarrhea, vomiting, joint or muscle pain, erectile dysfunction, decreased libido, or fatigue.

CASPOFUNGIN

(cas-po-fun′gin)

Cancidas

Classification: ECHINOCANDIN ANTIBIOTIC ANTIFUNGAL; ECHINOCANDIN

Therapeutic: ANTIFUNGAL

AVAILABILITY Powder for injection

ACTION & *THERAPEUTIC EFFECT* Caspofungin is an antifungal agent that inhibits the synthesis of an integral component of the fungal cell wall of susceptible species. *Interferes with reproduction and growth of susceptible fungi.*

USES Treatment of invasive aspergillosis in those refractory to or intolerant of other antifungal therapies; empirical therapy for presumed fungal infection with febrile neutropenia; treatment of candidemia and intra-abdominal abscesses, peritonitis, and pleural space infections due to *Candida*.

UNLABELED USES Treatment of esophageal candidiasis with or without oropharyngeal candidiasis (thrush).

CONTRAINDICATIONS Hypersensitivity (e.g., anaphylaxis) to any component of this product; mannitol; not studied in patients with ESRF. Lactation: Infant risk cannot be ruled out.

CAUTIOUS USE Patients with moderate hepatic insufficiency; cholestasis; older adults; pregnancy (category C); children younger than 18 yr. Not recommended for adults with severe hepatic impairment and children 3 mo to 18 yr with any degree of hepatic impairment.

ROUTE & DOSAGE

Invasive *Aspergillosis*, Empirical Therapy, *Candida*

Adult: **IV** 70 mg on day 1, then 50 mg daily thereafter

Hepatic Impairment Dosage Adjustment

Child–Pugh Class B: 70 mg initially then 35 mg daily

ADMINISTRATION

Intravenous

Allow vial to come to room temperature.

PREPARE: **IV Infusion:** Reconstitute a 50- or 70-mg vial with 10.8 mL of NS, sterile water for injection, or bacteriostatic water for injection to yield 5 mg/mL and 7 mg/mL, respectively. Mix gently until clear. ▪ Withdraw the required dose of reconstituted solution and add to 250 mL of NS, ½ NS, or ¼ NaCl, or LR. **Do not** use diluents or IV solutions containing dextrose.

ADMINISTER: **IV Infusion:** Give slowly over at least 1 h. Do not co-infuse with any other medication.

INCOMPATIBILITIES: **Solution/additive:** Any **dextrose**-containing solution. Do not mix or co-infuse with any other medications. **Y-site:** **Aminocaproic acid, amphotericin B, ampicillin, atenolol, bivalirudin, blinatumomab, cefazolin, cefepime, cefoperazone, cefotaxime, cefotetan, cefoxitin, ceftaroline, ceftazidime, ceftobiprole, ceftolozane-tazobactam, ceftriaxone, cefuroxime, chloramphenicol, clindamycin, dantrolene,**

C

dexamethasone, diazepam, digoxin, doxacurium, enalaprilat, ephedrine, ertapenem, fluorouracil, foscarnet, fosphenytoin, furosemide, gemtuzumab, heparin, ketorolac, lansoprazole, lidocaine, methotrexate, methylprednisolone, mivacurium, nafcillin, nitroprusside, pamidronate, pancuronium, pemetrexed, pentobarbital, phenobarbital, phenytoin, piperacillin/tazobactam, potassium phosphate, sodium acetate, sodium bicarbonate, sodium phosphate, sulfamethoxazole-trimethoprim, tedizolid phosphate, ticarcillin disodium-clavulanate potassium.

▪ Reconstituted solution should be stored at or below 25°C (77°F) for 1 h prior to preparing the IV solution for infusion. ▪ Store IV solution for up to 24 h at or below 25°C (77°F) or 48 h at 2°–8°C (36°–46°F).

ADVERSE EFFECTS **CV:** Hypotension, hypertension, peripheral edema, tachycardia. **Respiratory:** Pleural effusion, dyspnea, respiratory distress, respiratory failure, cough, pneumonia. **CNS:** Chills, headache. **Endocrine:** Hypomagnesemia, hyperglycemia, hypokalemia. **Skin:** Rash, erythema. **Hepatic:** ALT/SGPT elevation, AST/SGOT elevation, increased serum alkaline phosphatase, decreased albumin. **GI:** *Diarrhea*, vomiting, abdominal pain, nausea. **GU:** Increased serum creatinine, hematuria. **Hematologic:** Decreased hemoglobin, decreased hematocrit, decreased WBCs, anemia. **Other:** *Fever*, shivering, phlebitis, septic shock.

INTERACTIONS **Drug: Cyclosporine** increases overall systematic exposure to caspofungin; inducers of drug clearance or mixed inducer/inhibitors (e.g., **carbamazepine, dexamethasone, efavirenz, nelfinavir, nevirapine, phenytoin, rifampin**) can decrease caspofungin levels; caspofungin decreases the overall systematic exposure to **tacrolimus.**

PHARMACOKINETICS **Distribution:** 97% protein bound. **Metabolism:** Liver and plasma to inactive metabolites. **Elimination:** Both in urine and feces. **Half-Life:** 9–11 h.

NURSING IMPLICATIONS

Assessment & Drug Effects

- Monitor for S&S of hypersensitivity during IV infusion; frequently monitor IV site for thrombophlebitis.
- Monitor for and report S&S of fluid retention (e.g., weight gain, swelling, peripheral edema), especially with known cardiovascular disease.
- Monitor blood levels of tacrolimus with concurrent therapy.
- Monitor lab tests: Baseline and periodic LFTs; periodic kidney function tests, serum electrolytes, CBC with differential, and platelet count.

Patient & Family Education

- Report immediately any of the following: Facial swelling, wheezing, difficulty breathing or swallowing, tightness in chest, rash, hives, itching, or sensation of warmth.

CEFACLOR

(sef'a-klor)

Ceclor ♣

Classification: CEPHALOSPORIN ANTIBIOTIC

Therapeutic: ANTIBIOTIC

AVAILABILITY Capsule; sustained release tablet; suspension

Common adverse effects in *italic;* life-threatening effects underlined; generic names in **bold;** classifications in SMALL CAPS; ♣ Canadian drug name; Prototype drug; Alert

ACTION & *THERAPEUTIC EFFECT*

Preferentially binds to one or more of the penicillin-binding proteins (PBPs) located on cell walls of susceptible organisms. This inhibits third and final stages of bacterial cell wall synthesis, thus killing bacterium. *Effective in treating acute otitis media and acute sinusitis where causative agent is resistant to other antibiotics. Useful in treating respiratory and urinary tract infections.*

USES Treatment of otitis media and infections of upper and lower respiratory tract, urinary tract, and uncomplicated skin and skin structures.

CONTRAINDICATIONS Hypersensitivity to cephalosporins and related antibiotics.

CAUTIOUS USE History of sensitivity to penicillins or other drug allergies; GI disease, colitis; markedly impaired renal function; older adults; coagulopathy; pregnancy (category B); lactation.

ROUTE & DOSAGE

Mild to Moderate Infections

Adult: **PO** 250–500 mg q8h, or **Extended release** 500 mg/q12h
Child (1 mo or older): **PO** 20–40 mg/kg/day divided q8h (max: 2 g/day)

Otitis Media

Child (1 mo or older): **PO** 40 mg/kg/day divided q12h

ADMINISTRATION

Oral

- Give sustained release tablets with food to enhance absorption. Food does not affect absorption of capsules.
- Ensure that sustained release tablets are not chewed or crushed. They **must be** swallowed whole.
- After stock oral suspension is prepared, it should be kept refrigerated. Expiration date should appear on label. Discard unused portion after 14 days. Shake well before pouring.
- Store Pulvules in tightly closed container unless otherwise directed. Capsules and tablets should be stored at room temperature, 15°–30°C (59°–86°F).

ADVERSE EFFECTS None reported greater than 5%.

DIAGNOSTIC TEST INTERFERENCE

May produce positive ***direct Coombs test***. False-positive ***urine glucose*** determinations may result with use of ***copper sulfate reduction methods*** (e.g., ***Clinitest*** or ***Benedict reagent***).

INTERACTIONS Drug: Avoid LIVE VACCINES.

PHARMACOKINETICS Absorption: Well absorbed; acid stable. **Peak:** 30–60 min. **Elimination:** 60% of dose eliminated renally in 8 h; crosses placenta; excreted in breast milk. **Half-Life:** 0.5–1 h.

NURSING IMPLICATIONS

Assessment & Drug Effects

- Determine previous hypersensitivity to cephalosporins, penicillins, and other drug allergies before therapy is initiated.
- Report persistent diarrhea, as interruption of therapy may be necessary.
- Monitor for manifestations of drug hypersensitivity (see Appendix F). Discontinue drug and promptly report them if they appear.

C

- Monitor for manifestations of superinfection (see Appendix F). Promptly report their appearance.
- Monitor lab tests: Baseline C&S prior to initiation of therapy, CBC, hepatic/renal function.

Patient & Family Education

- Report promptly any signs or symptoms of superinfection (see Appendix F).
- Report severe diarrhea to provider.
- Yogurt or buttermilk (if allowed) may serve as a prophylactic against intestinal superinfections by helping to maintain normal intestinal flora.

CEFADROXIL

(sef-a-drox′ill)

Classification: CEPHALOSPORIN ANTIBIOTIC; FIRST-GENERATION CEPHALOSPORIN
Therapeutic: ANTIBIOTIC
Prototype: Cefazolin

AVAILABILITY Capsule; tablet; oral suspension

ACTION & *THERAPEUTIC EFFECT*
Drug penetrates bacterial cell wall, resists beta-lactamases, and inactivates enzymes essential to cell wall synthesis thus killing the bacterium. *Active against organisms that liberate cephalosporinase and penicillinase (beta-lactamases). Effective in reducing signs and symptoms of urinary tract infections, bone and joint infections, skin and soft tissue infections, and pharyngitis.*

USES Urinary tract infections, infections of skin and skin structures, pharyngitis, and tonsillitis.

UNLABELED USES Endocarditis prophylaxis, prosthetic joint infection.

CONTRAINDICATIONS Hypersensitivity to cephalosporins; drug-induced seizure activity.

CAUTIOUS USE Sensitivity to penicillins or other drug allergies; markedly impaired renal function, older adults; GI disease, history of GI disease particularly colitis, coagulopathy; pregnancy (category B); lactation; children less than 2 yr.

ROUTE & DOSAGE

Uncomplicated Urinary Tract Infection

Adult: **PO** 1 g bid × 10–14 days
Child: **PO** 30 mg/kg/day in 2 divided doses

Skin and Skin Structure Infections, Streptococcal Pharyngitis, or Tonsillitis

Adult: **PO** 1 g/day in 1–2 divided doses
Child: **PO** 30 mg/kg/day in 1–2 divided doses

Renal Impairment Dosage Adjustment

CrCl less than 25 mL/min:
Adult: **PO** 500 mg q24h

ADMINISTRATION

Oral

- Give with food or milk to reduce nausea. If nausea persists, termination of therapy may be necessary.
- Follow directions for mixing oral suspension found on drug label. Reconstituted suspension contains 125 or 250 mg cefadroxil/5 mL.
- Shake suspension well before use; discard after 14 days.
- Store in tight container unless otherwise directed. Oral suspensions are stable for 14 days under refrigeration at 2°–8°C (36°–46°F). Avoid freezing. Note expiration date on label. Store capsules and tablets at 15°–30°C (59°–86°F).

ADVERSE EFFECTS GI: Diarrhea.

DIAGNOSTIC TEST INTERFERENCE False-positive ***urine glucose*** determinations using ***copper sulfate reduction reagents***, such as ***Clinitest*** or ***Benedict reagent, Positive direct Coombs test*** may interfere with ***cross-matching procedures*** and ***hematologic studies.*** False-positive **serum/urine creatinine** with **Jaffé** reaction.

INTERACTIONS **Drug: Probenecid** decreases renal excretion of cefadroxil. Do not use with **BCG.**

PHARMACOKINETICS **Absorption:** Acid stable; rapidly absorbed from GI tract. **Peak:** 1 h. **Elimination:** 90% unchanged in urine within 8 h; bacterial inhibitory levels persist 20–22 h; crosses placenta; excreted in breast milk. **Half-Life:** 1–12 h.

NURSING IMPLICATIONS

Assessment & Drug Effects

- Determine previous hypersensitivity to cephalosporins, penicillins, and other drug allergies, before therapy is initiated.
- Monitor for manifestations of drug hypersensitivity (see Signs & Symptoms, Appendix F). Discontinue drug and promptly report them if they appear.
- Monitor for manifestations of superinfection (see Signs & Symptoms, Appendix F). Promptly report their appearance.
- Monitor I&O ratio and pattern.
- Monitor lab tests: Baseline C&S prior to initiation of therapy; CBC, baseline and periodic hepatic and renal function studies.

Patient & Family Education

- Report promptly the onset of rash, urticaria, pruritus, or fever, as the possibility of an allergic reaction is high, if you are allergic to penicillin.
- Take medication for the full course of therapy as directed by your prescriber.
- Report promptly S&S of superinfections (see Appendix F).

CEFAZOLIN SODIUM

(sef-a'zoe-lin)

Ancef

Classification: CEPHALOSPORIN ANTIBIOTIC; FIRST-GENERATION CEPHALOSPORIN

Therapeutic: ANTIBIOTIC

AVAILABILITY Solution for injection

ACTION & THERAPEUTIC EFFECT Preferentially binds to one or more of the penicillin-binding proteins (PBPs) located on cell walls of susceptible organisms. This inhibits third and final stages of bacterial cell wall synthesis, thus killing the bacterium. *Effective treatment for bone and joint infections, biliary tract infections, endocarditis prophylaxis and treatment, respiratory tract and genital tract infections, septicemia and skin infections, and surgical prophylaxis.*

USES Severe infections of urinary and biliary tracts, skin, soft tissue, and bone, and for bacteremia and endocarditis caused by susceptible organisms; respiratory tract infection; also perioperative prophylaxis in patients undergoing procedures associated with high risk of infection (e.g., open heart surgery).

CONTRAINDICATIONS Hypersensitivity to any cephalosporin and related antibiotics.

CAUTIOUS USE History of penicillin sensitivity, impaired renal or hepatic function, patients on sodium restriction; seizure disorders; coagulopathy; GI disease, colitis; pregnancy (category B); lactation: infant risk minimal.

ROUTE & DOSAGE

Moderate to Severe Infections

Adult: **IV/IM** 1–1.5 g q8h depending on severity (max: 12 g/day)
Child: **IV/IM** 25–100 mg/kg/day in 3–4 divided doses, up to 100 mg/kg/day (not to exceed adult doses)

Surgical Prophylaxis

Adult: **IV/IM** 1–2 g 30–60 min before surgery, then 0.5–1 g q8h
Child: **IV/IM** 25–50 mg/kg 30–60 min before surgery, then q8h for 24 h

Renal Impairment Dosage Adjustment

CrCl 11–34 mL/min: Administer 50% q12h; *less than 10 mL/min:* administer 50% q18–24 h

ADMINISTRATION

Intramuscular

- Preparation of IM solution: Reconstitute with sterile water for injection, bacteriostatic water for injection, or 0.9% sodium chloride injection.
- Reconstituted solutions are stable for 24 h at room temperature and for 10 days refrigerated.
- IM injections should be made deep into large muscle mass. Pain on injection is usually minimal. Rotate injection sites.

Intravenous

IV administration to neonates, infants, and children: Verify correct IV concentration and rate of infusion with prescriber.

PREPARE: **Direct:** Add 2 mL sterile water for injection to the 500-mg vial to yield 225 mg/mL, or add 2.5 mL to the 1-g vial to yield 330 mg/mL. Shake well to dissolve. ▪ Further dilute with 5 mL sterile water for injection. **Intermittent:** After initial vial reconstitution, add required dose to 50–100 mL of NS or D5W.

ADMINISTER: **Direct/Intermittent:** Infuse 1 g over 5 min or longer as determined by the amount of solution. ▪ The risk of IV site reactions may be reduced by proper dilution of IV solution, use of small-bore IV needle in a large vein, and by rotating injection sites.

INCOMPATIBILITIES: **Solution/additive: Atracurium, bleomycin, cimetidine, clindamycin, gentamicin, metronidazole, rocuronium, vancomycin. Y-site: Alemtuzumab, amiodarone, amphotericin B cholesteryl complex, ampicillin, azathioprine, calcium chloride, caspofungin, cefotaxime, chlorpromazine, cisatracurium, dacarbazine, dantrolene, danorubicin, diazepam, diazoxide, diphenhydramine, dobutamine, dolasetron, dopamine, doxorubicin, doxycycline, erythromycin, ganciclovir, garenoxacin, gemtuzumab, haloperidol, hydralazine, hydromorphone, hydroxyzine, idarubicin, inamrinone, lansoprazole, levofloxacin, minocycline, mitomycin, mitoxantrone, mivacurium, mycophenolate, netilmicin, papaverine, pemetrexed, pentamidine, pentazocine, pentobarbital, pentamidine, phentolamine, phenytoin, prochlorperazine,**

promethazine, protamine, pyridoxine, quinupristin/dalfopristin, sodium citrate, SMZ/TMP, tobramycin, high-dose **vancomycin, vinorelbine.**

ADVERSE EFFECTS Skin: *Pruritus.* **GI:** *Diarrhea.* **Hematologic:** *Drug-induced eosinophilia.*

DIAGNOSTIC TEST INTERFERENCE Because of cefazolin effect on the ***direct Coombs test***, transfusion ***cross-matching procedures*** and ***hematologic studies*** may be complicated. False-positive ***urine glucose*** determinations are possible with use of ***copper sulfate tests*** (e.g., ***Clinitest*** or ***Benedict reagent***).

INTERACTIONS Drug: Probenecid decreases renal elimination of cefazolin.

PHARMACOKINETICS Peak: 1–2 h after IM; 5 min after IV. **Distribution:** Poor CNS penetration even with inflamed meninges; high concentrations in bile and in diseased bone; crosses placenta. **Elimination:** 70% unchanged in urine in 6 h; small amount excreted in breast milk. **Half-Life:** 90–130 min.

NURSING IMPLICATIONS

Assessment & Drug Effects

- Determine history of hypersensitivity to cephalosporins, penicillins, and other drugs, before therapy is initiated.
- Monitor I&O rates and pattern: Be alert to changes in BUN, serum creatinine.
- Prompt attention should be given to onset of signs of hypersensitivity (see Appendix F).
- Promptly report the onset of diarrhea. Pseudomembranous colitis, a potentially life-threatening condition, starts with diarrhea.
- Monitor lab tests: Baseline C&S prior to initiation of therapy. Renal function tests in the elderly.

Patient & Family Education

- Report promptly any signs or symptoms of superinfection (see Appendix F).
- Report signs of coagulation problems such as easy bruising and nosebleeds.

CEFDINIR

(cef′di-nir)

Omnicef

Classification: CEPHALOSPORIN ANTIBIOTIC; THIRD-GENERATION CEPHALOSPORIN

Therapeutic: ANTIBIOTIC

Prototype: Cefotaxime sodium

AVAILABILITY Capsule; powder for suspension

ACTION & *THERAPEUTIC EFFECT* Has bactericidal activity resulting from the inhibition of cell wall synthesis through an affinity for penicillin binding proteins (PBPs). Stable in the presence of a variety of bacterial beta-lactamase enzymes. *Effective against a wide variety of gram-positive and gram-negative bacteria.*

USES Community-acquired pneumonia, acute exacerbations of chronic bronchitis, acute maxillary sinusitis, pharyngitis, tonsillitis, uncomplicated skin infections, bacterial otitis media.

CONTRAINDICATIONS Hypersensitivity to cefdinir and other cephalosporins.

CAUTIOUS USE Hypersensitivity to penicillins, penicillin derivatives; renal impairment; ulcerative colitis or antibiotic-induced colitis; bleeding disorders; GI disorders; liver or kidney disease; pregnancy (category B); lactation. Safety and efficacy in neonates and infants younger than 6 mo old not established.

ROUTE & DOSAGE

Community-Acquired Pneumonia

Adult: **PO** 300 mg q12h × at least 5 days

Skin Infections

Adult: **PO** 300 mg q12h × 10 days *Child/Infant (6 mo–12 yr):* **PO** 7 mg/kg q12h × 10 days

Chronic Bronchitis, Maxillary Sinusitis, Pharyngitis, Tonsillitis

Adult/Adolescent: **PO** 600 mg daily × 5–7 days or 300 mg q12h × 5–7 days
Child/Infant (6 mo–12 yr): **PO** 14 mg/kg q24h × 10 d or 7 mg/kg q12h × 5–10 days

Renal Impairment Dosage Adjustment

Adult: CrCl less than 30 mL/min: 300 mg daily *Child:* 7 mg/kg daily

Hemodialysis Dosage Adjustment

300 mg or 7 mg/kg dose PO every other day; dose given at the end of each session

ADMINISTRATION

Oral

- Do not give within 2 h of aluminum- or magnesium-containing antacids or iron supplements.
- Reconstitute oral suspension to 125 mg/mL by adding water (38 to 60 mL bottle or 63 to 100 mL bottle). Shake well before each use.
- Store in tightly closed container at 20°–25°C (68°–77°F). Store reconstituted suspension at room temperature at 20°–25°C (68°–77°F) for 10 days.

ADVERSE EFFECTS **GI:** Diarrhea.

DIAGNOSTIC TEST INTERFERENCE False positive for ***ketones*** or ***glucose*** in urine using ***nitroprusside*** or ***Clinitest***; may cause false-positive ***Direct Coombs test.***

INTERACTIONS **Drug: Probenecid** prolongs cefdinir elimination; **iron** decreases absorption. Do not use with LIVE VACCINES.

PHARMACOKINETICS **Absorption:** 16–25% bioavailability. **Peak:** 2–4 h. **Distribution:** 60–70% protein bound; penetrates sinus tissue, blister fluid, lung tissue, middle ear fluid. **Metabolism:** Hepatic. **Elimination:** In urine. **Half-Life:** 1.6 h.

NURSING IMPLICATIONS

Assessment & Drug Effects

- Determine previous hypersensitivity to cephalosporins, penicillins, and other drug allergies before therapy is initiated.
- Carefully monitor for and immediately report S&S of: Hypersensitivity, superinfection, or pseudomembranous colitis (see Appendix F).
- Discontinue drug and notify prescriber if seizures associated with drug therapy occur.
- Monitor lab tests: CBC, hepatic, and renal function tests.

Patient & Family Education

- Allow a minimum of 2 h between cefdinir and antacids containing aluminum or magnesium, or drugs containing iron.

- Immediately contact prescriber if a rash, diarrhea, fever or new infection (e.g., yeast infection) develops.

CEFDITOREN PIVOXIL

(cef-di-tor′en)

Spectracef

Classification: CEPHALOSPORIN ANTIBIOTIC; THIRD-GENERATION CEPHALOSPORIN

Therapeutic: ANTIBIOTIC

Prototype: Cefotaxime sodium

AVAILABILITY Tablet

ACTION & *THERAPEUTIC EFFECT* Has bactericidal activity resulting from the inhibition of cell wall synthesis through an affinity for penicillin-binding proteins (PBPs). Stable in the presence of a variety of bacterial beta-lactamase enzymes, including penicillinases and some cephalosporinases. *Antibacterial activity is effective against both aerobic gram-positive and aerobic gram-negative bacteria.*

USES Acute exacerbation of bacterial chronic bronchitis, pharyngitis, tonsillitis, community-acquired pneumonia, uncomplicated skin and skin-structure infections.

CONTRAINDICATIONS Known allergy to cephalosporins or cefditoren; carnitine deficiency; milk protein hypersensitivity (not lactose intolerance).

CAUTIOUS USE History of hypersensitivity to penicillin; renal or hepatic impairment; poor nutritional status; coagulopathy; diabetes mellitus; colitis, GI disease; older adults; concurrent anticoagulant therapy; pregnancy (category B); lactation. Safety and efficacy in children younger than 12 yr not established.

ROUTE & DOSAGE

Chronic Bronchitis/Pneumonia

Adult/Adolescent: **PO** 400 mg bid × 10–14 days

Pharyngitis, Tonsillitis, Skin Infections, Uncomplicated Skin/Soft Tissue Infections

Adult: **PO** 200 mg bid × 10 days

Renal Impairment Dosage Adjustment

CrCl 30–49 mL/min: 200 mg bid; *less than 30 mL/min:* 200 mg daily

ADMINISTRATION

Oral

- Give with food to enhance absorption.
- Do not give within 2 h of an antacid or H_2-receptor antagonist (such as cimetidine).
- Store at 15°–30°C (58°–86°F). Protect from light and moisture.

ADVERSE EFFECTS **GI:** Diarrhea, nausea. **GU:** Candida vaginitis.

DIAGNOSTIC TEST INTERFERENCE May cause false-negative ***ferricyanide test***, may induce positive ***Direct Coombs test.***

INTERACTIONS **Drug:** ANTACIDS, H_2-RECEPTOR ANTAGONISTS may decrease absorption; **probenecid** will decrease elimination.

PHARMACOKINETICS **Absorption:** 14% reaches systemic circulation. **Distribution:** 88% protein bound, distributes into blister fluid, tonsils. **Metabolism:** Hydrolyzed. **Elimination:** Primarily in urine. **Half-Life:** 1.6 h.

C

NURSING IMPLICATIONS

Assessment & Drug Effects

- Obtain history of hypersensitivity to cephalosporins, penicillins, and other drug allergies.
- Monitor for manifestations of drug hypersensitivity (see Appendix F). Withhold drug and report promptly to prescriber if they appear.
- Monitor for and report promptly manifestations of superinfection (see Appendix F), especially diarrhea. Diarrhea may indicate a change in intestinal flora and development of enterocolitis.
- Monitor for and report immediately signs of seizure activity or loss of seizure control.
- Monitor lab tests: Baseline C&S prior to initiating therapy. Baseline and periodic renal function tests; frequent PT in those at risk for increased prothrombin time; as indicated, Hct and Hgb, CBC with differential, urinalysis, serum electrolytes, and LFTs.

Patient & Family Education

- Do not take within 2 h of antacids or other drugs used to reduce stomach acids.
- Discontinue drug and report to prescriber signs of an allergic reaction (e.g., rash, urticaria, pruritus, fever).
- Report promptly S&S of superinfection (see Appendix F), especially unexplained diarrhea. Antibiotic-associated colitis is a superinfection that may occur in 4–9 days or as long as 6 wk after drug is discontinued.
- Use daily yogurt or buttermilk (if allowed) as a prophylactic against intestinal superinfections.

CEFEPIME HYDROCHLORIDE

(cef′e-peem)

Classification: CEPHALOSPORIN ANTIBIOTIC; FOURTH-GENERATION CEPHALOSPORIN

Therapeutic: ANTIBIOTIC; CEPHALOSPORIN

Prototype: Cefotaxime sodium

AVAILABILITY Solution for injection

ACTION & *THERAPEUTIC EFFECT* Cefepime preferentially binds to one or more of the penicillin-binding proteins (PBPs) located on cell walls of susceptible organisms. This inhibits the third and final stages of bacterial cell wall synthesis, thus killing the bacteria (bactericidal). *Cefepime is similar to third-generation cephalosporins with respect to broad gram-negative coverage; however, cefepime has broader gram-positive coverage than third-generation cephalosporins.*

USES Intra-abdominal infections, UTI, skin and soft tissue infections, pneumonia. Empiric monotherapy for febrile neutropenic patients.

CONTRAINDICATIONS Hypersensitivity to cefepime, other cephalosporins, severe reaction to penicillins, or other beta-lactam antibiotics; hypersensitivity to corn products (solutions containing dextrose only); development of neurotoxicity from use of drug.

CAUTIOUS USE Patients with history of GI disease, particularly colitis;

renal insufficiency; CrCl of 60 mL/min or less; diabetics; older adults; pregnancy (category B); lactation.

ROUTE & DOSAGE

UTI

Adult: **IV** 1–2 g q12h for 10–14 days

Febrile Neutropenia

Adult/Adolescent/Child (weight greater than 40 kg): **IV** 2 g q8h until resolution of neutropenia
Child (weight less than 40 kg)/Infant (older than 2 mo): **IV** 50 mg/kg q8h until resolution of neutropenia

Community-Acquired Pneumonia

Adult: **IV** 2 g q8h

Intra-Abdominal Infection

Adult: **IV** 2 g q8–12h × 4–7 d

Skin Infection

Adult: **IV** 2 g q12h × 5–14 days
Adolescent/Child/Infant (over 2 mo): **IV** 50 mg/kg/dose q12h × 10 d

Renal Impairment Dosage Adjustment

See package insert

ADMINISTRATION

Intramuscular

- Reconstitute the 1-g vial with 2.4 mL of one of the following: Sterile water for injection, 0.9% NaCl injection, bacteriostatic water for injection with parabens or benzyl alcohol, or other compatible solution to yield 280 mg/mL.
- Store reconstituted solution up to 24 h at room temperature 20°–25°C (68°–77°F).

Intravenous

PREPARE: **Intermittent:** Dilute 1- or 2-g vial with 10 mL of a compatible diluent to yield 100 mg/mL for 1-g vial and 160 mg/mL for 2-g vial. Further dilute in one of the following: NS, D5W, D5/NS, or other compatible solution.

ADMINISTER: **Intermittent:** Infuse over 30 min; with Y-type administration set, discontinue other compatible solutions while infusing cefepime.

INCOMPATIBILITIES: **Solution/additive:** AMINOGLYCOSIDES, **aminophylline, gentamicin sulfate, sodium citrate, tobramycin sulfate. Y-site: Acetylcysteine, acyclovir, alemtuzumab, amphotericin B, amphotericin B cholesteryl complex, amphotericin B liposomal, argatroban, asparaginase, caspofungin, chlordiazepoxide, chlorpromazine, cimetidine, ciprofloxacin, cisplatin, dacarbazine, daunorubicin, dexrazoxane, diazepam, diltiazem, diphenhydramine, dolasetron, doxorubicin, droperidol, enalaprilat, epirubicin, erythromycin, etoposide, famotidine, filgrastim, floxuridine, gallium, ganciclovir, garenoxacin mesylate, gatifloxacin, gemcitabine, gemtuzumab ozogamicin, haloperidol, hydroxyzine, idarubicin, ifosfamide, irinotecan, isavuconazonium sulfate, labetalol hydrochloride, lansoprazole, letermovir, magnesium sulfate,**

C

mannitol, mechlorethamine, meperidine, metoclopramide, midazolam, mitomycin, mitoxantrone, morphine, nalbuphine, ofloxacin, ondansetron, oxaliplatin, pantoprazole, pemetrexed, phenytoin, piritramide, plicamycin, prochlorperazine, promethazine, propofol, quinupristin-dalfopristin, streptozocin, tacrolimus, temocillin, theophylline, topotecan, vecuronium, vinblastine, vincristine, vinorelbine, voriconazole.

- Store reconstituted solution at 20°–25°C (68°–77°F) for 24 h or in refrigerator at 2°–8°C (36°–46°F) for 7 days. Protect from light.

ADVERSE EFFECTS **Hematologic:** Direct Coombs test positive.

DIAGNOSTIC TEST INTERFERENCE

Positive ***Coombs test*** without hemolysis. May cause false-positive ***urine glucose test*** with ***Clinitest.***

INTERACTIONS **Drug:** May decrease efficacy of ORAL CONTRACEPTIVES. **Probenecid** may increase levels. Do not administer with LIVE VACCINES.

PHARMACOKINETICS **Absorption:** Well absorbed after IM administration; serum levels significantly lower than after equivalent IV dose. **Distribution:** Widely distributed, may cross inflamed meninges; crosses placenta, secreted into breast milk. **Metabolism:** In liver. **Elimination:** In urine. **Half-Life:** 2 h.

NURSING IMPLICATIONS

Assessment & Drug Effects

- Determine history of hypersensitivity reactions to cephalosporins, penicillins, or other drugs before therapy is initiated.
- Monitor for S&S of hypersensitivity (see Appendix F). Report their appearance promptly and discontinue drug.
- Monitor for S&S of superinfection or pseudomembranous colitis (see Appendix F); immediately report either to prescriber.
- With concurrent high-dose aminoglycoside therapy, closely monitor for nephrotoxicity and ototoxicity.
- Monitor lab tests: Baseline C&S before initiation of therapy; WBCs, prothrombin time in patients at risk (patients with poor nutritional status, renal or hepatic impairment or receiving long-term treatment). Frequent renal function tests, especially with known renal impairment.

Patient & Family Education

- Promptly report S&S of hypersensitivity (e.g., rash) or superinfection, especially unexplained diarrhea (see Appendix F).
- Report immediately any S&S of encephalopathy (confusion, hallucinations, stupor, coma), myoclonus, and seizures.
- Report severe diarrhea.

CEFIXIME

(ce-fix′ime)

Suprax

Classification: CEPHALOSPORIN ANTIBIOTIC; THIRD-GENERATION CEPHALOSPORIN

Therapeutic: ANTIBIOTIC

Prototype: Cefotaxime sodium

AVAILABILITY Reconstituted suspension; chewable tablet; capsule

ACTION & THERAPEUTIC EFFECT It inhibits the third and final stages of bacterial cell wall synthesis by preferentially binding to specific penicillin-binding proteins (PBPs) located inside the bacterial cell wall. *Cefixime is highly stable in the presence of beta-lactamases (penicillinases and cephalosporinases) and therefore has excellent activity against a wide range of gram-negative bacteria. It is bactericidal against susceptible bacteria.*

USES Uncomplicated UTI, otitis media, pharyngitis, tonsillitis, and bronchitis.

CONTRAINDICATIONS Patients with known allergy to the cephalosporin group of antibiotics, severe reaction to penicillin.

CAUTIOUS USE Allergy to penicillin, history of colitis, renal insufficiency, seizure disorders; GI disease, coagulopathy, pregnancy (category B), children younger than 6 mo; lactation.

ROUTE & DOSAGE

Infection

Adult/Adolescent/Child (greater than 45kg): **PO** 400 mg/day in 1–2 divided doses × 10–14 days
Child (6 mo and older, weight 45 kg and greater): **PO** 8 mg/kg/day in 1–2 divided doses

Renal Impairment Dosage Adjustment

See package insert, varies based on dosage form

ADMINISTRATION

Oral

- Take with or without food.
- Do not substitute tablets for liquid in treatment of otitis media because of lack of bioequivalence.
- Ensure that chewable tablets are chewed or crushed before swallowing.
- After reconstitution, suspension may be kept for 14 days at room temperature or refrigerated. Store away from heat and light. Keep tightly closed and shake well before using.
- Store at controlled room temperature between 20° and 25°C (68° and 77°F).

ADVERSE EFFECTS **GI:** Diarrhea, loose stool, nausea.

DIAGNOSTIC TEST INTERFERENCE Positive ***Coombs test*** without hemolysis. May cause false-positive ***urine glucose test*** with Clinitest.

INTERACTIONS **Drug:** May decrease efficacy of ORAL CONTRACEPTIVES. **Probenecid** may increase levels. Avoid LIVE VACCINES.

PHARMACOKINETICS **Absorption:** 40–50% from GI tract. **Peak:** 2–6 h. **Distribution:** Into breast milk. **Elimination:** 50% in urine, 50% in bile. **Half-Life:** 3–4 h.

NURSING IMPLICATIONS

Assessment & Drug Effects

- Determine previous hypersensitivity reactions to cephalosporins, penicillins, and history of other allergies, particularly to drugs prior to initiation of therapy.

- Monitor for superinfections (see Appendix F) caused by overgrowth of nonsusceptible organisms, particularly during prolonged use.
- Monitor I&O rates and pattern: Nephrotoxicity occurs more frequently in patients older than 50 yr, with impaired renal function, in the debilitated, and in patients receiving high doses or other nephrotoxic drugs.
- Carefully monitor anyone with a history of allergies. Report manifestations of hypersensitivity (see Appendix F).
- Promptly report loose stools or diarrhea, which may indicate pseudomembranous colitis (see Appendix F). Discontinuation of drug may be necessary.
- Monitor dialysis patients closely.
- Monitor lab tests: Baseline C&S prior to initiation of therapy, prothrombin time in high-risk patients with renal or hepatic impairment, poor nutritional status or prolonged therapy.

Patient & Family Education

- Report loose stools or diarrhea during drug therapy and for several weeks after. Older adult patients are especially susceptible to pseudomembranous colitis.

CEFOTAXIME SODIUM (Pr)

(sef-oh-taks'eem)

Classification: CEPHALOSPORIN ANTIBIOTIC; THIRD-GENERATION CEPHALOSPORIN
Therapeutic: ANTIBIOTIC

AVAILABILITY Solution for injection

ACTION & *THERAPEUTIC EFFECT* Preferentially binds to one or more of the penicillin-binding proteins (PBPs) located on cell walls of susceptible organisms. This inhibits third and final stages of bacterial cell wall synthesis, thus killing the bacteria. *Generally active against a wide variety of gram-positive and gram-negative bacteria including most of the Enterobacteriaceae. Also active against some organisms resistant to first- and second-generation cephalosporins, and aminoglycoside antibiotics and penicillins.*

USES Serious infections of lower respiratory tract, skin and skin structures, bones, and joints, CNS (including meningitis and ventriculitis), gynecologic and GU tract infections, including uncomplicated gonococcal infections caused by penicillinase-producing *Neisseria gonorrhoeae* (PPNG). Also used to treat bacteremia or septicemia, intra-abdominal infections, and for perioperative prophylaxis.

UNLABELED USES Treatment of disseminated gonococcal infections (gonococcal arthritis-dermatitis syndrome), Lyme disease, typhoid fever.

CONTRAINDICATIONS Hypersensitivity to cefotaxime, or cephalosporins antibiotics.

CAUTIOUS USE History of Type I hypersensitivity reactions to penicillin; history of allergy to other beta-lactam antibiotics; coagulopathy; renal impairment; older adults; history of colitis or other GI disease; pregnancy (category B); lactation.

C

ROUTE & DOSAGE

Uncomplicated Infection

Adult: **IV/IM** 1 g q12h

Moderate to Severe Infections

Adult: **IV/IM** 1–2 g q8–12h, up to 2 g q4h (max: 12 g/day)
Child (1 mo–12 yr): **IV/IM** 50–180 mg/kg/day divided q6–8h (max: 6 g/day)

Rhinositus

Adult: **IV** 2 g q4–6h × 5–7 days

Sepsis

Adult: **IV** 2 g q6–8h

Renal Impairment Dosage Adjustment

CrCl less than 20 mL/min: Reduce dose by 50%

ADMINISTRATION

Intramuscular

- Dilute with SW for injection as follows: 2 mL for the 500-mg vial to yield 230 mg/mL; 3 mL for the 1-g vial to yield 300 mg/mL; 5 mL for the 2-g vial to yield 330 mg/mL.
- Administer IM injection deeply into large muscle mass (e.g., upper outer quadrant of gluteus maximus). Aspirate to avoid inadvertent injection into blood vessel. If IM dose is 2 g, divide dose and administer into 2 different sites.
- Store intact vials below 30°C (86°F). Reconstituted solution is stable for 12–24 h at room temperature and 7–10 days when refrigerated.

Intravenous

IV administration to neonates, infants, and children: Verify correct IV concentration and rate of infusion with prescriber.

- Do not admix cefotaxime with sodium bicarbonate or any fluid with a pH greater than 7.5. ▪ Risk of phlebitis may be reduced by use of a small needle in a large vein.

PREPARE: **Direct:** Add 10 mL diluent to vial with 1 or 2 g drug providing a solution containing 95 or 180 mg/mL, respectively. **Intermittent:** To 1 or 2 g drug add 50 or 100 mL D5W, NS, D5/NS, D5/.45% NaCl, LR, or other compatible diluent. **Continuous:** Dilute in 500–1000 mL compatible IV solution.

ADMINISTER: **Direct:** Give over 3–5 min. **Intermittent:** Give over 15–30 min, preferably via butterfly or scalp vein-type needles. **Continuous:** Infuse over 6–24 h.

INCOMPATIBILITIES: **Amikacin sulfate, gentamicin sulfate, metronidazole, vancomycin.** **Y-site:** **Alemtuzumab, allopurinol, amiodarone, amphotericin B liposome, ampicillin, azathioprine, caspofungin, cefazolin, ceftazidime, ceftizoxime, chloramphenicol, chlorpromazine, dacarbazine, dantrolene, danorubicin, diazepam, diazoxide, diphenhydramine, dobutamine, dolasetron, doxorubicin, filgrastim, fluconazole, ganciclovir, garenoxacin mesylate, gemcitabine, gemtuzumab, haloperidol, hydralazine, hydroxyzine, idarubicin, inamrinone lactate, irinotecan, labetalol, hydrochloride, levofloxacin, methylprednisolone, minocycline, mitomycin, mitoxantrone, mycophenolate, pantoprazole, papaverine, pemetrexed, pentamidine, pentazocine, pentobarbital sodium,**

C

phenobarbital sodium, phentolamine mesylate, phenytoin, prochlorperazine, promethazine, protamine, quinupristin/dalfopristin, sodium bicarbonate, sulfamethoxazole/trimethoprim, trastuzumab, vecuronium.

- Protect from excessive light. Reconstituted solutions may be stored in original containers for 24 h at room temperature; for 10 days under refrigeration at or below 5°C (41°F); or for at least 13 wk in frozen state.

DIAGNOSTIC TEST INTERFERENCE

May cause falsely elevated ***serum*** or ***urine creatinine*** values ***(Jaffé reaction)***. Positive ***direct antiglobulin (Coombs) test***; false-positive urinary glucose test using cupric sulfate.

INTERACTIONS

Drug: Probenecid decreases renal elimination.

PHARMACOKINETICS

Peak: 30 min after IM; 5 min after IV. **Distribution:** CNS penetration except with inflamed meninges; also penetrates aqueous humor, ascitic and prostatic fluids; crosses placenta. **Metabolism:** In liver to active metabolites. **Elimination:** 50–60% unchanged in urine in 24 h; small amount excreted in breast milk. **Half-Life:** 1 h.

NURSING IMPLICATIONS

Assessment & Drug Effects

- Determine previous hypersensitivity reactions to cephalosporins and penicillins, and history of other allergies, particularly to drugs, before therapy is initiated.
- Monitor I&O rates and patterns, especially with higher doses or concurrent aminoglycoside therapy. Report significant changes in I&O.
- Superinfection due to overgrowth of nonsusceptible organisms may occur, particularly with prolonged therapy.
- Report onset of diarrhea promptly. Check for fever. If diarrhea is mild, discontinuation of cefotaxime may be sufficient.
- If diarrhea is severe, suspect antibiotic-associated pseudomembranous colitis, a life-threatening superinfection (may occur in 4–9 days or as long as 6 wk after cephalosporin therapy is discontinued).
- Monitor lab tests: Baseline C&S before initiation of therapy; periodic renal function tests; periodic CBC with differential with high doses or prolonged therapy.

Patient & Family Education

- Report any early signs or symptoms of superinfection promptly. Superinfections caused by overgrowth of nonsusceptible organisms may occur, particularly during prolonged use.
- Yogurt or buttermilk, 120 mL (4 oz) of either (if allowed), may serve as a prophylactic against intestinal superinfection by helping to maintain normal intestinal flora.
- Report loose stools, diarrhea, or fever.

CEFOTETAN DISODIUM

(se-fo-tee'tan)

Cefotan

Classification: CEPHALOSPORIN ANTIBIOTIC; SECOND-GENERATION CEPHALOSPORIN

Therapeutic: ANTIBIOTIC

Prototype: Cefotaxime sodium

C

AVAILABILITY Solution for injection

ACTION & *THERAPEUTIC EFFECT*
Preferentially binds to one or more of the penicillin-binding proteins (PBPs) located on cell walls of susceptible organisms. This inhibits third and final stages of bacterial cell wall synthesis, thus killing the bacterium. *Generally less active against susceptible Staphylococci than first-generation cephalosporins, but has broad spectrum of activity against gram-negative bacteria when compared to first- and second-generation cephalosporins. It also shows moderate activity against gram-positive organisms. It is active against the Enterobacteriaceae and anaerobes.*

USES Infections caused by susceptible organisms in urinary tract, lower respiratory tract, skin and skin structures, bones and joints, gynecologic tract; also intra-abdominal infections, bacteremia, and perioperative prophylaxis.

CONTRAINDICATIONS Known allergy to cephalosporins and individuals who have experienced a cephalosporin-associated hemolytic anemia; pseudomembranous colitis.

CAUTIOUS USE Hypersensitivity to cefotetan, penicillins, or other drugs; preexisting coagulopathy; colitis, GI disease; renal impairment; cancer patients; patients in debilitated state; older adults; pregnancy (category B); lactation. Safety and efficacy in children not established.

ROUTE & DOSAGE

Moderate to Severe Skin Infections

Adult: **IV/IM** 1 g q12h or **IV** 2 g q24h

UTI

Adult: **IV** 500 mg q12h or 1–2 g/day q12–24h

Pelvic Inflammatory Disease

Adult: **IV** 2 g q12h

Surgical Prophylaxis

Adult/Adolescent: **IV** 2 g within 60 min before surgery

Renal Impairment Dosage Adjustment

CrCl 10–30 mL/min: Regular dose q24h or 50% of dose q12h; *less than 10 mL/min:* Regular dose q48h

Hemodialysis Dosage Adjustment

Give ¼ dose q24h on days between sessions, ½ dose on day of dialysis

ADMINISTRATION

Intramuscular

- For IM reconstitution (follow manufacturer's directions for selection of diluent), add 2 mL diluent to 1-g vial or 3 mL to the 2-g vial; yields approximately 400 or 500 mg/mL, respectively.
- For IM administration, inject well into body of large muscle such as upper outer quadrant of buttock (gluteus maximus).

Intravenous

IV administration to infants and children: Verify correct IV concentration and rate of infusion with prescriber.

C

PREPARE: **Direct:** Dilute each 1 g with 10 mL of sterile water for injection. **Intermittent:** Dilute each 1 g with 50–100 mL of D5W or NS.
ADMINISTER: **Direct:** Give over 3–5 min. **Intermittent:** Give a single dose over 30 min. ▪ For IV infusion, solution may be given for longer period of time through tubing system through which other IV solutions are being given.
INCOMPATIBILITIES: **Solution/additive:** **Promethazine** **Y-site:** **Alemtuzumab, amiodarone hydrochloride, amphotericin B conventional colloidal, amphotericin B liposome, ampicillin, atracurium, azathioprine sodium, caspofungin acetate, chlorpromazine hydrochloride, dantrolene sodium, daunorubicin citrate liposome, daunorubicin hydrochloride, diazepam, diazoxide, diphenhydramine hydrochloride, dobutamine hydrochloride, dolasetron mesylate, doxorubicin hydrochloride, doxycycline hyclate, epirubicin hydrochloride, erythromycin lactobionate, esmolol hydrochloride, famotidine, ganciclovir, garenoxacin mesylate, gemtuzumab hydrochloride, gemtuzumab ozogamicin, gentamicin sulfate, haloperidol lactate, hydralazine hydrochloride, hydroxyzine hydrochloride, idarubicin hydrochloride, inamrinone lactate, indomethacin sodium trihydrate, insulin, meperidine hydrochloride, midazolam hydrochloride, minocycline hydrochloride, mitomycin, mycophenolate mofetil hydrochloride, netilmicin sulfate, ondansetron hydrochloride, pantoprazole sodium, papaverine hydrochloride, pentamidine isethionate, pentazocine lactate, pentobarbital sodium, phenobarbital sodium, phentolamine mesylate, prochlorperazine edisylate, protamine sulfate, quinupristin-dalfopristin, sodium bicarbonate, sulfamethoxazole-trimethoprim, tobramycin sulfate, tolazoline hydrochloride, trastuzumab.**

▪ Protect sterile powder from light; store at or below 22°C (71.6°F); remains stable 24 mo after date of manufacture. May darken with age, but potency is unaffected. ▪ Reconstituted solutions: Stable for 24 h at 25°C (77°F); 96 h when refrigerated at 5°C (41°F); or at least 30 wk when frozen at –20°C (–4°F).

ADVERSE EFFECTS No side effects listed with over 5% incidence.

DIAGNOSTIC TEST INTERFERENCE May cause falsely elevated ***serum*** or ***urine creatinine*** values ***(Jaffé reaction)***. False-positive reactions for ***urine glucose*** using ***copper sulfate reduction methods*** (e.g., ***Benedict, Clinitest***); Positive ***direct antiglobulin (Coombs) test*** results may interfere with ***hematologic studies*** and ***cross-matching*** procedures.

INTERACTIONS **Drug: Probenecid** decreases renal elimination of cefotetan; **alcohol** produces disulfiram reaction.

PHARMACOKINETICS **Peak:** 1.5–3 h after IM. **Distribution:** Poor CNS penetration; widely distributed to body tissues and fluids, including bile, sputum, prostatic and peritoneal fluids; crosses placenta. **Elimination:** 51–81% unchanged in urine; 20% in bile; small amount in breast milk. **Half-Life:** 180–270 min.

NURSING IMPLICATIONS

Assessment & Drug Effects

- Determine history of hypersensitivity to cephalosporins and penicillins, and other drug allergies, before therapy begins.
- Report onset of loose stools or diarrhea. If diarrhea is severe, suspect pseudomembranous colitis (see Appendix F) caused by *Clostridium difficile*. Check temperature. Report fever and severe diarrhea to prescriber; drug should be discontinued.
- Monitor lab tests: Baseline C&S before initiation of therapy. Periodic hematologic studies and renal function tests, especially if cefotetan dose is high or if therapy is prolonged. Monitor prothrombin time in patients at risk of prolongation during cephalosporin therapy (nutritionally deficient, prolonged treatment, renal or hepatic disease).

Patient & Family Education

- Do not drink alcohol while taking this drug.
- Report promptly S&S of superinfection (see Appendix F).
- Report loose stools or diarrhea.

CEFOXITIN SODIUM

(se-fox'i-tin)

Classification: CEPHALOSPORIN ANTIBIOTIC; SECOND-GENERATION CEPHALOSPORIN

Therapeutic: ANTIBIOTIC

Prototype: Cefaclor

AVAILABILITY Solution for injection

ACTION & *THERAPEUTIC EFFECT*

Preferentially binds to one or more of the penicillin-binding proteins (PBPs) located on cell walls of susceptible organisms, thus making it bactericidal. *It shows enhanced activity against a wide variety of gram-negative organisms and is effective for mixed aerobic-anaerobic infections.*

USES Infections caused by susceptible organisms in the lower respiratory tract, urinary tract, skin and skin structures, bones and joints; also intra-abdominal infection, gynecologic infections, septicemia, and perioperative prophylaxis in GI, abdominal or vaginal hysterectomy.

CONTRAINDICATIONS Known hypersensitivity to cefoxitin or cephalosporins.

CAUTIOUS USE History of sensitivity to penicillin, or other drugs; impaired renal function; coagulopathy; GI disease, colitis; seizure disorders; patients with overt or subclinical diabetes; older adults; pregnancy (category B); children younger than 3 mo.

ROUTE & DOSAGE

Moderate to Severe Infections

Adult: **IV** 1–2 g q6–8h (max: 12 g/day)
Child (3 mo or older): **IV** 80 mg/kg/day q6–8h (max: 4000 mg/day)

Surgical Prophylaxis

Adult: **IV** 2 g 30–60 min before surgery, then 2 g q6h for 24 h
Child: **IV** 40 mg/kg 30–60 min before surgery, may repeat in 2 h

C

Pelvic Inflammatory Disease

Adult/Adolescent: **IV** 2 g q6h (with **doxycycline**)

Cesarean Surgery

Adult: **IV/IM** 2 g after clamping umbilical cord

Renal Impairment Dosage Adjustment

CrCl 30–50 mL/min: 1–2 g q8–12h; *10–29 mL/min:* 1–2 g q12–24h; *5–9 mL/min:* 0.5–1 g q12–24h; *greater than 5 mL/min:* 0.5–1 g q24–48h

Hemodialysis Dosage Adjustment

Dose of 1–2 g postdialysis

ADMINISTRATION

Intravenous

IV administration to neonates, infants, and children: Verify correct IV concentration and rate of infusion/injection with prescriber.

PREPARE: **Direct:** Reconstitute each 1 g with 10 mL sterile water, D5W, or NS. **Intermittent:** Following reconstitution, dilute 1–2 g in 50–100 mL of D5W or NS. **Continuous:** Dilute large doses in 1000 mL of D5W, D10W, or NS.

ADMINISTER: **Direct:** Give over 3–5 min. **Intermittent:** Give over 10–60 min. **Continuous:** Give at a rate determined by the volume of solution. ▪ Reconstituted solution may become discolored (usually light yellow to amber) if exposed to high temperatures; however, potency is not affected. ▪ Solution may be cloudy immediately after reconstitution; let stand and it will clear.

INCOMPATIBILITIES: **Y-site:** **Alemtuzumab, amphotericin B conventional colloidal, azathioprine, caspofungin, ceftizoxime, chloramphenicol, cisatracurium, dantrolene, danorubicin, diazepam, diazoxide, diphenhydramine, dobutamine, dolasetron, doxorubicin, doxycycline, epirubicin, erythromycin, famotidine, fenoldopam, filgrastim, ganciclovir, garenoxacin, gatifloxacin, gemtuzumab, haloperidol, hydroxyzine, idarubicin, inamrinone, insulin, labetalol, lansoprazole, levofloxacin, methylprednisolone, minocycline, mitoxantrone, mycophenolate, pantoprazole sodium, papaverine, pemetrexed, pentamidine, pentazocine, pentobarbital, phenobarbital, phentolamine, phenytoin sodium, polymyxin B sulfate prochlorperazine, promethazine, protamine, quinupristin/dalfopristin, sodium bicarbonate, SMZ/TMP, trastuzumab, vinorelbine.**

▪ Store powder for solution between 2° and 25°C (36° and 77°F). Dry materials or solution may darken, but potency is not affected. Discard vial within 4 h of entry. After dilution solutions are stale for an additional 18 h at room temperature or an additional 48 h under refrigeration.
▪ Store frozen premix solutions below –20°C (–4°F) or under refrigeration (2°–8°C; 36°–46°F). Thawed solutions is stable for 24 h at room temperature or 21 days at refrigerated temperatures.

ADVERSE EFFECTS

GI: Diarrhea.

DIAGNOSTIC TEST INTERFERENCE

Cefoxitin causes false-positive

C

(black-brown or green-brown color) ***urine glucose*** reaction with ***copper reduction reagents*** such as ***Benedict*** or ***Clinitest***, but not with ***enzymatic glucose oxidase reagents (Clinistix, TesTape)***. With high doses, falsely elevated ***serum and urine creatinine*** (with ***Jaffé reaction***) reported. False-positive ***direct Coombs test*** has also been reported.

INTERACTIONS Drug: Probenecid decreases renal elimination of cefoxitin. Avoid LIVE VACCINES.

PHARMACOKINETICS Peak: 20–30 min after IM; 5 min after IV. **Distribution:** Poor CNS penetration even with inflamed meninges; widely distributed in body tissues including pleural, synovial, and ascitic fluid and bile; crosses placenta. **Elimination:** 85% unchanged in urine in 6 h, small amount in breast milk. **Half-Life:** 45–60 min.

NURSING IMPLICATIONS

Assessment & Drug Effects

- Determine previous hypersensitivity to cephalosporins, penicillins, and other drug allergies before therapy is initiated.
- Monitor I&O rates and pattern: Nephrotoxicity occurs most frequently in patients older than 50 yr, in patients with impaired renal function, the debilitated, and in patients receiving high doses or other nephrotoxic drugs.
- Be alert to S&S of superinfections (see Appendix F). This condition is most apt to occur in older adult patients, especially when drug has been used for prolonged period.
- Report onset of diarrhea (may be dose related). If severe, pseudomembranous colitis (see Signs & Symptoms, Appendix F) **must be** ruled out. Older adult patients are especially susceptible.
- Monitor lab tests: Baseline C&S prior to therapy; CBC with differential, periodic renal function tests, test for *clostridium difficile* if patient develops diarrhea.
- Hematopoietic and hepatic function should be monitored in prolonged therapy.

Patient & Family Education

- Report promptly S&S of superinfection (see Appendix F).
- Report watery or bloody loose stools or severe diarrhea.
- Report severe vomiting or stomach pain.
- Report infusion site swelling, pain, or redness.
- Report development of fever.

CEFPODOXIME

(cef-po-dox'eem)

Classification: CEPHALOSPORIN ANTIBIOTIC; THIRD-GENERATION CEPHALOSPORIN
Therapeutic: ANTIBIOTIC
Prototype: Cefotaxime sodium

AVAILABILITY Tablet; liquid suspension

ACTION & THERAPEUTIC EFFECT Inhibits the final stage of bacterial cell wall synthesis by preferentially binding to specific penicillin-binding proteins (PBPs) within the bacterial cell wall. *Widely active against gram-positive and gram-negative bacteria and resistant beta-lactamase enzymes.*

USES Gonorrhea, otitis media, lower and upper respiratory tract infections, urinary tract infections, community-acquired pneumonia, skin/soft tissue infection.

C

CONTRAINDICATIONS Known hypersensitivity to cephalosporins. Safety and efficacy not established in infants younger than 2 mo.

CAUTIOUS USE History of Type I hypersensitivity reactions to penicillins; renal impairment; coagulopathy; history of colitis or other GI disease; pregnancy (category B); lactation; children.

ROUTE & DOSAGE

Respiratory Tract, Skin, and Soft Tissue Infections

Adult: **PO** 200 mg q12h for 10 days
Child: **PO** 5 mg/kg q12h × 10d

Urinary Tract Infections

Adult: **PO** 100 mg q12h × 5–7d

Community-Acquired Pneumonia

Adult: **PO** 200 mg q12h × 14 d

Gonorrhea

Adult: **PO** 200 mg as single dose

Otitis Media

Child (5 mo–12 yr): **PO** 5 mg/kg/dose q12h × 5d

ADMINISTRATION

Oral

- Give tablet with food to enhance absorption. Give suspension without regard to food.
- Give 1 h before or 2 h after an antacid.
- Consult prescriber regarding patients with renal impairment (i.e., creatinine clearance less than 30 mL/min); dosage intervals should be every 12 h.
- Preparation of suspension: To either the 50-mg/5-mL strength or the 100-mg/5-mL strength, add 25 mL of distilled water, then shake vigorously for 15 seconds. Next, to the 50-mg/5-mL strength add 33 mL, or to the 100-mg/5-mL strength add 32 mL of distilled water, and shake for at least 3 minutes.
- Store suspension for up to 14 days in a refrigerator [2°–8°C (36°–46°F)]. Shake well before using.

ADVERSE EFFECTS **Skin:** Diaper rash. **GI:** Diarrhea.

INTERACTIONS **Drug:** ANTACIDS may decrease absorption. May increase levels/effects of AMINOGLYCOSIDES, Vitamin K, or antagonists. Concurrent administration with cholera vaccine may reduce immune response. Avoid LIVE VACCINES. **Food:** Food may increase the absorption.

DIAGNOSTIC TEST INTERFERENCE Positive ***direct Coombs, false-positive urinary glucose test*** using cupric sulfate (Benedict solution, Clinitest, Fehling solution), false-positive serum or urine creatinine with Jaffé reaction.

PHARMACOKINETICS **Absorption:** 40–50% absorbed from GI tract. **Onset:** Therapeutic effect in 3 days. **Distribution:** Distributes well into inflammatory, pulmonary, and pleural fluid, and tonsils. Some distribution into prostate. 40% bound to plasma proteins. Distributed into breast milk. **Elimination:** 80% in urine. **Half-Life:** 2–3 h.

NURSING IMPLICATIONS

Assessment & Drug Effects

- Determine history of hypersensitivity reactions to cephalosporins and penicillins, and history of allergies, particularly to drugs, before therapy is initiated.

- Report onset of loose stools or diarrhea. Although pseudomembranous enterocolitis (see Appendix F) rarely occurs, this potentially life-threatening complication should be ruled out.
- Monitor for manifestations of hypersensitivity (see Appendix F). Discontinue drug and report S&S of hypersensitivity promptly.
- Monitor I&O (especially with high doses). Report significant changes.
- Monitor lab tests: Baseline C&S before initiation of therapy, CBC, hepatic and renal function.

Patient & Family Education

- Report any signs or symptoms of hypersensitivity immediately.
- Report loose stools or diarrhea.

CEFPROZIL

(cef′pro-zil)

Classification: CEPHALOSPORIN ANTIBIOTIC; SECOND-GENERATION CEPHALOSPORIN
Therapeutic: ANTIBIOTIC
Prototype: Cefaclor

AVAILABILITY Tablet; suspension

ACTION & THERAPEUTIC EFFECT

Generally resistant to hydrolysis by beta-lactamases. Preferentially binds to proteins in cell walls of susceptible organisms, thus killing gram-positive and gram-negative bacteria. *Third-generation cephalosporins are more active and have a broader spectrum against gram-negative bacteria than first- or second-generation of cephalosporins.*

USES Upper and lower respiratory tract infections, skin infections.

CONTRAINDICATIONS Known hypersensitivity to cephalosporin.

CAUTIOUS USE Hypersensitivity to penicillins, or other drugs; coagulopathy; renal impairment, renal disease; GI disease, especially colitis; suspension used in caution with patients with phenylketonuria; pregnancy (category B); infants (approved for use in children 6 mo and older).

ROUTE & DOSAGE

Pharyngitis/Tonsillitis/Acute Sinusitis

Adult: **PO** 500 mg q24h for 10 days
Child (2–12 yr): **PO** 7.5 mg/kg q12h × 10 d

Chronic Bronchitis

Adult: **PO** 500 mg q12h × 10 d

Otitis Media

Child (6 mo to 12 yr): **PO** 15 mg/kg q12h × 10 d

Skin Infection

Adult: **PO** 250–500 mg q12h or 500 q24h
Child (2–12 yr): **PO** 20 mg/kg q24h

Renal Impairment Dosage Adjustment

CrCl less than 29 mL/min: Reduce dose 50%

ADMINISTRATION

Oral

- Drug may be given without regard to meals.
- Consult prescriber for patients with impaired renal function. Dose is reduced by 50% when creatinine clearance is 0–29 mL/min.
- Administer after hemodialysis because drug is partially removed by dialysis.

C

- After reconstitution, oral suspension is refrigerated. Discard unused portion after 14 days.
- Store tablets between 15° and 30°C (59° and 86°F). Store powder for suspension between 15° and 25°C (59° and 77°F).

DIAGNOSTIC TEST INTERFERENCE

May cause a positive ***direct Coombs test***; false-positive reactions for ***urine glucose*** with ***copper reduction tests*** such as ***Benedict*** or ***Fehling solution*** or ***Clinitest tablets***.

INTERACTIONS **Drug: Probenecid** prolongs the elimination of cefprozil.

PHARMACOKINETICS **Absorption:** Readily from GI tract. **Peak:** 1–2 h. **Distribution:** Distributes into blister fluid at 50% of the serum level. **Elimination:** Primarily by kidneys. **Half-Life:** 1–2 h.

NURSING IMPLICATIONS

Assessment & Drug Effects

- Determine previous hypersensitivity to cephalosporins or penicillins before treatment.
- Withhold drug and notify prescriber if hypersensitivity occurs (e.g., rash, urticaria).
- Monitor for and report diarrhea, as pseudomembranous colitis is a potential adverse effect.
- Monitor for and report signs of superinfection (see Appendix F).
- When given concurrently with other cephalosporins or aminoglycosides, monitor for signs of nephrotoxicity.
- Monitor lab tests: Baseline C&S before therapy, renal function at baseline and during therapy for elderly or those with known or suspected renal impairment.

Patient & Family Education

- Report rash or other signs of hypersensitivity immediately.
- Report signs of superinfection (see Appendix F).
- Report loose stools and diarrhea even after completion of drug therapy.

CEFTAROLINE

(cef-tar′o-line)

Teflaro

Classification: CEPHALOSPORIN ANTIBIOTIC; THIRD-GENERATION CEPHALOSPORIN

Therapeutic: ANTIBIOTIC

Prototype: Cefotaxime

AVAILABILITY Powder for injection

ACTION & *THERAPEUTIC EFFECT*

It preferentially binds to one or more of the penicillin-binding proteins (PBPs) located on the cell walls of susceptible organisms. This inhibits the third and final stages of cell wall synthesis, thus destroying the bacterium. *Effective against certain gram-positive and gram-negative bacteria responsible for complicated, acute skin infections and community-acquired pneumonia.*

USES Treatment of acute bacterial skin and skin structure infections (ABSSSI) and community-acquired bacterial pneumonia (CABP) caused by susceptible microorganisms.

CONTRAINDICATIONS Known hypersensitivity to ceftaroline or other cephalosporins; *C. difficile*–associated diarrhea.

CAUTIOUS USE Previous hypersensitivity to penicillins or carbapenems; renal impairment; direct

Coombs test seroconversion; fetal risk cannot be ruled out; lactation. Safety and efficacy in children younger than 2 mo not established.

ROUTE & DOSAGE

Acute Bacterial Skin and Skin Structure Infections (ABSSSI) or Community-Acquired Bacterial Pneumonia (CABP)

Adult: **IV** 600 mg q12h for 5–14 days

Renal Impairment Dosage Adjustment

CrCl greater than 30 to 50 mL/min: 400 mg q12h; *15–30 mL/min:* 300 mg q12h; *less than 15 mL/min:* 200 mg q12h

Hemodialysis Dosage Adjustment

Administer dose after hemodialysis

ADMINISTRATION

Intravenous

PREPARE: **Intermittent:** Reconstitute the 400- or 600-mg vial with 20 mL of sterile water to yield 20 or 30 mg/mL, respectively. ▪ Mix gently then withdraw the required dose and add to at least 250 mL of NS, D5W, 2.5% DW, 0.45% NaCl, or LR. ▪ Do not mix with or add to solutions containing other drugs. ▪ Store diluted solution within the solution bag within 6 h when stored at room temperature or within 24 h when refrigerated at 2°–8°C (36°–46°F).

ADMINISTER: **Intermittent:** Slow IV infusion over 5–60 minutes. ▪ Monitor closely for S&S of hypersensitivity (see Appendix F). If suspected, stop infusion and notify prescriber immediately.

INCOMPATIBILITIES: **Y-site: Amphotericin B, caspofungin acetate, diazepam, dobutamine hydrochloride, filgrastim, isavuconazonium sulfate, labetalol hydrochloride, magnesium sulfate, potassium phosphate, sodium phosphate, tedizolid phosphate.**

ADVERSE EFFECTS **Skin:** Rash. **GI:** Diarrhea, vomiting. **Hematologic:** Positive direct Coombs test with no evidence of hemolysis.

DIAGNOSTIC TEST INTERFERENCE Ceftaroline can cause false-positive results for a ***Direct Coombs Test***.

INTERACTIONS **Drug: Probenecid** may decrease the renal excretion of ceftaroline. Do not give with LIVE VACCINES.

PHARMACOKINETICS **Peak:** 1 h. **Distribution:** Approximately 20% plasma protein bound. **Metabolism:** Dephosphorylated to active metabolite; hydrolyzed to inactive metabolite. **Elimination:** Primarily renal (88%) with minor fecal (6%). **Half-Life:** 1.6 h.

NURSING IMPLICATIONS

Assessment & Drug Effects

- Determine previous hypersensitivity reactions to cephalosporins and penicillins, and history of other allergies, particularly to drugs, before therapy is initiated.
- Monitor closely for S&S of hypersensitivity (see Appendix F).
- Monitor I&O rates and patterns, especially with concurrent aminoglycoside therapy. Report significant changes in I&O.
- Report promptly onset of diarrhea. If fever is present and diarrhea is severe, suspect antibiotic-associated pseudomembranous colitis (may occur during therapy

or following discontinuation of ceftaroline).

- Monitor lab tests: Baseline C&S before initiation of therapy; baseline and periodic kidney function tests, especially in the older adult; periodic serum electrolytes, CBC with differential, platelet count, and LFTs.

Patient & Family Education

- Report promptly frequent watery stools or bloody diarrhea.
- Yogurt or buttermilk may serve as a prophylactic against mild forms of diarrhea.
- Report any signs of hypersensitivity (see Appendix F).

CEFTAZIDIME

(sef′taz-i-deem)

Fortaz, Tazicef

Classification: CEPHALOSPORIN ANTIBIOTIC; THIRD-GENERATION CEPHALOSPORIN

Therapeutic: ANTIBIOTIC

Prototype: Cefotaxime sodium

AVAILABILITY Solution for injection; powder for solution for injection

ACTION & *THERAPEUTIC EFFECT* Preferentially binds to one or more of the penicillin-binding proteins (PBPs) located on cell walls of susceptible microbes; this inhibits the final stage of bacterial cell wall synthesis, leading to cell death of gram-negative and gram-positive bacterium. *More active and has a broader spectrum against aerobic gram-negative bacteria than do either first- or second-generation agents.*

USES To treat infections of lower respiratory tract, skin and skin structures, urinary tract, bones, and joints; also used to treat bacteremia, gynecologic, intra-abdominal, and CNS infections (including meningitis); management of pulmonary infections in patients with cystic fibrosis.

UNLABELED USES Surgical prophylaxis.

CONTRAINDICATIONS Hypersensitivity to ceftazidime or cephalosporins; viral disease.

CAUTIOUS USE Hypersensitivity to penicillins, or other drugs; coagulopathy, renal disease, renal or hepatic impairment; GI disease; colitis; older adults; pregnancy (category B); lactation, infant risk is minimal.

ROUTE & DOSAGE

Infection in Cystic Fibrosis

Adult: **IV** 90–150 mg/kg/day q8h
Child: **IV** 150–200 mg/kg/day divided q6–8h

Empiric Therapy

Adult: **IV** 2 g q8h

Uncomplicated Pneumonia/Skin or Soft Tissue Infection

Adult: **IM/IV** 500 mg –1 g q8h

Prosthetic Joint Infection

Adult: **IV** 2 g q8h × 4–6 wk

Severe Infection

Adult: **IV** 2 g q8h

Renal Impairment Dosage Adjustment

Adult: **IV/IM**
CrCl 31–50 mL/min: 1 g q12h; *CrCl 16–30 mL/min:* 1 g q24h; *CrCl 6–15 mL/min:* 500 mg q24h; *CrCl less than 5 mL/min:* 500 mg q48h

C

ADMINISTRATION

Intramuscular

- Reconstitute 500 mg by adding 3 mL sterile water or bacteriostatic water for injection or 0.5% or 1% lidocaine HCl injection to 1-g vial to yield 280 mg/mL.
- Inject into large muscle mass (e.g., upper outer quadrant of gluteus maximus or lateral part of thigh).

Intravenous

PREPARE: **Direct:** Using SW for injection: Add 5.3 mL to 500-mg vial then withdraw 5 mL for a 500-mg dose; or add 10 mL to 1-g vial then withdraw 10 mL for a 1-g dose; **Intermittent:** Prepare as for direct injection then further dilute with 50–100 mL of D5W, NS, D5NS, D10W, D5-0.225%NaCl, D5-0.45%NaCl, Ringer injection, 10% invert sugar water, Normosol(R)-M in D5W, 1/6M sodium lactate injection, or LR.

ADMINISTER: **Direct:** Give over 3–5 min. **Intermittent:** Give over 15–30 min. ▪ If given through a Y-type set, discontinue other solutions during infusion of ceftazidime.

INCOMPATIBILITIES: **Solution/additive:** **Amikacin, aminophylline, ranitidine, teicoplanin.** **Y-site:** **Acetylcysteine, alatrofloxacin, alemtuzumab, amiodarone, amphotericin B, ampicillin sodium, amsacrine, ascorbic acid, atracurium, azathioprine, azithromycin, blinatumomab, calcium chloride, caspofungin, cefotaxime, chloramphenicol, chlorpromazine, cisatracurium besylate, clarithromycin, dobutamine, dantrolene, danorubicin, diazepam, diazoxide, diphenhydramine, dobutamine, doxorubicin liposome, doxycycline, epirubicin, ganciclovir, garenoxacin mesylate, gemtuzumab, haloperidol, hydralazine hydrochloride, hydroxyzine, idarubicin, inamrinone lactate, isavuconazonium sulfate, lansoprazole, midazolam, minocycline, mitoxantrone, mycophenolate, nitroprusside, papaverine, pemetrexed, pentamidine, pentazocine, pentobarbital, phenytoin, piritramide, prochlorperazine, promethazine, protamine, quinupristin/dalfopristin, sulfamethoxazole/trimethoprim, temocillin, thiamine, ticarcillin, topotecan hydrochloride, verapamil, warfarin.**

- Store intact vials at 20°–25°C (68°–77°F). Protect sterile powder from light. Reconstituted solution is stable 7 days when refrigerated at 4°–5°C (39°–41°F); for 18–24 h when stored at 15°–30°C (59°–86°F). Stable for 24 wk if immediately frozen at –20° C (–4°F).

ADVERSE EFFECTS

Endocrine: Increased lactate dehydrogenase, increased gamma-glutamyl transferase. **Hepatic:** Increased ALT and serum AST. **Hematologic:** Eosinophilia.

DIAGNOSTIC TEST INTERFERENCE

False-positive reactions for ***urine glucose*** have been reported using ***copper sulfate*** (e.g., ***Benedict solution, Clinitest***). May cause positive ***direct antiglobulin (Coombs) test*** results, which can interfere with ***hematologic studies*** and ***transfusion cross-matching procedures***; false-positive serum or urine creatinine with Jaffé reaction.

C

INTERACTIONS **Drug: Probenecid** decreases renal elimination of ceftazidime. May reduce efficacy of bowel preparation kits. May impact efficacy of ORAL CONTRACEPTIVES. May increase bleeding risk with **warfarin.**

PHARMACOKINETICS **Peak:** 1 h. **Distribution:** CNS penetration with inflamed meninges; also penetrates bone, gallbladder, bile, endometrium, heart, skin, and ascitic and pleural fluids; crosses placenta. **Metabolism:** Not metabolized. **Elimination:** 80–90% unchanged in urine in 24 h; small amount in breast milk. **Half-Life:** 1.5–2 h.

NURSING IMPLICATIONS

Assessment & Drug Effects

- Determine history of hypersensitivity to cephalosporins and penicillins, and other drug allergies, before therapy begins.
- If administered concomitantly with another antibiotic, monitor renal function and report if symptoms of dysfunction appear (e.g., changes in I&O ratio and pattern, dysuria).
- Be alert to onset of rash, itching, and dyspnea. Check patient's temperature. If it is elevated, suspect onset of hypersensitivity reaction (see Appendix F).
- Monitor for superinfection. (See Appendix F).
- If diarrhea occurs and is severe, suspect pseudomembranous colitis (caused by *Clostridium difficile*). Report severe diarrhea to prescriber.
- Monitor lab tests: Baseline C&S before initiation of therapy; serum BUN/creatinine, prothrombin time in patients with renal or hepatic impairment, poor nutritional state, or receiving prolonged therapy.

Patient & Family Education

- Report loose stools or diarrhea promptly.
- Report any signs or symptoms of superinfection promptly (see Appendix F).

CEFTAZIDIME AND AVIBACTAM

(cef-ta-zi′deem and a-vi-bac′tam)

Avycaz

Classification: THIRD-GENERATION CEPHALOSPORIN (CEFTAZIDIME); NON-BETA-LACTAM BETA-LACTAMASE INHIBITOR (AVIBACTAM)

Therapeutic: ANTIBIOTIC

AVAILABILITY Sterile powder for reconstitution and injection

ACTION & *THERAPEUTIC EFFECT* Bactericidal action of **ceftazidime** is mediated through binding to essential penicillin-binding proteins (PBPs); **avibactam** inactivates some beta-lactamases and protects **ceftazidime** from degradation by certain beta-lactamases. *Drug has antibacterial activity against certain gram-negative and gram-positive bacteria.*

USES In combination with metronidazole for the treatment of complicated intra-abdominal infections as a single combination agent for the treatment of complicated urinary tract infections; hospital-acquired and ventilator-associated pneumonia.

CONTRAINDICATIONS Known serious hypersensitivity to ceftazidime, avibactam, or other members of the cephalosporin class.

CAUTIOUS USE History of penicillin allergy; renal impairment; seizures or other neurologic events. Pregnancy (category B); lactation (infant risk cannot be ruled out). Safety and efficacy in children younger than 18 yr not established.

ROUTE & DOSAGE

Complicated Infections

Adult: **IV** 2.5 g q8h for 5–14 days

Renal Impairment Dosage Adjustment

CrCL 31–50 mL/min: 1.25 g q8h
CrCL 16–30 mL/min: 0.94 g q12h
CrCL 6–15 mL/min: 0.94 g q24h
CrCL less than 6 mL/min: 0.94 g q48h

ADMINISTRATION

Intravenous

PREPARE: **Intermittent:** Reconstitute with 10 mL of one of the following: SW, NS, D5W, LR. Mix gently to yield ceftazidime 0.167 g/mL and avibactam 0.042 g/mL. Further dilute in NS, D5W, or LR to a total volume of 50–250 mL.
ADMINISTER: **Intermittent:** Infuse over 2 h. Monitor closely for anaphylaxis during the first dose.

- Store powder for solution at controlled temperature between 15° and 30°C (59° and 77°F).
- Store mixture at room temperature for up to 12 h and refrigerated for up to 24 h.

ADVERSE EFFECTS **GI:** Constipation, diarrhea, nausea, vomiting.

DIAGNOSTIC TEST INTERFERENCE Ceftazidime may cause a false-positive reaction for ***glucose tests*** in the urine. Use glucose tests based on enzymatic glucose oxidase reactions.

INTERACTIONS **Drug: Probenecid** decreases the elimination of avibactam. Do not use with LIVE VACCINES. May increase serum concentration of **tolvaptan.**

PHARMACOKINETICS **Distribution:** Minimal plasma protein binding. **Metabolism:** Minimal. **Elimination:** Renal excretion. **Half-Life:** 2.2 h (avibactam) and 3.3 h (ceftazidime).

NURSING IMPLICATIONS

Assessment & Drug Effects

- Monitor for and report promptly signs of hypersensitivity, including skin reactions. Stop infusion and contact prescriber if a hypersensitivity reaction is suspected.
- Report promptly the onset of diarrhea. Check for fever and monitor fluid and electrolyte balance.
- Monitor for and report promptly signs of adverse nervous system reactions (i.e., confusion, hallucinations, stupor, seizures, impaired motor activity).
- Monitor lab test: Baseline renal function tests, and repeat daily with renal impairment.

Patient & Family Education

- Report immediately if watery or bloody diarrhea develop up to 2 mo after treatment.
- Report immediately the following: Muscle rigidity, tremors, or difficulty with motor activity.
- Do not breastfeed while taking this drug without consulting a prescriber.

CEFTRIAXONE SODIUM

(sef-try-ax'one)

Classification: CEPHALOSPORIN ANTIBIOTIC; THIRD-GENERATION CEPHALOSPORIN
Therapeutic: ANTIBIOTIC
Prototype: Cefotaxime sodium

C

AVAILABILITY Solution for injection

ACTION & *THERAPEUTIC EFFECT* Preferentially binds to one or more of the penicillin-binding proteins (PBPs) located on cell walls of susceptible organisms. This inhibits third and final stages of bacterial cell wall synthesis, thus killing the bacterium. *Similar to other third-generation cephalosporins, ceftriaxone is effective against serious gram-negative organisms and also penetrates the CSF in concentrations useful in treatment of meningitis.*

USES Infections caused by susceptible organisms in lower respiratory tract, skin and skin structures, urinary tract, bones and joints; also intra-abdominal infections, pelvic inflammatory disease, uncomplicated gonorrhea, meningitis, and surgical prophylaxis.

CONTRAINDICATIONS Known hypersensitivity to cephalosporins; viral infections; neonates with hyperbilirubinemia 28 days or younger; neonates with calcium-containing infusions; signs and symptoms of gallbladder disease.

CAUTIOUS USE Hypersensitivity to penicillin or other drugs; impaired vitamin K synthesis; coagulopathy; hepatic or renal disease; history of GI disease, colitis; malnutrition, older adults; pregnancy (category B); lactation risk is minimal to infant.

ROUTE & DOSAGE

Moderate to Severe Infections, CAP, UTI

Adult: **IV/IM** 1–2 g q12–24h × 4–14 days (max: 4 g/day)
Child: **IV/IM** 50–75 mg/kg/day in 1–2 divided doses × 4–14 days (max: 2 g/day)

Bacterial Otitis Media

Child: **IM** 50 mg/kg (max: 1 g)

Prosthetic Joint Infection

Adult: **IV** 2 g q24h × 4–6 wk

Meningitis

Adult: **IV/IM** 2 g q12h
Child: **IV/IM** 100 mg/kg/day in 2 divided doses (max: 4 g/day)

Surgical Prophylaxis

Adult: **IV/IM** 1 g 30–120 min before surgery

ADMINISTRATION

Intramuscular

- Reconstitute the 1- or 2-g vial by adding 3.6 or 7.2 mL, respectively, of sterile water, NS, D5W, bacteriostatic water (with 0.9% benzyl alcohol), and 1% lidocaine solution (without epinephrine) for injection. Yields 350 mg/mL. See manufacturer's directions for other dilutions.
- Give deep IM into a large muscle.

Intravenous

IV administration to infants and children: Verify correct IV concentration and rate of infusion with prescriber.

PREPARE: **Intermittent:** Reconstitute each 250 mg with 2.4 mL of sterile water, D5W, NS, or D5/NS to yield 100 mg/mL. ▪ Further dilute with 50–100 mL of the selected IV solution.

ADMINISTER: **Intermittent:** Give over 30 min. Do not administer simultaneously with calcium-containing IV solutions, including infusions via a Y-site. In patients other than neonates (28 days and younger), ceftriaxone- and calcium-containing solutions may be administered sequentially if infusion lines are thoroughly flushed between infusions with a compatible fluid.

INCOMPATIBILITIES: **Solution/additive:** **Aminophylline, clindamycin, linezolid, theophylline, calcium**-containing products such as parenteral nutrition. **Y-site: Alatrofloxacin, alemtuzumab, amiodarone hydrochloride, amphotericin B cholesteryl complex, amsacrine, anakinra, ascorbic acid, blinatumomab, calcium**-containing products, **capreomycin, caspofungin, chloramphenicol, chlorpromazine, clindamycin, dacarbazine, dantrolene, daunorubicin, diazepam, diazoxide, diphenhydramine, dobutamine, dolasetron, doxorubicin, epirubicin, famotidine, filgrastim, fluconazole, ganciclovir, garenoxacin, gemtuzumab, haloperidol, hetastarch 6%, hydralazine, hydroxyzine, idarubicin, imipenem-cilastin, inamrinone lactate, irinotecan, labetalol, isavuconazonium sulfate, labetalol hydrochloride, leucovorin, magnesium sulfate, minocycline, mitoxantrone, mycophenolate, ondansetron hydrochloride, papaverine, pentamidine, pentazocine, pentobarbital, phenytoin, prochlorperazine, promethazine, propofol, protamine, quinupristin/dalfopristin, SMZ/TMP, tobramycin, vinorelbine.**

- Protect sterile powder from light. Store at 15°–25°C (59°–77°F).
- Reconstituted solutions: Diluent, concentration of solutions are determinants of stability. See manufacturer's instructions for storage.

ADVERSE EFFECTS

Skin: Warmth, tightness, or induration at injection site. **GI:** Diarrhea. **Hematologic:** Eosinophilia, thrombocythemia.

DIAGNOSTIC TEST INTERFERENCE

Positive ***direct Coombs***, false-positive urinary ***glucose test*** using nonenzymatic methods.

INTERACTIONS

Drug: Probenecid decreases renal elimination of ceftriaxone; effect of **warfarin** may be increased.

PHARMACOKINETICS

Peak: 1.5–4 h after IM; immediately after IV. **Distribution:** Widely in body tissues and fluids; good CNS penetration; crosses placenta. **Metabolism:** Not metabolized. **Elimination:** 33–65% unchanged in urine; also in bile and breast milk. **Half-Life:** 5–10 h.

NURSING IMPLICATIONS

Assessment & Drug Effects

- Determine history of hypersensitivity reactions to cephalosporins and penicillins and history of other allergies, particularly to drugs, before therapy is initiated.

C

- Inspect injection sites for induration and inflammation. Rotate sites. Note IV injection sites for signs of phlebitis (redness, swelling, pain).
- Monitor for manifestations of hypersensitivity (see Appendix F). Report promptly.
- Watch for and report: Petechiae, ecchymotic areas, epistaxis, or any unexplained bleeding. Ceftriaxone appears to alter vitamin K–producing gut bacteria; therefore, hypoprothrombinemic bleeding may occur.
- Report promptly development of diarrhea. The incidence of antibiotic-produced pseudomembranous colitis (see Appendix F) is higher than with most cephalosporins.
- Monitor lab tests: Baseline C&S before initiation of therapy, CBC, hepatic and renal function. PT and INR with concurrent warfarin.

Patient & Family Education

- Report any signs of bleeding.
- Report loose stools or diarrhea promptly.

CEFUROXIME SODIUM

(se-fyoor-ox'eem)

Zinacef

CEFUROXIME AXETIL

Ceftin ♣

Classification: CEPHALOSPORIN ANTIBIOTIC; SECOND-GENERATION CEPHALOSPORIN

Therapeutic: ANTIBIOTIC

Prototype: Cefaclor

AVAILABILITY Tablet; liquid suspension; solution for injection

ACTION & *THERAPEUTIC EFFECT* Preferentially binds to one or more of the penicillin-binding proteins (PBPs) located on cell walls of susceptible organisms. This inhibits third and final stages of bacterial cell wall synthesis, thus killing the bacterium. *Similar to other second-generation cephalosporins, cefuroxime is more active against gram-negative bacteria than are first-generation cephalosporins but not as active as third-generation cephalosporins.*

USES Infections caused by susceptible organisms in the lower respiratory tract, urinary tract, skin, and skin structures; also used for treatment of meningitis, gonorrhea, and otitis media and for perioperative prophylaxis (e.g., open-heart surgery), early Lyme disease.

CONTRAINDICATIONS Known hypersensitivity to cephalosporins; viral infections.

CAUTIOUS USE History of allergy, particularly to drugs; penicillin sensitivity; patients on anticoagulant therapy, renal insufficiency; history of seizures; history of poor nutritional status, colitis or other GI disease; suspension contains phenylalanine therefore cautious use in patients with PKU; pregnancy (category B); lactation.

ROUTE & DOSAGE

Bacterial Exacerbation of Chronic Bronchitis

Adult: **PO** 250–500 mg q12h × 10 d; **IV** 500–750 mg q8h

Bone/Joint Infections

Adult: **IV/IM** 1.5 g q8h

Pneumonia (Community-Acquired)

Adult: **IV/IM** 0.75–1.5 g q8h

Severe/Complicated Infections

Adult: **IV** 1.5 g q8h

Uncomplicated UTI

Adult: **PO** 250 bid × 7–10 days; **IV/IM** 750 mg q8h

Surgical Prophylaxis

Adult/Adolescent: **IV/IM** 1.5 g 30–60 min before surgery, then 750 mg q8h for 24 h
Child: **IV** 50 mg/kg within 60 min prior to surgery

Lyme Disease

Adult/Adolescent: **PO** 500 mg bid × 20 days

Renal Impairment Dosage Adjustment

CrCl 10–30 mL/min: **PO** Give q24h; *less than 10 mL/min:* Give q48h
CrCl 10–20 mL/min: **IV** give q12h; *less than 10 mL/min:* give q24h

ADMINISTRATION

Oral

- Cefuroxime tablets and oral suspension are not substitutable on a mg-for-mg basis and can be taken with or without food.
- The oral suspension is for infants and children 3 mo to 12 yr. Each teaspoon (5 mL) contains the equivalent of 125 mg cefuroxime. Shake oral suspension well before each use.

Intramuscular

- Shake IM suspension gently before administration. IM injections should be made deeply into large muscle mass. Rotate injection sites.

Intravenous

IV administration to neonates, infants, and children: Verify correct IV concentration and rate of infusion/injection with prescriber.

PREPARE: **Direct:** Dilute each 750 mg with 3 mL sterile water. **Intermittent:** Further dilute in 50–100 mL of D5W, 0.9% NS, or 0.45% NS. **Continuous:** May be added to 1000 mL of IV compatible solution.

ADMINISTER: **Direct:** Give slowly over 3–5 min. **Intermittent:** Give over 15–30 min. **Continuous:** Give over 6–24 h.

INCOMPATIBILITIES: **Solution/additive:** **Ciprofloxacin, sodium bicarbonate.** **Y-site:** **Alemtuzumab, amiodarone hydrochloride, amphotericin B conventional colloidal, ampicillin sodium, anakinra, azathioprine sodium, azathioprine, calcium chloride, caspofungin, chlorpromazine, clarithromycin, dantrolene, daunorubicin, dexamethasone, diazepam, diazoxide, diphenhydramine, dobutamine, dolasetron, doxorubicin, doxycycline, epirubicin, filgrastim, ganciclovir, garenoxacin, haloperidol, hydralazine, hydroxyzine, idarubicin, inamrinone, isavuconazonium sulfate, labetalol, magnesium, midazolam, minocycline, mitomycin, mitoxantrone, mycophenolate, nicardipine pantoprazole sodium, papaverine, pentamidine, pentazocine, pentobarbital, phenobarbital,**

phentolamine, phenytoin, piritramide, polymyxin B, prochlorperazine, promethazine, protamine, quinupristin/dalfopristin, sodium bicarbonate, SMZ/TMP, vinorelbine.

- Store powder protected from light unless otherwise directed between 20° and 25°C (68° and 77°F). After reconstitution, store suspension at room temperature for up to 24 h and up to 7 days when refrigerated at 5°C (41°F).

ADVERSE EFFECTS **GI:** Diarrhea, vomiting. **Hematologic:** Eosinophilia. **Other:** Jarisch–Herxheimer reaction.

DIAGNOSTIC TEST INTERFERENCE Cefuroxime causes false-positive (black-brown or green-brown color) ***urine glucose*** reaction with ***copper reduction reagents*** (e.g., ***Benedict*** or ***Clinitest***) but not with ***enzymatic glucose oxidase reagents*** (e.g., ***Clinistix, TesTape***). False-positive ***direct Coombs test*** (may interfere with ***cross-matching procedures*** and ***hematologic studies***) has been reported.

INTERACTIONS **Drug: Probenecid** decreases renal elimination of cefuroxime, thus prolonging its action. PROTON PUMP INHIBITORS or H_2-RECEPTOR ANTAGONISTS may decrease absorption of cefuroxime.

PHARMACOKINETICS **Absorption:** Well absorbed from GI tract; hydrolyzed to active drug in GI mucosa. **Peak:** PO 2 h; IM 30 min. **Distribution:** Widely distributed in body tissues and fluids; adequate CNS penetration with inflamed meninges; crosses placenta. **Elimination:** 66–100% in 24 h; in breast milk. **Half-Life:** 1–2 h.

NURSING IMPLICATIONS

Assessment & Drug Effects

- Determine history of hypersensitivity reactions to cephalosporins, penicillins, and history of allergies, particularly to drugs, before therapy is initiated.
- Report onset of loose stools or diarrhea. Pseudomembranous colitis (see Signs & Symptoms, Appendix F) should be ruled out as the cause of diarrhea during and after antibiotic therapy.
- Monitor for manifestations of hypersensitivity (see Appendix F). Discontinue drug and report their appearance promptly.
- Monitor lab tests: Baseline C&S before initiation of therapy, CBC, prothrombin time in patients at risk. Periodic renal function tests.

Patient & Family Education

- Report loose stools or diarrhea promptly.
- Report any signs or symptoms of hypersensitivity (see Appendix F).
- Combined estrogen and progesterone oral contraceptives may have reduced efficacy; choose alternative birth control methods.

CELECOXIB (Pr)

(cel-e-cox′ib)

Celebrex

Classification: ANALGESIC, NONSTEROIDAL ANTI-INFLAMMATORY DRUG (NSAID); CYCLOOXYGENASE-2 (COX-2) INHIBITOR; ANTI-INFLAMMATORY

Therapeutic: ANALGESIC, NSAID; COX-2 INHIBITOR; ANTIINFLAMMATORY; ANTIRHEUMATIC

C

AVAILABILITY Capsule

ACTION & *THERAPEUTIC EFFECT*
Inhibits prostaglandin synthesis by inhibiting cyclooxygenase-2 (COX-2) but does not inhibit cyclooxygenase-1 (COX-1). *Exhibits anti-inflammatory, analgesic, and antipyretic activities. Reduces or eliminates the pain of rheumatoid and osteoarthritis.*

USES Relief of S&S of osteoarthritis and rheumatoid arthritis. Treatment of acute pain and primary dysmenorrhea; ankylosing spondylitis, juvenile idiopathic arthritis.

CONTRAINDICATIONS Hypersensitivity to celecoxib, salicylate, or sulfonamide; asthmatic patients with aspirin triad; GI bleeding; advanced renal disease; development of S&S of renal impairment due to drug; severe hepatic impairment; development of S&S of hepatic impairment due to drug; anemia; pain from CABG surgery; pregnancy—fetal risk cannot be ruled out; lactation—infant risk cannot be ruled out.

CAUTIOUS USE Patients who are CYP2C9 poor metabolizers; patients who weigh less than 50 kg; mild or moderate hepatic impairment; elevated LTFs; renal insufficiency; prior history of GI bleeding or peptic ulcer disease; alcoholics; asthmatics; bone marrow suppression; CVA; PVD; fluid retention and/or HF; known risks for cardiovascular disease; kidney disease; hypertension; fluid retention; older adults; children with systemic-onset juvenile rheumatoid arthritis younger than 2 yr.

ROUTE & DOSAGE

Osteoarthritis/ Ankylosing Spondylitis

Adult: **PO** 100 mg bid or 200 mg daily

Rheumatoid Arthritis

Adult: **PO** 100–200 mg bid

Acute Pain, Dysmenorrhea

Adult: **PO** 400 mg 1st dose, then 200 mg same day if needed, then 200 mg bid prn

Juvenile Idiopathic Arthritis

Adolescent/Child (2 yr or older, weight greater than 25 kg): **PO** 100 mg bid
Child (2 yr or older, weight 10–25 kg): **PO** 50 mg bid

Hepatic Dosage Adjustment

Child–Pugh class B: Reduce dose by 50%

Pharmacogenetic Dosage Adjustment

Poor CYP2C9 metabolizers: Start with ½ normal dose

ADMINISTRATION

Oral

- Give 2 h before/after magnesium- or aluminum-containing antacids.
- Higher doses (400 mg twice daily) should be given with food to improve absorption.
- Contents of capsules can be added to a teaspoon of applesauce and ingested immediately with water.
- Store in tightly closed container and protect from light. Capsule and

solution can be stored at controlled room temperature between 20° and 25°C (68° and 77°F), with excursions permitted between 15° and 30°C (59° and 86°F)

ADVERSE EFFECTS (≥ 5%) **CV:** Familial adenomatous polyposis. **CNS:** Headache. **GI:** Diarrhea, nausea.

INTERACTIONS **Drug:** May diminish effectiveness of ACE INHIBITORS; **fluconazole** increases celecoxib concentrations; may increase **lithium** concentrations; may increase INR in older patients on **warfarin.** Do not use with **acemetacin,** PHOTOSENSITIZING AGENTS, **aspirin**, other NSAIDS, **cyclosporine.** Can enhance anticoagulant effect of other agents.

PHARMACOKINETICS **Peak:** 3 h. **Distribution:** 97% protein bound; crosses placenta. **Metabolism:** In liver by CYP2C9. **Elimination:** Primarily in feces (57%), 27% in urine. **Half-Life:** 11 h (adult); 6 h (child).

NURSING IMPLICATIONS

Black Box Warning

Celecoxib may increase the risk of serious, potentially fatal thrombosis (e.g., MI and stroke) and GI adverse events (e.g., bleeding, ulceration, and perforation).

Assessment & Drug Effects

- Monitor for S&S of GI bleeding that may occur suddenly and without warning, especially in older patients.
- Monitor blood pressure during initiation and throughout treatment course.
- Monitor for development of thrombotic events, even in those with no prior history of cardiovascular problems.
- Monitor closely lithium levels when the two drugs are given concurrently.
- Monitor closely PT/INR when used concurrently with warfarin.
- Monitor for fluid retention and edema, especially in those with a history of hypertension or CHF.
- Monitor lab tests: Periodic Hct and Hgb, LFTs, CBC, renal function tests, and serum electrolytes.

Patient & Family Education

- Seek immediate medical attention for any of the following: Chest pain, shortness of breath, sudden weakness, slurring of speech, or other S&S of a stroke.
- Promptly report any of the following: Unexplained weight gain, edema, skin rash.
- Stop taking celecoxib and promptly report to prescriber if any of the following occurs: S&S of liver dysfunction including nausea, fatigue, lethargy, itching, jaundice, abdominal pain, and flulike symptoms; S&S of GI ulceration including black, tarry stools and upper GI distress.
- Avoid use of nonprescription aspirin products or other NSAIDs.

CEPHALEXIN

(sef-a-lex′in)

Keflex

Classification: CEPHALOSPORIN ANTIBIOTIC; FIRST-GENERATION CEPHALOSPORIN

Therapeutic: ANTIBIOTIC

Prototype: Cefazolin

AVAILABILITY Capsule; oral suspension

ACTION & *THERAPEUTIC EFFECT* Preferentially binds to one or more of the penicillin-binding proteins

(PBPs) located on cell walls of susceptible organisms. This inhibits third and final stages of bacterial cell wall synthesis, thus killing the bacterium. *Broad-spectrum, first-generation cephalosporin active against many gram-positive aerobic cocci and much less active against gram-negative bacteria or anaerobic organisms.*

USES To treat infections caused by susceptible pathogens in respiratory and urinary tracts, middle ear, skin, soft tissue, and bone.

CONTRAINDICATIONS Known hypersensitivity to cephalosporin antibiotics; viral infections; prophylactic use.

CAUTIOUS USE History of hypersensitivity to penicillin or other drug allergy; severely impaired renal function; GI disease, colitis; hepatic disease; coagulopathy; pregnancy (category B); lactation. Safe use in younger than 1 yr not established.

ROUTE & DOSAGE

Cellulitis

Adult: **PO** 500 mg 4 × daily × 5 days
Child: **PO** 25–50 mg/kg/day in divided doses

Cystitis

Adult/Adolescent: **PO** 500 mg q12h × 5–7 days

Impetigo

Adult: **PO** 250–500 mg 4 × daily × 7 days
Child: **PO** 25–50 mg/kg/day in 3–4 divided doses

Streptococcal Pharyngitis

Adult: **PO** 500 q12h × 10 days
Child: **PO** 25–50 mg/kg/day divided q12h

Otitis Media

Child: **PO** 75–100 mg/kg/day in 4 divided doses

ADMINISTRATION

Oral

- Capsules should be stored at room temperature 15°–30°C (59°–86°F).
- Cephalexin oral suspension should be refrigerated; discard unused portions 14 days after preparation. Label should indicate expiration date. Keep tightly covered. Shake suspension well before pouring.

ADVERSE EFFECTS **CNS:** Dizziness, headache, fatigue. **Skin:** rash, urticaria. **GI:** Diarrhea, nausea, vomiting anorexia, abdominal pain. **Musculoskeletal:** Arthralgia. **Other:** Angioedema, anaphylaxis, superinfections.

DIAGNOSTIC TEST INTERFERENCE False-positive ***urine glucose*** determinations using ***copper sulfate reagents*** (e.g., ***Clinitest, Benedict reagent***). Positive ***direct Coombs test*** may complicate transfusion ***cross-matching procedures*** and ***hematologic studies***; false-positive serum or urine creatinine with ***Jaffé reaction***, false-positive urinary proteins and steroids.

INTERACTIONS **Drug: Probenecid** decreases renal elimination of cephalexin. **Metformin** can decrease absorption of cephalexin;

C

MULTIVITAMINS may decrease cephalexin concentration.

PHARMACOKINETICS

Absorption: Rapidly from GI tract; stable in stomach acid. **Peak:** 1 h. **Distribution:** Widely distributed in body fluids with highest concentration in kidney; crosses placenta. **Elimination:** 80–100% unchanged in urine in 8 h; excreted in breast milk. **Half-Life:** 38–70 min.

NURSING IMPLICATIONS

Assessment & Drug Effects

- Determine history of hypersensitivity reactions to cephalosporins and penicillin and history of other drug allergies before therapy is initiated.
- Monitor for manifestations of hypersensitivity (see Signs & Symptoms, Appendix F). Discontinue drug, and report their appearance promptly.
- Monitor lab tests: Periodic renal function tests, CBC, and LFTs with prolonged therapy.

Patient & Family Education

- Keep prescriber informed if adverse reactions appear.
- Be alert to S&S of superinfections (see Appendix F). These symptoms should be reported promptly and appropriate therapy instituted.

CERITINIB

(ce-ri'ti-nib)

Zykadia

Classification: ANTINEOPLASTIC; KINASE INHIBITOR

Therapeutic: ANTINEOPLASTIC

Prototype: Erlotinib

AVAILABILITY

Capsule

ACTION & THERAPEUTIC EFFECT

Potent inhibitor of anaplastic lymphoma kinase (ALK), an enzyme involved in the pathogenesis of non-small-cell lung cancer. ALK gene mutations may result in expression of oncogenic fusion proteins that increase cellular proliferation and survival of tumor cells that express these fusion proteins. *ALK inhibition reduces proliferation of lung cancer cells expressing the genetic alteration.*

USES

Treatment of anaplastic lymphoma kinase (ALK) positive metastatic non-small-cell lung cancer (NSCLC) in patients who have progressed on or are intolerant to crizotinib.

CONTRAINDICATIONS

Severe hepatotoxicity, severe QTc prolongation, or interstitial lung disease (ILD)/pneumonitis due to drug use; pregnancy (category D); lactation.

CAUTIOUS USE

GI, hepatic, or pulmonary toxicity; QTc prolongation; CHF; bradycardia; DM, hyperglycemia. Safety and efficacy in children younger than 18 yr not established.

ROUTE & DOSAGE

Non-Small-Cell Lung Cancer (NSCLC)

Adult: **PO** 750 mg daily

Concomitant Use of Strong CYP3A4 Inducers/Inhibitors Dosage Adjustment

Reduce dose by approximately one-third, rounded to nearest 150-mg dosage strength if taken with a strong CYP3A4 inhibitor. If strong CYP3A4 inhibitor is discontinued, resume previous dose. Avoid concomitant use with strong CYP3A4 inducers

Hepatic Impairment Dosage Adjustment

ALT or AST elevation greater than 5 × ULN with total bilirubin 2 × ULN or less: Withhold until recovery or 3 × ULN or less, resume with 150-mg dose reduction
ALT or AST elevation greater than 3 × ULN with total bilirubin 2 × ULN or greater in the absence of cholestasis or hemolysis: Permanently discontinue

Treatment-Related Toxicity Dosage Adjustment

Any grade interstitial lung disease (ILD) or pneumonitis: Permanently discontinued
Cardiac (QT prolongation, bradycardia), metabolic (hyperglycemia) and GI toxicities: See manufacturer's guidelines.

ADMINISTRATION

Oral

- Give on an empty stomach at least 2 h before/after a meal.
- Store at 15°–30°C (59°–86°F).

ADVERSE EFFECTS **CV:** Bradycardia, prolonged QT interval. **Respiratory:** Interstitial pulmonary disease. **HEENT:** Visual disturbances. **Endocrine:** Decreased serum phosphate, hyperglycemia, *increased serum ALT and AST*, increased serum bilirubin, increased serum creatinine, increased serum lipase. **Skin:** Acneiform dermatitis, maculopapular rash. **GI:** Abdominal pain, constipation, decreased appetite, *diarrhea*, dyspepsia, dysphagia, gastroesophageal reflux disease, *nausea, vomiting*. **Hematological:** Decreased hemoglobin. **Other:** Fatigue, neuropathy.

INTERACTIONS **Drug:** Strong CYP3A4 inhibitors (e.g., **ketoconazole**, MACROLIDE ANTIBIOTICS, **nefazodone, ritonavir**) increase the levels of ceritinib. Strong CYP3A4 inducers (e.g., **carbamazepine, phenytoin, rifampin**) decrease the levels of ceritinib. **Food:** Grapefruit and grapefruit juice may increase the levels of ceritinib. **Herbal: St. John's wort** decreases the levels of ceritinib.

PHARMACOKINETICS **Peak:** 4–6 h. **Distribution:** 97% plasma protein bound. **Metabolism:** Hepatic oxidation. **Elimination:** Primarily fecal (92%). **Half-Life:** 41 h.

NURSING IMPLICATIONS

Assessment & Drug Effects

- Monitor diabetics or those with glucose intolerance for loss of glycemic control (i.e., hyperglycemia).
- Monitor for and report promptly S&S of GI or hepatic toxicity, pneumonitis (e.g., shortness of breath, chest pain, cough with/without mucus), or cardiac arrhythmias (e.g., QTc prolongation and bradycardia with heart rate less than 50).
- Monitor lab tests: Baseline and periodic CBC with differential, LFTs, renal function tests, and blood glucose.

C

Patient & Family Education

- Do not drink grapefruit juice or eat grapefruit during treatment.
- Report promptly to prescriber if you experience any of the following: Severe or persistent GI distress or signs of liver toxicity (e.g., excessive fatigue, jaundice, loss of appetite, itchy skin, nausea and vomiting, abdominal pain); shortness of breath or chest pain; abnormal heartbeats (palpitations), light-headedness, or dizziness.
- Tell prescriber if you are taking any OTC drugs for reflux or acid stomach.
- Women of reproductive age should avoid pregnancy during treatment with this drug.
- Do not breastfeed while taking this drug.

CERTOLIZUMAB PEGOL

(cer-to'li-zu-mab)

Cimzia

Classification: BIOLOGIC RESPONSE MODIFIER; IMMUNOMODULATOR; DISEASE-MODIFYING ANTIRHEUMATIC (DMARD)

Therapeutic: DMARD; ANTIRHEUMATIC

Prototype: Etanercept

AVAILABILITY Powder for injection

ACTION & *THERAPEUTIC EFFECT*

A fragment of an antibody Fab fragment with specificity for tumor necrosis factor (TNF)-alpha. This causes a reduction in the production of proinflammatory cytokines including interleukin-1 beta as well as TNF-alpha. Increased levels of TNF-alpha are found in the bowel wall areas that are affected by Crohn disease and RA. *Reduces inflammatory cytokine production in Crohn disease. It also decreases the serum level of C-reactive protein, a direct measure of the inflammatory process related to Crohn disease. Effective for treatment of adults with moderately to severely active rheumatoid arthritis.*

USES Treatment of moderately to severely active Crohn disease; ankylosing spondylitis; moderate to severely active rheumatoid arthritis; plaque psoriasis, psoriatic arthritis, nonradiographic axial spondyloarthritis.

CONTRAINDICATIONS Active chronic or localized infections (e.g., TB, histoplasmosis, other fungal infections); hypersensitivity to certolizumab pegol or any component of the product, HBV reactivation; lupus-like syndrome; pregnancy—fetal risk cannot be ruled out; lactation—infant risk cannot be ruled out.

CAUTIOUS USE History of recurrent infection; concurrent immunosuppressive therapy; past/current residence in region where TB and histoplasmosis are endemic; CNS demyelinating disease; neurologic disorders, including seizure disorder, optic neuritis, peripheral neuropathy; recurrent/previous hematologic disorders; heart failure; hypersensitivity response to other TNF blocker(s); latex sensitivity, older adults. Safety and efficacy in children not established.

ROUTE & DOSAGE

Crohn Disease

Adult: **Subcutaneous** 400 mg (two 200-mg injections) at wk 0, 2, and 4, then 400 mg q4wk

Ankylosing Spondylitis, Nonradiographic Axial Spondyloarthritis
Adult: **Subcutaneous** 400 mg, repeat 2 and 4 weeks after initial dose; then 200 mg q2w OR 400 mg q4w.

Plaque Psoriasis
Adult: **Subcutaneous** 400 mg every other week

Rheumatoid Arthritis
Adult: **Subcutaneous** Two 200-mg injections, at wk 0, 2, and 4, then 200 mg every other week

ADMINISTRATION

Subcutaneous

- Reconstitute two 200-mg vials by adding 1 mL sterile water to each using a 20-gauge needle. Swirl gently then allow to sit to dissolve (may require up to 30 min); yields 200 mg/mL. Use within 2 h of reconstitution or refrigerate for up to 24 h.
- Use two separate syringes with 20-gauge needles; withdraw 1 mL from each vial. Change to 23-gauge needles and inject into two separate sites on the abdomen or thigh.
- Store reconstituted solution. May be kept at room temperature for no longer than 2 h and refrigerated for up to 24 h. Protect from light. Do not freeze.

ADVERSE EFFECTS (≥ 5%) Respiratory: Upper respiratory infection. **GU:** Pyelonephritis. **Musculoskeletal:** *Arthralgia*. **Other:** *Increased risk of serious infections (bacterial, mycobacterial, fungal, viral).*

DIAGNOSTIC TEST INTERFERENCE Certolizumab may cause erroneously elevated ***activated partial thromboplastin time (aPTT)*** assay results; can cause false-negative in tests for latent tuberculosis.

INTERACTIONS Drug: Coadministration of **anakinra, abatacept** may cause increased risks of serious infections and neutropenia. Do not use with TNF ALPHA BLOCKERS, LIVE VACCINES, DMARDS, IMMUNOSUPPRESANTS. **Herbal:** Recommend not using **echinacea**.

PHARMACOKINETICS Absorption: 80% bioavailable. **Peak:** 54–171 h. **Half-Life:** 14 days.

NURSING IMPLICATIONS

Black Box Warning

Certolizumab has been associated with serious, potentially fatal, infections.

Assessment & Drug Effects

- Prior to initiating therapy, patient should be evaluated for TB risk factors and latent TB. Monitor for S&S of TB throughout therapy.
- Report promptly any S&S of infection or hypersensitivity reaction. (See Appendix F for S&S.)
- Monitor closely carriers of HBV for signs of active infection. If suspected, withhold injection and notify prescriber.
- Monitor closely patients with heart failure for worsening cardiac status.
- Monitor for and report promptly any abnormal neurologic finding or unexplained bruising or bleeding.
- Monitor lab tests: Baseline TB test; periodic CBC with platelet count.

C

Patient & Family Education

- Report promptly any of the following: S&S of infections, such as persistent fever; signs of an allergic reaction (e.g., hives, itching, swelling); unexplained bleeding or bruising.
- Do not accept vaccination with live (or attenuated) vaccines while on certolizumab.
- Counsel, instruct patient regarding proper subcutaneous injection technique and rotation.

CETIRIZINE

(ce-tir'i-zeen)

Reactine ♣, Zyrtec

LEVOCETIRIZINE

(LEV-O-CE-TIR'I-ZEEN)

Xyzal

Classification: ANTIHISTAMINE; H_1-RECEPTOR ANTAGONIST; NONSEDATING

Therapeutic: ANTIHISTAMINE, NONSEDATING

Prototype: Loratadine

AVAILABILITY Tablet; chewable tablet; syrup. **Levocetirizine:** Syrup; tablet

ACTION & *THERAPEUTIC EFFECT* A potent H_1-receptor antagonist and an antihistamine without significant anticholinergic or CNS activity. Low lipophilicity combined with its H_1-receptor selectivity probably accounts for its relative lack of anticholinergic and sedative properties. *Effectively treats allergic rhinitis and chronic urticaria by eliminating or reducing the local and systemic effects of histamine release.*

USES Seasonal and perennial allergic rhinitis and chronic idiopathic urticaria.

CONTRAINDICATIONS Hypersensitivity to H_1-receptor antihistamines or hydroxyzine; lactation.

CAUTIOUS USE Moderate to severe renal impairment, hepatic impairment, pregnancy (category B), children.

ROUTE & DOSAGE

Allergic Rhinitis

Adult: **PO** 5–10 mg once/day
Child (2 to younger than 6 yr): **PO** 2.5 mg daily (max: 5 mg/day); *6 yr or older:* 5–10 mg daily

Allergic Rhinitis (Levocetirizine)

Adult/Adolescent/Child (6 yr or older): **PO** 2.5–5 mg once/day
Child (2 to younger than 6 yr): **PO** 1.25 mg each evening

Chronic Urticaria

Adult: **PO** 10 mg daily or bid

Chronic Urticaria (Levocetirizine)

Adult/Adolescent/Child (6 yr or older): **PO** 2.5–5 mg each evening
Child (6 mo to younger than 6 yr): **PO** 1.25 mg each evening

Renal Impairment Dosage Adjustment (Levocetirizine)

CrCl 51–80 mL/min: 2.5 mg daily; *30–50 mL/min:* 2.5 mg every other day; *10–29 mL/min:* 2.5 mg twice a week; *less than 10 mL/min:* Do not use

ADMINISTRATION

Oral

- May be administered with or without food.
- Consult prescriber about dosage if significant adverse effects appear. As elimination half-life is prolonged in the older adult, dosage adjustments may be warranted.
- Store at 20°–25°C (68°–77°F); excursions at 15°–30°C (59°–86°F).

ADVERSE EFFECTS **CV:** Syncope. **CNS:** *Drowsiness, sedation, headache*, depression. **GI:** Constipation, diarrhea, dry mouth.

INTERACTIONS **Drug: Theophylline** may decrease cetirizine clearance leading to toxicity. Use with **scopolamine** or **atropine** may cause anticholinergic effects. Alcohol may enhance the CNS depressant effect. May enhance the depressant effect of CNS depressants.

PHARMACOKINETICS **Absorption:** Readily from GI tract. **Peak:** 1 h. **Distribution:** 93% protein bound; minimal CNS concentrations. **Metabolism:** Minimal (by CYP3A4). **Elimination:** 60% unchanged in urine within 24 h, 5% in feces. **Half-Life:** 7.4 h (cetirizine), 8–9 h (levocetirizine).

NURSING IMPLICATIONS

Assessment & Drug Effects

- Monitor for drug interactions. As the drug is highly protein bound, the potential for interactions with other protein-bound drugs exists.
- Monitor for sedation, especially the older adult.

Patient & Family Education

- Do not use in combination with OTC antihistamines.
- Do not engage in driving or other hazardous activities, before experiencing your responses to the drug.

CETRORELIX

(ce-tro-re'lix)

Cetrotide

Classification: GONADOTROPIN-RELEASING HORMONE (GnRH) ANTAGONIST

Therapeutic: LUTEINIZING HORMONE-RELEASING HORMONE RECEPTOR ANTAGONIST

AVAILABILITY Solution for injection

ACTION & *THERAPEUTIC EFFECT* Competes with natural GnRH for binding to membrane receptors on pituitary cells and thus controls the release of LH and FSH. *Prevents premature LH surges in patients undergoing controlled ovarian hyperstimulation for assisted reproduction.*

USES Treatment of infertility as part of an assisted reproduction program.

UNLABELED USES BPH, endometriosis.

CONTRAINDICATIONS Hypersensitivity to cetrorelix, extrinsic peptide hormones, mannitol, gonadotropin-releasing hormone analogs; primary ovarian failure; renal failure; pregnancy (category X);

known or suspected pregnancy; lactation.

C

CAUTIOUS USE Hepatic insufficiency; polycystic ovary syndrome.

ROUTE & DOSAGE

Infertility

Adult: **Subcutaneous** 0.25 mg/days during early to mid-follicular phase of the cycle (stimulation day 5 or 6) following the initiation of FSH or 3 mg as a single dose is administered when the serum estradiol level is indicative of an appropriate stimulation response, usually on FSH stimulation day 7 (range day 5–9). If HCG has not been administered within 4 days after the injection of 3 mg, then 0.25 mg should be administered once daily until HCG administration.

ADMINISTRATION

Subcutaneous

- Reconstitute the 0.25- or 3-mL vial with 1 or 3 mL, respectively, of sterile water for injection.
- Inject into lower abdominal wall following reconstitution. Rotate injection sites.
- Store the 3-mg dose at room temperature, 15°–30°C (59°–86°F). Store the 0.25-mg dose in the refrigerator.

ADVERSE EFFECTS **CNS:** Headache. **Endocrine:** Hot flashes. **Skin:** Pruritus at injection site. **GI:** Nausea, vomiting, abdominal pain. **GU:** Ovarian enlargement, ovarian hyperstimulation syndrome, pelvic pain.

INTERACTIONS **Drug: Cimetidine, methyldopa, metoclopramide**, PHENOTHIAZINES may interfere with fertility efforts. **Herbal: Black cohosh, DHEA** may antagonize fertility efforts.

PHARMACOKINETICS **Absorption:** 85% absorbed from subcutaneous injection site. **Peak:** 1–2 h. **Metabolism:** Metabolized by peptidases. **Elimination:** 2–4% in urine, 5–10% in bile. **Half-Life:** 62 h after single dose, 20 h after multiple doses.

NURSING IMPLICATIONS

Assessment & Drug Effects

- Monitor weight and report development of edema and/or shortness of breath.
- Monitor lab tests: Routine blood chemistries.

Patient & Family Education

- Contact prescriber immediately for any of the following: Abdominal or stomach pain, persistent or severe nausea, vomiting or diarrhea; decreased urination; pelvic pain; moderate to severe bloating, rapid weight gain; shortness of breath; swelling of lower legs.

CETUXIMAB

(ce-tux′i-mab)

Erbitux

Classification: ANTINEOPLASTIC; MONOCLONAL ANTIBODY; EPIDERMAL GROWTH FACTOR RECEPTOR (EGFR) INHIBITOR
Therapeutic: ANTINEOPLASTIC
Prototype: Erlotinib

C

AVAILABILITY Solution for injection

ACTION & THERAPEUTIC EFFECT Cetuximab is a recombinant, monoclonal antibody that binds specifically to the epidermal growth factor receptor (EGFR, HER1, c-ErbB-1) on both normal and tumor cells. Binding to the EGFR results in inhibition of cell growth, induction of apoptosis, and decreased vascular endothelial growth factor production. *Overexpression of EGFR is detected in many human cancers, including those of the colon and rectum. Cetuximab inhibits the growth and survival of tumor cells that overexpress the EGFR.*

USES Metastatic colorectal cancer, squamous cancer of head and neck.

CONTRAINDICATIONS Lactation within 60 days of using cetuximab; worsening of preexisting pulmonary edema or interstitial lung disease; serious infusion reaction to drug.

CAUTIOUS USE Infusion reaction, especially with first-time users; history of hypersensitivity to murine proteins or cetuximab; cardiac disease, coronary artery disease, CHF, arrhythmias; pulmonary disease, pulmonary fibrosis; UV exposure, radiation therapy; older adults; pregnancy (category C). Safety in children not established.

ROUTE & DOSAGE

Colorectal Cancer/Head and Neck Cancer

Adult: **IV** Start with 400 mg/m^2 over 2 h; continue with 250 mg/m^2 over 1 h weekly

ADMINISTRATION

Intravenous

Administer with full resuscitation equipment available and under the supervision of a prescriber experienced with chemotherapy. ▪ Premedication with an H_1-receptor antagonist (e.g., diphenhydramine 50 mg IV) is recommended. ▪ Monitor for an infusion reaction for at least 1 h following completion of infusion.

PREPARE: **IV Infusion:** ▪ Do not shake or further dilute vial. Do not mix with other medication. ▪ Inject cetuximab solution into a sterile, evacuated container or bag (i.e., glass, polyolefin, ethylene vinyl acetate, DEHP plasticized PVC, or PVC); repeat until needed dose has been added to container, using a new needle for each vial. ▪ Attach to infusion set with a low-protein-binding 0.22-micron filter and prime line with cetuximab. May also administer by syringe and syringe pump; use a new needle and filter for each vial.

ADMINISTER: **IV Infusion: Do not** administer a bolus dose. ▪ Give IV infusion via an infusion pump or syringe pump; use a low-protein-binding 0.22-micron in-line filter. Give initial infusion over 120 min and subsequent infusions over 60 min. Do not exceed 10 mg/min. ▪ Flush line with NS after infusion.

INCOMPATIBILITIES: **Solution/additive:** Do not mix with other additives.

▪ Store unopened vials at 2°–8°C (36°–46°F). Note: Vials may contain a small amount of easily visible, white particles. ▪ Cetuximab in IV bag is stable for up to 12 h

C

refrigerated and up to 8 h at 20°–25°C (68°–77°F).

ADVERSE EFFECTS **CV:** Cardiopulmonary arrest. **Respiratory:** Pulmonary embolism, pulmonary fibrosis (rare), *dyspnea,* cough. **CNS:** *Headache,* insomnia, depression, fatigue. **Endocrine:** Weight loss, peripheral edema, dehydration, hypomagnesemia, hypokalemia. **Skin:** *Rash,* alopecia, pruritus, desquamation, radiodermatitis, changes in nails, acne vulgaris. **Hepatic:** Increased AST, ALT, ASP. **GI:** *Nausea, vomiting, diarrhea, abdominal pain, constipation,* stomatitis, dyspepsia. **GU:** Kidney failure. **Hematologic:** Leukopenia, anemia, neutropenia. **Other:** Infusion reactions (allergic reaction, anaphylactoid reaction, fever, chills, dyspnea, bronchospasm stridor, hoarseness, urticaria, hypotension), *fever,* sepsis, *asthenia, malaise,* pain, infection.

INTERACTIONS Do not use with **penicillamine.**

PHARMACOKINETICS **Half-Life:** 114 h (75–188 h).

NURSING IMPLICATIONS

Black Box Warning

Cetuximab has been associated with severe, potentially fatal, infusion reactions, and with cardiopulmonary arrest.

Assessment & Drug Effects

- Monitor throughout infusion and for 1 h after completion of infusion for development of an infusion reaction.
- Discontinue infusion immediately and notify prescriber for S&S of a severe infusion reaction: Chills, fever, bronchospasm, stridor, hoarseness, urticaria, and/or hypotension. Carefully monitor until complete resolution of all S&S.
- Monitor pulmonary status and report onset of acute or worsening pulmonary symptoms.
- Premedication with antihistamines is recommended.
- Monitor lab tests: Periodic serum magnesium, calcium, and potassium over 8 wk.

Patient & Family Education

- Report immediately: Difficulty breathing, wheezing, shortness of breath, hives, faintness and/or dizziness anytime during IV infusion.
- Report promptly any of the following: Eye inflammation, mouth sores, skin rash, redness, or severe dry skin.
- Wear sunscreen and a hat and limit sun exposure while being treated with this drug.

CEVIMELINE HYDROCHLORIDE

(cev-i-may'leen)

Evoxac

Classification: CHOLINERGIC AGONIST; CHOLINERGIC ENHANCER

Therapeutic: CHOLINERGIC RECEPTOR ENHANCER

AVAILABILITY Capsule

ACTION & *THERAPEUTIC EFFECT* Cholinergic agent that binds to muscarinic receptors. *Increases secretion of exocrine glands, such as salivary and sweat glands. It relieves severe dry mouth.*

USES Treatment of dry mouth in patients with Sjögren syndrome.

CONTRAINDICATIONS Hypersensitivity to cevimeline; uncontrolled asthma; acute iritis; narrow-angle glaucoma; lactation.

CAUTIOUS USE Controlled asthma; chronic bronchitis, COPD; cardiac disease, cardiac arrhythmias, myocardial infarction; history of nephrolithiasis or cholelithiasis; older adults; pregnancy (category C). Safety and efficacy in children not established.

ROUTE & DOSAGE

Dry Mouth

Adult: **PO** 30 mg tid

ADMINISTRATION

Oral

- May be administered with food to decrease GI upset.
- Store refrigerated at 2°–8°C (35.6°–46.4°F) with occasional fluctuations at 15°–30°C (59°–86°F).

ADVERSE EFFECTS **CV:** Peripheral edema, chest pain, palpitations. **Respiratory:** *Rhinitis, sinusitis, upper respiratory tract infection,* pharyngitis, bronchitis. **CNS:** Insomnia, anxiety, vertigo, depression, hyporeflexia. **HEENT:** Abnormal vision. **Skin:** Rash, conjunctivitis, pruritus. **GI:** *Nausea, diarrhea,* excessive salivation, dyspepsia, abdominal pain, coughing, vomiting, constipation, anorexia, dry mouth, hiccup. **GU:** Urinary tract infection. **Other:** *Excessive sweating, headache,* back pain, dizziness, fatigue, pain, hot flushes, rigors, tremor, hypertonia, myalgia, fever, eye pain, earache, flulike symptoms.

INTERACTIONS **Drug:** BETA-ADRENERGIC AGONISTS may cause conduction disturbances; PARASYMPATHOMIMETIC DRUGS may have additive effects.

PHARMACOKINETICS **Absorption:** Rapidly absorbed. **Peak:** 1.5–2 h. **Distribution:** Less than 20% protein bound. **Metabolism:** In liver by CYP2D6 and 3A3/4. **Elimination:** Primarily in urine. **Half-Life:** 5 h.

NURSING IMPLICATIONS

Assessment & Drug Effects

- Monitor for S&S of increased airway resistance, especially in patient with asthma, bronchitis, emphysema, or COPD.
- Report S&S of excess cholinergic activity (e.g., diaphoresis, frequent urge to urinate, nausea and/or diarrhea).
- Monitor lab tests: Routine blood chemistry during long-term therapy.

Patient & Family Education

- Do not drive or engage in potentially hazardous activities until response to drug is known.
- Consult prescriber if confusion, dizziness, or faintness occur.
- Report diminished night vision or depth perception.
- Drink fluids liberally (2000–3000 mL/day) in the event of excessive sweating.

CHARCOAL, ACTIVATED (LIQUID ANTIDOTE)

Actidose, CharcoAid, Charcocaps, Charcodote, Insta-Char

Classification: ANTIDOTE; ADSORBENT

Therapeutic: ANTIDOTE

AVAILABILITY Liquid suspension

ACTION & THERAPEUTIC EFFECT Acts by binding (adsorbing) toxic substances, thereby inhibiting their GI absorption, enterohepatic circulation, and thus bioavailability. *Action appears to result from drug diffusion from plasma into GI tract, where it is adsorbed by activated charcoal. Effectively adsorbs toxins in the gut preventing their systemic absorption and impact.*

USES General-purpose emergency antidote in the treatment of poisonings by most drugs and chemicals. Gastric dialysis (repetitive doses) in uremia to adsorb various waste products from GI tract; severe acute poisoning. Has been used to adsorb intestinal gases in treatment of dyspepsia, flatulence, and distention (value in these conditions not established). Sometimes used topically as a deodorant for foul-smelling wounds and ulcers.

CONTRAINDICATIONS Reportedly not effective for poisonings by cyanide, mineral acids, caustic alkalis, organic solvents, iron, ethanol, methanol; gag reflex depression, coma; GI obstruction; quinidine or quinine hypersensitivity.

CAUTIOUS USE Pregnancy (category C); lactation.

ROUTE & DOSAGE

Acute Poisonings

Adult: **PO** 30–100 g in at least 180–240 mL (6–8 oz) of water or 1 g/kg
Child (1–12 yr): **PO** 1–2 g/kg or 15–30 g in at least 6–8 oz of water
Infant (younger than 1 yr): **PO** 1 g/kg

Gastric Dialysis

Adult: **PO** 20–40 g q6h for 1 or 2 days

GI Disturbances

Adult: **PO** 520–975 mg p.c. up to 5 g/day

ADMINISTRATION

Oral

- In an emergency, dose may be approximated by stirring sufficient activated charcoal into tap water to make a slurry the consistency of soup (about 20–30 g in at least 240 mL of water).
- Activated charcoal can be swallowed or given through a nasogastric tube. If administered too rapidly, patient may vomit.
- Store in tightly covered container.

ADVERSE EFFECTS **GI:** Vomiting (rapid ingestion of high doses), constipation, diarrhea (from sorbitol).

INTERACTIONS **Drug:** May decrease absorption of all other oral medications—administer at least 2 h apart.

PHARMACOKINETICS **Absorption:** Not absorbed. **Elimination:** In feces.

NURSING IMPLICATIONS

Assessment & Drug Effects

- Record appearance, color, consistency, frequency, and relative amount of stools. Inform patient that activated charcoal will color feces black.

CHLORAMBUCIL

(klor-am′byoo-sil)

Leukeran

Classification: ANTINEOPLASTIC; ALKYLATING AGENT
Therapeutic: ANTINEOPLASTIC; NITROGEN MUSTARD
Prototype: Cyclophosphamide

AVAILABILITY Tablet

ACTION & THERAPEUTIC EFFECT Alkylating agent that interferes with DNA replication and RNA transcription by alkylation and cross-linking the strands of DNA, inducing cellular apoptosis. *Lymphocytic effect is marked; thus it is effective in treatment of various lymphomas.*

USES Management of chronic lymphocytic leukemia, non-Hodgkin lymphoma, Hodgkin lymphoma.

UNLABELED USES Idiopathic membranous nephropathy, necrobiotic xanthogranuloma, Waldenstrom macroglobulinemia.

CONTRAINDICATIONS Hypersensitivity to chlorambucil or to other alkylating agents; administration within 4 wk of a full course of radiation or chemotherapy; full dosage if bone marrow is infiltrated with lymphomatous tissue or is hypoplastic; smallpox and other vaccines; pregnancy (may result in adverse renal effects in the newborn); lactation.

CAUTIOUS USE Excessive or prolonged dosage, pneumococcus vaccination, history of seizures or head trauma.

ROUTE & DOSAGE

Palliative Treatment of CLL

Adult: **PO** 0.1 mg/kg/day for 3 to 6 weeks **or** 0.4 mg/kg pulsed doses administered intermittently

Hodgkin Lymphoma

Adult/Adolescent/Child: **PO** 6 mg/m^2 once daily (max 10 mg/day) on days 1 to 14 every 28 days

Non-Hodgkin Lymphoma

Adult/Adolescent/Child: **PO** 0.1mg/kg/day × 3–6 wk

Renal Impairment Dosage Adjustment

CrCl 10–50 mL/min: reduce to 75% or dose; *CrCl less than 10 mL/min:* administer 50% of dose.

ADMINISTRATION

Oral

- Control nausea and vomiting by giving entire daily dose at one time, 1 h before breakfast or 2 h after evening meal, or at bedtime. Consult prescriber.
- Store in tightly closed, light-resistant container.

ADVERSE EFFECTS **Endocrine:** Sterility, hyperuricemia. **GI:** Low incidence of gastric discomfort, hepatotoxicity. **Hematologic:** Bone marrow depression: *Leukopenia, thrombocytopenia*, anemia. **Other:** Drug fever, skin rashes, papilledema, alopecia, peripheral neuropathy, sterile cystitis, pulmonary complications, seizures (high doses).

INTERACTIONS **Drug** Avoid concurrent use with LIVE VACCINES or IMMUNOSUPPRESSANTS. Increased monitoring required with other MYELOSUPPRESSIVE AGENTS.

PHARMACOKINETICS **Absorption:** Rapidly and completely from GI tract. **Peak:** 1 h. **Distribution:** 99% protein binding; crosses placenta. **Metabolism:** In liver. **Elimination:** 60% in urine as metabolites within 24 h. **Half-Life:** 1.5–2.5 h.

C

NURSING IMPLICATIONS

Black Box Warning

Chlorambucil has been associated with severe bone marrow suppression and with infertility and severe fetal abnormalities.

Assessment & Drug Effects

- Leukopenia usually develops after the third week of treatment; it may continue for up to 10 days after last dose, then rapidly return to normal.
- Avoid or reduce to minimum injections and other invasive procedures (e.g., rectal temperatures, enemas) when platelet count is low.
- Monitor lab tests: Baseline and weekly CBC with differential; liver function tests.

Patient & Family Education

- Do not take chlorambucil if you are or suspect you are pregnant.
- Notify prescriber if the following symptoms occur: Unusual bleeding or bruising, sores on lips or in mouth; flank, stomach, or joint pain; fever, chills, or other signs of infection, sore throat, cough, dyspnea.
- Report immediately the onset of a skin reaction.
- Drink at least 10–12 glasses [240 mL (8 oz) each] of fluid/day, if not contraindicated.

CHLORAMPHENICOL SODIUM SUCCINATE

(klor-am-fen′i-kole)

Classification: ANTIBIOTIC
Therapeutic: BROAD-SPECTRUM ANTIBIOTIC

AVAILABILITY Solution for injection

ACTION & *THERAPEUTIC EFFECT* Synthetic broad-spectrum antibiotic believed to act by binding to the 50S ribosome of bacteria and thus interfering with protein synthesis. *Effective against a wide variety of gram-negative and gram-positive bacteria and most anaerobic microorganisms.*

USES Severe infections when other antibiotics are ineffective or are contraindicated.

CONTRAINDICATIONS History of hypersensitivity or toxic reaction to chloramphenicol; influenza; treatment of minor infections, prophylactic use; typhoid carrier state, history or family history of drug-induced bone marrow depression lactation.

CAUTIOUS USE Impaired hepatic or renal function, premature and full-term infants, children; intermittent porphyria; patients with G6PD deficiency; patient or family history of drug-induced bone marrow depression; pregnancy (category C).

ROUTE & DOSAGE

Serious Infections
Adult: **IV** 50–100 mg/kg/day in 4 divided doses
Adolescent/Child/Infant: **IV** 50 mg/kg/day in 4 divided doses

ADMINISTRATION

Intravenous

IV administration to neonates, infants, children: Verify correct IV concentration and rate of infusion with prescriber.

PREPARE: **Direct:** Dilute each 1 g with 10 mL of sterile water or D5W.

C

ADMINISTER: **Direct:** Give slowly over a period of at least 1 min.

INCOMPATIBILITIES: **Solution/additive:** **Chlorpromazine, erythromycin, hydroxyzine, metronidazole, glycopyrrolate, polymyxin B, prochlorperazine, promethazine, vancomycin.** **Y-site:** **Ascorbic acid, azathioprine, benztropine, butorphanol, caspofungin, cefotaxime, ceftazidime, ceftizoxime, ceftriaxone, chlorpromazine, cimetidine, dantrolene, diazepam, diazoxide, diltiazem, diphenhydramine, dobutamine, dopamine, doxycycline, erythromycin, esmolol, famotidine, fluconazole, ganciclovir, gatifloxacin, gemcitabine, gentamicin, haloperidol, hydralazine, hydroxyzine, idarubicin, irinotecan, labetalol, mechlorethamine, meperidine, metaraminol, midazolam, minocycline, mycophenolate, nafcillin, nalbuphine, ondansetron, pantoprazole, papaverine, pemetrexed, pentamidine, pentazocine, phentolamine, phenytoin, polymyxin B, procainamide, prochlorperazine, promethazine, protamine, pyridoxine, sulfamethoxazole/trimethoprim, thiamine, tigecycline, tolazoline, vancomycin, vecuronium, verapamil, vinorelbine.**

- Solution for infusion may form crystals or a second layer when stored at low temperatures. Solution can be clarified by shaking vial. ▪ Do not use cloudy solutions.

ADVERSE EFFECTS

CNS: Neurotoxicity: Headache, mental depression, confusion, delirium, digital paresthesias, peripheral neuritis. **HEENT:** Visual disturbances, optic neuritis, optic nerve atrophy, contact conjunctivitis. **Skin:** Urticaria, contact dermatitis, maculopapular and vesicular rashes, fixed-drug eruptions. **GI:** Nausea, vomiting, diarrhea, perianal irritation, enterocolitis, glossitis, stomatitis, unpleasant taste, xerostomia. **Hematologic:** Bone marrow depression (dose-related and reversible): Reticulocytosis, leukopenia, granulocytopenia, thrombocytopenia, increased plasma iron, reduced Hgb, hypoplastic anemia, hypoprothrombinemia. Non-dose-related and irreversible pancytopenia, agranulocytosis, aplastic anemia, paroxysmal nocturnal hemoglobinuria, leukemia. **Other:** Hypersensitivity, angioedema, dyspnea, fever, anaphylaxis, superinfections, Gray syndrome.

DIAGNOSTIC TEST INTERFERENCE

Possibility of false-positive results for ***urine glucose*** by ***copper reduction methods*** (e.g., ***Benedict solution, Clinitest***).

INTERACTIONS

Drug: The metabolism of **chlorpropamide, dicumarol, phenytoin, tolbutamide** may be decreased, prolonging their activity. **Phenobarbital** decreases chloramphenicol levels. The response to **iron** preparations, **folic acid,** and **vitamin B_{12}** may be delayed. Do not use with **ranolazine.** Monitor INR when using with **warfarin.** Do not use with LIVE VACCINES. Avoid use with **deferiprone.**

PHARMACOKINETICS

Peak: 1 h. **Distribution:** Widely distributed to most body tissues; concentrates in liver and kidneys; penetrates CNS; crosses placenta.

C

Metabolism: Inactivated in liver. **Elimination:** Much longer in neonates; metabolite and free drug excreted in urine; excreted in breast milk. **Half-Life:** 1.5–4.1 h.

NURSING IMPLICATIONS

Black Box Warning

Chloramphenicol has been associated with serious and potentially fatal blood dyscrasias.

Assessment & Drug Effects

- Check temperature at least q4h. Usually chloramphenicol is discontinued if temperature remains normal for 48 h.
- Monitor I&O ratio or pattern: Report any appreciable change.
- Withhold drug and notify prescriber if lab values indicate bone marrow suppression.
- Monitor for S&S of gray syndrome, which has occurred 2–9 days after initiation of high-dose chloramphenicol therapy in premature infants and neonates and in children 2 yr or younger. Report early signs: Abdominal distention, failure to feed, pallor, changes in vital signs.
- Monitor lab tests: Baseline C&S, CBC, platelets, serum iron, and reticulocyte cell counts q48h during therapy, and periodically thereafter. Weekly chloramphenicol blood levels or more frequently with hepatic dysfunction and in patients receiving therapy for longer than 2 wk.

Patient & Family Education

- A bitter taste may occur 15–20 sec after IV injection; it usually lasts only 2–3 min.
- Report immediately sore throat, fever, fatigue, petechiae, nosebleeds, bleeding gums, or other unusual bleeding or bruising, or any other suspicious sign or symptom.
- Watch for S&S of superinfection (see Appendix F).
- Notify prescriber immediately if signs of hypersensitivity reaction (see Appendix F), irritation, superinfection, or other adverse reactions appear.

CHLORDIAZEPOXIDE HYDROCHLORIDE

(klor-dye-az-e-pox′ide)

Classification: ANXIOLYTIC; SEDATIVE-HYPNOTIC; BENZODIAZEPINE

Therapeutic: ANTIANXIETY; SEDATIVE-HYPNOTIC

Prototype: Lorazepam

Controlled Substance: Schedule IV

AVAILABILITY Capsule

ACTION & *THERAPEUTIC EFFECT*

Benzodiazepine derivative that acts on the limbic, thalamic, and hypothalamic areas of the CNS. Has long-acting hypnotic properties. Causes mild suppression of REM sleep and of deeper phases, particularly stage 4, while increasing total sleep time. *Produces mild anxiolytic (reduces anxiety), sedative, anticonvulsant, and skeletal muscle relaxant effects.*

USES

Management of anxiety disorders or short-term relief of anxiety symptoms and for management of alcohol withdrawal.

CONTRAINDICATIONS

Hypersensitivity to chlordiazepoxide and other benzodiazepines; narrow-angle glaucoma, prostatic hypertrophy, shock, comatose states, primary depressive disorder or psychoses, acute alcohol intoxication; pregnancy (teratogenic effects have been observed with some benzodiazepines; neonatal withdrawal symptoms may occur within days to weeks after birth); lactation.

CAUTIOUS USE Anxiety states associated with impending depression, history of impaired hepatic or renal function; addiction-prone individuals, blood dyscrasias; in the older adult, debilitated patients, children; aggressive or hyperactive children; hyperkinesis; children younger than 6 yr.

ROUTE & DOSAGE

Anxiety Disorder

Adult: **PO** 5–25 mg bid or qid
Geriatric: **PO** 5 mg bid to qid

Alcohol Withdrawal Syndrome

CIWA-Ar score, symptom presentation and concurrent disease states impact dosage; see package insert for table of dosing regimens

Renal Impairment Dosage Adjustment

CrCl less than 10mL/min: Administer 50% of dose

ADMINISTRATION

Oral

- Give with or immediately after meals or with milk to reduce GI distress. If an antacid is prescribed, it should be taken at least 1 h before or after chlordiazepoxide to prevent delay in drug absorption.
- Store in tight, light-resistant containers at 25°C (77°F) unless otherwise specified by manufacturer.

ADVERSE EFFECTS **CV:** Edema, syncope. **CNS:** *Drowsiness*, changes in EEG pattern; confusion, drug-induced extrapyramidal reaction, ataxia. **Endocrine:** Change in libido, menstrual disease. **Skin:** Skin rash. **GI/Hepatic:** Nausea, constipation, hepatic insufficiency, jaundice. **Hematologic:** Agranulocytosis, bone marrow depression. **Other:** Paradoxical reaction.

DIAGNOSTIC TEST INTERFERENCE Chlordiazepoxide increases ***serum bilirubin, AST*** and ***ALT.***

INTERACTIONS **Drug: Alcohol,** CNS DEPRESSANTS, ANTICONVULSANTS potentiate CNS depression; may increase **phenytoin** levels; smoking decreases sedative and antianxiety effects. **Herbal: Kava, valerian** may potentiate sedation.

PHARMACOKINETICS **Absorption:** Well absorbed from GI tract. **Peak:** 1–4 h. **Distribution:** Widely distributed throughout body; crosses placenta; 96% protein bound. **Metabolism:** In liver via CYP3A4 to long-acting active metabolite. **Elimination:** Slowly excreted in urine (may last several days); excreted in breast milk. **Half-Life:** 5–30 h.

NURSING IMPLICATIONS

Assessment & Drug Effects

- Monitor for S&S of orthostatic hypotension and tachycardia; observe closely and monitor vital signs.
- Check BP and pulse before giving benzodiazepine in early part of therapy. If blood pressure falls 20 mmHg or more or if pulse rate is above 120 bpm, notify prescriber.
- Monitor I&O until drug dosage is stabilized. Report changes in I&O ratio and dysuria to prescriber.
- Monitor for S&S of paradoxic reactions—excitement, stimulation, disturbed sleep patterns, acute rage—which may occur

during first few weeks of therapy in psychiatric patients and in hyperactive and aggressive children receiving chlordiazepoxide. Withhold drug and report to prescriber.

- Assess patient's sleep pattern. If dreams or nightmares interfere with rest, notify prescriber.
- Supervise ambulation, especially with older adults and debilitated patients.

Patient & Family Education

- Abrupt discontinuation of drug in patients receiving high doses for long periods (4 mo or longer) has precipitated withdrawal symptoms, but not for at least 5–7 days because of slow elimination.
- Long-term use of this drug may cause mouth soreness. Good oral hygiene can alleviate the discomfort.
- Avoid activities requiring mental alertness until reaction to the drug has been evaluated.
- Avoid drinking alcoholic beverages. When combined with chlordiazepoxide, effects of both are potentiated.
- Avoid excessive sunlight. Use sunscreen lotion (SPF 12 or above) if allowed.

CHLOROQUINE PHOSPHATE

(klor′oh-kwin)

Aralen

Classification: ANTIMALARIAL

Therapeutic: ANTIMALARIAL; AMEBICIDE

AVAILABILITY Tablet

ACTION & THERAPEUTIC EFFECT Antimalarial activity is believed to be based on its ability to form complexes with DNA of parasite, thereby inhibiting replication and transcription to RNA and nucleic acid synthesis. *Acts as a suppressive agent in patient with* P. vivax *or* P. malariae *malaria; terminates acute attacks and increases intervals between treatment and relapse of malaria. Abolishes the acute attack of* P. falciparum *malaria but does not prevent the infection.*

USES Treatment and prophylaxis of malaria, extraintestinal amebiasis.

UNLABELED USES Discoid lupus erythematosus

CONTRAINDICATIONS Hypersensitivity to 4-aminoquinolines, psoriasis; ocular disease, porphyria, renal disease, 4-aminoquinoline-induced retinal or visual field changes.

CAUTIOUS USE Impaired hepatic function, alcoholism, eczema, patients with G6PD deficiency, infants and children, hematologic, GI, cardiac disease, diabetes, and neurologic disorders; pregnancy (recommended for the treatment of pregnant women with uncomplicated malaria); children. Safe use in women of childbearing potential not established.

ROUTE & DOSAGE

Acute Malaria

Adult (weight 60 kg or more): **PO** 1 gram on day 1 followed by 500-mg base at 6, 24, and 48 h

Adult (less than 60 kg)/Child: **PO** 16.6 mg/kg (max 1000 mg), then 8.3 mg/kg at 6, 24, and 48 h

Malaria Prevention

Adult: **PO** 500 mg base the same day each week starting 1–2 wk before exposure and continuing for 4–6 wk after leaving the area of exposure (max: 300 mg base/wk)

Child: **PO** 8.3 mg/kg the same day each week starting 1–2 wk before exposure and continuing for 4 wk after leaving the area of exposure (max: 300 mg base/wk)

Extraintestinal Amebiasis

Adult: **PO** 1 g daily for 2 days, then 500 mg/day for 2–3 wk
Child: **PO** 16.6 mg/kg/day x 21days

ADMINISTRATION

Oral

- Give immediately before or after meals to minimize GI distress.
- Monitor child's dose closely. Children are extremely susceptible to overdosage.

ADVERSE EFFECTS **CV:** Hypotension; ECG changes. **CNS:** Mild transient headache, fatigue, irritability, confusion, nightmares, skeletal muscle weakness, paresthesias, reduced reflexes, vertigo, suicidal ideation. **HEENT:** (Usually reversible): Blurred vision, disturbances of accommodation, night blindness, scotomas, visual field defects, photophobia, corneal edema, opacity or deposits, ototoxicity (rare). **Endocrine:** Hypoglycemia. **Skin:** Bleaching of scalp, eyebrows, body hair, and freckles, pruritus, patchy alopecia (reversible). **GI:** *Diarrhea*, abdominal cramps, *nausea*, vomiting, anorexia. **Hematologic:** Hemolytic anemia in patients with G6PD deficiency. **Other:** Slight weight loss, myalgia, lymphedema of upper limbs.

INTERACTIONS **Drug:** ANTACIDS decrease chloroquine absorption, so separate administration by at least 4 h; chloroquine may interfere with response to **rabies vaccine.** Use caution with ANTIDIABETES medications due to increased risk of hypoglycemia. Do not use with **posaconazole** or **fluconazole** other QT-PROLONGING AGENTS due to risk of arrhythmias. Avoid use with **cimetidine**, **dapsone. Food:** Taking **lemon juice** decreases therapeutic effect.

PHARMACOKINETICS **Absorption:** Rapidly and almost completely absorbed. **Peak:** 1–2 h. **Distribution:** Widely distributed; concentrates in lungs, liver, erythrocytes, eyes, skin, and kidneys; crosses placenta. **Metabolism:** Partially in liver to active metabolites. **Elimination:** In urine. **Half-Life:** 70–120 h.

NURSING IMPLICATIONS

Assessment & Drug Effects

- Monitor for changes in ECG, especially with a preexisting cardiac condition.
- Obtain baseline ophthalmologic exam and monitor for changes in vision. Retinopathy (generally irreversible) can be progressive even after termination of therapy. Patient may be asymptomatic or complain of night blindness, scotomas, visual field changes, blurred vision, or difficulty in focusing. Withhold drug and report immediately to prescriber.
- Monitor lab tests: Baseline CBC before initiation of therapy and periodically in patients on long-term therapy.

Patient & Family Education

- Report promptly visual or hearing disturbances, muscle weakness, or loss of balance, symptoms of blood dyscrasia (fever, sore mouth or throat, unexplained fatigue, easy bruising or bleeding).
- Use of dark glasses in sunlight or bright light may provide comfort

C

(because of photophobia) and reduce risk of ocular damage.
- Avoid driving or other potentially hazardous activities until reaction to drug is known.
- May cause rusty yellow or brown discoloration of urine.
- Do not drink lemon juice along with chloroquine. It decreases the drug's effectiveness.

CHLOROTHIAZIDE
(klor-oh-thye'a-zide)

CHLOROTHIAZIDE SODIUM
Diuril

Classification: ELECTROLYTE AND WATER BALANCE AGENT; THIAZIDE DIURETIC; ANTIHYPERTENSIVE
Therapeutic: THIAZIDE DIURETIC; ANTIHYPERTENSIVE
Prototype: Hydrochlorothiazide

AVAILABILITY Oral suspension; tablet; solution for injection

ACTION & *THERAPEUTIC EFFECT* Inhibits sodium and chloride reabsorption in the distal tubules causing increased excretion of sodium, chloride, and water resulting in diuresis. *Promotes renal excretion of sodium (and water), bicarbonate, magnesium, hydrogen ions, and potassium. Antihypertensive mechanism is due to decreased peripheral resistance and reduced blood pressure.*

USES Edema associated with CHF, hypertension.

CONTRAINDICATIONS Hypersensitivity to thiazide or sulfonamides; anuria; hypokalemia; hyponatremia; hypercalcemia; renal failure; jaundiced neonates.

CAUTIOUS USE History of sulfa allergy; impaired renal or hepatic function or gout; SLE; diabetes mellitus, older adult or debilitated patients, pancreatitis, sympathectomy; pregnancy (category C).

ROUTE & DOSAGE

Hypertension

Adult: **PO** 500 mg–2 g/day in 1–2 divided doses
Child (6 mo or older): **PO** 10–20 mg/kg/day in 1–2 doses (max: 375 mg)
Infant (younger than 6 mo): **PO** 10–30 mg/kg/day divided in 2 doses

Edema

Adult: **PO** 250–500 mg once or twice daily; **IV** 500–1000 mg daily

ADMINISTRATION

Oral
- Give with or after food to prevent gastric irritation. Extent of absorption appears to be increased by taking it with food.
- Schedule daily doses to avoid nocturia and interrupted sleep.

Intravenous

▪ Reserve for emergency or when patient unable to take oral medication. ▪ IV administration to infants and children: Verify correct IV concentration and rate of infusion with prescriber.

PREPARE: **Intermittent** Reconstitute the 500-mg vial with at least 18 mL sterile water for injection. ▪ May be further diluted with D5W or NS. **Must be** prepared immediately before use.

ADMINISTER: **Intermittent:** Give at a rate of 500 mg over 5 min. ▪ Thiazide preparations are extremely irritating to the tissues, and great care **must be** taken to

C

avoid extravasation. ▪ If infiltration occurs, stop medication, remove needle, and apply ice if area is small.

INCOMPATIBILITIES: Solution/additive: **Amikacin, chlorpromazine, hydralazine, insulin, levorphanol, morphine, norepinephrine, polymyxin B, procaine, prochlorperazine, promazine, promethazine, streptomycin, triflupromazine, vancomycin.** Y-site: **Chlorpromazine, codeine, hydralazine, prochlorperazine, promazine, promethazine.**

▪ Store tablets, PO solutions, and parenteral dosage forms at 15°–30°C (59°–86°F) unless otherwise directed by manufacturer. ▪ Unused reconstituted IV solutions may be stored at room temperature up to 24 h. Use only clear solutions.

ADVERSE EFFECTS **CV:** Hypotension, necrotizing angiitis, orthostatic hypotension. **Respiratory:** Pneumonitis, pulmonary edema, respiratory distress. **CNS:** Dizziness, headache, paresthesia, restlessness, vertigo. **HEENT:** Blurred vision, xanthopsia. **Endocrine:** Glycosuria, hypercalcemia, hyperglycemia, hyperuricemia, hypokalemia, hypomagnesemia, hyponatremia, increased serum cholesterol, increased serum triglycerides. **Hepatic/GI:** Jaundice, abdominal cramps, anorexia, constipation, diarrhea, nausea, pancreatitis. **GU:** Hematuria, impotence, interstitial nephritis, renal failure, renal insufficiency. **Musculoskeletal:** Muscle spasm, systemic lupus erythematosus, weakness. **Hematologic:** Agranulocytosis, aplastic anemia, hemolytic anemia, leukopenia, purpura, thrombocytopenia. **Other:** Fever, anaphylaxis.

DIAGNOSTIC TEST INTERFERENCE May interfere with ***parathyroid function tests.***

INTERACTIONS **Drug:** CORTICOSTEROIDS, **topiramate** increase hypokalemic effects of chlorothiazide; the hypoglycemic effects of SULFONYLUREAS and **insulin** may be antagonized; intensifies hypoglycemic and hypotensive effects of **diazoxide;** increased potassium and magnesium loss may cause **digoxin** toxicity; decreases **lithium** excretion, increasing its toxicity; increases risk of NSAID-induced renal failure and may attenuate diuresis. Use with **amifostine** or **bromperidol** may have increased risk of hypotension.

PHARMACOKINETICS **Absorption:** Incompletely absorbed PO. **Onset:** 2 h PO; 15 min IV. **Peak:** 3–6 h PO; 30 min IV. **Duration:** 6–12 h PO; 2 h IV. **Distribution:** Throughout extracellular tissue; concentrates in kidney; crosses placenta. **Metabolism:** Does not appear to be metabolized. **Elimination:** In urine and breast milk. **Half-Life:** 45–120 min.

NURSING IMPLICATIONS

Assessment & Drug Effects

- Monitor for therapeutic effect. Antihypertensive action of a thiazide diuretic requires several days before effects are observed; usually optimum therapeutic effect is not established for 3–4 wk.
- Monitor for hyperglycemia. Thiazide therapy can cause hyperglycemia (see Appendix F) and glycosuria in diabetic and diabetic-prone individuals.
- Monitor patients with gout. Asymptomatic hyperuricemia can be produced because of interference with uric acid excretion.

C

- Establish baseline weight before initiation of therapy. Weigh patient at the same time each a.m. under standard conditions. A gain of more than 1 kg (2.2) within 2 or 3 days and a gradual weight gain over the week's period is reportable.
- Monitor BP closely during early drug therapy.
- Inspect skin and mucous membranes daily for evidence of petechiae in patients receiving large doses and those on prolonged therapy.
- Monitor I&O rates and patterns: Excessive diuresis may cause electrolyte imbalance and necessitate prompt dosage adjustment.
- Monitor patients on digitalis therapy for S&S of hypokalemia (see Appendix G), which can precipitate digitalis intoxication.
- Monitor lab tests: Baseline and periodic serum electrolytes and renal function tests, and blood glucose.

Patient & Family Education

- Urination will occur in greater amounts and with more frequency than usual, and there will be an unusual sense of tiredness. With continued therapy, diuretic action decreases; BP lowering effects usually are maintained, and sense of tiredness diminishes.
- Make position changes slowly to minimize risks associated with orthostatic hypotension.
- Report to prescriber any illness accompanied by prolonged vomiting or diarrhea.
- Avoid drinking large quantities of coffee or other caffeine drinks. Caffeine has a diuretic effect.
- Report S&S of hypokalemia, hypercalcemia, or hyperglycemia (see Appendix F).
- Hypokalemia may be prevented if the daily diet contains potassium-rich foods. Eat a banana and drink at least 6 oz orange juice every day.
- Report photosensitivity reaction to prescriber. Photosensitivity may occur 1½–2 wk after initial sun exposure.

CHLORPHENIRAMINE MALEATE

(klor-fen-eer′a-meen)

Aller-Chlor, Chlo-Amine, Chlor-Trimeton, Chlor-Tripolon ◆, Novo-Pheniram ◆, Phenetron, Telachlor, Teldrin, Trymegan

Classification: ANTIHISTAMINE (H_1-RECEPTOR ANTAGONIST)

Therapeutic: ANTIHISTAMINE

Prototype: Diphenhydramine

AVAILABILITY Tablet; sustained release tablet; syrup

ACTION & *THERAPEUTIC EFFECT* Competes with histamine for H_1-receptor sites on effector cells; thus it promotes capillary permeability and edema formation and constrictive action on respiratory, gastrointestinal, and vascular smooth muscles. *Has effective antihistamine reaction resulting in decreasing allergic symptomatology.*

USES Symptomatic relief of various uncomplicated allergic conditions; to prevent transfusion and drug reactions in susceptible patients, and as adjunct to epinephrine and other standard measures in anaphylactic reactions.

CONTRAINDICATIONS Hypersensitivity to antihistamines of similar structure; lower respiratory tract symptoms, narrow-angle glaucoma, obstructive prostatic hypertrophy or other bladder neck obstruction, GI obstruction or stenosis; premature and newborn infants; during or within 14 days of MAO INHIBITOR therapy.

CAUTIOUS USE Convulsive disorders, increased intraocular pressure, hyperthyroidism, cardiovascular disease, hepatic disease; BPH; GI obstruction; hypertension, diabetes mellitus, history of bronchial asthma, COPD, older adult patients, patients with G6PD deficiency; pregnancy (category C), lactation.

ROUTE & DOSAGE

Symptomatic Allergy Relief

Adult: **PO** 2–4 mg tid or qid *or* 8–12 mg bid or tid (max: 24 mg/day)

Geriatric: **PO** 4 mg daily or bid *or* 8 mg sustained release at bedtime

Child (6–12 yr): **PO** 2 mg q4–6h (max: 12 mg/day); *2 to younger than 6 yr:* 1 mg q4–6h

ADMINISTRATION

Oral

- Give on an empty stomach for fastest response.
- Sustained release tablets should be swallowed whole and not crushed or chewed.
- Ensure that chewable tablets are chewed or crushed before being swallowed with a liquid.

ADVERSE EFFECTS **CV:** Palpitation, tachycardia, mild hypotension or hypertension. **CNS:** *Drowsiness,* sedation, headache, dizziness, vertigo, fatigue, disturbed coordination, tremors, euphoria, nervousness, restlessness, insomnia. **HEENT:** *Dryness of mouth,* nose, and throat, tinnitus, vertigo, acute labyrinthitis, thickened bronchial secretions, blurred vision, diplopia. **GI:** Epigastric distress, anorexia, nausea, vomiting, constipation, or diarrhea. **GU:** Urinary frequency or retention, dysuria. **Other:** Sensation of chest tightness.

DIAGNOSTIC TEST INTERFERENCE Antihistamines should be discontinued 4 days before ***skin testing*** procedures for allergy because they may obscure otherwise positive reactions.

INTERACTIONS **Drug: Alcohol (ethanol)** and other CNS DEPRESSANTS produce additive sedation and CNS depression.

PHARMACOKINETICS **Absorption:** Well absorbed from GI tract; about 45% of dose reaches systemic circulation intact. **Onset:** Within 6 h. **Peak:** 2–6 h. **Distribution:** Highest concentrations in lung, heart, kidney, brain, small intestine, and spleen. **Metabolism:** By CYP3A4. **Half-Life:** 12–43 h.

NURSING IMPLICATIONS

Assessment & Drug Effects

- Monitor for CNS depression and sedation, especially when chlorpheniramine is given in combination with other CNS depressants.
- Monitor BP in hypertensive patients because chlorpheniramine may elevate BP.

Patient & Family Education

- Avoid driving a car and other potentially hazardous activities until drug response has been determined.

C

- Avoid or minimize alcohol intake. Antihistamines have additive effects with alcohol.
- Report any of the following: Tinnitus or palpitations.
- Consult prescriber before taking additional OTC drugs for allergy relief.

CHLORPROMAZINE

(klor-proe′ma-zeen)

CHLORPROMAZINE HYDROCHLORIDE

Classification: ANTIPSYCHOTIC, PHENOTHIAZINE; ANTIEMETIC

Therapeutic: ANTIPSYCHOTIC; ANTIEMETIC

AVAILABILITY Tablet; solution for injection

ACTION & *THERAPEUTIC EFFECT* Phenothiazine derivative with actions at all levels of CNS with a mechanism that produces strong antipsychotic effects. Antiemetic effect due to suppression of the chemoreceptor trigger zone (CTZ). Mechanism thought to be related to blockade of postsynaptic dopamine receptors in the brain. *Effective in decreasing psychotic symptoms. Also has antiemetic effects due to its action on the CTZ.*

USES Symptomatic management of bipolar disorder, psychotic disorders, including schizophrenia, in management of nausea and vomiting, to control excessive anxiety and agitation before surgery, and for treatment of severe behavior problems in children (e.g., attention-deficit/hyperactivity disorder). Also used for treatment of acute intermittent porphyria, intractable hiccups, and as adjunct in treatment of tetanus.

UNLABLED USES Nausea and vomiting of pregnancy

CONTRAINDICATIONS Hypersensitivity to phenothiazine derivatives, sulfite, or benzyl alcohol; withdrawal states from alcohol; CNS depression; comatose states, brain damage, bone marrow depression, Reye syndrome; lactation.

CAUTIOUS USE Agitated states accompanied by depression, seizure disorders, dementia-related psychosis in the older adult, respiratory impairment due to infection or COPD; glaucoma, diabetes, hypertensive disease, peptic ulcer, prostatic hypertrophy; thyroid, cardiovascular, and hepatic disorders; patients exposed to extreme heat or organophosphate insecticides; previously detected breast cancer; pregnancy (may be considered for the adjunctive treatment of nausea and vomiting in pregnant women); children younger than 6 mo.

ROUTE & DOSAGE

Bipolar disorder/psychotic disorder/schizophrenia

Adult: **PO** 30–800 mg divided in 2–4 doses; titrate as needed
IM 25 mg, may repeat 25–50 mg in 1 hour if needed

Nausea and Vomiting

Adult/Adolescent (over 45.5 kg): **PO** 10–25 mg q4–6h prn; **IM/IV** 25–50 mg q3–4h prn
Adolescent/Child (6 mo or older; less than 45.5 kg): **PO/IV/IM** 0.55 mg/kg q6–8h prn up to 500 mg/day

Intractable Hiccups

Adult: **PO/IM** 25–50 mg tid or qid

Tetanus

Adult: **IM/IV 25–50 mg q6–8h**
Child: **IM/IV 0.55 mg/kg q6–8h**

Porphyria

Adult: **PO/IM 25 mg 3–4 times/day**

ADMINISTRATION

Oral

- Give with food or a full glass of fluid to minimize GI distress.
- Mix chlorpromazine concentrate just before administration in at least ½ glass juice, milk, water, coffee, tea, carbonated beverage, or with semisolid food.
- Ensure that sustained release form of drug is not chewed or crushed. It **must be** swallowed whole.

Intramuscular/Intravenous

- Avoid parenteral drug contact with skin, eyes, and clothing because of its potential for causing contact dermatitis.
- Keep patient recumbent for at least 30 min after parenteral administration. Observe closely. Report hypotensive reactions.

Intramuscular

- Inject IM preparations slowly and deep into upper outer quadrant of buttock. If irritation is a problem, consult prescriber about diluting medication with normal saline or 2% procaine. Rotate injection sites.

Intravenous

PREPARE: **Direct:** Dilute 25 mg with 24 mL of NS to yield 1 mg/mL. **Continuous:** May be further diluted in up to 1000 mL of NS.
ADMINISTER: **Direct:** Administer 1 mg or fraction thereof over 1 min for adults and over 2 min for children. **Continuous:** Give slowly at a rate not to exceed 1 mg/min.

- Lemon yellow color of parenteral preparation does not alter potency; if otherwise colored or markedly discolored, solution should be discarded.

INCOMPATIBILITIES: **Solution/additive:** **Acetaminophen, aminophylline, amphotericin B, ampicillin, cefodizime, chloramphenicol, chlorothiazide, furosemide, methohexital, penicillin G, phenobarbital.** **Y-site:** **Acetaminophen, acyclovir, allopurinol, amifostine, aminocaproic acid, amphotericin B cholesteryl complex, ampicillin, asparaginase, azathioprine, azithromycin, aztreonam, bivalirudin, bretylium, bumetanide, cangrelor, carboplatin, cefamandole, cephazolin, cefepime, cefoperazone, cefotaxime, cefotetan, cefoxitin, ceftazidime, ceftizoxime, ceftriaxone, cefuroxime, chloramphenicol, chlorothiazide, clindamycin, dantrolene, diazepam, epoetin, eptifibatide, ertapenem, etoposide, fludarabine, fluorouracil, folic acid, foscarnet, fosfomycin, fosphenytoin, gallium, ganciclovir, garenoxacin, gemtuzumab, imipenem/cilastin, inamrinone, indomethacin, insulin, irinotecan, ketorolac, lansoprazole, leucovorin, linezolid, melphalan, methohexital, methotrexate, nitroprusside, paclitaxel, pantoprazole, pemetrexed, pentobarbital, phenobarbital, phenytoin, piperacillin/tazobactam, sargramostim, sodium bicarbonate, streptokinase, sulfamethoxazole/trimethoprim, ticarcillin, tigecycline, trastuzumab.**

C

- All forms are stored preferably at 15°–30°C (59°–86°F) protected from light, unless otherwise specified by the manufacturer. Avoid freezing.

ADVERSE EFFECTS **CV:** Orthostatic hypotension, palpitation, tachycardia, ECG changes (usually reversible): Prolonged QT and PR intervals, blunting of T waves, ST depression. **Respiratory:** Laryngospasm. **CNS:** *Sedation, drowsiness,* dizziness, restlessness, neuroleptic malignant syndrome, tardive dyskinesias, tumor, syncope, headache, weakness, insomnia, reduced REM sleep, bizarre dreams, cerebral edema, convulsive seizures, hypothermia, inability to sweat, depressed cough reflex, *extrapyramidal symptoms,* EEG changes. **HEENT:** Blurred vision, lenticular opacities, mydriasis, photophobia. **Endocrine:** Weight gain, hypoglycemia, hyperglycemia, glycosuria (high doses), enlargement of parotid glands. **Skin:** Fixed-drug eruption, urticaria, reduced perspiration, contact dermatitis, exfoliative dermatitis, photosensitivity, eczema, anaphylactoid reactions, hypersensitivity vasculitis; hirsutism (long-term therapy). **GI:** Dry mouth; constipation, adynamic ileus, cholestatic jaundice, aggravation of peptic ulcer, dyspepsia, increased appetite. **GU:** Anovulation, infertility, pseudopregnancy, menstrual irregularity, gynecomastia, galactorrhea, priapism, inhibition of ejaculation, reduced libido, urinary retention and frequency. **Hematologic:** Agranulocytosis, thrombocytopenic purpura, pancytopenia (rare). **Other:** Idiopathic edema, muscle necrosis (following IM), SLE-like syndrome, sudden unexplained death.

DIAGNOSTIC TEST INTERFERENCE May cause false-positive with urine detection of amphetamine/methamphetamine and methadone. False-positive result may occur for ***amylase, 5-hydroxyindole acetic acid, phenylketonuria, porphobilinogens, urobilinogen (Ehrlich reagent),*** and ***urine bilirubin (Bili-Labstix).*** False-positive ***pregnancy test*** results possibly caused by a metabolite of phenothiazines, which discolors urine depending on test used.

INTERACTIONS **Drug:** **Alcohol,** CNS DEPRESSANTS increase CNS depression; could increase the risk of QT prolongation when used with other agents that also have this effect (e.g., **amiodarone**); **phenobarbital** increases metabolism of phenothiazine; GENERAL ANESTHETICS increase excitation and hypotension; TRICYCLIC ANTIDEPRESSANTS intensify hypotensive and anticholinergic effects; ANTICONVULSANTS decrease seizure threshold—may need to increase anticonvulsant dose; may enhance the adverse effects of ANTICHOLINERGIC AGENTS. Avoid **eluxadoline.** **Herbal:** **Kava** increases risk and severity of dystonic reaction.

PHARMACOKINETICS **Absorption:** Rapid absorption with considerable first-pass metabolism in liver; rapid absorption after IM. **Onset:** 30–60 min (PO); 15 min (IM). **Peak:** 2–4 h PO; 15–20 min IM. **Duration:** 4–6 h. **Distribution:** Widely distributed; accumulates in brain; crosses placenta. **Metabolism:** In liver by CYP2D6. **Elimination:** In urine as metabolites; excreted in breast milk. **Half-Life:** Biphasic 2 and 30 h.

NURSING IMPLICATIONS

Black Box Warning

Chlorpromazine has been associated with increased mortality in the older adult with dementia-related psychosis.

Assessment & Drug Effects

- Note that this drug is not approved for use in older adults with dementia-related psychosis.
- Establish baseline BP (in standing and recumbent positions), and pulse, before initiating treatment.
- Monitor BP frequently. Hypotensive reactions, dizziness, and sedation are common during early therapy, particularly in patients on high doses and in the older adult receiving parenteral doses.
- Monitor cardiac status with baseline ECG in patients with preexisting cardiovascular disease.
- Be alert for signs of neuroleptic malignant syndrome (see Appendix G). Report immediately.
- Report extrapyramidal symptoms that occur most often in patients on high dosage, the pediatric patient with severe dehydration and acute infection, the older adult, and women. Reduce smoking, if possible.
- Monitor I&O ratio and pattern: Urinary retention due to mental depression and compromised renal function may occur.
- Be alert to complaints of diminished visual acuity, reduced night vision, photophobia, and a perceived brownish discoloration of objects. Patient may be more comfortable with dark glasses.
- Monitor diabetics or prediabetics on long-term, high-dose therapy for reduced glucose tolerance and loss of diabetes control.
- Ocular examinations and EEG (in patients older than 50 yr) are recommended before and periodically during prolonged therapy.
- Monitor lab tests: Periodic CBC with differential, electrolytes, lipid panel, LFTs, and blood glucose.

Patient & Family Education

- Take medication as prescribed and keep appointments for follow-up evaluation of dosage regimen. Improvement may not be experienced until 7 or 8 wk into therapy.
- May cause pink to red-brown discoloration of urine.
- Wear protective clothing and sunscreen lotion with SPF above 12 when outdoors, even on dark days. Photosensitivity causes exposed skin areas to have appearance of an exaggerated sunburn. If reaction occurs, report to prescriber.
- Practice meticulous oral hygiene. Oral candidiasis occurs frequently in patients receiving phenothiazines.
- Avoid driving a car or undertaking activities requiring precision and mental alertness until drug response is known.
- Do not abruptly stop this drug. Abrupt withdrawal of drug or deliberate dose skipping, especially after prolonged therapy with large doses, can cause onset of extrapyramidal symptoms (see Appendix F) and severe GI disturbances. When drug is to be discontinued, dosage **must be** tapered off gradually over a period of several weeks.

C

CHLORPROPAMIDE

(klor-proe′pa-mide)

Classification: ANTIDIABETIC; SULFONYLUREA

Therapeutic: ANTIDIABETIC

Prototype: Glyburide

AVAILABILITY Tablet

ACTION & *THERAPEUTIC EFFECT* Lowers blood glucose by stimulating beta cells in pancreas to synthesize and release endogenous insulin. *Antidiabetic effect is due to the ability of the drug to stimulate beta cells of the pancreas to manufacture and release insulin. Therapeutic effectiveness is indicated by HbA1C level in normal range.*

USES Type 2 diabetes mellitus.

UNLABELED USES Neurogenic diabetes insipidus.

CONTRAINDICATIONS Known hypersensitivity to sulfonyl-ureas and sulfonamides; type I diabetes mellitus; diabetic ketoacidosis; lactation.

CAUTIOUS USE Older adult patients, cardiovascular mortality; hypoglycemia; pregnancy (category C). Safe use in children not established.

ROUTE & DOSAGE

Type 2 Diabetes Mellitus

Adult: **PO** Initial: 250 mg/day with breakfast, adjust by 50–125 mg/day q3–5 days until glycemic control is achieved (max: 750 mg/day)

ADMINISTRATION

Oral

- Give as a single morning dose with breakfast or 3 doses and taken with meals.
- Store at 15°–30°C (59°–86°F) in a tightly closed container, unless otherwise directed.

ADVERSE EFFECTS **CNS:** Disulfiram-like reaction, dizziness, headache. **Endocrine:** Hypoglycemia, weight gain. **Hepatic/GI:** Hepatic failure, jaundice, nausea. **Hematologic:** Agranulocytosis, aplastic anemia.

INTERACTIONS **Drug:** Adverse effects of ORAL ANTICOAGULANTS, **phenytoin,** SALICYLATES, NSAIDS may be increased along with those of chlorpropamide; THIAZIDE DIURETICS may increase blood sugar; may increase risk of **methotrexate** toxicity; use with THIAZOLIDINEDIONES increases risk of hypoglycemia; **probenecid,** MAO INHIBITORS may increase hypoglycemic effects; avoid use with **fluconazole.** **Herbal:** **Garlic, ginseng** may increase hypoglycemic effects.

PHARMACOKINETICS **Absorption:** Readily from GI tract. **Onset:** 1 h. **Peak:** 3–6 h. **Distribution:** Highly protein bound; distributed into breast milk. **Metabolism:** In liver. **Elimination:** 80–90% in urine in 96 h. **Half-Life:** 36 h.

NURSING IMPLICATIONS

Assessment & Drug Effects

- Report dizziness, shortness of breath, malaise, fatigue.
- Monitor for S&S of hypoglycemia (see Appendix F).
- Monitor lab tests: Periodic fasting and postprandial blood glucose; HbA1C every 3 mo; baseline and periodic hematologic tests

and LFTs, particularly in patients receiving high doses.

Patient & Family Education

- Report hypoglycemic episodes to prescriber. Because chlorpropamide has a long half-life, hypoglycemia can be severe.
- Report any of the following immediately to prescriber: Skin eruptions, malaise, fever, or photosensitivity. A change to another hypoglycemic agent may be indicated.

CHLORTHALIDONE

(klor-thal′i-done)

Classification: ELECTROLYTE & WATER BALANCE AGENT; DIURETIC; ANTIHYPERTENSIVE

Therapeutic: DIURETIC; ANTIHYPERTENSIVE

Prototype: Hydrochlorothiazide

AVAILABILITY Tablet

ACTION & *THERAPEUTIC EFFECT* Sulfonamide derivative that increases excretion of sodium and chloride by inhibiting their reabsorption in the distal convoluted tubule. *Antihypertensive effect is correlated to the decrease in extracellular and intracellular volumes. Decreased volume results in reduced cardiac output with subsequent decrease in peripheral resistance.*

USES Hypertension, refractory edema.

UNLABELED USE Prevention of calcium nephrolithiasis.

CONTRAINDICATIONS Hypersensitivity to sulfonamide or thiazide derivatives; anuria, hypokalemia; toxemia; hyperparathyroidism; lactation; neonates with jaundice.

CAUTIOUS USE History of renal and hepatic disease, hyponatremia, hypochloremia; gout, SLE, diabetes mellitus; history of allergy or bronchial asthma; pregnancy (maternal use may cause fetal or neonatal jaundice, thrombocytopenia, hypoglycemia, or electrolyte imbalance).

ROUTE & DOSAGE

Hypertension

Adult: **PO** 12.5–25 mg/day
Child: **PO** 0.3 mg/kg/dose daily (max 50 mg/day)

Edema

Adult: **PO** 12.5–25 mg/day, may be increased to 100 mg/day if needed

ADMINISTRATION

Oral

- Administer as single dose in a.m. to reduce potential for interrupted sleep because of diuresis.
- Consult prescriber when chlorthalidone is used as a diuretic; an intermittent dose schedule may reduce incidence of adverse reactions.
- Store tablets in tightly closed container at 15°–30°C (59°–86°F) unless otherwise advised.

ADVERSE EFFECTS **CV:** Orthostatic hypotension. **CNS:** Dizziness, vertigo, paresthesias, headache. **Endocrine:** *Hypokalemia,* hyponatremia, hypochloremia, hypercalcemia, glycosuria, hyperglycemia, exacerbation of gout. **Skin:** Rash, urticaria, photosensitivity, vasculitis. **GI:** Anorexia, nausea, vomiting, diarrhea, constipation, cramping, jaundice. **GU:** Impotence. **Hematologic:** Agranulocytosis, thrombocytopenia, aplastic anemia.

C

INTERACTIONS Drug: CORTICOSTEROIDS, increases hypokalemia; decreases **lithium** elimination; **dofetilide** or other QT PROLONGING AGENTS may have increased potential for arrhythmia; may antagonize the hypoglycemic effects of SULFONYLUREAS; NSAIDS may attenuate diuretic effects; increases concentration of **topiramate.** Use caution with other ANTIHYPERTENSIVES. Can enhance photosensitivity when used with other agents causing that effect.

PHARMACOKINETICS Absorption: Readily from GI tract. **Onset:** 2 h. **Peak:** 2–6 h. **Duration:** 24–72 h. **Distribution:** Crosses placenta; appears in breast milk. **Metabolism:** Hepatic **Elimination:** 30–60% in urine in 24 h. **Half-Life:** 54 h.

NURSING IMPLICATIONS

Assessment & Drug Effects

- Establish baseline BP measurements and check at regular intervals during period of dosage adjustment when chlorthalidone is used for hypertension.
- Be alert to signs of hypokalemia (see Appendix F). Older adult patients are more sensitive to adverse effects of drug-induced diuresis because of age-related changes in the cardiovascular and renal systems.
- Monitor lithium and digoxin levels closely when either of these drugs is used concurrently.
- Monitor weight and intake and output daily.
- Monitor lab tests: Baseline and periodic serum electrolytes, renal function tests, uric acid, and blood glucose (especially in patients with diabetes).

Patient & Family Education

- Maintain adequate potassium intake, monitor weight, and make a daily estimate of I&O ratio.

CHLORZOXAZONE

(klor-zox′a-zone)

Classification: CENTRALLY ACTING SKELETAL MUSCLE RELAXANT

Therapeutic: SKELETAL MUSCLE RELAXER; ANTISPASMODIC

Prototype: Cyclobenzaprine

AVAILABILITY Tablet

ACTION & *THERAPEUTIC EFFECT* Centrally acting skeletal muscle relaxant that acts indirectly by depressing nerve transmission through polysynaptic pathways in spinal cord, subcortical centers, and brain stem. *Effectively controls muscle spasms and pain associated with musculoskeletal conditions.*

USES Symptomatic treatment of muscle spasm and pain associated with various musculoskeletal conditions.

CONTRAINDICATIONS Hypersensitivity to chlorzoxazone or any component of the formulation; impaired liver function; alcoholism; hepatic disease, jaundice; lactation.

CAUTIOUS USE Patients with known allergies or history of drug allergies; renal impairment or failure; CNS depression; older adult patients; pregnancy (no evidence available).

ROUTE & DOSAGE

Skeletal Muscle Relaxant

Adult: **PO** 250–500 mg tid or qid
Child: **PO** 20 mg/kg/day in 3–4 divided doses (max: 750 mg/dose)

ADMINISTRATION

Oral

- Give with food or meals to prevent gastric distress. If necessary, tablet may be crushed and mixed with food or liquid (e.g., milk, fruit juice).
- Store in tight container at 20°–25°C (68°–77°F) unless otherwise directed.

ADVERSE EFFECTS **CNS:** *Drowsiness, dizziness,* malaise, paradoxical nervous system stimulation. **Skin:** Rash. **GU:** Urine discoloration.

INTERACTIONS **Drug: Alcohol,** CNS DEPRESSANTS add to CNS depression.

PHARMACOKINETICS **Absorption:** Readily absorbed from GI tract. **Onset:** 1 h. **Peak:** 1–4 h. **Duration:** 4–6 h. **Distribution:** Not known if crosses placenta or distributed into breast milk. **Metabolism:** In liver. **Elimination:** In urine. **Half-Life:** 66 min.

NURSING IMPLICATIONS

Assessment & Drug Effects

- Monitor ambulation during early drug therapy; some patients may require supervision.
- Monitor for signs/symptoms of hepatotoxicity.
- Monitor lab tests: Periodic LFTs in patients receiving long-term therapy.

Patient & Family Education

- Avoid activities requiring mental alertness, judgment, and physical coordination until reaction to drug is known because sedation, drowsiness, and dizziness may occur.
- Drug may discolor urine orange to purplish red, but this is of no clinical significance.
- Discontinue drug and notify prescriber if signs of hypersensitivity (see Appendix F) or of liver dysfunction appear (abdominal discomfort, yellow sclerae or skin, pruritus, malaise, nausea, vomiting).
- Check with prescriber before taking an OTC depressant (e.g., antihistamine, sedative, alcohol) because effects may be additive.

CHOLESTYRAMINE RESIN

(koe-less-tear'a-meen)

Questran, Questran Light, Prevalite

Classification: ANTILIPEMIC; BILE ACID SEQUESTRANT

Therapeutic: CHOLESTEROL-LOWERING

AVAILABILITY Powder for suspension

ACTION & *THERAPEUTIC EFFECT* Forms a nonabsorbable complex with bile acids in the intestine, releasing chloride ions in the process; inhibits enterohepatic reuptake of intestinal bile salts thereby increasing the fecal loss of bile salt-bound low-density lipoprotein cholesterol. *The resin anion-exchange agent increases fecal loss of bile acids, which leads to lowered serum total cholesterol by decreasing (LDL) cholesterol, and reducing bile acid deposit in dermal tissues (decreasing pruritus). Serum triglyceride levels may increase or remain unchanged.*

USES As adjunct to diet therapy in management of patients with primary hypercholesterolemia; for relief of pruritus associated with elevated levels of bile acids; regression of arteriosclerosis.

UNLABELED USES To control diarrhea caused by excess bile acids in colon; enhance elimination of digoxin when non-life-threatening toxicity occurs; hyperthyroidism.

CONTRAINDICATIONS Complete biliary obstruction or biliary cirrhosis, cholelithiasis; hypersensitivity to bile acid sequestrants; coagulopathy; lactation.

CAUTIOUS USE Bleeding disorders; hemorrhoids; impaired GI function, decreased GI motility; peptic ulcer, malabsorption states (e.g., steatorrhea); phenylketonuria (**Questran Light** only); renal disease; pregnancy (category C). Safe use in children 6 yr or younger not established.

ROUTE & DOSAGE

Hypercholesterolemia/Pruritus with Biliary Stasis

Adult: **PO** 4 g 1–2 × day; increase gradually; *maintenance dose:* 8–16 g/day divided in 2 doses (max: 24 g/day)
Child: **PO** 240 mg/kg/day in 2–3 divided doses (max: 8 g/day)

ADMINISTRATION

Oral

- Place contents of one packet or one level scoopful on surface of at least 60–180 mL (2–6 oz) of water or other preferred liquid. Mix well. Rinse glass with small amount of liquid and have patient drink remainder to ensure entire dose is taken. Administer before meals.
- Store in tightly closed container at 15°–30°C (59°–86°F) unless otherwise specified.

ADVERSE EFFECTS **CV:** Edema, syncope. **HEENT:** Tinnitus, tooth enamel decay. **Endocrine:** Hyperchloremic metabolic acidosis (children), increased libido, weight gain or loss. **GI:** Constipation, abdominal pain, abdominal distention, flatulence, nausea, vomiting, diarrhea, dyspepsia. **GU:** Diuresis, dysuria, hematuria. **Integumentary:** Perianal skin irritation, skin rash, urticaria.

DIAGNOSTIC TEST INTERFERENCE Cholestyramine therapy may be increased ***prothrombin time.***

INTERACTIONS **Drug:** Decreases the absorption of ORAL ANTICOAGULANTS, **digoxin,** TETRACYCLINES, **penicillins, mycophenolate, phenobarbital,** THYROID HORMONES, THIAZIDE DIURETICS, IRON SALTS, FAT-SOLUBLE VITAMINS (A, D, E, K) from the GI tract—administer cholestyramine 4 h before or 2 h after these drugs. Can bind to and affect absorption of any drug.

PHARMACOKINETICS **Absorption:** Not absorbed from GI tract. **Elimination:** Excreted in feces as insoluble complex.

NURSING IMPLICATIONS

Assessment & Drug Effects

- Be alert to early symptoms of hypoprothrombinemia (petechiae, ecchymoses, abnormal bleeding from mucous membranes, tarry stools) and report their occurrence promptly. Long-term use of cholestyramine resin can increase bleeding tendency.
- Monitor bowel function. Preexisting constipation may be worsened in the older adult and women.
- Consult prescriber regarding supplemental vitamins A and D and folic acid that may be required by patient on long-term therapy.

- Monitor lab tests: Periodic CBC, platelet count, serum electrolytes, and lipid profile.

Patient & Family Education

- Report constipation to prescriber. High-bulk diet with adequate fluid intake is an essential adjunct to cholestyramine treatment and generally resolves the problems of constipation and bloating sensation.
- Do not omit doses. Sudden withdrawal can promote uninhibited absorption of other drugs taken concomitantly, leading to toxicity or overdosage.
- GI adverse effects usually subside after the first month of drug therapy.
- The following symptoms may be drug-induced and should be reported promptly: Severe gastric distress with nausea and vomiting, unusual weight loss, black stools, severe hemorrhoids (GI bleeding), sudden back pain.

CHOLINE MAGNESIUM TRISALICYLATE

(cho'leen mag-ne'si-um tri-sal'i-ci-late)

Classification: ANALGESIC (SALICYLATE), NONSTEROIDAL ANTI-INFLAMMATORY DRUG (NSAID)

Therapeutic: ANALGESIC, NSAID

Prototype: Aspirin

AVAILABILITY Tablet; liquid

ACTION & *THERAPEUTIC EFFECT* Inhibits prostaglandin synthesis by reversibly inhibiting cyclooxygenase (both COX-1 and COX-2), resulting in its anti-inflammatory properties as well as its analgesic property. *Has anti-inflammatory, analgesic, and antipyretic action.*

USES Osteoarthritis, rheumatoid arthritis, and other arthrides; analgesia, antipyresis; juvenile idiopathic arthritis.

CONTRAINDICATIONS Hypersensitivity to nonacetylated salicylates; children and teenagers with chickenpox, influenza, or flu symptoms because of the potential for Reye syndrome; coagulopathy, anticoagulant therapy, G6PD deficiency; pregnancy (category D third trimester); contraindicated in late pregnancy, near term, or in labor and delivery; children younger than 6 yr.

CAUTIOUS USE Chronic renal and hepatic failure, history of GI disease, peptic ulcer; patients on Coumadin or heparin, anemia; hypovolemic states; older adults; pregnancy (category C first and second trimester); lactation.

ROUTE & DOSAGE

Arthritis

Adult: **PO** 1500 mg bid or 3000 mg daily; adjust to maximal response

Juvenile Idiopathic Arthritis

Child/Adolescent (weight greater than 37 kg): **PO** 1125 mg bid

ADMINISTRATION

Oral

- Give with food or large volume of water or milk to reduce gastric upset.
- Store at 15°–30°C (59°–86°F).

ADVERSE EFFECTS **HEENT:** Tinnitus. **GI:** Constipation, diarrhea, dyspepsia, epigastric pain, nausea, vomiting.

C

INTERACTIONS Drug: Aminosalicylic acid increases risk of salicylate toxicity; **acidifying agents** decrease its renal elimination, increasing risk of salicylate toxicity; ANTICOAGULANTS increase risk of bleeding; CARBONIC ANHYDRASE INHIBITORS enhance salicylate toxicity; CORTICOSTEROIDS compound ulcerogenic effects; increases **methotrexate** toxicity; low doses of salicylates may antagonize uricosuric effects of **probenecid, sulfinpyrazone.** Do not use live influenza vaccine or VARICELLA VACCINE due to risk of Reye syndrome.

PHARMACOKINETICS Absorption: Readily absorbed from small intestine. **Onset:** 30 min. **Peak:** 1–3 h. **Metabolism:** In liver. **Elimination:** In urine. **Half-Life:** 2–3 h.

NURSING IMPLICATIONS

Assessment & Drug Effects

- As with other NSAIDS, the antipyretic and anti-inflammatory effects may mask usual S&S of infection or other diseases.
- Assess for GI discomfort; nausea, gastric irritation, indigestion, diarrhea, and constipation are frequent complaints.
- Monitor for S&S of bleeding. Closely monitor PT if used concurrently with warfarin.
- Monitor serum salicylate levels, renal function, hearing changes or tinnitus, abnormal bruising, and pain response.

Patient & Family Education

- Avoid taking aspirin, NSAIDS, or acetaminophen concurrently with drug.
- Avoid dangerous activities until reaction to drug is determined, due to possible CNS effects (e.g., vertigo, drowsiness).
- Report tinnitus or persistent gastric irritation and epigastric pain.
- Report any unexplained bruising or bleeding to prescriber.
- Hypoglycemic effects may be enhanced for those with type 2 diabetes taking an oral hypoglycemic agent (OHA).
- Do not give to children or teenagers with chickenpox, influenza, or flu symptoms because of association with Reye syndrome.

CHORIONIC GONADOTROPIN

(go-nad′oh-troe-pin)

Pregnyl

Classification: HUMAN CHORIONIC GONADOTROPIN (HCG) HORMONE

Therapeutic: HCG HORMONE

AVAILABILITY Solution for injection

ACTION & THERAPEUTIC EFFECT Promotes production of gonadal steroid hormones by stimulating interstitial cells of the testes to produce androgen and the corpus luteum of the ovary to produce progesterone. *Administration of HCG to women of childbearing age with normal functioning ovaries causes maturation of the ovarian follicle and triggers ovulation.*

USES Prepubertal cryptorchidism not due to anatomic obstruction and male hypogonadism secondary to pituitary deficiency. Also used in conjunction with menotropins to induce ovulation and pregnancy in infertile women in whom the cause of anovulation is secondary; ovulation usually occurs within 18 h. To stimulate spermatogenesis in males with hypogonadism.

UNLABELED USES Corpus luteum dysfunction.

C

CONTRAINDICATIONS Known hypersensitivity to HCG, hypogonadism of testicular origin, hamster protein hypersensitivity; hypertrophy or tumor of pituitary, prostatic carcinoma or other androgen-dependent neoplasms, precocious puberty; ovarian failure; dysfunctional uterine bleeding; adrenal insufficiency; uncontrolled thyroid disease; pregnancy (category X).

CAUTIOUS USE Epilepsy, migraine, asthma, cardiac or renal disease; endometriosis; thrombophlebitis; lactation. Safe use in children younger than 4 yr has not been established.

ROUTE & DOSAGE

Prepubertal Cryptorchidism

Child: **IM** 4000 units 3 × wk for 3 wk, *or* 5000 units every other day for 4 doses, *or* 500–1000 units 3 × wk for 4–6 wk

Hypogonadotropic Hypogonadism

Adult: **IM** 500–1000 units 3 × wk for 3 wk, then 2 × wk for 3 wk *or* 4000 units 3 × wk for 6–9 mo followed by 2000 units 3 × wk for 3 mo

Stimulation of Spermatogenesis

Adult: **IM** 5000 units 3 × wk until normal testosterone levels are achieved (4–6 mo), then 2000 units 2 × wk with menotropins for 4 mo

Induction of Ovulation

Adult: **IM** 500–1000 units 1 day following last dose of menotropins

ADMINISTRATION

Intramuscular

- Reconstitute only with diluent supplied by manufacturer.
- Following reconstitution solution is stable for 30–90 day, depending on manufacturer, when refrigerated; thereafter potency decreases.
- Give IM into a large muscle.
- Store powder for injection at 15°–30°C (59°–86°F) unless otherwise directed.

ADVERSE EFFECTS **CNS:** Headache, irritability, restlessness, depression, fatigue. **Endocrine:** Gynecomastia, precocious puberty, increased urinary steroid excretion, ectopic pregnancy (incidence low). When used with menotropins (human menopausal gonadotropin): Ovarian hyperstimulation (ascites with or without pain, pleural effusion, ruptured ovarian cysts with resultant hemoperitoneum, multiple births). **Other:** Edema, pain at injection site, arterial thromboembolism.

DIAGNOSTIC TEST INTERFERENCE ***Pregnancy tests:*** Possibility of false results.

INTERACTIONS **Herbal:** **Black cohosh** may antagonize fertility effects.

PHARMACOKINETICS **Onset:** 2 h. **Peak:** 6 h. **Distribution:** Testes in males, ovaries in females. **Elimination:** 10–12% in urine within 24 h. **Half-Life:** 23 h.

NURSING IMPLICATIONS

Assessment & Drug Effects

- Assess prepubescent males for development of secondary sex characteristics.

- Assess females for and report excessive menstrual bleeding, irregular menstrual cycles, and abdominal/pelvic distention or pain.

Patient & Family Education

- Report promptly onset of abdominal pain and distension (ovarian hyperstimulation syndrome).
- Report to prescriber if the following appear: Axillary, facial, pubic hair; penile growth; acne; deepening of voice. Induction of androgen secretion by HCG may induce precocious puberty in patient treated for cryptorchidism.
- Observe for signs of fluid retention. A weight chart should be maintained for a biweekly record. Report to prescriber if weight gain is associated with edema.

CICLESONIDE

(ci-cle-so′nide)

Alvesco, Omnaris, Zetonna

See Appendix A-3.

CICLOPIROX

(sye-kloe-peer′ox)

Ciclodan, Loprox

Classification: ANTIFUNGAL ANTIBIOTIC

Therapeutic: ANTIFUNGAL ANTIBIOTIC

AVAILABILITY Cream; gel; nail lacquer; shampoo; topical solution

ACTION & *THERAPEUTIC EFFECT* Inhibits transport of amino acids within fungal cell, thereby interfering with synthesis of fungal protein, RNA, and DNA. *Effective against the following organisms: Dermatophytes, yeasts, some species of* Mycoplasma *and* Trichomonas vaginalis, *and certain strains of gram-positive and gram-negative bacteria.*

USES Topically for treatment of tinea pedis, tinea cruris, and tinea corporis (ringworm) due to *Trichophyton rubrum, Trichophyton mentagrophytes, Epidermophyton floccosum,* and *Microsporum canis,* and for tinea (pityriasis) versicolor due to *M. furfur;* also cutaneous candidiasis (moniliasis) caused by *Candida albicans.* Nail lacquer indicated for onychomycosis of fingernails and toenails due to *T. rubrum;* seborrheic dermatitis of the scalp.

CONTRAINDICATIONS Hypersensitivity to ciclopirox or to any component in the formulation.

CAUTIOUS USE Type 1 diabetic patient; history of seizure disorder; immunosuppression; pregnancy (adverse events not observed in animal reproduction studies); lactation. Safe use in children younger than 10 yr not established.

ROUTE & DOSAGE

Tinea

Adult: **Topical** Massage cream into affected area and surrounding skin twice daily, morning and evening

Onychomycosis

Adult/Adolescent/Child (10 yr or older): **Topical** Paint affected nail(s) under the surface of the nail and on the nail bed once daily at bedtime (at least 8 h before washing). After 7 days, remove lacquer with alcohol and remove or trim away unattached nail. Continue up to 48 wk.

C

Seborrheic Dermatitis

Adult/Adolescent: **Topical** Wet hair and apply approximately 1 tsp (5 mL) to the scalp (may use up to 10 mL for long hair), leave on scalp for 3 min, then rinse. Repeat treatment twice/wk × 4 wk, with a minimum of 3 days between applications.

ADMINISTRATION

Topical

- Wash hands thoroughly before and after treatments.
- Consult with prescriber about specific procedure for cleansing the skin before medication is applied. Regardless of method used, dry skin thoroughly before drug application. Not for ophthalmic, oral, or intravaginal use.
- Avoid occlusive dressing, wrapping, or clothing over site where cream is applied.
- Store at 15°–30°C (59°–86°F) unless otherwise directed.

ADVERSE EFFECTS **Cardiac:** Facial edema, ventricular tachycardia (with shampoo). **CNS:** Headache. **Integumentary:** Irritation, pruritus, burning, worsening of clinical condition.

PHARMACOKINETICS **Absorption:** 1.3% absorbed through intact skin. **Distribution:** Distributed to epidermis, corium (dermis), including hair and hair follicles and sebaceous glands; **Elimination:** Urine 3–10%. **Half-Life:** 1.7 h.

NURSING IMPLICATIONS

Assessment & Drug Effects

- Monitor for therapeutic effectiveness. Tinea versicolor generally responds to drug treatment in about 2 wk. Tinea pedis ("athlete's foot"), tinea corporis (ringworm), tinea cruris ("jock itch"), and candidiasis (moniliasis) require about 4 wk of therapy.

Patient & Family Education

- Use medication for the prescribed time even though symptoms improve.
- Report skin irritation or other possible signs of sensitization. A reaction suggestive of sensitization warrants drug discontinuation.
- Do not use occlusive dressings or wrappings.
- Avoid contact of drug in or near the eyes.
- Wear light clothing and footwear that will allow ventilation. Loose-fitting cotton underwear or socks are preferred.

CIDOFOVIR

(cye-do'fo-ver)

Classification: ANTIVIRAL
Therapeutic: ANTIVIRAL
Prototype: Acyclovir

AVAILABILITY Solution for injection

ACTION & *THERAPEUTIC EFFECT* Cidofovir reduces the rate of viral DNA synthesis of cytomegalovirus (CMV). *It is limited for use in treating CMV retinitis in patients with AIDS. Also effective against herpes viruses and other viruses.*

USES Treatment/prophylaxis of CMV retinitis in patients with AIDS.

UNLABELED USES Herpes simplex resistant to acyclovir.

CONTRAINDICATIONS Hypersensitivity to cidofovir, history of severe hypersensitivity to probenecid or other sulfa-containing

C

medications; childbearing women and men without barrier contraception; acute renal failure; serum creatinine more than 1.5 mg/dL, creatinine clearance 55 mL/min or less, or urine protein 100 mg/dL or more; lactation.

CAUTIOUS USE Renal function impairment, DM, myelosuppression, previous hypersensitivity to other nucleoside analogs; older adults; pregnancy (systemic therapy should be avoided during the first trimester when possible). Safety and efficacy in children not established.

ROUTE & DOSAGE

CMV Retinitis: Induction and Maintenance

Adult: **IV** 5 mg/kg once weekly for 2 wk then continue every 2 wk. Administer probenecid concomitantly.

Renal Impairment Dosage Adjustment

If serum Cr increases by 0.3–0.4, lower dose to 3 mg/kg

ADMINISTRATION

- Pretreatment: Prehydrate with IV of 1 L NS infused over 1–2 h immediately before cidofovir infusion. If able to tolerate fluid load, infuse second liter over 1–3 h starting at beginning (or end) of cidofovir infusion.

Intravenous

PREPARE: **IV Infusion:** Dilute the calculated dose in 100 mL of NS. ***ADMINISTER:*** **IV Infusion:** Give over 1 h at constant rate. ▪ Do not coadminister with other agents with significant nephrotoxic potential.

- Store vials at 20°–25°C (68°–77°F); may store diluted IV solution at 2°–8°C (36°–46°F) for up to 24 h.

ADVERSE EFFECTS **Respiratory:** Dyspnea, pneumonia. **CNS:** *Fever, headache,* asthenia. **HEENT:** Ocular hypotony. **Endocrine:** Metabolic acidosis. **GI:** Nausea, vomiting, diarrhea. **GU:** *Nephrotoxicity, proteinuria*. **Hematologic:** Neutropenia. **Other:** Infection, allergic reactions.

INTERACTIONS **Drug:** Do not use with **cladribine**.

PHARMACOKINETICS **Duration:** Probenecid increases serum levels and area under concentration–time curve. **Elimination:** 70-80% unchanged in urine.

NURSING IMPLICATIONS

Black Box Warning

Cidofovir has been associated with severe renal impairment and neutropenia.

Assessment & Drug Effects

- Periodic visual acuity tests and measurement of intraocular pressure are recommended.
- Note that probenecid is typically given concurrently to minimize potential nephrotoxicity. Potential adverse effects of probenecid include headache, nausea, vomiting, hypersensitivity reactions.
- Monitor for S&S of hypersensitivity (see Appendix F). Report their appearance promptly.
- Monitor lab tests: Serum creatinine and urine protein within 48 h prior to each dose. CBC with differential prior to each dose.

Patient & Family Education

- Initiate or continue regular ophthalmologic exams.

- Be alert to potential adverse reactions caused by probenecid (e.g., headache, nausea, vomiting, hypersensitivity reactions) and cidofovir.

CILOSTAZOL

(sil-os′tah-zol)

Classification: ANTIPLATELET; PHOSPHODIESTERASE INHIBITOR
Therapeutic: PERIPHERAL VASODILATOR; PLATELET AGGREGATION INHIBITOR

AVAILABILITY Tablet

ACTION & *THERAPEUTIC EFFECT* Suppresses degradation of cyclic AMP leading to reversible inhibition of platelet aggregation, vasodilation, and inhibition of vascular smooth muscle cell proliferation. *Increases the skin temperature of the extremities and improves claudication. Effectiveness is indicated by increased ability to walk further without claudication.*

USES Intermittent claudication.

UNLABELED USES Elective PCI with stent placement; secondary prevention of noncardioembolic ischemic stroke or transient ischemic attack (TIA); prevention of stent thrombosis and restenosis after coronary stent placement.

CONTRAINDICATIONS CHF of any severity; hypersensitivity to cilostazol; acute MI; hemostatic disorders or pathologic bleeding; lactation.

CAUTIOUS USE Cardiac arrhythmias, MI within 6 mo; valvular heart disease; peptic ulcer disease; renal failure; hepatic impairment; pregnancy (category C). Safety and efficacy in children younger than 18 yr not established.

ROUTE & DOSAGE

Intermittent Claudication

Adult: **PO** 100 mg bid, may need to reduce to 50 mg bid with concomitant CYP3A4 or CYP2C19 inhibitors

ADMINISTRATION

Oral

- Give at least 30 min before or 2 h after a meal. Do not give with grapefruit juice.
- Store at 20°–25°C (68°–77°F).

ADVERSE EFFECTS **CV:** Palpitations. **Respiratory:** Rhinitis, pharyngitis. **CNS:** *Headache*, dizziness. **GI:** Diarrhea, abnormal stools. **Other:** Infection.

INTERACTIONS **Drug:** **Diltiazem, erythromycin, anagrelide, conivaptan, idelalisib, fluconazole, fluvoxamine, fluoxetine, ketoconazole, itraconazole,** MACROLIDE ANTIBIOTICS, **nefazodone, omeprazole, sertraline,** PROTEASE INHIBITORS may increase cilostazol levels and adverse effects. Do not use with **defibrotide**. **Herbal:** **Evening primrose oil** may increase bleeding risk. **Food:** High-fat meals may increase peak concentrations. **Grapefruit juice** may increase concentration.

PHARMACOKINETICS **Onset:** 2–4 wk. **Distribution:** 95–98% protein- bound. May be excreted in breast milk. **Metabolism:** Metabolized by CYP3A4 and CYP 2C19 to active metabolites. **Elimination:** Metabolites primarily excreted in urine and feces. **Half-Life:** 11–13 h.

C

NURSING IMPLICATIONS

Assessment & Drug Effects

- Monitor therapeutic effectiveness indicated by ability to walk farther without leg pain.
- Monitor for S&S of CHF. Do not give cilostazol to patients with preexisting CHF.
- Monitor platelet and WBC counts periodically.

Patient & Family Education

- Avoid grapefruit or grapefruit juice while taking cilostazol.
- Allow 2–12 wk for therapeutic response.
- Monitor for signs of abnormal bleeding.

CIMETIDINE

(sye-met′i-deen)

Tagamet HB

Classification: ANTISECRETORY (H_2-RECEPTOR ANTAGONIST)

Therapeutic: ANTISECRETORY

AVAILABILITY Tablet; oral solution

ACTION & *THERAPEUTIC EFFECT* Has high selectivity for inhibition of histamine H_2-receptors on parietal cells of the stomach, thus suppressing all phases of daytime and nocturnal basal gastric acid secretion in the stomach. Indirectly reduces pepsin secretion. *Blocks the H_2-receptors on the parietal cells of the stomach, thus decreasing gastric acid secretion; raises the pH of the stomach and thereby reduces pepsin secretion.*

USES Short-term treatment of erosive gastroesophageal reflux disease and relief and prevention of heartburn.

UNLABELED USES Prophylaxis of stress-induced ulcers, upper GI bleeding, chronic urticaria; interstitial cystitis.

CONTRAINDICATIONS Known hypersensitivity to cimetidine or other H_2-receptor antagonists.

CAUTIOUS USE Older adults or critically ill patients; impaired renal or hepatic function; organic brain syndrome; gastric ulcers; immunocompromised patients, pregnancy (cimetidine crosses the placenta); children younger than 12 yr.

ROUTE & DOSAGE

GERD

Adult/Adolescent: **PO** 800 mg bid or 400 mg qid × 12 w
Child: **PO** 20–40 mg/kg/day in 3–4 divided doses

Heartburn

Adult: **PO** 200 mg 2–4 × day

Renal Impairment Dosage Adjustment

CrCl less than 30 mL/min: Reduce daily dose by 50%

ADMINISTRATION

Oral

- Administer with meals.

ADVERSE EFFECTS **CV (rare):** Cardiac arrhythmias and cardiac arrest after rapid IV bolus dose. **CNS:** Headache. **GU:** Gynecomastia, increased serum creatinine.

DIAGNOSTIC TEST INTERFERENCE Cimetidine may cause false-positive ***Hemoccult test***

for gastric bleeding if test is performed within 15 min of oral cimetidine administration.

INTERACTIONS **Drug:** Cimetidine may increase activity of **warfarin;** ANTACIDS may decrease absorption of cimetidine. Do not use with **dasatinib.** May decrease the effect of **mesalamine.** May decrease concentration of **acalabrutinib, atazanavir, bosutinib, cefditoren, cefuroxime, dacomitinib, delavirdine, erlotinib, gefitinib, ketoconazole, ledipasvir, neratinib, nilotinib, pazopanib, pexidartinib, rilpivirine, risedronate, selpercatinib.** May increase concentration of **amiodarone,** CALCIUM CHANNEL BLOCKERS, **chloroquine, citalopram, clozapine, dofetilide, epirubicin, fosphenytoin, phenytoin, itraconazole, lasmiditan, lemborexant, lomitapide, metformin, moclobemide, posaconazole, procainamide, quinidine, quinine, tizanidine, tolvaptan, ubrogepant, zolmitriptan.**

PHARMACOKINETICS **Absorption:** 70% from GI tract. **Peak:** 1–1.5 h. **Distribution:** Widely distributed; crosses blood–brain barrier and placenta. **Metabolism:** In liver by CYP1A2 and 3A4. **Elimination:** Most of drug excreted in urine in 24 h; excreted in breast milk. **Half-Life:** 2 h.

NURSING IMPLICATIONS

Assessment & Drug Effects

- Monitor pulse of patient during first few days of drug regimen. Bradycardia should be reported. Pulse usually returns to normal within 24 h after drug discontinuation.
- Monitor I&O ratio and pattern: Particularly in the older adult, severely ill, and in patients with impaired renal function.
- Be alert to onset of confusional states, particularly in the older adult or severely ill patient. Symptoms occur within 2–3 days after first dose; report immediately. Symptoms usually resolve within 3–4 days after therapy is discontinued.
- Check BP and report an elevation to the prescriber, if patient complains of severe headache.
- Monitor lab tests: Periodic CBC and renal function tests.

Patient & Family Education

- Seek advice about self-medication with any OTC drug.
- Report breast tenderness or enlargement. Mild bilateral gynecomastia and breast soreness may occur after 1 mo or more of therapy. It may disappear spontaneously or remain throughout therapy.
- Report recurrence of gastric pain or bleeding (black, tarry stools or "coffee ground" vomitus) immediately, and notify prescriber if diarrhea continues more than 1 day.
- Avoid driving and other potentially hazardous activities until reaction to drug is known.
- Duodenal or gastric ulcer is a chronic, recurrent condition that requires long-term maintenance drug therapy.

CINACALCET HYDROCHLORIDE

(sin-a-kal′set)

Sensipar

Classification: PARATHYROID HORMONE; CALCIUM RECEPTOR AGONIST

Therapeutic: PARATHYROID HORMONE

C

AVAILABILITY Tablet

ACTION & *THERAPEUTIC EFFECT* Directly lowers parathyroid hormone (PTH) levels by increasing sensitivity of calcium-sensing receptors on parathyroid gland to extracellular calcium. This causes decreased calcium and phosphate adsorption from bone, and thus decreased serum calcium and phosphate levels. *Lowers PTH production; this also decreases rate of bone turnover and bone fibrosis in chronic renal failure disease (CRFD).*

USES Primary or secondary hyperparathyroidism; hypercalcemia in patients with parathyroid cancer.

CONTRAINDICATIONS Hypersensitivity to cinacalcet; hypocalcemia or lower limit of normal serum calcium; chronic kidney disease patients not on dialysis; lactation.

CAUTIOUS USE Moderate and severe hepatic impairment, history of seizures; hypotension; heart failure; history of QT prolongation; history of arrhythmias; pregnancy (category C); children younger than 18 yr.

ROUTE & DOSAGE

Hyperparathyroidism

Adult: **PO** Start with 30 mg once daily; may increase q2–4wk until target iPTH of 150–300 pg/mL (max: 300 mg/day)

Hypercalcemia

Adult: **PO** 30 mg twice daily; titrate q2–4wk as 60 mg bid, 90 mg bid, then 90 mg 3–4 × daily as needed to normalize calcium concentrations

ADMINISTRATION

Oral

- Give with food or shortly after a meal.
- Tablets should be swallowed whole and not divided, crushed, or chewed.
- Do not give to patient with hypocalcemia.
- Store at 15°–30°C (59°–86°F).

ADVERSE EFFECTS **CV:** Hypertension. **Endocrine:** Hypocalcemia. **GI:** *Nausea, vomiting, diarrhea,* anorexia, constipation. **Musculoskeletal:** *Myalgia,* adynamic bone disease (renal osteo-dystrophy). **Other:** Dizziness, asthenia, noncardiac chest pain, dialysis access infection.

INTERACTIONS **Drug:** May increase **amoxapine, atomoxetine, carvedilol, clozapine, codeine, cyclobenzaprine, dexfenfluramine, dextromethorphan, donepezil, fenfluramine, flecainide, fluoxetine, haloperidol, hydrocodone, maprotiline, meperidine, methadone, methamphetamine, metoprolol, mexiletine, morphine, oxycodone, paroxetine, perphenazine, propafenone, propranolol, risperidone, thioridazine** (use may be contraindicated with cinacalcet), **timolol, tramadol, trazodone,** TRICYCLIC ANTIDEPRESSANTS, **venlafaxine, zolpidem** levels; cinacalcet levels may be increased by strong CYP3A4 inhibitors such as **amiodarone, aprepitant, clarithromycin, dalfopristin, diltiazem, erythromycin, fluconazole, fluvoxamine, itraconazole, ketoconazole, miconazole, nefazodone, quinupristin, troleandomycin, verapamil, voriconazole.** **Food: Grapefruit juice** may increase cinacalcet levels.

PHARMACOKINETICS **Peak:** 2–6 h. **Distribution:** 93–97% protein bound. **Metabolism:** In liver by CYP3A4. **Elimination:** 80% by kidneys, 15% in feces. **Half-Life:** 30–40 h.

NURSING IMPLICATIONS

Assessment & Drug Effects

- Monitor for S&S of hypocalcemia (e.g., paresthesias, myalgias, cramping, tetany, convulsions).
- Withhold drug and notify prescriber for serum calcium less than 7.5 mg/dL or symptoms of hypocalcemia. Drug should not be resumed until serum calcium levels reach 8 mg/dL, and/or symptoms of hypocalcemia resolve.
- Closely monitor iPTH and serum calcium with concurrent administration of a strong CYP3A4 (e.g., ketoconazole, erythromycin, itraconazole).
- Monitor lab tests: Baseline serum calcium, repeat within a week of initiation or dosage adjustment, and iPTH 1–4 wk after initiation of drug or dose adjustment; thereafter, monthly serum calcium and phosphorus (more often with a history of a seizure disorder), and iPTH every 1–3 mo.

Patient & Family Education

- Report promptly any of the following: Seizure or convulsion; muscle spasms or cramping of the abdomen, back, legs, face; burning, numbness, pricking, tickling, or tingling of the face, lips, tongue, hands, or feet; changes in mental status.

CIPROFLOXACIN HYDROCHLORIDE (Pr)

(ci-pro-flox'a-cin)

Cetraxal, Cipro, Cipro XR, OTIPRIO

CIPROFLOXACIN OPHTHALMIC

Ciloxan

Classification: QUINOLONE ANTIBIOTIC

Therapeutic: ANTIBIOTIC

AVAILABILITY Tablet; extended release tablet; suspension; solution for injection; ophthalmic solution; otic drops

ACTION & *THERAPEUTIC EFFECT* Inhibits DNA-gyrase, an enzyme necessary for bacterial DNA replication and some aspects of transcription, repair, recombination, and transposition. *Effective against many gram-positive and aerobic gram-negative organisms.*

USES UTIs, lower respiratory tract infections, skin and skin structure infections, bone and joint infections, GI infection or infectious diarrhea, chronic bacterial prostatitis, gonorrhea, urethritis, nosocomial pneumonia, acute sinusitis. Postexposure prophylaxis for anthrax. **Ophthalmic:** Corneal ulcers, bacterial conjunctivitis caused by *Staphylococci, Streptococci,* and *Pseudomonas aeruginosa.* **Otic:** Otitis externa.

CONTRAINDICATIONS Known hypersensitivity to ciprofloxacin or other quinolones, concurrent administration of tizanidine, syphilis, viral infection; history of myasthenia gravis; peripheral neuropathy; tendon inflammation or tendon pain; lactation.

CAUTIOUS USE Known or suspected CNS disorders (i.e., severe cerebral arteriosclerosis or seizure disorders); myocardial ischemia, atrial fibrillation, QT prolongation, CHF; GI disease, colitis; CVA; uncorrected hypokalemia; severe renal impairment and crystalluria during ciprofloxacin therapy; pregnancy (category C); children.

ROUTE & DOSAGE

Uncomplicated UTI

Adult: **PO** 250 mg q12h or 500 mg XR daily × 3 days; **IV** 200 mg q12h × 7–14 days

Complicated UTI

Adult: **PO** 250–500 mg q12h or 1000 mg XR daily × 7–14 days; **IV** 200–400 mg q12h × 7–14 days

Respiratory Tract Infections

Adult: **IV** 400 mg q8–12h × 7–14 days; **PO** 500–750 q12h × 7–14 days

Pneumonia

Adult: **IV** 400 mg q8–12h × 10–14 days

Acute Sinusitis

Adult: **PO** 500 mg bid × 10 days

Moderate to Severe Systemic Infection

Adult: **PO** 500–750 mg q12h; **IV** 200–400 mg q8–12h

Skin/Skin Structure Infection

Adult: **PO** 500–750 mg q12h × 7–14 days; **IV** 400 mg q8–12h × 7–14 days

Renal Impairment Dosage Adjustment

Adult (CrCl 30–50 mL/min): **PO** 250–500 mg q12h; **IV** No change in dose; *less than 30 mL/min:* **PO** 250–500 mg q18h; **IV** 200–400 mg q18–24h

Bacterial Conjunctivitis

Adult: **Ophthalmic** 1–2 drops in conjunctival sac q2h while awake for 2 days, then 1–2 drops q4h while awake for the next 5 days **Ointment** ½-inch ribbon into conjunctival sac tid × 2 days, then bid × 5 days

Corneal Ulcers

Adult: **Ophthalmic** 2 drops q15min for 6 h, 2 drops q30min for the next 18 h, then 2 drops q1h for 24 h, then 2 drops q4h for 14 days

Otitis Externa

Adult/Adolescent/Child (1 yr or older): 0.25 mL into affected ears q12h × 7 days

ADMINISTRATION

- For patients with renal impairment, oral and IV doses are lowered according to creatinine clearance.

Ophthalmic

- Apply ointment or solution directly into the conjunctival sac when treating conjunctivitis.

Oral

- Do not give an antacid within 4 h of the oral ciprofloxacin dose. May administer with food to minimize GI upset.
- Swallow whole; do not split, crush, or chew.

Otic

- Warm solution by holding container in hands for at least 1 min to minimize dizziness.
- Patient should lie on opposite side and remain for 1 min after instillation.

C

Intravenous

PREPARE: **Intermittent:** Dilute in NS or D5W to a final concentration of 0.5–2 mg/mL. ▪ Typical dilutions are 200 mg in 100–250 mL and 400 mg in 250–500 mL.

ADMINISTER: **Intermittent:** Give slowly over 60 min. Avoid rapid infusion and use of a small vein.

INCOMPATIBILITIES: **Solution/additive:** **Aminophylline, amoxicillin, amoxicillin/clavulanate potassium, amphotericin B, ampicillin/sulbactam, ceftazidime, cefuroxime, clindamycin, heparin, metronidazole, piperacillin, sodium bicarbonate, ticarcillin.** **Y-site:** **Aminophylline, ampicillin, ampicillin/sulbactam, azithromycin, cefepime, dexamethasone, furosemide, heparin, hydrocortisone, lansoprazole, phenytoin, propofol, sodium bicarbonate, theophylline, TPN, warfarin.**

▪ Discontinue other IV infusion while infusing ciprofloxacin or infuse through another site.

▪ Reconstituted IV solution is stable for 14 days refrigerated.

ADVERSE EFFECTS

Respiratory: Rhinitis, pharyngitis. **CNS:** Headache, vertigo, malaise, peripheral neuropathy, nervousness, insomnia seizures (especially with rapid IV infusion). **HEENT:** *Local burning and discomfort, crystalline precipitate on superficial portion of cornea,* lid margin crusting, scales, foreign body sensation, itching, and conjunctival hyperemia. **Endocrine:** Transient increases in liver transaminases, alkaline phosphatase, lactic dehydrogenase, and eosinophilia count. **Skin:** Rash, phlebitis, pain, burning, pruritus, and erythema at infusion site; photosensitivity. **GI:** Nausea, vomiting, diarrhea, cramps, gas, pseudomembranous colitis. **Musculoskeletal:** Tendon rupture, cartilage erosion.

DIAGNOSTIC TEST INTERFERENCE

May cause false positive on ***opiate screening tests.***

INTERACTIONS

Drug: May increase **theophylline** levels 15–30%; ANTACIDS, **sucralfate, iron** decrease absorption of ciprofloxacin; may increase PT for patients on **warfarin.** Do not use with **dofetilide, dronedarone, ziprasidone** due to risk of increased QT prolongation. Do not use with **tizanidine**. Avoid use with **zolpidem** due to increased exposure. **Food:** **Calcium** decreases the levels of ciprofloxacin.

PHARMACOKINETICS

Absorption: 60–80% from GI tract; ophthalmic: Minimal absorption through cornea or conjunctiva. **Onset:** Topical 0.5–2 h. **Duration:** Topical 12 h. **Peak:** Immediate release: 0.5–2 h; Cipro XR: 1–2.5 h; **Distribution:** Widely distributed including prostate, lung, and bone; crosses placenta; distributed into breast milk. **Elimination:** Primarily in urine with some biliary excretion. **Half-Life:** 3.5–4 h.

NURSING IMPLICATIONS

Black Box Warning

Ciprofloxacin (oral and IV) has been associated with increased risk of tendinitis and tendon rupture, and with exacerbations of muscle weakness in persons with myasthenia gravis.

Assessment & Drug Effects

- Report tendon inflammation or pain. Drug should be discontinued.
- Monitor I&O ratio and patterns: Patients should be well hydrated; assess for S&S of crystalluria.
- Monitor persons with myasthenia gravis for exacerbations of muscle weakness.
- Monitor plasma theophylline concentrations with concurrent use because drug may interfere with half-life.
- Administration with theophylline derivatives or caffeine can cause CNS stimulation.
- Assess for S&S of GI irritation (e.g., nausea, diarrhea, vomiting, abdominal discomfort) in clients receiving high dosages and in older adults.
- Monitor PT and INR in patients receiving coumarin therapy.
- Assess for S&S of superinfections (see Appendix F).
- Monitor lab tests: Baseline C&S, periodic LFTs, renal function tests, and CBC with differential with prolonged therapy.

Patient & Family Education

- Immediately report tendon inflammation or pain. Drug should be discontinued.
- Fluid intake of 2–3 L/day is advised, if not contraindicated.
- Report sudden, unexplained joint pain.
- Restrict caffeine due to the following effects: Nervousness, insomnia, anxiety, tachycardia.
- Use sunscreen and avoid overexposure to sunlight.
- Report nausea, diarrhea, vomiting, and abdominal pain or discomfort.
- Use caution with hazardous activities until reaction to drug is known. Drug may cause light-headedness.

CISATRACURIUM BESYLATE

(cis-a-tra-kyoo-ri′um)

Nimbex

Classification: NONDEPOLARIZING SKELETAL MUSCLE RELAXANT; NEUROMUSCULAR BLOCKER

Therapeutic: SKELETAL MUSCLE RELAXANT

Prototype: Atracurium

AVAILABILITY Solution for injection

ACTION & *THERAPEUTIC EFFECT* It binds competitively to cholinergic receptors on the motor endplate of neurons, antagonizing the action of acetylcholine. *Blocks neuromuscular transmission of nerve impulses.*

USES Adjunct to general anesthesia to facilitate tracheal intubation and provide skeletal muscle relaxation during surgery or mechanical ventilation.

CONTRAINDICATIONS Hypersensitivity to cisatracurium or other related agents; rapid-sequence endotracheal intubation.

CAUTIOUS USE History of hemiparesis, electrolyte imbalances, burn patients, pulmonary disease, COPD; neuromuscular diseases (e.g., myasthenia gravis), older adults, renal function impairment, pregnancy (category B), lactation. Safe use in children younger than 1 mo not established.

ROUTE & DOSAGE

Intubation

Adult: **IV** 0.15 or 0.20 mg/kg
Child (2–12 yr): **IV** 0.1–0.15 mg/kg; *Infant (1 mo or older):* **IV** 0.15 mg/kg

Maintenance

Adult: **IV** 0.03 mg/kg q20min prn *or* 1–2 mcg/kg/min
Child (2 yr or older): **IV** 1–2 mcg/kg/min

Mechanical Ventilation in ICU

Adult: **IV** 3 mcg/kg/min (can range from 0.5 to 10.2 mcg/kg/min)

ADMINISTRATION

- Administer carefully adjusted, individualized doses using a peripheral nerve stimulator to evaluate neuromuscular function.
- Given only by or under supervision of expert clinician familiar with the drug's actions and potential complications.
- Have immediately available personnel and facilities for resuscitation and life support and an antagonist of cisatracurium.
- Note that 10-mL multiple-dose vials contain benzyl alcohol and should not be used with neonates.

Intravenous

PREPARE: **Direct:** Give undiluted. **IV Infusion:** Dilute 10 mg in 95 mL or 40 mg in 80 mL of compatible IV fluid to prepare 0.1 mg/mL or 0.4 mg/mL, respectively, IV solution. ▪ Compatible IV fluids include D5W, NS, D5/NS, D5/LR. **ICU IV Infusion (Mechanical Ventilation):** Dilute the contents of the 200-mg vial (i.e., 10 mg/mL) in 1000 mL or 500 mL of compatible IV fluid to prepare 0.2-mg/mL or 0.4-g/mL, respectively, IV solutions.

ADMINISTER: **Direct:** Give a single dose over 5–10 sec. **IV Infusion:** Adjust the rate based on patient's weight.

INCOMPATIBILITIES: **Solution/additive:** **Ketorolac, propofol (dose dependent).** **Y-site:** **Amphotericin B, amphotericin B cholesteryl complex, ampicillin, cefazolin, cefotaxime, cefotetan, cefuroxime, diazepam, furosemide, ganciclovir, heparin, methylprednisolone, sodium bicarbonate, trimethoprim/sulfamethoxazole.**

- Refrigerate vials at 2°–8°C (36°–46°F). Protect from light. Diluted solutions may be stored refrigerated or at room temperature for 24 h.

ADVERSE EFFECTS **CV:** Bradycardia, hypotension, flushing. **Respiratory:** Bronchospasm. **Skin:** Rash.

PHARMACOKINETICS **Onset:** Varies from 1.5 to 3.3 min (higher dose has faster onset). **Peak:** Varies from 1.5 to 3.3 min (higher dose has faster peak). **Duration:** Varies with dose from 46 to 121 min (higher dose, longer recovery time). **Metabolism:** Undergoes Hoffman elimination (pH- and temperature-dependent degradation) and hydrolysis by plasma esterases. **Elimination:** In urine. **Half-Life:** 22 min.

NURSING IMPLICATIONS

Assessment & Drug Effects

- Time-to-maximum neuromuscular block is ≈1 min slower in the older adult.
- Monitor for bradycardia, hypotension, and bronchospasms; monitor ICU patients for spontaneous seizures.

C

CISPLATIN (*cis*-DDP, *cis*-PLATINUM II)

(sis′pla-tin)

Classification: ANTINEOPLASTIC; ALKYLATING AGENT

Therapeutic: ANTINEOPLASTIC

Prototype: Cyclophosphamide

AVAILABILITY Solution for injection

ACTION & THERAPEUTIC EFFECT
A heavy metal complex that produces cross linkage in DNA of rapidly dividing cells, thus preventing DNA, RNA, and protein synthesis. *Cell cycle-nonspecific (i.e., effective throughout the entire cell life cycle).*

USES Established combination therapy (cisplatin, vinblastine, bleomycin) in patient with advanced bladder cancer, ovarian cancer, or testicular cancer.

UNLABELED USES Carcinoma of endometrium, head, and neck, adrenocortical carcinoma, biliary tract cancer, cervical cancer, esophageal cancer, gastric cancer, malignant pleural mesothelioma, multiple myeloma, non-small-cell lung cancer, osteosarcoma, small-cell lung cancer.

CONTRAINDICATIONS History of hypersensitivity to cisplatin or other platinum-containing compounds; impaired renal function of CrCl below 30 mL/min; severe myelosuppression; impaired hearing; active infection; history of gout and urate renal stones, renal failure; hypomagnesia; Raynaud syndrome; pregnancy (cisplatin crosses the placenta; may cause fetal harm if administered to a pregnant female).

CAUTIOUS USE Previous cytotoxic drug or radiation therapy with other ototoxic and nephrotoxic drugs; peripheral neuropathy; hyperuricemia; electrolyte imbalances, moderate renal impairment; hepatic impairment; history of circulatory disorders. Safe use in children not established.

ROUTE & DOSAGE

Testicular Neoplasms

Adult: **IV** 20 mg/m²/day for 5 days q3wk

Ovarian Neoplasms

Adult: **IV** 75–100 mg/m² once q3–4wk; or 75 mg/m² q3wk (with paclitaxel)

Advanced Bladder Cancer

Adult: **IV** 50–75 mg/m² q3–4 wk

ADMINISTRATION

- Usually a parenteral antiemetic agent is administered 30 min before cisplatin therapy is instituted and given on a scheduled basis throughout day and night as long as necessary.
- Before the initial dose is given, hydration is started with 1–2 L IV infusion fluid to reduce risk of nephrotoxicity and ototoxicity.

Intravenous

PREPARE: **IV Infusion:** Use disposable gloves when preparing cisplatin solutions. If drug accidentally contacts skin or mucosa, wash immediately and thoroughly with soap and water. ▪ Do not use any equipment containing aluminum. ▪ Withdraw required dose and dilute in 2 L D5W 5% dextrose in ½ or ⅓ normal saline containing 37.5 g mannitol.

Common adverse effects in *italic;* life-threatening effects underlined; generic names in **bold;** classifications in SMALL CAPS; ♣ Canadian drug name; Prototype drug; Alert

ADMINISTER: **IV Infusion:** Infuse over 30 min to 4 h at rate of 1 mg/minute. Do not administer as a rapid IV injection. Avoid extravasation.

INCOMPATIBILITIES: **Solution/additive: fluorouracil, mesna, sodium bicarbonate, thiotepa. Y-site: Amifostine, amphotericin B cholesteryl, cefepime, dantrolene, diazepam, gallium, garenoxacin, insulin, lansoprazole, pantoprazole, piperacillin/tazobactam, thiotepa, TPN.**

- Hydration and forced diuresis are continued for at least 24 h after drug administration to ensure adequate urinary output.
- Store at 15°–30°C (59°–86°F). Do not refrigerate. Protect from light. Once vial is opened, solution is stable for 28 days protected from light or 7 days in fluorescent light.

ADVERSE EFFECTS **CNS:** Neurotoxicity, peripheral neuropathies (may be irreversible). **HEENT:** Ototoxicity. **Hepatic:** Elevated liver enzymes. **GI:** *Marked nausea, vomiting.* **GU:** Nephrotoxicity. **Hematologic:** Leukopenia, thrombocytopenia; hemolytic anemia.

INTERACTIONS **Drug:** AMINOGLYCOSIDES, **amphotericin B, vancomycin,** other **nephrotoxic drugs** increase nephrotoxicity and acute renal failure—try to separate by at least 1–2 wk. Avoid LIVE VACCINES, **cladribine, dipyrone, leflunomide, lenograstim, lipegfilgrastim, nivolumab, pimecrolimus, tacrolimus** (topical), **tofacitinib, topotecan.**

PHARMACOKINETICS **Peak:** Immediately after infusion. **Distribution:** Widely distributed in body fluids and tissues; concentrated in kidneys, liver, and prostate; accumulated in tissues. **Metabolism:** Nonenzymatic. **Half-Life:** 20–30 min.

NURSING IMPLICATIONS

Black Box Warning

Cisplatin has been associated with severe renal toxicity, ototoxicity, and anaphylactic reactions.

Assessment & Drug Effects

- Obtain baseline ECG and cardiac monitoring during induction therapy because of possible myocarditis or focal irritability.
- Monitor for anaphylactoid reactions (particularly in patient previously exposed to cisplatin), which may occur within minutes of drug administration.
- Audiometric testing should be performed before the first dose and before each subsequent dose. Ototoxicity (reported in 31% of patients) may occur after a single dose of 50 mg/m^2. Children who receive repeated doses are especially susceptible.
- Monitor closely for dose-related adverse reactions. Drug action is cumulative; therefore severity of most adverse effects (such as neurotoxicity) increases with repeated doses.
- Suspect ototoxicity if patient manifests tinnitus or difficulty hearing in the high-frequency range.
- Monitor lab tests: Baseline and before each cycle, renal function tests and serum electrolytes; weekly CBC with differential and platelet count; periodic LFTs.

Patient & Family Education

- Continue maintenance of adequate hydration (at least 3000 mL/24 h oral fluid if prescriber agrees) and report promptly: Reduced urinary output, flank pain, anorexia, nausea, vomiting, dry mucosae, itching skin, urine odor on breath, fluid retention, and weight gain.
- Avoid rapid changes in position to minimize risk of dizziness or falling.
- Tingling, numbness, and tremors of extremities, loss of vision, sense, and taste, and constipation are early signs of neurotoxicity. Report their occurrence promptly to prevent irreversibility.
- Report tinnitus or any hearing impairment.
- Report promptly evidence of unexplained bleeding and easy bruising.
- Report unusual fatigue, fever, sore mouth and throat, abnormal body discharges.

CITALOPRAM HYDROBROMIDE

(cit-a-lo′pram)

Celexa

Classification: SELECTIVE SEROTONIN-REUPTAKE INHIBITOR (SSRI)

Therapeutic: ANTIDEPRESSANT

Prototype: Fluoxetine

AVAILABILITY Tablet; oral solution

ACTION & *THERAPEUTIC EFFECT* Selective serotonin reuptake inhibitor (SSRI) with an antidepressant effect presumed to be linked to its inhibition of CNS presynaptic neuronal uptake of serotonin. *Selective-serotonin reuptake inhibition mechanism results in the antidepressant activity of citalopram.*

USES Major depressive disorder (unipolar).

UNLABELED USES Aggressive or agitated behavior associated with dementia, binge eating, hot flashes, obsessive-compulsive disorder, premenstural dysphoric disorder, social anxiety disorder posttraumatic stress disorder.

CONTRAINDICATIONS Hypersensitivity to citalopram; congenital QT prolongation; concurrent use of MAOIs or use within 14 days of discontinuing MAOIs; initiation of citalopram in a patient receiving linezolid or IV methylene blue; concomitant use with pimozide.

CAUTIOUS USE Hypersensitivity to other SSRIs; hepatic insufficiency; history of potential suicide; dehydration; severe renal impairment or renal failure; cardiovascular disease (e.g., dysrhythmias, conduction defects, myocardial ischemia); history of QT prolongation; history of drug abuse; history of seizure disorders or suicidal tendencies; history of mania; ECT treatments; narrow-angle glaucoma; volume depleted, hyponatremia; bipolar depression; older adults; pregnancy (use with caution during pregnancy); lactation; children younger than 18 yr.

ROUTE & DOSAGE

Depression

Adult: **PO** Start at 20 mg daily, may increase to max of 40 mg daily if needed

Geriatric: **PO** Do not exceed 20 mg daily

 Common adverse effects in *italic*; life-threatening effects underlined; generic names in **bold**; classifications in SMALL CAPS; ♣ Canadian drug name; ⊙ Prototype drug; ⚠ Alert

ADMINISTRATION

Oral

- Do not begin this drug within 14 days of stopping an MAOI.
- Reduced doses are advised for the older adult and those with hepatic or renal impairment.
- Dose increments should be separated by at least 1 wk.
- Store at 25°C (77°F) in a tightly closed container and protect from light.

ADVERSE EFFECTS **Respiratory:** Rhinitis. **CNS:** Drowsiness, *insomnia, somnolence*. **Skin:** Diaphoresis. **GI:** *Nausea,* vomiting, diarrhea, dyspepsia, *dry mouth*. **GU:** Ejaculation disorder.

INTERACTIONS **Drug:** Combination with MAOIS, **linezolid** or SEROTONERGIC AGENTS could result in serotonin syndrome; **cimetidine** may increase citalopram levels; Do not use with QT prolonging agents. CYP2C19 inhibitors may increase risk of adverse effects. Monitor for adverse effects with concurrent **esomeprazole** use. The antiplatelet effects of NSAIDS can be increased. Do not use with **bretylium**. **Herbal: St. John's wort** may cause serotonin syndrome.

PHARMACOKINETICS **Absorption:** Rapidly absorbed from GI tract; approximately 80% reaches systemic circulation. **Peak:** Steady-state serum concentrations in 1 wk; peak blood levels at 4 h. **Distribution:** 80% protein bound; crosses placenta; distributed into breast milk. **Metabolism:** In liver by CYP3A4 and CYP2C9 enzymes. **Elimination:** 20% in urine, 80% in bile. **Half-Life:** 35 h.

NURSING IMPLICATIONS

Black Box Warning

Citalopram has been associated with increased suicidal thinking and behavior, especially in children, adolescents, and young adults.

Assessment & Drug Effects

- Watch closely for worsening of depression or emergence of suicidal ideations.
- Monitor for therapeutic effectiveness: Indicated by elevation of mood; 1–4 wk may be needed before improvement is noted.
- Monitor periodically HR and BP, and carefully monitor complete cardiac status in person with known or suspected cardiac disease.
- Monitor closely older adult patients for adverse effects, especially with doses greater than 20 mg/day.
- Monitor lab tests: Periodic LFTs, CBC, renal function tests, electrolytes.

Patient & Family Education

- Report immediately worsening of clinical condition, including suicidal ideation or other unusual changes in behavior.
- Do not engage in hazardous activities until reaction to this drug is known.
- Do not abruptly stop taking this drug. It should be gradually tapered to minimize withdrawal symptoms.
- Avoid using alcohol while taking citalopram.
- Report distressing adverse effects including any changes in sexual functioning or response.
- Periodic ophthalmology exams are advised with long-term treatment.

C

CLADRIBINE

(cla′dri-been)

Classification: ANTINEOPLASTIC; ANTIMETABOLITE, PURINE ANTAGONIST

Therapeutic: ANTINEOPLASTIC; ANTIMETABOLITE

Prototype: 6-Mercaptopurine

AVAILABILITY Solution for injection

ACTION & *THERAPEUTIC EFFECT*

Cladribine is a synthetic antineoplastic agent with selective toxicity toward certain normal and malignant lymphocytes and monocytes. It accumulates intracellularly, preventing repair of single-stranded DNA breaks and ultimately interfering with cellular metabolism and DNA synthesis. *Cladribine is cytotoxic to both actively dividing and quiescent lymphocytes and monocytes, inhibiting both DNA synthesis and repair.*

USES Treatment of hairy cell leukemia; multiple sclerosis.

UNLABELED USES Advanced cutaneous T-cell lymphomas, acute myeloid leukemia, autoimmune hemolytic anemia, mycosis fungoides, chronic lymphocytic leukemia, non-Hodgkin lymphomas.

CONTRAINDICATIONS Hypersensitivity to cladribine; severe bone marrow suppression; severe neurologic toxicity; acute nephrotoxicity; pregnancy (category D); lactation.

CAUTIOUS USE Hepatic or renal impairment; previous radiation therapy or chemotherapy; bone marrow depression. Safety and efficacy in children not established.

ROUTE & DOSAGE

Hairy Cell Leukemia

Adult: **IV** 0.09–0.1 mg/kg/day by 7 days continuous infusion

Renal Impairment Dosage Adjustment

CrCl 10–50 mL/min: Administer 75% of dose; *less than 10 mL/min:* Administer 50% of dose

ADMINISTRATION

- Use disposable gloves and protective clothing when handling the drug.
- Wash immediately if skin contact occurs.

Intravenous

PREPARE: **IV Infusion reservoir usually prepared by pharmacists as follows:** Add the calculated dose of cladribine through a sterile 0.22-micron disposable hydrophilic syringe filter to an infusion bag containing 500 mL of NS.
ADMINISTER: **IV Infusion:** Give through a central line and control by a pump device as a continuous infusion or over 2 h.
INCOMPATIBILITIES: **Solution/additive:** Do not mix with any other diluents or drugs.

- Diluted solutions of cladribine may be stored refrigerated for up to 8 h prior to administration.
- Store unopened vials in refrigerator [2°–8°C (36°–46°F)], and protect from light.

ADVERSE EFFECTS **Respiratory:** Abnormal breath sounds, cough. **CNS:** Fatigue, headache. **Skin:** Skin rash, injection site reaction, purpura.

GI: Nausea, decreased appetite, vomiting. **Hematologic:** Neutropenia, febrile neutropenia, anemia, *bone marrow depression*, thrombocytopenia. **Other:** *Infection, fever.*

INTERACTIONS **Drug:** Additive risk of bleeding with ANTICOAGULANTS, NSAIDS, PLATELET INHIBITORS, SALICYLATES. May increase risk of adverse effects if used with **dipyrone, pimecrolimus, tacrolimus.** Do not use with LIVE VACCINES.

PHARMACOKINETICS **Onset:** Therapeutic effect 10 days to 4 mo. **Duration:** 7–25+ mo. **Distribution:** Crosses placenta; distributed into breast milk. **Metabolism:** In malignant leukocytes, cladribine is phosphorylated to active forms, which are subsequently incorporated into cellular DNA. **Half-Life:** 6.7 h.

NURSING IMPLICATIONS

Black Box Warning

Cladribine has been associated with severe bone marrow suppression and acute nephrotoxicity.

Assessment & Drug Effects

- Monitor vital signs during and after drug infusion. Fever (above 100°F) is common during the 5th to 7th day in patients with hairy cell leukemia, and severe fever (above 104°F) may develop within the first month of therapy.
- Closely monitor hematologic status; myelosuppression is common during the first month after starting therapy.
- Monitor for and report S&S of infection. Note that within the first month, fever may occur in the absence of infection.
- With high doses of cladribine, monitor for neurologic toxicity and acute nephrotoxicity.
- Monitor lab tests: CBC with differential, renal and hepatic function, bone marrow biopsy.

Patient & Family Education

- Be fully informed regarding adverse responses to the drug.
- Understand the need for close follow-up during and after treatment with the drug.

CLARITHROMYCIN

(clar′i-thro-my-sin)

Biaxin XL

Classification: MACROLIDE ANTIBIOTIC

Therapeutic: ANTIBIOTIC

Prototype: Erythromycin

AVAILABILITY Tablet; sustained release tablet; oral suspension

ACTION & *THERAPEUTIC EFFECT* A semisynthetic macrolide antibiotic that binds to the 50S ribosomal subunit of susceptible bacterial organisms and, thereby, blocks RNA-mediated bacterial protein synthesis of bacteria. *It is active against both aerobic and anaerobic gram-positive and gram-negative organisms.*

USES Treatment of community-acquired pneumonia; otitis media; and skin and soft-tissue infections, acute exacerbation of COPD, mycobacterial (nontuberculosis) infection.

UNLABELED USES Endocarditis, *Mycobacterium abscessus* infection, pertussis, Q fever.

CONTRAINDICATIONS Hypersensitivity to clarithromycin,

erythromycin, or any other macrolide antibiotics; history of cholestatic jaundice/hepatic dysfunction with previous use of clarithromycin; S&S of hepatitis; acute porphyria; congenital QT prolongation or history of QT prolongation; ventricular cardiac arrhythmia including torsades de pointes; viral infections.

CAUTIOUS USE Renal impairment, older adults, GI disease, colitis; myasthenia gravis; pregnancy (clarithromycin crosses the placenta; not recommended as a first-line treatment in pregnant women); lactation. Safety and efficacy in infants younger than 6 mo not established.

ROUTE & DOSAGE

Community-Acquired Pneumonia

Adult: **PO** 500 mg bid (immediate release)

MAC Infections (with Other Agents)

Adult: **PO** 500 mg q12h
Child /Adolescent/Infant (6 mo or older): **PO** 7.5 mg/kg q12h

COPD Exacerbation

Adult: **PO** 500 mg (immediate release) q12h x3–7 days

Renal Impairment Dosage Adjustment

CrCl less than 30 mL/min: Decrease dose by 50%

ADMINISTRATION

Oral

- Ensure that sustained release form of drug is not chewed or crushed. It **must be** swallowed whole.
- Shake suspension well before use.
- May be administered with or without food. Administer every 12 hours rather than twice daily to avoid peak and trough variation.
- Store at 15°–30°C (59°–86°F).

ADVERSE EFFECTS **CNS:** Headache. **Skin:** Rash, urticaria. **GI:** Diarrhea, abdominal discomfort, nausea, abnormal taste, dyspepsia. **Hematologic:** Eosinophilia.

INTERACTIONS **Drug:** May increase **theophylline** levels; drugs known to interact with **erythromycin** (i.e., **carbamazepine,** QT prolonging drugs) should be used with caution; decreases metabolism of CALCIUM CHANNEL BLOCKERS. May increase concentration of drugs metabolized by CYP3A4 or OATP1B1. ANTIHEPACIVIRAL drugs may increase concentration of clarithromycin. Do not use with LIVE VACCINES. May increase toxicity of **cobicistat, cyclosporine, edoxaban**, ERGOT DERIVATIVES, **lopinavir, lovastatin, midazolam, pimozide, rilpivirine, tacrolimus. Food: Grapefruit juice** increases risk of adverse effects.

PHARMACOKINETICS **Absorption:** Readily from GI tract; 50% reaches the systemic circulation. **Peak:** 2–3 h (immediate release); 5–8 (extended release). **Distribution:** Into most body tissue (excluding CNS); high pulmonary tissue concentrations. **Metabolism:** Partially in the liver via CYP3A4; active 14-OH metabolite acts synergistically with the parent compound against *H. influenzae*. **Elimination:** 20% unchanged in urine; 10–15% of 14-OH metabolite excreted in urine. **Half-Life:** 3–7 h.

C

NURSING IMPLICATIONS

Assessment & Drug Effects

- Inquire about previous hypersensitivity to other macrolides (e.g., erythromycin) before treatment.
- Withhold drug and notify prescriber, if hypersensitivity occurs (e.g., rash, urticaria).
- Monitor for and report loose stools or diarrhea because pseudomembranous colitis **must be** ruled out.
- When clarithromycin is given concurrently with anticoagulants, digoxin, or theophylline, blood levels of these drugs may be elevated. Monitor appropriate serum levels, and assess for S&S of drug toxicity.
- Monitor lab results: BUN, creatinine.

Patient & Family Education

- Complete prescribed course of therapy.
- Report rash or other signs of hypersensitivity immediately.
- Report loose stools or diarrhea even after completion of drug therapy.

CLASCOTERONE

(klas-KOE-ter-one)

Winlevi

Classifications: ANDROGEN RECEPTOR INHIBITOR

Therapeutic: ANTIACNE; ANDROGEN RECEPTOR INHIBITOR

AVAILABILITY Cream

ACTION & *THERAPEUTIC EFFECT*

An androgen receptor inhibitor that decreases sebum production and inflammation. *Works to control symptoms of acne.*

USES Used to treat acne vulgaris in patients 12 years and older.

CONTRAINDICATIONS There are no contraindications listed in the manufacturer labeling.

CAUTIOUS USE HPA axis suppression; pediatric patients; pregnancy (use with caution; adverse effects were observed in animal reproduction studies); lactation.

ROUTE & DOSAGE

Acne vulgaris

Adult/Adolescent: **Topical** Apply thin layer (1 g) to affected areas of the skin twice a day.

ADMINISTRATION

Topical

- Clean and dry skin prior to applying. Apply a thin, uniform layer.
- For topical external use only. Avoid contact with eyes, mouth, or other mucous membranes. Rinse thoroughly if accidental contact with these areas occurs. Avoid use on cuts, abrasions, and eczematous or sunburned skin.
- Store at 20°–25°C (68°–77°F).

ADVERSE EFFECTS **Skin:** Erythema, dryness, scaling, pruritus, exfoliation of skin.

INTERACTIONS No clinically relevant interactions reported.

PHARMACOKINETICS **Distribution:** 84–89% protein-bound

NURSING IMPLICATIONS

Assessment & Drug Effects

- Monitor for skin reaction or irritation.
- Assess for signs or symptoms of HPA axis suppression or adrenal insufficiency.

C

Patient & Family Education

- Call your doctor or seek medical help if any of these side effects or any other side effects bother you or do not go away: dryness, itching, redness, scaling, or other irritation where this drug is used.

CLEMASTINE FUMARATE

(klem'as-teen)

Tavist-1

Classification: ANTIHISTAMINE (H_1-RECEPTOR ANTAGONIST)

Therapeutic: ANTIHISTAMINE

Prototype: Diphenhydramine

AVAILABILITY Tablet; syrup

ACTION & THERAPEUTIC EFFECT

An antihistamine (H_1-receptor antagonist) that competes for H_1-receptor sites on cells, thus blocking histamine effectiveness. Has greater selectivity for peripheral H_1-receptors and, consequently, it produces little sedation. Has prominent antipruritic activity and low incidence of unpleasant adverse effects. *Effective in controlling various allergic reactions (e.g., nasal congestion, sneezing, itching).*

USES Symptomatic relief of allergic rhinitis and mild uncomplicated allergic skin manifestations such as urticaria and angioedema.

CONTRAINDICATIONS Hypersensitivity to clemastine or to other antihistamines of similar chemical structure; lower respiratory tract symptoms, including acute asthma; concomitant MAOI therapy; closed-angle glaucoma; lactation.

CAUTIOUS USE History of bronchial asthma, COPD; increased intraocular pressure; GI or GU obstruction; hyperthyroidism; hepatic disease; cardiovascular disease, hypertension, older adults; pregnancy (category B). Safety and efficacy in children younger than 5 yr not established.

ROUTE & DOSAGE

Allergic Rhinitis

Adult: **PO** 1.34 mg bid, may increase up to 8.04 mg/day
Child (6 yr or older): **PO** 0.67 mg bid, may increase up to 4.02 mg/day; *younger than 6 yr:* 0.335–0.67 mg/kg/day in 2 divided doses (max: 1.34 mg/day)

Allergic Urticaria

Adult: **PO** 2.68 mg bid or tid, may increase up to 8.04 mg/day
Child: **PO** 1.34 mg bid, may increase up to 4.02 mg/day

ADMINISTRATION

Oral

- Drug may be administered with food, water, or milk to reduce possibility of gastric irritation.
- Older adult patients usually require less than average adult dose.
- Store at 15°–30°C (59°–86°F) unless otherwise directed.

ADVERSE EFFECTS **CV:** Hypotension, palpitation, tachycardia, extrasystoles. **Respiratory:** Dry nose and throat, thickening of bronchial secretions, tightness of chest, wheezing, nasal stuffiness. **CNS:** Sedation, *transient drowsiness,* dry nose and throat, headache, dizziness, weakness, fatigue, disturbed coordination; confusion, restlessness, nervousness, hysteria, convulsions, tremors, irritability, euphoria, insomnia, paresthesias, neuritis. **HEENT:** Vertigo, tinnitus, acute labyrinthitis, blurred vision, diplopia. **Skin:** Urticaria, rash, photosensitivity. **GI:** *Dry mouth,* epigastric distress, anorexia, nausea, vomiting, diarrhea, constipation. **GU:** Difficult urination, urinary retention, early menses. **Hematologic:** Hemolytic anemia, thrombocytopenia, agranulocytosis. **Other:** Anaphylaxis, excess perspiration, chills.

INTERACTIONS **Drug: Alcohol** and other CNS DEPRESSANTS increase sedation; MAO INHIBITORS may prolong and intensify anticholinergic effects.

PHARMACOKINETICS **Absorption:** Readily from GI tract. **Peak:** 5–7 h. **Duration:** 10–12 h. **Distribution:** Into breast milk. **Metabolism:** In liver. **Elimination:** In urine.

NURSING IMPLICATIONS

Assessment & Drug Effects

- Monitor for drowsiness, poor coordination, or dizziness, especially in the older adult or debilitated. Supervision of ambulation may be warranted.
- Assess for symptomatic relief with use of the medication.
- Monitor lab tests: Periodic hematologic studies with long-term use.

Patient & Family Education

- Check with prescriber before taking alcohol or other CNS depressants because effects may be additive.
- Clemastine may cause lethargy and drowsiness; therefore, necessary safety precautions should be taken.
- Older adults should make position changes slowly and in stages, particularly from recumbent to upright posture, as dizziness and hypotension occur more frequently than in younger patients.
- Avoid driving and other potentially hazardous activities until response to the drug has been established.

CLEVIDIPINE BUTYRATE

(cle-vi-di'peen bu-ti'rate)

Cleviprex

Classification: CALCIUM CHANNEL BLOCKER; ANTIHYPERTENSIVE

Therapeutic: ANTIHYPERTENSIVE

Prototype: Nifedipine

AVAILABILITY Emulsion for injection

ACTION & *THERAPEUTIC EFFECT* A calcium channel blocker that interferes with the influx of calcium during depolarization of arterial smooth muscle. Decreases systemic vascular resistance, thus lowering mean arterial pressure. *Decreases blood pressure.*

USES Treatment of hypertension, hypertensive emergency/urgency when oral administration is neither feasible nor desired.

CONTRAINDICATIONS Hypersensitivity to soybeans, soy products, eggs/egg products; defective lipid metabolism (e.g., pathologic hyperlipidemia, lipid nephrosis, acute pancreatitis); severe aortic stenosis.

CAUTIOUS USE Reflex tachycardia, hypotension, heart failure; lipid intake restriction; rebound hypertension following drug discontinuation; elderly; pregnancy (category C); lactation. Safety and efficacy in children not established.

C

ROUTE & DOSAGE

Hypertension

Adult: **IV** Initial dose of 1–2 mg/h. Titrate dose to desired BP: May initially double dose every 90 sec; as BP approaches goal, decrease dose increments to less than double the previous dose and lengthen time intervals between doses to q5–10min.

ADMINISTRATION

Intravenous

PREPARE: **IV Infusion:** Supplied premixed, ready to use. Invert vial gently to produce a uniform emulsion.

ADMINISTER: **IV Infusion:** Use infusion device that permits calibrated rates. ▪ May infuse through a central or peripheral line using NS, D5W, D5W/NS, D5W/LR, LR, or 10% amino acid solution. ▪ Complete infusion within 12 h of entering vial.

INCOMPATIBILITIES: **Solution/additive:** Do not dilute in any IV solution. **Y-site:** Unknown; do not mix.

▪ Store refrigerated at 2°–8°C (36°–46°F). Do not return unopened vials to refrigeration once they have reached room temperature.

ADVERSE EFFECTS **CV:** Hypotension, reflex tachycardia. **CNS:** Headache. **GI:** Nausea, vomiting. **Other:** Acute renal failure.

PHARMACOKINETICS **Distribution:** 99.5% plasma protein bound. **Metabolism:** In the plasma. **Elimination:** Renal (63–74%) and fecal (7–22%). **Half-Life:** 15 min.

NURSING IMPLICATIONS

Assessment & Drug Effects

- Monitor HR and BP continuously during infusion. Increases in HR is a normal response to vasodilation, and rebound hypertension may occur for at least 8 h after infusion is stopped.
- Monitor cardiac status continuously during infusion, especially with preexisting HF. Clevidipine may have a negative inotropic effect and exacerbate HF.

Patient & Family Education

- Report promptly any of the following: Signs of heart failure; visual changes, weakness, or other signs of neurologic impairment.

CLINDAMYCIN HYDROCHLORIDE (Pr)

(klin-da-mye'sin)

Cleocin, Dalacin C ♣

CLINDAMYCIN PALMITATE HYDROCHLORIDE

Cleocin Pediatric

CLINDAMYCIN PHOSPHATE

Cleocin Phosphate, Cleocin T, Dalacin C, Evoclin, Cleocin Vaginal Ovules or Cream

Classification: LINCOSAMIDE ANTIBIOTIC

Therapeutic: ANTIBIOTIC

AVAILABILITY Capsule; oral suspension; solution for injection; vaginal cream; suppository; gel, lotion; foam

ACTION & *THERAPEUTIC EFFECT* Suppresses protein synthesis by preventing peptide bond formation in bacterial ribosomes. *Particularly*

effective against susceptible strains of anaerobic streptococci as well as aerobic gram-positive cocci.

USES Serious infections when less toxic alternatives are inappropriate. Topical applications are used in treatment of acne vulgaris. Vaginal applications are used in treatment of bacterial vaginosis in nonpregnant women.

UNLABELED USES In combination with pyrimethamine for toxoplasmosis in patients with AIDS.

CONTRAINDICATIONS History of hypersensitivity to clindamycin or lincomycin; meningitis; history of ulcerative colitis, or antibiotic-associated colitis; viral infection; UGI infections due to nonbacterial infections.

CAUTIOUS USE History of GI disease, severe hepatic disease; atopic individuals (history of eczema, asthma, hay fever); older adults; pregnancy (category B); lactation; children.

ROUTE & DOSAGE

Moderate to Severe Infections

Adult: **PO** 150–450 mg q6h; **IM/IV** 600–1200 mg/day in divided doses (max: 2700 mg/day)
Child: **PO** 8–20 mg/kg/day q6–8h; **IM/IV** 20–40 mg/kg/day in divided doses
Neonate (7 days or younger, weight 2000 g or less): **IM/IV** 10 mg/kg/day q12h; *7 days or younger, weight greater than 2000 g:* 15 mg/kg/day q8h; *7 days or older, weight less than 1200 g:* 10 mg/kg/day q12h; *7 days or older, weight 1200 g–2000 g:* 15 mg/kg/day q8h; *7 days or older, weight greater than 2000 g:* 20 mg/kg/day q6–8h

Acne Vulgaris

Adult: **Topical** Apply to affected areas bid; 1% foam used for once daily application

Bacterial Vaginosis

Adult: **Topical** Insert 1 suppository intravaginally at bedtime × 3 days, or insert 1 applicator full of cream intravaginally at bedtime × 7 days

ADMINISTRATION

Oral

- Administer clindamycin capsules with a full [240 mL (8 oz)] glass of water to prevent esophagitis. May administer with or without food.
- Note expiration date of oral solution; retains potency for 14 days at room temperature. Do not refrigerate, as chilling causes thickening and thus makes pouring it difficult.

Topical

- Gel (except Clindagel), lotion, pledget, solution: Apply thin film twice daily to affected area. More than 1 pledget may be used.
- Clindagel, foam: Apply once daily to affected area.

Intramuscular

- Deep IM injection is recommended. Rotate injection sites and observe daily for evidence of inflammatory reaction. Single IM doses should not exceed 600 mg.

C

Intravenous

IV administration to neonates, infants, and children: Verify correct IV concentration and rate of infusion with prescriber.

PREPARE: **Intermittent: ADD-Vantage System:** Clindamycin may be reconstituted in 50 or 100 mL, respectively, of D5W or NS in the ADD diluent container. Refer to manufacturer's instructions for the ADD-Vantage system guidelines.

ADMINISTER: **Intermittent:** Never give a bolus dose. ▪ Do not give more than 1200 mg in a single 1-h infusion. ▪ Infusion rate should not exceed 30 mg/min.

INCOMPATIBILITIES: **Solution/additive:** **Aminophylline,** BARBITURATES, **calcium gluconate, ceftriaxone, ciprofloxacin, gentamicin, magnesium sulfate. Y-site: Allopurinol, amphotericin B, azathioprine, azithromycin, caspofungin, ceftriaxone, chlorpromazine, dantrolene, daunorubicin, diazepam, diazoxide, doxapram, filgrastim, fluconazole, ganciclovir, haloperidol, hydroxyzine, idarubicin, lansoprazole, minocycline, mitomycin, mitoxantrone, mycophenolate, oritavancin, papaverine, pentamidine, pentobarbital, phentolamine, phenytoin, prochlorperazine, promethazine, quinupristin/dalfopristin, SMZ/TMP, temocillin.**

▪ Store in tight containers at 15°–30°C (59°–86°F) unless otherwise directed.

ADVERSE EFFECTS

CV: Hypotension (following IM), cardiac arrest (rapid IV). **Skin:** *Skin rashes,* urticaria, pruritus, dryness, contact dermatitis, gram-negative folliculitis, irritation, oily skin. **GI:** *Diarrhea,* abdominal pain, flatulence, bloating, *nausea, vomiting,* pseudomembranous colitis; esophageal irritation, loss of taste, medicinal taste (high IV doses), jaundice, abnormal liver function tests. **Hematologic:** Leukopenia, eosinophilia, agranulocytosis, thrombocytopenia. **Other:** Fever, serum sickness, sensitization, swelling of face (following topical use), generalized myalgia, superinfections, proctitis, vaginitis, pain, induration, sterile abscess (following IM injections); thrombophlebitis (IV infusion).

DIAGNOSTIC TEST INTERFERENCE

Clindamycin may cause increases in ***serum alkaline phosphatase, bilirubin, creatine phosphokinase (CPK)*** from muscle irritation following IM injection; ***AST, ALT.***

INTERACTIONS

Drug: Chloramphenicol, erythromycin possibly are mutually antagonistic to clindamycin; neuromuscular blocking action enhanced by NEUROMUSCULAR BLOCKING AGENTS **(atracurium, tubocurarine, pancuronium).**

PHARMACOKINETICS

Absorption: Approximately 90% absorbed from GI tract; 10% of topical application is absorbed through skin. **Peak:** 45–60 min PO; 3 h IM. **Duration:** 6 h PO; 8–12 h IM. **Distribution:** Widely distributed except for CNS; crosses placenta; distributed into breast milk. **Metabolism:** In liver. **Elimination:** In urine and feces. **Half-Life:** 2–3 h.

NURSING IMPLICATIONS

Black Box Warning

Clindamycin has been associated with severe, potentially fatal, Clostridium difficile-associated diarrhea (CDAD)

Assessment & Drug Effects

- Monitor BP and pulse in patients receiving drug parenterally. Hypotension has occurred following IM injection. Advise patient to remain recumbent following drug administration until BP has stabilized.
- Severe diarrhea and colitis, including pseudomembranous colitis (i.e., *Clostridium difficile*–associated diarrhea or CDAD), have been associated with oral (highest incidence), parenteral, and topical clindamycin. Report immediately the onset of watery diarrhea, with or without fever. Symptoms may appear within a few days to 2 wk after therapy is begun or up to several weeks following cessation of therapy.
- Be alert to signs of superinfection (see Appendix F).
- Be alert for signs of anaphylactoid reactions (see Appendix F), which require immediate attention.
- Monitor lab tests: Baseline C&S; periodic CBC with differential, LFTs, and renal function tests.

Patient & Family Education

- Report loose stools or diarrhea promptly.
- Stop drug therapy if significant diarrhea develops (more than 5 loose stools daily) and notify prescriber.
- Do not self-medicate with antidiarrheal preparations. Antiperistaltic agents may prolong and worsen diarrhea by delaying removal of toxins from colon.

CLOBETASOL PROPIONATE

(cloe-bay'ta-sol)

Clobex, Temovate, Embeline gel; Olux Foam

See Appendix A-4.

CLOBAZAM

(kloe'ba-zam)

Onfi, Sympazan

Classification: BENZODIAZEPINE; ANTICONVULSANT

Therapeutic: ANTICONVULSANT

Prototype: Diazepam

Controlled Substance: Schedule IV

AVAILABILITY Tablet; oral suspension; oral film

ACTION & *THERAPEUTIC EFFECT* Mechanism of action believed to involve potentiation of GABAergic neurotransmission resulting from binding at the benzodiazepine site of the $GABA_A$ receptor. *Helps inhibit development of seizures associated with Lennox–Gastaut syndrome.*

USES Adjunctive treatment of seizures associated with Lennox-Gastaut syndrome (LGS).

UNLABLED USES Treatment of refractory seizures.

CONTRAINDICATIONS Hypersensitivity to clobazam; severe hepatic impairment; signs and symptoms of Stevens–Johnson syndrome; suicidal ideation; lactation.

CAUTIOUS USE Hepatic impairment; severe renal impairment; history of substance abuse; history of suicidal thoughts or behaviors; pregnancy (exposure

C

to benzodiazepines immediately prior to or during birth may result in hypothermia, hypotonia, respiratory depression, and difficulty feeding in the neonate; exposed neonates may develop dependence and withdrawal); depression; drug withdrawal; older adults. Safety and efficacy in patients younger than 2 yr not established.

ROUTE & DOSAGE

Adjunctive Treatment of Lennox-Gastaut Seizures

Adult and Children (2 yr or older, weight over 30 kg): **PO** 5 mg bid, increase to 10 mg bid on day 7, then increase to 20 mg bid on day 14; *weight 30 kg or less:* 5 mg once daily, increase to 5 mg bid, on day 7, then increase to 10 mg bid on day 14
Geriatric Patients 5 mg once daily × 1 w then increase to 5 mg bid × 1 w then increase to 10 mg bid × 1 w; may increase to 20 mg twice daily

Pharmacogenetic Dosage Adjustment

Poor CYP2C19 metabolizers: Starting dose should be 5 mg/day; dose titration should proceed slowly according to weight, but to half the normal dose regimen. If necessary, additional titration to the 20 mg/day or 40 mg/day (depending on weight) may be started on day 21.

Hepatic Impairment Dosage Adjustment

Mild to moderate impairment (Child–Pugh score 5 to 9): Use geriatric dosing regimen
Severe impairment: Not recommended

ADMINISTRATION

Oral

- May give tablet whole or crushed and mixed in applesauce.
- Oral suspension: Insert provided adapter firmly into neck of bottle before first use and keep in place throughout use. Shake bottle well before every use. Use only the dosing syringe provided to measure dose.
- Give without regard to timing of meals.
- Abrupt discontinuation of this drug should be avoided. Drug should be tapered off by decreasing the daily dose every week by 5 to 10 mg.
- Store at 20°–25°C (68°–77°F).

ADVERSE EFFECTS **Respiratory:** Bronchitis, cough, pneumonia, upper respiratory tract infection. **CNS:** Aggression, ataxia, drooling, dysarthria, fatigue, drowsiness, insomnia, *lethargy*, psychomotor agitation, sedation, *somnolence*. **Endocrine:** Alterations in appetite. **GI:** Constipation, decreased appetite, dysphagia, *vomiting*. **GU:** Urinary tract infection. **Other:** *Fever*.

INTERACTIONS **Drug:** Clobazam may decrease the effectiveness of ORAL CONTRACEPTIVES and other drugs requiring CYP2D6 (e.g., **metoprolol, propranolol, aripiprazole, clozapine**). Strong and moderate inhibitors of CYP2C19 (e.g., **fluconazole, fluvoxamine, ticlopidine, omeprazole**) may result in increased levels of the active metabolite of clobazam. CNS DEPRESSANTS increase risk of adverse events.

PHARMACOKINETICS **Absorption:** Approximately 100% bioavailable. **Peak:** 0.5–4 h. **Distribution:** 80–90% plasma protein bound.

Metabolism: Extensive hepatic oxidation to active and inactive metabolites via CYP 3A4 or CYP2C19. **Elimination:** Renal (82%) and fecal (11%). **Half-Life:** 36–42 h.

NURSING IMPLICATIONS

Assessment & Drug Effects

- Monitor for adverse CNS effects (e.g., somnolence, sedation, new or worsening depression, impaired judgment, impaired motor skills), especially when used concurrently with other CNS depressants.
- Monitor for and report promptly suicidal thoughts or behaviors, or thoughts of self-harm.

Patient & Family Education

- Promptly notify prescriber of suicidal ideation or thoughts of self-harm.
- Avoid potentially hazardous tasks, such as driving, until response to the drug is known.
- Do not drink alcohol while taking clobazam.
- Abruptly stopping clobazam may increase the risk of seizure activity.
- Women of childbearing age who use hormonal contraceptives should use alternative nonhormonal methods during and for 28 days after discontinuing clobazam.
- Notify prescriber immediately if you become pregnant or intend to become pregnant, or if you are breastfeeding or intend to breastfeed.

CLOCORTOLONE PIVALATE

(kloe-kor′toe-lone)

Cloderm

See Appendix A-4.

CLOFARABINE

(clo-fa-ra′been)

Clolar

Classification: ANTINEOPLASTIC; PURINE ANTIMETABOLITE

Therapeutic: ANTINEOPLASTIC

Prototype: 6-Mercaptopurine

AVAILABILITY Solution for injection

ACTION & *THERAPEUTIC EFFECT* Clofarabine inhibits DNA repair within cancer cells, thus interfering with mitosis; it also disrupts the mitochondrial membrane, leading to cancer cell death. *Cytotoxic to rapidly proliferating and quiescent cancer cells.*

USES Relapsed or refractory acute lymphocytic leukemia (ALL) after at least 2 prior regimens.

CONTRAINDICATIONS Severe bone marrow suppression; active infection; venous occlusive liver disease; severe hepatotoxicity; pregnancy (category D); lactation.

CAUTIOUS USE Renal or hepatic function impairment; thrombocytopenia; neutropenia; previous chemotherapy or radiation therapy; history of viral infections such as herpes; history of cardiac disease or hypotension; females of childbearing age; older adults.

ROUTE & DOSAGE

Acute Lymphocytic Leukemia

Adolescent/Child: **IV** 52 mg/m²/day for 5 days q2–6w

Renal Impairment Dosage Adjustment

CrCl 30–60 mL/min: Reduce dose by 50%

C

Toxicity Dosage Adjustment

Grade 4 neutropenia lasting at least 4 wk: Reduce dose by 25%

Obesity Dosage Adjustment

Use actual body weight for calculation of BSA

ADMINISTRATION

- Do not give drugs with known renal toxicity during the 5 days of clofarabine administration.

Intravenous

PREPARE: **IV Infusion:** Withdraw required dose from vial using a 0.2-micron filter syringe. ▪ Further dilute in 100 mL or more of D5W or NS prior to infusion to a final concentration between 0.15 and 0.4 mg/mL.

ADMINISTER: **IV Infusion:** Give over 2 h.

- Store diluted solution at room temperature. Use within 24 h of mixing.

ADVERSE EFFECTS **CV:** *Tachycardia, hypotension,* flushing, hypertension, edema. **Respiratory:** *Epistaxis,* dyspnea, pleural effusion. **CNS:** *Headache, fatigue,* anxiety, pain. **Endocrine:** *Fever.* **Hepatic/GI:** *Increased serum ALT, increased serum AST, increased bilirubin, vomiting, nausea, diarrhea, abdominal pain, anorexia,* gingival bleeding, mucosal inflammation, oral candidiasis. **GU:** *Hematuria, increased serum creatinine.* **Musculoskeletal:** *Limb pain,* myalgia. **Hematologic:** *Leukopenia, anemia, lymphocytopenia, thrombocytopenia,* neutropenia, *febrile neutropenia.* **Integumentary:** *Pruritus, skin rash,* palmar-plantar erythrodysesthesia, erythema, *petechia.* **Other:** *Fever,* infection, sepsis.

DRUG INTERACTIONS May increase risk of adverse effects if used with **dipyrone, pimecrolimus, tacrolimus.** Do not use with LIVE VACCINES.

PHARMACOKINETICS **Distribution:** 47% protein bound. **Metabolism:** Negligible. **Elimination:** Primarily unchanged in the urine. **Half-Life:** 5.2 h.

NURSING IMPLICATIONS

Assessment & Drug Effects

- Monitor vital signs frequently during infusion of clofarabine.
- Monitor closely for S&S of capillary leak syndrome or systemic inflammatory response syndrome (e.g., tachypnea, tachycardia, hypotension, pulmonary edema). If either is suspected, immediately DC IV, institute supportive measures and notify prescriber.
- Monitor I&O rates and pattern and watch for S&S of dehydration, including dizziness, lightheadedness, fainting spells, or decreased urine output.
- Withhold drug and notify prescriber if hypotension develops for any reason during 5-day period of drug administration.
- Monitor lab tests: Baseline and periodic CBC and platelet counts; frequent LFTs; renal function tests; and coagulation parameters during therapy.

Patient & Family Education

- Report any distressing adverse effect of therapy to prescriber.
- Use effective measures to avoid pregnancy while taking this drug.

C

CLOMIPHENE CITRATE

(kloe′mi-feen)

Classification: OVULATION STIMULANT; NONSTEROID SELECTIVE ESTROGEN RECEPTOR MODULATOR (SERM)

Therapeutic: OVULATION STIMULANT; ANTIESTROGENIC

AVAILABILITY Tablet

ACTION & THERAPEUTIC EFFECT Induces ovulation in selected infrequently ovulating or anovulatory women, blocking the normal negative feedback of circulating estradiol on the hypothalamus, thus preventing estrogen from lowering the output of gonadotropin-releasing hormone (GnRH). *Stimulates pituitary release of luteinizing hormone (LH), follicle-stimulating hormone (FSH), and gonadotropins, leading to ovarian stimulation.*

USES Treatment of ovulatory dysfunction.

UNLABELED USES Male infertility, persistent lactation.

CONTRAINDICATIONS Hypersensitivity to clomiphene citrate or any of its components, neoplastic lesions, ovarian cyst; hepatic disease or dysfunction; abnormal uterine bleeding; endometriosis; primary ovarian failure; men with testicular failure; untreated thyroid disease; visual abnormalities; major depression or psychosis; thrombophlebitis; pregnancy (use is contraindicated in pregnant females); lactation.

CAUTIOUS USE Polycystic ovarian enlargement, pelvic discomfort, sensitivity to pituitary gonadotropins.

ROUTE & DOSAGE

Infertility

Adult (first course): **PO** 50 mg/day for 5 days; start on 5th day of cycle following start of spontaneous or induced bleeding (with progestin) or at any time in the patient who has had no recent uterine bleeding

ADMINISTRATION

Oral

- Each course of therapy should start on or about the 5th cycle day once ovulation has been established. Total daily dose should be taken at one time to maximize effectiveness.
- Store at 15°–30°C (59°–86°F) in tightly capped, light-resistant container.

ADVERSE EFFECTS **Endocrine:** *Enlarged ovaries with multiple follicular cysts, hot flash.* **GI:** Nausea, vomiting, bloating, abdominal distension, abdominal distress.

DIAGNOSTIC TEST INTERFERENCE Clomiphene may increase BSP retention; ***plasma transcortin, thyroxine*** and ***sex hormone binding globulin*** levels. Also increases ***follicle-stimulating*** and ***luteinizing hormone*** secretion in most patients.

INTERACTIONS **Drug:** Do not use with **ospemifene. Herbal: Black cohosh** may antagonize infertility treatments.

C

PHARMACOKINETICS **Absorption:** Readily absorbed from GI tract. **Metabolism:** In liver. **Elimination:** Primarily in feces. **Half-Life:** 5 days.

NURSING IMPLICATIONS

Assessment & Drug Effects

- Monitor for abnormal bleeding. Report it immediately.
- Monitor for visual disturbances. Their occurrence indicates the need for a complete ophthalmologic evaluation. Drug will be stopped until symptoms subside.
- Pelvic pain indicates the need for immediate pelvic examination for diagnostic purposes.
- Monitor lab results: Serum estrogen, serum triglycerides.

Patient & Family Education

- Take the medicine at same time every day to maintain drug levels and prevent forgetting a dose.
- Missed dose: Take drug as soon as possible. If not remembered until time for next dose, double the dose, then resume regular dosing schedule. If more than one dose is missed, check with prescriber.
- Report these symptoms: Hot flushes resembling those associated with menopause; nausea, vomiting, headache.
- Report promptly yellowing of eyes, light-colored stools, yellow, itchy skin, and fever symptomatic of jaundice.
- Stop taking clomiphene if pregnancy is suspected.
- Because of the possibility of lightheadedness, dizziness, and visual disturbances, do not perform hazardous tasks requiring skill and coordination in an environment with variable lighting.
- Report promptly excessive weight gain, signs of edema, bloating, decreased urinary output.
- If clomiphene is continued more than 1 yr, patient should have an ophthalmologic examination at regular intervals.

CLOMIPRAMINE HYDROCHLORIDE

(clo-mi′pra-meen)

Anafranil

Classification: TRICYCLIC ANTIDEPRESSANT

Therapeutic: ANTIPSYCHOTIC

Prototype: Imipramine

AVAILABILITY Capsule

ACTION & *THERAPEUTIC EFFECT* Inhibits reuptake of norepinephrine and serotonin at the presynaptic neuron. *The basis of its antidepressant effects is thought to be due to the elevated serum levels of norepinephrine and serotonin.*

USES Obsessive-compulsive disorder (OCD).

UNLABELED USES Panic disorder, major depressive disorder.

CONTRAINDICATIONS Hypersensitivity to clomipramine or other tricyclic agents; MAOI therapy; acute recovery period after MI, QT elongation, cardiac arrhythmias (AV block, bundle-branch block); suicidal ideation.

CAUTIOUS USE History of convulsive disorders, prostatic hypertrophy, urinary retention, cardiovascular, hepatic, GI, or blood disorders; history of seizure disorder; respiratory depression; diabetes mellitus; GERD; Parkinson disease; closed-angle glaucoma; asthma; bipolar disorder; history of suicidal tendencies; older adults; pregnancy (withdrawal symptoms have been observed in neonates whose mothers took clomipramine up to delivery); lactation; children younger than 10 yr.

ROUTE & DOSAGE

Obsessive-Compulsive Disorder

Adult: **PO** 25 mg daily, gradually increase to 100 mg daily as tolerated over 2 wk (max: 250 mg/day)
Adolescent/Child (10 yr or older): **PO** 25 mg daily, gradually increase to 100 mg daily or 3 mg/kg (whichever is less) in divided doses

Pharmacogenetic Dosage Adjustment

Poor CYP2D6 metabolizers should receive 50% of normal dose

ADMINISTRATION

Oral

- Give with meals to reduce GI adverse effects.
- Following titration to the full dose, drug may be given as a single dose at bedtime to reduce daytime sedation.
- Store at 15°–30°C (59°–86°F).

ADVERSE EFFECTS **CV:** Orthostatic hypotension, chest pain, flushing. **Respiratory:** Pharyngitis, rhinitis, sinusitis, bronchospasm. **CNS:** Drowsiness, headache, insomnia, fatigue, dizziness, nervousness, myoclonus, anxiety, paresthesia, memory impairment, sleep disorder, twitching, depression, lack of concentration. **HEENT:** Visual disturbances, tinnitus. **Endocrine:** *Weight gain,* change in libido, weight loss, hot flash. **GI:** Constipation, *dry mouth,* nausea, dyspepsia, anorexia, diarrhea, abdominal pain, vomiting, increased appetite, dysgeusia, flatulence. **GU:** Ejaculation failure, impotence, difficulty in micturition, urinary retention, urinary tract infection, urinary frequency. **Hematologic:** Leukopenia, agranulocytosis, thrombocytopenia, anemia. **Integumentary:** Skin rash, pruritus, diaphoresis. **Musculoskeletal:** Myalgia, tremor.

DIAGNOSTIC TEST INTERFERENCE

Increased glucose may interfere with urine detection of **methadone.**

INTERACTIONS **Drug:** MAO INHIBITORS may precipitate hyperpyrexic crisis, tachycardia, or seizures; ANTIHYPERTENSIVE AGENTS potentiate orthostatic hypotension; CNS DEPRESSANTS, **alcohol** add to CNS depression; **norepinephrine** and other SYMPATHOMIMETICS may increase cardiac toxicity; ANTICHOLINERGIC AGENTS increase risk of adverse effects. TCAs may increase risk of neuromalignant syndrome. **amoxapine, bromopride** may increase risk of side effects; may enhance effect of ANTICHOLINERGICS. Do not use with **dofetilide, dronedarone,** or **ziprasidone** due to increased risk of QT prolongation. SEROTONERGIC AGENTS increase risk of serotonin syndrome. **Herbal: Ginkgo** may decrease seizure threshold; **St. John's wort** may cause serotonin syndrome.

PHARMACOKINETICS **Absorption:** Rapidly from GI tract; 20–78% reaches systemic circulation. **Onset:** Approx 2–6 wk. **Distribution:** Distributes into CSF; crosses placenta; 97% protein binding. **Metabolism:** Extensive first-pass metabolism in the liver; active metabolite is desmethylclomipramine. **Elimination:** 50–60% in urine, 24–32% in feces. **Half-Life:** 36 h.

NURSING IMPLICATIONS

Black Box Warning

Clomipramine has been associated with increased suicidal thinking and behavior especially in children, adolescents, and young adults.

Assessment & Drug Effects

- Monitor for and report promptly suicidal thinking and behavior.
- Monitor for seizures, especially in those with predisposing factors or concurrent therapy with other drugs that lower seizure threshold.
- Monitor for and report signs of neuroleptic malignant syndrome (see Appendix F).
- Monitor for sedation and vertigo, especially at the beginning of therapy and following dosage increases. Supervision of ambulation may be indicated.
- Notify prescriber of fever and complaints of sore throat because these may indicate need to rule out adverse hematologic changes.
- Taper dosage slowly when discontinuing.
- Monitor lab tests: Periodic CBC, serum sodium in at-risk populations, LFTs, especially with long-term therapy. ECG/cardiac status in older adults and patients with cardiac disease.

Patient & Family Education

- Discontinue drug and report promptly to prescriber if suicidal ideation or behavior occurs.
- Do not take nonprescribed drugs or discontinue therapy without consent of prescriber. Abrupt discontinuation may cause nausea, headache, malaise, or seizures.
- Men should understand that the drug may cause impotence or ejaculation failure.
- Report promptly a sore throat accompanied by fever.
- Use caution with ambulation until response to drug is known.
- Moderate alcohol intake because it may potentiate adverse drug effects.

CLONAZEPAM

(kloe-na′zi-pam)

Klonopin, Rivotril ♣

Classification: ANTICONVULSANT; BENZODIAZEPINE

Therapeutic: ANTICONVULSANT; ANTIANXIETY

Prototype: Diazepam

Controlled Substance: Schedule IV

AVAILABILITY Tablet; orally disintegrating tablet

ACTION & *THERAPEUTIC EFFECT*

Benzodiazepine derivative with strong anticonvulsant activity that prevents seizures by potentiating the effects of GABA, an inhibitory neurotransmitter. Suppresses spread of seizure activity in the cortex, thalamus, and limbic regions of the brain. *Suppresses spike and wave discharge in absence seizures (petit mal) and decreases amplitude, frequency, duration, and spread of discharge in minor motor seizures.*

USES Seizure disorders, panic disorder.

UNLABELED USES Insomnia, nystagmus, restless leg syndrome, complex partial seizure pattern, and acute vertigo episodes.

C

CONTRAINDICATIONS Hypersensitivity to benzodiazepines; significant liver disease; acute narrow-angle glaucoma; pulmonary disease; coma or CNS depression; suicidal ideation; pregnancy (teratogenic effects have been observed with some benzodiazepines).

CAUTIOUS USE Renal or hepatic impairment; COPD; drug-controlled open-angle glaucoma; bipolar disorder, preexisting depression; history of suicidal thoughts; addiction-prone individuals; neuromuscular disease; mixed seizure disorders; debilitated individuals; older adults; children younger than 10 yr; lactation.

ROUTE & DOSAGE

Seizure Disorders

Adult: **PO** When used as monotherapy 0.5–1.5 mg/day in 3 divided doses, when used as adjunctive therapy 0.5–1 mg/day in 3 divided doses. In both cases can be increased by 0.5–1 mg q3days until seizures are controlled or until intolerable adverse effects (max dose: 20 mg/day)
Adolesecent/Child (greater than 10 yr, weight over 30 kg): **PO** 0.01–0.05 mg/kg/day in 2–3 divided doses, may increase by 25% q3–7 days until seizures are controlled.
Child (younger than 10 yr, weight 30 kg or less): **PO** 0.01–0.03 mg/kg/day (not to exceed 0.05 mg/kg/day) in 3 divided doses; may increase by 0.25–0.5 mg q3days until seizures are controlled or until intolerable adverse effects (max recommended dose: 0.2 mg/kg/day)

Panic Disorders

Adult/Adolescent: **PO** 0.25 mg bid initially, increase to 1 mg/day (max: 4 mg/day)

ADMINISTRATION

Oral

- Give largest dose at bedtime if daily dose cannot be equally divided.
- Place wafer form on tongue to dissolve.
- May be swallowed with or without water.
- Store in tightly closed container protected from light at 20°–25°C (68°–77°F) unless otherwise specified.

ADVERSE EFFECTS **CV:** Palpitations. **Respiratory:** Upper respiratory infection, sinusitis, influenza. **CNS:** *Drowsiness, sedation, ataxia,* panic disorder, insomnia, dizziness, aphonia, choreiform movements, coma, "glassy-eyed" appearance, headache, hemiparesis, hypotonia, slurred speech, tremor, vertigo, confusion, depression, suicide attempt. **GI:** Constipation. **GU:** Dysmenorrhea. **Hematologic:** Anemia, leukopenia, thrombocytopenia.

INTERACTIONS **Drug: Alcohol** and other CNS DEPRESSANTS increase sedation and CNS depression; may increase **phenytoin** levels. CYP34A inhibitors may increase risk of toxicity. **Herbal: Kava, valerian** may potentiate sedation. Avoid use with marijuana due to exaggerated sedation.

C

PHARMACOKINETICS Absorption: Readily absorbed from GI tract. **Onset:** 20–40 min. **Peak:** 1–2 h. **Duration:** Up to 12 h in adults; 6–8 h in children. **Distribution:** Crosses placenta; distributed into breast milk. **Metabolism:** In liver (via CYP3A4). **Elimination:** In urine primarily as metabolites. **Half-Life:** 18–40 h.

NURSING IMPLICATIONS

Assessment & Drug Effects

- Monitor for signs of suicidal ideation in depressive individuals.
- Both psychological and physical dependence may occur in the patient on long-term, high-dose therapy.
- Monitor for S&S of overdose, including somnolence, confusion, irritability, sweating, muscle and abdominal cramps, diminished reflexes, coma.
- Monitor lab tests: Periodic LFTs, CBC, and renal function tests.

Patient & Family Education

- Report loss of seizure control promptly. Anticonvulsant activity is often lost after 3 mo of therapy; dosage adjustment may reestablish efficacy.
- Do not abruptly discontinue this drug. Abrupt withdrawal can precipitate seizures. Other withdrawal symptoms include convulsion, tremor, abdominal and muscle cramps, vomiting, sweating.
- Do not drive a car or engage in other activities requiring mental alertness and physical coordination until reaction to the drug is known. Drowsiness occurs in approximately 50% of patients.

CLONIDINE HYDROCHLORIDE

(kloe′ni-deen)

Catapres, Catapres-TTS, Dixaril ♣, Duraclon, Kapvay

Classification: ANTIADRENERGIC; CENTRAL-ACTING ANTIHYPERTENSIVE; ANALGESIC

Therapeutic: ANTIHYPERTENSIVE; ANALGESIC

Prototype: Methyldopa

AVAILABILITY Tablet; transdermal patch; solution for injection; extended release tablet

ACTION & *THERAPEUTIC EFFECT* Centrally acting receptor agonist that stimulates alpha$_2$-adrenergic receptors in CNS to inhibit sympathetic cardioaccelerator and vasomotor centers. Central actions reduce plasma concentrations of norepinephrine. It decreases systolic and diastolic BP and heart rate. *Decreases systolic and diastolic BP and heart rate. Reportedly minimizes or eliminates many of the common clinical S&S associated with withdrawal of heroin, methadone, or other opiates.*

USES Hypertension, treatment of severe pain, ADHD.

UNLABELED USES Prophylaxis for migraine; treatment of dysmenorrhea, menopausal flushing, diarrhea, paroxysmal localized hyperhidroses, neuropathic pain; alcohol, smoking, opiate, and benzodiazepine withdrawal; Tourette syndrome.

CONTRAINDICATIONS Hypersensitivity to clonidine; first-line treatment of hypertension; coagulopathy. **Extended release:** Children younger than 6 yr. **Patch:** Polyarteritis nodosa, scleroderma, SLE on affected areas. **Epidural:** Severe cardiovascular disease, or those who are hemodynamically unstable; infection at injection site; obstetric, postpartum, perioperative pain management; use above the C_4 dermatome.

CAUTIOUS USE Severe coronary insufficiency, recent MI, sinus node dysfunction, cerebrovascular disease; diabetes mellitus; renal impairment; chronic renal failure; Raynaud disease, thromboangiitis obliterans; history of hypotension, heart block, bradycardia, or CVD; history of syncope; history of depression; addictive disorders; older adults; pregnancy (category C); lactation; children younger than 12 yr. **Extended release:** Children younger than 18 yr and over 6 yr. Adult use in ADHD of **Clonidine ER** has not been studied.

ROUTE & DOSAGE

Hypertension

Adult: **PO** 0.1 mg bid, may increase by 0.1–0.2 mg/day until desired response is achieved (max: 2.4 mg/day); **Transdermal** 0.1 mg patch once q7days, may increase by 0.1 mg q1–2wk; **Extended release** 0.1 mg daily
Geriatric: **PO** Start with 0.1 mg once daily
Child (12 yr or older): **PO** 0.2–0.6 mg/day in divided doses

Severe Pain

Adult: **Epidural** Start infusion at 30 mcg/h and titrate to response. Use rates greater than 40 mcg/h with caution.
Child: **Epidural** Start infusion at 0.5 mcg/kg/h and titrate to response.

ADHD

Adolescent/Child (6 yr or older): **PO Extended release** 0.1 mg qhs increase weekly to desired response

ADMINISTRATION

Oral

- Ensure that extended release tablets are swallowed whole. They should not be crushed or chewed.
- Give last PO dose immediately before patient retires to ensure overnight BP control and to minimize daytime drowsiness.
- Oral dosage is increased gradually over a period of weeks so as not to lower BP abruptly (especially important in the older adult).
- During change from PO clonidine to transdermal system, PO clonidine should be maintained for at least 24 h after patch is applied. Consult prescriber.
- Do not abruptly discontinue drug. It should be withdrawn over a period of 2–4 days. Abrupt withdrawal may result in a hypertensive crisis within 8–18 h.
- Store in tightly closed container at 15°–30°C (59°–86°F) unless otherwise directed.

Transdermal

- Apply transdermal patch to dry skin, free of hair and rash. Avoid irritated, abraded, or scarred skin. Recommended areas for applying transdermal patch are upper outer arm and anterior chest. Rotate application sites, and keep a record.

ADVERSE EFFECTS **CV:** *Hypotension (epidural),* postural hypotension (mild), peripheral edema, ECG changes, tachycardia, bradycardia, flushing, rapid increase in BP with abrupt withdrawal. **CNS:** *Drowsiness, sedation, dizziness,* headache, fatigue, weakness, sluggishness, dyspnea, vivid dreams, nightmares, insomnia, behavior changes, agitation, hallucination, nervousness, restlessness, anxiety, mental depression. **HEENT:** Dry eyes. **Skin:** Rash, pruritus, thinning of hair, exacerbation of psoriasis; with transdermal patch: Hyperpigmentation, recurrent herpes simplex, skin irritation, contact dermatitis, mild erythema. **GI:** *Dry mouth, constipation,* abdominal pain, pseudo-obstruction of large bowel, altered taste, nausea, vomiting, hepatitis, hyperbilirubinemia, weight gain (sodium retention). **GU:** Impotence, loss of libido.

DIAGNOSTIC TEST INTERFERENCE Avoid use of transdermal patch during ***MRI.*** Possibility of decreased urinary excretion of ***aldosterone, catecholamines,*** and ***VMA*** (however, sudden withdrawal of clonidine may cause increases in these values); transient increases in ***blood glucose;*** weakly positive ***direct antiglobulin (Coombs) tests.***

INTERACTIONS **Drug: Alcohol** and other CNS DEPRESSANTS add to CNS depression; TRICYCLIC ANTIDEPRESSANTS may reduce antihypertensive effects. OPIATE ANALGESICS increase hypotension with epidural clonidine. Increased risk of bradycardia or AV block when epidural clonidine is used with **digoxin,** CALCIUM CHANNEL BLOCKERS, or BETA BLOCKERS. Use with other ANTIHYPERTENSIVES can have added effect. Avoid with MAO INHIBITORS and **guanethidine.** Mirtazapine may antagonize antihypertensive effects.

PHARMACOKINETICS **Absorption:** Readily from GI tract. **Onset:** 30–60 min PO; 1–3 days transdermal. **Peak:** 2–4 h PO; 2–3 days transdermal. **Duration:** 8 h PO; 7 days transdermal. **Distribution:** Widely distributed; crosses blood–brain barrier; not known if crosses placenta or distributed into breast milk. **Metabolism:** In liver. **Elimination:** 80% in urine, 20% in feces. **Half-Life:** 6–20 h.

NURSING IMPLICATIONS

Assessment & Drug Effects

- Monitor BP closely. Determine positional changes (supine, sitting, standing).
- With epidural administration, frequently monitor BP and HR. Hypotension is a common side effect that may require intervention.
- Monitor BP closely whenever a drug is added to or withdrawn from therapeutic regimen.
- Monitor I&O during period of dosage adjustment. Report change in I&O ratio or change in voiding pattern.
- Determine weight daily. Patients not receiving a concomitant diuretic agent may gain weight, particularly during first 3 or 4 days of therapy, because of marked sodium and water retention.
- Supervise closely patients with history of mental depression, as

they may be subject to further depressive episodes.

Patient & Family Education

- Although postural hypotension occurs infrequently, make position changes slowly, and in stages, particularly from recumbent to upright position, and dangle and move legs a few minutes before standing. Lie down immediately if faintness or dizziness occurs.
- Avoid potentially hazardous activities until reaction to drug has been determined due to possible sedative effects.
- Do not omit doses or stop the drug without consulting the prescriber.
- Do not take OTC medications, alcohol, or other CNS depressants without prior discussion with prescriber.
- Avoid becoming overheated or dehydrated.
- Examine site when transdermal patch is removed and report to prescriber if erythema, rash, irritation, or hyperpigmentation occurs.
- If transdermal patch loosens, tape it in place with adhesive. The patch should never be cut or trimmed.

CLOPIDOGREL BISULFATE (Pr)

(clo-pi′do-grel)

Plavix

Classification: ANTIPLATELET

Therapeutic: PLATELET AGGREGATION INHIBITOR; ANTITHROMBOTIC

AVAILABILITY Tablet

ACTION & *THERAPEUTIC EFFECT* Inhibits platelet aggregation by selectively preventing the binding of adenosine diphosphate to its platelet receptor. The drug's effect on the adenosine diphosphate receptor of a platelet is irreversible. *Clopidogrel prolongs bleeding time, thereby reducing atherosclerotic events in high-risk patients.*

USES Acute coronary syndrome (ST or non-ST elevations). Secondary prevention of MI, stroke, and vascular death.

UNLABELED USES Reduction of restenosis after stent placement; atrial fibrillation.

CONTRAINDICATIONS Hypersensitivity to clopidogrel; intracranial hemorrhage, peptic ulcer, or any other active pathologic bleeding; lactation. Discontinue clopidogrel 5 days before elective surgery including CABG. Discontinue for at least 24 h for emergency on pump CABG.

CAUTIOUS USE GI bleeding, peptic ulcer disease; patients at risk for increased bleeding; hepatic impairment; renal impairment; pregnancy (category B). Safety and efficacy not established in children.

ROUTE & DOSAGE

Secondary Prevention Post Recent MI/Stroke/PAD

Adult: **PO** 75 mg daily

Secondary Prevention in Patients with STEMI (ST segment Elevated MI)

Adult: **PO** 75 mg daily with aspirin

Acute Coronary Syndrome (Non-ST Elevation MI)

Adult: **PO** 300 mg loading dose then 75 mg daily (use with aspirin)

C

Pharmacogenetic Dosage Adjustment

Poor CYP2C19 metabolizers: May need a higher initial dose or another treatment strategy.

ADMINISTRATION

Oral

- Administer without regard to meals. Avoid or minimize consumption of grapefruit juice.
- Do not administer to persons with active pathologic bleeding.
- Discontinue drug 7 days prior to surgery.
- Store at 15°–30°C (59°–86°F) in tightly closed container and protect from light.

ADVERSE EFFECTS **Respiratory:** Epistaxis. **Hematologic:** Hematoma, hemorrhage.

INTERACTIONS **Drug:** NSAIDS may increase risk of bleeding events. PROTON PUMP INHIBITORS may decrease effectiveness. **Fluoxetine, citalopram,** or **fluvoxamine, cangrelor** may decrease effectiveness. **Herbal: Garlic, ginger, ginkgo, evening primrose oil** may increase risk of bleeding. **Food:** Avoid grapefruit juice consumption.

PHARMACOKINETICS **Absorption:** Rapidly from GI tract. **Onset:** 2 h; reaches steady state in 3–7 days. **Distribution:** 94–98% protein bound. **Metabolism:** Via CYP2C19. **Elimination:** 50% in urine and 50% in feces. **Half-Life:** 8 h.

NURSING IMPLICATIONS

Black Box Warning

Clopidogrel has diminished efficacy in patients who are CYP2C19 poor metabolizers.

Assessment & Drug Effects

- Carefully monitor for and immediately report S&S of GI bleeding, especially when coadministered with NSAIDS, aspirin, heparin, or warfarin.
- Evaluate patients with unexplained fever or infection for myelotoxicity.
- Monitor lab tests: Baseline test for CYP2C19 genotype; periodic platelet count, hemoglobin, and hematocrit.

Patient & Family Education

- Report promptly any unusual bleeding (e.g., black, tarry stools).
- Avoid omeprazole, esomeprazole, or other over-the-counter acid-reducing drugs; do not take aspirin or NSAID use unless approved by prescriber.

CLORAZEPATE DIPOTASSIUM

(klor-az′e-pate)

Tranxene

Classification: ANXIOLYTIC; ANTICONVULSANT; BENZODIAZEPINE
Therapeutic: ANTIANXIETY; ANTICONVULSANT
Prototype: Lorazepam
Controlled Substance: Schedule IV

AVAILABILITY Tablet

ACTION & *THERAPEUTIC EFFECT* Exerts its effects through enhancement of GABA-benzodiazepine receptor complex, an inhibitory neurotransmitter. Clorazepate has depressant effects on the CNS, thus controlling anxiety associated with stress and also resulting in sedative effects. *Effective in controlling anxiety and withdrawal symptoms of alcohol.*

USES Management of anxiety disorders, adjunct therapy in management of focal (partial) onset seizure.

CONTRAINDICATIONS

Hypersensitivity to clorazepate; acute—narrow-angle glaucoma; depressive neuroses; pulmonary disease, COPD; psychotic reactions, drug abusers. Safe use during pregnancy (teratogenic effects have been observed with some benzodiazepines); lactation.

CAUTIOUS USE

Hypersensitivity to other benzodiazepines; older adults; debilitated patients; hepatic disease; kidney disease; Parkinson disease; neuromuscular disease; seizure disorders; bipolar disorder, mania, history of suicidal tendencies. Safe use in children younger than 9 yr not established.

ROUTE & DOSAGE

Anxiety Disorders

Adult: **PO** 15 mg daily may increase gradually up to 60 mg/day in divided doses (max: 60 mg/day)

Focal (partial) onset Seizures (Adjunctive)

Adult/Adolescent: **PO** 7.5 mg tid, may increase at weekly intervals (max dose: 90mg/day)
Child (9–12 yr): **PO** up to 7.5 mg bid, may increase in weekly intervals (max: 60 mg/day)

ADMINISTRATION

Oral

- Give with food or water to minimize gastric distress.
- Ensure that sustained-release form of drug is not chewed or crushed. It **must be** swallowed whole.
- Taper drug dose gradually over several days when drug is to be discontinued.
- Store in a light-resistant container at 20°–25°C (68°–77°F) unless otherwise specified.

ADVERSE EFFECTS

CV: Hypotension. **CNS:** *Drowsiness,* ataxia, dizziness, headache, paradoxical excitement, confusion, insomnia, anxiety, depression, dysarthria, nervousness, slurred speech, suicidal ideation. **Skin:** Rash. **HEENT:** Diplopia, blurred vision. **Endocrine:** Decreased libido. **GI/Hepatic:** Constipation, decreased appetite, diarrhea, nausea, vomiting, increased serum transaminase, jaundice, xerostomia. **Musculoskeletal:** Tremor.

INTERACTIONS

Drug: Alcohol and other CNS DEPRESSANTS compound CNS depression; avoid **olanzapine** due to additive adverse effects. **Herbal:** Kava, melatonin, marijuana, valerian may increase adverse effects.

PHARMACOKINETICS

Absorption: Decarboxylated in stomach; absorbed as active metabolite, desmethyldiazepam. **Peak:** 1 h. **Duration:** 24 h. **Distribution:** Crosses placenta; distributed into breast milk; 98% protein bound. **Metabolism:** In liver to oxazepam by CYP2C19 and CYP3A4. **Elimination:** Primarily in urine. **Half-Life:** 30–200 h.

NURSING IMPLICATIONS

Assessment & Drug Effects

- Drowsiness, a common side effect, is more likely to occur at initiation of therapy and with dose increments on successive days.

C

- Monitor patient with history of cardiovascular disease in early therapy for drug-induced responses. If systolic BP drops more than 20 mmHg or if there is a sudden increase in pulse rate, withhold drug and notify prescriber.
- Monitor for signs and symptoms of suicidal tendencies (anxiety, depression, behavior changes).
- Monitor lab tests: Periodic CBC, renal function tests, and LFTs throughout therapy.

Patient & Family Education

- Take drug as prescribed and do not change dose or abruptly stop taking the drug without prescriber's approval.
- Do not self-dose with OTC drugs (cold remedies, sleep medications, antacids) without consulting prescriber.
- Avoid driving and other potentially hazardous activities until reaction to drug is known.
- Do not use alcohol and other CNS depressants while on clorazepate therapy.
- If a woman becomes pregnant during therapy or intends to become pregnant, communicate with prescriber about the desirability of discontinuing the drug.

CLOTRIMAZOLE

(kloe-trim'a-zole)

Canesten ♣, Gyne-Lotrimin, Gyne-Lotrimin-3, Lotrimin, Mycelex, Mycelex-G

Classification: ANTIBIOTIC; AZOLE ANTIFUNGAL

Therapeutic: ANTIFUNGAL

Prototype: Fluconazole

AVAILABILITY Cream; solution; lotion; troches; vaginal tablet; vaginal cream

ACTION & THERAPEUTIC EFFECT

Acts by altering fungal cell membrane permeability, permitting loss of phosphorous compounds, potassium, and other essential intracellular constituents with consequent loss of ability to replicate. *Has broad-spectrum fungicidal activity. Active against a wide variety of fungi, yeast, dermatophytes and certain gram-positive bacteria.*

USES Dermal infections including tinea pedis, tinea cruris, tinea corporis, tinea versicolor; also vulvovaginal and oropharyngeal candidiasis.

UNLABELED USES Trichomoniasis.

CONTRAINDICATIONS Ophthalmic uses; systemic mycoses.

CAUTIOUS USE Hypersensitivity to other azole antifungals; hepatic impairment, diabetes mellitus; HIV; recurrent infections; pregnancy (category C for oral troches; category B for topical use); lactation. **Troches:** Safe use in children younger than 12 yr has not been established. **Oral:** Safe use in children younger than 3 yr not established. **Topical:** Cautious use in children younger than 2 yr.

ROUTE & DOSAGE

Dermal Infections

Adult: **Topical** Apply small amount onto affected areas bid a.m. and p.m.

Vulvovaginal Infections

Adult: **Intravaginal** Insert 1 applicator full or one 100-mg vaginal tablet into vagina at bedtime for 7 days, or one 500-mg vaginal tablet at bedtime for 1 dose

Oropharyngeal Candidiasis
Adult/Child (older than 3 yr): **PO** 1 troche (lozenge) 4–5 × day q3h for 14 days

ADMINISTRATION

Oral

- Instruct patient taking the oral lozenge to allow it to dissolve slowly in mouth over 15–30 min for maximum effectiveness.

Topical

- Apply skin cream and solution preparations sparingly. Protect hands with latex gloves when applying medication.
- Avoid contact of clotrimazole preparations with the eyes.
- Do not use occlusive dressings unless directed by prescriber to do so.
- Consult prescriber about skin cleansing procedure before applying medication. Regardless of procedure used, dry skin thoroughly.

Vaginal

- Apply small amount of cream to irritated area of vulva for relief of external vulvar itching associated with vaginal yeast infection.
- Store cream and solution formulations at 15°–30°C (59°–86°F); do not store troches or vaginal tablets above 35°C (95°F) unless otherwise directed.

ADVERSE EFFECTS **Skin:** Stinging, erythema, edema, vesication, desquamation, pruritus, urticaria, skin fissures. **GI:** Abnormal liver function tests; occasional nausea and vomiting (with oral troche). **GU:** Mild burning sensation, lower abdominal cramps, bloating, cystitis, urethritis, mild urinary frequency, vulval erythema and itching, pain and vaginal soreness during intercourse.

INTERACTIONS **Drug:** Intravaginal preparations may inactivate SPERMICIDES.

PHARMACOKINETICS **Absorption:** Minimal systemic absorption; minimally absorbed topically. **Peak:** High saliva concentrations less than 3 h; high vaginal concentrations in 8–24 h. **Metabolism:** In liver. **Elimination:** Eliminated as metabolite in bile.

NURSING IMPLICATIONS

Assessment & Drug Effects

- Evaluate effectiveness of treatment. Report any signs of skin irritation with dermal preparations.
- Anticipate signs of clinical improvement within the first week of drug use.

Patient & Family Education

- Use clotrimazole as directed and for the length of time prescribed by prescriber.
- Generally, clinical improvement is apparent during first week of therapy. Report to prescriber if condition worsens or if signs of irritation or sensitivity develop, or if no improvement is noted after 4 wk of therapy.
- If receiving the drug vaginally, your sexual partner may experience burning and irritation of penis or urethritis; refrain from sexual intercourse during therapy or have sexual partner wear a condom.

C

CLOZAPINE

(clo′za-pin)

Clozaril, Versacloz

Classification: ATYPICAL ANTIPSYCHOTIC

Therapeutic: ANTIPSYCHOTIC

AVAILABILITY Tablet; orally disintegrating tablet; oral suspension

ACTION & *THERAPEUTIC EFFECT* Interferes with the binding of dopamine type 2 (D_2) and the serotonin type 2A (5-HT_{2A}) receptors; also acts as an antagonist at adrenergic, cholinergic, histaminergic and other dopaminergic and serotonergic receptors. *Improves symptoms in patients with treatment-resistant schizophrenia.*

USES Management of schizophrenia and suicidal behavior in schizoaffective disorder.

UNLABELED USES Bipolar disorder, dementia-related behavioral disorders, psychosis in Parkinson disease.

CONTRAINDICATIONS Hypersensitivity to clozapine; history of clozapine-induced agranulocytosis or severe granulocytopenia; severe CNS depression, blood dyscrasia, patients with myeloproliferative disorders, uncontrolled epilepsy; chemotherapy, coma, leukemia, leukopenia, neutropenia, myocarditis; renal failure, dialysis, hepatitis, jaundice; suicidal ideation; dementia-related psychosis; neuroleptic malignant syndrome (NMS); infants; lactation. Discontinue clozapine if QTc interval is more than 500 msec.

CAUTIOUS USE Arrhythmias, GI disorders, history of bone marrow depression; narrow-angle glaucoma, hepatic and renal impairment, prostatic hypertrophy, history of seizures; DM; patients at risk for diabetes; cardiovascular and/or pulmonary disease; cerebrovascular disease, cardiac arrhythmias, tachycardia, dehydration, neurologic disease, tardive dyskinesia, patients at risk for aspiration pneumonia due to drug-induced esophageal dysmotility; history of suicidal thoughts; history of seizures or predisposition for seizures; previous history of agranulocytosis; surgery, glaucoma, infection, older adults; pregnancy (use with caution and individualized therapy during pregnancy). Safety and efficacy in children younger than 16 yr not established.

ROUTE & DOSAGE

Schizophrenia

Adult (16 yr or older): **PO** Initiate at 12.5 mg daily or bid, then increase by 25–50 mg/day and titrate to a target dose of 350–450 mg/day in 3 divided doses, further increases (not more than twice weekly) can be made if necessary (max: 900 mg/day)

ADMINISTRATION

Oral

- Drug is usually withdrawn gradually over 1–2 wk if therapy must be discontinued.
- May be given without regard to food.
- Store the drug away from heat or light.

ADVERSE EFFECTS **CV:** Orthostatic hypotension, *tachycardia,* syncope, hypertension. **CNS:** Drowsiness, sedation, dizziness, insomnia, vertigo, headache. **GI:** Nausea, dry mouth, constipation, weight gain, dyspepsia. **Musculoskeletal:** Tremor. **Other:** Fever, diaphoresis.

INTERACTIONS **Drug:** **Alcohol** and other CNS DEPRESSANTS compound depressant effects; ANTICHOLINERGIC AGENTS potentiate anticholinergic effects; ANTIHYPERTENSIVE AGENTS may potentiate hypotension; ANTINEOPLASTIC AGENTS may potentiate bone marrow suppression. Can have increased risk of QT prolongation, avoid use with **saquinavir. Amisulpride, bromopride, carbamazepine, metoclopramide, eluxadoline,** may increase side effects. May have increased risk of ulcer formation when used with potassium. **Herbal:** **St. John's wort** may decrease concentration of clozapine.

PHARMACOKINETICS **Absorption:** Readily absorbed from GI tract. **Onset:** 2–4 wk. **Peak:** 2.5 h. **Distribution:** Possibly distributed into breast milk. **Metabolism:** In liver via CYP1A2, 2C19, 3A4, and 2D6. **Elimination:** 50% in urine, 30% in feces. **Half-Life:** 12 h.

NURSING IMPLICATIONS

Black Box Warning

Clozapine has been associated with a significant risk of severe neutropenia, seizures (especially at higher doses), potentially fatal myocarditis (especially during, but not limited to, the first month of therapy), and orthostatic hypotension (especially during initial titration with dose acceleration). Elderly patients with dementia-related psychosis treated with antipsychotic drugs are at an increased risk of death.

Assessment & Drug Effects

- Monitor cardiovascular and respiratory status, especially during the first month of therapy. Report promptly S&S of potential cardiac problems.
- Monitor blood pressure and heart rate for development of tachycardia or hypotension, which may pose a serious risk for patients with compromised cardiovascular function.
- Monitor diabetics for loss of glycemic control.
- Monitor for seizure activity; seizure potential increases at the higher dose level.
- Monitor for S&S of NMS (see Appendix F) and tardive dyskinesia.
- Closely monitor for recurrence of psychotic symptoms if the drug is being discontinued.
- Monitor lab tests: Baseline CBC and absolute neutrophil count, then qwk × 6 mo, then q2wk for next 6 mo, then q4wk throughout therapy, and after drug discontinued, qwk × 4 wk; periodic blood glucose; electrolytes, liver function tests.

Patient & Family Education

- Carefully monitor blood glucose levels if diabetic.
- Do not engage in any hazardous activity until response to the drug is known. Drowsiness and sedation are common adverse effects.
- Due to the risk of agranulocytosis (see Appendix F), it is important to comply with blood test

regimen. Report flulike symptoms, fever, sore throat, lethargy, malaise, or other signs of infection.

- Rise slowly to avoid orthostatic hypotension.
- Report immediately any of the following: Unexplained fatigue, especially with activity; shortness of breath, sudden weight gain or edema of the lower extremities.
- Take drug exactly as ordered.
- Do not use OTC drugs or alcohol without permission of prescriber.

CODEINE

(koe'deen)

CODEINE SULFATE

Classification: NARCOTIC (OPIATE AGONIST) ANALGESIC; ANTITUSSIVE

Therapeutic: NARCOTIC ANALGESIC; ANTITUSSIVE

Prototype: Morphine

Controlled Substance: Schedule II

AVAILABILITY Tablet; oral solution

ACTION & *THERAPEUTIC EFFECT* Opium agonist in the CNS. Analgesia is mediated through changes in the perception of pain at the spinal cord and higher levels in the CNS. The antitussive effects are mediated through direct action on receptors in the cough center of the medulla. *Analgesic potency is about one-sixth that of morphine; antitussive activity is also a little less than that of morphine.*

USES Symptomatic relief of mild to moderately severe pain when control cannot be obtained by nonnarcotic analgesics and to suppress hyperactive or nonproductive cough.

CONTRAINDICATIONS Hypersensitivity to codeine or other morphine derivatives; increased intracranial pressure, head injury, acute alcoholism; use during labor.

CAUTIOUS USE Prostatic hypertrophy, G6PD deficiency; GI disease; COPD, acute asthma; hepatic or renal disease; hepatitis; immunosuppression; hypothyroidism; debilitated patients, very young and very old patients; history of drug abuse; pregnancy (category C); lactation; children/adolescent.

ROUTE & DOSAGE

Analgesic

Adult: **PO** 15–60 mg qid
Child: 0.5–1 mg/kg q4–6h prn (max: 60 mg/dose)

Antitussive

Adult: **PO** 10–20 mg q4–6h prn (max: 120 mg/24 h)
Child (6–12 yr): **PO** 5–10 mg q4–6h (max: 60 mg/24 h); *2 to younger than 6 yr:* 2.5–5 mg q4–6h (max: 30 mg/24 h)

ADMINISTRATION

Oral

- Administer codeine with milk or other food to reduce possibility of GI distress.

ADVERSE EFFECTS **CV:** Palpitation, hypotension, orthostatic hypotension, bradycardia, tachycardia, circulatory collapse. **CNS:** *Dizziness,* light-headedness, *drowsiness,* sedation, lethargy, euphoria, agitation; restlessness, exhilaration, convulsions, narcosis, respiratory depression. **HEENT:** Miosis. **Skin:** Diffuse erythema, rash, urticaria, *pruritus,* excessive perspiration, facial flushing, fixed-drug eruption.

GI: *Nausea,* vomiting, *constipation.* **GU:** Urinary retention. **Other:** Shortness of breath, anaphylactoid reaction.

INTERACTIONS **Drug: Alcohol** and other CNS DEPRESSANTS augment CNS depressant effects. **Herbal: St. John's wort** may cause increased sedation.

PHARMACOKINETICS **Absorption:** Readily from GI tract. **Onset:** 15–30 min. **Peak:** 1–1.5 h. **Duration:** 4–6 h. **Distribution:** Crosses placenta; distributed into breast milk. **Metabolism:** In liver. **Elimination:** In urine. **Half-Life:** 2.5–4 h.

NURSING IMPLICATIONS

Black Box Warning

Codeine has been associated with respiratory depression and death in children who are ultra-rapid metabolizers of codeine when used following tonsillectomy or adenoidectomy.

Assessment & Drug Effects

- Monitor closely for signs of respiratory depression. Withhold drug and notify prescriber if respiratory depression develops.
- Record relief of pain and duration of analgesia.
- Evaluate effectiveness as cough suppressant. Treatment of cough is directed toward decreasing frequency and intensity of cough without abolishing cough reflex, need to remove bronchial secretions.
- Supervise ambulation and use other safety precautions as warranted because drug may cause dizziness and light-headedness.
- Monitor for nausea, a common side effect. Report nausea accompanied by vomiting. Change to another analgesic may be warranted.

Patient & Family Education

- Make position changes slowly and in stages, particularly from recumbent to upright posture. Lie down immediately if lightheadedness or dizziness occurs.
- Lie down when feeling nauseated, and notify prescriber if this symptom persists. Nausea appears to be aggravated by ambulation.
- Avoid driving and other potentially hazardous activities until reaction to drug is known. Codeine may impair ability to perform tasks requiring mental alertness.
- Do not take alcohol or other CNS depressants unless approved by prescriber.

COLCHICINE

(kol'chi-seen)

Colcrys, Novocolchine ♣

Classification: ANTIGOUT

Therapeutic: ANTIGOUT

AVAILABILITY Tablet

ACTION & *THERAPEUTIC EFFECT* In gout anti-inflammatory action may involve a reduction in lactic acid production by leukocytes resulting in decreased uric acid deposition and a reduction in phagocytosis. Effect on fever may be due to preventing activation of neutrophils and monocytes. *Inhibition of inflammation and reduction of pain and swelling, which occurs in gouty arthritis. Colchicine is nonanalgesic and nonuricosuric.*

C

USES Prophylactically for recurrent gouty arthritis or for acute gout, treatment or prevention of Mediterranean fever.

UNLABELED USES Sarcoid arthritis, chondrocalcinosis (pseudogout), arthritis associated with erythema nodosum, leukemia, adenocarcinoma, acute calcific tendonitis, multiple sclerosis, primary biliary cirrhosis, mycosis fungoides, and Paget disease.

CONTRAINDICATIONS Hypersensitivity to the drug; blood dyscrasias; severe GI, renal, hepatic, or cardiac disease.

CAUTIOUS USE Early manifestations of GI, renal, hepatic, or cardiac disease; hematologic disorders; debilitated patients and older adults; pregnancy (category C). Safe use in children not established.

ROUTE & DOSAGE

Acute Gouty Flare

Adult: **PO** 1.2 mg followed by 0.6 mg one hour later (max: 1.8 mg in one hour).

Prophylaxis

Adult: **PO** 0.6 mg once or twice daily. *Adult with concurrent CYP3A4 inhibitor use:* **PO** 0.3 mg every day or every other day

Familial Mediterranean Fever

Adult: **PO** 1.2–2.4 mg in 1 or 2 doses.

Renal Impairment Dosage Adjustment

CrCl 30 mL/min: Use 50% of normal dose

ADMINISTRATION

Oral

- Administer oral drug with milk or food to reduce possibility of GI upset.
- Preserve in tight, light-resistant containers preferably at 15°–30°C (59°–86°F), unless otherwise directed by manufacturer.

ADVERSE EFFECTS **CNS:** Mental confusion, peripheral neuritis, syndrome of muscle weakness (accompanied by elevated serum creatine kinase). **Skin:** Severe irritation and tissue damage if IV administration leaks around injection site. **GI:** *Nausea, vomiting, diarrhea, abdominal pain,* anorexia, hemorrhagic gastroenteritis, steatorrhea, hepatotoxicity, pancreatitis. **GU:** Azotemia, proteinuria, hematuria, oliguria. **Hematologic:** Neutropenia, <u>bone marrow depression</u>, <u>thrombocytopenia</u>, <u>agranulocytosis</u>, <u>aplastic anemia</u>.

DIAGNOSTIC TEST INTERFERENCE False-positive ***urine tests for RBCs and Hgb*** reported.

INTERACTIONS **Drug:** May decrease intestinal absorption of vitamin B_{12}. Do not use with PROTEASE INHIBITORS. Avoid CYP3A4 inhibitors. **Food:** **Grapefruit juice** may increase adverse effects.

PHARMACOKINETICS **Absorption:** Rapidly from GI tract. **Peak:** 0.5–2 h; multiple peaks because of enterohepatic cycling. **Distribution:** Widely distributed; concentrates in leukocytes, kidney, liver, spleen, and intestinal tract. **Metabolism:** By P-glycoprotein and CYP3A4. **Elimination:** Primarily in feces.

NURSING IMPLICATIONS

Assessment & Drug Effects

- Monitor for dose-related adverse effects; they are most likely to occur during the initial course of treatment.
- Monitor for early signs of colchicine toxicity including weakness, abdominal discomfort, anorexia, nausea, vomiting, and diarrhea. Report to prescriber. To avoid more serious toxicity, drug should be discontinued promptly until symptoms subside.
- Monitor I&O ratio and pattern (during acute gouty attack): High fluid intake promotes excretion and reduces danger of crystal formation in kidneys and ureters.
- Monitor lab tests: Baseline and periodic serum uric acid and creatinine, CBC, platelet count, serum electrolytes, and urinalysis.

Patient & Family Education

- Withhold drug and report to the prescriber the onset of GI symptoms or signs of bone marrow depression (nausea, sore throat, bleeding gums, sore mouth, fever, fatigue, malaise, unusual bleeding or bruising).
- Avoid fermented beverages such as beer, ale, and wine as they may precipitate gouty attack.

COLESEVELAM HYDROCHLORIDE

(co-less′e-ve-lam)

Welchol

Classification: ANTIHYPERLIPIDEMIC; BILE ACID SEQUESTRANT

Therapeutic: CHOLESTEROL-LOWERING; BILE ACID SEQUESTRANT

Prototype: Cholestyramine resin

AVAILABILITY
Tablet; powder for suspension

ACTION & THERAPEUTIC EFFECT
Binds with bile salts in the intestinal tract to form an insoluble complex that is excreted in the feces, thus reducing circulating cholesterol and increasing serum LDL removal rate. Serum triglyceride levels may increase slightly. *Decreases serum LDL and total cholesterol level. Removes bile salts from the intestine.*

USES
Hypercholesterolemia, hyperlipoproteinemia, type 2 diabetes.

CONTRAINDICATIONS
Hypersensitivity to colesevelam; complete biliary obstruction; history of hypertriglyceridemia-induced pancreatitis; serum triglyceride concentrations greater than 500 mg/dL; bowel obstruction.

CAUTIOUS USE
Preexisting GI disorders or bowel disease, primary biliary cirrhosis, partial biliary obstruction, biliary atresia; diabetes mellitus; hypertriglyceridemia; older adults, malabsorption states; bleeding disorders; pregnancy (category B).

ROUTE & DOSAGE

Hypercholesterolemia; Type 2 Diabetes

Adult: **PO** 3 tablets (1.875 g powder) bid with meals or 6 tablets (3.75 g powder) daily with a meal.

C

ADMINISTRATION

Oral

- Give with meals (mandatory) and adequate liquid (e.g., 8 oz).
- Administer concurrently ordered drugs at least 4 h prior to colesevelam.
- Store at 15°–30°C (59°–86°F) with occasional fluctuations to 40°C (90°F); protect from moisture.

ADVERSE EFFECTS **CV:** Hypertension. **Respiratory:** Pharyngitis, flulike symptoms, nasopharyngitis, rhinitis. **Endocrine:** Hypoglycemia. **GI:** Constipation, dyspepsia, nausea.

INTERACTIONS **Drug:** May decrease absorption of **verapamil.** Can bind and affect absorption of any drug.

PHARMACOKINETICS **Absorption:** Not absorbed. **Metabolism:** Not metabolized. **Elimination:** 0.05% in urine.

NURSING IMPLICATIONS

Assessment & Drug Effects

- Withhold drug and notify prescriber for triglycerides greater than 300 mg/dL.
- Monitor lab tests: Baseline lipid profile, repeat at 3 mo, then q6–12 mo thereafter.

Patient & Family Education

- Report S&S of GI distress (see Appendix F), especially constipation.

COLESTIPOL HYDROCHLORIDE

(koe-les′ti-pole)

Colestid

Classification: ANTIHYPERLIPIDEMIC; BILE ACID SEQUESTRANT
Therapeutic: CHOLESTEROL-LOWERING AGENT; BILE ACID SEQUESTRANT
Prototype: Cholestyramine

AVAILABILITY Tablet; powder for suspension

ACTION & THERAPEUTIC EFFECT Binds with bile acids to form an insoluble complex that is eliminated in the feces thereby increasing the fecal loss of bile acid-bound LDL cholesterol. *Reduces circulating cholesterol and increases serum LDL removal rate. Serum triglycerides are not affected or are minimally increased.*

USES Primary hypercholesterolemia.

UNLABELED USES Digitoxin overdose and hyperoxaluria and to control postoperative diarrhea caused by excess bile acids in colon; pruritus associated with partial biliary obstruction.

CONTRAINDICATIONS Complete biliary obstruction, biliary cirrhosis; hypersensitivity to bile acid sequestrants; renal disease.

CAUTIOUS USE Hemorrhoids; bleeding disorders; malabsorption states; GI motility disorders, dysphagia; older adult; pregnancy (category C). Safe use in children not established.

ROUTE & DOSAGE

Hypercholesterolemia

Adult: **PO** 15–30 g (powder)/day in 2–4 doses a.c. and at bedtime, or 1–2 tabs 1–2 × day

ADMINISTRATION

Oral

- Give 30 min before a meal when ordered a.c.
- Ensure that tablets are not chewed or crushed. They **must be** swallowed whole.
- Always mix granule form with liquids, juices, soups, cereals, or

pulpy fruits. Add powder to at least 90 mL fluid. When carbonated drink is used, slowly stir in a large glass because excess foaming may occur. Rinse glass with small amount extra fluid to be sure all the drug is taken.

- Drugs given concomitantly should be scheduled at least 1 h before or 4 h after ingestion of colestipol to reduce interference with their absorption (see drug interactions).
- Store at 15°–30°C (59°–86°F) in tightly closed container unless otherwise instructed.

ADVERSE EFFECTS **CV:** Angina, peripheral edema, tachycardia. **Respiratory:** Dyspnea. **CNS:** Dizziness, fatigue, headache, insomnia. **Skin:** Dermatitis, rash, urticaria. **Hepatic/GI:** Increased serum ALP, increased serum ALT, increased serum AST, abdominal cramps, anorexia, constipation, diarrhea, dyspepsia, flatulence, nausea. **Musculoskeletal:** Arthralgia, arthritis, back pain, myalgia, weakness.

INTERACTIONS **Drug:** Because it decreases the absorption from the GI tract of ORAL ANTICOAGULANTS, **digoxin,** TETRACYCLINES, PENICILLINS, **phenobarbital,** THYROID HORMONES, THIAZIDE DIURETICS, IRON SALTS, FAT-SOLUBLE VITAMINS (A, D, E, K), administer cholestyramine 4 h before or 2 h after these drugs. Can bind and affect absorption of any drug.

PHARMACOKINETICS **Absorption:** Not absorbed from GI tract. **Elimination:** In feces as insoluble complex.

NURSING IMPLICATIONS

Assessment & Drug Effects

- Watch for changes in bowel elimination pattern. Constipation should not be allowed to persist without medical attention.
- Monitor lab tests: Baseline lipid profile, repeat at 3 mo, then q6–12 mo thereafter.

Patient & Family Education

- To prevent drug interactions, it is important to keep to established schedule for taking colestipol and other drugs. See Drug Interactions.
- If receiving prolonged therapy, report unusual bleeding (vitamin K deficiency). Colestipol prevents absorption of fat-soluble vitamins (A, D, E, K).

COLISTIMETHATE SODIUM

(koe-lis-ti-meth'ate)

Coly-Mycin M

Classification: URINARY TRACT ANTIINFECTIVE; ANTIBIOTIC

Therapeutic: URINARY TRACT ANTIINFECTIVE

Prototype: Trimethoprim

AVAILABILITY Solution for injection

ACTION & *THERAPEUTIC EFFECT* Acts by affecting phospholipid component in bacterial cytoplasmic membranes with resulting damage and leakage of essential intracellular components. *Bactericidal against most gram-negative organisms, but not effective against* Proteus *or* Neisseria *species.*

USES Severe, acute, and chronic UTIs caused by organisms resistant to other antibiotics.

CONTRAINDICATIONS Hypersensitivity to polypeptide antibiotics; concurrent use of nephrotoxic and ototoxic drugs.

CAUTIOUS USE Impaired renal function; myasthenia gravis; older adult patients; pregnancy (category C); lactation; infants.

C

ROUTE & DOSAGE

Urinary Tract Infections

Adult/Child: **IM/IV** 2.5–5 mg/kg/day divided in 2–4 doses (max: 5 mg/kg/day)

Renal Impairment Dosage Adjustment

CrCl 50–79 mL/min: Colistimethate sodium equivalent to 2.5–3.8 mg/kg/day of colistin base divided in 2 doses
CrCl 30–49 mL/min: Colistimethate sodium equivalent to 2.5 mg/kg/day of colistin base in 1–2 divided doses
CrCl 10–29 mL/min: Colistimethate sodium equivalent to 1.5 mg/kg of colistin base every 36 h

ADMINISTRATION

Intramuscular

- Reconstitute each 150-mg vial with 2 mL of sterile water for injection to yield a concentration of 75 mg/mL. Swirl vial gently during reconstitution to avoid bubble formation.
- IM injection should be made deep into upper outer quadrant of buttock.
- Patients commonly experience pain at injection site. Rotate sites.

Intravenous

PREPARE: **Direct/Intermittent:** Prepare first half of total daily dose as directed for IM then further dilute with 20 mL sterile water for injection. ▪ Prepare second half of total daily dose by diluting further in 50 mL or more of D5W, NS, D5/NS, LR, or other compatible solution. ▪ IV infusion solution should be freshly prepared and used within 24 h.

ADMINISTER: **Direct/Intermittent:** First half of total daily dose: Give slowly over 3–5 min. ▪ Second half of total daily dose: Starting 1–2 h after the first half dose has been given, infuse the second half dose over the next 22–23 h.

INCOMPATIBILITIES: **Solution/additive: Cefazolin, cephapirin, erythromycin, hydrocortisone, hydroxyzine, kanamycin, lincomycin.**

▪ Reconstituted solution may be stored in refrigerator at 2°–8°C (36°–46°F) or at controlled room temperature of 15°–30°C (59°–86°F). Use within 7 days. ▪ Store unopened vials at controlled room temperature.

ADVERSE EFFECTS **Respiratory-:** Respiratory arrest after IM injection. **CNS:** Circumoral, lingual, and peripheral paresthesias; visual and speech disturbances, neuromuscular blockade- (generalized muscle weakness, dyspnea, respiratory depression or paralysis), seizures, psychosis. **HEENT:** Ototoxicity-. **Skin:** Pruritus, urticaria, dermatoses. **GI:** GI disturbances. **GU:** Nephrotoxicity. **Other:** Drug fever, pain at IM site.

INTERACTIONS **Drug: Tubocurarine, pancuronium, atracurium,** AMINOGLYCOSIDES may compound and prolong respiratory depression; AMINOGLYCOSIDES, **amphotericin B, vancomycin** augment nephrotoxicity.

PHARMACOKINETICS **Peak:** 1–2 h IM. **Duration:** 8–12 h. **Distribution:** Widely distributed in most tissues except CNS; crosses placenta; distributed into breast milk in low concentrations. **Metabolism:** In liver. **Elimination:** 66–75% in urine within 24 h. **Half-Life:** 2–3 h.

NURSING IMPLICATIONS

Assessment & Drug Effects

- Report restlessness or dyspnea promptly. Respiratory arrest has been reported after IM administration.
- Monitor I&O ratio and patterns: Decrease in urine output or change in I&O ratio and rising BUN, serum creatinine, and serum drug levels (without dosage increase) are indications of renal toxicity. If they occur, withhold drug and report to prescriber.
- Be alert to neurologic symptoms: Changes in speech and hearing, visual changes, drowsiness, dizziness, ataxia, and transient paresthesias, and keep prescriber informed.
- Monitor closely postoperative patients who have received curariform muscle relaxants, ether, or sodium citrate for signs of neuromuscular blockade (delayed recovery, muscle weakness, depressed respiration).
- Monitor lab tests: Baseline C&S; periodic renal function tests and urine drug levels.

Patient & Family Education

- Avoid operating a vehicle or other potentially hazardous activities while on drug therapy because of the possibility of transient neurologic disturbances.

CONIVAPTAN HYDROCHLORIDE ⓟ

(con-i-vap'tin)

Vaprisol

Classification: ELECTROLYTIC & WATER BALANCE AGENT; DIURETIC; VASOPRESSIN ANTAGONIST

Therapeutic: VASOPRESSIN ANTAGONIST; DIURETIC

AVAILABILITY Solution for injection

ACTION & *THERAPEUTIC EFFECT*

Conivaptan is a vasopressin receptor (V2) antagonist that reduces the effect of vasopressin in the kidney, thus increasing the excretion of free water into the renal collecting ducts. *Conivaptan increases urine output and decreases urine osmolality in patients with euvolemic hyponatremia, thus restoring serum sodium balance.*

USES Treatment of euvolemic and hypervolemic hyponatremia in hospitalized patients.

CONTRAINDICATIONS Hypersensitivity to conivaptan; CHF; hyponatremia associated with hypovolemia; hypotension, syncope; lactation.

CAUTIOUS USE Renal or hepatic function impairment; pregnancy (category C). Safety and efficacy in children not established.

ROUTE & DOSAGE

Hyponatremia

Adult: **IV** 20 mg loading dose followed by 20 mg IV over 24 h. May repeat 20 mg/day dose for 1–3 days, or may titrate up to 40 mg/day based on response. Total duration of infusion should not exceed 4 days.

ADMINISTRATION

Intravenous

PREPARE: **IV Infusion:** Packaged as 20-mg/100-mL IV solution. No further preparation is necessary. ***ADMINISTER:*** **IV Infusion:** Give via a large vein and change infusion site every 24 h. *Loading dose:* Give over 30 min. *Maintenance dose:* Give over 24 h. ▪ Frequently monitor the serum sodium level. A reduction in dose or discontinuation of infusion may be required if the serum sodium rises too rapidly. Discontinue infusion immediately and notify prescriber of a rise in serum sodium greater than 12 mEq/L/24 h. **Do not** resume infusion if serum sodium continues to rise. ▪ Infusion may be resumed ONLY if hyponatremia persists or reoccurs and patient demonstrates no indication of neurologic impairment. If the serum sodium rises too slowly, the dose may be titrated up to 40 mg over 24 h.

INCOMPATIBILITIES: **Solution/additive:** **Lactated Ringer solution, sodium chloride 0.9%.**

▪ Store vials at 25°C (77°F). Ampules should be stored in the original container and protected from light until ready for use. ▪ After diluting with D5W, the solution should be used immediately, with infusion completed within 24 h of mixing.

ADVERSE EFFECTS **CV:** Atrial fibrillation, hypertension, hypotension, orthostatic hypotension, phlebitis. **Respiratory:** Pneumonia. **CNS:** Confusional state, *headache,* insomnia. **HEENT:** Oral candidiasis. **Skin:** Erythema. **Endocrine:** Dehydration, hyperglycemia, hypoglycemia, *hypokalemia,* hypomagnesemia, hyponatremia. **GI:** Constipation, diarrhea, dry mouth, nausea, vomiting. **Hematologic:** Anemia. **Other:** Cannula-site reaction, *infusion-site reaction,* pain, peripheral edema, pyrexia, *thirst.*

INTERACTIONS **Drug:** Compounds that inhibit CYP3A4 (e.g., **ketoconazole, itraconazole, clarithromycin, ritonavir, indinavir**) can increase conivaptan levels. Conivaptan can increase the levels of **digoxin** and drugs that require CYP3A4 for metabolism (e.g., **midazolam,** HMG COA REDUCTASE INHIBITORS, **amlodipine**). **Food: Grapefruit juice** may increase the level of conivaptan. **Herbal: St. John's wort** may decrease the level of conivaptan.

PHARMACOKINETICS **Distribution:** 99% protein bound. **Metabolism:** Extensive hepatic metabolism. **Elimination:** Primarily fecal elimination (83%) with minor renal elimination. **Half-Life:** 5 h.

NURSING IMPLICATIONS

Assessment & Drug Effects

- Monitor infusion site for erythema, phlebitis, or other site reaction.
- Monitor vital signs and neurologic status frequently; report immediately S&S of hypernatremia (see Appendix F).
- Monitor digoxin blood levels with concurrent therapy and assess for S&S of digoxin toxicity.

- Monitor I&O closely. Effective treatment is accompanied by increased urine output, whereas decreasing urine output and oliguria may indicate developing hypernatremia.
- Monitor lab tests: Baseline and frequent serum sodium, serum potassium, and urine osmolality.

Patient & Family Education

- Report any of the following to a healthcare provider: Pain at the infusion site, dizziness, confusion, palpitations, swelling of hands or feet.

CORTISONE ACETATE

(kor′ti-sone)

Classification: ADRENOCORTICAL STEROID; ANTI-INFLAMMATORY **Therapeutic:** ANTI-INFLAMMATORY; GLUCOCORTICOID REPLACEMENT; IMMUNOSUPPRESSANT. **Prototype:** Prednisone

AVAILABILITY Tablet

ACTION & *THERAPEUTIC EFFECT* Short-acting synthetic steroid with prominent glucocorticoid activity and minimal mineralocorticoid effects. Cortisone is converted in the body to cortisol, resulting in metabolic effects including promotion of protein, carbohydrate, and fat metabolism and interference with linear growth in children. *Has anti-inflammatory and immunosuppressive actions. Suppresses inflammation caused by radiant, mechanical, chemical, and infectious stimuli. Also suppress immune responses in diseases, such as in asthma, urticaria, or renal allograft.*

USES Replacement therapy for primary or secondary adrenocortical insufficiency and inflammatory and allergic disorders.

CONTRAINDICATIONS Hypersensitivity to glucocorticoids; psychoses; viral, fungal, or bacterial diseases of skin; Cushing syndrome, immunologic procedures; pregnancy (category D); lactation.

CAUTIOUS USE Diabetes mellitus; hypertension, CHF; older adults; active or arrested tuberculosis; coagulopathy; hepatic disease; psychosis, emotional instability; renal disease, seizure disorders; active or latent peptic ulcer.

ROUTE & DOSAGE

Anti-inflammatory

Adult: **PO** 20–300 mg/day in 1 or more divided doses, try to reduce periodically by 10–25 mg/day to lowest effective dose

ADMINISTRATION

Oral

- Administer cortisone (usually in a.m.) with food or fluid of patient's choice to reduce gastric irritation.
- Sodium chloride and a mineralocorticoid are usually given with cortisone as part of replacement therapy.

ADVERSE EFFECTS **CV:** CHF, hypertension, *edema*. **CNS:** Euphoria, insomnia, vertigo, nystagmus. **HEENT:** *Cataracts*, glaucoma, blurred vision. **Endocrine:** Hyperglycemia. **Skin:** Impaired wound healing, petechiae, ecchymosis, acne. **GI:** *Nausea*, peptic ulcer, pancreatitis. **Musculoskeletal:** *Compression fracture*, osteoporosis, muscle weakness. **Hematologic:** <u>Thrombocytopenia</u>.

C

INTERACTIONS **Drug:** BARBITURATES, **phenytoin, rifampin** decrease effects of cortisone. Do not use with other IMMUNOSUPRESSANTS.

PHARMACOKINETICS **Absorption:** Readily absorbed from GI tract. **Onset:** Rapid PO; 24–48 h IM. **Peak:** 2 h PO; 24–48 h IM. **Duration:** 1.25–1.5 days. **Distribution:** Concentrated in many tissues; crosses placenta; distributed into breast milk. **Metabolism:** In liver. **Elimination:** In urine. **Half-Life:** 0.5 h; HPA suppression: 8–12 h.

NURSING IMPLICATIONS

Assessment & Drug Effects

- Monitor for S&S of Cushing syndrome (see Appendix F), especially in patients on long-term therapy.
- Cortisone may mask some signs of infection, and new infections may appear.
- Be alert to clinical indications of infection: Malaise, anorexia, depression, and evidence of delayed healing. (Classic signs of inflammation are suppressed by cortisone.)
- Report ecchymotic areas, unexplained bleeding, and easy bruising.
- Monitor lab tests: Periodic blood glucose and CBC with platelet count.

Patient & Family Education

- Take drug exactly as prescribed. Do not alter dose intervals or stop therapy abruptly.
- Monitor weight and report a steady gain, especially if it is accompanied by signs of fluid retention (e.g., edema of ankles or hands).
- Report changes in visual acuity, including blurring, promptly.
- Inform prescriber or dentist that cortisone is being taken.

CRIZANLIZUMAB - TMCA

(kriz-an-liz-ue-mab)

Adakveo

Classifications: MONOCLONAL ANTIBODY, SELECTIN BLOCKER

Therapeutic: BLOOD FORMATION, COAGULATION

AVAILABILITY Solution for injection

ACTION & *THERAPEUTIC EFFECT* A selectin blocker monoclonal antibody that binds to P-selectin and blocks interactions with its ligands causing a blockage of the interactions between endothelial cells, platelets, red blood cells, and leukocytes. *Decreases or prevents sickle cell vasoocclusive crisis.*

USES Reduce frequency of sickle cell-associated vasoocclusive crisis.

UNLABELED USES None.

CONTRAINDICATIONS Specific contraindications have not been determined.

CAUTIOUS USE No preexisting diseases or populations listed for cautious use.

ROUTE & DOSAGE

Sickle cell disease

Adult and Child (16 y or older): **IV** 5 mg/kg on week 0, week 2, then repeated every 4 weeks

ADMINISTRATION

Intravenous

PREPARE: Obtain the number of vials required based upon the patient's weight, 1 vial is needed for every 10 mL of medication. Bring vials to room temperature for a maximum of 4 hours prior to piercing the first vial. Dilute in NS or D5W up to a total of 100 mL; infusion bags or containers must be made of either polyvinyl chloride (PVC), polyethylene (PE), or polypropylene (PP); the volume of crizanlizumab-tmca added to the infusion bag or container should not exceed 96 mL. Gently invert the infusion bag to mix the diluted solution. Do not shake. Visually inspect for discoloration or particulate matter. Solution should be clear to opalescent, colorless, or may have a slightly brownish-yellow tint. Discard if particles are present in the solution.

ADMINISTER: **IV Infusion:** Administer as soon as possible once prepared. Administer diluted solution over 30 minutes through an IV line, which must contain a sterile, nonpyrogenic 0.2-micron in-line filter. After administration, flush the line with at least 25 mL of NS or D5W.

INCOMPATIBILITIES: Do not mix or coadminister with any other drugs in the same line.

- Storage: If solution is not administered immediately, store the prepared solution at room temperature (up to 25°C or 77°F) for no more than 4.5 hours from the start of preparation of the infusion, or under refrigeration (2°–8°C or 36°–46°F) for no more than 24 hours from the start of the time of preparation to completion of infusion. This includes storage of diluted solution and the time to warm up to room temperature. Protect the diluted solution from light during storage under refrigeration.

ADVERSE EFFECTS (>5%) **GI:** Nausea **Musculoskeletal:** Joint and back pain **Other:** Fever or infusion reaction

INTERACTIONS None known

PHARMACOKINETICS **Distribution:** 4 L **Metabolism:** Nonspecific proteolysis. **Half-Life:** 7.6 d

NURSING IMPLICATIONS

Assessment & Drug Effects

- Monitor for an infusion reaction: Fever, chills, nausea, vomiting, fatigue, dizziness, itching, hives, shortness of breath, or wheezing.
- Decreased frequency of vasoocclusive crises for patient with sickle cell disease

Patient & Family Education

- Report immediately any symptoms of an infusion reaction: Fever, chills, nausea, vomiting, fatigue, dizziness, itching, hives, shortness of breath, or wheezing.
- Inform all healthcare providers of treatment with this drug prior to any blood tests.

CROFELEMER

(kroe-fel′e-mer)

Mytesi

Classification: ANTIDIARRHEAL

Therapeutic: ANTIDIARRHEAL

AVAILABILITY Delayed-release tablet

ACTION & THERAPEUTIC EFFECT Crofelemer blocks chloride ion secretion in the intestine and accompanying high-volume water loss in diarrhea, normalizing the flow of chloride ions and water in the GI tract. *By decreasing water loss via the GI tract, diarrhea is substantially diminished.*

USES Symptomatic relief of noninfectious diarrhea in patients with HIV/AIDS on antiretroviral therapy.

C

CONTRAINDICATIONS Diarrhea caused by infection; pregnancy – fetal risk cannot be ruled out; lactation – infant risk cannot be ruled out.

CAUTIOUS USE Worsening infection, older adults. Safety and efficacy in children younger than 18 yr not established.

ROUTE & DOSAGE

Diarrhea
Adult: PO 125 mg bid

ADMINISTRATION

Oral

- May be given without regard to food.
- Tablets must be swallowed whole. They should not be crushed or chewed.
- Store at 20°–25°C (68°–77°F), excursions permitted between 15° and 30°C (59° and 86°F).

ADVERSE EFFECTS (≥5%) **Respiratory:** *Upper respiratory tract infection.*

INTERACTIONS **Drug:** Crofelemer may have additive effects with other antidiarrheal agents or those who produce constipation (i.e., OPIOIDS). Constipation and bowel obstruction have been reported in IBS patients taking **alosetron** in combination with other agents to control diarrhea.

PHARMACOKINETICS **Absorption:** Minimal oral absorption. **Metabolism:** Not metabolized.

NURSING IMPLICATIONS

Assessment & Drug Effects

- Monitor bowel elimination. Report to prescriber if the number of daily episodes of watery diarrhea does not diminish.
- Note that infectious diarrhea will not respond to this therapy.

Patient & Family Education

- Contact prescriber if diarrhea does not substantially diminish.
- Contact prescriber if development of a cough, runny nose, congestion, sore throat, body aches, or fever.

CROMOLYN SODIUM

(kroe′moe-lin)

Crolom, Fivent ♣, Gastrocrom, Intal, Opticrom, Rynacrom ♣, Vistacrom ♣

Classification: RESPIRATORY AGENT; MAST CELL STABILIZER; ANTI-INFLAMMATORY; ANTIASTHMATIC

Therapeutic: ANTIASTHMATIC; ANTI-INFLAMMATORY

AVAILABILITY Solution for nebulization; spray; nasal solution; ophthalmic solution; oral concentrate

ACTION & *THERAPEUTIC EFFECT* Inhibits release of bronchoconstrictors, histamine and slow-reacting substance of anaphylaxis, from sensitized pulmonary mast cells, thereby suppressing an allergic response. Additionally, cromolyn may also reduce the release of inflammatory leukotrienes. *Particularly effective for IgE-mediated or "extrinsic asthma" precipitated by exposure to specific allergen (e.g., pollens, dust, animal dander), by inhibiting the release of bronchoconstrictors.*

USES Primarily for prophylaxis of mild to moderate seasonal and perennial bronchial asthma and allergic rhinitis. Also used for prevention of exercise-related bronchospasm, prevention of acute bronchospasm induced by known pollutants or antigens, and for prevention and treatment of allergic rhinitis. Orally for systemic mastocytosis. **Ophthalmic:** Allergic ocular disorders, conjunctivitis, vernal keratoconjunctivitis.

UNLABELED USES Orally for prophylaxis of GI and systemic reactions to food allergy.

CONTRAINDICATIONS Use of aerosol (because of fluorocarbon propellants) in patients with coronary artery disease or history of arrhythmias; dyspnea, acute asthma, status asthmaticus, or acute bronchospasm; patients unable to coordinate actions or follow instructions.

CAUTIOUS USE Renal or hepatic dysfunction; pregnancy (category B); lactation. **Inhalation and nasal spray:** Safe use in children younger than 6 yr not established. **Ophthalmic:** Safe use under 2 yr not established.

ROUTE & DOSAGE

Allergies

Adult: **Inhalation** Metered dose inhaler or capsule: 1 spray or 1 capsule inhaled qid; nasal solution: 1 spray in each nostril 3–6 × day at regular intervals
Child (6 yr or older): **Inhalation** Metered dose inhaler or capsule, same as for adult; *6 yr or older:* Nasal solution, same as for adult

Conjunctivitis

Adult: **PO** 2 ampules qid 30 min a.c. and at bedtime
Child (2–12 yr): **PO** 1 ampule qid 30 min a.c. and at bedtime

Mastocytosis

See Appendix A-1.

ADMINISTRATION

Oral

- Give at least 30 min before meals.

Inhalation

- Patients should receive detailed instructions for each inhalation device. See manufacturer's instructions. Therapeutic effect is dependent on proper inhalation technique.
- Advise patient to clear as much mucus as possible before inhalation treatments.
- Instruct patient to exhale as completely as possible before placing inhaler mouthpiece between lips, tilt head backward and inhale rapidly and deeply with steady, even breaths. Remove inhaler from mouth, hold breath for a few seconds, then exhale into the air. Repeat until entire dose is taken.
- Protect cromolyn from moisture and heat. Store in tightly closed, light-resistant container at 15°–30°C (59°–86°F) unless otherwise directed.

ADVERSE EFFECTS **CNS:** Headache, dizziness, peripheral neuritis. **HEENT:** *Sneezing, nasal stinging and burning,* dryness and *irritation of throat and trachea; cough;* nasal congestion, itchy, puffy eyes, lacrimation, *transient ocular burning, stinging.* **Skin:** Erythema, urticaria, rash, contact dermatitis. **GI:** Swelling of parotid glands, dry mouth, slightly bitter aftertaste, *nausea,* vomiting, esophagitis. **Other:** Peripheral eosinophilia, <u>angioedema, bronchospasm, anaphylaxis</u> (rare).

PHARMACOKINETICS **Absorption:** Approximately 8% of dose absorbed from lungs. **Onset:** 1 wk with regular use. **Peak:** 15 min. **Duration:** 4–6 h; may last as long as 2–3 wk. **Elimination:** In bile and urine in equal amounts. **Half-Life:** 80 min.

C

NURSING IMPLICATIONS

Assessment & Drug Effects

- Withhold drug and notify prescriber if any of the following occur: Angioedema or bronchospasm.
- Monitor for exacerbation of asthmatic symptoms including breathlessness and cough that may occur in patients receiving cromolyn during corticosteroid withdrawal.
- For patients with asthma, therapeutic effects may be noted within a few days but generally not until after 1–2 wk of therapy.

Patient & Family Education

- Throat irritation, cough, and hoarseness can be minimized by gargling with water, drinking a few swallows of water, or by sucking on a lozenge after each treatment.
- Talk to your prescriber about what to do in the event of an acute asthmatic attack. Cromolyn is of no value in acute asthma.
- Cromolyn does not eliminate the continued need for therapy with bronchodilators, expectorants, antibiotics, or corticosteroids, but the amount and frequency of use of these medications may be appreciably reduced.
- Report any unusual signs or symptoms. Hypersensitivity reactions (see Signs & Symptoms, Appendix F) can be severe and life threatening. Drug should be discontinued if an allergic reaction occurs.

CROTAMITON

(kroe-tam′i-ton)

Crotan

Classification: SCABICIDE; ANTIPRURITIC

Therapeutic: SCABICIDE; ANTIPRURITIC

Prototype: Lindane

AVAILABILITY Lotion

ACTION & *THERAPEUTIC EFFECT* By unknown mechanisms, drug eradicates *Sarcoptes scabiei* and *effectively relieves itching.*

USES Treatment of scabies and for symptomatic treatment of pruritus.

CONTRAINDICATIONS Application to acutely inflamed skin, raw or weeping surfaces, eyes, or mouth; history of previous sensitivity to crotamiton; pregnancy – fetal risk cannot be ruled out; lactation – infant risk cannot be ruled out.

CAUTIOUS USE Not FDA approved for children.

ROUTE & DOSAGE

Scabies

Adult: **Topical** Apply a thin layer of cream from neck to toes; apply a second layer 24 h later; bathe 48 h after last application to remove drug

Pruritus

Adult: **Topical** Massage into affected areas until medication is completely absorbed; repeat PRN

ADMINISTRATION

Topical

- Shake container well before use of solution.
- The skin **must be** thoroughly dry before applying medication.
- If drug accidentally contacts eyes, thoroughly flush out medication with water.
- Pruritus treatment: Massage medication gently into affected areas until it is completely absorbed. Repeat as needed (usually effective for 6–10 h).

- Store in tightly closed containers at 15°–30°C (59°–86°F). Do not freeze.

ADVERSE EFFECTS **Skin:** Skin irritation (particularly with prolonged use), rash, erythema, sensation of cooling, allergic sensitization.

NURSING IMPLICATIONS

Assessment & Drug Effects

- Monitor for and report significant skin irritation or allergic sensitization.

Patient & Family Education

- Review package insert before treatment begins.
- Discontinue medication and report to prescriber if irritation or sensitization develops.

CYANOCOBALAMIN

(sye-an-oh-koe-bal'a-min)

Cobex, Nascobal

Classification: VITAMIN B_{12}

Therapeutic: VITAMIN B_{12}

AVAILABILITY Tablet; nasal spray; sublingual tablet

ACTION & THERAPEUTIC EFFECT Vitamin B_{12} is a cobalt-containing B complex vitamin essential for normal growth, cell reproduction, maturation of RBCs, nucleoprotein synthesis, maintenance of nervous system (myelin synthesis), and believed to be involved in protein and carbohydrate metabolism. *Therapeutically effective for treatment of vitamin B_{12} deficiency and pernicious anemia.*

USES Vitamin B_{12} deficiency due to malabsorption, dietary deficiency, inadequate utilization of B_{12}; treatment of increased vitamin B_{12} requirements.

CONTRAINDICATIONS History of sensitivity to vitamin B_{12}, other cobalamins, or cobalt; early Leber disease (hereditary optic nerve atrophy).

CAUTIOUS USE Heart disease, concurrent folic acid or iron deficiency, patients with infection, renal impairment, patients with nasal pathology or chronic nasal symptoms, neonates, anemia, pulmonary disease; pregnancy—fetal risk cannot be ruled out; lactation—infant risk is minimal.

ROUTE & DOSAGE

Vitamin B_{12} Deficiency

Adult: **IM/Deep Subcutaneous** 100 mcg daily × 6–7 days **PO** 1000 to 2000 mcg daily for 1–2 weeks; then 1000 mcg daily **Intranasal** 500 mcg in 1 nostril weekly.

Child: **IM/Deep Subcutaneous** 250–1000 mcg daily or every other day × 1 week then weekly × 4–8 weeks then monthly.

Pernicious Anemia ?

Adult: **IM** 1000 mcg daily or every other day × 1 week then 1000 mcg weekly × 4–8w then 1000 mcg monthly. **PO** 1000–2000 mcg daily

Child: **IM** 100 mcg daily × 6–7d; if improvement then 100 mcg on alternate days × 7 doses then q3–4 days × 2 weeks; when hematologic values are normal administer 100 mcg monthly

Nutritional Supplement

Adult: **PO** 1–25 mcg/day

Child (younger than 1 yr): **PO** 0.3 mcg/day; *1 yr or older:* 1 mcg/day

C

ADMINISTRATION

Oral

- PO preparations may be mixed with fruit juices. However, administer promptly because ascorbic acid affects the stability of vitamin B_{12}.
- Administration of oral vitamin B_{12} with meals increases its absorption.
- Tablets should be stored in a tight container at room temperature between 15–30°C (59–86°F) and protected from light.

Sublingual

- Place tablet under the tongue for 30 seconds before swallowing.

Nasal

- Administer at least 1 hours before or 1 hour after ingestion of hot foods or liquids.
- Follow manufacturer's directions for priming or re-priming pump.
- Separate administration with other intranasal medication by several hours.
- Nasal spray should be stored in an upright position at controlled room temperature 15–30°C (59–86°F). Protect from light and freezing.

Subcutaneous/Intramuscular

- Give deep subcutaneous by slightly tenting the skin at the injection site.
- IM may be given into any normal IM injection site.
- Preserved in light-resistant containers at room temperature preferably at 15°–30°C (59°–86°F) unless otherwise directed by manufacturer.

ADVERSE EFFECTS (≥ 5%) CNS: Physical weakness, fatigue.

DIAGNOSTIC TEST INTERFERENCE Most antibiotics, methotrexate, and pyrimethamine may produce invalid diagnostic ***blood assays for vitamin B_{12}***.

INTERACTIONS Drug: Alcohol, aminosalicylic acid, neomycin, colchicine may decrease absorption of oral cyanocobalamin; **chloramphenicol** may interfere with therapeutic response to cyanocobalamin.

PHARMACOKINETICS Absorption: Intestinal absorption requires presence of intrinsic factor in terminal ileum. **Distribution:** Widely distributed; principally stored in liver, kidneys, and adrenals; crosses placenta, excreted in breast milk. **Metabolism:** Converted in tissues to active coenzymes; enterohepatically cycled. **Elimination:** 50–95% of doses 100 mcg or more are excreted in urine in 48 h. **Half-Life:** 6 days (400 days in liver).

NURSING IMPLICATIONS

Assessment & Drug Effects

- Obtain a careful history of sensitivities. Sensitization to cyanocobalamin can take as long as 8 yr to develop.
- Monitor vital signs in patients with cardiac disease and in those receiving parenteral cyanocobalamin, and be alert to symptoms of pulmonary edema, which generally occur early in therapy.
- Characteristically, reticulocyte concentration rises in 3–4 days, peaks in 5–8 days, and then gradually declines as erythrocyte count and Hgb rise to normal levels (in 4–6 wk).
- Obtain a complete diet and drug history and inquire into alcohol drinking patterns for all patients receiving cyanocobalamin to identify and correct poor habits.
- Monitor lab tests: Baseline reticulocyte and erythrocyte counts,

Hgb, Hct, vitamin B_{12}, and serum folate levels; then repeated between 5 and 7 days after start of therapy and at regular intervals during therapy. Monitor potassium levels during the first 48 h.

Patient & Family Education

- Notify prescriber of any intercurrent disease or infection. Increased dosage may be required.
- To prevent irreversible neurologic damage resulting from pernicious anemia, drug therapy **must be** continued throughout life.
- Rich food sources of B_{12} are nutrient-added breakfast cereals, vitamin B_{12}-fortified soy milk, organ meats, clams, oysters, egg yolk, crab, salmon, sardines, muscle meat, milk, and dairy products.
- If taking nasal spray, report to healthcare provider any nasal congestion, upper respiratory infection or allergic rhinitis. Another route may have to be prescribed to insure absorption of the medication.
- Avoid alcohol while taking this drug.

CYCLOBENZAPRINE HYDROCHLORIDE (Prototype drug)

(sye-kloe-ben′za-preen)

Amrix, Fexmid

Classification: CENTRAL ACTING SKELETAL MUSCLE RELAXANT

Therapeutic: SKELETAL MUSCLE RELAXANT; ANTISPASMODIC

AVAILABILITY Tablet; extended release capsule

ACTION & *THERAPEUTIC EFFECT* Relieves skeletal muscle spasm of local origin without interfering with muscle function. Believed to act primarily within CNS at brainstem. Depresses tonic somatic motor activity, although both gamma and alpha motor neurons are affected. *Relieves muscle spasm associated with acute, painful musculoskeletal conditions.*

USES Short-term adjunct to rest and physical therapy for relief of muscle spasm associated with acute musculoskeletal conditions.

UNLABELED USES Fibromyalgia.

CONTRAINDICATIONS Acute recovery phase of MI, cardiac arrhythmias, heart block or conduction disturbances, QT prolongation; CHF, hyperthyroidism; moderate or severe hepatic impairment; MAOI therapy within 14 days of use; cerebral palsy. **Extended release:** Do not use capsule for older adults; Hypersensitivity to cyclobenzaprine or any component of the product; pregnancy – fetal risk cannot be rule out; lactation – infant risk cannot be ruled out.

CAUTIOUS USE Prostatic hypertrophy, history of urinary retention, seizures; cardiovascular disease; mild hepatic impairment; closed-angle glaucoma; increased intraocular pressure; older adults, debilitated patients; history of psychiatric illness. Pregnancy—fetal risk cannot be ruled out; lactation—infant risk cannot be ruled out. Safe use in children younger than 15 yr not established.

ROUTE & DOSAGE

Muscle Spasm

Adult/Adolescent (15 yr or older): **PO** 5 mg tid may increase dose based on response (max: 30 mg/day); **Extended release** 15 mg daily, may increase to 30 mg once daily

C

Hepatic Impairment Dosage Adjustment

Mild: Start with 5 mg
Moderate to Severe: Not recommended

ADMINISTRATION

Oral

- Do not administer drug if patient is receiving an MAO inhibitor (e.g., furazolidone, isocarboxazid, pargyline, tranylcypromine).
- Do not break or crush extended release capsules. They **must be** swallowed whole.
- Take extended-release capsule at approximately the same time every day.
- Cyclobenzaprine is intended for short-term (2 or 3 wk) use.
- Store capsule, extended release in tightly closed container that is light-resistant, preferably at 25°C (77°F), with excursions permitted to 15°–30°C (59°–86°F) unless otherwise directed by manufacturer. Tablets should be in a tightly closed, light-resistant container away from moisture and direct light in a controlled room temperature 20°–25°C (68°–77°F).

ADVERSE EFFECTS (≥5%) CNS: *Drowsiness, dizziness.* **GI:** *Dry mouth.* **Other:** Fatigue.

DIAGNOSTIC TEST INTEFERENCE May cause false-positive serum TCA screen.

INTERACTIONS Drug: Alcohol, BARBITURATES, other CNS DEPRESSANTS enhance CNS depression; potentiates anticholinergic effects of **phenothiazine** and other ANTICHOLINERGICS; MAO INHIBITORS may precipitate hypertensive crisis – use with extreme caution. Use with **potassium chloride** increases risk of ulcer formation. Avoid use with **clozapine, eluxadoline** to decrease risk of GI adverse effects.

PHARMACOKINETICS Absorption: Well absorbed from GI tract with some first-pass elimination in liver. **Onset:** 1 h. **Peak:** 3–8 h. **Duration:** 12–24 h. **Distribution:** 93% protein bound. **Metabolism:** In liver to inactive metabolites via CYP3A4, 1A2, and 2D6. **Elimination:** Slowly in urine with some elimination in feces; may be excreted in breast milk. **Half-Life:** 8–37 h.

NURSING IMPLICATIONS

Assessment & Drug Effects

- Supervision of ambulation may be indicated, especially in the older adult, because of risk of drowsiness and dizziness.
- Withhold drug and notify prescriber if signs of hypersensitivity (e.g., pruritus, urticaria, rash) appear.
- Assess passive limb movement.

Patient & Family Education

- Avoid driving and other potentially hazardous activities until reaction to drug is known. Adverse effects include drowsiness and dizziness.
- Avoid alcohol and other CNS depressants (unless otherwise directed by prescriber) because cyclobenzaprine enhances their effects.
- Instruct patient to take at the same time every day
- Dry mouth may be relieved by increasing total fluid intake (if not contraindicated).
- Keep prescriber informed of therapeutic effectiveness. Spasmolytic effect usually begins within 1 or 2 days and may be manifested by lessening of pain and tenderness, increase in range of motion, and ability to perform ADL.

- Report to prescriber any racing heartbeat, development of rash or hives.
- Do not take medication with any over-the-counter medication without checking with prescriber first.

CYCLOPHOSPHAMIDE

(sye-kloe-foss′fa-mide)

Procytox ♣

Classification: ANTINEOPLASTIC; NITROGEN MUSTARD; ALKYLATING AGENT

Therapeutic: ANTINEOPLASTIC

AVAILABILITY Capsule; solution for injection

ACTION & THERAPEUTIC EFFECT Cell-cycle–nonspecific alkylating agent that causes cross-linkage of DNA strands, thereby blocking synthesis of DNA, RNA, and protein. *Has pronounced antineoplastic effects and immunosuppressive activity.*

USES Treatment of acute lymphoblastic leukemia (ALL), acute myelocytic leukemia (AML), breast cancer, chronic lymphocytic leukemia (CLL), chronic myeloid leukemia (CML), Hodgkin lymphoma, mycosis fungoides, multiple myeloma, neuroblastoma, non-Hodgkin lymphomas (including Burkitt lymphoma), ovarian adenocarcinoma, and retinoblastoma, nephrotic syndrome.

UNLABELED USES Refractory immune thrombocytopenia, lupus nephritis, systemic sclerosis-related interstitial lung disease, Waldenstrom macroglobulinemia.

CONTRAINDICATIONS Absolute contraindication with bladder or urinary tract obstruction. Hypersensitivity to cyclophosphamide; serious infections (including chickenpox, herpes zoster); live virus vaccines; severe myelosuppression; dehydration; severe hemorrhagic cystitis; pregnancy – fetal risk has been demonstrated; lactation – infant risk has been demonstrated.

CAUTIOUS USE History of radiation or cytotoxic drug therapy; hepatic and renal impairment, elderly; recent history of steroid therapy; history of cardiac disease or arrhythmias, bone marrow infiltration with tumor cells; history of urate calculi and gout; patients with leukopenia, wound healing in process, thrombocytopenia; history of respiratory disease; men and women of childbearing age.

ROUTE & DOSAGE

Neoplasm (dose may vary based on concurrent antineoplastic agents; see institution protocol)

Adult: **PO Initial** 1–5 mg/kg/day **IV** 40–50 mg/kg in divided doses over 2–5 days or 10–15 mg/kg q7–19 days or 3–5 mg/kg twice weekly

Renal Impairment Dosage Adjustment

CrCl less than 10 mL/min: Give 75% of dose

Hepatic Impairment Dosage Adjustment

Serum bilirubin 3.1–5 mg/dL: Give 75% of dose

ADMINISTRATION

Oral

- NIOSH: Always wear gloves when handling containers, vials,

C

capsules, or tablets to minimize risk of dermal exposure. Use single gloves when handling intact tablets, or capsules or administering from a unit-dose package.
- Use double gloves and a gown when administering injections. Eye/face and respiratory protection recommended if the substance could splash or if the patient may resist
- Administer in the morning PO drug on empty stomach. Do not cut, crush, or chew tablets. Wash hands immediately if contact with broken tablet occurs. If nausea and vomiting are severe, however, it may be taken with food. An antiemetic medication may be prescribed to be given before the drug.
- Coadminister with adequate amounts of fluids to force diuresis and reduce the risk of urinary tract toxicity.
- Store cyclophosphamide tablet in temperatures up to 25°C (77°F). Protect from temperatures above 30°C (86°F). Storage of oral solutions is dependent on concentration – follow manufacturer's instructions. Powder for IV route can be stored in vials up to 25°C (77°F). Excessive heat and storage may lead to melting of the powder. Do not use the vials if melting has occurred.

Intravenous

PREPARE: **Direct:** Add 5 mL NS for each 100 mg and shake gently to dissolve. **Do not** reconstitute with sterile water for injection if giving direct IV. **Intermittent:** May be further diluted for infusion with 100–250 mL D5W, D5/NS, or 0.45% NaCl.

ADMINISTER: **Direct/Intermittent:** Give each 100 mg or fraction thereof over 10–15 min.

INCOMPATIBILITIES: **Y-site: Amphotericin B cholesteryl complex, amphotericin B colloidal, asparaginase, diazepam, gemtuzumab, lansoprazole, phenytoin.**

- If mixed with 5% dextrose or 5% dextrose and 0.9% sodium chloride for injection, store at room temperature for up to 24 h and refrigerated for up to 36 h.

ADVERSE EFFECTS **CV:** *cardiac tamponade, cardiotoxicity, CHF, pericardial effusion.* **Respiratory:** Pulmonary emboli and edema, pneumonitis, interstitial pulmonary fibrosis. **Skin:** *Alopecia* (reversible), transverse ridging of nails, pigmentation of nail beds and skin (reversible), nonspecific dermatitis, erythema multiforme, malignant tumor or dermis, toxic epidermal necrolysis, Stevens–Johnson syndrome. **Hepatic:** Angiosarcoma of the liver. **GI:** *Nausea, vomiting,* mucositis, *anorexia, abdominal pain* diarrhea. **GU:** Sterile hemorrhagic and nonhemorrhagic cystitis, bladder fibrosis, nephrotoxicity, bladder cancer, pyelitis, hematuria. **Hematologic:** Leukopenia, *neutropenia,* acute myeloid leukemia, anemia, thrombophlebitis, interference with normal healing, myelodysplastic syndrome. **Other:** Anaphylaxis, secondary neoplasia, infectious disease.

INTERACTIONS **Drug: Succinylcholine** causes prolonged neuromuscular blocking activity; IMMUNOSUPRESSANTS and MYLEOSUPPRESIVE AGENTS should be avoided. Do not use with etanercept or **natalizumab** or LIVE VACCINES. **Herbal:** Avoid use of echinacea.

PHARMACOKINETICS **Absorption:** Readily from GI tract. **Peak:** 1 h PO. **Distribution:** Widely distributed, including brain, breast milk; crosses placenta. **Metabolism:** In liver by CYP3A4. **Elimination:** In urine as active metabolites and unchanged drug. **Half-Life:** 4–8 h.

NURSING IMPLICATIONS

Assessment & Drug Effects

- Assess for signs of unexplained bleeding or easy bruising, which could indicate thrombocytopenia.
- Marked leukopenia is the most serious side effect. It can be fatal. Nadir may occur in 2–8 days after first dose but may be as late as 1 mo after a series of several daily doses. Leukopenia usually reverses 7–10 days after therapy is discontinued.
- During severe leukopenic period, protect patient from infection and trauma and from visitors and medical personnel who have colds or other infections.
- Report onset of unexplained chills, sore throat, tachycardia. Monitor temperature carefully, and report an elevation immediately. The development of fever in a neutropenic patient (granulocyte count less than 1000) is a medical emergency because sepsis can develop quickly in these patients.
- Observe and report character of wound drainage. During period of neutropenia, purulent drainage may become serosanguineous because there are not enough WBC to create pus. Because of suppressed immune mechanisms, wound healing may be prolonged or incomplete.
- Monitor I&O ratio and patterns: Because the drug is a chemical irritant, PO and IV fluid intake is generally increased to help prevent renal irritation and hemorrhagic cystitis. Have patient void frequently, especially after each dose and just before retiring to bed.
- Watch for symptoms of water intoxication or dilutional hyponatremia; patients are usually well hydrated as part of the therapy.
- Promptly report hematuria or dysuria. Drug schedule is usually interrupted, and fluids are forced.
- Record body weight at least twice weekly (basis for dose determination). Alert prescriber to sudden change or slow, steady weight gain or loss over a period of time that appears inconsistent with caloric intake.
- Diarrhea may signal onset of hyperkalemia, particularly if accompanied by colicky pain, nausea, bradycardia, and skeletal muscle weakness. These symptoms warrant prompt reporting to prescriber.
- Monitor for hyperuricemia, which occurs commonly during early treatment period in patients with leukemias or lymphoma. Report edema of lower legs and feet; joint, flank, or stomach pain.
- Protect patient from potential sources of infection. Cyclophosphamide makes the patient particularly susceptible to varicella-zoster infections (chickenpox, herpes zoster).
- Report any sign of overgrowth with opportunistic organisms, especially in patient receiving corticosteroids or who has recently been on steroid therapy.
- Report fever, dyspnea, and nonproductive cough. Pulmonary toxicity is not common, but the already debilitated patient is particularly susceptible.
- Monitor lab tests: Baseline CBC, total and differential leukocyte count, platelet count, and Hct, and repeat at least 2 × wk during

maintenance period. Baseline and periodic LFTs, renal function, and serum electrolytes.

Patient & Family Education

- Adhere to dosage regimen, and do not omit, increase, decrease, or delay doses. If for any reason drug cannot be taken, notify prescriber. Take with plenty of fluids.
- Review proper safe handling of the drug.
- Avoid driving and any activity that requires clear vision until effects of the drug are realized.
- Report any symptoms of delayed wound healing or infections.
- Report blood in the urine or pain while urinating, swelling in extremities.
- Alopecia occurs in about 33% of patients on cyclophosphamide therapy. Hair loss may be noted 3 wk after therapy begins; regrowth (often differs in texture and color) usually starts 5–6 wk after drug is withdrawn and may occur while on maintenance doses.
- Use adequate means of contraception during and for at least 4 mo after termination of drug treatment. Breastfeeding should be discontinued before cyclophosphamide therapy is initiated.
- Amenorrhea may last up to 1 yr after cessation of therapy in 10–30% of women.

CYCLOSERINE

(sye-kloe-ser′een)

Classification: ANTITUBERCULOSIS

Therapeutic: ANTITUBERCULOSIS

AVAILABILITY Capsule

ACTION & *THERAPEUTIC EFFECT* Inhibits cell wall synthesis in susceptible strains of bacteria. It competitively interferes with the incorporation of D-alanine into the bacterial cell wall, resulting in cell death. *Effective against gram-positive and gram-negative bacteria and* Mycobacterium tuberculosis.

USES Treatment of tuberculosis, urinary tract infections.

CONTRAINDICATIONS Uncontrolled epilepsy; depression, severe anxiety, history of psychoses; severe renal insufficiency, excessive use of alcohol, pregnancy – fetal risk cannot be ruled out.

CAUTIOUS USE Renal impairment, anemia; chronic alcoholism; lactation – infant risk is minimal. Safe use in children not established.

ROUTE & DOSAGE

Tuberculosis

Adult: **PO** 250 mg q12h × 14 days, increase to 500–1000 mg/day in divided doses

ADMINISTRATION

Oral

- Pyridoxine 200–300 mg/day may be ordered concurrently to prevent neurotoxic effects of cycloserine.
- Store in tightly closed container at 15°–30°C (59°–86°F) unless otherwise directed.

ADVERSE EFFECTS CNS: *Drowsiness, headache,* vertigo, confusion.

INTERACTIONS Drug: Alcohol increases risk of seizures; **ethionamide, isoniazid** potentiates neurotoxic effects; avoid LIVE VACCINES.

PHARMACOKINETICS Absorption: 70–90% from GI tract. **Peak:** 3–4 h. **Distribution:** Distributed to lung, ascitic, pleural and synovial fluids, and CSF; crosses placenta; distributed into breast milk. **Metabolism:** Hepatic. **Elimination:** 60–70% in urine within 72 h; small amount in feces. **Half-Life:** 12 h.

NURSING IMPLICATIONS

Assessment & Drug Effects

- Maintenance of blood–drug level below 30 mg/mL considerably reduces incidence of neurotoxicity. Possibility of neurotoxicity increases when dose is 500 mg or more or when renal clearance is inadequate.
- Observe patient carefully for signs of hypersensitivity and neurologic effects. Neurotoxicity generally appears within first 2 wk of therapy and disappears after drug is discontinued.
- Drug should be withheld and prescriber notified or dosage reduced if symptoms of CNS toxicity or hypersensitivity reaction (see Appendix F) develop.
- Monitor lab tests: Baseline C&S; weekly plasma drug levels; hematologic, renal function studies and LFTs at regular intervals.

Patient & Family Education

- Take cycloserine after meals to prevent GI irritation.
- Notify prescriber immediately of the onset of skin rash and early signs of CNS toxicity (see Appendix F).
- Review adverse effects and warn of confusion, dizziness, sleepiness, or seizure.
- Avoid potentially hazardous tasks such as driving until reaction to cycloserine has been determined.
- Instruct patient to report depression, suicidal ideation, or unusual changes in behavior.
- Avoid alcohol.
- Take drug precisely as prescribed and keep follow-up appointments. Continuous therapy may extend into months or years.

CYCLOSPORINE

(sye'kloe-spor-een)

Gengraf, Neoral, Restasis, Sandimmune

Classification: CALCINEURIN INHIBITOR; IMMUNOSUPPRESSANT

Therapeutic: IMMUNOSUPPRESSANT; ANTIRHEUMATIC; ANTIPSORIATIC

AVAILABILITY **Gengraf:** Capsule, oral solution. **Neoral:** Capsule; oral solution; solution for injection. **Restasis:** Ophthalmic emulsion. **Sandimmune:** Capsule; oral solution; solution for injection.

ACTION & *THERAPEUTIC EFFECT* Suppresses certain humoral immunity reactions (i.e., antigen-antibody reactions) and, to a greater extent, cell-mediated immune reactions. T-lymphocytes are preferentially inhibited (the T-helper cell is the main target, although the T-suppressor cell also may be suppressed). *Prevents allograft rejection in transplant patients. Additionally, it is a disease-modifying antirheumatic drug (DMARD) in RA patients that have not responded on methotrexate alone.*

USES In conjunction with adrenal corticosteroids to prevent organ rejection after kidney, liver, and heart transplants; rheumatoid arthritis, severe psoriasis. Ophthalmic emulsion for the treatment of xerophthalmia.

UNLABELED USES Prophylaxis of acute graft-versus-host disease, treatment of chronic graft-versus-host disease, refractory immune thrombocytopenia, interstitial cystitis, lupus nephritis, refractory ulcerative colitis,

CONTRAINDICATIONS Hypersensitivity to cyclosporine; recent contact with or bout of chickenpox, herpes zoster; administration of live virus vaccines to patient or family members; **Gengraf** and **Neoral** in psoriasis or RA patients with abnormal renal function, uncontrolled hypertension, or malignancies; ocular infection. **PO form:** Pregnancy – fetal risk cannot be ruled out; Lactation – infant risk cannot be ruled out.

CAUTIOUS USE Renal, hepatic, pancreatic, or bowel dysfunction; biliary tract disease, jaundice, hyperkalemia; electrolyte imbalance, hyperuricemia, hypertension; infection; radiation therapy, older adults, encephalopathy, fungal or viral infection, gout, herpes infection, lymphoma; neoplastic disease, malabsorption problems (e.g., liver transplant patients); older adults; females of childbearing age.

ROUTE & DOSAGE

Neoral/Gengraf (cyclosporine modified) and Sandimmune (cyclosporine nonmodified) are not bioequivalent and cannot be used interchangeably. In general, cyclosporine (modified) is more commonly used clinically

Prevention of Organ Rejection

Can vary depending on transplanted organ and concurrent immunosuppressive use: See package insert for details

Rheumatoid Arthritis (Neoral)

Adult: **PO** 2.5 mg/kg/day divided into 2 doses. May increase by 0.5–0.75 mg/kg/day q4wk to (max: 4 mg/kg/day)

Severe Psoriasis (Neoral/Gengraf)

Adult: **PO** 1.25 mg/kg bid If significant improvement has not occurred after 4 wk, may increase dose by 0.5 mg/kg/day every 2 wk (max: 4 mg/kg/day); discontinue if no benefit at 6 weeks of max dose therapy.

Nephrotic Syndrome (Neoral/Gengraf)

Adult: **PO** 3.5 mg/kg/day in divided doses, may adjust to patient response (max 5 mg/kg/day)

Keratoconjunctivitis Sicca

Adult: **Ophthalmic** 1 drop in affected eye(s) twice daily approximately 12 h apart

ADMINISTRATION

Oral

- Do not dilute oral solution with grapefruit juice. Dilute with orange or apple juice, stir well, then administer immediately.
- The various product brands may not be bioequivalent on a mg for mg basis. Do not interchange without prescriber supervision.
- Store capsules at controlled room temperature, 25°C (77°F), excursions permitted between 15° and 30°C (59° and 86°F). Store solution in original container at a temperature below 30°C (86°F) and use within 2 months of opening. Do not refrigerate, and protect from freezing.

Intravenous

PREPARE: **IV Infusion:** Dilute each 1 mL immediately before administration in 20–100 mL of D5W or NS.

ADMINISTER: **IV Infusion:** Give by slow infusion over approximately 2–6 h. ▪ Rapid IV can result in nephrotoxicity. Discard diluted infusion solution after 24 hours.

▪ Store at temperatures below 30°C (86°F) and protect from light.

INCOMPATIBILITIES: **Solution/additive: Magnesium sulfate. Y-site: Amphotericin B cholesteryl complex, ceftolozane/tazobactam, cyanocobalamin, dantrolene, diazepam, diazoxide, drotrecogin, gemtuzumab, idarubicin, isavuconazonium, letermovir, nalbuphine, pentobarbital, phenobarbital, phenytoin, rituximab, sulfamethoxazole/trimethoprim, tedizolid, trastuzumab, voriconazole.**

ADVERSE EFFECTS (≥5%) CV: *Hypertension*. **CNS:** *Tremor*, convulsions, headache. **HEENT:** (ophthalmic route) Blepharitis, burning sensation. Sinusitis, tinnitus, hearing loss, sore throat. **Skin:** *Hirsutism*. **GI:** Gingival hyperplasia. **GU:** *Nephrotoxicity (oliguria)*. **Other:** Infectious disease.

DIAGNOSTIC TEST INTERFERENCE Cyclosporine metabolites cross-react with radioimmunoassay and fluorescence polarization immunoassay.

INTERACTIONS Drug: AMINOGLYCOSIDES, **danazol, diltiazem, doxycycline, erythromycin, ketoconazole, methylprednisolone, metoclopramide, nicardipine,** NSAIDS, **prednisolone, verapamil** may increase cyclosporine levels; **carbamazepine, isoniazid, octreotide, phenobarbital, phenytoin, rifampin,** ANTIFUNGAL AGENTS, may decrease cyclosporine levels; **acyclovir,** AMINOGLYCOSIDES, **amphotericin B, cidofovir, cimetidine, erythromycin, ketoconazole, melphalan, cotrimoxazole, trimethoprim** may increase risk of nephrotoxicity; POTASSIUM-SPARING DIURETICS, ACE INHIBITORS **(captopril, enalapril)** may potentiate hyperkalemia. Avoid use with HMG-COA REDUCTASE INHIBITORS, LIVE VACCINES, **aliskiren, alpelisib, bilastine, carbamazepine, cladribine, conivaptan, disulfiram, doxorubicin, dronedarone, enzalutamide, eplerenone, foscarnet, fusidic acid, grazoprevir, idelalisib, lasmiditan, lercanidipine, methotrimeprazine, ozanimod, pazopanib, pimecrolimus, pimozide, revefenacin, rimegepant, tacrolimus, topotecan, upadacitinib, voxilaprevir. Food: Grapefruit juice** may increase concentration. **Herbal: St. John's wort** may decrease cyclosporine levels; **berberine** may increase toxicities.

PHARMACOKINETICS Absorption: Variable and incomplete **Peak:** 3–4 h. **Distribution:** Widely distributed; 33–47% distributed to plasma; 41–50% to RBCs; crosses placenta; distributed into breast milk; 90–98% protein bound. **Metabolism:** In liver by CYP3A4, including significant first-pass metabolism; considerable enterohepatic circulation. **Elimination:** Primarily in bile and feces; 6% in urine. **Half-Life:** 19–27 h.

NURSING IMPLICATIONS

Assessment & Drug Effects

▪ Observe patients receiving the drug parenterally for at least 30 min continuously after start of

C

IV infusion, and at frequent intervals thereafter to detect allergic or other adverse reactions.
- Monitor I&O ratio and pattern: Nephrotoxicity has been reported in about one-third of transplant patients. It has occurred in mild forms as late as 2–3 mo after transplantation. In severe form, it can be irreversible, and therefore early recognition is critical.
- Monitor vital signs. Be alert to indicators of local or systemic infection that can be fungal, viral, or bacterial. Also report significant rise in BP.
- Periodic tests should be made of neurologic function. Neurotoxic effects generally occur over 13–195 days after initiation of cyclosporine therapy. Signs and symptoms are reportedly fully reversible with dosage reduction or discontinuation of drug.
- Monitor blood or plasma drug concentrations at regular intervals, particularly in patients receiving the drug orally for prolonged periods, as drug absorption is erratic.
- Monitor lab tests: Baseline and periodic renal function, LFTs, and serum potassium. In psoriasis patients, CBC, BUN, uric acid, potassium, lipids, and magnesium biweekly during first 3 mo.

Patient & Family Education

- Take medication with meals to reduce nausea or GI irritation. Avoid grapefruit juice
- Dosing syringe should be completely dry before use.
- Enhance palatability of oral solution by mixing it with milk, chocolate milk, or orange juice, preferably at room temperature. Mix in a glass rather than a plastic container. Stir well, drink immediately, and rinse glass with small quantity of diluent to ensure getting entire dose.
- Take medication at same time each day to maintain therapeutic blood levels.
- Practice good oral hygiene. Inspect mouth daily for white patches, sores, swollen gums.
- Hirsutism is reversible with discontinuation of drug.
- Avoid excess exposure to ultraviolet light.

CYPROHEPTADINE HYDROCHLORIDE

(si-proe-hep′ta-deen)

Classification: ANTIHISTAMINE; ANTIPRURITIC

Therapeutic: ANTIHISTAMINE

Prototype: Diphenhydramine

AVAILABILITY Tablet

ACTION & *THERAPEUTIC EFFECT*

Competes with histamine for serotonin and H_1-receptor sites, thus preventing histamine-mediated responses. *Has significant antipruritic, local anesthetic, and antiserotonin activity.*

USES Symptomatic relief of various allergic conditions.

UNLABELED USES Appetite stimulant, spasticity associated with spine cord damage.

CONTRAINDICATIONS Hypersensitivity to cyproheptadine; MAOI therapy within 14 days; angle closure glaucoma; stenosing peptic ulcer, symptomatic BPH, bladder neck obstruction, pyloroduodenal obstruction; elderly debilitated patients; acute asthma attack; newborns, premature infants; pregnancy – fetal risk cannot be

Common adverse effects in *italic;* life-threatening effects underlined; generic names in **bold;** classifications in SMALL CAPS; ♣ Canadian drug name; ⊙ Prototype drug; ⚠ Alert

ruled out; lactation – infant risk cannot be ruled out.

CAUTIOUS USE Patients predisposed to urinary retention; glaucoma; asthma; COPD; increased intraocular pressure; hyperthyroidism; cardiovascular or hepatic disease, hypertension; elderly; children with a family history of SIDS. Safe use in children younger than 2 yr not established.

ROUTE & DOSAGE

Allergies

Adult: **PO** 4 mg tid max: 0.5 mg/kg/day
Child: **PO** 0.25 mg/kg/day or 8 mg/m^2/day in 2–3 divided doses (max dose: age 2–6 yr is 12 mg/day; age 7–14 yr is 16 mg/day)

ADMINISTRATION

Oral

- GI adverse effects may be minimized by administering drug with food or milk.
- Store tablets in tightly covered container at 15°–30°C (59°–86°F) unless otherwise directed. Store syrup at temperatures between 15° and 30°C (59° and 86°F) in a tightly closed container; avoid freezing the bottle.

ADVERSE EFFECTS **Respiratory:** Thickened bronchial secretions. **CNS:** *Drowsiness,* dizziness, faintness, headache, tremulousness, fatigue, disturbed coordination. **HEENT:** Dry nose and throat. **GI:** *Dry mouth,* nausea, vomiting, epigastric distress, appetite stimulation, weight gain, transient decrease in fasting blood sugar level, increased serum amylase level, cholestatic jaundice.

DIAGNOSTIC TEST INTERFERENCE Antigen skin test results may be suppressed; false-positive serum TCA screen.

INTERACTIONS **Drug: Alcohol** and CNS DEPRESSANTS add to CNS depression; TRICYCLIC ANTIDEPRESSANTS and other ANTICHOLINERGICS have additive anticholinergic effects; may inhibit pressor effects of **epinephrine.** Do not use with **eluxadoline** or MAO INHIBITORS.

PHARMACOKINETICS **Absorption:** Readily absorbed from GI tract. **Duration:** 6–9 h. **Distribution:** Distribution into breast milk not known. **Metabolism:** In liver. **Elimination:** In urine.

NURSING IMPLICATIONS

Assessment & Drug Effects

- Monitor level of alertness. In some patients, the sedative effect disappears spontaneously after 3–4 days of drug administration.
- Because drug may cause dizziness, supervision of ambulation and other safety precautions may be warranted.

Patient & Family Education

- Avoid activities requiring mental alertness and physical coordination, such as driving a car, until reaction to the drug is known.
- Drug causes sedation, dizziness, and hypotension in older adults. Report these symptoms. Children are more apt to manifest CNS stimulation (e.g., confusion, agitation, tremors, hallucinations). Reduction in dosage may be indicated.
- Cyproheptadine may increase and prolong the effects of alcohol, barbiturates, narcotic analgesics, and other CNS depressants.
- Maintain sufficient fluid intake to help to relieve dry mouth and reduce risk of cholestatic jaundice.

C

CYTARABINE

(sye-tare′a-been)

Classification: PURINE ANTIMETABOLITE

Therapeutic: ANTINEOPLASTIC

Prototype: 6-Mercaptopurine

AVAILABILITY Liposomal; powder for injection

ACTION & *THERAPEUTIC EFFECT* Cell cycle-specific for the S phase of cell division. Activity occurs as a result of activation of cytarabine in the triphosphate in the tissues and inhibits incorporation of cytarabine into DNA and RNA. *Antineoplastic agent, which has strong myelosuppressant activity. Immunosuppressant properties are exhibited by obliterated cell-mediated immune responses, such as delayed hypersensitivity skin reactions.*

USES To induce and maintain remission in acute myelocytic leukemia, acute lymphocytic leukemia, and meningeal leukemia and for treatment of lymphomas. Used in combination with other antineoplastics in established chemotherapeutic protocols.

CONTRAINDICATIONS History of drug-induced myelosuppression; immunization procedures; active meningeal infection (**liposomal cytarabine**); pregnancy (category D); lactation.

CAUTIOUS USE Impaired renal, cardiac, or hepatic function, elderly; neurologic disease; gout, drug-induced myelosuppression. Safe use in infants and children not established

ROUTE & DOSAGE

Leukemias

Adult/Child: **IV** 100–200 mg/m^2/day by continuous infusion over 24 h

Renal Impairment Dosage Adjustment

Serum Cr of 1.5–1.9 mg/dL (or increase from baseline of 0.5–1.2 mg/dL): Reduce to 1 g/m^2/dose

Serum Cr of 2 mg/dL or more (or greater than 1.2 mg/dL change): reduce dose to 0.1 g/m^2/day

ADMINISTRATION

- NIOSH recommends the use of double gloves and protective gown. During administration if there is any chance that the substance could splash or the patient may resist, use eye/face protection.

Intrathecal

- For intrathecal injection, reconstitute with an isotonic, buffered diluent without preservatives. Follow manufacturer's recommendations.

Subcutaneous

- Reconstitute sterile powder with bacteriostatic water for injection with benzyl alcohol (**without** benzyl alcohol for neonates).

Intravenous

PREPARE: **Direct:** Reconstitute with bacteriostatic water for injection (without benzyl alcohol for neonates) as follows: Add 5 mL to the 100-mg vial to yield 20 mg/mL; add 10 mL to the 500-mg vial to yield 50 mg/mL. Further dilute with 100 mL or more of D5W or NS.

ADMINISTER: **Continuous:** Give over 24 h.

INCOMPATIBILITIES: **Solution/additive: Fluorouracil, heparin, insulin, methotrexate sodium, methylprednisolone, nafcillin, oxacillin, penicillin G. Y-site: Allopurinol, amiodarone hydrochloride, amphotericin B cholesteryl sulfate complex, caspofungin acetate, daptomycin, diazepam, gallium, ganciclovir, lansoprazole, phenytoin sodium, TPN.**

- Store cytarabine in refrigerator until reconstituted. ▪ Reconstituted solutions may be stored at 15°–30°C (59°–86°F) for 48 h. Discard solutions with a slight haze.

ADVERSE EFFECTS **CV:** Thrombophlebitis. **Respiratory:** Pulmonary toxicity. **Endocrine:** Hyperuricemia. **Hepatic:** Decreased liver function. **GI:** Anal inflammation, diarrhea, anorexia, nausea, stomatitis, ulcer of anus, ulcer of mouth, vomiting. **GU:** Kidney disease. **Hematologic:** Anemia, decreased reticulocyte count, hemorrhage, leukopenia, megablastic anemia, myelosuppression, thrombocytopenia. **Other:** Fever, sepsis.

INTERACTIONS **Drug:** GI toxicity may decrease **digoxin** absorption; decreases AMINOGLYCOSIDES activity against *Klebsiella pneumoniae*. Do not use with **deferiprone, dipyrone, fingolimod, pimecrolimus, topical tacrolimus.** Do not use with LIVE VACCINES.

PHARMACOKINETICS **Peak:** 20–60 min subcutaneous. **Distribution:** Crosses blood–brain barrier and placenta. **Metabolism:** In liver. **Elimination:** 80% in urine in 24 h. **Half-Life:** 1–3 h.

NURSING IMPLICATIONS

Black Box Warning

Must be ordered by an experienced chemotherapy physician. Drug toxicities resulting in bone marrow suppression.

Assessment & Drug Effects

- Inspect patient's mouth before the administration of each dose. Toxicity necessitating dosage alterations almost always occurs. Report adverse reactions immediately.
- Hyperuricemia due to rapid destruction of neoplastic cells may accompany cytarabine therapy. A regimen that includes a uricosuric agent such as allopurinol, urine alkalinization, and adequate hydration may be started. To reduce potential for urate stone formation, fluids are forced in excess of 2 L, if tolerated. Consult prescriber.
- Monitor I&O ratio and pattern.
- Monitor body temperature. Be alert to the most subtle signs of infection, especially low-grade fever, and report promptly.
- When platelet count falls below 50,000/mm^3 and polymorphonuclear leukocytes to below 1000/mm^3, therapy may be suspended. WBC nadir is usually reached in 5–7 days after therapy has been stopped. Therapy is restarted with appearance of bone marrow recovery and when preceding cell counts are reached.
- Provide good oral hygiene to diminish adverse effects and chance of superinfection. Stomatitis and cheilosis usually appear 5–10 days into the therapy.
- Monitor lab tests: Periodic LFTs, CBC with differential, platelet count, serum creatinine, BUN, serum uric acid.

C

Patient & Family Education

- Report promptly protracted vomiting or signs of nephrotoxicity (see Appendix F).
- Flulike syndrome occurs usually within 6–12 wk after drug administration and may recur with successive therapy. Report chills, fever, achy joints and muscles.
- Practice good oral hygiene to minimize discomfort from stomatitis.
- Report any S&S of superinfection (see Appendix F).

CYTOMEGALOVIRUS IMMUNE GLOBULIN (CMVIG, CMV-IgIV)

(cy-to-meg'a-lo-vi-rus)

CytoGam

Classification: BIOLOGICAL RESPONSE MODIFIER; IMMUNOGLOBULIN

Therapeutic: IMMUNOGLOBULIN

Prototype: Peginterferon alfa-2a

AVAILABILITY Solution for injection

ACTION & *THERAPEUTIC EFFECT*
Cytomegalovirus immune globulin (CMVIG) is a preparation of immunoglobulin G (IgG) antibodies with high concentrations of antibodies directed against cytomegalovirus (CMV). *The CMV antibodies attenuate or reduce the incidence of serious CMV disease, such as CMV-associated pneumonia, CMV-associated hepatitis, and concomitant fungi and parasitic superinfections.*

USES Attenuation of primary cytomegalovirus (CMV) disease associated with kidney transplantation.

UNLABELED USES Prevention of CMV disease in other organ transplants (especially heart) when the recipient is seronegative for CMV and the donor is seropositive.

CONTRAINDICATIONS History of previous severe reactions associated with CMVIG or other human immunoglobulin preparations, selective immunoglobulin A (IgA) deficiency.

CAUTIOUS USE Myelosuppression, maltose or sucrose hypersensitivity; renal insufficiency; DM; older adults; volume depletion; sepsis; paraproteinemia; cardiac disease; pregnancy (category C); lactation.

ROUTE & DOSAGE

Prevention of CMV Disease

Adult: **IV** 150 mg/kg within 72 h of transplantation, then 100 mg/kg 2, 4, 6, and 8 wk posttransplant, then 50 mg/kg 12 and 16 wk posttransplant

ADMINISTRATION

Intravenous

CMVIG should be administered through a separate IV line using an infusion pump. See manufacturer's directions if this is not possible.

PREPARE: **IV Infusion:** Do not shake vial; avoid foaming. Predilution of CMV-IgIV (human) before infusion is not recommended. ▪ **Must be** completely infused within 12 h of entering the vial because solution contains no preservative.

ADMINISTER: **IV Infusion:** Use a constant infusion pump and give at rate of 15, 30, 60 mg/kg/h over first 30 min, second 30 min, third 30 min, respectively. Monitor closely during and after each rate change. ▪ If flushing, nausea, back pain,

fever, or chills develops, slow or temporarily discontinue infusion. ▪ If BP begins to decrease, stop infusion and institute emergency measures. **Infusion of Subsequent IV Doses:** The intervals for increasing the dose from 15 to 30 to 60 mg may be shortened from 30 to 15 min.
- Never infuse more than 75 mL/h of CMVIG.

ADVERSE EFFECTS **CV:** Hypotension, palpitations. **Respiratory:** Shortness of breath, wheezing. **CNS:** Headache, anxiety. **Skin:** Flushing. **GI:** Nausea, vomiting, metallic taste. **Other:** Muscle aches, back pain, anaphylaxis (rare), fever and chills during infusion.

INTERACTIONS **Drug:** May interfere with the immune response to LIVE VIRUS VACCINES **(BCG, measles/mumps/rubella, live polio),** defer vaccination with live viral vaccines for approximately 3 mo after administration of CMVIG; revaccination may be necessary if these vaccines were given shortly after CMVIG.

NURSING IMPLICATIONS

Assessment & Drug Effects

- Monitor vital signs preinfusion, before increases in infusion rate, periodically during infusion, and postinfusion.
- Notify prescriber immediately if any of the following occur: Flushing, nausea, back pain, fall in BP, other signs of anaphylaxis.
- Emergency drugs should be available for treatment of acute anaphylactic reactions.
- Monitor for CMV-associated syndromes (e.g., leukopenia, thrombocytopenia, hepatitis, pneumonia) and for superinfections.

Patient & Family Education

- Familiarize yourself with potential adverse effects and know which to report to prescriber.
- Defer vaccination with live viral vaccines for 3 mo after administration of CMVIG.

D

DABIGATRAN ETEXILATE

(dab-i-ga′tran e-tex′i-late)

Pradaxa

Classification: ANTICOAGULANT; DIRECT THROMBIN INHIBITOR

Therapeutic: ANTITHROMBOTIC; THROMBIN INHIBITOR

Prototype: Argatroban

AVAILABILITY Capsule

ACTION & THERAPEUTIC EFFECT A direct inhibitor of thrombin, which prevents thrombin-induced platelet aggregation and conversion of fibrinogen into fibrin during the coagulation cascade. *It prolongs the aPTT and TT, and it prevents development of a thrombus.*

USES DVT and pulmonary embolism treatment and prevention; prevention of stroke and systemic embolism in patients with nonvalvular atrial fibrillation; prophylaxis of DVT and PE in total hip arthroplasty.

CONTRAINDICATIONS History of serious hypersensitivity to dabigatran etexilate; active pathological bleeding; mechanical prosthetic heart valve; acute renal failure; CrCl less than 15 mL/min; triple-positive antiphospholipid syndrome; pregnancy – fetal risk cannot be ruled out; lactation – infant risk cannot be ruled out.

CAUTIOUS USE Medications or conditions (e.g., labor and delivery, chronic NSAID use, use of antiplatelet agents) that predispose to bleeding; severe renal impairment; spinal procedures; surgical procedures; older adults, children. Safety and efficacy in children less than 3 months of age not established.

ROUTE & DOSAGE

Nonvalvular atrial fibrillation (stroke prevention)/DVT or PE Reduction/Treatment

Adult: PO 150 mg bid

VTE Prophylaxis in Patients Undergoing Hip Replacement

Adult: PO 110 mg 1–4 hours after surgery and establishment of hemostatis then 220 mg daily × 14–35 days

Renal Impairment Dosage Adjustment (nonvalvular atrial fibrillation)

CrCl greater than or equal to 15 to less than or equal to 30 mL/min: 75 mg bid; *CrCl less than 15 mL/min:* Not recommended

ADMINISTRATION

Oral

- Ensure that capsule is swallowed whole. It should not be broken or chewed and should be swallowed with a full glass of water without regard to food.
- Swallow capsules whole; do not break, chew, or empty contents.
- Do not administer oral pellets using a syringe and do not administer via a feeding tube.
- Oral pellets should not be administered with milk, milk products, or soft foods that contain milk products.
- Oral pellets can be mixed with 2 teaspoons of specific, room temperature soft food (baby rice cereal with water, mashed carrots, apple sauce, or mashed banana).
- Oral pellets can be spooned into patient's mouth and swallowed with apple juice or mixed in approximately 1–2 oz. of apple juice for drinking.
- Oral pellets must be administered immediately or within 30 minutes after mixing.
- If a dose of oral pellets is missed, administer a dose as soon as possible the same day. Skip the missed dose if it cannot be taken at least 6 hours before the next scheduled dose. Do not double a dose to make up for a missed dose.
- Converting from a parenteral anticoagulant: Start dabigatran up to 2 h before the next dose of parenteral drug was due or at time of discontinuation of an IV anticoagulant.
- Withhold drug and report to prescriber if active bleeding is suspected.
- Store capsules at 20°C (77°F), excursions permitted between 15 and 30°C (59 and 86°F). Store in original package to protect from moisture. Once bottle is opened, close tightly and use contents within 4 mo of opening.

ADVERSE EFFECTS (≥ 5%) **GI:** Gastroesophageal reflux disease in patient's with atrial fibrillation, gastrointestinal hemorrhage in pediatric patients and adults with atrial fibrillation, gastrointestinal ulcer, indigestion. **Hematological:** *Increased risk of bleeding.*

INTERACTIONS **Drug:** Concomitant use with P-GLYCOPROTEIN INDUCERS (**rifampin, carbamazepine, phenobarbital, tipranavir**) reduces the levels of dabigatran. **Ketoconazole** increases levels and subsequent bleeding risk. Monitor when starting SSRI. ESTROGEN or PROGESTINS may reduce anticoagulant effects. Do not use with ANTICOAGULANTS, ANTIPLATELETS, nonselective NSAIDS due to increased bleeding risk.

PHARMACOKINETICS **Absorption:** 3–7% bioavailable. **Peak:** 1 h. **Distribution:** 35% plasma protein bound. **Metabolism:** Hepatic to active metabolites. **Elimination:** Primarily renal; unabsorbed drug excreted in feces. **Half-Life:** 12–17 h.

NURSING IMPLICATIONS

Black Box Warning

Discontinuation of dabigatran without coverage with another anticoagulant poses a risk of thrombotic events. Concomitant epidural/spinal anesthesia or puncture may cause epidural or spinal hematoma, which may result in long-term or permanent paralysis.

Assessment & Drug Effects

- Monitor for and promptly report S&S of active bleeding.
- Monitor for and report promptly adverse GI effects including: Epigastric pain or discomfort, GERD, or abdominal pain or discomfort.
- Monitor lab tests: Periodic aPTT and PT; baseline and periodic renal function; LFTs; CBC with differential as needed.

Patient & Family Education

- Seek emergency care for any of the following: Unusual bruising; pink or brown urine; red or black, tarry stools; coughing up blood; vomiting blood, or vomit that looks like coffee grounds.
- Report promptly to prescriber any of the following: Pain, swelling or discomfort in a joint; nosebleeds or bleeding from gums; headaches, dizziness, or weakness; menstrual bleeding or vaginal bleeding that is heavier than normal; indigestion, gastric reflux, or nausea.
- Alert all healthcare providers that you are taking dabigatran before any invasive procedure, including dental procedures.
- Do not stop taking medication without consulting healthcare provider.
- Instruct patient to take a missed dose as soon as possible, but if the next dose is less than 6 hours, skip the missed dose. Patient should not take 2 doses at the same time.
- Do not take any over-the-counter medications without checking with prescriber.

DABRAFENIB MESYLATE

(da-braf′-e-nib)

Tafinlar

Classification: ANTINEOPLASTIC; BRAF TYROSINE KINASE INHIBITOR

Therapeutic: ANTINEOPLASTIC

AVAILABILITY Capsule

ACTION & THERAPEUTIC EFFECT Dabrafenib inhibits tyrosine kinases, which are enzymes required for cancer cell formation (oncogenesis), metastasis, tumor angiogenesis, and maintenance of the tumor microenvironment. *Slows BRAF V600 mutation–positive melanoma cell growth resulting in decreased tumor cell growth.*

USES Treatment of patients with unresectable or metastatic melanoma with BRAF V600E mutation as detected by an FDA-approved test; non-small-cell lung cancer; thyroid cancer with BRAF V600E mutation.

CONTRAINDICATIONS Wild-type BRAF melanoma; serious fever reactions to dabrafenib (104°F or greater); palmar-plantar erythrodysesthesia syndrome (PPES); pregnancy; lactation.

CAUTIOUS USE DM; history of hyperglycemia; G6PD deficiency history of cardiomyopathy. Safety and efficacy in children not established.

ROUTE & DOSAGE

Metastatic Melanoma; Thyroid Cancer

Adult: PO 150 mg every 12 h

Non-Small-Cell Lung Cancer

Adult: PO 150 mg q12h in combination with **trametinib** 2 mg daily

Toxicity Dosage Adjustment

See package insert for details

Recommended Dosage Reductions

First reduction: 100 mg every 12 h
Second reduction: 75 mg every 12 h
Third reduction: 50 mg every 12 h
Permanently discontinue: Patient is unable to tolerate 50 mg every 12 h

ADMINISTRATION

Oral

- Give 1 h before or at least 2 h after a meal.
- Capsules must be swallowed whole. They must not be opened or crushed.
- Store at 15°–30°C (59°–86°F).

ADVERSE EFFECTS **CV:** *Peripheral edema*. **Respiratory:** Cough. **CNS:** *Headache*. **Endocrine:** *Hyperglycemia, hypoalbuminemia, hypokalemia, hypophosphatemia*. **Skin:** Alopecia, hand-foot syndrome, *hyperkeratosis, night sweats, papilloma, rash*. **Hepatic:** *ALT/SGPT elevation, AST/SGOT elevation, gamma-glutamyl transferase elevation*. **GI:** *Abdominal pain*, constipation, decreased appetite, *diarrhea, nausea, vomiting*. **Musculoskeletal:** *Joint pain*, muscle pain. **Hematologic:** *Anemia, leukopenia, neutropenia, thrombocytopenia*.

INTERACTIONS **Drug:** Strong inhibitors of CYP3A4 or CYP2C8 (e.g., **clarithromycin, gemfibrozil, ketoconazole, nefazodone**) may increase the levels of dabrafenib. Strong inducers of CYP3A4 or CYP2C8 (e.g., **carbamazepine, phenobarbital, phenytoin, rifampin**) may decrease the levels of dabrafenib. **Herbal: St. John's wort** may decrease the levels of dabrafenib.

PHARMACOKINETICS **Absorption:** 95% bioavailable. **Peak:** 2 h. **Distribution:** 99.7% plasma protein bound. **Metabolism:** Hepatic oxidation. **Elimination:** Fecal (71%) and renal (23%). **Half-Life:** 8 h.

NURSING IMPLICATIONS

Assessment & Drug Effects

- Monitor existing melanoma lesions; report new lesions or changes in existing lesions.
- Monitor for and report S&S of uveitis (e.g., change in vision, photophobia, eye pain).
- Monitor diabetics for loss of glycemic control.
- Monitor skin.
- Monitor EKG at baseline and periodically.

- Monitor for S&S hemorrhage and thromboembolism.
- Monitor lab tests: Periodic blood glucose with preexisting diabetes, LFTs.

Patient & Family Education

- Report to prescriber: Changes in vision or eye pain; symptoms of severe hyperglycemia (e.g., excessive thirst, increase in volume or frequency of urination).
- Diabetics should monitor blood glucose frequently for loss of glycemic control.
- Women should use highly effective means of nonhormonal contraception during and for 2 wk after treatment.
- Do not breastfeed while taking this drug.

DACARBAZINE

(da-kar'ba-zeen)

Classification: ANTINEOPLASTIC; ALKYLATING AGENT
Therapeutic: ANTINEOPLASTIC

AVAILABILITY Solution for injection

ACTION & *THERAPEUTIC EFFECT* Although exact mechanism of action is unknown, it may have alkylating properties and may inhibit DNA synthesis by acting as a purine analog. It is cell cycle nonspecific. Either mechanism would interfere with DNA replication, RNA transcription, and protein synthesis in rapidly proliferating cells. *Has carcinogenic, mutagenic, and teratogenic effects.*

USES Metastatic malignant melanoma, refractory Hodgkin lymphoma.

UNLABELED USES Advanced medullary thyroid cancer, soft-tissue sarcoma.

CONTRAINDICATIONS Hypersensitivity to dacarbazine; severe bone marrow suppression; active infection; live vaccine; pregnancy – fetal risk cannot be ruled out; lactation – infant risk cannot be ruled out.

CAUTIOUS USE Hepatic or renal impairment; previous radiation or chemotherapy.

ROUTE & DOSAGE

Metastatic malignant melanoma

Adult: **IV** 250 mg/m^2 daily on days 1 to 5 q3w

Hodgkin Lymphoma

Adult: **IV** 375 mg/m^2 on days 1 and 15 every 4 weeks × 2–6 cycles

ADMINISTRATION

Intravenous ONLY

IV ADMINISTRATION TO INFANTS AND CHILDREN: Verify correct IV concentration and rate of infusion with prescriber.

- Wear double gloves and protective gown when handling this drug. If solution gets into the eyes, wash them with soap and water immediately, then irrigate with water or isotonic saline. If there is a potential that the substance could splash or if the patient may resist, use eye/face protection.

PREPARE: **Direct:** Reconstitute drug with sterile water for injection to make a solution containing 10 mg/mL dacarbazine (pH 3.0–4.0) by adding 9.9 mL to 100 mg or 19.7 mL to 200 mg. **IV Infusion:** Further dilute reconstituted solution in 50–250 mL of D5W or NS.

ADMINISTER: **Direct:** Give by direct IV into a freely running IV over 5 min. **IV Infusion** *(preferred):* Infuse IV over 30–60 min. ▪ If possible, avoid using antecubital vein or veins on dorsum of hand or wrist where extravasation could lead to loss of mobility of entire limb. ▪ Avoid veins in extremity with compromised venous or lymphatic drainage and veins near joint spaces.

INCOMPATIBILITIES: **Solution/additive:** **Doxorubicin, ondansetron.** **Y-site:** **Acyclovir, allopurinol, amikacin, amphotericin B, ampicillin, cefazolin, cefepime, cefoperazone, cefotaxime, ceftizoxime, ceftriaxone, chloramphenicol, dantrolene, dexamethasone, diazepam, dobutamine, dopamine, epinephrine, ganciclovir, garenoxacin, gentamicin, imipenem/cilastatin, ketorolac, meropenem, mesna, methohexital, methotrexate, methylprednisolone, minocycline, mitomycin, nafcillin, norepinephrine, pantoprazole, pemetrexed, pentazocine, phenytoin, piperacillin/tazobactam, sulfamethoxazole/trimethoprim, thiopental, ticarcillin, tobramycin.**

▪ Administer dacarbazine only to patients under close supervision because close observation and frequent laboratory studies are required during and after therapy. ▪ **IV Extravasation:** Monitor injection site frequently (instruct patient to do so, if able). Give prompt attention to patient's complaint of swelling, stinging, and burning sensation around injection site. ▪ Extravasation can occur painlessly and without visual signs. Danger areas for extravasation are dorsum of hand or ankle (especially if peripheral arteriosclerosis is present), joint spaces, and previously irradiated areas. ▪ If extravasation is suspected, infusion should be stopped immediately and restarted in another vein. Report to the prescriber. Prompt institution of local treatment is IMPERATIVE.

▪ Store reconstituted solution up to 72 h at 4°C (39°F). ▪

ADVERSE EFFECTS **CV:** Hypotension. **CNS:** Headache, polyneuropathy. **Skin:** Alopecia. **GI:** *Anorexia, nausea, vomiting.* **Hematologic:** Severe leukopenia and thrombocytopenia, mild anemia. **Other:** Hypersensitivity (erythematosus, urticarial rashes, hepatotoxicity, photosensitivity); facial paresthesia and flushing, flulike syndrome, myalgia, malaise, anaphylaxis. *Pain along injected vein.*

INTERACTIONS **Drug:** Avoid LIVE VACCINES, IMMUNOSUPPRESSANTS, MYELOSUPPRESSIVE AGENTS.

PHARMACOKINETICS **Distribution:** Localizes primarily in liver. **Metabolism:** In liver by CYP1A2. **Elimination:** 35–50% in urine in 6 h. **Half-Life:** 5 h.

NURSING IMPLICATIONS

Black Box Warning

Dacarbazine has been associated with hemopoietic depression and hepatic necrosis.

Assessment & Drug Effects

- Monitor IV site carefully for extravasation; if suspected, discontinue IV immediately and notify prescriber.
- Note: Skin damage by dacarbazine can lead to deep necrosis requiring surgical debridement, skin grafting, and even amputation. Older adults, the very young, comatose, and debilitated patients are especially at risk. Other risk factors include establishing an IV line in a vein previously punctured several times and the use of nonplastic catheters.
- Avoid, if possible, all tests and treatments during platelet nadir requiring needle punctures (e.g., IM). Observe carefully and report evidence of unexplained bleeding.
- Monitor for severe nausea and vomiting (greater than 90% of patients) that begin within 1 h after drug administration and may last for as long as 12 h.
- Check patient's mouth for ulcerative stomatitis prior to the administration of each dose.
- Monitor I&O ratio and pattern and daily temperature. Renal impairment extends the half-life and increases danger of toxicity. Report symptoms of renal dysfunction and even a slight elevation of temperature.
- Monitor lab tests: Baseline and periodic CBC with differential and Hct and Hgb.

Patient & Family Education

- Learn about all potential adverse drug effects.
- Report flulike syndrome that may occur during or even a week after treatment is terminated and last 7–21 days. Symptoms frequently recur with successive treatments.
- Avoid prolonged exposure to sunlight or to ultraviolet light during treatment period and for at least 2 wk after last dose. Protect exposed skin with sunscreen lotion (SPF 15), and avoid exposure in midday.
- Report promptly the onset of blurred vision or paresthesia.

D

DACLATASVIR

(da-cla-tas′vir)

Classification: ANTIVIRAL; DIRECT-ACTING ANTIVIRAL; VIRAL PROTEIN INHIBITOR ANTIHEPATITIS

Therapeutic: ANTIHEPATITIS

AVAILABILITY Tablets

ACTION & *THERAPEUTIC EFFECT* A direct-acting antiviral agent (DAA) that inhibits a nonstructural protein (i.e., NS5A) encoded by HCV. *Inhibits both viral RNA replication and virion assembly.*

USES In combination with sofosbuvir for the treatment of patients with chronic hepatitis C virus (HCV) genotype 1 or genotype 3 infections.

UNLABELED USES Chronic hepatitis C genotype 2, 4, 5, or 6.

CONTRAINDICATIONS Concurrent use with drugs that strongly induce CYP3A (e.g., phenytoin, carbamazepine, rifampin, St. John's wort).

CAUTIOUS USE Cardiac morbidities or advanced hepatic disease and concomitant use of amiodarone; pregnancy; lactation. Safety and efficacy in children not established.

D

ROUTE & DOSAGE

Hepatitis C Infection

Adult: **PO** 60 mg once daily in combination with sofosbuvir for 12 wk

ADMINISTRATION

Oral

- May be given without regard to food.
- Store at 25°C (77°F); excursions permitted between 15° and 30°C (59° and 86°F).

ADVERSE EFFECTS **CNS:** *Headache.* **Endocrine:** Elevated lipase enzymes. **GI:** Nausea. **Other:** *Fatigue.*

INTERACTIONS **Drug:** Strong and moderate inducers of CYP3A4 (e.g., **bosentan, dexamethasone, efavirenz, etravirine, modafinil, nafcillin, rifapentine**) may decrease the levels of daclatasvir. Strong inhibitors of CYP3A4 (e.g., **atazanavir, clarithromycin, indinavir, itraconazole, ketoconazole, nefazodone, nelfinavir, posaconazole, ritonavir, saquinavir, telithromycin, voriconazole**) may increase the levels of daclatasvir. Daclatasvir may increase the levels of **dabigatran, digoxin,** and HMG-COA REDUCTASE INHIBITORS. Daclatasvir may increase the levels of other drugs that are substrates of P-glycoprotein transporter (P-gp), organic anion transporting polypeptide (OATP), and/or breast cancer resistance protein (BCRP). **Herbal: St. John's wort** may decrease the levels of daclatasvir.

PHARMACOKINETICS **Absorption:** 67% bioavailable. **Peak:** 2 h. **Distribution:** 99% plasma protein bound. **Metabolism:** Hepatic via CYP3A4. **Elimination:** Fecal (88%) and renal (6.6%). **Half-Life:** 12–15 h.

NURSING IMPLICATIONS

BLACK BOX WARNING

Test all patients for evidence of current or prior hepatitis B virus (HBV) infection before initiating treatment. HBV reactivation has been reported in HCV/HBV coinfected patients who were undergoing or had completed treatment. Some cases resulted in fulminant hepatitis, hepatic failure, and death.

Assessment & Drug Effects

- Monitor cardiac status with ECG during first 48 h if coadministered with amiodarone, or if amiodarone discontinued just prior to initiation of therapy with daclatasvir. Report immediately development of bradycardia.
- Ensure that all medications (prescription and OTC) the patient is taking are known to prescriber.
- Monitor lab tests: Baseline and periodic LFTs and serum creatinine, hepatitis C virus viral load.

Patient & Family Education

- Inform prescriber of all prescription and nonprescription drugs being taken. Potentially serious drug interaction may require dosage adjustments.
- If taking amiodarone, monitor heart rate daily for the first 2 wk of therapy. If a slow heart rate develops, seek medical evaluation immediately. Symptoms may include near-fainting or fainting, dizziness or lightheadedness, weakness, excessive tiredness, shortness of breath, chest pain, confusion, or memory problems.

- Take appropriate precautions to prevent transmission of the hepatitis C virus during treatment because effect of treatment on transmission of the virus is unknown.

DACTINOMYCIN

(dak-ti-noe-mye′sin)

Cosmegen

Classification: ANTINEOPLASTIC; ANTHRACYCLINE (ANTIBIOTIC)

Therapeutic: ANTINEOPLASTIC

Prototype: Doxorubicin

AVAILABILITY Solution for injection

ACTION & *THERAPEUTIC EFFECT* Complexes with DNA, thereby inhibiting DNA, RNA, and protein synthesis in actively proliferating cells. Potentiates effects of x-ray therapy, and the converse also appears likely. *Has antineoplastic properties that result from inhibiting DNA and RNA synthesis.*

USES To treat Wilms tumor, rhabdomyosarcoma, carcinoma of testes and uterus, Ewing sarcoma, solid malignancies, gestational trophoblastic neoplasia, and sarcoma botryoides.

UNLABELED USES Malignant melanoma, Kaposi sarcoma, osteogenic sarcoma, among others.

CONTRAINDICATIONS Acute infection; pregnancy (category D); lactation.

CAUTIOUS USE Previous therapy with antineoplastics or radiation within 3–6 wk, bone marrow depression; infections; history of gout; impairment of kidney or liver function; obesity; chickenpox, herpes zoster, and other viral infections. Safe use in infants younger than 6 mo is not known.

ROUTE & DOSAGE

Neoplasms

Adult/Adolescent/Child/Infant (6 mo or older): **IV** 500 mcg/day for 5 days max, may repeat at 2–4 wk intervals if tolerated (if patient is obese or edematous, give 400–600 mcg/m^2/day to relate dosage to lean body mass); monitor for symptoms of toxicity from overdosage

Wilms Tumor, Childhood Rhabdomyosarcoma, Ewing Sarcoma, Nephroblastoma

Adult/Child: **IV** 15 mcg/kg/day × 5 days with other agents

Gestational Trophoblastic Neoplasia

Adult: **IV** 12 mcg/kg/day × 5 days or 500 mcg × 2 days with other agents

Solid Tumor

Adult/Adolescent/Child/Infant (6 mo or older): **IV** 50 mcg/kg (lower extremity) or 35 mcg/kg (upper extremity)

ADMINISTRATION

Intravenous

Use gloves and eye shield when preparing solution. If skin is contaminated, rinse with running water for 10 min; then rinse with buffered phosphate solution. ▪ If solution gets into the eyes, wash with water immediately; then irrigate with water or isotonic saline for 10 min.

D

PREPARE: **Direct:** Reconstitute 0.5 mg vial by adding 1.1 mL sterile water (without preservative) for injection; the resulting solution will contain approximately 0.5 mg/mL. **IV Infusion:** Further dilute reconstituted solution in 50 mL of D5W or NS for infusion.

ADMINISTER: **Direct:** Use two-needle technique for direct IV: Withdraw calculated dose from vial with one needle, change to new needle to give directly into vein without using an infusion. Give over 2–3 min. ▪ Or give directly into an infusing solution of D5W or NS, or into tubing or side arm of a running IV infusion. **IV Infusion:** Give diluted solution as a single dose over 15–30 min.

INCOMPATIBILITIES: **Y-site: Filgrastim.**

- Store drug at 15°–30°C (59°–86°F) unless otherwise directed. Protect from heat and light.

ADVERSE EFFECTS **Skin:** Acne, desquamation, hyperpigmentation and reactivation of erythema especially over previously irradiated areas, *alopecia* (reversible). **GI:** *Nausea, vomiting*, anorexia, abdominal pain, diarrhea, proctitis, GI ulceration, *stomatitis*, cheilitis, glossitis, dysphagia, hepatitis. **Hematologic:** Anemia (including aplastic anemia), agranulocytosis, *leukopenia, thrombocytopenia*, pancytopenia, reticulopenia. **Other:** Malaise, fatigue, lethargy, fever, myalgia, anaphylaxis, gonadal suppression, hypocalcemia, hyperuricemia, thrombophlebitis; *necrosis, sloughing, and contractures at site of extravasation;* hepatitis, hepatomegaly.

INTERACTIONS **Drug:** Elevated **uric acid** level produced by dactinomycin may necessitate dose adjustment of ANTIGOUT AGENTS; effects of both dactinomycin and other MYELOSUPPRESSANTS are potentiated; effects of both **radiation** and dactinomycin are potentiated, and dactinomycin may reactivate erythema from previous radiation therapy; **vitamin K** effects (antihemorrhagic) decreased, leading to prolonged clotting time and potential hemorrhage.

PHARMACOKINETICS **Distribution:** Concentrated in liver, spleen, kidneys, and bone marrow; does not cross blood–brain barrier; crosses placenta. **Elimination:** 50% unchanged in bile and 10% in urine; only 30% in urine over 9 days. **Half-Life:** 36 h.

NURSING IMPLICATIONS

Black Box Warning

Dactinomycin is highly toxic and extremely corrosive to soft tissue. Extravasation will cause severe tissue damage.

Assessment & Drug Effects

- Observe injection site frequently; if extravasation occurs, stop infusion immediately. Restart infusion in another vein. Report to prescriber. Institute prompt local treatment to prevent thrombophlebitis and necrosis.
- Monitor for severe toxic effects that occur with high frequency. Effects usually appear 2–4 days after a course of therapy is stopped and may reach maximal severity 1–2 wk following discontinuation of therapy.
- Use antiemetic drugs to control nausea and vomiting, which often occur a few hours after drug administration. Vomiting may be severe enough to require

intermittent therapy. Observe patient daily for signs of drug toxicity.

- Monitor temperature and inspect oral membranes daily for stomatitis.
- Monitor for stomatitis, diarrhea, and severe hematopoietic depression. These may require prompt interruption of therapy until drug toxicity subsides.
- Report onset of unexplained bleeding, jaundice, and wheezing. Also, be alert to signs of agranulocytosis (see Appendix F). Report to prescriber. Antibiotic therapy, protective isolation, and discontinuation of the antineoplastic are indicated.
- Observe and report symptoms of hyperuricemia (see Appendix F). Urge patient to increase fluid intake up to 3000 mL/day if allowed.
- Monitor lab tests: Frequent renal, hepatic, and bone marrow function tests. Frequent WBC counts and platelet counts.

Patient & Family Education

- Note: Infertility is a possible, irreversible adverse effect of this drug.
- Learn preventative measures to minimize nausea and vomiting.
- Note: Alopecia (hair loss) is an anticipated reversible adverse effect of this drug. Seek appropriate supportive guidance.

DALBAVANCIN HYDROCHLORIDE

(dal-ba'van-sin)

Dalvance

Classification: ANTIBIOTIC; GLYCOPROTEIN

Therapeutic: ANTIBIOTIC

Prototype: Vancomycin

AVAILABILITY Single-use vials containing sterile powder

ACTION & THERAPEUTIC EFFECT Binds to components required for the bacterial cell wall preventing cell wall synthesis. *It is bactericidal against* Staphylococcus aureus *and* Streptococcus pyogenes.

USES Parenterally for the treatment of acute bacterial skin and skin structure infections (ABSSSI) caused by designated susceptible strains of gram-positive microorganisms.

CONTRAINDICATIONS Hypersensitivity to dalbavancin or to any component of the formulation; pseudomembranous colitis due to drug.

CAUTIOUS USE Known hypersensitivity to other glycopeptide antibiotics; moderate to severe hepatic impairment; severe renal impairment; colitis; elderly; pregnancy—fetal risk cannot be ruled out; lactation—infant risk cannot be ruled out. Safety and efficacy in children younger than 18 yr not established. Orphan drug designation for children 0–16 years for treatment of osteomyelitis.

ROUTE & DOSAGE

Acute Bacterial Skin and Skin Structure Infection

Adult: **IV** 1.5 g as single dose OR 1000 mg followed by 500 mg one wk later
Adolescent/Child (at least 6 y) **IV** 18 mg/kg as single dose (max 1500 mg)
Infant/Child (under 6 y) **IV** 22.5 mg/kg as single dose (max 1500 mg)

D

Renal Impairment Dosage Adjustment

CrCl less than 30 mL/min in patients not on hemodialysis: Reduce to 750 mg initially and follow with 375 mg (2 dose regimen) or 1.125 g (single dose regimen)

ADMINISTRATION

Intravenous

PREPARE: **IV Infusion:** Reconstitute with 25 mL of SW for each 500-mg vial to yield 20 mg/mL. Swirl gently and invert vial several times until completely dissolved. Do not shake. Further dilute in D5W to a final concentration of 1–5 mg/mL.

ADMINISTER: **IV Infusion:** Infuse over 30 min. If using IV line for other drugs, flush before/after with D5W. Total time from reconstitution to administration should not exceed 48 hours. Do not infuse at the same time with other medications or electrolytes.

INCOMPATIBILITIES: **Solution/additive:** Normal saline. **Y-site:** Flush before/after infusion.

- Store vials at 15–30°C (59–86°F). Store reconstituted vial or IV solution up to 48 h at controlled room temperature 20–25°C (68–77°F). or under refrigeration 2–8°C (36–46°F). Do not freeze.

ADVERSE EFFECTS (≥ 5%) **GI:** Nausea.

INTERACTIONS **Drug:** Do not use with LIVE VACCINES.

PHARMACOKINETICS **Distribution:** 93% plasma protein bound. **Metabolism:** Minor. **Elimination:** Renal (45%) and fecal (20%). **Half-Life:** 8.5 days.

NURSING IMPLICATIONS

Assessment & Drug Effects

- Monitor patients for any infusion-related reactions.
- Monitor for S&S of superinfection, including *C. difficile*–associated diarrhea (CDAD) and pseudomembranous colitis, which may develop within days or up to several months after completion of therapy.
- If superinfection is suspected, withhold drug and contact prescriber.
- Monitor lab tests: Baseline serum urea nitrogen, serum creatinine, CBC, and LFTs.

Patient & Family Education

- Report promptly to prescriber if you develop nausea, vomiting or frequent watery or bloody diarrhea.
- Consult with prescriber if you are a female who is or plans to become pregnant.
- Do not breastfeed without consulting prescriber.

DALFAMPRIDINE

(dal-fam'pri-deen)

Ampyra

Classification: NEUROLOGIC; POTASSIUM CHANNEL BLOCKER

Therapeutic: NEUROLOGIC

AVAILABILITY Extended release tablet

ACTION & *THERAPEUTIC EFFECT* The mechanism by which it exerts its therapeutic effect is not fully understood. *Improves walking speed in persons with multiple sclerosis.*

USES To improve walking speed in patients with multiple sclerosis.

D

CONTRAINDICATIONS History of seizures; moderate or severe renal impairment; concurrent use of other forms of 4-aminopyridine (4-AP, fampridine); lactation.

CAUTIOUS USE Mild renal impairment; urinary tract infections. Safe use in children younger than 18 yr is not established.

ROUTE & DOSAGE

Multiple Sclerosis

Adult: **PO** 10 mg q12h

Renal Impairment Dosage Adjustment

CrCl 50 mL/min or less: Dalfampridine is contraindicated

ADMINISTRATION

Oral

- Ensure that extended release tablet is swallowed whole. It should not be crushed or chewed.
- Store at 15°–30°C (59°–86°F).

ADVERSE EFFECTS **Respiratory:** Nasopharyngitis, pharyngolaryngeal pain. **CNS:** Asthenia, balance disorder, dizziness, headache, *insomnia*, MS relapse, paresthesia. **GI:** Constipation, dyspepsia, nausea. **GU:** *Urinary tract infection*. **Musculoskeletal:** Back pain.

PHARMACOKINETICS **Absorption:** 96% bioavailability. **Peak:** 3–4 h. **Metabolism:** Minimal. **Elimination:** Renal as unchanged drug. **Half-Life:** 5.2–6.5 h.

NURSING IMPLICATIONS

Assessment & Drug Effects

- Monitor closely for signs of seizure activity. Withhold drug and notify prescriber if a seizure occurs.
- Monitor for and report signs of urinary tract infection.
- Monitor I&O and report significant changes in output.
- Monitor lab tests: Baseline and periodic renal function tests.

Patient & Family Education

- Stop taking drug and notify prescriber immediately if a seizure occurs.
- Tablets must be taken whole. Breaking the tablet may allow too much medication to be released too quickly increasing the risk of a seizure.
- Do not take more than 2 tablets in a 24-h period, and maintain an approximate 12-h interval between doses.
- If you take too much dalfampridine, immediately call your prescriber or go to the nearest emergency room.

DALTEPARIN SODIUM

(dal-tep-a'rin)

Fragmin

See Appendix A-2.

DANAZOL

(da'na-zole)

Cyclomen ♣

Classification:

ANDROGEN/ANABOLIC STEROID

Therapeutic: ANABOLIC STEROID

Prototype: Testosterone

AVAILABILITY Capsule

ACTION & *THERAPEUTIC EFFECT*

Suppresses pituitary output of FSH and LH, resulting in anovulation and associated amenorrhea. Has mild androgenic effects. *Interrupts progress and pain of endometriosis by causing atrophy and involution of both normal and ectopic endometrial tissue.*

D

USES Palliative treatment of endometriosis. Also used to treat fibrocystic breast disease and hereditary angioedema.

UNLABELED USES To treat precocious puberty, gynecomastia, menorrhagia, premenstrual syndrome (PMS), chronic immune thrombocytopenic purpura (ITP), autoimmune hemolytic anemia, hemophilia A and B.

CONTRAINDICATIONS Undiagnosed abnormal genital bleeding; porphyria; markedly impaired hepatic, renal, or cardiac function; peripheral neuropathy; vaginal bleeding; pregnancy (category X); lactation.

CAUTIOUS USE Migraine headache, epilepsy; seizure disorders; renal impairment; history of strokes; history of thrombotic disorders; CAD atherosclerosis; fibrocystic disease; older adults.

ROUTE & DOSAGE

Endometriosis

Adult: **PO** 200–400 mg bid for 3–6 mo

Fibrocystic Breast Disease

Adult: **PO** 100–400 mg in 2 divided doses

Hereditary Angioedema

Adult: **PO** 200 mg bid or tid, may decrease by 50% at intervals of 1–3 mo or longer

ADMINISTRATION

Oral

- Start therapy during menstruation, or after a negative pregnancy test.
- Store capsules at 15°–30°C (59°–86°F) in a tightly closed container.

ADVERSE EFFECTS **CV:** Elevated BP. **CNS:** Dizziness, sleep disorders, fatigue, tremor, irritability. **HEENT:** Conjunctival edema. **Endocrine:** Androgenic effects (acne, mild hirsutism, deepening of voice, oily skin and hair, hair loss, edema, weight gain, pitch breaks, voice weakness, decrease in breast size); hypoestrogenic effects (*hot flashes*; sweating; emotional lability; nervousness; vaginitis with itching, drying, burning, or bleeding; *amenorrhea, irregular menstrual patterns*); impairment in glucose tolerance, rare splenic peliosis. **GI:** Gastroenteritis, hepatic damage (rare), increased LDL, decreased HDL. **GU:** Decreased libido. **Musculoskeletal:** Joint lock-up, joint swelling. **Other:** Hypersensitivity (skin rashes, nasal congestion).

INTERACTIONS **Herbal:** **Echinacea** possibility of increased hepatotoxicity.

PHARMACOKINETICS **Elimination:** Other pharmacokinetic information is not known. **Half-Life:** 4.5 h.

NURSING IMPLICATIONS

Black Box Warning

Danazol may cause fetal harm and should never be given to a pregnant woman. Danazol has been associated with thrombosis, emboli, phlebitis, potentially fatal strokes, and benign intracranial hypertension.

Assessment & Drug Effects

- Routine breast examinations should be carried out during therapy. Carcinoma of the breast should be ruled out prior to start of therapy for fibrocystic breast disease. Advise patient to report to prescriber if any nodule enlarges or becomes tender or hard during therapy.

- Because danazol may cause fluid retention, patients with cardiac or renal dysfunction, epilepsy, or migraine should be observed closely during therapy, as these problems could worsen. Monitor weight.
- Drug-induced edema may compress the median nerve, producing symptoms of carpal tunnel syndrome. If patient complains of wrist pain that worsens at night, paresthesias in radial palmar aspect of the hand and fingers, consult prescriber.
- Monitor diabetics for loss of glycemic control.
- Monitor lab tests: Baseline and periodic LFTs. Patients with diabetes should be monitored for loss of glycemic control.

Patient & Family Education

- Note: Pain and discomfort of endometriosis are usually relieved in 2 or 3 mo; the nodularity in 4–6 mo. Menses may be regular or irregular in pattern during therapy.
- Note: Drug-induced amenorrhea is reversible. Ovulation and cyclic bleeding usually return within 60–90 days after therapeutic regimen is discontinued as well as the potential for conception.
- Use a reliable nonhormonal contraceptive during treatment because ovulation may not be suppressed until 6–8 wks after therapy is begun. If pregnancy occurs while taking this drug, contact prescriber immediately.
- Report voice changes or other masculinizing effects promptly. Virilizing adverse effects may persist even after drug therapy is terminated.

DANTROLENE SODIUM

(dan'troe-leen)

Dantrium, Revonto, Ryanodex

Classification: DIRECT-ACTING SKELETAL MUSCLE RELAXANT

Therapeutic: SKELETAL MUSCLE RELAXANT; ANTISPASMODIC

AVAILABILITY Capsule; solution for injection; suspension for injection

ACTION & THERAPEUTIC EFFECT Hydantoin derivative with peripheral skeletal muscle relaxant action. Directly relaxes spastic muscle by interfering with calcium ion release from sarcoplasmic reticulum within skeletal muscle. *Relief of muscle spasticity, however, may be accompanied by muscle weakness sufficient to affect overall functional capacity of the patient. Dantrolene also can attenuate or prevent development of malignant hyperthermia.*

USES Orally for spasticity. Used intravenously for the management of malignant hyperthermia.

UNLABELED USES Neuroleptic malignant syndrome, exercise-induced muscle pain, and flexor spasms.

CONTRAINDICATIONS Active hepatic disease such as hepatitis and cirrhosis; drug-induced hepatitis; when spasticity is necessary to sustain upright posture and balance in locomotion or to maintain increased body function; spasticity due to rheumatic disorders; pregnancy – fetal risk cannot be ruled out; lactation – infant risk cannot be ruled out.

CAUTIOUS USE Impaired cardiac or pulmonary function, muscular sclerosis; neuromuscular disease; myopathy; history of liver disease or dysfunction; patients older than 35 yr, especially women; long-time use in children. Safe use in children younger than 5 yr is not established.

D

ROUTE & DOSAGE

Chronic Spasticity

Adult/Adolescent/Child (over 5 yr and over 50 kg): **PO** 25 mg once/day, increase to 25 mg tid, may increase q7days up to 100 mg tid (max dose 400 mg/day)

Child (5 yr or older less than 50 kg): **PO** 0.5 mg/kg bid × 7 days, increase to 0.5 mg/kg tid × 7 days, may increase to 2 mg/kg/dose tid (max: 400 mg/day.)

Malignant Hyperthermia Treatment

Adult/Child: **IV** 2.5 mg/kg; monitor and can repeat dose of 1 mg/kg up to cumulative dose of 10 mg/kg; **PO** 4–8 mg/kg/day in 4 divided doses × *1–3 days*

Hepatic Impairment Dosage Adjustment

Do not use in active liver disease

ADMINISTRATION

Oral

- Prepare oral suspension for a single dose, when necessary, by emptying contents of capsule(s) into fruit juice or other liquid. Shake suspension well before pouring.
- Avoid contamination, keep suspension refrigerated, and use within several days because it does not contain a preservative.
- Store capsules in controlled room temperature, between 20° and 25°C (68° and 77°F).

Intravenous

PREPARE: **Direct:** Dilute each 20 mg with 60 mL sterile water without preservatives. Shake until clear. **Infusion:** Large volume used for prophylaxis may be transferred to plastic (not glass) infusion bags.

ADMINISTER: **Direct:** Give by rapid direct IV push. Avoid extravasation; solution has a high pH and therefore is extremely irritating to tissue. ▪ Ensure IV patency prior to giving drug direct IV. **Infusion:** Give over 1 h.

INCOMPATIBILITIES: **Y-site:** Do not administer with other medications.

- Store contents of vial (for IV use) at controlled room temperature between 20° and 25°C (68° and 77°F) and **must be** protected from direct light. Reconstituted vials can also be stored at controlled room temperature and used within 6 h after reconstitution.

ADVERSE EFFECTS **CNS:** Drowsiness. **Skin:** Flushing. **GI:** *Diarrhea,* nausea, anorexia, swallowing difficulty, GI bleeding. **Musculoskeletal:** Muscle weakness. **Other:** Fatigue, malaise.

INTERACTIONS **Drug: Alcohol** and other CNS DEPRESSANTS compound CNS depression; **estrogens** increase risk of hepatotoxicity in women older than 35 yr; IV use with **verapamil** and other CALCIUM CHANNEL BLOCKERS increase risk of hyperkalemia. Use caution with CYP3A4 inducers.

PHARMACOKINETICS **Absorption:** Incompletely absorbed from

GI tract. **Peak:** 5 h. **Distribution:** Crosses placenta. **Metabolism:** In liver. **Elimination:** In urine chiefly as metabolites. **Half-Life:** 4–11 h.

NURSING IMPLICATIONS

Black Box Warning

Dantrolene has been associated with severe hepatic damage. Risk is greater in patients taking higher doses, in females, in patients older than 35 yr, and in patients taking additional medications.

Assessment & Drug Effects

- Monitor for and report promptly S&S of hepatotoxicity (see Appendix F) that are more common in females and in those older than 35 yr.
- Monitor vital signs during IV infusion. Also monitor ECG, CVP, and serum potassium.
- Supervise ambulation until patient's reaction to drug is known. Relief of spasticity may be accompanied by some loss of strength.
- Monitor patients with impaired cardiac or pulmonary function closely for cardiovascular or respiratory symptoms such as tachycardia, BP changes, feeling of suffocation.
- Monitor for and report symptoms of allergy and allergic pleural effusion: Shortness of breath, pleuritic pain, dry cough.
- Monitor for difficulty swallowing.
- Alert prescriber if improvement is not evident within 45 days. Drug may be discontinued because of the possibility of hepatotoxicity (see Appendix F).
- Monitor bowel function. Persistent diarrhea may necessitate drug withdrawal. Severe constipation with abdominal distention and signs of intestinal obstruction have been reported.
- Monitor lab tests: Baseline and periodic LFTs, blood cell counts, and renal function tests.

Patient & Family Education

- Report promptly the onset of jaundice: Yellow skin or sclerae; dark urine, clay-colored stools, itching, abdominal discomfort. Hepatotoxicity frequently occurs between the 3rd and 12th mo of therapy.
- Do not drive or engage in other potentially hazardous activities until response to drug is known.
- Oral forms of medication can have photosensitivity reaction; sun protection is advised.
- Do not use OTC medications, alcoholic beverages, or other CNS depressants unless otherwise advised by prescriber. Liver toxicity occurs more commonly when other drugs are taken concurrently.

DAPAGLIFLOZIN

(dap-a-gli-flo'sin)

Farxiga

Classification: ANTIDIABETIC; SODIUM-GLUCOSE COTRANSPORTER 2 (SGLT2) INHIBITOR

Therapeutic: ANTIDIABETIC

Prototype: Canagliflozin

AVAILABILITY

Tablets

ACTION & THERAPEUTIC EFFECT

Inhibits the sodium-glucose cotransporter 2 (SGLT2) in the proximal renal tubules that is responsible for the majority of the reabsorption of filtered glucose in the kidney. *Dapagliflozin inhibits SGLT2 thus allowing more glucose to be removed from the bloodstream and excreted by the kidney.*

D

USES An adjunct to diet and exercise to improve glycemic control in adults with type 2 diabetes mellitus. To reduce the risk of sustained eGFR decline, end-stage kidney disease, cardiovascular death, in adults with chronic kidney disease at risk of progression. To reduce the risk of cardiovascular death and hospitalization for heart failure in adults with heart failure with reduced ejection fraction.

CONTRAINDICATIONS History of serious hypersensitivity reaction to dapagliflozin; severe renal impairment, end-stage renal disease, or dialysis; active bladder cancer, pregnancy—fetal risk cannot be ruled out; lactation—infant risk cannot be ruled out.

CAUTIOUS USE Risk factors for hypotension; impaired renal function; urinary tract infection (UTI) hypoglycemia; ketoacidosis, genital mycotic infections; increased LDL-C; history of bladder cancer; DM; older adults. Safety and efficacy in children younger than 18 yr not established.

ROUTE & DOSAGE

Type 2 Diabetes Mellitus

Adult: **PO** 5 mg once daily; may increase to 10 mg

Chronic Kidney Disease/Heart Failure

Adult: **PO** 10 mg daily

Renal Impairment Dosage Adjustment

eGFR less than 45 mL/min/1.73 m²: See package insert for adjustments based on concurrent disease states.

ADMINISTRATION

Oral

- Give in the morning with/without food.
- Store at 15° C–30°C (59°F–86°F).

ADVERSE EFFECTS (≥ 5 %) **Respiratory:** Nasopharyngitis. **GU:** Urinary tract infection. **Other:** Female genital infection.

INTERACTIONS **Drug:** May potentiate the hypoglycemia effect of **insulin** and INSULIN SECRETAGOGUES, SULFONYLUREAS.

PHARMACOKINETICS **Absorption:** 78% bioavailable after oral dose. **Peak:** 2 h. **Distribution:** 9 1% plasma protein bound. **Metabolism:** In liver. **Elimination:** Renal (75%) and fecal (21%). **Half-Life:** 12.9 h.

NURSING IMPLICATIONS

Assessment & Drug Effects

- Monitor blood sugars (hypo/hyperglycemia).
- Monitor fluids.
- Monitor BP throughout therapy as drug causes intravascular volume depletion.
- Monitor for symptomatic hypotension, especially at the initiation of therapy and in the older adult or those taking other drugs that lower BP.
- Monitor for S&S of genital fungal infections and urinary tract infections.
- Monitor lab tests: Baseline and periodic renal function tests; periodic HbA1C; periodic lipid profile.

Patient & Family Education

- Monitor blood sugar as directed by prescriber. Note that this drug will cause sugar to appear in your urine.
- Report to prescriber if you experience S&S of hypoglycemia (see Appendix F).

- Report to prescriber any S&S of an allergic reaction (e.g., rash, hives).
- Maintain adequate fluid intake as drug can cause dehydration. Inform prescriber if you experience dizziness upon standing.
- Yeast infections of the vagina and penis (especially in uncircumcised men) may occur. Report promptly for treatment.
- Report to prescriber if a pregnancy is suspected.
- Discontinue breastfeeding while taking this drug.
- Take a missed dose as soon as possible, but if it is almost time for the next dose, skip missed dose. Do not double the dose.

DAPSONE

(dap'sone)

Aczone, Avlosulfon ♣

Classification: ANTILEPROSY (SULFONE)

Therapeutic: ANTILEPROSY

AVAILABILITY Tablet; gel

ACTION & *THERAPEUTIC EFFECT* Has bacteriostatic and bactericidal activity. Interferes with bacterial cell growth by competitive inhibition of folic acid synthesis by susceptible organisms. It also interferes with alternative pathways of complement system. *Effective against dapsone-sensitive multibacillary (borderline, borderline lepromatous, or lepromatous) leprosy, and dapsone-sensitive paucibacillary (indeterminate, tuberculoid, or borderline tuberculoid) leprosy.* ***Gel form*** *is effective against acne vulgaris.*

USES All forms of leprosy. Used in dapsone-sensitive multibacillary leprosy (with clofazimine and rifampin) and in dapsone-sensitive paucibacillary leprosy (with rifampin, clofazimine, or ethionamide). Also used prophylactically in contacts of patients with all forms of leprosy except tuberculoid and indeterminate leprosy. Used for treatment of dermatitis herpetiformis. **Gel** used for acne vulgaris.

UNLABELED USES Chemoprophylaxis of malaria (with pyrimethamine), systemic and discoid lupus erythematosus, pemphigus vulgaris, dermatosis (especially those associated with bullous eruptions, mucocutaneous lesions, inflammation, or pustules); rheumatoid arthritis, allergic vasculitis; treatment of initial episodes of *P. carinii* pneumonia (with trimethoprim) in limited number of adults with AIDS.

CONTRAINDICATIONS Hypersensitivity to sulfones or its derivatives; advanced renal amyloidosis, anemia, methemoglobin reductase deficiency.

CAUTIOUS USE Sulfonamide hypersensitivity; chronic renal, hepatic, pulmonary, or cardiovascular disease, refractory anemias, albuminuria, G6PD deficiency; pregnancy (category C); lactation.

ROUTE & DOSAGE

Tuberculoid and Indeterminate-Type Leprosy

Adult: **PO** 100 mg/day (with 6 mo of rifampin 600 mg/day) for a minimum of 3 yr

Lepromatous and Borderline Lepromatous Leprosy

Adult: **PO** 100 mg/day for 10 yr or more

D

Child: **PO** 1–2 mg/kg/day once daily in combination therapy (max: 100 mg/day)

Dermatitis Herpetiformis

Adult: **PO** 50 mg/day, may be increased to 300 mg/day if necessary (max: 500 mg/day)

Prophylaxis for Close Contacts of Patient with Multibacillary Leprosy

Adult: **PO** 50 mg/day
Child (younger than 6 mo): **PO** 6 mg 3 × wk; *6–23 mo:* 12 mg 3 × wk; *2–5 yr:* 25 mg 3 × wk; *6–12 yr:* 25 mg/day

***P. carinii* Pneumonia Prophylaxis**

Adult: **PO** 50 mg bid or 100 mg daily
Child: **PO** 2 mg/kg once daily (max: 100 mg/day)

Acne

Topical Apply pea-sized amount of gel to affected area bid

ADMINISTRATION

Oral

- Give with food to reduce possibility of GI distress.
- Store in tightly covered, light-resistant containers at 15°–30°C (59°–86°F). Drug discoloration apparently does not indicate a chemical change.

Topical

- Clean skin with soap and water before application.

ADVERSE EFFECTS **CV:** Tachycardia. **CNS:** Headache, nervousness, insomnia, vertigo; paresthesia, *muscle weakness*. **HEENT:** Blurred vision, tinnitus. **Skin:** Drug-induced lupus erythematosus, phototoxicity. **GI:** Anorexia, nausea, vomiting, abdominal pain; toxic hepatitis, cholestatic jaundice (reversible with discontinuation of drug therapy); increased ALT, AST, LDH; hyperbilirubinemia. **Hematologic:** In patient with or without G6PD deficiency; *dose-related hemolysis,* Heinz body formation, *methemoglobinemia with cyanosis,* hemolytic anemia; aplastic anemia (rare), agranulocytosis. **Other:** Hypersensitivity (cutaneous reactions); erythema multiforme, exfoliative dermatitis, toxic epidermal necrolysis (rare), allergic rhinitis, urticaria, fever, infectious mononucleosis-like syndrome. Male infertility; sulfone syndrome (fever, malaise, exfoliative dermatitis, hepatic necrosis with jaundice, lymphadenopathy, methemoglobinemia, anemia).

INTERACTIONS **Drug: Activated charcoal** decreases dapsone absorption and enterohepatic circulation; **pyrimethamine, trimethoprim** increase risk of adverse hematologic reactions; **rifampin** decreases dapsone levels 7- to 10-fold.

PHARMACOKINETICS **Absorption:** Rapidly and nearly completely absorbed from GI tract. **Peak:** 2–8 h. **Distribution:** Distributed to all body tissues; high concentrations in kidney, liver, muscle, and skin; crosses placenta; distributed into breast milk. **Metabolism:** In liver by CYP3A4. **Elimination:** 70–85% in urine; remainder in feces; traces of drug may be found in body for 3 wk after repeated doses. **Half-Life:** 20–30 h.

NURSING IMPLICATIONS

Assessment & Drug Effects

- Monitor for therapeutic effectiveness that may not appear for leprosy until after 3–6 mo of therapy.

- Determine periodic dapsone blood levels.
- Perform liver function tests in patients who complain of malaise, fever, chills, anorexia, nausea, vomiting, and have jaundice.
- Monitor severity of anemia. Nearly all patients demonstrate hemolysis.
- Monitor temperature during first few weeks of therapy. If fever is frequent or severe, leprosy reactional state should be ruled out.
- Monitor lab tests: Baseline then weekly CBC during the first month of therapy, at monthly intervals for at least 6 mo, and semiannually thereafter.

Patient & Family Education

- Report symptoms of leprosy that do not improve within 3 mo or that get worse to prescriber.
- Report the appearance of a rash with bullous lesions around elbows and other joints promptly. Drug-induced or worsening skin lesions require withdrawal of dapsone.
- Report symptoms of peripheral neuropathy with motor loss (muscle weakness) promptly.

DAPTOMYCIN

(dap-to-my′sin)

Cubicin

Classification: ANTIBIOTIC; LIPOPEPTIDE

Therapeutic: ANTIBIOTIC

AVAILABILITY Solution for injection

ACTION & *THERAPEUTIC EFFECT* It binds to bacterial membranes of gram-positive bacteria causing rapid depolarization of the membrane potential leading to inhibition of protein, DNA, and RNA synthesis and bacterial cell death. *Daptomycin is effective against a broad spectrum of gram-positive organisms, including both susceptible and resistant strains of* S. aureus.

USES Complicated skin and skin structure infections, bacteremia, endocarditis.

UNLABELED USES Vancomycin-resistant enterococci, MRSA-associated bone/joint infections, febrile neutropenia.

CONTRAINDICATIONS Hypersensitive reaction to daptomycin; pseudomembranous colitis; myopathy; eosinophilic pneumonia; nonbacterial infection.

CAUTIOUS USE Severe renal or hepatic impairment, end-stage renal failure; peripheral neuropathy; GI disease; history of rhabdomyolysis, or myopathy; older adults; pregnancy (category B); lactation. Safe use in infants is not established.

ROUTE & DOSAGE

Skin Infections

Adult: **IV** 4 mg/kg q24h × 7–14 days
Adolescent: **IV** 5 mg/kg q24h × 14 d
Children (7–11 yr): **IV** 7 mg/kg q24h × 14 d; *(2–6 yr)*: 9 mg/kg q24h × 14 d; *(1–2 yr)*: 10 mg/kg q24h × 14 d

Bacteremia *(S. aureus)*

Adult: **IV** 6 mg/kg daily × 2–6 wk
Adolescent: **IV** 7 mg/kg every 24 h
Children (7–11 yr): **IV** 9 mg/kg every 24 h; *(1–6 yr)*: 12 mg/kg every 24 h

D

Endocarditis

Adult: **IV** 6 mg/kg q24h × 2–6 wk

Renal Impairment Dosage Adjustment

CrCl less than 30 mL/min: administer q48h

Hemodialysis Dosage Adjustment

Dose by CrCl, administer after dialysis

ADMINISTRATION

Intravenous

PREPARE: **IV Direct:** Note: Double-check manufacturer's guidelines for reconstitution, not all recommend normal saline – varies by product. Slowly add 10 mL of NS to the 500-mg vial, pointing needle toward the wall of the vial. Gently rotate vial to wet the powder, then allow to stand for 10 min. Gently rotate vial to completely dissolve. Yields 50 mg/mL. **IV Infusion:** Further dilute the 50-mg/mL solution in 50 mL of NS.

ADMINISTER: **Direct:** Inject over 2 min. **IV Infusion:** Infuse over 30 min; if same IV line is used for infusion of other drugs, flush line before/after with NS.

INCOMPATIBILITIES: **Solution/additive:** **Dextrose**-containing solutions. **Y-site:** **Acyclovir, alemtuzumab, allopurinol, amphotericin B, amphotericin B liposomal, blinatumomab, cytarabine, dantrolene, gemcitabine, gemtuzumab, imipenem/cilastin, methotrexate, metronidazole, minocycline, mitomycin, nitroglycerin, pantoprazole, pentazoine, pentobarbital, phenytoin, remifentanil, streptozocin, sufentanil, thiopental, vancomycin.**

- Store unopened vials in 2°–8°C (36°–46°F). Avoid excessive heat.
- Refer to manufacturer's labeling for specific storage and reconstitution guidelines – varies by product.

ADVERSE EFFECTS

CV: Hypotension, hypertension, peripheral edema, chest pain, atrial fibrillation. **Respiratory:** Dyspnea, pharyngolaryngeal pain. **CNS:** Headache, anxiety, *insomnia*, dizziness. **HEENT:** Tinnitus. **Endocrine:** Elevated CPK, hypokalemia, elevated hepatic enzymes. **Skin:** Rash, diaphoresis, erythema, pruritus, hyperhidrosis. **GI:** Nausea, vomiting, diarrhea, abdominal pain, abnormal liver function tests. **GU:** UTIs, renal failure. **Musculoskeletal:** Limb pain, arthralgia, uncontrolled muscle movement. **Hematologic:** Anemia, eosinophilia, leukocytosis, <u>thrombocytopenia</u>. **Other:** Injection site reactions, fever, fungal infections.

INTERACTIONS

Do not use with bowel preparation kits. Use caution when also administering **tobramycin**.

PHARMACOKINETICS

Elimination: Primarily renal. **Distribution:** 90% protein bound. **Half-Life:** 8 h.

NURSING IMPLICATIONS

Assessment & Drug Effects

- Monitor for and report: Muscle pain or weakness, especially with concurrent therapy with HMG-CoA reductase inhibitors (statin drugs); S&S of peripheral neuropathy, superinfection such as candidiasis, irregular pulse.

- Withhold drug and notify prescriber if S&S of myopathy develop with CPK elevation greater than 1000 units/L (~5 × ULN), or if CPK level is 10 × ULN or greater.
- Monitor lab tests: Baseline C&S and renal function tests.

Patient & Family Education

- Report any of the following to the prescriber: Muscle pain, weakness or unusual tiredness; numbness or tingling; difficulty breathing or shortness of breath; severe diarrhea or vomiting; skin rash or itching, dark urine, jaundice.

DARBEPOETIN ALFA

(dar-be-po-e'tin)

Aranesp

Classification: BLOOD FORMER; ERYTHROPOIESIS-STIMULATING AGENT

Therapeutic: ANTIANEMIC

Prototype: Epoetin alfa

AVAILABILITY Solution for injection

ACTION & *THERAPEUTIC EFFECT* An erythropoiesis-stimulating protein that stimulates red blood cell production in the bone marrow in response to hypoxia. *Darbepoetin stimulates release of reticulocytes from the bone marrow into the bloodstream where they mature into RBCs.*

USES Treatment of anemia in patients with chronic renal failure or chemotherapy-associated anemia.

CONTRAINDICATIONS Patients with uncontrolled hypertension; serious hypersensitivity to darbepoetin or human albumin; antibody-mediated anemia due to antierythropoietin antibodies; pure red cell aplasia that begins after treatment with darbepoetin alfa or other related drugs.

CAUTIOUS USE Controlled hypertension, elevated hemoglobin, folic acid or vitamin B_{12} deficiencies, hematologic diseases; cardiovascular disease, stroke, anemia, latex allergy, history of seizures, infections, inflammatory or malignant processes, osteofibrosis, occult blood loss, hemolysis, severe aluminum toxicity, bone marrow fibrosis, chronic renal failure patients not on dialysis; pregnancy (category C); lactation.

ROUTE & DOSAGE

Anemia

Adult: **IV/Subcutaneous** See package insert for dosage table. Dose varies based on current laboratory data and patient specific changes each week.

ADMINISTRATION

All Routes

- Correct deficiencies of folic acid or vitamin B_{12} prior to initiation of therapy.

Subcutaneous

- Do not shake solution. Shaking may denature the darbepoetin, rendering it biologically inactive.
- Inspect solution for particulate matter prior to use. Do not use if solution is discolored or if it contains particulate matter.
- Use only one dose per vial, and do not reenter vial.
- Administer subq injection in upper arm, abdomen, or anterior thigh surface and alternate site of injection with each administration.
- Do not give with any other drug solution.

D

Intravenous

PREPARE: **Direct:** Do not shake or dilute vials or prefilled syringes. Do not use vials or prefilled syringes that have been shaken. ***ADMINISTER:*** **Direct:** Give direct IV as a bolus dose over 1 min. ▪ Discard any unused portion of the vial or syringe. It contains no preservatives.
▪ May be administered at any stage during dialysis session.
▪ Store injection solution between 2 and 8°C (36–46°F) in original carton protected from light. Do not freeze or shake.

ADVERSE EFFECTS (≥ 5%) **CV:** Edema, hypotension, peripheral edema. **Respiratory:** *Dyspnea, cough.* **GI:** Abdominal pain.

DIAGNOSTIC TEST INTERFERENCE May artificially lower ***HbA1c***.

PHARMACOKINETICS **Absorption:** 37% absorbed from subcutaneous site. **Peak:** 24–72 h subcutaneous. **Distribution:** Distribution confined primarily to intravascular space. **Elimination:** 10% in urine. **Half-Life:** 21 h IV, 49 h subcutaneous.

NURSING IMPLICATIONS

Black Box Warning

Darbepoetin has been associated with increased risk of MI, stroke, venous thromboembolism, thrombosis of vascular access, and tumor progression or recurrence.

Assessment & Drug Effects

- Control BP adequately prior to initiation of therapy and closely monitor and control during therapy. Report immediately S&S of CHF, cardiac arrhythmias, or sepsis. Note that hypertension is an adverse effect that **must be** controlled.
- Notify prescriber of a rapid rise in Hgb as dosage will need to be reduced because of risk of serious hypertension and other adverse events. Note that BP may rise during early therapy as Hgb increases.
- Monitor for premonitory neurologic symptoms (i.e., aura, and report their appearance promptly). The potential for seizures exists during periods of rapid Hgb increase (e.g., greater than 1.0 g/dL in any 2-wk period).
- Monitor closely and report immediately S&S of thrombotic events (e.g., MI, CVA, TIA), especially for patients with CRF.
- Monitor lab tests: Baseline and periodic transferrin and serum ferritin; Hgb twice weekly until stabilized and maintenance dose is established, then weekly for at least 4 wk, and at regular intervals thereafter; periodic CBC with differential and platelet count; periodic BUN, creatinine, serum phosphorus, and serum potassium.

Patient & Family Education

- Adhere closely to antihypertensive drug regimen and dietary restrictions.
- Monitor BP as directed by prescriber.
- Avoid activities requiring coordination until drug effects are realized, as the drug may cause dizziness.
- Do not drive or engage in other potentially hazardous activity during the first 90 days of therapy because of possible seizure activity.
- Report any of the following to the prescriber: Chest pain, difficulty

breathing, shortness of breath, severe or persistent headache, fever, muscle aches and pains, or nausea.

DARIFENACIN HYDROBROMIDE

(dar-i-fen′a-sin)

Enablex

Classification: ANTICHOLINERGIC; MUSCARINIC RECEPTOR ANTAGONIST; BLADDER ANTISPASMODIC

Therapeutic: BLADDER ANTISPASMODIC

Prototype: Oxybutynin

AVAILABILITY Extended release tablet

ACTION & *THERAPEUTIC EFFECT* Darifenacin is a selective M_3 muscarinic receptor antagonist. Muscarinic M_3 receptors play an important role in contraction of the urinary bladder smooth muscle and stimulation of salivary secretion. *Control of urinary incontinence due to urgency and frequency.*

USES Overactive bladder with symptoms of urge urinary incontinence, urgency, and frequency.

CONTRAINDICATIONS Hypersensitivity to darifenacin; angioedema; severe hepatic impairment (Child–Pugh C class); patients at risk of urinary retention, gastric retention; pyloric stenosis, ileus; urinary retention; uncontrolled narrow-angle glaucoma; pregnancy – fetal risk cannot be ruled out; lactation – infant risk cannot be ruled out.

CAUTIOUS USE Risk of urinary retention, clinically significant bladder outflow obstruction, renal disease; mild to moderate hepatic impairment; decreased GI motility, GERD, severe constipation, ulcerative colitis; myasthenia gravis; controlled narrow-angle glaucoma. Safety and efficacy in patients with severe hepatic impairment is unknown.

ROUTE & DOSAGE

Overactive Bladder

Adult: **PO** 7.5–15 mg daily

Moderate Hepatic Impairment Dosage Adjustment

Child–Pugh B Class: Max: 7.5 mg daily

ADMINISTRATION

Oral

- Ensure that the drug is not chewed or crushed. It **must be** swallowed whole.
- Can be given with or without food.
- Note: Dosage should not exceed 7.5 mg daily with moderate hepatic impairment (i.e., Child–Pugh B class) or concurrent therapy with potent inhibitors of CYP3A4 (e.g., itraconazole, clarithromycin, nefazodone, nelfinavir, ritonavir).
- Store at controlled room temperature of 25°C (77°F), excursions permitted between 15° and 30°C (59°and 86°F). Protect from light.

ADVERSE EFFECTS (≥5%) **CNS:** *Headache.* **GI:** *Constipation, dry mouth.*

INTERACTIONS Drug: Potent inhibitors of CYP3A4 (e.g., **clarithromycin, erythromycin, itraconazole, ketoconazole,**

nefazodone, nelfinavir, and **ritonavir**) increase darifenacin levels. Darifenacin will cause additive anticholinergic effects with other ANTICHOLINERGIC drugs. Darifenacin can increase **digoxin** concentrations. DIURETICS can increase bladder symptoms. May increase concentrations of other medications metabolized by CYP2D6 (e.g., **doxorubicin, doxepin, amitriptyline**). **Food: Grapefruit juice** may increase darifenacin levels.

PHARMACOKINETICS Absorption: 15–19% bioavailability. **Peak:** 7 h. **Distribution:** 98% protein bound. **Metabolism:** Extensive hepatic metabolism. **Elimination:** Renal and fecal. **Half-Life:** 13–19 h.

NURSING IMPLICATIONS

Assessment & Drug Effects

- Monitor for adverse effects of concurrently used drugs that have a narrow therapeutic window and are metabolized by CYP26D (e.g., flecainide, thioridazine, or TRICYCLIC ANTIDEPRESSANTS).
- Monitor I and O to confirm urine output.
- Signs of toxicity: headache, confusion, hallucinations, and somnolence.
- Monitor lab tests: Frequent digoxin levels with concurrent therapy.

Patient & Family Education

- Do not crush, chew or divide drug tablets.
- Do not drive or engage in potentially hazardous activities until response to drug is known.
- Use caution in hot environments to minimize the risk of heat prostration.
- Report any of the following to a healthcare provider: Difficulty passing urine, unexplained nausea, or persistent constipation.

DARUNAVIR

(da-run′a-ver)

Prezista

Classification: ANTIRETROVIRAL; PROTEASE INHIBITOR

Therapeutic: HIV PROTEASE INHIBITOR

Prototype: Saquinavir

AVAILABILITY Tablet; oral suspension

ACTION & *THERAPEUTIC EFFECT* Darunavir is an inhibitor of HIV-1 protease that selectively inhibits the cleavage of HIV polyproteins in infected cells, thereby preventing the maturation of virus particles. *Darunavir reduces viral load (decreases the number of RNA copies) and increases the number of T helper CD4 cells.*

USES Treatment of HIV infection with other antiretroviral agents.

UNLABELED USES HIV prophylaxis.

CONTRAINDICATIONS Hypersensitivity to darunavir or protease inhibitors, ritonavir; severe hepatic impairment; pancreatitis; pregnancy (fetal risk cannot be ruled out); lactation (infant risk cannot be ruled out).

CAUTIOUS USE Hypersensitivity to sulfa drugs; hepatic function impairment, hepatitis B or C; patients at risk for pancreatitis; severe renal impairment, chronic renal failure; hemophilia A or B; concurrent autoimmune disease; sulfonamide allergy; DM; diabetes ketoacidosis; hyperglycemia; older adults; children.

ROUTE & DOSAGE

HIV Infection, Treatment Naive

Adult: **PO** 800 mg daily with 100 mg ritonavir or cobicistat 150 mg PO

HIV Infection, Treatment Experienced

Adult: **PO** 600 mg bid with 100 mg ritonavir bid PO (genetic screening to determine if 800 mg daily is needed)

Adolescent/Child: Weight, genetic screen, and previous drug exposure all affect dose; see package insert for dosing table.

Pregnancy Dosage Adjustment

Decrease to 600 mg bid

ADMINISTRATION

Oral

- Give with food and coadminister with 100 mg ritonavir (adult dose).
- Suspension shake well before use.
- Tablets **must be** swallowed whole.
- Store at 15°–30°C (59°–86°F). Protect from light, excessive heat, and moisture.

ADVERSE EFFECTS **CNS:** Headache. **Endocrine:** Hypertriglyceridemia, *serum cholesterol raised*. **Skin:** Rash. **GI:** Abdominal pain, diarrhea, nausea, vomiting.

INTERACTIONS **Drug:** AZOLE ANTIFUNGALS and **indinavir** increase the levels of darunavir. Coadministration of other inhibitors of CYP3A4 may also increase darunavir. ANTICONVULSANTS (e.g., **carbamazepine, phenobarbital, phenytoin**), CORTICOSTEROIDS (e.g., **dexamethasone**), **efavirenz,** RIFAMYCINS (e.g., **rifampin, rifabutin**), and **saquinavir** may decrease darunavir levels. Darunavir may increase the levels of AZOLE ANTIFUNGALS, CORTICOSTEROIDS, **efavirenz, indinavir,** RIFAMYCINS, **amiodarone, bepridil, lidocaine, quinidine,** CALCIUM CHANNEL BLOCKERS (e.g., **nifedipine, nicardipine, felodipine**), **clarithromycin,** IMMUNOSUPPRESSANTS (e.g., **cyclosporine, sirolimus, tacrolimus**), PHOSPHODIESTERASE TYPE 5 INHIBITORS (e.g., **sildenafil, tadalafil, vardenafil**), and trazodone, due in part to its ability to inhibit CYP3A4. Darunavir decreases the levels of the **lopinavir/ritonavir** combination, ORAL CONTRACEPTIVES (e.g., **norethindrone**), **methadone,** SELECTIVE SEROTONIN REUPTAKE INHIBITORS [SSRIS (e.g., **paroxetine, sertraline**)]. Use of BENZODIAZEPINES (e.g., **midazolam, triazolam**) increases the risk of prolonged or increased sedation or respiratory depression. Use of ERGOT ALKALOIDS may increase ergot toxicity. Coadministration with HMG-COA REDUCTASE INHIBITORS increases the risk of myopathy. Combination use with **pimozide** increases the risk of cardiac arrhythmias. **Food:** Food enhances the bioavailability of darunavir. **Herbal:** **St. John's wort** decreases the level of darunavir.

PHARMACOKINETICS **Absorption:** 82% absorbed (in combination with ritonavir). **Peak:** 2.5–4 h. **Distribution:** 95% protein bound. **Metabolism:** In the liver. **Elimination:** Primarily fecal (80%) with minor elimination in urine. **Half-Life:** 15 h.

NURSING IMPLICATIONS

Assessment & Drug Effects

- Monitor for and report S&S of pancreatitis, as this may be an indication for discontinuation of darunavir.

D

- Monitor for S&S of skin rash. Notify prescriber immediately if a severe rash appears.
- Monitor diabetics for loss of glycemic control.
- Increase monitoring of INR with concurrent warfarin therapy.
- Monitor for adverse effects or loss of efficacy of concurrent medications, as many drug interactions occur with darunavir.
- Monitor lab tests: Periodic CD4+ cell count, plasma HIV-RNA, lipid profile, LFTs, and plasma glucose.

Patient & Family Education

- Follow directions for taking the drug (see Administration). If a dose is missed by more than 6 h, wait until the next regularly scheduled dose. If a dose is missed by less than 6 h, take a dose and continue with the next regularly scheduled dose.
- Ensure that you know which medicines should **not** be taken with darunavir, as serious consequences could occur.
- Report any of the following to a healthcare provider: Blistering, redness, or peeling skin or mucous membranes; severe skin rash.
- Use or add a barrier contraceptive if using an estrogen-containing oral contraceptive if you wish to prevent pregnancy.

DASATINIB

(das-a'ti-nib)

Sprycel

Classification: ANTINEOPLASTIC BIOLOGIC RESPONSE MODIFIER; TYROSINE KINASE INHIBITOR

Therapeutic: ANTINEOPLASTIC

Prototype: Erlotinib

AVAILABILITY Tablet

ACTION & *THERAPEUTIC EFFECT* Dasatinib is a BCR-ABL tyrosine kinase inhibitor. BCR-ABL tyrosine kinase is an enzyme produced by a chromosomal translocation associated with chronic myeloid leukemia (CML) and certain types of acute lymphocytic leukemias (Ph^+ ALL). *Dasatinib inhibits the growth of CML and ALL cell lines overexpressing BCR-ABL kinase.*

USES Treatment of chronic, accelerated, or myeloid or lymphoid blast phase chronic myelogenous leukemia (CML). Treatment of Philadelphia chromosome–positive (Ph^+) acute lymphocytic leukemia (ALL) in adults.

CONTRAINDICATIONS Hypersensitivity to dasatinib; active bleeding; pulmonary arterial hypertension; hypokalemia; hypomagnesemia; pregnancy (fetal risk has been demonstrated); lactation (infant risk cannot be ruled out).

CAUTIOUS USE Hepatic impairment; bacterial or viral infection; history of GI bleeding; interstitial pneumonia; pleural effusion; bone marrow suppression; patients at risk for QT prolongation including patients with long QT syndrome; older adults. Safe use in children younger than 18 yr not established.

ROUTE & DOSAGE

CML and Philadelphia Chromosome–Positive ALL

Adult: **PO** 100 mg once daily; may increase dose to 180 mg once daily.

Chronic Phase CML

Adult: **PO** 100 mg daily

Acute Lymphoblastic Leukemia

Adult: PO 140 mg daily until disease progression

D

Toxicity Dosage Adjustment

See package insert for dosage adjustments and adjustment for concomitant strong CYP3A4 inhibitors

ADMINISTRATION

Oral

- NIOSH recommends use of single gloves by anyone handling intact tablets or capsules or administering from a unit-dose package.
- Do not crush or break tablets. They should be swallowed whole.
- Take with or without food.
- Take antacids at least 2 h prior or 2 h after dose.
- Ensure that hypokalemia and hypomagnesemia are corrected prior to administering dasatinib.
- Store at 15°–30°C (59°–86°F).

ADVERSE EFFECTS **CV:** Localized edema. **Respiratory:** Dyspnea, *pleural effusion,* pulmonary hypertension. **CNS:** *Headache.* **Endocrine:** *Body fluid retention.* **GI:** Abdominal pain, *diarrhea,* nausea, vomiting, gastrointestinal hemorrhage. **Musculoskeletal:** Pain. **Hematologic:** *Anemia,* neutropenia, *hemorrhage, neutropenia, thrombocytopenia.* **Other:** *Fatigue,* fever, sepsis.

INTERACTIONS **Drug:** AZOLE ANTIFUNGAL AGENTS (e.g., **ketoconazole, itraconazole**), MACROLIDE ANTIBIOTICS (e.g., **clarithromycin, erythromycin, telithromycin**), HIV PROTEASE INHIBITORS (e.g., **indinavir, nelfinavir, ritonavir, saquinavir**), **nefazodone,** and other inhibitors of CYP3A4 may increase dasatinib levels. Compounds that induce CYP3A4 (e.g., **carbamazepine, dexamethasone, phenobarbital, phenytoin, rifampin**) may decrease dasatinib levels. PROTON PUMP INHIBITORS may decrease dasatinib concentrations. Dasatinib may alter the plasma concentrations of other drugs that require CYP3A4 and have a narrow therapeutic window (e.g., **cyclosporine,** ERGOT ALKALOIDS). Dasatinib increases the levels of **simvastatin**. May have additive effects with QT-PROLONGING AGENTS. **Food:** Food enhances the bioavailability of dasatinib. Avoid grapefruit and grapefruit juice. **Herbal: St. John's wort** may decrease the level of dasatinib.

PHARMACOKINETICS **Peak:** 0.5–6 h. **Distribution:** 93–96% protein bound. **Metabolism:** Extensive hepatic metabolism. **Elimination:** Fecal. **Half-Life:** 3–5 h.

NURSING IMPLICATIONS

Assessment & Drug Effects

- Monitor for and report S&S of fluid retention (e.g., pleural or pericardial effusion, peripheral or pulmonary edema, ascites).
- Monitor for S&S of cardiac dysfunction (e.g., heart failure, arrhythmias). ECG monitoring may be needed to evaluate potential QT interval prolongation.
- Monitor for numerous adverse side effects of dasatinib. Immediately report suspected bleeding or infection.
- Monitor lab tests: Baseline and periodic serum potassium and magnesium; baseline CBC with differential (including ANC and platelet count), then weekly for first 2 mo, then monthly; periodic LFTs.

Patient & Family Education

- Take antacids (if needed for GI distress) 2 h before or after dasatinib.
- Do not use OTC medications for heartburn (other than antacids) without consulting prescriber.

D

- Women should use effective means of contraception to avoid pregnancy during treatment.
- Inform your prescriber if you are pregnant or planning to become pregnant, as dasatinib may harm the fetus.
- Discontinue breastfeeding as it is not known if drug is excreted in breast milk.
- Report immediately to your healthcare provider any of the following: Bleeding (including wine- or coke-colored urine, or black tarry stools) or easy bruising, fever or other signs of an infection, severe lethargy or weakness.

DASIGLUCAGON

(DAS-i-GLOO-ka-gon)

Zegalogue

Classifications: ANTIHYPOGLYCEMIC

Therapeutic: ANTIDOTE; ANTIHYPOGLYCEMIC

AVAILABILITY Single-use subcutaneous injection

ACTION & THERAPEUTIC EFFECT A glucagon receptor agonist, which stimulates glycogenolysis and hepatic gluconeogenesis, causing an increase in blood glucose levels; antihypoglycemic effect requires preexisting hepatic glycogen stores. *Increases serum glucose levels to manage hypoglycemia.*

USES Used to treat severe hypoglcemia.

CONTRAINDICATIONS Pheochromocytoma; insulinoma.

CAUTIOUS USE Hypersensitivity reaction; adrenal insufficiency; chronic hypoglycemia; starvation; pediatric patients; pregnancy (adverse events not observed in animal reproduction studies); lactation.

ROUTE & DOSAGE

Hypoglycemia

Adult/Adolescent/Child (greater than 6yo): **Subcutaneous** 0.6 mg; can repeat as needed after 15 minutes with a new device.

ADMINISTRATION

Subcutaneous

- May administer SC injection in the outer upper arms, lower abdomen, thighs, or buttocks; do not inject through clothing. If patient is unconscious, place in lateral recumbent position after injecting to prevent choking when consciousness returns.
- Administer fast-acting and long-acting oral carbohydrates to patient as soon as possible after response to treatment.
- Autoinjector: Push the device straight down into the skin until the needle guard is fully pressed down; hold the device in the skin to a count of 10 (until the medicine window is red) before removing to ensure the full dose has been administered.
- Prefilled syringe: Pinch skin and insert needle at a 45-degree angle. After inserting needle, release pinched skin and slowly depress plunger until fully depressed and syringe is empty before removing.
- Store at 20°–25°C (68°–77°F).

ADVERSE EFFECTS **CNS:** Headache. **Endocrine:** Hyperglycemia. **GI:** Nausea, vomiting, diarrhea.

INTERACTIONS Drug: Concomitant use with BETA-BLOCKERS (e.g., metoprolol) may increase pulse and blood pressure; may enhance the effects of **warfarin;** concomitant use with **indomethacin** may decrease dasiglucagon's effect on blood sugar.

PHARMACOKINETICS **Peak:** 21–35 min. **Distribution:** 47–57 L. **Metabolism:** Nonspecific proteolysis. **Half-Life:** 30 min.

NURSING IMPLICATIONS

Assessment & Drug Effects

- Monitor Bp, blood glucose, and mentation.
- Monitor for signs and symptoms of hypersensitivity reaction.

Patient & Family Education

- Call your doctor or seek medical help if any of these side effects or any other side effects bother you or do not go away: Upset stomach, throwing up, headache, diarrhea, pain where the shot was given.

DAUNORUBICIN HYDROCHLORIDE

(daw-noe-roo'bi-sin)

Cerubidine

DAUNORUBICIN CITRATED LIPOSOMAL

DaunoXome

Classification: ANTINEOPLASTIC; ANTHRACYCLINE (ANTIBIOTIC)

Therapeutic: ANTINEOPLASTIC

Prototype: Doxorubicin HCl

AVAILABILITY **Daunorubicin HCl:** Solution for injection. **Daunorubicin Citrated Liposomal:** Solution for injection

ACTION & *THERAPEUTIC EFFECT* Cytotoxic and antimitotic anthracycline antibiotic that is cell cycle specific for S-phase of cell division. Has rapid interaction with the DNA molecule changing its shape, thus resulting in inhibition of DNA, RNA, and protein synthesis. *Antineoplastic effects against acute leukemias with decreased incidence of cardiotoxicity than doxorubicin.*

D

USES To induce remission in acute nonlymphocytic/lymphocytic leukemia, advanced HIV-associated Kaposi sarcoma.

UNLABELED USES Non-Hodgkin lymphoma.

CONTRAINDICATIONS Severe myelosuppression; immunizations (patient, family), and preexisting cardiac disease unless risk-benefit is evaluated; uncontrolled systemic infection; pregnancy (category D); lactation.

CAUTIOUS USE History of gout, urate calculi, hepatic or renal function impairment; older adults with inadequate bone reserve due to age or previous cytotoxic drug therapy, radiation therapy, tumor cell infiltration of bone marrow, patient who has received potentially cardiotoxic drugs or related antineoplastics; children.

ROUTE & DOSAGE

Neoplasms

Adult (younger than 60 yr): **IV** 45 mg/m²/day on days 1, 2, and 3 of first course then days 1 and 2 of subsequent courses (max total cumulative dose: 500–600 mg/m²); *60 yr or older:* 30 mg/m²/day on days 1, 2, and 3 of first course then days 1 and 2 of subsequent courses
Child (2 yr or older): **IV** As combination therapy, 25 mg/m² weekly; *Younger than 2 yr:* 1 mg/kg

Kaposi Sarcoma (DaunoXome)

Adult: **IV** 40 mg/m² over 1 h, repeat q2wk (withhold therapy if granulocyte count less than 750 cells/mm^3)

Renal Impairment Dosage Adjustment

If serum Cr greater than 3 mg/dL: Give 50% of dose

Hepatic Impairment Dosage Adjustment

Total bilirubin 1.2–3 mg/dL: Give 50% of dose
Greater than 3–5 mg/dL: Give 25% of dose
Greater than 5 mg/dL: Omit dose

ADMINISTRATION

Intravenous

Hazardous Agent: Use double gloves and gown during preparation and administration for infusion to prevent skin contact with this drug. If contact occurs, decontaminate skin with copious amounts of water with soap.

Daunorubicin HCl

PREPARE: **Direct:** Reconstitute 20-mg vial with 4 mL sterile water for injection. The concentration of the solution will be 5 mg/mL. ▪ Withdraw dose into syringe containing 10–15 mL normal saline. **IV Infusion:** Dilute further in 100 mL NS or D5W as required.

ADMINISTER: **Direct:** Inject over approximately 3 min into the tubing or side arm of a rapidly flowing IV infusion of D5W or NS. **Infusion:** Give a single dose over 30–45 min.

DaunoXome

PREPARE: **IV Infusion:** Each vial of **DaunoXome** contains the equivalent of 50 mg daunorubicin base. Dilute with enough D5W to produce a concentration of 1 mg/1 mL.

ADMINISTER: **IV Infusion:** Give **DaunoXome** over 60 min. Do not use a filter with **DaunoXome.**

INCOMPATIBILITIES: **Solution/additive:** **Dexamethasone, heparin.** **Y-site:** **Acyclovir, allopurinol, aminophylline, amphotericin B, ampicillin, aztreonam, cefazolin sodium, cefepime, cefoperazone, cefotaxime, cefotetan disodium, cefoxitin, ceftazidime, ceftriaxone, cefuroxime, chloramphenicol, dantrolene, dexamethasone, diazepam, ertapenem sodium, fludarabine phosphate, foscarnet sodium, fosphenytoin sodium, furosemide, gallium nitrate, ganciclovir, sodium, heparin sodium, indomethacin sodium, ketorolac tromethamine, lansoprazole, levofloxacin, methohexital sodium, methylprednisolone sodium succinate, mitoxantrone hydrochloride, nafcillin sodium, nitroprusside sodium, pantoprazole sodium, pemetrexed disodium, pentobarbital sodium, phenobarbital sodium, piperacillin/tazobactam, sulfamethoxazole-trimethoprim, thiopental sodium.**

- Avoid extravasation because it can cause severe tissue necrosis.
- Store reconstituted solution at room temperature (15°–30°C; 59°–86°F) for 24 h and under refrigeration at 2°–8°C (36°–46°F) for 48 h. Protect from light.

ADVERSE EFFECTS

CV: Pericarditis, myocarditis, arrhythmias, chest pain, EKG abnormality, cardiac arrest, peripheral edema, CHF, hypertension, tachycardia. **CNS:** Amnesia, anxiety, ataxia, confusion, hallucinations, emotional lability, tremors. **Endocrine:** Hyperuricemia, gonadal suppression. **Skin:** Generalized *alopecia* (reversible), transverse pigmentation of nails, discoloration of sweat and tears, severe cellulitis or tissue necrosis at site of drug extravasation. **GI:** *Acute nausea and vomiting* (mild), anorexia, *stomatitis,* mucositis, discoloration of saliva, diarrhea (occasionally), hemorrhage. **GU:** Dysuria, red urine discoloration, nocturia, polyuria, dry skin. **Hematologic:** Bone marrow depression thrombocytopenia, leukopenia, anemia. **Other:** Fever.

PHARMACOKINETICS **Distribution:** Highest concentrations in spleen, kidneys, liver, lungs, and heart; does not cross blood–brain barrier; crosses placenta. **Metabolism:** In liver to active metabolite. **Elimination:** 25% in urine, 40% in bile. **Half-Life:** 18.5–26.7 h.

NURSING IMPLICATIONS

Black Box Warning

Daunorubicin has been associated with cardiac toxicity and CHF, severe local tissue necrosis, bone marrow suppression, dosages reduced with impaired renal or hepatic function.

Assessment & Drug Effects

- Monitor infusion site closely. With daunorubicin hydrochloride severe local tissue necrosis will result if extravasation occurs. In the event of extravasation, stop the infusion and do not flush. Leave the catheter or needle in place. Note that liposomal daunorubicin is not known to cause tissue damage with extravasation.
- Monitor during infusion of liposomal daunorubicin for back pain, flushing, and chest tightness. These symptoms may occur during the first 5 min of infusion. They subside when infusion is stopped and typically do not return if infusion resumed at a slower rate.
- Monitor serum bilirubin; drug dose needs to be reduced when bilirubin is greater than 1.2 mg/dL.
- Monitor BP, temperature, pulse, and respiratory function during treatment.
- Monitor for S&S of acute CHF. It can occur suddenly or in patients with compromised heart function because of previous radiation therapy to heart area.
- Report immediately: Breathlessness, orthopnea, change in pulse and BP parameters. Early clinical diagnosis of drug-induced CHF is essential for successful treatment.
- Report promptly S&S of superinfections including elevation of temperature, chills, upper respiratory tract infection, tachycardia, overgrowth with opportunistic organisms because myelosuppression imposes risk of superimposed infection (see Appendix F).
- Control nausea and vomiting (usually mild) by antiemetic therapy.
- Inspect oral membranes. Mucositis may occur 3–7 days after drug is administered.
- Monitor lab tests: Baseline and periodic Hct, platelet count, total and differential leukocyte count, serum uric acid, LFTs, and renal function tests.

Patient & Family Education

- Avoid contact with persons with infections. The most hazardous period is when the WBC count is most suppressed.
- Use barrier contraceptives during treatment because this drug is teratogenic. Tell your prescriber immediately if you become pregnant during therapy.

▪ Note: A transient effect of the drug is to turn urine red on the day of infusion.

D

DECITABINE

(de-sit'a-bine)

Dacogen

Classification: ANTINEOPLASTIC; ANTIMETABOLITE; PYRIMIDINE

Therapeutic: ANTINEOPLASTIC

Prototype: 5-Fluorouracil

AVAILABILITY Lyophilized powder for injection

ACTION & *THERAPEUTIC EFFECT* An antimetabolite that exerts antineoplastic effects after its direct incorporation into DNA and inhibition of DNA transferase, causing loss of cell differentiation and cell death. Nonproliferating cells are resistant to the effects of decitabine. *Decitabine-induced changes in neoplastic cells may restore normal function to genes that are critical for control of cellular differentiation and proliferation.*

USES Treatment of patients with myelodysplastic syndrome (MDS).

UNLABELED USES Treatment of chronic myelogenous leukemia (CML).

CONTRAINDICATIONS Pregnancy (category D); lactation.

CAUTIOUS USE Moderate to severe renal failure; hepatic impairment; older adults. Safety and efficacy in children not established.

ROUTE & DOSAGE

Myelodysplastic Syndrome

Adult: **IV** 15 mg/m^2 q8h × 3 days; repeat q6w for at least 4 cycles; or 20 mg/m^2 × 5 days q4w.

ADMINISTRATION

Intravenous

PREPARE: **IV Infusion:** Caution should be exercised when handling and preparing decitabine. Procedures for proper handling and disposal of antineoplastic drugs should be applied. ▪ Reconstitute each vial with 10 mL sterile water for injection to yield approximately 5-mg/mL at pH 6.7–7.3. Immediately after reconstitution, further dilute with NS, D5W, or LR to a final drug concentration of 0.1–1 mg/mL. ▪ Use within 15 min of reconstitution (see Storage).

ADMINISTER: **IV infusion:** Premedicate with standard antiemetic therapy. Give 15 mg/m^2 dose over 3 h and 20-mg/m^2 dose over 1 h.

▪ Store vials at 15°–30°C (59°–86°F). Unless used within 15 min of reconstitution, the diluted solution **must be** prepared using cold (2°–8°C) infusion fluids and stored at 2°–8°C (36°–46°F) for up to a maximum of 7 h until administration.

ADVERSE EFFECTS **CV:** Edema, heart murmur, *peripheral edema,* congestive heart failure. **Respiratory:** *Cough,* decreased breath sounds, epistaxis, <u>hypoxia</u>, pharyngitis, URI, pneumonia, pulmonary edema. **CNS:** Weakness, dizziness, *headache,* reduced touch sensation, *insomnia,* lethargy, shivering. **Endocrine:** *Hyperglycemia,* hyperkalemia, hypoalbuminemia, hypokalemia, hypomagnesemia, hyponatremia, abnormal serum bicarbonate. **Skin:** Cellulitis, bruising, erythema, pruritus, rash, skin lesions. **Hepatic:** Increased alkaline phosphatase, ascites, hyperbilirubinemia, increased liver aminotransferase. **GI:** Abdominal pain, *constipation,* decreased appetite, *diarrhea,* indigestion, *nausea,* stomatitis, *vomiting.* **GU:** Frequent urination, increased BUN. **Musculoskeletal:** Joint pain, backache, limb pain. **Hematologic:** *Leukopenia, anemia, febrile neutropenia, neutropenia, thrombocytopenia.* **Other:** *Fatigue, fever,* pain, tenderness, anxiety, confusion.

INTERACTIONS Drug: Avoid LIVE VACCINES. Use with **deferiprone, dipyrone,** or **palifermin** may increase adverse effects.

PHARMACOKINETICS Distribution: Negligible plasma protein binding. **Half-Life:** 0.2–0.8 h.

NURSING IMPLICATIONS

Assessment & Drug Effects

- Withhold dose and notify prescriber of any of the following: Absolute neutrophil count (ANC) less than 1000/mcL; platelet count less than 50,000/mcL; serum creatinine at 2 mg/dL or higher; ALT, total bilirubin 2 × ULN or more; or an active or uncontrolled infection.
- Monitor for and report S&S of pulmonary or peripheral edema, cardiac arrhythmias, new-onset depression, or infection.
- Avoid IM injections with platelet counts less than 50,000/mcL.
- Monitor diabetics for loss of glycemic control.
- Monitor lab tests: CBC with differentials and platelet count prior to each chemotherapy cycle; baseline and periodic LFTs and serum creatinine.

Patient & Family Education

- Do not accept vaccinations during treatment with decitabine.
- Avoid contact with anyone who recently received the oral poliovirus vaccine.
- Women of childbearing age should avoid becoming pregnant while receiving decitabine.
- Men should not father a child while receiving decitabine and for 2 mo after the end of therapy.
- Report any of the following to a healthcare provider: Signs of infection such as fever, chills, sore throat; signs of bleeding such as easy bruising, black tarry stools, blood in the urine; irregular heart rate; significant tiredness or weakness.

DEFEROXAMINE MESYLATE

(de-fer-ox′a-meen)

Desferal

Classification: CHELATING AGENT; ANTIDOTE

Therapeutic: ANTIDOTE

AVAILABILITY Powder for injection

ACTION & *THERAPEUTIC EFFECT* Chelating agent with specific affinity for ferric ion and low affinity for calcium. Binds ferric ions to form a stable water-soluble chelate readily excreted by kidneys. *Main effect is removal of iron from ferritin, hemosiderin, and transferrin in iron toxicity.*

USES Adjunct in treatment of acute iron intoxication or iron overload.

UNLABELED USES Aluminum toxicity.

CONTRAINDICATIONS Severe renal disease, anuria, pyelonephritis; primary hemochromatosis; acute infection.

CAUTIOUS USE History of pyelonephritis; cardiac dysfunction; aluminum overload; older adults; pregnancy (category C); lactation; infants and children younger than 3 yr.

ROUTE & DOSAGE

Acute Iron Intoxication

Adult: **IM/IV** 1 g followed by 500 mg at 4 h intervals for 2 doses, subsequent doses of 500 mg

q4–12h may be given if necessary (max: 6 g/24 h), infuse at 15 mg/kg/h or less
Child (3 yr or older): **IV** 15 mg/kg/h (max: 6 g/24 h); **IM** 40–90 mg/kg (up to 1 g) q4–8h

Chronic Iron Overload

Adult: **IM** 500 mg–1 g/day; **Subcutaneous** 1–2 g/day (20–40 mg/kg/day) infused over 8–24 h
Child (3 yr or older): **IM** 500 mg–1 g/day; **Subcutaneous** 20–40 mg/kg/day over 8–12 h

ADMINISTRATION

Subcutaneous

- Reconstitute by adding 5 mL sterile water for injection to each 500-mg vial or 20 mL to each 2-gram vial to yield 100 mg/mL. Dissolve completely.
- Give subcutaneously over 8–24 h using a portable minipump device.

Intramuscular

- Reconstitute by adding 2 mL sterile water for injection to 500-mg vial or 8 mL to the 2-g vial to yield 250 mg/mL. Dissolve completely.
- Use IM route for all patients not in shock; preferred route for acute intoxication.

Intravenous

For infants and children: Verify correct IV concentration and rate with prescriber.

PREPARE: **IV Infusion:** Reconstitute by adding 5 mL sterile water for injection to 500-mg vial to yield 100 mg/mL. ▪ After drug is completely dissolved, withdraw prescribed amount from vial and add to NS, D5W, or LR solution.

ADMINISTER: **IV Infusion:** *Adult:* Give initial dose at a rate not to exceed 15 mg/kg/h; give two subsequent 500-mg doses at 125 mg/h; give any additional doses over 4–12 h. *Child:* Give at 15 mg/kg/h. ▪ Do not infuse IV rapidly; such infusion is associated with the occurrence of more adverse effects.

INCOMPATIBILITIES: **Solution/additive: Iron dextran.**

- Store at room temperature 15°–30°C (59°–86°F) for not longer than 1 wk. Protect from light.

ADVERSE EFFECTS **CV:** Hypotension, tachycardia. **HEENT:** Decreased hearing; blurred vision, decreased visual acuity and visual fields, color vision abnormalities, night blindness, retinal pigmentary degeneration. **GI:** Abdominal discomfort, diarrhea. **GU:** Dysuria, exacerbation of pyelonephritis, orange-rose discoloration of urine. **Other:** Hypersensitivity (generalized itching, cutaneous wheal formation, rash, fever, <u>anaphylactoid reaction</u>). *Pain and induration at injection site.*

INTERACTIONS **Drug:** Use with **ascorbic acid** increases cardiac risk, **prochlorperazine** may cause loss of consciousness.

PHARMACOKINETICS **Distribution:** Widely distributed in body tissues. **Metabolism:** Forms nontoxic complex with iron. **Elimination:** Primarily in urine; some in feces.

NURSING IMPLICATIONS

Black Box Warning

Deferoxamine has been associated with potentially fatal acute renal failure, hepatic failure, and GI hemorrhage.

Assessment & Drug Effects

- Monitor injection site. If pain and induration occur, move infusion to another site.

- Monitor I&O ratio and pattern. Report any change. Observe stools for blood (iron intoxication frequently causes necrosis of GI tract).
- Monitor for S&S of GI bleeding and/or ulceration; older adults are especially at risk when they have conditions causing low platelet counts.
- Note: Periodic ophthalmoscopic (slit lamp) examinations and audiometry are advised for patients on prolonged or high-dose therapy for chronic iron overload.
- Monitor lab tests: Baseline and periodic renal function tests.

Patient & Family Education

- Deferoxamine chelate makes urine turn a reddish color.
- Report promptly signs of GI bleeding.
- Consult prescriber if you are concurrently taking drugs than can cause GI bleeding such as NSAIDs, corticosteroids, oral osteoporosis drugs, or anticoagulants.
- Report blurred vision or any other visual abnormality.

DEGARELIX ACETATE

(de-ga′re-lix)

Firmagon

Classification: GONADOTROPIN-RELEASING HORMONE (GNRH) ANTAGONIST

Therapeutic: GNRH ANTAGONIST

Prototype: Ganirelix acetate

AVAILABILITY Powder for injection

ACTION & *THERAPEUTIC EFFECT* It binds reversibly to pituitary GnRH receptors, reducing release of gonadotropins and, consequently, testosterone. *Testosterone suppression slows growth of androgen-sensitive prostate cancer cells as indicated by decrease in PSA values.*

USES Treatment of advanced prostate cancer.

CONTRAINDICATIONS Hypersensitivity to degarelix; women who are or may become pregnant (category X); lactation.

CAUTIOUS USE Congenital long QT syndrome; electrolyte abnormalities; CHF; older adults. Safety and efficacy in children not established.

ROUTE & DOSAGE

Prostate Cancer

Adult: **Subcutaneous** Initial dose of 240 mg in two 120-mg injections, followed by 80 mg q28days

ADMINISTRATION

Subcutaneous

- Glove should be worn for reconstitution. Follow carefully manufacturer's guidelines for reconstitution of the powder vial.
- Administer into the abdominal area within 1 h of reconstitution.
- Initial dose: Give as 2 subcutaneous injections of 120 mg each (at a concentration of 40 mg/mL).
- Maintenance dose: Give 1 subcutaneous injection of 80 mg (at a concentration of 20 mg/mL).
- Store at 25°C (77°F), excursions permitted at 15°–30°C (59°–86°F).

ADVERSE EFFECTS **CV:** *Hot flashes*, hypertension. **CNS:** Asthenia, chills, dizziness, fatigue, fever, headache, insomnia. **Endocrine:** Increases in ALT, AST, and GGT,

D

weight gain. **GI:** Constipation, nausea, diarrhea. **GU:** Erectile dysfunction, gynecomastia, testicular atrophy, urinary tract infections. **Musculoskeletal:** Arthralgia, back pain. **Other:** *Injection-site reactions*, night sweats.

INTERACTIONS Drug: Degarelix may cause an additive effect with other drugs that prolong the QT interval prolongation (e.g., ANTIARRHYTHMIC AGENTS, **chlorpromazine, dolasetron, droperidol, mefloquine, mesoridazine, moxifloxacin, pentamidine, pimozide, tacrolimus, thioridazine, ziprasidone**).

PHARMACOKINETICS Peak: 2 days. **Distribution:** 90% plasma protein bound. **Metabolism:** Hepatobiliary. **Elimination:** Biliary excretion 70–80%; urinary excretion 20–30%. **Half-Life:** 53 days.

NURSING IMPLICATIONS

Assessment & Drug Effects

- Monitor ECG and QT interval, especially with electrolyte imbalances, a history of CHF, and concurrent Class IA (e.g., quinidine) or III (e.g., amiodarone) antiarrhythmics.
- Monitor lab tests: Baseline and periodic PSA and serum testosterone; periodic LFTs.

Patient & Family Education

- Hot flashes are a common side effect that usually subside spontaneously.
- Degarelix can decrease bone density leading to osteoporosis. With long-term therapy, bone density tests are advisable, and supplemental calcium and vitamin D may reduce the risk of osteoporosis.

DELAFLOXACIN

(del-a-floks′a-sin)

Baxdela

Classification: QUINOLONE ANTIBIOTIC; ANTIBIOTIC

Therapeutic: ANTIBIOTIC

Prototype: Ciprofloxacin

AVAILABILITY Tablet; powder for injection

ACTION & *THERAPEUTIC EFFECT* Inhibits DNA gyrase and topoisomerase enzymes, which are required for bacterial DNA replication, transcription, repair, and recombination. *Used to treat acute bacterial skin infections.*

USES Treatment of bacterial skin and skin structure infections.

CONTRAINDICATIONS Hypersensitivity to delafloxacin, quinolone antibiotics, or components of the tablet or powdered injection.

CAUTIOUS USE Hypersensitivity to delafloxacin, other fluoroquinolones, or any component of the formulation; myasthenia gravis; renal impairment; elderly; pregnancy; lactation. Safety and efficacy in patients younger than 18 yr not established.

ROUTE & DOSAGE

Infection

Adult: **PO** 450 mg bid for 5–14 days; **IV** 300 mg bid for 5–14 days

Renal Impairment Dosage Adjustment

CrCL 15–29 mL/min: **IV** 200 mg bid; **PO** No adjustment
CrCL less than 15 mL/min: **IV** Do not use; **PO** No adjustment

ADMINISTRATION

Oral

- Administer with or without food at least 2 h before or 6 h after antacids containing magnesium or aluminum, sucralfate, metal cations, or multivitamins containing zinc or iron.

Intravenous

PREPARE: **IV Infusion:** Reconstitute 300-mg vials with 10.5 mL of D5W or NS, and shake vigorously until completely dissolved. Then dilute to a total volume of 250 mL with NS or D5W.
ADMINISTER: Administer intravenously over 60 min. Do not administer with any solution containing multivalent cations (calcium or magnesium) through the same IV line. Do not infuse with other medications.
INCOMPATIBILITIES: Not compatible with solutions containing multivalent cations (e.g., calcium or magnesium).

ADVERSE EFFECTS **CNS:** Headache. **GI:** *Nausea, diarrhea*. **Hepatic:** Increased serum transaminase.

INTERACTIONS **DRUG: Magnesium** or **aluminum-**containing antacids, **sucralfate, iron, calcium, zinc** may decrease absorption of delafloxacin. NSAIDS may increase risk of CNS reactions, including seizures; may cause hyper- or hypoglycemia in patients on ORAL HYPOGLYCEMIC AGENTS. Do not use with agents known to prolong QT interval **(bepridil, dofetilide, dronedarone, thioridazine, ziprasidone).**

PHARMACOKINETICS **Absorption: PO** 59% bioavailability, unaffected by food. **Distribution:** 84% protein (albumin) bound. **Metabolism:** Glucuronidation through UGT_1A_1, UGT_1A_3, and UGT_2B_{15}. **Elimination: PO** 50% in urine, 48% in feces; **IV** 65% in urine, 28% in feces. **Half-Life: PO** 4–8 h (multiple dose); **IV** 4 h.

NURSING IMPLICATIONS

Black Box Warning

Quinolone antibiotics have been associated with tendinitis and tendon rupture; drug may exacerbate muscle weakness in those with MG. Quinolone antibiotics are also associated with peripheral neuropathy and central nervous system effects.

Assessment & Drug Effects

- Monitor for signs of infection.
- Routine monitoring of WBC and serum creatinine.

Patient & Family Education

- Notify prescriber if you have symptoms of irritated or torn tendons or nerve problems in the arms, hands, legs, or feet.
- Notify prescriber if you experience signs or symptoms of allergic reaction such as rash, hives, itching, shortness of breath, wheezing, cough, swelling of the face, lips, tongue, or throat; or any other signs.

DELAVIRDINE MESYLATE

(del-a-vir′deen)

Rescriptor

Classification: ANTIVIRAL; NONNUCLEOSIDE REVERSE TRANSCRIPTASE INHIBITOR (NNRTI)

Therapeutic: ANTIVIRAL; NNRTI

Prototype: Efavirenz

D

AVAILABILITY Tablet

ACTION & *THERAPEUTIC EFFECT* Nonnucleoside reverse transcriptase inhibitor (NNRTI) of HIV-1 binds directly to reverse transcriptase (RT) and disrupts RNA- and DNA-dependent DNA polymerase activities. *Prevents replication of the HIV-1 virus; resistant strains appear rapidly.*

USES Treatment of HIV infection in combination with other antiretroviral agents.

UNLABELED USES HIV prophylaxis.

CONTRAINDICATIONS Hypersensitivity to delavirdine; lactation.

CAUTIOUS USE Impaired liver function; older adults; autoimmune disorders, achlorhydria; pregnancy (category C). Safety and efficacy in combination with other antiretroviral agents not established in children younger than 16 yr.

ROUTE & DOSAGE

HIV Infection

Adult/Adolescent: **PO** 400 mg tid

ADMINISTRATION

Oral

- Disperse in water by adding a single dose to at least 3 oz of water, let it stand for a few minutes, then stir to create a uniform suspension just prior to administration.
- Administer with or without food.
- Antacids should be given 1 h before or 1 h after the dose.
- Give drug to patients with achlorhydria with an acid beverage such as orange or cranberry juice.
- Store at 20°–25°C (68°–77°F) and protect from high humidity in a tightly closed container.

ADVERSE EFFECTS **Respiratory:** Bronchitis. **CNS:** Headache, depression, anxiety. **Skin:** *Rash*. **GI:** *Nausea*, vomiting, abdominal pain. **Other:** Fever.

INTERACTIONS **Drug:** ANTACIDS, H_2-RECEPTOR ANTAGONISTS decrease absorption; **didanosine** and **delavirdine** should be taken 1 h apart to avoid decreased delavirdine levels; **clarithromycin, fluoxetine, ketoconazole** may increase delavirdine levels; **carbamazepine, phenobarbital, phenytoin, rifabutin, rifampin** may decrease delavirdine levels; delavirdine may increase levels of **clarithromycin, indinavir, saquinavir, dapsone, rifabutin, alprazolam, midazolam, triazolam,** DIHYDROPYRIDINE, CALCIUM CHANNEL BLOCKERS (e.g., **nifedipine, nicardipine,** etc.), **quinidine, warfarin.** Use with HMG-COA REDUCTASE INHIBITORS may increase the risk of rhabdomyolysis. Use with **pimozide** may cause cardiac arrhythmias. Use with HYPNOTICS, **alprazolam, midazolam, triazolam** can cause respiratory depression. **Herbal: St. John's wort** may decrease antiretroviral activity.

PHARMACOKINETICS Absorption: Rapidly from GI tract, 80% reaches systemic circulation. **Peak:** 1h. **Distribution:** 98% protein bound. **Metabolism:** In the liver by CYP3A4. **Elimination:** Half in urine, 44% in feces. **Half-Life:** 2–11 h.

NURSING IMPLICATIONS

Assessment & Drug Effects

- Therapeutic effectiveness: Indicated by decreased viral load.
- Monitor for and immediately report appearance of a rash, generally within 1–3 wk of starting therapy; rash is usually diffuse, maculopapular, erythematous, and pruritic.

Patient & Family Education

- Take this drug exactly as prescribed. Missed doses increase risk of drug resistance.
- Do not take antacids and delavirdine at the same time; separate by at least 1 h.
- Report all prescription and nonprescription drugs used to prescriber because of multiple drug interactions.
- Discontinue medication and notify prescriber if rash is accompanied by any of the following: Fever, blistering, oral lesions, conjunctivitis, swelling, muscle or joint pain.

DEMECLOCYCLINE HYDROCHLORIDE

(dem-e-kloe-sye'kleen)

Declomycin

Classification: ANTIBIOTIC; TETRACYCLINE

Therapeutic: ANTIBIOTIC

Prototype: Tetracycline

AVAILABILITY Capsule; tablet

ACTION & *THERAPEUTIC EFFECT* Demeclocycline blocks the binding of transfer RNA (tRNA) to messenger RNA (mRNA) of bacteria. Therefore, bacterial protein synthesis is inhibited and bacterial cells are destroyed. *Effective against both gram-positive and gram-negative bacteria.*

USES Similar to those of tetracycline.

UNLABELED USES Treatment of chronic SIADH (syndrome of inappropriate antidiuretic hormone) secretion.

CONTRAINDICATIONS Hypersensitivity to any of the tetracyclines; severe renal or hepatic disease; cirrhosis, common bile duct obstruction; period of tooth development in fetus; pregnancy (category D); lactation; children younger than 8 yr (causes permanent yellow discoloration of teeth, enamel hypoplasia, and retarded bone growth).

CAUTIOUS USE Mild or moderate impaired renal or hepatic function; nephrogenic diabetes insipidus.

D

ROUTE & DOSAGE

Anti-Infective

Adult: **PO** 150 mg q6h or 300 mg q12h (max: 2.4 g/day)
Child (8 yr or older): **PO** 8–12 mg/kg/day divided q8–12h

Gonorrhea

Adult: **PO** 600 mg followed by 300 mg q12h for 4 days

SIADH

Adult: **PO** 600–1200 mg/day in 3–4 divided doses

ADMINISTRATION

Oral

- Give not less than 1 h before or 2 h after meals. Foods rich in iron (e.g., red meat or dark green vegetables) or calcium (e.g., milk products) impair absorption.
- Concomitant therapy: Do not give antacids with tetracyclines.
- Check expiration date before giving drug. Renal damage and death have resulted from use of outdated tetracyclines.
- Store in tight, light-resistant containers, preferably at 15°–30°C (59°–86°F) unless otherwise directed. Tetracyclines form toxic products when outdated or exposed to light, heat, or humidity.

ADVERSE EFFECTS **Skin:** Pruritus, erythematous eruptions, exfoliative dermatitis. **GI:** *Nausea,* vomiting, *diarrhea,* esophageal irritation or ulceration, enterocolitis, abdominal cramps, anorexia. **GU:** Diabetes insipidus, azotemia, hyperphosphatemia. **Other:** Hypersensitivity [*photosensitivity,* pericarditis, anaphylaxis (rare)].

DIAGNOSTIC TEST INTERFERENCE

Like other tetracyclines, demeclocycline may cause false increases in ***urine catecholamines*** (***fluorometric*** methods); false decreases in ***urine urobilinogen;*** and false-negative ***urine glucose*** with ***glucose oxidase*** methods (e.g., ***Clinistix, TesTape***).

INTERACTIONS **Drug:** ANTACIDS, IRON PREPARATION, **calcium, magnesium, zinc, kaolin pectin, sodium bicarbonate** can significantly decrease demeclocycline absorption; effects of **desmopressin** and demeclocycline antagonized; increases **digoxin** absorption, increasing risk of **digoxin** toxicity; **methoxyflurane** increases risk of renal failure. **Food: Dairy** products significantly decrease demeclocycline absorption; food may decrease drug absorption also.

PHARMACOKINETICS **Absorption:** 60–80% absorbed from GI tract. **Peak:** 3–4 h. **Distribution:** Concentrated in liver; crosses placenta; distributed into breast milk. **Metabolism:** In liver; enterohepatic circulation. **Elimination:** 40–50% excreted in urine and 31% in feces in 48 h. **Half-Life:** 10–17 h.

NURSING IMPLICATIONS

Assessment & Drug Effects

- Monitor I&O ratio and pattern and record weights in patients with impaired kidney or liver function, or on prolonged or high-dose therapy.
- Monitor lab tests: Baseline C&S and, with prolonged therapy, periodic serum electrolytes, kidney function, and LFTs.

Patient & Family Education

- Do not use antacids while taking this drug.
- Take drug on an empty stomach to enhance absorption. Because esophageal irritation and ulceration have been reported, take each dose with a full glass (240 mL) of water; remain upright for at least 90 sec after taking medication; and avoid taking drug within 1 h of lying down or bedtime.
- Notify prescriber if gastric distress is a problem; a snack or light meal free of dairy products may be added to the regimen.
- Report symptoms of superinfections (see Appendix F).
- Demeclocycline-induced phototoxic reaction can be unusually severe. Avoid sunlight as much as possible, and use sunscreen.

DENOSUMAB

(den-o′su-mab)

Prolia, Xgeva

Classification: MONOCLONAL ANTIBODY; RANK LIGAND INHIBITOR; BONE RESORPTION INHIBITOR

Therapeutic: MONOCLONAL ANTIBODY; BONE RESORPTION INHIBITOR

AVAILABILITY Solution for injection

ACTION & *THERAPEUTIC EFFECT* Denosumab prevents RANKL (receptor activator of nuclear factor κB ligand, a protein essential for survival of osteoclasts) from activating its receptor, RANK, on the surface of osteoclasts. Prevention of the RANKL/RANK interaction inhibits osteoclast formation, function, and survival. *Decreases bone resorption and increases bone mass and strength.*

USES Treatment of osteoporosis; prevention of bone loss in patients with prostate or breast cancer, giant cell tumor of bone, hypercalcemia; bone metastases from solid tumor, multiple myeloma.

CONTRAINDICATIONS Preexisting hypocalcemia; lactation; pregnancy (category X) for **Prolia** and pregnancy (category D) for **Xgeva.**

CAUTIOUS USE Predisposition to hypocalcemia and electrolyte imbalance (e.g., history of hypoparathyroidism, thyroid or parathyroid surgery, malabsorption syndromes, removal of small intestine, severe renal impairment [(creatinine clearance less than 30 mL/min) or on dialysis]; dental work such as tooth extraction and/or infection; poor dental hygiene, or use of a dental appliance; any serious infection; older adults; presence of bone fractures. Safety and efficacy in children younger than 18 yr not established. **Xgeva** has been used in children older than 13 yr with skeletally mature status.

ROUTE & DOSAGE

Osteoporosis, Bone Loss in Cancer Patients

Adult: **Subcutaneous** 60 mg every 6 m

Hypercalcemia of Malignancy/ Giant Cell Tumor/Bone Metastases from Solid Tumor

Adult: **Subcutaneous** 120 mg every 4 wk (additional 120 mg on day 8 and 15 in first mo)

D

ADMINISTRATION

Subcutaneous

- Ensure that hypocalcemia is corrected prior to initiation of therapy.
- Bring syringe to room temperature by removing from refrigeration 15–30 min prior to injection. Do not warm any other way.
- Inject into upper arm, upper thigh, or abdomen.
- Store refrigerated.

ADVERSE EFFECTS **CV:** Peripheral edema, hypertension. **Respiratory:** Dyspnea, cough, upper respiratory tract. **CNS:** *Fatigue,* headache. **Endocrine:** Hypophosphatemia, hypocalcemia. **Skin:** Skin rash, dermatitis, eczema. **GI:** Diarrhea, *nausea,* decreased appetite, vomiting, constipation. **Musculoskeletal:** *Weakness,* back pain, arthralgia, limb pain. **Hematologic:** Anemia, thrombocytopenia.

INTERACTIONS Do not use with MONOCLONAL ANTIBODIES as that can increase toxic effect.

PHARMACOKINETICS **Peak:** 10 day. **Half-Life:** 25.4 day.

NURSING IMPLICATIONS

Assessment & Drug Effects

- Monitor for S&S of hypocalcemia (see Appendix F) and report immediately if any of these appear.
- Monitor for and report promptly any of the following: S&S of infection; skin reaction such as dermatitis, eczema, rash; or jaw pain.
- Monitor lab tests: Baseline and periodic serum creatinine, calcium, phosphorus, and magnesium.

Patient & Family Education

- Ensure that calcium and vitamin D supplements (usually 1000 mg calcium and at least 400 IU vitamin D daily) are taken exactly as ordered.
- Notify your prescriber immediately if you develop any of the following: S&S of low calcium (e.g., spasms, twitches, cramps; numbness or tingling in your fingers, toes, or around your mouth); S&S of infection (e.g., fever or chills; skin that is red, hot, or swollen; abdominal pain; frequency, urgency, or burning with urination); signs of skin irritation (e.g., rash, itching, peeling); jaw pain.
- Practice meticulous oral hygiene while you are taking this drug.
- Inform prescriber if you become pregnant while taking this drug.

DESIPRAMINE HYDROCHLORIDE

(dess-ip′ra-meen)

Norpramin

Classification: TRICYCLIC ANTIDEPRESSANT

Therapeutic: TRICYCLIC ANTIDEPRESSANT

Prototype: Imipramine

AVAILABILITY Tablet

ACTION & *THERAPEUTIC EFFECT* Antidepressant activity appears to be related to blocking reuptake of norepinephrine and serotonin in the CNS, thus increasing their levels. *Has antidepressant activity.*

USES Treatment of depression.

UNLABELED USES Irritable bowel syndrome, bulimia,

diabetic neuropathy, panic disorder, postherpetic neuralgia.

CONTRAINDICATIONS Hypersensitivity to tricyclic compounds; recent MI, QT prolongation, cardiac arrhythmias, AV block, bundle branch block; concurrent use of MAOI therapy; suicidal ideation; lactation.

CAUTIOUS USE Urinary retention, prostatic hypertrophy; narrow-angle glaucoma; epilepsy; alcoholism; adolescents, older adults; bipolar disease; thyroid; cardiovascular, renal, and hepatic disease; suicidal tendency; ECT; elective surgery; pregnancy (may be associated with irritability, jitteriness, and convulsions in the neonate). Safe use in children younger than 6 yr is not established.

ROUTE & DOSAGE

Depression

Adult/Adolescent: **PO** 25–50 mg/day at bedtime or in divided doses, may gradually increase to 150–300 mg/day (use lower doses in older adult patients)

Child (6–12 yr): **PO** 1–3 mg/kg/day in divided doses (max: 5 mg/kg/day)

Pharmacogenetic Dosage Adjustment

CYP2D6 poor metabolizers: Start with 40% of normal dose

ADMINISTRATION

Oral

- Give drug with food to reduce possibility of gastric irritation.
- Give maintenance dose at bedtime to minimize daytime sedation.
- Store drug in tightly closed container at 15°–30°C (59°–86°F) unless otherwise specified. Protect from excessive heat.

ADVERSE EFFECTS **CV:** *Postural hypotension,* hypotension, palpitation, tachycardia, cardiac arrhythmia, edema, flushing, heart block. **CNS:** *Drowsiness,* dizziness, fatigue, headache, insomnia, confusion, peripheral neuropathy, ataxia, agitation, anxiety, seizure, withdrawal syndrome. **HEENT:** Tinnitus, parotid swelling; blurred vision, disturbances in accommodation, mydriasis, increased IOP. **Endocrine:** Decreased libido, decreased serum glucose, gynecomastia, SIADH, weight gain/loss. **Skin:** Alopecia, diaphoresis, pruritis, skin photosensitivity,skin rash, urticaria. **GI:** *Dry mouth, constipation,* bad taste, diarrhea, nausea, anorexia. **GU:** *Urinary retention,* frequency, delayed micturition, nocturia; impaired sexual function, galactorrhea. **Hematologic:** Bone marrow depression and agranulocytosis (rare). **Other:** Hypersensitivity (rash, urticaria, photosensitivity). Sweating, craving for sweets, weight gain or loss, SIADH secretion, hyperpyrexia, eosinophilic pneumonia.

DIAGNOSTIC TEST INTERFERENCE May interfere with ***urine detection*** of amphetamines/methamphetamines.

INTERACTIONS **Drug:** May somewhat decrease response to ANTIHYPERTENSIVES; CNS DEPRESSANTS, **alcohol,** HYPNOTICS, BARBITURATES, SEDATIVES potentiate CNS depression; may increase hypoprothrombinemic effect of ORAL ANTICOAGULANTS; **levodopa,** SYMPATHOMIMETICS (e.g., **epinephrine, norepinephrine**) pose possibility of sympathetic hyperactivity with hypertension and hyperpyrexia; MAO INHIBITORS pose possibility of severe reactions, toxic psychosis, cardiovascular instability; use with drugs impacting QT interval (ex dronedarone) is contraindicated; minimize use with ANTICHOLINERGIC AGENTS; may increase vasopressor effects of ALPHA-BETA AGONISTS **methylphenidate** increases plasma TCA levels; THYROID AGENTS may increase possibility of arrhythmias; **cimetidine** may increase plasma TCA levels. **Herbal: Ginkgo** may decrease seizure threshold; **St. John's wort** may cause **serotonin** syndrome.

PHARMACOKINETICS **Absorption:** Rapidly from GI tract and injection sites. **Peak:** 6 h. **Distribution:** Crosses placenta. **Metabolism:** In liver (CYP2D6). **Elimination:** Primarily in urine. **Half-Life:** 15–24 h.

NURSING IMPLICATIONS

Black Box Warning

Desipramine has been associated with suicidal thinking and behavior in children, adolescents, and young adults.

Assessment & Drug Effects

- Monitor children, adolescents, and young adults for signs of suicidal ideation and behavior.
- Monitor for therapeutic effectiveness: Usually not realized until after at least 2 wk of therapy.
- Monitor BP and pulse rate during early phase of therapy, particularly in older adult, debilitated, or cardiovascular patients. If BP rises or falls more than 20 mmHg or if there is a sudden increase in pulse rate or change in rhythm, withhold drug and inform prescriber.
- Note: Drowsiness, dizziness, and orthostatic hypotension are signs of impending toxicity in patient on long-term, high-dosage therapy. Prolonged QT or QRS intervals indicate possible toxicity. Report to prescriber.
- Observe patient with history of glaucoma. Report symptoms that may signal acute attack: Severe headache, eye pain, dilated pupils, halos of light, nausea, vomiting.
- Monitor bowel elimination pattern and I&O ratio. Severe constipation and urinary retention are potential problems of TCA therapy.
- Monitor lab tests: CBC, blood glucose; serum sodium in at-risk populations.

Patient & Family Education

- Be alert for and promptly report unusual changes in behavior (e.g., anxiety, agitation, panic attacks, insomnia, irritability, hostility, aggressiveness), worsening of depression, or suicidal ideation.
- Make all position changes slowly and in stages, particularly from recumbent to standing position.
- Do not drive or engage in other potentially hazardous activities until reaction to drug is known.
- Take medication exactly as prescribed; do not change dose or dose intervals.
- Note: Patients who receive high doses for prolonged periods may experience withdrawal symptoms including headache, nausea, musculoskeletal pain, and weakness if drug is discontinued abruptly.
- Do not take OTC drugs unless prescriber has approved their use.
- Stop, or at least limit, smoking because it may increase the metabolism of desipramine, thereby diminishing its therapeutic action.

DESLORATADINE

(des-lor-a-ta′deen)

Clarinex, Clarinex Reditabs

Classification: NONSEDATING ANTIHISTAMINE, H_1-RECEPTOR ANTAGONIST

Therapeutic: ANTIHISTAMINE; ANTIALLERGIC

Prototype: Loratadine

AVAILABILITY Tablet; orally dissolving tablet; syrup

ACTION & *THERAPEUTIC EFFECT* A long-acting, nonsedating antihistamine with selective H_1-receptor antagonist properties. Reduces human mast cell release of inflammatory cytokines. Therefore, it also exhibits antiallergic effects. *Desloratadine is effective in controlling allergic rhinitis and inhibiting histamine-induced wheals and flare (hives).*

USES Treatment of seasonal or perennial allergic rhinitis and idiopathic urticaria.

CONTRAINDICATIONS Hypersensitivity to desloratadine or loratadine; neonates; infants.

CAUTIOUS USE Renal and hepatic insufficiencies; bladder neck obstruction or urinary retention; prostatic hypertrophy; asthma; glaucoma; pregnancy (category C); lactation. Safety and efficacy in children younger than 12 yr not established.

ROUTE & DOSAGE

Allergic Rhinitis, Idiopathic Urticaria

Adult: **PO** 5 mg daily

Renal Impairment Dosage Adjustment

CrCl less than 50 mL/min: 5 mg every other day

Hepatic Impairment Dosage Adjustment

5 mg every other day

ADMINISTRATION

Oral

- Note that drug should be given every other day to patients with significant renal or hepatic impairment.
- Store at 2°–25°C (36°–77°F).

ADVERSE EFFECTS **CNS:** Somnolence, dizziness. **GI:** Dry mouth, nausea, dry throat. **GU:** Dysmenorrhea. **Other:** Pharyngitis, fatigue, flulike symptoms, myalgia.

PHARMACOKINETICS **Absorption:** Well absorbed. **Peak:** 3 h. **Distribution:** 85–89% protein bound. **Metabolism:** Extensively metabolized in liver to 3-hydroxydesloratadine, an active metabolite. **Elimination:** Equally in urine and feces. **Half-Life:** 27 h.

NURSING IMPLICATIONS

Assessment & Drug Effects

- Monitor cardiovascular status and report significant changes in BP and palpitations or tachycardia.
- Concurrent drugs: Monitor ECG when used in combination with any other drug that can produce an additive effect causing QT interval prolongation.
- Monitor lab tests: Periodic renal function and LFTs.

D

Patient & Family Education

- Drug may cause significant drowsiness in older adult patients and those with liver or kidney impairment.
- Note: Concurrent use of alcohol and other CNS depressants may have an additive effect.
- Do not take this drug more often than every other day if you have renal impairment.

DESMOPRESSIN ACETATE

(des-moe-pres′sin)

DDAVP, Noctiva, Stimate

Classification: POSTERIOR PITUITARY HORMONE

Therapeutic: ANTIDIURETIC HORMONE (ADH); ANTIHEMOPHILIC FACTOR

Prototype: Vasopressin

AVAILABILITY Tablet; nasal spray; solution for injection

ACTION & *THERAPEUTIC EFFECT* Synthetic analog of natural posterior pituitary (antidiuretic) hormone, vasopressin. Reduces urine volume and osmolality of serum in patients with central diabetes insipidus by increasing reabsorption of water by kidney collecting tubules. Produces a dose-related increase in factor VIII (antihemophilic factor) and von Willebrand factor. *Desmopressin is an effective replacement for antidiuretic hormone. It also can shorten or normalize bleeding time and correct platelet adhesion abnormalities in certain patients with bleeding disorders.*

USES To control and prevent symptoms and complications of central (neurohypophyseal) diabetes insipidus, and to relieve temporary polyuria and polydipsia associated with trauma or surgery in the pituitary region; bleeding prophylaxis, enuresis.

UNLABELED USES To increase factor VIII activity in selected patients with mild to moderate hemophilia A and in type I von Willebrand disease or uremia, and to control enuresis in children.

CONTRAINDICATIONS Nephrogenic diabetes insipidus, type II B von Willebrand disease; CrCl less than 50 mL/min; hyponatremia, moderate to severe renal impairment. **PO:** Patients with fluid and electrolyte imbalance.

CAUTIOUS USE Coronary artery insufficiency, hypertensive cardiovascular disease; psychogenic polydipsia; severe CHF; older adults; history of thromboembolic disease; diarrhea, electrolyte imbalance, nasal trauma; pregnancy (category B). **PO:** Children younger than 6 yr. **Intranasal:** Children 3 mo and older.

ROUTE & DOSAGE

Diabetes Insipidus

Adult/Adolescent: **Intranasal** 0.1–0.4 mL (10–40 mcg) in 1–3 divided doses; **IV/Subcutaneous** 2–4 mcg in 2 divided doses; **PO** 0.05 mg bid titrate to response

Child (3 mo–12 yr): **Intranasal** 0.05–0.3 mL in 1–2 divided doses; **IV/Subcutaneous** 0.3 mcg/kg infused over 15–30 min; *younger than 4 yr:* **PO** 0.05 mg titrated to response

Enuresis

Adult/Adolescent/Child (6 yr or older): **PO** 0.2 mg at bedtime, may titrate up to 0.6 mg at bedtime

Nocturia

Adults (50–64 yr): **Intranasal** 1 spray (use 0.83 mcg strength in those at high risk for hyponatremia) in either nostril 30 min before bedtime

Bleeding Prophylaxis in Patients with Von Willebrand Disease

Adult/Child (3 mo or older): **IV/Subcutaneous** 0.3 mcg/kg 30 min preoperative, may repeat in 48 h if needed
Adult (over 50 kg): **Intranasal** 1 spray each nostril, repeat in 8–24 h if needed
Adult (50 kg or below)/Adolescent/Child: **Intranasal** 1 spray, may repeat in 8–24 h if needed

Renal Impairment Dosage Adjustment

CrCl less than 50 mL/min: Do not use

ADMINISTRATION

Oral

- Note that 0.2 mg PO is equivalent to 10 mcg (0.1 mL) intranasal. May administer with or without food.

Intranasal

- Follow manufacturer's instructions for proper technique with nasal spray.
- Give initial dose in the evening, and observe antidiuretic effect. Dose is increased each evening until uninterrupted sleep is obtained. If daily urine volume is more than 2 L after nocturia is controlled, morning dose is started and adjusted daily until urine volume does not exceed 1.5–2 L/24 h.

Subcutaneous

- Give undiluted as direct injection.

Intravenous

PREPARE: **Direct:** Give undiluted for diabetes insipidus. **IV Infusion:** Dilute 0.3 mcg/kg in 10 mL of NS (children weighing 10 kg or less) or 50 mL of NS (children greater than 10 kg and adults) for von Willebrand disease (type I).
ADMINISTER: **Direct:** Give direct IV over 30 sec for diabetes insipidus. **IV Infusion:** Give over 15–30 min for von Willebrand disease (type I).

- Store parenteral and nasal solution in refrigerator preferably at 4°C (39.2°F) unless otherwise directed. Avoid freezing. ▪ Nasal spray can be stored at room temperature. ▪ Discard solutions that are discolored or contain particulate matter.

ADVERSE EFFECTS **CV:** Hypertension. **CNS:** Transient headache, drowsiness, dizziness, listlessness. **HEENT:** Nasal congestion, rhinitis, nasal irritation. **GI:** Nausea, heartburn, mild abdominal cramps. **All:** Dose related. **Other:** Vulval pain, shortness of breath, facial flushing, pain and swelling at injection site, *hyponatremia*.

INTERACTIONS **Drug: Demeclocycline, lithium,** other VASOPRESSORS may decrease antidiuretic response; **carbamazepine, chlorpropamide, clofibrate** may prolong antidiuretic response. NSAIDs or CORTICOSTEROIDS may increase risk of hyponatremia.

PHARMACOKINETICS **Absorption:** 10–20% through nasal mucosa. **Onset:** 15–60 min.

D

Peak: 1–5 h. **Duration:** 5–21 h. **Distribution:** Small amount crosses blood–brain barrier; distributed into breast milk. **Half-Life:** 76 min.

NURSING IMPLICATIONS

Assessment & Drug Effects

- Monitor I&O ratio and pattern (intervals). Fluid intake **must be** carefully controlled, particularly in older adults and the very young to avoid water retention and sodium depletion.
- Weigh patient daily and observe for edema. Severe water retention may require reduction in dosage and use of a diuretic.
- Monitor BP during dosage-regulating period and whenever drug is administered parenterally.
- Monitor lab tests: Baseline and periodic urine and plasma osmolality.

Patient & Family Education

- Report upper respiratory tract infection or nasal congestion.
- Follow manufacturer's instructions for insertion to ensure delivery of drug high into nasal cavity and not down throat. A flexible calibrated plastic tube is provided.

DESONIDE

(dess′oh-nide)

DesOwen

See Appendix A-4.

DESOXIMETASONE

(des-ox-i-met′a-sone)

Topicort

See Appendix A-4.

DESVENLAFAXINE

(des-ven-la-fax′een)

Pristiq

See Venlafaxine

DEXAMETHASONE

(dex-a-meth′a-sone)

Maxidex

DEXAMETHASONE SODIUM PHOSPHATE

Classification: ADRENAL CORTICOSTEROID; GLUCOCORTICOID

Therapeutic: ADRENOCORTICAL STEROID; ANTI-INFLAMMATORY

Prototype: Prednisone

AVAILABILITY **Dexamethasone:** Tablet; oral solution; ophthalmic drops. **Dexamethasone sodium phosphate:** Solution for injection; ophthalmic solution; suspension

ACTION & *THERAPEUTIC EFFECT* Long-acting corticosteroid with minimal sodium-retaining potential. **Anti-inflammatory action:** Prevents accumulation of inflammatory cells at sites of infection; inhibits phagocytosis, lysosomal enzyme release, and synthesis of potent mediators of inflammation, prostaglandins, and leukotrienes; reduces capillary dilation and permeability. **Immunosuppression:** Probably due to prevention or suppression of delayed hypersensitivity immune reaction. *Has anti-inflammatory and immunosuppression properties.*

USES Adrenal insufficiency concomitantly with a mineralocorticoid; inflammatory conditions, allergic states, collagen diseases, hematologic disorders, cerebral edema, and addisonian shock. Also palliative treatment of neoplastic disease, as adjunctive short-term therapy in acute rheumatic disorders and GI diseases, and as a diagnostic test for Cushing syndrome and for differential diagnosis of adrenal hyperplasia and adrenal adenoma.

UNLABELED USES As an antiemetic in cancer chemotherapy; as treatment of severe/critical hospitalized patients with COVID-19; cancer related cachexia; acute asthma exacerbation; acute mountain sickness; acceleration of fetal lung maturation.

CONTRAINDICATIONS Hypersensitivity to any component of formulation, including sulfites; fungal infections; cerebral malaria; acute infections, active or resting tuberculosis, vaccinia, varicella, administration of live virus vaccines (to patient, family members), latent or active amebiasis; Cushing syndrome; Kaposi sarcoma; rupture of posterior ocular lens capsule; neonates or infants weighing less than 1300 g; lactation. **Topical use:** Rosacea, perioral dermatitis; venous stasis ulcers. **Ophthalmic use:** Primary open-angle glaucoma, eye infections, superficial ocular herpes simplex, keratitis, and tuberculosis of eye.

CAUTIOUS USE Hypersensitivity to corticosteroids; stromal herpes simplex, keratitis, GI disease; renal disease, DM; hypothyroidism, acute MI; myasthenia gravis, CHF, cirrhosis, psychiatric disorders; ocular disease such as cataracts, glaucoma, increased intraocular pressure, open-angle glaucoma; seizures; coagulopathy; older adults; pregnancy (some studies have shown an association between first trimester corticosteroid use and oral clefts or decreased birth weight); children.

ROUTE & DOSAGE

Allergies, Inflammation, Neoplasias (Note: Dosages are very individualized based on patient response and concurrent treatments consult current guidelines)

Adult: **PO/IV/IM:** 4–20 mg/day given in a single daily dose or in 2 to 4 divided doses
Child: **PO/IV/IM** 0.08–0.3 mg/kg/day divided q6–12h

Child: **Ophthalmic/ Topical/ Inhalation/Intranasal.** See Appendix A.

ADMINISTRATION

Oral

- Administer with meals to help prevent GI upset. If appropriate, may administer antacids between meals to help prevent peptic ulcers.
- For the oral concentrate, use the calibrated dropper provided. Draw dose into dropper and mix with liquid or semi-solid food. Administer entire mixed dose immediately.

Intramuscular

- Give IM injection deep into a large muscle mass (e.g., gluteus maximus). Avoid subcutaneous injection. Atrophy and sterile abscesses may occur.

Intravenous

PREPARE: **Direct:** Give undiluted. **Intermittent:** Dilute in D5W or NS for infusion.
ADMINISTER: **Direct:** Give direct IV push over 1 min or less. **Intermittent:** Set rate as prescribed or according to amount of solution to infuse.

INCOMPATIBILITIES: **Solution/additive:** **Daunorubicin, haloperidol, metaraminol, oxaliplatin, vancomycin.** **Y-site:** **Alemtuzumab, amiodarone, amphotericin B, blinatumomab, caspofungin, cefuroxime, ciprofloxacin, dacarbazine, dantrolene, daunorubicin, diazepam, diazoxide, diphenhydramine, dobutatmine, doxycycline, epirubicin, esmolol, fenoldopam, garenoxacin, gemtuzumab, haloperidol, hydroxyzine, idarubicin, labetalol, magnesium, midazolam, minocycline, mitxantrone, mycophenolate, netilimicin, nicardipine, pantoprazole, papaverine, pentamidine, pentazocine, phenytoin, prochlorperazine, protamine, quinupristine, sulfamethxazole-trimethoprim, tobramycin, topotecan.**

- Store at 15°–30°C (59°–86°F) unless otherwise directed.

ADVERSE EFFECTS **CV:** CHF, hypertension, *edema*. **Respiratory:** *Nasal irritation,* dryness, epistaxis, rebound congestion, bronchial asthma, anosmia, perforation of nasal septum. **CNS:** Euphoria, insomnia, convulsions, increased ICP, vertigo, headache, ptosis, psychic disturbances. **HEENT:** *Posterior subcapsular cataract,* increased IOP, glaucoma, exophthalmos, ocular hemorrhage. **Endocrine:** Menstrual irregularities, *hyperglycemia;* cushingoid state; growth suppression in children; hirsutism. **Skin:** Acne, *impaired wound healing,* petechiae, ecchymoses, diaphoresis, allergic dermatitis, hypo- or hyperpigmentation, subcutaneous and cutaneous atrophy, burning and tingling in perineal area (following IV injection). **GI:** Peptic ulcer with possible perforation, abdominal distension, nausea, increased appetite, heartburn, dyspepsia, pancreatitis, bowel perforation, *oral candidiasis.* **Musculoskeletal:** Muscle weakness, loss of muscle mass, vertebral compression fracture, pathologic fracture of long bones, tendon rupture.

DIAGNOSTIC TEST INTERFERENCE May suppress ***wheal and flare reaction*** to skin test antigens.

INTERACTIONS **Drug:** BARBITURATES, **phenytoin, rifampin** increase steroid metabolism—dosage of dexamethasone may need to be increased; may decrease effects of ANTINEOPLASTICS or IMMUNOSUPPRESSANTS **amphotericin B,** DIURETICS compound potassium loss; **neostigmine, pyridostigmine** may cause severe muscle weakness in patients with myasthenia gravis; may inhibit antibody response to VACCINES, TOXOIDS. ANTACIDS or CYP3A4 inducers may decrease effect of corticosteroids. May impact efficacy of hormonal CONTRACEPTIVES. Do not use with **dasabuvir, ritonavir, emtricitabine, tenofovir.**

PHARMACOKINETICS **Absorption:** Readily from GI tract. **Onset:** Rapid. **Peak:** 1–2 h PO; 8 h IM. **Duration:** 2.75 days PO; 6 days IM; 1–3 wk intralesional, intraarticular. **Distribution:** Crosses placenta; distributed into breast milk. **Metabolism:** Induces CYP3A4. **Elimination:** Hypothalamus-pituitary axis suppression: 36–54 h. **Half-Life:** 3–4.5 h.

NURSING IMPLICATIONS

Assessment & Drug Effects

- Monitor and report S&S of Cushing syndrome (see Appendix F) or other systemic adverse effects.
- Monitor neonates born to a mother who has been receiving a corticosteroid during pregnancy for symptoms of hypoadrenocorticism.
- Monitor intraocular pressure with systemic use > 6 weeks. Consider routine eye exams with chronic use.
- Monitor for S&S of a hypersensitivity reaction (see Appendix F). The acetate and sodium phosphate formulations may contain bisulfites, parabens, or both; these inactive ingredients are allergenic to some individuals.
- Monitor lab tests: Serum Hgb, potassium, glucose, creatine kinase, bone mineral density.

Patient & Family Education

- Take drug exactly as prescribed.
- Report lack of response to medication or malaise, orthostatic hypotension, muscular weakness and pain, nausea, vomiting, anorexia, hypoglycemic reactions (see Appendix F), ocular changes, or mental depression to prescriber.
- Report changes in appearance and easy bruising to prescriber.
- Add potassium-rich foods to diet; report signs of hypokalemia (see Appendix F). Concomitant potassium-depleting diuretic can enhance dexamethasone-induced potassium loss.
- Note: Dexamethasone dose regimen may need to be altered during stress (e.g., surgery, infections, emotional stress, illness, acute bronchial attacks, trauma). Consult prescriber if change in living or working environment is anticipated.
- Discontinue drug gradually under the guidance of the prescriber.
- Note: It is important to prevent exposure to infection, trauma, and sudden changes in environmental factors, as much as possible, because drug is an immunosuppressor.

D

DEXMEDETOMIDINE HYDROCHLORIDE (Pr)

(dex-med-e-to′mi-deen)

Precedex

Classification: ALPHA$_2$-ADRENERGIC AGONIST; NONBARBITURATE SEDATIVE-HYPNOTIC

Therapeutic: SEDATIVE-HYPNOTIC

AVAILABILITY Solution for injection

ACTION & *THERAPEUTIC EFFECT* Stimulates alpha$_2$-adrenergic receptors in the CNS (primarily in the medulla oblongata) causing inhibition of the sympathetic vasomotor center of the brain resulting in sedative effects. *Sedative properties utilized in intubating patients and for initially maintaining them on a mechanical ventilator.*

USES Sedation of initially intubated or mechanically ventilated patients.

CONTRAINDICATIONS Hypersensitivity to dexmedetomidine.

CAUTIOUS USE Cardiac arrhythmias or cardiovascular disease, uncontrolled hypertension; hypotension; cerebrovascular disease; renal or hepatic insufficiency; signs of light anesthesia; older adults; pregnancy (limited information related to use during pregnancy; use with caution); lactation. Safety and efficacy in children younger than 18 yr not established.

D

ROUTE & DOSAGE

Sedation of Mechanically Ventilated Patients

Adult: **IV** 1 mcg/kg loading dose infused over 10 min, then continue with infusion of 0.2–1.5 mcg/kg/h for up to 24 h adjusted to maintain sedation

Hepatic Impairment Dosage Adjustment

Reduce initial dosage

ADMINISTRATION

Intravenous

PREPARE: **Continuous:** Withdraw 2 mL of dexmedetomidine and add to 48 mL of NS to yield 4 mcg/mL. Shake gently to mix.
ADMINISTER: **Continuous:** Administer using a controlled infusion device. ▪ A loading dose of 1 mcg/kg is infused over 10 min followed by the ordered maintenance dose. **Do not** use administration set containing natural rubber. **Do not** infuse longer than 24 h.
INCOMPATIBILITIES: Y-site: **Amphotericin B, diazepam, garenoxacin, gemtuzumab, irinotecan, pantoprazole, phenytoin.**

- Store unopened vials at room temperature.

ADVERSE EFFECTS **CV:** *Hypotension,* bradycardia, tachycardia, atrial fibrillation, hypertension, peripheral edema. **Respiratory:** Respiratory depression, respiratory failure. **CNS:** Agitation, anxiety. **Endocrine:** Hypokalemia, hyperglycemia, hypoglycemia. **GI:** *Nausea,* constipation, thirst. **Other:** Fever.

INTERACTIONS **Drug:** BARBITURATES, BENZODIAZEPINES, GENERAL ANESTHETICS, OPIATE AGONISTS, ANXIOLYTICS, SEDATIVES/HYPNOTICS, **ethanol,** TRICYCLIC ANTIDEPRESSANTS, **tramadol,** PHENOTHIAZINES, SKELETAL MUSCLE RELAXANTS, **azatadine, brompheniramine, carbinoxamine, chlorpheniramine, clemastine, cyproheptadine, dexchlorpheniramine, dimenhydrinate, diphenhydramine, doxylamine, hydroxyzine, methdilazine, phenindamine, promethazine, tripelennamine** enhance CNS depression possibly prolong recovery from anesthesia. **Fexinidazole** may increase significant bradycardia.

PHARMACOKINETICS **Metabolism:** Extensively in liver (CYP2A6). **Elimination:** Primarily in urine. **Half-Life:** 2 h.

NURSING IMPLICATIONS

Assessment & Drug Effects

- Monitor for hypertension during loading dose; reduction of loading dose may be required.
- Monitor Bp, heart rate, respiratory rate; notify prescriber immediately if hypotension or bradycardia occurs.

DEXMETHYLPHENIDATE

(dex-meth-ill-fen′i-date)

Focalin, Focalin XR

Classification: CEREBRAL STIMULANT
Therapeutic: CEREBRAL STIMULANT
Prototype: Amphetamine
Controlled Substance: Schedule II

AVAILABILITY Tablet; extended release capsule

D

ACTION & *THERAPEUTIC EFFECT*

Thought to block reuptake of norepinephrine and dopamine into presynaptic neurons and thereby increases release of these substances into the synapse. *Is effective in controlling ADHD syndrome in conjunction with other measures (psychological, educational, and social).*

USES Attention-deficit/hyperactivity disorder (ADHD).

CONTRAINDICATIONS Hypersensitivity to methylphenidate; known structural cardiac abnormalities in children or adults, cardiomyopathy, congenital heart disease; coronary heart disease; severe agitation, marked anxiety, or tension; psychotic symptomatology; glaucoma; motor tics; family history of or diagnosis of Tourette syndrome; concurrent MAOI therapy or within 14 days of discontinuation; occurrence of seizures without a history.

CAUTIOUS USE Moderate to severe hepatic insufficiency; depression; preexisting psychosis; emotional instability, bipolar disorder, history of suicides; alcoholism or drug dependence; history of seizure disorders; hypertension, CHF, cardiac arrhythmias; hyperthyroidism; older adults; pregnancy (category C); lactation. Safe use in children younger than 6 yr is not established.

ROUTE & DOSAGE

Attention-Deficit/Hyperactivity Disorder

Adult: **PO** 2.5 mg bid, may increase by 2.5–5 mg/day at weekly intervals (max: 20 mg/day). If converting from methylphenidate, start with ½ of methylphenidate dose. **Extended release** 10 mg daily, may increase by 5 mg at weekly intervals (max: 40 mg/day)

Child (6 yr or older): **PO** 2.5 mg bid, may increase by 2.5–5 mg/day at weekly intervals (max: 20 mg/day). If converting from methylphenidate, start with ½ of methylphenidate dose. **Extended release** 5 mg daily, may increase by 5 mg at weekly intervals (max: 20 mg/day)

ADMINISTRATION

Oral

- Do not administer with or within 14 days following discontinuation of an MAO inhibitor.
- Give sustained release capsules whole. They should not be crushed or chewed.
- Give bid doses at least 4 h apart.
- Store at 15°–30°C (59°–86°F).

ADVERSE EFFECTS **CV:** Hypertension, tachycardia. **CNS:** Dizziness, insomnia, nervousness, tics, abnormal thinking, hallucinations, emotional lability, CNS overstimulation or sympathomimetic effects [angina, anxiety, agitation, biting, blurred vision, delirium, diaphoresis, flushing or pallor, hallucinations, hyperthermia, labile blood pressure and heart rate (hypotension or hypertension), mydriasis, palpitations, paranoia, purposeless movements, psychosis, sinus tachycardia, tachypnea, or tremor]. **GI:** *Abdominal pain,* anorexia, nausea, vomiting. **Other:** Fever, allergic reactions.

INTERACTIONS **Drug:** Additive stimulant effects with other STIMULANTS (including **amphetamine, caffeine**); increased vasopressor effects with **dopamine, epinephrine, norepinephrine,**

D

phenylpropanolamine, pseudoephedrine; MAO INHIBITORS may cause hypertensive crisis; antagonizes hypotensive effects of **guanethidine,** may inhibit metabolism and increase serum levels of **fosphenytoin, phenytoin, phenobarbital,** and **primidone, warfarin,** TRICYCLIC ANTIDEPRESSANTS.

PHARMACOKINETICS Absorption: Well absorbed. **Peak:** 1–1.5 h. **Metabolism:** De-esterified in liver. No interaction with CYP450 system. **Elimination:** Primarily in urine. **Half-Life:** 2.2 h.

NURSING IMPLICATIONS

Black Box Warning

Use dexmethylphenidate with extreme caution in those with a history of drug dependence or alcoholism.

Assessment & Drug Effects

- Monitor for potential abuse and dependence on this drug. Careful supervision is needed during drug withdrawal because severe depression may occur.
- Withhold drug and notify prescriber if patient has a seizure. Monitor closely for loss of seizure control with a prior history of seizures.
- Monitor BP in all patients receiving this drug. Monitor cardiac status and report palpitations or other signs of arrhythmias.
- Monitor for signs of aggression or psychotic behavior in adolescents and children.
- Concurrent drugs: Monitor patients on BP-lowering drugs for loss of BP control. Monitor plasma levels of oral anticoagulants and anticonvulsants; doses of these drugs may need to be decreased.
- Monitor lab tests: Periodic CBC with differential and platelet count, and LFTs during prolonged therapy.

Patient & Family Education

- Withhold drug and report immediately any of the following signs of overdose: Vomiting, agitation, tremors, muscle twitching, convulsions, confusion, hallucinations, delirium, sweating, flushing, headache, or high temperature.
- Note that drug is usually discontinued if improvement is not observed after appropriate dosage adjustment over 1 mo.

DEXRAZOXANE

(dex-ra-zox'ane)

Totect, Zinecard

Classification: ANTINEOPLASTIC; CYTOPROTECTIVE AGENT; CARDIOPROTECTIVE

Therapeutic: CARDIOPROTECTIVE FOR DOXORUBICIN

AVAILABILITY Solution for injection

ACTION & *THERAPEUTIC EFFECT* A derivative of EDTA that readily penetrates cell membranes. Dexrazoxane is converted intracellularly to a chelating agent that interferes with iron-mediated free radical generation thought to be partially responsible for one form of cardiomyopathy. *Cardioprotective effect is related to its chelating activity.*

USES Reduction of cardiomyopathy associated with a cumulative doxorubicin dose of 300 mg/m^2; extravasation due to anthracycline therapy.

CONTRAINDICATIONS Zinecard, generic products; use with chemotherapy regimens that do not contain an anthracycline; pregnancy (category D); lactation.

D

CAUTIOUS USE Myelosuppression, prior radiation or chemotherapy; renal failure or moderate to severe renal impairment; hepatic or cardiac impairment; older adults. Safety and efficacy in children not established.

ROUTE & DOSAGE

Cardiomyopathy

Adult: **IV** 10:1 ratio of dexrazoxane to doxorubicin

Extravasation (Totect)

Adult: **IV** 1000 mg/m^2 on day 1 and day 2, then 500 mg/m^2 on day 3

Renal Impairment Dosage Adjustment

CrCl less than 40 mL/min: Reduce dose by 50%

ADMINISTRATION

Intravenous

Wear gloves when handling dexrazoxane. Immediately wash with soap and water if drug contacts skin or mucosa.

- Doxorubicin dose **must be** started within 30 min of beginning dexrazoxane.

PREPARE: **Direct:** Reconstitute by adding 25 or 50 mL of 0.167 M sodium lactate injection (provided by manufacturer) to the 250- or 500-mg vial, respectively, to produce a 10-mg/mL solution. **IV Infusion:** Further dilute reconstituted solution with NS or D5W to a concentration of 1.3–5 mg/mL for infusion.

ADMINISTER: **Direct:** Give bolus dose slowly. **IV Infusion:** Give over 10–15 min.

INCOMPATIBILITIES: **Y site: Acyclovir, allopurinol, aminophylline, amphotericin B, cefepime, dantrolene, diazepam, dobutamine, furosemide, ganciclovir, gemtuzumab, methotrexate, methylprednisolone, mitomycin, nafcillin, pantoprazole, pentobarbital, phenytoin, sodium phosphate, SMZ/TMP, thiopental, zidovudine.**

- Store reconstituted solutions for 6 h at 15°–30°C (59°–86°F).

ADVERSE EFFECTS **CV:** Phlebitis. **Skin:** Erythema. Adverse effects of dexrazoxane are difficult to distinguish from those of the chemotherapeutic agents but are dose related and include pain at injection site, leukopenia, granulocytopenia, and thrombocytopenia. **Other:** Fatigue, neurotoxicity, fever, infection, sepsis, bone marrow depression.

PHARMACOKINETICS **Distribution:** Not protein bound. **Metabolism:** In liver. **Elimination:** 42% in urine. **Half-Life:** 2–4 h.

NURSING IMPLICATIONS

Assessment & Drug Effects

- Monitor cardiac function. Drug does not eliminate risk of doxorubicin cardiotoxicity.
- Note: Adverse effects are likely due to concurrent cytotoxic drugs rather than dexrazoxane.
- Assess infusion site frequently; avoid extravasation.
- Monitor lab tests: Baseline and periodic blood cell counts; periodic LFTs and renal function tests.

Patient & Family Education

- Report any of the following to prescriber: Worsening shortness of breath, swelling extremities, or chest pains.

D

DEXTRAN 40

(dex′tran)

Classification: PLASMA VOLUME EXPANDER
Therapeutic: PLASMA VOLUME EXPANDER
Prototype: Albumin

AVAILABILITY Solution for injection

ACTION & *THERAPEUTIC EFFECT*
A hypertonic colloidal solution that produces immediate and short-lived expansion of plasma volume by increasing colloidal osmotic pressure and drawing fluid from interstitial to intravascular space. *Cardiovascular response to volume expansion includes increased BP, pulse pressure, CVP, cardiac output, venous return to heart, and urinary output.*

USES Adjunctively to expand plasma volume and provide fluid replacement in treatment of shock or impending shock. Also used in prophylaxis and therapy of venous thrombosis and pulmonary embolism. Used as priming fluid or as additive to other primers during extracorporeal circulation.

CONTRAINDICATIONS Hypersensitivity to dextrans, severe renal failure, hypervolemic conditions, severe CHF, significant anemia, hypofibrinogenemia or other marked hemostatic defects including those caused by drugs (e.g., heparin, warfarin); lactation.

CAUTIOUS USE Active hemorrhage; severe dehydration; chronic liver disease; impaired renal function; thrombocytopenia; patients susceptible to pulmonary edema or CHF; pregnancy (category C).

ROUTE & DOSAGE

Shock

Adult/Adolescent/Child: **IV** Up to 20 mL/kg in the first 24 h (doses up to 10 mL/kg/day may be given for a maximum of 4 additional days if needed)

Prophylaxis for Thromboembolic Complications

Adult: **IV** 500–1000 mL (10 mL/kg) on the day of operation followed by 500 mL/day for 2–3 days, may continue with 500 mL q2–3 days for up to 2 wk if necessary

Priming for Extracorporeal Circulation

Adult: **IV** 10–20 mL/kg added to perfusion circuit

ADMINISTRATION

Intravenous

If blood is to be administered, draw a cross-match specimen before dextran infusion.
PREPARE: **IV Infusion:** Use only if seal is intact, vacuum is detectable, and solution is absolutely clear. ▪ No dilution required.
ADMINISTER: **IV Infusion:** Specific flow rate should be prescribed by prescriber. ▪ For emergency treatment of shock in adults give first 500 mL rapidly (e.g., 20–40 mL/min); give remaining portion of the daily dose over 8–24 h or at the rate prescribed.
INCOMPATIBILITIES: **Solution/additive: Amoxicillin, ampicillin, oxacillin, penicillin.**

▪ Store at a constant temperature, preferably 25°C (77°F). Once opened, discard unused portion because dextran contains no preservative.

ADVERSE EFFECTS Other: Hypersensitivity (mild to generalized urticaria, pruritus, anaphylactic shock (rare), angioedema, dyspnea), renal tubular vacuolization (osmotic nephrosis), stasis, and blocking; oliguria, renal failure; increased AST and ALT, interference with platelet function, prolonged bleeding and coagulation times.

DIAGNOSTIC TEST INTERFERENCE When blood samples are drawn for study, notify laboratory that patient has received dextran. ***Blood glucose:*** False increases (utilizing ***ortho-toluidine methods*** or ***sulfuric*** or ***acetic acid*** hydrolysis). ***Urinary protein:*** False increases (utilizing ***Lowry method***). ***Bilirubin assays:*** False increases when alcohol is used. ***Total protein assays:*** False increases using ***biuret reagent. Rh testing, blood typing*** and ***cross-matching*** procedures: Dextran may interfere with results (by inducing rouleaux formation) when ***proteolytic enzyme techniques*** are used (***saline agglutination*** and ***indirect antiglobulin methods*** reportedly not affected).

INTERACTIONS Drug: May potentiate ANTICOAGULANT effects.

PHARMACOKINETICS Onset: Volume expansion within minutes of infusion. **Duration:** 12 h. **Metabolism:** Degraded to glucose and metabolized to CO_2 and water over a period of a few weeks. **Elimination:** 75% excreted in urine within 24 h; small amount excreted in feces.

NURSING IMPLICATIONS

Assessment & Drug Effects

- Evaluate patient's state of hydration before dextran therapy begins. Administration to severely dehydrated patients can result in renal failure.
- Monitor vital signs and observe patient closely for at least the first 30 min of infusion. Hypersensitivity reaction is most likely to occur during the first few minutes of administration. Terminate therapy at the first sign of a hypersensitivity reaction (see Appendix F).
- Monitor CVP as an estimate of blood volume status and a guide for determining dosage. Normal CVP: 5–10 cm H_2O.
- Observe for S&S of circulatory overload (see Appendix F).
- Note: When sodium restriction is indicated, know that 500 mL of dextran 40 in 0.9% normal saline contains 77 mEq of both sodium and chloride.
- Monitor I&O ratio and check urine specific gravity at regular intervals. Low urine specific gravity may signify failure of renal dextran clearance and is an indication to discontinue therapy.
- Report oliguria, anuria, or lack of improvement in urinary output (dextran usually causes an increase in urinary output). Discontinue dextran at first sign of renal dysfunction.
- High doses are associated with transient prolongation of bleeding time and interference with normal blood coagulation.
- Monitor lab tests: Baseline Hct and repeat Hct as needed.

Patient & Family Education

- Report immediately S&S of bleeding: Easy bruising, blood in urine, or dark tarry stool.

D

DEXTROAMPHETAMINE SULFATE

(dex-troe-am-fet'a-meen)

Classification: RESPIRATORY AND CEREBRAL STIMULANT; AMPHETAMINE; ANOREXIANT

Therapeutic: AMPHETAMINE; ANOREXIANT

Prototype: Amphetamine

Controlled Substance: Schedule II

AVAILABILITY Tablet; sustained release capsule

ACTION & *THERAPEUTIC EFFECT* A CNS stimulant that may cause diminished appetite through loss of acuity of smell and taste. *Is a more potent appetite suppressant than amphetamine. In hyperkinetic children, amphetamines reduce motor restlessness by an unknown mechanism.*

USES Adjunct in short-term treatment of exogenous obesity, narcolepsy, and attention-deficit disorder with hyperactivity in children (also called minimal brain dysfunction or hyperkinetic syndrome).

UNLABELED USES Adjunct in epilepsy to control ataxia and drowsiness induced by barbiturates; to combat sedative effects of trimethadione in absence seizures.

CONTRAINDICATIONS Hypersensitivity to sympathomimetic amines, closed-angle glaucoma, agitated states, psychoses (especially in children), structural cardiac abnormalities, valvular heart disease; congenital heart disease, coronary heart disease, advanced arteriosclerosis, symptomatic heart disease, moderate to severe hypertension, hyperthyroidism, history of drug abuse, during or within 14 days of MAOI therapy; children younger than 3 yr; lactation.

CAUTIOUS USE Bipolar disease; salicylate hypersensitivity; seizure disorders; suicidal ideation, depression; salicylate hypersensitivity; pregnancy (category C). Safety and efficacy in children younger than 6 yr for narcolepsy and younger than 3 yr for attention-deficit/hyperactivity disorder not established.

ROUTE & DOSAGE

Narcolepsy

Adult: **PO** 5–20 mg 1–3 × day at 4–6 h intervals
Child (6 to younger than 12 yr): **PO** 5 mg/day, may increase by 5 mg at weekly intervals; *12 yr or older:* 10 mg/day, may increase by 10 mg at weekly intervals

Attention-Deficit/Hyperactivity Disorder

Child (3–5 yr): **PO** 2.5 mg 1–2 × day, may increase by 2.5 mg at weekly intervals; *6 yr or older:* 5 mg 1–2 × day, may increase by 5 mg at weekly intervals (max: 40 mg/day)

Obesity

Adult: **PO** 5–10 mg 1–3 × day or 10–15 mg of sustained release once/day 30–60 min a.c.

ADMINISTRATION

Oral

- Ensure that sustained release capsule is not chewed or crushed. It **must be** swallowed whole.

- Give 30–60 min before meals for treatment of obesity. Give long-acting form in the morning.
- Give last dose no later than 6 h before patient retires (10–14 h before bedtime for sustained release form) to avoid insomnia.
- Store in tightly closed containers at 15°–30°C (59°–86°F) unless otherwise directed.

ADVERSE EFFECTS **CV:** Palpitations, tachycardia, elevated BP. **CNS:** Nervousness, *restlessness,* hyperactivity, *insomnia,* euphoria, dizziness, headache; ***with prolonged use:*** Severe depression, psychotic reactions. **GI:** Dry mouth, unpleasant taste, anorexia, weight loss, diarrhea, constipation, abdominal pain. **Other:** Impotence, changes in libido, unusual fatigue, increased intraocular pressure, marked dystonia of head, neck, and extremities; sweating.

DIAGNOSTIC TEST INTERFERENCE Dextroamphetamine may cause significant elevations in ***plasma corticosteroids*** (evening levels are highest) and increases in ***urinary epinephrine*** excretion (during first 3 h after drug administration).

INTERACTIONS **Drug: Acetazolamide, sodium bicarbonate** decrease dextroamphetamine elimination; **ascorbic acid** increase dextroamphetamine elimination; effects of both BARBITURATES and dextroamphetamine may be antagonized; **furazolidone** may increase BP effects of AMPHETAMINES—interaction may persist for several weeks after discontinuing **furazolidone;** antagonizes antihypertensive effects of **guanethidine;** MAO INHIBITORS, **selegiline** can cause—hypertensive crisis (fatalities reported)—do not administer AMPHETAMINES during or within 14 days of these drugs; PHENOTHIAZINES may inhibit mood-elevating effects of AMPHETAMINES; TRICYCLIC ANTIDEPRESSANTS enhance dextroamphetamine effects because of increased **norepinephrine** release; BETA-ADRENERGIC AGONISTS increase cardiovascular adverse effects.

PHARMACOKINETICS **Absorption:** Rapid. **Peak:** 1–5 h. **Duration:** Up to 10 h. **Distribution:** All tissues, especially the CNS. **Metabolism:** In liver. **Elimination:** Renal elimination; excreted in breast milk. **Half-Life:** 10–30 h.

Black Box Warning

Dextroamphetamine has been associated with fatal respiratory depression in children younger than 2 yr ***(do not use*** *in this age group). Children older than 2 yr may experience serious adverse effects.*

NURSING IMPLICATIONS
Assessment & Drug Effects

- Monitor children, adolescents, and adults for signs and symptoms of respiratory depression and adverse cardiac reactions (e.g., arrhythmias).
- Monitor growth rate closely in children.
- Monitor children and adolescents for development of aggressive or abnormal behaviors.
- Note: Tolerance to anorexiant effects may develop after a few weeks; however, tolerance does not appear to develop when dextroamphetamine is used to treat narcolepsy.

Patient & Family Education

- Swallow sustained release capsule whole with a liquid; do not chew or crush.
- Do not drive or engage in other potentially hazardous activities until response to drug is known.
- Drug is usually tapered off gradually following long-term use to avoid extreme fatigue, mental depression, and prolonged sleep pattern.

DEXTROMETHORPHAN HYDROBROMIDE

(dex-troe-meth-or'fan)

Balminil DM ♣, Benylin DM, Cremacoat 1, Delsym, DM Cough, Hold, Koffex ♣, Mediquell, Neo-DM ♣, Ornex DM ♣, Pedia Care, Pertussin 8 Hour Cough Formula, Robidex ♣, Robitussin DM, Romilar CF, Romilar Children's Cough, Sedatuss ♣, Sucrets Cough Control

Classification: ANTITUSSIVE
Therapeutic: ANTITUSSIVE
Prototype: Benzonatate

AVAILABILITY Capsule; liquid; syrup

ACTION & *THERAPEUTIC EFFECT* Chemically related to morphine but without central hypnotic or analgesic effect. Controls cough spasms by depressing the cough center in medulla. Antitussive activity comparable to that of codeine. *Temporarily relieves coughing spasm.*

USES Temporary relief of cough spasms in nonproductive coughs.

CONTRAINDICATIONS Asthma, COPD, productive cough, persistent or chronic cough; severe hepatic function impairment. Concurrent administration with or within 2 wk of discontinuing an MAO inhibitor.

CAUTIOUS USE Chronic pulmonary disease; enlarged prostate; mild or moderate hepatic impairment; pregnancy (category C); lactation. Safe use in children younger than 2 yr not established.

ROUTE & DOSAGE

Cough

Adult:/Adolescent: **PO** 10–20 mg q4h or 30 mg q6–8h (max: 120 mg/day) or 60 mg of sustained action liquid bid
Child (2 to younger than 6 yr): **PO** 2.5–5 mg q4h or 7.5 mg q6–8h (max: 30 mg/day) or 15 mg sustained action liquid bid; *6–11 yr:* 5–10 mg q4h or 15 mg q6–8h (max: 60 mg/day) or 30 mg sustained action liquid bid

ADMINISTRATION

Oral

- Do not give lozenges to children younger than 6 yr.
- Ensure that extended release form of drug is not chewed or crushed. It **must be** swallowed whole.
- Note: Although soothing local effect of the syrup may be enhanced if given undiluted, depression of cough center depends only on systemic absorption of drug.

ADVERSE EFFECTS **CNS:** Dizziness, drowsiness, CNS depression with very large doses; excitability, especially in children. **GI:** GI upset, constipation, abdominal discomfort.

INTERACTIONS **Drug:** High risk of excitation, hypotension, and hyperpyrexia with MAO INHIBITORS. Due to potential of serotonin syndrome use caution with SSRIs.

PHARMACOKINETICS Absorption: Readily from GI tract. **Onset:** 15–30 min. **Duration:** 3–6 h. **Metabolism:** In liver. **Elimination:** In urine.

NURSING IMPLICATIONS

Black Box Warning

Do not use in children younger than 2 yr due to risk of fatal respiratory depression.

Assessment & Drug Effects

- Monitor for dizziness and drowsiness, especially when concurrent therapy with CNS depressant is used.

Patient & Family Education

- Note: Treatment aims to decrease the frequency and intensity of cough without completely eliminating protective cough reflex.
- While dextromethorphan is available OTC, any cough persisting longer than 1 wk–10 days needs to be medically diagnosed.

DIAZEPAM

(dye-az′e-pam)

Diastat, Valium

Classification: BENZODIAZEPINE ANTICONVULSANT; ANXIOLYTIC

Therapeutic: ANTICONVULSANT; ANTIANXIETY

Controlled Substance: Schedule IV

AVAILABILITY Tablet; oral solution; solution for injection; rectal gel

ACTION & THERAPEUTIC EFFECT Acts at the limbic, thalamic, and hypothalamic regions of the CNS and produces CNS depression resulting in sedation, hypnosis, skeletal muscle relaxation, and anticonvulsant activity dependent on the dosage. *Has antianxiety, anticonvulsant, and skeletal muscle relaxation properties.*

USES Drug of choice for acute active seizures. Management of anxiety disorders, for short-term relief of anxiety symptoms, to relieve anxiety and tension prior to surgery, cardioversion and endoscopic procedures. Also used to alleviate acute withdrawal symptoms of alcoholism, voiding problems in older adults, and adjunctively for relief of skeletal muscle spasm and or rigidity.

CONTRAINDICATIONS Acute narrow-angle glaucoma, untreated open-angle glaucoma; during or within 14 days of MAOI therapy; pregnancy (teratogenic effects have been observed with diazepam use); lactation. **Injectable form:** Shock, coma, acute alcohol intoxication, depressed vital signs, obstetric patients.

CAUTIOUS USE Epilepsy, psychoses, mental depression; myasthenia gravis; impaired hepatic or renal function; neuromuscular disease; bipolar disorder, dementia, Parkinson disease; organic brain syndrome, psychosis, suicidal ideation; drug abuse, addiction-prone individuals. **Injectable form:** Extreme caution in older adults, the very ill, and patients with COPD, or asthma; infant.

D

ROUTE & DOSAGE

Acute Active Seizure (non status epilepticus)

Adult: **IV/IM** 5–10 mg, repeat if needed at 3–5 min intervals up to 30 mg, **Intranasal** 0.2mg/kg as single dose; may repeat after 4 hours (max: two doses)
Child (age 6–11) **Intranasal:** see weight based dosing table in package insert.

Status Epilepticus

Child (5 yr or older): **IV** 1 mg/kg q2–5min (max: 10 mg), may repeat in 2–4 h
Child/Infant (1 mo to younger than 5 yr): **IV** 0.2–0.5 mg slowly q2–5min (max dose: 5 mg)

Muscle Spasm

Adult/Adolescent/Child (5 yr or older): **PO** 2 mg bid or 5 mg at bedtime
Adolescent/Child (5 yr or older): **PO** 0.12–0.8 mg/kg/day in divided doses q6–8h (max 10 mg/dose)

Anxiety

Adult/Adolescent: **IV/PO** 2–10 mg q 3–6 hours (max: 40 mg/day)

Alcohol Withdrawal

Adult: **IV/PO** 10–20 mg q 6–12 hours on day 1; for the next 3 to 5 days, decrease the total daily dose by 25% to 50% each day

Procedural Anxiety

Adult: **IV** 2–10 mg mg 5–15 min before procedure

ADMINISTRATION

Oral

- Ensure that sustained release form is not chewed or crushed. It **must be** swallowed whole. Give other tablets crushed with fluid or mixed with food if necessary.
- Supervise oral ingestion to ensure drug is swallowed.
- Avoid abrupt discontinuation of diazepam. Taper doses to termination.

Intramuscular

- Give undiluted deep into large muscle mass. Inject slowly. Rotate injection sites.

Intravenous

PREPARE: **Direct:** Do not dilute or mix with any other drug.
ADMINISTER: **Direct:** Administer undiluted by slow IV push; do not mix with other solutions or medications. ▪ The emulsion form is incompatible with PVC infusion sets. ▪ Avoid small veins and take extreme care to avoid intra-arterial administration or extravasation.
INCOMPATIBILITIES: **Solution/additive: Bleomycin, dobutamine, doxorubicin, fluorouracil, furosemide, ketamine.** Emulsion also incompatible with **morphine. Y-site: Acyclovir, alemtuzumab, alfentanil, amikacin, aminocaproic acid, aminophylline, amiodarone, amphotericin B cholesteryl complex, amophtericin B lipid, amphotericin B liposome, ampicillin, anidulafungin, argatroban, ascorbic acid, asparaginase, atenolol, atracurium, atropine, azathioprine,**

azithromycin, aztreonam, benztropine, bivalirudin, bleomycin, bretylium, bumetanide, buprenorphine, butorphanol, calcium chloride, calcium gluconate, cangrelor, capreomycin, carboplatin, carmustine, caspofungin, cefamandole, cefazolin, cefepime, cefoperazone, cefotaxime, cefotetan, cefoxitin, ceftaroline, ceftazidime, ceftobiprole, ceftriaxone, cefuroxime, chloramphenicol, chlorpromazine, cisplatin, clindamycin, cloxacillin, cyanocobalamine, cyclophosphamide, cyclosporine, cytarabine, dacarbazine, dactinomycin, dantrolene, dexamethaxome, dexmedetomidine, dexrazoxane, diazoxide, digoxin, diltiazem, dimenhydrinate, diphenhydramine, dolasetron, dopamine, doripenem, doxorubicin, doxycycline, enalaprilat, ephedrine, epirubicin, epoetin, eptifibatide, ertapenem, erythromycin, esmolol, etoposide, famotidine, fenoldopam, fluconazole, fludarabine, fluorouracil, folic acid, foscarnet, fosphenytoin, furosemide, gallium, ganciclovir, garenoxacin, gemcitabine, gemtuzumab, gentamicin, glycopyrrolate, granisetron, haloperidol, heparin, hydralazine, hydrocortisone, hydroxocobalamin, idarubicin, ifsosfamide, imipenem/cilastatin, indomethacin, insulin, irinotecan, isoproterenol, ketorolac, labetalol, lansoprazole, lepirudin, leucoforin, levofloxacin, lidocaine, linezolid, magnesium sulfate, mannitol, mechlorethamine, meperidine, meropenem, methotrexate, methyldopate, methylprednisolone, metoclopramide, metoprolol, metronidazole, midazolam, milrinone, minocycline, mitomycin, mitoxantrone, mivacurium, mycophenolate, nalbuphin, naloxone, nesiritide, metilmicin, nicardipine, nitroglycerin, nitroprusside, norepinephrine, octreotde, oxacillin, oxaliplatin, oxytocin, paclitaxel, palonosetron, pamidronate, pancuronium, pantoprazole, papaverine, premetrexed, pencillin G, pentamidine, pentazocine, penobarbital, phenobarbital, phentolamine, phenylephrine, phenytoin, phytonadione, piperacillin, polymyxin B, potassium acetate, procainamide, prochlorperazine, propofol, propranolol, protamine, pyridoxine, quinupristin, rocuronium, sodium acetate, streptokinase, succinylcholine, tacrolimus, theophylline, thiamine, thiotepa, ticarcillin, tigecycline, tirofiban, tobramycin, tolazoline, topotecan, urokinase, vancomycin, vasopressin, vecuronium, verapamil, vinblastine, vincristine, vinorelbine, vitamin B complex with C, voriconazole, zoledronic acid. Do not mix emulsion with any other drugs. Do not administer through **polyvinyl chloride (PVC)** infusion sets.

- Store in tight, light-resistant containers at 20°–25°C (68°–77°F), unless otherwise specified by manufacturer.

ADVERSE EFFECTS **CV:** <u>Cardiovascular shock</u>. **CNS:** *Drowsiness*, headache.

DIAGNOSTIC TEST INTERFERENCE
Can cause false negative ***urine***

D

glucose determinations using Clinstix or Diastix.

INTERACTIONS **Drug: Alcohol,** CNS DEPRESSANTS, ANTICONVULSANTS potentiate CNS depression; **cimetidine** increases diazepam plasma levels, increases toxicity; may decrease antiparkinson effects of **levodopa;** may increase **phenytoin** levels; smoking decreases sedative and antianxiety effects. Strong CYP3A4 inducers may decrease efficacy; strong CYP2C19 inhibitors may increase risk of adverse effects. **Herbal: Kava, valerian** may potentiate sedation.

PHARMACOKINETICS **Absorption:** Readily from GI tract; erratic IM absorption. **Onset:** 30–60 min PO; 15–30 min IM; 1–3 min IV; 2–10 min rectal. **Peak:** 1–2 h PO. **Duration:** 15 min–1 h IV; up to 3 h PO. **Distribution:** Crosses blood-brain barrier and placenta; distributed into breast milk. **Metabolism:** In liver (via CYP3A4 and CYP2C19) to active metabolites. **Elimination:** Primarily in urine. **Half-Life:** 20–50 h.

NURSING IMPLICATIONS

Assessment & Drug Effects

- Monitor for therapeutic effectiveness. Maximum effect may require 1–2 wk; patient tolerance to therapeutic effects may develop after 4 wk of treatment.
- Monitor for and report promptly signs of suicidal ideation especially in those treated for anxiety states accompanied by depression.
- Observe patient closely and monitor vital signs when diazepam is given parenterally; hypotension, muscular weakness, tachycardia, and respiratory depression may occur.
- Supervise ambulation. Adverse reactions such as drowsiness and ataxia are more likely to occur in older adults and debilitated or those receiving larger doses. Dosage adjustment may be necessary.
- Monitor I&O ratio, including urinary and bowel elimination.
- Monitor lab tests: Periodic LFTs, CBC, serum creatinine, BUN, serum lactate, osmol gap with long term use.

Patient & Family Education

- Avoid alcohol and other CNS depressants during therapy unless otherwise advised by prescriber. Concomitant use of these agents can cause severe drowsiness, respiratory depression, and apnea.
- Do not drive or engage in other potentially hazardous activities or those requiring mental precision until reaction to drug is known.
- Tell prescriber if you become or intend to become pregnant during therapy; drug may need to be discontinued.
- Take drug as prescribed; do not change dose or dose intervals.

DIAZOXIDE

(dye-az-ox′ide)

Proglycem

Classification: GLUCOSE ELEVATING AGENT

Therapeutic: HYPOGLYCEMIC

AVAILABILITY Oral suspension

ACTION & *THERAPEUTIC EFFECT* Causes dose-related increase in blood glucose level caused by inhibition of insulin release from the pancreas. *Increases blood glucose level.*

USES Orally in treatment of various diagnosed hypoglycemic states due to hyperinsulinism when other medical treatment or surgical management has been unsuccessful or is not feasible.

CONTRAINDICATIONS Hypersensitivity to diazoxide or other thiazides; cerebral bleeding, eclampsia; aortic coarctation; AV shunt, significant coronary artery disease; pheochromocytoma; functional hypoglycemia; lactation. Use in presence of increased bilirubin in newborns.

CAUTIOUS USE Diabetes mellitus; impaired cerebral or cardiac circulation; impaired renal function; patients taking corticosteroids or estrogen–progestogen combinations; hyperuricemia, history of gout, uremia; pregnancy (category C).

ROUTE & DOSAGE

Hypoglycemia

Adult/Child: **PO** 3–8 mg/kg divided every 8–12 h
Neonate/Infant: **PO** 8–15 mg/kg/day divided q8–12h

ADMINISTRATION

Oral

- Do not give darkened solutions. Store at 2°–30°C (36°–86°F) unless otherwise directed. Protect from light, heat, and freezing.

ADVERSE EFFECTS **CV:** Palpitations, atrial and ventricular arrhythmias, flushing, shock; *orthostatic hypotension,* CHF, transient hypertension. **CNS:** Headache, weakness, malaise, *dizziness,* polyneuritis, sleepiness, insomnia, euphoria, anxiety, extrapyramidal signs. **HEENT:** Tinnitus, momentary hearing loss; blurred vision, transient cataracts, subconjunctival hemorrhage, ring scotoma, diplopia, lacrimation, papilledema. **Endocrine:** Advance in bone age (children), *hyperglycemia, sodium and water retention, edema,* hyperuricemia, glycosuria, enlargement of breast lump, galactorrhea; decreased immunoglobulinemia, hirsutism. **Skin:** Monilial dermatitis, herpes, hirsutism; loss of scalp hair, sweating, sensation of warmth, burning, or itching. **GI:** *Nausea, vomiting,* abdominal discomfort, diarrhea, constipation, ileus, anorexia, transient loss of taste, impaired hepatic function. **GU:** Decreased urinary output, nephrotic syndrome (reversible), hematuria, increased nocturia, proteinuria, azotemia; inhibition of labor. **Hematologic:** Transient neutropenia, eosinophilia, decreased Hgb/Hct, decreased IgG. **Other:** Hypersensitivity (rash, fever, leukopenia); chest and back pain, muscle cramps.

DIAGNOSTIC TEST INTERFERENCE Diazoxide can cause false-negative response to ***glucagon.***

INTERACTIONS **Drug:** SULFONYLUREAS antagonize effects; THIAZIDE DIURETICS may intensify hyperglycemia and antihypertensive effects; **phenytoin** increases risk of hyperglycemia, and diazoxide may increase **phenytoin** metabolism, causing loss of seizure control.

PHARMACOKINETICS **Onset:** 1 h. **Duration:** 8 h. **Distribution:** Crosses blood–brain barrier and placenta. **Metabolism:** Partially metabolized in the liver. **Elimination:** In urine. **Half-Life:** 21–45 h.

D

NURSING IMPLICATIONS

Assessment & Drug Effects

- Monitor closely for S&S of CHF (e.g., development of edema, weight gain). Sodium and fluid retention may precipitate CHF in those with preexisting cardiac disease.
- Report promptly any change in I&O ratio.
- Oral administration usually does not produce marked effects on BP. However, do make periodic measurements of BP and vital signs.
- Monitor lab tests: Baseline and periodic blood glucose, urine for glucose and ketones, serum electrolytes, CBC with differential, Hct, platelet count, AST, and serum uric acid.

Patient & Family Education

- Note: Drug may cause hyperglycemia and glycosuria. Closely monitor blood and urine glucose; report any abnormalities to prescriber.
- Report palpitations, chest pain, dizziness, fainting, or severe headache.

DIBUCAINE

(dye'byoo-kane)

Nupercainal

Classification: ANESTHETIC, LOCAL (AMIDE-TYPE)

Therapeutic: LOCAL ANESTHETIC

Prototype: Procaine

AVAILABILITY Ointment

ACTION & *THERAPEUTIC EFFECT* Inhibits initiation and conduction of nerve impulses by reducing permeability of nerve cell membrane to sodium ions. *Relief of pain and itching due to inhibiting conduction of nerve impulses.*

USES Fast, temporary relief of pain and itching due to hemorrhoids and other anorectal disorders, nonpoisonous insect bites, sunburn, minor burns, cuts, and scratches.

CONTRAINDICATIONS Hypersensitivity to amide-type anesthetics.

CAUTIOUS USE Pregnancy (category C); lactation; children younger than 12 yr.

ROUTE & DOSAGE

Itching Due to Insect Bites or Hemorrhoids

Adult: **Topical** Apply skin cream or ointment to affected area as needed [max: 1 oz (28 g)/24 h]; insert rectal ointment morning and evening and after each bowel movement

Child: **Topical** Apply skin cream or ointment to affected area as needed [max: ¼ oz (7 g)/24 h]

ADMINISTRATION

Topical

- Apply cream preparation after bathing or swimming (water soluble).
- Store at 15°–30°C (59°–86°F) in tight, light-resistant containers.

ADVERSE EFFECTS **Skin:** Irritation, contact dermatitis; rectal bleeding (suppository).

PHARMACOKINETICS **Absorption:** Poorly absorbed from intact skin; readily absorbed from mucous membranes or abraded skin. **Onset:** 15 min. **Duration:** 2–4 h.

D

NURSING IMPLICATIONS

Patient & Family Education

- Discontinue if irritation or rectal bleeding (following use of rectal preparations) develops and consult prescriber.
- Prescriber may prescribe sitz baths 3–4 × day to reduce the swelling and pain of hemorrhoids.
- Note: Medication is intended for temporary relief of mild to moderate itching or pain. Seek medical advice for continuing discomfort, pain, bleeding, or sensation of rectal pressure.

DICLOFENAC

(di-klo′fen-ak)

Zorvolex

DICLOFENAC SODIUM

PENNSAID, Solaraze, Voltaren

DICLOFENAC POTASSIUM

Cambia, Cataflam, Zipsor

DICLOFENAC EPOLAMINE

Flector, Licart

Classification: NONSTEROIDAL ANALGESIC, ANTI-INFLAMMATORY DRUG (NSAID)

Therapeutic: ANALGESIC, NSAID; ANTIPYRETIC

Prototype: Ibuprofen

AVAILABILITY **Diclofenac:** Capsule. **Diclofenac Sodium:** Delayed release tablet; sustained release tablet; ophthalmic solution; gel; transdermal solution. **Diclofenac Potassium:** Tablet; powder for solution. **Diclofenac Epolamine:** Transdermal patch

ACTION & *THERAPEUTIC EFFECT* Diclofenac competitively inhibits both cyclooxygenase (COX) isoenzymes, COX-1, and COX-2, enzymes resulting in decreased formation of prostaglandin precursors. *Nonsteroidal anti-inflammatory drug (NSAID) with analgesic and antipyretic activity.*

USES Analgesic and antipyretic effects in symptomatic treatment of rheumatoid arthritis, osteoarthritis, and ankylosing spondylitis; dysmenorrhea, and migraine treatment. **Ophthalmic:** Postoperative ocular inflammation photophobia associated with refractive surgery. **Topical:** Relief of pain in joints, actinic keratosis. **Transdermal:** Acute pain.

CONTRAINDICATIONS Hypersensitivity to diclofenac, NSAIDS, or salicylate or bovine protein; patients in whom asthma, urticaria, angioedema, bronchospasm results from use of aspirin or other NSAIDs; GI bleeding or ulcer; hepatic porphyria; perioperative CABG pain; pregnancy (use of NSAIDs close to conception may be associated with an increased risk of miscarriage; birth defects have been observed following in utero NSAID exposure); 30 wk gestation or more with use of **PO** form; lactation; **gelatin** form use in individuals with previous history of hypersensitivity.

CAUTIOUS USE Patients receiving anticoagulant therapy; DM; asthma; history of GI disease or bleeding; hepatic disease; GU tract problems such as dysuria, cystitis, hematuria, impaired renal function; nephritis, nephrotic syndrome, patients who must restrict their sodium intake; dehydration; impaired hepatic function; SLE; heart failure or reduced left ventricular ejection fraction; cardiac disease; fluid retention; hypertension; older adults; pregnancy (category C), children.

D

ROUTE & DOSAGE

Mild/Moderate Pain

Adult: **PO** 100–150 mg/day in divided doses

Rheumatoid Arthritis

Adult: **PO** 100 mg/day in divided doses or 75 mg delayed release daily or 100 mg sustained release daily

Juvenile idiopathic arthritis

Child: **PO** 2–3 mg/kg/day in divided doses

Osteoarthritis

Adult: **PO** 50 mg 2 to 3 X daily; 75 mg delayed release bid; 100 mg sustained release daily; **Topical (gel)** apply to affected area qid **(solution)** 40 drops to each affected knee qid

Dysmenorrhea

Adult: **PO** 150mg/day in divided doses

Migraine

Adult: **PO** 50–100 mg as single dose (powder or IR tablet)

Ankylosing Spondylitis

Adult: **PO** 100–150 mg/day in divided doses.

Actinic Keratosis

Adult: **Topical** Apply to affected area bid for 60–90 days

Acute Pain

Adult: **Transdermal** Apply one patch to most painful area bid (Flector) or daily (Licart)

Renal Impairment Dosage Adjustment

eGFR 30–60 mL/min: temporarily discontinue use

ADMINISTRATION

Oral

- Ensure that sustained release forms of drug are not chewed or crushed. **Must be** swallowed whole.
- Minimize gastric irritation by administering it with a full glass of milk or food.
- Store at 20°–25°C (68°–77°F) away from heat and direct light.

Topical/Transdermal

- Do not apply gel or patch to areas of skin irritation.
- Massage gel into skin of entire affected area. Do not wash area within 1 h of application.
- Avoid application of any other topical products to treated area.
- Do not apply external heat or occlusive dressing to treated area.

Intravenous

- Administer as an IV bolus over 15 seconds.

ADVERSE EFFECTS **CV:** Edema. **CNS:** Headache, dizziness. **Skin:** Pruritus. **Hepatic/GI:** Increased liver enzymes, constipation, nausea, abdominal pain, diarrhea, vomiting. **Hematologic:** Anemia, prolonged bleeding time, infusion site pain, impaired wound healing.

DIAGNOSTIC TEST INTERFERENCE

May lead to false-positive ***aldosterone/renin ratio***.

INTERACTIONS **Drug:** Increases **cyclosporine**-induced nephrotoxicity; increases **methotrexate** levels (increases toxicity); do not use with other NSAIDS; may decrease BP-lowering effects of DIURETICS; may increase levels and toxicity of **lithium;** may decrease renal function when used with ARB or ACE INHIBITOR; may increase **digoxin** levels. **Herbal: Feverfew, garlic,**

ginger, ginkgo may increase risk of bleeding.

PHARMACOKINETICS

Absorption: Readily absorbed from GI tract; 50–60% reaches systemic circulation. **Peak:** 2–3 h. **Distribution:** Widely distributed including synovial fluid and into breast milk; 99% protein bound. **Metabolism:** Extensively metabolized in liver. **Elimination:** 50–70% in urine, 30–35% in feces. **Half-Life:** 1.2–2 h (PO); 12 h (transdermal).

NURSING IMPLICATIONS

Black Box Warning

Diclofenac has been associated with increased risk of serious, potentially fatal, CV thrombotic events (i.e., MI and stroke). Risk may increase with duration of use and may be greater in those with risk factors for CV disease.

Assessment & Drug Effects

- Monitor for signs and symptoms of GI irritation and ulceration especially in the older adult.
- Monitor for and report promptly S&S of CV thrombotic events (i.e., angina, MI, TIA, or stroke).
- Monitor BP for new onset or worsening of preexisting hypertension.
- Monitor diabetics closely for loss of diabetic glycemic control.
- Monitor for increased serum sodium and potassium in patients receiving potassium-sparing diuretics.
- Monitor for S&S of CHF, including weight gains greater than 1 kg (2 lb)/24 h.
- Monitor lab tests: Periodic LFTs, CBC, chemistry profile, and renal function tests.

Patient & Family Education

- Seek immediate medical attention if you experience S&S of adverse cardiovascular effects, such as chest pain, shortness of breath, weakness, or slurring of speech.
- Report immediately to prescriber S&S of serious GI irritation, such as stomach pain, frequent indigestion, tarry stools, or vomiting blood.
- Be alert for S&S of adverse skin reactions. Report promptly development of rash, blisters, or other skin reactions.
- Do not take aspirin or other OTC analgesics without permission of the prescriber.
- Avoid alcohol or other CNS depressants.
- Do not drive or engage in other potentially hazardous activities until reaction to drug is known.
- Diabetics should monitor blood glucose carefully for loss of glycemic control.

DICLOXACILLIN SODIUM

(dye-klox-a-sill'in)

Classification: PENICILLIN ANTIBIOTIC, PENICILLINASE-RESISTANT PENICILLIN
Therapeutic: PENICILLIN ANTIBIOTIC
Prototype: Oxacillin sodium

AVAILABILITY

Capsule

ACTION & *THERAPEUTIC EFFECT*

Inhibits the final stage of bacterial cell wall synthesis by preferentially binding to specific penicillin-binding proteins (PBPs) that are located inside bacterial cell wall; this leads to cell death. *Effective against penicillinase-producing staphylococci.*

D

USES Systemic infections caused by penicillinase-producing staphylococci.

UNLABLED USES Animal bite wounds, impetigo.

CONTRAINDICATIONS Hypersensitivity to dicloxacillin, other penicillins, and any component of the formulation.

CAUTIOUS USE History of or suspected allergy (asthma, eczema, hives, hay fever); history of hypersensitivity to cephalosporins or carbapenem; GI disease, colitis; renal or hepatic impairment; pregnancy (maternal use has generally not resulted in an increased risk of birth defects); lactation.

ROUTE & DOSAGE

Mild to Moderate Infections

Adult: **PO** 125–250 mg q6h
Child (weight less than 40 kg): **PO** 12–25 mg/kg/day divided q6h (max: 4 g/day)

ADMINISTRATION

Oral

- Give on an empty stomach at least 1 h before or 2 h after meals. Food reduces drug absorption. Should not be administered in the supine position or immediately before going to bed.
- Store capsules at room temperature in tight containers unless otherwise directed.

ADVERSE EFFECTS **GI:** Nausea, *diarrhea,* abdominal pain. **Other:** Hypersensitivity (pruritus, urticaria, rash, wheezing, sneezing, anaphylaxis; eosinophilia).

DIAGNOSTIC TEST INTERFERENCE May interfere with urinary glucose tests, may cause false positive for urine/serum proteins, may cause false positive in uric acid.

INTERACTIONS **Drug:** **Probenecid** decreases dicloxacillin elimination. Avoid LIVE VACCINES.

PHARMACOKINETICS **Absorption:** 35–76% absorbed from GI tract. **Peak:** 0.5–2 h. **Duration:** 4–6 h. **Distribution:** Distributed throughout body with highest concentrations in liver and kidney; low CSF penetration; crosses placenta; distributed into breast milk. Highly protein bound. **Metabolism:** In liver. **Elimination:** Primarily in urine with some elimination through bile. **Half-Life:** 30–60 min.

NURSING IMPLICATIONS

Assessment & Drug Effects

- Note: Take care to establish previous exposure and sensitivity to penicillins and cephalosporins as well as other allergic reactions of any kind before initiating therapy.
- Obtain C&S prior to initiation of therapy to determine susceptibility of causative organism. Therapy may begin pending test results.
- Monitor lab tests: Baseline C&S; periodic CBC with differential, and periodic LFTs.

Patient & Family Education

- Take medication around the clock. Do not miss a dose, and continue taking medication until it is all gone, unless otherwise directed by prescriber.
- Check with prescriber if GI side effects appear.
- Watch for and report the signs of hypersensitivity reactions and superinfections (see Appendix F).

DICYCLOMINE HYDROCHLORIDE

(dye-sye'kloe-meen)

Bentyl

Classification: ANTICHOLINERGIC; ANTISPASMODIC

Therapeutic: GI ANTISPASMODIC

Prototype: Atropine

AVAILABILITY Capsule; tablet; oral solution; solution for injection

ACTION & *THERAPEUTIC EFFECT* Relieves smooth muscle spasm by blocking the action of acetylcholine at parasympathetic sites in the smooth muscles, secretory glands, and the CNS. *Exerts antispasmodic effect on the GI tract.*

USES Irritable bowel syndrome.

CONTRAINDICATIONS Hypersensitivity to anticholinergic drugs; obstructive diseases of GU and GI tracts, paralytic ileus, intestinal atony, biliary tract disease; closed-angle glaucoma; unstable cardiovascular status; severe ulcerative colitis, toxic megacolon, esophagitis; myasthenia gravis; peripheral neuropathy; lactation; infants younger than 6 mo.

CAUTIOUS USE Prostatic hypertrophy; autonomic neuropathy; hyperthyroidism; coronary heart disease, CHF, arrhythmias, hypertension; hepatic or renal disease; GERD, hiatal hernia associated with esophageal reflux; older adults; pregnancy (use with caution in pregnant women); children.

ROUTE & DOSAGE

Irritable Bowel Syndrome

Adult/Adolescent: **PO** 20 mg up to qid

ADMINISTRATION

Oral

- Give 30 min before meals and at bedtime. May be taken with or without food.

Intramuscular

- Give deep IM into a large muscle. **Do not** give IV.
- Store below 30°C (86°F) unless otherwise directed.

ADVERSE EFFECTS **CNS:** Dizziness, drowsiness, nervousness. **HEENT:** Blurred vision. **GI:** *Dry mouth,* nausea. **Musculoskeletal:** Weakness.

INTERACTIONS **Drugs:** Avoid ANTICHOLINERGIC AGENTS, do not use with potassium citrate.

PHARMACOKINETICS **Absorption:** Readily from GI tract. **Onset:** 1–2 h. **Duration:** 4 h. **Metabolism:** In liver. **Elimination:** 80% in urine, 10% in feces. **Half-Life:** 2 h.

NURSING IMPLICATIONS

Assessment & Drug Effects

- Monitor for adverse effects especially in infants. Treatment of infant colic with dicyclomine includes some risk, especially in infants younger than 2 mo of age. Infants younger than 6 wk have developed respiratory symptoms as well as seizures, fluctuations in heart rate, weakness, and coma within minutes after taking syrup formulation. Symptoms generally last 20–30 min and are believed to be due to local irritation.
- Monitor for anticholinergic effects, decreased urine output, urinary retention, GI symptoms.
- If drug produces drowsiness and lightheadedness, supervision of ambulation and other safety precautions are warranted.

D

Patient & Family Education

- Exercise caution in hot weather. Dicyclomine may increase risk of heatstroke by decreasing sweating, especially in older adults.
- Do not drive or engage in other potentially hazardous activities until reaction to drug is known.
- Report changes in urine volume, voiding pattern.

DIDANOSINE (DDI)

(di-dan′o-sine)

Classification: ANTIRETROVIRAL; NUCLEOSIDE REVERSE TRANSCRIPTASE INHIBITOR (NRTI)
Therapeutic: ANTIRETROVIRAL (NRTI)
Prototype: Lamivudine

AVAILABILITY Delayed release capsule; powder for oral solution

ACTION & *THERAPEUTIC EFFECT* DDI interferes with the HIV RNA-dependent DNA polymerase (reverse transcriptase), thus preventing replication of the virus. *Synthetic purine nucleotide that inhibits replication of HIV.*

USES Treatment of HIV-1 infection with didanosine is not recommended in current guidelines.

CONTRAINDICATIONS Hypersensitivity to any of the components in the formulation; suspected or confirmed pancreatitis; lactic acidosis; severe hepatomegaly; portal hypertension; development of peripheral neuropathy; PKU; lactation; concurrent use with allopurinol, ribavirin, or stavudine.

CAUTIOUS USE Individuals with peripheral vascular disease, history of neuropathy, chronic pancreatitis, renal impairment, or any liver impairment; risk of liver disease; patients on sodium restriction; renal failure, renal impairment; alcoholism; older adults; gout; pregnancy (use not recommended during pregnancy due to risk of toxicity).

ROUTE & DOSAGE

HIV Infection

Adult/Adolescent/Child: **PO** *Weight 60 kg or more:* 400 mg daily; *weight 25–60 kg:* 250 mg daily; *weight 20–25 kg:* 200 mg daily

Renal Impairment Dosage Adjustment

Varies based on patient weight and dosage form used; see package insert

ADMINISTRATION

Oral

- Give drug on an empty stomach. Food should not be consumed within 15–30 min of drug administration.
- Give with water. **Do not** give with fruit juice or any other acid-containing liquid.
- Ensure that delayed release forms are swallowed whole. They must not be crushed or chewed.
- Mix powder for oral solution (buffered) with at least 120 mL (4 oz) of water, stir until dissolved (requires 2–3 min), and immediately swallow.
- Dosage reduction may be indicated in those with renal impairment.
- Store reconstituted liquid in a tightly closed container in refrigerator for up to 30 days.

ADVERSE EFFECTS **CNS:** *Peripheral neuropathy.* **Endocrine:** Hyperuricemia, lactic acidosis, increased amylase. **Skin:** Rash, *pruritus.* **GI:** *Abdominal pain,* *diarrhea*, pancreatitis, increased liver enzymes, hepatomegaly.

INTERACTIONS **Drug:** Do not use with alcohol, **allopurinol, febuxostat, hydroxyurea, ribavirin, stavudine** due to increased adverse effects. May decrease efficacy of **atazanavir, cladribine, darunavir, indinavir, itraconazole, ketoconazole, lopinavir.** Reduce dose when used with **tenofovir**. **Food:** Absorption is significantly decreased by food. Take on an empty stomach.

PHARMACOKINETICS **Absorption:** Rapidly absorbed from GI tract when administered to fasting patient with antacids; 23–40% reaches systemic circulation. **Peak:** 0.6–1 h. **Distribution:** Distributed primarily to body water; 21% reaches CSF; crosses placenta. **Elimination:** 36% in urine. **Half-Life:** 0.8–1.5 h.

NURSING IMPLICATIONS

Black Box Warning

Didanosine has been associated with fatal and nonfatal pancreatitis, lactic acidosis, and hepatomegaly with steatosis.

Assessment & Drug Effects

- Monitor for S&S of pancreatitis (e.g., abdominal pain, nausea, vomiting, elevated serum amylase). Report immediately to prescriber and withhold drug until ruled out.
- Monitor for S&S of peripheral neuropathy (e.g., numbness, tingling, burning, pain in hands or feet). Report to prescriber; dose reduction may be indicated.
- Monitor patients with renal impairment for drug toxicity and hypermagnesemia manifested by muscle weakness and confusion.
- Perform dilated retinal exam every 6 months.
- Monitor lab tests: Periodic CBC with differential, platelet count, CD4 cells, serum electrolytes, creatinine, uric acid, liver function tests, and lipid profile.

Patient & Family Education

- Report immediately to prescriber any of the following: Abdominal pain, nausea, or vomiting.
- Do not breastfeed while taking this drug.

DIETHYLPROPION HYDROCHLORIDE

(dye-eth-il-proe′pee-on)

Nobesine ♣

Classification: ANOREXIANT

Therapeutic: ANOREXIANT

Controlled Substance: Schedule IV

AVAILABILITY Tablet; sustained release tablet

ACTION & *THERAPEUTIC EFFECT* Anorexigenic action is probably secondary to direct (CNS) stimulation of appetite control center in hypothalamus and limbic regions. *Suppresses appetite as a result of drug action on CNS appetite control center.*

USES As short-term (a few weeks) adjunct in a regimen of weight reduction based on caloric restriction in obesity management.

CONTRAINDICATIONS Known hypersensitivity or idiosyncrasy to sympathomimetic amines; severe hypertension, advanced arteriosclerosis, hyperthyroidism; glaucoma; history of drug abuse; agitated states; within 14 days of MAOI therapy; pulmonary hypertension.

CAUTIOUS USE Hypertension, valvular heart disease; cardiac arrhythmia; symptomatic cardiovascular disease; psychosis, mania, epilepsy; diabetes mellitus; older adults; renal failure or impairment; seizure disorder; pregnancy (category B); lactation. Safe use in children younger than 16 yr is not known.

ROUTE & DOSAGE

Obesity

Adult/Adolescent: **PO** 25 mg tid 30–60 min a.c. or 75 mg sustained release daily midmorning

ADMINISTRATION

Oral

- Give on an empty stomach, 30 min–1 h before meals.
- Store at 15°–30°C (59°–86°F) in well-closed container unless otherwise specified.

ADVERSE EFFECTS **CV:** Palpitation, tachycardia, precordial pain, rise in BP. **CNS:** Mild euphoria, restlessness, *nervousness,* dizziness, headache, irritability, hyperactivity, insomnia, drowsiness, mood changes, lethargy, increase in convulsive episodes in patients with epilepsy. **GI:** Nausea, vomiting, diarrhea, constipation, dry mouth, unpleasant taste. **GU:** Impotence, changes in libido, gynecomastia, menstrual irregularities; polyuria, dysuria. **Other:** Hypersensitivity (urticaria, rash, erythema); muscle pain, dyspnea, hair loss, blurred vision, severe dermatoses (chronic intoxication), increased sweating.

INTERACTIONS **Drug: Acetazolamide, sodium bicarbonate** decreases diethylpropion elimination; **ascorbic acid** increases diethylpropion elimination; a BARBITURATE and diethylpropion taken together may antagonize the effects of both drugs; **furazolidone** may increase blood pressure effects of AMPHETAMINES, and interaction may persist for several weeks after discontinuation of **furazolidone; guanethidine** antagonizes antihypertensive effects; MAO INHIBITORS, **selegiline** can cause hypertensive crisis (fatalities reported)—AMPHETAMINES should not be administered at the same time or within 14 days of these drugs; PHENOTHIAZINES may inhibit mood-elevating effects of AMPHETAMINES; TRICYCLIC ANTIDEPRESSANTS enhance AMPHETAMINES' effects by increasing **norepinephrine** release; BETA AGONISTS increase cardiovascular adverse effects.

PHARMACOKINETICS **Absorption:** Readily from GI tract. **Duration:** 4 h, regular tablets; 10–14 h, sustained release. **Elimination:** In urine. **Half-Life:** 4–6 h.

NURSING IMPLICATIONS

Assessment & Drug Effects

- Observe patients with epilepsy closely for reduction in seizure control.
- Monitor diabetics for loss of glycemic control.
- Note: Varying degrees of psychologic and rarely physical dependence can occur.

Patient & Family Education

- Swallow sustained release tablets whole; **do not** chew.
- Do not drive or engage in other potentially hazardous activities until reaction to drug is known.
- If diabetic, closely monitor blood glucose values.

D

DIFLORASONE DIACETATE

(dye-flor′a-sone)

Maxiflor, Psorcon

See Appendix A-4.

DIFLUNISAL

(dye-floo′ni-sal)

Classification: ANALGESIC, NONSTEROIDAL ANTI-INFLAMMATORY DRUG (NSAID)

Therapeutic: ANALGESIC, NSAID; ANTIRHEUMATIC

Prototype: Ibuprofen

AVAILABILITY Tablet

ACTION & *THERAPEUTIC EFFECT* Has peripheral analgesic properties due to interfering with prostaglandin synthesis by inhibiting cyclooxygenase (COX) isoenzymes, COX-1 and COX-2. *Has analgesic and anti-inflammatory properties.*

USES Treatment of osteoarthritis and rheumatoid arthritis; mild to moderate pain.

CONTRAINDICATIONS Patients in whom aspirin or other NSAIDs precipitate an acute asthmatic attack (bronchospasm), urticaria, angioedema, severe rhinitis, or shock; active peptic ulcer, GI bleeding; severe salicylate hypersensitivity; treatment of perioperative pain in CABG care; pregnancy (category D third trimester).

CAUTIOUS USE History of upper GI disease; preexisting renal disease; impaired renal or hepatic function; alcoholics; compromised cardiac function, and other conditions associated with fluid retention; bone marrow suppression; geriatric patients; hypertension; patients who may be adversely affected by prolonged bleeding time; elderly; pregnancy (category C first and second trimester); lactation. Safe use in children younger than 12 yr not established.

ROUTE & DOSAGE

Arthritis

Adult: **PO** 250–500 bid (max: 1500 mg/day)

Pain

Adult: **PO** 1000 mg initial dose then 500 mg q12h

ADMINISTRATION

Oral

- Give with water, milk, or food to reduce GI irritation. Food causes slight reduction in absorption rate, but does not affect total amount absorbed.
- Store at 15°–30°C (59°–86°F) in tightly closed containers unless otherwise directed.

ADVERSE EFFECTS **CNS:** Headache. **Skin:** Rash, toxic epidermal necrolysis, exfoliative dermatitis, urticaria. **GI:** Dyspepsia, diarrhea, nausea, eructation, cholestatic jaundice. **GU:** Hematuria, proteinuria, interstitial nephritis, <u>renal failure</u>. **Hematologic:** Prolonged PT, anemia, decreased serum uric acid, transient elevations of liver function tests. **Other:** Weight gain, hyperventilation, dyspnea, photosensitivity.

DIAGNOSTIC TEST INTERFERENCE False elevation of **serum salicylate levels;** may lead to false-positive **aldosterone/renin ratio.**

INTERACTIONS **Drug:** ANTACIDS decrease diflunisal absorption;

D

aspirin and other NSAIDS increase risk of GI bleeding; increases risk of **warfarin**-induced hypoprothrombinemia; increases **methotrexate** levels and toxicity; may decrease renal function when used with ARB or ACE INHIBITOR.

PHARMACOKINETICS **Absorption:** Readily from GI tract. **Onset:** 1 h. **Peak:** 2–3 h. **Duration:** 12 h. **Distribution:** Probably crosses placenta; distributed into breast milk. **Metabolism:** In liver. **Elimination:** In urine. **Half-Life:** 8–12 h.

NURSING IMPLICATIONS

Black Box Warning

Diflunisal has been associated with increased risk of serious, potentially fatal, CV thrombotic events (i.e., MI and stroke). Risk may increase with duration of use and may be greater in those with risk factors for CV disease.

Assessment & Drug Effects

- Monitor for and report promptly S&S of CV thrombotic events (i.e., angina, MI, TIA, or stroke).
- Note: Although the antipyretic effect is mild, chronic or high doses may mask fever in some patients.
- Monitor lab tests: Periodic CBC, chemistry profile, liver function, PT/INR, and renal function tests with prolonged use.

Patient & Family Education

- Seek immediate medical attention if you experience S&S of adverse cardiovascular effects, such as chest pain, shortness of breath, weakness, or slurring of speech.
- Report to prescriber onset of visual or auditory problems.
- Check for and report peripheral edema and unusual weight gain.
- Report immediately to prescriber S&S of serious GI irritation, such as stomach pain, frequent indigestion, tarry stools, or vomiting blood.
- Be alert for S&S of adverse skin reactions. Report promptly development of rash, blisters, or other skin reactions.
- Do not drive or engage in other potentially hazardous activities until reaction to drug is known.
- Do not take aspirin or other OTC analgesics without permission of the prescriber.

DIGOXIN (Pr)

(di-jox'in)

Lanoxin

Classification: CARDIAC GLYCOSIDE; INOTROPIC

Therapeutic: CARDIAC GLYCOSIDE; ANTIARRHYTHMIC

AVAILABILITY Tablet; oral solution; solution for injection

ACTION & *THERAPEUTIC EFFECT*

Inhibits the sodium pump (NaK-ATPase), causing increased availability of intracellular calcium in the myocardium and conduction system, resulting in increased inotropy and automaticity, and reduced conduction velocity; indirectly causes parasympathetic stimulation of the autonomic nervous system resulting in a variety of effects on the CV system (e.g., decreased conduction through the AV node). *Increases contractility of heart muscle (positive inotropic effect). Has antiarrhythmic properties that result from its effects on the AV node.*

USES Rapid digitalization and for maintenance therapy in CHF, atrial fibrillation, atrial flutter, paroxysmal atrial tachycardia.

D

CONTRAINDICATIONS Digitalis hypersensitivity, sick sinus syndrome, Wolff–Parkinson–White syndrome; ventricular fibrillation, ventricular tachycardia unless due to CHF; hypocalcemia; myocarditis. Full digitalizing dose not given if patient has received digoxin during previous week or if slowly excreted cardiotonic glycoside has been given during previous 2 wk.

CAUTIOUS USE Renal insufficiency, hypokalemia, advanced heart disease, cardiomyopathy, acute MI, incomplete AV block, cor pulmonale; hypothyroidism; lung disease; older adults, or debilitated patients; pregnancy (category C); lactation; premature, children.

ROUTE & DOSAGE

Atrial Fibrillation/Digitalizing Dose

Give ½ dose initially followed by ¼ at 8–12 h intervals
Adult: **PO** 0.75–1.5 mg; **IV** 0.5–1 mg
Child (2 to younger than 10 yr): **IV** 20–35 mcg/kg; *10 yr or older:* 8–12 mcg/kg; **PO** *2 to younger than 10 yr:* 30–40 mcg/kg; *10 yr or older:* 10–15 mcg/kg
Infant: **IV** 30–50 mcg/kg; **PO** 35–60 mcg/kg
Neonate (Preterm): **IV** 15–25 mcg/kg; *full-term:* 20–30 mcg/kg

Maintenance Dose

Adult/Adolescent/Child (10 yr or older): **IV** 2.4–3.6 mcg/kg/day; **PO** 3.4–5.1 mcg/kg/day
Child (5 to younger than 10 yr): **IV** 4.6–9 mcg/kg/day in divided doses; **PO** 6.4–12 mcg/kg/day in divided doses
Child (2–4 yr): **IV** 7.6–10.6 mcg/kg/day in divided doses
Child (younger than 2 yr): 9–15 mcg/kg/day in divided doses

Renal Impairment Dosing Adjustment

See package insert for adjustment based on CrCl and lean body weight

ADMINISTRATION

Oral

- Give without regard to food. Administration after food may slightly delay rate of absorption, but total amount absorbed is not affected.
- Crush and mix with fluid or food if patient cannot swallow it whole.

Intravenous

PREPARE: **Direct:** Give undiluted or diluted in 4 mL of sterile water, D5W, or NS (using less diluent than 4 mL per 1 mL digoxin may cause precipitation).
ADMINISTER: **Direct:** Give each dose over at least 5 min. ▪ Monitor IV site frequently. Infiltration of parenteral drug into subcutaneous tissue can cause local irritation and sloughing.
INCOMPATIBILITIES: **Solution/additive:** **Dobutamine.** **Y-site:** **Amiodarone, amphotericin B cholesteryl complex, caspofungin, dantrolene, daunorubicin, diazepam, diazoxide, doxorubicin, fluconazole, foscarnet, gemtuzumab, idarubicin, lansoprazole, minocycline, mitoxantrone, paclitaxel, pentamidine, phenytoin, propofol, quinupristin/dalfopristin, sulfamethoxazole/trimethoprim, telavancin, propofol.**

- Store tablets, elixir, and injection solution at 25°C (77°F) or at 15°–30°C (59°–86°F).

D

ADVERSE EFFECTS CV: Arrhythmias, hypotension, AV block. **CNS:** Fatigue, muscle weakness, headache, facial neuralgia, mental depression, paresthesias, hallucinations, confusion, drowsiness, agitation, dizziness. **HEENT:** Visual disturbances. **GI:** Anorexia, *nausea,* vomiting, diarrhea. **Other:** Diaphoresis, recurrent malaise, dysphagia.

INTERACTIONS Drug: ANTACIDS, **cholestyramine, colestipol** decrease digoxin absorption; DIURETICS, CORTICOSTEROIDS, **amphotericin B,** LAXATIVES, **sodium polystyrene sulfonate** may cause hypokalemia, increasing the risk of digoxin toxicity; **calcium IV** may increase risk of arrhythmias if administered together with digoxin; **quinidine, verapamil, amiodarone, atorvastatin, captopril, diltiazem, erythromycin, alprazolam,** BETA BLOCKERS, **cyclosporine, ranolazine, SSRIS, telmisartan flecainide** significantly increase digoxin levels, and digoxin dose should be decreased; **succinylcholine** may potentiate arrhythmogenic effects; **nefazodone** may increase digoxin levels. **Food:** High fiber intake may decrease absorption. **Herbal: Ginseng** increase digoxin toxicity; **ma huang, ephedra** may induce arrhythmias; **St. John's wort** decreases plasma concentration. **Lab Test: Panax ginseng** can falsely elevate concentrations with fluorescence polarization immunoassay (FPIA) or falsely lower concentrations with microparticle enzyme immunoassay (MEIA).

PHARMACOKINETICS Absorption: 70% **Onset:** 1–2 h PO; 5–30 min IV. **Peak:** 6–8 h PO; 1–5 h IV. **Duration:** 3–4 days in fully digitalized patient. **Distribution:** Widely distributed; tissue levels significantly higher than plasma levels; crosses placenta. **Metabolism:** 14% in liver. **Elimination:** 80–90% by kidneys; may appear in breast milk. **Half-Life:** 34–44 h.

NURSING IMPLICATIONS

Assessment & Drug Effects

- Take apical pulse for 1 full min, noting rate, rhythm, and quality before administering drug.
- Withhold medication and notify prescriber if apical pulse falls below ordered parameters (e.g., less than 50 or 60/min in adults and less than 60 or 70/min in children).
- Be familiar with patient's baseline data (e.g., quality of peripheral pulses, blood pressure, clinical symptoms, serum electrolytes, creatinine clearance) as a foundation for making assessments.
- Monitor for S&S of drug toxicity: In children, cardiac arrhythmias are usually reliable signs of early toxicity. Early indicators in adults (anorexia, nausea, vomiting, diarrhea, visual disturbances) are rarely initial signs in children.
- Monitor I&O ratio during digitalization, particularly in patients with impaired renal function. Also monitor for edema daily and auscultate chest for rales.
- Monitor serum digoxin levels closely during concurrent antibiotic–digoxin therapy, which can precipitate toxicity because of altered intestinal flora.
- Observe patients closely when being transferred from one preparation (tablet, parenteral) to another.
- Monitor lab tests: Baseline and periodic serum digoxin, potassium, magnesium, and calcium.

Patient & Family Education

- Report to prescriber if pulse falls below 60 or rises above 110 or if you detect skipped beats or other changes in rhythm, when digoxin is prescribed for atrial fibrillation.
- Suspect toxicity and report to prescriber if any of the following occur: Anorexia, nausea, vomiting, diarrhea, or visual disturbances.
- Weigh each day under standard conditions. Report weight gain greater than 1 kg (2 lb)/day.
- Take digoxin PRECISELY as prescribed. Do not skip or double a dose or change dose intervals, and take it at same time each day.
- Do not take OTC medications, especially those for coughs, colds, allergy, GI upset, or obesity, without prior approval of prescriber.
- Continue with brand originally prescribed unless otherwise directed by prescriber.

DIGOXIN IMMUNE FAB (OVINE)

(di-jox′in)

Digibind, DigiFab

Classification: ANTIDOTE
Therapeutic: ANTIDOTE

AVAILABILITY Solution for injection

ACTION & *THERAPEUTIC EFFECT* Fab acts by selectively complexing with circulating digoxin or digitoxin, thereby preventing drug from binding at receptor sites; the complex is then eliminated in urine. *Used as an antidote for digitalis toxicity.*

USES Treatment of potentially life-threatening digoxin or digitoxin intoxication in carefully selected patients.

CONTRAINDICATIONS Hypersensitivity to sheep products; renal or cardiac failure.

CAUTIOUS USE Prior treatment with sheep antibodies or ovine Fab fragments; mannitol hypersensitivity; history of allergies; impaired renal function or renal failure; older adults; pregnancy (category C); lactation.

ROUTE & DOSAGE

Serious Digoxin Toxicity Secondary to Overdose

Adult/Child: **IV** Dosages vary according to amount of digoxin to be neutralized; dosages are based on total body load or steady-state serum digoxin concentrations (see package insert); some patients may require a second dose after several hours

ADMINISTRATION

Intravenous

PREPARE: **Direct:** Dilute each vial with 4 mL of sterile water for injection to yield 9.5 mg/mL for Digibind and 10 mg/mL for DigiFab; mix gently. **IV Infusion:** Dilute further with any volume of NS compatible with cardiac status. ▪ For those receiving less than 3 mg, further dilute to a concentration of 1 mg/mL by adding an additional 34 mL of NS to Digibind or 36 mL of NS to DigiFab. ▪ For very small doses for infants, reconstitute to a concentration of 10 mg/mL.

ADMINISTER: **Direct:** Give undiluted bolus only if cardiac arrest is imminent. **IV Infusion:** Give IV infusion over 30 min, preferably through a 0.22-micron membrane filter if Digibind is being infused.

D

- For administration to infants: Reconstitute as for direct IV and administer with a tuberculin syringe. ▪ For small doses (e.g., 2 mg or less), dilute the reconstituted 40-mg vial with 36 mL of NS to yield 1 mg/mL. ▪ Closely monitor for fluid overload.
- Use reconstituted solutions promptly or refrigerate at 2°–8°C (36°–46°F) for up to 4 h.

ADVERSE EFFECTS Adverse reactions associated with use of digoxin immune Fab are related primarily to the effects of **digitalis** withdrawal on the heart (see Nursing Implications). Allergic reactions have been reported rarely. Hypokalemia.

DIAGNOSTIC TEST INTERFERENCE Digoxin immune Fab may interfere with ***serum digoxin*** determinations by immunoassay tests.

PHARMACOKINETICS **Onset:** Less than 1 min after IV administration. **Elimination:** In urine over 5–7 days. **Half-Life:** 14–20 h.

NURSING IMPLICATIONS

Assessment & Drug Effects

- Perform skin testing for allergy prior to administration of immune Fab, particularly in patients with history of allergy or who have had previous therapy with immune Fab.
- Keep emergency equipment and drugs immediately available before skin testing is done or first dose is given and until patient is out of danger.
- Monitor for therapeutic effectiveness: Reflected in improvement in cardiac rhythm abnormalities, mental orientation and other neurologic symptoms, and GI and visual disturbances. S&S of reversal of digitalis toxicity occurs in 15–60 min in adults and usually within minutes in children.
- Baseline and frequent vital signs and EGG during administration.
- Note: Serum potassium is particularly critical during first several hours following administration of immune Fab. Monitor closely.
- Monitor closely: Cardiac status may deteriorate as inotropic action of digitalis is withdrawn by action of immune Fab. CHF, arrhythmias, increase in heart rate, and hypokalemia can occur.
- Make sure serum digoxin levels and ECG readings are obtained for at least 2–3 wk.
- Monitor lab tests: Baseline serum digoxin and serum creatinine; baseline serum potassium, then hourly for 4–6 h, and at least daily thereafter.

Patient & Family Education

- Tell prescriber about all other medications you are taking, including nonprescription medications, nutritional supplements, or herbal products.
- Check with your prescriber before stopping or starting any of your medicines.

DIHYDROERGOTAMINE MESYLATE

(dye-hye-droe-er-got′a-meen)

D.H.E. 45, Migranal

Classification: ALPHA-ADRENERGIC ANTAGONIST; ERGOT ALKALOID

Therapeutic: ANTIMIGRAINE

Prototype: Ergotamine

AVAILABILITY Nasal spray; solution for injection

ACTION & *THERAPEUTIC EFFECT* Alpha-adrenergic blocking agent and ergot alkaloid with direct constricting effect on smooth muscle of peripheral and cranial blood vessels. Acts as selective serotonin agonists at the 5-HT_1 receptors located on intracranial blood vessels, which may also cause vasoconstriction of large intracranial conductance arteries. *Reduces rate of serotonin-induced platelet aggregation. Has somewhat weaker vasoconstrictor action than ergotamine but greater adrenergic blocking activity, resulting in relief from migraine headaches.*

USES To prevent or abort headache or migraine; intractable migraine.

UNLABELED USES To treat postural hypotension; pelvic congestion with pain.

CONTRAINDICATIONS History of hypersensitivity to ergot preparations; peripheral vascular disease, coronary heart disease, MI, hypertension; peptic ulcer; severely impaired hepatic or renal function; sepsis; concurrent treatment with potent CYP3A4 inhibitors, including protease inhibitors, and macrolide antibiotics; within 48 h of surgery; pregnancy (category X); lactation.

CAUTIOUS USE Moderate or mild renal or hepatic impairment; obesity; diabetes mellitus; postmenopausal women; males older than 40 yr; pulmonary heart disease; valvular heart disease; smokers. Safe use in children younger than 6 yr is not established.

ROUTE & DOSAGE

Migraine Headache

Adult: **IV/IM/Subcutaneous** 1 mg, may be repeated at 1 h intervals to a total of 3 mg **IM** or 2 mg **IV/ Subcutaneous Intranasal** 1 spray (0.5 mg) in each nostril, may repeat with additional spray in 15 min if no relief (max: 4 sprays/attack); wait 6–8 h before treating another attack (max: 8 sprays/24 h, 24 sprays/wk)

ADMINISTRATION

Intranasal

- Give at first warning of migraine headache.
- Prior to administration of nasal spray, applicator must be primed with 4 pumps.

Intramuscular/Subcutaneous

- Give at first warning of migraine headache.
- Withdraw IM or subcutaneous dose directly from ampule. Do not dilute.
- Note: Onset of action is about 20 min; when rapid relief is required, the IV route is prescribed.

Intravenous

PREPARE: **Direct:** Give undiluted.
ADMINISTER: **Direct:** Over 2 to 3 min.

- Store at 15°–30°C (59°–86°F) unless otherwise directed. ▪ Protect ampules from heat and light; do not freeze. ▪ Discard ampule if solution appears discolored.

ADVERSE EFFECTS **Respiratory:** *Rhinitis.* **GI:** Nausea.

INTERACTIONS **Drug:** BETA BLOCKERS, ALPHA-BLOCKERS, **erythromycin** increase peripheral vasoconstriction with risk of ischemia; increased **ergotamine** toxicity with drugs that inhibit CYP3A4 (e.g., PROTEASE INHIBITORS, **amprenavir, ritonavir, nelfinavir, indinavir,**

saquinavir), MACROLIDE ANTIBIOTICS **(erythromycin, azithromycin, clarithromycin),** AZOLE ANTIFUNGALS **(ketoconazole, itraconazole, fluconazole, clotrimazole), nefazodone, fluoxetine, fluvoxamine. Food: Grapefruit juice** may increase toxicity.

PHARMACOKINETICS **Onset:** 15–30 min IM; less than 5 min IV. **Duration:** 3–4 h. **Distribution:** Probably distributed into breast milk. **Metabolism:** In liver by CYP3A4. **Elimination:** Primarily in urine; some in feces. **Half-Life:** 21–32 h.

NURSING IMPLICATIONS

Black Box Warning

Serious and life-threatening peripheral ischemia have been associated with concurrent administration of dihydroergotamine with potent CYP3A4 inhibitors such as protease inhibitors and macrolide antibiotics.

Assessment & Drug Effects

- Monitor cardiac status including hypertension and cardiac events.
- Monitor for and report numbness and tingling of fingers and toes, extremity weakness, muscle pain, or intermittent claudication.

Patient & Family Education

- Take at first warning of migraine headache.
- Lie down in a quiet, darkened room for several hours after drug administration for best results.
- Report immediately if any of the following S&S develop: Chest pain, nausea, vomiting, change in heartbeat, numbness, tingling, pain or weakness of extremities, edema, or itching.
- Women should use effective means of contraception while using this drug. Notify prescriber if you become pregnant.

DILTIAZEM

(dil-tye′a-zem)

Cardizem, Cardizem CD, Cardizem LA, Cartia XT, Dilacor XR, Dilt-CD, Dilt-XR, Matzim LA, Taztia XT, Tiazac

Classification: CALCIUM CHANNEL BLOCKING AGENT; ANTIANGINAL; ANTIHYPERTENSIVE

Therapeutic: ANTIANGINAL; ANTIARRHYTHMIC; ANTIHYPERTENSIVE

Prototype: Verapamil

AVAILABILITY Tablet; sustained release tablet; extended release capsule; extended release tablet; solution for injection

ACTION & *THERAPEUTIC EFFECT* Inhibits calcium ion influx through slow channels into cell of myocardial and arterial smooth muscle. Improves myocardial perfusion, and reduces left ventricular workload. *Slows SA and AV node conduction (antiarrhythmic effect). Dilates coronary arteries and arterioles and inhibits coronary artery spasm; thus myocardial oxygen delivery is increased (antianginal effect). By vasodilation of peripheral arterioles, drug decreases total peripheral vascular resistance and reduces arterial BP at rest (antihypertensive effect).*

USES Vasospastic angina (Prinzmetal variant or at rest angina), chronic stable (classic effort-associated) angina, essential hypertension. **IV:** Atrial fibrillation, atrial flutter, supraventricular tachycardia.

UNLABELED USES Prevention of reinfarction in non-Q-wave MI.

CONTRAINDICATIONS Known hypersensitivity to drug; sick sinus syndrome (unless pacemaker is in place and functioning); acute MI; pulmonary congestion; severe hypotension (systolic less than 90 mmHg or diastolic less than 60 mmHg); heart failure; patients undergoing intracranial surgery; bleeding aneurysms; lactation.

CAUTIOUS USE Sinoatrial nodal dysfunction, sick sinus syndrome with functioning pacemaker; left ventricular dysfunction, CHF, severe bradycardia; hypertrophic obstructive cardiomyopathy; conduction abnormalities; renal or hepatic impairment; older adults; pregnancy (category C); children.

ROUTE & DOSAGE

Angina

Adult: **PO** 30 mg qid, may increase q1–2 days as required (usual range: 180–360 mg/day in divided doses); **PO Extended release** 120–180 mg daily **PO (Cardizem LA)** 180 mg daily

Hypertension

Adult/Adolescent: **PO Extended release (once daily formulations)** 120–240 mg daily or 20–120 mg bid

Atrial Fibrillation/Flutter

Adult: **IV** 0.25 mg/kg IV bolus over 2 min, if inadequate response, may repeat in 15 min with 0.35 mg/kg, followed by a continuous infusion of 5–10 mg/h (max: 15 mg/h for 24 h)

ADMINISTRATION

Oral

- Do not crush sustained release capsules or tablets. They **must be** swallowed whole.
- Withhold if systolic BP is less than 90 mmHg or diastolic is less than 60 mmHg.
- Give before meals and at bedtime.
- Store at 15°–30°C (59°–86°F).

Intravenous

PREPARE: **Direct:** Give undiluted. **Continuous:** For IV infusion, add to a volume of D5W, NS, or D5/0.45% NaCl (e.g., 100–500 mL) that can be administered in 24 h or less.

ADMINISTER: **Direct:** Give as a bolus dose over 2 min. A second bolus may be given after 15 min. **Continuous:** Give at a rate 10–15 mg/h. Infusion duration longer than 24 h and infusion rate greater than 15 mg/h are not recommended.

INCOMPATIBILITIES: **Y-site:** **Acetazolamide, acyclovir, allopurinol, aminophylline, amphotericin B, ampicillin, ampicillin/sulbactam, cefepime, cefoperazone, ceftobiprole, chloramphenicol, dantrolene, diazepam, doxorubicin, fluorouracil, furosemide, ganciclovir, gemtuzumab, heparin, hydrocortisone, insulin, ketorolac, lansoprazole, methotrexate, methylprednisolone, micafungin, mitomycin, nafcillin, pantoprazole, pentobarbital, phenobarbital, phenytoin, piperacillin/tazobactam, procainamide, rifampin, sodium bicarbonate.**

D

ADVERSE EFFECTS **CV:** Edema, arrhythmias, angina, second- or third-degree AV block, bradycardia, CHF, flushing, hypotension, syncope, palpitations. **CNS:** *Headache,* fatigue, dizziness, asthenia, drowsiness, nervousness, insomnia, confusion, tremor, gait abnormality. **Skin:** Rash. **GI:** Nausea, constipation, anorexia, vomiting, diarrhea, impaired taste, weight increase.

INTERACTIONS **Drug:** BETA BLOCKERS, **digoxin** may have additive effects on av node conduction prolongation; may increase **digoxin** or **quinidine** levels; **cimetidine** may increase diltiazem levels, thus increasing effects; may increase **cyclosporine** levels. May increase STATIN levels, monitor closely. Do not use more than 10 mg of **simvastatin** concurrently. Do not use with **lomitapide**. **Herbal:** Monitor carefully if used with hawthorn.

PHARMACOKINETICS **Absorption:** Approximately 80% from GI tract, with 40% reaching systemic circulation. **Peak:** 2–3 h; 6–11 h sustained release; 11–18 h Cardizem LA. **Distribution:** Into breast milk. **Metabolism:** In liver (CYP3A4). **Elimination:** Primarily in urine with some elimination in feces. **Half-Life:** Oral 3.5–9 h, IV 2 h.

NURSING IMPLICATIONS

Assessment & Drug Effects

- Check BP and ECG before initiation of therapy and monitor particularly during dosage adjustment period.
- Monitor for and report S&S of CHF.
- Monitor for headache. An analgesic may be required.
- Supervise ambulation as indicated.

Patient & Family Education

- Make position changes slowly and in stages; light-headedness and dizziness (hypotension) are possible.
- Do not drive or engage in other potentially hazardous activities until reaction to drug is known.

DIMENHYDRINATE

(dye-men-hye′dri-nate)

Dramamine

Classification: ANTIHISTAMINE (H_1-RECEPTOR ANTAGONIST); ANTIVERTIGO

Therapeutic: ANTIVERTIGO; ANTIEMETIC

Prototype: Diphenhydramine

AVAILABILITY Tablet; chewable tablet; solution for injection

ACTION & *THERAPEUTIC EFFECT* H_1-receptor antagonist with antiemetic action thought to involve ability to inhibit cholinergic stimulation in vestibular and associated neural pathways. *Has antiemetic and antivertigo activity.*

USES Prevention and treatment of motion sickness.

UNLABELED USES Nausea and vomiting of pregnancy.

CONTRAINDICATIONS Hypersensitivity to dimenhydrinate or any component of the formulation, narrow-angle glaucoma, BPH; GI obstruction; urinary tract obstruction; CNS depression; lactation, neonates.

CAUTIOUS USE Convulsive disorders; asthma, COPD; severe hepatic disease; PKU; history of porphyria; closed-angle glaucoma; older adults; pregnancy (use with caution in pregnant women).

Safe use in children younger than 2 yr not established.

ROUTE & DOSAGE

Motion Sickness

Adult: **PO** 50–100 mg q4–6h (max: 400 mg/24 h); **IV/IM** 50 mg q4h
Child (2–6 yr): **PO** up to 25 mg q6–8h (max: 75 mg/24 h); *6–12 yr:* 25–50 mg q6–8h (max: 150 mg/24 h); **IM** 1.25 mg/kg qid up to 300 mg/day

ADMINISTRATION

- First dose should be given 30–60 min before starting activity.

Oral

- Ensure that chewable tablets are chewed and not swallowed whole.

Intramuscular

- Give undiluted and inject deep IM into a large muscle.

Intravenous

PREPARE: **Direct:** Dilute each 50 mg in 10 mL of NS.
ADMINISTER: **Direct:** Give each 50 mg or fraction thereof over 2 min.

- Store preferably at 15°–30°C (59°–86°F), unless otherwise directed by manufacturer. ▪ Examine parenteral preparation for particulate matter and discoloration. Do not use unless absolutely clear.

ADVERSE EFFECTS

CV: Tachycardia. **Respiratory:** Thickening of bronchial secretions. **CNS:** *Drowsiness,* headache, incoordination, dizziness, blurred vision, nervousness, restlessness, *insomnia (especially children).* **Integumentary:** Skin rash. **GI:** Dry mouth, epigastric distress, nausea, anorexia. **GU:** Dysuria.

INTERACTIONS

Drug: Alcohol and other CNS DEPRESSANTS enhance CNS depression, drowsiness; TRICYCLIC ANTIDEPRESSANTS, ANTICHOLINERGIC AGENTS compound anticholinergic effects.

PHARMACOKINETICS

Absorption: Readily absorbed from GI tract. **Onset:** 15–30 min PO; immediate IV; 20–30 min IM. **Duration:** 4–6 h. **Distribution:** Distributed into breast milk. **Elimination:** In urine.

NURSING IMPLICATIONS

Assessment & Drug Effects

- Use fall precautions and supervise ambulation; drug produces high incidence of drowsiness.
- Note: Tolerance to CNS depressant effects usually occurs after a few days of drug therapy; some decrease in antiemetic action may result with prolonged use.
- Monitor for dizziness, nausea, and vomiting; these may indicate drug toxicity.

Patient & Family Education

- Do not drive or engage in other potentially hazardous activities until response to drug is known.
- Take 30–60 min before departure to prevent motion sickness; repeat before meals and upon retiring.

DIMERCAPROL

(dye-mer-kap'role)

BAL in Oil

Classification: CHELATING AGENT; ANTIDOTE
Therapeutic: ANTIDOTE

AVAILABILITY

Solution for injection

ACTION & THERAPEUTIC EFFECT

Combines with ions of various heavy metals to form relatively stable, nontoxic, soluble complexes called chelates, which can be excreted; inhibition of enzymes by toxic metals is thus prevented. *Neutralizes the effects of various heavy metals.*

D

USES Acute poisoning by arsenic, gold, and mercury; as adjunct to edetate calcium disodium (EDTA) in treatment of lead encephalopathy.

UNLABELED USES Chromium dermatitis; ocular and dermatologic manifestations of arsenic poisoning, as adjunct to penicillamine to increase rate of copper excretion in Wilson disease, and for poisoning with heavy metals.

CONTRAINDICATIONS Hepatic insufficiency (with exception of postarsenical jaundice); history of peanut oil hypersensitivity; severe renal insufficiency; poisoning due to cadmium, iron, selenium, or uranium; lactation.

CAUTIOUS USE Hypertension; oliguria; patients with G6PD deficiency; preexisting renal disease; rheumatoid arthritis; pregnancy (category C).

ROUTE & DOSAGE

Arsenic or Gold Poisoning

Adult/Child: **IM** 2.5–3 mg/kg q4h for first 2 days, then qid on 3rd day, then bid for 10 days

Mercury Poisoning

Adult/Child: **IM** 5 mg/kg initially, followed by 2.5 mg/kg 1–2 × day for 10 days

Acute Lead Encephalopathy

Adult/Child: **IM** 4 mg/kg initially, then 3–4 mg/kg q4h with EDTA for 2–7 days depending on response

ADMINISTRATION

Intramuscular

- Initiate therapy ASAP (within 1–2 h) after ingestion of the poison because irreversible tissue damage occurs quickly, particularly in mercury poisoning.
- Give by deep IM injection only. Local pain, gluteal abscess, and skin sensitization possible. Rotate injection sites, and observe daily.
- Determine if a local anesthetic may be given with the injection to decrease injection site pain.
- Handle with caution; contact of drug with skin may produce erythema, edema, dermatitis.

ADVERSE EFFECTS **CV:** *Elevated BP,* tachycardia. **CNS:** Headache, anxiety, muscle pain or weakness, restlessness, paresthesias, tremors, *convulsions,* shock. **HEENT:** Rhinorrhea; burning sensation, feeling of pain and constriction in throat. **GI:** Nausea, *vomiting;* burning sensation in lips and mouth, halitosis, salivation; abdominal pain, metabolic acidosis. **GU:** Burning sensation in penis, <u>renal damage</u>. **Other:** Pain in chest or hands, pain and sterile abscess at injection site, sweating, reduction in polymorphonuclear leukocytes, dental pain.

DIAGNOSTIC TEST INTERFERENCE ***I^{131} thyroid uptake*** values may be decreased if test is done during or immediately following dimercaprol therapy.

INTERACTIONS **Drug:** **Iron, cadmium, selenium, uranium** form toxic complexes with dimercaprol.

PHARMACOKINETICS **Peak:** 30–60 min. **Distribution:** Distributed mainly in intracellular spaces, including brain; highest concentrations in liver and kidneys.

Elimination: Completely excreted in urine and bile within 4 h. **Half-Life:** Short.

NURSING IMPLICATIONS

Assessment & Drug Effects

- Monitor vital signs. Elevations of systolic and diastolic BPs accompanied by tachycardia frequently occur within a few minutes following injection and may remain elevated up to 2 h.
- Note: Fever occurs in approximately 30% of children receiving treatment and may persist throughout therapy.
- Monitor I&O. Drug is potentially nephrotoxic. Report oliguria or change in I&O ratio to prescriber.
- Check urine daily for albumin, blood, casts, and pH. Blood and urinary levels of the metal serve as guides for dosage adjustments.
- Minor adverse reactions generally reach maximum 15–20 min after drug administration and subside in 30–90 min.

Patient & Family Education

- Drink as much fluid as the prescriber will permit.

DIMETHYL FUMARATE

(dye-meth′il fue′ma-rate)

Tecfidera

Classification: NEUROPROTECTIVE; ANTI-INFLAMMATORY

Therapeutic: NEUROPROTECTIVE; ANTI-INFLAMMATORY

AVAILABILITY Delayed release capsule

ACTION & THERAPEUTIC EFFECT Mechanism of action is unknown but believed to be associated with activation of a pathway involved in the cellular response to oxidative stress. *DMF decreases inflammation in neurologic tissue thus exerting a protective effect.*

USES Treatment of patients who have relapsing forms of multiple sclerosis.

CONTRAINDICATIONS Serious infections.

CAUTIOUS USE Drug-related lymphopenia; QT prolongation; pregnancy (category C); lactation.

ROUTE & DOSAGE

Multiple Sclerosis

Adult: PO 120 mg bid for 7 days, then 240 mg bid

ADMINISTRATION

Oral

- May be given irrespective of food.
- Capsules **must be** swallowed whole. They should not be opened or chewed.
- Store at 15°–30°C (59°–86°F). Protect from light.

ADVERSE EFFECTS **Endocrine:** ALT/AST increased. **Skin:** Erythema, pruritus, rash. **GI:** *Abdominal pain, diarrhea*, dyspepsia, *nausea, vomiting.* **Hematological:** Lymphopenia. **Other:** *Flushing, infection.*

PHARMACOKINETICS **Peak:** 2–2.5 h. **Distribution:** 27–45% plasma protein bound. **Metabolism:** In liver to active metabolite, monomethyl fumarate (MMF). **Elimination:** Exhalation of CO_2 (60%) and renal (16%). **Half-Life:** 1 h.

NURSING IMPLICATIONS

Assessment & Drug Effects

- Monitor response to therapy.
- Monitor for adverse events: Flushing and GI reactions (abdominal pain, diarrhea, and nausea) are

D

the most common reactions, especially in early therapy, and may decrease over time.
- Monitor lab tests: Baseline CBC (within first 6 mo), then annually thereafter.

Patient & Family Education
- Store in original container.
- Discard opened container of medication after 90 days.
- Inform prescriber if you are pregnant or plan to become pregnant.

DIMETHYL SULFOXIDE
(dye-meth′il sul-fox′ide)

DMSO, Rimso-50

Classification: GENITOURINARY; LOCAL ANTI-INFLAMMATORY

Therapeutic: INTERSTITIAL CYSTITIS AGENT

AVAILABILITY Solution

ACTION & *THERAPEUTIC EFFECT* Reported effects include anti-inflammatory effects, membrane penetration, collagen dissolution, vasodilation, muscle relaxation, diuresis, initiation of histamine release at administration site, cholinesterase inhibition. *Has symptomatic relief of interstitial cystitis with local anti-inflammatory properties.*

USES Symptomatic treatment of interstitial cystitis.

UNLABELED USES Topical treatment of a variety of musculoskeletal disorders, arthritis, scleroderma, tendinitis, breast and prostate malignancies, retinitis pigmentosa, herpesvirus infections, head and spinal cord injuries, shock, and as a carrier to enhance penetration and absorption of other drugs. Also used to protect living cells and tissues during cold storage (cryoprotection). Widely used as an industrial solvent and in veterinary medicine for treatment of musculoskeletal injuries.

CONTRAINDICATIONS Urinary tract malignancy; lactation.

CAUTIOUS USE Hepatic or renal dysfunction; pregnancy (category C). Safe use in children is not established.

ROUTE & DOSAGE

Interstitial Cystitis

Adult: **Instillation** 50 mL of 50% solution instilled slowly into urinary bladder and retained for 15 min; may repeat q2wk until maximum relief obtained, then increase intervals between treatments

ADMINISTRATION

Instillation
- Apply analgesic lubricant such as lidocaine jelly to urethra to facilitate insertion of catheter.
- Instruct patient to retain instillation for 15 min and then expel it by spontaneous voiding.
- Note: Discomfort associated with instillation usually lessens with repeated administration. Prescriber may prescribe an oral analgesic or suppository containing belladonna and an opiate prior to instillation to reduce bladder spasm.
- Store at 15°–30°C (59°–86°F) unless otherwise directed. Protect from strong light. Avoid contact with plastics.

ADVERSE EFFECTS **HEENT:** Transient disturbances in color vision, photophobia. **GI:** Nausea, diarrhea. Hypersensitivity: Local or generalized rash, erythema, pruritus, urticaria, swelling of face, dyspnea (anaphylactoid reaction). **Other:** Nasal congestion, headache, sedation, drowsiness. *Following instillation: Garlic-like odor on breath and skin; garlic-like taste;* discomfort during administration; transient cystitis. *Following topical application:* Vesicle formation.

INTERACTIONS **Drug:** Decreases effectiveness of **sulindac,** possibly causing severe peripheral neuropathy.

PHARMACOKINETICS **Absorption:** Readily absorbed systemically. **Peak:** 4–8 h. **Distribution:** Widely distributed in tissues and body fluids; penetrates blood–brain barrier; distributed into breast milk. **Metabolism:** Metabolized to dimethyl sulfide (garlic breath) and dimethyl sulfone. **Elimination:** Dimethyl sulfide excreted through lungs and skin; dimethyl sulfone may remain in serum longer than 2 wk and is excreted in urine and feces.

NURSING IMPLICATIONS

Assessment & Drug Effects

- Monitor and report level of bladder discomfort. In cases of severe discomfort prescriber may elect to do instillation under anesthesia.
- Monitor for visual disturbances. Complete eye evaluation, including slit-lamp examination, is recommended prior to and at regular intervals during therapy.

Patient & Family Education

- Note: Garlic-like taste may be experienced within minutes after drug instillation and may last for several hours. Garlic-like odor on breath and skin may last as long as 72 h.

DINOPROSTONE (PGE$_2$, PROSTAGLANDIN E$_2$)

(dye-noe-prost'one)

Cervidil, Prostin E$_2$, Prepidil

Classification: OXYTOCIC

Therapeutic: PROSTAGLANDIN; OXYTOCIC

Prototype: Oxytocin

AVAILABILITY Vaginal suppository; **Prepidil:** Vaginal gel; **Cervidil:** Vaginal insert

ACTION & *THERAPEUTIC EFFECT* Synthetic prostaglandin E$_2$ that appears to act directly on myometrium and vascular smooth muscle. Stimulation of gravid uterus in early weeks of gestation is more potent than that of oxytocin. *Contractions are qualitatively similar to those that occur during term labor. Has high success rate when used as abortifacient before 20th week and for stimulation of labor in cases of intrauterine fetal death.*

USES To terminate pregnancy from 12th week through second trimester; cervical ripening prior to labor induction.

CONTRAINDICATIONS Acute pelvic inflammatory disease; abnormal fetal position; history of pelvic surgery, cervical stenosis, active cardiac, pulmonary, renal, or hepatic disease.

CAUTIOUS USE History of hypertension, hypotension, asthma, epilepsy, anemia, diabetes mellitus; jaundice, history of hepatic, renal, or cardiovascular disease; glaucoma or raised intraocular pressure; cervicitis, acute vaginitis, infected endocervical lesion; previous history of caesarean section; pregnancy (category C). Safety and efficacy in children or adolescents not established.

ROUTE & DOSAGE

Induction of Labor

Adult: **Endocervical** Place **Prepidil** 0.5 mg endocervically, may repeat q6h (max: 1.5 mg); place **Cervidil** insert 10 mg transversely in the posterior fornix of the vagina, remove on onset of active labor or 12 h after insertion

Evacuation of Uterus/Abortion

Adult: **Intravaginal** Insert 20 mg suppository high in vagina, repeat q3–5h until abortion occurs or membranes rupture (max total dose: 240 mg)

ADMINISTRATION

Endocervical & Intravaginal

- **Do not** exceed recommended dose.
- Antiemetic and antidiarrheal medication may be prescribed to be given before dinoprostone to minimize GI side effects.
- Place vaginal insert in the vagina immediately after removal from the foil package. **Do not** use without retrieval system.
- Keep patient in supine position for 10 min after administration of suppository to prevent expulsion and enhance absorption.
- Store suppositories in freezer at temperature not exceeding −20°C (−4°F) unless otherwise specified.

ADVERSE EFFECTS **CV:** Transient hypotension, flushing, cardiac arrhythmias. **Respiratory:** Dyspnea, cough, hiccups. **CNS:** Headache, tremor, tension. **GI:** *Nausea, vomiting, diarrhea.* **GU:** Vaginal pain, endometritis, uterine contractions, uterine rupture. **Other:** *Chills, fever,* dehydration, diaphoresis, rash, localized warm feeling, back pain.

INTERACTIONS **Drug:** OXYTOCICS used with extreme caution.

PHARMACOKINETICS **Absorption:** Slowly absorbed from vagina; Cervidil insert releases approximately 0.3 mg/h. **Onset:** 10 min. **Duration:** 2–3 h. **Distribution:** Widely distributed in body. **Metabolism:** Rapidly metabolized in lungs, kidneys, spleen, and other tissues. **Elimination:** Mainly in urine; some in feces.

NURSING IMPLICATIONS

Black Box Warning

Recommended doses of dinoprostone should not be exceeded.

Assessment & Drug Effects

- Observe patient carefully, after insertion of the drug. Rupture of the membranes is not a contraindication to drug, but be aware that profuse bleeding may result in expulsion of the suppository. Report wheezing, chest pain, dyspnea, and significant changes in BP and pulse to the prescriber.
- Monitor uterine contractions and observe for and report excessive vaginal bleeding and cramping pain.
- Monitor vital signs. Fever is a physiologic response of the hypothalamus to use of dinoprostone and occurs within 15–45 min after insertion of suppository. Temperature returns to normal within 2–6 h after discontinuation of medication.

Patient & Family Education

- Continue taking your temperature (late afternoon) for a few days after discharge. Contact prescriber with onset of fever, bleeding, abdominal cramps, abnormal or foul-smelling vaginal discharge.

- Avoid douches, tampons, intercourse, and tub baths for at least 2 wk. Clarify with prescriber.

DINUTUXIMAB

(di-nu-tux'i-mab)

Unituxin

Classification: ANTINEOPLASTIC; IMMUNOMODULATOR; MONOCLONAL ANTIBODY

Therapeutic: ANTINEOPLASTIC

Prototype: Basiliximab

AVAILABILITY Solution for injection

ACTION & *THERAPEUTIC EFFECT* Binds to the glycolipid GD2 that is expressed on neuroblastoma cells and induces cell lysis of GD2-expressing cells through antibody-dependent cell-mediated cytotoxicity (ADCC) and complement-dependent cytotoxicity (CDC). *Kills neuroblastoma cells and slows tumor growth.*

USES Treatment of pediatric patients with high-risk neuroblastoma who achieve at least a partial response to prior first-line multiagent, multimodality therapy; used in combination with granulocyte-macrophage colony-stimulating factor (GM-CSF), interleukin-2 (IL-2), and 13-*cis*-retinoic acid (RA).

CONTRAINDICATIONS History of anaphylaxis to dinutuximab; severe unresponsive pain, severe sensory neuropathy, or moderate to severe peripheral motor neuropathy; atypical hemolytic uremic syndrome; severe capillary leak syndrome; pregnancy; lactation.

CAUTIOUS USE Infusion reactions; pain and peripheral neuropathy; capillary leak syndrome; hypotension; infection; neurologic disorders of the eye; electrolyte imbalance.

ROUTE & DOSAGE

Neuroblastoma

Child/Adolescent: **IV** 17.5 mg/m²/d for 10–20 h for 4 consecutive days; repeat for a total of 5 cycles (max infusion rate: 1.75 mg/m²/h); cycles 1, 3, and 5 are 24 days with infusions on days 4–7; cycles 2–4 are 32 days with infusions on days 8–11

Adverse Reactions/Toxicity Dosage Adjustments

See manufacturer's information for adjustments

ADMINISTRATION

Intravenous

PRETREATMENT:

- Hydration: Administer IV NS 10 mL/kg over 1 h just prior to initiating each infusion.
- Analgesics: Morphine sulfate or similar opioid is required before/during dinutuximab infusion to control pain.
- Antihistamine: Diphenhydramine or similar antihistamine is required before/during dinutuximab infusion to reduce risk of infusion reaction.
- Antipyretics: Acetaminophen is required before/during dinutuximab infusion to control fever.

PREPARE: **IV Infusion:** Withdraw required volume from vial and inject into a 100-mL bag of NS. Mix by gentle inversion but do not shake. Discard unused contents of the vial.

ADMINISTER: **IV Infusion:** Initiate at 0.875 mg/m²/h for 30 min; then rate can be gradually increased as tolerated (max: 1.75 mg/m²/h).

- Store undiluted vials under refrigeration. Initiate infusion within 4 h of preparation.

ADVERSE EFFECTS

CV: *Capillary leak syndrome*, hemorrhage, hypotension, hypertension, tachycardia, angioedema. **Respiratory:** *Hypoxia*, bronchospasm, wheezing. **CNS:** Peripheral neuropathy. **Endocrine:** Hyperglycemia, hypertriglyceridemia, *hypoalbuminemia, hypocalcemia, hypokalemia*, hypomagnesemia, *hyponatremia, hypophosphatemia, increased ALT/AST*, increased serum creatinine, increased weight. **Skin:** *Urticaria*. **GI:** *Diarrhea*, nausea, anorexia, *vomiting, abdominal pain*. **GU:** Proteinuria. **Hematological:** *Anemia, lymphopenia, neutropenia, thrombocytopenia*. **Other:** Device-related infection, *arthralgia*, back pain, *angioedema, infusion reactions, pain, pyrexia*, sepsis.

PHARMACOKINETICS

Half-Life: 10 d.

NURSING IMPLICATIONS

Black Box Warning

Dinutuximab has been associated with potentially life-threatening infusion reactions and is known to cause severe neuropathic pain.

Assessment & Drug Effects

- Monitor patients closely for S&S of an infusion reaction or other serious adverse effects during and for at least 4 h after infusion. Immediately interrupt infusion and notify prescriber for severe infusion reactions (see Adverse Effects).
- Monitor vital signs during and for at least 4 h after infusion. Stop infusion and notify prescriber for symptomatic hypotension, systolic BP less than lower limit of normal for age or decreased by more than 15% of baseline.
- Monitor pain level frequently.
- Monitor for signs of severe motor neuropathy or ocular neurological disorders (e.g., blurred vision, photophobia, mydriasis, fixed or unequal pupils, eyelid ptosis).
- Monitor lab tests: Baseline and periodic CBC with differential, serum electrolytes, renal function tests, and LFTs.

Patient & Family Education

- Report immediately symptoms such as facial or lip swelling, hives, difficulty breathing, lightheadedness or dizziness that occur during or within 24 h following the infusion.
- Report promptly severe or worsening pain and S&S of neuropathy (e.g., numbness, tingling, burning, or weakness).
- Report promptly problems with the eyes (e.g., blurred vision, photophobia, double vision, drooping eyelid).
- Women should use effective contraception during therapy and for 2 mo after the last dose.
- Do not breastfeed while taking this drug.

DIPHENHYDRAMINE HYDROCHLORIDE (Pr)

(dye-fen-hye'dra-meen)

Allerdryl ♣, Benadryl

Classification: CENTRALLY ACTING CHOLINERGIC ANTAGONIST; ANTIHISTAMINE; H_1-RECEPTOR ANTAGONIST
Therapeutic: ANTIHISTAMINE; SEDATIVE-HYPNOTIC; ANTIPARKINSON; ANTIDYSKINETIC; NONNARCOTIC ANTITUSSIVE

AVAILABILITY Capsules; tablet; syrup; solution for injection; cream

ACTION & *THERAPEUTIC EFFECT* Competes for H_1-receptor sites on effector cells in the GI tract, blood vessels, and respiratory tract; also has anticholinergic and sedative effects. *Has antihistamine, antivertigo, antiemetic, antianaphylactic, antitussive, antidyskinetic, and sedative effects.*

USES Temporary symptomatic relief of various allergic conditions and to treat or prevent motion sickness, vertigo, and reactions to blood or plasma in susceptible patients. Also used in anaphylaxis as adjunct to epinephrine and other standard measures after acute symptoms have been controlled; in treatment of parkinsonism and drug-induced extrapyramidal reactions; as a sedative-hypnotic; occasional insomnia.

CONTRAINDICATIONS Hypersensitivity to antihistamines of similar structure; lower respiratory tract symptoms (including acute asthma); narrow-angle glaucoma; prostatic hypertrophy, bladder neck obstruction; GI obstruction or stenosis; lactation, premature neonates, and neonates.

CAUTIOUS USE History of asthma; COPD; convulsive disorders; increased IOP; hyperthyroidism; hypertension, cardiovascular disease; hepatic disease; diabetes mellitus; older adults, infants, and young children; pregnancy (use with caution in pregnant women). Use as a nighttime sleep aid in children younger than 2 yr not established.

ROUTE & DOSAGE

Allergy Symptoms, Motion Sickness

Adult: **PO** 25 mg q4–6h or 50 mg q6–8h prn (max: 300 mg/day)
Child: 6–12 yr: **PO** 5 mg/kg/day in divided doses q6–8h mg q4–6h (max: 50 mg/dose)

Adjunct to anaphylaxis

Adult: **IV** 25–50 mg after administering epinephrine then q4–6h as needed

Dystonic reaction

Adult: **IM/IV** 25–50 mg initially then **PO** 25 mg q4–6h or 50 mg q6–8h

Occasional Insomnia

Adult: **PO** 25–50 mg at bedtime (occasional use only)

ADMINISTRATION

Oral

- Give with food or milk to lessen GI adverse effects.
- For motion sickness: Give the first dose 30 min before exposure to motion.
- When used for occasional insomnia, dose should be given 30 minutes before bedtime.

Intramuscular

- Give IM injection deep into large muscle mass; alternate injection sites. Avoid perivascular or subcutaneous injections because of localized necrosis effects.
- Note: Hypersensitivity reactions (including anaphylactic shock) are more likely to

occur with parenteral than PO administration.

Intravenous

PREPARE: **Direct:** Give undiluted.
ADMINISTER: **Direct:** Give at a rate of 25 mg or less over 1 min.
INCOMPATIBILITIES: **Solution/additive:** **Amphotericin B, iodipamide, lorazepam, thiopental.** **Y-site:** **Allopurinol, aminophylline, amphotericin B cholesteryl complex, ampicillin, azathioprine, cefamandole, cefazolin, cefepime, cefiderocol, cefoperazone, cefotaxime, cefotetan, cefoxitin, ceftazidime, ceftobiprole, ceftriaxone, cefuroxime, chloramphenicol, dantrolene, dexamethasone, diazepam, diazoxide, fluorouracil, foscarnet, fosfomycin, furosemide, ganciclovir, indomethacin, insulin, ketorolac, lansoprazole, meropenem/vaborbactam, methylprednisolone, nitroprusside, oxacillin, pantoprazole, pentobarbital, phenobarbital, phenytoin, sodium bicarbonate, sulfamethoxazole/trimethoprim.**

- Store in tightly covered containers at 20°–25°C (68°–77°F) unless otherwise directed by manufacturer. Keep injection and elixir formulations in light-resistant containers.

ADVERSE EFFECTS **CV:** Palpitation, *tachycardia,* hypotension, chest tightness. **Respiratory:** Thickened bronchial secretions, wheezing, nasal congestion, pharyngeal edema. **CNS:** *Drowsiness,* dizziness, headache, fatigue, ataxia, neuritis, paresthesia, tremors, euphoria, nervousness, restlessness, excitement, fever. **HEENT:** Tinnitus, vertigo; blurred vision, diplopia. **GI:** *Dry mouth,* nausea, epigastric distress, anorexia, vomiting, constipation, or diarrhea. **GU:** Urinary frequency or retention, dysuria. **Hematologic:** Agranulocytosis, hemolytic anemia, thrombocytopenia. **Other:** Hypersensitivity (skin rash, urticaria, photosensitivity, diaphoresis, anaphylactic shock).

DIAGNOSTIC TEST INTERFERENCE Diphenhydramine should be discontinued 4 days prior to ***skin testing*** procedures for allergy because it may suppress wheal and flare reactions may cause false-positive with urine detection of methadone and phencyclidine; may cause false-positive serum TCA screen.

INTERACTIONS **Drug:** **Alcohol** and other CNS DEPRESSANTS compound CNS depression. Avoid use with ANTICHOLINERGIC AGENTS.

PHARMACOKINETICS **Absorption:** Readily absorbed from GI tract but only 40–60% reaches systemic circulation. **Onset:** 15–30 min. **Peak:** 1–4 h. **Duration:** 4–7 h. **Distribution:** Crosses placenta; distributed into breast milk. **Metabolism:** In liver; some degradation in lung and kidney. **Elimination:** Mostly in urine within 24 h.

NURSING IMPLICATIONS

Assessment & Drug Effects

- Monitor cardiovascular status especially with preexisting cardiovascular disease.
- Monitor for adverse effects especially in children and the older adult.
- Supervise ambulation and institute fall precautions as necessary. Drowsiness is most prominent during the first few days of

therapy and often disappears with continued therapy. Older adults are especially likely to manifest dizziness, sedation, and hypotension.

Patient & Family Education

- Do not use alcohol and other CNS depressants because of the possible additive CNS depressant effects with concurrent use.
- Do not drive or engage in other potentially hazardous activities until the response to drug is known.
- Increase fluid intake, if not contraindicated; drug has an atropine-like drying effect (thickens bronchial secretions) that may make expectoration difficult.

DIPHENOXYLATE HYDROCHLORIDE WITH ATROPINE SULFATE

(dye-fen-ox'i-late)

Diphenatol, Lofene, Lomanate, Lomotil, Lonox, Lo-Trol, Low-Quel, Nor-Mil

Classification: ANTIDIARRHEAL

Therapeutic: ANTIDIARRHEAL

Controlled Substance: Schedule V

AVAILABILITY Tablet; liquid

ACTION & *THERAPEUTIC EFFECT* A synthetic narcotic opiate agonist that inhibits mucosal receptors responsible for peristaltic reflex, thereby reducing GI motility. *Reduces peristalsis thereby stopping or diminishing diarrhea*.

USES Adjunct in symptomatic management of diarrhea.

CONTRAINDICATIONS Hypersensitivity to diphenoxylate or atropine; severe dehydration or electrolyte imbalance, advanced liver disease, obstructive jaundice, diarrhea caused by pseudomembranous enterocolitis; diarrhea induced by poisons; glaucoma; lactation.

CAUTIOUS USE Advanced hepatic disease, abnormal liver function tests; renal function impairment, MAOI therapy; addiction-prone individuals, or those whose history suggests drug abuse; ulcerative colitis; children; pregnancy (category C). Safe use in children younger than 2 yr not established.

ROUTE & DOSAGE

Diarrhea

Adult: **PO** 1–2 tablets or 1–2 teaspoons full (5 mL) 3–4 × day (each tablet or 5 mL contains 2.5 mg diphenoxylate HCl and 0.025 mg atropine sulfate)
Child (2–12 yr): **PO** 0.3–0.4 mg/kg/day of liquid in divided doses

ADMINISTRATION

Oral

- Crush tablet if necessary and give with fluid of patient's choice.
- Reduce dosage as soon as initial control of symptoms occurs.
- Withhold drug in presence of severe dehydration or electrolyte imbalance until appropriate corrective therapy has been initiated.
- Note: Treatment is generally continued for 24–36 h before it is considered ineffective.
- Store in tightly covered, light-resistant container, preferably 15°–30°C (59°–86°F), unless otherwise directed by manufacturer.

ADVERSE EFFECTS **CV:** Flushing, palpitation, tachycardia. **CNS:** Headache, sedation, drowsiness, dizziness, lethargy, numbness of extremities; restlessness, euphoria, mental depression, weakness, general malaise. **HEENT:** Nystagmus, mydriasis, blurred vision, miosis (toxicity). **GI:** Nausea, vomiting, anorexia, dry mouth, abdominal discomfort or distension, paralytic ileus, toxic megacolon. **Other:** Hypersensitivity (pruritus, angioneurotic edema, giant urticaria, rash). Urinary retention, swelling of gums.

INTERACTIONS Drug: MAO INHIBITORS may precipitate hypertensive crisis; **alcohol** and other CNS DEPRESSANTS may enhance CNS effects; also see **atropine.**

PHARMACOKINETICS Absorption: Readily absorbed from GI tract. **Onset:** 45–60 min. **Peak:** 2 h. **Duration:** 3–4 h. **Distribution:** Distributed into breast milk. **Metabolism:** Rapidly metabolized to active and inactive metabolites in liver. **Elimination:** Slowly through bile into feces; small amount in urine. **Half-Life:** 4.4 h.

NURSING IMPLICATIONS

Assessment & Drug Effects

- Assess GI function; report abdominal distention and signs of decreased peristalsis.
- Monitor for S&S of dehydration (see Appendix F). It is essential to monitor young children closely; dehydration occurs more rapidly in this age group and may influence variability of responses to diphenoxylate and predispose patient to delayed toxic effects.
- Monitor frequency and consistency of stools.

Patient & Family Education

- Take medication only as directed by prescriber.
- Notify prescriber if diarrhea persists or if fever, bloody stools, palpitation, or other adverse reactions occur.
- Do not drive or engage in other potentially hazardous activities until response to drug is known.

DIPYRIDAMOLE

(dye-peer-id′a-mole)

Classification: ANTIPLATELET; PLATELET AGGREGATE INHIBITOR

Therapeutic: PLATELET AGGREGATE INHIBITOR

AVAILABILITY Tablet; solution for injection

ACTION & *THERAPEUTIC EFFECT* Nonnitrate coronary vasodilator that increases coronary blood flow by selectively dilating coronary arteries, thereby increasing myocardial oxygen supply. Additionally, it exhibits antiplatelet aggregation activity. *Reduces the risk of thromboembolism.*

USES To prevent postoperative thromboembolic complications associated with prosthetic heart valves and as adjunct for thallium stress testing.

UNLABELED USES To reduce rate of reinfarction following MI; to prevent TIAs (transient ischemic attacks) and coronary bypass graft occlusion.

CAUTIOUS USE Hypotension, anticoagulant therapy; aspirin sensitivity; elderly; severe hepatic dysfunction; syncope; pregnancy (category B); lactation. Safety and efficacy in children younger than 12 yr not established.

ROUTE & DOSAGE

Prevention of Thromboembolism in Cardiac Valve Replacement

Adult: **PO** 75–100 mg qid

Thallium Stress Test

Adult: **IV** 0.56 mg/kg over 4 min (max: 70 mg)

ADMINISTRATION

Oral

- Give on an empty stomach at least 1 h before or 2 h after meals, with a full glass of water. Prescriber may prescribe with food if gastric distress persists.

Intravenous

PREPARE: **Direct:** Dilute to at least a 1:2 ratio with 0.45% NaCl, NS, or D5W to yield a final volume of 20–50 mL.
ADMINISTER: **Direct:** Give a single dose over 4 min (0.142 mg/kg/min).
INCOMPATIBILITIES: **Y-Site:** Fosfomycin admixture: **Lysine**.

- Store in a tightly closed container at 15°–30°C (59°–86°F) unless otherwise directed. Protect injection from direct light.

ADVERSE EFFECTS **CV:** Angina pectoris, flushing, tachycardia, hypotension. **CNS:** Dizziness, headache, fatigue. **Hepatic:** Hepatic insufficiency.

INTERACTIONS **Drug:** Other ANTICOAGULANTS can increase bleeding risk. **Herbal: Evening primrose oil, ginseng** can increase bleeding risk.

PHARMACOKINETICS **Absorption:** Readily absorbed from GI tract. **Peak:** 45–150 min. **Distribution:** Small amount crosses placenta. **Metabolism:** In liver. **Elimination:** Mainly in feces. **Half-Life:** 10–12 h.

NURSING IMPLICATIONS

Assessment & Drug Effects

- Monitor therapeutic effectiveness. Clinical response may not be evident before second or third month of continuous therapy. Effects include reduced frequency or elimination of anginal episodes, improved exercise tolerance, reduced requirement for nitrates.
- Monitor Bp, Hr, ECG, respirations. Monitor for signs of poor perfusion (pallor, cyanosis, cold skin).

Patient & Family Education

- Notify prescriber of any adverse effects.
- Make all position changes slowly and in stages, especially from recumbent to upright posture, if postural hypotension or dizziness is a problem.

DISOPYRAMIDE PHOSPHATE

(dye-soe-peer'a-mide)

Norpace, Norpace CR, Rythmodan ♣, Rythmodan-LA ♣

Classification: CLASS IA ANTIARRHYTHMIC

Therapeutic: CLASS IA ANTIARRHYTHMIC

Prototype: Procainamide

AVAILABILITY Capsule; sustained release capsule

ACTION & *THERAPEUTIC EFFECT* Decreases myocardial conduction velocity and excitability in the atria, ventricles, and accessory pathways. It prolongs the QRS and QT intervals in normal sinus rhythm and atrial arrhythmias. *Acts as myocardial depressant by reducing rate of*

D

spontaneous diastolic depolarization in pacemaker cells, thereby suppressing ectopic focal activity.

USES Treatment of ventricular tachycardia.

UNLABELED USES To treat or prevent serious refractory arrhythmias. To convert atrial fibrillation, atrial flutter, and paroxysmal atrial tachycardia to normal sinus rhythm.

CONTRAINDICATIONS Cardiogenic shock, preexisting second- or third-degree AV block (if no pacemaker is present); sick sinus syndrome (bradycardia-tachycardia); Wolff–Parkinson–White (WPW) syndrome or bundle branch block, history of torsades de pointes; cardiogenic shock; QT prolongation; uncompensated or inadequately compensated CHF, hypotension (unless secondary to cardiac arrhythmia), hypokalemia.

CAUTIOUS USE Myocarditis or other cardiomyopathy, underlying cardiac conduction abnormalities; hepatic or renal impairment; urinary tract disease (especially prostatic hypertrophy); diabetes mellitus; myasthenia gravis; older adults; narrow-angle glaucoma; family history of glaucoma; pregnancy (category C); lactation.

ROUTE & DOSAGE

Arrhythmias

Adult (weight greater than 50 kg): **PO** 100–200 mg q6h or 300 mg loading dose; *weight less than 50 kg:* 100 mg q6h
Adolescent: **PO** 6–15 mg/kg/day in divided doses q6h
Child (younger than 1 yr): **PO** 10–30 mg/kg/day in divided doses q6h; *1 to younger than 4 yr:* 10–20 mg/kg/day in divided doses q6h; *4–12 yr:* 10–15 mg/kg/day in divided doses q6h

ADMINISTRATION

Oral

- Start drug 6–12 h after last quinidine dose and 3–6 h after last procainamide dose for patients who have been receiving either quinidine or procainamide.
- Give sustained release capsules whole.
- Do not use sustained release capsules in loading doses when rapid control is required or in patients with creatinine clearance of 40 mL/min or less.
- Start sustained release capsules 6 h after last dose of conventional capsule if change in drug form is made.
- Store at 15°–30°C (59°–86°F) unless otherwise directed.

ADVERSE EFFECTS **CV:** *Hypotension,* chest pain, edema, dyspnea, syncope, bradycardia, tachycardia; worsening of CHF or cardiac arrhythmia; <u>cardiogenic shock, heart block</u>; edema with weight gain. **CNS:** Dizziness, headache, fatigue, muscle weakness, convulsions, paresthesias, nervousness, acute psychosis, peripheral neuropathy. **HEENT:** *Blurred vision,* dry eyes, increased IOP, precipitation of acute angle-closure glaucoma. **GI:** *Dry mouth, constipation,* epigastric or abdominal pain, cholestatic jaundice. **GU:** *Hesitancy* and *retention,* urinary frequency, urgency, renal insufficiency. **Other:** Dry nose and throat, drying of bronchial secretions, initiation of uterine contractions (pregnant patient); muscle aches, precipitation of myasthenia gravis, <u>agranulocytosis</u> (rare), thrombocytopenia. Hypersensitivity (pruritus, urticaria, rash, photosensitivity, laryngospasm).

INTERACTIONS **Drug:** ANTICHOLINERGIC DRUGS (e.g., TRICYCLIC ANTIDEPRESSANTS, ANTIHISTAMINES) compound anticholinergic effects; other ANTIARRHYTHMICS compound toxicities; **phenytoin, rifampin** may increase disopyramide metabolism and decrease levels; may increase **warfarin**-induced hypoprothrombinemia.

PHARMACOKINETICS **Absorption:** Readily from GI tract; 60–83% reaches systemic circulation. **Onset:** 30 min–3.5 h. **Peak:** 1–2 h. **Duration:** 1.5–8.5 h. **Distribution:** Distributed in extracellular fluid; crosses placenta; distributed into breast milk. **Metabolism:** In liver. **Elimination:** 80% in urine, 10% in feces. **Half-Life:** 4–10 h.

NURSING IMPLICATIONS

Black Box Warning

Disopyramide should only be used in patients with life-threatening ventricular arrhythmias.

Assessment & Drug Effects

- Check apical pulse before administering drug. Withhold drug and notify prescriber if pulse rate is slower than 60 bpm, faster than 120 bpm, or if there is any unusual change in rate, rhythm, or quality.
- Monitor ECG closely. The following signs are indications for drug withdrawal: Prolongation of QT interval and worsening of arrhythmia interval, QRS widening (greater than 25%).
- Monitor for rapid weight gain or other signs of fluid retention.
- Monitor BP closely in all patients during periods of dosage adjustment and in those receiving high dosages.
- Monitor I&O, particularly in older adults and patients with impaired renal function or prostatic hypertrophy. Persistent urinary hesitancy or retention may necessitate lower dosage or discontinuation of drug.
- Report S&S of hyperkalemia (see Appendix F); it enhances drug's toxic effects.
- Monitor for S&S of CHF.
- Monitor lab tests: Baseline and periodic blood glucose and serum potassium.

Patient & Family Education

- Take drug precisely as prescribed to maintain regularity of heartbeat.
- Weigh daily under standard conditions and check ankles for edema. Report to prescriber a weekly weight gain of 1–2 kg (2–4 lb) or more.
- Make position changes slowly, particularly when getting up from lying down because of the possibility of hypotension; dangle legs for a few minutes before walking, and do not stand still for prolonged periods.
- Do not drive or engage in other potentially hazardous activities until response to drug is known.

DISULFIRAM

(dye-sul'fi-ram)

Antabuse

Classification: ENZYME INHIBITOR; ANTIALCOHOL AGENT

Therapeutic: ALCOHOL ABUSE DETERRENT

D

AVAILABILITY Tablet

ACTION & *THERAPEUTIC EFFECT* Inhibits the enzyme acetaldehyde dehydrogenase, which normally metabolizes alcohol in the body. *When a small amount of alcohol is ingested, a complex of highly unpleasant symptoms known as the disulfiram reaction occurs, which serves as a deterrent to further drinking.*

USES Management of chronic alcoholism.

CONTRAINDICATIONS Severe myocardial disease; cardiac disease; psychosis; patients who have recently ingested alcohol, metronidazole, paraldehyde; multiple drug dependence.

CAUTIOUS USE Diabetes mellitus; epilepsy; seizure disorders; hypothyroidism; coronary artery disease, cerebral damage; chronic and acute nephritis; renal disease; hepatic cirrhosis or insufficiency; abnormal EEG; pregnancy (category B); lactation.

ROUTE & DOSAGE

Alcoholism
Adult: **PO** 500 mg/day for 1–2 wk, then 125–500 mg/day (max: 500 mg/day)

ADMINISTRATION

Oral

- Daily dose may be given at bedtime to minimize sedative effect of the drug. Decrease in dose may also reduce sedative effect.
- Make sure patient has abstained from alcohol and alcohol-containing preparations for at least 12 h and preferably 48 h before initiating therapy. **Never** give to a person who is intoxicated.
- Store at 15°–30°C (59°–86°F) unless otherwise directed. Protect tablets from light.

ADVERSE EFFECTS **CNS:** Drowsiness, fatigue, restlessness, headache, tremor, psychoses (usually with high doses), polyneuritis, peripheral neuropathy, optic neuritis. **GI:** Mild GI disturbances, garlic-like or metallic taste, hepatotoxicity, hypersensitivity hepatitis. **Reaction with alcohol ingestion:** Flushing of face, chest, arms, pulsating headache, nausea, violent vomiting, thirst, sweating, marked uneasiness, confusion, weakness, vertigo, blurred vision, pruritic skin rash, hyperventilation, abnormal gait, slurred speech, disorientation, confusion, personality changes, bizarre behavior, psychoses, tachycardia, palpitation, chest pain, hypotension to shock level arrhythmias, acute congestive failure. **Severe reactions:** Marked respiratory depression, unconsciousness, convulsions, sudden death. **Other:** Hypersensitivity (allergic or acneiform dermatitis; urticaria, fixed-drug eruption).

DIAGNOSTIC TEST INTERFERENCE Disulfiram can reduce ***uptake of*** I^{131}; or decreases ***PBI*** test results (rare).

INTERACTIONS **Drug: Alcohol** (including in liquid OTC drugs, **IV nitroglycerin, IV cotrimoxazole**), **metronidazole, paraldehyde** will produce disulfiram reaction; **isoniazid** can produce neurologic symptoms; may increase blood levels and toxicity of **warfarin, paraldehyde**, BARBITURATES, **phenytoin.** Do not use with **tinidazole.**

D

PHARMACOKINETICS Absorption: Slowly absorbed from GI tract. **Onset:** Up to 12 h. **Duration:** Up to 2 wk after last dose. **Distribution:** Initially deposited in fat. **Metabolism:** Metabolized slowly in liver. **Elimination:** 5–20% excreted in feces; 20% remains in body for 1–2 wk; some may be excreted in breath as carbon disulfide.

NURSING IMPLICATIONS

Black Box Warning

Disulfiram should not be given to anyone in a state of alcohol intoxication or without their full knowledge.

Assessment & Drug Effects

- Note: Disulfiram reaction occurs within 5–10 min following ingestion of alcohol and may last 30 min to several hours. Intensity of reaction varies with each individual, but is generally proportional to the amount of alcohol ingested.
- Treat patient with severe disulfiram reaction as though in shock. Monitor potassium levels, especially if patient has diabetes mellitus.
- Monitor lab tests: Baseline and periodic LFTs.

Patient & Family Education

- Patient should understand fully the possible dangers if alcohol is ingested during disulfiram treatment. Carry identification card indicating use of disulfiram.
- Report promptly to prescriber the onset of nausea with right upper quadrant pain or discomfort, itching, jaundiced sclerae or skin, dark urine, clay-colored stools. Withhold drug pending liver function tests.
- Note: Ingestion of even small amounts of alcohol or use of external applications that contain alcohol may be sufficient to produce a reaction. Read all labels and avoid use of anything containing alcohol.
- Alcohol sensitivity may last as long as 2 wk after disulfiram has been discontinued.
- Note: Adverse effects of drug are often experienced during first 2 wk of therapy; symptoms usually disappear with continued therapy or with dose reduction.
- Do not drive or engage in other potentially hazardous activities until response to drug is known.

DOBUTAMINE HYDROCHLORIDE

(doe-byoo'ta-meen)

Dobutrex

Classification: ADRENERGIC AGONIST; VASOPRESSOR

Therapeutic: CARDIAC STIMULANT; IONOTROPIC

Prototype: Isoproterenol

AVAILABILITY Solution for injection

ACTION & *THERAPEUTIC EFFECT*

Stimulates $beta_1$-receptors in the heart, increasing contractility and cardiac output. It also has weak $beta_2$ activity, and $alpha_1$ selective activity. Sympathetic nervous system effects increase cardiac output and decrease pulmonary wedge pressure and total systemic vascular resistance. Also increases conduction through AV node, and has lower potential for precipitating arrhythmias than dopamine. *In CHF or cardiogenic shock it increases cardiac output, enhances renal perfusion, increases renal output and renal sodium excretion.*

D

USES Inotropic support in short-term treatment of adults with cardiac decompensation due to depressed myocardial contractility (cardiogenic shock) resulting from either organic heart disease or from cardiac surgery.

UNLABELED USES To augment cardiovascular function in children undergoing cardiac catheterization, stress thallium testing.

CONTRAINDICATIONS History of hypersensitivity to other sympathomimetic amines or sulfites, ventricular tachycardia, idiopathic hypertrophic subaortic stenosis; hypovolemia.

CAUTIOUS USE Preexisting hypertension, hypotension; atrial fibrillation; acute MI; unstable angina, severe coronary artery disease; pregnancy (category C). Safe use in children younger than 2 yr is not established.

ROUTE & DOSAGE

Cardiac Decompensation

Adult: **IV** 0.5–1 mcg/kg/min then titrate up to 2.5–15 mcg/kg/min (max: 40 mcg/kg/min)
Adolescent/Child: **IV** 2–20 mcg/kg/min

ADMINISTRATION

Intravenous

PREPARE: **Continuous:** Dilute 250-mg/20-mL vial or 500-mg/40-mL vial of dobutamine in at least 50 mL or 100 mL, respectively, of compatible IV solution. ▪ Use IV solutions within 24 h.
ADMINISTER: **Continuous:** Rate of infusion is determined by body weight and controlled by an infusion pump (preferred) or a microdrip IV infusion set. ▪ IV infusion rate and duration of therapy are determined by heart rate, blood pressure, ectopic activity, urine output, and whenever possible, by measurements of cardiac output and central venous or pulmonary wedge pressures.
INCOMPATIBILITIES: **Solution/additive:** **Acyclovir, alteplase, aminophylline, bumetanide, calcium chloride, calcium gluconate, diazepam, digoxin, furosemide, heparin, insulin, magnesium sulfate, phenytoin, potassium chloride, potassium phosphate, sodium bicarbonate.** **Y-site:** **Acyclovir, alteplase, aminophylline, amphotericin B cholesteryl sulfate, cefepime, foscarnet, furosemide, heparin, indomethacin, lansoprazole, pantoprazole, pemetrexed, phytonadione, piperacillin/tazobactam, warfarin.**

▪ Refrigerate reconstituted solution at 2°–15°C (36°–59°F) for 48 h or store for 6 h at room temperature.

ADVERSE EFFECTS Generally dose related. **CV:** *Increased heart rate and BP,* premature ventricular beats, palpitation, *anginal pain.* **CNS:** Headache, tremors, paresthesias, mild leg cramps, nervousness, fatigue (with overdosage). **GI:** Nausea, vomiting. **Other:** Nonspecific chest pain, shortness of breath.

INTERACTIONS **Drug:** GENERAL ANESTHETICS (especially **cyclopropane** and **halothane**) may sensitize myocardium to effects of CATECHOLAMINES such as dobutamine and lead to serious arrhythmias—use with extreme caution; BETA-ADRENERGIC BLOCKING AGENTS (e.g., **metoprolol, propranolol**) may make dobutamine ineffective in increasing cardiac output, but total peripheral resistance may increase—concomitant use generally avoided; MAO INHIBITORS, TRICYCLIC ANTIDEPRESSANTS potentiate pressor effects—use with extreme caution.

PHARMACOKINETICS **Onset:** 2–10 min. **Peak:** 10–20 min. **Metabolism:** Metabolized in liver and other tissues by COMT. **Elimination:** In urine. **Half-Life:** 2 min.

NURSING IMPLICATIONS

Assessment & Drug Effects

- Correct hypovolemia by administration of appropriate volume expanders prior to initiation of therapy.
- Monitor therapeutic effectiveness. At any given dosage level, drug takes 10–20 min to produce peak effects.
- Monitor ECG and BP continuously during administration.
- Note: Marked increases in blood pressure (systolic pressure is the most likely to be affected) and heart rate, or the appearance of arrhythmias or other adverse cardiac effects, are usually reversed promptly by reduction in dosage.
- Observe patients with preexisting hypertension closely for exaggerated pressor response.
- Monitor I&O ratio and pattern. Urine output and sodium excretion generally increase because of improved cardiac output and renal perfusion.

Patient & Family Education

- Report anginal pain to prescriber promptly.

DOCETAXEL

(doc-e-tax′el)

Taxotere

Classification: ANTINEOPLASTIC; TAXANE

Therapeutic: ANTINEOPLASTIC

Prototype: Paclitaxel

AVAILABILITY Solution for injection

ACTION & *THERAPEUTIC EFFECT* A semisynthetic analog of paclitaxel that binds to the microtubule network essential for interphase and mitosis of the cell cycle. *Docetaxel stabilizes the microtubules involved in cell division and prevents their normal functioning; this results in inhibited mitosis in cancer cells.*

USES Breast cancer, gastric cancer, prostate cancer, head/neck cancer, non-small-cell lung cancer.

CONTRAINDICATIONS Hypersensitivity to docetaxel or other drugs formulated with polysorbate 80, paclitaxel; neutrophil count less than 1500 cells/mm^3, biliary tract disease, hepatic disease, jaundice, intramuscular injections, thrombocytopenia, acute infection, pregnancy (category D); lactation.

CAUTIOUS USE Bone marrow suppression, bone marrow transplant patients; CHF, ascites, peripheral edema, pleural effusion; radiation therapy; pulmonary disorders, acute bronchospasm; cardiac tamponade; dental disease, dental work, herpes infection; hypotension, elderly; infection. Safety and efficacy in children younger than 18 yr not established.

D

ROUTE & DOSAGE

Breast Cancer

Adult: **IV** 60–100 mg/m^2 q3wk (premedicate patients with dexamethasone 8 mg bid × 5 days, starting 1 day prior to docetaxel)

Prostate Cancer

Adult: **IV** 75 mg/m^2 q21 days plus prednisone

Non-Small-Cell Lung Cancer

Adult: **IV** 75 mg/m^2 q3wk

Head/Neck Cancer

Adult: **IV** 75 mg/m^2 q21 days × 4 cycles

ADMINISTRATION

- Note: If drug contacts skin during preparation, wash immediately with soap and water.

Intravenous

PREPARE: **IV Infusion:** Preparation instructions vary by manufacturer; refer to specific prescribing information.

ADMINISTER: **IV Infusion** Give at a constant rate over 1 h. ▪ Administer ONLY after premedication with corticosteroids to prevent hypersensitivity. ▪ Reduce dose by 25% following severe neutropenia (less than 500 cells/mm^3) for 7 days or longer for febrile neutropenia, severe cutaneous reactions, or severe peripheral neuropathy.

INCOMPATIBILITIES: **Y-site: Amphotericin B, dantrolene, doxorubicin, methylprednisolone, mitomycin, nalbuphine, phenytoin.**

- Refrigerate vials at 2°–8°C (36°–46°F). Protect from light. Do not store in PVC bags. ▪ Store diluted solutions in refrigerator or at room temperature for 8 h.

ADVERSE EFFECTS

Respiratory: *Pulmonary reaction.* **CNS:** Neurotoxicity. **Endocrine:** *Fluid retention.* **Skin:** *Alopecia,* dermatologic reaction, nail disease. **Hepatic/GI:** Increased serum transaminase, *stomatitis,* diarrhea, *nausea,* vomiting. **Musculoskeletal:** *Weakness,* myalgia. **Hematologic:** *Neutropenia, leukopenia, anemia,* thrombocytopenia, febrile neutropenia. **Other:** *Fever,* infection.

INTERACTIONS

Drug: Possible interaction with other drugs metabolized by CYP3A4. Do not use LIVE VACCINES. Increases serum concentration of **conivaptan.** Increases adverse effects of **deferiprone.** Increases adverse effects of MYELOSUPPRESSIVE AGENTS.

PHARMACOKINETICS

Distribution: 97% protein bound. **Metabolism:** In liver by CYP3A4. **Elimination:** 80% in feces, 20% renally. **Half-Life:** 11.1 h.

NURSING IMPLICATIONS

Black Box Warning

Docetaxel has been associated with increased mortality in persons with abnormal liver function, non-small-cell lung cancer, and those receiving higher doses. Docetaxel can cause severe neutropenia, hypersensitivity reactions, and marked fluid retention.

Assessment & Drug Effects

- Monitor for S&S of hypersensitivity (see Appendix F), which may develop within a few minutes of initiation of infusion. It is usually not necessary to discontinue infusion for minor reactions (i.e., flushing or local skin reaction).

- Assess throughout the course of therapy, and report cardiovascular dysfunction, respiratory distress; fluid retention; development of neurosensory symptoms; severe, cutaneous eruptions on feet, hands, arms, face, or thorax; and S&S of infection.
- Monitor lab tests: LFTs prior to each drug cycle; renal function; frequent CBCs with differential.

Patient & Family Education

- Learn common adverse effects and measures to control or minimize them when possible. Report immediately any distressing adverse effects.
- Report promptly to prescriber any of the following: Fever, edema in lower extremities, weight gain, shortness of breath, muscle pain, or skin reactions.
- Note: It is extremely important to comply with corticosteroid therapy and monitoring of lab values.
- Avoid pregnancy during therapy.

DOCOSANOL

(doc′os-a-nol)

Abreva

Classification: ANTIVIRAL

Therapeutic: ANTIVIRAL

AVAILABILITY Cream

ACTION & THERAPEUTIC EFFECT Docosanol inhibits viral replication by interfering with the early intracellular events surrounding viral entry into target cells. *Believed to exert its antiviral effect by inhibiting fusion of the HSV (herpes virus) envelope with the human cell plasma membrane, therefore making it difficult for the virus to enter the cell and replicate.*

USES Treatment of herpes simplex infections of the face and lips (i.e., cold sores).

CONTRAINDICATIONS Hypersensitivity to docosanol or any of the inactive ingredients in the cream; immunosuppressant patients; lactation.

CAUTIOUS USE Pregnancy (insufficient information related to use in pregnant women). Safety and efficacy in children not established.

ROUTE & DOSAGE

Herpes Simplex Infections

Adult/Adolescent: **Topical** Apply to lesions 5 × day for up to 10 days, starting at onset of symptoms

ADMINISTRATION

Topical

- Apply cream only to the affected areas using a gloved finger. Rub in gently but completely.
- Do not apply near or in the eyes.
- Avoid application to the mucous membranes inside of the mouth.
- Store at 20°–25°C (68°–77°F).

ADVERSE EFFECTS Other: Hypersensitivity reaction.

INTERACTIONS Drug: No clinically significant interactions established.

NURSING IMPLICATIONS

Assessment & Drug Effects

- Monitor severity and extent of infection.
- Notify prescriber if improvement is not seen within 10 days of initiating treatment

D

Patient & Family Education

- Wash hands before and after applying cream.
- Do not share this cream with any other individual as this may spread the herpes virus.
- Report to prescriber if your condition worsens or does not improve within 10 days of beginning treatment.

DOCUSATE CALCIUM (DIOCTYL CALCIUM SULFOSUCCINATE) Pr

(dok'yoo-sate)

DCS, PMS-Docusate Calcium, Pro-Cal-Sof, Surfak

DOCUSATE POTASSIUM

Dialose, Diocto-K, Kasof

DOCUSATE SODIUM

Colace, Colace Enema, Dio Sul, Disonate, DGSS, D-S-S, Duosol, Lax-gel, Laxinate 100, Modane, Pro-Sof, Regulax ♣, Regutol, Therevac-Plus, Therevac-SB

Classification: STOOL SOFTENER

Therapeutic: STOOL SOFTENER

AVAILABILITY **Docusate Calcium:** Capsule. **Docusate Potassium:** Tablet; capsule. **Docusate Sodium:** Tablet; capsule; syrup

ACTION & *THERAPEUTIC EFFECT* Anionic surface-active agent with emulsifying and wetting properties. *Detergent action lowers surface tension, permitting water and fats to penetrate and soften stools for easier passage.*

USES Prophylactically in patients who should avoid straining during defecation and for treatment of constipation associated with hard, dry stools (e.g., following anorectal surgery, MI).

CONTRAINDICATIONS Atonic constipation, nausea, vomiting, abdominal pain, fecal impaction, structural anomalies of colon and rectum, intestinal obstruction or perforation; use of docusate sodium in patients on sodium restriction; use of docusate potassium in patients with renal dysfunction.

CAUTIOUS USE History of CHF, edema, diabetes mellitus; pregnancy (category C).

ROUTE & DOSAGE

Stool Softener

Adult: **PO** 50–500 mg/day **PR** 50–100 mg added to enema fluid
Child (younger than 3 yr): **PO** 10–40 mg/day; *3 to younger than 6 yr:* 20–60 mg/day; *6–12 yr:* 40–120 mg/day

ADMINISTRATION

Oral

- Give with a full glass of water if allowed.
- Store syrup formulations in tight, light-resistant containers at 15°–30°C (59°–86°F) unless directed otherwise.

Rectal

- Microenema: Insert full length of nozzle (half length for children) into the rectum. Squeeze entire contents of tube and remove completely before releasing grip on tube.
- Store in tightly covered containers.

ADVERSE EFFECTS **GI:** Occasional mild abdominal cramps, *diarrhea*, nausea, bitter taste. **Other:** Throat irritation (liquid preparation), rash.

INTERACTIONS **Drug:** Docusate will increase systemic absorption of **mineral oil.**

 Common adverse effects in *italic*; life-threatening effects underlined; generic names in **bold**; classifications in SMALL CAPS; ♣ Canadian drug name; Pr Prototype drug; ⚠ Alert

NURSING IMPLICATIONS

Assessment & Drug Effects

- Withhold drug if diarrhea develops and notify prescriber.
- Therapeutic effectiveness: Usually apparent 1–3 days after first dose.

Patient & Family Education

- Take sufficient liquid with each dose and increase fluid intake during the day, if allowed. Oral liquid (**not** syrup) may be administered in milk, fruit juice, or infant formula to mask bitter taste.
- Do not take concomitantly with mineral oil.
- Do not take for prolonged periods in lieu of proper dietary management or treatment of underlying causes of constipation.

DOFETILIDE

(do-fe-ti'lyde)

Tikosyn

Classification: CLASS III ANTIARRHYTHMIC, POTASSIUM CHANNEL BLOCKER

Therapeutic: CLASS III ANTIARRHYTHMIC

Prototype: Amiodarone HCl

AVAILABILITY Capsule

ACTION & *THERAPEUTIC EFFECT* Prolongs the cardiac action potential by blocking potassium channels and thus one or more potassium currents. Action results in suppression of arrhythmias dependent upon reentry of potassium ions. *Effectiveness indicated by correction of atrial arrhythmias.*

USES Symptomatic atrial fibrillation and flutter.

CONTRAINDICATIONS Hypersensitivity to dofetilide; QT prolongation; ventricular arrhythmias; history of torsades de pointes; electrolyte imbalances (e.g., hypokalemia, hypomagnesemia); renal failure; lactation.

CAUTIOUS USE Atrioventricular block, bradycardia, CHF, concurrent administration of potassium-depleting diuretics, hepatic or renal impairment; history of moderate QT_c interval prolongation; moderate to severe hypertension; recent MI or unstable angina; vascular heart disease; older adults; pregnancy (category C). Safety and efficacy in children younger than 18 yr not established.

ROUTE & DOSAGE

Dosing of dofetilide must be done very carefully. Dofetilide can cause serious cardiac arrhythmias, particularly, ventricular tachycardia of the torsades de pointes type. Ecg and renal function must be assessed prior to beginning therapy. Clinicians who are unfamiliar with the use of this drug should read the package insert.

Atrial Fibrillation/Flutter

Adult: **PO** Based on creatinine clearance (CrCl) and QT_c interval, if QT_c increases by more than 15% from baseline or is greater than 500 milliseconds 2–3 h after initial dose. Decrease subsequent doses by 50%.

Renal Impairment Dosage Adjustment

CrCl greater than 60 mL/min: 500 mcg bid; *40–60 mL/min:* 250 mcg bid; *20–39 mL/min:* 125 mcg bid

D

ADMINISTRATION

Oral

- Administer with or without food.
- Do not give dofetilide if QT/QT_C interval greater than 420 milliseconds (or greater than 500 milliseconds with ventricular conduction abnormalities).
- Administer only with continuous ECG monitoring.
- Do not initiate therapy until 3 mo after withdrawal of previous antiarrhythmic therapy.
- Do not initiate therapy until 3 mo after amiodarone has been withdrawn or plasma level is less than 0.3 mcg/mL.
- Store at 15°–30°C (59°–86°F); protect from moisture and humidity.

ADVERSE EFFECTS **CV:** *Torsades de pointes arrhythmia*, *ventricular arrhythmias*, AV block, *chest pain* v. tach, v. fibrillation, **Respiratory:** Respiratory infection, dyspnea. **CNS:** *Headache*, dizziness, insomnia. **Skin:** Rash. **GI:** Nausea, diarrhea, abdominal pain. **Other:** Flulike syndrome, back pain.

INTERACTIONS **Drug: Dofetilide** levels increased by **verapamil, cimetidine, trimethoprim, ketoconazole, prochlorperazine, megestrol;** do not give with drugs known to increase the QT_C interval such as **bepridil,** PHENOTHIAZINES, TRICYCLIC ANTIDEPRESSANTS, ORAL MACROLIDES, other ANTIARRHYTHMICS. Do not use with BETA-AGONISTS.

PHARMACOKINETICS **Absorption:** Greater than 90% bioavailable. **Peak:** 2–3 h. **Distribution:** 60–70% protein bound. **Metabolism:** In liver. **Elimination:** Primarily excreted unchanged in urine. **Half-Life:** 10 h.

NURSING IMPLICATIONS

Assessment & Drug Effects

- Monitor ECG continuously during first 3 days of therapy; then periodically.
- Do not discharge patient until 12 h after conversion to normal sinus rhythm.
- Notify prescriber immediately of electrolyte imbalances, especially hypokalemia and hypomagnesemia.
- Monitor lab tests: Baseline and periodic serum electrolytes and creatinine clearance; periodic CBC and routine blood chemistry.

Patient & Family Education

- Report immediately conditions that cause potassium loss (e.g., prolonged vomiting, diarrhea, excessive sweating).
- **Do not** take concurrently cimetidine, verapamil, ketoconazole, trimethoprim.

DOLASETRON MESYLATE

(dol-a-se'tron)

Anzemet

Classification: SELECTIVE SEROTONIN ($5\text{-}HT_3$) RECEPTOR ANTAGONIST; ANTIEMETIC

Therapeutic: ANTIEMETIC

Prototype: Ondansetron

AVAILABILITY Solution for injection

ACTION & *THERAPEUTIC EFFECT* A selective serotonin ($5\text{-}HT_3$) receptor antagonist. Serotonin receptors affected are located in the chemoreceptor trigger zone (CTZ) of the brain and peripherally on the vagal nerve terminal. Serotonin, released from the cells of the small intestine, activate $5\text{-}HT_3$ receptors located on vagal efferent neurons, thus initiating the vomiting reflex. *Has effective antiemetic properties.*

USES Prevention of nausea and vomiting from emetogenic chemotherapy, prevention and treatment of postoperative nausea and vomiting.

CONTRAINDICATIONS Hypersensitivity to dolasetron. **IV route:** Nausea and vomiting associated with cancer chemotherapy; congenital QT prolongation syndrome; uncorrected hypokalemia or hypomagnesemia.

CAUTIOUS USE Patients who have or may develop prolongation of cardiac conduction intervals, particularly QT_c (i.e., patients with potential hypokalemia, hypomagnesemia, diuretics; patients taking antiarrhythmic drugs and high-dose anthracycline therapy, etc.), pregnancy (category B); lactation. Safety and efficacy in children younger than 2 yr not established.

ROUTE & DOSAGE

Prevention of Chemotherapy-Induced Nausea and Vomiting

Adult/Child (2 yr or older): **PO** 100 mg 1 h prior to chemotherapy

Pre-/Postoperative Nausea and Vomiting

Adult: **IV** 12.5 mg 15 min before cessation of anesthesia or when postoperative nausea and vomiting occurs; **PO** 100 mg within 2 h prior to surgery

Child (2 yr or older): **IV** 0.35 mg/kg up to 12.5 mg 15 min before cessation of anesthesia or when postoperative nausea and vomiting occurs; **PO** 1.2 mg/kg up to 100 mg starting 2 h prior to surgery (may also mix IV formulation in apple or apple-grape juice and administer orally)

ADMINISTRATION

Oral

- Give within 2 h before surgery, when used for postoperative nausea.

Intravenous

PREPARE: **Direct:** Give undiluted. **IV Infusion:** Dilute in 50 mL of any of the following: NS, D5W, D5/0.45% NaCl, LR.

ADMINISTER: **Direct:** Inject undiluted drug over 30 sec. **IV Infusion:** Infuse diluted drug over 15 min.

INCOMPATIILITIES: **Solution/additive:** **Potassium chloride.**

- Store at 20°–25°C (66°–77°F) and protect from light. ▪ Diluted IV solution may be stored refrigerated up to 48 h.

ADVERSE EFFECTS **CV:** Hypertension. **CNS:** *Headache,* dizziness, drowsiness. **GI:** *Diarrhea,* increased LFTs, abdominal pain. **Genitourinary:** Urinary retention. **Other:** Fever, fatigue, pain, chills or shivering.

INTERACTIONS **Drug:** Avoid use with **apomorphine** due to hypotension; **ziprasidone** may prolong QT interval.

PHARMACOKINETICS **Absorption:** Rapidly absorbed from GI tract. **Peak:** 0.6 h IV, 1 h PO. **Distribution:** Crosses placenta, distributed into breast milk. **Metabolism:** Metabolized to hydrodolasetron by carbonyl reductase. Hydrodolasetron is metabolized in the liver by CYP2D6. **Elimination:** Primarily in urine as hydrodolasetron. **Half-Life:** 10 min dolasetron, 7.3 h hydrodolasetron.

D

NURSING IMPLICATIONS

Assessment & Drug Effects

- Monitor closely cardiac status especially with vomiting, excess diuresis, or other conditions that may result in electrolyte imbalances.
- Monitor lab results and report promptly development of hypokalemia or hypomagnesemia.
- Monitor ECG, especially in those taking concurrent antiarrhythmic or other drugs that may cause QT prolongation.
- Monitor for and report signs of bleeding (e.g., hematuria, epistaxis, purpura, hematoma).
- Monitor lab tests: Baseline serum electrolytes before initiating drug.

Patient & Family Education

- Headache requiring analgesic for relief is a common adverse effect.

DOLUTEGRAVIR

(doe'loo-teg'ra-vir)

Tivicay

Classification: ANTIRETROVIRAL; INTEGRASE INHIBITOR

Therapeutic: ANTIRETROVIRAL

Prototype: Raltegravir

AVAILABILITY Tablet

ACTION & *THERAPEUTIC EFFECT* Dolutegravir binds to an enzyme (integrase) necessary for HIV-1 viral DNA integration and HIV replication. *Inhibits the HIV viral replication cycle.*

USES In combination with other retroviral agents for the treatment of HIV-1 infection in adults and children age 12 yr and older and weighing at least 40 kg.

CONTRAINDICATIONS Hypersensitivity to dolutegravir; coadministration with dofetilide; severe hepatic impairment; lactation.

CAUTIOUS USE Patients with hepatitis B or C coinfections; mild-to-moderate hepatic impairment; older adults; children younger than 12 yr or weighing less than 40 mg; pregnancy (category B).

ROUTE & DOSAGE

HIV-1 Infection

Adult: PO 50 mg once daily
Child (12 yr or older and weight at least 40 kg): PO 50 mg once daily

Concurrent Potent UGT1A/CYP3A Inducer Dosage Adjustment

50 mg bid

Known or Suspected INSTI Resistance Dosage Adjustment

50 mg bid

Hepatic Impairment Dosage Adjustment

Severe hepatic impairment (Child–Pugh class C): Not recommended

ADMINISTRATION

Oral

- May be given without regard to food.
- Store at 15°–30°C (59°–86°F).

ADVERSE EFFECTS **CNS:** Dizziness, headache, insomnia **Endocrine:** Hyperglycemia, increased ALT/AST, increased bilirubin, increased cholesterol, increased creatine kinase, increased lipase, increased triglycerides. **Skin:** Pruritus. **GI:** Abdominal pain, abdominal discomfort, flatulence, nausea, vomiting. **GU:** Renal impairment. **Musculoskeletal:** Abdominal discomfort, myositis, upper abdominal pain. **Hematological:** Neutropenia. **Other:** Fatigue, hepatitis, hypersensitivity reactions.

INTERACTIONS **Drug:** Dolutegravir may increase the levels of coadministered drugs that require the renal organic cation transporter (OCT2). Coadministration of UGT inhibitors and inducers may increase or decrease the levels of dolutegravir, respectively. **Carbamazepine, efavirenz, etravirine, fosamprenavir, nevirapine, oxcarbazepine, phenobarbital, phenytoin, rifampin, ritonavir, tipranavir** decrease the levels of dolutegravir. **Metformin** increases the levels of dolutegravir. BUFFERED MEDICATIONS, **calcium supplements**, CATION-CONTAINING ANTACIDS or LAXATIVES, **iron supplements, sucralfate. Herbal: St. John's wort** decreases the levels of dolutegravir.

PHARMACOKINETICS **Peak:** 2–3 h. **Distribution:** Greater than 98.9% plasma protein bound. **Metabolism:** In liver. **Elimination:** Fecal (53%) and renal (31%). **Half-Life:** 14 h.

NURSING IMPLICATIONS

Assessment & Drug Effects

- Monitor for S&S of hypersensitivity (see Appendix F).
- Withhold drug and notify prescriber if a rash appears.
- Monitor for S&S of hepatotoxicity (see Appendix F).
- Monitor lab tests: Baseline and periodic LFTs, viral load, CD4 count, and lipid profile.

Patient & Family Education

- Report promptly development of a rash accompanied by any of the following: Fever, extreme tiredness, muscle or joint aches, blisters, swelling about the face, difficulty breathing.
- Report promptly S&S of liver damage: Yellowing of skin or whites of eyes, dark urine, pale stools, nausea or vomiting, loss of appetite, right-sided abdominal pain.
- Notify prescriber immediately if you suspect a pregnancy.
- Do not breastfeed while taking this drug.

DONEPEZIL HYDROCHLORIDE

(don-e′pe-zil)

Aricept

Classification: CENTRAL ACTING CHOLINERGIC; CHOLINESTERASE INHIBITOR

Therapeutic: ANTIDEMENTIA; ALZHEIMER AGENT

AVAILABILITY Tablet; orally disintegrating tablet

ACTION & *THERAPEUTIC EFFECT* A cholinesterase inhibitor, presumably elevates acetylcholine concentration in the cerebral cortex by slowing degrading acetylcholine released by remaining intact neurons. *Improves global function, cognition, and behavior of patients with mild to moderate Alzheimer disease.*

USES Mild, moderate, or severe dementia of Alzheimer type.

UNLABELED USES Vascular dementia, Parkinson-related dementia.

CONTRAINDICATIONS Hypersensitivity to donepezil, or piperidine derivatives; GI bleeding, jaundice; lactation; children.

CAUTIOUS USE Anesthesia, sick sinus rhythm, AV block,

D

bradycardia, cardiac arrhythmias, cardiac disease, hypotension; hyperthyroidism, history of ulcers, abnormal liver function; history of asthma or obstructive pulmonary disease, history of seizures, urinary tract obstruction, intestinal obstruction; diarrhea, emesis, GI disease, renal failure, renal impairment, surgery; pregnancy (adverse effects have been observed in some animal reproduction studies).

ROUTE & DOSAGE

Alzheimer Disease-Related Dementia

Adult: **PO** 5 mg daily, may increase after 4–6 weeks to 10 mg daily (may increase to 23 mg daily after 3 mo of 10 mg daily)

ADMINISTRATION

Oral

- Give immediately before going to bed with or without food.
- Dosage increase from 5 to 10 mg is usually made only after 4–6 wk of therapy.
- Store at 15°–30°C (59°–86°F).

ADVERSE EFFECTS **CV:** Syncope. **CNS:** *Insomnia,* dizziness. **Skin:** Pruritus, sweating, urticaria. **GI:** *Nausea, diarrhea, vomiting, anorexia.* **Other:** Accidental injury, ecchymoses.

INTERACTIONS **Drug:** Donepezil may interfere with the action of ANTICHOLINERGIC AGENTS. May increase bradycardic effect of other medications (e.g., **ceritinib,** **BETA BLOCKERS**).

PHARMACOKINETICS **Absorption:** Rapidly from GI tract. **Peak:** 3–4 h. **Distribution:** 96% protein bound. **Metabolism:** In liver by CYP2D6 and CYP3A4. **Elimination:** Primarily in urine. **Half-Life:** 70 h.

NURSING IMPLICATIONS

Assessment & Drug Effects

- Monitor closely for S&S of GI ulceration and bleeding, especially with concurrent use of NSAIDs.
- Monitor mental status/cognitive status.
- Monitor carefully patients with a history of asthma or obstructive pulmonary disease.
- Monitor cardiovascular status; drug may have vagotonic effect on the heart, causing bradycardia, especially in presence of conduction abnormalities.
- Assess bladder adequacy prior to treatment.

Patient & Family Education

- Exercise caution. Fainting episodes related to slowing the heart rate may occur.
- Report immediately to prescriber any S&S of GI ulceration or bleeding (e.g., "coffee-ground" emesis, tarry stools, epigastric pain).

DOPAMINE HYDROCHLORIDE

(doe′pa-meen)

Classification: ALPHA- AND BETA-ADRENERGIC AGONIST; IONOTROPIC

Therapeutic: CARDIAC STIMULANT; VASOPRESSOR

Prototype: Epinephrine

AVAILABILITY Solution for injection

ACTION & *THERAPEUTIC EFFECT*

Major cardiovascular effects produced by direct action on alpha- and beta-adrenergic receptors and on specific dopaminergic receptors in mesenteric and renal vascular beds. Positive inotropic effect on myocardium increases cardiac output with increase in systolic and pulse pressure. Improves circulation to renal vascular bed by decreasing renal vascular resistance with resulting increase in GFR and urinary output. *Due to its potential for inotropic, chronotropic, and vasopressor effects, dopamine has several clinical uses, including decreased cardiac output as well as correction of hypotension associated with cardiogenic and septic shock.*

USES To correct hemodynamic imbalance in shock syndrome due to MI (cardiogenic shock), trauma, endotoxic septicemia (septic shock), open heart surgery, and heart failure.

UNLABELED USES Acute renal failure; cirrhosis; hepatorenal syndrome; barbiturate intoxication.

CONTRAINDICATIONS Pheochromocytoma; uncorrected tachyarrhythmias or ventricular fibrillation; persistent hypotension.

CAUTIOUS USE Patients with history of occlusive vascular disease (e.g., Buerger or Raynaud disease); CAD; cold injury; acute MI; diabetic endarteritis, arterial embolism; pregnancy (category C); lactation, children younger than 2 yr.

ROUTE & DOSAGE

Shock/Surgery

Adult: **IV** 2–5 mcg/kg/min increased gradually up to 20 mcg/kg/min if necessary
Adolescent/Child: **IV** 1–5 mcg/kg/min increased gradually up to 20 mcg/kg/min

Heart Failure

Adult: **IV** 3–10 mcg/kg/min

ADMINISTRATION

Intravenous

PREPARE: **Continuous:** Dilute just prior to administration. ▪ Dilute contents of 1 or more vials in either 250 or 500 mL of the following: D5W, D5/NS, D5/LR, D5/0.45% NaCl, NS.

ADMINISTER: **Continuous:** Infusion rate is based on body weight. ▪ Infusion rate and guidelines for adjusting rate relative changes in blood pressure are prescribed by prescriber. ▪ Microdrip and other reliable metering device should be used for accuracy of flow rate.

INCOMPATIBILITIES: **Solution/additive: Acyclovir, alteplase, amphotericin B, ampicillin, metronidazole, penicillin G, sodium bicarbonate. Y-site: Acyclovir, alteplase, amphotericin B cholesteryl complex, cefepime, doxycycline, furosemide, indomethacin, insulin, lansoprazole, sodium bicarbonate.**

▪ Correct hypovolemia, if possible, with either whole blood or plasma before initiation of dopamine therapy. ▪ Monitor infusion continuously for free flow, and take care to avoid extravasation, which can result in tissue sloughing and gangrene. Use a large vein of the antecubital fossa. ▪ Antidote for extravasation: Stop infusion promptly and remove needle. Immediately infiltrate the ischemic area with 5–10 mg phentolamine mesylate in 10–15 mL of NS, using syringe and fine needle. Pediatric dosage of phentolamine should be 0.1–0.2 mg/kg (max: 10 mg per dose). ▪ Protect dopamine from light. Discolored solutions should not be used.

▪ Store reconstituted solution for 24 h at 2°–15°C (36°–59°F) or 6 h at room temperature, 15°–30° C.

D

ADVERSE EFFECTS CV: *Hypotension,* ectopic beats, *tachycardia,* anginal pain, palpitation, vasoconstriction (indicated by disproportionate rise in diastolic pressure), cold extremities; aberrant conduction, bradycardia, widening of QRS complex, elevated blood pressure. **CNS:** Headache, anxiety. **Skin:** Necrosis, tissue sloughing with extravasation, gangrene, piloerection. **GI:** Nausea, vomiting. **Other:** Azotemia, dyspnea, dilated pupils (high doses), increased serum glucose.

DIAGNOSTIC TEST INTERFERENCE Dopamine may modify test response when histamine is used as a control for ***intradermal skin tests.***

INTERACTIONS Drug: MAO INHIBITORS, ERGOT ALKALOIDS, increase alpha-adrenergic effects (headache, hyperpyrexia, hypertension); **guanethidine, phenytoin** may decrease dopamine action; BETA BLOCKERS antagonize cardiac effects; ALPHA BLOCKERS antagonize peripheral vasoconstriction; **halothane, cyclopropane** increase risk of hypertension and ventricular arrhythmias.

PHARMACOKINETICS Onset: Less than 5 min. **Duration:** Less than 10 min. **Distribution:** Widely distributed; does not cross blood–brain barrier. **Metabolism:** Inactive in the liver, kidney, and plasma by monoamine oxidase and COMT. **Elimination:** In urine. **Half-Life:** 2 min.

NURSING IMPLICATIONS

Black Box Warning

Dopamine extravasation may cause necrosis and sloughing of surrounding tissue.

Assessment & Drug Effects

- Monitor infusion continuously for free flow, and take care to avoid extravasation, which can result in tissue sloughing and gangrene.
- Monitor blood pressure, pulse, peripheral pulses, and urinary output at intervals prescribed by prescriber. Precise measurements are essential for accurate titration of dosage.
- Report the following indicators promptly to prescriber for use in decreasing or temporarily suspending dose: Reduced urine flow rate in absence of hypotension; ascending tachycardia; dysrhythmias; disproportionate rise in diastolic pressure (marked decrease in pulse pressure); signs of peripheral ischemia (pallor, cyanosis, mottling, coldness, complaints of tenderness, pain, numbness, or burning sensation).
- Monitor therapeutic effectiveness. In addition to improvement in vital signs and urine flow, other indices of adequate dosage and perfusion of vital organs include loss of pallor, increase in toe temperature, adequacy of nail bed capillary filling, and reversal of confusion or comatose state.

DORAVIRINE

(DOR-a-VIR-een)

Pifeltro

Classifications: ANTIRETROVIRAL, NONNUCLEOSIDE REVERSE TRANSCRIPTASE INHIBITOR

Therapeutic: ANTIRETROVIRAL NNRTI

Prototype: Efavirenz

AVAILABILITY Tablet

ACTION & *THERAPEUTIC EFFECT* A nonnucleoside reverse transcriptase inhibitor (NNRTI) of human immunodeficiency virus type 1 (HIV-1). *Inhibits HIV-1 replication and slows/prevents disease progression.*

USES HIV-1 infection in combination with other antiretroviral agents.

CONTRAINDICATIONS Concurrent administration of strong CYP3A inducers including, but not limited to, carbamazepine, oxcarbazepine, phenobarbital, phenytoin, enzalutamide, rifampin, rifapentine, mitotane, and St. John's wort.

CAUTIOUS USE Risk for immune reconstitution syndrome; pregnancy (inefficient data related to use during pregnancy); lactation.

ROUTE & DOSAGE

HIV-1 Infection (with Other Agents)

Adult: **PO** 100 mg once daily

ADMINISTRATION

ORAL

- Administer with or without food.
- Store at 20°–25°C (68°–77°F). Store in original blister bottle; protect from moisture. Do not remove desiccant.

ADVERSE EFFECTS [no need to indicate (>1% or 2%) anymore] Follow the order below: **CV:** Increased serum creatine kinase. **CNS:** Fatigue, headache. **Hepatic:** Increased serum bilirubin. **GI:** Nausea, increased serum lipase, diarrhea, abdominal pain.

INTERACTIONS **Drug:** Strong CYP3A4 inducers (e.g., **rifampin, phenytoin, carbamazepine, efavirenz**, and **phenobarbital**) can decrease **doravirine** levels. **Herbal: St. John's wort** may decrease the levels of doravirine.

PHARMACOKINETICS **Absorption:** 64% bioavailability **Peak:** 2 h **Distribution:** 60.5 L; 76% protein bound **Metabolism:** In the liver; primarily through CYP3A4 **Elimination:** 6% excreted unchanged in urine **Half-Life:** 15 h

NURSING IMPLICATIONS

Assessment & Drug Effects

- Monitor lab tests: Viral load, CD4 count.

Patient & Family Education

- Notify your doctor or get medical help right away if you have any of the following signs or symptoms of allergic reaction such as rash, hives, itching; red, swollen, blistered, or peeling skin with or without fever; wheezing; tightness in the chest or throat; trouble

D

breathing, swallowing, or talking; unusual hoarseness; or swelling of the mouth, face, lips, tongue, or throat; or any dizziness or passing out.

DORIPENEM

(dor-i-pen′em)

Doribax

Classification: BETA-LACTAM ANTIBIOTIC; CARBAPENEM ANTIBIOTIC

Therapeutic: ANTIBIOTIC

Prototype: Imipenem-cilastatin

AVAILABILITY Powder for injection

ACTION & *THERAPEUTIC EFFECT* Inhibits essential penicillin-binding proteins resulting in inhibition of bacterial cell wall synthesis, resulting in bacterial cell death. *Bactericidal against aerobic and anaerobic gram-negative and gram-positive bacteria, and effectively resolves infection.*

USES Single-agent treatment of complicated intra-abdominal infections and urinary tract infections, including pyelonephritis caused by susceptible organisms.

UNLABELED USES Hospital-acquired pneumonia.

CONTRAINDICATIONS Hypersensitivity to doripenem, or beta-lactam antibiotics; multiple allergies; ventilator-assisted pneumonia; inhalation route.

CAUTIOUS USE Hypersensitivity to cephalosporins, penicillins; moderate to severe renal impairment; GI disease, colitis, IBD; history of a seizure disorder; stroke; bacterial meningitis; older adults; pregnancy (category B); lactation. Safe use in children and adolescents is not established.

ROUTE & DOSAGE

Complicated Intra-Abdominal Infection

Adult: **IV** 500 mg q8h × 5–14 days

Complicated UTI, Including Pyelonephritis

Adult: **IV** 500 mg q8h × 10 days

Renal Impairment Dosage Adjustment

CrCl 30–50 mL/min: 250 mg q8h; *greater than 10 mL/min but less than 30 mL/min:* 250 mg q12h

ADMINISTRATION

Intravenous

PREPARE: **Intermittent:** Add 10 mL of sterile water for injection or NS to the 500-mg or 250-mg vial, gently shake to form suspension; yields 50 mg/mL (500-mg vial) or 25 mg/mL (250-mg vial). ▪ **Preparation of 500-mg dose:** Withdraw contents of 500-mg vial with a 21-gauge needle and add to infusion bag of 100 mL of NS or D5W, gently shake until clear. Final concentration is approximately 4.5 mg/mL. ▪ **Preparation of 250-mg dose:** Withdraw contents of 250-mg vial with a 21-gauge needle and add to infusion bag of 50 or 100 mL of NS or D5W, gently shake

until clear. Final concentration is approximately 4.2 mg/mL (50-mL bag) or 2.3 mg/mL (100-mL bag). ***ADMINISTER:*** **Intermittent:** Infuse over 60 min.
INCOMPATIBILITIES: **Solution/additive:** Do not combine with any other drug. **Y-site: Amphotericin B, amphotericin B lipid, diazepam, potassium, propofol**. ▪ Transfer reconstituted suspension to IV bag within 1 h of preparation.

ADVERSE EFFECTS **CV:** Phlebitis. **CNS:** *Headache,* seizures. **Endocrine:** Elevated hepatic enzymes. **Skin:** Rash. **GI:** Diarrhea, nausea, oral candidiasis. **GU:** Vulvomycotic infection. **Hematologic:** Anemia. **Other:** Anaphylaxis, hypersensitivity reactions.

INTERACTIONS **Drug:** Doripenem decreases plasma levels of **valproic acid. Probenecid** increases doripenem plasma levels.

PHARMACOKINETICS **Distribution:** Minimal protein binding. **Metabolism:** In liver (18%) to inactive metabolite. **Elimination:** Urine (primarily unchanged). **Half-Life:** 1 h.

NURSING IMPLICATIONS

Assessment & Drug Effects

- Determine history of hypersensitivity reactions to other beta-lactams, cephalosporins, penicillins, or other drugs.
- Discontinue drug and immediately report S&S of hypersensitivity (see Appendix F).
- Report S&S of superinfection or pseudomembranous colitis (see Appendix F).
- Monitor lab tests: Baseline C&S; periodic LFTs, Hct, and Hgb.

Patient & Family Education

- Learn S&S of hypersensitivity, superinfection, and pseudomembranous colitis; report any of these to prescriber promptly.

D

DORNASE ALFA

(dor′naze)

Pulmozyme

Classification: RESPIRATORY ENZYME; MUCOLYTIC

Therapeutic: MUCOLYTIC

AVAILABILITY Solution for inhalation

ACTION & *THERAPEUTIC EFFECT* In cystic fibrosis (CF) viscous, purulent secretions in the airway reduce pulmonary function and lead to exacerbations of infection. Purulent pulmonary secretions contain very high concentrations of DNA released by degenerating leukocytes that are present in response to infection. Dornase alfa hydrolyzes the DNA present in sputum/mucus of cystic fibrosis patients and reduces viscosity in the lungs. *Promotes improved clearance of secretions from the respiratory tract.*

USES In combination with standard therapies to reduce the frequency of respiratory infections in patients with CF and to improve pulmonary function.

D

UNLABELED USES Chronic bronchitis, management of atelectasis.

CONTRAINDICATIONS Hypersensitivity to dornase or hamster protein; lactation.

CAUTIOUS USE Decreased pulmonary function; pregnancy (category B). Safe use in children younger than 3 mo not established.

ROUTE & DOSAGE

Cystic Fibrosis

Adult/Child (3 mo or older): **Inhalation** 2.5 mg (1 ampule) inhaled once daily using a recommended nebulizer, may increase to twice daily (do not mix with other agents in nebulizer)

ADMINISTRATION

Inhalation

- Do not dilute or mix with any other drugs or solutions in the nebulizer.
- Use only with nebulizer systems recommended by the drug manufacturer.
- Do not shake ampules; do not use ampules that have been at room temperature longer than 24 h or have become cloudy or discolored.
- Store refrigerated at 2°–8°C (36°–46°F) in protective foil pouch.

ADVERSE EFFECTS **Respiratory:** Hoarseness, sore throat, voice alterations, pharyngitis, laryngitis, cough, rhinitis. **Other:** Conjunctivitis, chest pain, rash.

PHARMACOKINETICS **Absorption:** Minimal systemic absorption. **Onset:** 3–8 days. **Duration:** Benefit lasts up to 4 days after discontinuing treatment.

NURSING IMPLICATIONS

Assessment & Drug Effects

- Monitor for improvement in dyspnea and sputum clearance.
- Monitor for S&S of hypersensitivity (see Appendix F). Patients with a history of hypersensitivity to bovine pancreatic dornase are at high risk.
- Monitor for adverse effects; rarely, dosage adjustments may be required.

Patient & Family Education

- Report rash, hives, itching, or other S&S of hypersensitivity to prescriber immediately.
- Know potential adverse effects and report those that are bothersome or do not disappear.
- Take a missed dose as soon as possible; if it is almost time for the next dose, skip the missed dose.

DORZOLAMIDE HYDROCHLORIDE

(dor-zol'a-mide)

Trusopt

Classification: EYE PREPARATION; CARBONIC ANHYDRASE INHIBITOR

Therapeutic: ANTIGLAUCOMA; OCULAR ANTIHYPERTENSIVE
Prototype: Acetazolamide

AVAILABILITY Ophth solution

ACTION & *THERAPEUTIC EFFECT* Dorzolamide is a sulfonamide that inhibits carbonic anhydrase in the eye, thus reducing the rate of aqueous humor formation with subsequent lowering of IOP. Elevated IOP is a major risk factor in the pathogenesis of optic nerve damage and visual field loss due to glaucoma. *Lowers IOP in glaucoma or ocular hypertension.*

USES Ocular hypertension, open-angle glaucoma.

CONTRAINDICATIONS Previous hypersensitivity to dorzolamide.

CAUTIOUS USE History of hypersensitivity to other carbonic anhydrase inhibitors, sulfonamides, or thiazide diuretics; ocular infection or inflammation; recent ocular surgery; moderate to severe renal or hepatic insufficiency; angle-closure glaucoma; corneal abrasion; older adults, pregnancy (category C).

ROUTE & DOSAGE

Glaucoma, Ocular Hypertension

Adult/Adolescent/Child/Infant: **Ophthalmic** 1 drop in affected eye tid

ADMINISTRATION

Instillation

- Apply gentle pressure to lacrimal sac during and immediately following drug instillation for about 1 min to lessen degree of systemic absorption.
- Administer at least 10 min apart, if another ophthalmic drug is being used concurrently.
- Store at 15°–30°C (59°–86°F).

ADVERSE EFFECTS **CNS:** Headache. **HEENT:** *Transient burning or stinging, transient blurred vision,* superficial punctate keratitis, tearing, dryness, photophobia, ocular allergic reaction. **Skin:** Rash. **GI:** Bitter taste, nausea.

PHARMACOKINETICS **Absorption:** Some systemic absorption. **Onset:** 2 h. **Duration:** 8–12 h. **Distribution:** Into red blood cells. **Elimination:** In urine. **Half-Life:** RBC elimination about 4 mo.

NURSING IMPLICATIONS

Assessment & Drug Effects

- Inquire about previous hypersensitivity to sulfonamides prior to therapy.
- Withhold drug and notify prescriber if S&S of local or systemic hypersensitivity occur (see Appendix F).
- Withhold the drug and notify the prescriber if ocular irritation occurs.

Patient & Family Education

- Learn proper technique for applying eyedrops.
- Do not allow tip of drug dispenser to come in contact with the eye.
- Discontinue drug and report to prescriber: Ocular irritation, infection, or S&S of systemic hypersensitivity occur (see Appendix F).

DOXAPRAM HYDROCHLORIDE

(dox′a-pram)

Dopram

Classification: CEREBRAL STIMULANT; RESPIRATORY STIMULANT
Therapeutic: CEREBRAL STIMULANT; RESPIRATORY STIMULANT
Prototype: Caffeine

D

AVAILABILITY Solution for injection

ACTION & *THERAPEUTIC EFFECT* Short-acting stimulant capable of stimulating all levels of the cerebrospinal axis. Respiratory stimulation by direct medullary action increases tidal volume and slightly increases respiratory rate. Decreases PCO_2 and increases PO_2 by increasing alveolar ventilation. *Effectively used to stimulate respiration postanesthesia, for drug-induced CNS depression, and for chronic pulmonary disease associated with acute hypercapnia.*

USES Short-term adjunctive therapy to alleviate postanesthesia and drug-induced respiratory depression. Also as a temporary measure (approximately 2 h) in hospitalized patients with COPD associated with acute respiratory insufficiency as an aid to prevent elevation of $PaCO_2$ during administration of oxygen. (Not used with mechanical ventilation.)

UNLABELED USES Neonatal apnea refractory to xanthine therapy.

CONTRAINDICATIONS Epilepsy and other convulsive disorders; head injury, cerebral edema; ventilatory disorders, pulmonary fibrosis, flail chest, pneumothorax, airway obstruction, extreme dyspnea, or acute bronchial asthma; severe hypertension, severe coronary artery disease, uncompensated heart failure, CVA; lactation.

CAUTIOUS USE History of bronchial asthma, COPD; cardiac disease, severe tachycardia, arrhythmias, hypertension; renal or hepatic impairment; hyperthyroidism; pheochromocytoma; increased intracranial pressure; peptic ulcer, patients undergoing gastric surgery; acute agitation; older adults; pregnancy (category C). Safe use in children younger than 12 yr not established.

ROUTE & DOSAGE

Postanesthesia

Adult: **IV** 0.5–1 mg/kg single injection (not more than 1.5 mg/kg), may repeat q5min up to 2 mg/kg total dose; infusion of 0.5–1 mg/kg (max total dose: 4 mg/kg)

Drug-Induced CNS Depression

Adult: **IV** 1–2 mg/kg repeat in 5 min, then q1–2h until patient awakens [if relapse occurs, resume q1–2h injections (max total dose: 3 g), if no response after priming dose, may give 1–3 mg/min for up to 2 h until patient awakens]

Chronic Obstructive Pulmonary Disease

Adult: **IV** 0.5–2 mg/kg OR 1–2 mg/min for a max of 2 h (max rate: 3 mg/min)

ADMINISTRATION

- IV administration to neonates: Verify correct IV concentration and rate of infusion with prescriber. Generally do not use in newborns because doxapram contains benzyl alcohol.
- Ensure adequacy of airway and oxygenation before initiation of doxapram therapy.

Intravenous

PREPARE: **Direct:** Give undiluted. **IV Infusion for CNS Depression:** Dilute 250 mg (12.5 mL) in

250 mL of D5W or NS. **IV Infusion for COPD:** Add 400 mg doxapram to 180 mL of D5W, D10W, or NS to yield 2 mg/mL.

ADMINISTER: **Direct for CNS Depression:** Give undiluted over 5 min. **IV Infusion for CNS Depression:** Give at a rate of 1–3 mg/min, depending on patient response. Never exceed 3 mg/min.

- Infusion should not be administered for longer than 2 h. **IV Infusion for COPD:** Infuse at 0.5–1.5 mL/min.

INCOMPATIBILITIES: **Solution/additive:** **Aminophylline, ascorbic acid**, CEPHALOSPORINS, **dexamethasone, diazepam, digoxin, dobutamine, folic acid, furosemide, hydrocortisone, ketamine, methylprednisolone, minocycline, ticarcillin.** **Y-site:** **Clindamycin.**

- Store at 15°–30°C (59°–86°F) unless otherwise directed.

ADVERSE EFFECTS

CV: *Mild to moderate increase in BP, sinus tachycardia*, bradycardia, extrasystoles, lowered T waves, PVCs, chest pains, tightness in chest. **Respiratory:** Dyspnea, tachypnea, cough, laryngospasm, bronchospasm, hiccups, rebound hypoventilation, hypocapnia with tetany. **CNS:** Dizziness, sneezing, apprehension, confusion, *involuntary movements*, hyperactivity, paresthesias; feeling of warmth and burning, especially of genitalia and perineum; flushing, sweating, hyperpyrexia, headache, pilomotor erection, pruritus, muscle tremor, rigidity, convulsions, *increased deep-tendon reflexes*, bilateral Babinski sign, *carpopedal spasm*, pupillary dilation, mild delayed narcosis. **GI:** Nausea, vomiting, diarrhea, salivation, sour taste. **GU:** Urinary retention, frequency, incontinence. **Other:** Local skin irritation, thrombophlebitis with extravasation; decreased Hgb, Hct, and RBC count; elevated BUN; albuminuria.

INTERACTIONS

Drug: MAO INHIBITORS, SYMPATHOMIMETIC AGENTS add to pressor effects.

PHARMACOKINETICS

Onset: 20–40 sec. **Peak:** 1–2 min. **Duration:** 5–12 min. **Metabolism:** Rapidly metabolized. **Elimination:** In urine as metabolites.

NURSING IMPLICATIONS

Assessment & Drug Effects

- Monitor IV site frequently. Extravasation or use of same IV site for prolonged periods can cause thrombophlebitis (see Appendix F) or tissue irritation.
- Monitor carefully and observe accurately: BP, pulse, deep tendon reflexes, airway, and arterial blood gases. All are essential guides for determining minimum effective dosage and preventing overdosage. Make baseline determinations for comparison.
- Discontinue doxapram if arterial blood gases show evidence of deterioration and when mechanical ventilation is initiated.
- Observe patient continuously during therapy, and maintain vigilance until patient is fully alert (usually about 1 h) and protective pharyngeal and laryngeal reflexes are completely restored.
- Notify prescriber immediately of any adverse effects. Be alert for early signs of toxicity: Tachycardia, muscle tremor, spasticity, hyperactive reflexes.
- Note: A mild to moderate increase in BP commonly occurs.
- Discontinue if sudden hypotension or dyspnea develops.

D

- Monitor lab tests: Arterial PO_2, PCO_2, and O_2 saturation prior to both initiation of doxapram infusion and oxygen administration in patients with COPD, and then at least every 30 min during infusion.

DOXAZOSIN MESYLATE

(dox-a′zo-sin)

Cardura, Cardura XL

Classification: ALPHA$_1$-ADRENERGIC ANTAGONIST

Therapeutic: ANTIHYPERTENSIVE

Prototype: Prazosin

AVAILABILITY Tablet; extended release tablet

ACTION & *THERAPEUTIC EFFECT* By selective competitive inhibition of alpha$_1$-adrenoreceptors, it produces vasodilation in both arterioles and veinous vessels, resulting in both peripheral vascular resistance and reduced blood pressure. *Long-acting effect of lowering blood pressure in supine or standing individuals with most pronounced effect on diastolic pressure. Also used for benign prostatic, hyperplasia.*

USES Mild to moderate hypertension, benign prostatic hyperplasia.

UNLABELED USES Ureteral calculi expulsion.

CONTRAINDICATIONS Hypersensitivity to doxazosin, prazosin, and terazosin; hypotension, syncope; pregnancy—fetal risk cannot be ruled out; lactation—infant risk cannot be ruled out.

CAUTIOUS USE Hepatic impairment or disease; renal disease, impairment, or failure; history of cardiac disease, preexisting gastrointestinal narrowing, older adults due to high incidence of orthostatic hypotension. Safe use in children not established.

ROUTE & DOSAGE

Hypertension

Adult: **PO Immediate release** Start with 1 mg at bedtime and titrate as needed up to maximum of 16 mg/day in 1–2 divided doses

BPH

Adult: **PO Immediate release** 1 mg daily, may titrate to max of 8/day; **Extended release** 4 mg daily may titrate to max of 8 mg/day

ADMINISTRATION

Oral

- Give extended release tablet at breakfast.
- Swallow tablets whole; do not chew, divide, cut or crush.
- Individualize maintenance dose according to the standing BP response.
- Store at controlled room temperature of 25°C (77°F), excursions permitted between 15° and 30°C (59° and 86°F).

ADVERSE EFFECTS (≥5%) **CV:** *Orthostatic hypotension.* **CNS:** Vertigo, *headache, dizziness*, somnolence, fatigue.

INTERACTIONS **Drug: Sildenafil, vardenafil, avanafil, nifedipine**, and **tadalafil** may enhance hypotensive effects. Do not use with ALPHA BLOCKERS **abametapir, idelalisib, fusidic acid, conivaptan, bromperidol**. Other ANTIHYPERTENSIVES increase the risk of hypotension. **Herbal: Ma huang** or **yohimbine** may decrease effect.

PHARMACOKINETICS Absorption: Readily from GI tract; 62–69% reaches systemic circulation. **Peak:** 2–6 h. **Duration:** Up to 24 h. **Distribution:** Highly protein bound (98–99%). **Metabolism:** In liver via CYP3A4. **Elimination:** 9% in urine, 63% in feces. **Half-Life:** 22 h (immediate release).

NURSING IMPLICATIONS

Assessment & Drug Effects

- Monitor BP with patient lying down and standing; doses above 4 mg increase the risk of postural hypotension.
- Monitor BP 2–6 h after initial dose or any dose increase. This is when postural hypotension is most likely to occur.

Patient & Family Education

- Do not drive or engage in other potentially hazardous activities for 12–24 h after the first dose or an increase in dosage or when medication is restarted after an interruption in dosage.
- Use caution when rising from a sitting or supine position in order to avoid orthostatic hypotension and syncope; make position and directional changes slowly and in stages.
- Report to the prescriber episodes of dizziness or palpitations. These will require a dosage adjustment.
- Report priapism.
- Instruct patient to take the extended-release dose with breakfast.

DOXEPIN HYDROCHLORIDE

(dox′e-pin)

Prudoxin, Silenor, Triadapin ♣, Zonalon

Classification: TRICYCLIC ANTIDEPRESSANT; ANXIOLYTIC

Therapeutic: ANTIDEPRESSANT; ANTIANXIETY

Prototype: Imipramine

AVAILABILITY Capsule; oral concentrate; tablet, cream

ACTION & *THERAPEUTIC EFFECT* Dibenzoxepin is a tricyclic antidepressant (TCA) that inhibits serotonin reuptake from the synaptic gap; also inhibits norepinephrine reuptake to a moderate degree. *Effective for treatment of both depression and anxiety.*

USES Depression; insomnia; atopic dermatitis; eczema; lichen simplex.

UNLABELED USES Migraine prophylaxis, neuralgia, irritable bowel syndrome.

CONTRAINDICATIONS Hypersensitivity to doxepin, dibenzoxepins; urinary retention; tendency toward urinary retention; glaucoma; suicidal ideation; within 14 days of MAOI drug use; pregnancy—fetal risk cannot be ruled out; lactation—infant risk has been demonstrated.

CAUTIOUS USE Patients receiving electroconvulsive therapy, history of suicidal tendency, head trauma; alcoholism; bipolar disorder, schizophrenia, psychosis; depression; risk factors for bone fractures; risk factors for orthostatic hypotension; severe sleep apnea; Safe use in children younger than 18 yr not established.

ROUTE & DOSAGE

Depression

Adult: **PO** 25–50 mg/day at bedtime, may increase in 25–50 mg increments up to 300 mg/day (use lower doses in older adult patients)

D

Insomnia (Silenor)

Adult: **PO** 3–6 mg at bedtime
Geriatric: **PO** 3 mg at bedtime

Pruritus

Adult: **Topical** Apply a thin film qid with at least 3–4 h between applications, may use up to 8 days

Pharmacogenetic Dosage Adjustment

CYP2D6 Poor metabolizers: Give 40% of normal starting oral dose

ADMINISTRATION

Oral

- Give oral concentrate diluted with approximately 120 mL water, milk, or fruit juice.
- Empty capsule and swallow contents with fluid or mix with food as necessary if it cannot be swallowed whole.
- Inform prescriber if daytime sedation is pronounced. Entire daily dose (up to 150 mg) may be prescribed for bedtime administration. Store at controlled temperature between 20 and 25°C (68–77°F). Protect from light.

Topical

- Apply a thin film to affected areas; allow 3–4 h between applications.
- Do not use occlusive dressings over the medication.
- Store at or below 27°C (80°F).

ADVERSE EFFECTS (≥5%) **CNS:** *Drowsiness*, dizziness. **GU:** Urinary retention.

INTERACTIONS **Drug:** May decrease some antihypertensive response to ANTIHYPERTENSIVES; CNS DEPRESSANTS, **alcohol**, HYPNOTICS, BARBITURATES, SEDATIVES potentiate CNS depression; may increase hypoprothrombinemic effect of ORAL ANTICOAGULANTS; **levodopa**, SYMPATHOMIMETICS (e.g., **epinephrine, norepinephrine**) introduce possibility of sympathetic hyperactivity with hypertension and hyperpyrexia; MAO INHIBITORS introduce possibility of severe reactions, toxic psychosis, cardiovascular instability; **methylphenidate** or **cimetidine** increases plasma levels; THYROID AGENTS may increase possibility of arrhythmias; be cautious with other drugs that prolong the QT interval (e.g., ANTIARRHYTHMICS); ANTICHOLINERGIC AGENTS may have additive effects. **Herbal: Ginkgo** may decrease seizure threshold; **St. John's wort** may cause **serotonin** syndrome.

PHARMACOKINETICS **Absorption:** Rapidly from GI sites and through intact skin. **Peak:** 2 h. **Distribution:** Crosses placenta; distributed into breast milk. **Metabolism:** In liver. via CYP2C19 and CYP2D6. **Elimination:** Primarily in urine. **Half-Life:** 6–8 h.

NURSING IMPLICATIONS

Black Box Warning

Doxepin has been associated with increased risk of suicidal thinking and behavior in children, adolescents, and young adults.

Assessment & Drug Effects

- Monitor for clinical worsening, suicidality, or unusual changes in behavior, especially at initiation of therapy and with children, adolescents, and young adults.

- Monitor use of other CNS depressants, including alcohol. Danger of overdosage or suicide attempt is increased when patient uses excessive amounts of alcohol.
- Monitor sleep maintenance.
- Monitor blood pressure at baseline and with dosage changes and every 3–6 months once stabilized.
- ECG for QT prolongation at baseline, steady state, initial dose, and dose changes.
- Monitor weight gain at 3, 6, 12 months and then annually.
- Be alert to changes in voiding and evaluate patient for constipation and abdominal distention; drug has moderate to strong anticholinergic effects.
- Monitor labs: Sodium level at baseline and after 3–4 weeks.

Patient & Family Education

- Monitor closely during initial treatment and when the dose is adjusted up or down for worsening of depression or suicidal thoughts and behavior. Report promptly to prescriber.
- Be alert for and report to prescriber emergence of anxiety, agitation, panic attacks, insomnia, irritability, hostility, aggressiveness, restlessness, or other unusual changes in behavior.
- Maintain established dosage regimen and avoid change of intervals, doubling, reducing, or skipping doses.
- Patient should not drink alcohol while taking this drug.
- Report insomnia that worsens or persists longer than 7 to 10 days.
- Improvement in depression may not be seen for a few weeks.
- Do not suddenly discontinue the drug.
- Do not place an occlusive dressing over a topical cream.
- Do not drive or engage in other potentially hazardous activities until response to drug is known.

D

DOXERCALCIFEROL

(dox-er-kal′si-fe-rol)

Hectorol

Classification: VITAMIN D ANALOG

Therapeutic: ANTIHYPERPARATHYROID; VITAMIN D ANALOG

Prototype: Calcitriol

AVAILABILITY Capsule; solution for injection

ACTION & *THERAPEUTIC EFFECT*

Vitamin D_2 analog that is activated by the liver. Activated vitamin D is needed for absorption of dietary calcium in the intestine, and the parathyroid hormone (PTH), which mobilizes calcium from the bone tissue. *Regulates the blood calcium level.*

USES Hyperparathyroidism.

CONTRAINDICATIONS Hypersensitivity to doxercalciferol or other vitamin D analogs; recent hypercalcemia, recent hyperphosphatemia, hypervitaminosis D.

CAUTIOUS USE Renal or hepatic insufficiency; renal osteodystrophy with hyperphosphatemia, prolonged hypercalcemia; oversuppression of parathyroid hormone; pregnancy (category B); lactation (infant risk cannot be ruled out). Safety and efficacy in children not established.

ROUTE & DOSAGE

Secondary Hyperparathyroidism

Adult: **PO** 10 mcg 3 × wk at dialysis, adjust dose as needed

D

to lower iPTH into the range of 150–300 pg/mL by increasing the dose in 2.5-mcg increments every 8 wk (max: 60 mcg/wk) **IV** 4 mcg 3 × wk at end of dialysis (max: 18 mcg/wk)

ADMINISTRATION

Oral

- Give at time of dialysis.
- Withhold drug and notify prescriber if any of the following occurs: iPTH less than 100 pg/mL, hypercalcemia, hyperphosphatemia, or product of serum calcium × serum phosphorus greater than 70.
- Store at 20°–25°C (66°–77°F); excursions to 15°–30°C (59°–86°F) are permitted.

Intravenous

PREPARE: **Direct:** No dilution is needed.
ADMINISTER: **Direct:** Give a bolus injection at the end of dialysis sessions.

- Store at 15°–20°C (59°–77°F); protect from light.

ADVERSE EFFECTS **CV:** *Edema*. **Respiratory:** Dyspnea. **CNS:** Dizziness, *headache*. **Skin:** Pruritus. **GI:** Nausea, vomiting. **Other:** *Malaise*.

INTERACTIONS **Drug: Cholestyramine, mineral oil** may decrease absorption; MAGNESIUM-CONTAINING ANTACIDS may cause hypermagnesemia; other VITAMIN D ANALOGS may increase toxicity and hypercalcemia. **Aluminum** absorption may be increased. **Multivitamins** may increase adverse effects.

PHARMACOKINETICS **Absorption:** Absorbed from GI tract and is activated in the liver. **Peak:** 11–12 h. **Metabolism:** Activated by CYP27 to form 1alpha, 25-$(OH)_2D_2$ (major metabolite) and 1alpha, 24-dihydroxy vitamin D_2 (minor metabolite). **Half-Life:** 32–37 h.

NURSING IMPLICATIONS

Assessment & Drug Effects

- Monitor for S&S of hypercalcemia (see Appendix F).
- Monitor lab tests: Baseline and weekly during dose titration iPTH, serum calcium, serum phosphorus; then periodically thereafter.

Patient & Family Education

- Do not take antacids without consulting the prescriber.
- Notify the prescriber if you become pregnant while taking this drug.
- Do not use mineral oil on the days doxercalciferol is taken. Mineral oil may decrease absorption of drug.
- Do not take nonprescription drugs containing magnesium while taking doxercalciferol.
- Report S&S of hypercalcemia immediately: Bone or muscle pain, dry mouth with metallic taste, rhinorrhea, itching, photophobia, conjunctivitis, frequent urination, anorexia, and weight loss.

DOXORUBICIN HYDROCHLORIDE

(dox-oh-roo'bi-sin)

Adriamycin

DOXORUBICIN LIPOSOME

Doxil

Classification: ANTINEOPLASTIC; ANTHRACYCLINE

Therapeutic: ANTINEOPLASTIC

 Common adverse effects in *italic*; life-threatening effects underlined; generic names in **bold**; classifications in SMALL CAPS; ♣ Canadian drug name; Prototype drug; Alert

AVAILABILITY Powder for injection; solution for injection; liposomal injection

ACTION & *THERAPEUTIC EFFECT* Cytotoxic agent with wide spectrum of antitumor activity. Intercalates with preformed DNA residues, blocking effective DNA and RNA transcription. A potent radiosensitizer capable of enhancing radiation reactions. *Highly destructive to rapidly proliferating cells and slowly developing carcinomas; selectively toxic to cardiac tissue.*

USES Adjuvant therapy in breast cancer, disseminated neoplastic conditions.

CONTRAINDICATIONS History of hypersensitive reactions to conventional or liposomal doxorubicin; severe hepatic impairment; severe myelosuppression; severe arrhythmias, recent MI; obstructive jaundice, previous treatment with complete cumulative doses of doxorubicin or daunorubicin; pregnancy (category D); lactation.

CAUTIOUS USE Impaired hepatic or renal function; patients who have received cyclophosphamide or pelvic irradiation or radiotherapy to areas surrounding heart; preexisting heart disease; history of atopic dermatitis; children.

ROUTE & DOSAGE

CONVENTIONAL DOXORUBICIN

Acute Lymphatic Leukemia

Adult/Child: **IV** 30 mg/m^2 weekly × 4 wk

Acute Myelogenous Leukemia

Adult/Child: **IV** 30 mg/m^2 × 3 days (with cytarabine)

Breast Cancer

Adult: **IV** 60 mg/m^2 on day 1 of 21-day cycle × 4 cycles.

Transitional Bladder Cell Cancer

Adult: **IV** 30 mg/m^2/dose once monthly

Hodgkin Disease

Adult/Child: **IV** 25 mg/m^2 days 1 and 15, repeat q28days

Thyroid Cancer

Adult/Child: **IV** 60–75 mg/m^2 q3wk

Other Neoplasms

Adult: **IV** 40–50 mg/m^2 usually in combination with other agents (max total cumulative lifetime dose: 500–550 mg/m^2)
Child: **IV** 35–75 mg/m^2 as single dose, repeat at 21-day interval, or 20–30 mg/m^2 once weekly (max total cumulative lifetime dose: 500–550 mg/m^2)

Hepatic Impairment Dosage Adjustment

Bilirubin 1.2–3 mg/dL: Reduce dose by 50%; bilirubin 3–5 mg/dL: Reduce dose by 75%
Bilirubin greater than 5 mg/dL: Stop therapy

DOXORUBICIN LIPOSOME

Kaposi Sarcoma

Adult: **IV** 20 mg/m^2 q3wk. Infuse over 30 min (do not use in-line filters).

Progressive/Refractory Ovarian Cancer

Adult: **IV** 50 mg/m^2 q4wk, minimum of 4 courses

D

Relapsed/Refractory Multiple Myeloma

Adult: IV 45 mg/m^2 q4wk, up to 6 cycles

Hepatic Impairment Dosage Adjustment

Bilirubin 1.2–3 mg/dL: Reduce dose 50%; *bilirubin 3–5 mg/dL:* Reduce dose by 75%

ADMINISTRATION

Intravenous

▪ IV administration to children: Verify correct IV concentration and rate of infusion with prescriber. ▪ Wear gloves and use caution when preparing drug solution. If powder or solution contacts skin or mucosa, wash copiously with soap and water.

Conventional Doxorubicin

PREPARE: **Direct:** *Vial reconstitution:* Dilute with 1 mL of nonbacteriostatic NS for each 2 mg of doxorubicin to yield a final concentration of 2 mg/mL. ▪ For each mL of NS added, withdraw an equal volume of air from vial to minimize pressure buildup. Shake to dissolve. ▪ *Doxorubicin solutions:* Solutions of 2 mg/mL are available that can be further diluted in 50 mL or more of NS or D5W.

ADMINISTER: **Direct:** Give bolus dose slowly into Y-site of freely running IV infusion of NS or D5W. ▪ If possible, use IV tubing attached to a needle inserted into a larger vein with a butterfly needle. ▪ Usually infused over 3–10 min or longer. ▪ Monitor for red streaking along vein or facial flushing, which indicates need to slow infusion rate.

Lyophilized Doxorubicin

PREPARE: **IV Infusion:** Dilute doses up to 90 mg in 250 mL of D5W and doses greater than 90 mg in 500 mL D5W. Solution will be translucent but not clear and will be red in color. ▪ **Do not** use filters during preparation or administration.

ADMINISTER: **IV Infusion: Do not** give bolus injection or undiluted solution. ▪ Infuse at 1 mg/min initially; may increase rate to complete infusion in 1 h if no adverse reactions occur. Slow infusion rate as warranted if an adverse reaction occurs. ▪ Do not use a filter.

INCOMPATIBILITIES: **Solution/additive:** *Conventional doxorubicin:* **Aminophylline, diazepam, fluorouracil.** **Y-site:** *Conventional doxorubicin:* **Allopurinol, amphotericin B cholesteryl sulfate, cefepime, gallium ganciclovir, lansoprazole, pemetrexed, prochlorperazine, propofol, TPN.** *Doxorubicin liposome:* **Amphotericin B, amphotericin B cholesteryl complex, hydroxyzine, mannitol, meperidine, metoclopramide, mitoxantrone, morphine, paclitaxel, piperacillin/tazobactam, promethazine, sodium bicarbonate.**

▪ Facial flushing and local red streaking along the vein may occur if drug is administered too rapidly. ▪ Avoid using antecubital vein or veins on dorsum of hand or wrist, if possible, where extravasation could damage underlying tendons and nerves. ▪ Also avoid veins in extremity with compromised venous or lymphatic drainage.

▪ Store reconstituted solution for 24 h at room temperature;

refrigerated at 4°–10°C (39°–50°F) for 48 h. Protect from sunlight; discard unused solution.

ADVERSE EFFECTS CV: Serious, irreversible myocardial toxicity with delayed CHF, ventricular arrhythmias, acute left ventricular failure, hypertension, hypotension, cardiomyopathy. **Skin:** Hyperpigmentation of nail beds, tongue, and buccal mucosa (especially in blacks); *complete alopecia* (reversible), hyperpigmentation of dermal creases (especially in children), rash, *recall phenomenon (skin reaction due to prior radiotherapy)*. **GI:** *Stomatitis*, esophagitis with ulcerations; nausea, vomiting, anorexia, inanition, diarrhea. **Hematologic:** *Severe myelosuppression* (60–85% of patients); leukopenia *(principally granulocytes)*, thrombocytopenia, anemia. **Other:** Lacrimation, drowsiness, fever, facial flush with too rapid IV infusion rate, microscopic hematuria, hyperuricemia, *hand-foot syndrome*, *severe cellulitis, vesication, tissue necrosis*, lymphangitis, phlebosclerosis with extravasation. Hypersensitivity (red flare around injection site, erythema, skin rash, pruritus, angioedema, urticaria, eosinophilia, fever, chills, anaphylactoid reaction).

INTERACTIONS Drug: BARBITURATES may decrease effects by increasing its hepatic metabolism; **streptozocin** may prolong doxorubicin half-life; agents affecting QT interval (e.g., **Bepridil, droperidol, erythromycin, haloperidol, methadone**, PHENOTHIAZINES, etc.) may increase risk of cardiac side effects. Conventional doxorubicin: Avoid use with **zidovudine**, monitor **warfarin** carefully.

PHARMACOKINETICS Distribution: Widely distributed; does not cross blood–brain barrier; 75% protein binding; does not cross placenta; passes into breast milk. **Metabolism:** In liver to active metabolite. **Elimination:** Primarily in bile. **Half-Life:** 30–50 h. *Doxorubicin Liposome:* **Distribution:** Vascular fluid. **Metabolism:** In plasma and liver. **Elimination:** In urine. **Half-Life:** 44–55 h.

NURSING IMPLICATIONS

Black Box Warning

Doxorubicin can cause severe local tissue necrosis if extravasation occurs. Doxorubicin has been associated with cardiotoxicity, severe bone marrow suppression, and development of secondary malignancies (i.e., acute myelogenous leukemia or myelodysplastic syndrome).

Assessment & Drug Effects

- Care should be taken to avoid extravasation. Stop infusion, remove IV needle, and notify prescriber promptly if patient complains of stinging or burning sensation at the injection site.
- Monitor any area of extravasation closely for 3–4 wk. If ulceration begins (usually 1–4 wk after extravasation), a plastic surgeon should be consulted.
- Establish baseline data. Include temperature, pulse, respiration, BP, body weight, laboratory values, and I&O ratio and pattern.
- Cardiac function must be evaluated prior to initiation of therapy, at regular intervals, and at end of therapy.
- Be alert to and report early signs of cardiotoxicity (see Appendix F).

Acute life-threatening arrhythmias may occur within a few hours of drug administration.

- Report promptly objective signs of hepatic dysfunction (jaundice, dark urine, pruritus) or kidney dysfunction (altered I&O ratio and pattern, local discomfort with voiding).
- Report signs of superinfection (see Appendix F) promptly; these may result from antibiotic therapy during leukopenic period.
- Avoid rectal medications and use of rectal thermometer; rectal trauma is associated with bloody diarrhea resulting from an antiblastic effect on rapidly growing intestinal mucosal cells.
- Monitor lab tests: Baseline and periodic LFTs, renal function, CBC with differential.

Patient & Family Education

- Complete loss of hair (reversible) is an expected adverse effect. It may also involve eyelashes and eyebrows, beard and mustache, pubic and axillary hair. Regrowth of hair usually begins 2–3 mo after drug is discontinued.
- Drug turns urine red for 1–2 days after administration.
- Keep hands away from eyes to prevent conjunctivitis. Increased tearing for 5–10 days after a single dose is possible.
- Maintain fastidious oral hygiene, especially before and after meals. Stomatitis, generally maximal in second week of therapy, frequently begins with a burning sensation accompanied by erythema of oral mucosa that may progress to ulceration and dysphagia in 2 or 3 days.
- Exposure to doxorubicin during the first trimester of pregnancy can result in fetal abnormalities or fetal loss.

DOXYCYCLINE HYCLATE

(dox-i-sye′kleen)

Apo-Doxy ♣, Doryx, Doxy, Doxycin ♣, Monodox, Vibramycin

Classification: ANTIBIOTIC; TETRACYCLINE

Therapeutic: ANTIBIOTIC

Prototype: Tetracycline

AVAILABILITY Capsule, tablet; solution for injection

ACTION & *THERAPEUTIC EFFECT* Semisynthetic broad-spectrum long-acting tetracycline antibiotic that is more lipophilic than the other tetracyclines, allowing it to pass through the lipid layer of bacteria where reversible binding to the 30 S ribosomal subunits of bacteria occurs. This blocks the binding of transfer RNA (tRNA) to the messenger RNA (mRNA) of bacteria, resulting in inhibition of bacterial protein synthesis. *Primarily bacteriostatic against both gram-positive and gram-negative bacteria.*

USES Similar to those of tetracycline (e.g., chlamydial and mycoplasmal infections); gonorrhea, syphilis in penicillin-allergic patients; rickettsial diseases; acute exacerbations of chronic bronchitis.

UNLABELED USES Treatment of acute PID, leptospirosis, prophylaxis for rape victims, suppression and chemoprophylaxis of chloroquine-resistant *Plasmodium falciparum* malaria, short-term prophylaxis and treatment of travelers' diarrhea caused by enterotoxigenic strains of *Escherichia coli*. Intrapleural administration for malignant pleural effusions, postexposure anthrax treatment and prophylaxis.

CONTRAINDICATIONS Sensitivity to any of the tetracyclines; use during period of tooth development including last half of pregnancy; pregnancy (category D); lactation, infants, and children younger than 8 yr except for use in anthrax exposure (causes permanent yellow discoloration of teeth, enamel hypoplasia, and retardation of bone growth).

CAUTIOUS USE Alcoholism; hepatic disease; GI disease; sulfite hypersensitivity; sunlight (UV) exposure.

ROUTE & DOSAGE

Skin/Skin Structure Infections

Adult/Adolescent/Child (8 yr or older, weight 45 kg or more): **IV** 200 mg on day 1 then 100–200 mg daily
Child (8 yr or older, weight 45 kg or less): **IV** 4.4 mg/kg on day 1 then 2.2–4.4 mg/kg/day in divided doses

UTI

Adult/Adolescent: **PO** 100 mg q12h × 1 day then 100 mg daily; **IV** 200 mg on day 1 then 100–200 mg daily

Gonorrhea

Adult: **PO** 100 mg bid × 7 days

Primary and Secondary Syphilis

Adult: **PO** 100 mg bid × 14 days

Acute Pelvic Inflammatory Disease

Adult: **IV** 100 mg q12h until improved, then 100 mg **PO** bid to complete 14 days

Acne

Adult: **PO** 100 mg q12h on day 1, then 100 mg daily
Child (8 yr or older, weight greater than 45 kg): **PO** 100 mg q12h on day 1, then 100 mg daily; *weight less than 45 kg:* **PO** 2.2 mg/kg q12h on day 1, then 2.2 mg/kg/daily

Anthrax Postexposure

Adult/Adolescent/Child (8 yr or older, weight greater than 45 kg): **IV** 100 mg q12h, then switch to **PO** for a total of 60
Child (8 yr or less or weight 45 kg or less) **IV** 2.2 mg/kg q12h, then switch to **PO** for a total of 60

ADMINISTRATION

Oral

- Check expiration date. Degradation products of tetracycline are toxic to the kidneys.
- Give with food or a full glass of milk to minimize nausea without significantly affecting bioavailability of drug (unlike most **tetracyclines**). Patient should sit up for at least 30–120 min after administration to reduce the risk of esophageal irritation and ulceration.
- Consult prescriber about ordering the oral suspension for patients who are bedridden or have difficulty swallowing.

Intravenous

PREPARE: **Intermittent:** Reconstitute by adding 10 mL sterile water for injection, or D5W, NS, LR, D5/LR, or other diluent recommended by manufacturer, to

D

each 100 mg of drug. ▪ Further dilute with 100–1000 mL (per 100 mg of drug) of compatible infusion solution to produce concentrations ranging from 0.1 to 1 mg/mL.

ADMINISTER: **Intermittent:** Duration of infusion varies with dose but is usually 1–4 h. ▪ Recommended minimum infusion time for 100 mg of 0.5 mg/mL solution is 1 h. Infusion should be completed within 12 h of dilution. ▪ When diluted with LR or D5/LR, infusion **must be** completed within 6 h to ensure adequate stability. ▪ Protect all solutions from direct sunlight during infusion.

INCOMPATIBILITIES: **Solution/additive:** **Potassium phosphate.** **Y-site:** **Allopurinol, heparin, meropenem, pemetrexed disodium, piperacillin/tazobactam, TPN.**

▪ Store oral and parenteral forms (prior to reconstitution) in tightly covered, light-resistant containers at 15°–30°C (59°–86°F) unless otherwise directed. ▪ Refrigerate reconstituted solutions for up to 72 h. After this time, infusion **must be** completed within 12 h.

ADVERSE EFFECTS

CV: Hypertension. **Respiratory:** Nasopharyngitis, bronchitis, sinusitis, nasal congestion. **CNS:** Pain, anxiety. **HEENT:** Interference with color vision. **Skin:** Rashes, photosensitivity reaction. **GI:** Anorexia, *nausea*, vomiting, diarrhea, enterocolitis; esophageal irritation (oral capsule and tablet). **GU:** Dysmenorrhea. **Musculoskeletal:** Arthralgia. **Other:** Thrombophlebitis (IV use), superinfections.

DIAGNOSTIC TEST INTERFERENCE

Like other ***tetracyclines***, doxycycline may cause false increases in ***urinary catecholamines*** (fluorometric methods); false decreases in ***urinary urobilinogen***; false-negative ***urine glucose*** with ***glucose oxidase methods*** (e.g., ***Clinistix, Tes-Tape***); parenteral doxycycline (containing ascorbic acid) may cause false-positive determinations using ***Benedict reagent*** or ***Clinitest***.

INTERACTIONS

Drug: ANTACIDS, **iron** preparation, **calcium, magnesium, zinc, kaolin pectin, sodium bicarbonate** can significantly decrease absorption; effects of both doxycycline and **desmopressin** antagonized; increases **digoxin** absorption, thus increasing risk of **digoxin** toxicity; **methoxyflurane** increases risk of renal failure. Do not use with **acitretin** or **isotretinoin**.

PHARMACOKINETICS

Absorption: Completely absorbed from GI tract. **Peak:** 1.5–4 h. **Distribution:** Penetrates eye, prostate, and CSF; crosses placenta; distributed into breast milk. **Metabolism:** In GI tract. **Elimination:** Mainly in feces. **Half-Life:** 14–24 h.

NURSING IMPLICATIONS

Assessment & Drug Effects

- Report sudden onset of painful or difficult swallowing promptly to prescriber. Doxycycline (capsule and tablet forms) is associated with a comparatively high incidence of esophagitis, especially in patients older than 40 yr.
- Report evidence of superinfections (see Appendix F).

Patient & Family Education

- Take capsule or tablet forms with a full glass (240 mL) of water to ensure passage into stomach and prevent esophageal ulceration. Avoid taking capsule or tablet within 1 h of lying down or retiring.

- Avoid exposure to direct sunlight and ultraviolet light during and for 4 or 5 days after therapy is terminated to reduce risk of phototoxic reaction. Phototoxic reaction appears like an exaggerated sunburn. Sunscreens provide little protection.

DRONABINOL

(droe-nab′i-nol)

Marinol, Syndros

Classification: CANNABINOID; ANTIEMETIC

Therapeutic: ANTIEMETIC; APPETITE STIMULANT

Controlled Substance: Schedule III (Marinol)/Schedule II (Syndros)

AVAILABILITY Capsule, oral solution

ACTION & *THERAPEUTIC EFFECT*
Synthetic derivative of tetrahydrocannabinol (THC), the principal psychoactive constituent of marijuana (*Cannabis sativa*). Inhibits vomiting through the control mechanism in the medulla oblongata, producing potent antiemetic effect. Risk of drug abuse is high. *Produces potent antiemetic effect and is used to treat chemotherapy-induced nausea and vomiting. For use of appetite stimulant in the treatment of anorexia associated with weight loss.*

USES To treat chemotherapy-induced nausea and vomiting; anorexia in patients with AIDS.

CONTRAINDICATIONS Nausea and vomiting caused by other than chemotherapeutic agents; hypersensitivity to dronabinol or sesame oil; pregnancy—fetal risk cannot be ruled out; lactation—infant risk cannot be ruled out. Safety and effectiveness not established in pediatric patients.

CAUTIOUS USE First exposure, especially in the older adult or cardiac patient; hypertension, hypotension, cardiovascular disorders; epilepsy; psychiatric illness, patient receiving other psychoactive drugs; severe hepatic dysfunction.

ROUTE & DOSAGE

Chemotherapy-Induced Nausea

Adult/Child(over 9y): **PO** capsule 5 mg/m^2 1–3 h prior to chemotherapy, then q2–4h after chemotherapy for a total of 4–6 doses, dose may be increased by 2.5 mg/m^2 (max: 15 mg/m^2/dose if necessary); solution 4.2 mg/m^2 1–3 h prior to chemotherapy then q2–4h after chemotherapy for a total of 4–6 doses, titrate in 2.1 mg/m^2 doses (max: 12.6 mg/m^2/dose)

Anorexia in AIDS

Adult: **PO** capsule: 2.5 mg bid, before lunch and dinner; solution: 2.1 mg bid, before lunch and dinner, may titrate up to 4.2 mg bid if needed

ADMINISTRATION

Oral

- Do not repeat dose following a CNS adverse reaction until patient's mental state has returned to normal and the circumstances have been evaluated.
- Take each dose with 6 to 8 ounces of water.

D

- Take first dose on an empty stomach at least 30 minutes before eating; subsequent doses can be taken without regard to meals.
- Store capsules in a cool place at 8°–15°C (46°–59°F) or refrigerate. Protect from freezing.

ADVERSE EFFECTS (≥5%)

CV: Tachycardia, orthostatic hypotension. **CNS:** *Drowsiness*, dizziness, confusion, euphoria, sensory or perceptual difficulties, impaired coordination, depression, ataxia. **GI:** Dry mouth, abdominal pain, nausea, vomiting, diarrhea.

INTERACTIONS

Drug: Alcohol and other CNS DEPRESSANTS may exaggerate effects of dronabinol; do not use with **disulfiram, methotrimeprazine, metronidazole** due to increased toxic effects.

PHARMACOKINETICS

Absorption: Rapidly absorbed from GI tract, with bioavailability of 10–20%. **Peak:** 2–4 h. **Distribution:** Fat soluble; distributed to many organs; distributed into breast milk; 97% protein bound. **Metabolism:** In liver; extensive first-pass metabolism. **Elimination:** 50% in feces; 10–15% in urine. **Half-Life:** 25–36 h.

NURSING IMPLICATIONS

Assessment & Drug Effects

- Monitor patients with hypertension or heart disease for BP and cardiac status.
- Response to dronabinol is varied, and previous uneventful use does not guarantee that adverse reactions will not occur. Effects of drug may persist an unpredictably long time (days). Extended use at therapeutic dosage may cause accumulation of toxic amounts of dronabinol and its metabolites.
- Watch for disturbing psychiatric symptoms if dose is increased: Altered mental state, loss of coordination, evidence of a psychologic high (easy laughing, elation and heightened awareness), or depression.
- Note: Abrupt withdrawal is associated with symptoms (within 12 h) of irritability, insomnia, restlessness. Peak intensity occurs at about 24 h: Hot flashes, diaphoresis, rhinorrhea, watery diarrhea, hiccups, anorexia. Usually, syndrome is over in 96 h.

Patient & Family Education

- Do not drive or engage in other potentially hazardous activities that require alertness and judgment because of high incidence of dizziness and drowsiness.
- Understand potential (reversible) for drug-induced mood or behavior changes that may occur during dronabinol use.
- Do not ingest alcohol during period of systemic dronabinol effect. Effect on blood ethanol levels is complex and unpredictable.
- Report worsening nausea, vomiting, and abdominal pain.

DRONEDARONE

(dro-ne′da-rone)

Multaq

Classification: CLASS III ANTIARRHYTHMIC

Therapeutic: CLASS III ANTIARRHYTHMIC

AVAILABILITY

Tablet

ACTION & THERAPEUTIC EFFECT

Antiarrhythmic class III drug known to inhibit potassium currents, sodium channels, and slow-L type calcium channels. *Reduces risk of hospitalization in patients with recent paroxysmal or persistent atrial fibrillation (AF).*

USES Recent episode of paroxysmal or persistent atrial fibrillation.

CONTRAINDICATIONS NYHA Class IV HF or NYHA Class II–III HF with a recent decompensation requiring hospitalization or referral to a specialized HF clinic; permanent atrial fibrillation; second- and third-degree AV block or sick sinus syndrome (except with used in conjunction with a functioning pacemaker); bradycardia less than 40 bpm; QT_c interval elongation; severe hepatic impairment; pregnancy (category X); lactation.

CAUTIOUS USE HF; prolonged QT interval; hypokalemia, hypomagnesium; potassium-depleting diuretics; moderate liver impairment; women of childbearing age. Safety and efficacy in children younger than 18 yr not established.

ROUTE & DOSAGE

Atrial Fibrillation

Adult: **PO** 400 mg bid with meals

ADMINISTRATION

Oral

- Give with morning and evening meal. **Do not** give with grapefruit juice.
- Store at 15°–3°C (56°–89°F).

ADVERSE EFFECTS CV: Bradycardia, *QT_c prolongation*. **Endocrine:** *Increased serum creatinine*, hepatic injury. **Skin:** Dermatitis, eczema, erythematous, macula-papular rash, pruritus. **GI:** Abdominal pain, diarrhea, dyspepsia, nausea, vomiting. **Other:** Asthenia.

INTERACTIONS Drug: Concomitant use of CYP3A4 inducers (e.g., **rifampin, phenobarbital, carbamazepine, phenytoin**) can increase the levels of dronedarone. **Ketoconazole, itraconazole, clarithromycin**, and other inhibitors of CYP3A4 can increase the levels of dronedarone. Dronedarone can increase the levels of **digoxin** and other compounds requiring P-glycoprotein (P-gp) transport. BETA BLOCKERS may provoke excessive bradycardia. **Verapamil** and **diltiazem** can potentiate dronedarone's effects on conduction. Use cautiously with **dabigatran. Food: Grapefruit juice** can increase the levels of dronedarone. **Herbal: St. John's wort** can decrease the levels of dronedarone.

PHARMACOKINETICS Peak: 3–6 h. **Distribution:** 98% plasma protein bound. **Metabolism:** Extensive hepatic metabolism to active and inactive compounds. **Elimination:** 84% in the feces; 6% in the urine. **Half-Life:** 13–19 h.

NURSING IMPLICATIONS

Assessment & Drug Effects

- Monitor vital signs and ECG. Report promptly prolongation of the QT_c interval.
- Monitor for S&S of hepatic toxicity (see Appendix F).
- Report promptly S&S of worsening HF (e.g., rapid weight gain, dependent edema, increasing shortness of breath).
- Withhold drug and notify prescriber if hypokalemia or hypomagnesemia develops.
- Monitor lab tests: Baseline and periodic potassium and magnesium levels; periodic serum creatinine.

D

Patient & Family Education

- Report immediately any of the following: Shortness of breath, wheezing, chest tightness, coughing up frothy sputum, rapid weight gain, requiring more pillows to sleep at night.
- Women of childbearing age should use effective contraception while on this drug.
- Avoid grapefruit and grapefruit juice while taking this drug.

DROPERIDOL

(droe-per'i-dole)

Classification: BUTYROPHENONE; MISCELLANEOUS ANTIEMETIC; ANXIOLYTIC
Therapeutic: ANTIEMETIC; ANTIANXIETY
Prototype: Chlorpromazine

AVAILABILITY Solution for injection

ACTION & *THERAPEUTIC EFFECT* The mechanism of action is not known. It has been be theorized that it antagonizes emetic effects of morphine-like analgesics and other drugs that act on chemoreceptor trigger zone. *Sedative property reduces anxiety and motor activity without necessarily inducing sleep; patient remains responsive. Has antiemetic properties.*

USES Postoperative nausea/vomiting.

UNLABELED USES Acute agitation.

CONTRAINDICATIONS Known or suspected QT elongation; history of torsades de pointes; known intolerance to droperidol; pregnancy—fetal risk cannot be ruled out; lactation infant risk cannot be ruled out.

CAUTIOUS USE Older adult, debilitated, alcoholism, and other poor-risk patients; MAOI therapy; liver and kidney impairment or disease; pheochromocytoma. Safe use in children younger than 2 yr is not established.

ROUTE & DOSAGE

Postoperative Nausea and Vomiting Prevention

Adult: **IV/IM** 2.5 mg; additional doses of 1.25 mg may be given
Child: **IV/IM** 0.01–0.015 mg/kg/dose (max: 2.5 mg)

ADMINISTRATION

Intramuscular

- Give undiluted.
- Give deep IM into a large muscle.

Intravenous

IV administration to children: Verify correct rate of IV injection with prescriber.

PREPARE: **Direct:** Give undiluted.
ADMINISTER: **Direct:** *Adult:* Give at a rate of 2.5 mg or fraction thereof over 1–2 min. *Child:* Give a single dose over at least 2 min. Administer slowly.
INCOMPATIBILITIES: **Solution/additive:** **Lornoxicam.** **Y-site:** **Allopurinol, amphotericin B cholesteryl complex, cangrelor, cefepime, cloxacillin, ertapenem, fluorouracil, foscarnet, fosphenytoin, furosemide, gallium, gemtuzumab, irinotecan, lansoprazole, leucovorin, nafcillin, pantoprazole, pemetrexed, piperacillin/tazobactam, potassium acetate.**

- Store at controlled room temperature between 20° and 25°C

(68° and 77°F); excursions permitted to 15°–30°C (59°–86°F), unless otherwise directed by manufacturer. Protect from light.

ADVERSE EFFECTS (≥5%) **CV:** *Hypotension, tachycardia*, irregular heartbeats *(prolonged QT_c interval even at low doses)*. **CNS:** *Postoperative drowsiness*. **Other:** Anxiety, dysphoric mood, hyperactivity, restlessness.

INTERACTIONS **Drugs:** Additive effect with CNS depressants, **metoclopramide** may increase extrapyramidal symptoms, closely monitor or avoid other drugs affecting QT interval. ANTIHCOLINERGIC AGENTS may have increased risk of adverse effects. Concurrent use of POTASSIUM SALTS increases risk of ulcer formation. ANTIPARKSINSON AGENTS may decrease efficacy of droperidol. May increase adverse effects of **eluxadoline**, **iomeprol** or **iopamidol.**

PHARMACOKINETICS **Onset:** 3–10 min. **Peak:** 30 min. **Duration:** 2–4 h; may persist up to 12 h. **Distribution:** Crosses placenta and blood–brain barrier. **Metabolism:** In liver. **Elimination:** In urine and feces.

NURSING IMPLICATIONS

Black Box Warning

Droperidol has been associated with development of QT prolongation and/or torsade de pointes, some fatal.

Assessment & Drug Effects

- Monitor 12-lead ECG throughout therapy and 2–3 h after treatment is completed. Report immediately prolongation of QT_c interval.
- Monitor vital signs closely. Hypotension and tachycardia are common adverse effects.
- Exercise care in moving medicated patients because of possibility of severe orthostatic hypotension. Avoid abrupt changes in position.
- Observe patients for signs of impending respiratory depression carefully when receiving a concurrent narcotic analgesic.
- Note: EEG patterns are slow to return to normal during the postoperative period.
- Observe carefully and report promptly to prescriber early signs of acute dystonia: Facial grimacing, restlessness, tremors, torticollis, oculogyric crisis. Extrapyramidal symptoms may occur within 24–48 h postoperatively.
- Note: Droperidol may aggravate symptoms of acute depression.

Patient & Family Education

- Report excessive drowsiness, anxiety, or change in mood; increased restlessness or frustration.
- Report any light-headedness, or slowed respiratory rate.

DROXIDOPA

(drox-i-dop'a)

Northera

Classification: DOPAMINE RECEPTOR AGONIST; HYPERTENSIVE

Therapeutic: HYPERTENSIVE

Prototype: Carbidopa

AVAILABILITY Gelatin capsules

ACTION & THERAPEUTIC EFFECT Droxidopa is directly metabolized to norepinephrine. Believed to exert its pharmacological effects through norepinephrine, which *increases BP by inducing peripheral arterial and venous vasoconstriction*.

D

USES Treatment of neurogenic orthostatic hypotension caused by primary autonomic failure (Parkinson disease, multiple system atrophy, and pure autonomic failure), dopamine beta-hydroxylase deficiency, and nondiabetic autonomic neuropathy.

CONTRAINDICATIONS Lactation.

CAUTIOUS USE Supine hypertension; neuroleptic malignant syndrome; ischemic heart disease; CHF; arrhythmias; hypersensitivity to tartrazine (especially in those with aspirin hypersensitivity); severe renal impairment; pregnancy (category C).

ROUTE & DOSAGE

Neurogenic Orthostatic Hypotension

Adult: **PO** 100 mg tid initially; can titrate in 100 mg increments q24–48h (max: 600 mg tid)

ADMINISTRATION

Oral

- Give capsule whole. It should not be crushed or chewed.
- Give consistently with/without food, upon arising in a.m., at midday, and in late afternoon at least 3 h before bedtime (to reduce risk of supine hypertension during sleep).
- Store at 15°C–30°C (59°F–86°F).

ADVERSE EFFECTS **CV:** Hypertension, *syncope*. **CNS:** Dizziness. **GI:** Nausea. **GU:** *Urinary tract infection*. **Other:** *Falling*, headache.

INTERACTIONS **Drug: Carbidopa** may decrease the levels of droxidopa's active metabolite. Other drugs that increase blood pressure (**ephedrine, midodrine**, SEROTONIN 5-HT1D RECEPTOR AGONISTS).

PHARMACOKINETICS **Peak:** 1–4 h. **Distribution:** Plasma protein binding is dose related. **Metabolism:** Bioactivated to norepinephrine. **Elimination:** Primarily renal. **Half-Life:** 2.5 h.

NURSING IMPLICATIONS

Black Box Warning

Droxidopa has been associated with severe, potentially fatal supine hypertension.

Assessment & Drug Effects

- Elevate the head of the bed to lessen risk of supine hypertension.
- Monitor supine BP (with head of bed elevated) prior to and during treatment and more frequently when increasing doses.
- If supine hypertension cannot be managed by elevating head of the bed, report to prescriber, as dose should be reduced or drug discontinued.

Patient & Family Education

- Rest and sleep in an upper-body elevated position.
- Monitor blood pressure and report promptly to prescriber significant elevations when supine.
- Be consistent when taking drug with respect to food (see ADMINISTRATION).

DULAGLUTIDE

(du-la-glu'tide)

Trulicity

Classification: ANTIDIABETIC; INCRETIN MIMETIC; GLUCAGON-LIKE PEPTIDE-1

Therapeutic: ANTIDIABETIC

Prototype: Exenatide

AVAILABILITY Subcutaneous injection

ACTION & *THERAPEUTIC EFFECT* Improves glycemic control in type 2 diabetes mellitus by mimicking the functions of incretin, a glucagon-like peptide-1 (GLP-1), which enhances glucose-dependent insulin secretion by pancreatic beta cells, suppresses inappropriately elevated glucagon secretion, and slows gastric emptying. *Improves glycemic control by reducing fasting and postprandial glucose concentrations.*

USES Type 2 diabetes mellitus in combination with diet and exercise.

CONTRAINDICATIONS Serious hypersensitivity to dulaglutide or component of the formulation; personal or family history of medullary thyroid carcinoma; multiple endocrine neoplasia (MEN); pancreatitis; pregnancy—fetal risk cannot be ruled out; lactation—infant risk cannot be ruled out.

CAUTIOUS USE Hepatic impairment; renal impairment; severe GU disease; gastroparesis; history of pancreatitis. Safety and efficacy in children younger than 18 yr not established.

ROUTE & DOSAGE

Type 2 Diabetes Mellitus

Adult: **Subcutaneous** 0.75 mg once weekly; may increase to 1.5 mg once weekly

ADMINISTRATION

Subcutaneous only

- Administer weekly on the same day each wk, without regard to meals or time of day.
- May change injection day as long as the last dose was administered at least 3 days prior.
- Avoid administering adjacent to insulin injections.
- Inject into the upper arm, thigh, or abdomen.
- Use a different injection site each week.
- Store at 2°–8°C (36°–46°F). Do not freeze. Protect from light. Single-dose pen or prefilled syringe can be kept at room temperature, up to 30°C (86°F), for 14 days.

ADVERSE EFFECTS (≥5%) **Endocrine:** Increased amylase and lipase levels, *hypoglycemia*. **GI:** Abdominal pain, decreased appetite, diarrhea, nausea, vomiting.

INTERACTIONS **Drug:** Concomitant use with **insulin** or an INSULIN SECRETAGOGUE may result in additive effects on blood glucose. Dulaglutide slows gastric emptying and has the potential to decrease the rate of absorption of other coadministered oral drugs. SULFONYLUREAS have increased risk of hypoglycemia.

PHARMACOKINETICS **Peak:** 24–72 h. **Metabolism:** In liver. **Elimination:** Primarily in urine. **Half-Life:** 5 days.

NURSING IMPLICATIONS

Black Box Warning

Dulaglutide may pose a risk of thyroid C-cell tumor development, although a direct link has not been established.

Assessment & Drug Effects

- Monitor for and report S&S of significant GI distress, including nausea, vomiting, and diarrhea.
- Monitor for S&S of hypoglycemia and S&S of acute pancreatitis (acute abdominal pain

with/without vomiting). If pancreatitis is suspected, withhold drug and notify prescriber immediately.

- Monitor for and report immediately site injection reactions such as cellulitis, abscess, and skin necrosis.
- Monitor progression of diabetic retinopathy.
- Monitor lab tests: Frequent fasting and postprandial plasma glucose and periodic HbA1C; baseline and periodic renal function tests.

Patient & Family Education

- If a weekly dose is missed, administer it as soon as possible as long as next scheduled dose is due at least 3 days later
- Maintain adequate hydration.
- Dulaglutide may cause decreased appetite and some weight loss.
- Patient or family member demonstrate correct administration of subcutaneous injection.
- Report significant GI distress to prescriber. Report promptly persistent, severe abdominal pain that may be accompanied by vomiting.
- Report symptoms of thyroid tumors (e.g., a lump in the neck, hoarseness, dysphagia, dyspnea).
- Avoid pregnancy while taking medication; discuss birth control options.
- Do not breastfeed while taking this drug.

DULOXETINE HYDROCHLORIDE

(du-lox′e-teen)

Cymbalta, Drizalma Sprinkle, Irenka

Classification: ANTIDEPRESSANT; SEROTONIN NOREPINEPHRINE REUPTAKE INHIBITOR (SNRI)

Therapeutic: ANTIDEPRESSANT; SNRI; ANTIANXIETY; NEUROPATHIC PAIN RELIEVER

Prototype: Venlafaxine

AVAILABILITY Delayed-release capsule

ACTION & *THERAPEUTIC EFFECT* Potentiates serotonergic and noradrenergic activity in the CNS. Antidepressant and antianxiety effects are presumed to be due to its dual inhibition of CNS presynaptic neuronal uptake of serotonin and norepinephrine, thus increasing the serum levels of both substances. *Effective as an antidepressant, antianxiety, and neuropathic pain reliever.*

USES Treatment of major depressive disorder, generalized anxiety, fibromyalgia, diabetic peripheral neuropathy, musculoskeletal pain.

UNLABELED USES Stress urinary incontinence, chemotheraphy-induced peripheral neuropathy.

CONTRAINDICATIONS Concurrent administration of MAOI therapy or within 14 days of use; initiation of MAOI within 5 days of starting duloxetine; pregnancy—fetal risk cannot be ruled out; lactation—infant risk cannot be ruled out.

CAUTIOUS USE Bipolar disease; history of mania, history of suicidal tendencies; cardiac disease; history of seizures; renal impairment or renal failure; hepatic impairment; impaired gastric motility; DM; hypertension; risk factors for hyponatremia or SIADH; older adults; Safe use in children younger than 7 yr not established.

ROUTE & DOSAGE

Depression

Adult: **PO** 40–60 mg/day in 1 or 2 divided doses

Generalized Anxiety/Diabetic Neuropathy

Adult: **PO** 60 mg once daily

Musculoskeletal Pain

Adult: **PO** 30 mg daily then increase to 60 mg daily

Fibromyalgia

Adult: **PO** 30 mg/day × 1 wk then 60 mg/day

ADMINISTRATION

Oral

- Do not initiate therapy within 14 days of the last dose of an MAOI.
- **Must be** swallowed whole. Do not cut, chew, or crush. Do not sprinkle on food or mix with liquids.
- Store at 15°–30°C (59°–86°F).

ADVERSE EFFECTS (≥5%) **CNS:** Dizziness, somnolence. **Endocrine:** Decreased appetite, weight loss. **Skin:** Increased sweating. **GI:** *Nausea, dry mouth, constipation*, anorexia, diarrhea, vomiting. **Other:** Fatigue.

INTERACTIONS **Drug:** **Alcohol** may result in increased liver function tests; MAOIS may result in hyperthermia, rigidity, mental status changes, myoclonus, autonomic instability, features resembling neuroleptic malignant syndrome; **cimetidine, fluoxetine, fluvoxamine, paroxetine, quinidine,** QUINOLONES or CYP1A2 inhibitors may increase levels and half-life of duloxetine; may increase levels and toxicity of **thioridazine**, TRICYCLIC ANTIDEPRESSANTS. **Amphetamine, dextroamphetamine, buspirone, cocaine, dexfenfluramine, fenfluramine, lithium, phentermine, sibutramine, nefazodone**, SSRIS, TRIPTANS, **tramadol, trazodone** may cause serotonin syndrome. May increase ANTIPLATELET or ANTICOAGULANT effects. **Herbal:** **St. John's wort, tryptophan** may cause serotonin syndrome.

PHARMACOKINETICS **Peak:** 6 h. **Metabolism:** In the liver by CYP2D6 and CYP1A2. **Elimination:** 70% in urine, 20% in feces. **Half-Life:** 12 h (8–17 h).

NURSING IMPLICATIONS

Black Box Warning

Suicidal thoughts and behaviors in patients under 24 years of age.

Assessment & Drug Effects

- Ensure that a complete list of all concurrent medications is obtained.
- Monitor for S&S of numerous drug-drug interactions (see Interaction section).
- Monitor closely for and report suicide ideation, especially when drug is initiated or dosage changed.
- Report emergence of any of the following: Anxiety, agitation, panic attacks, insomnia, irritability, hostility, psychomotor restlessness, hypomania, and mania.
- Monitor BP, especially in those being treated for hypertension.
- Monitor lab tests: Periodic serum creatinine, electrolytes, blood urea nitrogen, and LFTs.

Patient & Family Education

- The beneficial effects of this drug may not be felt for approximately 4 wk.
- Avoid activities requiring mental alertness or coordination until the drug effects are realized.
- Report any of the following: Suicidal ideation (especially early in treatment or when dosage is changed), palpitations, anxiety, hyperactivity, agitation, panic

attacks, insomnia, irritability, hostility, restlessness.

- Do not abruptly discontinue taking this drug. Notify prescriber if side effects are bothersome.
- Avoid or minimize use of alcohol while taking this drug.
- Report difficulty urinating, changes in sexual function.
- Avoid use of aspirin or NSAIDS to to potential bleeding.
- Do not self-treat for coughs, colds, or allergies. Consult prescriber.

DUPILUMAB

(doo-pil´ue-mab)

Dupixent

Classification: SKIN AND MUCOUS MEMBRANE AGENT; MONOCLONAL ANTIBODY; INTERLEUKIN-4 RECEPTOR ANTAGONIST

Therapeutic: ANTIECZEMA AGENT

AVAILABILITY Subcutaneous injection; prefilled syringe

ACTION & *THERAPEUTIC EFFECT* Human monoclonal IgG4 antibody that inhibits interleukin-4 and interleukin-13 signaling by binding to the subunit, thus inhibiting the cytokine-induced responses including proinflammatory cytokines. *Reduces inflammatory response in moderate to severe eczema (atopic dermatitis).*

USES Treatment of moderate to severe eczema (atopic dermatitis) when topical therapies have failed or contraindicated.

CONTRAINDICATIONS Hypersensitivity to dupilumab or components of the injection.

CAUTIOUS USE Hypersensitivity to dupilumab; pregnancy; lactation. Safety and efficacy in children not established.

ROUTE & DOSAGE

Atopic Dermatitis

Adult: **Subcutaneous** 600 mg at first dose, then 300 mg every other wk

ADMINISTRATION

Subcutaneous

- Allow prefilled syringe to reach room temperature for approx 45 min prior to use.
- Administer subcutaneously into the thigh, lower abdomen, or outer upper arm. Do not inject into tissue that is tender, bruised, red, hard, scaly, or affected by psoriasis.
- Rotate injection sites.

ADVERSE EFFECTS **Skin:** *Injection site reaction.* **GI:** Oral herpes. **Other:** Antibody development, *conjunctivitis,* eye pruritus.

INTERACTIONS **DRUG:** Avoid use with live vaccines; avoid use with other monoclonal antibodies.

PHARMACOKINETICS **Absorption:** 64% bioavailability. **Onset:** Peak effect in 1 wk. **Metabolism:** Catabolism to small peptides and amino acids, similar to endogenous IgG. **Elimination:** Nondetectable 10 wk post discontinuation.

NURSING IMPLICATIONS

Assessment & Drug Effects

- Monitor for signs of hypersensitivity reaction and ocular adverse effects.

Patient & Family Education

- Notify prescriber if you experience signs or symptoms of allergic reaction such as rash, hives, itching, shortness of breath, wheezing, cough, swelling of the face, lips, tongue, or throat; or any other signs.

DUTASTERIDE

(du-tas′ter-ide)

Avodart

Classification: ANTIANDROGEN; 5-ALPHA REDUCTASE INHIBITOR

Therapeutic: BENIGN PROSTATIC HYPERPLASIA (BPH) AGENT

Prototype: Finasteride

AVAILABILITY
Capsule

ACTION & THERAPEUTIC EFFECT
Specific inhibitor of the steroid 5-alpha-reductase, an enzyme necessary to convert testosterone into the potent androgen 5-alpha-dihydrotestosterone (DHT) in the prostate gland. *Decreases the production of testosterone in the prostate gland.*

USES
Treatment of benign prostatic hypertrophy (BPH).

UNLABELED USES
Alopecia.

CONTRAINDICATIONS
Hypersensitivity to dutasteride or finasteride; women of childbearing potential; pregnancy; lactation—infant risk cannot be ruled out; pediatric patients.

CAUTIOUS USE
Hepatic impairment, obstructive uropathy; history of prostate cancer; older adult males; effects of male fertility unknown.

ROUTE & DOSAGE

BPH

Adult: **PO** 0.5 mg once daily

ADMINISTRATION

Oral

- NIOSH recommends the use of single gloves by anyone handling intact tablets or capsules or administering from a unit-dose package.
- Do not handle capsules if you are or may become pregnant or are breastfeeding because of the potential for absorption of dutasteride and the subsequent risk to a developing male fetus.
- This drug poses a hazard to men and women actively trying to conceive.
- Take with or without food.
- Do not open or crush capsules. They **must be** swallowed whole.
- Store at 15°–30°C (59°–86°F).

ADVERSE EFFECTS (≥5%)
GU: Erectile dysfunction.

DIAGNOSTIC TEST INTERFERENCE
Dutasteride affects the ***serum PSA levels***, so levels should be established after 3 mo of therapy.

INTERACTIONS
Drug: CYP3A4 inhibitors (ex **itraconazole, lopinavir**) may increase concentration of dutasteride. **Herbal: Saw palmetto** may increase adverse effects.

PHARMACOKINETICS
Absorption: Rapidly; 60% bioavailability. **Peak:** 2–3 h. **Distribution:** 99% protein bound. **Metabolism:** In liver by CYP3A4. **Elimination:** Primarily in feces. **Half-Life:** 5 wk.

NURSING IMPLICATIONS

Assessment & Drug Effects

- Monitor voiding patterns, assessing for ease of starting a stream, frequency, and urgency.
- Monitor lab tests: Baseline and periodic PSA.

Patient & Family Education

- Do not donate blood until at least 6 mo following last dose to prevent administration of dutasteride to a pregnant female transfusion recipient.
- Men and women assisting with care should wear one pair of gloves when handling the

capsule. Men and women trying to conceive should avoid contact with the drug.

- Make sure to swallow the capsule whole. Do not chew or open contents.
- Ejaculate volume might be decreased during treatment but this does not seem to interfere with normal sexual function.
- Note that the incidence of most drug-related sexual adverse events (impotence, decreased libido, and ejaculation disorder) typically decrease with duration of treatment.

CONTRAINDICATIONS Hypersensitivity to xanthine compounds; apnea in newborns.

CAUTIOUS USE Severe cardiac disease, hypertension, acute myocardial injury; renal or hepatic dysfunction; glaucoma; seizure disorders; hyperthyroidism; peptic ulcer; older adults; children; pregnancy (category C); lactation. Safe use in children is not established.

ROUTE & DOSAGE

Asthma

Adult: **PO** Up to 15 mg/kg qid

ADMINISTRATION

Oral

- Give oral preparation with a full glass of water on an empty stomach (e.g., 1 h before or 2 h after meals) to enhance absorption. However, administration after meals may help to relieve gastric discomfort.
- Store between 20° and 25°C (68° and 77°F).

ADVERSE EFFECTS **CV:** Tachycardia, ventricular arrhythmia, **CNS:** Headache, seizure. **GI:** Diarrhea, nausea, vomiting, agitation, feeling excited, irritability.

INTERACTIONS **Drug:** BETA BLOCKERS may antagonize bronchodilating effects of dyphylline; **halothane** increases risk of cardiac arrhythmias; **probenecid** may decrease dyphylline elimination.

PHARMACOKINETICS **Absorption:** Readily from GI tract. **Peak:** 1 h. **Metabolism:** In liver (but not to theophylline). **Elimination:** In urine. **Half-Life:** 2 h.

NURSING IMPLICATIONS

Assessment & Drug Effects

- Monitor therapeutic effectiveness; usually occurs at a blood level of at least 12 mcg/mL.
- Note: Toxic dyphylline plasma levels, although rare with normal dosage, are a risk in patients with a diminished capacity for dyphylline clearance (e.g., those with CHF or hepatic impairment or who are older than 55 yr).

Patient & Family Education

- Take medication consistently with or without food at the same time each day.
- Notify prescriber of adverse effects: Nausea, vomiting, insomnia, jitteriness, headache, rash, severe GI pain, restlessness, convulsions, or irregular heartbeat.
- Avoid alcohol and also large amounts of coffee and other xanthine-containing beverages (e.g., tea, cocoa, cola) during therapy.
- Consult prescriber before taking OTC preparations. Many OTC drugs for coughs, colds, and allergies contain nervous system stimulants.

E

ECONAZOLE NITRATE

(e-kone′a-zole)

Ecostatin ♣, Spectazole

Classification: ANTIBIOTIC; AZOLE ANTIFUNGAL

Therapeutic: ANTIFUNGAL

Prototype: Fluconazole

AVAILABILITY Cream

ACTION & *THERAPEUTIC EFFECT* Disrupts normal fungal cell membrane permeability resulting in cell death. *Active against dermatophytes, yeasts, and many other fungi.*

USES Topically for treatment of tinea pedis (athlete's foot or ringworm of foot), tinea cruris ("jock itch" or ringworm of groin), tinea corporis (ringworm of body), tinea versicolor, and cutaneous candidiasis (moniliasis).

UNLABELED USES Has been used for topical treatment of erythrasma and with corticosteroids for fungal or bacterial dermatoses associated with inflammation.

CONTRAINDICATIONS Infants younger than 3 mo.

CAUTIOUS USE Pregnancy (category C); lactation.

ROUTE & DOSAGE

Tinea Cruris, Tinea Corporis, Tinea Pedis, Cutaneous Candidiasis

Adult/Child: **Topical** Apply sufficient amount to affected areas twice daily, morning and evening

Tinea Versicolor

Adult: **Topical** Apply sufficient amount to affected areas once daily

ADMINISTRATION

Topical

- Cleanse skin with soap and water and dry thoroughly before applying medication (unless otherwise directed by prescriber). Wash hands thoroughly before and after treatments.
- Do not use occlusive dressings unless prescribed by prescriber.
- Store at less than 30°C (86°F) unless otherwise directed.

ADVERSE EFFECTS **Skin:** Burning, stinging sensation, pruritus, erythema.

PHARMACOKINETICS **Absorption:** Minimal percutaneous absorption through intact skin; increased absorption from denuded skin. **Peak:** 0.5–5 h. **Elimination:** Less than 1% of applied dose is eliminated in urine and feces.

NURSING IMPLICATIONS

Patient & Family Education

- Use medication for the prescribed time even if symptoms improve and report to prescriber skin reactions suggestive of irritation or sensitization.
- Notify prescriber if full course of therapy does not result in improvement. Diagnosis should be re-evaluated.
- Do not apply the topical cream in or near the eyes or intravaginally.

EDETATE CALCIUM DISODIUM

(ed′e-tate)

Classification: CHELATING AGENT

Therapeutic: CHELATING AGENT; ANTIPOISON

E

AVAILABILITY Solution for injection

ACTION & *THERAPEUTIC EFFECT* Combines with divalent and trivalent metals to form stable, nonionizing soluble complexes that can be readily excreted by kidneys. Action is dependent on ability of heavy metal to displace the less strongly bound calcium in drug molecules. *Chelating agent that binds with heavy metals such as lead to form a soluble complex that can be excreted through the kidney, thereby ridding the body of the poisonous substance.*

USES As adjunct in treatment of acute and chronic lead poisoning (plumbism).

UNLABELED USES Treatment of poisoning from other heavy metals such as chromium, manganese, nickel, zinc, and possibly vanadium.

CONTRAINDICATIONS Severe kidney disease, active renal disease, anuria, oliguria; hepatitis; IV use in patients with lead encephalopathy not generally recommended (because of possible increase in intracranial pressure); pregnancy—fetal risk cannot be ruled out; lactation—infant risk cannot be ruled out.

CAUTIOUS USE Kidney dysfunction; active tubercular lesions; history of gout; cardiac arrhythmias.

ROUTE & DOSAGE

Lead Poisoning

Adult/Adolescent/Child: (Blood lead levels less than 70 mcg/dL and asymptomatic): **IV/IM** 1000 mg/m²/day × 5 days; *(Lead levels over 70 mcg/dL and symptomatic):* IV/IM 1000 mg/m²/day or 25–50 mg/kg/day × 5 days (max 3000 mg)

ADMINISTRATION

- **Never** give higher than recommended doses.

Intramuscular

- IM route preferred for symptomatic children and recommended for patients with incipient or overt lead-induced encephalopathy.
- Give total daily dose in equally divided doses IM every 8–12 hours.
- Add Procaine HCl to minimize pain at injection site (usually 1 mL of procaine 1% to each 1 mL of concentrated drug). Consult prescriber.

Intravenous

PREPARE: **IV Infusion:** Dilute the total daily dose in 250–500 mL of NS or D5W.
ADMINISTER: **IV Infusion:** Warning: Rapid IV infusion may be LETHAL by suddenly increasing intracranial pressure in patients who already have cerebral edema. ▪ Manufacturer recommends total daily dose over 8–12 h. Consult prescriber for specific rate.
INCOMPATIBILITIES: **Solution/additive: D10W hydralazine, lactated Ringer. Y-site: Amphotericin B.**

ADVERSE EFFECTS **CV:** Cardiac dysrhythmia. **Hepatic:** Elevated enzyme levels. **GU:** Nephrotoxicity (renal tubular necrosis). **Hematologic:** Transient bone marrow depression, depletion of blood metals.

INTERACTIONS **Drugs:** avoid use with LIVE VACCINES and MYELOSUPPRESSIVE AGENTS.

PHARMACOKINETICS **Absorption:** Well absorbed IM. **Onset:** 1 h. **Peak:** Peak chelation 24–48 h.

Distribution: Distributed to extracellular fluid; does not enter CSF. **Metabolism:** Not metabolized. **Elimination:** Chelated lead excreted in urine; 50% excreted in 1 h. **Half-Life:** 20–60 min IV.

NURSING IMPLICATIONS

Black Box Warning

Edeta calcium has been associated with potentially fatal effects, especially when higher doses are used or when it is continued after toxic effects appear.

Assessment & Drug Effects

- Determine adequacy of urinary output prior to therapy. This may be done by administering IV fluids before giving first dose.
- Monitor ECG during IV administration.
- Increase fluid intake to enhance urinary excretion of chelates. Avoid excess fluid intake, however, in patients with lead encephalopathy because of the danger of further increasing intracranial pressure. Consult prescriber regarding allowable intake.
- Monitor I&O. Because drug is excreted almost exclusively via kidneys, toxicity may develop if output is inadequate. Stop therapy if urine flow is markedly diminished or absent. Report any change in output or I&O ratio to prescriber.
- Be alert for occurrence of febrile reaction that may appear 4–8 h after drug infusion.
- Monitor lab tests: Before each course of therapy, urinalysis and urine sediment, renal and hepatic function, and serum electrolytes, repeat after the 2nd and 5th day of therapy, or daily in severe cases.

EDOXABAN

(e-dox'a-ban)

Savaysa

Classification: ANTICOAGULANT; ANTITHROMBOTIC; SELECTIVE FACTOR XA INHIBITOR

Therapeutic: ANTITHROMBOTIC

Prototype: Rivaroxaban

AVAILABILITY Tablet

ACTION & THERAPEUTIC EFFECT Inhibits free FXa and prothrombinase activity, and inhibits thrombin-induced platelet aggregation. *Inhibition of FXa in the coagulation cascade reduces thrombin generation, which reduces thrombus formation.*

USES Treatment of deep vein thrombosis (DVT) and pulmonary embolism (PE) and reduction of the risk of stroke and systemic embolism (SE) in patients with nonvalvular atrial fibrillation (NVAF).

CONTRAINDICATIONS Active pathological bleeding; atrial fibrillation if CrCl greater than 95 mL/min; severe renal impairment; CrCl less than 15 mL/min; concomitant use of rifampin or other anticoagulants; patients with triple positive antiphospholipid syndrome; pregnancy—fetal risk cannot be ruled out; lactation—infant risk cannot be ruled out.

CAUTIOUS USE Nonvalvular atrial fibrillation; moderately impaired renal function (dose adjustment for CrCl 15–50 mL/min); moderate or severe hepatic impairment (Child–Pugh class B and C); patients with low body weight, 60 kg or less; concomitant use of drugs affecting hemostasis;

spinal/epidural anesthesia or spinal/epidural puncture; mechanical heart valves or moderate to severe mitral stenosis. Elderly patients should have renal function monitored closely. Safety and efficacy in children not established.

ROUTE & DOSAGE

Nonvalvular Atrial Fibrillation

Adult: **PO** 60 mg once daily

Deep Vein Thrombosis and Pulmonary Embolism

Adult (60 kg or less): **PO** 30 mg daily following at least 5 days of therapy with a parenteral anticoagulant
Adult (over 60 kg): **PO** 60 mg once daily following at least 5 days of therapy with a parenteral anticoagulant

Renal Impairment Dosage Adjustment

CrCl 15 to 50 mL/min: 30 mg once daily
CrCl greater than 95 mL/min: Avoid use for VTE treatment

ADMINISTRATION

Oral

- May be given without regard to food.
- May crush tablet and combine with 2–3 ounces of water or applesauce and consume immediately.
- Store at controlled room temperature at 20°–25°C (68°–77°F), excursions permitted between 15°and 30°C (59°and 86°F).

ADVERSE EFFECTS (≥5%)

Skin: Rash. **Hepatic:** Abnormal liver function tests, pulmonary embolism. **Hematological:** Anemia, increased bleeding tendencies.

INTERACTIONS

Drug: Concurrent use of other ANTICOAGULANTS, ANTIPLATELETS, and THROMBOLYTICS, NSAIDs, **mifepristone** may increase the risk of bleeding. ESTROGENS or PROGESTINS may decrease therapeutic effect. **Itraconazole, ketoconazole, lasmiditan** may increase serum concentration. **Rifampin** should not be used with edoxaban.

PHARMACOKINETICS

Absorption: 62% bioavailable. **Peak:** 1–2 h. **Metabolism:** Minimal, primarily excreted unchanged. **Elimination:** Primarily renal. **Half-Life:** 10–14 h.

NURSING IMPLICATIONS

Black Box Warning

Edoxaban has reduced efficacy in nonvalvular atrial fibrillation patients with CrCl greater than 95 mL/min; it should not be used in these patients. Premature discontinuation of edoxaban increases the risk of ischemic events. Edoxaban has been associated with hematomas that may result in long-term or permanent paralysis when used in patients treated with spinal or epidural anesthesia or puncture.

Assessment & Drug Effects

- Monitor closely for S&S of frank or occult bleeding.
- Monitor for and report promptly S&S of neurologic impairment, especially following any invasive spinal or epidural procedure.
- Monitor lab tests: Baseline and periodic CrCl; baseline LFTs; CBC upon initiation and at regular intervals (at least yearly) to assess Hgb and Hct.

Patient & Family Education

- Report promptly S&S of bleeding.
- Do not abruptly stop taking this drug unless advised to do so by prescriber.

- Take a missed dose as soon as possible on the same day and then resume normal schedule.
- Do not take aspirin-containing products or nonsteroidal anti-inflammatory drugs (NSAIDs) without discussing their use with your prescriber.
- Following spinal anesthesia or spinal puncture while taking edoxaban: Report immediately back pain, tingling, numbness (especially in your legs and feet), muscle weakness, loss of control of the bowels or bladder.
- Women of childbearing age should discuss with prescriber potential risks associated with pregnancy and use birth control.
- Do not breastfeed while taking this drug without consulting prescriber.

EFAVIRENZ

(e-fa'vi-renz)

Sustiva

Classification: ANTIRETROVIRAL; NONNUCLEOSIDE REVERSE TRANSCRIPTASE INHIBITOR (NNRTI)
Therapeutic: ANTIRETROVIRAL; NNRTI

AVAILABILITY Capsule; tablet

ACTION & *THERAPEUTIC EFFECT* Binds directly to reverse transcriptase and blocks RNA polymerase activities of the HIV-1 virus, thus preventing replication of the virus. *Prevents replication of the HIV-1 virus. Resistant strains appear rapidly. Effectiveness is indicated by reduction in viral load (plasma level HIV RNA).*

USES HIV-1 infection in combination with other antiretroviral agents.

CONTRAINDICATIONS Hypersensitivity to efavirenz; suicidal ideation; pregnancy (fetal harm has been demonstrated), lactation (infant risk cannot be ruled out).

CAUTIOUS USE Liver disease, alcoholism, hepatitis B or C, hypertriglyceridemia, hypercholesterolemia, substance abuse; moderate to severe hepatic impairment; antimicrobial resistance, bipolar disorder, depression, suicidal tendencies, psychiatric disorders related to use of efavirenz; drug or alcohol abuse; exfoliative dermatitis; females of childbearing age, CNS disorders; history of seizures; older adults. Safety and efficacy in children younger than 3 mo or who weigh less than 3.5 kg (8 lb) not established.

ROUTE & DOSAGE

HIV Infection (with other antiretrovirals)

Adult/Adolescent: **PO** 600 mg daily
Child/Infant: See package insert for weight-based dosing

ADMINISTRATION

Oral

- Take on an empty stomach.
- Use bedtime dosing to increase tolerability of CNS adverse effects.
- Give exactly as ordered. Do not skip a dose or discontinue therapy without consulting the prescriber.
- Do not give efavirenz following a high-fat meal.
- Capsules should be swallowed whole but may be opened and contents administered in 1–2 teaspoons of age-appropriate food or reconstituted infant formula.

E

- Store at 15°–30°C (59°–86°F) in a tightly closed container and protect from light.

ADVERSE EFFECTS **Respiratory:** Cough. **CNS:** *Dizziness*, fever, depression, insomnia, pain, anxiety, headache. **Endocrine:** *Increased cholesterol, increased HDL cholesterol*, increased serum triglycerides. **Skin:** *Rash*. **Hepatic:** Increased AST, increased ALT. **GI:** Diarrhea, nausea, vomiting.

DIAGNOSTIC TEST INTERFERENCE False-positive ***urine tests*** for **marijuana**; false-positive tests for BENZODIAZEPINES have been reported.

INTERACTIONS **Drug:** Can decrease serum concentration of any CYP 3A4 substrate. Decreased concentrations of **atazanavir, clarithromycin, indinavir, nelfinavir, saquinavir, voriconazole, ponatinib, ketoconazole, amprenavir, saquinavir**, increased concentrations of **ritonavir, azithromycin**. Efavirenz levels are increased by **ritonavir, fluconazole, voriconazole** and decreased by **saquinavir, rifampin, carbamazepine, nevirapine**. Additional drugs not recommended for administration with efavirenz include **midazolam, triazolam**, ERGOT DERIVATIVES, **warfarin**. May enhance CNS DEPRESSANT effects. Avoid use with **darunavir. Herbal: St. John's wort** may decrease antiretroviral activity.

PHARMACOKINETICS **Peak:** 5 h; steady-state 6–10 days. **Distribution:** 99% protein bound. **Metabolism:** In liver by cytochrome P450 3A4 and 2B6; can induce (increase) its own metabolism. **Elimination:** 14–34% in urine, 16–61% in feces. **Half-Life:** 52–76 h after single dose, 40–55 h after multiple doses.

NURSING IMPLICATIONS

Assessment & Drug Effects

- Monitor for suicidal ideation in patients who are depressed, or who have a history of depression.
- Monitor GI status and evaluate ability to maintain a normal diet.
- Monitor lab tests: Periodic LFTs CBC with differential, CD4 counts, urinalysis, and lipid profile.

Patient & Family Education

- Contact prescriber promptly if any of the following occurs: Skin rash, delusions, inappropriate behavior, suicidal ideation.
- Avoid pregnancy.
- Use or add barrier contraception if using hormonal contraceptive.
- Notify prescriber immediately if you become pregnant.
- Do not drive or engage in potentially hazardous activities until response to the drug is known. Dizziness, impaired concentration, and drowsiness usually improve with continued therapy.

EFLORNITHINE HYDROCHLORIDE

(e-flor'ni-theen)

Vaniqa

Classification: DERMATOLOGIC
Therapeutic: FACIAL HIRSUTISM AGENT

AVAILABILITY Cream

ACTION & *THERAPEUTIC EFFECT* Inhibits enzyme activity in the skin that is required for hair growth. *Results in retarding the rate of facial hair growth.*

USES Reduction of unwanted facial hair in women.

CONTRAINDICATIONS Hypersensitivity to eflornithine or its components.

CAUTIOUS USE Bone marrow suppression; HIV; hearing impairment, renal impairment or failure; pregnancy (category C); lactation. Safe use in children younger than 12 yr is not established.

ROUTE & DOSAGE

Hair Removal

Adult: **Topical** Apply thin layer bid (at least 8 h apart) to affected areas of the face

ADMINISTRATION

Topical

- Apply thin layer to affected skin areas on face and under chin and rub in thoroughly.
- Do not wash treated areas for at least 8 h after application.
- Store at 15°–30°C (59°–86°F).

ADVERSE EFFECTS **CNS:** Dizziness, headache. **Skin:** *Acne, pseudofolliculitis barbae,* stinging, burning, pruritus, erythema, tingling, irritation, rash, alopecia, folliculitis, ingrown hair. **GI:** Dyspepsia, anorexia. **Other:** Facial edema.

PHARMACOKINETICS **Absorption:** Less than 1% absorbed through intact skin. **Metabolism:** Not metabolized. **Elimination:** Primarily in urine. **Half-Life:** 8 h.

NURSING IMPLICATIONS

Assessment & Drug Effects

- Monitor for and report skin irritation.
- Note: Drug slows growth of facial hair, but is not a depilatory.

Patient & Family Education

- Note: Effect of drug is usually not apparent for 4–8 wk.
- Reduce frequency of drug application to once daily if skin irritation occurs. If irritation continues, contact prescriber.

ELAGOLIX

(el'a-goe'lix)

Orilissa

Classification: GONADOTROPIN-RELEASING HORMONE (GNRH) ANTAGONIST

Therapeutic: LUTEINIZING HORMONE-RELEASING HORMONE RECEPTOR ANTAGONIST

AVAILABILITY Tablet

ACTION & THERAPEUTIC EFFECT Elagolix works by inhibiting endogenous GnRH signaling through competitively binding to GnRH receptors in the pituitary gland, which suppresses luteinizing hormone and follicle-stimulating hormone. *Therapy decreases blood concentration of ovarian sex hormones, lessening symptoms of endometriosis.*

USES Management of moderate to severe pain associated with endometriosis.

CONTRAINDICATIONS Patients who are pregnant (category X); history of severe hepatic impairment; severe bone loss or history of osteoporosis.

CAUTIOUS USE Use of elagolix leads to dose-dependent decrease in bone mineral density; may impact menstrual bleeding pattern; suicidal ideation and behavior increase in patients being treated with elagolix;

patients currently taking estrogen-containing contraceptives; patients with history of hepatic injury or cirrhosis.

ROUTE & DOSAGE

E

Endometriosis Pain

Adult: **PO** 150 mg once a day, for no more than 24 mo

Hepatic Impairment Dosage Adjustment

Moderate impairment (Child–Pugh class B): 150 mg once a day, for no more than 6 mo
Severe impairment (Child–Pugh class C): Use is not recommended

ADMINISTRATION

Oral

- Given with or without food, at approximately the same time every day.
- Treatment should be started within 7 days of onset of menses.
- Patients should have a negative pregnancy test prior to start of therapy with elagolix.
- Women should be advised to begin nonhormonal contraception during treatment with elagolix and confirm negative pregnancy test prior to administration.
- Store at 2°–8°C (36°–46°F) within supplied blister packs.

ADVERSE EFFECTS **CNS:** Headache, insomnia, dizziness. **Endocrine:** Bone loss, change in menstrual bleeding patterns, amenorrhea. **Skin:** *Flushing, night sweats.* **Hepatic:** Increase in hepatic enzymes, increased cholesterol (HDL, LDL), increased triglycerides. **GI:** Nausea, diarrhea, abdominal pain, constipation. **Musculoskeletal:** Arthralgia, *decreased bone mineral density.* **Other:** Increase in suicidal ideation and behavior, mood disturbances, hot flashes, depressed mood, anxiety, weight gain.

INTERACTIONS **Drugs:** Elagolix is a substrate of CYP3A4, OATP1B1/SLCO1B1, and P glycoprotein. Avoid use with strong CYP3A4 inducers (e.g., **carbamazepine**, **phenytoin**, **rifampin**). If used with strong CYP3A4 inhibitors (e.g., **clarithromycin, itraconazole, ketoconazole**), dose elagolix 150 mg once a day for only 6 mo. Use with strong OATP1B1 inhibitors (e.g., **cyclosporine**, **gemfibrozil**) is not recommended.

PHARMACOKINETICS **Peak:** 1 h. **Distribution:** 80% protein bound. **Metabolism:** Metabolized through CYP3A4 (major), CYP2D6, CYP2C8, and UGTs. **Elimination:** Primarily secreted through feces; 90% feces, 3% urine. **Half-Life:** 4–6 h.

NURSING IMPLICATIONS

Assessment & Drug Effects

- Exclude positive pregnancy before initiating treatment.
- Relief of endometrial pain.
- Assess for jaundice.
- Worsening of depression, anxiety, or other mood changes.
- Monitor lab tests: LFTs.

Patient & Family Education

- Reduced efficacy of estrogen-containing contraceptive. Use nonhormonal contraceptive methods during therapy and for 1 wk after discontinuation of therapy.
- Notify prescriber right away of positive pregnancy test.
- Notify prescriber right away if S&S of depression, mood changes, or suicidal ideation develop.
- Report to prescriber any low-trauma fracture.

ELETRIPTAN HYDROBROMIDE

(e-le-trip′tan)

Relpax

Classification: SEROTONIN 5-HT_1 RECEPTOR AGONIST

Therapeutic: ANTIMIGRAINE

Pregnancy Category: C

AVAILABILITY Tablet

ACTION & *THERAPEUTIC EFFECT* Eletriptan stimulates presynaptic 5-HT_{1D} receptors inhibiting dural vasodilation and agonizes vascular 5-HT_{1B} receptors causing vasoconstriction of intracranial extracerebral vessels. *Inhibits dural vasodilation and inflammation, and causes vasoconstriction of painfully dilated intracranial extracerebral vessels, thus relieving the migraine headache. Also relieves photophobia, phonophobia, and nausea and vomiting associated with migraine attacks.*

USES Acute treatment of migraine attacks with or without aura.

CONTRAINDICATIONS Hypersensitivity to eletriptan; history of CAD; ischemic or vasospastic CAD, arteriosclerosis, history of MI; ischemic colitis, Raynaud disease, uncontrolled hypertension; CVA or TIA; within 24 h of administering of another ergotamine; lactation within 24 h after dose; severe hepatic insufficiency; hemiplegic or basilar migraine; peripheral vascular disease; concurrent MAOI therapy.

CAUTIOUS USE Hypotension in the elderly; older adults; mild to moderate hepatic impairment; diabetes, obesity, smoking, high cholesterol; men older than 40 yr; postmenopausal women; pregnancy (category C); lactation—infant risk cannot be ruled out. Safe use in children younger than 18 yr not established.

ROUTE & DOSAGE

Acute Migraine

Adult: **PO** 20 mg or 40 mg at onset of migraine (max: 40 mg/dose), may repeat dose in 2 h if partial response (max: 80 mg/day)

Hepatic Impairment Dosage Adjustment

Severe Hepatic Impairment: Not recommended

ADMINISTRATION

Oral

- Give one tablet as soon as the migraine begins.
- May give 2nd tablet if headache improves but returns after 2 h.
- If 1st tablet is ineffective, do not give a 2nd without consulting prescriber.
- Do not give within 72 h of potent CYP3A4 inhibitors (see INTERACTIONS).
- Store at 15°–30°C (59°–86°F). Protect from light and moisture.

ADVERSE EFFECTS **CNS:** Weakness, dizziness, sleepiness. **GI:** Nausea.

INTERACTIONS **Drug:** Avoid drugs that inhibit CYP3A4, as they may increase eletriptan levels and toxicity, do not administer eletriptan within 72 h of AZOLE ANTIFUNGALS (especially **itraconazole, ketoconazole, voriconazole**), **amiodarone, cimetidine, dalfopristin, quinupristin, diltiazem, metronidazole, nicardipine, norfloxacin, quinine, verapamil, zafirlukast, zileuton**, MACROLIDE ANTIBIOTICS,

E

NONNUCLEOTIDE REVERSE TRANSCRIPTASE INHIBITORS, PROTEASE INHIBITORS, SELECTIVE SEROTONIN REUPTAKE INHIBITORS, MONOAMINE OXIDASE INHIBITORS, **sibutramine**; ERGOT ALKALOIDS may prolong vasospastic adverse reactions (do not use within 24 h of ergot-containing drugs); do not administer within 24 h of other 5-HT_1 AGONISTS (increases adverse effects). **Food: Grapefruit juice** may increase eletriptan levels and toxicity. **Herbal: Echinacea, St. John's wort** may increase triptan toxicity.

PHARMACOKINETICS

Absorption: Rapid with 50% reaching systemic circulation. **Onset:** 1–2 h. **Peak:** 1.5 h. **Distribution:** 85% protein bound. **Metabolism:** In liver by CYP3A4. **Elimination:** Nonrenal routes. **Half-Life:** 4–5 h.

NURSING IMPLICATIONS

Assessment & Drug Effects

- Monitor CV status carefully following first dose in patients at risk for coronary artery disease (e.g., history of hypertension, postmenopausal women, men older than 40 yr, persons with known CAD risk factors) or who have coronary artery vasospasms.
- Report immediately chest pain, tightness in chest or throat that is severe or does not quickly resolve following a dose of eletriptan.
- Monitor therapeutic effectiveness. Pain relief is usually achieved within 1 h.

Patient & Family Education

- Note: If first dose is ineffective, take a second dose two or more hours after the first, if needed and do not exceed 80 mg a day.
- Inform prescriber of all prescription, nonprescription, and herbal drugs you are taking. Do not add additional drugs without informing prescriber, as many drugs interact with eletriptan.
- Report promptly any of the following: Headache more severe than usual, migraine; dizziness, faintness, blurred vision; chest, neck, or throat pain; irregular heartbeat, palpitations; shortness of breath, wheezing, difficulty breathing; tingling, pain, or numbness in the face, hands, or feet; seizures; severe stomach pain, cramping, or bloody diarrhea.
- Do not drive or engage in any potentially hazardous task until reaction to drug is known.

ELUXADOLINE

(e-lux'a-do-line)

Viberzi

Classification: PERIPHERAL MU-RECEPTOR AGONIST; ANTISECRETORY AGENT

Therapeutic: ANTISECRETORY AGENT

AVAILABILITY

Tablet

ACTION & *THERAPEUTIC EFFECT*

A mixed mu-opioid receptor agonist, delta opioid receptor antagonist, and kappa opioid receptor agonist. *Acts locally to reduce abdominal pain and diarrhea in patients with IBS-D without constipating side effects.*

USES

Indicated for the treatment of irritable bowel syndrome with diarrhea (IBS-D) in adults.

CONTRAINDICATIONS

Severe hepatic impairment (Child–Pugh class C); known hypersensitivity to eluxadoline; history of chronic or severe constipation or sequelae from constipation, or known or suspected mechanical GI obstruction; known or suspected biliary duct obstruction or sphincter of Oddi disease or dysfunction; patients without a gallbladder; history of pancreatitis or structural diseases of the pancreas, including known or suspected pancreatic duct obstruction; alcoholism, alcohol abuse, or alcohol addiction, or consumption of more than three alcoholic beverages per day; pregnancy—fetal risk cannot be ruled out; lactation—infant risk cannot be ruled out

CAUTIOUS USE Older adults; severe constipation; patients with a history of substance abuse; concomitant use of strong CYP inhibitors. Safety and efficacy in children not established.

ROUTE & DOSAGE

Irritable Bowel Syndrome

Adult: **PO** 100 mg bid; decrease to 75 mg bid if not tolerated

ADMINISTRATION

Oral

- Give with food.
- Store at controlled room temperature between 20° and 25°C (68° and 77°F), excursions permitted between 15° and 30°C (59° and 86°F).

ADVERSE EFFECTS (≥5%) **Respiratory:** Upper respiratory tract infection. **Endocrine:** Increased ALT/AST. **Skin:** Rash. **GI:** Abdominal pain, *constipation*, nausea.

INTERACTIONS **Drug:** There are many significant interactions, please check package insert or drug interaction database.

PHARMACOKINETICS **Peak:** 1.5 h. **Distribution:** 81% plasma protein bound. **Metabolism:** In liver. **Elimination:** Primarily fecal (82%). **Half-Life:** 3.7–6 h.

NURSING IMPLICATIONS

Assessment & Drug Effects

- Monitor for and report promptly S&S of symptoms of sphincter of Oddi spasm (e.g., acute worsening of epigastric or biliary-type abdominal pain, increased pancreatic enzymes, or increased hepatic transaminases).
- Monitor patients with hepatic impairment for impaired mental or physical abilities and other adverse drug reactions.
- Monitor lab tests: Baseline and periodic LFTs; periodic pancreatic enzymes.

Patient & Family Education

- Stop taking this drug and notify prescriber if experiencing new or worsening abdominal pain or pain in the upper right side of abdomen that radiates to the back or shoulder, with or without nausea and vomiting.
- Limit use of alcohol while taking this drug.
- Stop taking this drug and notify prescriber if experiencing constipation that lasts more than 4 days.
- Advise patient to skip a missed dose and continue with the regular dosing schedule.
- In cases with liver impairment, do not drive or engage in other dangerous activities until response to drug is known.
- Women of childbearing age should discuss with prescriber potential risks associated with taking this drug.
- Do not breastfeed while taking this drug without consulting prescriber.

E

ELVITEGRAVIR/COBICISTAT/EMTRICITABINE/TENOFOVIR DISOPROXIL FUMARATE

(el-vi-te-gra′vir) (co-bi-ci′stat) (em-tri′ci-ta-been) (ten-o-fo′vir)

Stribild

Classification: ANTIRETROVIRAL; INTEGRASE STRAND INHIBITOR; NUCLEOSIDE REVERSE TRANSCRIPTASE INHIBITOR

Therapeutic: ANTIRETROVIRAL

Prototype: Raltegravir and zidovudine

AVAILABILITY Elvitegravir 150 mg/cobicistat 150 mg/emtricitabine 200 mg/tenofovir disoproxil fumarate 300 mg tablets

ACTION & *THERAPEUTIC EFFECT* **Elvitegravir:** Inhibits activity of HIV-1 integrase, an HIV-1 encoded enzyme that is required for viral replication. *Blocks formation of the HIV-1 provirus and propagation of the viral infection.* **Cobicistat:** Inhibits CYP3A-mediated metabolism of elvitegravir, thus increasing the bioavailability and prolonging the half-life of elvitegravir. *Increases the efficacy of elvitegravir.* **Emtricitabine:** See separate monograph for emtricitabine. **Tenofovir:** See separate monograph for tenofovir.

USES Used for the treatment of HIV-1 infection in adults who are antiretroviral treatment-naive.

CONTRAINDICATIONS Lactic acidosis; coinfection with chronic hepatitis B virus (HBV); severe hepatic impairment; acute renal failure; creatinine clearance below 50 mL/min; lactation.

CAUTIOUS USE Mild-to-moderate hepatic impairment; renal impairment; history of or risk for pancreatitis; older adults; pregnancy (category B). Safety and efficacy in children younger than 18 yr not established.

ROUTE & DOSAGE

HIV-1 Infection

Adult: One combination tablet daily

Hepatic Impairment Dosage Adjustment

Child–Pugh class C (Severe impairment): Not recommended

Renal Impairment Dosage Adjustment

CrCl less than 70 mL/min: Do not initiate treatment.
CrCl less than 50 mL/min: Discontinue if CrCl falls below 50 mL/min during treatment

ADMINISTRATION

Oral

- Give with food.
- Store at 15°–30°C (59°–86°F).

ADVERSE EFFECTS **Respiratory:** Increased cough, nasopharyngitis, pneumonia, rhinitis, sinusitis, upper respiratory tract infection. **CNS:** Abnormal dreams, anxiety, depression, dizziness, fatigue, headache, insomnia, somnolence. **Endocrine:** Alterations in serum glucose, decreased bone mineral density, elevated amylase, elevated alkaline phosphatase, elevated ALT and AST, elevated bilirubin, elevated creatine kinase, elevated cholesterol, elevated creatinine, glycosuria, elevated triglycerides, hematuria, neutropenia. **Skin:** Rash. **GI:** *Diarrhea*, flatulence, dyspepsia, *nausea*, vomiting. **GU:** Onset or worsening of renal impairment. **Musculoskeletal:** Abdominal pain, arthralgia, back pain, myalgia. **Hematological:** Immune reconstitution syndrome. **Other:** Fever, lactic acidosis, paresthesia, peripheral neuropathy, severe acute exacerbations of hepatitis B, pain, severe hepatomegaly with stenosis.

INTERACTIONS **Drug:** Elvitegravir/cobicistat/emtricitabine/tenofovir disoproxil fumarate can increase the levels of other compounds that require CYP3A4 (**amiodarone, disopyramide**) or CYP2D6 (**paroxetine**, BETA BLOCKERS, **risperidone**) for metabolism or are substrates for P-glycoprotein. Strong (i.e., **atazanavir, clarithromycin, indinavir, itraconazole, ketoconazole, nefazodone, nelfinavir, ritonavir, saquinavir, telithromycin**) and moderate (i.e., **aprepitant, diltiazem, erythromycin, fluconazole, fosamprenavir, verapamil**) inhibitors of CYP3A4 can increase the levels of elvitegravir and cobicistat. Strong (i.e., **carbamazepine, dexamethasone, phenobarbital, phenytoin, rifabutin, rifampin, rifapentine**) and moderate (i.e., **bosentan, efavirenz, etravirine, modafinil, nafcillin**) CYP3A4 inducers may decrease the levels of elvitegravir and cobicistat. Elvitegravir levels are lowered if used in combination with ANTACIDS. Elvitegravir/cobicistat/emtricitabine/tenofovir disoproxil fumarate can increase the levels of **warfarin, colchicine, fluticasone**, and **norgestimate**. Elvitegravir/cobicistat/emtricitabine/tenofovir disoproxil fumarate can increase adverse effects associated with PHOSPHODIESTERASE-5 INHIBITORS (**sildenafil, tadalafil, vardenafil**). **Food: Grapefruit** or **grapefruit juice** may increase the levels of elvitegravir and cobicistat. **Herbal: St. John's wort** may decrease the levels of elvitegravir and cobicistat.

PHARMACOKINETICS **Peak:** Elvitegravir 4 h; cobicistat and emtricitabine 3 h; tenofovir 2 h. **Distribution:** Elvitegravir and cobicistat 97–99% plasma protein bound; emtricitabine and tenofovir minimally bound to plasma proteins. **Metabolism:** Cobicistat, elvitegravir, and emtricitabine in the liver; tenofovir is not significantly metabolized. **Elimination:** Elvitegravir and cobicistat primarily fecal; emtricitabine and tenofovir primarily renal. **Half-Life:** 12.6 h. (elvitegravir); 3.5 h. (cobicistat); 10 h. (emtricitabine); 17 h. (tenofovir).

NURSING IMPLICATIONS

Note: Consult individual monographs for emtricitabine and tenofovir disoproxil fumarate for additional nursing implications.

Black Box Warning

This combination of drugs has been associated with severe, and potentially fatal, lactic acidosis and hepatomegaly.

Assessment & Drug Effects

- Monitor for and report S&S of lactic acidosis and hepatic impairment. Withhold drug and report to prescriber if either is suspected.
- Monitor for signs of bone fractures as bone mineral density may be diminished.
- Monitor lab tests: Baseline and periodic renal function tests, urine for glucose and protein, serum electrolytes, alkaline phosphatase, LFTs, and parathyroid hormone.

Patient & Family Education

- Ensure that prescriber has a complete list of all prescription and OTC drugs you are taking.

E

- Exercise caution with potentially harmful physical activities as decreased bone density may predispose to fractures.
- Notify prescriber if you experience unexplained nausea, vomiting, or stomach discomfort.
- Do not breastfeed while taking this drug.

EMEDASTINE DIFUMARATE

(em-e-das'teen di-foom'a-rate)

Emadine

Classification: OCULAR; ANTIHISTAMINE; H_1-RECEPTOR ANTAGONIST

Therapeutic: OCULAR ANTIHISTAMINE

AVAILABILITY Ophthalmic solution

ACTION & *THERAPEUTIC EFFECT* It blocks H_1-receptors and inhibits histamine-stimulated vascular permeability in the conjunctiva. *Relieves ocular pruritus related to allergic response to histamine.*

USES Temporary relief of seasonal allergic conjunctivitis.

CONTRAINDICATIONS Hypersensitivity to emedastine.

CAUTIOUS USE Hypersensitivity to other antihistamines, soft contact lenses; pregnancy (category B); lactation. Safety and efficacy in children younger than 3 yr not established.

ROUTE & DOSAGE

Allergic Conjunctivitis

Adult/Adolescent/Child (older than 3 yr): **Ophthalmic** 1 drop in affected eye qid

ADMINISTRATION

Instillation

- Wash hands before and after use.
- Shake well before using. Apply drops in the center of the lower conjunctional sac. Do not touch eyelids with dropper.
- Gently close eyes for 1–2 min after installation of drops.
- Wait 10 min after installation of drug before inserting soft lenses into eyes.
- Store in a tightly closed bottle. Protect the solution from light.
- Do not use if discolored.

ADVERSE EFFECTS **CNS:** Headache. **HEENT:** *Ocular irritation, mild transient stinging and burning*, conjunctival congestion, eyelid edema, eye pain, photophobia, abnormal lacrimation.

INTERACTIONS **Drug:** No clinically significant interactions established.

PHARMACOKINETICS **Absorption:** Minimal. **Half-Life:** 3–4 h.

NURSING IMPLICATIONS

Assessment & Drug Effects

- Monitor for S&S of hypersensitivity to the drug (see Appendix F).
- Evaluate safety of engaging in hazardous activities because drowsiness is a potential adverse effect.

Patient & Family Education

- Learn potential adverse responses to emedastine.
- Eye drops contain benzalkonium chloride, which may damage soft contact lenses. After instillation of drops, wait 10 min before inserting these contact lenses into the eye.
- Contact your prescriber if symptoms do not start to improve in 2 or 3 days.

EMLA (EUTECTIC MIXTURE OF LIDOCAINE AND PRILOCAINE)

EMLA Cream

Classification: LOCAL ANESTHETIC
Therapeutic: LOCAL ANESTHETIC
Prototype: Procaine

AVAILABILITY Cream

ACTION & *THERAPEUTIC EFFECT* EMLA cream is a mixture of lidocaine and prilocaine. *EMLA is a topical analgesic.*

USES Topical anesthetic on normal intact skin for local anesthesia.

UNLABELED USES Topical anesthetic prior to leg ulcer debridement; treatment of postherpetic neuralgia.

CONTRAINDICATIONS Patients with known sensitivity to local anesthetics; patients with congenital or idiopathic methemoglobinemia; tympanic membrane perforation.

CAUTIOUS USE Acutely ill, debilitated, or older adult patients; severe liver disease; pregnancy (category B); lactation. Safe use in children younger than 1 mo not established.

ROUTE & DOSAGE

Topical Anesthetic

Adult/Child (1 mo or older): **Topical** Apply 2.5 g of cream (½ of 5-g tube) over 20–25 cm^2 of skin, cover with occlusive dressing and wait at least 1 h, then remove dressing and wipe off cream, cleanse area with an antiseptic solution and prepare patient for the procedure.

ADMINISTRATION

Topical

- Apply a thick layer to skin (approximately ½ of 5-g tube/20–25 cm^2 or 2 × 2 in) at site of procedure. Apply an occlusive dressing. Do not spread out cream. Seal edges of dressing well to avoid leakage.
- Apply EMLA cream 1 h before routine procedure and 2 h before painful procedure.
- Remove EMLA cream prior to skin puncture, and clean area with an aseptic solution.
- Store at room temperature 15°–30°C (59°–86°F).

ADVERSE EFFECTS **Skin:** *Blanching and redness,* itching, heat sensation. **Hematologic:** Methemoglobinemia, especially in infants, small children, and patients with G6PD deficiency. **Other:** The adverse effects of lidocaine could occur with large doses or if there is significant systemic absorption. Edema, soreness, aching, numbness, heaviness.

INTERACTIONS **Drug:** May cause additive toxicity with CLASS I ANTIARRHYTHMICS; may increase risk of developing methemoglobin when used with **acetaminophen, chloroquine, dapsone, fosphenytoin**, NITRATES and NITRITES, **nitric oxide, nitrofurantoin, nitroprusside, pamaquine, phenobarbital, phenytoin, primaquine, quinine**, or SULFONAMIDES.

PHARMACOKINETICS **Absorption:** Penetrates intact skin. **Onset:** 15–60 min. **Peak:** 2–3 h. **Duration:** 1–2 h after removal of cream. **Distribution:** Crosses blood–brain barrier and placenta, distributed into breast milk. **Metabolism:** In liver. **Elimination:** 98% of absorbed dose is excreted in urine. **Half-Life:** 60–150 min.

E

E

NURSING IMPLICATIONS

Assessment & Drug Effects

- Monitor for local skin reactions including erythema, edema, itching, abnormal temperature sensations, and rash. These reactions are very common and usually disappear in 1–2 h.
- Note: Patients taking Class I antiarrhythmic drugs may experience toxic effects on the cardiovascular system. EMLA should be used with caution in these patients.
- Wash immediately with water or saline if contact with the eye occurs; protect the eye until sensation returns.

Patient & Family Education

- Skin analgesia lasts for 1 h following removal of the occlusive dressing. Analgesia may be accompanied by temporary loss of all sensation in the treated skin. Advise caution until sensation returns.

EMPAGLIFLOZIN

(em-pa-gli-flo'sin)

Jardiance

Classification: ANTIDIABETIC; SODIUM-GLUCOSE COTRANSPORTER 2 (SGLT2) INHIBITOR

Therapeutic: ANTIDIABETIC

Prototype Canagliflozin

AVAILABILITY Tablet

ACTION & *THERAPEUTIC EFFECT* Inhibits the sodium-glucose cotransporter 2 (SGLT2) in the proximal renal tubules that is responsible for the majority of the reabsorption of filtered glucose in the kidney. *Empagliflozin inhibits SGLT2, thus allowing more glucose to be removed from the bloodstream and excreted by the kidney.*

USES An adjunct to diet and exercise to improve glycemic control in adults with type 2 diabetes mellitus; heart failure with reduced ejection fraction.

CONTRAINDICATIONS Hypersensitivity to canagliflozin or any component of the formulation; severe renal impairment (GFR less than 30 mL/minute/1.73 m^2), end-stage renal disease, or on dialysis; lactation.

CAUTIOUS USE Mild or moderate renal impairment; low systolic pressure; increased LDL-C; older adults; pregnancy (category C). Safety and efficacy in children younger than 18 yr not established.

ROUTE & DOSAGE

Type 2 Diabetes Mellitus

Adult: **PO** 10 mg once daily; can increase to 25 mg once daily

Heart Failure with Reduced Ejection Fraction

Adult: **PO** 10 mg daily

Renal Impairment Dosage Adjustment

GFR less than 30 mL/min/1.73 m^2: Do not exceed 10 mg daily

ADMINISTRATION

Oral

- Give in the morning without regard to food.
- Store at 15°–30°C (59°–86°F).

ADVERSE EFFECTS **Endocrine:** Dyslipidemia, hypoglycemia, increased serum creatinine. **GI:** Nausea. **GU:** Genital mycotic infections, increased urination, *urinary tract infection*. **Musculoskeletal:** Arthralgia.

Hematological: Decreased hematocrit. **Other:** Polydipsia, volume depletion.

DIAGNOSTIC TEST INTERFERENCE Empagliflozin increases urinary glucose excretion and will lead to positive **urine glucose tests**. Empagliflozin will interfere with a 1,5-anhydroglucitol (1,5-AG) assay.

INTERACTIONS **Drug:** Coadministration with DIURETICS may cause volume depletion. Coadministration with **insulin** or INSULIN SECRETAGOGUES increases the risk for hypoglycemia. Avoid use with **fexinidazole.**

PHARMACOKINETICS **Peak:** 1.5 h. **Distribution:** 86% plasma protein bound. **Metabolism:** In liver. **Elimination:** Renal (54%) and fecal (41%). **Half-Life:** 12.4 h.

NURSING IMPLICATIONS

Assessment & Drug Effects

- Monitor BP throughout therapy as drug causes intravascular volume depletion.
- Monitor for symptomatic hypotension, especially at the initiation of therapy and in the older adult or those taking other drugs that lower BP.
- Monitor for S&S of genital fungal infections.
- Monitor lab tests: Baseline and periodic renal function tests; periodic HbA1C and lipid profile.

Patient & Family Education

- Monitor blood sugar as directed by prescriber. Note that this drug will cause sugar to appear in your urine.
- Report to prescriber if you experience S&S of hypoglycemia (see Appendix F).
- Report to prescriber any S&S of an allergic reaction (e.g., rash, hives).
- Maintain adequate fluid intake as drug can cause dehydration. Inform prescriber if you experience dizziness upon standing.
- Yeast infections of the vagina and penis (especially in uncircumcised men) may occur. Report promptly for treatment.
- Report to prescriber if a pregnancy is suspected.
- Discontinue breastfeeding while taking this drug.

E

EMTRICITABINE

(em-tri′ci-ta-been)

Emtriva

Classification: ANTIRETROVIRAL; NUCLEOSIDE REVERSE TRANSCRIPTASE INHIBITOR (NRTI)

Therapeutic: ANTIRETROVIRAL, NRTI

Prototype: Zidovudine

AVAILABILITY Capsule; oral solution

ACTION & *THERAPEUTIC EFFECT* It inhibits HIV-1 reverse transcriptase (RT), both by competing with the natural DNA nucleoside and by incorporation into viral DNA, which terminates the formation of the viral DNA chain. *The viral load is decreased as measured by an increase in CD4 leukocyte count and suppression of viral RNA.*

USES Treatment of HIV-1 in combination with other antiretroviral agents.

UNLABELED USES HIV prophylaxis.

CONTRAINDICATIONS Hypersensitivity to emtricitabine; suicidal ideation; chronic HBV infection; development of lactic acidosis or hepatomegaly; pregnancy (category B); lactation.

E

CAUTIOUS USE Renal impairment, and with end-stage renal disease; hepatic impairment; history of mental illness, including bipolar disorder, psychosis; history of suicidal tendencies; alcoholism; substance abuse; seizure disorders; hypercholesterolemia, hypertriglyceridemia; older adults; children less than 3 mo.

ROUTE & DOSAGE

HIV

Adult/Adolescent/Child (weight greater than 33 kg): **PO** 200 mg (capsule) or 240 mg (solution) once/day
Child (3 mo–17 yr): **PO** 6 mg/kg/day (solution) (max: 240 mg/day)
Neonate/Infant (younger than 3 mo): 3 mg/kg daily

Renal Impairment Dosage Adjustment

CrCl 30–49 mL/min: 200 mg (capsule) q48h or 120 mg (solution) q24h; *15–29 mL/min:* 200 mg (capsule) q72h or 80 mg (solution) q24h; *less than 15 mL/min:* 200 mg (capsule) q96h or 60 mg (solution) q24h

ADMINISTRATION

Oral

- Give at the same time daily with or without food.
- Store capsules at 25°C (77°F), with excursions permitted between 15° and 30°C (59° and 86°F).

ADVERSE EFFECTS **Respiratory:** Cough, rhinitis. **CNS:** *Headache*, depression, dizziness, insomnia. **Endocrine:** Lactic acidosis. **Skin:** *Rash, hyperpigmentation* of palms and soles of feet. **GI:** *Diarrhea, nausea*, abdominal pain. **Other:** Asthenia *infection in pediatric patients.*

INTERACTIONS **Drugs:** Do not use with **cladribine** or **lamivudine**.

PHARMACOKINETICS **Absorption:** 93% reaches systemic circulation. **Peak:** 1–2 h. **Distribution:** 4% protein bound. **Metabolism:** In liver. **Elimination:** Urine. **Half-Life:** 10 h (single dose).

NURSING IMPLICATIONS

Black Box Warning

Severe acute exacerbation of hepatitis B (HBV) has been reported in patients who are coinfected with HIV-1 and HBV and discontinued emtricitabine. Hepatic function should be monitored closely with both clinical and laboratory follow-up for at least several months in patients coinfected with HIV-1 and HBV and discontinue emtricitabine. If appropriate, initiation of antihepatitis B therapy may be warranted.

Assessment & Drug Effects

- Monitor closely for S&S of lactic acidosis, especially in persons with known risk factors such as female gender, obesity, alcoholism, or hepatic disease.
- Withhold drug and notify prescriber if S&S suggestive of lactic acidosis or hepatotoxicity occur.
- Monitor closely for severe exacerbation of hepatitis B in coinfected patients if this drug is discontinued.
- Monitor lab tests: Baseline renal function tests; frequent LFTs and serum electrolytes; pregnancy test prior to therapy initiation;

complete blood chemistry if lactic acidosis is suspected; viral loads at baseline and with modifications; Hepatitis C antibody testing prior or when initiating treatment; and periodic lipid profile.

Patient & Family Education

- May cause serious CNS effects. Avoid driving or operating machinery until individual reaction to the drug is known.
- Report any of the following to the prescriber: Difficulty breathing, shortness of breath, fast or irregular heartbeat; weight gain with fullness around waist and/or face; vomiting or diarrhea; unexplained muscle aches, pains, fever, weakness, or fatigue; yellow eyes or skin.
- Avoid alcoholic drinks while taking this drug.
- Do not self-treat nausea, vomiting, or stomach pain. Contact prescriber for guidance.
- Advise patient against sudden discontinuation of the drug.

ENALAPRIL MALEATE (Pr)

(e-nal'a-pril)

Epaned, Vasotec

ENALAPRILAT

Classification: ANGIOTENSIN-CONVERTING ENZYME (ACE) INHIBITOR; ANTIHYPERTENSIVE

Therapeutic: ANTIHYPERTENSIVE

AVAILABILITY Tablet; oral solution; solution for injection

ACTION & THERAPEUTIC EFFECT Angiotensin-converting enzyme (ACE) inhibitor that catalyzes the conversion of angiotensin I to angiotensin II, therefore decreases angiotensin II levels, thus decreasing vasopressor activity and aldosterone secretion. Both actions achieve an antihypertensive effect by suppression of the renin–angiotensin–aldosterone system. ACE inhibitors also reduce peripheral arterial resistance (afterload), pulmonary capillary wedge pressure (PCWP), a measure of preload, pulmonary vascular resistance, and improve cardiac output. *Antihypertensive effect lowers blood pressure. Improvement in cardiac output results in increased exercise tolerance.*

USES Management of hypertension, heart failure.

UNLABELED USES Proteinuric chronic kidney disease, stable coronary artery disease, ST elevation MI.

CONTRAINDICATIONS Hypersensitivity to enalapril or captopril; uncorrected hypotension; heredity of idiopathic angioedema; history of angioedema related to an ACE inhibitor; acute renal failure; coadministration of aliskiren in diabetics. There has been evidence of fetotoxicity and kidney damage in newborns exposed to ACE inhibitors during pregnancy including first trimester; lactation—infant risk cannot be ruled out.

CAUTIOUS USE Renal impairment, renal artery stenosis; history of angioedema; patients with hypovolemia, receiving diuretics; undergoing dialysis; hepatic disease; bone marrow suppression; patients in whom excessive hypotension would present a hazard (e.g., cerebrovascular insufficiency); CHF; aortic stenosis, cardiomyopathy; hepatic impairment; DM; women of childbearing age; infants and children with CrCl less than 30 mL/min/1.73 m^2.

E

ROUTE & DOSAGE

Hypertension

Adult: **PO** 5 mg/day in 1 to 2 doses, may increase as needed q4–6w up to 40 mg/day in 1–2 divided doses; **IV** 1.25 mg q6h, may give up to 5 mg q6h in hypertensive emergencies
Child/Infant (1 mo or older): **PO** 0.08 mg/kg/day, may increase (max: 5 mg/kg/day)

Heart Failure

Adult: **PO** 2.5 mg bid, may increase up to target dose of 10–20 mg/day in 1–2 divided doses (max: 40 mg/day).

Renal Impairment Dosage Adjustment

Enalapril: *CrCl less than 30 mL/min:* Start with 2.5-mg dose then titrate
Enalaprilat: *CrCl less than 30 mL/min:* Start with dose of 0.625 mg q6h then titrate

ADMINISTRATION

Oral

- Discontinue diuretics, if possible, for 2–3 days prior to initial oral dose to reduce incidence of hypotension. If the diuretic cannot be discontinued, give an initial dose of 2.5 mg. Keep patient under medical supervision for at least 2 h and until BP has stabilized for at least an additional hour.
- Give with food or drink of patient's choice.
- Protect from heat and light. Expiration date: 30 mo following date of manufacture if stored at less than 30°C.
- Store suspensions at 2 to 8°C (36 to 46°F); stable for 30 days when refrigerated.

Intravenous

Note: Verify correct IV concentration and rate of infusion/injection with prescriber for neonates, infants, children.

PREPARE: **Direct:** May be given undiluted or diluted with up to 50 mL of a compatible diluent. For neonates, mix 1 mL (1.25 mg) in 49 mL D5W or NS to yield 0.025 mg/mL. **Intermittent:** Dilute in 50 mL of D5W, NS, D5/NS, D5/LR.

ADMINISTER: **Direct/Intermittent:** Give direct IV slowly over at least 5 min through a port of a free-flowing infusion of D5W or NS or as an infusion over 5 min. ▪ Longer infusion time decreases risk of severe hypotension.

INCOMPATIBILITIES: **Y-site: Amphotericin B, amphotericin B cholesteryl, caspofungin, cefepime, dantrolene, diazepam, diazoxide, gemtuzumab, lansoprazole, phenytoin.**

ADVERSE EFFECTS **CV:** *Hypotension, including postural hypotension*, syncope. **CNS:** *Dizziness.* **GU:** Acute kidney failure, deterioration in kidney function.

INTERACTIONS **Drug: Indomethacin** and other NSAIDS may decrease antihypertensive activity; POTASSIUM SUPPLEMENTS, POTASSIUM-SPARING DIURETICS may cause hyperkalemia; use with other ACE INHIBITORS or ARBS does not provide additional benefit compared to monotherapy; other ANTIHYPERTENSIVES may increase risk of hypotension; may increase **lithium** levels and toxicity. **Pregabalin,**

sacubitril may cause angioedema. Do not use with **azathioprine.**

PHARMACOKINETICS

Absorption: 50–70% from GI tract. **Onset:** 1 h PO; 15 min IV. **Peak:** 4–6 h PO; **Duration:** 12–24 h PO; 6 h IV. **Distribution:** Limited amount crosses blood–brain barrier; crosses placenta. **Metabolism:** PO dose undergoes first-pass metabolism in liver to active form, enalaprilat. **Elimination:** 60% in urine, 33% in feces within 24 h. **Half-Life:** 2 h.

NURSING IMPLICATIONS

Black Box Warning

Enalapril has been associated with fetal injury and death.

Assessment & Drug Effects

- Monitor for therapeutic effectiveness. Peak effects after the first IV dose may not occur for up to 4 h; peak effects of subsequent doses may exceed those of the first.
- Maintain bedrest and monitor BP for the first 3 h after the initial IV dose. First-dose phenomenon (i.e., a sudden exaggerated hypotensive response) may occur within 1–3 h of first IV dose, especially in the patient with very high blood pressure or one on a diuretic and controlled salt intake regimen. An IV infusion of normal saline for volume expansion may be ordered to counteract the hypotensive response. This initial response is not an indicator to stop therapy.
- Monitor BP for first several days of therapy. If antihypertensive effect is diminished before 24 h, the total dose may be given as 2 divided doses.
- Report transient hypotension with light-headedness. Older adults are particularly sensitive to drug-induced hypotension. Supervise ambulation until BP has stabilized.
- Monitor for hyperkalemia. Patients who have diabetes, impaired kidney function, or CHF are at risk of developing hyperkalemia during enalapril treatment.
- Consider ECG at baseline in patients initiating therapy.
- Monitor lab tests: Baseline and periodic serum potassium and renal function tests.

Patient & Family Education

- Notify prescriber immediately if a pregnancy is suspected. Drug should be discontinued as soon as possible.
- Full antihypertensive effect may not be experienced until several weeks after enalapril therapy starts.
- When drug is discontinued due to severe hypotension, the hypotensive effect may persist a week or longer after termination because of long duration of drug action.
- Instruct patient to change positions slowly from sitting or lying down positions.
- Do not follow a low-sodium diet (e.g., low-sodium foods or low-sodium milk) without approval from prescriber.
- Avoid use of salt substitute (principal ingredient: potassium salt) and potassium supplements because of the potential for hyperkalemia.
- Notify prescriber of a persistent nonproductive cough, especially at night, accompanied by nasal congestion or sore throat.
- Report to prescriber promptly if swelling of face, eyelids, tongue, lips, or extremities occurs. Angioedema is a rare adverse effect

and, if accompanied by laryngeal edema, may be fatal.

- Do not drive or engage in other potentially hazardous activities until response to drug is known.

E

ENASIDENIB

(en-a-sid´a-nib)

Idhifa

Classification: ANTINEOPLASTIC AGENT; IDH2 INHIBITOR

Therapeutic: ANTINEOPLASTIC AGENT

AVAILABILITY Tablet

ACTION & THERAPEUTIC EFFECT Small-molecule inhibitor that reduces abnormal histone hypermethylation, restores myeloid differentiation, reduces blast counts, and increases percentages of mature myeloid cells. *Antineoplastic agent used to treat relapsed or refractory acute myeloid leukemia.*

USES For the treatment of relapsed or refractory acute myeloid leukemia in patients with isocitrate dehydrogenase-2 (IDH2) mutation.

CAUTIOUS USE Pregnancy; lactation. Safety and efficacy in children not established.

ROUTE & DOSAGE

Acute Myeloid Leukemia

Adult: **PO** 100 mg daily

Hepatic Impairment Dosage Adjustment

Total bilirubin greater than 3 × ULN for more than 2 wk: 50 mg daily; *once bilirubin decreases to less than 2 × ULN:* Resume 100 mg daily

ADMINISTRATION

Oral

- Administer orally once daily with or without food at approximately the same time each day.
- Swallow whole with a glass of water.
- Do not split or crush tablets.

ADVERSE EFFECTS Respiratory: Acute respiratory distress, pulmonary edema. **Endocrine:** *Decreased serum calcium, decreased serum potassium.* **Hepatic:** *Increased serum bilirubin.* **GI:** *Nausea, diarrhea, decreased appetite, vomiting, dysgeusia.* **Hematologic:** *Abnormal phosphorus levels, leukocytosis,* tumor lysis syndrome. **Other:** *Cytokine release syndrome.*

PHARMACOKINETICS Absorption: 57% bioavailability, 98.5% protein bound. **Onset:** Peak effect in 4 h. **Metabolism:** Hepatic via multiple CYP enzymes and UGTs. **Elimination:** 89% in feces, 11% in urine. **Half-Life:** 137 h.

NURSING IMPLICATIONS

Black Box Warning

Enasidenib has been associated with symptoms of differentiation syndrome, which if left untreated is fatal. Symptoms include fever, hypotension, and dyspnea.

Assessment & Drug Effects

- Monitor for signs of differentiation syndrome including fever, cough, dyspnea, bone pain, rapid weight gain, edema, and lymphadenopathy as well as tumor lysis syndrome.
- Obtain CBC and electrolytes prior to therapy and every 2 wk for the first 3 mo of therapy.
- Monitor lab tests: Baseline and routine monitoring of IDH2

mutation, LFTs, renal function tests, and pregnancy tests.

Patient & Family Education

- Notify prescriber if you have signs of differentiation syndrome, including bone pain, cough, fever, shortness of breath, sudden weight gain, swelling in the arms or legs, or swollen gland(s).
- Notify prescriber right away if you have signs of kidney problems such as inability to urinate, change in appearance of urine, change in amount of urine, or blood in the urine.
- Call prescriber if you have signs of liver problems, including dark urine, feeling tired, upset stomach, stomach pain, light-colored stools, vomiting, or yellow skin or eyes.
- Notify prescriber if you experience signs or symptoms of allergic reaction such as rash, hives, itching, shortness of breath, wheezing, cough, swelling of the face, lips, tongue, or throat; or any other signs.
- Use effective birth control while on this medication and for 1 mo after stopping this drug.

ENFUVIRTIDE

(en-fu-vir′tide)

Fuzeon

Classification: ANTIRETROVIRAL; FUSION INHIBITOR

Therapeutic: ANTIRETROVIRAL

AVAILABILITY Solution for injection

ACTION & *THERAPEUTIC EFFECT*

Enfuvirtide interferes with entry of HIV-1 into host cells by inhibiting fusion of the virus with the host cell membranes. In order for HIV-1 to enter and infect a human cell, the viral surface glycoprotein (gp41) must bind to the host CD4+ cells. Then, the viral glycoprotein undergoes a change in shape facilitating the fusion of viral membranes with the host cell membrane. Prevents entry of the HIV-1 virus into host cells. *Effectiveness is measured in reduction of viral load as measured by an increase in CD4 leucocyte count and suppression of viral RNA.*

USES Treatment of HIV-1 infection disease with evidence of resistance to other therapies.

CONTRAINDICATIONS Hypersensitivity to enfuvirtide or any of its components; HIV/HBV coinfected patients; severe hepatomegaly; pregnancy—fetal risk cannot be ruled out; lactation—infant risk cannot be ruled out.

CAUTIOUS USE Renal and hepatic impairment; renal clearance of less than 35 mL/min; bacterial pneumonia, low initial CD4 count, past history of lung disease, high initial viral load, IV drug use; history of pulmonary disease.

ROUTE & DOSAGE

Advanced HIV Disease

Adult/Adolescent (16 yr or older or weight 42.6 kg or more): **Subcutaneous** 90 mg bid
Child/Adolescent (6–16 yr or over 11 kg): **Subcutaneous** 2 mg/kg (up to 90 mg) bid; package insert provides weight-based dosing

ADMINISTRATION

Subcutaneous

- Reconstitute by adding 1.0 mL sterile water for injection into vial. Mix by gently tapping vial for 10 sec, then gently rolling in palms of hands. Ensure that no drug is remaining on vial wall. Allow vial to stand until powder completely dissolves (up to 45 min). Solution should be clear, colorless, and without bubbles or particulate matter.

- Vial contains no preservatives; use immediately or refrigerate; bring refrigerated reconstituted solution to room temperature before injection. Ensure that powder is fully dissolved and solution is clear, colorless, and without bubbles or particulate matter.
- Inject into upper arm, abdomen, or anterior thigh.
- Rotate injection sites, and inject in an area with no current injection site reaction.
- Store unreconstituted vials at 25°C (77°F), excursions permitted between15° and 30°C (59° and 86°F) or refrigerated at 2°–6°C (3°–46°F); do not freeze. Reconstituted solution should be stored at 2°–8°C (36°–46°F); use within 24 hours.

ADVERSE EFFECTS (≥5%) **Respiratory:** Bacterial pneumonia. **Skin:** Injection site reaction (pain, induration, erythema, nodules, cysts, pruritus, ecchymoses). **GI:** Diarrhea, nausea. **Other:** Injection site reactions, fatigue.

INTERACTIONS Monitor concentrations when used with PROTEASE INHIBITORS.

PHARMACOKINETICS **Absorption:** 84.3% absorbed from subcutaneous site. **Peak:** Average 4–8 h. **Distribution:** 92% protein bound. **Metabolism:** Catabolized into constituent amino acids. **Half-Life:** 4 h.

NURSING IMPLICATIONS

Assessment & Drug Effects

- Inspect subcutaneous sites for S&S of site reactions (e.g., itching, swelling, redness, pain, tenderness, or hardened skin) that usually last for less than 7 days postinjection.
- Monitor closely for S&S of pneumonia, especially with low initial CD4 count, high initial viral load, IV drug use, smoking, or prior history of lung disease.
- Monitor lab tests: Periodic LFTs, serum lipase and amylase, lipid profile, and CBC with differential, fasting blood glucose or HbA1c at baseline and with modification, urinalysis at baseline and with modification, pregnancy test for women with reproductive potential prior to therapy initiation.

Patient & Family Education

- Report promptly S&S of infection at subcutaneous injection sites: Increased heat, redness, pain, or oozing.
- Report promptly S&S of pneumonia: Cough with fever, rapid breathing, shortness of breath.
- Instruct and provide opportunity for a return demonstration of correct subcutaneous injection technique.

ENOXAPARIN

(e-nox′a-pa-rin)

Lovenox

Classification: ANTICOAGULANT; LOW-MOLECULAR-WEIGHT HEPARIN
Therapeutic: ANTICOAGULANT; ANTITHROMBOTIC

AVAILABILITY Solution for injection

ACTION & *THERAPEUTIC EFFECT* Low-molecular-weight heparin with antithrombotic properties. Does affect thrombin time (TT) and activated thromboplastin time (aPTT) up to 1.8 × the control value. Antithrombotic properties are due to its antifactor Xa and antithrombin (antifactor IIa) in the coagulation activities. *An effective anticoagulation agent, it is used for prophylactic treatment as an antithrombotic agent following certain types of surgery.*

USES Venous thromboembolism prophylaxis after hip, knee, or abdominal surgery, treatment of DVT management of acute ST-elevation myocardial infarction (STEMI), unstable angina, non-Q wave MI.

UNLABELED USES Bridging anticoagulation in mechanical heart valve, acute PE, VTE prophylaxis in bariatric surgery.

CONTRAINDICATIONS Hypersensitivity to enoxaparin, porcine protein hypersensitivity, active major bleeding, GI bleeding, hemophilia, heparin hypersensitivity, heparin-induced thrombocytopenia (HIT), thrombocytopenia associated with an antiplatelet antibody in the presence of enoxaparin, bleeding disorders, idiopathic thrombocytopenic purpura (ITP), pregnancy—fetal risk cannot be ruled out; lactation—infant risk cannot be ruled out.

CAUTIOUS USE Uncontrolled arterial hypertension, recent history of GI disease, conditions or surgery with increased risk of bleeding; history of spinal deformity or spinal surgery; percutaneous coronary revascularization procedures; hepatic disease, hypertension, coagulopathy, thrombocytopenia; dental disease; diabetic retinopathy; dialysis, diverticulitis, inflammatory bowel disease, peptic ulcer disease; endocarditis; renal impairment, stroke, surgery, older adults. Safe use in neonates, infants, and children has not been established.

ROUTE & DOSAGE

Prevention of DVT after Hip or Knee Surgery

Adult: **Subcutaneous** 30 mg bid for 10–14 days starting 12–24 h postsurgery

Prevention of DVT after Abdominal Surgery

Adult: **Subcutaneous** 40 mg daily starting 2 h before surgery and continuing for 7–10 days (max: 12 days)

Treatment of DVT

Adult: **Subcutaneous** 1 mg/kg q12h or 1.5 mg/kg/day

Non-ST-elevation acute coronary syndrome

Adult: **Subcutaneous** 1 mg/kg q12h with antiplatelet regimen

Acute STEMI/Unstable Angina

Adult (under 75 yr): **IV** 30 mg bolus plus 1 mg/kg subcutaneously, then 1 mg/kg q12h subcutaneously; *(75 yr or older):* No bolus; 0.75 mg/kg (max 75 mg for the first 2 doses) q12h

Renal Impairment Dosage Adjustment

CrCl less than 30 mL/min: 30 mg or 1 mg/kg q24h

E

ADMINISTRATION

Subcutaneous

- Use a TB syringe or prefilled syringe to ensure accurate dosage.
- Do not expel the air bubble from the 30- or 40-mg prefilled syringe before injection.
- Place patient in a supine position for injection of the drug.
- Alternate injections between left and right anterolateral and posterolateral abdominal wall.
- Hold the skinfold between the thumb and forefinger and insert the whole length of the needle into the skinfold. Hold skinfold throughout the injection. Do not rub site postinjection.
- Store at controlled room temperature, 25°C (77°F), with excursions permitted between 15° and 30°C (59° and 86°F). Do not store multiple vials beyond 28 days after first use.

Intravenous

PREPARE: **Direct:** Give undiluted.
ADMINISTER: **Direct:** Give bolus dose direct IV through an IV line. Flush before and after with NS or D5W to ensure that the IV line has been cleared. Do not mix with any other drugs or solutions.

ADVERSE EFFECTS (≥5%) **Hematologic:** *Hemorrhage*, anemia. **Other:** Fever.

DIAGNOSTIC TEST INTERFERENCE May cause falsely elevated free thyrotropin and free triiodothyronine levels.

INTERACTIONS **Drug:** Aspirin, NSAIDS, **warfarin**, ANTICOAGULANTS, ANTIPLATELTS can increase risk of hemorrhage. ESTROGEN and PROGESTIN may decrease therapeutic effects. **Herbal: Garlic, ginger, ginkgo, feverfew** may increase risk of bleeding.

PHARMACOKINETICS **Absorption:** 91% from subcutaneous injection site. **Peak:** 3–5 h. **Duration:** 4.6 h. **Distribution:** Accumulates in liver, kidneys, and spleen. Does not cross placenta. **Elimination:** Primarily in urine. **Half-Life:** 4.6 h.

NURSING IMPLICATIONS

Black Box Warning

Epidural or spinal hematomas, which may result in long-term or permanent paralysis, may occur in patients who are anticoagulated with low-molecular-weight heparins or heparinoids and are receiving neuraxial anesthesia or undergoing spinal puncture. Factors that can increase the risk of developing these hematomas include use of indwelling epidural catheters, concomitant use of drugs affecting hemostasis such as NSAIDs, platelet inhibitors or other anticoagulants, or history of traumatic or repeated epidural or spinal puncture, spinal deformity, or spinal surgery.

Assessment & Drug Effects

- Monitor platelet count closely. Withhold drug and notify prescriber if platelet count less than 100,000/mm^3.
- Monitor closely patients with renal insufficiency and older adults who are at higher risk for thrombocytopenia.
- Monitor for and report immediately any sign or symptom of unexplained bleeding.
- Monitor for and report promptly S&S of neurological impairment (midline back pain, sensory and

motor deficits, numbness or weakness in lower limbs, bowel and/or bladder dysfunction).

- Monitor lab tests: Periodic CBC, platelet count, anti-Factor Xa levels, urine and stool for occult blood.

Patient & Family Education

- Report to prescriber promptly signs of unexplained bleeding such as: Pink, red, or dark brown urine; red or dark brown vomitus; bleeding gums or bloody sputum; dark, tarry stools.
- Do not take any OTC drugs without first consulting prescriber.
- Instruct and provide opportunities for return demonstrations of subcutaneous injections and instruct patient to lie down for injection and rotate injection sites in the abdomen.
- Report to prescriber if a dose is missed.

ENTACAPONE

(en-ta'ca-pone)

Comtan

Classification: CATECHOLAMINE O-METHYLTRANSFERASE (COMT) INHIBITOR; ANTIPARKINSON

Therapeutic: ANTIPARKINSON

Prototype: Tolcapone

AVAILABILITY Tablet

ACTION & *THERAPEUTIC EFFECT* Selective inhibitor of catecholamine O-methyltransferase (COMT). COMT is responsible for metabolizing levodopa to an intermediate compound 3-O-methyldopa, a chemical that interferes with the availability of levodopa to the brain. Therefore, it increases availability of levodopa in CNS. *Taken with levodopa, it decreases formation of 3-O-methyldopa, thus increasing the duration of the motor response of the brain to levodopa in Parkinson disease, diminishing its manifestations.*

USES Adjunct to levodopa/carbidopa to treat Parkinson disease.

CONTRAINDICATIONS Hypersensitivity to entacapone; concurrent use of nonselective MAOI inhibitors; major psychiatric disorders; individuals with suspicious, undiagnosed skin lesions or history of melanoma; children; pregnancy—fetal risk cannot be ruled out; lactation—infant risk cannot be ruled out.

CAUTIOUS USE Hepatic impairment; biliary obstruction; renal impairment; history of hypotension or syncope; sleep disorders; history of obsessive-compulsive disorder.

ROUTE & DOSAGE

Parkinson Disease

Adult: **PO** 200 mg administered with each dose of levodopa/carbidopa, up to max of 8 times daily (max: 1600 mg/day)

ADMINISTRATION

Oral

- Give simultaneously with each levodopa/carbidopa dose.
  - May be taken with or without food.
- **Must be** tapered if discontinued. Never discontinue abruptly.
- Do not administer to patients receiving nonselective MAOI inhibitors.
- Store at controlled room temperature 25°C (77°F), with excursions permitted to 15°–30°C (59°–86°F).

ADVERSE EFFECTS (≥5%) **CNS:** *Dyskinesia, hyperkinesia,* hypokinesia, hyperactive behavior. **GI:** *Nausea, diarrhea,* abdominal pain. **GU:** *Urine discoloration.* **Other:** Fatigue.

E

INTERACTIONS Drug: Extreme caution **must be** used if administered with a nonselective MAOI; may increase heart rates, possibly cause arrhythmias, excessive changes in BP. May increase risk of bleeding when used with **warfarin**. May enhance effect of CNS DEPRESSANTS. Increases toxicity risk of **lofepramine. Iron** may decrease concentration of entacapone.

PHARMACOKINETICS Absorption: Rapidly absorbed, 35% bioavailable. **Peak:** 1 h. **Distribution:** Highly protein bound. **Metabolism:** Extensively metabolized in plasma and erythrocytes. **Elimination:** Primarily in feces. **Half-Life:** 2.4 h (terminal).

NURSING IMPLICATIONS

Assessment & Drug Effects

- Monitor carefully for hyperpyrexia, confusion, or emergence of Parkinson S&S during drug withdrawal.
- Monitor for orthostatic hypotension and worsening of dyskinesia or hyperkinesia.

Patient & Family Education

- Take with levodopa/carbidopa; not effective alone.
- Do not discontinue abruptly; gradually reduce dosage.
- Exercise caution when rising from a sitting or lying position because faintness/dizziness can occur.
- Exercise caution with hazardous activities until reaction to the drug is known.
- Harmless brownish-orange discoloration of urine is possible.
- Report unusual adverse effects (e.g., hallucinations unexplained diarrhea, compulsive behaviors, impaired impulse control).

ENTECAVIR

(en-te′ca-vir)

Baraclude

Classification: ANTIRETROVIRAL; NUCLEOSIDE REVERSE TRANSCRIPTASE INHIBITOR (NRTI)

Therapeutic: ANTIRETROVIRAL; NRTI

Prototype: Lamivudine

AVAILABILITY Tablet; oral solution

ACTION & *THERAPEUTIC EFFECT* Inhibits hepatitis B viral (HBV) DNA polymerase by inhibiting viral reverse transcriptase of messenger RNA that ultimately results in inhibiting the synthesis of HBV DNA. *The antiviral activity of entecavir inhibits HBV DNA synthesis.*

USES Chronic hepatitis B infection.

CONTRAINDICATIONS Hypersensitivity to entecavir; lactic acidosis; severe hepatomegaly; HIV/HVB coinfected patients, if HIV is not being treated with highly active antiretroviral therapy; pregnancy—fetal risk cannot be ruled out; lactation—infant risk cannot be ruled out.

CAUTIOUS USE Liver transplant patients; liver disease; HIV patients; renal impairment, ESRF, dialysis; older adults; women, obesity, labor and delivery. Safety and efficacy in children younger than 2 yr not established.

ROUTE & DOSAGE

Chronic Hepatitis B (nucleoside-treatment–naïve patients)

Adult/Adolescent (16 yr or older): **PO** 0.5 mg daily

Chronic Hepatitis B (lamivudine- or telbivudine-resistant patients/ chronic hepatitis B with decompensated liver disease)

Adult/Adolescent (16 yr or older): **PO** 1 mg daily

Renal Impairment Dosage Adjustment

CrCl 30–49 mL/min: Decrease dose by 50% or administer q48 h; *10–29 mL/min:* Decrease dose by 70% or administer q72 h; *less than 10 mL/min:* Decrease dose by 90% or administer q7days

ADMINISTRATION

Oral

- Give on an empty stomach (at least 2 h before/after a meal).
- NIOSH recommends use of single gloves by anyone handling the intact tablets or capsules or administering from a unit-dose package. Use double gloves, protective gown if cutting, crushing, or manipulating uncoated tablets. Wear single gloves and eye/face protection if the formulation is hard to swallow or if the patient may resist, vomit, or spit up.
- Do not dilute or mix water or any other liquid with solution.
- Use the calibrated dosing spoon supplied with the solution; hold in a vertical position and gradually fill; rinse spoon with water after each dose.
- Administer after hemodialysis.
- Store tablets and solution in a tightly closed container at 25°C (77°F) with excursions permitted between 15° and 30°C (59° and 86°F). Store in outer carton to protect from light. Solution can be used up to the expiration date on the bottle.

ADVERSE EFFECTS (≤4%) CNS: Headache.

INTERACTIONS Drug: Use of entecavir with drugs that reduce renal function or compete for active tubular secretion may increase serum concentrations of either drug. Do not use with **cladribine. Food:** ***High-fat*** meal reduces oral absorption.

PHARMACOKINETICS Peak: 0.5–1 h. **Distribution:** 13% protein bound. **Metabolism:** Minimal. **Elimination:** Primarily in the urine. **Half-Life:** 5–6 days.

NURSING IMPLICATIONS

Black Box Warning

Severe acute exacerbations of hepatitis B have been reported in patients who have discontinued antihepatitis B therapy. Entecavir has been associated with severe, and potentially fatal, lactic acidosis and hepatomegaly.

Assessment & Drug Effects

- Monitor closely for adverse reactions when drugs that are known to affect renal function are taken concurrently.
- Monitor for S&S of lactic acidosis, including respiratory distress, tachycardia, and irregular HR.
- Monitor lab tests: Periodic LFTs during treatment and for several months after drug is discontinued; renal function tests; periodic fasting plasma glucose, Hepatitis B envelope antigen, hepatitis B surface antigen, HBV DNA levels.

E

Patient & Family Education

- Follow directions for taking the drug (see ADMINISTRATION). Review correct measurement technique if solution is prescribed.
- Do not discontinue medication without consent of prescriber.
- Do not drive or engage in potentially hazardous activities until response to drug is known.
- Inform prescriber if you are or plan to become pregnant.
- Report any of the following to a healthcare provider: Unexplained tiredness or weakness, unusual muscle pain, difficulty breathing, cold extremities, dizziness or light-headedness, irregular heartbeat, loss of appetite, stomach pain, nausea, vomiting, clay-colored stool, dark urine, or jaundice.

ENZALUTAMIDE

(en-za-loo'ta-mide)

Xtandi

Classification: ANTINEOPLASTIC; ANDROGEN RECEPTOR INHIBITOR; ANTIANDROGEN

Therapeutic: ANTINEOPLASTIC

Prototype: Flutamide

AVAILABILITY Capsule

ACTION & THERAPEUTIC EFFECT Competitively inhibits androgen binding to androgen receptors and inhibits androgen receptor-mediated nuclear translocation and interaction with DNA. *Decreases proliferation and induces cell death of prostate cancer cells.*

USES Metastatic castration-resistant prostate cancer in patients who have previously received docetaxel.

CONTRAINDICATIONS Pregnancy—fetal risk cannot be ruled out; fetal harm and loss of pregnancy have been reported; lactation—infant risk cannot be ruled out.

CAUTIOUS USE History of seizures, TIA within 12 mo, or CVA; history of heart disease; brain metastases; severe renal or hepatic impairment. Safety and efficacy in children younger than 18 yr not established.

ROUTE & DOSAGE

Prostate Cancer

Adult: **PO** 160 mg once daily

Toxicity Adjustment

Grade 3 or Greater Toxicity: Withhold drug for 1 wk or until symptoms improve to Grade 2 or better; resume at the same or a reduced dose

Concomitant Therapy with a Strong CYP2C8 Inhibitor: Decrease dose to 80 mg once daily

ADMINISTRATION

Oral

- Give without regard to food.
- NIOSH recommends the use of single gloves by anyone handling intact tablets, capsules, or administering from a unit-dose package.
- Take at the same time every day.
- Ensure that capsules and tablets are swallowed whole and not chewed or opened.
- Store in a dry location at a temperature between 20° and 25°C (68° and 77°F), with excursions permitted between 15° and 30°C (59° and 86°F). Keep container tightly closed.

ADVERSE EFFECTS (≥5%) **CV:** Hypertension, peripheral edema. **Respiratory:** Lower respiratory tract and lung infection, *upper* *respiratory tract infection*, dyspnea. **CNS:** Dizziness, *headache*, weakness, and fatigue. **Endocrine:** Weight loss. **Skin:** Flushing. **GI:** *Diarrhea, constipation, anorexia, altered sense of taste.* **Musculoskeletal:** *Arthralgia, back pain.*

INTERACTIONS **Drug:** Significant drug interactions exist, requiring dose/frequency adjustment or avoidance. Consult drug interactions database for more information. Examples of some interactions: Strong inhibitors of CYP2C8 (e.g., **gemfibrozil**) or CYP3A4 (e.g., **itraconazole**) increase the levels of enzalutamide. Strong or moderate inducers of CYP2C8 (e.g., **rifampin**) or CYP3A4 (e.g., **carbamazepine, phenobarbital, phenytoin, rifabutin, rifampin, rifapentine, bosentan, efavirenz, etravirine, modafinil, nafcillin**) may decrease the levels of enzalutamide. Enzalutamide may decrease the levels of other drugs that require CYP2C9, CYP2C19, or CYP3A4 for metabolism; therefore drugs with narrow therapeutic indexes that require these isoforms for metabolism (e.g., **alfentanil, cyclosporine, dihydroergotamine, ergotamine, fentanyl, phenytoin, pimozide, quinidine, sirolimus, tacrolimus, warfarin**) should not be used in combination with enzalutamide. **Food: Grapefruit** or **grapefruit juice** may increase the levels of enzalutamide. **Herbal: St. John's wort** may decrease the levels of enzalutamide.

PHARMACOKINETICS **Peak:** 1 h. **Distribution:** 97–98% plasma protein bound. **Metabolism:** In liver via CYP2C8. **Elimination:** Renal (71%) and fecal (14%). **Half-Life:** 5.8 days.

NURSING IMPLICATIONS

Assessment & Drug Effects

- Monitor ambulation, as drug may cause dizziness and predisposition to falls.
- Monitor signs of ischemic heart disease (dizziness, fainting, shortness of breath, chest pain).
- Monitor cognitive status and report signs of mental impairment.
- Monitor lab tests: Baseline and periodic CBC with differential, renal function tests, and LFTs.

Patient & Family Education

- Take drug at the same time each day.
- Exercise caution with potentially dangerous activities until response to drug is known.
- Report to provider any symptoms of dizziness, fainting, seizures, shortness of breath or chest pain.
- Use a condom and another effective method of birth control during and for 3 mo after treatment if having sex with a woman of childbearing potential.

EPHEDRINE SULFATE

(e-fed′rin sul-fate)

Classification: ALPHA- AND BETA-ADRENERGIC AGONIST; BRONCHODILATOR

Therapeutic: BRONCHODILATOR

Prototype: Epinephrine HCl

AVAILABILITY Solution for injection

ACTION & *THERAPEUTIC EFFECT* Both indirect- and direct-acting sympathomimetic amine thought to act indirectly by releasing tissue stores of norepinephrine and directly by stimulation of alpha-, beta$_1$-, and beta$_2$-adrenergic receptors. Like epinephrine, contracts dilated arterioles of nasal mucosa, thus reducing engorgement and edema and facilitating ventilation and drainage. *Ephedrine relaxes bronchial smooth muscle, relieving mild bronchospasm, improving air exchange and increasing vital capacity.*

E

USES Anesthesia-induced hypotension.

CONTRAINDICATIONS History of hypersensitivity to ephedrine or other sympathomimetics; narrow-angle glaucoma; angina pectoris, coronary insufficiency, chronic heart disease, uncontrolled hypertension, cardiac arrhythmias, cardiomyopathy; hypovolemia; concurrent MAOI therapy; pregnancy (fetal risk cannot be ruled out); lactation (infant risk cannot be ruled out).

CAUTIOUS USE Hypertension, arteriosclerosis, closed-angle glaucoma; diabetes mellitus; hyperthyroidism; prostatic hypertrophy; renal impairment; unstable vasomotor symptoms.

ROUTE & DOSAGE

Hypotension

Adult: **IM/Subcutaneous/IV** 5–25 mg slow IV, may repeat if necessary (max: 50 mg)

ADMINISTRATION

Subcutaneous/Intramuscular

- Give undiluted.

Intravenous

PREPARE: **Direct:** Dilute in 5 or 10 mg/mL with D5W or NS.
ADMINISTER: **Direct:** Direct IV at a rate of 10 mg or fraction thereof over 30–60 sec.
INCOMPATIBILITIES: **Solution/additive: Pentobarbital, phenobarbital, thiopental. Y-site: Amphotericin B liposome, ampicillin, azathioprine, caspofungin, dantrolene, diazepam, diazoxide, ganciclovir, garenoxacin mesylate, haloperidol lactate, hydralazine hydrochloride, pantoprazole, pentamidine, phenytoin sodium, SMZ/TMP, thiopental sodium.**

- Store in tightly closed, light-resistant containers. Do not use liquid formulation unless it is absolutely clear.

ADVERSE EFFECTS **CV:** Hypertension, palpitations, tachycardia, arrhythmia, bradycardia. **CNS:** Dizziness, anxiety, insomnia, hallucination, restlessness. **GI:** Nausea, vomiting.

DIAGNOSTIC TEST INTERFERENCE Can cause a false-positive **amphetamine EMIT assay.**

INTERACTIONS **Drug:** TRICYCLIC ANTIDEPRESSANTS, **furazolidone, guanethidine** may increase alpha-adrenergic effects (headache, hyperpyrexia, hypertension); **sodium bicarbonate** decreases renal elimination of ephedrine, increasing its CNS effects; **epinephrine, norepinephrine** compound sympathomimetic effects; effects of ALPHA and BETA BLOCKERS and ephedrine antagonized. Do not use with ERGOT derivatives or MAO INHIBITORS.

PHARMACOKINETICS **Absorption:** Readily absorbed from GI tract. **Peak:** 15 min–1 h. **Duration:** Bronchodilation 2–4 h; cardiac and pressor effects up to 4 h PO and 1 h IV. **Distribution:** Widely distributed; crosses blood–brain barrier and placenta; distributed into breast milk. **Metabolism:** Small amounts metabolized in liver. **Elimination:** In urine. **Half-Life:** 3–6 h.

NURSING IMPLICATIONS

Assessment & Drug Effects

- Supervise continuously patients receiving ephedrine IV. Take baseline BP and other vital signs. Check BP repeatedly during first 5 min, then q3–5min until stabilized.
- Monitor I&O ratio and pattern, especially in older male patients. Encourage patient to void before taking medication (see ADVERSE EFFECTS).

Patient & Family Education

- Note: Ephedrine is a commonly abused drug. Learn adverse effects and dangers; take medication ONLY as prescribed.
- Do not take OTC medications for coughs, colds, allergies, or asthma unless approved by prescriber. Ephedrine is a common ingredient in these preparations.

EPINASTINE HYDROCHLORIDE

(e-pi-nas′teen)

Elestat

See Appendix A-1.

EPINEPHRINE ⚠

(ep-i-ne′frin)

Akovaz, EpiPen Auto-Injector, Symjepi

EPINEPHRINE BITARTRATE

EPINEPHRINE HYDROCHLORIDE

Adrenalin, Sus-Phrine ♣

EPINEPHRINE, RACEMIC

Classification: ALPHA- AND BETA-ADRENERGIC AGONIST; CARDIAC STIMULANT; VASOPRESSOR

Therapeutic: ANTIANAPHYLACTIC; VASOPRESSOR

AVAILABILITY Solution for inhalation; spray; suspension; nasal solution; solution for injection

ACTION & *THERAPEUTIC EFFECT* A catecholamine that acts directly on both alpha and beta receptors; it is the most potent activator of alpha receptors. Strengthens myocardial contraction; increases systolic but may decrease diastolic blood pressure; increases cardiac rate and cardiac output. Constricts bronchial arterioles and inhibits histamine release, thus reducing congestion and edema and increasing tidal volume and vital capacity. Relaxes uterine smooth musculature and inhibits uterine contractions. *Reverses anaphylactic reactions and provides temporary relief from acute asthmatic attack. Restores normal cardiac rhythm.*

USES Temporary relief of bronchospasm, acute asthmatic attack, hypotension during anesthesia, hypersensitivity and anaphylactic reactions, hypotension or shock, syncope due to heart block or carotid sinus hypersensitivity, and to restore cardiac rhythm in cardiac arrest.

CONTRAINDICATIONS There are no absolute contraindications to the use of injectable epinephrine in a life-threatening situation. Hypersensitivity to sympathomimetic amines; narrow-angle glaucoma; hemorrhagic, traumatic, or cardiogenic shock; cardiac dilatation, cerebral arteriosclerosis, coronary insufficiency, arrhythmias, organic heart or brain disease; during second stage of labor; for local anesthesia of fingers, toes, ears, nose, genitalia.

CAUTIOUS USE Older adults or debilitated patients; prostatic hypertrophy; hypertension; diabetes mellitus; hyperthyroidism; pheochromocytoma; Parkinson disease; tuberculosis; psychoneurosis; in patients with spinal cord injury; in patients with long-standing bronchial asthma and emphysema with degenerative heart disease; pregnancy (fetal risk cannot be ruled out); lactation (infant risk cannot be ruled out).

E

ROUTE & DOSAGE

Anaphylaxis

Adult: **Subcutaneous/IM** 0.3 or 0.5 mg using the 1 mg/mL solution; may repeat q5–15 min.
Child: **Subcutaneous/IM** 0.01 mg/kg not to exceed 0.3 mg (prepubertal child) to 0.5 mg (adolescent) every 5 to 15 min

Asystole/Pulseless VT/VF

Child: **IV** 0.01 mg/kg immediately after initiating CPR (max: 1 mg/dose)

Septic Shock (adjunct)

Adult: **IV** 1–15 mcg/minute; titrate to goal MAP.

Bradycardia

Child: **IV** 0.01 mg/kg (max: 1 mg/dose) q3–5 min prn

Asthma

Adult: **Inhalation** 1 inhalation of metered dose inhaler q4h prn
Child: (over 4 y)/Adolescent **Inhalation** Add 0.5 mL to nebulizer; 1 to 3 inhalations; may repeat dose in 3 h prn (max: 12 inhalations in 24 h)

Decongestant

Adult/Child: **Topical** Apply 1 mg/mL solution locally

ADMINISTRATION

Inhalation

- Have patient in an upright position when aerosol preparation is used. The reclining position can result in overdosage by producing large droplets instead of fine spray.
- Instruct patient to rinse mouth and throat with water immediately after inhalation to avoid swallowing residual drug (may cause epigastric pain and systemic effects from the propellant in the aerosol preparation) and to prevent dryness of oropharyngeal membranes.

Instillation (Nasal)

- Instill nose drops with head in lateral, head-low position to prevent entry of drug into throat.
- Instruct patient to rinse nose dropper or spray tip with hot water after each use to prevent contamination of solution with nasal secretions.

Instillation (Ocular)

- Remove soft contact lenses before instilling eye drops.
- Instruct patient to apply gentle finger pressure against nasolacrimal duct immediately after drug is instilled for at least 1 or 2 min following instillation to prevent excessive systemic absorption.

Subcutaneous

- Use tuberculin syringe to ensure greater accuracy in measurement of parenteral doses.
- Auto-injector: For single use only into anterolateral aspect of the thigh.
- Protect epinephrine injection from exposure to light at all times. Do not remove ampule or vial from carton until ready to use.
- Shake vial or ampule thoroughly to disperse particles before

withdrawing epinephrine suspension into syringe; then inject promptly.

- Aspirate carefully before injecting epinephrine. Inadvertent IV injection of usual subcutaneous doses can result in sudden hypertension and possibly cerebral hemorrhage.
- Rotate injection sites and observe for signs of blanching. Vascular constriction from repeated injections may cause tissue necrosis.

Intravenous

Note: Verify correct rate of IV injection to neonates, infants, children with prescriber.
Note: 1:1000 solution contains 1 mg/1 mL. 1:10,000 solution contains 0.1 mg/1 mL.
PREPARE: **Direct:** Dilute each 1 mg/mL yield 1 mcg/mL dilution.
- The 1:10,000 solution may be given undiluted. **IV Infusion:** Dilute required dose in D5W and NS or D5W.

ADMINISTER: **Direct:** Give each 1 mg over 1 min or longer; may give more rapidly in cardiac arrest. **IV Infusion:** 1–10 mcg/min titrated according to patient's condition.
INCOMPATIBILITIES: Admixtures and Y-site not tested. If extravasation occurs, stop infusion immediately and disconnect (leave cannula/needle in place); gently aspirate extravasated solution (**do not** flush the line); remove needle/cannula; elevate extremity. Initiate antidote, and apply dry warm compresses.

ADVERSE EFFECTS **CV:** Palpitations. **Respiratory:** Difficulty breathing. **CNS:** Decreased sensation, dizziness, headache, tremor, anxiety, apprehension, restlessness. **Skin:** Pallor, sweating. **GI:** Nausea, vomiting.

INTERACTIONS **Drug:** May increase hypotension in circulatory collapse or hypotension caused by PHENOTHIAZINES, **oxytocin, entacapone**. Additive toxicities with other SYMPATHOMIMETICS (**albuterol, dobutamine, dopamine, isoproterenol, metaproterenol, norepinephrine, phenylephrine, phenylpropanolamine, pseudoephedrine, ritodrine, salmeterol, terbutaline**), MAO INHIBITORS, TRICYCLIC ANTIDEPRESSANTS. ALPHA- AND BETA-ADRENERGIC BLOCKING AGENTS (e.g., **ergotamine, propranolol**) antagonize effects of epinephrine. GENERAL ANESTHETICS increase cardiac irritability. Do not use with **bromocriptine, bromperidol, cabergoline, methylergonovine**.

PHARMACOKINETICS **Absorption:** Inactivated in GI tract. **Onset:** subcutaneous 5–10 min; **IV** 3–5 min, 1 h on conjunctiva. **Peak:** 20 min, 4–8 h on conjunctiva. **Duration:** 12–24 h topically. **Distribution:** Widely distributed; does not cross blood–brain barrier; crosses placenta. **Metabolism:** In tissue and liver by monoamine oxidase (MAO) and catecholamine-methyltransferase (COMT). **Elimination:** Small amount unchanged in urine; excreted in breast milk.

NURSING IMPLICATIONS

Assessment & Drug Effects

- Check BP repeatedly when epinephrine is administered IV during first 5 min, then q3–5min until stabilized.
- Monitor BP, pulse, respirations, and urinary output and observe patient closely following IV administration. Continuous cardiac monitoring is

recommended during IV infusion. If disturbances in cardiac rhythm occur, withhold epinephrine and notify prescriber immediately.

- Monitor infusion site frequently to ensure free flow and avoid extravasation.
- Keep prescriber informed of any changes in intake-output ratio.
- Advise patient to report bronchial irritation, nervousness, or sleeplessness. Dosage should be reduced.

Patient & Family Education

- Report to prescriber if symptoms of asthma are not relieved in 20 min or if they become worse following inhalation.
- Be aware intranasal application may sting slightly.
- Administer ophthalmic drug at bedtime or following prescribed miotic to minimize mydriasis, with blurred vision and sensitivity to light (possible in some patients being treated for glaucoma).
- Transitory stinging may follow initial ophthalmic administration, and headache and browache occur frequently at first but usually subside with continued use. Notify prescriber if symptoms persist.
- Discontinue epinephrine eyedrops and consult a prescriber if signs of hypersensitivity develop (edema of lids, itching, discharge, crusting eyelids).
- Learn how to administer epinephrine subcutaneously. Keep medication and equipment available for home emergency. Confer with prescriber.
- Advise patient to report bronchial irritation, nervousness, or sleeplessness. Dosage should be reduced.
- Report tolerance to prescriber; may occur with repeated or prolonged use. Continued use of epinephrine in the presence of tolerance can be dangerous.
- Take medication only as prescribed, and immediately notify prescriber of onset of systemic effects of epinephrine.
- Instruct caregiver and patient to periodically review user instructions, practice using auto-injector trainer, and inspect auto-injector to ensure the blue safety release is not raised and that the device can easily be removed from the carrier tube.
- Discard discolored or precipitated solutions.
- Dispose of blue safety release immediately after administration as the small part may pose a choking hazard for children.

EPIRUBICIN HYDROCHLORIDE

(e-pi-roo′bi-sin)

Ellence

Classification: ANTINEOPLASTIC; ANTHRACYCLINE

Therapeutic: ANTINEOPLASTIC

Prototype: Doxorubicin HCl

AVAILABILITY Intravenous solution

ACTION & *THERAPEUTIC EFFECT*

Cytotoxic antibiotic with wide spectrum of antitumor activity and strong immunosuppressive properties. Complexes with DNA causing the DNA helix to change shape, thus blocking effective DNA and RNA transcription. *Highly destructive to rapidly proliferating cells. Effectiveness indicated by tumor regression.*

USES Adjunctive therapy for axillary node-positive breast cancer.

CONTRAINDICATIONS

Hypersensitivity to epirubicin and other related drugs; marked myelosuppression with neutrophil count less than 1500 cells/mm^3; severely impaired cardiac function, cardiomyopathy; severe cardiac arrhythmias, recent MI; severe hepatic disease, jaundice; previous treatment with maximum doses of epirubicin, doxorubicin, or daunorubicin; pregnancy (category D); lactation.

CAUTIOUS USE

Arrhythmias, CHF; mild or moderate liver dysfunction; severe renal insufficiency or renal failure; females 70 yr and older.

ROUTE & DOSAGE

Breast Cancer

Adult: IV 100–120 mg/m^2 infused on day 1 of a 3–4 wk cycle or 50–60 mg/m^2 on day 1 and 8 of a 3–4 wk cycle (max cumulative dose: 900 mg/m^2)

Hepatic Impairment Dosage Adjustment

Bilirubin 1.2–3 mg/dL: Give 50% of dose; *bilirubin over 3 mg/dL:* Give 25% of dose; *bilirubin greater than 5 mg/dL:* Skip dose

Toxicity Dosage Adjustment

Reduce dose by 25% if platelets less than 50,000/mm^3, ANC less than 250/mm^3, neutropenic fever, or Grade 3 or 4 hematologic toxicity

ADMINISTRATION

Intravenous

Note: Pregnant women **should not** prepare or administer this drug. Wear protective goggles, gowns and disposable gloves and masks when handling this drug. **Discard all** equipment used in preparation of this drug in high-risk, waste-disposal bags for incineration. Treat accidental contact with skin or eyes by rinsing with copious amounts of water followed by prompt medical attention.

PREPARE: **IV Infusion:** Epirubicin is manufactured as a preservative-free ready-to-use solution. The contents of a vial **must be** used within 24 h of first penetrating the rubber stopper. Discard unused solution.

ADMINISTER: **IV Infusion:** Measure ordered dose and inject into a port of a freely flowing IV solution of D5W or NS over 3–20 min. ▪ **Do not** give by direct IV push into a vein. ▪ Avoid IV sites that enter small veins or repeated injections into the same vein. ▪ Monitor IV site closely for S&S of extravasation, and if suspected, notify prescriber immediately.

INCOMPATIBILITIES: **Solution/additive:** ALKALINE SOLUTIONS (including **sodium bicarbonate**), **fluorouracil, heparin. Y-site: Acyclovir, allopurinol, aminophylline, amphotericin B, ampicillin, azithromycin, cefepime, cefoperazone, cefotetan, cefoxitin, ceftazidime, ceftriaxone, cefuroxime, dexamethasone, diazepam, ertapenem, fluorouracil, foscarnet, fosphenytoin, furosemide, gallium, ganciclovir, gemtuzumab, heparin, hydrocortisone, ketorolac, leucovorin, magnesium, meropenem, methohexital, methylprednisolone, nafcillin, pantoprazole, pemetrexed, pentobarbital, phenobarbital, phenytoin, piperacillin, potassium,**

sodium bicarbonate, sulfamethoxazole/trimethoprim, thiopental, ticarcillin, tigecycline.

- Store at 2°–8°C (36°–46°F). Protect from light.

E

ADVERSE EFFECTS **CV:** Asymptomatic decrease in LVEF, CHF. **Skin:** *Alopecia, injection site reaction,* rash, itching, skin changes. **GI:** *Nausea, vomiting, mucositis, diarrhea,* anorexia. **Hematologic:** Leukopenia, neutropenia, anemia, thrombocytopenia, AML. **Other:** *Amenorrhea, hot flashes, infection, conjunctivitis/keratitis,* secondary acute myelogenous leukemia (related to cumulative dose). *Lethargy,* fever.

INTERACTIONS **Drug: Cimetidine** increases epirubicin levels; concomitant use with cardioactive drugs (e.g., CALCIUM CHANNEL BLOCKERS) may affect cardiac function.

PHARMACOKINETICS **Distribution:** Widely distributed, 77% protein bound, concentrated in red blood cells. **Metabolism:** Extensively in liver, blood, and other organs. Clearance is reduced in patients with hepatic impairment. **Elimination:** Primarily in bile, some urinary excretion; clearance decreases in older adult female patients. **Half-Life:** 33 h.

NURSING IMPLICATIONS

Black Box Warning

Epirubicin extravasation can cause severe local tissue necrosis. Epirubicin has been associated with cardiac toxicity (including fatal CHF during or long after termination of therapy), hepatic impairment, myelosuppression, and secondary AML.

Assessment & Drug Effects

- Withhold drug and notify prescriber of any of the following: Neutrophil count less than 1500 cells/mm^3, recent MI, suspicion of severe myocardial insufficiency.
- Obtain baseline and periodic (before each cycle of therapy) cardiac evaluation: Left ventricular ejection fraction, ECG and ECHO (tests are recommended especially in the presence of risk factors of cardiac toxicity).
- Monitor cardiac status closely throughout therapy as the risk of developing severe CHF increases rapidly when cumulative doses approach 900 mg/m^2. Report significant ECG changes immediately. Report immediately S&S of the following: Tachycardia, gallop rhythm, pleural effusion, pulmonary edema, dependent edema, ascites, or hepatomegaly.
- Monitor lab tests: Baseline and before each cycle of therapy CBC with differential and platelet count, serum electrolytes, LFTs, and serum creatinine.

Patient & Family Education

- Review all literature regarding the adverse effects of epirubicin therapy carefully.
- Report any of the following to prescriber immediately: Pain at the site of IV infusion, chest pain, palpitations, shortness of breath or difficulty breathing, sudden weight gain, swelling of hands, feet, or legs, or any unexplained bleeding.
- Be aware that your urine may turn red for 1–2 days after receiving this drug. This change is expected and harmless.
- Do not take OTC cimetidine or any other OTC drug without consulting prescriber.

- Use effective means of contraception (both men and women) while on epirubicin therapy.

EPLERENONE

(e-ple're-none)

Inspra

Classification: POTASSIUM SPARING DIURETIC; SELECTIVE ALDOSTERONE RECEPTOR ANTAGONIST (SARA); ANTIHYPERTENSIVE

Therapeutic: ANTIHYPERTENSIVE; DIURETIC; SARA

Prototype: Spironolactone

AVAILABILITY Tablet

ACTION & THERAPEUTIC EFFECT Binds to mineralocorticoid receptors and blocks the binding of aldosterone, a component of the renin–angiotensin–aldosterone system (RAAS). Thus, eplerenone blocks the primary effect of aldosterone, which is sodium reabsorption. *Lowers blood pressure by inhibiting sodium and water retention, thus reducing total plasma volume.*

USES Treatment of hypertension. Adjunctive therapy for post MI heart failure.

CONTRAINDICATIONS Serum potassium greater than 5.5 mEq/L; type 2 diabetes with microalbuminuria; serum creatinine greater than 2 mg/dL in males or greater than 1.8 mg/dL in females; CrCl less than 30 mL/min; type II diabetics do not use if CrCl is less than 50 mL/min; severe hepatic impairment; lactation.

CAUTIOUS USE Hepatic impairment; hepatic disease; diabetics with CHF post-MI; CHF; renal impairment; older adults; pregnancy (fetal risk cannot be ruled out); lactation (infant risk cannot be ruled out). Safety and efficacy in children, infants, or neonates not established.

ROUTE & DOSAGE

Hypertension

Adult: **PO** 50 mg once daily, may be increased to 50 mg bid, if inadequate response after 4 wk

Heart Failure/Post MI

Adult: **PO** 25 mg then titrate to 50 mg daily; see package insert to adjust for serum potassium

Renal Impairment Dosage Adjustment

CrCl less than 50 mL/min (hypertension patient): Do not administer

CrCl less than 30 mL/min (heart failure patients): Do not administer

ADMINISTRATION

Oral

- May be taken with or without food.
- Do not administer in combination with potassium supplements or potassium-sparing diuretics.
- Manufacturer recommends dosage reduction to 25 mg once daily with concurrent administration of erythromycin, saquinavir, verapamil, or fluconazole.
- Store at 15°–30°C (59°–86°F).

ADVERSE EFFECTS **Endocrine:** Hyperkalemia, hypertension, hypertriglyceridemia.

INTERACTIONS **Drug:** ACE INHIBITORS, ANGIOTENSIN II RECEPTOR BLOCKERS, AZOLE ANTIFUNGALS (e.g., **fluconazole**), **erythromycin, saquinavir, verapamil, spironolactone** may increase risk of

E

hyperkalemia. CYP3A4 INHIBITORS may increase concentration of eplerenone and increase risk of ADRs. Do not use with **atazanavir, bromperidol, clarithromycin, cobicistat, conivaptan, cyclosporine, darunavir, fusidic acid, idelalisib, indinavir, itraconazole, ketoconazole, lopinavir, mifepristone, nelfinavir, ritonavir, saquinavir, tacrolimus, voriconazole. Food: Potassium**-containing SALT SUBSTITUTES may increase risk of hyperkalemia.

PHARMACOKINETICS **Absorption:** Rapidly absorbed. **Peak:** 1.5 h. **Distribution:** 50% protein bound, primarily to alpha$_1$-acid glycoproteins. **Metabolism:** In liver by CYP3A4. **Elimination:** 32% in feces, 67% in urine. **Half-Life:** 3–6 h.

NURSING IMPLICATIONS

Assessment & Drug Effects

- Monitor cardiovascular status with frequent BP determinations. Note that BP lowering usually occurs within 2 wk with maximal antihypertensive effects achieved within 4 wk.
- Concurrent drugs: Monitor serum potassium levels more frequently when patient also receiving an ACE inhibitor or an angiotensin II receptor antagonist. Monitor frequently for lithium toxicity with concurrent use.
- Withhold drug and notify prescriber for any of the following: Serum potassium greater than 5.5 mEq/L, serum creatinine greater than 2 mg/dL in males or greater than 1.8 mg/dL in females, creatinine clearance less than 50 mL/min, microalbuminuria in type 2 diabetics.
- Monitor lab tests: Baseline serum potassium, repeat within the 1st wk, again at 1 mo or after dosage adjustment, then periodically thereafter.

Patient & Family Education

- Do not use potassium supplements, salt substitutes containing potassium, or contraindicated drugs (e.g., ketoconazole, itraconazole) without consulting prescriber.
- Do not use OTC nonsteroidal anti-inflammatory drugs without consulting prescriber.
- Do not drive or operate machinery until reaction to drug is known. It may cause dizziness.

EPOETIN ALFA (HUMAN RECOMBINANT ERYTHROPOIETIN) (Pr)

(e-po-e-tin)

Epogen, Eprex ♣, Procrit, Retacrit

Classification: HEMATOPOIETIC GROWTH FACTOR

Therapeutic: ANTIANEMIC; HUMAN ERYTHROPOIETIN

AVAILABILITY Solution for injection

ACTION & *THERAPEUTIC EFFECT* Human erythropoietin is produced in the kidney and stimulates bone marrow production of RBCs (erythropoiesis). Hypoxia and anemia generally increase the production of erythropoietin. Epoetin alpha stimulates RBC production. *Stimulates the production of RBCs in the bone marrow of severely anemic patients.*

USES Treatment of anemia due to CKD, chemotherapy, zidovudine treatment.

CONTRAINDICATIONS Uncontrolled hypertension and known hypersensitivity to mammalian cell–derived products and albumin (human); hamster protein hypersensitivity; uncontrolled hypertension; iron-deficiency anemia; pure red cell aplasia associated with erythropoietin protein drugs.

CAUTIOUS USE Leukemia, sickle cell disease; coagulopathy; seizure disorders; history of coronary artery bypass graft surgery (CABG); infection; pregnancy—fetal risk cannot be ruled out; lactation—infant risk cannot be ruled out; infants; neonates.

ROUTE & DOSAGE

Anemia of CKD

Adult: **Subcutaneous/IV** Start with 50–100 units/kg/dose three times a week until target Hct range of 30–33% (max: 36%) is reached; if Hgb increases more than 1 g/dL and approaches 12 g/dL, reduce dose by 25%. If after 4 wk there is less than 1 g/dL, increase dose by 25%.
Child/Infant: **IV/Subcutaneous** 50 units/kg 3 × wk (adjust as above)

Anemia Related to Chemotherapy

Adult: **Subcutaneous** 150 units/kg 3 × wk or 40,000 units once/wk when Hgb below 10 g/dL
Adolescent/Child (older than 5 yr): **IV** 600 units/kg/wk when Hgb below 10 g/dL

ADMINISTRATION

Subcutaneous

- Do not shake solution. Shaking may denature the glycoprotein, rendering it biologically inactive.
- Inspect solution for particulate matter prior to use. Do not use if solution is discolored or if it contains particulate matter.
- Use only one dose/vial, and do not reenter vial.
- Do not give with any other drug solution.

Intravenous

PREPARE: **Direct:** Give undiluted.
ADMINISTER: **Direct:** Give direct IV as a bolus dose over 1 min.
INCOMPATIBILITIES: **Solution/additive:** D10W, normal saline. **Y-site: Amphotericine B, chlorpromazine, dantrolene, diazepam, diazoxide, haloperidol, inamrinone, midazolam, minocycline, pentamidine, phenytoin, prochlorperazine, sulfamethoxazole-trimethoprim, vancomycin.** ▪ Discard any unused portion of the vial. It contains no preservatives.

- Store at 2°–8°C (36°–46°F). Do not freeze or shake.

ADVERSE EFFECTS (≥5%) **Respiratory:** Cough. **CNS:** Dizziness and *headache*. **Skin:** Injection site pain, itching. **GI:** Nausea, *vomiting*. **Musculoskeletal:** Joint pain, muscle pain. **Other:** Fever.

DIAGNOSTIC TEST INTERFERENCE May artificially lower ***HbA1C.***

INTERACTIONS **Drug:** Do not give concurrently with **darbepoetin alfa.** Monitor when used with **lenalidomide, nandrolone, pomalidomide, thalidomide.**

PHARMACOKINETICS **Onset:** within 10 days. **Metabolism:** In serum. **Elimination:** Minimal recovery in urine. **Half-Life:** 4–13 h.

NURSING IMPLICATIONS

Black Box Warning

Epoetin Alfa has been associated with increased risk of death, MI, stroke, venous thrombosis, vascular access thrombosis, and tumor progression.

E

Assessment & Drug Effects

- Control BP adequately prior to initiation of therapy and closely monitor and control during therapy. Hypertension is an adverse effect that **must be** controlled.
- Be aware that BP may rise during early therapy as Hct increases. Notify prescriber of a rapid rise in Hct (more than 4 points in 2 wk). Dosage will need to be reduced because of risk of serious hypertension.
- Monitor for hypertensive encephalopathy in patients with CRF during period of increasing Hct.
- Monitor for premonitory neurologic symptoms (i.e., aura, and report their appearance promptly). The potential for seizures exists during periods of rapid Hct increase (more than 4 points in 2 wk).
- Monitor closely for thrombotic events (e.g., MI, CVA, TIA), especially for patients with CRF.
- Monitor lab tests: Baseline transferrin and serum ferritin; Hgb at least weekly; periodic CBC with differential and platelet count, BUN, creatinine, and serum electrolytes.

Patient & Family Education

- Important for those with CDK to comply with antihypertensive medication and dietary restrictions.
- Do not drive or engage in other potentially hazardous activity during the first 90 days of therapy because of possible seizure activity.
- Report an unusual tiredness or lack of energy.
- Rotate injection sites when administering.
- Understand that headache is a common adverse effect. Report if severe or persistent, may indicate developing hypertension.

EPOPROSTENOL SODIUM (Pr)

(e-po-pros′te-nol)

Flolan

Classification: PROSTAGLANDIN; PULMONARY ANTIHYPERTENSIVE

Therapeutic: PULMONARY ANTIHYPERTENSIVE

AVAILABILITY Powder for injection

ACTION & *THERAPEUTIC EFFECT*

Naturally occurring prostaglandin that reduces right and left ventricular afterload, increases cardiac output, and increases stroke volume through its vasodilation effect. Potent pulmonary vasodilator that reduces pulmonary hypertension. *Potent vasodilator of pulmonary and systemic arterial vascular beds and an inhibitor of platelet aggregation.*

USES Long-term treatment of primary pulmonary hypertension in NYHA Class III and IV patients.

CONTRAINDICATIONS Hypersensitivity to **epoprostenol** or related compounds; chronic use with left ventricular systolic dysfunction in CHF patients; long-term use in patients who develop pulmonary edema during dose initiation; lactation.

CAUTIOUS USE Patients with risk factors for bleeding; older adults, pregnancy (category B). Safety and efficacy in children not established.

ROUTE & DOSAGE

Primary Pulmonary Hypertension

Adult (acute dose): **IV** Initiate with 2 ng/kg/min, increase by

2 ng/ kg/min q15min until dose-limiting effects occur (e.g., nausea, vomiting, headache, hypotension, flushing); **Chronic administration** Start infusion at 4 ng/kg/min less than the maximum tolerated infusion; if maximum tolerated infusion is 5 ng/ kg/min or less, start *maintenance infusion* at 50% of maximum tolerated dose

Intravenous

PREPARE: **Continuous** Note: **Must be** reconstituted using sterile diluent for epoprostenol; must not be mixed with any other medications or solution prior to or during administration. ▪ To make 100 mL of 3000 ng/mL, add 5 mL of the supplied diluent to one 0.5-mg vial; withdraw 3 mL, and add to enough diluent to make a total of 100 mL. ▪ To make 100 mL of 5000 ng/mL, add 5 mL of diluent to one 0.5-mg vial; withdraw contents of vial, and add to enough diluent to make a total of 100 mL. ▪ To make 100 mL of 10,000 ng/ mL, add 5 mL of diluent to each of two 0.5-mg vials; withdraw contents of each vial, and add to enough diluent to make a total of 100 mL. ▪ To make 100 mL of 15,000 ng/mL, add 5 mL of diluent to a 1.5-mg vial; withdraw contents of vial, and add to enough diluent to make a total of 100 mL.

ADMINISTER: **Continuous:** Give at ordered rate using an infusion control device. Avoid abrupt infusion interruption or large dosage reduction.

INCOMPATIBILITIES: **Solution/ additive:** Do not mix or infuse with any other parenteral drugs or solutions prior to or during administration.

▪ Store unopened vials at 15°–25°C (59°–77°F). Protect from light. ▪ See manufacturer's directions for stability or storage of reconstituted solutions.

ADVERSE EFFECTS **CV:** *Tachycardia, hypotension, flushing, chest pain*, bradycardia. **Respiratory:** Dyspnea. **CNS:** *Chills, fever, flu-like syndrome, dizziness*, syncope, *headache, anxiety/ nervousness*, agitation, hyperesthesia, paresthesia, dizziness. **GI:** *Diarrhea, nausea, vomiting, anorexia*, abdominal pain. **Musculoskeletal:** *Jaw pain, myalgia, nonspecific musculoskeletal pain*. **Dermatologic:** Dermal ulcer, eczema, skin rash, urticaria. **Other:** Dose-limiting effects.

INTERACTIONS **Drug:** Hypotension if administered with other VASODILATORS or ANTIHYPERTENSIVES.

PHARMACOKINETICS **Peak:** Approximately 15 min. **Metabolism:** Rapidly hydrolyzed at neutral pH in blood; also subject to enzyme degradation. **Elimination:** 82% in urine. **Half-Life:** Approximately 6 min.

NURSING IMPLICATIONS

Assessment & Drug Effects

- Assess carefully for development of pulmonary edema during dose ranging.
- Monitor respiratory and cardiovascular status frequently during entire period of chronic use of epoprostenol.
- Monitor for and report recurrence or worsening of symptoms associated with primary pulmonary hypertension (e.g., dyspnea, dizziness, exercise intolerance) or adverse effects of drug; dosage adjustments may be needed.

Patient & Family Education

- Learn correct techniques for storage, reconstitution, and

administration of drug, and maintenance of catheter site (see ADMINISTRATION).
- Notify prescriber immediately of S&S of worsening primary pulmonary hypertension, adverse drug reactions, and S&S of infection at catheter site or sepsis.

EPROSARTAN MESYLATE

(e-pro-sar'tan)

Classification: ANGIOTENSIN II RECEPTOR BLOCKER; ANGIOTENSIN II RECEPTOR ANTAGONIST, ANTIHYPERTENSIVE

Therapeutic: ANTIHYPERTENSIVE

Prototype: Losartan potassium

AVAILABILITY Tablet

ACTION & *THERAPEUTIC EFFECT* Selectively blocks the binding of angiotensin II to the AT_1 receptors found in many tissues. This blocks vasoconstricting and aldosterone-secreting effects of angiotensin II, thus resulting in an antihypertensive effect. *It decreases both the systolic and diastolic BP.*

USES Treatment of hypertension.

CONTRAINDICATIONS Hypersensitivity to eprosartan, losartan, or other angiotensin II receptor antagonists; pregnancy (category D); lactation.

CAUTIOUS USE Angioedema, aortic or mitral value stenosis, coronary artery disease, cardiomyopathy, hypotension, CHF; biliary obstruction; older adults; severe hepatic dysfunction, renal artery stenosis, renal disease, renal impairment. Safe use in children younger than 18 yr not established.

ROUTE & DOSAGE

Hypertension

Adult: **PO** 600 mg daily titrate based on patient response up to 800 mg/day in 1–2 divided doses

ADMINISTRATION

Oral

- May be taken with or without food.
- Correct volume depletion prior to therapy to prevent hypotension.
- Store at 20°–25°C (68°–77°F).

ADVERSE EFFECTS **Respiratory:** URI.

INTERACTIONS **Drug:** Use of another ARB does not provide any additional benefits. Use caution with **lithium** due to increased lithium toxicity risk. Use of DIURETICS or other ANTIHYPERTENSIVES may increase hypotension risk; do not use with **aliskiren.**

PHARMACOKINETICS **Absorption:** Only 13% of oral dose reaches systemic circulation. **Peak:** 1–2 h. **Metabolism:** Minimal metabolism. **Elimination:** 61% in feces and 37% in urine. **Half-Life:** 5–9 h.

NURSING IMPLICATION

Black Box Warning

Eprosartan has been associated with fetal injury and death.

Assessment & Drug Effects

- Monitor BP periodically; do trough readings just before scheduled dose when possible.
- Monitor for S&S of angioedema (may occur within 30 min or as long as 30 days after initial dose).

- Monitor lab tests: Periodic LFTs, BUN and creatinine, serum potassium, sodium, CBC with differential.

Patient & Family Education

- Inform prescriber immediately of pregnancy. Drug should be discontinued as soon as possible.
- Report episodes of dizziness especially associated with position changes.
- Report swelling of lips, tongue, face, or feeling of obstruction in neck immediately.

EPTIFIBATIDE

(ep-ti-fib′a-tide)

Integrilin

Classification: ANTIPLATELET; PLATELET GLYCOPROTEIN (GP IIB/IIIA) INHIBITOR

Therapeutic: ANTIPLATELET

AVAILABILITY Solution for injection

ACTION & *THERAPEUTIC EFFECT* Binds to the glycoprotein IIb/IIIa (GPIIb/IIIa) receptor sites of platelets. *Inhibits platelet aggregation by preventing fibrinogen, von Willebrand factor, and other molecules from adhering to GPIIb/IIIa receptor sites on platelets.*

USES Treatment of acute coronary syndromes (unstable angina, non-ST-element MI) and patients undergoing percutaneous coronary interventions (PCIs).

UNLABELED USES ST-elevation MI

CONTRAINDICATIONS Hypersensitivity to eptifibatide; active bleeding; GI or GU bleeding within 6 wk; thrombocytopenia; renal failure requiring dialysis; coagulopathy; recent major surgery or trauma within the last 6 weeks; intracranial neoplasm, history of stroke within 30 days or any history of hemorrhagic stroke; severe hypertension (systolic blood pressure greater than 200 mmHg or diastolic blood pressure greater than 110 mmHg), aneurysm; pregnancy—fetal risk cannot be ruled out; lactation—infant risk cannot be ruled out.

CAUTIOUS USE Hypersensitivity to related compounds (e.g. tirofiban, lamifiban); elderly; safety and efficacy in children not established.

ROUTE & DOSAGE

Acute Coronary Syndromes (ACS)

Adult: **IV** 180-mcg/kg initial bolus (max: 22.6 mg) followed by 2 mcg/kg/min (max 15 mg/h); after 10 min, a second 180-mcg/kg bolus should be given

Percutaneous Coronary Interventions (PCI)

Adult: **IV** 180-mcg/kg initial bolus followed by 2 mcg/kg/min (max 15 mg/h); after 10 min, a second 180-mcg/kg bolus should be given; the infusion should continue up to 24 h after the end of the procedure

Renal Impairment Dosage Adjustment

CrCl 10–49 mL/min: Give 1 mcg/kg/min continuous infusion

ADMINISTRATION

- Note: Review contraindications to administration prior to giving this drug.

E

Intravenous

PREPARE: **Direct:** Give undiluted.
ADMINISTER: **Direct:** Give bolus doses IV push over 1–2 min. **Continuous** Start continuous infusion immediately following bolus dose. ▪ Give undiluted directly from the 100-mL vial (at a rate based on patient's weight) using a vented infusion set. ▪ May be given in the same IV line with NS or D5/NS (either solution may contain up to 60 mEq KCl).

▪ Store unopened vials at 2°–8°C (36°–46°F) and protect from light. Vials may be stored for up to 2 mo under controlled room temperature at 25°C (77°F) with excursions permitted between 15° and 30°C (59° and 86°F). Discard any unused portion in opened vial.

ADVERSE EFFECTS (≥5%) **CV:** Hypotension. **Hematologic:** *Bleeding* (minor bleeding 3% to 13.1%; major bleeding 1.3% to 10.8%), thrombocytopenia.

INTERACTIONS **Drug:** ORAL ANTICOAGULANTS, NSAIDS, **dipyridamole, ticlopidine**, may increase risk of bleeding.

PHARMACOKINETICS **Duration:** 6–8 h after stopping infusion. **Metabolism:** Minimally metabolized. **Elimination:** 50% in urine. **Half-Life:** 2.5 h.

NURSING IMPLICATIONS

Assessment & Drug Effects

- Prior to infusion determine PT/aPTT and INR, activated clotting time (ACT) for those undergoing percutaneous coronary intervention (PCI); Hct or Hgb; platelet count; and serum creatinine.
- Minimize all vascular and other trauma during treatment. When obtaining IV access, avoid using a noncompressible site such as the subclavian vein.
- Monitor carefully for and immediately report S&S of bleeding (e.g., femoral artery access site bleeding, intracerebral hemorrhage, GI bleeding).
- Immediately stop infusion of eptifibatide and heparin if bleeding at the arterial access site cannot be controlled by pressure.
- Achieve hemostasis at the arterial access site by standard compression for a minimum of 4 h prior to hospital discharge following discontinuation of eptifibatide and heparin.
- Monitor lab tests: Baseline and periodic aPTT and INR (target aPPT, 50–70 sec); Hgb, Hct, during PCI (target ACT, 300–350 sec); serum creatinine baseline.

Patient & Family Education

- Advise patient that bleeding may take longer to stop after the infusion. Pressure may be applied to bleeding sites postinfusion.
- Bedrest may be required during and several hours postinfusion.
- Report uncontrolled bleeding and any dizziness, fainting, or light-headedness.
- Instruct and provide demonstration of taking blood pressure for at-home monitoring.

EPTINEZUMAB-JJMR

(ep-ti-nez-ue-mab)

Vyepti

Classification: CALCITONIN GENE-RELATED PEPTIDE RECEPTOR ANTAGONIST
Therapeutic: ANTIMIGRAINE

AVAILABILITY Solution for injection

ACTION & *THERAPEUTIC EFFECT* A humanized monoclonal antibody that binds to calcitonin gene-related peptide (CGRP) ligand and blocks its binding to the receptor. The mechanism by which it exerts its clinical effects is unknown. *Used to prevent migraines.*

USES Prevention of migraine.

CONTRAINDICATIONS Hypersensitivity to eptinezumab-jjmr or any of the inactive substances in the drug.

CAUTIOUS USE No disease processes or population cautions listed.

ROUTE & DOSAGE

Migraine prophylaxis

Adult: **IV** 100 mg or 300 mg every 3 mo

ADMINISTRATION

Intravenous Infusion—ONLY; Do not give by IV push or bolus.

PREPARE: Vial solution is clear to slightly opalescent and colorless to brownish-yellow; do not use if discolored or cloudy. Requires dilution prior to administration. Withdraw 1 mL of either the 100- or 300-mg vial and dilute only in NS bags made of polyvinyl chloride (PVC), polyethylene (PE), or polyolefin (PO). Single-dose vials contain no preservative; discard unused portion. Gently invert diluted solution to mix; do not shake. Diluted solution must be infused within 8 h; during this time, it can be stored at room temperature, 20°–25°C (68°–77°F); do not freeze.

ADMINISTER: **IV Infusion:** Administer IV over 30 min using an infusion set with a 0.2-micron or 0.22-micron in-line or add-on sterile filter. No other medications should be administered through the infusion set with eptinezumab-jjmr.

- Store refrigerated between 2° and 8°C (36° and 46°F) in the original carton; protect from light. Do not freeze or shake.

ADVERSE EFFECTS (>5%) **Respiratory:** Nasopharyngitis. **Other:** Antibody development.

INTERACTIONS None defined by the manufacturer.

PHARMACOKINETICS **Distribution:** 3.7 L. **Metabolism:** Nonspecific proteolysis. **Half-Life:** 27 d.

NURSING IMPLICATIONS

Assessment & Drug Effects

- Monitor frequency of migraines.
- Monitor for signs and symptoms of nasopharygitis: Nasal congestion, runny nose, sneezing, coughing, sore or scratchy throat, itchy watery eyes, or tiredness.

Patient & Family Education

- Report to healthcare provider development of nasal congestion, runny nose, sneezing, coughing, sore or scratchy throat, itchy watery eyes, or tiredness.

ERAVACYCLINE

(er-a-va-sye-kleen)

Xerava

Classification: TETRACYCLINE ANTIBIOTICS

Therapeutic: ANTIBIOTICS

Prototype: Tetracycline

E

AVAILABILITY Solution for injection

ACTION & *THERAPEUTIC EFFECT* A synthetic fluorocycline antibacterial within the tetracycline class. It disrupts the bacterial protein synthesis. Bacteriostatic against gram-positive bacteria and potentially bactericidal against some strains of *E. coli* and *Klebsiella pneumoniae*. *Helpful in treating complicated intrabdominal infections.*

USES Treatment of complicated intra-abdominal infections caused by susceptible organisms.

UNLABELED USES Treatment of infections caused by susceptible organisms.

CONTRAINDICATIONS Known hypersensitivity to eravacycline, tetracycline-class antibacterial drugs, or to any of the inactive substances in the drug.

CAUTIOUS USE Patients with history of decreased liver function or immunosuppression.

ROUTE & DOSAGE

Intra-abdominal Infections

Adult: **IV** 1 mg/kg q12h over 60 minutes × 4–14 days

Hepatic Impairment Dosage Adjustment

Child–Pugh class C: Initial dose 1 mg/kg q12h on day 1, followed by 1 mg/kg q24h for total treatment duration

ADMINISTRATION

Intravenous use only

PREPARE: Reconstitute each vial with 5 mL of sterile water for injection. Swirl vial gently until powder dissolves completely; avoid shaking or rapid movement to prevent foaming. Further dilute reconstituted solution in NS infusion bag to a final concentration of 0.3 mg/mL.

ADMINISTER: **IV Infusion:** May be administered IV through a dedicated line or through a Y-site. Infuse diluted solution over approximately 60 min. If the IV line is used for several drugs, the line should be flushed before and after eravacycline administration with NS.

INCOMPATIBILITIES: Do not mix with other drugs or solutions containing other drugs.

- Use reconstituted vial within 6 h if stored at room temperature (not to exceed 36°C or 77°F) or within 24 h if stored refrigerated (2°–8°C/36°–46°F). Do not freeze.

ADVERSE EFFECTS (>5%) **Skin:** *Infusion reaction.* **GI:** *Nausea, vomiting.*

INTERACTIONS **Drug:** Depressed plasma prothrombin activity may require decreased dose of anticoagulant medications (**warfarin**). Strong CYP3A4 inducers (e.g., **rifampin, phenytoin, carbamazepine, efavirenz,** and **phenobarbital**) can decrease efficacy and require increased dose of eravacycline.

PHARMACOKINETICS **Distribution:** 321 L; 79–100% protein bound. **Metabolism:** In the liver; primarily through CYP3A4 and FMO-mediated oxidation. **Elimination:** 34% and 47% excreted unchanged in urine and feces, respectively. **Half-Life:** 20 h.

NURSING IMPLICATIONS

Assessment & Drug Effects

- Development of diarrhea, consider *C. diff* associated.
- Improvement of intra-abdominal infection.
- Monitor lab tests: CBC, blood culture, and susceptibility studies.

Patient & Family Education

- Most likely side effects are nausea and vomiting.
- Contact healthcare provider if diarrhea develops prior to taking any over-the-counter antidiarraheal medication.

ERENUMAB-AOOE

(e-ren'ue mab-aooe)

Aimovig

Classification: CGRP RECEPTOR ANTAGONIST; MONOCLONAL ANTIBODY

Therapeutic: ANTIMIGRAINE

AVAILABILITY Subcutaneous injection; single-dose prefilled syringe; autoinjector

ACTION & THERAPEUTIC EFFECT Erenumab is a human immunoglobulin G2 (IgG2) monoclonal antibody that binds to calcitonin gene-related peptide receptors and antagonizes their function. *It is thought that this activity helps to prevent migraine headaches.*

USES Preventative treatment of migraines.

CONTRAINDICATIONS Hypersensitivity to erenumab-aooe or any component of the product.

CAUTIOUS USE Prefilled syringe and autoinjector both contain a derivative of latex, which may cause an allergic reaction in patients sensitive to latex.

ROUTE & DOSAGE

Migraine Prophylaxis

Adult: **Subcutaneous** 70 mg once a mo

ADMINISTRATION

Subcutaneous

- Intended for self-administration.
- Subcutaneous injection should be allowed to warm at room temperature 30 min prior to injection.
- Protect from direct sunlight. Do not warm by using heat source such as hot water or microwave. Do not shake. Do not use if solution is cloudy, discolored or contains flakes or particles.
- Syringe or autoinjectors should not be shaken prior to use.
- Injection should be given in abdomen, thigh, or upper arm; avoid injecting erenumab in areas where the skin is compromised or bruised.
- Store in refrigerator at 2°–8°C (36°–46°F) in original carton protected from light; may be kept at room temperature for up to 7 days.

ADVERSE EFFECTS **Skin:** Injection site reactions, erythema, pruritus. **GI:** Constipation, cramps. **Musculoskeletal:** Muscle spasms. **Other:** Antibody formation.

E

PHARMACOKINETICS Absorption: 82% bioavailability. **Peak:** 6 days. **Metabolism:** Reaches peak saturation at CGRP receptors, then elimination depends on proteolytic pathways similar to endogenous proteins. **Half-Life:** 28 days.

NURSING IMPLICATIONS

Assessment & Drug Effects

- New onset or worsening of hypertension may occur at any time. Cases of hypertension were reported after the first dose. Monitor blood pressure before administering and after administration.
- Monitor frequency and consistency of stools. Severe constipation is a risk. Encourage plenty of fluids, high fiber diet and regular exercise for patients that have no orders to the contrary.
- Patient to monitor number of monthly migraine days.

Patient & Family Education

- Notify prescriber if you have a latex allergy.
- Notify prescriber if you plan to become pregnant or are pregnant or breastfeeding.
- Notify prescriber if you experience any signs of an allergic reaction: Wheezing, tightness in the chest or throat, swelling of the mouth, face, lips, tongue, or throat, rash, hives, itching, or blistering skin.
- Teach patient or family member how to take blood pressure for monitoring at home. Patients should report and new or worsening hypertension to healthcare provider.
- Report any episodes of severe constipation to healthcare provider.
- Provide opportunity for patient or family member to demonstrate correct technique for subcutaneous injection.
- Report any injection pain accompanied by severe muscle cramps or spasms.

ERGOCALCIFEROL

(er-goe-kal-si'fe-role)

Calcidol, Calciferol, Drisdol, D-Forte ♣, Vitamin D_2

Classification: VITAMIN D ANALOG

Therapeutic: VITAMIN D ANALOG

Prototype: Calcitriol

AVAILABILITY Oral liquid; capsule, tablet

ACTION & *THERAPEUTIC EFFECT* The name vitamin D encompasses two related fat-soluble substances. Vitamin D acts like a hormone in that it is distributed through the circulation and plays a major regulatory role. Responsible for regulation of serum calcium level. *Maintains normal blood calcium and phosphate ion levels by enhancing their intestinal absorption and by promoting mobilization of calcium from bone and renal tubular resorption of phosphate.*

USES Vitamin D insufficiency/deficiency, rickets, osteoporosis prevention, hypoparathyroidism.

CONTRAINDICATIONS Hypersensitivity to vitamin D, hypervitaminosis D, hypercalcemia, hyperphosphatemia, renal osteodystrophy with hyperphosphatemia, malabsorption syndrome, decreased kidney function.

CAUTIOUS USE Coronary disease; arteriosclerosis (especially in older adults); history of kidney stones; biliary tract disease; pregnancy—fetal risk cannot be ruled out; lactation (infant risk is minimal).

E

ROUTE & DOSAGE

Prevention of Osteoporosis

Adult: **PO** 800–1000 units/day

Vitamin D Insufficiency

Adult/Adolescent/Child/Infant: **PO** Varies depended on target serum 25 (OH) D levels, see package insert

ADMINISTRATION

Oral

- Swallow tablets; do not chew.
- Store at 2°–8°C (35.6°–46.4°F). Preserve in tightly covered, light-resistant containers. Drug decomposes when exposed to light and air.

ADVERSE EFFECTS (common)

GI: Constipation, loss of appetite, nausea.

INTERACTIONS **Drug: Cholestyramine, colestipol, mineral oil, orlistat**, may decrease absorption of vitamin D. Avoid use of **sucralfate** or **aluminum hydroxide** due to increased aluminum serum levels. Other sources of vitamin D (multivitamins) may increase risk of adverse effects.

PHARMACOKINETICS **Absorption:** Readily from GI tract. **Peak:** After 4 wk. **Duration:** 2 mo or more. **Distribution:** Most of drug first appears in lymph, stored chiefly in liver and in skin, brain, spleen, and bones. **Metabolism:** In liver and kidney to active metabolites. **Elimination:** Fecal; but may be stored in tissues for months. **Half-Life:** 12–24 h.

NURSING IMPLICATIONS

Assessment & Drug Effects

- Monitor closely patients receiving therapeutic doses of vitamin D; must remain under close medical supervision.
- Monitor for hypercalcemia; in patients with osteomalacia a decrease in serum alkaline phosphatase may signal the onset of hypercalcemia.
- Expect monthly bone x-rays.
- Monitor lab tests: Baseline and periodic serum calcium and phosphorus.

Patient & Family Education

- Avoid magnesium-containing antacids and laxatives with chronic kidney failure when receiving vitamin D preparations because vitamin D increases the risk of magnesium intoxication.
- Maintain adequate intake of calcium with drug.
- Do not use OTC medications unless approved by prescriber.
- Avoid using any additional Vitamin D supplements.

ERGOTAMINE TARTRATE

(er-got′a-meen)

Ergomar

Classification: ALPHA-ADRENERGIC ANTAGONIST; ERGOT ALKALOID

Therapeutic: ANTIMIGRAINE

AVAILABILITY Sublingual tablet

ACTION & *THERAPEUTIC EFFECT*

Natural amino acid alkaloid of ergot. Alpha-adrenergic blocking agent with direct-stimulating action on cranial and peripheral vascular smooth muscles and depressant effect on central vasomotor centers.

In vascular headache, exerts vasoconstrictive action on previously dilated cerebral vessels, reduces amplitude of arterial pulsations, and antagonizes effects of serotonin.

E

USES As single agent or in combination with caffeine to prevent or abort migraine, cluster headache (histamine cephalalgia), and other vascular headaches.

CONTRAINDICATIONS Hypersensitivity to ergotamine; sepsis, obliterative vascular disease, thromboembolic disease, prolonged use of excessive dosage, liver and kidney disease, severe pruritus, diabetes mellitus; marked arteriosclerosis, history of MI, peripheral vascular disease; coronary artery disease, angina; basilar/hemiplegic migraine; hepatic disease; biliary tract disease; cholestasis; hypertension; infectious states, anemia, malnutrition; concurrent administration of potent CYP3A4 inhibitors (e.g., protease inhibitors and macrolide antibiotics); pregnancy (category X).

CAUTIOUS USE Older adult patients; lactation (infant risk cannot be ruled out). Safe use in children not established.

ROUTE & DOSAGE

Vascular Headaches

Adult: **SL** 2 mg followed by 2 mg q30min until headache abates or until max of 6 mg/24 h or 10 mg/wk

ADMINISTRATION

Sublingual

- For best results, take at the first sign of a migraine attack.
- Instruct patient to allow sublingual (SL) tablet to dissolve under tongue and not to drink, eat, or smoke while tablet is in place. Do not crush SL tablets.
- Store at 20°–25°C (68°–77°F). Excursions permitted from 15°–30°C (59°–86°C). Protect from heat and light.

ADVERSE EFFECTS **CV:** Absent pulse, bradycardia, edema, hypertension, tachycardia, cold extremities, cyanosis, abnormal ECG, gangrenous disorder, ischemia. **CNS:** Numbness, vertigo. **Skin:** Gangrene, pruritus. **GI:** Nausea, vomiting. **Musculoskeletal:** Weakness. **Other:** Withdrawal symptoms.

INTERACTIONS **Drug:** With high doses of BETA-ADRENERGIC BLOCKERS, SYMPATHOMIMETICS, possibility of additive vasoconstrictor effects; **erythromycin, troleandomycin** may cause severe peripheral vasospasm. **Eletriptan, naratriptan, rizatriptan, sumatriptan, or zolmitriptan** may increase risk of coronary ischemia, separate drugs by 24 h; AZOLE ANTIFUNGALS **(ketoconazole, itraconazole, fluconazole, clotrimazole), nefazodone, fluoxetine, fluvoxamine, amprenavir, delavirdine, efavirenz, indinavir, nelfinavir, ritonavir, and saquinavir**, may inhibit ergot metabolism and increase toxicity; **sibutramine, dexfenfluramine, nefazodone, fluvoxamine**, 5HT3 ANTAGONISTS may increase risk of serotonin syndrome. **Food: Grapefruit juice** may increase toxicity.

PHARMACOKINETICS **Absorption:** Variable. **Peak:** 0.5–3 h. **Distribution:** Crosses blood–brain barrier. **Metabolism:** Extensive first-pass metabolism in liver. **Elimination:** 96% in feces; excreted in breast milk. **Half-Life:** 2.7 h initial phase, 21 h terminal phase.

NURSING IMPLICATIONS

Assessment & Drug Effects

- Monitor adverse GI effects. Nausea and vomiting are adverse reactions that occur in about 10% of patients after they take ergotamine. Patient may need an antiemetic. Consult with prescriber.
- Drug abuse and psychological dependence have been reported.
- Monitor patients with PVD carefully for development of peripheral ischemia.
- Monitor long-term effectiveness. Patients receiving high ergotamine doses for prolonged periods may experience increased frequency of headaches, fatigue, and depression. Discontinuation of the drug in these patients results in severe withdrawal headache that may last a few days.
- Withdrawal symptoms (rebound headache) with long-term chronic use have been reported.
- Overdose symptoms: Nausea, vomiting, weakness, and pain in legs, numbness and tingling in fingers and toes, tachycardia or bradycardia, hypertension or hypotension, and localized edema.

Patient & Family Education

- Begin drug therapy as soon after onset of migraine attack as possible, preferably during migraine prodrome (scintillating scotomas, visual field defects, nausea, paresthesias usually on side opposite to that of the migraine).
- Notify prescriber if migraine attacks occur more frequently or are not relieved.
- Lie down in a quiet, dark room for 2–3 h after drug administration.
- Report muscle pain or weakness of extremities, cold or numb digits, irregular heartbeat, nausea, or vomiting. Carefully protect extremities from exposure to cold temperatures; provide warmth, but not heat, to ischemic areas.
- **Do not** increase dosage without consulting prescriber; overdosage is the chief cause of adverse effects from the drug.

E

ERIBULIN MESYLATE

(er-e-bu′lin)

Halaven

Classification: ANTINEOPLASTIC; MITOTIC INHIBITOR

Therapeutic: ANTINEOPLASTIC

AVAILABILITY Solution for injection

ACTION & *THERAPEUTIC EFFECT*

A microtubule inhibitor that blocks completion of the cell cycle and prevents cell replication resulting in apoptotic cell death. *Interferes with mitosis and cell replication thus reducing growth and metastatic spread of cancer cells.*

USES Treatment of metastatic breast cancer in patients; Unresectable or Metastatic Liposarcoma

CONTRAINDICATIONS Congenital long QT syndrome; ANC less than 1000 mm^3; platelets less than 75,000 mm^3; Grade 3 or 4 nonhematologic toxicities; pregnancy—fetal risk cannot be ruled out; lactation—infant risk cannot be ruled out.

CAUTIOUS USE Neutropenia; peripheral neuropathy; QT prolongation; hepatic impairment; renal impairment. Safety and efficacy in children not established.

ROUTE & DOSAGE

Metastatic Breast Cancer; Liposarcoma

Adult: **IV** 1.4 mg/m^2 days 1 and 8 of a 21-day cycle. Repeat cycle as needed or until unacceptable toxicities arise

Delay Doses for Any of the Following

If ANC less than 1000/mm^3, platelets less than 75,000/mm^3, or Grade 3 or 4 nonhematological toxicities: Do not administer eribulin; the day 8 dose may be delayed a max of 1 wk *If toxicities do not resolve to Grade 2 or better by day 15:* Omit the dose *If toxicities resolve or improve to Grade 2 or better by day 15:* Administer eribulin at a reduced dose and initiate the next cycle no sooner than 2 wk later

Hematologic Toxicity Dosage Adjustment

If ANC less than 500/mm^3 for more than 7 days, ANC less than 1000/mm^3 with fever or infection, platelets less than 25,000/mm^3 or less than 50,000/mm^3 requiring transfusion or day 8 of previous cycle omitted or delayed: Permanently reduce dose to 1.1 mg/m^2
If while receiving 1.1 mg/m^2, recurrence of hematologic event occurs, or if day 8 of previous cycle omitted or delayed: Permanently reduce dose to 0.7 mg/m^2
If while receiving 0.7 mg/m^2, recurrence of hematologic event occurs, or if day 8 of previous cycle omitted or delayed: Discontinue eribulin

Nonhematologic Toxicity Dosage Adjustment

If Grade 3 or 4 nonhematologic toxicity or if day 8 of previous cycle omitted or delayed: Permanently reduce dose to 1.1 mg/m^2
While receiving 1.1 mg/m^2, if recurrence of Grade 3 or 4 nonhematologic toxicity occurs, or if day 8 of previous cycle omitted or delayed: Permanently reduce dose to 0.7 mg/m^2
While receiving 0.7 mg/m^2, if recurrence of Grade 3 or 4 nonhematologic toxicity occurs, or if day 8 of previous cycle omitted or delayed: Discontinue eribulin

Hepatic Impairment Dosage Adjustment

Mild hepatic impairment (Child–Pugh class A): Reduce dose to 1.1 mg/m^2
Moderate hepatic impairment (Child–Pugh class B): Reduce dose to 0.7 mg/m^2

Renal Impairment Dosage Adjustment

CrCl 30–50 mL/min: Reduce dose to 1.1 mg/m^2

ADMINISTRATION

Intravenous

- Correct hypokalemia or hypomagnesemia prior to initiating eribulin.
- NIOSH: In preparation and administration of injections, use double gloves and protective gown. Eye/face and respiratory protection may be needed. If there is a potential that the substance could splash or if the patient may resist, use eye/face protection.

PREPARE: **IV Infusion:** May be given undiluted or diluted in 100 mL of NS. Do not dilute with dextrose. ***ADMINISTER:*** **IV Infusion:** Give over 2–5 min. Do not administer in same IV line as dextrose or any other required medication. ***INCOMPATIBILITIES:*** **Solution/additive:** Incompatible with D5W for dilution.

- Undiluted or diluted eribulin may be stored in a syringe or IV bag for up to 4 hours at room temperature or up to 24 hours under refrigeration.

- Store in original carton at 25°C (77°F), with excursions permitted between 15° and 30°C (59° and 86°F).

ADVERSE EFFECTS (≥5%) **CNS:** *Peripheral neuropathy.* **Endocrine:** Hypokalemia, hypocalcemia. **Skin:** *Alopecia.* **GI:** *Constipation.* **Hematological:** *Anemia, neutropenia.*

INTERACTIONS **Drug:** Eribulin has been associated with QT prolongation. Coadministration of another drug that prolongs the QT interval (e.g., **disopyramide, procainamide, amiodarone, bretylium, clarithromycin, levofloxacin**) may cause additive effects. Do not administer with LIVE VACCINES, MYELOSUPPRESSSIVE AGENTS.

PHARMACOKINETICS **Distribution:** 49–65% plasma protein bound. **Metabolism:** Minimal. **Elimination:** Fecal (82%) and renal (9%). **Half-Life:** 40 h.

NURSING IMPLICATIONS

Assessment & Drug Effects

- Monitor ECG in those with CHF, bradyarrhythmias, concurrent use of Class Ia and III antiarrhythmics, and electrolyte imbalances.
- Monitor closely for S&S of peripheral motor and sensory neuropathy.
- Monitor temperature. Report fever and/or S&S of infection.
- Withhold drug and notify prescriber of the following: Grade 3 or 4 peripheral neuropathy; hypokalemia or hypomagnesemia; prolonged QT interval.
- Monitor lab tests: Baseline and periodic serum electrolytes; CBC with differential prior to each dose and more often with Grade 3 or 4 cytopenia; periodic LFTs.

Patient & Family Education

- Report promptly fever (100.5°F or greater) or other S&S of infection.
- Report S&S of peripheral neuropathy, including: Tingling, numbness, deep pain in the feet, legs, or arms; weakness or problems with balance; or difficulty with fine motor skills.
- Effective methods of birth control are recommended during therapy. Notify prescriber immediately if a pregnancy develops.
- Do not breastfeed while taking this drug without consulting prescriber.

ERLOTINIB (Pr)

(er-lo'ti-nib)

Tarceva

Classification: ANTINEOPLASTIC; TYROSINE KINASE INHIBITOR; EPIDERMAL GROWTH FACTOR RECEPTOR INHIBITOR

Therapeutic: ANTINEOPLASTIC

AVAILABILITY Tablet

ACTION & *THERAPEUTIC EFFECT*

Erlotinib is a human epidermal growth factor receptor type 1 (HER1/EGFR) inhibitor. Antitumor action is believed to be due to inhibition of phosphorylation of tyrosine kinase associated with the EGFR present on the cell surface of both normal and cancer cells. *Inhibition of EGFR in cancer cells diminishes their capacity for cell proliferation, cell survival, and decreases metastases.*

USES Treatment of patients with locally advanced or metastatic non-small-cell lung cancer (NSCLC), pancreatic cancer.

E

CONTRAINDICATIONS Hypersensitivity to erlotinib; severe hepatic impairment; acute/worsening of ocular disorders such as eye pain; GI perforation; interstitial lung disease; severe renal impairment; exfoliative skin reaction; pregnancy (fetal risk has been demonstrated); lactation (infant risk cannot be ruled out).

CAUTIOUS USE Mild or moderate hepatic or renal impairment; history of peptic ulcers or diverticular disease; myelosuppression; ocular toxicities (corneal ulcer). Safety and efficacy in children not established.

ROUTE & DOSAGE

Metastatic Non-Small-Cell Lung Cancer

Adult: **PO** 150 mg once daily

Pancreatic Cancer (with Gemcitabine)

Adult: **PO** 100 mg daily

Hepatic Impairment Dosage Adjustment

Discontinue use in patient with severe change in liver function

Concomitant Smoking Dosage Adjustment

Increase dose at 2 wk intervals by 50 mg (max dose: 300 mg)

Concomitant CYP Inhibitor/Inducer Dosage Adjustment

See package insert

Renal Toxicity Dosage Adjustment

Grade 3 or 4 toxicity: Withhold treatment; if treatment is resumed reinitiate with a 50-mg dose reduction

ADMINISTRATION

Oral

- NIOSH recommends the use of single gloves by anyone handling intact tablets or capsules or administering from a unit-dose package.
- If crushing or cutting tablets, use of double gloves and protective gown. Wear additional eye/face protection if the formulation is difficult to swallow or if the patient may resist, vomit, or spit up.
- Give at least 1 h before or 2 h after eating.
- Separate administration time from concurrent antacid by several hours.
- Administer 10 h after a dose of an H_2 blocker and at least 2 h before the next dose of the 2 blocker.
- Store at 15°–30°C (59°–86°F). Keep container tightly closed. Protect from light.

ADVERSE EFFECTS **CV:** *Edema.* **Respiratory:** *Cough, shortness of breath.* **CNS:** Headache, anxiety, depression. **HEENT:** Conjunctivitis, keratoconjunctivitis. **Endocrine:** *Weight loss.* **Skin:** Alopecia, pruritus, *rash.* **GI:** *Abdominal pain, diarrhea,* flatulence, indigestion, inflammatory disease of mucous membranes, *loss of appetite, nausea, vomiting.* **Musculoskeletal:** *Bone pain,* muscle pain. **Other:** *Fatigue, fever.*

INTERACTIONS **Drug:** Dose will need to be adjusted with concurrent strong **CYP3A4 inducers**

(e.g., **carbamazepine, nevirapine, phenobarbital, phenytoin**). **Atazanavir, clarithromycin, conivaptan, fluvoxamine, idelalisib, indinavir, itraconazole, ketoconazole, nefazodone, nelfinavir, ritonavir, saquinavir, telithromycin, troleandomycin, voriconazole** may increase erlotinib levels and toxicity; increased bleeding with **warfarin.** Do not use with PROTON PUMP INHIBITORS. **Herbal: St. John's wort** may decrease erlotinib levels. **Food:** Avoid grapefruit juice.

PHARMACOKINETICS **Absorption:** 60% absorbed; food can increase to 100%. **Peak:** 4 h. **Metabolism:** In liver by CYP3A4. **Elimination:** In feces (83%). **Half-Life:** 36.2 h.

NURSING IMPLICATIONS

Assessment & Drug Effects

- Monitor closely changes in pulmonary function.
- Withhold drug and notify prescriber for acute onset of new or progressive pulmonary symptoms (e.g., dyspnea, cough, or fever) or significant changes in liver functions as indicated by elevated transaminases, bilirubin, and alkaline phosphatase.
- Monitor lab tests: Periodic LFTs, renal function, and serum electrolytes.

Patient & Family Education

- Report promptly any of the following: Severe or persistent diarrhea, nausea, anorexia, or vomiting; onset or worsening of unexplained shortness of breath or cough; eye irritation.
- Sun exposure can create or worsen skin reactions. Use sunscreen or avoid sun exposure.
- Monitor closely PT/INR values with concurrent warfarin therapy.
- Do not eat grapefruit or drink grapefruit juice with the drug.
- Cigarette smokers should report change in smoking routine as it impacts dosing.
- Women should use effective means to avoid pregnancy while taking this drug.

E

ERTAPENEM SODIUM

(er-ta-pen'em)

Invanz

Classification: BETA-LACTAM ANTIBIOTIC

Therapeutic: ANTIBIOTIC

Prototype: Imipenem-cilastatin

AVAILABILITY Solution for injection

ACTION & THERAPEUTIC EFFECT Broad-spectrum carbapenem antibiotic that inhibits the cell wall synthesis of gram-positive and gram-negative bacteria by its strong affinity for penicillin-binding proteins (PBPs) of the bacterial cell wall. *Effective against both gram-positive and gram-negative bacteria. Highly resistant to most bacterial beta-lactamases.*

USES Complicated intra-abdominal infections, complicated skin and skin structure infections, community-acquired pneumonia, complicated UTI (including pyelonephritis), and acute pelvic infections due to susceptible bacteria.

CONTRAINDICATIONS Hypersensitivity to ertapenem, penicillins, or carbapenem antibiotics; hypersensitivity to amide-type local anesthetics such as lidocaine; hypersensitivity to meropenem or imipenem.

CAUTIOUS USE Hypersensitivity to other beta-lactam antibiotics (penicillins, cephalosporins);

hypersensitivity to other allergens; renal impairment; history of CNS disorders; history of seizures; meningitis; older adults; pregnancy (category B); lactation (bottle feed during and for 5 days after therapy ends). Safe use in infants younger than 3 mo not established.

E

ROUTE & DOSAGE

Community-Acquired Pneumonia; Complicated UTI

Adult/Adolescent: **IV/IM** 1 g daily × 10–14 days; may switch to appropriate **PO** antibiotic after 3 days if responding
Child/Infant (3 mo or older): **IV/IM** 15 mg/kg q12h × 10–14 days (max: 1 g/day)

Intra-Abdominal Infection

Adult/Adolescent: **IV/IM** 1 g daily × 5–14 days
Child/Infant (3 mo or older): **IV/IM** 15 mg/kg bid × 5–14 days (max: 1 g/day)

Skin and Skin Structure Infections

Adult/Adolescent: **IV/IM** 1 g daily × 7–14 days
Child/Infant (3 mo or older): **IV/IM** 15 mg/kg bid × 7–14 days (max: 1 g/day)

Acute Pelvic Infections

Adult: **IV/IM** 1 g daily × 3–10 days

Renal Impairment Dosage Adjustment

CrCl less than 30 mL/min: Reduce dose to 500 mg daily

ADMINISTRATION

Intramuscular

- Reconstitute 1 g vial with 3.2 mL of 1% lidocaine HCl injection (without epinephrine). Shake vial thoroughly to form solution. Use immediately.
- Inject deep IM into a large muscle mass (such as the gluteal muscles or lateral part of the thigh).
- The reconstituted IM solution should be used within 1 h after preparation. Note: **Do not** use this solution for IV administration.

Intravenous

PREPARE: **Intermittent for Adult/Child:** Reconstitute 1-g vial with 10 mL of sterile water for injection, NS, or bacteriostatic water for injection. Shake well to dissolve. **Intermittent for Adult/Child (13 yr or older):** Immediately after reconstitution, transfer contents to 50 mL of NS injection solution. **Intermittent for Child (3 mo–12 yr):** Immediately after reconstitution, transfer required dose to enough NS injection solution to yield a final concentration of 20 mg/mL or less.
ADMINISTER: **Intermittent:** Infuse over 30 min. Note: Infusion should be completed within 6 h of reconstitution.
INCOMPATIBILITIES: **Solution/additive:** **Mannitol, sodium bicarbonate.** **Y-site:** **Alemtuzumab, allopurinol, amiodarone, amphotericin B, anidulafungin, caspofungin, chlorpromazine, dantrolene, daunorubicin, diazepam, dobutamine, doxorubicin, droperidol, epirubicin, hydralazine, hydroxyzine, idarubicin, midazolam, minocycline, mitoxantrone, nicardipine, ondansetron, pentamidine, phenytoin, prochlorperazine, promethazine, quinupristin/dalfopristin, thiopental, topotecan, verapamil.**

▪ Store lyophilized powder above 25°C (77°F). ▪ Must use reconstituted solution stored at room temperature (not above 25°C/77°F) within 6 h. ▪ May store for 24 h under refrigeration. Use within 4 h of removal from refrigeration. ▪ Do not freeze.

ADVERSE EFFECTS **CV:** Chest pain, hypertension, hypotension, tachycardia, edema. **Respiratory:** Cough, dyspnea, pharyngitis, rales/rhonchi, and respiratory distress. **CNS:** Anxiety, altered mental status, dizziness, headache, insomnia. **Skin:** Erythema, pruritus, rash. **GI:** Abdominal pain, *diarrhea*, acid regurgitation, constipation, dyspepsia, nausea, vomiting, increased AST and ALT. **GU:** Vaginitis. **Other:** Phlebitis or thrombosis at injection site, asthenia, fatigue, <u>death</u>, fever, leg pain.

INTERACTIONS **Drug:** **Probenecid** decreases renal excretion. **Valproic acid** levels may be decreased.

PHARMACOKINETICS **Absorption:** 90% from IM site. **Peak:** 2.3 h. **Distribution:** 95% protein bound, distributes into breast milk. **Metabolism:** Hydrolysis of beta-lactam ring. **Elimination:** 80% in urine, 10% in feces. **Half-Life:** 4.5 h.

NURSING IMPLICATIONS

Assessment & Drug Effects

- Determine history of hypersensitivity reactions to other beta-lactams, cephalosporins, penicillins, or other drugs.
- Discontinue drug and immediately report S&S of hypersensitivity (see Appendix F).
- Report S&S of superinfection or pseudomembranous colitis (see Appendix F).
- Monitor for seizures especially in older adults and those with renal insufficiency.
- Monitor lab tests: Periodic LFTs, CBC, platelet count, and routine blood chemistry during prolonged therapy.

Patient & Family Education

- Learn S&S of hypersensitivity, superinfection, and pseudomembranous colitis (see Appendix F); report any of these to prescriber promptly.

E

ERTUGLIFLOZIN

(er-too-gli-floe′zin)

Steglatro

Classification: ANTIDIABETIC; SODIUM-GLUCOSE COTRANSPORTER 2 (SGLT2) INHIBITOR

Therapeutic: ANTIDIABETIC; SGLT2 INHIBITOR

Prototype: Canagliflozin

AVAILABILITY Tablet

ACTION & *THERAPEUTIC EFFECT* Inhibits the sodium-glucose cotransporter 2 (SGLT2) in the proximal renal tubules that is responsible for the majority of the reabsorption of filtered glucose in the kidneys. *Inhibits SGLT2 thus allowing more glucose to be removed from the bloodstream and excreted by the kidneys.*

USES Adjunct therapy for the treatment of type 2 diabetes mellitus in combination with diet and exercise.

CONTRAINDICATIONS History of serious hypersensitivity reaction to ertugliflozin; Type 1 DM; severe renal impairment (eGFR of 30 mL/min/1.73m^2), ESRD, or on dialysis; severe hepatic impairment; lactation.

E

CAUTIOUS USE Hypotension; cardiovascular disease; diabetic ketoacidosis renal impairment; low systolic blood pressure; increases in low-density cholesterol; moderate hepatic impairment; renal insufficiency, reduced intravascular volume; history of genital mycotic infections; older adults; pregnancy (category C). Safety and efficacy in children younger than 18 yr not established; history of pancreatitis.

ROUTE & DOSAGE

Type 2 Diabetes Mellitus

Adult: **PO** 5 mg once a day (max: 15 mg once a day)

ADMINISTRATION

Oral

- Taken with or without food.
- Store tablets at 2°–8°C (36°–46°F), protect from moisture.

ADVERSE EFFECTS **CV:** Hypotension. **Respiratory:** Nasopharyngitis. **CNS:** Headache. **Endocrine:** Increased LDL, Hypoglycemia, ketoacidosis, weight loss, kidney injury, hypovolemia, increased serum phosphate. **GU:** Genital candidiasis, urinary tract infections, increased urinary frequency, increased serum creatinine. **Musculoskeletal:** Back pain, bone fractures. **Other:** increased risk of lower limb amputation, thirst.

INTERACTIONS **Drug:** May enhance the hypoglycemic effects of SULFONYLUREAS and insulins.

PHARMACOKINETICS **Absorption:** Roughly 100% bioavailability at highest dose. **Peak:** 1 h. **Distribution:** 93.6% protein bound. **Metabolism:** Primarily metabolized by O-glucuronidation through UGT1A9 and UGT2B-7; CYP-mediated metabolism is minimal. **Elimination:** 50% feces and 41 % urine. **Half-Life:** 16.6 h.

NURSING IMPLICATIONS

Assessment & Drug Effects

- Monitor for S&S of genital mycotic infection or urinary tract infection.
- Obtain baseline blood pressure and evaluate for changes.
- Monitor for lower limb and feet sores, ulcers, or infection.
- Monitor lab tests: Plasma glucose (HbA1C) at least twice yearly, renal function tests, serum phosphate, serum LDL.

Patient & Family Education

- Check your blood sugar as you have been told by prescriber.
- Do not drive if your blood sugar has been low.
- Have your bloodwork checked as ordered by prescriber.
- Talk with prescriber before drinking alcohol.

ERYTHROMYCIN (Pr)

(er-ith-roe-mye′sin)

Ery-Tab, Erythromid ♣, Erythromycin Base, Novo-Rythro ♣

ERYTHROMYCIN STEARATE

Classification: MACROLIDE ANTIBIOTIC

Therapeutic: ANTIBIOTIC

AVAILABILITY **Erythromycin:** Tablet; delayed release tablet; capsule; topical solution; gel; ointment pledgets; ophthalmic ointment. **Erythromycin Stearate:** Tablet

ACTION & *THERAPEUTIC EFFECT* Macrolide antibiotic that binds to the 50S ribosomal subunit, thus inhibiting bacterial protein synthesis. *More active against gram-positive organisms than against gram-negative organisms due to its superior penetration into gram-positive organisms.*

USES Bacterial infections; colorectal decontamination prior to surgery. **Topical applications:** Pyodermas, acne vulgaris, and external ocular infections, including neonatal chlamydial conjunctivitis and gonococcal ophthalmia.

CONTRAINDICATIONS Hypersensitivity to erythromycins or other macrolide antibiotics; congenital QT prolongation; electrolyte imbalances.

CAUTIOUS USE Impaired liver function; seizure disorders; history of GI disorders; lactation—infant risk is minimal.

ROUTE & DOSAGE

Moderate to Severe Infections

Adult: **PO** 250–500 mg q6–12h (max 4 g daily)
Child: **PO** 30–50 mg/kg/day divided q6–8h; **Topical** Apply ointment to infected eye 1 or more × day

ADMINISTRATION

Oral

- Erythromycin base or stearate should be given on an empty stomach 2 h before or after a meal. Do not give with, or immediately before or after, fruit juices.
- Enteric-coated tablets may be given without regard to meals.
- Ensure that capsules and tablets are not chewed or crushed. They **must be** swallowed whole.
- Store tablets and capsules and powder suspension below 30°C (86°F). Protect from freezing and avoid excessive heat.

Topical

- Prophylaxis for neonatal eye infection: Ribbon of ointment approximately 1 cm long is placed into lower conjunctival sac of neonate shortly after birth. Use a new tube of erythromycin for each neonate.
- Store all forms at 20°–25°C (68°–77°F) in tightly capped containers unless otherwise directed by manufacturer. Keep away from heat and flames.

ADVERSE EFFECTS **CV:** Torsade de pointes, <u>ventricular arrhythmia</u>, ventricular tachycardia. **CNS:** Seizures. **HEENT:** Ototoxicity: Reversible bilateral hearing loss, tinnitus, vertigo. **Skin:** (Topical use) Erythema, desquamation, burning, tenderness, dryness or oiliness, pruritus. **Hepatic:** Hepatitis. **GI:** *Nausea, vomiting, abdominal cramping*, diarrhea, heartburn, anorexia. (Estolate) Cholestatic hepatitis syndrome, pancreatitis. **GU:** Interstitial nephritis. **Other:** Fever, eosinophilia, urticaria, skin eruptions, fixed drug eruption, anaphylaxis. Superinfections by nonsusceptible bacteria, yeasts, or fungi.

DIAGNOSTIC TEST INTERFERENCE False elevations of ***urinary catecholamines, urinary steroids.***

INTERACTIONS **Drug:** There are many drug interactions, some significant interactions are listed here, consult a drug interaction resource for a complete list. Serum levels and toxicities of CYP3A4 substrates (ex **alfentanil, bexarotene, carbamazepine, cevimeline, cilostazol, clozapine, cyclosporine, disopyramide, estazolam, fentanyl, midazolam, methadone, modafinil, quinidine, sirolimus, digoxin, theophylline, triazolam, warfarin)** are increased. Use is contraindicated with **eliglustat, ezetimibe, flibanserin, itraconazole, ketoconazole, lomitapide, lovastatin, pimozide, simvastatin, ergotamine, dihydroergotamine** may increase peripheral vasospasm. Do not use with drugs that prolong QT interval (e.g., **abarelix, asenapine, bepridil, chloroquine, clozapine, disopyramide, dofetilide, dronedarone, droperidol, fluconazole, levomethadyl, nilotinib, posaconazole, saquinavir, thioridazine, ziprasidone**). Do not use with LIVE VACCINES. **Food: Grapefruit juice** may increase side effects.

PHARMACOKINETICS Absorption: Most erythromycins are absorbed in small intestine. **Peak:** 1–4 h PO. **Distribution:** Widely distributed to most body tissues; low concentrations in CSF; concentrates in liver and bile; crosses placenta. **Metabolism:** Partially in liver via CYP3A4. **Elimination:** Primarily in bile; excreted in breast milk. **Half-Life:** 1.5–2 h.

NURSING IMPLICATIONS

Assessment & Drug Effects

- Report onset of GI symptoms after PO administration. These are dose related; if symptoms persist after dosage reduction, prescriber may prescribe drug to be given with meals despite impaired absorption.
- Monitor for adverse GI effects. Pseudomembranous enterocolitis (see Appendix F), a potentially life-threatening condition, may occur during or after antibiotic therapy.
- Observe for S&S of superinfection by overgrowth of nonsusceptible bacteria or fungi. Emergence of resistant staphylococcal strains is highly predictable during prolonged therapy.
- Monitor for S&S of hepatotoxicity. Premonitory S&S include: Abdominal pain, nausea, vomiting, fever, leukocytosis, and eosinophilia; jaundice may or may not be present. Symptoms may appear a few days after initiation of drug but usually occur after 1–2 wk of continuous therapy. Symptoms are reversible with prompt discontinuation of erythromycin.
- Monitor for ototoxicity that appears to develop most frequently in patients receiving 4 g/day or more, older adults, female patients, and patients with kidney or liver dysfunction. It is reversible with prompt discontinuation of drug.
- Monitor lab tests: Periodic LFTs during prolonged therapy.

Patient & Family Education

- Notify prescriber for S&S of superinfection (see Appendix F).
- Notify prescriber immediately for S&S of pseudomembranous enterocolitis (see Appendix F), which may occur even after the drug is discontinued.
- Report any ototoxic effects including dizziness, vertigo, nausea, tinnitus, roaring noises, hearing impairment (see Appendix F).
- Elderly patients with history of renal or hepatic disease are more at risk for ototoxicity and cardiac events.

ERYTHROMYCIN ETHYLSUCCINATE

(er-ith-roe-mye′sin)

Apo-Erythro-ES ♣, E.E.S., EryPed

Classification: MACROLIDE ANTIBIOTIC

Therapeutic: ANTIBIOTIC

Prototype: Erythromycin

AVAILABILITY Tablet

ACTION & THERAPEUTIC EFFECT Macrolide antibiotic that binds to the 50S ribosomal subunit of bacteria, thus inhibiting bacterial protein synthesis. *More active against gram-positive than gram-negative bacteria.*

USES See ERYTHROMYCIN.

CONTRAINDICATIONS Hypersensitivity to erythromycins or any macrolide antibiotic; history of erythromycin-associated hepatitis; preexisting liver disease; congenital QT prolongation; electrolyte imbalances; pregnancy—fetal risk cannot be ruled out.

CAUTIOUS USE Myasthenia gravis; history of GI disease; seizure disorders; lactation: infant risk is minimal.

ROUTE & DOSAGE

Infection

Adult: **PO** 400–800 mg q6–12h (max 4 g/day)
Child: **PO** 30–50 mg/kg/day divided q6–8 h (max: 400 mg/day)

ADMINISTRATION

- Note: 400 mg erythromycin ethylsuccinate is approximately equal to 250 mg erythromycin base.

Oral

- Administer with or without food.
- Refrigerate after mixing and use within 10 days. Note expiration date.
- Store tablets, capsules, and powder for suspension below 30°C (86°F) in tight containers unless otherwise directed. Protect from excessive heat and moisture.

ADVERSE EFFECTS **CV:** Torsades de point. **CNS:** Seizure. **Skin:** Skin eruptions. **Hepatic:** Hepatotoxicity. **GI:** Diarrhea, nausea, vomiting, stomatitis, abdominal cramps, anorexia, pancreatitis. **GU:** Interstitial nephritis.

INTERACTIONS **Drug:** see ERYTHROMYCIN monograph

PHARMACOKINETICS **Absorption:** Readily absorbed from GI tract. **Peak:** 2 h. **Distribution:** Concentrates in liver; crosses placenta; distributed into breast milk. **Metabolism:** In liver via CYP 3A4. **Elimination:** Primarily in bile and feces. **Half-Life:** 2–5 h.

NURSING IMPLICATIONS

Assessment & Drug Effects

- Cholestatic hepatitis syndrome is most likely to occur in adults who have received erythromycin estolate for more than 10 days or who have had repeated courses of therapy. The condition generally clears within 3–5 days after cessation of therapy.
- Monitor lab tests: Baseline C&S.

Patient & Family Education

- Advise patient to report immediately the onset of adverse reactions and to be on the alert for signs and symptoms associated with jaundice (see Appendix F).

- Report immediately watery and bloody stools (with or without stomach cramps and fever). May occur up to 2 mo after drug discontinuation.
- Significant drug-to-drug interactions. Consult healthcare provider for all new medications, over-the-counter and herbal drugs.

E

ERYTHROMYCIN LACTOBIONATE

(er-ith-roe-mye′sin lak′toe-bye′oh-nate)

Erythrocin

Classification: MACROLIDE ANTIBIOTIC

Therapeutic: ANTIBIOTIC

Prototype: Erythromycin

AVAILABILITY Solution for injection

ACTION & THERAPEUTIC EFFECT Soluble salt of erythromycin that binds to the 50S ribosome subunits of susceptible bacteria, resulting in the suppression of protein synthesis of bacteria. *More active against gram-positive than gram-negative bacteria.*

USES When oral administration is not possible or the severity of infection requires immediate high serum levels. See erythromycin monograph.

CONTRAINDICATIONS Hypersensitivity to erythromycin or macrolide antibiotics; congenital QT prolongation; electrolyte imbalances; pregnancy—fetal risk cannot be ruled out.

CAUTIOUS USE Impaired liver function; seizure disorders; myasthenia gravis; lactation—infant risk is minimal: children.

ROUTE & DOSAGE

Infections

Adult/Child: **IV** 15–20 mg/kg/day divided q6h or 500–1000 mg q6h (max 4 g/day)

ADMINISTRATION

Intravenous

PREPARE: **Intermittent/Continuous:** Initial solution is prepared by adding 10 mL sterile water for injection without preservatives to each 500 mg or fraction thereof. ▪ Shake vial until drug is completely dissolved. **Intermittent:** Further dilute each 1-g dose in 100–250 mL of LR or NS. **Continuous (*preferred*):** Further dilute each 1 g in 1000 mL LR or NS. ▪ Give within 8 h.

ADMINISTER: **Intermittent:** Give 1 g or fraction thereof over 20–60 min. ▪ Slow rate if pain develops along course of vein. **Continuous (*preferred*):** Continuous infusion is administered slowly, usually over 6–8 h.

INCOMPATIBILITIES: **Solution/additive:** **Dextrose**-containing solutions, **ascorbic acid, colistimethate, clindamycin, furosemide, heparin, linezolid, metaraminol, metoclopramide, tetracycline, vitamin B complex with C.** **Y-site:** **Amphotericin B, ascorbic acid, aztreonam, cefamandole, cefazolin, cefepime, cefotetan, cefoxitin, ceftizoxime, dantrolene, diazepam, diazoxide, doxycycline, ganciclovir, gemtuzumab, indomethacin, ketorolac, metaraminol, minocycline, nitroprusside, pemetrexed, pentobarbital, phenytoin, sulfamethoxazole/trimethoprim, ticarcillin.**

- Store vials at controlled room temperature from 20°–25°C (68°–66°F). When reconstituted to 50 mg/mL, solution may be stored up to 2 weeks when refrigerated or up to 24 hours at room temperature. Administer the final diluted solution within 8 hours.

ADVERSE EFFECTS **CV:** Venous Irritation. **HEENT:** Hearing loss. **Skin:** Urticaria, erythema multiforme, Stevens–Johnson syndrome.

INTERACTIONS **Drug:** See erythromycin monograph.

PHARMACOKINETICS **Peak:** 1 h. **Distribution:** Concentrates in liver; crosses placenta; distributed into breast milk. **Metabolism:** In liver via CYP3A4. **Elimination:** Primarily in bile and feces; 12–15% in urine. **Half-Life:** 3–5 h.

NURSING IMPLICATIONS

Assessment & Drug Effects

- Monitor for hearing impairment, which may occur with large doses of this drug. It may occur as early as the second day and as late as the third week of therapy.
- Monitor for S&S of thrombophlebitis (see Appendix F). IV infusion of large doses is reported to increase risk.
- Monitor lab tests: Baseline C&S, LFTs.

Patient & Family Education

- Notify prescriber immediately of tinnitus, dizziness, or hearing impairment.
- Patient with myasthenia gravis should report signs/symptoms of disease exacerbation during therapy.

ESCITALOPRAM OXALATE

(es-ci-tal′o-pram)

Lexapro

Classification: ANTIDEPRESSANT; SELECTIVE SEROTONIN REUPTAKE INHIBITOR (SSRI)

Therapeutic: ANTIDEPRESSANT; SSRI

Prototype: Fluoxetine

AVAILABILITY Liquid, tablet

ACTION & *THERAPEUTIC EFFECT* Selective serotonin reuptake inhibitor (SSRI) in the CNS. Antidepressant effect is presumed to be linked to its inhibition of CNS presynaptic neuronal uptake of serotonin. *Selective serotonin reuptake inhibition mechanism results in the antidepressant activity with or without anxiety symptoms.*

USES Depression, generalized anxiety disorder.

UNLABELED USES Treatment of panic disorders, PTSD, bulimia, OCD, panic disorder.

CONTRAINDICATIONS Hypersensitivity to citalopram; concurrent use of MAOIS or use within 14 days of discontinuing MAOIS; concomitant use of pimozide; abrupt discontinuation; suicidal ideations; mania; bipolar depression; volume depleted; lactation—infant risk has been demonstrated.

CAUTIOUS USE Hypersensitivity to other SSRIs; suicidal tendencies; bipolar disorder; obsessive-compulsive disorder, major depressive disorder, all major psychiatric disorders especially pediatric patients; depression, history of mania, hypomania; hyponatremia, ethanol intoxication, ECT, dehydration, severe renal impairment, hepatic disease; older adults; history of seizure disorders; pregnancy—fetal risk cannot be ruled out; lactation (not within 4 h of drug ingestion). Safety and efficacy in children younger than 12 yr not established.

E

ROUTE & DOSAGE

Depression, Generalized Anxiety

Adult/Adolescent: **PO** 10 daily, may increase to 20 mg daily if needed after 1 wk
Geriatric: **PO** 5–10 mg daily

Renal Impairment Dosage Adjustment

CrCl less than 20 mL/min: 5 mg daily

Hepatic Impairment Dosage Adjustment

Adult: **PO** 10 daily

ADMINISTRATION

Oral

- Do not begin this drug within 14 days of stopping an MAOI.
- Dose increments should be separated by at least 1 wk.
- May take without regard to meals.
- Store at 20–25°C (68–77°F); excursions permitted between 15 and 30°C (59 to 86°F) in tightly closed container and protect from light.

ADVERSE EFFECTS (≥5%) **CNS:** Dizziness, *insomnia, somnolence*, migraine. **Skin:** Increased sweating. **GI:** *Nausea*, diarrhea, dyspepsia, dry mouth. **GU:** Decreased libido, ejaculation disorder, impotence, Orgasm incapacity (females), reduced libido. **Other:** Fatigue, withdrawal symptoms.

INTERACTIONS **Drug:** Combination with MAOI could result in hypertensive crisis, hyperthermia, rigidity, myoclonus, autonomic instability; use with **bromopride** may cause extrapyramidal reactions; **cimetidine** may increase escitalopram levels; **linezolid**, SSRIS may cause serotonin syndrome; may increase risk of bleeding when used with ANTICOAGULANTS. Use with drugs affecting hemostasis (**aspirin, warfarin**) increases bleeding risk. **Food:** Use with alcohol increases risk of psychomotor impairment. **Herbal: St. John's wort** may cause serotonin syndrome.

PHARMACOKINETICS **Absorption:** Rapidly absorbed from GI tract. **Onset:** Approximately 2 wk. **Peak:** 3 h. **Distribution:** 80% protein bound; crosses placenta; distributed into breast milk. **Metabolism:** In liver by CYP3A4, 2C19, and 2D6 enzymes. **Elimination:** 20% in urine, 80% in bile. **Half-Life:** 25 h.

NURSING IMPLICATIONS

Black Box Warning

Escitalopram has been associated with suicidal thinking and behavior in children, adolescents, and young adults.

Assessment & Drug Effects

- Closely observe for worsening of depression or emergence of suicidality, especially in adolescents or children.
- Monitor periodically HR and BP, and carefully monitor complete cardiac status in person with known or suspected cardiac disease.
- Monitor closely older adult patients for adverse effects, especially with doses greater than 20 mg/day.

- Monitor lab tests: Periodic lithium levels when given concurrently, sodium levels at baseline and after 3-4 weeks of therapy.

Patient & Family Education

- Report promptly changes in behavior such as anxiety, agitation, depression, mania, hypomania, panic attacks, aggressiveness, and suicidal ideation.
- Do not engage in hazardous activities until reaction to this drug is known.
- Avoid using alcohol while taking escitalopram.
- Inform prescriber of commonly used OTC drugs as there is potential for drug interactions. The use of aspirin and NSAIDs can affect coagulation and cause increased risk of bleeding.
- Report distressing adverse effects including any changes in sexual functioning or response.
- Avoid sudden discontinuation of the drug.
- Periodic ophthalmology exams are advised with long-term treatment.

ESLICARBAZEPINE ACETATE

(es-li-car'ba-ze-peen)

Aptiom

Classification: ANTICONVULSANT; TRICYCLIC

Therapeutic: ANTICONVULSANT

Prototype: Carbamazepine

AVAILABILITY Tablet

ACTION & *THERAPEUTIC EFFECT*

Inhibits voltage-gated sodium channels. *Decreases frequency of partial-onset seizures.*

USES Adjunctive treatment of partial-onset seizures.

CONTRAINDICATIONS Hypersensitivity to eslicarbazepine or oxcarbazepine including anaphylactic reactions and angioedema; drug reaction with eosinophilia and systemic symptoms (DRESS)/multi-organ reaction; hypersensitivity or previous such reaction with oxcarbazepine; severe hematologic reactions; jaundice and drug-induced hepatic injury; severe hepatic impairment; severe hyponatremia; pregnancy—fetal risk cannot be ruled out; lactation—infant risk cannot be ruled out.

CAUTIOUS USE Depression or other psychiatric conditions; history of suicidal thoughts; renal impairment; hyponatremia or patients at risk for hyponatremia symptoms; mild to moderate hepatic impairment; thyroid disorders.

ROUTE & DOSAGE

Partial-Onset Seizures

Adult/Adolescent: **PO** 400 mg daily, may increase to 800 mg and then by 400–600 mg increments to maintenance dose of 800–1600 mg daily.
Child (over 4 yr and 11 kg): **PO** see package insert for weight-based dosing table.

Hepatic Impairment Dosage Adjustment

Severe Impairment: Not recommended

Renal Impairment Dosage Adjustment

Moderate to Severe Impairment (CrCl less than 50 mL/min): Reduce dosage by 50%

E

ADMINISTRATION

Oral

- NIOSH presents a potential occupational hazard to men and women actively trying to conceive and women who are pregnant or may become pregnant and are breastfeeding. Use single gloves for anyone handling intact tablets or capsules or administering unit-dose package. Use double gloves and protective gown if cutting, crushing, manipulating or handling of uncoated tablets. During administration, wear single gloves and wear eye/face protection if the formulation is hard to swallow or if the patient may resist, vomit, or spit up.
- May give without regard to food.
- Tablets must be swallowed whole. They should not be crushed or chewed.
- When drug is discontinued, dose should be reduced gradually.
- Store tablets at 20°–25°C (68°–77°F), with excursions permitted to between 15° and 30°C (59° and 86°F).

ADVERSE EFFECTS (≥5%) **CNS:** *Ataxia, dizziness, headache, somnolence, vertigo.* **HEENT:** *Blurred vision, diplopia.* **Endocrine:** Hyponatremia. **GI:** *Nausea, vomiting.* **Other:** Suicidal ideation, *fatigue.*

INTERACTIONS **Drug:** Significant drug interactions exist, requiring dose/frequency adjustment or avoidance. Consult drug interactions database for more comprehensive information. Other ANTIEPILEPTIC DRUGS (e.g., **carbamazepine, phenobarbital, phenytoin, primidone**) may decrease the levels of eslicarbazepine. Eslicarbazepine can increase the levels of other drugs that are metabolized by CYP2C19 (e.g., **clobazam, omeprazole, phenytoin**). Eslicarbazepine can decrease the levels of other drugs that are metabolized by CYP3A4 (e.g., **rosuvastatin, simvastatin**). Eslicarbazepine decreases the levels of **ethinyl estradiol** and **levonorgestrel.**

PHARMACOKINETICS **Absorption:** Greater than 90% bioavailable. **Peak:** 1–4 h. **Distribution:** Less than 40% plasma protein bound. **Metabolism:** Rapidly hydrolyzed to active metabolite; inactivated via conjugation. **Elimination:** Primarily renal. **Half-Life:** 13–20 h.

NURSING IMPLICATIONS

Assessment & Drug Effects

- Monitor for and report promptly suicidal thoughts or behavioral or mood changes.
- Withhold drug and notify prescriber immediately for any of the following: Manifestations of hypersensitivity (e.g., swelling of the face, eyes, lips, tongue, or difficulty in swallowing or breathing, fever, lymphadenopathy), rash or any other dermatologic reaction.
- Monitor for dizziness, ataxia, vertigo, balance disorder, gait disturbance, and abnormal coordination. Institute safety precautions as needed.
- Monitor for and report promptly signs of hyponatremia (see Appendix F).
- Monitor lab tests: Periodic serum sodium and chloride, saliva levels, plasma levels, and LFTs.

Patient & Family Education

- Do not abruptly stop taking this drug. Doing so may trigger increased seizure frequency and status epilepticus.
- Report immediately emergence or worsening of depression, unusual changes in mood or behavior,

or the emergence of suicidal thoughts or behavior.

- Report promptly to prescriber: Development of a rash or other skin reaction; signs of low serum sodium (e.g., tiredness, irritability, confusion, muscle weakness spasms, more frequent or more severe seizures), or fever.
- Report any signs of jaundice (yellowing of skin or whites of the eye).
- Do not drive or engage in other potentially dangerous activities until response to drug is known.
- Notify prescriber immediately if you become or suspect you are pregnant. Women who do not wish to become pregnant should use additional or alternative nonhormonal birth control.
- Do not breastfeed while taking this drug.

ESMOLOL HYDROCHLORIDE

(ess′moe-lol)

Brevibloc

Classification: BETA BLOCKER; CLASS II

Therapeutic: ANTIARRHYTHMIC

Prototype: Propranolol

AVAILABILITY Solution for injection

ACTION & *THERAPEUTIC EFFECT* Ultrashort-acting $beta_1$-adrenergic blocking agent with cardioselective properties. Inhibits the agonist effect of catecholamines by competitive binding at beta-adrenergic receptors. Antiarrhythmic properties occur at the AV node. *Effective as an antiarrhythmic agent on the AV-nodal conduction system. Blocks sympathetically mediated increases in cardiac rate and BP because it binds predominantly to* $beta_1$*-receptors in cardiac tissue. At higher doses, it inhibits* $beta_2$*-receptors located in bronchi and blood vessels.*

USES Supraventricular tachyarrhythmias (SVT) in perioperative and postoperative periods or in other critical situations. Also short-term treatment of noncompensating sinus tachycardia.

UNLABELED USES Treatment of intense transient adrenergic response to surgical stress in cardiac as well as noncardiac surgery.

CONTRAINDICATIONS Hypersensitivity to esmolol; heart block greater than first degree, severe sinus bradycardia, sick sinus syndrome, cardiogenic shock; decompensated HF or cardiac shock; pulmonary hypertension, acute bronchospasm.

CAUTIOUS USE History of allergy; CHF; pulmonary disease such as bronchial asthma, COPD, or pulmonary edema; diabetes mellitus; pheochromocytoma; renal impairment; hyperthyroidism; older adults; pregnancy (category C); lactation (infant risk cannot be ruled out). Safe use in children younger than 18 yr not established.

ROUTE & DOSAGE

Supraventricular Tachyarrhythmias

Adult: **IV** 500-mcg/kg loading dose followed by 50 mcg/kg/min × 4 min; infusion may be continued at 50 mcg/kg/min or, if the response is inadequate, titrated up in 50-mcg/

kg/min increments (increased no more frequently than every 4 minutes) (max dose 200 mcg/kg/min)

Intraoperative/Postoperative Tachycardia

Adult: **IV** 80-mg bolus followed by 150 mcg/kg/min; increase if needed (max: 300 mcg/kg/min)

ADMINISTRATION

Intravenous

PREPARE: **Direct:** Use the 10-mg/mL vial undiluted for the loading dose. **IV Infusion:** Prepare maintenance infusion by adding 2.5 g to 250 mL or 5 g to 500 mL or 10 mg to 1000 mL of IV solution to yield 10 mg/mL. Compatible diluents include D5W, D5/LR, D5/NS, D5/.45NS, LR, NS, potassium chloride (40 mEq/L) D5W.

ADMINISTER: **Direct:** Give loading dose over 1 min. **IV Infusion:** ▪ Give maintenance infusion over 4 min. ▪ If adequate response is noted, continue maintenance infusion with periodic adjustments as needed. ▪ Avoid infusion into small veins through butterfly catheter.

INCOMPATIBILITIES: **Solution/additive: Procainamide. Y-site: Acyclovir, amphotericin B cholesteryl, amphotericin B conventional, amphotericin B colloidal, and amphotericin lipid complex, ampicillin sodium, ampicillin sodium-sulbactam sodium, azathioprine, cefamandole, cefoperazone, cefotetan, chloramphenicol sodium succinate, ciprofloxacin, dantrolene, dexamethasone, diazepam, diazoxide, esomeprazole sodium, furosemide, ganciclovir, gemtuzumab, haloperidol lactate, hydralazine hydrochloride, hydrocortisone sodium succinate, ibuprofen arginine, inamrinone, indomethacin, ketorolac, lansoprazole, methylprednisolone sodium succinate, milrinone, minocycline, mitomycin, nafcillin, oxacillin, pantoprazole, pentobarbital sodium, phenobarbital, phenytoin sodium, sulfamethoxazole-trimethoprim, tedizolid phosphate, warfarin.**

▪ Diluted infusion solution is stable for at least 24 h at room temperature. ▪ Store between 15° and 30°C (59° and 86°F). Avoid exposure to excessive heat and protect from freezing.

ADVERSE EFFECTS **CV:** *Hypotension.* **Skin:** Injection site reaction. **GI:** Nausea.

INTERACTIONS **Drug: Morphine** IV may increase esmolol levels by 45%; **succinylcholine** may prolong neuromuscular blockade. ALPHA$_2$ AGONISTS may cause additive effects. ANTIHYPERTENSIVES can enhance hypotensive effects. Use with dronedarone can increase adverse effects. Do not use with ERGOT derivatives, **fingolimod, methacholine, obinutuzumab, rivastigmine.**

PHARMACOKINETICS **Onset:** Less than 5 min. **Peak:** 10–20 min. **Duration:** 10–30 min. **Metabolism:** Hydrolyzed by RBC esterases. **Elimination:** In urine. **Half-Life:** 9 min.

NURSING IMPLICATIONS

Assessment & Drug Effects

- Monitor BP, pulse, ECG, during esmolol infusion. Hypotension may have its onset during the initial titration phase; thereafter the risk increases with increasing doses. Usually the hypotension experienced during esmolol infusion is resolved within 30 min after infusion is reduced or discontinued.
- Change injection site if local reaction occurs. IV site reactions (burning, erythema) or diaphoresis may develop during infusion. Both reactions are temporary. Blood chemistry abnormalities have not been reported.
- Overdose symptoms: Discontinue administration if the following symptoms occur: Bradycardia, severe dizziness or drowsiness, dyspnea, bluish-colored fingernails or palms of hands, seizures.

ESOMEPRAZOLE MAGNESIUM

(e-so-me′pra-zole)

Nexium

Classification: PROTON PUMP INHIBITOR

Therapeutic: ANTIULCER

Prototype: Omeprazole

AVAILABILITY Capsule; powder for injection; oral suspension

ACTION & *THERAPEUTIC EFFECT* Isomer of omeprazole, a weak base that is converted to the active form in the highly acidic environment of the gastric parietal cells. Inhibits the enzyme H^+K^+-ATPase (the acid pump), thus suppressing gastric acid secretion. *Due to inhibition of the H^+K^+-ATPase, esomeprazole substantially decreases both basal and stimulated acid secretion through inhibition of the acid pump in parietal cells.*

USES Erosive esophagitis, gastrointestinal reflux disease (GERD), hypersecretory diseases, duodenal ulcer associated with *H. pylori* in combination with antibiotics, prevention of gastric ulcer associated with continuous NSAID use in patients at risk, Zollinger–Ellison syndrome, heartburn, risk reduction of ulcer rebleeding postprocedure.

CONTRAINDICATIONS Hypersensitivity to esomeprazole, magnesium, omeprazole, or other proton pump inhibitors; gastric malignancy; pregnancy (fetal risk cannot be ruled out); lactation (infant risk cannot be ruled out).

CAUTIOUS USE Severe renal insufficiency; severe hepatic impairment; treatment for more than a year; gastric ulcers; elderly; IBD, GI disease; safe use in infants younger than 1 mo has not been established.

ROUTE & DOSAGE

Healing of Erosive Esophagitis

Adult/Adolescent: **PO** 20–40 mg daily at least 1 h before meals × 4–8 wk

Child/Infant: **PO** 2.5–10 mg daily × 6 wk (see package insert for weight-based dose)

Heartburn

Adult: **PO** 20 mg daily × 14 d

E

GERD, Erosive Esophagitis Maintenance

Adult/Adolescent: **PO/IV** 20–40 mg daily at least 1 h before meals × 4–8 wk
Child (1 yr or older): **PO** *55 kg or greater:* 20 mg daily at least 1 h before meals up to 8 wk; *weight less than 55 kg:* 10 mg daily at least 1 h before meals up to 8 wk

Duodenal Ulcer

Adult: **PO** 40 mg daily × 10 days

Hypersecretory Disease (Zollinger–Ellison)

Adult: **PO** 40 mg bid, adjust if needed (max: 240 mg daily)

NSAID Ulcer Prophylaxis

Adult: **PO** 20–40 mg daily

Prevention of Recurrent Gastric/Duodenal Ulcer

Adult: **IV** 80 mg over 30 min then 8 mg/hour × 72 h then 40 mg; **PO** daily × 27 days

Hepatic Impairment Dosage Adjustment

Child–Pugh class C: Do not exceed 20 mg/day

ADMINISTRATION

Oral

- Give at least 1 h before eating.
- Do not crush or chew capsule. **Must be** swallowed whole.
- Open capsule and mix pellets with applesauce (cold or room temperature) if patient cannot swallow capsules. **Do not** crush pellets. Applesauce should be swallowed immediately after mixing without chewing.
- May take with antacids.
- Store in the original blister package 15°–30°C (59°–86°F).

Intravenous

PREPARE: **Direct:** Reconstitute powder with 5 mL of NS. **IV Infusion:** Further dilute reconstituted solution in 50 mL of NS, LR, or D5W.
ADMINISTER: **Direct:** Withdraw required dose from reconstituted solution and give over no less than 3 min. **Do not** give direct IV to children. **IV Infusion:** Give IV solution over 10–30 min.
INCOMPATIBILITIES: Do not give simultaneously with any other medication through the same IV site or line.
- Flush IV line with NS, LR, or D5W before/after infusion.

- Store reconstituted solution at room temperature up to 30°C (86°F); give within 12 h of reconstitution with NS or LR and within 6 h of reconstitution with D5W.

ADVERSE EFFECTS **CNS:** Headache. **GI:** Diarrhea, flatulence, abdominal pain, nausea.

INTERACTIONS **Drug:** May increase **diazepam, phenytoin, warfarin** levels. Use caution with **clopidogrel.** May decrease levels of **atazanavir** and **nelfinavir.** Do not use with **acalabrutinib, cefuroxime, dacomitinib, dasatinib, delavirdine, erlotinib, nelfinavir, neratinib, rifampin, rilpivirine, velpatasvir.** **Food:** Prolonged use may lead to Vitamin B_{12} deficiency. **Herbal:** Do not use with St. John's wort.

DIAGNOSTIC TEST INTERFERENCE Esomeprazole may falsely elevate serum chromogranin A (CgA) levels.

PHARMACOKINETICS Absorption: Destroyed in acidic environment, therefore capsules are designed for delayed absorption in the small intestine. 70% reaches systemic circulation. **Metabolism:** In liver by CYP2C19. **Elimination:** Inactive metabolites excreted in both urine and feces. **Half-Life:** 1.5 h.

NURSING IMPLICATIONS

Assessment & Drug Effects

- Monitor for S&S of adverse CNS effects (vertigo, agitation, depression) especially in severely ill patients.
- Monitor phenytoin levels with concurrent use.
- Monitor INR/PT with concurrent warfarin use.
- Monitor lab tests: Periodic serum magnesium with drugs, such as diuretics, that might lower magnesium levels, vitamin B_{12}.

Patient & Family Education

- Report any changes in urinary elimination such as pain or discomfort associated with urination to prescriber.
- Report S&S hypomagnesemia: muscle weakness, spasm, cramps, or abnormal eye movements.
- Report severe diarrhea. Drug may need to be discontinued.

ESTAZOLAM

(es-ta-zo′lam)

Classification: SEDATIVE-HYPNOTIC, NONBARBITURATE; BENZODIAZEPINE
Therapeutic: SEDATIVE
Prototype: Triazolam
Controlled Substance: Schedule IV

AVAILABILITY Tablet

ACTION & THERAPEUTIC EFFECT Benzodiazepine whose effects (anxiolytic, sedative, hypnotic, skeletal muscle relaxant) are mediated by the inhibitory neurotransmitter gamma-aminobutyric acid (GABA). GABA acts at the thalamic, hypothalamic, and limbic levels of CNS. *Benzodiazepines generally decrease the number of awakenings from sleep. Stage 2 sleep is increased with all benzodiazepines. Estazolam shortens stages 3 and 4 (slow-wave sleep), and REM sleep is shortened. The total sleep time, however, is increased.*

USES Short-term management of insomnia.

CONTRAINDICATIONS Known sensitivity to benzodiazepines; acute closed-angle glaucoma, primary depressive disorders or psychosis; abrupt discontinuation; coma, shock, acute alcohol intoxication; pregnancy—fetal harm demonstrated; lactation—Infant risk cannot be ruled out.

CAUTIOUS USE Renal and hepatic impairment, renal failure; organic brain syndrome, alcoholism, benzodiazepine dependence, suicidal ideations, CNS depression, seizure disorder, status epilepticus, persistent insomnia; substance abuse; shock, coma; dementia, mania, psychosis; myasthenia gravis, Parkinson disease; sleep apnea; open-angle glaucoma, GI disorders, compromised respiratory function, older adult and debilitated patients; limited pulmonary reserve, pulmonary disease, COPD. Safe use in children younger than 18 yr not established.

E

ROUTE & DOSAGE

Insomnia

Adult: **PO** 1 mg at bedtime, may increase up to 2 mg if necessary (older adult patients may start with 0.5 mg at bedtime)

ADMINISTRATION

Oral

- For older adult patients in good health, a 1-mg dose is indicated; reduce initial dose to 0.5 mg for debilitated or small older adult patients.
- Dosage reduction also may be needed in the presence of hepatic impairment.
- Store tablets below 30°C (86°F).

ADVERSE EFFECTS (≥5%) **CNS:** Dizziness, impaired coordination, hypokinesia, *somnolence*, hangover, weakness. **GI:** Constipation, xerostomia. **Other:** Anxiety.

INTERACTIONS **Drug: Alcohol** and other CNS DEPRESSANTS may increase drowsiness; CYP3A4 inhibitors **(ketoconazole, itraconazole, nefazodone, diltiazem, fluvoxamine, cimetidine, isoniazid, erythromycin)** can increase concentrations and toxicity of estazolam; **carbamazepine, phenytoin, rifampin**, BARBITURATES may decrease estazolam concentrations; may increase respiratory depression when used with **clozapine. Food: Grapefruit juice** greater than 1 quart may increase toxicity. **Herbal: Kava, valerian** may potentiate sedation.

PHARMACOKINETICS **Absorption:** Rapidly absorbed from GI tract. **Onset:** 20–30 min. **Peak:** 2 h. **Distribution:** Crosses rapidly into brain; crosses placenta; distributed into breast milk. **Metabolism:** Extensively in liver (via CYP3A4). **Elimination:** In urine. **Half-Life:** 10–24 h.

NURSING IMPLICATIONS

Black Box Warning

Concomitant use with opioids can lead to abuse, misue, and addiction and dependence with withdrawal reactions. Concomitant use of benzodiazipines and opioids may result in profound sedation, respiratory depression, coma, and death.

Assessment & Drug Effects

- Monitor for improvement in S&S of insomnia.
- Assess for excess CNS depression or daytime sedation.
- Assess for safety, especially with older adult or debilitated patients, as dizziness and impaired coordination are known adverse effects.
- Monitor labs: CBC, urinalysis, and blood chemistry periodically during prolonged therapy.

Patient & Family Education

- Learn adverse effects, and report those experienced to the prescriber.
- Avoid using this drug in combination with other CNS depressant drugs or alcohol.
- High risk of abuse, misuse and addiction. Make sure to report any symptoms to provider.
- Do not drive or engage in other potentially hazardous activities until response to drug is known.
- Driving while asleep, preparing food, making calls, having sex when not fully awake and have no recall. Report behavior to healthcare provider.

- Report worsening depression, suicidal ideation, or unusual changes in behavior.
- Do not suddenly stop taking the medication due to potential withdrawal reaction.

ESTRADIOL

(ess-tra-dye′ole)

Alora, Climara, Divigel, Elestrin, Estrace, Estring, EstroGel, Evamist, Menostar, Minivelle, DOT, Vagifem

ESTRADIOL ACETATE

Femring

ESTRADIOL CYPIONATE

Depo-Estradiol

ESTRADIOL VALERATE

Delestrogen

Classification: ESTROGEN

Therapeutic: ESTROGEN REPLACEMENT

AVAILABILITY **Estradiol:** Oral tablet; topical gel; topical spray; transdermal patch; vaginal cream; vaginal tablet. **Cypionate:** Solution for injection. **Valerate:** Solution for injection

ACTION & *THERAPEUTIC EFFECT* Estrogens exert their effects by binding to and activating intracellular estrogen receptors, which modulate expression of many genes. Estradiol is the predominant estrogen during reproductive years. It acts as a growth hormone that stimulates and maintains tissue in reproductive organs, and it reduces bone resorption and increases bone formation. *Estradiol is effective in controlling symptoms of menopause due to natural decline of circulating endogenous estrogens.*

USES Metastatic breast cancer in selected patients, vasomotor symptoms or vaginal atrophy associated with menopause, hypoestrogenism due to castration, hypogonadism, primary ovarian failure, prevention of postmenopausal osteoporosis, advanced prostrate cancer. Combined with progestins in many oral contraceptive formulations.

UNLABELED USES Functional hypothalamic amenorrhea with low bone density; hormone therapy for transgender females.

CONTRAINDICATIONS Estrogenic-dependent neoplasms, breast cancer (except in selected patients being treated for metastatic disease). History of thromboembolic disorders; history of stroke; active arterial thrombosis, antithrombin deficiency, or thrombophilic disorders; undiagnosed abnormal genital bleeding; uterine fibroids; endometriosis; history of cholestatic disease; hepatic dysfunction or disease; thyroid dysfunction; blood dyscrasias; known protein C, protein S, or antithrombin deficiency; hypercalcemia; known or suspected pregnancy Known to cause harm to the fetus; lactation—Avoid breastfeeding if possible. Infant risk cannot be ruled out.

CAUTIOUS USE Adolescents with incomplete bone growth; endometriosis; hypertension, cardiac insufficiency; diseases of calcium and phosphate metabolism (metabolic bone disease); cerebrovascular disease; mental depression; benign breast disease, family history of breast or genital tract neoplasm; DM; CAD; SLE; gallbladder disease; preexisting leiomyoma, abnormal mammogram, history of idiopathic jaundice of pregnancy; varicosities; asthma; diabetes mellitus; hypothyroidism; hypertriglyceridemia; systemic lupus erythematosus; history of retinal thrombosis; history of endometriosis, vaginal infection, history of asthma; epilepsy; migraine headaches; liver or kidney dysfunction; jaundice, acute intermittent porphyria, pyridoxine deficiency.

ROUTE & DOSAGE

Menopause, Atrophic Vaginitis

Adult: **PO** 0.5–2 mg/day; **Topical** 2–4 g vaginal cream intravaginally once/day for 1–2 wk, then 1–2 g/day for 1–2 wk, then 1 g 1–3 × wk; **Transdermal patch** Weekly or twice a week depending on product directions; **IM Cypionate** 1–5 mg once q3–4wk; **Valerate** 10–25 mg once q4wk; **Topical Divigel** Apply 0.25 g/day, adjust to patient response (alternate legs); **EstroGel** Apply 1.25 g every day (usually in the morning). **Evamist** Apply one spray to inner forearm daily, dose may be increased to 2–3 sprays daily

Metastatic Breast Cancer

Adult: **PO** 10 mg tid

Prostatic Cancer

Adult: **PO** 1–2 mg tid **IM Valerate** 30 mg q1–2wk

Hypoestrogenism

Adult: **PO** 1–2 mg/day **IM:** 10–20 mg q4w **Transdermal:** refer to product specific information

ADMINISTRATION

Oral

- NIOSH: Use of single gloves by anyone handling intact tablets or capsules or administering from unit-dose package. Use double gloves, protective gown and respiratory protections if cutting, crushing or manipulating uncoated tablets. During administration, wear single gloves, eye/face protection if the formulation is hard to swallow or if the patient may resist, vomit, or spit up.
- Give with or immediately after solid food to reduce nausea.
- Protect tablets from light and moisture in well-closed container. Protect from freezing, unless otherwise directed by manufacturer.
- Store tablets at controlled room temperature 20–25°C (68–77°F).

Intravaginal

- Insert calibrated dosage applicator approximately 5 cm (2 in.) into vagina, directing it slightly back toward sacrum. Instill medication by pushing plunger. Patient should remain in recumbent position about 30 min to prevent losing the medication. Observe perineal area before each administration: If mucosa is red, swollen, or excoriated or if there is a change in vaginal discharge, report to prescriber.
- Store cream at room temperature and protect from temperatures above 40°C (104°F).

Topical

- Cleanse and dry selected skin area. Apply as directed under Route & Dosage.
- Store gel/jelly at controlled room temperature 20–25°C (68–77°F). Excursions permitted between 15–30°C (59–86°F).

E

Transdermal

- Cleanse and dry selected skin area on trunk of body, preferably the abdomen, upper quadrant of the buttock, or outer aspect of the hip. Avoid application to the breasts, waistline, to an irritated, abraded, oily area, or to the waistline. If system falls off, it may be reapplied, or if necessary, a new one can be applied. Return to original treatment schedule. Rotate application site with an interval of at least 1 wk between applications to a particular site.
- Store patch between 20 and 25°C (66–77°F). Store in protective pouch and apply immediately after removal. Excursions permitted between 15–30°C (59–86°F).

Intramuscular

- Give deep with at least a 21-gauge needle in the gluteal muscle.
- Store estradiol cypionate at controlled room temperature 20–25°C (68–77°F). Store estradiol valerate at room temperature; protect from light and freezing.

ADVERSE EFFECTS (≥5%) CV: Edema. **Respiratory:** Upper respiratory infection. **CNS:** Headache. **Endocrine:** Weight increase. **Skin:** Dermatitis, pruritus, chloasma, loss of scalp hair, hirsutism. **GI:** Abdominal cramps or pain, constipation, bloating. **GU:** Mastodynia, spotting, changes in menstrual flow, in women: Gynecomastia, testicular atrophy, feminization, impotence (reversible). **Other:** Pain.

DIAGNOSTIC TEST INTERFERENCE Estradiol reduces response of ***metyrapone*** test and excretion of ***pregnanediol.*** May increase ***cortisol-binding globulin levels*** and elevate plasma cortisol levels.

INTERACTIONS Drug: BARBITURATES, **bosentan, phenytoin, rifampin** decrease estrogen effect by increasing its metabolism; ORAL ANTICOAGULANTS may decrease hypoprothrombinemic effects; interfere with effects of **bromocriptine**; may increase levels and toxicity of **cyclosporine**, TRICYCLIC ANTIDEPRESSANTS, **theophylline**; decrease effectiveness of **amprenavir, clofibrate.** CYP3A4 inhibitors may increase serum concentrations and risk of adverse drug reactions. Do not use with **anastrozole** or ESTROGEN derivatives.

PHARMACOKINETICS Absorption: Rapid from GI tract; readily through skin and mucous membranes; slow from IM injections. **Distribution:** Throughout body tissues, especially in adipose tissue; crosses placenta. **Metabolism:** Primarily in liver via CYP 3A4. **Elimination:** In urine; in breast milk.

NURSING IMPLICATIONS

Black Box Warning

Estrogen use in postmenopausal women has been associated with increased risk of endometrial cancer, MI, stroke, breast cancer, PE, DVT, and dementia.

Assessment & Drug Effects

- Monitor for and promptly report any of the following: Abnormal vaginal bleeding; S&S of CV problems (e.g., shortness of breath, chest pain, calf tenderness, dizziness, visual changes); abdominal pain or other signs of gallbladder disease.

- Monitor adverse GI effects. Nausea, frequently at breakfast time, usually disappears after 1 or 2 wk of drug use.
- Check BP on a regular basis in patients with cardiac or kidney dysfunction or hypertension; monitored carefully.
- Postmenopausal osteoporosis prevention indicated. Periodic bone mineral density and biochemical marker measurements.
- Note: Severe hypercalcemia (greater than 15 mg/dL) may be caused by estradiol therapy in patients with breast cancer and bone metastasis.
- Monitor triglycerides, thyroid function tests.

Patient & Family Education

- Notify prescriber of intermittent breakthrough bleeding, spotting, bleeding, or unexplained and sudden pain.
- Determine weight under standard conditions 1 or 2 × wk; report sudden weight gain or other signs of fluid retention.
- Notify prescriber of calf pain upon flexing foot and the following symptoms of thromboembolic disorders: Tenderness, swelling, and redness in extremity; sudden, severe headache or chest pain; slurring of speech; change in vision; tenderness, pain, sudden shortness of breath.
- Learn breast self-examination and perform every month.
- Report persistent or recurrent upper abdominal pain, as it may indicate gallbladder problems.
- Monitor blood glucose for loss of glycemic control if diabetic.
- Decrease caffeine intake because estrogen depresses caffeine metabolism.
- Notify healthcare provider 4–6 weeks before a scheduled surgery.
- Avoid eating grapefruit or drinking grapefruit juice while taking the oral form.
- Learn self-examination of breasts, and follow a monthly schedule.
- Estrogen-induced feminization and impotence in male patients are reversible with termination of therapy.

ESTRAMUSTINE PHOSPHATE SODIUM

(ess-tra-muss′teen)

Emcyt

Classification: ANTINEOPLASTIC; ALKYLATING AGENT; NITROGEN MUSTARD

Therapeutic: ANTINEOPLASTIC

AVAILABILITY Capsule

ACTION & *THERAPEUTIC EFFECT*

Conjugate of estradiol and the carbamate of nitrogen mustard. Incorporation of estramustine in tumor tissues is probably due to the presence of estramustine-binding protein (EMBP), which is found in prostate carcinoma, glioma, melanoma, and breast carcinoma. Binds to proteins and microtubulin resulting in microtubule changes in the cell division cycle, thus arresting cell division in the G2/M phase of the cell cycle. *Major effectiveness reported to be in patients who have been refractory to estrogen therapy alone.*

USES Prostate cancer.

CONTRAINDICATIONS Hypersensitivity to either estradiol or nitrogen mustard; active thrombophlebitis or thromboembolic disorders; pregnancy (category D); lactation (infant risk cannot be ruled out).

 Common adverse effects in *italic*; life-threatening effects underlined; generic names in **bold**; classifications in SMALL CAPS; ♣ Canadian drug name; Prototype drug; Alert

CAUTIOUS USE History of thrombophlebitis, thromboses, or thromboembolic disorders; cerebrovascular or coronary artery disease; gallstones or peptic ulcer; impaired liver function; metabolic bone diseases associated with hypercalcemia; diabetes mellitus; hypertension, conditions that might be aggravated by fluid retention (e.g., epilepsy, migraine, kidney dysfunction); prostate cancer and osteoblastic metastases, older adults.

ROUTE & DOSAGE

Prostate Cancer

Adult: **PO** 14 mg/kg/day in 3–4 divided doses

ADMINISTRATION

Oral

- NIOSH Group 1 use single gloves when handling intact tablets or capsules or administering form a unit-dose package. If cutting, crushing, manipulating, or handling uncoated tablets, use double gloves and protective gown. Wear single gloves during administration, and wear eye/face protection if the formulation is hard to swallow or if the patient may resist, vomit, or spit up.
- Take at least 1 hour before or 2 hours after meals.
- Do not administer with milk, milk products, or calcium-rich food or drugs.
- Store at 2°–8°C (38°–46°F) in tight, light-resistant containers, unless otherwise directed by manufacturer.

ADVERSE EFFECTS **CV:** *Peripheral edema, CHF, MI.* **Respiratory:** Dyspnea. **CNS: CVA. Endocrine:** Breast tenderness. **GI:** *Nausea*, diarrhea. **GU:** Hemolytic uremic syndrome. **Musculoskeletal:** Leg cramps. **Hematologic:** Thrombocytopenia, thrombophlebitis.

INTERACTIONS **Food:** Milk, dairy products, calcium supplements may decrease estramustine absorption. **Drug:** Do not use with **lenograstim, lipegfilgrastim, palifermin.**

PHARMACOKINETICS **Absorption:** Readily absorbed from GI tract. **Peak:** 2–3 h. **Metabolism:** Dephosphorylated in intestines to estramustine, estradiol, and nitrogen mustard; further metabolized in liver. **Elimination:** In feces via bile. **Half-Life:** 20 h.

NURSING IMPLICATIONS

Assessment & Drug Effects

- Monitor weight and examine for peripheral edema. Be mindful that drug can cause CHF.
- Monitor I&O ratio and pattern to prevent dehydration and electrolyte imbalance, especially with vomiting or diarrhea.
- Observe diabetics closely because of possibility of estramustine-induced reduction in glucose tolerance.
- Monitor lab tests: Baseline and periodic LFTs and bilirubin; repeat after drug has been discontinued for 2 mo, calcium levels, testosterone levels.

Patient & Family Education

- Eat small meals at frequent intervals to reduce drug-induced nausea, eat slowly, and try cold food if food odors are offensive.
- Review proper handling and disposal of chemotherapy.
- Drink liquids 1 h before or 2 h after rather than with meals; clear liquids may be more palatable.

- Avoid milk, dairy products, and calcium-rich foods and drugs.
- Avoid live vaccines during therapy.
- Use reliable contraception (men and women).
- Review adverse reactions.

E

ESTROGEN-PROGESTIN COMBINATIONS (CONTRACEPTIVES)

Oral
Monophasic: **Apri, Annovera, Aviane, Balziva, Brevicon, Cryselle, Junel, Lessina, Levora, Loestrin, Low-Ogestrel, Microgestin, Nordette, Norethin, Norinyl, Nortrel, Ogestrel, Ovcon, Portia, Previfem, Seasonale, Sprintec, Yasmin, Yaz, Zovia**
Biphasic: **LoSeasonique, Kariva**
Triphasic: **Aranelle, Cyclessa, Enpresse, Estrostep, Estrostep Fe, Lybrel, Tri-Norinyl, Tri-Previfem, Tri-Sprintec, Triphasil, Trivora, Velivet**
Four-Phasic: **Natazia, Quartette**
Postcoital Contraceptives (levonorgestrel): **Plan B, MyWay, Next Choice One Dose**
Transdermal
Ortho Evra
Intravaginal
NuvaRing
Classification: ESTROGEN-PROGESTIN COMBINATIONS
Therapeutic: CONTRACEPTIVE
Prototype: Estradiol, Norethindrone

AVAILABILITY Oral tablet; transdermal; intravaginal

ACTION & *THERAPEUTIC EFFECT* Three types of estrogen-progestin combinations are available: (1) monophasic, fixed dosage of estrogen-progestin throughout the cycle; (2) biphasic, amount of estrogen remains the same throughout cycle, less progestin in first half of cycle and increased progestin in second half; (3) triphasic, estrogen amount is the same or varies throughout cycle, progestin amount varies. *Fixed combination of estrogen and progestin produces contraception by preventing ovulation and rendering reproductive tract structures hostile to sperm penetration and zygote implantation.*

USES To prevent conception, postcoital contraceptive or "morning after pill"; moderate acne in females 15 yr or older.

UNLABELED USES Abnormal uterine bleeding, dysmenorrhea, hirsutism, pain associated with endometriosis, polycystic ovary syndrome.

CONTRAINDICATIONS Familial or personal history of or existence of breast or other estrogen-dependent neoplasm, recurrent chronic cystic mastitis, patients at high risk of arterial or venous thrombotic diseases; DM with vascular disease; history of or existence of thrombophlebitis or thromboembolic disorders, cerebral vascular or coronary artery disease, MI, hepatic tumor or disease; family history of hepatic porphyria, renal impairment, adrenal insufficiency, undiagnosed abnormal vaginal bleeding, women age 35 and over who smoke, adolescents with incomplete epiphyseal closure; pregnancy. Fetal risk cannot be ruled out; lactation—Infant risk cannot be ruled out.

CAUTIOUS USE History of depression, preexisting hypertension, or cardiac or renal disease; impaired liver function, history of migraine, convulsive disorders, or asthma; multiparous women with grossly irregular menses, DM, or familial history of diabetes; gallbladder disease, lupus erythematosus, heredity angioedema; rheumatic disease, varicosities, smokers.

ROUTE & DOSAGE

Contraception

Adult: **PO** 1 tablet daily, see product specific information. **Topical** Apply one patch once weekly for 3 wk, then have 1 wk patch-free before repeating the cycle; **Intravaginal** Insert 1 ring on or before day 5 of the cycle. Remove ring after 3 wk, followed by a 1 wk rest. Then insert new ring.

Postcoital Contraception (levonorgestrel)

Adult: **PO** 1 tablet within 72 h of intercourse, some products also require a second dose 12 h later

ADMINISTRATION

Oral

- Give without regard to meals.
- Do not exceed 24-h intervals between the daily doses; taking with a meal or at bedtime is a helpful reminder.
- Missed doses follow manufacturer instructions. Alternate forms of contraception may need to be used.
- Vomiting and diarrhea occur within 3–4 hours of a dose, take the tablet scheduled for the next day as soon as possible; backup contraception should be use d if 2 or more doses are missed.

Topical

- Apply transdermal patch immediately after removing from pouch.
- Apply the adhesive side to a clean, dry area of the lower abdomen or upper quadrant of buttock.

E

ADVERSE EFFECTS (>5%)

Endocrine: Weight increase. **GU:** Dysmenorrhea, *menstrual disorders.* Breast signs and symptoms, reduced libido.

DIAGNOSTIC TEST INTERFERENCE ORAL CONTRACEPTIVES (OCS) may change the results of some laboratory tests (e.g., ***coagulation factors, lipids, glucose tolerance, thyroxine-binding globulin, sex hormone-binding globulin, and cortisol-binding globulin***) and reduce the ***metyrapone*** test response.

INTERACTIONS **Drug: Aminocaproic acid** may increase clotting factors, leading to hypercoagulable state; CYP3A4 inducers including BARBITURATES, ANTICONVULSANTS, ANTIBIOTICS, **rifampin**, ANTIFUNGALS reduce efficacy of OCS and increase incidence of breakthrough bleeding and risk of pregnancy. May decrease efficacy of **lamotrigine.** Do not use with **dehydroepiandrosterone, exemestane. Herbal: St. John's wort** may decrease efficacy of OCS.

PHARMACOKINETICS **Absorption:** Oral: Readily from GI tract; or from transdermal patch placed on abdomen, buttock, upper outer arm, and upper torso (excluding breast). Vaginal insert: Norgestrel 100% absorbed. **Peak:** Patch: 48 h. **Duration:** Patch: 1 wk. **Distribution:**

Widely distributed; crosses placenta; small amount distributed into breast milk. **Metabolism:** In liver. **Elimination:** In urine and feces. **Half-Life:** 6–45 h oral. Following removal of the patch: Norelgestromin 28 h, vaginal ring: Norgestrel 29 h.

NURSING IMPLICATIONS

Black Box Warning

Estrogen use in postmenopausal women has been associated with increased risk of endometrial cancer, MI, stroke, breast cancer, PE, DVT, and dementia. Cigarette smoking increases the risk of serious cardiovascular events and increases with age particularly in women over 35 yr and with number of cigarettes smoked.

Assessment & Drug Effects

- Monitor for and promptly report any of the following: Abnormal vaginal bleeding; S&S of CV problems (e.g., shortness of breath, chest pain, calf tenderness, dizziness, visual changes); abdominal pain or other signs of gallbladder disease.
- Check BP periodically. In some women, changes in BP occur within each cycle; in others, slow increase of pressure, particularly diastolic, over several months is significant. Drug-induced BP elevation is usually reversible with cessation of OCs.
- Nausea with or without vomiting occurs in approximately 10% of patients during the first cycle and is reportedly one of the major reasons for voluntary discontinuation of therapy. Most adverse effects tend to disappear in third or fourth cycle of use. Instruct patient to report symptoms that persist after fourth cycle. Dose adjustment or a different product may be indicated.
- Hirsutism and loss of hair are reversible with discontinuation of OCs or by change of selected combination.
- Acne may improve, worsen, or develop for first time. In women on OCs for at least 1 yr, postcontraceptive acne sometimes occurs 3–4 mo after stopping drug and may continue for 6–12 mo.
- Anovulation or amenorrhea following termination of OC regimen may persist more than 6 mo. The user with pretreatment oligomenorrhea or secondary amenorrhea is most apt to have oversuppression syndrome.
- Monitor blood glucose in females with DM or prediabetes, and TSH.

Patient & Family Education

- Use an additional method of birth control during the first week of the initial cycle.
- Consult patient information supplied with drug for management of missed doses.
- Ovulation is unlikely with omission of 1 daily dose; however, the possibility of escaped ovulation, spotting, or breakthrough bleeding increases with each missed dose.
- Discontinue medication if intracycle bleeding resembling menstruation occurs. Begin taking tablets from a new compact on day 5. If bleeding persists, see prescriber.
- Transdermal patches: Apply only one patch at a time, and never cut or otherwise alter a patch prior to application.

- See prescriber to rule out pregnancy if 2 consecutive periods are missed, before continuing on OCs.
- Learn breast self-examination, and do every month.
- Monitor blood pressure.
- Report symptoms of hyperkalemia: belly pain, diarrhea, chest pain, heart palpitations, muscle weakness, nausea and vomiting.
- Record frequent weight checks to permit early recognition of fluid retention.
- Understand the increased risk of thromboembolic and cardiovascular problems and increased incidence of gallbladder disease with OC use. Be alert to manifestations of thrombotic or thromboembolic disorders: Severe headache (especially if persistent and recurrent), dizziness, blurred vision, leg or chest pain, respiratory distress, unexplained cough. Discontinue drug if any of these symptoms appear, and report them promptly to prescriber.
- Report sudden abdominal pain immediately to prescriber in order to rule out ectopic pregnancy.
- Stop drug and contact prescriber if unexplained partial or complete, sudden or gradual loss of vision, protrusion of eyeballs, or blurred vision occurs.
- If OC use is accompanied by vaginal itching and irritation, report to prescriber promptly to rule out candidiasis.
- Monitor blood glucose closely if diabetic. Adjustment of antidiabetic medication may be necessary.
- Use alternate method of birth control when breastfeeding until infant is weaned.

ESTROGENS, CONJUGATED

(ess′tro-jenz)

C.E.S. ♣, Premarin

Classification: ESTROGENS

Therapeutic: FEMALE HORMONE REPLACEMENT THERAPY (HRT)

Prototype: Estradiol

AVAILABILITY Tablet; solution for injection; vaginal cream

ACTION & *THERAPEUTIC EFFECT* Circulating estrogens modulate the pituitary secretion of the gonadotropins luteinizing hormone (LH) and follicle-stimulating hormone (FSH) through a negative feedback mechanism. Estrogens act to reduce the elevated levels of these gonadotropins seen in postmenopausal women. *Binds to intracellular receptors that stimulate DNA and RNA to synthesize proteins responsible for effects of estrogen.*

USES Genitourinary syndrome of menopause, and abnormal bleeding (hormonal imbalance); also female hypoestrogenism, primary ovarian failure, vasomotor symptoms associated with menopause; to retard progression of osteoporosis and as palliative therapy of breast and advanced prostate cancer.

UNLABELED USES Uremic bleeding.

CONTRAINDICATIONS History of breast cancer, except for palliative therapy; known anaphylactic reaction or angioedema to conjugated estrogens; vaginal

E

and cervical cancers; endometrial cancer; endometrial hyperplasia; abnormal vaginal bleeding; hepatic disease or cancer; CAD; hepatic impairment; history of cholestatic jaundice associated with use of estrogen or pregnancy; hypercalcemia; ovarian cancer; history of thromboembolic disease; thrombophilic disorders; known protein C, protein S, or antithrombin deficiency; known or suspected pregnancy—known to cause fetal harm; lactation—avoid breastfeeding drug may inhibit lactation and milk effects are possible.

CAUTIOUS USE Hypertension; gallbladder disease; DM; heart failure; kidney dysfunction; elderly patients; thyroid and parathyroid disease; hepatic disease; history of asthma.

ROUTE & DOSAGE

Menopause, Atrophic Vaginitis, Kraurosis Vulvae

Adult: **PO** 0.3 mg/day for 21 days each month, adjust to lowest level that gives symptom control
Topical 0.5 g/day administered cyclically

Female Hypoestrogenism

Adult: **PO** 1.25 mg/day given cylically; adjust for symptoms

Breast Cancer

Adult: **PO** 10 mg tid for at least 3 mo

Prostatic Cancer Palliation

Adult: **PO** 1.25–2.5 mg tid

Abnormal uterine bleeding

Adult: **IM/IV** 25 mg may repeat q 6–12 hours

Osteoporosis Prevention

Adult: **PO** 0.3 mg/day cyclically or daily, depending on patient assessment.

ADMINISTRATION

Oral

- Give at the same time each day.
- NIOSH: Use of single gloves by anyone handling intact tablets or capsules or administering from a unit-dose package. If cutting, crushing, or handling uncoated tablets, use double gloves and protective gown. During administration, wear single gloves and wear eye/face protections if the patient may resist. Use respiratory protection if there is an inhalation potential.
- Store tablets at 20 to 25°C (68 to 77°F); excursions permitted between 15 and 30°C (59 and 86°F).

Topical

- Use calibrated dosage applicator dispensed with the cream.
- Store vaginal cream at 20 to 25°C (68 to 77°F); excursions permitted between 15 and 30°C (59 and 86°F).

Intramuscular

- Reconstitute by first removing approximately 5 mL of air from the dry-powder vial, then slowly inject the supplied diluent to the vial by aiming it at the side of the vial. Gently agitate to dissolve but **do not shake.**
- NIOSH: Use double gloves and wear a gown to prepare injection. Wear eye/face protections if the patient may resist. Use respiratory

protection if there is an inhalation potential.
- Use within a few hours of reconstitution.

Intravenous

PREPARE: **Direct:** Reconstitute as for IM injection.
ADMINISTER: **Direct:** Give slowly at a rate of 5 mg/min. ▪ Estrogen solution is compatible with D5W and NS and may be added to IV tubing just distal to the needle if necessary.
INCOMPATIBILITIES: **Y-site: Pantoprazole.**

- Store ampule and reconstituted solution at 2°–8°C (38°–46°F) and protected from light; stable for 60 days. ▪ Discard precipitated or discolored solution.

ADVERSE EFFECTS (≥5%) **CV:** Edema, vasodilation. **Respiratory:** Cough, sore throat. **CNS:** Headache, weakness. **Endocrine:** Reduced carbohydrate tolerance, fluid retention. **Skin:** Itching. **GI:** *Nausea*, flatulence, diarrhea, bloating, abdominal pain. **GU:** Breast pain, spotting, changes in menstrual flow, dysmenorrhea, amenorrhea. **Musculoskeletal:** Backache. **Other:** Leg cramps, psychiatric depression.

DIAGNOSTIC TEST INTERFERENCE Reduces response of ***metyrapone*** test.

INTERACTIONS **Drug:** BARBITURATES, **carbamazepine, phenytoin, rifampin** decrease estrogen effect by increasing its metabolism; ORAL ANTICOAGULANTS may decrease hypoprothrombinemic effects; interfere with effects of **bromocriptine**; may increase levels and toxicity of **cyclosporine**, TRICYCLIC ANTIDEPRESSANTS, **theophylline**; decrease effectiveness of **clofibrate.** CYP3A4 inhibitors may increase serum concentrations and risk of adverse drug reactions. Do not use with **anastrozole** or ESTROGEN DERIVATIVES.

PHARMACOKINETICS **Absorption:** Rapid absorption from GI tract; readily absorbed through skin and mucous membranes (including vaginal mucosa); slow absorption from IM injections. **Distribution:** Distributed throughout body tissues, especially in adipose tissue; crosses placenta, excreted in breast milk. Conjugated estrogens are bound primarily to albumin. **Metabolism:** Metabolized primarily in liver to glucuronide and sulfate conjugates of estradiol, and estriol. **Elimination:** In urine. **Half-Life:** 4–18 h.

NURSING IMPLICATIONS

Black Box Warning

Estrogen use in postmenopausal women has been associated with increased risk of endometrial cancer, MI, stroke, breast cancer, PE, DVT, and dementia.

Assessment & Drug Effects

- See additional implications under estradiol.
- Monitor for and report breakthrough vaginal bleeding.
- Monitor blood pressure.
- Monitor for fluid retention.
- Assess for relief of menopausal symptoms.
- Monitor bone density annually when used for osteoporosis prophylaxis.

E

- Monitor lab tests: Periodic serum phosphatase levels with prostate cancer, serum calcium for hypocalcemic patients, thyroid function studies for hypothyroid patients.

Patient & Family Education

- Be aware of importance of taking drug exactly as prescribed: Specifically, do not omit, increase, or decrease doses without advice of prescriber.
- Intravaginal administration: For self-administration, wash hands well before and after application, and avoid contact of denuded areas with the cream. Do not use tampons while on vaginal cream therapy.
- Notify prescriber promptly of adverse symptoms.
- Know signs of thrombophlebitis (see Appendix F) and report promptly if suspected.
- Review package insert to ensure understanding of estrogen therapy.

ESTROGENS, ESTERIFIED

(ess′tro-jenz)

Menest, Neo-Estrone ♣

Classification: ESTROGEN

Therapeutic: ESTROGEN; FEMALE HORMONE REPLACEMENT THERAPY (HRT)

Prototype: Estradiol

AVAILABILITY Tablet

ACTION & *THERAPEUTIC EFFECT* At the cellular level, estrogens increase cervical secretions, result in proliferation of the endometrium, and increase uterine tone. Estrogens also can affect bone calcium deposition and accelerate epiphyseal closure. Estrogens appear to prevent osteoporosis associated with the onset of menopause; they generally do not reverse bone density loss that has already developed. *Binds to intracellular receptors that stimulate DNA and RNA to synthesize proteins responsible for effects of estrogen.*

USES Metastatic breast cancer in selected patients, vasomotor symptoms or vaginal atrophy associated with menopause, hypoestrogenism due to castration, hypogonadism, primary ovarian failure, prevention of postmenopausal osteoporosis, advanced prostate cancer. Atrophic vaginitis, kraurosis vulvae and abnormal bleeding (hormonal imbalance), female hypogonadism, castration, primary ovarian failure, vasomotor symptoms associated with menopause, palliative therapy of breast and prostatic carcinomas; prevention of osteoporosis.

CONTRAINDICATIONS Breast cancer except as treatment; cervical cancer; endometrial cancer; endometrial hyperplasia; prostate cancer; hepatic disease or cancer; hypercalcemia; lupus (SLE); abnormal genital bleeding; thromboembolic disorders; known or suspected pregnancy—known to cause fetal harm; lactation—milk effects on the infant are possible.

CAUTIOUS USE Hypertension; history of depression; gallbladder disease; DM; heart failure; risk of thromboembolic or thrombotic disease; impaired liver function; kidney dysfunction; history of asthma; migraine headaches; seizure disorders; elderly; women over 65 yr.

ROUTE & DOSAGE

Vasomotor or Vaginal Atrophy/Menopause

Adult: **PO** 0.3–1.25 mg/day for 21 days each month, adjust to lowest level that gives symptom control

Female Hypoestrogenism due to hypogonadism

Adult: **PO** 2.5–7.5 mg/day in 1–3 divided doses for 20 days followed by a 10-day rest period

Breast Cancer

Adult: **PO** 10 mg tid for 2–3 mo

Prostatic Cancer (palliation)

Adult: **PO** 1.25–2.5 mg tid for several weeks

ADMINISTRATION

Oral

- Give with food or fluid of patient's choice.
- NIOSH: Use single gloves when handling intact tablets, capsules or when administering from a unit-dose package. Double glove and wear a protective gown when cutting, crushing or manipulating uncoated tablets. During administration, wear single gloves, wear eye/face protection if the patient may resist, vomit or spit up.
- Store tablets below 35° (77°F) in a tightly closed container.

ADVERSE EFFECTS (common)

CV: Edema. **CNS:** Headache, migraine. **Skin:** Chloasma, hirsutism. **GI:** *Nausea*, vomiting, bloating, stomach cramping. **GU:** Breast pain, spotting, changes in menstrual flow, dysmenorrhea, amenorrhea. **Other:** Psychiatric depression, disturbance in mood.

DIAGNOSTIC TEST INTERFERENCE

Reduces response of ***metyrapone*** test.

INTERACTIONS

Drug: BARBITURATES, **phenytoin, rifampin** decrease estrogen effect by increasing its metabolism; ORAL ANTICOAGULANTS may decrease hypoprothrombinemic effects; interfere with effects of **bromocriptine**; may increase levels and toxicity of **cyclosporine**, TCAS, **theophylline**; decrease effectiveness of **clofibrate.** CYP3A4 inhibitors may increase serum concentrations and risk of adverse drug reactions. Do not use with **anastrozole** or estrogen derivatives.

PHARMACOKINETICS

Absorption: Well absorbed with first-pass metabolism. **Metabolism:** Metabolized in GI mucosa and liver to estrone, further metabolized to inactive metabolites. **Elimination:** In urine and bile. **Half-Life:** 4–18.5 h.

E

NURSING IMPLICATIONS

Black Box Warning

Estrogen use in postmenopausal women has been associated with increased risk of endometrial cancer, MI, stroke, breast cancer, PE, DVT, and dementia.

Assessment & Drug Effects

- See nursing implications under estradiol.
- Monitor for and report breakthrough vaginal bleeding.
- Assess for relief of menopausal symptoms.
- Monitor bone density annually when used for osteoporosis prophylaxis.
- Monitor lab tests: Periodic serum phosphatase levels with prostate cancer, renal function tests, serum calcium, thyroid function for hypothyroid patients.

Patient & Family Education

- Be aware of importance of taking drug exactly as prescribed: Specifically, do not omit, increase, or decrease doses without advice of prescriber. Know what to do when a dose is missed.
- Do not smoke during therapy.
- Notify healthcare provider of any abnormal vaginal bleeding.
- Review package insert to ensure understanding of estrogen therapy.

ESZOPICLONE

(es-zo′pi-clone)

Lunesta

Classification: SEDATIVE-HYPNOTIC

Therapeutic: SEDATIVE-HYPNOTIC

Controlled Substance: Schedule IV

AVAILABILITY Tablet

ACTION & *THERAPEUTIC EFFECT* Mechanism of action believed to result from its interaction with GABA-receptor complexes at binding sites close to or coupled to benzodiazepine receptors in the brain. *Improves sleep maintenance in transient insomnia.*

USES Treatment of insomnia.

CONTRAINDICATIONS Hypersensitivity to eszopiclone; alcohol intoxication; alcoholism; eszopiclone-induced angioedema; suicidal tendencies or ideation; pregnancy—fetal risk cannot be ruled out; lactation—infant risk cannot be ruled out.

CAUTIOUS USE Hepatic impairment; debilitated patients; signs and symptoms of depression; compromised respiratory function; COPD; persistent insomnia, older adults. Safe use in children younger than 18 yr is not established.

ROUTE & DOSAGE

Insomnia

Adult: **PO** 1 mg at bedtime; may increase if needed

Severe Hepatic Impairment Dosage Adjustment

Max dose: 2 mg

ADMINISTRATION

Oral

- Give immediately prior to bedtime.
- Store at 15°–30°C (59°–86°F).

ADVERSE EFFECTS (≥5%) **Respiratory:** Infection. **CNS:** dizziness. **GI:** Disorder of taste.

INTERACTIONS Drug: Do not use with CYP3A4 inhibitors **amiodarone,** ANTIRETROVIRAL PROTEASE INHIBITORS, **aprepitant, clarithromycin, dalfopristin/quinupristin, delavirdine, diltiazem, efavirenz, erythromycin, fluconazole, fluoxetine, fluvoxamine, itraconazole, ketoconazole, mifepristone, nefazodone, norfloxacin,** other systemic AZOLE ANTIFUNGALS (**miconazole** and **voriconazole**), **troleandomycin, zafirlukast** due to increased eszopiclone levels. **Ethanol** and other CNS DEPRESSANT agents can produce additive effects in combination with eszopiclone. CYP3A4 inducers may decrease concentration of eszopiclone. **Herbal: St. John's wort** can increase eszopiclone levels.

PHARMACOKINETICS Absorption: Rapidly absorbed from GI tract. **Distribution:** 52–59% protein bound. **Peak:** 1 h. **Metabolism:** Extensive hepatic metabolism. **Elimination:** Primarily in the urine. **Half-Life:** 5–6 h.

NURSING IMPLICATIONS

Black Box Warning

Complex sleep behaviors including sleep-walking, sleep-driving, and engaging in other activities while not fully awake may occur. Some of these events my result in serious injuries, including death. Discontinue immediately if a patient experiences a complex sleep behavior.

Assessment & Drug Effects

- Monitor for and report worsening insomnia and cognitive or behavioral changes.
- Monitor for suicidal ideation in depressive patients.
- Monitor for S&S of CNS depression when other CNS depressants are used concurrently.
- Supervise ambulation if patient is out of bed after taking eszopiclone.

Patient & Family Education

- Follow directions for taking the drug (see Administration).
- Do not take this drug unless you can get at least 8 h of sleep.
- Do not consume alcohol while taking this drug.
- Do not drive or engage in potentially hazardous activities until response to drug is known.
- Report any of the following to a healthcare provider: Worsening insomnia, cognitive or behavioral changes, suicidal thoughts, problem with reproductive function.

ETANERCEPT

(e-tan′er-cept)

Enbrel

Classification: BIOLOGIC RESPONSE MODIFIER; IMMUNOMODULATOR; TUMOR NECROSIS FACTOR (TNF) MODIFIER

Therapeutic: DISEASE-MODIFYING ANTIRHEUMATIC (DMARD); ANTIPSORIATIC

AVAILABILITY Solution for injection; prefilled syringe

ACTION & *THERAPEUTIC EFFECT* A recombinant DNA-derived protein that binds specifically to tumor necrosis factor (TNF) and blocks it from attaching to cell surface TNF receptors. TNF plays an important role in the inflammatory processes and the resulting joint pathology of rheumatoid arthritis, juvenile idiopathic arthritis, ankylosing spondylitis, and plaque psoriasis. *Effectiveness is indicated by* *improved RA symptomatology and/or decreased inflammation in other inflammatory disorders.*

USES Reduction of the signs and symptoms of RA and psoriatic RA in adults, and polyarticular juvenile idiopathic arthritis in children. Treatment of ankylosing spondylitis, moderate-severe chronic plaque psoriasis.

E

CONTRAINDICATIONS Hypersensitivity to etanercept; malignancy; benzyl alcohol hypersensitivity; patients with sepsis or other active infection; agranulocytosis; malignancy; bleeding, hematologic disease, intramuscular administration, intravenous administration; latex hypersensitivity; sepsis; varicella; lactation.

CAUTIOUS USE Immunosuppression; autoimmune disease, bone marrow suppression; diabetes mellitus; hamster protein hypersensitivity; heart failure; multiple sclerosis, neoplastic disease, neurologic disease, seizure disorder, seizures; vaccination, varicella, vasculitis; pregnancy (category B). Safety and efficacy in children younger than 2 yr not established.

ROUTE & DOSAGE

Rheumatoid Arthritis, Psoriatic Arthritis, Ankylosing Spondylitis

Adult: **Subcutaneous** 50 mg once weekly

Juvenile RA

Adolescent/Child (2–17 yr): **Subcutaneous** 0.8 mg/kg weekly (max: 50 mg/week); *weight over 63 kg:* 50 mg once weekly

Plaque Psoriasis

Adult/Adolescent/Child (4 yr and older, weight over 63 kg): **Subcutaneous** 50 mg twice weekly (3–4 days apart) for 3 mo, then 50 mg weekly; *younger than 4 yr, weight less than 63 kg:* 0.8 mg/kg once wk (max: 50 mg)

ADMINISTRATION

Subcutaneous

- Reconstitute by slowly injecting the supplied diluent into the vial. Swirl gently to dissolve and do not shake. Reconstituted solution should be clear and colorless. Use within 6 h.
- Inject into thigh, abdomen, upper arm; rotate injection sites and never inject into an old injection site or where skin is tender, bruised, red, or hard.
- Store reconstituted solution up to 6 h refrigerated at 2°–8°C (36°–46°F). Store unopened dose tray refrigerated at 2°–8°C (36°–46°F).

ADVERSE EFFECTS **Respiratory:** *Respiratory tract infection.* **Skin:** Skin rash, injection site reaction. **GI:** Diarrhea. **Other:** *Infection,* antibody development, positive ANA titer.

INTERACTIONS **Drug:** Concurrent or recent use with **azathioprine, cyclophosphamide, leflunomide, methotrexate** has been associated with pancytopenia. Do not use with DMARDS due to increased risk of infection. Do not use with **certolizumab, leflunomide, tocilizumab.** Avoid use with LIVE VACCINES.

PHARMACOKINETICS **Onset:** 1–2 wk. **Peak:** 72 h. **Half-Life:** 115 h.

NURSING IMPLICATIONS

Black Box Warning

Etanercept has been associated with serious, potentially fatal infections, especially in those taking immunosuppressants, and with development of lymphomas and other malignancies in children and adolescents.

Assessment & Drug Effects

- Monitor carefully for and immediately report S&S of infection.
- Monitor CBC with differential.

Patient & Family Education

- A PPD test is recommended before starting therapy to check for TB.
- Discard all needles and syringes after use; do not reuse.
- Withhold etanercept and notify prescriber before resuming drug if you develop an infection or are exposed to varicella virus.
- Avoid vaccinations, in general, and live vaccines, in particular, while on etanercept.
- Note: Injection site reactions (e.g., redness, pain, swelling) are common in the first month of therapy but generally decrease over time.

ETELCALCETIDE

(e-tel-kals′se-tide)

Parsabiv

Classification: CALCIMIMETIC; ENDOCRINE AGENT

Therapeutic: ANTIPARATHYROID AGENT

AVAILABILITY Solution for injection

ACTION & *THERAPEUTIC EFFECT* A synthetic peptide calcimimetic that activates the calcium-sensing receptor of the parathyroid gland. *Results in decreased PTH secretion, serum calcium, and serum phosphorus levels in patients with secondary hyperparathyroidism on hemodialysis.*

USES Treatment of secondary hyperparathyroidism in patients with chronic kidney disease on hemodialysis.

CONTRAINDICATIONS Hypersensitivity to etelcalcetide or components of the injection.

CAUTIOUS USE Hypersensitivity to etelcalcetide; heart failure; seizure disorder; pregnancy; lactation. Safety and efficacy in children not established.

ROUTE & DOSAGE

Hyperparathyroidism

Adult: **IV** 5-mg bolus 3 × wk at the end of hemodialysis; titration scenarios available in package insert (max: 15 mg 3 × wk)

ADMINISTRATION

Intravenous

PREPARE: Do not mix or dilute prior to administration. Do not use vial if particulate matter or discoloration is observed.
ADMINISTER: Administer intravenously as an undiluted IV bolus into venous line of the dialysis circuit at the end of hemodialysis during or after rinse back.
INCOMPATIBILITIES: Do not mix with other IV medications.

- Store in original carton in refrigerator at 2°–8°C (36°–46°F) to protect from light. Do not expose to temperatures greater than 25°C

(77°F). Use within 7 days if stored in the original carton. Use within 4 h and do not expose to direct sunlight if removed from the original carton.

E

ADVERSE EFFECTS CV: Prolonged QT interval, cardiac failure. **CNS:** Headache, paresthesia. **Endocrine:** *Decreased serum calcium, hypophosphatemia,* hypocalcemia, hyperkalemia. **GI:** *Nausea, diarrhea,* vomiting. **Musculoskeletal:** *Muscle spasm,* myalgia. **Other:** Antibody development.

PHARMACOKINETICS Onset: Effect seen within 30 min. **Metabolism:** Biotransformed in blood; forms conjugates with serum albumin. **Elimination:** 60% in dialysate, 3% in urine, 4.5% in feces. **Half-Life:** 3–4 days (hemodialysis patients).

NURSING IMPLICATIONS

Assessment and Drug Effects

- Monitor for signs of hypocalcemia, worsening of heart failure, GI bleeding or ulceration, QT interval prolongation, and ventricular arrhythmia.
- Monitor lab tests: Baseline and routine monitoring of serum calcium and PTH levels.

Patient & Family Education

- Notify prescriber if you have symptoms of low calcium levels such as muscle cramps or spasms, numbness or tingling, or seizures.
- Notify prescriber if you experience signs or symptoms of allergic reaction such as rash, hives, itching, shortness of breath, wheezing, cough, swelling of the face, lips, tongue, or throat; or any other signs.

ETHACRYNIC ACID

(eth-a-krin′ik)

Edecrin

ETHACRYNATE SODIUM

Classification: ELECTROLYTIC AND WATER BALANCE AGENT; LOOP DIURETIC

Therapeutic: LOOP DIURETIC

Prototype: Furosemide

AVAILABILITY Tablet; solution for injection

ACTION & *THERAPEUTIC EFFECT* Inhibits sodium and chloride reabsorption in the ascending loop of Henle and distal renal tubule interfering with the chloride-binding cotransport system, thus causing increased excretion of water, sodium, chloride, magnesium, and calcium. *Rapid and potent diuretic effect resulting in hypotensive effect.*

USES Management of severe edema.

CONTRAINDICATIONS History of hypersensitivity to ethacrynic acid; increasing azotemia, anuria; hepatic coma; severe diarrhea, dehydration, electrolyte imbalance, hypotension; lactation.

CAUTIOUS USE Hepatic cirrhosis, history of hepatic encephalopathy; severe myocardial disease; older adults, cardiac patients; diabetes mellitus; history of gout; pulmonary edema associated with acute MI; diabetic mellitus; hyperaldosteronism; nephrotic syndrome; history of pancreatitis; pregnancy (category B). **IV:** Safe use in children, infants, and neonates not established.

ROUTE & DOSAGE

Edema

Adult: **PO** 50–200 mg/day in 1–2 divided doses, may increase by 25–50 mg prn (max: 400 mg/day); **IV** 0.5–1 mg/kg (max: 100 mg/dose), may repeat q8–12h if necessary
Child: **PO** 1 mg/kg daily, may increase to 3 mg/kg/day

ADMINISTRATION

Oral

- Give after a meal or food to prevent gastric irritation.
- Schedule doses to avoid nocturia and thus sleep interference. Avoid administration within at least 4 h of bedtime, if possible. This recommendation may not apply to the patient who accumulates fluid and develops respiratory symptoms during sleep.

Intravenous

PREPARE: **Direct:** Reconstitute by adding 50 mL of D5W or NS to vial. ▪ Use solution within 24 h. ▪ Vials reconstituted with D5W may turn cloudy; if so, discard the vial.
ADMINISTER: **Direct:** Give at a rate of 10 mg/min. May give through tubing of a freely flowing, compatible infusion. ▪ If a second IV dose is required, a new site should be selected to prevent thrombophlebitis.
INCOMPATIBILITIES: **Solution/additive:** **Hydralazine, procainamide, tolazoline, triflupromazine.**

- Store oral and parenteral form at 15°–30°C (59°–86°F) unless otherwise directed.

ADVERSE EFFECTS **CV:** Thrombophlebitis. **CNS:** Apprehension, chills, confusion, fatigue, headache, vertigo. **HEENT:** Blurred vision, deafness, tinnitus. **Endocrine:** Abnormal phosphorus levels, abnormal serum calcium, hyperglycemia, hyperuricemia. **Skin:** Skin rash. **Hepatic/GI:** Abnormal hepatic function tests, jaundice, abdominal pain, anorexia, diarrhea, dysphagia, gastrointestinal hemorrhage, nausea, vomiting. **GU:** Hematuria, increased serum creatinine. **Hematologic:** Agranulocytosis, severe neutropenia, thrombocytopenia. **Other:** Fever, chills, acute gout; local irritation and thrombophlebitis with IV injection.

INTERACTIONS **Drug:** THIAZIDE DIURETICS increase potassium loss; increased risk of **digoxin** toxicity from hypokalemia; CORTICOSTEROIDS, **amphotericin B** increases risk of hypokalemia; decreased **lithium** clearance, so increased risk of lithium toxicity; SULFONYLUREA effect may be blunted, causing hyperglycemia; NSAIDS may decrease effect, ANTIHYPERTENSIVE AGENTS increase risk of orthostatic hypotension; AMINOGLYCOSIDES may increase risk of ototoxicity; **warfarin** potentiates hypoprothrombinemia. Do not use with **desmopressin, furosemide, levosulpiride, promazine.**

DIAGNOSTIC TEST INTERFERENCE May lead to false-negative **aldosterone/renin ratio.**

PHARMACOKINETICS **Absorption:** Rapidly absorbed from GI tract. **Onset:** 30 min PO; 5 min IV. **Peak:** 2 h PO; 15–30 min IV. **Duration:** 6–8 h PO; 2 h IV. **Distribution:** Does not cross CSF. **Metabolism:** Metabolized to cysteine conjugate. **Elimination:** 30–65% in urine; 35–40% in bile. **Half-Life:** 30–70 min.

E

NURSING IMPLICATIONS

Assessment & Drug Effects

- Observe closely following IV infusion. Rapid, copious diuresis following IV administration can produce hypotension.
- Monitor IV site closely. Extravasation of IV drug causes local pain and tissue irritation from dehydration and blood volume depletion.
- Monitor BP during initial therapy. Because orthostatic hypotension can occur, supervise ambulation.
- Monitor BP and pulse throughout therapy in patients with impaired cardiac function. Diuretic-induced hypovolemia may reduce cardiac output, and electrolyte loss promotes cardiotoxicity in those receiving digitalis (cardiac) glycosides.
- Establish baseline weight prior to start of therapy; weigh patient under standard conditions. Keep prescriber informed of weight loss or gain in excess of 1 kg (2 lb)/day.
- Monitor I&O ratio. Report promptly excessive diuresis, oliguria, hematuria, or sudden profuse diarrhea. Report signs to prescriber.
- Observe for and report S&S of electrolyte imbalance: Anorexia, nausea, vomiting, thirst, dry mouth, polyuria, oliguria, weakness, fatigue, dizziness, faintness, headache, muscle cramps, paresthesias, drowsiness, mental confusion.
- Report immediately possible signs of thromboembolic complications (see Appendix F).
- Impaired glucose tolerance with hyperglycemia and glycosuria has occurred in patients receiving doses in excess of 200 mg/day.
- Monitor lab tests: Baseline and periodic serum electrolytes, BUN, and creatinine.

Patient & Family Education

- Learn S&S of hypokalemia and hyponatremia (see Appendix F), and report any of these promptly to prescriber.
- Make position changes slowly, particularly from lying to upright posture.
- Notify prescriber immediately of any evidence of impaired hearing. Hearing loss may be preceded by vertigo, tinnitus, or fullness in ears; it may be transient, lasting 1–24 h, or it may be permanent.

ETHAMBUTOL HYDROCHLORIDE

(e-tham′byoo-tole)

Etibi ✦, Myambutol

Classification: ANTITUBERCULOSIS

Therapeutic: ANTITUBERCULAR

Prototype: Isoniazid

AVAILABILITY Tablet

ACTION & *THERAPEUTIC EFFECT* Inhibits arabinosyl transferase resulting in impaired mycobacterial cell wall synthesis. *Synthetic antituberculosis agent that is also effective against atypical mycobacterial infections.*

USES In conjunction with other antituberculosis agents in treatment of pulmonary tuberculosis.

UNLABELED USES Mycobacterium avium complex disease, tuberculous meningitis.

CONTRAINDICATIONS Hypersensitivity to ethambutol; optic neuritis, patients unable to report changes in vision (young children or unconscious patients).

CAUTIOUS USE Renal impairment, hepatic disease; gout; ocular defects (e.g., cataract, recurrent ocular inflammatory conditions, diabetic retinopathy); pregnancy (use with caution in pregnant women). Safe use in children younger than 6 yr not established.

ROUTE & DOSAGE

Tuberculosis

Adult/Adolescent/Child (over 40 kg): **PO** once daily weight based therapy; *40–55 kg:* 800 mg; *56–75 kg:* 1200 mg; *76–90 kg:* 1600 mg

Child (under 40 kg): **PO** 20 mg/kg/dose daily

ADMINISTRATION

Oral

- Give with food if GI irritation occurs. Tablet may be crushed and mixed with apple juice or applesauce if needed.
- Protect ethambutol from light, moisture, and excessive heat. Store at 15°–30°C (59°–86°F) in tightly closed container unless otherwise directed.

ADVERSE EFFECTS **CNS:** Headache, dizziness, confusion, hallucinations, paresthesias, joint pain. **HEENT:** Ocular toxicity: *Retrobulbar optic neuritis;* possibility of anterior optic neuritis with decrease in visual acuity, temporary loss of vision, constriction of visual fields, red–green color blindness, central and peripheral scotomas, eye pain, photophobia; retinal hemorrhage and edema. **GI:** Anorexia, nausea, vomiting, abdominal pain. **Other:** Hypersensitivity (pruritus, dermatitis, anaphylaxis).

INTERACTIONS **Drug: Aluminum-containing antacids** can decrease absorption. Do not give with LIVE VACCINES.

PHARMACOKINETICS **Absorption:** 80% from GI tract. **Peak:** 2–4 h. **Distribution:** Distributes to most body tissues; highest concentrations in erythrocytes, kidney, lungs, saliva; crosses placenta; distributed into breast milk. **Metabolism:** In liver. **Elimination:** 50% in urine within 24 h; 20–22% in feces. **Half-Life:** 3–4 h.

NURSING IMPLICATIONS

Assessment & Drug Effects

- Baseline and periodic (monthly) visual testing.
- Monitor I&O ratio in patients with renal impairment. Report oliguria or any significant changes in ratio or in laboratory reports of kidney function. Systemic accumulation with toxicity can result from delayed drug excretion.
- Monitor lab tests: Periodic LFTs, renal function tests, and CBC.

Patient & Family Education

- Adhere to drug regimen exactly and keep follow-up appointments.
- Notify prescriber promptly of the onset of blurred vision, changes in color perception, constriction of visual fields, or any other visual symptoms. Have eyes checked periodically. Ethambutol can cause irreversible blindness due to optic neuritis.

ETHIONAMIDE

(e-thye-on-am′ide)

Trecator

Classification: ANTITUBERCULOSIS

Therapeutic: ANTITUBERCULAR

Prototype: Isoniazid

AVAILABILITY Tablet

ACTION & *THERAPEUTIC EFFECT*

Inhibits peptide synthesis, which disrupts the formation of the mycobacterial cell wall; bacteriostatic. *Effective against human and bovine strains of* Mycobacterium tuberculosis *and* M. kansasii *and some strains of* Mycobacterium avium-intracellulare *complex. Also active against* M. leprae.

USES Active tuberculosis infection (with other agents).

E

CONTRAINDICATIONS Hypersensitivity to ethionamide and chemically related drugs [e.g., isoniazid, niacin (nicotinamide)]; severe liver damage; hepatic encephalopathy.

CAUTIOUS USE Diabetes mellitus, liver dysfunction, history of psychiatric illnesses including depression; history of thyroid disease; pregnancy (use during pregnancy is not recommended); lactation, children younger than 12 yr.

ROUTE & DOSAGE

Tuberculosis

Adult: **PO** 15–20 mg/kg/day in 1–2 divided doses

ADMINISTRATION

Oral

- Give with or after meals to minimize GI adverse effects. Some patients tolerate ethionamide best when it is taken as a single dose after the evening meal or as a single dose at bedtime.
- Directly observed therapy (DOT) is recommended.
- Store in a cool, dry place at 8°–15°C (46°–59°F) in a tightly closed container unless otherwise directed.

ADVERSE EFFECTS **CNS:** Headache, restlessness, mental depression, drowsiness, dizziness, ataxia, hallucinations, paresthesias, convulsions, postural hypotension. **Endocrine:** Elevated ALT, AST; hepatitis (with jaundice), hypothyroidism. **GI:** Dose-related and frequent; symptoms may be due to CNS stimulation rather than to GI irritation: Anorexia, *epigastric distress, nausea, vomiting,* metallic taste, *diarrhea,* stomatitis, sialorrhea. **GU:** Menorrhagia, impotence.

INTERACTIONS **Drug: Cycloserine, isoniazid** may increase neurotoxic effects. Do not use with LIVE VACCINES. May decrease effect of **sodium picosulfate.**

PHARMACOKINETICS **Absorption:** 80% absorbed from GI tract. **Peak:** 3 h. **Distribution:** Widely distributed including CSF; crosses placenta; distribution into breast milk unknown. **Metabolism:** In liver. **Elimination:** In urine. **Half-Life:** 2 h.

NURSING IMPLICATIONS

Assessment & Drug Effects

- Report onset of skin rash. Progression to exfoliative dermatitis can occur if drug is not promptly discontinued.
- Monitor blood glucose closely in the diabetic until response to drug is established. Diabetics appear to be especially prone to hepatotoxicity (see Appendix F).
- Monitor baseline and periodic ophthalmic exams.
- Monitor lab tests: Baseline C&S. Baseline and periodic LFTs, TSH, and serum glucose.

Patient & Family Education

- Avoid alcohol or use in moderation because ethionamide may increase potential for liver dysfunction.
- Notify prescriber of S&S of hepatotoxicity (see Appendix F);

generally reversible if drug is promptly withdrawn.

- Make position changes slowly and in stages, particularly from lying to upright posture if experiencing hypotension.

ETHOSUXIMIDE

(eth-oh-sux'i-mide)

Zarontin

Classification: SUCCINIMIDE ANTICONVULSANT

Therapeutic: ANTICONVULSANT

AVAILABILITY Capsule; oral solution

ACTION & *THERAPEUTIC EFFECT* Increases the seizure threshold and suppresses paroxysmal spike-and-wave pattern in absence seizures; depresses nerve transmission in the motor cortex. *Reduces frequency of epileptiform attacks, apparently by depressing motor cortex and elevating CNS threshold to stimuli.*

USES Management of absence (petit mal) seizures.

CONTRAINDICATIONS Hypersensitivity to succinimides; severe liver or kidney disease; bone marrow suppression; use alone in mixed types of epilepsy (may increase frequency of grand mal seizures).

CAUTIOUS USE Hematologic disease; preexisting hepatic disease; intermittent porphyria; renal disease; pregnancy (may increase the risk of congenital malformations; use with caution and close monitoring). Safe use in children younger than 3 yr not established.

ROUTE & DOSAGE

Absence Seizures

Adult/ Adolescent/Child (over 6 yr): **PO** 500 mg/day; individualize dose based on patient response (max: 1.5 g/day)
Child (3–6 yr): **PO** 250 mg/day, may increase by small increments (max: 1.5 g/day)

ADMINISTRATION

Oral

- Give with food or milk to decrease GI upset.
- Store all forms at 20°–25°C (68°–77°F); capsules in tight containers, and syrup in light-resistant containers; avoid freezing.

ADVERSE EFFECTS **CNS:** Drowsiness, hiccups, ataxia, dizziness, headache, euphoria, restlessness, irritability, hyperactivity, aggressiveness, inability to concentrate, lethargy, sleep disturbances, night terrors, fatigue. **HEENT:** Myopia. **Endocrine:** Hirsutism, increased libido. **Skin:** Pruritis, urticaria, alopecia, Stevens–Johnson syndrome. **GI:** Nausea, vomiting, *anorexia, epigastric distress,* abdominal pain, *weight loss,* diarrhea, gingival hyperplasia. **GU:** Vaginal bleeding. **Hematologic:** Eosinophilia, leukopenia, agranulocytosis, pancytopenia, **Musculoskeletal:** Systemic lupus erythematosus. **Other:** Hypersensitivity reaction, DRESS syndrome.

INTERACTIONS **Drug:** **Carbamazepine** decreases ethosuximide levels; **isoniazid** significantly increases ethosuximide levels; levels of both **phenobarbital** and ethosuximide may be altered with increased seizure frequency.

E

CNS DEPRESSANTS may increase sedation. **Herbal: Ginkgo** may decrease anticonvulsant effectiveness.

PHARMACOKINETICS Absorption: Readily from GI tract. **Peak:** 4 h; steady state: 4–7 days. **Metabolism:** In liver (via CYP3A4). **Elimination:** In urine; small amounts in bile and feces. **Half-Life:** 30 h (child), 60 h (adult).

NURSING IMPLICATIONS

Assessment & Drug Effects

- Monitor adverse drug effects. GI symptoms, drowsiness, ataxia, dizziness, and other neurologic adverse effects occur frequently and indicate the need for dosage adjustment.
- Observe closely during period of dosage adjustment and whenever other medications are added or eliminated from the drug regimen. Therapeutic serum levels: 40–80 mcg/mL.
- Observe patients with prior history of psychiatric disturbances for behavioral changes. Close supervision is indicated. Drug should be withdrawn slowly if these symptoms appear.
- Monitor lab tests: Baseline and periodic serum concentrations, CBC, platelets, LFTs and urinalysis tests.

Patient & Family Education

- Discontinue drug only under prescriber supervision; abrupt withdrawal of ethosuximide (whether used alone or in combination therapy) may precipitate seizures or petit mal status.
- Do not drive or engage in other potentially hazardous activities until response to drug is known.
- Monitor weight on a weekly basis. Report anorexia and weight loss to prescriber; may indicate need to reduce dosage.

ETIDRONATE DISODIUM Pr

(e-ti-droe′nate)

Classification: BISPHOSPHONATE; BONE METABOLISM REGULATOR

Therapeutic: BONE METABOLISM REGULATOR

AVAILABILITY Tablet

ACTION & *THERAPEUTIC EFFECT* Inhibits bone resorption by inhibiting osteocytic osteolysis; decreases mineral release and matrix or collagen breakdown in bone. *Inhibits bone resorption and increases bone mass.*

USES Symptomatic Paget disease, and heterotopic ossification.

UNLABELED USES Prevention and treatment of corticosteroid-induced osteoporosis; hypercalcemia due to malignant neoplasm.

CONTRAINDICATIONS Hypersensitivity to etidronate; clinically overt osteomalacia, abnormalities of the esophagus; enterocolitis; pathologic fractures; renal failure; osteonecrosis of the jaw.

CAUTIOUS USE Renal impairment; asthma; colitis; dysphagia; esophagitis; gastritis; patients on restricted calcium and vitamin D intake; older adults; pregnancy (category C); lactation. Safe use in children younger than 18 yr not established.

ROUTE & DOSAGE

Paget Disease

Adult: **PO** 5–10 mg/kg/day for up to 6 mo or 11–20 mg/kg/day for up to 3 mo, may repeat after 3 mo off the drug if necessary

Heterotopic Ossification Due to Spinal Cord Injury

Adult: **PO** 20 mg/kg/day for 2 wk, then 10 mg/kg/day for an additional 10 wk

Heterotopic Ossification Due to Total Hip Arthroplasty

Adult: **PO** 20 mg/kg/day starting 1 mo before the procedure and continuing for 3 mo after

ADMINISTRATION

Oral

- Give as single dose on empty stomach 2 h before meals with full glass of water or juice to reduce gastric irritation. Instruct patient to stay upright after taking the medication.
- Relieve GI adverse effects by dividing total oral daily dose.

ADVERSE EFFECTS **GI:** Diarrhea, nausea. **Musculoskeletal:** Ostealgia.

INTERACTIONS **Drug:** CALCIUM SUPPLEMENTS, ANTACIDS, IRON, AND OTHER MINERAL SUPPLEMENTS may decrease absorption of etidronate (give etidronate 2 h before other drugs). **Food:** Food will decrease bioavailability of etidronate (give 2 h before meals).

DIAGNOSTIC TEST INTERFERENCE May interfere with diagnostic imaging agents such as technetium–99m–diphosphonate in bone scans.

PHARMACOKINETICS **Absorption:** Variably from GI tract. **Distribution:** 50% distributed to bone. **Metabolism:** Not metabolized. **Elimination:** 50% in urine. **Half-Life:** 6 h.

NURSING IMPLICATIONS

Assessment & Drug Effects

- Report persistent nausea or diarrhea; GI adverse effects may interfere with adequate nutritional status and need to be treated promptly.
- Monitor I&O ratio, serum creatinine, or BUN of patient with impaired renal function.
- Monitor for signs of hypocalcemia. Latent tetany (hypocalcemia) may be detected by Chvostek and Trousseau signs and a serum calcium value of 7–8 mg/dL.
- Note: Serum phosphate levels generally return to normal 2–4 wk after medication is discontinued.
- Monitor lab tests: Periodic serum calcium and phosphate.

Patient & Family Education

- Avoid eating 2 h before or after taking etidronate. Drug absorption is decreased by food, especially milk, milk products, and other foods high in calcium, mineral supplements, and antacids.
- Notify prescriber promptly of sudden onset of unexplained pain. Risk of pathological fractures increases when daily dose of 20 mg/kg is taken longer than 3 mo.
- Report promptly if bone pain, restricted mobility, heat over involved bone site occur.

ETODOLAC

(e-to′do-lac)

Classification: ANALGESIC, NONSTEROIDAL ANTI-INFLAMMATORY AGENT (NSAID)

Therapeutic: ANALGESIC, NSAID; ANTIPYRETIC

Prototype: Ibuprofen

E

AVAILABILITY Tablet; capsule; sustained release tablet

ACTION & *THERAPEUTIC EFFECT* Inhibits cyclooxygenase (COX-1 and COX-2) enzyme activity and prostaglandin synthesis. NSAIDs may also suppress production of rheumatoid factor. *Produces analgesic, antipyretic, and anti-inflammatory effects of an NSAID.*

USES Osteoarthritis and acute pain, rheumatoid arthritis, arthralgia, juvenile rheumatoid arthritis; management of acute pain.

CONTRAINDICATIONS Hypersensitivity to NSAIDS, salicylates; ulceration or inflammation; perioperative CABG pain; asthma, urticaria, or other allergic reactions to aspirin or other NSAIDs; S&S of developing liver disease; use in labor and delivery; pregnancy (category D third trimester).

CAUTIOUS USE Renal impairment, liver function impairment, GI disorders, history of GI ulceration, GI bleeding; cardiac disorders including fluid retention, hypertension, heart failure; dehydration; asthma; preexisting hematologic diseases (e.g., coagulopathy and hemophilia) or thrombocytopenia; IM injections; dental work; DM; surgery when hemostasis is required; immunosuppression, neutropenia; patients over 65 yr, pregnancy (category C first and second trimester); lactation. Safe use in children younger than 6 yr not established.

ROUTE & DOSAGE

Acute Pain

Adult: **PO** 200–400 mg q6–8h prn

Osteoarthritis/Rheumatoid Arthritis

Adult: **PO Immediate release** 600–1200 mg/day in divided doses (max: 1200 mg/day); **Extended release** 400–1000 mg daily

Juvenile Rheumatoid Arthritis

Adolescent/Child (6 yr or older), weight 20–30 kg: **PO** *20–30 kg:* 400 mg daily; *31–45 kg:* 600 mg daily; *46–60 kg:* 800 mg daily; *over 60 kg:* 1000 mg daily

ADMINISTRATION

Oral

- Give with food or milk to reduce risk of GI ulceration.
- Ensure that sustained release form of drug is not chewed or crushed. It **must be** swallowed whole.
- Store at 15°–25°C (59°–77°F); tablets and capsules in bottles; sustained release capsules in unit-dose packages. Protect all forms from moisture.

ADVERSE EFFECTS **GI:** Dyspepsia, nausea.

DIAGNOSTIC TEST INTERFERENCE May cause a false-positive ***urinary bilirubin*** test and a false-positive ***ketone*** test done with the dipstick method. May lead to false-positive ***aldosterone/renin ratio.***

INTERACTIONS **Drug:** May reduce effects of **diuretics** and antihypertensive effects of **beta blockers** and other ANTIHYPERTENSIVE MEDICATIONS. May increase **digoxin** and **lithium** levels and nephrotoxicity due to **cyclosporine.** Increased risk of bleeding with ANTICOAGULANTS or

ANTIPLATELETS. Do not use with **cidofovir, acemetacin, aminolevulinic acid, dexketoprofen, mifamurtide,** or with other NSAIDs. **Herbal: Feverfew, garlic, ginger, ginkgo** may increase bleeding.

PHARMACOKINETICS **Absorption:** Readily from GI tract. **Onset:** 30 min. **Peak:** 1–2 h. **Duration:** 4–12 h. **Distribution:** Widely distributed; 99% protein bound; not known if crosses placenta or if distributed into breast milk. **Metabolism:** Extensively in liver. **Elimination:** 72% in urine, 16% in feces. **Half-Life:** 6–7 h.

NURSING IMPLICATIONS

Black Box Warning

Etodolac has been associated with increased risk of serious, potentially fatal GI bleeding and cardiovascular events (e.g., MI & CVA); risk may increase with duration of use and may be greater in the older adult and those with risk factors for CV disease.

Assessment & Drug Effects

- Assess for signs of GI ulceration and bleeding. Risk factors include high doses of etodolac, history of peptic ulcer disease, alcohol use, smoking, and concomitant use of aspirin.
- Monitor for and report promptly S&S of CV thrombotic events (i.e., angina, MI, TIA, or stroke).
- Assess carefully for fluid retention by monitoring weight and observing for edema in patients with a history of CHF.
- Monitor for decreased BP control in hypertensive patients.
- Monitor for drug toxicity when used concurrently with either digoxin or lithium.
- Monitor for rhinitis, urticaria, or other signs of allergic reactions.
- Monitor carefully increases in etodolac dosage with older adult patients; adverse effects are more pronounced.
- Monitor lab tests: Periodic CBC, chemistry panel, renal function tests, and LFTs.

Patient & Family Education

- Learn S&S of GI ulceration. Stop medication in presence of bleeding and contact the prescriber immediately.
- Stop taking drug and report promptly to prescriber if you experience chest pain, shortness of breath, weakness, slurring of speech, or other signs of a cardiac or neurologic problem.
- Do not take aspirin, which may potentiate ulcerogenic effects.

ETOPOSIDE

(e-toe-po′side)

Toposar

Classification: ANTINEOPLASTIC; MITOTIC INHIBITOR

Therapeutic: ANTINEOPLASTIC, CELL-CYCLE SPECIFIC

Prototype: Vincristine

AVAILABILITY Capsule; solution for injection

ACTION & *THERAPEUTIC EFFECT* Produces cytotoxic action by arresting G_2 (resting or premitotic) phase of cell cycle; also acts on S phase of DNA synthesis. High doses cause lysis of cells entering mitotic phase, and lower doses inhibit cells from entering prophase. *Antineoplastic effect is due to its ability to arrest mitosis (cell division).*

USES Testicular cancer, small-cell lung cancer.

UNLABELED USES Hodgkin and non-Hodgkin lymphoma, non-small-cell lung cancer, ovarian cancer, soft-tissue sarcoma, advanced adrenocortical carcinoma, breast metastases, hemophagocytic lymphohistiocytosis, multiple myeloma.

CONTRAINDICATIONS Severe bone marrow depression; severe hepatic or renal impairment; existing or recent viral infection, bacterial infection; intraperitoneal, intrapleural, or intrathecal administration; pregnancy (fetal growth restriction and newborn myelosuppression risk when administered during pregnancy); lactation.

CAUTIOUS USE Impaired kidney or liver function; gout; radiation therapy. Safe use in children not established.

ROUTE & DOSAGE

Testicular Carcinoma

Adult: **IV** 100 mg/m²/day for 5 consecutive days q3w for 4 cycles

Small-Cell Lung Carcinoma

Adult: **IV** multiple regimen options 100 or 120 mg/m² on days 1, 2, 3 q3–4wk; **PO** Twice the IV dose rounded to the nearest 50 mg

Hepatic Impairment Dosage Adjustment

Total bilirubin 1.5–3 mg/dL: Decrease by 50%;

Renal Impairment Dosage Adjustment

CrCl 15–50 mL/min: Administer 75% of dose

ADMINISTRATION

Oral

- Refrigerate capsules at 2°–8°C (36°–46°F) unless otherwise directed. Do not freeze.

Intravenous

This drug is a cytotoxic agent, and caution should be used to prevent any contact with the drug. Follow institutional or standard guidelines for preparation, handling, and disposal of cytotoxic agents.

PREPARE: **IV Infusion:** *Etoposide concentration for injection:* Each 100 mg **must be** diluted with 250–500 mL of D5W or NS to produce final concentrations of 0.2–0.4 mg/mL. *Etoposide phosphate:* Add 5 or 10 mL of sterile water for injection, D5W, NS, bacteriostatic water for injection, or bacteriostatic NS for injection to yield 20 or 10 mg/mL etoposide, respectively. ▪ May be given as prepared or further diluted to as low as 0.1 mg/mL in either D5W or NS.

ADMINISTER: **IV Infusion:** Give by slow IV infusion over 30–60 min to reduce risk of hypotension and bronchospasm. ▪ Before administration, inspect solution for particulate matter and discoloration. Solution should be clear and yellow. If crystals are present, discard.

INCOMPATIBILITIES: **Y-site: Cefepime, dantrolene, diazepam, filgrastim, gallium, gemtuzumab, idarubicin, indomethacin, lansoprazole, mitomycin, pantoprazole, phenytoin, thiopental.**

- Diluted solutions with concentration of 0.2 mg/mL are stable for 96 h, and the 0.4 mg/mL solutions are stable for 24 h under normal room fluorescent light in glass or plastic (PVC) containers. ▪ Phosphate solution is stable for 24 h at room temperature or refrigerated.

ADVERSE EFFECTS **Skin:** *Alopecia.* **GI:** *Nausea, vomiting,* anorexia, diarrhea. **Hematologic:** *Leukopenia (principally granulocytopenia), thrombocytopenia, anemia.*

INTERACTIONS **Drug:** ANTICOAGULANTS, ANTIPLATELET AGENTS, NSAIDS, **aspirin** may increase risk of bleeding. May enhance the effect of MYELOSUPRESSIVE AGENTS or IMMUNOSUPPRESANTS. Avoid concurrent use of LIVE VACCINES, use caution with INACTIVATED VACCINES. CYP3A4 INDUCERS may decrease concentration of etoposide.

PHARMACOKINETICS **Absorption:** Approximately 50% from GI tract. **Peak:** 1–1.5 h. **Distribution:** Variable penetration into CSF, 95–98% protein bound. **Metabolism:** In liver via CYP3A4 and 3A5. **Elimination:** 44–60% in urine, 2–16% in feces over 3 days. **Half-Life:** 5–10 h (adult).

NURSING IMPLICATIONS

Black Box Warning

Etoposide has been associated with severe myelosuppression with resulting infection and/or bleeding.

Assessment & Drug Effects

- Check IV site during and after infusion. Extravasation can cause thrombophlebitis and necrosis.
- Be prepared to treat an anaphylactoid reaction (see Appendix F). Stop infusion immediately if the reaction occurs.
- Monitor vital signs during and after infusion. Stop infusion immediately if hypotension or tachycardia develop.
- Withhold therapy when an absolute neutrophil count is below 500/mm^3 or a platelet count below 50,000/mm^3.
- Be alert to evidence of patient complaints that might suggest development of leukopenia (see Appendix F), infection (immunosuppression), and bleeding.
- Protect patient from any trauma that might precipitate bleeding during period of platelet nadir particularly. Withhold invasive procedures if possible.
- Monitor lab tests: Prior to each cycle and at frequent intervals CBC with platelet count; periodic renal function, LFTs, and albumin.

Patient & Family Education

- Learn possible adverse effects of etoposide, such as blood dyscrasias, alopecia, carcinogenesis, before treatment begins.
- Make position changes slowly, particularly from lying to upright position, because transient hypotension after therapy is possible.
- Inspect mouth daily for ulcerations and bleeding. Avoid obvious irritants such as hot or spicy foods, smoking, and alcohol.

ETRAVIRINE

(e-tra'vi-reen)

Intelence

Classification: ANTIRETROVIRAL; NONNUCLEOSIDE REVERSE TRANSCRIPTASE INHIBITOR (NNRTI)
Therapeutic: ANTIRETROVIRAL; NNRTI
Prototype: Efavirenz

E

AVAILABILITY Tablet

ACTION & *THERAPEUTIC EFFECT* Prevents replication of HIV-1 viruses by binding directly to reverse transcriptase, thus blocking RNA- and DNA-dependent polymerase activities. *Effectiveness is indicated by reduction in viral load (plasma level HIV RNA).*

USES HIV-1 infection in combination with other antiretroviral agents.

CONTRAINDICATIONS Severe skin reactions; lactation.

CAUTIOUS USE Severe hepatic impairment (Child–Pugh class C); concurrent hepatitis B or C, dyslipidemia; older adults; pregnancy (category B). Safety and efficacy in children not established.

ROUTE & DOSAGE

HIV Infection

Adults/Adolescent/Child (6 yr or older, weight 30 kg or more): **PO** 200 mg bid

Adolescent/Child (6 yr or older, weight 25–29 kg): **PO** 150 mg bid; *weight 20–24 kg:* 125 mg bid; *weight 10–19 kg:* 100 mg bid

ADMINISTRATION

Oral

- Give after a meal. Ensure that tablets are not chewed.
- May dissolve in water if patient cannot swallow tablets. Once dissolved, should be swallowed immediately. Rinse glass several times and instruct to swallow each time to ensure entire dose has been administered.
- Store at 15°–30°C (59°–86°F). Keep bottles closed tightly to protect from moisture. Do not remove desiccant pouches from bottle.

ADVERSE EFFECTS **CV:** Hypertension, hemorrhagic stroke. **CNS:** Fatigue, headache. **Endocrine:** Elevated creatinine, elevated LDL, elevated total cholesterol, elevated triglycerides, elevated glucose, elevated ALT, hepatic failure. **Skin:** *Rash*. **GI:** Abdominal pain, *diarrhea, nausea*, vomiting. **Other:** Peripheral neuropathy, rhabdomyolysis.

INTERACTIONS **Drug:** Compounds that inhibit CYP3A4, CYP2C9, and/or CYP2C19 (e.g., **itraconazole, ketoconazole**) may increase plasma levels of etravirine. Compounds that induce CYP3A4, CYP2C9, and/or CYP2C19 (e.g., **carbamazepine, phenobarbital, phenytoin**) may decrease plasma levels of etravirine. Etravirine may decrease the plasma levels of other compounds that require CYP3A4 for metabolism (e.g., HIV PROTEASE INHIBITORS) and may increase the plasma levels of other compounds that require CYP2C9 and/or CYP2C19 for metabolism (e.g., **diazepam, warfarin**). **Herbal:** **St. John's wort, echinacea** may decrease etravirine efficacy.

PHARMACOKINETICS **Peak:** 2.5 to 4 h. **Distribution:** 99.9% protein bound. **Metabolism:** In liver by CYP2C9, CYP2C19, and CYP3A4. **Elimination:** 93.7% in feces, 1.2% in urine. **Half-Life:** 41 h.

NURSING IMPLICATIONS

Assessment & Drug Effects

- Monitor for and report promptly potentially serious adverse reactions, including skin hypersensitivity reactions, muscle pain indicative of rhabdomyolysis, and S&S of hepatic dysfunction.
- Monitor for and report S&S of opportunistic infections.
- Monitor lab tests: Periodic CD4+ T cell count, plasma HIV RNA,

CBC with platelet count, serum amylase, LFTs, renal function tests, and lipid profile.

Patient & Family Education

- Do not take on an empty stomach.
- Do not remove drying-agent pouches from medication bottle.
- Report promptly any of the following: Rash, S&S of infection, or unexplained muscle pain.
- Report use of all prescription and nonprescription medications, as well as herbs, to prescriber.

EVEROLIMUS

(e-ver-o-li′mus)

Afinitor, Zortress

Classification: BIOLOGIC RESPONSE MODIFIER; IMMUNOMODULATOR; ANTINEOPLASTIC; KINASE INHIBITOR

Therapeutic: ANTINEOPLASTIC; IMMUNOSUPPRESSANT

Prototype: Erlotinib

AVAILABILITY Tablet; oral suspension

ACTION & *THERAPEUTIC EFFECT* Binds to an intracellular protein of several types of cancer cells and inhibits a major dysfunctional kinase pathway in cancer development. It also reduces the expression of vascular endothelial growth factor (VEGF) in these cells. *Reduces cell proliferation, angiogenesis, and glucose uptake in renal and several other types of carcinoma cells.*

USES **Zortress** only: Prophylaxis of kidney/liver transplant rejection **Afinitor** only: HER2 negative breast cancer, astrocytoma, pancreatic tumors, advanced renal carcinoma, renal angiomyolipoma with tuberous sclerosis.

CONTRAINDICATIONS Hypersensitivity to everolimus, or other rapamycin derivatives; use in heart transplants, hypersensitivity to sirolimus (**Zortress**) only. Severe hepatic impairment (Child–Pugh class C); acute renal failure; within 30 days of liver transplant; severe noninfection pneumonitis; fungal infection; live vaccine; severe hereditary problems of galactose intolerance; pregnancy (category D); lactation.

CAUTIOUS USE Child–Pugh class B hepatic impairment; renal impairment; severe refractory hyperlipidemia; DM; older adults.

ROUTE & DOSAGE

Renal Cell Cancer (Afinitor)

Adult: **PO** 10 mg once daily; 15–20 mg daily for patients taking a strong CYP3A4 inducer

PNET/HERS 2 Negative Breast Cancer

Adult: **PO** 10 mg daily

Astrocytoma (Afinitor only)

Adult/Adolescent/Child (3 yr or older): **PO** 4.5 mg/m^2 qd

Hepatic Impairment Dosage Adjustment

Moderate impairment (Child–Pugh class B): Reduce to 5 mg once daily

Kidney Transplant Rejection Prophylaxis (Zortress only)

Adult: **PO** 0.75 mg q12h

Liver Transplant (Zortress only)

Adult: **PO** 1 mg bid

E

ADMINISTRATION

Oral

- Give at the same time each day with/without food.
- Ensure that the tablet is swallowed whole. It should not be crushed or chewed.
- Store at 15°–30°C (59°–86°F). Protect from light and moisture.

ADVERSE EFFECTS **CV:** Hypertension, tachycardia. **Respiratory:** Alveolitis, bronchitis, *cough, dyspnea,* interstitial lung disease, lung infiltration, nasopharyngitis, pneumonia, *pneumonitis*, pulmonary alveolar hemorrhage, pulmonary effusion, pharyngolaryngeal pain, rhinorrhea, sinusitis. **CNS:** Dizziness, dysgeusia, headache, insomnia, paresthesia. **HEENT:** Eyelid edema. **Endocrine:** Decreased weight, elevated AST and ALT, elevated bilirubin, elevated creatinine, *hypercholesterolemia, hypertriglyceridemia, hyperglycemia, hypophosphatemia.* **Skin:** Acneiform dermatitis, dry skin, erythema, hand-foot syndrome, nail disorder, onychoclasis, pruritus, *rash*, skin lesion. **GI:** Abdominal pain, *diarrhea,* dry mouth, dysphagia, hemorrhoids, *mucosal inflammation,* nausea, *stomatitis,* vomiting. **GU:** Renal failure. **Musculoskeletal:** Jaw pain, pain in extremity. **Hematologic:** *Anemia, decreased hemoglobin,* decreased neutrophils, decreased platelets, *lymphopenia,* hemorrhage. **Other:** *Asthenia,* chest pain, chills, epistaxis, *fatigue, infection,* peripheral edema, pyrexia.

INTERACTIONS **Drug:** Strong inhibitors of CYP3A4 and P-glycoprotein (e.g., **ketoconazole, erythromycin, verapamil**) increase everolimus levels. Strong inducers (e.g., **rifampin**) decrease everolimus levels.

PHARMACOKINETICS **Peak:** 1–2 h. **Distribution:** 74% plasma protein bound. **Metabolism:** In liver to inactive metabolites. **Elimination:** Fecal (80%) and renal (5%). **Half-Life:** 30 h.

NURSING IMPLICATIONS

Black Box Warning

Everolimus has been associated with increased risk of malignancies, graft thrombosis, nephrotoxicity, and serious infection following heart transplant.

Assessment & Drug Effects

- Monitor for and promptly report S&S of a hypersensitivity reaction (e.g., anaphylaxis, dyspnea, flushing, chest pain, angioedema).
- Monitor renal function and promptly report S&S of nephrotoxicity.
- Monitor pulmonary status and report promptly unexplained cough, shortness of breath, pain on inspiration, or diminished breath sounds.
- Monitor for and promptly report S&S of infection.
- Monitor lab tests: Baseline and periodic CBC with differential, renal function tests, blood glucose, and lipid profile.

Patient & Family Education

- Report promptly any signs of infections, including sore throat, fever, and flulike symptoms.
- Avoid live vaccinations and close contact with those who have received live vaccines.
- Practice meticulous oral hygiene. Do not use mouthwashes that contain alcohol or peroxide.
- Women should use adequate means of contraception to avoid pregnancy while on this drug and for 8 wk after ending treatment.

EVINACUMAB-DGNB

(E vin AK ue mab)

Evkeeza

Classifications: ANTILIPEMIC AGENT; ANGIOPOIETIN-LIKE PROTEIN 3 INHIBITOR

Therapeutic: ANTILIPEMIC AGENT

AVAILABILITY Solution for infusion

ACTION & THERAPEUTIC EFFECT

A recombinant human monoclonal antibody that binds to and inhibits angiopoietin-like protein 3 (ANGPTL3) thereby inhibiting lipoprotein lipase (LPL) and endothelial lipase (EL). *Results in increased lipid metabolism leading to decreased low-density lipoprotein-cholesterol (LDL-C), high-density lipoprotein-cholesterol (HDL-C), and triglycerides.*

USES Treatment of homozygous familial hypercholesterolemia in conjunction with other low-density lipoprotein lowering therapies.

CONTRAINDICATIONS Serious hypersensitivity to evinacumab or any component of the formulation.

CAUTIOUS USE Pregnancy (in utero exposure to evinacumab can cause fetal harm); lactation.

ROUTE & DOSAGE

Homozygous Familial Hypercholesterolemia

Adult /Children (12 years old or greater): **IV Infusion:** 15mg/kg every four weeks

ADMINISTRATION

Intravenous

PREPARE: Do not shake. If refrigerated, allow diluted solution to come to room temperature prior to administration. Otherwise administer immediately after preparation.

ADMINISTER: Administer IV infusion over 60 minutes through an IV line containing a sterile, in-line or add-on, 0.2 to 5 micron. Rate may be slowed, interrupted, or discontinued if patient develops any adverse reactions.

- Store at 2°-8° C (36°-46°F).

ADVERSE EFFECTS **Respiratory:** Nasopharyngitis, flu-like symptoms, rhinorrhea. **CNS:** Dizziness **Skin:** Infusion site pruritus **GU:** Nausea **Other:** Infusion-related reaction.

INTERACTIONS **Drug:** No described interactions

PHARMACOKINETICS **Peak:** 60 minutes (end of infusion) **Metabolism:** Similar to IgG, undergoes catabolic metabolism to small peptides and amino acids **Half-Life:** 21 h

NURSING IMPLICATIONS

Assessment & Drug Effects

- Monitor for signs/symptoms of hypersensitivity reaction.
- Rule out pregnancy prior to initiating therapy.
- Monitor lab results: Baseline LDL-C when clinically appropriate and 2 weeks after initiating therapy.

E

Patient & Family Education

- Seek medical help immediately if you have any of the following signs or symptoms of an allergic reaction such as rash; hives; itching; red, swollen, blistered, or peeling skin with or without fever; wheezing; tightness in the chest or throat; trouble breathing, swallowing, or talking; unusual hoarseness; or swelling of the mouth, face, lips, tongue, or throat.
- This drug may be harmful to an unborn baby. A pregnancy test may be done before starting this drug to ensure that you are not pregnant. If you may become pregnant, you must use birth control while taking this drug and for sometime after the last dose. If you get pregnant, call your doctor right away.

EVOLOCUMAB

(e-vo-loc′u-mab)

Repatha

Classification: MONOCLONAL ANTIBODY; PROPROTEIN CONVERTASE SUBTILISIN KEXIN TYPE 9 (PCSK9) INHIBITOR; ANTILIPIDEMIC; LIPID LOWERING

Therapeutic: ANTILIPIDEMIC

AVAILABILITY Prefilled syringe for injection

ACTION & *THERAPEUTIC EFFECT* Binds to the enzyme, human proprotein convertase subtilisin kexin 9 (PCSK9), and inhibits circulating PCSK9 from binding to the LDL receptor (LDLR), preventing PCSK9-mediated LDLR degradation. *Increases the number of LDLRs available to clear LDL from the blood, thereby lowering LDL-C levels.*

USES Homozygous familial hypercholesterolemia (HoFH), prevention of CV events in patients with CVD, primary hyperlipidemia.

CONTRAINDICATIONS History of a serious hypersensitivity reaction to evolocumab; concomitant use of belimumab; pregnancy (limited information available).

CAUTIOUS USE Allergic reactions (e.g., rash, urticaria), pregnancy (first trimester); lactation. Safety and efficacy not established in children with HoFH who are younger than 13 yr or who have primary hyperlipidemia or HeFH.

ROUTE & DOSAGE

Heterozygous Familial Hypercholesterolemia or Atherosclerotic Disease

Adult: **Subcutaneous** 140 mg q2wk or 420 mg once monthly

Homozygous Familial Hypercholesterolemia

Adult: **Subcutaneous** 420 mg once monthly, may increase to 420 mg q2w if no meaningful clinical response

ADMINISTRATION

Subcutaneous

- Allow evolocumab to warm to room temperature for at least 30 min if refrigerated. ▪ Administer into abdomen, thigh, or upper arm; avoid areas that are tender, bruised, red, or indurated. Rotate injection sites.
- To administer the 420-mg dose, give three 140-mg injections consecutively within 30 min.
- Store refrigerated or at room temperature [up to 20°–25°C (68°–77°F) 25°C (77°F)] in the original

carton. If kept at room temperature, must be used within 30 days.

ADVERSE EFFECTS **Respiratory:** Cough, *nasopharyngitis*, sinusitis, upper respiratory tract infection. **Endocrine:** Diabetes mellitus. **GI:** Gastroenteritis. **GU:** Urinary tract infection. **Other:** Influenza, injection site reactions.

PHARMACOKINETICS **Peak:** 3–4 days. **Metabolism:** Peptide degradation. **Half-Life:** 11–17 days.

NURSING IMPLICATIONS

Assessment & Drug Effects

- Monitor for and report S&S of an allergic reaction. Withhold drug and notify prescriber for S&S of a serious allergic reaction.
- Monitor lab tests: Baseline and periodic lipid profile.

Patient & Family Education

- If a dose is missed, administer as soon as possible if there are more than 7 days until the next scheduled dose, or omit the missed dose and administer the next dose according to the original schedule.
- Women of childbearing age should discuss potential risks of pregnancy with prescriber.
- Do not breastfeed without consulting prescriber.

EXEMESTANE

(ex-e-mes′tain)

Aromasin

Classification: ANTINEOPLASTIC; AROMATASE INHIBITOR

Therapeutic: ANTINEOPLASTIC

Prototype: Anastrozole

AVAILABILITY Tablet

ACTION & *THERAPEUTIC EFFECT* Steroidal aromatase inhibitor that suppresses the plasma estrogens, estradiol and estrone. The enzyme, aromatase, converts estrone to estradiol. *Tumor regression is possible in postmenopausal women with estrogen-dependent breast cancer. Effectiveness is indicated by evidence of reduction in tumor size.*

E

USES Estrogen-receptor positive early breast cancer following treatment with tamoxifen, treatment of advanced breast cancer in postmenopausal women whose disease has progressed following tamoxifen therapy.

UNLABELED USES Risk reduction for invasive breast cancer in postmenopausal women.

CONTRAINDICATIONS Hypersensitivity to exemestane; coadministration of estrogen-containing drugs; women who are or may become pregnant; premenopausal women; lactation; pregnancy (category X).

CAUTIOUS USE Hepatic or renal insufficiency; GI disorders; cardiovascular disease; hyperlipidemia. Safe use in children not established.

ROUTE & DOSAGE

Early and Advanced Breast Cancer

Adult: PO 25 mg daily

ADMINISTRATION

Oral

- Give following a meal.
- Store at 15°–30°C (59°–86°F).

ADVERSE EFFECTS **CV:** Hypertension. **Respiratory:** Dyspnea. **CNS:** Fatigue, insomnia, pain, headache, depression, dizziness, anxiety. **Endocrine:** Hot flash. **Integumentary:** Alopecia. **Hepatic/GI:** Increased serum ALP, nausea, abdominal pain, diarrhea. **Musculoskeletal:** Arthralgia. **Hematologic:** Lymphedema.

INTERACTIONS Drugs: CYP3A4 inducers (e.g., **bosentan, dabrafenib**) may decrease concentration of exemestane. Do not use with ESTROGEN derivatives

PHARMACOKINETICS Absorption: Rapidly, approximately 42% reaches systemic circulation. **Distribution:** Extensive tissue distribution, 90% protein bound. **Metabolism:** Extensively in liver (CYP3A4). **Elimination:** Equally in urine and feces. **Half-Life:** 24 h.

NURSING IMPLICATIONS

Assessment & Drug Effects

- Monitor lab tests: Baseline LFTs, BUN and creatinine; periodic WBC with differential, Monitor vitamin D levels and bone mineral density tests.

Patient & Family Education

- Review manufacturer's patient literature thoroughly to reinforce understanding of likely adverse effects.
- Report bothersome adverse effects to prescriber.

EXENATIDE

(e-xe'na-tide)

Byetta, Bydureon

Classification: ANTIDIABETIC, INCRETIN MIMETIC

Therapeutic: ANTIDIABETIC

AVAILABILITY Solution for injection, extended release suspension for injection

ACTION & *THERAPEUTIC EFFECT* Improves glycemic control in type 2 diabetes mellitus by mimicking the functions of the hormone incretin. Exenatide enhances glucose-dependent insulin secretion by pancreatic beta-cells, suppresses inappropriately elevated glucagon secretion, slows gastric emptying, and decreases food intake. These actions decrease glucagon stimulation of hepatic glucose output and decrease insulin demand. *Improves glycemic control by reducing fasting and postprandial glucose concentrations in patients with type 2 diabetes.*

USES Type 2 diabetes mellitus in combination with diet/exercise.

CONTRAINDICATIONS Hypersensitivity to exenatide; type I diabetes; severe GI disease, diabetic ketoacidosis; gastroparesis; history of pancreatitis; severe GI disease or gastroparesis; end-stage renal disease, severe renal impairment (CrCl less than 30 mL/min); history of drug-induced immune-mediated thrombocytopenia. Extend release exenatide is contraindicated in family/personal history of medullary thyroid carcinoma and multiple endocrine neoplasia syndrome type 2.

CAUTIOUS USE Renal impairment; renal disease; thyroid disease; older adults; pregnancy (use with caution in pregnant women; low potential to cross the placenta); lactation. Safety and efficacy in children not established.

ROUTE & DOSAGE

Type 2 Diabetes Mellitus

Adult: **Subcutaneous** Initial dose of 5 mcg bid, within 60 min prior to the morning and evening meal.

After 1 mo, may increase to 10 mcg bid, within 60 min prior to the morning and evening meal;
Adult/Adolescent/Child (at least 10 y):
Extended release 2 mcg each week.

Renal Impairment Dosage Adjustment

CrCl less than 30 mL/min:
Do not use.

ADMINISTRATION

Subcutaneous

- Give daily dose subcutaneously into thigh, abdomen, or upper arm within 60 min before the morning and evening meals. Do not administer after a meal.
- Extended release (ER) form: May be given any time of day without regard to meals. The day of weekly dosing may be changed as needed if last dose given at least 3 days prior.
- Do not give within 1 h of oral antibiotics or an oral contraceptive.
- Store at 2°–8°C (36°–46°F) and protect from light. Discard pen 30 days after first use. Do not use if pen has been frozen. After first use, pen may be kept at or below 25°C (77°F).

ADVERSE EFFECTS **CNS:** Headache. **Endocrine:** Hypoglycemia. **GI:** Nausea, diarrhea, constipation, dyspepsia. **Other:** Injection site reaction nodule, antibody development.

INTERACTIONS **Drug:** Owing to its ability to slow gastric emptying, exenatide can decrease the rate and/or serum levels of oral medications that require GI absorption, increased risk of hypoglycemia with other INSULIN OR ANTIDIABETES products.

PHARMACOKINETICS **Peak:** 2 h (immediate release); 2 wk (extended release). **Elimination:** Primarily in urine. **Half-Life:** 2.4 h (immediate release form).

NURSING IMPLICATIONS

Black Box Warning

Exenatide may pose a risk of thyroid C-cell tumor development, although a direct link has not been established.

Assessment & Drug Effects

- Monitor for and report S&S of significant GI distress, including NV&D.
- Monitor for S&S of hypoglycemia and S&S of acute pancreatitis (acute abdominal pain with/without vomiting). If pancreatitis is suspected, withhold drug and notify prescriber immediately.
- Monitor for and report immediately site injection reactions such as cellulitis, abscess, and skin necrosis.
- Monitor lab tests: Frequent fasting and postprandial plasma glucose, and periodic HbA1C; baseline and periodic renal function tests; triglycerides.

Patient & Family Education

- If a scheduled daily dose is missed, wait for the next scheduled dose.
- If a weekly dose is missed, administer it as soon as possible as long as next scheduled dose is due at least 3 days later.
- Discard any pen that has been in use for greater than 30 days.
- Exenatide may cause decreased appetite and some weight loss.
- Report significant GI distress to prescriber. Report promptly persistent, severe abdominal pain that may be accompanied by vomiting.

- Report promptly discomfort and/or irritation at injection sites.
- Report symptoms of thyroid tumors (e.g., a lump in the neck, hoarseness, dysphagia, dyspnea).

E

EZETIMIBE

(e-ze-ti′mibe)

Zetia, Ezetrol ♣

Classification: ANTILIPEMIC; CHOLESTEROL ABSORPTION INHIBITOR

Therapeutic: CHOLESTEROL LOWERING

AVAILABILITY Tablet

ACTION & *THERAPEUTIC EFFECT* Inhibits absorption of cholesterol at the brush border of the small intestine leading to a decreased delivery of cholesterol to the liver, reduction of hepatic cholesterol stores and an increased clearance of cholesterol from the blood. *Decreases total cholesterol, LDL cholesterol, apo B, and triglycerides while increasing HDL cholesterol.*

USES Treatment of primary hypercholesterolemia alone or with an HMG-CoA reductase inhibitor (statin); treatment of homozygous sitosterolemia as an adjunct to diet.

CONTRAINDICATIONS Hypersensitivity to ezetimibe; concurrent use with HMG-CoA reductase inhibitor (statin) in patients with active liver disease or elevated serum transaminases; moderate to severe hepatic disease; myopathy; lactation.

CAUTIOUS USE Mild hepatic insufficiency; severe renal impairment; older adults; pregnancy (category C). Safe use in children younger than 10 yr not established.

ROUTE & DOSAGE

Hypercholesterolemia

Adult: **PO** 10 mg daily

ADMINISTRATION

Oral

- Give no sooner than 2 h before or 4 h after administration of a bile acid sequestrant such as cholestyramine.
- Store at 15°–30°C (59°–86°F). Protect from moisture.

ADVERSE EFFECTS **Respiratory:** Pharyngitis, sinusitis, cough. **CNS:** Dizziness, headache. **Skin:** Rash. **GI:** Abdominal pain, diarrhea. **Hematologic:** Thrombocytopenia. **Other:** Fatigue, arthralgia, back pain, myalgia, angioedema, myopathy. Hepatitis, pancreatitis, rhabdomyolysis.

INTERACTIONS **Drug:** BILE ACID SEQUESTRANTS (e.g., **cholestyramine**) may decrease absorption (give ezetimibe 2 h before or 4 h after these drugs); **cyclosporine** or FIBRIC ACID DERIVATIVES can significantly increase ezetimibe levels.

PHARMACOKINETICS **Absorption:** Well absorbed from the small intestine. **Peak:** 4–12 h. **Distribution:** Ezetimibe-glucuronide is 99% protein bound. **Metabolism:** Extensively conjugated to an active glucuronide compound (ezetimibe-glucuronide). Metabolized in small intestine and liver. **Elimination:** Primarily in feces. **Half-Life:** 22 h.

NURSING IMPLICATIONS

Assessment & Drug Effects

- Assess for and report unexplained muscle pain, especially when used in combination with a statin drug.

- Monitor closely patients who take both ezetimibe and cyclosporine.
- Monitor lab tests: Baseline and periodic lipid profile; baseline LFTs and, when used with a statin, periodic LFTs in accordance with the monitoring schedule for that statin.

Patient & Family Education

- Report unexplained muscle pain, tenderness, or weakness.
- Females should use effective methods of contraception to prevent pregnancy while taking this drug in combination with a statin.

FAMCICLOVIR

(fam-ci′clo-vir)

Classification: ANTIVIRAL
Therapeutic: ANTIVIRAL
Prototype: Acyclovir

AVAILABILITY Tablet

ACTION & THERAPEUTIC EFFECT
Prodrug of the antiviral agent penciclovir that prevents viral replication by inhibition of DNA synthesis in herpes virus–infected cells. *Effectiveness is indicated by decreasing pain and crusting of lesions followed by loss of vesicles, ulcers, and crusts. Interferes with DNA synthesis of herpes simplex virus type 1 and 2 (HSV-1 and HSV-2) infections, varicella-zoster virus, and cytomegalovirus.*

USES Management of acute herpes zoster, recurrent episodes of genital herpes, herpes labialis, recurrent orolabial/genital herpes complex in immunocompromised adults.

UNLABELED USES general herpes simplex, varicella infection in patients with HIV.

CONTRAINDICATIONS Hypersensitivity to famciclovir; lactation.

CAUTIOUS USE Renal or hepatic impairment, carcinoma, older adults, pregnancy (use during pregnancy appears to be well tolerated). Safety in children younger than 18 yr not established.

ROUTE & DOSAGE

Herpes Zoster, Treatment

Adult: **PO** 500 mg q8h for 7 days, start within 48–72 h of onset of rash

Herpes Labialis/Orolabial

Adult: **PO** 1500 mg as single dose or 500 bid × 5–10 days

Genital Herpes

Adult: **PO** 125 mg bid × 5 days or 50 mg single dose followed by 250 mg bid × 2 days

Renal Impairment Dosage Adjustment

Varies based on use; see package insert

ADMINISTRATION

Oral

- Most effective when given within 72 h of appearance of a rash or within 6 h of onset of a genital lesion.
- May be given with or without food.
- Store at room temperature, 15°–30°C (59°–86°F).

ADVERSE EFFECTS **CNS:** *Headache,* fatigue. **GI:** Nausea, diarrhea, vomiting, flatulence. **GU:** Dysmenorrhea.

INTERACTIONS **Drug:** Do not use with LIVE VACCINES. Do not use with **cladribine.**

PHARMACOKINETICS Absorption: Readily absorbed from GI tract and rapidly converted to penciclovir in intestinal and liver tissue. **Onset:** Median times to full crusting of lesions, loss of vesicles, loss of ulcers, and loss of crusts were 6, 5, 7, and 19 days, respectively; median time to loss of acute pain was 21 days. **Peak:** 1 h. **Distribution:** Distributes into breast milk of animals. **Metabolism:** Metabolized in liver and intestinal tissue to penciclovir, which is the active antiviral agent. **Elimination:** Approximately 60% recovered in urine as penciclovir. **Half-Life:** Penciclovir 2–3 h.

F

NURSING IMPLICATIONS

Assessment & Drug Effects

- Monitor lab tests: Baseline and periodic CBC; renal function tests.

Patient & Family Education

- Learn potential adverse effects, and report those that are bothersome to prescriber.
- Be aware that a full therapeutic response may take several weeks.

FAMOTIDINE

(fa-moe'ti-deen)

Pepcid, Pepcid AC

Classification: ANTISECRETORY (H_2-RECEPTOR ANTAGONIST)

Therapeutic: ANTIULCER

Prototype: Cimetidine

AVAILABILITY Tablet; oral suspension; solution for injection

ACTION & THERAPEUTIC EFFECT Competitive inhibitor of histamine at H_2-receptor sites in gastric parietal cells. Inhibits gastric acid secretion as well as pepsin secretion. *Reduces parietal cell output of hydrochloric acid; thus, detrimental effects of acid on gastric mucosa are diminished.*

USES Treatment of gastroesophageal reflux disease (GERD), heartburn, peptic ulcer disease.

UNLABELED USES Stress ulcer prophylaxis, aspiration prophylaxis, spontaneous urticaria.

CONTRAINDICATIONS Hypersensitivity to famotidine or other H_2-receptor antagonists; sudden GI bleeding; lactation.

CAUTIOUS USE Renal insufficiency; renal failure; PKU; hepatic disease vitamin B_{12} deficiency; older adults; pregnancy (crosses the placenta; renal clearance of famotidine may be increased).

ROUTE & DOSAGE

GERD, Gastritis

Adult: **PO** 10 mg bid; increase to 20 mb bid if symptoms persist
Child/Adolescent (over 40 kg): PO 20 mg daily × 6 weeks
Infant (over 3 mo): **PO** 0.5 mg bid (max: 40 mg bid); *Infant (under 3 months):* **PO** 0.5 mg/ daily × 8 weeks
Infant (3 mo–1 yr): **PO** 0.5 mg/ kg bid for up to 8 wk

Heartburn/Dyspepsia Prevention (self-treatment)

Adult: **PO** 10–20 mg 10–60 min prior to meal (max dose: 20 mg/ day)

Hypersecretory Condition

Adolescent: **PO** 20 mg q6h; **IV** 20 mg q 12h

Peptic Ulcer Disease

Adolescent/Child (over 40 kg): **PO** 40 mg daily at bedtime; **IV** 0.25 mg/kg/dos q12h (max dose 20 mg/dose)

Renal Impairment Dosage Adjustment

CrCl 30–60 mL/min: 50% of usual dose or usual dose every other day; *CrCl:* 50% of usual dose every other day

ADMINISTRATION

Oral

- Give with liquid or food of patient's choice; an antacid may also be given if patient is also on antacid therapy.
- Shake suspension vigorously before use.
- Do not chew tablet; dose may be taken 10–60 min before eating food or drinking beverages known to cause heartburn.
- Store at 15°–30°C (59°–86°F). Protect from moisture and strong light; do not freeze.

Intravenous

Note: Verify correct IV concentration and rate of infusion/injection with prescriber before administration to infants or children.

PREPARE: **Direct:** Dilute each 20-mg (2 mL) famotidine IV solution (containing 10 mg/mL) with D5W, NS, or other compatible IV diluent (see manufacturer's directions) to a total volume of 5 or 10 mL. **Intermittent:** Dilute required dose with 100 mL compatible IV solution.

ADMINISTER: **Direct:** Give over not less than 2 min. **Intermittent:** Infuse over 15–30 min.

INCOMPATIBILITIES: **Y-site: Amphotericin B cholesteryl complex, azathioprine, cefamandole, cefepime, ceftobiprole, chloramphenicol, dantrolene, diazepam, ganciclovir, gemtuzumab, indomethacin, lansoprazole, minocycline, mitomycin, pantoprazole, piperacillin/tazobactam, sulfamethoxazole/trimethoprim.**

- Store IV solution at 2°–8°C (36°–46°F); reconstituted IV solution is stable for 48 h at room temperature 15°–30°C (59°–86°F).

ADVERSE EFFECTS **CNS:** Headache, agitation. **Hematologic:** Thrombocytopenia.

INTERACTIONS **Drug:** Do not use with **dasatinib, dichlorphenamide.** Can affect serum concentrations of other medications requiring acid environment for absorption (i.e., **atazanavir, budesonide, erlotinib, itraconazole ketoconazole**). Decreases absorption of **iron. Tafenoquine** may increase concentration of famotidine.

Food: Prolonged use may lead to vitamin B_{12} deficiency.

PHARMACOKINETICS **Absorption:** Incompletely from GI tract (40–50% reaches systemic circulation). **Onset:** 1 h. **Peak:** 1–3 h PO; 30 min IV. **Duration:** 10–12 h. **Metabolism:** In liver. **Elimination:** In urine. **Half-Life:** 2.5–4 h (adult).

NURSING IMPLICATIONS

Assessment & Drug Effects

- Monitor for improvement in GI distress.
- Monitor for signs of GI bleeding.
- Monitor CBC, gastric pH, occult blood with GI bleeding.

Patient & Family Education

- Be aware that pain relief may not be experienced for several days after starting therapy.

FAT EMULSION, INTRAVENOUS

(fat e-mul'sion)

Intralipid, Liposyn II, Nutrilipid, Smoflipid

Classification: CALORIC AGENT; LIPID EMULSION

Therapeutic: NUTRITIONAL SUPPLEMENT; LIPID

F

AVAILABILITY Emulsion

ACTION & *THERAPEUTIC EFFECT* Provides the essential fatty acids (e.g., linoleic acid and alpha linolenic acid) necessary for normal structure and function of cell membranes. *Used as a nutritional supplement.*

USES Fatty acid deficiency treatment or prophylaxis. Also to supply fatty acids and calories in high-density form to patients receiving prolonged TPN therapy who cannot tolerate high dextrose concentrations or when fluid intake **must be** restricted.

CONTRAINDICATIONS Hyperlipemia; bone marrow dyscrasias; impaired fat metabolism as in pathological hyperlipemia, lipoid nephrosis, acute pancreatitis accompanied by hyperlipemia.

CAUTIOUS USE Severe hepatic or pulmonary disease; coagulation disorders; anemia; when danger of fat embolism exists; history of gastric ulcers; diabetes mellitus; thrombocytopenia; newborns, premature neonates, infants with hyperbilirubinemia; pregnancy (category C); preterm neonates.

ROUTE & DOSAGE

Prevention of Essential Fatty Acid Deficiency

Adult: **IV** 500 mL of 10% or 250 mL of 20% solution twice/wk (max: rate of 100 mL/h)
Child: **IV** 5–10 mL/kg/day twice/wk (max: 3–4 g/kg/day; max: rate of 100 mL/h)

Essential Fatty Acid Deficiency Treatment

Adult/Child/Infant/Neonate: **IV** 8–10% of caloric intake

Calorie Source in Fluid-Restricted Patients

Adult: **IV** 1–2 g/kg/day up to 2.5 g/kg or no more than 60% of nonprotein calories daily (max: rate of 100 mL/h)
Child (11–17 yr): **IV** 1 g/kg/day up to 2.5 g/kg/day or no more than 60% of nonprotein calories daily (max: rate of 100 mL/h)
Child/Infant (1–10 yr): **IV** 1–2 g/kg/day, up to 3 g/kg/day (no more than 60% of nonprotein calories daily)
Neonate: **IV** 0.5–1 g/kg/day, increase by 0.5 g/kg/day (max: 3 g/kg/day; max: infusion 0.15 g/kg/h)

ADMINISTRATION

Intravenous

Do not use if oil appears to be separating out of the emulsion.

PREPARE: **IV Infusion** ▪ Allow preparations that have been refrigerated to stand at room temperature for about 30 min before using whenever possible. ▪ Check with a pharmacist before mixing fat emulsions with electrolytes, vitamins, drugs, or other nutrient solutions.

ADMINISTER: Check specific manufacturer's guidelines regarding use of in-line filter for infusion. **IV Infusion for Adult:** *10% emulsion:* Infuse at 1 mL/min for first 15–30 min; increase to 2 mL/min if no adverse reactions. ▪ *20% emulsion:* Infuse at 0.5 mL/min for first 15–30 min; increase to 2 mL/min if no adverse reactions occur. **IV Infusion for Child:** *10% emulsion:* Infuse at 0.1 mL/min for first 10–15 min; give as slow as possible and NEVER exceed 1 g/kg in 4 h. ▪ Do not exceed 100 mL/h. ▪ *20% emulsion:* Infuse at 0.05 mL/min for first 10–15 min; increase to 1 g/kg in 4 h if no adverse reactions occur. ▪ Do not exceed 50 mL/h. **IV Infusion for Premature Neonate:** Infuse at rate not to exceed 0.15 g/kg/h. **IV Infusion for All Patients:** Give fat emulsions via a separate peripheral site or by piggyback into same vein receiving amino acid injection and dextrose mixtures or give by piggyback through a Y-connector near infusion site so that the two solutions mix only in a short piece of tubing proximal to needle. ▪ Must hang fat emulsions higher than hyperalimentation solution bottle to prevent backup of fat emulsion into primary line. ▪ Do not use an in-line filter because size of fat particles is larger than pore size. ▪ Control flow rate of each solution by separate infusion pumps. ▪ Use a constant rate over 20–24 h to reduce risk of hyperlipemia in neonates and prematures because they tend to metabolize fat slowly.

INCOMPATIBILITIES: Solution/additive: **Aminophylline, amphotericin B, ampicillin, calcium chloride, calcium gluconate, dextrose 10%, gentamicin, hetastarch, magnesium chloride, penicillin G, phenytoin, vitamin B complex.** Y-site: **Acyclovir, albumin, amphotericin B, cyclosporine, doxorubicin, doxycycline, droperidol, ganciclovir, haloperidol, heparin, hetastarch, hydromorphone, levorphanol, lorazepam, midazolam, minocycline, nalbuphine, ondansetron, pentobarbital, phenobarbital, potassium phosphate, sodium phosphate.**

▪ Discard contents of partly used containers. ▪ Store, unless otherwise directed by manufacturer, Intralipid 10% and Liposyn 10% at room temperature [25°C (77°F) or below]; refrigerate Intralipid 20%. Do not freeze.

ADVERSE EFFECTS **GI:** *Nausea, transient increases in liver function tests, hypertriglyceridemia.* **Hematologic:** Hypercoagulability, thrombocytopenia in neonates. **Long-Term Administration:** Sepsis, jaundice (cholestasis), hepatomegaly, kernicterus (infants with hyperbilirubinemia), shock (rare), aluminum toxicity. **Other:** Hypersensitivity reactions (to egg protein), irritation at infusion site.

DIAGNOSTIC TEST INTERFERENCE Blood samples drawn during or shortly after fat emulsion infusion may produce abnormally high ***hemoglobin MCH and MCHC*** values. Fat emulsions may cause transient abnormalities in ***liver function tests*** and may interfere with estimations of ***serum bilirubin*** (especially in infants).

INTERACTIONS **Drug:** No clinically significant interactions established.

NURSING IMPLICATIONS

Black Box Warning

Fat emulsion infusion has been associated with deaths in preterm infants.

F

Assessment & Drug Effects

- Monitor closely infusion rate and total daily dose. Strict adherence to the recommended total daily dose is mandatory; hourly infusion rate should be as slow as possible and should not exceed 1 g/kg in 4 h.
- Observe patient closely. Acute reactions tend to occur within the first 2½ h of therapy.
- Note: Lipemia must clear after each daily infusion. Degree of lipemia is measured by serum triglycerides and cholesterol levels 4–6 h after infusion has ceased.
- Neonate lab tests: Obtain daily platelet counts in neonates during first week of therapy, then every other day during second week, and 3 × a week thereafter because newborns are prone to develop thrombocytopenia.
- Monitor lab tests: Baseline hematologic studies; baseline and periodic LFTs, renal function tests, and lipid profile.

Patient & Family Education

- Report difficulty breathing, nausea, vomiting, or headache to prescriber.

FEBUXOSTAT

(fee-bux'o-stat)

Uloric

Classification: ANTIGOUT; XANTHINE OXIDASE INHIBITOR

Therapeutic: ANTIGOUT

Prototype: Allopurinol

AVAILABILITY Tablet

ACTION & *THERAPEUTIC EFFECT*

Febuxostat decreases serum uric acid by inhibiting the enzyme needed to convert xanthine to uric acid (end product of protein catabolism). *Effectiveness is measured by decreasing serum uric acid level to less than 6 mg/dL.*

USES Management of hyperuricemia in patients with chronic gout.

CONTRAINDICATIONS Asymptomatic hyperuricemia; concurrent use with **azathioprine** or **mercaptopurine.**

CAUTIOUS USE History of MI or stroke; severe renal impairment (CrCl less than 30 mL/min); severe hepatic dysfunction (Child–Pugh class C); pregnancy (category C); lactation. Safety and efficacy in children younger than 18 yr not established.

ROUTE & DOSAGE

Gout

Adult: **PO** 40 mg once daily; can be increased to 80 mg once daily

Renal Impairment Dosage Adjustment

CrCl 15 to 29 mL/minute: Do not exceed 40 mg daily; *CrCl less than 15 mL/minute:* Use with caution

ADMINISTRATION

Oral

- Administer with or without food or antacids.
- Concurrent therapy with an NSAID or colchicine is recommended to prevent gout flares during the first 6 mo of therapy.
- Store at 15°–30°C (59°–86°F) away from light.

ADVERSE EFFECTS **CV:** Atrial fibrillation, AV block, thromboembolic events. **Endocrine:** Elevated AST and ALT levels. **Skin:** Rash. **GI:** Nausea. **Musculoskeletal:** Arthralgia. **Whole Body:** Rhabdomyolysis.

INTERACTIONS **Drug:** Febuxostat will increase the levels of drugs requiring xanthine oxidase for normal metabolism (e.g., **6-mercaptopurine, azathioprine**). Use with cytotoxic ANTINEOPLASTIC agents may cause nephropathy.

PHARMACOKINETICS **Absorption:** 49%. **Peak:** 1–1.5 h. **Distribution:** Greater than 99% plasma protein bound. **Metabolism:** Extensive hepatic metabolism via oxidation and glucuronide conjugation. **Elimination:** Renal (49%) and fecal (45%). **Half-Life:** 5–8 h.

NURSING IMPLICATIONS

Assessment & Drug Effects

- Monitor for and report gout flares.
- Monitor CV status throughout therapy.
- Monitor for signs/symptoms of hypersensitivity or severe skin reactions.
- Monitor lab tests: Baseline serum uric acid and at 2 wk, and periodically thereafter. Baseline and periodic LFTs.

Patient & Family Education

- Notify prescriber if you experience a gout flare, but do not stop taking this drug.
- NSAIDs are typically used to control gout flares. Consult prescriber.

FELBAMATE

(fel′ba-mate)

Felbatol

Classification: ANTICONVULSANT

Therapeutic: ANTICONVULSANT

AVAILABILITY Tablet; suspension

ACTION & *THERAPEUTIC EFFECT* Anticonvulsant that blocks repetitive firing of neurons and increases seizure threshold; prevents seizure spread. *Increases seizure threshold and prevents seizure spread.*

USES Treatment of Lennox–Gastaut syndrome and partial seizures.

CONTRAINDICATIONS Hypersensitivity to felbamate, history of blood dyscrasia or hepatic dysfunction; bone marrow depression; active liver disease; elevated serum AST or ALT; severe anemia.

CAUTIOUS USE Hypersensitivity to other carbamates; renal impairment, renal failure; thrombocytopenia; iron-deficiency anemia; older adults; pregnancy (may increase risk of fetal death, genital malformation, anencephaly, encephalocele, placental disorder); lactation. Safety and efficacy in children other than those with Lennox–Gastaut syndrome not established.

ROUTE & DOSAGE

Partial Seizures

Adult: **PO** Initiate with 1200 mg/day in 3–4 divided doses, may increase by 600 mg/day q2wk (max: 3600 mg/day)

Converting to Monotherapy

Reduce dose of concomitant anticonvulsants by one-third when initiating felbamate, then continue to decrease other anticonvulsants by one-third with each increase in felbamate q2wk

Lennox–Gastaut Syndrome

Child (2–14 yr): **PO** Start at 15 mg/kg/day in 3 or 4 divided doses, reduce concurrent antiepileptic drugs by 20–33%, further reductions may be required to minimize side effects due to drug interactions, may increase felbamate by 15 mg/kg/day at weekly intervals (max: 45 mg/kg/day)

F

ADMINISTRATION

Oral

- Administer with or without food.
- Shake suspension well prior to use.
- Store in airtight container at room temperature, 20°–25°C (68°–77°F).

ADVERSE EFFECTS **Respiratory:** *Upper respiratory infection.* **CNS:** *Drowsiness,* headache, dizziness, insomnia, fatigue, nervousness, abnormal gait, anxiety, depression. **HEENT:** Visual disturbances. **Integumentary:** Rash. **GI/Hepatic:** *Anorexia,* vomiting, *nausea,* dyspepsia, constipation, hiccups, abdominal pain, increased liver enzymes. **Hematologic:** Purpura. **Other:** Fever.

INTERACTIONS **Drug:** Felbamate reduces serum **carbamazepine** levels by a mean of 25%, but increases levels of its active metabolite, increases serum **phenytoin** levels approximately 20%, and increases **valproic acid** levels. Do not use with nasal **azelastine, bromperidol, conivaptan, fusidic acid, orphenadrine, oxomemazine, thalidomide, ulipristal**, or with CNS DEPRESSANTS. **Herbal: Gingko** may decrease anticonvulsant effectiveness.

PHARMACOKINETICS **Absorption:** 90% from GI tract. Absorption of tablet not affected by food. **Onset:** Therapeutic effect approximately 14 days. **Peak:** Peak plasma levels at 1–6 h. **Distribution:** 20–25% protein bound, readily crosses the blood–brain barrier. **Metabolism:** In the liver via the cytochrome P450 system. **Elimination:** 40–50% excreted unchanged in urine, rest excreted in urine as metabolites. **Half-Life:** 20–23 h.

NURSING IMPLICATIONS

Black Box Warning

Felbamate has been associated with a development of acute liver failure and a marked increase in risk of aplastic anemia.

Assessment & Drug Effects

- Report immediately any hematologic abnormalities.
- Note: When used concomitantly with either phenytoin or carbamazepine, carefully monitor serum levels of these drugs when felbamate is added, when adjustments in felbamate dosing are made, or when felbamate is discontinued.
- Monitor weight, because both weight gain and loss have been reported.
- Monitor for S&S of drug toxicity including GI distress, liver dysfunction, and CNS toxicity. Withhold drug and notify prescriber if any liver function test parameters exceed the ULN.
- Monitor lab tests: Baseline and periodic LFTs and CBC.

Patient & Family Education

- Report promptly signs of liver dysfunction including jaundice, anorexia, GI discomfort, and fatigue.
- Report promptly signs of bone marrow suppression including infection, bleeding, easy bruising, or signs of anemia.

FELODIPINE

(fel-o′di-peen)

Classification: CALCIUM CHANNEL BLOCKER; ANTIHYPERTENSIVE

Therapeutic: ANTIHYPERTENSIVE

Prototype: Nifedipine

AVAILABILITY Sustained release tablet

ACTION & *THERAPEUTIC EFFECT* Calcium channel antagonist with high vascular selectivity that reduces systolic, diastolic, and mean arterial pressure at rest and during exercise. Felodipine inhibits influx of extracellular calcium across myocardial and vascular smooth muscle cell membranes. Resultant decrease in intracellular calcium inhibits contractility of smooth muscle, resulting in dilation of coronary and systemic arteries. *BP reduction is due to reduction in peripheral vascular resistance (afterload) against which the heart works. This reduces oxygen demand by the heart and may account for its effectiveness in chronic stable angina.*

USES Treatment of hypertension.

UNLABELED USES Angina.

CONTRAINDICATIONS Hypersensitivity to felodipine; sick sinus rhythm or second- or third-degree heart block except with the use of a pacemaker; abnormal aortic stenosis; hypotension; bradycardia; cardiogenic shock; acute MI; left ventricular dysfunction.

CAUTIOUS USE Hypotension, CHF, angina; aortic stenosis, cardiomyopathy; older adults; GERD; hiatal hernia; hepatic impairment; older adults; pregnancy (category C); lactation. Safety and efficacy in children not established.

ROUTE & DOSAGE

Hypertension

Adult: **PO** 5 mg once/day can increase if needed (max: 10 mg/day)

Geriatric: **PO** 2.5 mg once daily; may increase if needed

ADMINISTRATION

Oral

- Give tablet whole. Do not crush or chew tablets.
- Store at or below 30°C (86°F) in a tightly closed, light-resistant container.

ADVERSE EFFECTS **CV:** Tachycardia, *palpitations, flushing, peripheral edema.* **CNS:** *Dizziness, fatigue,* headache. **GI:** Nausea, flatulence, diarrhea, dyspepsia. **Hematologic:** Small but significant decreases in Hct, Hgb, and RBC count. **Other:** Most adverse effects appear to be dose dependent.

DIAGNOSTIC TEST INTERFERENCE Serum ***alkaline phosphatase*** may be slightly but significantly increased. Plasma total and ionized ***calcium*** levels rise significantly. Serum ***gamma-glutamyl transferase*** may increase.

INTERACTIONS **Drug:** Do not use with **itraconazole, ketaconazole, clarithromycin** due to increased levels of felodipine. **Adenosine** may cause prolonged bradycardia if it is used to treat patients with toxic concentrations of CALCIUM CHANNEL BLOCKERS. **Carbamazepine,**

F

phenobarbital, phenytoin may decrease felodipine effect. **Cimetidine** may increase felodipine bioavailability and adverse effect risk. Concomitant felodipine and **digoxin** administration produces only transient increases in plasma **digoxin** concentrations (35–40% increase), which are not sustained with continued administration. **Food: Grapefruit juice** may increase adverse effects.

PHARMACOKINETICS **Absorption:** Completely from GI tract; it undergoes extensive first-pass metabolism with only about 15% of dose reaching systemic circulation. **Onset:** Less than 1 h. **Peak:** 2–4 h. **Duration:** 20–24 h (sustained release formulation). **Distribution:** Greater than 99% bound to plasma proteins. **Metabolism:** Metabolized via hepatic cytochrome P-450 mixed function oxidase system. **Elimination:** 60–70% of metabolites are excreted in urine within 72 h. **Half-Life:** 10 h.

NURSING IMPLICATIONS

Assessment & Drug Effects

- Monitor BP carefully, especially at initiation of drug therapy, in patients older than 64 yr, and in those with impaired liver function.
- Anticipate BP reduction with possible reflex heart rate increase (5–10 beats/min) 2–5 h after dosing.
- Report sustained hypotension promptly; more common with concurrent beta-blocker therapy.
- Assess for and report reflex tachycardia; may precipitate angina.
- Monitor patients for possible digoxin toxicity when taking concurrent digoxin.

Patient Education

- Report peripheral edema, headache, or flushing to prescriber. These may necessitate discontinuation of drug.
- Get up from lying down slowly and in stages; there is potential for dizziness and hypotension.

FENOFIBRATE

(fen-o-fi'brate)

Antara, Fenoglide, Lipofen, Tricor, TriLipix

Classification: ANTILIPEMIC; FIBRATE

Therapeutic: CHOLESTEROL-LOWERING

AVAILABILITY Tablet; capsule; delayed release capsule

ACTION & *THERAPEUTIC EFFECT* Fibric acid derivative with lipid-regulating properties. Lowers plasma triglycerides by inhibiting triglyceride synthesis and, as a result, lowers VLDL production as well as stimulates the catabolism of triglyceride-rich lipoprotein (e.g., VLDL). Produces a moderate increase in HDL cholesterol levels in most patients. *Effectiveness indicated by reduction in the level of serum triglycerides and VLDL production.*

USES Adjunctive therapy to diet for patients with hypercholesterolemia or mixed dyslipidemia.

CONTRAINDICATIONS Hypersensitivity to fenofibrate or other fibric acid derivatives (e.g., clofibrate, bezafibrate); liver or severe kidney dysfunction; unexplained liver function abnormality; preexisting hepatic disease; primary biliary cirrhosis; preexisting gallbladder disease; thrombocytopenia; lactation.

CAUTIOUS USE Renal impairment, older adults; history of bleeding disorders; myelosuppression;

pregnancy (use with caution). Safety and efficacy in children not established.

ROUTE & DOSAGE

Hypertriglyceridemia

Adult: **PO** 30–200 mg/day depending on product; see package insert for details.

ADMINISTRATION

Oral

- Drug is usually discontinued after 2 mo if adequate lipid reduction is not achieved with the maximum recommended dose.
- Give at least 1 h before or 4–6 h after cholestyramine.
- Administer with or without meals. Swallow whole; do not open, crush, dissolve, or chew.
- Store at 15°–30°C (59°–86°F) in a tightly closed container and protect from light.

ADVERSE EFFECTS **Respiratory:** Nasopharyngitis, sinusitis. **GI/hepatic:** Elevated liver enzymes, acute hepatotoxicity, abdominal pain. **Musculoskeletal:** Arthralgia, myalgia.

INTERACTIONS **Drug:** Do not use other FIBRIC ACID DERIVATIVES. May potentiate anticoagulant effects of **warfarin;** combination with an HMG-COA REDUCTASE INHIBITOR (STATIN) may result in rhabdomyolysis; **cholestyramine, colestipol** may decrease absorption (give fenofibrate 1 h before or 4–6 h after BILE ACID SEQUESTRANTS); may increase risk of nephrotoxicity of **cyclosporine.**

PHARMACOKINETICS **Absorption:** Well absorbed from the GI tract; increased with food. **Peak:** 6–8 h. **Distribution:** 99% protein bound; excreted in breast milk. **Metabolism:** Rapidly hydrolyzed by esterases to active metabolite, fenofibric acid. **Elimination:** 60% in urine, 25% in feces. **Half-Life:** 20 h.

NURSING IMPLICATIONS

Assessment & Drug Effects

- Assess for muscle pain, tenderness, or weakness and, if present, monitor CPK level. Withdraw drug with marked elevations of CPK or if myopathy is suspected.
- Monitor patients on coumarin-type drugs closely for prolongation of PT/INR.
- Monitor lab tests: Periodic lipid levels, LFTs, and renal function tests (in patients with renal impairment).

Patient & Family Education

- Contact prescriber immediately if any of the following develops: Unexplained muscle pain, tenderness, or weakness, especially with fever or malaise; yellowing of skin or eyes; nausea or loss of appetite; skin rash or hives.
- Inform prescriber regarding concurrent use of cholestyramine, oral anticoagulants, or cyclosporine.

FENOLDOPAM MESYLATE

(fen-ol'do-pam mes'y-late)

Corlopam

Classification: NONNITRATE VASODILATOR; DOPAMINE AGONIST; ANTIHYPERTENSIVE

Therapeutic: ANTIHYPERTENSIVE

AVAILABILITY Solution for injection

ACTION & *THERAPEUTIC EFFECT* Rapid-acting vasodilator that is a dopamine D_1-like receptor agonist. Exerts hypotensive effects by decreasing peripheral vascular resistance while increasing renal blood flow, diuresis, and natriuresis. Effectiveness *indicated by rapid reduction in BP. Decreases both systolic and diastolic pressures.*

F

USES Short-term (up to 48 h) management of severe hypertension.

CONTRAINDICATIONS Hypersensitivity to fenoldopam.

CAUTIOUS USE Asthmatic patients; hepatic cirrhosis, portal hypertension, or variceal bleeding; arrhythmias, tachycardia, or angina, particularly unstable angina; elevated IOP; angular-closure glaucoma; hypotension; hypokalemia; acute cerebral infarct or hemorrhage; pregnancy (category B); lactation.

ROUTE & DOSAGE

Severe Hypertension

Adult: **IV** 0.1–0.3 mcg/kg/min by continuous infusion for up to 48 h, may increase by 0.05–0.1 mcg/kg/min q15min (dosage range: 0.01–1.6 mcg/kg/min)
Child: **IV** 0.2 mcg/kg/min, may increase to 0.3–0.5 mcg/kg/min

ADMINISTRATION

Intravenous

PREPARE: **Continuous for Adult:** Dilute to a final concentration of 40 mcg/mL by adding 1 mL (10 mg), 2 mL (20 mg), or 3 mL (30 mg) of fenoldopam to 250, 500, or 1000 mL, respectively, of NS or D5W. **Continuous for Child:** Dilute to a final concentration of 60 mcg/mL by adding 0.6 mL (6 mg), 1.5 mL (15 mg), or 3 mL (3 mg) of fenoldopam to 100, 250, or 500 mL, respectively, of NS or D5W.

ADMINISTER: **Continuous for Adult/Child:** Give only by continuous infusion; never give a direct or bolus dose. ▪ Titrate initial dose up or down no more frequently than q15min.

INCOMPATIBILITIES: **Y-site: Acyclovir, aminophylline, amphotericin B, ampicillin, bumetanide, cefoxitin, dantrolene, dexamethasone, diazepam, fosphenytoin, furosemide, ganciclovir, gemtuzumab, hetastarch, ketorolac, meropenem, mesna, methohexital, methylprednisolone, mitomycin, pantoprazole, pentobarbital, phenytoin, prochlorperazine, sodium bicarbonate.**

▪ Note: Diluted solution is stable under normal room temperature and light for 24 h. Discard any unused solution after 24 h. ▪ Store at 15°–30°C (59°–86°F) in a tightly closed container and protect from light.

ADVERSE EFFECTS **CV:** *Hypotension, tachycardia,* T-wave inversion, flushing, postural hypotension, extrasystoles, palpitations, bradycardia, heart failure, ischemic heart disease, MI, angina. **Respiratory:** Nasal congestion, dyspnea, upper respiratory disorder. **CNS:** Headache, nervousness, anxiety, insomnia, dizziness. **Endocrine:** Increased creatinine, BUN, glucose, transaminases, LDH; hypokalemia. **Skin:** Sweating. **GI:** Nausea, vomiting, abdominal pain or fullness, constipation, diarrhea. **Other:** Injection site reaction, pyrexia, nonspecific chest pain. UTI, leukocytosis, bleeding.

INTERACTIONS Use with BETA BLOCKERS increases risk of hypotension.

PHARMACOKINETICS **Onset:** 5 min. **Peak:** 15 min. **Duration:** 15–30 min. **Distribution:** Crosses placenta. **Metabolism:** Conjugated in liver. **Elimination:** 90% in urine, 10% in feces. **Half-Life:** 5 min.

NURSING IMPLICATIONS

Assessment & Drug Effects

- Monitor BP and HR carefully at least q15min or more often as warranted; expect dose-related tachycardia.
- Monitor lab tests: Frequent serum electrolytes.

FENOPROFEN CALCIUM

(fen-oh-proe′fen)

Nalfon

Classification: ANALGESIC, NONSTEROIDAL ANTI-INFLAMMATORY DRUG (NSAID)

Therapeutic: ANALGESIC; NSAID; ANTIARTHRITIC; ANTIPYRETIC

Prototype: Ibuprofen

AVAILABILITY Tablet; capsule

ACTION & *THERAPEUTIC EFFECT*

Fenoprofen competitively inhibits both cyclooxygenase COX-1 and COX-2 enzymes by blocking arachidonate binding to prostaglandin G_2 resulting in its pharmacologic effects. *Has nonsteroidal, anti-inflammatory, antipyretic, antiarthritic properties that provide relief from mild to severe pain.*

USES Rheumatoid arthritis; osteoarthritis; relief of mild to moderate pain.

UNLABELED USES Juvenile rheumatoid arthritis, acute gouty arthritis, ankylosing spondylitis.

CONTRAINDICATION Hypersensitivity to fenoprofen or other NSAIDs; salicylate; history of nephrotic syndrome associated with aspirin or other NSAIDS; patient in whom urticaria, severe rhinitis, bronchospasm, angioedema, nasal polyps are precipitated by aspirin or other NSAIDS; preexisting asthma; severe renal or hepatic dysfunction; GI bleeding, ulceration, or perforation; perioperative pain associated in CABG; pregnancy (category D starting 30 wk gestation).

CAUTIOUS USE History of GI tract disorders; lupus; renal failure; renal impairment; hemophilia or other bleeding tendencies; compromised cardiac function, risk factors for CAD; CHF; hypertension; fluid retention; impaired hearing; older adults; pregnancy (category C before 30 wk gestation); lactation. Safety in children less than 18 yr not established.

ROUTE & DOSAGE

RA/OA

Adult: **PO** 400–600 mg tid or qid (max: 3200 mg/day)

Mild to Moderate Pain

Adult: **PO** 200 mg q4–6h prn

ADMINISTRATION

Oral

- Give with meals, milk, or antacid (prescribed) if patient experiences GI disturbances.
- May crush tablets or empty capsule and mix with fluid or mix with food.
- Store capsules and tablets in tightly closed containers at 15°–30°C (59°–86°F); avoid freezing.

ADVERSE EFFECTS **CNS:** Drowsiness. **GI:** Dyspepsia.

F

INTERACTIONS **Drug: Fenoprofen** may prolong bleeding time; should not be given with ORAL ANTICOAGULANTS, **heparin.** Concurrent use may potentiate action and side effects of **phenytoin,** SULFONYLUREAS, **cyclosporine,** SULFONAMIDES. Do not use with **aminolevulinic acid, floctafenine,** other NSAIDS, **phenylbutazone. Herbal: Feverfew, garlic, ginger, gingko** may increase bleeding potential.

DIAGNOSTIC TEST INTERFERENCE
May elevate Amerlex-M assay values for ***thyroid tests***; may lead to false-positive aldosterone/renin ratio.

PHARMACOKINETICS **Absorption:** 80% from GI tract, 99% protein bound. **Onset:** 2 h. **Peak:** 2 h. **Duration:** 4–6 h. **Distribution:** Small amounts into breast milk. **Metabolism:** In liver. **Elimination:** Primarily in urine; some biliary excretion. **Half-Life:** 3 h.

NURSING IMPLICATIONS

Black Box Warning

Etodolac has been associated with increased risk of serious, potentially fatal GI bleeding and cardiovascular events (e.g., MI & CVA); risk may increase with duration of use and may be greater in the older adult and those with risk factors for CV disease.

Assessment & Drug Effects

- Baseline and periodic auditory and ophthalmic examinations are recommended in patients receiving prolonged or high-dose therapy.
- Monitor for S&S of GI bleeding. Significant GI bleeding may occur without prior warning.
- Monitor for and report promptly S&S of CV thrombotic events (i.e., angina, MI, TIA, or stroke).
- Monitor lab tests: Baseline Hct and Hgb, renal function tests, and LFTs.

Patient & Family Education

- Do not drive or engage in potentially hazardous activities until response to drug is known; fenoprofen may cause dizziness and drowsiness.
- Report immediately the onset of unexplained fever, rash, arthralgia, oliguria, edema, weight gain to prescriber. Possible symptoms of nephrotic syndrome are rapidly reversible if drug is promptly withdrawn.
- Understand that alcohol and aspirin may increase risk of GI ulceration and bleeding tendencies; avoid both unless otherwise advised by prescriber.

FENTANYL CITRATE

(fen′ta-nil)

Abstral, Actiq, Duragesic, Fentora, Ionsys, Lazanda, Onsolis, Sublimaze, Subsys

Classification: ANALGESIC; NARCOTIC (OPIATE AGONIST)
Therapeutic: NARCOTIC ANALGESIC
Prototype: Morphine
Controlled Substance: Schedule II

AVAILABILITY Solution for injection; lozenge; lozenge on a stick; transdermal patch; buccal tablet; buccal film; sublingual tablet; nasal spray

ACTION & *THERAPEUTIC EFFECT*
Synthetic, potent narcotic agonist that causes analgesia and sedation. Its alterations in respiratory rate and alveolar ventilation may

persist beyond the analgesic effect. *Provides analgesia for moderate to severe pain as well as sedation.*

USES Short-acting analgesic during operative and perioperative periods, moderate or severe pain.

UNLABELED USES Dyspnea, sedation maintenance.

CONTRAINDICATIONS Hypersensitivity to **fentanyl;** patients who have received MAO inhibitors within 14 days; substance abuse; patients who are not opioid tolerant; acute pain; out-patient surgery; significant respiratory compromise including acute or severe bronchial asthma; myasthenia gravis; labor and delivery; have or are suspected of having paralytic ileus; lactation. **Transdermal patch:** Patients not opioid tolerant, acute pain or short-term use; postoperative pain; mild pain; intermittent pain. **Sublingual:** Acute or postoperative pain, including headache/migraine and in patients not opioid tolerant.

CAUTIOUS USE Head injuries, increased intracranial pressure; older adults, debilitated, poor-risk patients; cardiac diseases, angina, hypotension, or cardiac arrhythmias; COPD, other respiratory problems; liver and kidney dysfunction; history of drug addiction; family history of substance abuse; bradyarrhythmias; children; pregnancy (category C).

ROUTE & DOSAGE

General Anesthesia Induction

Adult: **IV** 50–100 mcg 30–60 min before surgery

Postoperative Pain Management

Adult/Adolescent/Child (1 yr or older): **IV/IM** 1–2 mcg/kg

Breakthrough Cancer Pain

Adult: **PO Actiq** only: 200 mcg over 15 min
Fentora only: 100 mcg over 30 min
Onsolis only: 200 mcg initial dose, may titrate up by 200 mcg in each subsequent episode (max: 4 simultaneous doses)
Abstral only: 100 mcg until dissolved, may repeat after 30 min, do not repeat for at least 2 h
Intranasal Lazanda only: 100-mcg spray, do not repeat for at least 2 h

Postoperative Pain in Recovery Room

Adult: **IM/IV** 50–100 mcg q1–2h prn

Chronic Pain

Adult: **Transdermal** Individualize and regularly reassess doses of transdermal fentanyl; for patient not already receiving an opioid, the initial dose is 25-mcg/h patch q3days; for patients already on opioids, see package insert for conversions; **Stick lozenge (Actiq)** 200 mcg (**Actiq** only) as breakthrough agent; **IV/IM** 50–110 mcg
Child (2 yr or older): **Transdermal** Individualize and reassess regularly

ADMINISTRATION

Buccal

- *Buccal tablet:* Do not push tablet through blister, as this may cause damage to tablet.
- *Buccal film:* Place film on inside of cheek with the pink side against the mucous membrane.

Hold film against cheek for 5 sec. Film should be left in place until it dissolves (15–30 min). Liquids may be consumed after 5 min, but solids should not be eaten until film dissolves.

Oral

- *Lozenge:* Place unit between cheek and lower gum, moving it from one side to the other using the handle. Instruct the patient to suck, not chew, the lozenge. Should be consumed over a 15-min period.

Sublingual

- *Sublingual tablet:* Note that Abstral tablets are not equivalent on a mcg/mcg basis with other fentanyl products. Place tablet under tongue immediately after removal from blister pack. Instruct patient not to chew, suck, or swallow tablet, and allow to completely dissolve in the sublingual cavity before eating or drinking.
- *Sublingual tablet and spray:* Note that the sublingual spray and tablet are not interchangeable on a dosage basis.

Intranasal

- *Nasal spray:* Lazanda is not equivalent to other fentanyl products on a mcg/mcg basis.

Intramuscular

- Inject undiluted into a large muscle.

Transdermal

- Place on nonirritated flat surface (e.g., chest, back, upper arm). The upper back is preferred to minimize unintended patch removal. Clip (not shave) hair at application site prior to system application. If needed, clean site prior to application only with clear water. Press patch in place for 30 sec. If gel from patch leaks out and contacts skin of patient or caregiver, wash thoroughly with water.
- Do not expose the fentanyl application site and surrounding area to any direct external heat source (e.g., heating pad or electric blanket, heat or tanning lamp, sauna, hot bath).

Intravascular

PREPARE: **Direct:** Give parenteral doses undiluted or diluted in 5 mL sterile water or NS.
ADMINISTER: **Direct:** Inject slowly over 1–3 min.
INCOMPATIBILITIES: **Solution/additive:** **Fluorouracil, levobupivacaine, lornoxicam, ropivacaine.** **Y-site:** **Amiodarone, amphotericin B conventional, ampicillin, azithromycin, dantrolene, diazepam, diazoxide, gemtuzumab, haloperidol, hydralazine, hydroxycobalamin, pantoprazole, phenytoin, SMZ/TMP.**

- Store at 15°–30°C (59°–86°F) unless otherwise directed. Protect drug from light.

ADVERSE EFFECTS **CV:** Hypotension, bradycardia, circulatory depression, cardiac arrest. **Respiratory:** Laryngospasm, bronchoconstriction, respiratory depression or arrest. **CNS:** *Sedation,* euphoria, dizziness, diaphoresis, delirium, convulsions with high doses. **HEENT:** Miosis, blurred vision. **Skin:** Rash, contact dermatitis from patch. **GI:** *Nausea,* vomiting, constipation, ileus. **Other:** Muscle rigidity, especially muscles of respiration after rapid IV infusion, urinary retention.

INTERACTIONS **Drug:** **Alcohol** and other CNS DEPRESSANTS potentiate effects; MAO INHIBITORS may precipitate hypertensive crisis.

PHARMACOKINETICS **Absorption:** Absorbed through the skin, leveling off between 12 and 24 h. **Onset:** Immediate IV; 7–15 min IM; 12–24 h transdermal. **Peak:** 3–5 min IV; 24–72 h transdermal. **Duration:** 30–60 min IV; 1–2 h IM; 72 h transdermal. **Metabolism:** In liver by CYP3A4. **Elimination:** In urine. **Half-Life:** 17 h transdermal.

NURSING IMPLICATIONS

Black Box Warning

Fentanyl has been associated with severe, potentially fatal, respiratory depression.

Assessment & Drug Effects

- Monitor vital signs and observe patient for signs of skeletal and thoracic muscle (depressed respirations) rigidity and weakness.
- Watch closely for respiratory depression and for movements of various groups of skeletal muscle in extremities, external eye, and neck during postoperative period. These movements may present patient management problems; report promptly.
- Note: Duration of respiratory depressant effect may be considerably longer than narcotic analgesic effect. Have immediately available oxygen, resuscitative and intubation equipment, and an opioid antagonist such as naloxone.

Patient & Family Education

- Follow exactly instructions for taking fentanyl and for disposal of unit provided in patient information.
- Exercise caution when engaging in hazardous activities until reaction to drug is known.
- Do not apply any source of direct, external heat to skin area to which patient is attached.
- Children exposed to buccal tablets are at high risk for respiratory depression. Keep out of reach of children.

FERROUS SULFATE (Pr)

(fer'rous sul'fate)

Feosol, Fer-In-Sol, Fer-Iron, Slow-Fe, Slow Iron

FERROUS FUMARATE

(fer'rous foo'ma-rate)

Femiron, Neo-Fer-50 ♣, Novofumar ♣, Palafer ♣

FERROUS GLUCONATE

(fer'rous gloo'koe-nate)

Ferate, Fertinic ♣, Novo Ferrogluc ♣

Classification: IRON PREPARATION

Therapeutic: ANTIANEMIC; IRON SUPPLEMENT

AVAILABILITY

Ferrous Sulfate: Tablet; sustained release tablet; syrup; elixir; **Ferrous Fumarate:** Tablet; extended release tablet; **Ferrous Gluconate:** Tablet

ACTION & *THERAPEUTIC EFFECT*

Replaces iron found in hemoglobin, myoglobin, and enzymes; allows the transportation of oxygen via hemoglobin. *Effectiveness is experienced within 48 h as a sense of well-being, increased vigor, improved appetite, and decreased irritability (in children). Reticulocyte response begins in about 4 days; it usually peaks in 7–10 days and returns to normal after 2 or 3 wk.*

USES

To correct simple iron deficiency and to treat iron deficiency anemias. May be used prophylactically during periods of increased iron needs, as in infancy, childhood, and pregnancy.

CONTRAINDICATIONS Peptic ulcer, regional enteritis, ulcerative colitis; hemolytic anemias (in absence of iron deficiency), hemochromatosis, cirrhosis of liver.

CAUTIOUS USE Hepatic disease; GI diseases; sulfite hypersensitivity; pregnancy (safe to use during pregnancy to meet maternal iron requirements).

F

ROUTE & DOSAGE

Ferrous Sulfate (20% elemental iron)

Ferrous Fumarate (33% elemental iron)

Ferrous Gluconate (12% elemental iron)

Treatment of Iron Deficiency Anemia

Adult: **PO** 65–200 mg **elemental** iron 1–3 × daily for 4 wk
Infant/Child: **PO** 10–12 mg **elemental** iron/kg/day (divide doses) for 3 months

ADMINISTRATION

Oral

- Give with water or juice on an empty stomach.
- Do not crush tablet or empty contents of capsule when administering.
- Do not give tablets or capsules within 1 h of bedtime.
- Consult prescriber about prescribing a liquid formulation or a less corrosive form, such as ferrous gluconate, if the patient experiences difficulty in swallowing tablet or capsule.
- Dilute liquid preparations well and give through a straw or placed on the back of tongue with a dropper to prevent staining of teeth and to mask taste. Instruct the patient to rinse mouth with clear water immediately after ingestion.
- Mix ferrosol elixir with water; not compatible with milk or fruit juice. Fer-In-Sol (drops) may be given in water or in fruit or vegetable juice, according to manufacturer.
- Do not use discolored tablets.
- Store in tightly closed containers and protect from moisture. Store at 15°–30°C (59°–86°F).

ADVERSE EFFECTS **HEENT:** Yellow-brown discoloration of teeth (liquid forms). **GI:** *Nausea, heartburn,* anorexia, *constipation,* stomach cramps, *dark stools.* **GU:** Urine discoloration.

DIAGNOSTIC TEST INTERFERENCE By coloring feces black, large iron doses may cause false-positive tests for ***occult blood with orthotoluidine (Hematest, Occultist, Labstix); guaiac reagent benzidine test*** is reportedly not affected.

INTERACTIONS **Drug:** ANTACIDS decrease iron absorption; iron decreases absorption of TETRACYCLINES, **ciprofloxacin, ofloxacin; chloramphenicol** may delay iron's effects; iron may decrease absorption of **penicillamine.** **Food:** Food decreases absorption of iron; **ascorbic acid (vitamin C)** may increase iron absorption.

PHARMACOKINETICS **Absorption:** 5–10% absorbed in healthy individuals; 10–30% absorbed in iron deficiency; food decreases amount absorbed. **Distribution:** Transported by transferrin to bone marrow, where it is incorporated into hemoglobin; crosses placenta. **Elimination:** Most of iron released from hemoglobin is reused in body; small amounts are lost in desquamation of skin, GI mucosa, nails, and hair; 12–30 mg/mo lost through menstruation.

NURSING IMPLICATIONS

Assessment & Drug Effects

- Continue iron therapy for 2–3 mo after the hemoglobin level has returned to normal (roughly twice the period required to normalize hemoglobin concentration).
- Monitor bowel movements, as constipation is a common adverse effect.
- Monitor lab tests: Periodic Hgb, Hct, RBC count, serum ferritin, transferrin saturation, total iron-binding capacity, serum iron concentration, and erythrocyte protophorphyrin concentration.

Patient & Family Education

- Note: Ascorbic acid increases absorption of iron. Consuming citrus fruit or tomato juice with iron preparation (except the elixir) may increase its absorption.
- Be aware that milk, eggs, or caffeine beverages when taken with the iron preparation may inhibit absorption.
- Be aware that iron preparations cause dark green or black stools.
- Report constipation or diarrhea to prescriber; symptoms may be relieved by adjustments in dosage or diet or by change to another iron preparation.

FESOTERODINE

(fes′oh-ter′oh-deen)

Toviaz

Classification: ANTICHOLINERGIC; MUSCARINIC RECEPTOR ANTAGONIST; BLADDER ANTISPASMODIC

Therapeutic: BLADDER ANTISPASMODIC

Prototype: Oxybutynin

AVAILABILITY Extended release tablet

ACTION & *THERAPEUTIC EFFECT* A muscarinic receptor antagonist that reduces urinary incontinence, urgency, and frequency. It helps regulate the involuntary contractions of the bladder associated with sudden urges to urinate. *It controls urinary incontinence or overactive bladder (OAB).*

USES Treatment of overactive bladder in patients with urinary incontinence, urgency.

CONTRAINDICATIONS Severe hepatic impairment (Child–Pugh class C); gastric obstruction, paralytic ileus, uncontrolled narrow-angle glaucoma; urinary retention; severe BPH; lactation.

CAUTIOUS USE Cross-sensitivity to tolterodine; mild to moderate hepatic impairment (Child–Pugh class A and B); renal insufficiency; history of constipation; bladder outlet obstruction; history of decreased GI motility; severe constipation; palpitations; narrow-angle glaucoma; myasthenia gravis; pregnancy (use with caution in pregnant women). Safe use in children not established.

ROUTE & DOSAGE

Overactive Bladder

Adult: **PO** 4 mg daily, may increase to 8 mg daily based on response. Do not exceed 4 mg daily with concurrent potent CYP3A4 inhibitors.

Hepatic Impairment Dosage Adjustment

Severe hepatic impairment (Child–Pugh class C): Not recommended

F

Renal Impairment Dosage Adjustment

CrCl less than 30 mL/min: Do not exceed 4 mg

ADMINISTRATION

Oral

- Give with water without regard to food.
- Do not break or crush extended release tablet. Ensure that it is swallowed whole.
- Store at 15°–30°C (59°–86°F).

ADVERSE EFFECTS **HEENT:** Dry eyes. **GI:** Constipation, *dry mouth*. **GU:** Urinary tract infection.

INTERACTIONS **Drug:** Potent CYP-3A4 INHIBITORS (e.g., **clarithromycin, ketoconazole, nefazodone, nelfinavir,** and **ritonavir**) increase fesoterodine levels. INDUCERS OF CYP3A4 (e.g., **rifampin**) can decrease fesoterodine levels. ANTICHOLINERGIC AGENTS can increase adverse effects. Can increase adverse effects of **clozapine, eluxadoline**, POTASSIUM SALTS. Limit **fesoterodine** dose to 4 mg when combined with **itraconazole.**

PHARMACOKINETICS **Absorption:** well absorbed. **Peak:** 5 h. **Distribution:** 50% plasma protein bound. **Metabolism:** Hepatic metabolism via CYP2D and CYP3A4 to active and inactive metabolites. **Elimination:** Renal (70%) and fecal (7%). **Half-Life:** 7 h.

NURSING IMPLICATIONS

Assessment & Drug Effects

- Monitor bowel and bladder function as urinary retention and constipation are potential adverse effects. Older adults are at greater risk for adverse effects, especially with the 8-mg dose.
- Monitor for and report bothersome anticholinergic effects (see Appendix F).

Patient & Family Education

- Use caution in hot environments to avoid heat prostration as fesoterodine causes decreased sweating and reduces body cooling in excessive heat.
- Exercise caution with hazardous activities until response to drug is known.
- Moderate alcohol consumption as it may enhance drowsiness caused by fesoterodine.

FEXOFENADINE

(fex-o-fen′a-deen)

Allegra

Classification: NONSEDATING; ANTIHISTAMINE; H_1-RECEPTOR ANTAGONIST

Therapeutic: NONSEDATING ANTIHISTAMINE

Prototype: Loratadine

AVAILABILITY Tablet; capsule; orally disintegrating tablet; oral suspension

ACTION & *THERAPEUTIC EFFECT* Competes with histamine for binding at the H_1-receptor. This blocks effects of histamine on H_1-receptors resulting in decreased formation of edema, flare, and pruritus. *Inhibits antigen-induced bronchospasm and histamine release from mast cells. Efficacy is indicated by reduction of the following: Nasal congestion and sneezing; watery or red eyes; itching nose, palate, or eyes.*

USES Relief of symptoms associated with seasonal allergic rhinitis, and chronic urticaria.

CONTRAINDICATIONS Hypersensitivity to fexofenadine or terfenadine; neonates.

CAUTIOUS USE Mild to severe renal and hepatic insufficiency, hypertension, diabetes mellitus, ischemic heart disease, increased ocular pressure, hyperthyroidism, renal impairment, prostatic hypertrophy; elderly, pregnancy (category C); lactation; young children.

ROUTE & DOSAGE

Allergic Rhinitis

Adult/Adolescent: **PO** 60 mg bid OR 180 mg daily
Child (2–11 yr): **PO** 30 mg bid
Child (6–11 yr): **PO (oral disintegrating tablet)** 30 mg bid

Chronic Urticaria

Adult: **PO** 60 mg bid OR 180 mg daily
Child (2–11 yr): **PO** 30 mg bid
Child (6–11 yr): **PO (oral disintegrating tablet)** 30 mg bid
Child (younger than 2 yr)/Infant (6 mo or older): **PO** 15 mg bid

Renal Impairment Dosage Adjustment

CrCl less than 80 mL/min: Give normal dose only once/day

ADMINISTRATION

Oral

- Reduce starting dose for those with decreased kidney function.
- Do not give within 15 min of an aluminum- or magnesium-containing antacid.
- Store at 20°–25°C (68°–77°F). Protect from excess moisture.

ADVERSE EFFECTS **CNS:** *Headache,* drowsiness, fatigue. **GI:** Nausea, dyspepsia, throat irritation.

INTERACTIONS **Drug:** ANTACIDS will decrease serum level of fexofenadine. **Herbal: St. John's wort** will decrease serum level of fexofenadine. **Food: Grapefruit juice** or **apple juice** may decrease efficacy.

PHARMACOKINETICS **Absorption:** Rapidly from GI tract, 33% reaches systemic circulation. **Onset:** 1 h. **Peak:** 2–3 h. **Duration:** At least 12 h. **Distribution:** 60–70% bound to plasma proteins. **Metabolism:** Only 5% of dose metabolized in liver. **Elimination:** 80% in urine, 11% in feces. **Half-Life:** 14.4 h.

NURSING IMPLICATIONS

Assessment & Drug Effects

- Monitor therapeutic effectiveness, which is indicated by decreased nasal congestion, sneezing, watery or red eyes, and itching nose, palate, or eyes.

Patient & Family Education

- Note: Drug is well tolerated and causes minimal adverse effects.

FIDAXOMICIN

(fye-dax'oh-mye'sin)

Dificid

Classification: MACROLIDE ANTIBIOTIC
Therapeutic: ANTIBIOTIC
Prototype: Erythromycin

AVAILABILITY Tablet

ACTION & THERAPEUTIC EFFECT Macrolide antibiotic that inhibits RNA-synthesis by RNA polymerases. *Bactericidal action on* Clostridioides difficile *in the GI tract.*

USES Treatment *Clostridioides* (formerly *Clostridium*) *difficile* infection.

CAUTIOUS USE Not for use in systemic infections; hyperglycemia; metabolic acidosis; pregnancy; lactation. Safety and efficacy in children younger than 18 yr not established.

F

ROUTE & DOSAGE

Clostridioides Difficile–Associated Diarrhea

Adult: **PO** 200 mg bid × 10 d

ADMINISTRATION

Oral

- May give without regard to food.
- Store at 15°–30°C (59°–86°F).

ADVERSE EFFECTS **Skin:** Pruritus. **Hepatic:** Increased liver enzymes. **GI:** Abdominal pain, constipation, diarrhea, *nausea, vomiting*. **Other:** Fever.

INTERACTIONS **Drug:** May decrease effect of **sodium picosulfate**, may increase concentration of **mizolastine**.

PHARMACOKINETICS **Absorption:** Minimal systemic absorption. **Peak:** 2 h. **Distribution:** Primarily confined to GI tract. **Metabolism:** Hydrolysis in GI tract to active metabolite. **Elimination:** Primarily fecal (92%).

NURSING IMPLICATIONS

Assessment & Drug Effects

- Note that fidaxomicin is not effective for treatment of systemic infections.
- Monitor GI symptoms of CDAD (*C. difficile*-associated disease) and report increasing GI distress.
- Effectiveness is indicated by decreasing diarrhea and improvement in other S&S of GI distress.
- Monitor lab tests: CBC with differential as needed.

Patient & Family Education

- It is common to feel better soon after beginning treatment; however, do not stop taking the drug until the full course of treatment is completed.

FILGRASTIM

(fil-gras′tim)

Granix, Neupogen, Nivestym, Zarxio

Classification: HEMATOPOIETIC GROWTH FACTOR

Therapeutic: ANTINEUTROPENIC; GRANULOCYTE COLONY-STIMULATING FACTOR (G-CSF)

AVAILABILITY Solution for injection

ACTION & *THERAPEUTIC EFFECT* Granulocyte colony stimulating factors (G–CSF) produced by recombinant DNA technology; G–CSFs stimulate production, maturation, and activation of neutrophils to increase both their migration and cytotoxicity. *Increases neutrophil proliferation and differentiation within the bone marrow.*

USES Treatment of chemotherapy-induced neutropenia, neutropenia, peripheral blood stem cell mobilization, radiation exposure.

CONTRAINDICATIONS Hypersensitivity to *Escherichia coli*–derived proteins, concurrent administration with chemotherapy, radiation; ARDS.

CAUTIOUS USE Sickle cell disease; renal impairment; respiratory insufficiency; pregnancy (category C); lactation.

ROUTE & DOSAGE

Neutropenia Prophylaxis

Adult/Adolescent/Child: **IV** 5 mcg/kg/day by 30-min infusion, may increase by 5 mcg/kg/day for up to 14 days (max: 30 mcg/kg/day); **Subcutaneous** 5 mcg/kg/day as single dose, may increase based on pt response

Bone Marrow Transplant

Adult: **IV** 10 mcg/kg/day given 24 h after cytotoxic therapy and 24 h after bone marrow transfusion

Radiation Exposure

Adult/Adolescent/Child/Infant (older than 7 mo): **Subcutaneous** 10 mcg/kg/day, continue until ANC remains above 1,000 m^3 for 3 consecutive CBCs

ADMINISTRATION

Subcutaneous & Intravenous

- Do not administer filgrastim 24 h before or after cytotoxic chemotherapy or while undergoing radiation therapy. ▪ Use only one dose/vial; do not reenter the vial. ▪ Prior to injection, filgrastim may be allowed to reach room temperature for a maximum of 6 h. ▪ Discard any vial left at room temperature for longer than 6 h.

Subcutaneous

- Inject into the outer upper arm, abdomen (except within 2 inches of navel), front middle thigh, or the upper outer buttocks area.

Intravenous

PREPARE: **Intermittent/Continuous:** May dilute with 10–50 mL D5W to yield 15 mcg/mL or greater. ▪ If more diluent is used to yield concentrations of 5–15 mcg/mL, 2 mL of 5% human albumin **must be** added for each 50 mL D5W (prior to adding filgrastim) to prevent adsorption to plastic IV infusion materials.

ADMINISTER: **Intermittent:** Give a single dose over 15–30 min. ▪ Flush line before/after with D5W. **Continuous:** Give a single dose over 4–24 h. ▪ Flush line before/after with D5W.

INCOMPATIBILITIES: **Y-site: Aminocaproic acid, amphotericin B, cefepime, cefoperazone, cefotaxime, cefoxitin, ceftaroline, ceftizoxime, ceftobiprole, ceftriaxone, cefuroxime, clindamycin, dactinomycin, etoposide, fluorouracil, furosemide, heparin, isavuconazonium, letermovir, mannitol, methylprednisolone, metronidazole, mitomycin, piperacillin, prochlorperazine, thiotepa.**

- Store refrigerated at 2°–8°C (36°–46°F). Do not freeze. Avoid shaking.

ADVERSE EFFECTS

CV: Chest pain. **CNS:** Fatigue, dizziness, pain, headache. **Skin:** Skin rash. **Hepatic/GI:** Increased serum ALP, *nausea*. **Musculoskeletal:** Ostealgia, back pain. **Hematologic:** Thrombocytopenia. **Other:** Fever.

DIAGNOSTIC TEST INTERFERENCE

May interfere with bone imaging studies.

INTERACTIONS

Drug: Can interfere with activity of CYTOTOXIC AGENTS, do not use 24 h before or after CYTOTOXIC AGENTS.

PHARMACOKINETICS

Absorption: Readily from subcutaneous site. **Onset:** 4 h. **Peak:** 1 h. **Elimination:** Probably in urine. **Half-Life:** 1.4–7.2 h.

NURSING IMPLICATIONS

Assessment & Drug Effects

- Discontinue filgrastim if absolute neutrophil count exceeds 10,000/mm^3 after the chemotherapy-induced nadir. Neutrophil counts should then return to normal.
- Assess degree of bone pain if present. Consult prescriber if nonnarcotic analgesics do not provide relief.
- Monitor lab tests: Baseline and twice weekly CBC with differential and platelet count.

Patient & Family Education

- Report bone pain and, if necessary, to request analgesics to control pain.
- Some patients (or caregivers) are candidates for self-administration using the prefilled syringe form with proper training.
- Note: Proper drug administration and disposal are important. A puncture-resistant container for the disposal of used syringes and needles should be available to the patient.

FINAFLOXACIN

(fin-a-flox′a-sin)

Xtoro

Classification: QUINOLONE ANTIBIOTIC

Therapeutic: ANTIBIOTIC

Prototype: Ciprofloxacin

AVAILABILITY Otic suspension

ACTION & *THERAPEUTIC EFFECT*

An antimicrobial effective against most strains of *Pseudomonas aeruginosa* and *Staphylococcus aureus*. *Effective in controlling external ear infections.*

USES Treatment of acute otitis externa caused by susceptible strains of *Pseudomonas aeruginosa* and *Staphylococcus aureus* in patients 1 yr and older.

CAUTIOUS USE Allergic reactions to finafloxacin or other quinolones; prolonged use (may lead to overgrowth of nonsusceptible organisms).

ROUTE & DOSAGE

Otitis Externa

Adult/Child (1 yr or older): **Otic** 4 drops bid into affected ear(s) for 7 days; if using OtoWick, initial dose can be doubled

ADMINISTRATION

Otic

- Warm suspension by holding bottle in the hand for 1–2 min prior to dosing. Shake bottle well before use.
- Place patient with the affected ear upward, instill the drops, and maintain the position for 60 sec.
- Store at 2°–25°C (36°–77°F).

ADVERSE EFFECTS **HEENT:** Ear pruritus. **GI:** Nausea.

NURSING IMPLICATIONS

Assessment & Drug Effects

- Monitor for and report promptly rash or other allergic reaction.

Patient & Family Education

- Warm by holding bottle in hand for 1–2 min before instillation. Instilling a cold solution may cause dizziness.
- Have patient lie with the affected ear upward, instill the drops, and maintain the position for 60 sec.
- Report promptly to prescriber if an allergic reaction occurs.

FINASTERIDE

(fin-as′te-ride)

Propecia, Proscar

Classification: ANTIANDROGEN; 5-ALPHA REDUCTASE INHIBITOR

Therapeutic: ANTIANDROGEN

AVAILABILITY Tablet

ACTION & *THERAPEUTIC EFFECT* Specific inhibitor of the steroid 5-alpha-reductase, an enzyme necessary to convert testosterone into potent androgen 5-alpha-dihydrotestosterone (DHT) in the prostate gland. *Decreases the production of testosterone in the prostate gland.*

USES Benign prostatic hypertrophy, male pattern hair loss (androgenetic alopecia).

CONTRAINDICATIONS Hypersensitivity to finasteride; females, pregnancy (use during pregnancy is contraindicated due to risk of abnormal development of male genital tract), lactation, children.

CAUTIOUS USE Hepatic impairment, obstructive uropathy.

ROUTE & DOSAGE

Benign Prostatic Hypertrophy

Adult: **PO** 5 mg/day

Male Pattern Hair Loss

Adult: **PO** 1 mg daily

ADMINISTRATION

Oral

- May be administered with or without food.
- Crush tablets if necessary. Pregnant women and women who could become pregnant should not handle the crushed drug.
- Store at 15°–30°C (59°–86°F) unless otherwise directed.

ADVERSE EFFECTS **CV:** Orthostatic hypotension. **Endocrine:** Decreased libido. **GU:** Impotence, ejaculatory disorder.

DIAGNOSTIC TEST INTERFERENCE Depresses levels of **DHT** and **prostate-specific antigen (PSA).**

INTERACTIONS **Drug:** No clinically significant interactions established. **Herbal: Saw palmetto** may potentiate effects of finasteride.

PHARMACOKINETICS **Absorption:** Readily from GI tract; 90% protein bound. **Onset:** 3–6 mo. **Duration:** 5–7 days. **Elimination:** 39% in urine, 57% in feces. **Half-Life:** 5–7 h.

NURSING IMPLICATIONS

Assessment & Drug Effects

- Evaluate carefully any sustained increase in serum PSA levels while patient is taking finasteride. It may indicate the presence of prostate cancer or noncompliance with the therapy.
- Monitor patients with a large residual urinary volume or decreased urinary flow. These patients may not be candidates for this therapy.
- Monitor lab results: Baseline and periodic PSA.

Patient & Family Education

- Use a barrier contraceptive to prevent pregnancy in a sexual partner.
- Be aware that impotence and decreased libido may occur with treatment.
- Report promptly any of the following: breast tenderness or enlargement; testicular pain; rash, itching, or swelling about the face and lips.

F

FINERENONE

(fin ER e none)

Kerendia

Classifications: MINERALOCORTICOID/ALDOSTERONE RECEPTOR ANTAGONIST

Therapeutic: MINERALCORTICOID RECEPTOR ANTAGONIST

AVAILABILITY
Oral tablet

ACTION & *THERAPEUTIC EFFECT*
Selectively blocks mineralocorticoid receptor-mediated sodium reabsorption and overactivation in both epithelial and nonepithelial tissues reducing fibrosis and inflammation. *Reduces the risk of sustained GFR decline in patients with type 2 diabetes and chronic kidney disease associated with type 2 diabetes.*

USES
For patients with chronic kidney disease secondary to type 2 diabetes, decreases risk of kidney function decline, CKD, cardiovascular death, myocardial infarction, and hospitalization due to heart failure.

CONTRAINDICATIONS
Concomitant therapy with strong CYP3A4 inhibitors; adrenal insufficiency.

CAUTIOUS USE
Hyperkalemia; hepatic impairment; renal impairment; pregnancy (developmental toxicity has been observed in animal reproduction studies); lactation.

ROUTE & DOSAGE

Chronic Kidney Disease in patients with Type 2 Diabetes

Adult: **Oral:** 20 mg once a day

Renal Impairment Dosage Adjustment

CrCl less than 60 mL/min: 10 mg once a day

CrCl less than 25 mL/min: Not recommended

Hepatic Impairment Dosage Adjustment

Child-Pugh class C (Severe impairment): Not recommended

ADMINISTRATION

Oral

- Administer with or without food.
- If unable to swallow tablet whole, tablet may be crushed and mixed with water or soft foods; administer immediately after mixing.
- Store at 20°–25° C (68°–77° F).

ADVERSE EFFECTS
CV: Hypotension. **Endocrine:** Hyperkalemia.

INTERACTIONS
Drug: Avoid combination with strong CYP3A4 inhibitors (eg. **ketoconazole, clarithyromycin**) or inducers (eg. **rifampin, phenobarbital, carbamazepine, phenytoin**). **Food: Grape-fruit juice** may increase levels, avoid combination.

PHARMACOKINETICS
Absorption: 44% bioavailability. **Peak:** 0.5–1.25 h. **Distribution:** 92% protein-bound. **Metabolism:** Primarily metabolized by CYP3A4. **Elimination:** 80% urine, 20% feces. **Half-Life:** 2–3 h.

NURSING IMPLICATIONS

Assessment & Drug Effects

- Monitor lab tests: Serum potassium and GFR at baseline, 4 weeks after therapy initiation or dosage adjustments, and periodically during therapy.

Patient & Family Education

- Seek medical help immediately if you have any of the following signs or symptoms of an allergic reaction such as rash; hives;

itching; red, swollen, blistered, or peeling skin with or without fever; wheezing; tightness in the chest or throat; trouble breathing, swallowing, or talking; unusual hoarseness; or swelling of the mouth, face, lips, tongue, or throat.

FINGOLIMOD

(fin-go′-li-mod)

Gilenya

Classification: BIOLOGIC RESPONSE MODIFIER; IMMUNOMODULATOR; SPHINGOSINE 1-PHOSPHATE RECEPTOR MODULATOR

Therapeutic: IMMUNOMODULATOR

AVAILABILITY Capsule

ACTION & *THERAPEUTIC EFFECT*

Reduces the number of lymphocytes leaving lymph nodes and entering the peripheral bloodstream. Mechanism of action in MS is unknown but may involve reduction in the migration of lymphocytes into the CNS. *Reduces the frequency of exacerbations in relapsing MS and slows development of physical disability.*

USES Treatment of relapsing forms of multiple sclerosis.

CONTRAINDICATIONS Sensitivity to fingolimod, MI, unstable angina, stroke, transient ischemic attack, decompensated heart failure requiring hospitalization, or class III/IV heart failure in the past 6 mo; Mobitz type II second-degree heart block and Mobitz type II third-degree heart block or sick sinus syndrome, unless patient has a functioning pacemaker; baseline QTc interval 500 msec or more; PML.

CAUTIOUS USE Bradyarrhythmia, sick sinus syndrome, prolonged QT interval, ischemic cardiac disease, congestive heart failure, or hypertension; risk factors for hypotension; concurrent immunosuppressive or immune modulating therapies; infection; varicella zoster antibody testing/vaccination; macula edema; decreased respiratory function; hepatic dysfunction; renal impairment; age 65 yr or older; pregnancy (category C); lactation. Safety and efficacy in children younger than 18 yr not established.

ROUTE & DOSAGE

Multiple Sclerosis

Adult: **PO** 0.5 mg once daily

Hepatic Impairment Dosage Adjustment

Mild or moderate hepatic impairment: No dosage adjustment needed

Severe hepatic impairment (Child–Pugh class C, total score greater than 10): Monitor closely due to increased risk of adverse effects.

ADMINISTRATION

Oral

- May be given with or without food.
- Monitor closely for 6 h after first dose for S&S of bradycardia. If fingolimod is discontinued for more than 2 wk then reinitiated, observe for bradycardia for 6 h following reinitiated dose.
- Store at 15°–30°C (59°–86°F).

ADVERSE EFFECTS **CV:** Bradycardia, hypertension, AV block. **Respiratory:** Bronchitis, cough, dyspnea, sinusitis. **CNS:** *Headache,* depression, dizziness, migraine, paresthesia. **HEENT:** Blurred vision, eye pain. **Endocrine:** *Increased ALT* *and AST,* increased GGT, increased triglycerides, weight loss. **Skin:** Alopecia, eczema, pruritus, tinea infections. **GI:** Diarrhea, nausea, abdominal pain, gastroenteritis. **Musculoskeletal:** Back pain, leg pain, weakness. **Hematologic:** Leukopenia, lymphopenia. **Other:** Asthenia, *infection,* influenza, herpes infections.

INTERACTIONS

Drug: Ketoconazole increases levels of fingolimod; ANTINEOPLASTIC, IMMUNOSUPPRESSIVE or IMMUNOMODULATING agents may increase the risk of immunosuppression; fingolimod causes an additional reduction of heart rate when used with **atenolol;** CLASS IA and CLASS III ANTIARRHYTHMICS may increase risk of serious rhythm disturbances, and BETA BLOCKERS may cause increased bradycardia during fingolimod initiation.

PHARMACOKINETICS

Absorption: 93% bioavailable. **Peak:** 12–16 h. **Distribution:** 99.7% plasma protein bound. **Metabolism:** Phosphorylated to active metabolite; oxidized by multiple CYP450 enzymes. **Elimination:** Renal (81%) and fecal (2.5%). **Half-Life:** 6–9 d.

NURSING IMPLICATIONS

Assessment & Drug Effects

- Baseline ECG is recommended to identify risk factors for bradycardia and AV block, especially in those with known cardiac risk factors or concurrent antiarrhythmic drugs including beta blockers and calcium channel blockers.
- Monitor HR and BP at baseline and for 6 h after the first dose. HR declines within 1 h and is maximal at approximately 6 h. Monitor HR during first month of therapy during which time a return to baseline should be seen.
- Monitor for and report promptly S&S of the following: Infection, hepatic dysfunction (e.g., unexplained nausea, vomiting, abdominal pain, fatigue, anorexia, or jaundice and/or dark urine), or dyspnea.
- Baseline ophthalmologic exam is recommended and should be performed if patient reports visual disturbances at any time while taking this drug.
- Monitor lab tests: Baseline and periodic CBC, bilirubin.

Patient & Family Education

- Those who have not had chickenpox or received the vaccination should consider receiving the VZV vaccine prior to starting treatment with fingolimod.
- Promptly report any of the following: S&S of infection; visual disturbances; new onset or worsening dyspnea; unexplained nausea, vomiting, abdominal pain, fatigue, loss of appetite, jaundice, and/or dark urine.
- Women of childbearing age should use effective contraception during and for 2 mo following discontinuation of fingolimod.
- Notify prescriber immediately if a pregnancy occurs.

FLAVOXATE HYDROCHLORIDE

(fla-vox′ate)

Classification: ANTICHOLINERGIC; SMOOTH MUSCLE RELAXANT

Therapeutic: URINARY TRACT ANTISPASMODIC

Prototype: Oxybutynin

AVAILABILITY

Tablet

ACTION & *THERAPEUTIC EFFECT*

Exerts spasmolytic action on smooth muscle. Increases urinary bladder capacity in patients with spastic bladder, possibly by direct action on detrusor muscle. Also demonstrates local anesthetic and analgesic action. *Has antispasmodic action on the urinary bladder.*

USES Symptomatic relief of dysuria, overactive bladder, urinary urgency/incontinence.

CONTRAINDICATIONS Pyloric or duodenal obstruction, obstructive intestinal lesions, ileus, achalasia, GI hemorrhage; obstructive uropathies of lower urinary tract.

CAUTIOUS USE Suspected or closed-angle glaucoma; myasthenia gravis; autonomic neuropathy; dehydration; older adults; pregnancy (use with caution; limited information regarding use in pregnant women). Safety in children younger than 12 yr not established.

ROUTE & DOSAGE

Dysuria, Nocturia, Incontinence/ OAB

Adult/Adolescent: **PO** 100–200 mg tid or qid, reduce when symptoms improve

ADMINISTRATION

Oral

- Give without regard to meals.
- Store at 15°–30°C (59°–86°F) unless otherwise directed.

ADVERSE EFFECTS **CV:** Palpitation, tachycardia. **CNS:** Headache, vertigo, drowsiness, mental confusion (especially in older adults), nervousness. **HEENT:** Blurred vision, increased intraocular tension, disturbances of eye accommodation. **Skin:** Rash, urticaria. **GI:** Nausea, vomiting, dry mouth (and throat), constipation (with high doses). **Other:** Dysuria, leukopenia (rare).

INTERACTIONS **Drug:** May antagonize the GI motility effects of **metoclopramide,** may add to GI slowing caused by ANTIDIARRHEALS. Use with other ANTICHOLINERGIC AGENTS may have increased adverse effects. Use with POTASSIUM SALTS increases risk of ulcer formation.

PHARMACOKINETICS **Onset:** 55 min **Elimination:** 10–30% in urine within 6 h.

NURSING IMPLICATIONS

Assessment & Drug Effects

- Monitor heart rate. Report tachycardia.
- Monitor for anticholinergic signs and symptoms including I&O.
- Those with suspected glaucoma should be closely monitored for increased intraocular tension.

Patient & Family Education

- Do not drive or engage in potentially hazardous activities until response to drug is known.
- Report adverse reactions to prescriber as well as clinical improvement or the lack of a favorable response.

FLECAINIDE

(fle-kay'nide)

Tambocor

Classification: CLASS IC ANTIARRHYTHMIC

Therapeutic: CLASS IC ANTIARRHYTHMIC

AVAILABILITY Tablet

ACTION & *THERAPEUTIC EFFECT*

Local (membrane) anesthetic and antiarrhythmic with electrophysiologic properties similar to other class IC antiarrhythmic drugs. Slows conduction velocity throughout myocardial conduction system, increases ventricular refractoriness.

Is an effective suppressant of PVCs and a variety of atrial and ventricular arrhythmias.

USES Life-threatening ventricular arrhythmias.

UNLABELED USES Atrial tachycardia and other arrhythmias unresponsive to standard agents (e.g., quinidine), Wolff–Parkinson–White syndrome, and recurrent ventricular tachycardias.

CONTRAINDICATIONS Hypersensitivity to flecainide; preexisting second- or third-degree AV block, right bundle branch block when associated with a left hemiblock unless a pacemaker is present; cardiogenic shock, left ventricular dysfunction; recent acute MI; QT prolongation syndromes; electrolyte imbalances.

CAUTIOUS USE Hypersensitivity to amide local anesthetics; atrial fibrillation; cardiac arrhythmias; cardiac disease; sick sinus syndrome; severe or moderate hepatic or renal impairment; older adults; pregnancy (category C); children and infants.

ROUTE & DOSAGE

Life-Threatening Ventricular Arrhythmias

Adult: **PO** 100 mg q12h, may increase by 50 mg bid q4days (max: 400 mg/day)
Child: **PO** 1–3 mg/kg/day in 3 divided doses (max: 8 mg/kg/day)

ADMINISTRATION

Oral

- Do not increase dosage more frequently than every 4 days.
- Store in tightly covered, light-resistant containers at 15°–30°C (59°–86°F) unless otherwise directed.

ADVERSE EFFECTS **CV:** Arrhythmias, chest pain, worsening of CHF. **CNS:** *Dizziness,* headache, lightheadedness, unsteadiness, paresthesias, fatigue. **HEENT:** *Blurred vision, difficulty in focusing,* spots before eyes. **GI:** *Nausea,* constipation, change in taste perception. **Other:** Dyspnea, fever, edema.

INTERACTIONS **Drug: Cimetidine** may increase flecainide levels; may increase **digoxin** levels 15–25%; BETA BLOCKERS may have additive negative inotropic effects.

PHARMACOKINETICS **Absorption:** Readily from GI tract. **Peak:** 2–3 h. **Distribution:** Crosses placenta; distributed into breast milk. **Metabolism:** In liver. **Elimination:** Mainly in urine. **Half-Life:** 7–22 h.

NURSING IMPLICATIONS

Black Box Warning

Flecainide has ventricular proarrhythmic effects in patients with atrial fibrillation/flutter.

Assessment & Drug Effects

- Correct preexisting hypokalemia or hyperkalemia before treatment is initiated.
- ECG monitoring, including Holter monitor for ambulating patients, is recommended because of the possibility of drug-induced arrhythmias.
- Note: Effective trough plasma levels are between 0.7 and 1 mcg/mL. The probability of adverse reactions increases when trough levels exceed 1 mcg/mL.
- Monitor carefully during period of dose adjustment.
- Monitor lab tests: Periodic flecainide plasma level, especially in patients with severe CHF or renal failure.

Patient & Family Education

- Note: It is VERY important to take this drug at the prescribed times.
- Report visual disturbances to prescriber.

FLOXURIDINE

(flox-yoor'i-deen)

Classification: ANTINEOPLASTIC; ANTIMETABOLITE, PYRIMIDINE

Therapeutic: ANTINEOPLASTIC

Prototype: Fluorouracil

AVAILABILITY Powder for injection

ACTION & *THERAPEUTIC EFFECT* Pyrimidine antagonist and cell-cycle specific that is catabolized to fluorouracil in the body; highly toxic because it blocks an enzyme essential to normal DNA and RNA synthesis. *Proliferative cells of neoplasms are affected more than healthy tissue cells.*

USES Colorectal cancer; hepatic metastases.

UNLABELED USES Carcinoma of breast, ovary, cervix, urinary bladder, and prostate not responsive to other antimetabolites.

CONTRAINDICATIONS Existing or recent viral infections; pregnancy (category D); lactation.

CAUTIOUS USE Bone marrow suppression; serious infections; high-risk patients: prior high-dose pelvic irradiation, impaired kidney or liver function.

ROUTE & DOSAGE

Carcinoma

Adult: **Intra-Arterial** 0.1–0.6 mg/kg/day by continuous intra-arterial infusion until intolerable toxicity

Obesity Dosage Adjustment

Use actual body weight

ADMINISTRATION

Intra-arterial Infusion

PREPARE: **Direct:** Reconstitute with 5 mL sterile distilled water for injection; further dilute with D5W or NS injection to a volume appropriate for the infusion apparatus to be used.

ADMINISTER: **Direct:** It is administered by pump to overcome pressure in large arteries and to ensure a uniform rate. ▪ Examine infusion site frequently for signs of extravasation. If this occurs, stop infusion and restart in another vessel.

INCOMPATIBILITIES: **Y-site: Allopurinol, cefepime.**

- Keep reconstituted solutions, which are stable at 2°–8°C (36°–46°F), for no more than 2 wk. ▪ Store at 15°–30°C (59°–86°F) unless otherwise directed.

ADVERSE EFFECTS **GI:** Diarrhea, stomatitis. **Hematologic:** Anemia, bone marrow depression (nadir 7–10 days), leukopenia, thrombocytopenia.

INTERACTIONS **Drug: Metronidazole** may increase general floxuridine toxicity; may increase or decrease serum levels of **phenytoin, fosphenytoin; hydroxyurea** can decrease conversion to active metabolite. Do not use with LIVE VACCINES, **deferiprone, dipyrone, gimeracil, tacrolimus.**

PHARMACOKINETICS **Distribution:** Distributed to tumor, intestinal mucosa, bone marrow, liver, and CSF; probably crosses placenta. **Metabolism:** Rapidly metabolized in liver to fluorouracil. **Elimination:** 15% in urine, 60–80% through lungs as carbon dioxide. **Half-Life:** 16 min.

NURSING IMPLICATIONS

Black Box Warning

Because floxuridine has been associated with severe toxic reactions, patient should be hospitalized for the first course of therapy.

Assessment & Drug Effects

- Discontinue therapy promptly with onset of any of the following: Stomatitis, esophagopharyngitis, intractable vomiting, diarrhea, leukopenia (WBC less than 3500/mm^3), or rapidly falling WBC count, thrombocytopenia (platelets 100,000/mm^3), GI bleeding, hemorrhage from any site.
- Monitor lab tests: Baseline and periodic total and differential WBC counts, LFTs, and platelet count.

Patient & Family Education

- Be aware that floxuridine sometimes causes temporary thinning of hair.

FLUCONAZOLE

(flu-con'a-zole)

Diflucan

Classification: AZOLE ANTIFUNGAL

Therapeutic: ANTIFUNGAL

AVAILABILITY Tablet; oral suspension; solution for injection

ACTION & THERAPEUTIC EFFECT Interferes with formation of ergosterol, the principal sterol in the fungal cell membrane leading to cell death. *Antifungal properties are related to the drug effect on the functioning of fungal cell membrane.*

USES Cryptococcal meningitis and oropharyngeal and systemic candidiasis, both commonly found in AIDS and other immunocompromised patients; vaginal candidiasis.

CONTRAINDICATIONS Hypersensitivity to fluconazole; S&S of drug-induced liver disease; lacatation.

CAUTIOUS USE Hypersensitivity to other azole antifungals; AIDS or malignancy; hepatic impairment; structural cardiac disease; history of torsades de pointes or QT prolongation; renal impairment or failure; pregnancy (category C).

ROUTE & DOSAGE

Oropharyngeal Candidiasis

Adult: **PO/IV** 200 mg day 1, then 100 mg/day × 14 days
Child: **PO/IV** 3–6 mg/kg/day × 14 days

Esophageal Candidiasis

Adult: **PO/IV** 200 mg day 1, then 100 mg daily × 3 wk
Child/Infant: **PO/IV** 3–6 mg/kg/day × 21 days

Systemic Candidemia

Adult: **PO/IV** 400 mg day 1, then 200 mg daily × 4 wk
Child/Infant/Neonate (14 days or older): **PO/IV** 6 mg/kg q12h × 28 days
Neonate (0–14 days): **IV** 6 mg/kg q72h

Vaginal Candidiasis

Adult: **PO** 150 mg × 1 dose

Cryptococcal Meningitis

Adult: **PO/IV** 400 mg day 1, then 200 mg daily × 10–12 wk
Child/Infant/Neonate: **PO/IV** 12 mg/kg day 1, then 6–12 mg/kg/day × 10–12 wk

Renal Impairment Dosage Adjustment

CrCl 50 mL/min or less (without concurrent dialysis): Give 50% of maintenance dose

Hemodialysis Dosage Adjustment

Administer full dose postdialysis

ADMINISTRATION

Oral

- Take this medication for the full course of therapy, which may take weeks or months.
- Take next dose as soon as possible if you miss a dose; however, do not take a dose if it is almost time for next dose. Do not double dose.

Intravenous

PREPARE: **Continuous:** Packaged ready for use as a 2-mg/mL solution. Remove wrapper just prior to use.
ADMINISTER: **Continuous:** Give at a maximum rate of approximately 200 mg/h. Give after hemodialysis is completed. ▪ Do not use IV admixtures of fluconazole and other medications.
INCOMPATIBILITIES: **Solution/additive:** **Trimethoprim-sulfamethoxazole.** **Y-site:** **Amphotericin B, amphotericin B cholesteryl, ampicillin, calcium gluconate, cefotaxime, ceftazidime, ceftriaxone, cefuroxime, chloramphenicol, clindamycin, dantrolene, diazepam, diazoxide, digoxin, furosemide, gemtuzumab, haloperidol, hydralazine, hydroxyzine, imipenem-cilastatin, pantoprazole, pentamidine, phenytoin, piperacillin, SMZ/TMP ticarcillin.**

ADVERSE EFFECTS **CNS:** Headache. **Skin:** Rash. **GI:** Nausea, vomiting, abdominal pain, diarrhea, increase in AST in patients with cryptococcal meningitis and AIDS.

INTERACTIONS **Drug:** Increased PT in patients on **warfarin;** may increase **alosetron, bexarotene, phenytoin, cevimeline, cilostazol, cyclosporine, dihydroergotamine, ergotamine, dofetilide, haloperidol, levobupivacaine, modafinil, zonisamide** levels and toxicity; hypoglycemic reactions with ORAL SULFONYLUREAS; decreased fluconazole levels with **rifampin, cimetidine;** may prolong the effects of **fentanyl, alfentanil, methadone.**

PHARMACOKINETICS **Absorption:** 90% from GI tract. **Peak:** 1–2 h. **Distribution:** Widely distributed, including CSF. **Metabolism:** 11% of dose metabolized in liver. **Elimination:** In urine. **Half-Life:** 20–50 h.

NURSING IMPLICATIONS

Assessment & Drug Effects

- Monitor for allergic response. Patients allergic to other azole antifungals may be allergic to fluconazole.
- Note: Drug may cause elevations of the following laboratory serum values: ALT, AST, alkaline phosphatase, bilirubin.
- Monitor for S&S of hepatotoxicity.
- Monitor lab tests: Periodic LFTs, renal function tests, and serum potassium.

Patient & Family Education

- Monitor carefully for loss of glycemic control if diabetic.
- Inform prescriber of all medications being taken.

FLUCYTOSINE

(floo-sye′toe-seen)

Ancobon

Classification: ANTIFUNGAL

Therapeutic: ANTIFUNGAL

Prototype: Fluconazole

F

AVAILABILITY Capsule

ACTION & *THERAPEUTIC EFFECT* Selectively penetrates fungal cell and is converted to fluorouracil, an antimetabolite believed to be responsible for antifungal activity. *Has antifungal activity against* Cryptococcus *and* Candida *as well as chromomycosis.*

USES Alone or in combination for serious systemic infections caused by susceptible strains of *Cryptococcus* and *Candida* species.

CONTRAINDICATIONS Hypersensitivity to flucytosine; lactation.

CAUTIOUS USE Hepatic disease; electrolyte imbalance; bone marrow depression, hematologic disorders, patients being treated with or having received radiation or bone marrow depressant drugs; dental disease; extreme caution in impaired kidney function; pregnancy (may cause adverse effects in fetus if taken during pregnancy); children.

ROUTE & DOSAGE

Fungal Infection

Adult: **PO** 50–150 mg/kg/day divided q6h

Renal Impairment Dosage Adjustment

CrCl 21–40 mL/min: 25 mg/kg/dose q12h; *CrCl 10–20 mL/min:* 25 mg/g/dose q24h; *CrCl less than 10 mL/min:* 25 mg/kg/dose q48h

ADMINISTRATION

Oral

- Lower dosages with longer dosage intervals are recommended in patients with serum creatinine of 1.7 mg/dL or higher. Check with prescriber.
- Give capsules a few at a time over 15 min to decrease incidence and severity of nausea and vomiting.
- Store in light-resistant containers at 15°–30°C (59°–86°F).

ADVERSE EFFECTS **Cardiac:** Cardiotoxicity, chest pain, ventricular dysfunction. **Respiratory:** Dyspnea. **CNS:** Confusion, ataxia, paresthesia, peripheral neuropathy, hallucinations, headache, sedation, vertigo. **Endocrine:** Elevated levels of serum alkaline phosphatase, AST, ALT, BUN, serum creatinine. **Skin:** Rash, pruritus. **GI:** Nausea, vomiting, diarrhea, abdominal bloating, enterocolitis. Hepatomegaly, hepatitis. **Hematologic:** Hypoplasia of bone marrow: Anemia, <u>leukopenia</u>, <u>thrombocytopenia</u>, <u>agranulocytosis</u>, eosinophilia.

DIAGNOSTIC TEST INTERFERENCE False elevations of ***serum creatinine.***

INTERACTIONS **Drug: Amphotericin B** can increase flucytosine toxicity. **Cytosine** may decrease activity of flucytosine. **Cladribine** can have increased myelosuppression. Avoid LIVE VACCINES. Do not use with **gimeracil** or *Saccharomyces boulardii.*

PHARMACOKINETICS **Absorption:** Readily from GI tract. **Peak:** 2 h.

Distribution: Widely distributed in body tissues including aqueous humor and CSF; crosses placenta. **Metabolism:** Minimal. **Elimination:** 90% in urine unchanged. **Half-Life:** 2–5 h (adult).

NURSING IMPLICATIONS

Black Box Warning

Flucytosine is associated with severe hematologic, renal, and hepatic adverse reactions.

Assessment & Drug Effects

- Monitor renal status closely because renal impairment can cause increased serum concentration of drug with greater adverse effects.
- Frequent assays of blood drug level are recommended, especially in patients with impaired kidney function to determine adequacy of drug excretion (therapeutic range: 25–120 mg/mL).
- Monitor I&O. Report change in I&O ratio or pattern. Because most of drug is eliminated unchanged by kidneys, compromised function can lead to drug accumulation.
- C&S tests should be performed before initiation of therapy and at weekly intervals during therapy. Organism resistance has been reported.
- Monitor lab tests: Baseline and periodic CBC with differential, renal function tests, electrolytes.

Patient & Family Education

- Report fever, sore mouth or throat, and unusual bleeding or bruising tendency to prescriber.
- Be aware that the general duration of therapy is 4–6 wk, but it may continue for several months.

FLUDROCORTISONE ACETATE (Pr)

(floo-droe-kor′ti-sone)

Florinef Acetate

Classification: ADRENOCORTICAL STEROID; MINERALOCORTICOID

Therapeutic: MINERALOCORTICOID; ANTI-INFLAMMATORY

AVAILABILITY Tablet

ACTION & *THERAPEUTIC EFFECT* Long-acting synthetic steroid with potent mineralocorticoid activity. Small doses produce marked sodium retention, increased urinary potassium excretion, and elevated BP. *Synthetic corticosteroid replacement product for adrenocortical insufficiency.*

USES Partial replacement therapy for adrenocortical insufficiency and for treatment of salt-losing forms of congenital adrenogenital syndrome.

UNLABELED USES To increase systolic and diastolic blood pressure in patients with severe hypotension secondary to diabetes mellitus or to levodopa therapy.

CONTRAINDICATIONS Hypersensitivity to glucocorticoids, idiopathic thrombocytopenic purpura, psychoses, acute glomerulonephritis, viral or bacterial diseases of skin, systemic fungal infections; infections not controlled by antibiotics, active or latent amebiasis, hypercorticism, smallpox vaccination, or other immunologic procedures.

CAUTIOUS USE Diabetes mellitus; chronic, active hepatitis positive for hepatitis B surface antigen;

hyperlipidemia; cirrhosis; stromal herpes simplex; glaucoma, tuberculosis of eye; osteoporosis; convulsive disorders; hypothyroidism; diverticulitis; nonspecific ulcerative colitis; fresh intestinal anastomoses; active or latent peptic ulcer; gastritis; esophagitis; thromboembolic disorders; CHF; metastatic carcinoma; hypertension; renal insufficiency; history of allergies; active or arrested tuberculosis; myasthenia gravis; history of psychosis; pregnancy (category C); lactation; children.

ROUTE & DOSAGE

Adrenocortical Insufficiency

Adult: **PO** 0.1 mg/day, may range from 0.1 mg 3 × wk to 0.2 mg/day
Child: **PO** 0.05–0.1 mg/day

Salt-Losing Adrenogenital Syndrome

Adult: **PO** 0.1–0.2 mg/day
Child: **PO** 0.05–0.1 mg/day

ADMINISTRATION

Oral

- Note: Concomitant oral cortisone or hydrocortisone therapy may be advisable to provide substitute therapy approximating normal adrenal activity.
- Store in airtight containers at 15°–30°C (59°–86°F). Protect from light.

ADVERSE EFFECTS **CV:** CHF, hypertension, thromboembolism (rare), tachycardia. **CNS:** Vertigo, headache, nystagmus, increased intracranial pressure with papilledema (usually after discontinuation of medication), mental disturbances, aggravation of preexisting psychiatric conditions, insomnia, ataxia (rare). **HEENT:** Posterior subcapsular cataracts (especially in children), glaucoma, exophthalmos, increased intraocular pressure with optic nerve damage, perforation of the globe. **Endocrine:** Suppressed linear growth in children, decreased glucose tolerance; hyperglycemia, manifestations of latent diabetes mellitus; hypocorticism; amenorrhea; and other menstrual difficulties. Hypocalcemia; *sodium and fluid retention;* hypokalemia and hypokalemic alkalosis, negative nitrogen balance, decreased serum concentration of vitamins A and C. **Skin:** Skin thinning and atrophy, *acne, impaired wound healing;* petechiae, ecchymosis, easy bruising; suppression of skin test reaction; hypopigmentation or hyperpigmentation, hirsutism, acneiform eruptions, subcutaneous fat atrophy; allergic dermatitis, urticaria, angioneurotic edema, increased sweating. **GI:** *Nausea,* increased appetite, ulcerative esophagitis, pancreatitis, abdominal distension, peptic ulcer with perforation and hemorrhage, melena. **GU:** Increased or decreased motility and number of sperm. **Musculoskeletal:** (Long-term use) Osteoporosis, compression fractures, muscle wasting and weakness, tendon rupture, aseptic necrosis of femoral and humeral heads. **Hematologic:** Thrombocytopenia. **Other:** Anaphylactoid reactions (rare), aggravation or masking of infections; malaise, weight gain, obesity.

INTERACTIONS **Drug:** The antidiabetic effects of **insulin** and SULFONYLUREAS may be diminished; **amphotericin B,** DIURETICS may increase **potassium** loss; **warfarin** may decrease prothrombin time; **indomethacin, ibuprofen** can potentiate the pressor effect of fludrocortisone; ANABOLIC STEROIDS increase risk of edema and acne; **rifampin** may increase the hepatic metabolism of fludrocortisone.

PHARMACOKINETICS **Absorption:** Readily from GI tract. **Peak:** 1.7 h. **Metabolism:** In liver. **Half-Life:** 3.5 h.

NURSING IMPLICATIONS

Assessment & Drug Effects

- Monitor weight and I&O ratio to observe onset of fluid accumulation, especially if patient is on unrestricted salt intake and without potassium supplement. Report weight gain of 2 kg (5 lb)/wk.
- Monitor and record BP daily. If hypertension develops as a consequence of therapy, report to prescriber. Usually, the dose will be reduced to 0.05 mg/day.
- Check BP q4–6h and weight at least every other day during periods of dosage adjustment.
- Monitor for S&S of hypokalemia and hyperkalemic metabolic alkalosis (see Appendix F).
- Monitor lab tests: Periodic serum electrolytes.

Patient & Family Education

- Report signs of hypokalemia (see Appendix F).
- Be aware of signs of potassium depletion associated with high sodium intake: Muscle weakness, paresthesias, circumoral numbness; fatigue, anorexia, nausea, mental depression, polyuria, delirium, diminished reflexes, arrhythmias, cardiac failure, ileus, ECG changes.
- Eat foods with high potassium content.
- Signs of edema should be reported immediately. Sodium intake may or may not require regulation, depending on individual needs and clinical situation.
- Weigh daily under standard conditions and report steady weight gain.
- Report intercurrent infection, trauma, or unexpected stress of any kind promptly when taking maintenance therapy.
- Carry medical identification at all times.

F

FLUMAZENIL

(flu-ma′ze-nil)

Classification: BENZODIAZEPINE ANTAGONIST

Therapeutic: BENZODIAZEPINE ANTIDOTE

AVAILABILITY Solution for injection

ACTION & *THERAPEUTIC EFFECT* Antagonizes the effects of benzodiazepine on the CNS, including sedation, impairment of recall, and psychomotor impairment. *Reverses the action of a benzodiazepine.*

USES Reversal of sedation induced by benzodiazepine for anesthesia or diagnostic or therapeutic procedures as well as through overdose.

CONTRAINDICATIONS Hypersensitivity to flumazenil or to benzodiazepines; patients given a benzodiazepine for control of a life-threatening condition; patients showing signs of cyclic antidepressant overdose; seizure-prone individuals; during labor and delivery.

CAUTIOUS USE Hepatic function impairment, older adults, intensive care patients, head injury, anxiety or pain disorder; drug- and alcohol-dependent patients, and physical dependence upon benzodiazepines; pregnancy (embryocidal effects seen at large doses; use during labor and delivery is not recommended); lactation; children.

F

ROUTE & DOSAGE

Reversal of Sedation

Adult: **IV** 0.2 mg over 15 sec, may repeat 0.2 mg each min for 4 additional doses or a cumulative dose of 1 mg
Child: **IV** 0.01 mg/kg may repeat each min (max: 1 mg)

Benzodiazepine Overdose

Adult: **IV** 0.2 mg over 30 sec, if no response after 30 sec, then 0.3 mg over 30 sec, may repeat with 0.5 mg each min (max cumulative dose: 3 mg)

ADMINISTRATION

- Use all diluted solutions within 24 h of dilution.

Intravenous

PREPARE: **Direct:** May give undiluted or diluted. If diluted use D5W, lactated Ringer, NS.
ADMINISTER: **Direct:** Ensure patency of IV before administration of flumazenil because extravasation will cause local irritation. ▪ Do not give as bolus dose. Give through an IV that is freely flowing into a large vein. **Direct for Reversal of Anesthesia or Sedation:** Give each dose slowly over 15 sec. ▪ In high-risk patients, slow the rate to provide the smallest effective dose. **Direct for Benzodiazepine Overdose:** Give each dose slowly over 30 sec.

ADVERSE EFFECTS **CV:** Palpitation. **Respiratory:** Dyspnea, hyperventilation. **CNS:** Emotional lability, *dizziness,* agitation, ataxia, anxiety, insomnia, nervousness, **HEENT:** Blurred vision. **GI:** *Vomiting,* xerostomia. **Other:** Pain at injection site.

INTERACTIONS **Drug:** May antagonize effects of **zaleplon, zolpidem;** may cause convulsions or arrhythmias with TRICYCLIC ANTIDEPRESSANTS.

PHARMACOKINETICS **Onset:** 1–5 min. **Peak:** 6–10 min. **Duration:** 2–4 h. **Metabolism:** In the liver to inactive metabolites. **Elimination:** 90–95% in urine, 5–10% in feces within 72 h. **Half-Life:** 54 min.

NURSING IMPLICATIONS

Black Box Warnings

Flumazenil has been associated with the occurrence of seizures.

Assessment & Drug Effects

- Monitor respiratory status carefully until risk of resedation is unlikely (up to 120 min). Drug may not fully reverse benzodiazepine-induced ventilatory insufficiency.
- Monitor carefully for seizures, and take appropriate precautions.

Patient & Family Education

- Do not drive or engage in potentially hazardous activities until at least 18–24 h after discharge following a procedure.
- Do not ingest alcohol or nonprescription drugs for 18–24 h after flumazenil is administered or if the effects of the benzodiazepine persist.

FLUNISOLIDE

(floo-niss′oh-lide)

See Appendix A-3.

FLUOCINOLONE ACETONIDE

(floo-oh-sin′oh-lone)

Fluoderm ♣, Synalar

Prototype: HYDROCORTISONE

See Appendix A-4.

FLUOCINONIDE

(floo-oh-sin'oh-nide)

Vanos

See Appendix A-4.

FLUOROMETHOLONE

(flure-oh-meth'oh-lone)

Flarex, FML Forte, FML Liquifilm

See Appendix A-1.

FLUOROURACIL [5-FLUOROURACIL (5-FU)]

(flure-oh-yoor'a-sil)

Carac, Efudex, Fluoroplex, Tolak

Classification: ANTINEOPLASTIC; ANTIMETABOLITE, PYRIMIDINE

Therapeutic: ANTINEOPLASTIC

AVAILABILITY Solution for injection; topical solution; topical cream

ACTION & *THERAPEUTIC EFFECT* Pyrimidine antagonist and cell cycle specific agent that blocks action of enzymes essential to normal DNA and RNA synthesis; unbalanced growth and death of cell follow. Exhibits higher affinity for tumor tissue than healthy tissue. *Highly toxic, especially to proliferative cells in neoplasms, bone marrow, and intestinal mucosa.*

USES Systemically as single agent or in combination with other antineoplastics for treatment of patients with inoperable neoplasms of breast, colon or rectum, stomach, pancreas.

UNLABELED USES Anal carcinoma, bladder cancer, cervical cancer, esophageal cancer, head and neck cancer, hepatobiliary cancers, nasopharyngeal carcinoma, neuroendocrine tumors, penile cancer, vulvar cancer, glaucoma surgery.

CONTRAINDICATIONS Hypersensitivity to any fluorouracil components; poor nutritional status; myelosuppression; patients with dihydropyrimidine dehydrogenase (DPD) enzyme deficiency; women who are or may become pregnant; pregnancy (category D); lactation.

CAUTIOUS USE Major surgery during previous month; history of high-dose pelvic irradiation, metastatic cell infiltration of bone marrow, previous use of alkylating agents; cardiac disease, CAD, angina; men and women in childbearing ages; hepatic or renal impairment. Safety and efficacy in children younger than 18 yr not established.

ROUTE & DOSAGE

Cancer Therapy

Dose depends on concurrent medication and stage/location of cancer. See package insert for specific dosing.

Actinic and Solar Keratosis

Adult: **Topical** Apply cream or solution bid for 2–6 wk; apply **Carac** or **Tolak** cream once daily

Superficial Basal Cell Carcinoma

Adult: **Topical** Apply 5% cream bid for 3–6 wk

Obesity Dosage Adjustment

Dose patient based on lean body mass

F

ADMINISTRATION

Topical

- Use gloved fingers to apply topical drug.
- Do not use occlusive dressings with topical drug. Use a porous gauze dressing for cosmetic purposes.
- Store at 15°–30°C (59°–86°F) unless otherwise directed. Protect from light and freezing.

Intravenous

This drug is a cytotoxic agent, and caution should be used to prevent any contact with the drug. Follow institutional or standard guidelines for preparation, handling, and disposal of cytotoxic agents.

PREPARE: **Direct/Infusion:** This drug may be given undiluted or further diluted in D5W or NS for infusion. ▪ If a precipitate forms, redissolve drug by heating to 60°C (140°F) and shake vigorously. Allow to cool to body temperature before administration.

ADMINISTER: **Direct/Infusion:** Give by direct IV injection over 1–2 min. ▪ Infuse over 2–24 h as ordered. **IV Extravasation:** Inspect injection site frequently; avoid extravasation. If it occurs, stop infusion and restart in another vein. ▪ Ice compresses may reduce danger of local tissue damage from infiltrated solution.

INCOMPATIBILITIES: **Solution/additive:** **Carboplatin, ciprofloxacin, cisplatin, cytarabine, diazepam, doxorubicin, epirubicin, morphine.** **Y-site:** **Aldesleukin, amiodarone, amphotericin B cholesteryl, buprenorphine, calcium chloride, caspofungin, chlorpromazine, ciprofloxacin, diazepam, diltiazem, diphenhydramine, dobutamine, dolasetron, doxycycline, droperidol, epinephrine, epirubicin, filgrastim, gallium, haloperidol, hydroxyzine, idarubicin, irinotecan, lansoprazole, levofloxacin, lorazepam, methadone, midazolam, minocycline, moxifloxacin, nicardipine, ondansetron, pentamidine, phenytoin, prochlorperazine, promethazine, quinupristin/dalfopristin, topotecan, vancomycin, verapamil, vinorelbine.**

- Fluorouracil solution is normally colorless to faint yellow. Slight discoloration during storage does not appear to affect potency or safety. ▪ Discard dark yellow solution.

ADVERSE EFFECTS **CV:** Angina, cardiac arrhythmia, ischemic heart disease, local thrombophlebitis, vasospasm. **Respiratory:** Epistaxis. **CNS:** Euphoria, confusion, headache, CVA. **HEENT:** Lacrimal stenosis, nystagmus, photophobia, visual disturbance. **Skin:** *Alopecia,* hyperpigmentation, pruritus, changes in nails, dermatitis, maculopapular rash, Stevens–Johnson syndrome, and xeroderma. **GI:** Anorexia, *nausea, vomiting, stomatitis,* esophagopharyngitis, *diarrhea,* gastrointestinal hemorrhage. **Hematologic:** Anemia, leukopenia, thrombocytopenia, pancytopenia. **Other:** Anaphylaxis, hypersensitivity reaction.

DIAGNOSTIC TEST INTERFERENCE Fluorouracil may decrease ***plasma albumin*** (because of drug-induced protein malabsorption).

INTERACTIONS **Drug:** **Metronidazole** may increase general floxuridine toxicity; may increase or decrease serum levels of

phenytoin, fosphenytoin; Avoid use with IMMUNOSUPPRESSANTS, MYELOSUPPRESSIVE agents (e.g., **deferiprone, dipyrone**) may enhance neutropenic effects.

PHARMACOKINETICS

Distribution: Distributed to tumor, intestinal mucosa, bone marrow, liver, and CSF; probably crosses placenta. **Metabolism:** In liver. **Elimination:** 15% in urine, 60–80% through lungs as carbon dioxide. **Half-Life:** 16 min.

NURSING IMPLICATIONS

Assessment & Drug Effects

- Use protective isolation of patient during leukopenic period (WBC less than 3500/mm^3).
- Watch for and report signs of abnormal bleeding from any source during thrombocytopenic period (day 7–17); inspect skin for ecchymotic and petechial areas. Protect patient from trauma.
- Report disorientation or confusion; drug should be withdrawn immediately.
- Indications to discontinue drug: Severe stomatitis, leukopenia (WBC less than 3500/mm^3 or rapidly decreasing count), intractable vomiting, diarrhea, thrombocytopenia (platelets less than 100,000/mm^3), and hemorrhage from any site.
- Inspect patient's mouth daily. Promptly report cracked lips, xerostomia, white patches, and erythema of buccal membranes.
- Report development of maculopapular rash; it usually responds to symptomatic treatment and is reversible.
- Be aware of expected response of lesion to topical 5-FU: Erythema followed in sequence by vesiculation, erosion, ulceration, necrosis, epithelialization. Applications of drug are continued until ulcerative stage is reached (2–6 wk after initial applications) and then discontinued.
- Monitor lab tests: CBC with differential and platelet counts before each dose. Baseline and periodic LFTs, renal function tests, INR, and prothrombin time.

Patient & Family Education

- Understand that it is very important to report the first signs of toxicity: Anorexia, vomiting, nausea, stomatitis, diarrhea, GI bleeding.
- Avoid exposure to sunlight or ultraviolet lamp treatments. Protect exposed skin. Photosensitivity usually subsides 2–3 mo after last dose.
- Report promptly to prescriber any difficulty in maintaining balance while ambulating.
- Use contraception during 5-FU treatment. If you suspect you are pregnant, tell your prescriber.

FLUOXETINE HYDROCHLORIDE

(flu′ox-e-tine)

Prozac

Classification: SELECTIVE SEROTONIN REUPTAKE INHIBITOR (SSRI); ANTIDEPRESSANT

Therapeutic: ANTIDEPRESSANT; SSRI

AVAILABILITY

Tablet; capsule; solution; sustained release capsule

ACTION & *THERAPEUTIC EFFECT*

A selective serotonin reuptake inhibitor (SSRI). Antidepressant effect is presumed to be linked to its inhibition of CNS neuronal uptake of serotonin, a neurotransmitter. *Effectiveness may take from several days to 5 wk to develop fully. Drug has antidepressant, antiobsessive-compulsive, and antibulimic actions.*

USES Major depressive disorder, obsessive-compulsive disorder (OCD), bipolar depression, bulimia nervosa, premenstrual dysphoric disorder, panic disorder, treatment-resistant depression.

F

UNLABELED USES Fibromyalgia, PTSD, social anxiety disorder.

CONTRAINDICATIONS Hypersensitivity to fluoxetine or other SSRI drugs; bipolar disorder; hyponatremia; concurrent administration with MAOIs, pimozide or thioridazine; children younger than 7 yr for OCD, children younger than 8 yr for depression.

CAUTIOUS USE Hepatic and renal impairment, renal failure, abrupt discontinuation, anorexia nervosa, mania, bleeding; hyponatremia, cardiac disease, dehydration, DM, patients with history of suicidal ideations or current suicidal \tendencies; history of QT prolongation, or congenital long QT syndrome; seizure disorders, ECT, hepatic disease. Older adults may require dose adjustments; pregnancy (use with caution during pregnancy); lactation.

ROUTE & DOSAGE

Depression

Adult: **PO Immediate release** 20 mg/day may increase by 20 mg/day at weekly intervals (max: 80 mg/day)
Child (12 yr or older): **PO** 10–20 mg/day in a.m.; may increase q1–2 weeks
Child (8 yr or older): **PO** 5–10 mg/day in a.m.
Geriatric: **PO** Start with 10 mg/day

Obsessive Compulsive Disorder

Adult: **PO** 10–20 mg daily may increase if needed (max: 80 mg/day)
Adolescent/Child (7 yr or older): **PO** 5–10 mg/day may increase to 20 mg/day

Premenstrual Dysphoric Disorder

Adult: **PO** 10 mg daily (max: 60 mg/day)

Bulimia Nervosa

Adult: **PO** 20 mg daily, increase dose gradually to target dose of 60 mg daily

Panic Disorder

Adult: **PO** 5–10 mg daily may increase to 20 mg daily

Pharmacogenetic Dosage Adjustment

CYP2D6 poor metabolizers: Start at 80% of normal dose

ADMINISTRATION

Oral

- Give as a single dose in morning. Give in two divided doses; one in a.m. and one at noon to prevent insomnia, when more than 20 mg/day prescribed. For Bipolar I disorder and treatment-resistant depression, take once daily in the evening.
- Provide suicidal or potentially suicidal patient with small quantities of prescription medication.
- Monitor for worsening of depression or expression of suicidal ideations.

- Store at controlled room temperature. Protect from light.

ADVERSE EFFECTS CV: Vasodilation. **Respiratory:** Pharyngitis, sinusitis, flu-like symptoms. **CNS:** *Headache, nervousness, anxiety, insomnia,* drowsiness, yawning, abnormal dreams. **HEENT:** Blurred vision. **Endocrine:** Decreased libido. **Skin:** Diaphoresis, rash. **GI:** *Nausea, diarrhea,* anorexia, constipation, dyspepsia, dry mouth. **GU:** Sexual dysfunction, ejaculatory disorder, impotence. **Musculoskeletal:** Asthenia, tremor.

INTERACTIONS Drug: Concurrent use of **tryptophan** may cause agitation, restlessness, and GI distress; MAO INHIBITORS, **selegiline** may increase risk of severe hypertensive reaction and death; increases half-life of **diazepam;** may increase toxicity of TRICYCLIC ANTIDEPRESSANTS; AMPHETAMINES, **cilostazol, linezolid, selegiline, nefazodone, pentazocine, propafenone, sibutramine, tramadol, venlafaxine** may increase risk of serotonin syndrome; do not use with **bromopride**; may inhibit metabolism of **carbamazepine, phenytoin, ritonavir;** increased ergotamine toxicity with **dihydroergotamine, ergotamine.** Do not use with agents that cause QT prolongation (**pimozide, ziprasidone**). **Herbal: St. John's wort** may cause serotonin syndrome.

PHARMACOKINETICS Absorption: 60–80% from GI tract. **Onset:** 1–3 wk. **Peak:** 4–8 h. **Distribution:** Widely distributed, including CNS. **Metabolism:** In liver to active metabolite, norfluoxetine. **Elimination:** Greater than 80% in urine; 12% in feces. **Half-Life:** Fluoxetine 2–3 days, norfluoxetine 7–9 days.

NURSING IMPLICATIONS

Assessment & Drug Effects

- Monitor children and adolescents for changes in behavior and suicidal ideation.
- Use with caution in the older adult patient or patient with impaired renal or hepatic function (may need lower dose).
- Supervise patients closely who are high suicide risks, especially during initial therapy.
- Monitor for S&S of anaphylactoid reaction (see Appendix F).
- Monitor serum sodium level for development of hyponatremia, especially in patients who are taking diuretics or are otherwise hypovolemic.
- Monitor diabetics for loss of glycemic control; hypoglycemia has occurred during initiation of therapy, and hyperglycemia during drug withdrawal.
- Weigh weekly to monitor weight loss, particularly in the older adult or nutritionally compromised patient. Report significant weight loss to prescriber.
- Observe for and promptly report rash or urticaria and S&S of fever, leukocytosis, arthralgias, carpal tunnel syndrome, edema, respiratory distress, and proteinuria.
- Observe for dizziness and drowsiness and employ safety measures as indicated.
- Monitor for and report increased anxiety, nervousness, or insomnia; may need modification of drug dose.
- Monitor for seizures in patients with a history of seizures. Use appropriate safety precautions.
- Taper dosage slowly when discontinuing.
- Baseline and periodic ECG in patients with risk factors for QT prolongation and ventricular arrhythmia.

- Monitor lab tests: Periodic serum electrolytes; frequent plasma glucose in diabetics, LFTs, renal function tests.

Patient & Family Education

- Notify prescriber of any rash; possible sign of a serious group of adverse effects.
- Do not drive or engage in potentially hazardous activities until response to drug is known, especially if dizziness noted.
- Monitor blood glucose for loss of glycemic control if diabetic.
- Note: Drug may increase seizure activity in those with history of seizure.

FLUPHENAZINE DECANOATE

(floo-fen′a-zeen)

Modecate Decanoate ♣

FLUPHENAZINE HYDROCHLORIDE

Moditen HCl ♣

Classification: ANTIPSYCHOTIC; PHENOTHIAZINE

Therapeutic: ANTIPSYCHOTIC

Prototype: Chlorpromazine

AVAILABILITY Tablet; elixir; oral concentrate; solution for injection; **Decanoate:** Solution for injection

ACTION & THERAPEUTIC EFFECT Potent phenothiazine, antipsychotic agent that blocks postsynaptic dopamine receptors in the brain. Similar to other phenothiazines with the following exceptions: More potent/weight, higher incidence of extrapyramidal complications, and lower frequency of sedative, hypotensive, and antiemetic effects. *Effective for treatment of antipsychotic symptoms including schizophrenia.*

USES Management of manifestations of psychotic disorders.

UNLABELED USES Chorea of Huntington disease; chronic tic disorder.

CONTRAINDICATIONS Known hypersensitivity to fluphenazine; older adults with dementia-related psychosis; suspected or subcortical brain damage, comatose or severely depressed states, blood dyscrasias, liver damage; renal or hepatic disease; NMS; lactation; children younger than 12 yr.

CAUTIOUS USE Older adults, previously diagnosed breast cancer; closed-angle glaucoma; GI disorders; significant pulmonary disease; renal failure; seizure disorders; history of suicidal ideation or high risk for suicide attempt; cardiovascular diseases; pheochromocytoma; history of convulsive disorders; patients exposed to extreme heat or phosphorous insecticides; peptic ulcer; respiratory impairment; older adults; pregnancy (use during third trimester of pregnancy has a risk for abnormal movements and withdrawal symptoms in newborns following delivery).

ROUTE & DOSAGE

Psychosis

Adult: **PO** 2.5–10 mg/day in 3–4 divided doses (max: of 40 mg/day); **IM** 1.25 mg single dose, may need 2.5–10 mg/day divided q6–8h (max: 10 mg/day); **Decanoate IM/Subcutaneous** 6.25–25 mg q2wk

ADMINISTRATION

Oral

- Immediately prior to administration, dilute oral concentrate in fruit juice, water, carbonated beverage, milk, soup.

Avoid caffeine-containing beverages (cola, coffee) as a diluent, also tannic acid (tea) or pectinates (apple juice).

- Protect all preparations from light and freezing. Solutions may safely vary in color from almost colorless to light amber. Discard dark or otherwise discolored solutions.
- Store in tightly closed container at 15°–30°C (59°–86°F) unless otherwise specified by manufacturer. Protect all forms from light.

Intramuscular/Subcutaneous

- Fluphenazine hydrochloride (HCl) is given IM, and fluphenazine decanoate may be given IM or subcutaneously.

ADVERSE EFFECTS **CV:** Tachycardia, cardiac arrhythmias, hypertension, hypotension. **CNS:** *Extrapyramidal symptoms* (resembling Parkinson disease), tardive dyskinesia, sedation, drowsiness, dizziness, headache, mental depression, catatonic-like state, impaired thermoregulation, grand mal seizures. **HEENT:** Nasal congestion, blurred vision, increased intraocular pressure, *photosensitivity*. **Endocrine:** Hyperprolactinemia. **Skin:** Contact dermatitis. **GI:** Dry mouth, nausea, epigastric pain, constipation, fecal impaction, cholecystic jaundice. **GU:** Urinary retention, polyuria, inhibition of ejaculation. **Hematologic:** Transient leukopenia, agranulocytosis. **Other:** Peripheral edema.

INTERACTIONS **Drug:** **Alcohol** and other CNS DEPRESSANTS may potentiate depressive effects; decreases seizure threshold, may need to adjust dosage of ANTICONVULSANTS. Do not use with drugs that prolong QT interval. ANTICHOLINERGIC AGENTS may increase adverse effects. PHOTOSENSITIZING AGENTS may have additive effects. **Amisulpride** can increase the risk of neuroleptic malignant syndrome. May decrease effect of ANTIPARKINSON AGENTS. **Herbal:** **Kava** may increase risk and severity of dystonic reactions.

PHARMACOKINETICS **Absorption:** HCl is readily absorbed PO and IM; decanoate has delayed IM absorption. **Onset:** 1 h HCl; 24–72 h decanoate. **Peak:** 0.5 h PO; 1.5–2 h IM HCl; 48–96 h decanoate. **Duration:** 6–8 h HCl; 4–6 wk decanoate. **Distribution:** Crosses blood–brain barrier and placenta. **Metabolism:** In liver. **Half-Life:** 15 h HCl; 14 days decanoate.

NURSING IMPLICATIONS

Black Box Warning

Fluphenazine has been associated with increased mortality in older adults with dementia-related psychosis.

Assessment & Drug Effects

- Monitor very closely older adults with dementia. Report immediately onset of mental depression and extrapyramidal symptoms.
- Be alert for appearance of acute dystonia (see Appendix F). Symptoms can be controlled by reducing dosage or by adding an antiparkinsonism drug such as benztropine.
- Monitor BP during early therapy. If systolic drop is more than 20 mmHg, inform prescriber.
- Monitor I&O ratio and bowel elimination pattern. Check for abdominal distension and pain. Monitor for xerostomia and constipation.

- Monitor lab tests: Periodic renal function tests with long-term treatment; periodic WBC with differential, and LFTs.

Patient & Family Education

- Do not drive or engage in potentially hazardous activities until response to drug is known.
- Do not stop taking drug abruptly.
- Inform prescriber promptly if following symptoms appear: Light-colored stools, changes in vision, sore throat, fever, cellulitis, rash, any interference with movement.
- Avoid exposure to sun; wear protective clothing, and cover exposed skin surfaces with sunscreen.
- Avoid alcohol while on fluphenazine therapy.
- Note: Fluphenazine may discolor urine pink to red or reddish brown.
- Periodic ophthalmologic exams are recommended.

FLURANDRENOLIDE

(flure-an-dren'oh-lide)

Cordran

See Appendix A-4.

FLURAZEPAM HYDROCHLORIDE

(flure-az'e-pam)

Classification: SEDATIVE-HYPNOTIC, NONBARBITURATE; BENZODIAZEPINE

Therapeutic: SEDATIVE

Prototype: Triazolam

Controlled Substance: Schedule IV

AVAILABILITY Capsule

ACTION & *THERAPEUTIC EFFECT* Benzodiazepine derivative that enhances the GABA-benzodiazepine receptor complex. GABA is an inhibitory neurotransmitter involved in anxiolytic and sedative effects. Flurazepam appears to act at the limbic and subcortical levels of CNS to produce sedation. *Reduces sleep induction time; produces marked reduction of stage 4 sleep (deepest sleep stage) while at the same time increasing duration of total sleep time.*

USES In management of all kinds of insomnia (e.g., difficulty in falling asleep, frequent nocturnal awakening or early morning awakening or both).

CONTRAINDICATIONS Prolonged administration; benzodiazepine hypersensitivity; ethanol intoxication; COPD, sleep apnea; respiratory depression; shock; coma; major depression or psychosis; intermittent porphyria; pregnancy (teratogenic effects have been observed with some benzodiazepines); lactation.

CAUTIOUS USE Impaired renal or hepatic function; glaucoma; mental depression, psychoses, history of suicidal tendencies, bipolar disorder; intermittent porphyria; addiction-prone individuals; older adult or debilitated patients; COPD; children younger than 15 yr.

ROUTE & DOSAGE

Sedative, Hypnotic

Adult (15 yr or older): **PO** 15–30 mg (men) or 15 mg (women) at bedtime

Geriatric: **PO** 15 mg at bedtime

ADMINISTRATION

Oral

- May be administered without regard to meals; administer dose at bedtime.

- Store in light-resistant container with childproof cap at 20°–25°C (68°–77°F) unless otherwise specified.

ADVERSE EFFECTS **Cardiovascular:** Chest pain, flushing, hypotension, palpitations, syncope. **CNS:** *Residual sedation, drowsiness,* dizziness, ataxia, headache, nervousness, apprehension, talkativeness, irritability, depression, hallucinations, confusion, paradoxic reactions: Excitement, euphoria, hyperactivity, disorientation, coma (overdosage). **HEENT:** Blurred vision, burning eyes. **GI:** Heartburn, nausea, vomiting, constipation, diarrhea, abdominal pain. **Other:** Immediate allergic reaction, hypotension, granulocytopenia (rare), jaundice (rare).

INTERACTIONS **Drug:** **Alcohol,** CNS DEPRESSANTS, ANTICONVULSANTS potentiate CNS depression; **cimetidine, disulfiram** may increase flurazepam levels, thus increasing its toxicity. **Herbal:** **Kava, valerian** may potentiate sedation.

PHARMACOKINETICS **Absorption:** Readily from GI tract; 97% protein bound. **Onset:** 15–45 min. **Duration:** 7–8 h. **Distribution:** Crosses blood–brain barrier and placenta; distributed into breast milk. **Metabolism:** In liver to active metabolites. **Elimination:** Primarily in urine. **Half-Life:** 47–100 h.

NURSING IMPLICATIONS

Assessment & Drug Effects

- Monitor effectiveness. Hypnotic effect is apparent on second or third night of consecutive use and continues 1–2 nights after drug is stopped (drug has a long half-life).
- Supervise ambulation. Residual sedation and drowsiness are relatively common. Excessive drowsiness, ataxia, vertigo, and falling occur more frequently in older adults or debilitated patients.
- Be aware that withdrawal symptoms have occurred 3 days after abrupt discontinuation after prolonged use and include worsening of insomnia, dizziness, blurred vision, anorexia, GI upset, nasal congestion, paresthesias.

Patient & Family Education

- Avoid potentially hazardous activities until response to drug is known.
- Avoid alcohol. Concurrent ingestion with flurazepam intensifies CNS depressant effects; symptoms may occur even when alcohol is ingested as long as 10 h after last flurazepam dose.
- Be aware of the possible additive depressant effects when drug is combined with barbiturates, tranquilizers, or other CNS depressants.

FLURBIPROFEN SODIUM

(flure-bi′proe-fen)

Classification: ANALGESIC, NONSTEROIDAL ANTI-INFLAMMATORY DRUG (NSAID); COX-1 AND COX-2 INHIBITOR; ANTIPYRETIC

Therapeutic: ANALGESIC, NSAID

Prototype: Ibuprofen

AVAILABILITY Tablet

ACTION & *THERAPEUTIC EFFECT* Inhibits prostaglandin synthesis including in the conjunctiva and uvea by inhibiting the COX-1 or COX-2 enzymes. Ocular flurbiprofen reduces miosis, permitting maintenance of drug-induced mydriasis during surgical procedures. *An anti-inflammatory, nonsteroidal*

analgesic. Inhibits chemotaxis, alters lymphocyte activity, inhibits neutrophil aggregation/activation, and decreases proinflammatory cytokine levels.

USES Inhibition of intraoperative miosis; rheumatoid arthritis; osteoarthritis.

UNLABELED USES Management of postoperative ocular inflammation, postoperative pain.

CONTRAINDICATIONS Hypersensitivity to NSAIDs, or salicylates; perioperative pain from CABG; pregnancy (category D third trimester); lactation.

CAUTIOUS USE Patient who may be adversely affected by prolonged bleeding time; patient in whom asthma, rhinitis, or urticaria is precipitated by aspirin or other NSAIDs; pregnancy (category B first and second trimester). Safe use in children not established.

ROUTE & DOSAGE

Inflammatory Disease

Adult: **PO** 200–300 mg/day in 2–4 divided doses

Mild to Moderate Pain

Adult: **PO** 50–100 mg q6–8h

ADMINISTRATION

Topical

- Instill ophthalmic preparation with great care to avoid contamination of solution. Do not touch eye surface with dropper.

Oral

- May be given with food, milk, or antacids.
- Store at 15°–30°C (59°–86°F) in tight, light-resistant container.

ADVERSE EFFECTS **CV:** Edema. **Respiratory:** Rhinitis. **CNS:** Amnesia, anxiety, depression, dizziness, headache, hyperreflexia, insomnia, nervousness, vertigo. **HEENT:** Tinnitus, visual disturbances. **Endocrine:** Weight changes. **Skin:** Skin rash. **Hepatic/GI:** Increased liver enzymes, abdominal pain, constipation, diarrhea, dyspepsia, flatulence, gastrointestinal bleeding, nausea, vomiting. **Musculoskeletal:** Tremor, weakness.

DIAGNOSTIC TEST INTERFERENCE May cause false-positive aldosterone/renin ratio.

INTERACTIONS **Drug:** ORAL ANTICOAGULANTS, **heparin** may prolong bleeding time; actions and side effects of **phenytoin,** SULFONYLUREAS, or SULFONAMIDES may be potentiated. Do not use with other NSAIDS. Do not use with cyclosporine. **Herbal:** **Feverfew, garlic, ginger, gingko** may increase bleeding potential.

PHARMACOKINETICS **Absorption:** 80% absorbed from GI tract. **Onset:** 2 h. **Peak:** 2 h. **Duration:** 6–8 h. **Distribution:** Small amounts distributed into breast milk. **Metabolism:** In liver. **Elimination:** Primarily in urine; some biliary excretion. **Half-Life:** 5 h.

NURSING IMPLICATIONS

Black Box Warning

Flurbiprofen has been associated with increased risk of serious, potentially fatal GI bleeding and cardiovascular events (e.g., MI & CVA); risk may increase with duration of use and may be greater in the older adult and those with risk factors for CV disease.

Assessment & Drug Effects

- Observe patients with history of cardiac decompensation closely for evidence of fluid retention and edema.
- Monitor for and report promptly S&S of CV thrombotic events (i.e., angina, MI, TIA, or stroke).
- Lab tests: Baseline and periodic evaluations of CBC, chemistry panel, renal function tests, LFTs.
- Auditory and ophthalmologic examinations are recommended with prolonged or high-dose therapy.
- Monitor for GI distress and S&S of GI bleeding.

Patient & Family Education

- Report ocular irritation that persists after flurbiprofen use during surgery (tearing, dry eye sensation, dull eye pain, photophobia) to prescriber.
- Be alert for bleeding tendency, and report unexplained bleeding, prolongation of bleeding time, or bruises.
- Notify prescriber immediately of passage of dark tarry stools, "coffee ground" emesis, frankly bloody emesis, or other GI distress, as well as blood or protein in urine, and onset of skin rash, pruritus, jaundice.
- Monitor for and report promptly S&S of CV thrombotic events (i.e., angina, MI, TIA, or stroke).
- Do not drive or engage in potentially hazardous activities until response to the drug is known.
- Avoid alcohol. Concurrent use may increase risk of GI ulceration and bleeding tendencies.

FLUTAMIDE ⓟ

(flu′ta-mide)

Eulexin

Classification: ANTINEOPLASTIC; ANTIANDROGEN

Therapeutic: ANTINEOPLASTIC; ANTIANDROGEN

AVAILABILITY Capsule

ACTION & *THERAPEUTIC EFFECT* Nonsteroidal, antiandrogenic drug that inhibits androgen uptake or binding of androgen to target tissues (i.e., prostatic cancer cells). *Interferes with the binding of both testosterone and dihydrotestosterone to target tissue (i.e., prostate cancer cells).*

USES In combination with luteinizing hormone-releasing hormone agonists (i.e., leuprolide) or castration for locally confined metastatic prostate cancer.

CONTRAINDICATIONS Hypersensitivity to flutamide; severe liver impairment if ALT is equal to twice the normal value; females; pregnancy (risk to fetus if used during pregnancy); lactation.

CAUTIOUS USE Lactase deficiency.

ROUTE & DOSAGE

Prostate Cancer

Adult: **PO** 250 mg q8h

ADMINISTRATION

Oral

- Use with caution in patients with severe hepatic impairment.
- May be given with or without food. Administer in 3 divided doses (every 8 hours).
- Store at 2°–30°C (36°–86°F) in a tightly closed, light-resistant container.

ADVERSE EFFECTS **CNS:** Drowsiness, confusion, depression, anxiety, nervousness, insomnia. **Endocrine:** Gynecomastia, breast tenderness, galactorrhea. **Skin:** Rash. **GI:** Diarrhea, nausea, vomiting, gastric distress, anorexia, proctitis, rectal hemorrhage, acute hepatic failure, increased serum AST. **GU:** *Hot flashes, loss of libido, impotence*, cystitis. **Hematologic:** Anemia. **Other:** Edema.

INTERACTIONS **Drug:** Do not use with **indium 111.**

F

PHARMACOKINETICS **Absorption:** Readily absorbed from GI tract. **Onset:** Antiandrogenic activity 2.2 h; symptomatic relief 2–4 wk. **Metabolism:** Metabolized in liver to at least 10 different metabolites; the major metabolite, 2-hydroxy-flutamide (SCH-16423), is an alpha-hydroxylated derivative that is biologically active. **Elimination:** 98% in urine. **Half-Life:** 6 h.

NURSING IMPLICATIONS

Black Box Warning

Flutamide has been associated with severe, potentially fatal, liver injury.

Assessment & Drug Effects

- Monitor for symptomatic relief of bone pain.
- Assess for development of gynecomastia and galactorrhea; if these become bothersome, dosage reduction may be warranted.
- Lab tests: Monitor LFTs, serum transaminases, CBC, and PSA periodically.
- Monitor for and report promptly S&S of liver dysfunction or development of a lupus-like syndrome.

Patient & Family Education

- Be aware of potential adverse effects of therapy.
- Notify prescriber immediately of the following: Pain in upper abdomen, yellowing of skin and eyes, dark urine, respiratory problems, rashes on face, difficulty urinating, sore throat, fever, chills.

FLUTICASONE

(flu-ti-ca′sone)

Advair, Flonase, Flovent, Flovent HFA, Cutivate

See Appendixes A-3, A-4.

FLUVASTATIN

(flu-vah-stat′in)

Lescol XL

Classification: HMG-COA REDUCTASE INHIBITOR (STATIN); ANTIHYPERLIDEMIC

Therapeutic: CHOLESTEROL-LOWERING (STATIN)

Prototype: Lovastatin

AVAILABILITY Capsule; extended release tablet

ACTION & *THERAPEUTIC EFFECT*

Inhibits reductase 3-hydroxy-3-methylglutaryl coenzyme A (HMG-CoA) that is essential to hepatic production of cholesterol. Cholesterol-lowering effect triggers induction of LDL receptors, which promotes removal of LDL and VLDL remnants (precursors of LDL) from plasma. *Results in an increase in plasma HDL concentration. HDLs collect excess cholesterol from body cells and transport it to the liver for excretion.*

USES Dyslipidemias and secondary prevention of cardiovascular disease.

UNLABELED USES Other types of hyperlipidemias.

CONTRAINDICATIONS Hypersensitivity to fluvastatin, lovastatin, pravastatin, or simvastatin; active liver disease or unexplained persistent elevated liver function tests; pregnancy (category X); lactation.

CAUTIOUS USE Patients who consume substantial quantities of alcohol; history of severe liver impairment; renal impairment. Safe use in children younger than 10 yr not established.

ROUTE & DOSAGE

Hypercholesterolemia

Adult/Adolescent: **PO** 40–80 mg at bedtime or 40 mg bid
Child (10 yr or older): **PO**
Immediate release capsule
20 mg daily (max dose: 40 mg/day)

ADMINISTRATION

Oral

- Administer without regard to meals.
- Ensure the extended release tablet is not chewed or crushed. It **must be** swallowed whole.
- Separate doses of this drug and bile-acid resin (e.g., cholestyramine) by at least 2 h when given concomitantly.
- Note: Dosage adjustments may be required in patients with significant renal or hepatic impairment.
- Store at room temperature, 15°–30°C (59°–86°F).

ADVERSE EFFECTS **CNS:** Headache. **GI:** Dyspepsia.

INTERACTIONS **Drug:** May increase risk of bleeding with **warfarin; cholestyramine** decreases fluvastatin absorption; **rifampin** increases metabolism of fluvastatin; may increase risk of myopathy and rhabdomyolysis with **gemfibrozil, fenofibrate, clofibrate. Atazanavir, cyclosporine, mifepristone** may increase concentration. **Daptomycin** increases risk of skeletal muscle toxicity.

PHARMACOKINETICS **Absorption:** Readily from GI tract; about 24% reaches systemic circulation after first-pass metabolism. **Onset:** 3–6 wk. **Peak:** Serum level 0.5–1 h. **Distribution:** 98% protein bound; distributed into breast milk. **Metabolism:** In liver. **Elimination:** 95% in bile; 5% in urine. **Half-Life:** 0.5–1 h.

F

NURSING IMPLICATIONS

Assessment & Drug Effects

- Lab tests: Monitor lipid panel; maximal lipid-lowering effect occurs in 4–6 wk. Monitor hepatic transaminase levels every 3–4 mo for the first year and periodically thereafter.

Patient & Family Education

- Take fluvastatin at bedtime.
- Be alert and report signs of bleeding immediately when also taking warfarin.
- Notify prescriber immediately of the following: Fever; rash; muscle pain, weakness, tenderness, or cramping.
- Reduce or eliminate alcohol consumption while taking fluvastatin.

FLUVOXAMINE

(flu-vox′a-meen)

Luvox

Classification: SELECTIVE SEROTONIN REUPTAKE INHIBITOR (SSRI); ANTIDEPRESSANT
Therapeutic: ANTIDEPRESSANT; SSRI
Prototype: Fluoxetine

AVAILABILITY Tablet; extended release capsule

ACTION & *THERAPEUTIC EFFECT*

Antidepressant with potent, selective, inhibitory activity on neuronal (5-HT) serotonin reuptake (SSRI). *Effective as an antidepressant and for control of obsessive-compulsive disorder and social anxiety.*

F

USES Treatment of obsessive-compulsive disorders.

UNLABELED USES Posttraumatic stress disorder, major depressive disorder, panic attacks, eating disorder, social anxiety disorder, major depressive disorder.

CONTRAINDICATIONS Hypersensitivity to fluvoxamine or fluoxetine; suicidal ideation; concurrent MAOI therapy or within 14 days of use; bipolar depression; lactation.

CAUTIOUS USE Liver disease, renal impairment, abrupt discontinuation; cardiac disease, dehydration, hyponatremia, older adults, ECT, seizure disorders, history of suicidal tendencies, tobacco smoking; pregnancy (use with caution during pregnancy). Safety and efficacy in children younger than 8 yr for obsessive compulsive disorder not established.

ROUTE & DOSAGE

Obsessive-Compulsive Disorder

Adult: **PO** Start with 50 mg daily, may increase slowly up to 100–300 mg/day given every night or divided bid OR; **Extended release** 100 mg every night, may increase up (max: 300 mg/day)

Adolescent/Child (over 8 yr): **PO** Start with 25 mg every night, may increase by 25 mg q4–7days (max: 200 mg/day in divided doses)

Pharmacogenetic Dosage Adjustment

Poor CYP2D6 metabolizers: Reduce starting dose by 25–50%

ADMINISTRATION

Oral

- May be administered with or without food.
- Do not open extended release capsules. They **must be** swallowed whole.
- Give starting doses at bedtime to improve tolerance to nausea and vomiting; both are common early in therapy.
- Store at room temperature, 15°–30°C (59°–86°F), away from moisture and light.

ADVERSE EFFECTS Respiratory: Upper respiratory tract infection, pharyngitis. **CNS:** *Drowsiness, pain, headache, nervousness, insomnia, dizziness*. **Skin:** <u>Diaphoresis.</u> **GI:** *Nausea, vomiting, dry mouth, constipation, anorexia,* dyspepsia, abdominal pain, diarrhea. **GU:** Ejaculatory disorder. **Musculoskeletal:** Weakness, tremor, myalgia.

INTERACTIONS Drug: Increases plasma levels of **amitriptyline, clomipramine,** and other TRICYCLIC ANTIDEPRESSANTS. Other agents affecting serotonin (e.g. SSRI) increase risk of serotonin syndrome. May antagonize the blood pressure-lowering effects of **atenolol** and other BETA BLOCKERS. May increase levels and toxicity of **carbamazepine, mexiletine.** May increase **lithium** levels causing neurotoxicity, serotonin syndrome, somnolence, and mania. Increases prothrombin time in patients on **warfarin;** increased ergotamine toxicity with **dihydroergotamine, ergotamine.** Use with CYP1A2 INHIBITORS **(thioridazine, pimozide, alosetron, tizanidine, ramelteon)** increases **fluvoxamine** levels and toxicity. Do not use with **theophylline. Food: Grapefruit juice** may increase risk of side effects. **Herbal: Melatonin**

may increase and prolong drowsiness; **St. John's wort** may cause serotonin syndrome.

PHARMACOKINETICS **Absorption:** Almost completely absorbed from GI tract. **Onset:** 4–7 days. **Distribution:** Approximately 80% bound to plasma proteins; excreted in human breast milk but in an amount that poses little risk to the nursing infant. **Metabolism:** In liver. **Elimination:** Completely in urine. **Half-Life:** 16–24 h.

NURSING IMPLICATIONS

Black Box Warning

Fluvoxamine has been associated with increased risk of suicidal thinking and behavior in children, adolescents, and young adults.

Assessment & Drug Effects

- Monitor for worsening of depression or emergence of suicidal ideations especially in adolescents and children.
- Monitor for significant nausea and vomiting, especially during initial therapy.
- Assess safety; drowsiness and dizziness are common adverse effects.
- Monitor lab tests: Baseline LFTs.

Patient & Family Education

- Note: Nausea and vomiting are common in early therapy. Notify prescriber if these adverse effects last more than a few days.
- Exercise caution with hazardous activity until response to the drug is known.

FOLIC ACID (VITAMIN B_9, PTEROYLGLUTAMIC ACID)

(fol'ic)

Apo-Folic ♣, Folacin, Novo Folacid ♣

FOLATE SODIUM

Classification: VITAMIN B_9
Therapeutic: VITAMIN SUPPLEMENT

AVAILABILITY Tablet; capsule; solution for injection

ACTION & *THERAPEUTIC EFFECT* Vitamin B_9 essential for nucleoprotein synthesis and maintenance of normal erythropoiesis. Acts to correct folic acid deficiency that results in production of defective DNA that leads to megaloblast formation and arrest of bone marrow maturation. *Stimulates production of RBCs, WBCs, and platelets in patients with megaloblastic anemias.*

USES Folate deficiency, macrocytic anemia, and megaloblastic anemias associated with malabsorption syndromes, alcoholism, primary liver disease, inadequate dietary intake, pregnancy, infancy, and childhood.

CONTRAINDICATIONS Folic acid alone for pernicious anemia or other vitamin B_{12} deficiency states; normocytic, refractory, aplastic, or undiagnosed anemia; neonates.

CAUTIOUS USE Pregnancy (safe for use during pregnancy).

ROUTE & DOSAGE

Megaloblastic and Macrocytic Anemia

Adult: **PO** 1–5 mg/day
Child: **PO/IM/Subcutaneous/IV** 0.5–1 mg/day × 3–4 w

Parenteral nutrition Maintenance

Adolescent/Child: **IV** 140 mcg/day; *Infant:* **IV** 56 mcg/kg/day

ADMINISTRATION

Oral

- Oral route is preferred to other routes.

Intramuscular

- Give undiluted. Use caution not to inject intradermally.

F

Intravenous

PREPARE: **Direct/Continuous:** Given undiluted.
ADMINISTER: **Direct/Continuous:** Give over 1 minute. ▪ May also add to a continuous infusion.
INCOMPATIBILITIES: **Solution/additive: Calcium gluconate, dextrose 40% in water, doxapram. Y-site: Amicackin, calcium chloride, chlorpromazine, dantolene, diazepam, diazoxide, dobutamine, doxycycline, gentamicin, haloperidol, hydralazine, inamrinone, isoproterneol, methydopate, minocycline, morphine, naficillin, netilmicin, norepinephrine, pentamidine, pentazocine, phenytoin, prochlorperazine, promethazine, protamine, pyridoxine, tacrolimus, tobramycin, tolazoline, verapamil.**

- Store at 20°–25°C (68°–77°F) in tightly closed containers protected from light, unless otherwise directed.

ADVERSE EFFECTS **Cardiovascular:** Flushing. **Respiratory:** Bronchospasm. **CNS:** Malaise. **Integumentary:** Erythema, pruritis, rash. **Other:** Hypersensitivity reaction.

DIAGNOSTIC TEST INTERFERENCE Falsely low serum ***folate levels*** may occur with ***Lactobacillus casei assay*** in patients receiving antibiotics such as TETRACYCLINES.

INTERACTIONS **Drug: Chloramphenicol** may antagonize effects of **folate** therapy; **phenytoin** metabolism may be increased, thus decreasing its levels.

PHARMACOKINETICS **Absorption:** Readily from proximal small intestine. **Peak:** 30–60 min PO. **Distribution:** Distributed to all body tissues; high concentrations in CSF; crosses placenta; distributed into breast milk. **Metabolism:** In liver to active metabolites. **Elimination:** Small amounts in urine in folate-deficient patients; large amounts excreted in urine with high doses.

NURSING IMPLICATIONS

Assessment & Drug Effects

- Obtain a careful history of dietary intake and drug and alcohol usage prior to start of therapy.
- Keep prescriber informed of patient's response to therapy.

Patient & Family Education

- Remain under close medical supervision while taking folic acid therapy. Adjustment of maintenance dose should be made if there is threat of relapse.

FONDAPARINUX SODIUM

(fon-da-par′i-nux)

Arixtra

Classification: ANTICOAGULANT, SELECTIVE FACTOR XA INHIBITOR
Therapeutic: ANTICOAGULANT; ANTITHROMBOTIC
Prototype: RIVAROXABAN

AVAILABILITY Solution for injection

ACTION & *THERAPEUTIC EFFECT* Fondaparinux sodium is a synthetic pentasaccharide that causes an antithrombin III-mediated selective inhibition of factor Xa thus interrupting the blood coagulation cascade, inhibiting thrombin formation and development. *Effective in the prevention and treatment of deep-vein thrombosis measured by the laboratory value of the amount of anti-Xa assay expressed in mg.*

USES Venous thromboembolism prophylaxis in patients undergoing hip or knee replacement surgery or abdominal surgery; treatment of acute DVT or PE with warfarin.

UNLABELED USES Acute coronary syndrome, unstable angina/non-ST-elevation MI, heparin-induced thrombocytopenia.

CONTRAINDICATIONS Hypersensitivity to fondaparinux; active bleeding; GI bleeding; severe renal impairment with a creatinine clearance of less than 30 mL/min; weight less than 50 kg; active major bleeding; bacterial endocarditis; intramuscular administration; thrombocytopenia associated with fondaparinux.

CAUTIOUS USE Renal impairment or disease; indwelling epidural catheter; dental disease, dental work; diabetic retinopathy; diverticulitis; endocarditis, epidural anesthesia; hemophilia, heparin-induced thrombocytopenia (HIT), hepatic impairment; hypertension, idiopathic thrombocytopenia purpura (ITP); inflammatory bowel disease, lumbar puncture, spinal anesthesia; stroke, surgery; thrombocytopenia, thrombolytic therapy; vaginal bleeding, menstruation; peptic ulcer disease; bleeding disorders including a history of GI ulceration, etc., history of heparin-induced thrombocytopenia; older adults; pregnancy (use of fondaparinux during pregnancy should be limited to women who have severe allergic reactions to heparin or HIT); lactation. Safety and efficacy in children not established.

ROUTE & DOSAGE

DVT, Pulmonary Embolism Prophylaxis

Adult (weight greater than 50 kg): **Subcutaneous** 2.5 mg daily starting at least 6 h postsurgery × 5–9 days; *for hip fracture patients:* up to 24 days additional use

Treatment of DVT, Pulmonary Embolism

Adult (weight less than 50 kg): **Subcutaneous** 5 mg daily; *weight 50–100 kg:* 7.5 mg daily; *weight greater than 100 kg:* 10 mg once daily

Renal Impairment Dosage Adjustment

CrCl 30–50 mL/min: Use with caution; *less than 30 mL/min:* Use is contraindicated

ADMINISTRATION

Subcutaneous

- Give no sooner than 6 h after surgery.
- Inspect visually for particulate matter and discoloration prior to administration.
- Do not expel the air bubble from the syringe before the injection.
- Use prefilled syringe to inject into fatty tissue, alternating injection sites (e.g., between L and R abdominal wall).
- Store at 25°C (77°F); excursions permitted to 15°–30°C (59°–86°F).

ADVERSE EFFECTS **CV:** Hypotension. **CNS:** Insomnia, dizziness. **Endocrine:** Hypokalemia. **Skin:** Irritation at injection site, rash, purpura. **Hepatic:** Elevated LFTs. **Hematologic:**

Hemorrhage, hematoma. **Other:** Postoperative wound infection.

INTERACTIONS **Drug:** ANTICOAGULANTS, ANTIPLATELETS, NSAIDS, **aspirin** may increase risk of bleeding. ESTROGEN and PROGESTINS can decrease therapeutic effect. **Mifepristone** increases the toxic effects of anticoagulants. **Herbal:** **Feverfew, ginkgo, ginger, evening primrose oil** may potentiate bleeding.

PHARMACOKINETICS **Absorption:** Rapidly and completely absorbed from subcutaneous injection site. **Peak:** 2–3 h. **Distribution:** Primarily in blood. **Metabolism:** Negligible metabolism. **Elimination:** In urine. **Half-Life:** 18 h.

NURSING IMPLICATIONS

Black Box Warning

Fondaparinux has been associated with development of epidural and spinal hematomas.

Assessment & Drug Effects

- Monitor frequently for S&S of neurologic impairment; if noted, urgent treatment is necessary.
- Monitor for S&S of bleeding or hemorrhage. If noted, withhold fondaparinux and notify prescriber immediately.
- Withhold fondaparinux and notify prescriber if platelet count falls below 100,000/mm^3.
- Monitor lab tests: Baseline and periodic renal function tests; periodic CBC with platelet count, occult blood testing of stool, and serum creatinine.

Patient & Family Education

- Report any of the following to a healthcare provider: Signs of unexplained bleeding such as: Pink, red, or dark brown urine; red or dark brown vomitus; bleeding gums or bloody sputum; dark, tarry stools.
- Learn proper injection technique if you are to self-administer this drug.
- Do not take any OTC drugs without first consulting prescriber.

FORMOTEROL FUMARATE

(for-mo-ter′ol)

Perforomist

Classification: BETA-ADRENERGIC AGONIST; BRONCHODILATOR

Therapeutic: BRONCHODILATOR

Prototype: Albuterol

AVAILABILITY Solution for inhalation

ACTION & *THERAPEUTIC EFFECT* Long-acting selective $beta_2$-adrenergic receptor agonist that stimulates production of intracellular cyclic AMP, which causes relaxation of bronchial smooth muscle. *Acts locally in lung as a bronchodilator; prevents bronchoconstriction that occurs during an asthma attack.*

USES Treatment of asthma, prevention of bronchospasm in COPD.

CONTRAINDICATIONS Hypersensitivity to formoterol; significantly worsening or acutely deteriorating asthma; status asthmaticus or other severe asthmatic attacks; acute episode of COPD where extensive measures are required; paradoxical bronchospasm.

CAUTIOUS USE Cardiovascular disorders (especially coronary insufficiency, cardiac arrhythmias, and hypertension), QT prolongation; convulsive disorders;

thyrotoxicosis; heightened responsiveness to sympathomimetic amines; diabetes mellitus; pregnancy (category C); lactation. Safe use in children younger than 5 yr has not been established.

ROUTE & DOSAGE

Treatment of Asthma, COPD, Bronchitis/Emphysema

Adult/Child (5 yr or older): **Inhaled** Nebulized solution 20 mcg bid

Adult: **Powder Inhaler** 12 mcg q12h

ADMINISTRATION

Oxeze Turbuhaler

- Hold inhaler upright, and turn colored grip as far as it will go in one direction, and then turn back to original position until a clicking sound is heard.
- Exhale fully. Do not exhale into mouthpiece of inhaler.
- Place mouthpiece to lips and inhale forcefully and deeply
- Clean outside of mouthpiece once weekly with a dry tissue.

Nebulization Solution

- Remove unit-dose vial from foil pouch immediately before use. Place contents of unit-dose vial into the reservoir of a standard jet nebulizer connected to an air compressor.
- Turn nebulizer on. Breathe deeply and evenly until all of the medication has been inhaled. Average inhalation time is 9 min.

ADVERSE EFFECTS Respiratory: Respiratory tract infection, exacerbation of asthma.

INTERACTIONS Drug: Effects may be antagonized by NONSELECTIVE BETA BLOCKERS; XANTHINES, STEROIDS; DIURETICS may potentiate hypokalemia. Avoid use with MAOIs. Use with **dronedarone** is contraindicated.

PHARMACOKINETICS Absorption: Rapidly absorbed. **Onset:** 1–3 min. **Peak:** 1–3 h. **Metabolism:** Metabolized by glucuronidation in the liver. **Elimination:** 60% in urine, 33% in feces. **Half-Life:** 10 h.

NURSING IMPLICATIONS

Black Box Warning

Formoterol has been associated with increased risk of asthma-related hospitalizations and deaths.

Assessment & Drug Effects

- Monitor cardiovascular status with periodic ECG, BP, and HR determinations.
- Withhold drug and notify prescriber immediately of S&S of bronchospasm.
- Monitor diabetics closely for loss of glycemic control.
- Monitor FEV1, peak flow, and/or other pulmonary function tests.

Patient & Family Education

- Do not take this drug more frequently than every 12 h.
- Use a short-acting inhaler if symptoms develop between doses of formoterol.
- Seek medical care immediately if a previously effective dosage regimen fails to provide the usual response, or if swelling about the face and neck and difficulty breathing develop.
- Report any of the following immediately to the prescriber: Rash, hives, palpitations, chest pain, rapid heart rate, tremor, or nervousness.

- Diabetics should monitor blood glucose levels carefully for hyperglycemia.

FOSAMPRENAVIR CALCIUM

(fos-am-pre′na-vir)

Lexiva

Classification: ANTIRETROVIRAL; PROTEASE INHIBITOR

Therapeutic: PROTEASE INHIBITOR

Prototype: Saquinavir

F

AVAILABILITY Tablet; oral suspension

ACTION & *THERAPEUTIC EFFECT* Amprenavir is an HIV-1 protease inhibitor that binds to the active site of HIV-1 protease. Binding prevents processing of viral Gag and Gag-Pol polyprotein precursors, resulting in formation of immature noninfectious viral particles. *Inhibits normal replication of the HIV virus rendering the virus noninfectious.*

USES Treatment of HIV infection in combination with other antiretroviral agents.

UNLABELED USES HIV prophylaxis (occupational exposure).

CONTRAINDICATIONS Hypersensitivity to amprenavir or sulfonamide severe or life-threatening skin reactions; severe hepatic impairment; lactation.

CAUTIOUS USE Sulfonamide allergy; mild to moderate hepatic impairment; hypercholesterolemia, hypertriglyceridemia; DM; diabetic ketoacidosis; older adults; autoimmune diseases; hemophilia; pregnancy (category C), children/infants.

ROUTE & DOSAGE

HIV Infection

Adult/Adolescent: **PO** 700 mg bid in combination with 100 mg **ritonavir** bid or 1400 mg daily in combination with 200 mg ritonavir daily; or 1400 mg bid (without ritonavir).
Child/Infant (6 mo or older, weight greater than 20 kg): (All with concurrent **ritonavir** use) **PO** 18 mg/kg bid; *weight 15–20 kg:* 23 mg/kg bid; *weight 11–14 kg:* 30 mg/kg bid; *weight less than 11 kg:* 45 mg/kg bid (max: 700 mg/dose)

Hepatic Impairment Dosage Adjustment

Mild to moderate impairment (Child–Pugh class A or B): Reduce dose to 700 mg bid without **ritonavir**; *Severe hepatic impairment (Child–Pugh class C):* 350 mg bid (without ritonavir) or 300 mg bid (with ritonavir).

ADMINISTRATION

Oral

- Ensure that patient is not receiving drugs contraindicated with fosamprenavir.
- Oral suspension should be administered to adults without food and to pediatric patients with food.
- Store at 15°–30°C (59°–86°F) in a tightly closed container.

ADVERSE EFFECTS **Endocrine:** Hypertriglyceridemia. **Skin:** Skin rash. **GI:** Diarrhea.

INTERACTIONS Note: Interaction profile can be significantly affected by coadministration with ritonavir. Metabolite is a strong inhibitor of

CYP3A4. **Drug:** Administration with **amiodarone, bepridil, dihydroergotamine, ergotamine, flecainide, itraconazole, ketoconazole, lidocaine, midazolam, pimozide, propafenone, quinidine, triazolam,** and TRICYCLIC ANTIDEPRESSANTS may cause life-threatening reactions; **rifampin, rifabutin,** ORAL CONTRACEPTIVES, **phenobarbital, phenytoin, carbamazepine** decrease **fosamprenavir** concentrations; **amprenavir** may increase **dihydroergotamine, ergotamine, sildenafil** concentrations and toxicity; **amprenavir** may decrease **methadone** levels; monitor INR with **warfarin;** increased risk of myopathy and rhabdomyolysis with **lovastatin, simvastatin;** may decrease antiviral effectiveness of **delavirdine** or **lopinavir/ritonavir. Herbal: St. John's wort** may decrease antiretroviral activity.

PHARMACOKINETICS Absorption: Rapidly hydrolyzed to amprenavir (active component) by gut enzymes. **Peak:** 2.5 h. **Metabolism:** In liver by CYP3A4 (major), CP2C9 (minor), CYP 2D6 (minor). **Elimination:** 14% in urine, 75% in feces. **Half-Life:** 7.7 h.

NURSING IMPLICATIONS

Assessment & Drug Effects

- Ensure that patient has provided a complete list of all prescription, nonprescription, or herbal drugs being used.
- Monitor closely diabetics for loss of glycemic control.
- Monitor males taking PDE5 inhibitors for erectile dysfunction for adverse events including hypotension, visual changes, and priapism. Report promptly.
- Monitor lab tests: Baseline and periodic LFTs and CD4 count; periodic lipid profile and blood glucose.

Patient & Family Education

- If you miss a dose by more than 4 h, wait and take the next dose at the regular time.
- Do not take other prescription, nonprescription, or herbal drugs without consulting prescriber.
- Monitor blood glucose more often than usual if diabetic.
- To prevent pregnancy, use a barrier contraceptive in addition to hormonal contraception.

FOSCARNET

(fos′car-net)

Classification: ANTIVIRAL

Therapeutic: ANTIVIRAL

AVAILABILITY Solution for injection

ACTION & *THERAPEUTIC EFFECT* Selectively inhibits the viral-specific DNA polymerases and reverse transcriptases of susceptible viruses, thus preventing elongation of the viral DNA chain. *Effective against cytomegalovirus (CMV), herpes simplex virus types 1 and 2 (HSV-1, HSV-2), human herpesvirus 6 (HHV-6), Epstein–Barr virus (EBV), and varicella-zoster virus (VZV).*

USES CMV retinitis, acyclovir-resistant HSV in immunocompromised patients.

UNLABELED USES Other CMV infections, herpes zoster infections in AIDS patients, CMV prevention.

CONTRAINDICATIONS Hypersensitivity to foscarnet; lactation.

CAUTIOUS USE Renal impairment, cardiac disease; mineral and electrolyte imbalances, seizures, older adults; pregnancy (limited information regarding use during pregnancy); children.

ROUTE & DOSAGE

CMV Retinitis

Adult: **IV Induction** 60 mg/kg q8h for 2–3 wk **or** 90 mg/kg q12h for 2–3 wk; induction may be repeated if relapse occurs

Recurrent CMV Retinitis

Adult: **IV** 90–120 mg/kg once daily

Acyclovir-Resistant HSV in Immunocompromised Patients

Adult: **IV** 40 mg/kg q8–12h for 14–21 days or until lesions heal

Renal Impairment Dosage Adjustment

See package insert.

ADMINISTRATION

- Note: Dose **must be** adjusted for renal insufficiency. See package insert for specific dosing adjustment.

Intravenous

PREPARE: **Direct:** Given undiluted (24 mg/mL) through a central line. ▪ For peripheral infusion, dilute to 12 mg/mL with D5W or NS. ▪ Do not give other IV solution or drug through the same catheter with foscarnet.

ADMINISTER: **Direct:** Give at a constant rate not to exceed 1 mg/kg/min over the specified period of infusion with an infusion pump. ▪ Do not increase the rate of infusion or shorten the specified interval between doses. ▪ Use prepared IV solutions within 24 h.

INCOMPATIBILITIES: **Solution/additive:** **Lactated Ringer. Y-site:** **Acyclovir, allopurinol, amiodarone, amphotericin B, calcium chloride, calcium gluconate, caspofungin, chlorpromazine, ciprofloxacin, dantrolene, daunorubicin, diazepam, digoxin, diphenhydramine, dobutamine, dolasetron, doxorubicin, droperidol, epirubicin, ganciclovir, garenoxacin, haloperidol, hydralazine, idarubicin, labetalol, lansoprazole, leucovorin, methylprednisolone, midazolam, minocycline, mitoxantrone, mycophenolate, nicardipine, norepinephrine, ondansetron, pentamidine, pentazocine, prochlorperazine, promethazine, quinupristin/dalfopristin, thiopental, topotecan, trimetrexate, vancomycin, verapamil, vinorelbine.**

- Prehydrate and continue daily hydration with 2.5 L of NS to reduce nephrotoxicity. ▪ Store according to manufacturer's directions.

ADVERSE EFFECTS **CV:** Chest pain, edema, facial edema, first-degree AV block, flushing, palpitations, sinus tachycardia. **CNS:** *Headache*, fatigue, confusion, anxiety, seizure, depression, dizziness. **Endocrine:** *Hypophosphatemia, hypokalemia, hypomagnesemia, hypocalcemia*. **Skin:** Diaphoresis, rash. **GI:** Nausea, vomiting, *diarrhea*, abdominal pain, stomatitis, cachexia. **GU:** Renal insufficiency, nephrotoxicity. **Hematologic:** *Anemia*, leukopenia, thrombocytopenia, granulocytopenia, fever, bone marrow suppression.

INTERACTIONS **Drug:** AMINOGLYCOSIDES, **amphotericin B**, acyclovir/valacyclovir, **vancomycin, cyclosporine, tacrolimus** may increase risk of nephrotoxicity. **Etidronate, pamidronate,**

pentamidine (IV) may exacerbate hypocalcemia. LOOP DIURETICS may increase concentration of foscarnet.

PHARMACOKINETICS **Onset:** 3–7 days. **Duration:** Relapse usually occurs 3–4 wk after end of therapy. **Distribution:** 3–28% of dose may be deposited in bone; variable penetration into CSF; crosses placenta; distributed into breast milk. **Metabolism:** Not metabolized. **Elimination:** 73–94% in urine. **Half-Life:** 3–4 h.

NURSING IMPLICATIONS

Black Box Warning

Foscarnet has been associated with severe renal impairment and seizures associated with mineral and electrolyte imbalances.

Assessment & Drug Effects

- Monitor for electrolyte imbalances.
- Monitor ECG.
- Monitor for seizures and take appropriate precautions.
- Monitor lab tests: Periodic CBC, serum electrolytes, serum creatinine, and creatinine clearance.

Patient & Family Education

- Report perioral tingling, numbness, and paresthesia to prescriber immediately.
- Understand that drug is not a cure for CMV retinitis; regular ophthalmologic exams are necessary.
- Note: Good hydration is important to maintain adequate output of urine.

FOSFOMYCIN TROMETHAMINE

(fos-fo-my′sin)

Monurol

Classification: ANTIBIOTIC

Therapeutic: URINARY TRACT ANTI-INFECTIVE

Prototype: Nitrofurantoin

AVAILABILITY Packets

ACTION & THERAPEUTIC EFFECT Synthetic, broad-spectrum, bactericidal agent that blocks the first steps in bacterial cell wall synthesis. *Acts as a bactericidal agent against* Enterococcus faecalis, E. faecium, *and* Escherichia coli. *In addition, it is effective against* Klebsiella, Proteus, *and* Serratia. *Effectiveness is indicated by improvement in cystitis symptoms within 2–3 days.*

USES Treatment of uncomplicated UTIs in women.

CONTRAINDICATIONS Hypersensitivity to fosfomycin.

CAUTIOUS USE Pregnancy (category B); lactation. Safety and efficacy in children younger than 12 yr not established.

ROUTE & DOSAGE

UTI

Adult: **PO** 3 g sachet dissolved in 3–4 oz of water as a single dose given once

ADMINISTRATION

Oral

- Pour entire contents of a single dose into 3–4 oz water (not hot), stir to dissolve completely, and give immediately. Drug must not be taken in the dry form.
- Store at 15°–30°C (59°–86°F).

ADVERSE EFFECTS **Respiratory:** Rhinitis, pharyngitis. **CNS:** *Headache*, dizziness. **GI:** *Diarrhea*, nausea, abdominal pain, dyspepsia. **GU:** Vaginitis, dysmenorrhea. **Other:** Pain.

INTERACTIONS **Drug: Metoclopramide** may decrease urinary excretion of fosfomycin.

PHARMACOKINETICS **Absorption:** Rapidly from GI tract, 37% of dose reaches systemic circulation as free acid. **Peak Urine Concentration:** 2–4 h. **Distribution:** Not protein bound, distributed to kidneys, bladder wall, prostate, and seminal vesicles. **Elimination:** Primarily in urine. **Half-Life:** 5.7 h.

F

NURSING IMPLICATIONS

Assessment & Drug Effects

- Monitor lab tests: Urine C&S before and after therapy.

Patient & Family Education

- Notify prescriber if symptoms do not improve in 2–3 days.

FOSINOPRIL

(fos-in'o-pril)

Classification: ANGIOTENSIN-CONVERTING ENZYME (ACE) INHIBITOR; ANTIHYPERTENSIVE

Therapeutic: ANTIHYPERTENSIVE; ACE INHIBITOR

Prototype: Enalapril

AVAILABILITY Tablet

ACTION & *THERAPEUTIC EFFECT* Lowers BP by interrupting conversion sequences initiated by renin that leads to formation of angiotensin II, a potent vasoconstrictor. Inhibition of ACE also leads to decreased circulating aldosterone, a secretory response to angiotensin II stimulation. *Lowers blood pressure and reduces peripheral arterial resistance (afterload) and improves cardiac output as well as activity tolerance.*

USES Mild to moderate hypertension, heart failure.

UNLABELED USES HIV-associated nephropathy, non-ST-elevation acute coronary syndrome.

CONTRAINDICATIONS Hypersensitivity to fosinopril or any other ACE inhibitor(s); angioedema; renal artery stenosis; lactation.

CAUTIOUS USE Impaired kidney function, autoimmune disease; collagen-vascular disease; hepatic disease; hyperkalemia, or surgery and anesthesia; history of angioedema; Black patients; aortic stenosis or cardiomyopathy; dialysis; older adult; pregnancy (risk to fetus in first trimester; discontinue as soon as pregnancy is suspected). Safety in children not established.

ROUTE & DOSAGE

Hypertension

Adult: **PO** 10 mg once/day, may increase to 20–40 mg (max: 80 mg/day)
Child (over 6 yr at least 50 kg): **PO** 5 mg daily (max 40 mg/day); *(over 6 yr less than 50 kg):* 0.1 mg/kg/dose daily (max 40 mg/day)

Heart Failure

Adult: **PO** 10 mg daily; may increase to 20–40 mg

ADMINISTRATION

Oral

- May be administered with or without food.
- Store at 15°–30°C (59°–86°F) and protect from moisture.

ADVERSE EFFECTS **CV:** Hypotension. **Respiratory:** Cough. **CNS:** Headache, dizziness. **Endocrine:** Hyperkalemia. **Skin:** Rash. **GU:** Increased serum creatinine.

INTERACTIONS **Drug:** NSAIDS may decrease antihypertensive effects of fosinopril. POTASSIUM

SUPPLEMENTS, POTASSIUM-SPARING DIURETICS increase risk of hyperkalemia. ANTIHYPERTENSIVES increase the risk of hypotension. ACE inhibitors may increase **lithium** levels and toxicity. **Aliskiren** enhances risk of hyperkalemia and nephrotoxicity. Increases risk of adverse effects when used with **iron dextran complex**. Do not use with **sacubitril**. **Herbal:** Increased risk of adverse reaction to grass pollen extract.

PHARMACOKINETICS **Absorption:** Readily absorbed from GI tract; converted to its active form, fosinoprilat, in the liver. **Peak:** 3 h. **Duration:** 24 h. **Distribution:** Approximately 99% protein bound; crosses placenta. **Metabolism:** Hydrolyzed by intestinal and hepatic esterases to its active form, fosinoprilat. **Elimination:** 44% in urine, 46% in feces. **Half-Life:** 12 h (adult)(fosinoprilat).

NURSING IMPLICATIONS

Black Box Warning

Fosinopril can cause fetal injury and death when used during the second and third trimesters.

Assessment & Drug Effects

- Monitor for at least 2 h after initial dose for first-dose hypotension, especially in salt- or volume-depleted patients.
- Monitor BP at the time of peak effectiveness, 2–6 h after dosing, and at the end of the dosing interval just before next dose.
- Report diminished antihypertensive effect toward the end of the dosing interval. An inadequate trough response may be an indication for dividing the daily dose.
- Observe for S&S of hyperkalemia (see Appendix F).
- Monitor lab tests: Periodic BUN, serum creatinine, serum potassium, and CBC with differential.

Patient & Family Education

- Discontinue fosinopril and report to prescriber any of the following: S&S of angioedema (e.g., swelling of face or extremities, difficulty breathing or swallowing); syncope; chronic, nonproductive cough.
- Maintain adequate fluid intake, and avoid potassium supplements or salt substitutes unless specifically prescribed by the prescriber.
- Report promptly if pregnancy is suspected.
- Report vomiting or diarrhea to prescriber immediately.

FOSNETUPITANT AND PALONOSETRON

(fos-net-UE-pi-tant & pal-oh-NOE-se-tron)

Akynzeo

Classification: ANTIEMETICS, 5-HT_3 ANTAGONISTS

Therapeutic: ANTIEMETIC

Prototype: Ondansetron

AVAILABILITY Oral capsule; solution for injection

ACTION & *THERAPEUTIC EFFECT* Palonosetron is a selective 5-HT_3 receptor antagonist that blocks serotonin, both on vagal nerve terminals in the periphery and centrally in the chemoreceptor zone. Fosnetupitant is a prodrug of netupitant that augments the antiemetic activity of 5-HT_3 receptor antagonists and corticosteroids to inhibit acute and delayed chemotherapy-induced emesis. *Works synergistically to inhibit chemotherapy-induced emesis.*

USES Prevention of acute and delayed nausea and vomiting associated with highly emetogenic cancer chemotherapy. Used with dexamethasone.

CONTRAINDICATIONS Hypersensitivity reaction to any component of the product.

CAUTIOUS USE Serotonin syndrome; impaired hepatic function; impaired renal function; geriatric population; pregnancy (use with caution in pregnant women); lactation.

ROUTE & DOSAGE

Prevention of Chemotherapy-Induced Nausea and Vomiting

Adult: **PO** 1 capsule 1 h prior to chemotherapy on day 1 of treatment; **IV** One vial infused over 30 min, 30 min prior to chemotherapy day 1

Renal Impairment Dosage Adjustment

CrCl less than or equal to 30 mL/min: Avoid use

ADMINISTRATION

Intravenous

PREPARE: For powder form, reconstitute by slowly adding 20 mL of D5W or NS to the vial, directing the solution toward the wall of the vial to avoid foaming. Swirl vial gently. Prepare an infusion vial or bag filled with 30 mL of D5W or NS. Add entire volume of medication from the vial into the infusion vial or bag to a total of 50 mL. Gently invert the vial or bag to mix completely.
ADMINISTER: **Direct: IV Infusion:** Infuse over 30 min starting 30 min before chemotherapy. Flush infusion line with the same solution used for dilution after administration. If same IV line is used for subsequent administration of other medications, flush the line with NS before and after fosnetupitant and palonosetron administration.
INCOMPATIBILITIES: Do not mix with any solution containing divalent cations (lactated Ringer) or other medications.

- Store at 20° to 25°C (68° to 77°F). Protect from light. Store solutions diluted for infusion at room temperature; the total time from infusion preparation to the start of the infusion should not exceed 24 hours.

ADVERSE EFFECTS [no need to indicate (>1% or 2%) anymore] Follow the order below: **CNS:** Headache. **GI:** Constipation.

INTERACTIONS **Drugs:** Can cause profound hypotension with **apomorphine.** May cause serotonin syndrome with other serotonergic drugs (e.g., SSRI). Strong CYP3A4 inducers (e.g., **rifampin**) may decrease netupitant concentrations. Netupitant may increase levels of other drugs that require CYP3A4 for their metabolism—consider dose reduction or avoidance of CYP3A4 substrates.

PHARMACOKINETICS **Absorption:** Netupitant: Absorbed within 15 min–3 h (oral route); Palonosetron: Well absorbed. **Peak:** Netupitant: 4–5 h; Palonosetron: 5 h. **Distribution:** Netupitant: 1982 L, 99% protein bound; Palonosetron: 663 L, 62% protein bound. **Metabolism:** Netupitant: In the liver, primarily via CYP3A4; Palonosetron: In liver to inactive megabolites. **Elimination:** Netupitant: 71% excreted in feces; Palonosetron: 85–93% excreted unchanged in urine. **Half-Life:** Netupitant: 80 h; Palonosetron: 50 h.

NURSING IMPLICATIONS

Assessment & Drug Effects

- Monitor for signs/symptoms of hypersensitivity and serotonin syndrome.
- Monitor lab tests: Liver function tests, renal function tests. Avoid use in severe impairment.

Patient & Family Education

- Notify your doctor or get medical help right away if you have any of the following signs or symptoms of allergic reaction such as rash, hives, itching; red, swollen, blistered, or peeling skin with or without fever; wheezing; tightness in the chest or throat; trouble breathing, swallowing, or talking; unusual hoarseness; or swelling of the mouth, face, lips, tongue, or throat; or any dizziness or passing out.

FOSPHENYTOIN SODIUM

(fos-phen'i-toin)

Cerebyx

Classification: ANTICONVULSANT; HYDANTOIN

Therapeutic: ANTICONVULSANT

Prototype: Phenytoin

AVAILABILITY Solution for injection

ACTION & *THERAPEUTIC EFFECT* Prodrug of phenytoin that converts to the anticonvulsant phenytoin that modulates the sodium channels of neurons, calcium flux across neuronal membranes, and enhances the sodium–potassium ATPase activity of neurons and glial cells. *Effective as an anticonvulsant agent by preventing seizure activity.*

USES Control of generalized tonic-clonic convulsive status epilepticus and the prevention and treatment of seizures during neurosurgery, or as a parenteral short-term substitute for oral phenytoin.

CONTRAINDICATIONS Hypersensitivity to hydantoin products, rash, seizures due to hypoglycemia, sinus bradycardia, heart block; Adams–Stokes syndrome; pregnancy (use during pregnancy increases risk of congenital malformations; requires close monitoring and altered pharmacokinetics).

CAUTIOUS USE Impaired liver or kidney function, alcoholism, hypotension, heart block, bradycardia, severe CAD, diabetes mellitus, hyperglycemia, respiratory depression, acute intermittent porphyria; children; lactation.

ROUTE & DOSAGE

Status Epilepticus

Adult: **IV Loading Dose** 20 mg PE/kg (PE = phenytoin sodium equivalents) administered at 100–150 mg PE/min;
IV Maintenance Dose 4–7 mg PE/kg/day in divided doses

Substitution for Oral Phenytoin Therapy

Adult: **IV/IM** Substitute fosphenytoin at the same total daily dose in mg PE as the oral dose at a rate of infusion not greater than 150 mg PE/min

ADMINISTRATION

- Note: All dosing is expressed in phenytoin sodium equivalents (PE) to avoid the need to calculate molecular weight adjustments between fosphenytoin and phenytoin sodium doses. **Always** prescribe and fill fosphenytoin in PE units.

F

Intramuscular

- Administer as a single dose using 1 to 4 injection sites (up to 20 mL per site).

Intravenous

PREPARE: **Direct:** Dilute in D5W or NS to a concentration of 1.5–25 mg PE/mL.
ADMINISTER: **Direct:** Give 100–150 mg PE/min. Do **NOT** administer at a rate greater than 150 mg PE/min.
INCOMPATIBILITIES: **Y-site:** **Amiodarone, amphotericin B, calcium, caspofungin, chlorpromazine, dantrolene, daunorubicin, diazepam, dobutamine, dolasetron, doxorubicin, droperidol, epirubicin, fenoldopam, haloperidol, hydralazine, hydroxyzine, idarubicin, irinotecan, isavuconazonium, midazolam, mitoxantrone, moxifloxacin, mycophenolate, nicardipine, pentamidine, pentazocine, phenytoin, polymyxin B, prochlorperazine, thiopental, topotecan, verapamil.**

- Store at 2°–8°C (36°–46°F); may store at room temperature not to exceed 48 h.

ADVERSE EFFECTS **CNS:** *Burning sensation, paresthesia, dizziness,* drowsiness, ataxia, tremor. **HEENT:** *Nystagmus.* **Skin:** *Pruritus.* **GI:** Nausea (IV).

DIAGNOSTIC TEST INTERFERENCE Fosphenytoin may produce lower-than-normal values for ***dexamethasone*** or ***metyrapone*** tests.

INTERACTIONS **Drug:** Extensive drug interactions (see package insert for more details). Partial list includes: Avoid use with drugs metabolized via CYP3A4. **Alcohol** decreases effects; OTHER ANTICONVULSANTS may increase or decrease fosphenytoin levels; fosphenytoin increases metabolism of CORTICOSTEROIDS, ORAL ANTICOAGULANTS, and ORAL CONTRACEPTIVES, decreasing their effectiveness; **amiodarone, chloramphenicol, omeprazole** increase fosphenytoin levels; antituberculosis agents, **voriconazole** decrease fosphenytoin levels. Do not use with **delavirdine.** May decrease concentration of ANTIFUNGAL agents. **Food:** **Folic acid** absorption may be decreased by fosphenytoin; fosphenytoin absorption may be decreased by enteral nutrition supplements. **Herbal:** **Ginkgo** may decrease anticonvulsant effectiveness.

PHARMACOKINETICS **Absorption:** Completely absorbed after IM administration. **Peak:** 30 min IM. **Distribution:** 95–99% bound to plasma proteins, displaces phenytoin from protein binding sites; crosses placenta, small amount in breast milk. **Metabolism:** Converted to phenytoin by phosphatases; phenytoin is oxidized in liver to inactive metabolites. **Elimination:** Half-life 15 min to convert fosphenytoin to phenytoin, 22 h phenytoin; phenytoin metabolites excreted in urine.

NURSING IMPLICATIONS

Black Box Warning

Fosphenytoin infusion has been associated with risk of severe hypotension and cardiac arrhythmias, especially if infusion rate exceeds 150 mg (PE)/min.

Note: See **phenytoin** for additional Nursing Implications.

Assessment & Drug Effects

- Monitor ECG, BP, heart rate, and respiratory function continuously during and for 10–20 min after infusion.
- Discontinue infusion and notify prescriber if rash appears. Be prepared to substitute alternative therapy rapidly to prevent withdrawal-precipitated seizures.
- Allow at least 2 h after IV infusion and 4 h after IM injection before monitoring total plasma phenytoin concentration.
- Monitor diabetics for loss of glycemic control.
- Monitor carefully for adverse effects, especially in patients with renal or hepatic disease or hypoalbuminemia.
- Monitor lab tests: Periodic CBC, hepatic function tests, and plasma phenytoin concentration.

Patient & Family Education

- Be aware of potential adverse effects. Itching, burning, tingling, or paresthesia are common during and for some time following IV infusion.

FOSTAMATINIB

(fos-ta-ma-ti-nib)

Tavalisse

Classification: TYROSINE KINASE INHIBITOR

Therapeutic: TYROSINE KINASE INHIBITOR; COAGULATION AND THROMBOSIS AGENT

AVAILABILITY Tablet

ACTION & THERAPEUTIC EFFECT Small-molecule spleen tyrosine kinase inhibitor, which inhibits signal transduction of F_c-activating receptors and B-cell receptor; this changes autoantibody production. *Reduces antibody-mediated destruction of platelets, to assist in the treatment of thrombocytopenia.*

USES Treatment of thrombocytopenia in patients with chronic immune thrombocytopenia who have failed other treatments.

CAUTIOUS USE Cautious use in patients experiencing neutropenia, unmanaged hypertension, or liver injury or history of hepatic disease. Avoid use in pregnancy, as animal studies show potential birth defect (pregnancy category C).

ROUTE & DOSAGE

Chronic Immune Thrombocytopenia

Adult: **PO** 100 mg bid; with insufficient response, dose is increased to 150 mg bid; dosing strategies to manage adverse reactions are listed in the package insert

ADMINISTRATION

Oral

- May be administered with or without food.
- Twice daily doses should be administered in the morning and evening. Once daily dose administered in the morning.
- Store at 20°–25°C (68°–77°F) with provided desiccant canisters.

ADVERSE EFFECTS **CV:** *Hypertension*. **Respiratory:** *Respiratory infection*, dyspnea, hypoxia. **CNS:** *Dizziness, fatigue*. **Skin:** *Rash*. **Hepatic:** *Liver enzyme elevation (ALT, AST)*. **GU:** *Diarrhea, nausea, GI pain*, nephrolithiasis. **Musculoskeletal:** Chest pain. **Hematologic:** Neutropenia.

INTERACTIONS Active metabolite is a CYP3A4 substrate; avoid use with strong CYP3A4 inhibitors (e.g., **clarithromycin, itraconazole, ketoconazole**). Avoid use with CYP3A4 inducers (e.g., **carbamazepine, phenytoin, rifampin**). Concomitant use with BCRP substrates (e.g., **rosuvastatin**) or P-Glycoprotein substrates (e.g., **digoxin**) may increase those drug concentrations.

PHARMACOKINETICS Absorption: Active metabolite is 55% bioavailable; administration with high-fat, high-calorie meal increases C_{max} by 15%. **Peak:** 1.5 h. **Distribution:** Active metabolite is 98.3% protein bound. **Metabolism:** Fostamatinib is metabolized in the gut to R406 (active metabolite); active metabolite is metabolized extensively via hepatic (CYP3A4 and UGT1A9) enzymes. **Elimination:** Primarily 80% through the feces; 20% urine. **Half-Life:** Active metabolite approximately 15 h.

NURSING IMPLICATIONS

Assessment & Drug Effects

- Monitor for blood pressure at baseline and every 2 wk until stable dose established.
- Monitor for diarrhea and hepatotoxicity.
- Monitor lab tests: CBC including platelets at baseline and monthly until a stable platelet count of greater than 50,000/mm^3, LFTs, pregnancy test.

Patient & Family Education

- Monitor blood pressure as directed by prescriber.
- Report any S&S such as diarrhea, dizziness, upset stomach, or feeling tired or weak.

FROVATRIPTAN

(fro-va-trip′tan)

Frova

Classification: SEROTONIN 5-HT_1 RECEPTOR AGONIST

Therdpeutic: ANTIMIGRAINE

Prototype: Sumatriptan

AVAILABILITY Tablet

ACTION & *THERAPEUTIC EFFECT* Selective agonist for 5-HT_{1D} and 5-HT_{1B} serotonin receptors, which are found on cranial arteries; and on other structures in the CNS. This results in vasoconstriction and agonist effects on nerve terminals in the trigeminal system. *Activation of 5-HT_1 receptors results in constriction of cranial vessels that become dilated during a migraine attack, and reduced signal transmission in the pain pathways.*

USES Treatment of migraine headache with or without aura.

CONTRAINDICATIONS Hypersensitivity to frovatriptan; significant cardiovascular disease such as ischemic heart disease, coronary artery vasospasms, peripheral vascular disease, history of cerebrovascular events, or uncontrolled hypertension; within 24 h of receiving another 5-HT_1 agonist or an ergotamine-containing or ergot-type drug; basilar or hemiplegic migraine.

CAUTIOUS USE Significant risk factors for coronary artery disease unless a cardiac evaluation has been done; hypertension; risk factors for cerebrovascular accident; impaired liver or kidney function; pregnancy (category C); lactation.

Safe use in children younger than 18 yr has not been established.

ROUTE & DOSAGE

Migraine Headache

Adult: **PO** 2.5 mg if headache returns, may repeat after at least 2 h (max: 7.5 mg/24 h).

ADMINISTRATION

Oral

- Do not give within 24 h of an ergot-containing drug.
- Administer any time after symptoms of migraine appear.
- Do not administer a second dose without consulting the prescriber for any attack during which the FIRST dose did **not** work.
- Give a second dose if headache was relieved by first dose but symptoms return; however, wait at least 2 h after the first dose before giving a second dose.
- Do not give more than two doses in 24 h.
- Store at 15°–30°C (59°–86°F).

ADVERSE EFFECTS **CV:** Flushing. **CNS:** Dizziness.

INTERACTIONS **Drug: Dihydroergotamine, methysergide,** other 5-HT_1 AGONISTS may cause prolonged vasospastic reactions; SSRIS, **sibutramine** have rarely caused weakness, hyperreflexia, and incoordination; MAOIS should not be used with 5-HT_1 AGONISTS. **Herbal: Gingko, ginseng, echinacea, St. John's wort** may increase triptan toxicity.

PHARMACOKINETICS **Absorption:** 20–30% bioavailability. **Peak:** 2–4 h. **Distribution:** 15% protein bound. **Metabolism:** In liver by CYP1A2. **Elimination:** 30% renally, 60% in feces. **Half-Life:** 26 h.

NURSING IMPLICATIONS

Assessment & Drug Effects

- Monitor cardiovascular status carefully following first dose in patients at relatively high risk for coronary artery disease (e.g., postmenopausal women, men older than 40 yr, persons with known CAD risk factors), or who have coronary artery vasospasms.
- Report to prescriber immediately chest pain or tightness in chest or throat that is severe, or does not quickly resolve following a dose of frovatriptan.
- Pain relief usually begins within 10 min of ingestion, with complete relief in approximately 65% of all patients within 2 h.
- Monitor BP, especially in those being treated for hypertension.

Patient & Family Education

- Review patient information leaflet provided by the manufacturer carefully.
- Notify prescriber immediately if symptoms of severe angina (e.g., severe or persistent pain or tightness in chest, back, neck, or throat) or hypersensitivity (e.g., wheezing, facial swelling, skin rash, itching, or hives) occur.
- Do not take any other serotonin receptor agonist (e.g., Imitrex, Maxalt, Zomig, Amerge) within 24 h of taking frovatriptan.
- Report any other adverse effects (e.g., tingling, flushing, dizziness) at next prescriber visit.

FULVESTRANT

(ful-ves'trant)

Faslodex

Classification: ANTINEOPLASTIC; ANTIESTROGEN

Therapeutic: ANTINEOPLASTIC; ANTIESTROGEN

Prototype: Tamoxifen citrate

F

AVAILABILITY Solution for injection

ACTION & THERAPEUTIC EFFECT Fulvestrant is an estrogen receptor antagonist that selectively binds to the estrogen receptors (ER) of breast cancer cells. Estrogen stimulates the tumor growth of estrogen-sensitive breast tissue cancer cells in postmenopausal women. *In postmenopausal women, many breast cancers have positive estrogen receptors (ERs), and the growth of these tumors is stimulated by estrogen. Therefore, fulvestrant decreases estrogen-sensitive breast tissue tumor growth.*

USES Treatment of hormone receptor-positive metastatic breast cancer in postmenopausal women.

CONTRAINDICATIONS Hypersensitivity to fulvestrant; pregnancy (may cause fetal harm if administered during pregnancy); lactation.

CAUTIOUS USE Moderate liver impairment; biliary disease; coagulopathy; anticoagulant therapy; older adults. Safety and efficacy in children not established.

ROUTE & DOSAGE

Metastatic Breast Cancer

Adult: **IM** 500 mg on days 1, 15, and 29; then 500 mg monthly

Hepatic Impairment Dosage Adjustment

Moderate hepatic impairment (Child–Pugh class B): **IM** administer 250 mg on days 1, 15, 29, and once monthly thereafter

ADMINISTRATION

Intramuscular

- Break the seal of the white plastic cover on the syringe Luer connector to remove the cover with the attached rubber tip cap. Twist to lock the needle to the Luer connector. Remove excess gas from the syringe (a small gas bubble may remain).
- Administer 500-mg dose as two 5-mL IM injections (one in each buttock slowly) over 1 to 2 minutes per injection.
- Immediately activate needle protection device upon withdrawal from patient by pushing lever arm completely forward until needle tip is fully covered.
- Store in a refrigerator, 2°–8°C (36°–46°F) in original container.

ADVERSE EFFECTS **CV:** *Peripheral edema.* **Respiratory:** *Dyspnea, cough.* **CNS:** Dizziness, headache, fatigue. **Endocrine:** Decreased serum glucose, hot flash, decreased serum albumin, decreased serum phosphate. **Skin:** Rash, pruritus, alopecia. **Hepatic:** Increased liver enzymes. **GI:** *Nausea, vomiting, constipation, diarrhea,* abdominal pain, anorexia, stomatitis, decreased appetite. **GU:** Increased serum creatinine. **Musculoskeletal:** *Arthralgia, back pain, myalgia.* **Hematologic:** Anemia, lymphocytopenia, leukopenia. **Other:** *Asthenia, injection site pain,* fever, infection.

DIAGNOSTIC TEST INTERFERENCE May interfere with estradiol immunoassay, resulting in falsely elevated estradiol levels.

PHARMACOKINETICS **Peak:** 7 days. **Duration:** 1 mo. **Distribution:** 99% protein bound. **Metabolism:** In liver via CYP3A4. **Elimination:** 90% in feces. **Half-Life:** 40 days (adult).

NURSING IMPLICATIONS

Assessment & Drug Effects

- Monitor for S&S of tumor progression.
- Monitor for S & S of bleeding.

- Monitor lab tests: Periodic CBC with differential, LFTs, and pregnancy testing.

Patient & Family Education

- Use two methods of contraception while taking this drug. Immediately notify prescriber if you think you are pregnant.
- Report vaginal bleeding to prescriber. Understand the possibility of drug-induced menstrual irregularities before starting treatment.

FUROSEMIDE

(fur-oh'se-mide)

Fumide ♣, Lasix

Classification: ELECTROLYTIC AND WATER BALANCE AGENT; LOOP DIURETIC; ANTIHYPERTENSIVE

Therapeutic: LOOP DIURETIC; ANTIHYPERTENSIVE

AVAILABILITY Tablet; oral solution; solution for injection

ACTION & *THERAPEUTIC EFFECT* Primarily inhibits reabsorption of sodium and chloride in the ascending loop of Henle and proximal and distal renal tubules, interfering with the chloride-binding cotransport system, thus causing its natriuretic effect. *An antihypertensive that decreases edema and intravascular volume, which lowers blood pressure.*

USES Treatment of edema associated with CHF, cirrhosis of liver, and kidney disease, including nephrotic syndrome. May be used for management of hypertension.

CONTRAINDICATIONS History of hypersensitivity to furosemide or sulfonamides; increasing oliguria, anuria, fluid and electrolyte depletion states; hepatic coma; preeclampsia, eclampsia.

CAUTIOUS USE Hepatic disease; hepatic cirrhosis; renal disease, nephrotic syndrome; cardiogenic shock associated with acute MI; ventricular arrhythmias, CHF, diarrhea; history of SLE, history of gout; DM; older adults; pregnancy (category C); lactation, infants.

ROUTE & DOSAGE

Edema

Adult: **PO** 20–80 mg in 1 dose, may repeat at intervals of 6–8 h or up to 600 mg/day if needed; **IV/IM** 20–40 mg in 1 dose if no adequate response may repeat dose (max 200 mg/dose)
Child: **PO** 0.5 to 2 mg/kg/dose every 6–24 h; may increase dose by 1–2 mg/kg/dose (max: 600 mg/day)

Hypertension

Adult: **PO** 20–40 mg bid (max: 480 mg/day)

ADMINISTRATION

Oral

- Give on an empty stomach; if patient has gastric irritation, can give with food or milk.
- Schedule doses to avoid sleep disturbance (e.g., a single dose is generally given in the morning; twice-a-day doses at 8 a.m. and 2 p.m.).
- Store tablets at controlled room temperature, preferably at 15°–30°C (59°–86°F) unless otherwise directed. Protect from light.
- Store oral solution in refrigerator, preferably at 2°–8°C (36°–46°F). Protect from light and freezing.

Intramuscular

- Protect syringes from light once they are removed from package.

- Discard yellow or otherwise discolored injection solutions.

Intravenous

Note: Verify correct IV concentration and rate of infusion/injection with prescriber before administration to infants or children.

PREPARE: **Direct:** Give undiluted. For high-dose therapy, dilute in NS or other compatible solution.

ADMINISTER: **Direct:** Give undiluted at a rate of 20–40 mg per min. ▪ With high doses a rate of 4 mg/min is recommended to decrease risk of ototoxicity.

INCOMPATIBILITIES: **Solution/additive:** **Chlorpromazine, conivaptan, diazepam, dobutamine, erythromycin, isoproterenol, meperidine, metoclopramide, netilmicin, ondansetron, papaveretum, prochlorperazine, promethazine.** **Y-site:** **Alemtuzumab, amphotericin B, amrinone, amsacrine, atracurium, benztropine, blinatumomab, butorphanol, caspofungin, cimetidine, ciprofloxacin, clarithromycin, codeine, dantrolene, daunorubicin, dexrazoxane, diazepam, diazoxide, diltiazem, dimenhydrinate, diphenhydramine, dolasetron, doxycycline, epirubicin, eptifibatide, esmolol, fenoldopam, filgrastim, garenoxacin, gatifloxacin, gemcitabine, gemtuzumab, gentamicin, glycopyrrolate, haloperidol, hydroxyzine, idarubicin, irinotecan, isavuconazonium, ketamine, lansoprazole, levofloxacin, milrinone, minocycline, mitoxantrone, mivacurium, mycophenolate, nalbuphine, nesiritide, nicardipine, ondansetron, oritavancin, pancuronium, pantoprazole, papaverine, pentamidine, pentazocine, phenytoin, potassium, prochlorperazine, protamine, pyridoxine, quinupristin/dalfopristin, rituximab, rocuronium, SMZ/TMP, telavancin, thiamine, trastuzumab, urapidil, vancomycin, vecuronium, verapamil, vinblastine, vinorelbine.**

- Use infusion solutions within 24 h.
- Store parenteral solution at controlled room temperature, preferably at 15°–30°C (59°–86°F) unless otherwise directed. Protect from light.

ADVERSE EFFECTS **CV:** Necrotizing angiitis, orthostatic hypotension, thrombophlebitis, vasculitis. **CNS:** Dizziness, headache, paresthesia, restlessness, vertigo. **HEENT:** Blurred vision, xanthopsia, deafness, tinnitus. **Endocrine:** Glycosuria, hyperglycemia, hyperuricemia, increased serum cholesterol, increased serum triglycerides, fever. **Integumentary:** Erythema multiforma, exfoliative dermatitis, pruritus, photosensitivity, skin rash, Stevens–Johnson syndrome, urticaria, DRESS syndrome. **Hepatic/GI:** Hepatic encephalopathy, intrahepatic cholestatic jaundice, elevated liver enzymes, abdominal cramps, anorexia, constipation, diarrhea, gastric irritation, oral irritation, nausea, pancreatitis, vomiting. **GU:** Bladder spasm, interstitial nephritis. **Musculoskeletal:** Muscle spasm, weakness. **Hematologic:** Agranulocytosis, anemia, leukopenia, purpura, thrombocytopenia.

DIAGNOSTIC TEST INTERFERENCE Furosemide may cause false-negative aldosterone/renin ratio.

INTERACTIONS Drug: OTHER DIURETICS enhance diuretic effects; NONDEPOLARIZING NEUROMUSCULAR BLOCKING AGENTS (e.g., **tubocurarine**) prolong neuromuscular blockage; CORTICOSTEROIDS, **amphotericin B** potentiate hypokalemia; decreased **lithium** elimination and increased toxicity; SULFONYLUREAS, **insulin** blunt hypoglycemic effects; NSAIDS may attenuate diuretic effects.

PHARMACOKINETICS Absorption: 60% PO dose from GI tract. **Peak:** 60–70 min PO; 20–60 min IV. **Onset:** 30–60 min PO; 5 min IV. **Duration:** 2 h. **Distribution:** Crosses placenta. **Metabolism:** Small amount in liver. **Elimination:** Rapidly in urine; 50% of oral dose and 80% of IV dose excreted within 24 h; excreted in breast milk. **Half-Life:** 30 min.

NURSING IMPLICATIONS

Black Box Warning

Furosemide has been associated with profound diuresis and water and electrolyte depletion.

Assessment & Drug Effects

- Observe patients receiving parenteral drug carefully; closely monitor BP and vital signs. Sudden death from cardiac arrest has been reported.
- Monitor for S&S of hypokalemia (see Appendix F).
- Monitor BP during periods of diuresis and through period of dosage adjustment.
- Observe older adults closely during period of brisk diuresis. Sudden alteration in fluid and electrolyte balance may precipitate significant adverse reactions. Report symptoms to prescriber.
- Monitor urine and blood glucose and HbA1C closely in diabetics and patients with decompensated hepatic cirrhosis. Drug may cause hyperglycemia.
- Monitor I&O ratio and pattern. Report decrease or unusual increase in output. Excessive diuresis can result in dehydration and hypovolemia, circulatory collapse, and hypotension. Weigh patient daily under standard conditions.
- Monitor lab tests: Frequent electrolytes and renal function tests.

Patient & Family Education

- Consult prescriber regarding allowable salt and fluid intake.
- Ingest potassium-rich foods daily (e.g., bananas, oranges, peaches, dried dates) to reduce or prevent potassium depletion.
- Learn S&S of hypokalemia (see Appendix F). Report muscle cramps or weakness to prescriber.
- Make position changes slowly because high doses of antihypertensive drugs taken concurrently may produce episodes of dizziness or imbalance.
- Avoid prolonged exposure to direct sun.

GABAPENTIN

(gab-a-pen′tin)

Gralise, Horizant, Neurontin

Classification: ANTICONVULSANT; GABA ANALOG

Therapeutic: ANTICONVULSANT; NEUROPATHY

G

AVAILABILITY Capsule; tablet; extended release tablet; oral solution

ACTION & *THERAPEUTIC EFFECT* Gabapentin is a GABA neurotransmitter analog; however, it does not inhibit GABA uptake or degradation. It appears to interact with GABA cortical neurons, but its relationship to functional activity as an anticonvulsant is unknown. *Used in conjunction with other anticonvulsants to control certain types of seizures in patients with epilepsy. Effective in controlling painful neuropathies.*

USES Adjunctive therapy for focal (partial) seizures with or without secondary generalization in adults, postherpetic neuralgia.

UNLABELED USES Alcohol use disorder, chronic pruritis, restless leg syndrome, vasomotor symptoms of menopause, peripheral neuropathy, migraine prophylaxis.

CONTRAINDICATIONS Hypersensitivity to gabapentin; suicidal ideations; lactation.

CAUTIOUS USE Status epilepticus, renal impairment, history of suicidal tendencies; psychiatric disorders; older adults; pregnancy (limited information related to use during pregnancy; use with caution). Safety and efficacy in infants and children younger than 3 yr not established.

ROUTE & DOSAGE

Seizure, focal (partial) onset

Adult/Child (12 yr or older): **PO Immediate Release** 300 mg tid, increase based on response, usual dose 300–600 mg tid
Child (3–12 yr): **PO** Start 10–15 mg/kg/day in 3 divided doses, titrate q3days to target dose of 40 mg/kg/day in pts 3–4 yr or 25–35 mg/kg/day in pts 5 yr or older in 3 divided doses

Postherpetic Neuralgia

Adult: **PO Immediate Release** Start 300 mg day 1, 300 mg bid day 2, and 300 mg tid day 3; may increase up to 1.8–3.6 mg/day in divided doses
Extended Release: 300 mg daily, increase by 300 mg each day up to 900 mg daily.

Restless Leg Syndrome (Horizant only)

Adult: **PO** 600 mg qd at 5 p.m.

Renal Impairment Dosage Adjustment

CrCl 30–49 mL/min: 50% reduction of dose; *15–29 mL/min:* 75% reduction of dose; *less than 15 mL/min:* 90% reduction in dose

ADMINISTRATION

Oral

- Ensure that extended release tablet is swallowed whole, and not crushed or chewed. Capsules may be opened and sprinkled on food.
- Immediate release: Administer first dose on first day at bedtime to avoid somnolence and dizziness. Maximum time between doses should not exceed 12 hours.
- Extended release: Administer with evening meal.
- Store at 15°–30°C (59°–86°F); protect from heat, moisture, and direct light.

ADVERSE EFFECTS **CNS:** *Drowsiness, fatigue,* ataxia, dizziness, tremor. **GI:** Diarrhea. **Other:** Infection. **Musculoskeletal:** Asthenia.

DIAGNOSTIC TEST INTERFERENCE May lead to false-positive with ***Ames N-Multistix SG dipstick*** test for urine protein.

INTERACTIONS **Drug:** CNS DEPRESSANTS enhance risk of sedation of other ANTICONVULSANTS. ANTACIDS reduce absorption of gabapentin. **Herbal:** **Ginkgo** may decrease effectiveness.

PHARMACOKINETICS **Absorption:** 50–60% from GI tract. **Peak:** Peak level 1–3 h; peak effect 2–4 wk. **Distribution:** Crosses the blood–brain barrier; readily passes into cerebrospinal fluid; not bound to plasma proteins; highest concentrations found in pancreas and kidneys. **Metabolism:** Does not appear to be metabolized. **Elimination:** 76–81% unchanged in 96 h; 10–23% recovered in feces. **Half-Life:** 5–6 h.

NURSING IMPLICATIONS

Assessment & Drug Effects

- Monitor for therapeutic effectiveness; may not occur until several weeks following initiation of therapy.
- In those treated for seizure disorders, assess frequency of seizures: In rare cases, the drug has increased the frequency of partial seizures.
- Monitor for and report dizziness, somnolence, or other signs of CNS depression. Assess safety: Vision, concentration, and coordination impairment increase the risk for injury.
- Monitor for changes in behavior that may be indicative of suicidal ideation.
- Monitor lab values: Periodic renal function.

Patient & Family Education

- Learn potential adverse effects of drug.
- Notify prescriber immediately if any of the following occur: Increased seizure frequency, visual changes, unusual bruising or bleeding.
- Do not drive or engage in other potentially hazardous activities until response to drug is known.
- Do not abruptly discontinue use of drug; do not take drug within 2 h of an antacid.

GALANTAMINE HYDROBROMIDE

(ga-lan′ta-meen)

Razadyne, Razadyne ER

Classification: CENTRALLY ACTING CHOLINERGIC; CHOLINESTERASE INHIBITOR; ANTIDEMENTIA
Therapeutic: ANTI-ALZHEIMER; ANTIDEMENTIA
Prototype: Donepezil HCl

AVAILABILITY Tablet; extended release capsule; oral solution

ACTION & *THERAPEUTIC EFFECT* Competitive and reversible inhibitor of acetylcholinesterase, which is the enzyme responsible for the hydrolysis (breakdown) of the neurotransmitter, acetylcholine. The cholinergic system is used in processing needed for attention, memory, as well as modulation of excitatory neurotransmission. *In Alzheimer disease cholinesterase inhibitors are designed to offset loss of presynaptic cholinergic function, slowing decline of memory and maintaining ability to perform functions of daily living.*

USES Treatment of mild to moderate Alzheimer-type dementia.

UNLABELED USES Vascular dementia, dementia associated with Parkinson disease.

CONTRAINDICATIONS Hypersensitivity to galantamine; CrCl less than 9 mL/min; severe hepatic impairment or in children.

CAUTIOUS USE Bradycardia, heart block, or other cardiac conduction disorders; asthma, COPD; potential bladder outflow obstruction; a history of seizures or GI bleeding; Alzheimer disease; renal impairment; mild or moderate hepatic impairment; pregnancy (adverse fetal effects have been seen in animal studies); lactation.

ROUTE & DOSAGE

Alzheimer Dementia

Adult: **PO immediate release** Initiate with 4 mg bid × at least 4 wks, if tolerated may increase by 4 mg bid q4wk to target dose of 12 mg bid; **Extended release:** 8 mg daily × 4 wks, increase to 16 mg daily then after 4 weeks increase to 24 mg daily

Hepatic Impairment Dosage Adjustment

Not recommended with severe hepatic impairment

Renal Impairment Dosage Adjustment

CrCl 9–59 mL/min: Max dose 16 mg/day; *CrCl less than 9 mL/min:* Not recommended

ADMINISTRATION

Oral

- Give with meals (breakfast and dinner) to reduce the risk of nausea.
- Extended release capsules should be swallowed whole and not crushed or chewed.
- Make increases in dosage increments at 4-wk intervals.
- If drug is interrupted for several days or more, restart at the lowest dose and gradually increase to the current dose.
- Store at 15°–30°C (59°–86°F).

ADVERSE EFFECTS CNS: Dizziness, headache, depression. **GI:** *Nausea, vomiting,* diarrhea, decreased appetite, abdominal pain, anorexia.

INTERACTIONS **Drug:** Additive effects with other CHOLINESTERASE INHIBITORS (e.g., **succinylcholine**); **cimetidine, erythromycin, ketoconazole, paroxetine** may increase levels and toxicity. **Ceritinib** has increased risk of bradycardia.

PHARMACOKINETICS **Absorption:** Rapidly and completely. **Peak:** 1 h. **Distribution:** Mainly distributes to red blood cells. **Metabolism:** In liver by CYP2D6 and CYP3A4. **Elimination:** 95% in urine. **Half-Life:** 7 h (4.4–10 h).

NURSING IMPLICATIONS

Assessment & Drug Effects

- Monitor cardiovascular status including baseline and periodic EKG and BP readings. Assess for postural hypotension.
- Monitor I&O rates and pattern for urinary incontinence or urinary retention.
- Monitor appetite and food intake. Weigh weekly and report significant weight loss.

Patient & Family Education

- Report any of the following to a healthcare provider immediately: Loss of weight, urinary retention, chest pain, palpitations, difficulty breathing, fainting, dark stools, blood in the urine.

GANCICLOVIR

(gan-ci'clo-vir)

Cytovene, Zirgan

Classification: ANTIVIRAL; PURINE NUCLEOSIDE

Therapeutic: ANTIVIRAL

Prototype: Acyclovir

AVAILABILITY Powder for injection; ophthalmic gel; solution for injection

ACTION & *THERAPEUTIC EFFECT* A synthetic purine nucleoside analog that inhibits the replication of CMV DNA. *Sensitive human viruses include CMV, herpes simplex virus-1 and -2 (HSV-1, HSV-2), Epstein–Barr virus, and varicella-zoster virus.*

USES CMV retinitis, prophylaxis and treatment of systemic CMV infections; herpetic keratitis (ophthalmic formulation).

UNLABELED USES CMV pneumonitis, encephalitis, herpes simplex virus, varicella infection.

CONTRAINDICATIONS Hypersensitivity to ganciclovir or acyclovir. **IV form:** Lactation.

CAUTIOUS USE Valacyclovir or penciclovir hypersensitivity; renal impairment, bone marrow suppression; chemotherapy; radiation therapy; dehydration; preexisting cytopenias; secondary malignancy; older adults; pregnancy (potential to cause birth defects in humans if administered during pregnancy).

ROUTE & DOSAGE

CMV Retinitis (Immunocompromised Patients)

Adult: **IV** 5 mg/kg/dose q12h 14–21 days followed by maintenance therapy

Maintenance Therapy for CMV

Adult: **IV** 5 mg/kg daily 7 days/wk or 6 mg/kg daily 5 days/wk

G

Herpetic Keratitis

Adult/Adolescent/Child (older than 2 yr): **Ophthalmic** 1 drop in affected eye 5 × daily until healed then 1 drop in affected eye tid × 7 days

Renal Impairment Dosage Adjustment

See package insert, varies based on use

ADMINISTRATION

- Avoid direct contact with skin and mucous membranes. Wash thoroughly with soap and water if contact occurs.

Ophthalmic

- Place one drop in the conjunctival sac.

Intravenous

- Note: Do not administer if neutrophil count falls below 500/mm^3 or platelet count falls below 25,000/mm^3.

PREPARE: **Intermittent** Reconstitute the 500-mg vial using only 10 mL of sterile water (supplied) for injection immediately before use to yield 50 mg/mL. ▪ Shake well to dissolve. ▪ Withdraw the ordered amount and add to 100 mL of NS, D5W, or LR (volume less than 100 mL may be used, but the final concentration should be less than 10 mg/mL).

ADMINISTER: **Intermittent:** Give at a slow rate over 1 h. ▪ Avoid rapid infusion or bolus injection.

INCOMPATIBILITIES: **Solution/additive:** Amino acid solutions (TPN). **Y-site:** **Aldesleukin, amifostine, amikacin, aminocaproic acid, aminophylline, amiodarone, amphotericin B colloidal, ampicillin, ampicillin/sulbactam, amsacrine, ascorbic acid, atracurium, azathioprine, aztreonam, benztropine, bumetanide, butorphanol, capreomycin, cefamandole, cefazolin, cefepime, cefoperazone, cefotaxime, cefotetan, cefoxitin, ceftazidime, ceftizoxime, ceftriaxone, cefuroxime, chloramphenicol, chlorpromazine, cimetidine, clindamycin, codeine, cytarabine, dacarbazine, dantrolene, daunorubicin, dexrazoxane, diazepam, diazoxide, diltiazem, diphenhydramine, dobutamine, dolasetron, dopamine, doxorubicin, doxycycline, ephedrine, epinephrine, epirubicin, erythromycin, esmolol, famotidine, fenoldopam, fludarabine, foscarnet, gemcitabine, gemtuzumab, gentamicin, haloperidol, hydralazine, hydrocortisone, hydroxyzine, idarubicin, imipenem/cilastin, Inamrinone, irinotecan, isoproterenol, ketorolac, levofloxacin, lidocaine, magnesium sulfate, meperidine, mesna, metaraminol, methadone, methylprednisolone, metoclopramide, metronidazole, midazolam, minocycline, mitomycin, morphine, mycophenolate, nalbuphine, netilmicin, nicardipine, norepinephrine, ondansetron, oxacillin, palonosetron, papaverine, penicillin G, pentamidine, pentazocine, phentolamine, phenylephrine, phenytoin, piperacillin/tazobactam, potassium**

acetate, procainamide, prochlorperazine, promethazine, pyridoxine, quinupristin/dalfopristin, sargramostim, sodium bicarbonate, streptokinase, succinylcholine, SMZ/TMP, theophylline, thiamine, ticarcillin, tobramycin, tolazoline, topotecan, vancomycin, vecuronium, verapamil, vinorelbine.

- Store reconstituted solutions refrigerated at 4°C; use within 12 h. ▪ Store infusion solution refrigerated up to 24 h of preparation.

ADVERSE EFFECTS **CV:** Edema, phlebitis. **CNS:** Chills, peripheral neuropathy, headache, disorientation, mental status changes, ataxia, coma, confusion, dizziness, paresthesia, nervousness, somnolence, tremor. **HEENT:** Retinal detachment. **Skin:** Pruritus, hyperhidrosis. **GI:** *Diarrhea,* anorexia, vomiting. **GU:** Increased serum creatinine. **Hematologic:** *Bone marrow suppression,* thrombocytopenia, leukopenia, neutropenia, anemia, sepsis, infection. **Other:** Fever, catheter infection, catheter site reaction.

INTERACTIONS **Drug:** ANTINEOPLASTIC AGENTS, **amphotericin B, didanosine, trimethoprim-sulfamethoxazole (TMP-SMZ), probenecid, zidovudine** may increase bone marrow suppression and other toxic effects of ganciclovir; may increase risk of nephrotoxicity from **cyclosporine;** may increase risk of seizures due to **imipenem-cilastatin.** Do not use with **cladribine.**

PHARMACOKINETICS **Onset:** 3–8 days. **Distribution:** Distributes throughout body including CSF, eyes, lungs, liver, and kidneys; crosses placenta in animals; not known if distributed into breast milk. **Metabolism:** Not metabolized. **Elimination:** Unchanged in urine. **Half-Life:** 2.5–4.2 h.

NURSING IMPLICATIONS

Black Box Warning

Ganciclovir has been associated with severe bone marrow suppression.

Assessment & Drug Effects

- Inspect IV insertion site throughout infusion for signs and symptoms of phlebitis.
- Monitor lab tests: CBC with differential and platelet count at baseline and twice weekly; serum creatinine at baseline and once weekly; pregnancy test prior to initiation in females of reproductive potential; frequent ophthalmic exams in patients with CMV retinitis.

Patient & Family Education

- Note: Drug is not a cure for CMV retinitis; follow regular ophthalmologic examination schedule.
- Drink lots of fluids during therapy.
- Use barrier contraception throughout therapy and for at least 90 days afterward.
- Maintain frequent hematologic monitoring.

GANIRELIX ACETATE

(gan-i-rel′ix)

Antagon

Classification: GONADOTROPIN-RELEASING HORMONE (GnRH) ANTAGONIST

Therapeutic: GnRH ANTAGONIST; INFERTILITY AGENT

Prototype: Ganirelix

AVAILABILITY Syringe

ACTION & *THERAPEUTIC EFFECT* It acts by competitively blocking the GnRH receptors on the pituitary inducing a rapid, reversible suppression of gonadotropin secretion, and subsequent suppression of pituitary LH and FSH secretion. *Upon discontinuation of the drug, LH and FSH levels are fully recovered within 48 h, increasing fertility.*

USES Infertility treatment.

CONTRAINDICATIONS Prior hypersensitivity to ganirelix, LHRH, or other LHRH analogs, mannitol hypersensitivity; ovarian cyst; primary ovarian failure; pregnancy (category X); lactation.

CAUTIOUS USE History of current allergic disorders (e.g., asthma, hay fever, urticaria, eczema) or a history of allergic reactions to medications; renal/hepatic dysfunction; endocrine disorders; alcohol consumption.

ROUTE & DOSAGE

Infertility

Adult: **Subcutaneous** After initiating follicle-stimulating hormone (FSH) therapy on day 2 or 3 of the cycle, give 250 mcg once daily during the early-to-mid-follicular phase

ADMINISTRATION

- Note: The packaging of the product, Antagon, contains natural rubber latex, which may cause allergic reactions.

Subcutaneous

- Inject into subcutaneous tissue in the abdomen around the umbilicus or into the upper thigh.
- Rotate injection sites.
- Store at 5°–30°C (59°–86°F) and protect from light.

ADVERSE EFFECTS **CNS:** Headache. **Endocrine:** Ovarian hyperstimulation syndrome. **Skin:** Injection site reaction. **GI:** Abdominal pain, nausea. **GU:** Vaginal bleeding.

PHARMACOKINETICS **Absorption:** 91% from subcutaneous site. **Peak:** 1 h. **Distribution:** 81% protein bound. **Elimination:** 75% in feces; 22% in urine. **Half-Life:** 13–16 h.

NURSING IMPLICATIONS

Assessment & Drug Effects

- Exercise caution with patients with hypersensitivity to GnRH or with known allergic disorders (e.g., asthma, hay fever). These patients should be carefully monitored after the first injection for S&S of an anaphylactic reaction.
- Monitor lab tests: Baseline and periodic CBC with differential, and periodic total bilirubin.

Patient & Family Education

- Report menstrual disorders (e.g., spotting, frank vaginal bleeding) to prescriber.
- Notify prescriber immediately if you think you are pregnant.

GEMCITABINE HYDROCHLORIDE

(gem-ci'ta-been)

Infugem

 Common adverse effects in *italic;* life-threatening effects underlined; generic names in **bold;** classifications in SMALL CAPS; ♣ Canadian drug name; ● Prototype drug; ⚠ Alert

Classification: PYRIMIDINE, ANTIMETABOLITE
Therapeutic: ANTINEOPLASTIC
Prototype: Fluorouracil

AVAILABILITY Solution for injection; powder for injection

ACTION & *THERAPEUTIC EFFECT* A pyrimidine analog that inhibits DNA polymerase and ribonucleotide reductase, enzymes necessary for DNA synthesis in tumor cells. It is also incorporated into tumor cell DNA causing the DNA to malfunction, resulting in the initiation of apoptotic cell death. *Gemcitabine induces DNA fragmentation in dividing cells, resulting in cell death of tumor cells.*

USES Locally advanced or metastatic adenocarcinoma of the pancreas, non–small-cell lung cancer, breast cancer, ovarian cancer.

CONTRAINDICATIONS Hypersensitivity to gemcitabine; drug-induced pulmonary toxicity; pregnancy (fetal risk cannot be ruled out); lactation (infant risk cannot be ruled out).

CAUTIOUS USE Myelosuppression, neutropenia; renal or hepatic dysfunction; history of bleeding disorders, infection, previous cytotoxic or radiation treatment; history of pulmonary disease; older adults. Safety and efficacy in children 18 y or younger not established.

ROUTE & DOSAGE

Pancreatic Cancer

Adult: **IV** 1000 mg/m^2 dose, frequency differs based on concurrent antineoplastic agents

Non–Small-Cell Lung Cancer

Adult: **IV** 1000 mg/m^2 on days 1, 8, 15 of 28-day cycle OR 1250 mg/m^2 on days 1 and 8 of 21-day cycle. Given with cisplatin.

Breast Cancer

Adult: **IV** 1250 mg/m^2 on days 1 and 8 of 21-day cycle. Given with paclitaxel.

Ovarian Cancer

Adult: **IV** 1000 mg/m^2 on days 1 and 8 of 21 day cycle

ADMINISTRATION

Intravenous

This drug is a cytotoxic agent and caution should be used to prevent any contact with the drug. Follow institutional or standard guidelines for preparation, handling, and disposal of cytotoxic agents. NIOSH recommends gloves (single) **must be** worn during receiving, unpacking, and placing in storage. Double glove and gown when administering. If there is potential that the substance could splash or the patient may resist, use eye/face protection. If solution comes into contact with skin or mucous membranes, immediately wash with soap and water or thoroughly rinse with copious amounts of water.

PREPARE: **IV Infusion:** Dilute with NS without preservatives by adding 5 mL or 25 mL to the 200 mg or 1 g vial, respectively, to yield 38 mg/mL. ▪ Shake to dissolve. ▪ Dilute further if necessary with NS to concentrations as low as 0.1 mg/mL.

G

***ADMINISTER:* IV Infusion:** Infuse over 30 min. Infusion time greater than 60 min is associated with increased toxicity.

***INCOMPATIBILITIES:* Y-site: Acyclovir, amphotericin B (conventional colloidal, lipid complex, liposome), cefepime hydrochloride, cefoperazone, cefotaxime, chloramphenicol, dantrolene, daptomycin, diazepam, doxorubicin hydrochloride liposomal, furosemide, ganciclovir, imipenem/cilastatin, irinotecan, ketorolac, lansoprazole, methotrexate, methylprednisolone, mitomycin, nafcillin, pantoprazole, pemetrexed, phenylephrine hydrochloride, phenytoin, piperacillin/tazobactam, prochlorperazine, thiopental sodium.**

- Store reconstituted solutions unrefrigerated at 20°–25° C (68°–77° F). Use within 24 h of reconstitution.

ADVERSE EFFECTS **CV:** Peripheral edema. **Respiratory:** Dyspnea. **CNS:** *Paresthesia, peripheral neuropathy, sensory neuropathy*. **Endocrine:** *Hyperglycemia, hypomagnesemia*. **Skin:** *Aolpecia, rash*. **Hepatic:** *Increased alkaline phosphatase, increased ALT/SGPT, & AST/SGOT.* **GI:** *Constipation, diarrhea, nausea, vomiting,* stomatitis. **GU:** *Hematuria, proteinuria, increased serum creatinine*. **Hematologic:** *Anemia, neutropenia, thrombocytopenia*. **Other:** *Fatigue, fever.*

INTERACTIONS **Drug:** May increase effect of **warfarin** or ORAL ANTICOAGULANTS or NSAIDS. Do not use with **sargramostin** or **filgrastim.** Neutropenic effect of **deferipone** may be enhanced.

PHARMACOKINETICS **Peak:** Peak concentrations reached 30 min after infusion; lower clearance in women and older adult results in higher concentrations at any given dose. **Distribution:** Crosses placenta, distributed into breast milk. **Metabolism:** Intracellularly by nucleoside kinases to active diphosphate and triphosphate nucleosides. **Elimination:** 92–98% recovered in urine within 1 wk. **Half-Life:** 32–94 min.

NURSING IMPLICATIONS

Assessment & Drug Effects

- Monitor lab tests: CBC with differential and platelet count prior to each dose. Baseline and periodic renal function tests and LFTs.

Patient & Family Education

- Learn about common adverse effects and measures to control or minimize when possible. Notify prescriber immediately of any distressing adverse effects.
- Note: Fever with flu-like symptoms, rash, and GI distress are very common.
- Females should use reliable contraception while taking this drug and for 6 months after the final dose.
- Male patients with a female partner should use effective contraception during therapy and for 3 months after the final dose.

GEMFIBROZIL

(gem-fi'broe-zil)

Lopid

Classification: ANTILIPEMIC; FIBRATE

Therapeutic: CHOLESTEROL-LOWERING

Prototype: Fenofibrate

AVAILABILITY Tablet

ACTION & *THERAPEUTIC EFFECT* Fibric acid derivative with lipid regulating properties. Blocks lipolysis of stored triglycerides in adipose tissue and inhibits hepatic uptake of fatty acids. *Decreases VLDL and therefore triglyceride synthesis. Produces a moderate increase in HDL cholesterol levels and reduces levels of total and LDL cholesterol and triglycerides.*

USES Patients with very high serum triglyceride levels (type IV and V hyperlipidemia) who have not responded to intensive diet restriction and are at risk of pancreatitis and abdominal pain. Also severe familial hypercholesterolemia (type IIa or IIb) that developed in childhood and has failed to respond to dietary control or to other cholesterol-lowering drugs.

CONTRAINDICATIONS Gallbladder disease, biliary cirrhosis, hepatic, or severe renal dysfunction.

CAUTIOUS USE Diabetes mellitus, hypothyroidism; renal impairment, anemia; history of cancer; cholelithiasis; pregnancy—fetal risk cannot be ruled out; lactation—infant risk cannot be ruled out. Safety and efficacy in children younger than 18 y not established.

ROUTE & DOSAGE

Hypertriglyceridemia

Adult: **PO** 600 mg bid 30 min before morning and evening meal, may increase up to 1500 mg/day

Renal Impairment Dosage Adjustment

GFR 10–50 mL/min: Administer 75% of dose; *GFR less than 10 mL/min:* Administer 50% of dose

ADMINISTRATION

Oral

- Give 30 min before breakfast and evening meal.
- Store at 20°–25° C (68°–77° F) unless otherwise directed. Protect from light and humidity.

ADVERSE EFFECTS (≥5%) GI: *Abdominal or epigastric pain,* indigestion.

INTERACTIONS Drug: Significant interactions exist, consult package insert for complete listing. May impact medications metabolized via CYP28. May potentiate hypoprothrombinemic effects of ORAL ANTICOAGULANTS; ANTIHYPERLIPIDEMICS, **lovastatin** increases risk of myopathy and rhabdomyolysis; may increase hypoglycemic effects of ANTIDIABETIC MEDICATIONS. **Cyclosporine** increases nephrotoxic effects. Do not use with **eluxadoline.**

PHARMACOKINETICS Absorption: Readily from GI tract; 99% protein bound. **Peak:** 1–2 h. **Metabolism:** Undergoes enterohepatic circulation. **Elimination:** In urine; 6% in feces. **Half-Life:** 1.3–1.5 h.

NURSING IMPLICATIONS

Assessment & Drug Effects

- Note: Mild decreases in WBC, Hgb, Hct may occur during early stage of treatment but generally stabilize with continued therapy.
- Note: Drug is usually withdrawn if lipid response is inadequate after 3 mo of therapy.
- Notify prescriber if patient presents S&S suggestive of cholelithiasis or cholecystitis; gallbladder studies may be indicated. Symptoms often occur during the night or early morning; jaundice may or may not be present.

- Monitor lab tests: Baseline and periodic lipid profile, CBC, blood glucose, and LFTs.

Patient & Family Education

- Report promptly if you develop jaundice, pruritus, or unexplained, upper abdominal discomfort, muscle weakness.

G

GEMIFLOXACIN

(gem-i-flox'a-cin)

Factive

Classification: QUINOLONE ANTIBIOTIC

Therapeutic: ANTIBIOTIC

Prototype: Ciprofloxacin HCl

AVAILABILITY Tablet

ACTION & *THERAPEUTIC EFFECT* Gemifloxacin inhibits bacterial DNA gyrases (topoisomerase II), enzymes essential in replication, transcription, and repair of bacterial DNA. *Gemifloxacin is active against a wide range of gram-positive and gram-negative bacteria.*

USES Treatment of acute exacerbations of chronic bronchitis, mild to moderate community-acquired pneumonia.

UNLABELED USES Acute sinusitis, UTI, acute pyelonephritis, gonorrhea.

CONTRAINDICATIONS Hypersensitivity to gemifloxacin or other fluoroquinolone antibiotics; known QT prolongation; tendon pain; viral disease; history of myasthenia gravis; history of peripheral neuropathy; lactation.

CAUTIOUS USE Hypokalemia, hypomagnesemia, or concurrent use of Class IA or III antiarrhythmic agents; history of OT prolongation; bradycardia, acute myocardial ischemia; renal disease or impairment; hepatic disease; central nervous system disorders such as epilepsy; glu-cose 6-phosphate dehydrogenase deficiency; tendinitis; older adults; pregnancy (category C). Safe use in children 18 y or younger not established.

ROUTE & DOSAGE

Acute Exacerbation of Chronic Bronchitis

Adult: **PO** 320 mg daily × 5 days

Community-Acquired Pneumonia

Adult: **PO** 320 mg daily × 5–7 days

Renal Impairment Dosage Adjustment

CrCl 40 mL/min or less: 160 mg daily

ADMINISTRATION

Oral

- Give 2 h before or 3 h after drugs containing aluminum, magnesium, iron, zinc, or buffered tablets of any type.
- Give at least 2 h before sucralfate.
- Store at 15°–30° C (59°–86° F) and protect from light.

ADVERSE EFFECTS **CNS:** Headache. **Skin:** Rash. **GI:** Nausea, vomiting, diarrhea, elevated liver enzymes.

INTERACTIONS **Drug:** ANTACIDS, **didanosine (tablets and powder), iron, sevelamer, sulcralfate** decrease absorption; may prolong the QT interval with **amiodarone, bepridil, bretylium, chloroprocaine, disopyramide, dofetilide,**

dronedarone, ibutilide, quinidine, pimozide, procainamide, sotalol, ziprasidone leading to arrhythmias; may augment phototoxicity of RETINOIDS.

PHARMACOKINETICS Absorption: 71% absorbed. **Distribution:** 50–75% protein bound. **Peak:** 0.5–2 h. **Metabolism:** Minimally in liver. **Elimination:** Primarily renal. **Half-Life:** 7 h.

NURSING IMPLICATIONS

Black Box Warning

Gemifloxacin has been associated with increased risk of tendinitis and tendon rupture, and with exacerbation of muscle weakness in those with MG.

Assessment & Drug Effects

- Monitor cardiac status with concurrent use of drugs that may prolong the QT interval. Report immediately bradycardia or S&S of heart failure.
- Withhold drug and report to prescriber any of the following: Tremors, restlessness, lightheadedness, confusion, hallucinations, paranoia, depression, nightmares, and insomnia.
- Lab tests: C&S prior to initiation of therapy; baseline and periodic serum electrolytes; serum creatinine, BUN; LFTs. frequent blood glucose levels in diabetics; CBC with differential and platelet count with prolonged treatment.

Patient & Family Education

- Warn patient to report hallucinations, depression, suicidal thoughts, or convulsions.
- Use sunscreen and protective clothing outdoors. Avoid sun lamps.
- Stop gemifloxacin and notify prescriber for pain or swelling of a tendon or around a joint.
- Drink fluid liberally (unless contraindicated) while taking this drug.
- Do not drive or engage in other hazardous activities until reaction to drug is known.

GENTAMICIN SULFATE (Pr)

(jen-ta-mye′sin)

Garamycin Ophthalmic, Genoptic

Classification: AMINOGLYCOSIDE ANTIBIOTIC

Therapeutic: ANTIBIOTIC

AVAILABILITY Ointment; cream; ophthalmic solution; ophthalmic ointment; solution for injection

ACTION & *THERAPEUTIC EFFECT* Broad-spectrum aminoglycoside antibiotic that binds irreversibly to 30S subunit of bacterial ribosomes, blocking a vital step in protein synthesis, and attachment of RNA molecules to bacterial ribosomes resulting in cell death. *Active against a wide variety of aerobic gram-negative but not anaerobic gram-negative bacteria. Also effective against certain gram-positive organisms, particularly penicillin-sensitive bacteria.*

USES Parenteral use restricted to treatment of serious infections of GI, respiratory, and urinary tracts, CNS, bone, skin, and soft tissue (including burns) when other less toxic antimicrobial agents are ineffective or are contraindicated. Has been used in combination with other antibiotics. Also used topically for primary and secondary skin infections and for superficial infections of external eye and its adnexa.

UNLABELED USES Prophylaxis of bacterial endocarditis in patients undergoing operative procedures or instrumentation.

CONTRAINDICATIONS History of hypersensitivity to, or toxic reaction with any aminoglycoside antibiotic; pregnancy (category D); lactation.

CAUTIOUS USE Impaired renal function; history of eighth cranial (acoustic) nerve impairment; preexisting vertigo or dizziness or tinnitus; dehydration, fever; renal impairment, dehydration; hypocalcemia; HF; Fabry disease; older adults, obesity, neuromuscular disorders: MG; parkinsonian syndrome; premature infants, neonates, infants; children. **Topical:** Applied to widespread areas.

ROUTE & DOSAGE

Moderate to Severe Infection

Adult: **IV/IM** 1–2 mg/kg loading dose followed by 3–5 mg/kg/day in 3 divided doses; **Intrathecal** 4–8 mg preservative free daily; **Ophthalmic** 1–2 drops of solution in eye q4h up to 2 drops q1h; **Topical** small amount of ointment bid or tid
Child: **IV/IM** 6–7.5 mg/kg/day in 3 divided doses; *3 mo or older:* **Intrathecal** 1–2 mg preservative free daily
Neonate: **IV/IM** 2.5 mg/kg/day

Prophylaxis of Bacterial Endocarditis

Adult: **IV/IM** 1.5 mg/kg 30 min before procedure, may repeat in 8 h
Child (weight less than 27 kg): **IV/IM** 2 mg/kg 30 min before procedure, may repeat in 8 h

Obesity Dosage Adjustment

Dose based on IBW, in morbid obesity use IBW + 0.4 (TBW–IBW)

Renal Impairment Dosage Adjustment

Reduce dose or extend dosing interval

ADMINISTRATION

Ophthalmic

- Apply pressure to inner canthus for 1 min immediately after instillation of drops.
- Have patient keep eyes closed for 1–2 min after administration of ophthalmic ointment to assure medication contact. Caution patient that vision will be blurred for a few minutes.

Topical

- Wash affected area with mild soap and water, rinse, and dry thoroughly. Gently apply small amount of medication to lesions; cover with sterile gauze.
- Do not apply topical preparations, particularly cream, to large denuded body surfaces because systemic absorption and toxicity are possible.

Intramuscular

- Give deep into a large muscle.
- Do not use solutions that are discolored or that contain particulate matter; drug for IV or IM is clear and colorless or slightly yellow.

Intrathecal

- Note: Intrathecal formulation is a clear and colorless solution.
- Use promptly after opening; contains no preservatives and any unused portion should be discarded.

Intravenous

PREPARE: **Intermittent:** Dilute a single dose with 50–200 mL of D5W or NS. ▪ For pediatric patients, amount of infusion fluid may be proportionally smaller depending on patient's needs but should be sufficient to be infused over the same time period as for adults. ▪ Note: Premixed, single-dose containers are ready to use and require no dilution.

ADMINISTER: **Intermittent:** Give over 30 min–1 h. May extend infusion time to 2 h for a child.

INCOMPATIBILITIES: **Solution/additive:** Fat emulsion, **TPN, amphotericin B, ampicillin,** CEPHALOSPORINS, **cytarabine, heparin, ticarcillin. Y-site: Allopurinol, amphotericin B cholesteryl, azithromycin, furosemide, heparin, hetastarch, idarubicin, indomethacin, iodipamide, propofol, warfarin.**

▪ Store all gentamicin solutions at 2°–30° C (36°–86° F) unless otherwise directed by manufacturer.

ADVERSE EFFECTS **CV:** Hypotension or hy-pertension. **CNS:** Neuromuscular blockade: Skeletal muscle weakness, apnea, respiratory paralysis (high doses); arachnoiditis (intra-thecal use). **HEENT:** Ototoxicity (vestibular disturbances, impaired hearing), optic neuritis. **GI:** Nausea, vomiting, transient increase in AST, ALT, and serum LDH and bilirubin; hepatomegaly, splenomegaly. **GU:** Nephrotoxicity: Proteinuria, tubular necrosis, cells or casts in urine, hematuria, rising BUN, nonprotein nitrogen, serum creatinine; *decreased creatinine clearance*. **Hematologic:** Increased or decreased reticulocyte counts; granulocytopenia, thrombocytopenia (fever, bleeding tendency), thrombocytopenic purpura, anemia. **Other:** Hypersensitivity (rash, pruritus, urticaria, exfoliative dermatitis, eosinophilia, burning sensation of skin, drug fever, joint pains, laryngeal edema, anaphylaxis). Local irritation and pain following IM use; thrombophlebitis, abscess, superinfections, syndrome of hypocalcemia (tetany, weakness, hypokalemia, hypomagnesemia), photosensitivity, sensitization, erythema, pruritus; burning, stinging, and lacrimation (ophthalmic formulation).

INTERACTIONS **Drug: Amphotericin B, capreomycin, cisplatin, methoxyflurane, polymyxin B, vancomycin, ethacrynic acid,** and **furosemide** increase risk of nephrotoxicity. GENERAL ANESTHETICS and NEUROMUSCULAR BLOCKING AGENTS (e.g., **succinylcholine**) potentiate neuromuscular blockade. **Indomethacin** may increase gentamicin levels in neonates.

PHARMACOKINETICS **Absorption:** Well absorbed from IM site. **Peak:** 30–90 min IM. **Distribution:** Widely distributed in body fluids, including ascitic, peritoneal, pleural, synovial, and abscess fluids; poor CNS penetration; concentrates in kidney and inner ear; crosses placenta. **Metabolism:** Not metabolized. **Elimination:** Excreted unchanged in urine; small amounts accumulate in kidney and are eliminated over 10–20 days; small amount excreted in breast milk. **Half-Life:** 2–4 h.

NURSING IMPLICATIONS

Black Box Warning

Gentamicin has been associated with nephrotoxicity and ototoxicity.

Assessment & Drug Effects

- Lab tests: Perform C&S and renal function tests prior to first dose and periodically during therapy. Determine creatinine clearance and serum drug concentrations at frequent intervals.
- Note: Dosages are generally adjusted to maintain peak serum gentamicin concentrations of 4–10 mcg/mL, and trough concentrations of 1–2 mcg/mL. Prolonged peak concentrations above 12 mcg/mL and trough concentrations above 2 mcg/mL are associated with toxicity.
- Draw blood specimens for peak serum gentamicin concentration 30 min–1h after IM administration, and 30 min after completion of a 30–60 min IV infusion. Draw blood specimens for trough levels just before the next IM or IV dose.
- Monitor vital signs and I&O. Keep patient well hydrated to prevent chemical irritation of renal tubules. Report oliguria, unusual appearance of urine, change in I&O ratio or pattern, and presence of edema (prolongs elimination time).
- Watch for S&S of bacterial overgrowth (opportunistic infections) with resistant or nonsusceptible organisms (diarrhea, anogenital itching, vaginal discharge, stomatitis, glossitis).

Patient & Family Education

- Report promptly S&S of ototoxic effect (e.g., headache, dizziness or vertigo, nausea and vomiting with motion, ataxia, nystagmus, tinnitus, roaring noises, sensation of fullness in ears, hearing impairment).
- Note: When using topical applications: Avoid excessive exposure to sunlight because of danger of photosensitivity; withhold medication and notify prescriber if condition fails to improve within 1 wk, worsens, or signs of irritation or sensitivity occur; and apply medication as directed and only for length of time prescribed (overuse can result in superinfections).

GLATIRAMER ACETATE

(gla-tir′a-mer)

Copaxone, Glatopa

Classification: BIOLOGIC RESPONSE MODIFIER; IMMUNOLOGIC

Therapeutic: IMMUNOSUPPRESSANT

AVAILABILITY Solution for injection

ACTION & *THERAPEUTIC EFFECT* Mechanism of action is not fully understood. Thought to modify immune processes that are responsible for the pathogenesis of multiple sclerosis. *Its function is to reduce the relapse rate of multiple sclerosis (MS), a demyelinating disease of the CNS.*

USES Reduce frequency of relapses in patients with relapsing–remitting multiple sclerosis.

CONTRAINDICATIONS Hypersensitivity to glatiramer acetate or mannitol.

CAUTIOUS USE Immunosuppression, history of asthma or other respiratory disorders; angina; pregnancy (category B); lactation. Safe use in children younger than 18 y has not been established.

ROUTE & DOSAGE

Multiple Sclerosis

Adult: **Subcutaneous** 20 mg daily or 40 mg 3 × wk at least 48 h apart

ADMINISTRATION

Subcutaneous

- Use recommended subcutaneous injection sites: Arms, abdomen, hips, and thighs.
- Give 40 mg dose on same 3 days each wk.
- Allow prefilled syringe to stand at room temperature for 20 min prior to injection.
- Note that glatiramer 20 mg/mL and 40 mg/mL formulations are not interchangeable.
- Store vials at –20° to –10° C (–4° to –14° F).

ADVERSE EFFECTS **CV:** *Chest pain, palpitations,* syncope, tachycardia, *vasodilation*. **Respiratory:** *Dyspnea, rhinitis,* bronchitis. **CNS:** Migraine, agitation, *anxiety, hypotonia*. **Skin:** *Rash, pruritus, sweating*. **GI:** *Diarrhea, nausea,* anorexia, gastroenteritis, vomiting. **Other:** *Asthenia, back pain,* chills, facial edema, fever, *flu-like syndrome, infection, pain, arthralgia. Postinjection reaction (flushing, chest pain, palpitations, anxiety, dyspnea, constriction of throat, urticaria), injection site reactions (erythema, hemorrhage, pain, pruritus, urticaria, swelling),* ecchymoses, *lymphadenopathy,* ear pain, dysmenorrhea, urinary urgency.

NURSING IMPLICATIONS

Assessment & Drug Effects

- Monitor for therapeutic effectiveness: Indicated by longer remission periods and reduced frequency of attacks.
- Assess for systemic postinjection reactions (see PATIENT & FAMILY EDUCATION). Assure patient that reaction is self-limiting. Assess for local reactions at injection sites including erythema, itching, induration, and soreness.
- Monitor for S&S of compromised immune response (e.g., increasing frequency of infections).

Patient & Family Education

- Note: Systemic postinjection reaction with chest pain, palpitations, flushing, urticaria, anxiety, dyspnea, and laryngeal constriction may occur immediately after injection. These symptoms are transient (lasting from 30 sec to 30 min), require no treatment, and resolve spontaneously.
- Report any distressing adverse drug effects.

G

GLIMEPIRIDE

(gli-me′pi-ride)

Amaryl

Classification: SULFONYLUREA

Therapeutic: ANTIDIABETIC

Prototype: Glyburide

AVAILABILITY Tablet

ACTION & *THERAPEUTIC EFFECT* Second-generation sulfonylurea hypoglycemic agent that directly stimulates functioning pancreatic beta cells to secrete insulin, leading to a direct drop in blood glucose. Indirect action leads to increased sensitivity of peripheral insulin receptors, resulting in increased insulin binding in peripheral tissues. *Lowers blood sugar by increasing secretion of insulin from pancreatic beta cells. Glimepiride improves postprandial glycemic control.*

USES Adjunct to diet and exercise in patients with type 2 diabetes.

CONTRAINDICATIONS Hypersensitivity to glimepiride, diabetic ketoacidosis; nondiabetic patients with renal glycosuria; lactation (infant risk cannot be ruled out).

G

CAUTIOUS USE Previous hypersensitivity to other sulfonylureas, sulfonamides, or thiazide diuretics; hypoglycemia or conditions predisposing to hypoglycemia (e.g., prolonged nausea and vomiting, alcohol ingestion, surgery; renal or hepatic function impairment, severe infections); older adults, pregnancy (category C). Safe use in children is not established.

ROUTE & DOSAGE

Type 2 Diabetes Mellitus

Adult: **PO** Start with 1–2 mg once daily with breakfast or first main meal, may increase to usual maintenance dose of 1–4 mg once daily (max: 8 mg/day)

ADMINISTRATION

Oral

- Give with breakfast or first main meal.
- Note: Maximum starting dose is 2 mg or less. With renal or hepatic insufficiency, initial recommended dose is 1 mg.
- Store in tightly closed container at 20°–25° C (68°–77° F).

ADVERSE EFFECTS **CNS:** Weakness, dizziness, headache. **Endocrine:** Hypoglycemia. **GI:** Nausea.

INTERACTIONS **Drug:** Hypoglycemic effects may be potentiated by other highly protein-bound drugs (e.g., ADRENERGIC ANTAGONISTS, **chloramphenicol,** MAO INHIBITORS, NSAIDS, **probenecid,** SALICYLATES, SULFONAMIDES, **warfarin**). CORTICOSTEROIDS, **phenytoin, isoniazid, nicotinic acid,** SYMPATHOMIMETIC AMINES, THIAZIDE DIURETICS may attenuate effects of glimepiride. Do not use with **mitiglinide.** **Herbal:** **Ginseng, garlic** may increase hypoglycemic effects.

PHARMACOKINETICS **Absorption:** Completely absorbed from GI tract. **Onset:** 1 h. **Peak:** 2–3 h. **Distribution:** Greater than 99.5% protein bound; probably secreted into breast milk. **Metabolism:** In liver by CYP2C9. **Elimination:** 60% in urine, 40% in feces. **Half-Life:** 5–9 h.

NURSING IMPLICATIONS

Assessment & Drug Effects

- Monitor for hypoglycemia especially with concurrent drugs which enhance hypoglycemic effects.
- Monitor lab tests: Frequent fasting and postprandial blood glucose, HgbA1C every 3–6 mo.

Patient & Family Education

- Take a missed dose as soon as possible unless it is almost time for next dose; NEVER take two doses at the same time.
- Avoid drinking alcohol or using OTC drugs without informing prescriber.
- Treat mild hypoglycemia (reaction without loss of consciousness or neurologic symptoms) with PO glucose and adjustment of dosage and meal pattern; monitor closely for at least 5–7 days to assure reestablishment of safe control. Severe hypoglycemia requires emergency hospitalization to permit treatment to maintain a blood glucose level above 100 mg/dL.

GLIPIZIDE

(glip'i-zide)

Glucotrol, Glucotrol XL

Classification: SULFONYLUREA

Therapeutic: ANTIDIABETIC

Prototype: Glyburide

AVAILABILITY Tablet; sustained release tablet

ACTION & *THERAPEUTIC EFFECT* Second-generation sulfonylurea hypoglycemic agent that directly stimulates functioning pancreatic-beta cells to secrete insulin, leading-to an acute drop in blood glucose. Indirect action leads to altered numbers and sensitivity of peripheral insulin receptors, resulting in increased insulin binding. It also causes inhibition of hepatic glucose production and reduction in serum glucagon- levels. *It lowers blood glucose level- by stimulating pancreatic beta cells. Glipizide improves postprandial glycemic control.*

USES Adjunct to diet for control of hyperglycemia in patient with type 2 diabetes mellitus.

CONTRAINDICATIONS Hypersensitivity to sulfonylureas; diabetic ketoacidosis; lactation. (infant risk cannot be ruled out).

CAUTIOUS USE Impaired renal and hepatic function; thyroid disease; debilitated, malnourished- patients; G6PD deficiency; trauma; surgery; patients with adrenal or pituitary insufficiency; older adults. **Extended release form:** Severe GI narrowing; pregnancy (category C). Safe use in children has not been established.

ROUTE & DOSAGE

Control of Hyperglycemia

Adult: **PO** 2.5–5 mg/day 30 min before breakfast, may increase by 2.5–5 mg q1–2wk; greater than 15 mg/day in divided doses 30 min before morning and evening meal (max: 40 mg/day); 5–10 mg sustained release tablets once/day

ADMINISTRATION

Oral

- Give once daily dosing 30 min before the first meal of the day.
- Ensure that sustained release form of drug is not chewed or crushed. It **must be** swallowed whole.
- Store in tightly closed, light-resistant container at 15°–30° C (59°–86° F).

ADVERSE EFFECTS CNS: Dizziness. **GI:** Diarrhea

INTERACTIONS Drug: Alcohol produces **disulfiram**-like reaction in some patients; ORAL ANTICOAGULANTS, **chloramphenicol, clofibrate, phenylbutazone,** MAO INHIBITORS, SALICYLATES, **probenecid,** SULFONAMIDES may potentiate hypoglycemic actions; THIAZIDES may antagonize hypoglycemic effects; **cimetidine** may increase glipizide levels, causing hypoglycemia. Do not use with **mitiglinide** or **mecamylamine. Herbal: Ginseng, garlic** may increase hypoglycemic effects.

PHARMACOKINETICS Absorption: Readily from GI tract. **Onset:** 15–30 min. **Peak:** 1–2 h. **Duration:** Up to 24 h. **Metabolism:** Metabolized extensively in liver. **Elimination:** Mainly in urine with some excretion via bile in feces. **Half-Life:** 3–5 h.

NURSING IMPLICATIONS

Assessment & Drug Effects

- Observe response to the initial dose, especially in older adult or debilitated patients; early signs of hypoglycemia are easily overlooked.
- Patients transferred from a sulfonylurea with a long half-life (e.g., chlorpropamide, half-life: 30–40 h) **must be** made aware of the potential for hypoglycemic responses (see Appendix F)

for 1–2 wk because of potential overlapping of drug effect.

- Note: The first signs of hypoglycemia may be hard to detect in patients receiving concurrent beta-blockers or older adults.
- Monitor lab tests: Periodic fasting and postprandial blood glucose, and HgbA1C.

Patient & Family Education

- Treat mild hypoglycemia (reaction without loss of consciousness or neurologic symptoms) with PO glucose and adjustment of dosage and meal pattern; monitor closely for at least 5–7 days to assure reestablishment of safe control. Severe hypoglycemia requires emergency hospitalization to permit treatment to maintain a blood glucose level above 100 mg/dL.
- Test fasting and postprandial blood glucose frequently.
- Keep all follow-up medical appointments and adhere to dietary instructions, regular exercise program, and scheduled and blood testing.
- When a drug that affects the hypoglycemic action of sulfonylureas (see DRUG INTERACTIONS) is withdrawn or added to the glipizide regimen, be alert to the added danger of loss of control. Urine and blood glucose tests and test for ketone bodies should be carefully monitored.
- Report promptly severe skin rash and pruritus as these may indicate a need for discontinuation of drug. Symptoms usually subside rapidly when drug is withdrawn.

GLUCAGON

(gloo′ka-gon)

GlucaGen

Classification: ANTIHYPOGLYCEMIC

Therapeutic: ANTIHYPOGLYCEMIC; DIAGNOSTIC TEST AID

AVAILABILITY Powder for injection

ACTION & *THERAPEUTIC EFFECT* Recombinant glucagon identical to glucagon produced by alpha cells of islets of Langerhans. Stimulates uptake of amino acids and their conversion to glucose precursors. Promotes lipolysis in liver and adipose tissue with release of free fatty acid and glycerol, which further stimulates ketogenesis and hepatic gluconeogenesis. Action in hypoglycemia relies on presence of adequate liver glycogen stores. *Increases blood glucose secondary to gluconeogenesis, which is the breakdown of glycogen to glucose in the liver.*

USES Hypoglycemia, radiologic studies of GI tract.

UNLABELED USES GI disturbances associated with spasm, cardiovascular emergencies, and to overcome cardiotoxic effects of beta-blockers, quinidine, tricyclic antidepressants; as an aid in abdominal imaging; choking due to esophageal foreign body impaction.

CONTRAINDICATIONS Hypersensitivity to glucagon or protein compounds; depleted glycogen stores in liver; insulinemia; pheochromocytoma.

CAUTIOUS USE Cardiac disease, CAD; adrenal insufficiency; malnutrition; children; pregnancy (category B); lactation.

ROUTE & DOSAGE

Hypoglycemia

Adult/Adolescent/Child (greater than 25 kg): **IM/IV/Subcutaneous** 1 mg, may repeat q5–20 min if no response for 1–2 more doses

 Common adverse effects in *italic*; life-threatening effects underlined; generic names in **bold**; classifications in SMALL CAPS; ♣ Canadian drug name; ◐ Prototype drug; ⚠ Alert

Child (younger than 8y, weight less than 25 kg): **IM/IV/Subcutaneous** 0.5 mg (max: 1 mg)

Diagnostic Aid to Relax Stomach or Upper GI Tract

Adult: **IV** 0.2–0.5 mg **IM** 1 mg

Diagnostic Aid for Colon Exam

Adult: **IV** 0.5–0.75 mg; **IM** 1–2 mg

ADMINISTRATION

Note: 1 mg = 1 unit

Subcutaneous/Intramuscular

- Dilute 1 unit (1 mg) of glucagon with 1 mL of diluent supplied by manufacturer.
- Use immediately after reconstitution of dry powder. Discard any unused portion.
- Note: Glucagon is incompatible in syringe with any other drug.

Intravenous

PREPARE: **Direct:** Prepare as noted for intramuscular injection. Do not use a concentration greater than 1 unit/mL.
ADMINISTER: **Direct:** ▪ Give 1 unit or fraction thereof over 1 min. ▪ May be given through a Y-site D5W (not NS) infusing. Note: Rapid injection may be associated with increased nausea and vomiting; place patient in lateral recumbent position to protect airway.
INCOMPATIBILITIES: **Solution/additive: Sodium chloride.**

- Store unreconstituted vials and diluent at 20°–25° C (68°–77° F).

ADVERSE EFFECTS **Endocrine:** Hyperglycemia, hypokalemia. **Skin:** Stevens–Johnson syndrome (erythema multiforme). **GI:** Nausea and vomiting. **Other:** Hypersensitivity reactions.

INTERACTIONS **Drug:** May enhance effect of ORAL ANTICOAGULANTS.

PHARMACOKINETICS **Onset:** 5–20 min. **Peak:** 30 min. **Duration:** 1–1.5 h. **Metabolism:** In liver, plasma, and kidneys. **Half-Life:** 3–10 min.

NURSING IMPLICATIONS

Assessment & Drug Effects

- Be prepared to give IV glucose if patient fails to respond to glucagon. Notify prescriber immediately.
- Note: Patient usually awakens from (diabetic) hypoglycemic coma 5–20 min after glucagon injection. Give PO carbohydrate as soon as possible after patient regains consciousness.
- Note: After recovery from hypoglycemic reaction, symptoms such as headache, nausea, and weakness may persist.

Patient & Family Education

- Note: Prescriber may request that a responsible family member be taught how to administer glucagon subcutaneously or IM for patients with frequent or severe hypogly-cemic reactions. Notify prescriber promptly whenever a hypoglycemic reaction occurs so the reason for the reaction can be determined.
- Review package insert and directions (see ADMINISTRATION).

GLYBURIDE (Pr)

(glye′byoor-ide)

Euglucon ♣, Glynase

Classification: SULFONYLUREA

Therapeutic: ANTIDIABETIC

AVAILABILITY Tablet

G

ACTION & THERAPEUTIC EFFECT

One of the most potent of the second-generation sulfonylurea hypoglycemic agents. Appears to lower blood sugar concentration by sensitizing pancreatic beta cells to release insulin in the presence of elevated serum glucose levels and by reducing glucose output from the liver as well as increasing insulin sensitivity in peripheral target sites. *Blood glucose-lowering effect persists during long-term glyburide treatment, but there is a gradual decline in meal-stimulated secretion of endogenous insulin toward pretreatment levels.*

USES Adjunct to diet and exercise to lower blood glucose in patients with type 2 diabetes mellitus.

CONTRAINDICATIONS Hypersensitivity to glyburide or sulfonylureas; concomitant use of bosentan; diabetic ketoacidosis; type I diabetes mellitus; major surgery; severe trauma; severe infection; withhold 14 days before labor and delivery; pregnancy—fetal risk cannot be ruled out; lactation (infant risk cannot be ruled out), older adults; safety and efficacy not established in children.

CAUTIOUS USE History of sulfonamide hypersensitivity; renal and hepatic impairment; cardiovascular disease; thyroid disease; mild renal impairment or hepatic disease; history of autonomic neuropathy, stress caused by infection, fever, trauma or recent surgery; adrenal or pituitary insufficiency; debilitated, or malnourished patients.

ROUTE & DOSAGE

Control of Hyperglycemia

Adult: **PO** 2.5–5 mg/day with breakfast, may increase by 2.5 mg q1–2wk; greater than 10 mg/day should be given in divided doses (max: 20 mg/day); **Micronized** 1.5–3 mg/day (max: 12 mg/day) with breakfast, may increase by 1.5 mg/day each week based on patient response (max: 12 mg/day)

ADMINISTRATION

Oral

- Give once daily in the morning with breakfast or with first main meal.
- Store in tightly closed, light-resistant container at 25°C (77°F); excursions permitted between 15 and 30°C (59 and 86°F).

ADVERSE EFFECTS Endocrine: Weight gain. **GI:** Epigastric fullness, heartburn, nausea.

INTERACTIONS Drug: Alcohol causes disulfiram-like reaction in some patients; ANTIDIABETIC medications, ORAL ANTICOAGULANTS, **chloramphenicol, clofibrate, phenylbutazone,** MAO INHIBITORS, SALICYLATES, **probenecid,** SULFONAMIDES, **clarithromycin** may potentiate hypoglycemic actions; THIAZIDES may antagonize hypoglycemic effects; **cimetidine** may increase glyburide levels, causing hypoglycemia. Contraindicated with **aminolevulinic acid, bosentan, mecamylamine, mitiglinide. Herbal: Ginseng, garlic** may increase hypoglycemic effects.

PHARMACOKINETICS Absorption: Readily absorbed from GI tract. **Onset:** 15–60 min. **Peak:** 1–2 h. **Duration:** Up to 24 h. **Distribution:** Distributed in highest concentrations in liver, kidneys, and intestines; crosses placenta. **Metabolism:** Extensively in liver.

Elimination: Equally in urine and feces. **Half-Life:** 10 h.

NURSING IMPLICATIONS

Assessment & Drug Effects

- Monitor blood glucose levels carefully during the dangerous early treatment period when dosage is being individualized. Older adults are especially vulnerable to glyburide-induced hypoglycemia (see Appendix F) because the antidiabetic agent is long-acting.
- Note: The first signs of hypoglycemia may be hard to detect when the patient is also receiving a beta-blocker or is an older adult.
- Monitor lab tests: Frequent fasting and postprandial blood glucose, periodic HbA1C, renal function tests.

Patient & Family Education

- Treat mild hypoglycemia (reaction without loss of consciousness or neurologic symptoms) with PO glucose and adjustment of dosage and meal pattern; monitor closely for at least 5–7 days to assure reestablishment of safe control. Severe hypoglycemia requires emergency hospitalization to permit treatment to maintain a blood glucose level above 100 mg/dL.
- Remember that loss of control of diabetes may result from stress such as fever, surgery, trauma, or infection. Check blood glucose more frequently during stress periods.
- Keep all follow-up medical appointments and adhere to dietary instructions, regular exercise program, and scheduled blood testing.
- Avoid alcohol while taking this drug.
- Report blurred vision to prescriber.

GLYCERIN

(gli′ser-in)

Fleet Babylax, Glycerol, Osmoglyn

Classification: HYPEROSMOTIC LAXATIVE; ANTIGLAUCOMA; DIURETIC

Therapeutic: HYPEROSMOTIC LAXATIVE; ANTIGLAUCOMA; OCULAR OSMOTIC DIURETIC

AVAILABILITY Oral solution; suppositories

ACTION & *THERAPEUTIC EFFECT*

Oral: Glycerin raises plasma osmotic pressure by withdrawing fluid from extravascular spaces; lowers ocular tension by decreasing volume of intraocular fluid. May also reduce CSF pressure. **Ocular topic application:** Reduces edema by hydroscopic effect. **Glycerin suppositories:** Apparently work by causing dehydration of exposed tissue, which produces an irritant effect, and by absorbing water from tissues, thus creating more bowel mass. Both actions stimulate peristalsis in the large bowel. *Reduces intraocular pressure by lowering intraocular fluid. Relieves constipation by absorption of water and stimulation of peristalsis.*

USES Orally to reduce elevated intraocular pressure (IOP) before or after surgery in patients with acute narrow-angle glaucoma, retinal detachment, or cataract and to reduce elevated CSF pressure. Used rectally (suppository or enema) to relieve constipation.

CONTRAINDICATIONS Diabetic ketoacidosis; moderate or severe renal impairment (CrCl less than 50 mL/min), renal failure.

CAUTIOUS USE Cardiac disease, mild renal impairment; hepatic disease; diabetes mellitus; thyroid disease; dehydrated or older adults; pregnancy (generally considered safe to use during pregnancy); lactation.

ROUTE & DOSAGE

Decrease IOP

Adult/Child: **PO** 1–1.8 g/kg 1–1.5 h before ocular surgery, may repeat q5h

Constipation

Adult/Child (6 y or older): **PR** Insert 1 suppository or 5–15 mL of enema high into rectum and retain for 15 min

Child (younger than 6 y): **PR** Insert 1 infant suppository or 2–5 mL of enema high into rectum and retain for 15 min

Neonate: **PR** 0.5 mL of rectal solution (enema)

ADMINISTRATION

Oral

- Pour oral solution over crushed ice and have patient sip through a straw.
- Prevent or relieve headache (from cerebral dehydration) by having patient lie down during and after administration of drug.

Rectal

- Ensure that suppository is inserted beyond rectal sphincter.

ADVERSE EFFECTS CV: Irregular heartbeat. **CNS:** Headache, confusion. **GI:** Abdominal cramps, diarrhea, nausea, vomiting, dry mouth, rectal irritation (suppository).

PHARMACOKINETICS Absorption: Readily absorbed from GI tract after oral administration; rectal preparations are poorly absorbed. **Onset:** 10 min PO. **Peak:** 30 min–2 h. **Duration:** 4–8 h. **Metabolism:** 80% metabolized in liver; 10–20% metabolized in kidneys to CO_2 and water or utilized in glucose or glycogen synthesis. **Elimination:** 7–14% excreted unchanged in urine. **Half-Life:** 30–40 min.

NURSING IMPLICATIONS

Assessment & Drug Effects

- Consult prescriber regarding fluid intake in patients receiving drug for elevated IOP. Although hypotonic fluids will relieve thirst and headache caused by the dehydrating action of glycerin, these fluids may nullify its osmotic effect.
- Monitor glycemic control in diabetics. Drug may cause hyperglycemia (see Appendix F).
- Monitor lab tests: Electrolytes.

Patient & Family Education

- Evacuation usually comes 15–30 min after administration of glycerin rectal suppository or enema.
- Note: Slight hyperglycemia and glycosuria may occur with PO use; adjustment in antidiabetic medication dosage may be required.

GLYCOPYRROLATE

(glye-koe-pye′roe-late)

Cuvposa, Glycate, Seebri Breezhaler

Classification: ANTICHOLINERGIC; ANTIMUSCARINIC; ANTISPASMODIC

Therapeutic: GI ANTISPASMODIC

Prototype: Atropine

AVAILABILITY Oral solution; tablet; solution for injection; oral inhaler

ACTION & *THERAPEUTIC EFFECT* An anticholinergic (antimuscarinic)

agent that inhibits the action of acetylcholine on smooth muscle, cardiac muscle, the SA and AV nodes, and exocrine glands (including salivary). Its effect on gastric glands diminishes the volume and acidity of gastric secretions and, in the respiratory tract, controls excessive pharyngeal, tracheal, and bronchial secretions. *Inhibits motility of GI and genitourinary tract; it also decreases volume of gastric and pan-creatic secretions, saliva, and perspiration.*

USES Reduction of secretions, reversal of bradycardia, reversal of muscarinic effects of cholinergic agents; chronic drooling (Cuvposa only), maintenance treatment of COPD (Seebri Breezhaler only)

CONTRAINDICATIONS Glaucoma; asthma; prostatic hypertrophy, obstructive uropathy; obstructive lesions or atony of GI tract; achalasia; severe ulcerative colitis; myasthenia gravis; BPH; urinary tract obstruction; during cyclopropane anesthesia; unstable cardiac status; pregnancy—fetal risk cannot be ruled out; lactation—infant risk cannot be ruled out.

CAUTIOUS USE Autonomic neuropathy, hepatic or renal disease; cardiac arrhythmias, coronary heart disease, hypertension, CHF; hyperthyroidism, constipation, diarrhea, hiatal hernia, spastic paralysis, brain damage; Down syndrome; elderly; children.

ROUTE & DOSAGE

Reduction of Secretions

Adult: **IM** 4 mcg/kg 30–60 min before anesthesia

Chronic Drooling (Cuvposa only)

Child/Adolescent (3 y or older): **PO** 0.02 mg/kg tid; titrate to response (max: 0.1 mg/kg)

Reversal of Cholinergic Agents

Adult/Child: **IV** 0.2 mg administered for each 1 mg of neostigmine or 5 mg pyridostigmine

COPD (Seebri Breezhaler only)
Adult: **PO** 1 capsule bid

ADMINISTRATION

Oral

- Take at least 1 hour before or 2 hours after meals

Inhalation

- Use Neohaler device; do not swallow.
- Remove capsule from blister immediately prior to administration.
- Remove vial from foil pouch immediately before use; unused unit-dose vials may be stored in foil pouch for up to 7 days.
- Only use vials with Magnair device; do not swallow solution.

Intramuscular

- Give diluted or undiluted, deep into a large muscle.

Intravenous

PREPARE: **Direct:** Give diluted or undiluted. ▪ Inspect for cloudiness and discoloration. Discard if present. May dilute in D5W, D10W, D5W/NS, D10W/NS, D5W/0.45%NS, NS, and Ringer injection; do not mix in LR.
ADMINISTER: **Direct:** Give 0.2 mg or fraction thereof over 1–2 min.
INCOMPATIBILITIES: **Solution/additive: Methylprednisolone. Y-site: Amphotericin B,**

dantrolene, diazepam, diazoxide, fluorescein, furosemide, indomethacin, insulin, irinotecan, mitomycin, pantoprazole, phenytoin, piperacillin, sulfamethoxazole/trimethoprim.

- Store capsule in blister pack at controlled room temperature at 25° C (77° F), with excursions permitted between 15 and 30 degrees C (59 and 86 degrees F) until immediately before use. Protect from moisture. Store inhalation, oral and injection solutions and tablets at controlled room temperature between 20 and 25 degrees C (68 and 77 degrees F)

G

ADVERSE EFFECTS (≥5%) **Respiratory:** *Nasal congestion, upper respiratory infection*. **Skin:** Flushing. **GI:** *Xerostomia, constipation, vomiting*. **GU:** *Urinary tract infection*.

INTERACTIONS **Drug:** **Amantadine,** TRICYCLIC ANTIDEPRESSANTS, **quinidine, disopyramide, procainamide** compound anticholinergic effects; decreases **levodopa** effects; **methotrimeprazine** may precipitate extrapyramidal effects; decreases antipsychotic effects (decreased absorption) of PHENOTHIAZINES. Do not use with **eluxadoline, levosulpiride,** POTASSIUM SALTS.

PHARMACOKINETICS **Absorption:** Poorly and incompletely absorbed. **Onset:** 1 min IV; 15–30 min IM; 1 h PO. **Peak:** 30–45 min IM; 1 h PO. **Duration:** 2–7 h IM; 8–12 h PO. **Distribution:** Crosses placenta. **Metabolism:** Minimally in liver. **Elimination:** 85% in urine. **Half-Life:** 30–70 min (adult), 20–99 min (child), 20–120 min (infant).

NURSING IMPLICATIONS

Assessment & Drug Effects

- Incidence and severity of adverse effects are generally dose related.
- Monitor I&O ratio and pattern particularly in older adults. Watch for urinary hesitancy and retention.
- Monitor for any red eyes, conjunctival congestion, eye pain, corneal edema and blurred vision
- Monitor vital signs, especially when drug is given parenterally. Report any changes in heart rate or rhythm.
- Monitor lab tests: LFTs and renal studies.

Patient & Family Education

- Avoid high environmental temperatures (heat prostration can occur because of decreased sweating).
- Administer the same time every day either 1 hour before or 2 hours after a meal.
- Do not drive or engage in other potentially hazardous activities requiring mental alertness until response to drug is known.
- Use good oral hygiene, rinse mouth with water frequently and use a saliva substitute to lessen effects of dry mouth.
- Report constipation or urinary retention.
- Review adverse effects.
- Protect eyes from light related to light sensitivity.

GOLD SODIUM THIOMALATE

(thye-oh-mah'late)

Classification: DISEASE-MODIFYING ANTIRHEUMATIC DRUG (DMARD)

Therapeutic: ANTIRHEUMATIC;GOLD COMPOUND

Prototype: Auranofin

AVAILABILITY Solution for injection

ACTION & *THERAPEUTIC EFFECT* Mechanism of action is unknown. Appears to act by suppression of phagocytosis, altered immune responses, and possibly by inhibition of prostaglandin synthesis. *Has immunomodulatory and anti-inflammatory effects.*

USES Selected patients (adults and juveniles) with acute rheumatoid arthritis.

UNLABELED USES Psoriatic arthritis, Felty's syndrome.

CONTRAINDICATIONS History of severe toxicity from previous exposure to gold or other heavy metals; severe debilitation; SLE, Sjögren's syndrome in rheumatoid arthritis; renal disease; hepatic dysfunction, history of systemic lupus erythematosus, history of infectious hepatitis; uncontrolled diabetes or CHF.

CAUTIOUS USE History of drug allergies or hypersensitivity; marked hypertension; history of blood dyscrasias such as granulocytopenia or anemia caused by drug sensitivity; CHF; diabetes mellitus; previous kidney or liver disease; colitis, IBD; compromised cerebral or cardiovascular circulation; older adults; pregnancy (category C); lactation (infant risk cannot be ruled out); children.

ROUTE & DOSAGE

Rheumatoid Arthritis

Adult: **IM** 10 mg wk 1, 25 mg wk 2, then 25–50 mg/wk to a cumulative dose of 1 g (if improvement occurs, continue at 25–50 mg q2wk for 2–20 wk, then q3–4wk indefinitely or until adverse effects occur)

Child: **IM** 10 mg test dose, then 1 mg/kg/wk then 1 mg/kg q1–4wk (max single dose: 50 mg)

ADMINISTRATION

Intramuscular

- Agitate vial before withdrawing dose to ensure uniform suspension.
- Give deep into upper outer quadrant of gluteus maximus with patient lying down. Patient should remain recumbent for at least 10 min after injection because of the danger of "nitritoid reaction" (transient giddiness, vertigo, facial flushing, fainting).
- Observe for allergic reactions.
- Store in tight, light-resistant containers at 15°–30° C (59°–86° F). Do not use if any darker than pale yellow.

ADVERSE EFFECTS **CV:** Bradycardia, syncopy, vasomotor symptoms. **Respiratory:** Bronchitis, dyspnea, pneumonitis, pulmonary fibrosis. **CNS:** Cerebral ischemia, encephalopathy. **HEENT:** Conjunctivitis, corneal ulcer, iritis. **Skin:** Alopecia, dermatitis, urticaria, itching. **Hepatic:** Jaundice, heptotoxicity. **GI:** Enterocolitis, abdominal pain, anorexia, diarrhea, dysphagia, gingivitis, nausea, vomiting, ulcerative colitis. **GU:** Acute renal failure, nephrotic syndrome, hematuria, proteinuria. **Musculoskeletal:** Joint pain. **Hematologic:** Agranulocytosis, aplastic anemia, pancytopenia, thrombocytopenia, leukopenia, purpura. **Other:** Fever.

INTERACTIONS **Drug:** ACE INHIBITORS may increase adverse effects.

PHARMACOKINETICS **Absorption:** Slowly and irregularly

absorbed from IM site. **Peak:** 3–6 h. **Distribution:** Widely distributed, especially to synovial fluid, kidney, liver, and spleen; does not cross blood–brain barrier; crosses placenta. **Metabolism:** Not studied. **Elimination:** 60–90% of dose ultimately excreted in urine; also eliminated in feces; traces may be found in urine for 6 mo. **Half-Life:** 3–168 days.

NURSING IMPLICATIONS

Black Box Warning

Gold sodium thiomalate has been associated with severe and potentially fatal adverse reactions.

Assessment & Drug Effects

- Note: Rapid reduction in hemoglobin level, WBC count below 4000/mm^3, eosinophil count above 5%, and platelet count below 100,000/mm^3 signify possible toxicity.
- Interview and examine patient before each injection to detect occurrence of transient pruritus or dermatitis (both are common early indications of toxicity), stomatitis (sore tongue, palate, or throat), metallic taste, indigestion, or other signs and symptoms of possible toxicity. Interrupt treatment immediately and notify prescriber if any of these reactions occurs.
- Observe for allergic reaction, which may occur almost immediately after injection, 10 min after injection, or at any time during therapy. Withhold drug and notify prescriber if observed. Keep antidote dimercaprol (BAL) on hand during time of injection.
- Monitor lab tests: Prior to each injection, urinalysis for protein, blood, and sediment. Baseline Hgb and CBC count with differential, and platelet count before initiation of therapy and at regular intervals, LFTs, pulmonary function tests.

Patient & Family Education

- Therapeutic effects may not appear until after 2 mo of therapy.
- Notify prescriber of rapid improvement in joint swelling; this is indicative that you are closely approaching drug tolerance level.
- Use protective measures in sunlight. Exposure to sunlight may aggravate gold dermatitis.
- Notify prescriber at the appearance of unexplained skin bruising; this is always an indication for doing a platelet count.
- Know possible adverse reactions and report any symptom suggestive of toxicity immediately to prescriber: weight gain, edema, decreased appetite or foamy urine.

GOLIMUMAB

(go-li-mu′mab)

Simponi, Simponi Aria

Classification: DISEASE-MODIFYING ANTIRHEUMATIC DRUG (DMARD)

Therapeutic: IMMUNOMODULATOR; ANTIRHEUMATIC (DMARD); ANTIPSORIATIC

Prototype: Etanercept

AVAILABILITY

Solution for injection

ACTION & *THERAPEUTIC EFFECT*

A monoclonal antibody that binds to TNF-alpha, thus preventing it from binding to its receptors. TNF is a cytokine that plays an important role in the immune and inflammatory responses. Elevated levels of TNF are found in the synovial fluids, joints, and blood of rheumatoid arthritis (RA) patients. *Effectiveness is indicated by improved RA symtomatology and/or decreased inflammation in other inflammatory disorders.*

USES Treatment of moderately to severely active rheumatoid arthritis, active ankylosing spondylitis, active psoriatic arthritis and ulcerative colitis.

CONTRAINDICATIONS Hypersensitivity to golimumab; serious infection or sepsis; live vaccines; agranulocytosis; lactation (infant risk cannot be ruled out).

CAUTIOUS USE History of hepatitis B; history of TB or opportunistic infection; chronic or recurrent infections; history of HBV infection or carriers of HBV; malignancy; CHF; central or peripheral demyelization disorders, MS; cytopenias; older adults; pregnancy (fetal risk cannot be ruled out). Safe use in children not established.

ROUTE & DOSAGE

Rheumatoid Arthritis/Anklyosing Spondylitis/Psoriatic Arthritis

Adult: **Subcutaneous** 50 mg qmo; **IV (Simponi Aria)** 2 mg/kg then repeat at 4 wk and then q8 wk

Ulcerative Colitis

Adult: **Subcutaneous** 200 mg then 100 mg 2 wk later for induction, then 100 mg q4wk (starting week 6)

Rheumatoid Arthritis (Simponi Aria)

Adult: **IV** 2 mg/kg, repeat at 4 wk then q8wk or 50 mg monthly

ADMINISTRATION

Subcutaneous

- Allow prefilled syringe/autoinjector to come to room temperature for 30 min prior to injection. Do not warm any other way.
- Do not shake the autoinjector at any time. After injection, do not pull autoinjector away from skin until a second click sound (3–15 sec after the first sound) is heard.
- Rotate injection sites. Do not inject into areas that are tender, bruised, red, or hard.
- Do not initiate treatment in anyone with an active infection.

Intravenous

PREPARE: **IV Infusion:** Dilute required volume of golimumab in NS to a final volume of 100 mL. Mix gently, do not shake. Diluted solution may be stored at room temperature for 4 h.

ADMINISTER: **IV Infusion:** Give over 30 min through a nonpyrogenic, low-protein-binding filter, pore size 0.22 micrometer or less.

INCOMPATIBILITIES: Do not infuse in same IV line with other agents.

- Store refrigerated at 2°–8° C (36°–46° F) and protect from light by keeping in carton until use.

ADVERSE EFFECTS **Respiratory:** URI. **Skin:** Injection site reaction. **Hepatic:** Increased ALT/SGPT, increased AST/SGOT. **Hematologic:** Positive ANA titer. **Other:** *Infection,* antibody development.

INTERACTIONS **Drug: Abatacept, anakinra** and other TNF-ALPHA BLOCKERS or other IMMUNOSUPPRESANTS may increase the risk of serious infection.

PHARMACOKINETICS **Peak:** 2–6 days. **Half-Life:** 2 wk.

G

NURSING IMPLICATIONS

Black Box Warning

Golimumab has been associated with severe, potentially fatal, infections, and development of malignancies in children and adolescents.

Assessment & Drug Effects

- Monitor closely for S&S of infection.
- Withhold drug and notify prescriber if symptoms of an infection develop.
- Monitor for and report new-onset and exacerbations of psoriasis.
- Monitor lab tests: Baseline and periodic TB tests, CBC with differential, periodic LFTs.

Patient & Family Education

- Contact prescriber immediately for any of the following: Symptoms of infection; jaundice; extreme fatigue; poor appetite or vomiting; or pain in the upper, right abdomen.
- If a case of pre-existing psoriasis worsens or if a new rash develops, contact prescriber.

GOSERELIN ACETATE

(gos-er′e-lin)

Zoladex

Classification: ANTINEOPLASTIC; GONADOTROPIN-RELEASING HORMONE (GnRH) ANALOG

Therapeutic: ANTINEOPLASTIC; GnRH ANALOG

Prototype: Leuprolide

AVAILABILITY Subcutaneous implant

ACTION & *THERAPEUTIC EFFECT* A synthetic form of luteinizing hormone-releasing hormone (LHRH or GnRH) that inhibits pituitary gonadotropin secretion. *With chronic administration, serum testosterone levels in males fall into the range normally seen with surgically castrated men.*

USES Prostate cancer, breast cancer. Endometrial thinning agent prior to endometrial ablation for dysfunctional uterine bleeding, endometriosis, prevention of early menopause during chemotherapy.

UNLABELED USES Benign prostatic hyperplasia, uterine leiomyomas, prevention of early menopause during chemotherapy.

CONTRAINDICATIONS Known hypersensitivity to an LHRH; hypercalcemia; pregnancy (category X for endometriosis, endometrial thinning, category D for breast cancer); lactation.

CAUTIOUS USE Renal impairment; family history of osteoporosis; prostate cancer; patients at risk for spinal cord compression; DM; CVD; obesity; low BMI. Safety and efficacy in children not established.

ROUTE & DOSAGE

Prostate Cancer, Breast Cancer, Endometriosis

Adult: **Subcutaneous** 3.6 mg q28days, 10.8 mg depot q12wk

Endometrial Thinning Prior to Endometrial Ablation

Adult: **Subcutaneous** 3.6 mg (procedure performed 4 wk after administration) if second injection required then surgery performed 2–4 wk after that dose

ADMINISTRATION

Subcutaneous

- Follow manufacturer's directions exactly for implanting the drug subcutaneously in the upper abdominal wall.
- Store at room temperature not to exceed 25° C (77° F).

ADVERSE EFFECTS **CV:** Increased risk of MI (men only), *peripheral edema, vasodilation*. **CNS:** Headache, tumor flare, depression, insomnia. **Endocrine:** Gynecomastia, breast swelling and tenderness, *postmenopausal symptoms* (*hot flashes*, vaginal dryness). **Skin:** *Acne, diaphoresis, seborrhea*. **GI:** Nausea. **GU:** Vaginal spotting, breakthrough bleeding, decreased libido, *impotence*. **Musculoskeletal:** Bone pain, bone loss.

DIAGNOSTIC TEST INTERFERENCE Interferes with pituitary gonadotropic and gonadal function tests during and for 12 wk after treatment.

PHARMACOKINETICS **Absorption:** Rapidly absorbed following subcutaneous administration. **Duration:** 29 days. **Elimination:** Excreted by kidneys. **Half-Life:** 4.9 h.

NURSING IMPLICATIONS

Assessment & Drug Effects

- Monitor carefully during the first month of therapy for S&S of spinal cord compression or ureteral obstruction in patients with prostate cancer. Report immediately to prescriber.
- Anticipate a transient worsening of symptoms (e.g., bone pain) during the first weeks of therapy in patients with prostate cancer.
- Monitor lab tests: Periodic fasting blood glucose.

Patient & Family Education

- Note: Sexual dysfunction in men and hot flashes may accompany drug use.
- Notify prescriber immediately of symptoms of spinal cord compression or urinary obstruction.

GRANISETRON

(gran'i-se-tron)

Sancuso, Sustol

Classification: ANTIEMETIC; 5-HT_3 ANTAGONIST

Therapeutic: ANTIEMETIC

Prototype: Ondansetron

AVAILABILITY Tablet; solution for injection; oral solution; transdermal patch; extended release injection

ACTION & *THERAPEUTIC EFFECT* Granisetron is a selective serotonin (5-HT_3) receptor antagonist. Serotonin receptors of the 5-HT_3 type are located centrally in the chemoreceptor trigger zone, and peripherally on the vagal nerve terminals. Serotonin released from the wall of the small intestine stimulates these vagal afferent neurons through the serotonin receptors, and initiates vomiting reflex. *Effective in preventing nausea and vomiting associated with cancer chemotherapy.*

USES Chemotherapy-induced nausea/vomiting treatment and prophylaxis; radiation-induced nausea/vomiting prophylaxis.

CONTRAINDICATIONS Hypersensitivity to granisetron, or benzyl alcohol; GI obstruction; neonates.

CAUTIOUS USE Hypersensitivity to ondansetron or similar drugs; liver disease; patients with long QT interval; pregnancy (category B); lactation; children 2 y or younger.

G

ROUTE & DOSAGE

Chemotherapy-Related Nausea and Vomiting

Adult/Child (2 y or older): **IV** 10 mcg/kg, beginning at least 30 min before initiation of chemotherapy (up to 40 mcg/kg/dose has been used); **PO** 1 mg bid, start 1 mg up to 1 h prior to chemotherapy, then second tab 12 h later OR 2 mg daily
Adult: **Transdermal** Apply 1 patch q5days

Radiation-Induced Nausea/Vomiting

Adult: **PO** 2 mg dose within 1 h of radiation

Renal Impairment Dosage Adjustment

Crl Cl 30–59 mL/min: **Extended release injection** Do not administer more frequently than every 14 days

ADMINISTRATION

Oral

- Give only on the day of chemotherapy. one hour prior to chemotherapy.

Transdermal

- Apply patch to upper outer arm 24–48 h before start of chemotherapy.
- Remove patch no sooner than 24 h after completion of chemotherapy.
- Patch may be left in place for up to 7 days.

Intravenous

PREPARE: **Direct:** Give undiluted. **IV Infusion:** ▪ Dilute in NS or D5W to a total volume of 20–50 mL. ▪ Prepare infusion at time of administration; do not mix in solution with other drugs.

ADMINISTER: **Direct:** Give a single dose over 30 sec. **IV Infusion:** Infuse diluted drug over 5 min or longer; complete infusion 20–30 min prior to initiation of chemotherapy.

INCOMPATIBILITIES: **Y-site: Amphotericin B, dantrolene sodium, diazepam, gemtuzumab ozogamcin, lansprazone, phenytoin sodium.**

- Store at 15°–30° C (59°–86° F)for 24 h after dilution under normal lighting conditions.

ADVERSE EFFECTS **CNS:** *Headache,* dizziness, *somnolence,* insomnia, labile mood, anxiety, fatigue. **GI:** *Constipation,* nausea, diarrhea, elevated liver function tests. **Other:** Injection site reaction.

INTERACTIONS **Drug: Ketoconazole** may inhibit metabolism. Contraindicated with medications that prolong the QT interval (e.g., **bepridil, dofetilide, fluconazole**).

PHARMACOKINETICS **Onset:** Several minutes. **Duration:** Approximately 24 h. **Distribution:** Widely distributed in body tissues. **Metabolism:** Appears to be metabolized in liver. **Elimination:** Excreted in urine as metabolites. **Half-Life:** 10–11 h in cancer patients, 4–5 h in healthy volunteers.

NURSING IMPLICATIONS

Assessment & Drug Effects

- Monitor the frequency and severity of nausea and vomiting.
- Monitor for constipation and for decreased bowel activity.
- Assess for headache, which usually responds to nonnarcotic analgesics.
- Monitor lab tests: Periodic LFTs.

Patient & Family Education

- Note: Headache requiring an analgesic for relief is a common adverse effect.
- Learn ways to manage constipation.

GRISEOFULVIN

(gri-see-oh-ful′vin)

Classification: ANTIFUNGAL ANTIBIOTIC

Therapeutic: ANTIFUNGAL

AVAILABILITY **Griseofulvin Microsize:** Suspension. **Griseofulvin Ultramicrosize:** Tablet

ACTION & *THERAPEUTIC EFFECT* Arrests metaphase of cell division by disrupting mitotic spindle structure in fungal cells. Deposits in keratin precursor cells and has special affinity for diseased tissue. It is tightly bound to new keratin of skin, hair, and nails that becomes highly resistant to fungal invasion. *Effective against various species of* Epidermophyton, Microsporum, *and* Trichophyton *(has no effect on other fungi, including* Candida, *bacteria, and yeasts).*

USES Mycotic disease of skin, hair, and nails not adequately treated by conventional topical measures.

CONTRAINDICATIONS Hypersensitivity to griseofulvin; porphyria; hepatocellular failure; SLE; serious skin reaction to drug; pregnancy (X) - may cause fetal harm; lactation—infant risk cannot be ruled out, prophylaxis against fungal infections.

CAUTIOUS USE Penicillin-sensitive patients (possibility if cross-sensitivity with penicillin exists; however, reportedly penicillin-sensitive patients have been treated without difficulty); hepatic impairment; existing lupus erythematosus, children 2 y or younger.

ROUTE & DOSAGE

Dermatophyte infection

Adult: **PO** 500 mg microsize or 375 mg ultramicrosize daily in single or divided doses
Child: **PO** 20–25 mg/kg/day microsize or 10–15 mg/kg/day ultramicrosize in single or divided doses

ADMINISTRATION

Oral

- Give with or after meals to allay GI disturbances.
- Give the microsize formulations with a high fat content meal (increases drug absorption rate) to enhance serum levels. Consult prescriber.
- Tablets may be swallowed whole or crushed and sprinkled over 1 tablespoonful of applesauce and swallowed immediately without chewing.
- Store at 15°–30° C (59°–86° F) in tightly covered containers unless otherwise directed.

ADVERSE EFFECTS **CNS:** *Severe headache.* **Skin:** Photosensitivity, rash and urticaria. **GI:** Nausea, vomiting, diarrhea.

INTERACTIONS **Drug: Alcohol** may cause flushing and tachycardia; BARBITURATES may decrease activity of griseofulvin; may decrease hypoprothrombinemic effects of ORAL ANTICOAGULANTS; may increase **estrogen** metabolism, resulting in breakthrough bleeding, and decrease contraceptive efficacy of ORAL CONTRACEPTIVES. Photosensitizing agents can have increased effect. Avoid use with **ulipristal**, Saccaromyces boulardii.

PHARMACOKINETICS **Absorption:** Absorbed primarily from duodenum; microsize is variably and unpredictably absorbed; ultramicrosize is almost completely absorbed. **Distribution:** Concentrates in skin, hair, nails, fat, and skeletal muscle; crosses placenta. **Metabolism:** In liver. **Elimination:** Mainly in urine and feces. **Half-Life:** 9–24 h.

NURSING IMPLICATIONS

G

Assessment & Drug Effects

- Inquire about history of sensitivity to griseofulvin, penicillins, or other allergies prior to initiating treatment.
- Monitor food intake. Drug may alter taste sensations, and this may cause appetite suppression and inadequate nutrient intake.
- Monitor lab tests: WBC with differential at least once weekly during first month of therapy; periodic renal function tests and LFTs.

Patient & Family Education

- Continuing treatment as prescribed to prevent relapse, even if you experience symptomatic relief after 48–96 h of therapy.
- Review adverse effects with patient and/or caregivers.
- Note: Duration of treatment depends on time required to replace infected skin, hair, or nails, and thus varies with infection site. Average duration of treatment for tinea capitis (scalp ringworm), 4–6 wk; tinea corporis (body ringworm), 2–4 wk; tinea pedis (athlete's foot), 4–8 wk; tinea unguium (nail fungus), at least 4 mo for fingernails, depending on rate of growth, and 6 mo or more for toenails.
- Avoid exposure to intense natural or artificial sunlight, because photo-sensitivity-type reactions may occur. Use sunscreen and avoid tanning beds.
- Note: Headaches often occur during early therapy but frequently disappear with continued drug administration.
- Avoid alcohol while taking this drug. Disulfiram-type reaction (see Appendix F) are possible with ingestion of alcohol during therapy.
- Pharmacologic effects of oral contraceptives may be reduced. Breakthrough bleeding and pregnancy may occur. Alternative forms of birth control should be used during therapy and for 1-month post therapy for females and 6 months post therapy for males.

GUAIFENESIN (Pr)

(gwye-fen′e-sin)

Anti-Tuss, GG-Cen, Glyceryl Guaiacolate, Glycotuss, Glytuss, Guiatuss, Humibid, Hytuss, Malotuss, Mytussin, Mucinex, Resyl ♣, Robitussin

Classification: EXPECTORANT

Therapeutic: EXPECTORANT

AVAILABILITY Syrup; oral liquid; tablet; sustained release tablet

ACTION & *THERAPEUTIC EFFECT* Reduces viscosity of respiratory secretions and increases sputum volume, thus increasing the efficiency of the cough reflex and of ciliary action in removing accumulated secretions from the trachea and bronchi. *Increases respiratory tract fluid secretions and helps to loosen phlegm and bronchial secretions.*

USES To combat dry, nonproductive cough associated with colds and bronchitis. A common ingredient in cough mixtures.

CONTRAINDICATIONS Hypersensitivity to guaifenesin; cough due to CHF, ACE inhibitor therapy, or tobacco smoking.

 Common adverse effects in *italic*; life-threatening effects underlined; generic names in **bold**; classifications in SMALL CAPS; ♣ Canadian drug name; (Pr) Prototype drug; ⚠ Alert

CAUTIOUS USE Chronic cough; asthma; pregnancy (category C); lactation; children younger than 6 y.

ROUTE & DOSAGE

Cough

Adult/Adolescent: **PO Immediate release** 200–400 mg q4h up to 2.4 g/day; **Extended release** 600–1200 mg q12h up to 2.4 g/day
Child (6–11 y): **PO** 100–200 mg q4h up to 1.2 g/day or **Extended release** 600 mg q12h
Child (2–5 y): **PO Immediate release** 50–100 mg q4h; **PO Extended release** 300 mg q12h

ADMINISTRATION

Oral

- Ensure that sustained release form of drug is not chewed or crushed. It **must be** swallowed whole.
- Follow dose with a full glass of water if not contraindicated.
- Carefully observe maximum daily doses for adults and children.

ADVERSE EFFECTS **CNS:** Drowsiness. **GI:** Low incidence of nausea.

DIAGNOSTIC TEST INTERFERENCE May produce color interference with determinations of ***urinary 5-hydro-xyindoleacetic acid (5-HIAA)*** and ***vanillylmandelic acid (VMA).***

PHARMACOKINETICS **Absorption:** Well absorbed. **Elimination:** In urine

NURSING IMPLICATIONS

Assessment & Drug Effects

- Monitor for therapeutic effectiveness. Persistent cough may indicate a serious condition requiring further diagnostic work.
- Notify prescriber if high fever, rash, or headaches develop.

Patient & Family Education

- Increase fluid intake to help loosen mucus; drink at least 8 glasses of fluid daily.
- Contact prescriber if cough persists beyond 1 wk.
- Contact prescriber if high fever, rash, or headache develops.

GUANFACINE HYDROCHLORIDE

(gwahn'fa-seen)

Intuniv, Tenex

Classification: ALPHA-ADRENERGIC AGONIST; CENTRAL-ACTING ANTIHYPERTENSIVE
Therapeutic: ANTIHYPERTENSIVE
Prototype: Methyldopa

AVAILABILITY Tablet; extended release tablet

ACTION & *THERAPEUTIC EFFECT* In cerebral cortex, stimulation of alpha$_2$-adrenoreceptors triggers inhibitory neurons to reduce central sympathetic outflow (i.e., impulses from vasomotor center to heart and blood vessels). **Extended release form:** Targets ADHD symptoms through central alpha$_2$-receptor activity in the prefrontal cortex. *Results in decreased peripheral vascular resistance, thus lowering blood pressure, and a slightly reduced (5 bpm) heart rate. Minimizes the signs and symptoms of ADHD in children.*

USES Management of mild-to-moderate hypertension; attention deficit hyperactivity disorder (ADHD) (**extended release form** only).

UNLABELED USES Adjunct in heroin withdrawal; Tourette's syndrome.

CONTRAINDICATIONS Hypersensitivity to guanfacine; treatment of acute hypertension associated with toxemia of pregnancy; psychiatric disorders that mimic ADHD.

CAUTIOUS USE Severe coronary insufficiency, recent MI, cerebrovascular disease; chronic renal or hepatic failure; older adult; pregnancy (category B); lactation; children younger than 6 y (**extended release form**).

ROUTE & DOSAGE

Hypertension

Adult: **PO** 1 mg/day at bedtime, may be gradually increased to 3 mg/day if needed

Attention Deficit Hyperactivity Disorder

Adolescent/Child (6 y or older): **PO Extended release** 1 mg daily, titrate up based on response (normal range: 1–4 mg daily)

ADMINISTRATION

Oral

- Ensure that extended release tablets are swallowed whole and not crushed or chewed.
- Usually given as a single dose at bedtime to reduce effect of somnolence.
- Discontinue treatment gradually with planned tapering of schedule.
- Store tablets at 15°–30° C (59°–86° F) in tightly closed container; protect from light.

ADVERSE EFFECTS **CV:** Bradycardia, palpitation, substernal pain, arrhythmia exacerbation. **Respiratory:** Bronchospasm. **CNS:** Confusion, amnesia, mental depression, drowsiness, *dizziness, sedation,* headache, asthenia, *fatigue,* insomnia, nightmares. **HEENT:** Rhinitis, tinnitus, taste change; vision disturbances, conjunctivitis, iritis. **Skin:** Dermatitis, pruritus, purpura, sweating. **GI:** *Dry mouth, constipation,* abdominal pain, diarrhea, dysphagia, nausea. **GU:** *Impotence,* testicular disorder, urinary incontinence. **Musculoskeletal:** Leg cramps, hypokinesia. **Other:** Dyspnea.

INTERACTIONS **Drug: Alcohol** and other CNS DEPRESSANTS compound sedation and CNS depression. May increase **valproic acid** levels. Use cautiously with MAO INHIBITORS or CYP3A4 INHIBITORS or INDUCERS. **Conivaptan** can cause increased hypotension.

PHARMACOKINETICS **Absorption:** Readily absorbed from GI tract; 70% protein bound. **Onset:** 2 h; 6 h (extended release). **Peak:** 6 h. **Duration:** Up to 24 h. **Distribution:** Crosses placenta. **Metabolism:** In liver. **Elimination:** 80% ActHIB, Hiberix, Liquid PedvaxHIB in the urine in 24 h. **Half-Life:** 17 h.

NURSING IMPLICATIONS

Assessment & Drug Effects

- Do not discontinue abruptly; may cause plasma and urinary catecholamine increases leading to symptoms of tachycardia, insomnia, anxiety, nervousness. Rebound hypertension (i.e., increases in BP to levels significantly greater than those before therapy) may occur 2–7 days after abrupt drug withdrawal, but serious effects rarely develop.
- Monitor BP until it is stabilized. Report a rise in pressure that occurs toward end of dose interval;

a divided dose schedule may be ordered.

- Assess mental status and alertness. Adverse effects tend to be dose-dependent, increasing significantly with doses above 3 mg/day.

Patient & Family Education

- Continue drug even after you feel well. This is a maintenance dosage regimen (dose and dose intervals). If 2 or more doses are missed, consult prescriber about how to re-establish dosage regimen.
- Employ measures to keep mouth moist; saliva substitutes (e.g., Moi-Stir, Xero-Lube) are available OTC. If dry mouth persists longer than 2 wk, patient should check with dentist.
- Do not drive or engage in other potentially hazardous tasks requiring alertness until response to drug is known.
- Avoid alcohol and do not self-medicate with OTC drugs such as sleeping medications, or cough medications without consulting prescriber.

GUSELKUMAB

(gue-sel-koo′mab)

Tremfya

Classification: ANTIPSORIATIC AGENT; MONOCLONAL ANTIBODY; INTERLEUKIN-23 INHIBITOR

Therapeutic: ANTIPSORIATIC

AVAILABILITY Subcutaneous injection, prefilled syringe

ACTION & *THERAPEUTIC EFFECT* Human monoclonal IgG1 antibody that selectively binds with interleukin-23 receptor to inhibit the release of proinflammatory cytokines and chemokines. *Reduces inflammatory response in adults with moderate to severe plaque psoriasis.*

USES Treatment of moderate to severe plaque psoriasis in patients who are candidates for systemic therapy or phototherapy. Treatment of psoriatic arthritis.

CONTRAINDICATION Patients with active TB, Patients with active infections.

CAUTIOUS USE Pregnancy—fetal risk cannot be ruled out; lactation—infant risk cannot be ruled out. Safety and efficacy in children not established.

ROUTE & DOSAGE

Psoriasis/Psoriatic Arthritis

Adult: **Subcutaneous** 100 mg at wk 0, 4, and then every 8 wk thereafter

ADMINISTRATION

Subcutaneous

- Allow prefilled syringe to reach room temperature for approximately 30 min prior to use.
- Administer subcutaneously into the thigh, abdomen more than 2 in from umbilicus, or outer upper arm.
- Do not inject into tissue that is tender, bruised, red, hard, scaly, or affected by psoriasis.
- Store in original carton in temperatures between 2 and 8°C (36 and 46°F). Protect from light. Do not freeze or shake.

ADVERSE EFFECTS (>5%) **Respiratory:** *URI.* **Other:** *Infection.*

INTERACTIONS **Drug:** Avoid use of LIVE VACCINES in patients treated with guselkumab. Potential interaction for drugs metabolized by CYP450 enzymes, however no specific medications identified in clinical studies. Do not use with IMMUNOSUPRESSANTS. **Herbal:** Do not use with Echinacea.

PHARMACOKINETICS **Absorption:** 49% bioavailability. **Onset:** Peak in 5.5 days. **Metabolism:** Similar to endogenous IgG. **Half-Life:** 15–18 days.

NURSING IMPLICATIONS

Assessment & Drug Effects

- Evaluate for tuberculosis infection prior to treatment.
- Monitor for signs of infection including active tuberculosis.

Patient & Family Education

- Notify prescriber if you experience signs or symptoms of allergic reaction such as rash, hives, itching, shortness of breath, wheezing, cough, swelling of the face, lips, tongue, or throat; or any other signs.
- Report any signs of infection: fever, malaise, inflammation, etc.
- Have patient perform return demonstration for correct subcutaneous injections.
- Avoid live vaccines during therapy.
- Prior to initiating treatment, notify prescriber if you have active TB.

HAEMOPHILUS b CONJUGATE VACCINE (Hib)

(hee-mof′il-us)

ActHIB, Hiberix, PedvaxHIB

See Appendix J.

HALCINONIDE

(hal-sin′oh-nide)

Halog

Classification: ANTI-INFLAMMATORY; FLUORINATED STEROID

Therapeutic: ANTI-INFLAMMATORY

Prototype: Hydrocortisone

AVAILABILITY Ointment; cream; external solution

ACTION & THERAPEUTIC EFFECT Fluorinated steroid with substituted 17-hydroxyl group. Crosses cell membranes, complexes with nuclear DNA and stimulates synthesis of enzymes thought to be responsible for anti-inflammatory effects. *Exhibits anti-inflammatory, antipyretic, and vasocontrictive properties.*

USES Relief of pruritic and inflammatory manifestations of corticosteroid-responsive dermatoses.

CONTRAINDICATIONS Hypersensitivity to drug or other corticosteroids; Use on large body surface area; uncontrolled infection; long-term use.

CAUTIOUS USE Diabetes mellitus; older adults; patients with liver failure; skin abrasion; children; pregnancy—fetal risk cannot be ruled out; lactation—infant risk cannot be ruled out.

ROUTE & DOSAGE

Inflammation

Adult: **Topical** Apply thin layer bid or tid

Child: **Topical** Apply thin layer once or twice per day for minimum number of days

ADMINISTRATION

Topical

- Wash skin gently and dry thoroughly before each application.
- Note: Ointment is preferred for dry scaly lesions. Moist lesions are best treated with solution.
- Do not apply in or around the eyes.
- Do not apply occlusive dressings over areas covered with halcinonide unless specifically prescribed.
- Store at 15°–30° C (59°–86° F). Do not refrigerate.

ADVERSE EFFECTS **Endocrine:** Reversible HPA axis suppression, hyperglycemia, glycosuria. **Skin:** Burning, itching, irritation, dryness.

INTERACTIONS **Drug:** Do not use with **aldesleukin.**

PHARMACOKINETICS **Absorption:** Depends on amount applied, skin integrity and use of occlusive dressing. **Metabolism:** Hepatic.

NURSING IMPLICATIONS

Assessment & Drug Effects

- Discontinue if signs of infection or irritation occur.
- Monitor for systemic corticosteroid effects that may occur with occlusive dressings or topical applications over large areas of skin.
- Monitor hypothalamic-pituitary-adrenal (HPA) axis suppression test.

Patient & Family Education

- Do not use an occlusive dressing with this drug unless specifically directed to do so by prescriber.
- Wash your hands before and after applying this topical medicine.
- Do not get any of the medication in your eyes. If you do, rinse it out with plenty of cool tap water.
- Report signs/symptom of HPA axis suppression: fatigue, anxiety, depression, hyperglycemia, muscle weakness.

HALOPERIDOL ⓟ

(ha-loe-per'i-dole)

Haldol, Peridol ♣

HALOPERIDOL DECANOATE

Classification: ANTIPSYCHOTIC; BUTYROPHENONE

Therapeutic: ANTIPSYCHOTIC

AVAILABILITY Tablet; oral solution; solution for injection

ACTION & THERAPEUTIC EFFECT It is theorized that haloperidol blocks postsynaptic dopamine (D_2) receptors in the limbic system of the brain. Decrease in dopamine neurotransmission has been correlated with its antipsychotic effects, and its higher instance of extrapyramidal effects. The exact mechanism of action is unknown. *Decreases psychotic manifestations and exerts strong antiemetic effect.*

USES Management of schizophrenia and Tourette's syndrome; nonpsychotic behavioral disorders; hyperactivity.

UNLABELED USES chemotherapy induced breakthrough nausea/vomiting; bipolar disorder.

CONTRAINDICATIONS Parkinson disease, seizure disorders, coma; hypersensitivity to haloperidol, older adults with dementia-related psychosis; severe toxic CNS depression; Parkinson disease; severe neutropenia (ANC less than 1000/mm^3); alcoholism; severe mental depression, CNS depression; signs and symptoms of neuroleptic malignant syndrome (NMS); bronchopneumonia; pregnancy—fetal risk cannot be ruled out; lactation—infant risk cannot be ruled out.

CAUTIOUS USE Cyclic mood disorders; older adult or debilitated patients, urinary retention, pulmonary disease; history of hypocalcemia; glaucoma, severe cardiovascular disorders, long QT syndrome, AV block, bundle-branch block, cardiac arrhythmias, uncompensated heart failure, recent acute MI; hematologic disease; thyrotoxicosis, hypothyroidism, hypokalemia, hypomagnesemia; debilitated patients; history of seizures. Safe use in children younger than 3 y is not established.

ROUTE & DOSAGE

Schizophrenia

Adult:/Adolescent **PO/IV/IM** 2–10 mg/day in single or divided doses **Decanoate:** 10–20 × daily oral dose **haloperidol** equivalents (see package insert for conversion tables)

Bipolar Disorder

Adult: **PO** 2–15 mg/day or 0.2 mg/kg/day (up to 15 mg/day) in 1–2 doses

Tourette's Disorder

Adult: **PO** 1–2 mg/day in 1–3 divided doses

Child(3–12 y and 15–40 kg): **PO** 0.5 mg/day in 2–3 divided doses; may be increased by 0.5 mg q5–7days to 0.05–0.075 mg/kg/day in divided doses

Nonpsychotic behavior disorders

Child (3–12 y and 15–40 kg): **PO** 0.5 mg/day in 2–3 divided doses, may be increased by 0.5 mg q5–7days to 0.05–0.15 mg/kg/day in divided doses

Pharmacogenetic Dosage Adjustment

CYP3D6 poor metabolizers: reduce dose by 50%

H

ADMINISTRATION

Oral

- Give with a full glass (240 mL) of water or with food or milk.
- Taper dosing regimen when discontinuing therapy. Abrupt termination can initiate extrapyramidal symptoms.
- Store at controlled room temperature between 20 and 25 degrees C (68 and 77 degrees F), in a tight, light-resistant container; do not freeze and protect from light.

Intramuscular

- Give by deep injection into a large muscle. Do not exceed 3 mL/injection site. A 21-guage needle is recommended. Initial doses greater than 100 mg should be administered 3–7 days apart.
- Have patient recumbent at time of parenteral administration and for about 1 h after injection. Assess for orthostatic hypotension.
- Store in light-resistant container at 15°–30° C (59°–86° F), unless otherwise specified by manufacturer. Discard darkened solutions. Do not freeze and protect from light.

ADVERSE EFFECTS **CV:** Hypotension. **CNS:** *Extrapyramidal reactions:* Parkinsonian symptoms, dystonia, akathisia, tardive dyskinesia (after long-term use); drowsiness, lethargy, fatigue. **HEENT:** *Blurred vision.* **GI:** *Dry mouth,* constipation.

INTERACTIONS **Drug:** CNS DEPRESSANTS, OPIATES, **alcohol** increase CNS depression; may antagonize activity of ORAL ANTICOAGULANTS; ANTICHOLINERGICS may have increased adverse effects; **methyldopa** may precipitate dementia. May increase concentration of CYP3A4 substrates. May reduce effect of ANTIPARKINSON AGENTS. **Cabergoline** may decrease effect of haldoperidol.

PHARMACOKINETICS **Absorption:** Well absorbed from GI tract; 60% reaches systemic circulation; 92% protein bound. **Onset:** 30 min IM. **Peak:** 4–6 h PO; 10–20 min IM; 6–7 days decanoate. **Distribution:** Distributes mainly to liver with lower concentration in brain, lung, kidney, spleen, heart. **Metabolism:** In liver via CYP 3A4. **Elimination:** 30% excreted in urine.

NURSING IMPLICATIONS

Black Box Warning

Haloperidol has been associated with increased mortality in older adults with dementia-related psychosis.

Assessment & Drug Effects

- Monitor for therapeutic effectiveness. Because of long half-life, therapeutic effects are slow to develop in early therapy or when established dosing regimen is changed. "Therapeutic window" effect (point at which increased dose or concentration actually decreases therapeutic response) may occur after long period of high doses. Close observation is imperative when doses are changed.
- Fall risk—particularly elderly patients.
- Monitor blood pressure, heart rate, and symptoms of hypotension.
- Monitor patient's mental status daily. Target symptoms expected to decrease with successful haloperidol treatment include hallucinations, insomnia, hostility, agitation, and delusions.
- Monitor for neuroleptic malignant syndrome (NMS) (see Appendix F), especially in those with hypertension or taking lithium. Symptoms of NMS can appear suddenly after initiation of therapy or after months or years of taking neuroleptic (antipsychotic) medication. Immediately discontinue drug if NMS suspected.
- Monitor for parkinsonism and tardive dyskinesia (see Appendix F). Risk of tardive dyskinesia appears to be greater in women receiving high doses and in older adults. It can occur after long-term therapy and even after therapy is discontinued.
- Monitor for extrapyramidal (neuromuscular) reactions that occur frequently during first few days of treatment. Symptoms are usually dose related and are controlled by dosage reduction or concomitant administration of antiparkinson drugs.
- Be alert for behavioral changes in patients who are concurrently receiving antiparkinson drugs.
- Monitor for exacerbation of seizure activity.
- Monitor for muscle rigidity.
- Observe patients closely for rapid mood shift to depression when haloperidol is used to control mania or cyclic disorders. Depression may represent a drug adverse effect or reversion from a manic state.
- Monitor lab tests: Periodic WBC with differential urinalysis and LFTs with prolonged therapy.

Patient & Family Education

- Avoid use of alcohol and other CNS depressants during therapy.
- Review adverse effects.
- Do not drive or engage in other potentially hazardous activities until response to drug is known.
- Discuss oral hygiene with healthcare provider; dry mouth may promote dental problems. Drink adequate fluids.
- Avoid activities that lead to an increase in core temperature: strenuous exercise, exposure to extreme heat, or dehydration.

- Move from lying to sitting to standing positions slowly
- Avoid overexposure to sun or sunlamp and use a sunscreen; drug can cause a photosensitivity reaction.
- Do not stop drug suddenly.

HEPARIN SODIUM

(hep′a-rin)

Hepalean ♣, Heparin Sodium Lock Flush Solution, Hep-Lock

Classification: ANTICOAGULANT

Therapeutic: ANTICOAGULANT

H

AVAILABILITY Solution for injection

ACTION & *THERAPEUTIC EFFECT* Exerts direct effect on the cascade of blood coagulation by enhancing the inhibitory actions of antithrombin III (heparin cofactor) on several factors essential to normal blood clotting. This blocks the conversion of prothrombin to thrombin and fibri-nogen to fibrin. *Inhibits formation of new clots. Has rapid anticoagulant effect. Does not lyse already existing thrombi but may prevent their extension and propagation.*

USES Prophylaxis and treatment of venous thrombosis and pulmonary embolism and to prevent thromboembolic complications arising from cardiac and vascular surgery, frostbite, and during acute stage of MI. Also used in treatment of disseminated intravascular coagulation (DIC), atrial fibrillation with embolization, and as anticoagulant in blood transfusions, extracorporeal circulation, and dialysis procedures.

UNLABELED USES Prophylaxis in hip and knee surgery. Heparin Sodium Lock Flush Solution is used to maintain potency of indwelling IV catheters in intermittent IV therapy or blood sampling. It is not intended for anticoagulant therapy.

CONTRAINDICATIONS History of hypersensitivity to heparin (white clot syndrome); uncontrollable bleeding state, except when due to DIC; active bleeding, severe thrombocytopenia; patients in whom suitable blood coagulation tests cannot be performed; ascorbic acid deficiency; active or angiodysplasitic GI disorders including ulcerative lesions; suspected intracranial hemorrhage, severe uncontrolled hypertension; shock; pregnancy when using formulation with bentyl alcohol; lactation for premature infants or neonates if using formulation with bentyl alcohol.

CAUTIOUS USE Alcoholism; history of allergy; immediate postpartum period; high risk factors for bleeding including subacute bacterial endocarditis, congenital or acquired bleeding disorders; history of hemorrhagic stroke; advanced kidney, liver, or biliary disease; active tuberculosis; bacterial endocarditis; recent GI bleeding; recent evasive surgery; recent surgery of eye, brain, spinal cord or spinal tap; patients older than 60 y especially women; reduced bone density; patients in hazardous occupations; cerebral embolism; pregnancy (category C); lactation; children.

ROUTE & DOSAGE

Treatment of Arterial Thromboembolism

Adult: **IV** 80 units/kg bolus then 18 units/kg/h infusion dose adjusted to maintain desired aPTT; **Subcutaneous**

10,000–20,000 units followed by 8000–20,000 units q8–12h
Child: **IV** 50 units/kg bolus, then 20,000 units/m^2/24 h or 50–100 units/kg q4h

Open Heart Surgery

Adult: **IV** 150–400 units/kg

Prophylaxis of Embolism

Adult: **Subcutaneous** 5000 units q8–12h until patient is ambulatory

ADMINISTRATION

- Note: Before administration, check coagulation test values; if results are not within therapeutic range, notify prescriber for dosage adjustment.
- Do not use solutions of heparin or heparin lock-flush that contain benzyl alcohol preservative in neonates.

Subcutaneous

- Use more concentrated heparin solutions for subcutaneous injection.
- Make injections into the fatty layer of the abdomen or just above the iliac crest. Avoid injecting within 5 cm (2 in.) of umbilicus or in a bruised area. Insert needle into tissue roll perpendicular to skin surface. Do not withdraw plunger to check entry into blood vessel.
- Systematically rotate injection sites and keep record.
- Exercise caution to avoid IM injection.

Intravenous

PREPARE: **Direct:** Give undiluted. **Intermittent/Continuous:** ▪ May add to any amount of NS, D5W, or LR for injection. ▪ Invert IV solution container at least 6 × to ensure adequate mixing.

ADMINISTER: **Direct:** Give a single dose over 60 sec. **Intermittent/Continuous (*preferred*):** Use infusion pump to give at ordered rate.

INCOMPATIBILITIES: **Solution/additive:** **Alteplase, amikacin, atracurium, ciprofloxacin, codeine, cytarabine, daunorubicin, dobutamine, epirubicin, erythromycin, gentamicin, hyaluronidase, hydrocortisone, kanamycin, levorphanol, meper-idine, morphine, netilmicin, polymyxin B, promethazine, streptomycin, tobramycin, vancomycin.** **Y-site:** **Alteplase, amiodarone, amphotericin B cholesteryl, amsacrine, capreomycin, caspofungin, ciprofloxacin, clarithromycin, dacarbazine, dantrolene, daunorubicin, diazepam, diazoxide, dimenhydrinate, dobutamine, dolasetron, doxorubicin, doxycycline, droperidol, epirubicin, ergotamine, filgrastim, garenoxacin, gatifloxacin, gentamicin, haloperidol, hydroxyzine, idarubicin, isosorbide, ketamine, levofloxacin, methotrimeprazine, mexiletine, mitoxantrone, mycophenolate, netilmicin, oritavancin, palifermin, papaverine, pentamidine, phenytoin, polymyxin B, posaconazole, propafenone, protamine, quinupristin/dalfoprisin, retaplase, streptomycin, tobramycin, tramadol, triflupromazine, vancomycin, vinorelbine.**

- Store at 15°–30° C (59°–86° F). Protect from freezing.

ADVERSE EFFECTS

Endocrine: Osteoporosis, hypoaldosteronism, suppressed renal function, hyperkalemia; rebound hyperlipidemia

H

(following termination of heparin therapy). **Skin:** Injection site reactions: Pain, itching, ecchymoses, tissue irritation and sloughing; cyanosis and pains in arms or legs (vasospasm), reversible transient alopecia (usually around temporal area). **GI:** Increased AST, ALT. **GU:** Priapism (rare). **Hematologic:** Spontaneous bleeding, *transient* thrombocytopenia, hypofibrinogenemia, "white clot syndrome." **Other:** Fever, chills, urticaria, pruritus, skin rashes, itching and burning sensations of feet, numbness and tingling of hands and feet, elevated BP, headache, nasal congestion, lacrimation, conjunctivitis, chest pains, arthralgia, bronchospasm, anaphylactoid reactions.

DIAGNOSTIC TEST INTERFERENCE Notify laboratory that patient is receiving heparin, when a test is to be performed. Possibility of false-positive rise in ***BSP*** test and in ***serum thyroxine;*** and increases in ***resin T_3 uptake;*** false-negative ***^{125}I fibrinogen uptake.*** Heparin prolongs ***PT.*** Valid readings may be obtained by drawing blood samples at least 4–6 h after an IV dose (but at any time during heparin infusion) and 12–24 h after a subcutaneous heparin dose.

INTERACTIONS Drug: May prolong PT, which is used to monitor therapy with ORAL ANTICOAGULANTS; **aspirin,** NSAIDS increase risk of bleeding; **nitroglycerin** IV may decrease anticoagulant activity; **protamine** antagonizes effects of heparin. **Herbal: Evening primrose oil, feverfew, ginkgo, ginger** may potentiate bleeding.

PHARMACOKINETICS Onset: 20–60 min subcutaneous. **Peak:** Within minutes. **Duration:** 2–6 h IV; 8–12 h subcutaneous. **Distribution:** Does not cross placenta; not distributed into breast milk. **Metabolism:** In liver and by reticuloendothelial system. **Elimination:** In urine. **Half-Life:** 90 min.

NURSING IMPLICATIONS

Assessment & Drug Effects

- Monitor aPTT levels closely.
- Note: In general, dosage is adjusted to keep aPTT between 1.5–2.5 × normal control level.
- Draw blood for coagulation test 30 min before each scheduled subcutaneous or intermittent IV dose and approximately q4h for patients receiving continuous IV heparin during dosage adjustment period. After dosage is established, tests may be done once daily.
- Patients vary widely in their reaction to heparin; risk of hemorrhage appears greatest in women, all patients older than 60 y, and patients with liver disease or renal insufficiency.
- Monitor vital signs. Report fever, drop in BP, rapid pulse, and other S&S of hemorrhage.
- Observe all needle sites daily for hematoma and signs of inflammation (swelling, heat, redness, pain).
- Antidote: Have on hand protamine sulfate (1% solution), specific heparin antagonist.
- Monitor lab tests: Baseline coagulation tests, Hct, Hgb, RBC, and platelet counts prior to initiation of therapy and at regular intervals throughout therapy.

Patient & Family Education

- Protect from injury and notify prescriber of pink, red, dark brown, or cloudy urine; red or dark brown vomitus; red or black stools; bleeding gums or oral mucosa; ecchymoses, hematoma, epistaxis, bloody sputum; chest pain; abdominal or lumbar pain or swelling; unusual increase in menstrual flow; pelvic pain; severe or continuous headache, faintness, or dizziness.

- Note: Menstruation may be somewhat increased and prolonged; usually, this is not a contraindication to continued therapy if bleeding is not excessive.
- Learn correct technique for subcutaneous administration if discharged from hospital on heparin.
- Engage in normal activities such as shaving with a safety razor in the absence of a low platelet (thrombocyte) count. Usually, heparin does not affect bleeding time.
- Caution: Smoking and alcohol consumption may alter response to heparin and are not advised.
- Do not take aspirin or any other OTC medication without prescriber's approval.

HEPATITIS A VACCINE

(hep'a-ti-tis)

Havrix, Vaqta

See Appendix J.

HEPATITIS B IMMUNE GLOBULIN

(hep'a-ti-tis)

HepaGam B, HyperHep, Nabi-HB

See Appendix J.

HEPATITIS B VACCINE (RECOMBINANT)

(hep'a-ti-tis)

Engerix-B, Recombivax HB

See Appendix J.

HETASTARCH

(het'a-starch)

Hespan

Classification: PLASMA EXPANDER

Therapeutic: PLASMA EXPANDER

Prototype: Albumin

AVAILABILITY Solution for injection

ACTION & *THERAPEUTIC EFFECT*

Synthetic starch closely resembling human glycogen. Acts much like albumin and dextran but is claimed to be less likely to produce anaphylaxis or to interfere with cross matching or blood typing procedures. *May prolong the aPTT and PT. In hypovolemic patients, it increases arterial and venous pressures, heart rate, cardiac output, urine output, as well as colloidal osmotic pressure.*

USES Treatment of hypovolemia, leukapheresis.

UNLABELED USES As a priming fluid in pump oxygenators for perfusion during extracorporeal circulation and as a cryoprotective agent for long-term storage of whole blood.

CONTRAINDICATIONS Hypersensitivity to hetastarch; severe bleeding disorders, CHF, severe liver disease; treatment of shock not accompanied by hypovolemia; critically ill adult patients; renal disease with oliguria or anuria not related to hypovolemia; intracranial bleeding; critically ill including those with sepsis.

CAUTIOUS USE Hepatic or renal insufficiency, pulmonary edema in the very young or older adults, fluid overload; CABG surgery; patients on sodium restriction; pregnancy (category C); lactation. Safe use in children is not established.

ROUTE & DOSAGE

Hypovolemia

Adult: **IV** 500–1000 mL or 20 mL/kg/day (max: 1500 mL/day)

Leukapheresis

Adult: **IV** 250–750 mL infused at a constant fixed ratio of 1:8 to venous whole blood

Renal Impairment Dosage Adjustment

CrCl less than 10 mL/min: Use original initial dose, then reduce doses by 25–50%

ADMINISTRATION

Intravenous

PREPARE: **IV Infusion:** Use undiluted as prepared by manufacturer. ***ADMINISTER:*** **IV Infusion:** Specific flow rate is prescribed by prescriber. Rate may be as high as 20 mL/kg/h in acute hemorrhagic shock. ▪ Rate is usually reduced in patients with burns or septic shock.
INCOMPATIBILITIES: **Y-site:** Varies based on manufacturer consult package insert.

▪ Store at room temperature; avoid extremes of heat or cold. ▪ Discard partially used bags.

ADVERSE EFFECTS **CV:** Peripheral edema, circulatory overload, heart failure. **Hematologic:** With large volumes, prolongation of PT, PTT, clotting time, and bleeding time; decreased Hct, Hgb, platelets, calcium, and fibrinogen; dilution of plasma proteins, hyperbilirubinemia, increased sedimentation rate. **Other:** Pruritus, anaphylactoid reactions (periorbital edema, urticaria, wheezing), vomiting, mild fever, chills, influenza-like symptoms, headache, muscle pains, submaxillary and parotid glandular swelling.

PHARMACOKINETICS **Duration:** 24–36 h. **Distribution:** Remains in intravascular space. **Metabolism:** In reticuloendothelial system. **Elimination:** In urine with some biliary excretion.

NURSING IMPLICATIONS

Assessment & Drug Effects

Black Box Warning

Hetastarch has been associated with increased mortality in critically ill patients, including those with sepsis.

- Monitor for S&S of hypersensitivity reaction (see Appendix F).
- Measure and record I&O. Report oliguria or significant changes in I&O ratio.
- Monitor BP and vital signs and observe patient for unusual bruising or bleeding.
- Observe for signs of circulatory overload (see Appendix F).
- Check laboratory reports of Hct values. Notify prescriber if there is an appreciable drop in Hct or if value approaches 30% by volume. Hct should not be allowed to drop below 30%.
- Monitor lab tests: Periodic WBC count with differential, platelet count; and PT & PTT during leukapheresis.

Patient & Family Education

- Notify prescriber for any of the following: Difficulty breathing, nausea, chills, headache, itching.

HOMATROPINE HYDROBROMIDE

(hoe-ma′troe-peen)

Isopto Homatropine

See Appendix A-1.

HUMAN PAPILLOMAVIRUS BIVALENT VACCINE

(hu′man pap-ih-lo′ma-vye′rus)

Cervarix

See Appendix J.

HUMAN PAPILLOMAVIRUS QUADRIVALENT VACCINE

(hu′man pap-ih-lo′ma-vye′rus)

Gardasil

See Appendix J.

HYALURONIDASE, OVINE

(hi-a-lu-ron′i-dase)

Amphadase, Hylenex, Vitrase

Classification: HYALURONIC ACID DERIVATIVE; ABSORPTION AND DISPERSING ENHANCER

Therapeutic: ABSORPTION AND DISPERSING ENHANCER

AVAILABILITY Solution for injection

ACTION & *THERAPEUTIC EFFECT* Hyaluronidase is a diffusing substance that modifies the permeability of connective tissue through the hydrolysis of hyaluronic acid found in the intercellular substance of connective tissue. *It increases the absorption and dispersion of solutions in the intercellular spaces.*

USES Adjuvant to increase the absorption and dispersion of other injected drugs; hypodermoclysis; adjunct in subcutaneous urography for improving resorption of radiopaque agents.

UNLABELED USES Management of extravastion.

CONTRAINDICATIONS Hypersensitivity to hyaluronidase or any other ingredient in formulation; injection into infected or acutely inflamed area, area of swelling due to bites or stings; corneal injection; injection by IV; pregnancy—fetal risk cannot be ruled out; lactation—infant risk cannot be ruled out.

CAUTIOUS USE None known.

ROUTE & DOSAGE

Adjuvant to Increase the Absorption and Dispersion of Other Drugs

Adult/Adolescent/Child: 50–300 units (usual dose 150 units) added to solution

Hypodermoclysis

Adult/Adolescent/Child: 150–200 units followed by isotonic fluid administration

ADMINISTRATION

Subcutaneous ONLY

- Give subcutaneously prior to contrast media. Do not inject near an infected or acutely inflamed area.
- Store unopened vial at 2°–8° C (36°–46° F). After reconstitution, store at 15°–25° C (59°–77° F), and use within 6 h. Protect from light. Do not freeze.

ADVERSE EFFECTS **CV:** Edema. **Other:** *Injection site reaction* (e.g., erythema, irritation); enhanced adverse events associated with coadministered drugs.

INTERACTIONS Drug: SALICYLATES, CORTICOSTEROIDS, ESTROGENS, or H_1-BLOCKERS may confer partial resistance to the action of hyaluronidase in some tissues. May increase vasoconstricting effects of ALPHA/BETA AGONISTS. May increase adverse effects of **dopamine.**

NURSING IMPLICATIONS

Assessment & Drug Effects

- Monitor for S&S of hypersensitivity: Urticaria, erythema, chills, nausea, vomiting, dizziness, tachy-cardia, and hypotension. With-hold and notify prescriber if hypersensitivity occurs.
- Note: Those receiving large doses of salicylates, cortisone, ACTH, estrogens, or antihistamines may require larger amounts of hyaluronidase for equivalent dispersing effect.

Patient & Family Education

- Report immediately any of the following: Rash, itching, chills, nausea, vomiting, dizziness, or palpitations.

HYDRALAZINE HYDROCHLORIDE (Pr)

(hye-dral'a-zeen)

Classification: NONNITRATE VASODILATOR; ANTIHYPERTENSIVE
Therapeutic: ANTIHYPERTENSIVE

AVAILABILITY Tablet; solution for injection

ACTION & *THERAPEUTIC EFFECT* Reduces BP mainly by direct effect on vascular smooth muscles of arterial-resistance vessels, resulting in vasodilatation. *Reduces BP with diastolic response often being greater than systolic response. Vasodilation reduces peripheral resistance and substantially improves cardiac output, and renal and cerebral blood flow.*

USES In management of hypertension.

UNLABELED USES Treatment of acute CHF.

CONTRAINDICATIONS Monotherapy for CHF, mitral valvular rheumatic heart disease, MI, tachycardia.

CAUTIOUS USE Coronary heart disease; cerebrovascular accident, advanced renal impairment, coronary heart disease, renal disease; renal failure; SLE; use with MAO inhibitors; pregnancy (category C); children; lactation.

ROUTE & DOSAGE

Hypertension

Adult: **PO** 10–50 mg qid; **IM** 10–50 mg q4–6h; **IV** 10–20 mg q4–6h, switch to oral ASAP

Renal Impairment Dosage Adjustment

CrCl 10–50 mL/min: Dose q8h

ADMINISTRATION

Oral

- Give with food; bioavailability is increased by taking it with food.
- Discontinue gradually to avoid sudden rise in BP and acute heart failure.
- Inform patients of the dangers of abrupt withdrawal.

Intramuscular

- Give deep into a large muscle.

Intravenous

PREPARE: **Direct:** Give undiluted. Use immediately after being drawn into syringe. ▪ Do not add to IV solutions.

ADMINISTER: **Direct:** Give each 10 mg or fraction thereof over 1 min.

INCOMPATIBILITIES: **Solution/additive:** **Aminophylline, ampicillin, chlorothiazide, edetate calcium disodium, ethacrynate, hydrocortisone, mephentermine, methohexital, nitroglycerin, phenobarbital, verapamil, D5W.** **Y-site:** **Acyclovr, alfetnanil, amikacin, aminophylline, amphotericin B, ampicillin, ascorbic acid, atracurium, atropine, azathioprine, aztreonam, benztropine, bretylium, bumetanide,** CEPHALOSPORINS, **chlorthiazide, dantrolene, diazepam, diazoxide, doxorubicin, ertapenem, folic acid, foscarent, furosemide, ganciclovir, gemtuzumab, haloperidol, indomethacin, lorazepam, methohexital, methylprendisolone, nafcillin, nitroprusside, oxacillin, pantoprazole, pemetrexed, pentobarbital, phenytoin, piperacillin/tazobactam, SMZ/TMP, ticarcillin, tigecycline.**

▪ Store at 15°–30° C (59°–86° F) in tight, light-resistant containers unless otherwise directed. Avoid freezing.

ADVERSE EFFECTS

CV: *Palpitation,* angina, *tachycardia,* flushing, paradoxical pressor response. Overdose: Arrhythmia, shock. **CNS:** *Headache,* dizziness, tremors. **HEENT:** Lacrimation, conjunctivitis. **GI:** Anorexia, nausea, vomiting, diarrhea, constipation, abdominal pain, paralytic ileus. **GU:** Difficulty in urination, glomerulonephritis. **Hematologic:** Decreased hematocrit and hemoglobin, anemia, agranulocytosis (rare). **Other:** Hypersensitivity (rash, urticaria, pruritus, fever, chills, arthralgia, eosinophilia, cholangitis, hepatitis, obstructive jaundice). Nasal congestion, muscle cramps, SLE-like syndrome, fixed drug eruption, edema.

DIAGNOSTIC TEST INTERFERENCE

Positive ***direct Coombs' tests*** in patients with hydralazine-induced SLE. Hydralazine interferes with urinary ***17-OHCS*** determinations ***(modified Glenn-Nelson technique).***

INTERACTIONS

Drug: BETA-BLOCKERS and other ANTIHYPERTENSIVE AGENTS compound hypotensive effects.

PHARMACOKINETICS

Absorption: Readily absorbed from GI tract. **Onset:** 20–30 min. **Peak:** 2 h. **Duration:** 2–6 h. **Distribution:** Crosses placenta; distributed into breast milk. **Metabolism:** In liver. **Elimination:** 90% in urine; 10% in feces. **Half-Life:** 2–8 h.

NURSING IMPLICATIONS

Assessment & Drug Effects

- Monitor BP and HR closely. Check every 5 min until it is stabilized at desired level, then every 15 min thereafter throughout hypertensive crisis.
- Monitor for S&S of SLE, especially with prolonged therapy.
- Monitor I&O when drug is given parenterally and in those with renal dysfunction.
- Monitor lab tests: Baseline and periodic BUN, creatinine clearance, uric acid, serum potassium,

and blood glucose. Baseline and periodic antinuclear antibody titer with prolonged therapy.

Patient & Family Education

- Monitor weight, check for edema, and report weight gain to prescriber.
- Note: Some patients experience headache and palpitations within 2–4 h after first PO dose; symptoms usually subside spontaneously.
- Make position changes slowly and avoid standing still, hot baths/showers, strenuous exercise, and excessive alcohol intake.
- Do not drive or engage in other potentially hazardous activities until response to drug is known.

H

HYDROCHLOROTHIAZIDE (HCTZ) Pr

(hye-droe-klor-oh-thye′a-zide)

Apo-Hydro ♣

Classification: ELECTROLYTIC AND WATER BALANCE; THIAZIDE DIURETIC

Therapeutic: DIURETIC

AVAILABILITY Capsule; tablet; oral solution

ACTION & *THERAPEUTIC EFFECT* Diuretic action is associated with drug interference with reabsorption of sodium ions across the distal renal tubular segment of the nephron. This enhances excretion of sodium, chloride, potassium, bicarbonates, and water. It also decreases cardiac output and reduces plasma and extracellular fluid volume. *Therapeutic effectiveness is measured by decrease in edema and lowering of blood pressure.*

USES Adjunct in treatment of edema associated with CHF, hepatic cirrhosis, renal failure, and in the management of hypertension.

UNLABELED USES Nephrogenic diabetes insipidus, hypercalciuria, and treatment of electrolyte disturbances associated with renal tubular acidosis.

CONTRAINDICATIONS Hypersensitivity to thiazides or other sulfonamides; anuria; electrolyte imbalance.

CAUTIOUS USE Bronchial asthma, allergy; hepatic cirrhosis; hepatic impairment; renal impairment; acid/base imbalance; CHF; stroke, CVA; history of gout, SLE; DM; latent DM; parathyroid disease, angle-closure glaucoma, post sympathectomy; older adults; excessive sunlight UV exposure; neonates with jaundice; pregnancy (category B); lactation (infant risk cannot be ruled out).

ROUTE & DOSAGE

Edema

Adult: **PO** 25–100 mg/day in 1–2 divided doses (max: 200 mg/day)

Hypertension

Adult/Adolescent: **PO** 12.5–25 mg/day in 1–2 divided doses; may titrate up

Child/Infant (6 mo and older): **PO** 1–2 mg/kg/day in 2 divided doses

Neonate (younger than 6 mo): **PO** 1–2 mg/kg/day in 2 divided doses

ADMINISTRATION

Oral

- Give with food or milk to reduce GI upset.

- Schedule doses to avoid nocturia and interrupted sleep. If given in 2 doses, schedule second dose no later than 3 p.m.
- Store tablets in tightly closed container at 15°–30° C (59°–86° F) unless otherwise directed.

ADVERSE EFFECTS **CV:** Hypotension, cardiac dysrhythmia. **Respiratory:** Respiratory distress, pneumonitis, pulmonary edema. **CNS:** Vertigo, headache, restlessness. **HEENT:** Transient blurred vision, predominance of yellow vision. **Endocrine:** Glycosuria, hyperglycemia, hyperuricemia, hypochloremic alkalosis, hypokalemia, hypomagnesemia, hyponatremia. **Skin:** Alopecia, erythema multiforme, exfoliative dermatitis, skin photosensitivity, rash, Stevens–Johnson syndrome, toxic epidermal necrolysis, urticaria. **Hepatic:** Jaundice. **GI:** Abdominal cramps, anorexia, constipation, diarrhea, gastric irritation, nausea, vomiting, pancreatitis, inflammation of salivary gland. **GU:** Impotence. **Musculoskeletal:** Muscle spasm, weakness. **Hematologic:** Agranulocytosis, aplastic anemia, hemolytic anemia, leukopenia, pupura, thrombocytopenia. **Other:** Fever.

DIAGNOSTIC TEST INTERFERENCE May interfere with ***parathyroid function tests, tyramine/phentolamine tests, histamine tests for pheochromocytoma.*** May lead to false-negative ***aldosterone/renin ratio.***

INTERACTIONS **Drug:** **Amphotericin B**, CORTICOSTEROIDS increase hypokalemic effects; SULFONYLUREAS, **insulin** may antagonize hypoglycemic effects; BILE ACID SEQUESTRANTS decrease THIAZIDE absorption; **diazoxide** intensifies hypoglycemic and hypotensive effects; increased **potassium** and **magnesium** loss may cause **digoxin** toxicity; decreases **lithium** excretion and increases toxicity; increases risk of NSAID-induced renal failure and may attenuate diuresis. Do not use with **dofetilide.** Withhold dose for 24 h prior to **amifostine** usage. Monitor with **topiramate.**

PHARMACOKINETICS **Absorption:** Incompletely absorbed. **Onset:** 2 h. **Peak:** 4 h. **Duration:** 6–12 h. **Distribution:** Distributed throughout extracellular tissue; concentrates in kidney; crosses placenta; distributed in breast milk. **Metabolism:** Does not appear to be metabolized. **Elimination:** In urine. **Half-Life:** 45–120 min.

NURSING IMPLICATIONS

Assessment & Drug Effects

- Monitor for therapeutic effectiveness. Antihypertensive effects may be noted in 3–4 days; maximal effects may require 3–4 wk.
- Check BP at regular intervals.
- Monitor closely for hypokalemia; it increases the risk of digoxin toxicity.
- Monitor I&O and check for edema.
- Note: Drug may cause hyperglycemia and loss of glycemic control in diabetics.
- Note: Drug may cause orthostatic hypotension, dizziness.
- Monitor lab tests: Baseline and periodic serum electrolytes, blood counts, BUN, blood glucose, uric acid, calcium levels, CO_2.

Patient & Family Education

- Monitor weight daily.
- Note: Diabetic patients need to monitor blood glucose closely. This drug causes impaired glucose tolerance.

- Report signs of hypokalemia (see Appendix F) to prescriber.
- Change positions slowly; avoid hot baths or showers, extended exposure to sunlight, and sitting or standing still for long periods.
- Note: Photosensitivity reaction may occur 10–14 days after initial sun exposure.

HYDROCODONE BITARTRATE

(hye-droe-koe'done)

Hysingla ER, Zohydro ER

Classification: NARCOTIC (OPIATE AGONIST) ANALGESIC; ANTITUSSIVE

Therapeutic: NARCOTIC ANALGESIC; ANTITUSSIVE

Prototype: Morphine

Controlled Substance: Schedule II

AVAILABILITY Usually formulated with acetaminophen, ibuprofen, or homatropine. Extended release tablet; extended release capsule

ACTION & *THERAPEUTIC EFFECT* CNS depressant with moderate to severe relief of pain. Suppresses cough reflex by direct action on cough center in medulla. *CNS depressant with moderate to severe relief of pain. Effective in cough suppression.*

USES Symptomatic relief of hyperactive or nonproductive cough and for relief of moderate to moderately severe pain. A common ingredient in a variety of proprietary mixtures.

CONTRAINDICATIONS Hypersensitivity to hydrocodone; acute or severe asthmatic bronchitis; COPD; upper airway obstruction; paralytic ileus (known or suspected), GI obstruction; lactation.

CAUTIOUS USE Respiratory depression, asthma, emphysema; history of drug abuse or dependence; postoperative patients; congenital long QT syndrome; drug-inducted QT prolongation; history of seizure disorder; BPH; adrenal insufficiency; hepatic impairment; renal impairment; G6PD deficiency; GI disease; patients with preexisting increased ICP, head trauma; CNS depression; older adults, debilitated patients; pregnancy (category C). Safety and efficacy in children not established.

ROUTE & DOSAGE

Chronic/Severe Pain

Adult: **PO** 10 mg q12h in opioid-tolerant patients

ADMINISTRATION

Oral

- Give with food or milk to prevent GI irritation.
- Preserve in tight, light-resistant containers.
- Do not crush, chew, or dissolve, as these actions may lead to an uncontrolled delivery of a fatal dose.

ADVERSE EFFECTS **CV:** Peripheral edema. **Respiratory:** *Respiratory depression*. **CNS:** Light-headedness, sedation, anxiety, dizziness, *drowsiness,* euphoria, anxiety dysphoria. **Skin:** Urticaria, rash, pruritus. **GI:** Dry mouth, *constipation, nausea,* vomiting, abdominal pain.

INTERACTIONS Drug: Alcohol and other CNS DEPRESSANTS compound sedation and CNS depression. **Herbal: St. John's wort** increases sedation.

PHARMACOKINETICS Onset: 10–20 min. **Duration:** 3–6 h. **Distribution:** Crosses placenta; distributed into breast milk. **Metabolism:** In liver. **Elimination:** In urine. **Half-Life:** 3.8 h.

NURSING IMPLICATIONS

Black Box Warning

Hydrocodone has been associated with high potential for abuse and addiction, life-threatening respiratory depression, and neonatal opioid withdrawal syndrome. The risk of potentially fatal overdose increases with coingestion of alcohol.

Assessment & Drug Effects

- Monitor for effectiveness of drug for pain relief.
- Monitor for nausea and vomiting, especially in ambulatory patients.
- Monitor respiratory status and bowel elimination.

Patient & Family Education

- Avoid hazardous activities until response to drug is determined.
- Do not use alcohol or other CNS depressants; may cause additive CNS depression.
- Drink plenty of liquids for adequate hydration.
- Do not take larger doses than prescribed since abuse potential is high.

HYDROCORTISONE (Pr)

(hye-droe-kor′ti-sone)

Cortenema, Rectocort ♣

HYDROCORTISONE ACETATE

Anusol HC, Cortifoam, Cortiment ♣, Epifoam

HYDROCORTISONE CYPIONATE

Cortef

HYDROCORTISONE SODIUM SUCCINATE

Solu-Cortef

HYDROCORTISONE VALERATE
HYDROCORTISONE BUTYRATE

Locoid

Classification: ADRENOCORTICAL STEROID

Therapeutic: ANTI-INFLAMMATORY; IMMUNOSUPPRESSANT; ANTIPSORIATIC

AVAILABILITY Hydrocortisone: Tablet; cream, lotion, ointment, spray; gel. **Hydrocortisone Acetate:** Oral suspension; cream; ointment; foam; lotion; suppository. **Hydrocortisone Cypionate:** Tablet. **Hydrocortisone Sodium Succinate:** Solution for injection. **Hydrocortisone Valerate:** ointment. **Hydrocortisone Butyrate:** Cream; ointment; topical solution; lotion.

ACTION & *THERAPEUTIC EFFECT* Short-acting synthetic steroid with both glucocorticoid and mineralocorticoid properties that affects nearly all systems of the body. **Anti-inflammatory (glucocorticoid) action:** Stabilizes leukocyte lysosomal membranes; inhibits phagocytosis and release of allergic substances; suppresses fibroblast formation and collagen deposition; reduces capillary dilation and permeability; and increases responsiveness of cardiovascular system to circulating catecholamines. **Immunosuppressive action:** Modifies immune response to various stimuli; reduces antibody titers; and suppresses cell-mediated hypersensitivity reactions. **Mineralocorticoid action:** Promotes sodium retention, but under certain circumstances (e.g., sodium loading), enhances sodium excretion; promotes potassium excretion; and increases glomerular filtration rate (GFR). **Metabolic action:** Promotes hepatic gluconeogenesis, protein catabolism, redistribution of body fat, and lipolysis. *Has anti-inflammatory, immunosuppressive, and metabolic functions in the body.*

USES Replacement therapy in adrenocortical insufficiency; to reduce serum calcium in hypercalcemia, to suppress undesirable inflammatory or immune responses, to produce temporary remission in nonadrenal disease, and to block ACTH production in diagnostic tests; to induce diuresis or remission of proteinuria in nephrotic syndrome, ulcerative colitis; palliative management of leukemias; asthma. Use as anti-inflammatory or immunosuppressive agent largely replaced by synthetic glucocorticoids that have minimal mineralocorticoid activity. Topically for atopic dermatitis or inflammatory conditions.

CONTRAINDICATIONS Hypersensitivity to glucocorticoids, idiopathic thrombocytopenic purpura, psychoses, acute glomerulonephritis, systemic fungal infections, viral or bacterial diseases of skin, infections not controlled by antibiotics, active or latent amebiasis, hypercorticism (Cushing's syndrome), smallpox vaccination or other immunologic procedures; acne; pregnancy—fetal risk cannot be ruled out; lactation—infant risk cannot be ruled out. **Topical steroids:** Presence of varicella, vaccinia, on surfaces with compromised circulation.

CAUTIOUS USE Diabetes mellitus; chronic, active hepatitis positive for hepatitis B surface antigen; hyperlipidemia; cirrhosis; stromal herpes simplex; glaucoma, tuberculosis of eye; osteoporosis; convulsive disorders; hypothyroidism; diverticulitis; nonspecific ulcerative colitis; fresh intestinal anastomoses; active or latent peptic ulcer; gastritis; esophagitis; thromboembolic disorders; CHF; metastatic carcinoma; hypertension; renal insufficiency; history of allergies; active or arrested tuberculosis; systemic fungal infection; myasthenia gravis; known Strongyloides (threadworm) infestation; ocular herpes; preexisting psychiatric conditions; older adults; children and infants.

ROUTE & DOSAGE

Anti-Inflammatory

Adult: **PO** 20–240 mg/day in divided doses; **IV/IM** 100–500 mg/dose at intervals of 2, 4, or 6 hours; **Topical** Apply a small amount to the affected area 1–2 × day
Adolescent: **PO/IM/IV:** 15–240 mg q12h
Child: **PO** 2.5–10 mg/kg/day in 3–4 divided doses; **IV/IM** 1–5 mg/kg/day divided q12–24h

Chronic Adrenal Insufficiency

Adult: **PO** 15–25 mg/day in 2–3 divided doses

Atopic Dermatitis

Adult/Adolescent/Child/Infant (3 mo or older): **Topical** Apply bid for 2–4 weeks

Hemorrhoids

Adult **PR** Insert 1% cream, 10% foam, 10–25 mg suppository

ADMINISTRATION

Note: Hydrocortisone succinate may be given IM or IV.

Oral

- Give oral drug with food.
- Take antacids between meals.
- Avoid grapefruit and grapefruit juice.

Rectal

- Administer retention enema preferably after a bowel movement; retain at least 1 h or all night if possible. Position preferably on the left side and for 30 minutes after.

Topical

- Shake well. Apply medication sparingly, rub until it disappears, and then reapply, leaving a thin coat over lesion. Cover area with transparent plastic or other occlusive device or vehicle only when so ordered.
- Avoid covering a weeping or exudative lesion.
- Note: Occlusive dressings usually are not applied to face, scalp, scrotum, axilla, and groin.
- Inspect skin carefully between applications for ecchymotic, petechial, and purpuric signs, maceration, secondary infection, skin atrophy, striae, or miliaria; if present, stop medication and notify prescriber.
- Store tablet, cream/ointment, rectal suspension at 20°–25° C (68°–77° F) unless otherwise directed by manufacturer; protect from light and freezing. Store spray at a temperature below 120 degrees F. Keep from heat or flame; product is flammable.

Intramuscular

- Inject deep into gluteal muscle.
    - Store powder before and after reconstitution at controlled room temperature between 20 and 25 degrees C (68–77 degrees F). Use reconstituted solution within 3 days. Protect from light.

Intravenous

IV administration to infants, children: Verify correct IV concentration and rate of infusion/injection with prescriber.

PREPARE: **Direct (preferred):** Give undiluted. May be reconstituted with no more than 2 mL of bacteriostatic water or bacteriostatic NS. Discard solution after 3 days. **Intermittent:** Dilute in 50–1000 mL of D5W, NS, or D5/NS.

ADMINISTER: **Direct:** Give over 30 sec (e.g., 100 mg) to 10 min (e.g., 500 mg or more). **Intermittent:** Give over 10 min.

INCOMPATIBILITIES: **Solution/additive:** **Bleomycin, colistimethate, hydralazine, linezolid, nafcillin, prochlorperazine, promethazine.** **Y-site:** **Amiodarone, amphotericin B, ampicillin, azathioprine, dantrolene, diazepam, diazoxide, dobutamine, dolasetron, doxycycline, epirubicin, ganciclovir, garenoxacin, gemtuzumab, haloperidol, idarubicin, labetalol, lansoprazole, mycophenolate,**

nalbuphine, netilmicin, nicardipine, oritavancin, pentamidine, phenytoin, protamine, pyridoxine, quinupristin/dalfopristin, rocuronium, sargramostim, sulfamethoxazole/trimethoprim, thiamine, topotecan.
- Administer solutions that have been diluted for IV infusion within 24 h.

ADVERSE EFFECTS (common)

CV: Increased blood pressure. **Endocrine:** Body fluid retention, impaired glucose tolerance, weight gain. **Other:** Altered behavior, disturbance in mood.

DIAGNOSTIC TEST INTERFERENCE

May suppress reactions to skin tests.

INTERACTIONS

Drug: BARBITURATES, **phenytoin, rifampin** may increase hepatic metabolism, thus decreasing cortisone levels; ESTROGENS potentiate the effects of hydrocortisone; NSAIDS compound ulcerogenic effects; **cholestyramine, colestipol** decrease hydrocortisone absorption; DIURETICS, **amphotericin B** exacerbate hypokalemia; desmopressin increases hyponatremic effect; **miferprisone** decreases effect; ANTICHOLINESTERASE AGENTS (e.g., **neostigmine**) may produce severe weakness; immune response to VACCINES and TOXOIDS may be decreased. May diminished effect of ANTINEOPLASTICS, IMMUNOSUPPRESSANTS, mifamurtide. ANTACIDS may decrease the bioavailability of oral hydrocortisone. **Aprepitant, fosaprepitant** may increase concentration of hydrocortisone.

PHARMACOKINETICS

Absorption: Rapid. **Onset:** 1 h. **Peak:** 1 h PO; 4–8 h IM. **Duration:** 1–1.5 days PO/IM; 0.5–4 wk intra-articular. **Distribution:** Distributed primarily to muscles, liver, skin, intestines, kidneys; crosses placenta. **Metabolism:** In liver. **Elimination:** metabolites excreted in urine; excreted in breast milk. **Half-Life:** 1.5–2 h.

NURSING IMPLICATIONS

Assessment & Drug Effects

- Establish baseline and continuing data on BP, weight, fluid and electrolyte balance, and blood glucose.
- Monitor for adverse effects. Older adults and patients with low serum albumin are especially susceptible to adverse effects.
- Be alert to signs of hypocalcemia (see Appendix F).
- Ophthalmoscopic examinations are recommended every 2–3 mo, especially if patient is receiving ophthalmic steroid therapy.
- Monitor for persistent backache or chest pain; compression and spontaneous fractures of long bones and vertebrae present hazards.
- Monitor for and report changes in mood and behavior, emotional instability, or psychomotor activity, especially with long-term therapy.
- Be alert to possibility of masked infection and delayed healing (anti-inflammatory and immunosuppressive actions).
- Note: Dose adjustment may be required if patient is subjected to severe stress (serious infection, surgery, or injury).
- Note: Single doses of corticosteroids or use for a short period (less than 1 wk) do not produce

withdrawal symptoms when discontinued, even with moderately large doses.

- Monitor growth and development in pediatric long-term therapy.
- Monitor lab tests: Periodic serum electrolytes, blood glucose, Hct and Hgb, platelet count, Urinary free cortisol test and ACTH stimulation test; periodic in large doses and long-term therapy. WBC with differential.

Patient & Family Education

- Expect a slight weight gain with improved appetite. After dosage is stabilized, notify prescriber of a sudden slow but steady weight increase [2 kg (5 lb)/wk].
- Avoid vaccines.
- Avoid alcohol and caffeine; may contribute to steroid-ulcer development in long-term therapy.
- Do not ignore dyspepsia with hyperacidity. Report symptoms to prescriber and **do not** self-medicate to find relief.
- **Do not** use aspirin or other OTC drugs unless prescribed specifically by the prescriber.
- Note: A high protein, calcium, and vitamin D diet is advisable to reduce risk of corticosteroid-induced osteoporosis.
- Notify prescriber of slow healing, any vague feeling of being sick, or return to pretreatment symptoms.
- Do not abruptly discontinue drug; doses are gradually reduced to prevent withdrawal symptoms.
- Report exacerbation of disease during drug withdrawal.
- Apply topical preparations sparingly in small children. The hazard of systemic toxicity is higher because of the greater ratio of skin surface area to body weight.

HYDROMORPHONE HYDROCHLORIDE

(hye-droe-mor'fone)

Dilaudid, Dilaudid-HP, Exalgo

Classification: NARCOTIC (OPIATE AGONIST); ANALGESIC

Therapeutic: NARCOTIC ANALGESIC; ANTITUSSIVE

Prototype: Morphine

Controlled Substance: Schedule II

H

AVAILABILITY Tablet; oral liquid; solution for injection; extended release tablet; rectal suppository

ACTION & *THERAPEUTIC EFFECT* Potent opiate receptor agonist that does not alter pain threshold but changes the perception of pain in the CNS. *An effective narcotic analgesic that controls mild to moderate pain. Also has antitussive properties.*

USES Relief of moderate to severe pain.

CONTRAINDICATIONS Intolerance to opiate agonists; opiate-naïve patients; severe respiratory depression; acute or severe asthma, bronchial asthma, status asthmaticus in an unmonitored setting or in absence of resuscitative equipment; upper airway obstruction, GI obstruction; ilieus; obstetrical analgesia; pregnancy (category D in high doses at term); lactation. **Extended release form:** Preexisting severe narrowing of any portion of GI tract.

CAUTIOUS USE Abrupt discontinuation, alcoholism or history of drug abuse; angina; biliary tract disease; epidural administration; GI disease; head trauma, other intracranial lesions, preexisting increase intracranial lesions; or increased ICP; heart failure; hepatic disease; hypotension, hypovolemia, oliguria, BPH; pulmonary disease; significant COPD; respiratory depression; disease, renal impairment; increased inflammatory bowel disease, ulcerative colitis; adrenal insufficiency; bladder obstruction; cardiac arrhythmias, cardiac disease; history of seizures; history of substance abuse; surgery of biliary tract, GI surgery; urethral stricture, urinary retention; debilitated patients; older adults; pregnancy (category C); children.

ROUTE & DOSAGE

Moderate to Severe Pain

Adult: **PO** 2–4 mg q4–6h prn in opioid naïve patients or 2.5–10 mg q3–6h (liquid form); **Subcutaneous/IM** 1–2 mg q2–3h depending on patient response and previous opioid exposure; **IV** 0.2–1 mg q2–3h; **Rectal** 3mg q6–8h titrate to relief

ADMINISTRATION

Oral

- Ensure that extended release tablet is swallowed whole and not crushed or chewed.
- For chronic pain, around-the-clock dosing is recommended.

Rectal

- Insert beyond the rectal sphincter to ensure retention.

Subcutaneous/Intramuscular

- **Do not** confuse Dilaudid-HP Injection (a concentrated formulation) with Dilaudid Injection. Overdose and death could result.
- Store at room 15°–30° C (59°–86° F) and protect from light.

Intravenous

IV administration to children: Verify correct IV concentration and rate of infusion with prescriber.

PREPARE: **Direct:** May be given undiluted or diluted in 5 mL of sterile water or NS. **IV Infusion:** Solution typically diluted to 1 mg/mL (specific concentration is ordered by prescriber) in D5W, NS, or other compatible solution. ▪ **For Dilaudid-HP:** Reconstitute 250 mg dry powder vial immediately prior to use with 25 mL sterile water for injection to yield 10 mg/mL. ▪ Final dilution of Dilaudid-HP 250 and HP 500 (supplied 500 mg/50 mL) **must be** ordered by prescriber.

ADMINISTER: **Direct:** Give 2 mg or fraction thereof over 3–5 min. **IV Infusion:** Both final volume and rate of infusion **must be** ordered by prescriber.

INCOMPATIBILITIES: **Solution/additive: Prochlorperazine, sodium bicarbonate, thiopental. Y-site: Amphotericin B cholesteryl, cefazolin, ceftobiprole, dantrolene, dimenhydrinate, diazepam, gallium, lansoprazole, minocycline, pantoprazole, phenobarbital, phenytoin, sargramostim, thiopental.**

- A slight discoloration in ampules or multidose vials causes no loss of potency. ▪ Store in tight, light-resistant containers at 15°–30° C (59°–86° F).

ADVERSE EFFECTS **CV:** Hypotension, bradycardia or tachycardia. **Respiratory:** Respiratory depression. **CNS:** Euphoria, dizziness, sedation, *drowsiness*. **HEENT:** Blurred vision. **GI:** Nausea, vomiting, constipation.

INTERACTIONS Drug: Alcohol and other CNS DEPRESSANTS compound sedation and CNS depression. **Herbal: St. John's wort, kava** may increase sedation.

PHARMACOKINETICS Absorption: 60% absorbed from GI tract. **Onset:** 15 min IV, 30 min PO. **Peak:** 30–90 min. **Duration:** 3–4 h; higher AUC in geriatric patients. **Distribution:** Crosses placenta; distributed into breast milk. **Metabolism:** In liver. **Elimination:** In urine. **Half-Life:** 2–3 h.

NURSING IMPLICATIONS

Black Box Warning

Hydromorphone has been associated with respiratory depression and substance abuse.

Assessment & Drug Effects

- Note baseline respiratory rate, rhythm, and depth and size of pupils before administration. Respirations of 12/min or less and mitosis are signs of toxicity. Withhold drug and promptly notify prescriber.
- Monitor vital signs at regular intervals. Drug-induced respiratory depression may occur even with small doses and increases progressively with higher doses.
- Assess effectiveness of pain relief 30 min after medication administration.
- Monitor drug effects carefully in older adult or debilitated patients and those with impaired renal and hepatic function.
- Assess effectiveness of cough. Drug depresses cough and sigh reflexes and may induce atelectasis, especially in postoperative patients and those with pulmonary disease.
- Note: Nausea and orthostatic hypotension most often occur in ambulatory patients or when a supine patient assumes the head-up position.
- Monitor I&O ratio and pattern. Assess lower abdomen for bladder distension. Report oliguria or urinary retention.
- Monitor bowel pattern; drug-induced constipation may require treatment.

Patient & Family Education

- Request medication at the onset of pain and do not wait until pain is severe.
- Use caution with activities requiring alertness; drug may cause drowsiness, dizziness, and blurred vision.
- Hydromorphone may be habit forming and has the potential for abuse.
- Avoid alcohol and other CNS depressants while taking this drug.

HYDROQUINONE

(hye′droe-kwin-one)

Aclaro, Eldopaque, Eldoquin, Esoterica Regular, Lustra, Melanex, Porcelana, Solaquin

Classification: PIGMENT AGENT; DEPIGMENTOR

Therapeutic: DEPIGMENTOR

AVAILABILITY Cream; gel; solution

ACTION & *THERAPEUTIC EFFECT*
Causes reversible bleaching of hyperpigmented skin due to increased melanin. Depresses melanin synthesis and melanocytic growth, possibly by increasing excretion of melanin from melanocytes. *Interferes with formation of new melanin but does not destroy existing pigment.*

USES Gradual bleaching of hyperpigmented skin conditions.

CONTRAINDICATIONS Hypersensitivity to hydroquinone, PABA, paraben, or sulfite; prickly heat, sunburn, irritated skin, depilatory usage.

CAUTIOUS USE Pregnancy (category C), lactation. Safe use in children younger than 12 y not established.

H

ROUTE & DOSAGE

Bleaching of Hyperpigmented Skin

Adult: **Topical** Apply thin layer and rub into hyperpigmented skin bid, a.m. and p.m.

ADMINISTRATION

Topical

- Test skin for sensitivity before treatment is initiated. Apply small amount of drug (about 25 mm in diameter) to an unbroken patch of skin and check in 24 h. Do not use drug if vesicle formation, itching, or excessive inflammation occur. Minor redness is not a contraindication.
- Limit applications to an area no larger than that of face and neck.

ADVERSE EFFECTS **Skin:** Dryness and fissuring of paranasal and infraorbital areas, inflammatory reaction, erythema; stinging, tingling, burning sensations; irritation, sensitization, and contact dermatitis.

NURSING IMPLICATIONS

Assessment & Drug Effects

- Monitor for therapeutic effectiveness: In general, complete depigmentation occurs in 1–4 mo and lasts 2–6 mo after hydroquinone is discontinued. Once desired results are obtained, reduce amount and frequency of applications to the least that will maintain depigmentation.
- Discontinue if bleaching or skin lightening does not occur after 2 or 3 mo of therapy.

Patient & Family Education

- Use a sunscreen agent or a hydroquinone formulation containing a sunscreen for daytime applications.
- Wash drug off if rash or irritation develops and consult prescriber.
- Avoid contact with the eyes and not to use on open lesions, sunburned, irritated, or otherwise damaged skin.
- Continue use of protective clothing and sunscreening agent after treatment is terminated to reduce possibility of repigmentation.

HYDROXOCOBALAMIN (VITAMIN B_{12} ALPHA)

(hye-drox-oh-koe-bal'a-min)

Cyanokit

Classification: VITAMIN SUPPLEMENT

Therapeutic: VITAMIN B_{12} REPLACEMENT

Prototype: Cyanocobalamin

AVAILABILITY Solution for injection

ACTION & *THERAPEUTIC EFFECT*

Cobalamin derivative similar to cyanocobalamin (vitamin B_{12}). Essential for normal cell growth, cell reproduction maturation of RBCs, myelin synthesis, and believed to be involved in protein synthesis. *Effective in vitamin B_{12} deficiency that results in megaloblastic anemia.*

USES Treatment of vitamin B_{12} deficiency; treatment of pernicious anemia; treatment of cyanide poisoning.

UNLABELED USES Vasoplegic syndrome.

CONTRAINDICATIONS History of sensitivity to vitamin B_{12}, other cobalamins, or cobalt; indiscriminate use in folic acid deficiency.

CAUTIOUS USE Hypertension; renal injury; pregnancy (limited data; cyanide poisoning can be fatal for the pregnant female and fetus if untreated; treatment should not be withheld during pregnancy); lactation; children.

ROUTE & DOSAGE

Vitamin B_{12} Deficiency

Adult: **IM** 1000 mcg weekly until deficiency is corrected and then 1000 mcg/mo
Child: **IM** 250–1000 mcg daily or every other day × 1 week; then weekly × 4–8 weeks, then monthly for life.

Cyanide Poisoning

Adult: **IV** 5 grams as single infusion, may repeat 1 time (max cumulative dose 10 g)

ADMINISTRATION

Intramuscular

- Give deep into a large muscle.

Intravenous

- ***CYANOKIT:*** Administer initial dose by IV infusion over 15 minutes; If a second dose is needed, administer second dose over 15 minutes to 2 hours. ▪ If given concomitantly with sodium thiosulfate or sodium nitrate, use separate IV lines.

INCOMPATIBILITIES: **Y-site: Ascorbic acid, diazepam, dobutamine, dopamine, fentanyl, nitroglycerin, pentobarbital, propofol, sodium nitrite, sodium thiosulfate, thiopental.**

- Store at 20°–25°C (68°–77°F).

ADVERSE EFFECTS **Cardiovascular:** Hypertension. **CNS:** Headache. **Integumentary:** Pruritis, rash, erythema. **GI:** Diarrhea, nausea. **GU:** Urine discoloration, calcium oxalate nephrolithiasis. **Hematologic:** Lymphocytopenia. **Other:** Anaphylaxis, pain at injection site, swelling (generalized).

DIAGNOSTIC TEST INTERFERENCE For 24 hours after last dose many test results can be impacted. May falsely elevate basophils, hemoglobin, albumin, bilirubin, urinalysis results (glucose, protein, erythrocytes, leukocytes, ketones, bilirubin). May falsely decrease ALT and amalyase. Has unpredictable impact on AST, CK, LDH, phosphate, uric acid, PT, aPTT, urine pH.

INTERACTIONS **Drug: Chloramphenicol** may interfere with therapeutic response to hydroxocobalamin.

PHARMACOKINETICS **Distribution:** Widely distributed; principally stored in liver, kidneys, and adrenals; crosses placenta. **Metabolism:** Converted in tissues to active coenzymes; enterohepatically cycled. **Elimination:** 50–95% of doses 100 mcg or greater are excreted in urine in 48 h; excreted in breast milk.

NURSING IMPLICATIONS

Assessment & Drug Effects

- Monitor for therapeutic effectiveness: Response to drug therapy is usually dramatic, occurring within

H

48 h. Effectiveness is measured by laboratory values and improvement in manifestations of vitamin B_{12} deficiency.

- Obtain a careful history of sensitivities. Sensitization can take as long as 8 y to develop.
- Monitor potassium levels during the first 48 h, particularly in patients with Addisonian pernicious anemia or megaloblastic anemia. Conversion to normal erythropoiesis can result in severe hypokalemia and sudden death.
- Monitor vital signs in patients with cardiac disease and be alert to symptoms of pulmonary edema; generally occur early in therapy.
- Monitor bowel function. Bowel regularity is essential for consistent absorption of oral preparations.
- Monitor lab tests: Prior to therapy reticulocyte, RBC count, Hgb, Hct, vitamin B_{12}, and serum folate and iron levels; repeated 5–7 days after start of therapy and at regular intervals during therapy.

Patient & Family Education

- Notify prescriber of any intercurrent disease or infection. Increased dosage may be required.
- Note: It is imperative to understand that drug therapy **must be** continued throughout life for pernicious anemia to prevent irreversible neurologic damage.
- Neurologic damage is considered irreversible if there is no improvement after 1–1.5 y of adequate therapy.
- Dietary deficiency of vitamin B_{12} has been observed in strict vegetarians (vegans) and their breast-fed infants as well as in the elderly.

HYDROXYCHLOROQUINE

(hye-drox-ee-klor′oh-kwin)

Plaquenil

Classification: BIOLOGIC RESPONSE MODIFIER; ANTIMALARIAL; DISEASE MODIFYING RHEUMATIC DRUG (DMARD)

Therapeutic: ANTIMALARIAL; ANTI-RHEUMATIC

Prototype: Chloroquine

AVAILABILITY Tablets

ACTION & *THERAPEUTIC EFFECT* Interferes with digestive vacuole function within sensitive malarial parasites by increasing the pH and interfering with lysosomal degradation of hemoglobin; inhibits locomotion of neutrophils and chemotaxis of eosinophils; impairs antigen-antibody reactions. *Effective against* Plasmodium vivax *and* Plasmodium malariae. *Also is effective as second line of defense for treatment of rheumatoid arthritis and SLE.*

USES Treatment of uncomplicated malaria; malaria prophylaxis in areas without resistance, treatment of lupus erythematous, rheumatoid arthritis.

UNLABELED USES Porphyria cutanea tarda; Q fever.

CONTRAINDICATIONS Known hypersensitivity to hydroxychloroquine; retinal or visual field changes associated with quinoline compounds; psoriasis, porphyria, G6PD deficiency; long-term therapy in children.

CAUTIOUS USE Hepatic disease; alcoholism, use with hepatotoxic drugs; impaired renal function,

 Common adverse effects in *italic;* life-threatening effects underlined; generic names in **bold;** classifications in SMALL CAPS; ♣ Canadian drug name; ● Prototype drug; ⚠ Alert

porphyria; metabolic acidosis; patients with tendency to dermatitis; pregnancy (potential benefits may warrant use of drug in pregnant women).

ROUTE & DOSAGE

Note: Doses are expressed in terms of hydroxychloroquine sulfate. Hydroxychloroquine sulfate 200 mg = hydroxychloquine base 155 mg

Acute Malaria Attack

Adult: **PO** 800 mg followed by 400 mg at 6, 24, and 48 h
Child (weight greater than 30 kg): **PO** 12.9 mg/kg (max initial dose 800 mg), then 6.5 mg base/kg at 6, 24, and 48 h (max dose 400 mg)

Malaria Prophylaxis

Adult: **PO** 400 mg weekly the same day each week starting 1–2 wk before exposure and continuing for 4 wk after leaving the area of exposure
Child: (weight greater than 30 kg): **PO** 6.5 mg/kg weekly the same day each week starting 1–2 wk before exposure and continuing for 4 wk after leaving the area of exposure

Lupus/Rheumatoid Arthritis:

Adult: **PO** 200–400 mg daily (max 5/mg/kg/day or 400 mg whichever is lower)

ADMINISTRATION

Oral

- Give drug with food or milk to reduce incidence of GI distress.
- Do not crush or divide film-coated tablets. In patients unable to swallow tablets, crush tablets in mix with a small amount of applesauce, chocolate syrup, or jelly.
- Store at 20°–25° C (68°–77° F). Protect from light.

ADVERSE EFFECTS **CNS:** Fatigue, vertigo, headache, mood or mental changes, anxiety, *retinopathy,* blurred vision, difficulty focusing, suicidal ideation. **Skin:** Bleaching or loss of hair, unusual pigmentation (blue-black) of skin or inside mouth, skin rash, itching. **GI:** Anorexia, nausea, vomiting, diarrhea, abdominal cramps, weight loss. **Hematologic:** Hemolysis in patients with G6PD deficiency, agranulocytosis (rare), aplastic anemia (rare), thrombocytopenia, cadiomyopathy. **Other:** Hepatic failure.

INTERACTIONS **Drug:** **Aluminum** and **magnesium**-containing ANTACIDS and LAXATIVES decrease hydroxychloroquine absorption; separate administrations by at least 4 h; hydroxychloroquine may interfere with response to **rabies vaccine.** Decreases effect of **remdesivir.** Do not use with other agents that prolong the QT interval; may increase adverse effect of **lumefantrine, dapsone, mefloquine.**

PHARMACOKINETICS **Absorption:** Rapidly and almost completely absorbed. **Peak:** 1–2 h. **Distribution:** Widely distributed; crosses placenta. **Metabolism:** Partially in liver to active metabolite. **Elimination:** In urine; excreted in breast milk. **Half-Life:** 40 days.

NURSING IMPLICATIONS

Assessment & Drug Effects

- Monitor for therapeutic effectiveness; may not appear for several weeks, and maximal benefit may not occur for 6 mo.

- Withhold drug and notify prescriber if weakness, visual symptoms, hearing loss, unusual bleeding, bruising, or skin eruptions occur.
- Baseline and annual ophthalmologic exam.
- Baseline and periodic ECG.
- Monitor lab tests: Baseline and periodic CBC with differential, liver function, renal function, blood glucose.

Patient & Family Education

- Learn about adverse effects and their symptoms when taking prolonged therapy.
- Follow drug regimen exactly as prescribed by the prescriber.

HYDROXYPROGESTERONE CAPROATE

(hye-drox'ee-proe-jes'ter-one kap'roe-ate)

Makena

Classification: HORMONE; PROGESTIN

Therapeutic: PROGESTIN

Prototype: Progesterone

AVAILABILITY Solution for injection

ACTION & *THERAPEUTIC EFFECT* The mechanism by which hydroxyprogesterone reduces the risk of preterm birth is unknown. *Decreases risk of recurrent preterm births.*

USES Decrease risk of premature birth in women with a singleton pregnancy who have a history of singleton spontaneous preterm birth.

UNLABELED USES Amenorrhea, dysfunctional uterine bleeding, endometrial cancer, test for endogenous estrogen production.

CONTRAINDICATIONS Current/history of thrombosis or thromboembolic disorders; current/history of breast cancer or other hormone-sensitive cancer; undiagnosed abnormal vaginal bleeding not related to pregnancy; cholestatic jaundice of pregnancy; benign or malignant liver tumors or other active liver disease; uncontrolled hypertension; postmenopausal status.

CAUTIOUS USE Hypersensitivity; diabetes or prediabetes; conditions exacerbated by fluid retention (e.g., preeclampsia, seizure disorder, migraine, asthma, cardiac or renal dysfunction); hypertension; jaundice; depression. Safety and efficacy in children under 16 y not established.

ROUTE & DOSAGE

Prevention of Premature Birth

Adult: IM 250 mg weekly. Begin between 16 wk 0 d to 20 wk 6 d of pregnancy. Continue until wk 37 or delivery whichever occurs first.

ADMINISTRATION

Intramuscular

- Draw up 1 mL using an 18-guage needle. Change to a 21-gauge 1½-inch needle.
- Slowly inject (over at least 1 min) into the upper outer quadrant of the gluteus maximus.
- Store at 15°–30° C (59°–86° F) upright and protect from light. Discard vial 5 wk after first use.

ADVERSE EFFECTS **CV:** Gestational hypertension or preeclampsia, <u>thromboembolic disorders</u>. **Endocrine:** Decreased glucose tolerance, fluid retention, gestational diabetes. **Skin:** Pruritus, *urticaria*. **GI:** Diarrhea, nausea. **Other:** Hypersensitivity reactions, injection-site nodule, *injection-site pain*, injection-site pruritus, *injection-site swelling*, miscarriage, stillbirth.

INTERACTIONS **Drug:** Hydroxyprogesterone can decrease the plasma levels of drugs that are substrates for CYP1A2 (e.g., **clozapine, theophylline, tizanidine**), CYP2A6 (e.g., **acetaminophen, nicotine**), or CYP2B6 (i.e., **bupropion, efavirenz, methadone**). Do not use with **bosentan.**

PHARMACOKINETICS **Peak:** 3–7 d. **Distribution:** Extensively bound to plasma proteins. **Metabolism:** In liver. **Elimination:** Fecal (50%) and renal (30%). **Half-Life:** 7.8 d.

NURSING IMPLICATIONS

Assessment & Drug Effects

- Monitor periodically: BP, weight, and mental status.
- Monitor diabetics closely for loss of glycemic control.
- Promptly report development of any of the following: New onset hypertension; S&S of thromboembolic disorder; unexplained vaginal bleeding; sudden weight gain; jaundice; depression; S&S of hypersensitivity (see Appendix F).

Patient & Family Education

- Report to prescriber if injection site becomes inflamed or increasingly painful over time.
- Diabetics should frequently monitor blood sugar and report significant changes to the prescriber.

HYDROXYUREA

(hye-drox′ee-yoo-ree-ah)

Hydrea, Droxia

Classification: ANTINEOPLASTIC; ANTIMETABOLITE

Therapeutic: ANTINEOPLASTIC

AVAILABILITY Capsule

ACTION & THERAPEUTIC EFFECT A cell-cycle-phase antineoplastic that causes an immediate inhibition of DNA synthesis by acting as an RNA reductase inhibitor necessary for DNA synthesis but without interfering with the synthesis of RNA or protein. *Cytotoxic effect limited to tissues with high rates of cell proliferation.*

USES Palliative treatment of metastatic melanoma, chronic myelocytic leukemia; recurrent metastatic, or inoperable ovarian cancer. Also used as adjunct to x-ray therapy for treatment of advanced primary squamous cell (epidermoid) carcinoma of head (excluding lip), neck, lungs.

UNLABELED USES Psoriasis; combination therapy with radiation of lung carcinoma; sickle cell anemia.

CONTRAINDICATIONS Severe myelosuppression; severe anemia, thrombocytopenia; pregnancy (category D); lactation.

CAUTIOUS USE Recent use of other cytotoxic drugs or irradiation; bone marrow depression; renal dysfunction; HIV patients; older adults; history of gout. Safe use in children not established.

ROUTE & DOSAGE

Palliative Therapy

Adult: **PO** 80 mg/kg q3days or 20–30 mg/kg/day

Sickle Cell Disease

Adult: **PO** 15 mg/kg/day, may increase by 5 mg/kg/day (max: 35 mg/kg/day or until toxicity develops)

Renal Impairment Dosage Adjustment

CrCl 10–50 mL/min: Administer 50% of dose; *less than 10 mL/min:* Administer 20% of dose

Hemodialysis Dosage Adjustment

Administer dose after hemodialysis; no supplemental dose needed

ADMINISTRATION

Oral

- Open, mix with water, and give immediately when patient has difficulty swallowing capsule.
- Store in tightly covered container at 15°–30° C (59°–86° F) unless otherwise directed.

ADVERSE EFFECTS **CNS:** Rare: Headache, dizziness, hallucinations, convulsions. **Skin:** Maculopapular rash, facial erythema, postirradiation erythema. **GI:** Stomatitis, anorexia, nausea, vomiting, diarrhea, constipation. **GU:** Renal tubular dysfunction, elevated BUN, serum, creatinine levels, hyperuricemia. **Hematologic:** Bone marrow suppression (leukopenia, anemia, thrombocytopenia), megaloblastic erythropoiesis. **Other:** Fever, chills, malaise.

INTERACTIONS **Drug:** No clinically significant interactions established.

PHARMACOKINETICS **Absorption:** Readily absorbed from GI tract. **Peak:** 2 h. **Distribution:** Crosses blood–brain barrier. **Metabolism:** In liver. **Elimination:** As respiratory CO_2 and as urea in urine.

NURSING IMPLICATIONS

Assessment & Drug Effects

- Interrupt therapy if WBC drops to 2500/mm^3 or platelets to 100,000/mm^3.
- Monitor I&O. Advise patients with high serum uric acid levels to drink at least 10–12 240 mL (8 oz) glasses of fluid daily to prevent uric acid nephropathy.
- Note: Patients with marked renal dysfunction may rapidly develop visual and auditory hallu-cinations and hematologic toxicity.
- Monitor lab tests: Baseline and periodic renal function tests, LFTs, and bone marrow function tests; hemoglobin, CBC with differential, platelet counts at least once weekly.

Patient & Family Education

- Notify prescriber of fever, chills, sore throat, nausea, vomiting, diarrhea, loss of appetite, and unusual bruising or bleeding.
- Use barrier contraceptive during therapy. Drug is teratogenic.

HYDROXYZINE HYDROCHLORIDE (Pr)

(hye-drox′i-zeen)

HYDROXYZINE PAMOATE

Vistaril

Classification: ANTIHISTAMINE; H_1-RECEPTOR ANTAGONIST

Therapeutic: ANTIPRURITIC; ANTI-ANXIETY; ANTIEMETIC

AVAILABILITY **Hydroxyzine HCl:** Tablet; syrup; solution for injection. **Hydroxyzine Pamoate:** Capsule

ACTION & *THERAPEUTIC EFFECT* H_1-receptor antagonist effective in treatment of histamine-mediated pruritus or other allergic reactions. Its tranquilizing effect is produced primarily by depression of hypothalamus and brainstem reticular formation, rather than cortical areas. *Effective as an antianxiety*

 Common adverse effects in *italic;* life-threatening effects underlined; generic names in **bold;** classifications in SMALL CAPS; ♣ Canadian drug name; (Pr) Prototype drug; ⚠ Alert

agent and sedative. Additionally, it is an effective agent for pruritus and as an antiemetic agent.

USES To relieve anxiety; perioperative adjunct, control nausea and emesis, and reduce narcotic requirements before or after surgery or delivery. Also used in management of pruritus due to allergic conditions, urticaria, atopic and contact dermatoses.

CONTRAINDICATIONS Hypersensitivity to hydroxyzine; early pregnancy; prolonged QT interval.

CAUTIOUS USE GI disorders; cardiac disease; COPD; older adults; pregnancy (crosses the placenta; possible withdrawal symptoms in neonates); lactation; children.

ROUTE & DOSAGE

Anxiety

Adult: **PO** 25–50 mg up to qid

Pruritus

Adult: **PO** 10–25 mg tid or qid
Child (6 y or older): **PO** 12.5 mg tid or qid

Peripartum management, adjunct to opioid

Adult: **IM** 25–50 mg; may repeat after 4 hours if needed

Renal Impairment Adjustment

CrCl 10–50 mL/min: administer 50% of dose; *CrCl less than 10 mL/min:* administer 25–50% of dose

ADMINISTRATION

Oral

- Note: Tablets may be crushed and taken with fluid of patient's choice. Capsule may be emptied and contents swallowed with water or mixed with food. Liquid formulations are available. Shake suspension vigorously prior to use.

Intramuscular

- Give deep into large muscle. The Z-track technique of injection is recommended to prevent subcutaneous infiltration. Aspirate before injection to avoid inadvertent injection into blood vessel.
- Recommended site: In adult, the gluteus maximus or vastus lateralis; in children, the vastus lateralis.
- Protect all forms from light. Store at 20°–25° C (68°–77° F). Protect from light.

ADVERSE EFFECTS CV: Hypotension. **Respiratory:** Respiratory depression. **CNS:** *Drowsiness*, cognitive dysfunction, hallucination, involuntary body movements, seizure, headache. **Skin:** Erythematous macular eruptions, erythema multiforme, urticaria, pruritis, rash. **GI:** *Dry mouth*. **Musculoskeletal:** Tremor.

DIAGNOSTIC TEST INTERFERENCE Possible false positive ***serum TCA screen.***

INTERACTIONS Drug: Alcohol and CNS DEPRESSANTS add to CNS depression; TRICYCLIC ANTIDEPRESSANTS and other ANTICHOLINERGICS have additive anticholinergic effects; may inhibit pressor effects of **epinephrine;** may enhance adverse effect of **eluxadoline.** Do not administer concurrently with COVID-19 vaccination because that might mask and delay treatment of adverse effects.

PHARMACOKINETICS Absorption: Readily from GI tract. **Onset:** 15–30 min PO. **Duration:** 4–6 h. **Distribution:** Not fully characterized.

Metabolism: In liver. **Elimination:** In urine.

NURSING IMPLICATIONS

Assessment & Drug Effects

- Evaluate alertness and mentation. Drowsiness may occur and usually disappears with continued therapy or following reduction of dosage.
- Reduce dosage of the depressant up to 50% when CNS depressants are prescribed concomitantly.
- Monitor blood pressure and for presence of hypersensitivity reaction.

Patient & Family Education

- Do not drive or engage in other potentially hazardous activities until response to drug is known.
- **Do not** take alcohol and hydroxyzine at the same time.
- Relieve dry mouth by frequent warm water rinses, increasing fluid intake, and use of a salivary substitute.
- Give teeth scrupulous care. Avoid irritation or abrasion of gums and other oral tissues.

HYOSCYAMINE SULFATE

(hye-oh-sye′a-meen)

Anaspaz, Levsin, Levsinex, NuLev

Classification: ANTICHOLINERGIC; ANTIMUSCARINIC; ANTISPASMODIC

Therapeutic: GI ANTISPASMODIC

Prototype: Atropine

AVAILABILITY Tablet; sublingual tablet; orally disintegrating tablet; oral solution; elixir; solution for injection; extended release tablet

ACTION & THERAPEUTIC EFFECT Blocks the action of acetylcholine at parasympathetic sites in smooth muscle, secretory glands, and the CNS. Increases cardiac output, dries secretions, and antagonizes histamine and serotonin. *Effective as a GI antispasmodic.*

USES GI tract disorders caused by spasm and hypermotility, as conjunct therapy with diet and antacids for peptic ulcer management, and as an aid in the control of gastric hypersecretion and intestinal hypermotility. Also symptomatic relief of biliary and renal colic, as a "drying agent" to relieve symptoms of acute rhinitis, to control preanesthesia salivation and respiratory tract secretions, to treat symptoms of parkinsonism, and to reduce pain and hypersecretion in pancreatitis; antidote for anticholinesterase agent poisoning; treat neurogenic bladder.

CONTRAINDICATIONS Hypersensitivity to belladonna alkaloids, prostatic hypertrophy, obstructive diseases of GI or GU tract, ulcerative colitis, paralytic ileus or intestinal atony; MG.

CAUTIOUS USE Diabetes mellitus, cardiac disease, cardiac arrhythmias; autonomic neuropathy; closed-angle glaucoma; GERD, hiatal hernia; pulmonary disease; renal or hepatic disease; elderly (avoid long-term use); pregnancy (crosses the placenta; unknown effect on the fetus); lactation; children younger than 2 y.

ROUTE & DOSAGE

GI Spasms

Adult: **IV/IM/Subcutaneous** 0.25–0.5 mg q4h (up to 4 times daily); **PO/Sublingual** 0.125–0.25 mg q4h prn (dose varies based on brand used)

Child (2–12 y): **PO** varies based on weight and brand used; consult package insert

Preanesthesia

Adult/Adolescent/Child over 2y): **IV/IM/Subcutaneous** 5 mcg/kg given 30–60 min before anesthesia

ADMINISTRATION

- Note: Dose for older adults may need to be less than the standard adult dose. Observe patient carefully for signs of paradoxic reactions.

Oral

- Give immediate release and sublingual tablets 30 min to 1 h ac.
- Orally disintegrating tablets may be chewed or placed on tongue for disintegration.
- Ensure that sustained release form of drug is not chewed or crushed. It **must be** swallowed whole.

Intramuscular/Subcutaneous

- May be given undiluted.

Intravenous

PREPARE: **Direct:** Give undiluted.
ADMINISTER: **Direct:** Give a single dose over 60 sec.

- Store at 20°–25°C (68°–77°F).

ADVERSE EFFECTS **CV:** Palpitations, tachycardia. **CNS:** Headache, unusual tiredness or weakness, confusion, *drowsiness,* excitement in older adult patients. **HEENT:** *Blurred vision,* increased intraocular tension, cycloplegia, mydriasis. **GI:** *Dry mouth, constipation,* paralytic ileus. **Other:** *Urinary retention,* anhidrosis, suppression of lactation.

INTERACTIONS **Drug: Amantadine,** ANTIHISTAMINES, TRICYCLIC ANTI-DEPRESSANTS, ANTICHOLINERGICS **disopyramide, procainamide** add anticholinergic effects; may decrease therapeutic effects of **levosulpiride;** decreases antipsychotic effects of PHENOTHIAZINES (decreased absorption).

PHARMACOKINETICS **Absorption:** Well absorbed from all administration sites. **Onset:** 2–3 min IV; **Duration:** 4–6 h (up to 12 h with extended release form). **Distribution:** Distributed in most body tissues; crosses blood–brain barrier and placenta; distributed in breast milk. **Metabolism:** In liver. **Elimination:** In urine. **Half-Life:** 2-4 h; 7h (extended release form).

NURSING IMPLICATIONS

Assessment & Drug Effects

- Monitor bowel elimination; may cause constipation.
- Monitor urinary output. Lessen risk of urinary retention by having patient void prior to each dose.
- Assess for excessive dryness of eyes, nose, mouth, or throat. Recommend good oral hygiene practices.

Patient & Family Education

- Avoid excessive exposure to high temperatures; drug-induced heatstroke can develop.
- Do not drive or engage in other potentially hazardous activities until response to drug is known.
- Use dark glasses if experiencing blurred vision, but if this adverse effect persists, notify prescriber for dose adjustment or possible drug change.

IBANDRONATE SODIUM

Boniva

Classification: BISPHOSPHONATE; BONE METABOLISM REGULATOR
Therapeutic: BONE METABOLISM REGULATOR
Prototype: Etidronate

AVAILABILITY Tablet

ACTION & *THERAPEUTIC EFFECT* It inhibits activity of osteoclasts and reduces bone resorption and turnover in the matrix of the bone. *In postmenopausal women, it reduces the rate of bone turnover, resulting in a net gain in bone mass.*

USES Prevention and treatment of osteoporosis in postmenopausal women.

UNLABELED USES Treatment of metastatic bone disease in breast cancer.

CONTRAINDICATIONS Hypersensitivity to ibandronate; severe renal impairment; hypocalcemia, vitamin D deficiency; inability to stand or sit up straight for 60 min; achalasia, esophageal stricture, dysphagia; signs and symptoms of bone fracture due to ibandromate use; severe renal impairment (CrCl less than 30 mL/min).

CAUTIOUS USE Hypersensitivity to other bisphosphanates; mild or moderate renal impairment; history of GI bleeding or disease, esophagitis, esophageal or gastric ulcers; older adults; pregnancy (category C); lactation. Safe use in children younger than 18 y not established.

ROUTE & DOSAGE

Postmenopausal Osteoporosis

Adult: **PO** 150 mg once monthly on the same day each month; **IV** 3 mg every 3 mo

Renal Impairment Dosage Adjustment

CrCl less than 30 mL/min: Use not recommended

ADMINISTRATION

Oral

- Correct hypocalcemia before administering ibandronate.
- Give at least 60 min before food, beverage, or other medications (including vitamins).
- Instruct to swallow whole with a full glass of plain water (180–240 mL; 6–8 oz) while standing or sitting in an upright position.
- Keep patient sitting up or ambulating for 60 min after taking drug.

Intravenous

PREPARE: **Direct:** Give undiluted.
ADMINISTER: **Direct:** Give over 15–30 sec.

- Store at 15°–30° C (59°–86° F).

ADVERSE EFFECTS **Respiratory:** *Upper respiratory infection,* bronchitis, **GI:** Dyspepsia. **Musculoskeletal:** Back pain.

DIAGNOSTIC TEST INTERFERENCE Interferes with the use of bone-imaging agents.

INTERACTIONS **Drug:** Concurrent administration of **calcium, magnesium,** or **iron** reduces ibandronate adsorption. **Food:** Food reduces ibandronate absorption (ibandronate should be taken in a fasting state).

PHARMACOKINETICS **Absorption:** Bioavailability poor (0.6%). **Peak:** 0.5–2 h. **Distribution:** 86–99% protein bound. **Metabolism:** None. **Elimination:** Renal. **Half-Life:** 10–60 h.

NURSING IMPLICATIONS

Assessment & Drug Effects

- Withhold drug and notify prescriber if the CrCl less than 30 mL/min.

- Diagnostic test: Bone density scan every 1–2 y after initiation.
- Monitor for S&S of upper GI distress, especially with concurrent use of NSAIDs or aspirin.
- Monitor lab tests: Periodic serum calcium. Obtain serum creatinine prior to each IV dose.

Patient & Family Education

- Take the monthly dose on the same day each month. Carefully follow directions for taking the drug (see ADMINISTRATION).
- If a monthly dose is missed, and the next scheduled dose is more than 7 days away, take one 150 mg tablet the next morning, then resume the original monthly schedule. Do not take two 150 mg tablets in the same week.
- Report to prescriber any of the following: Severe bone, joint, or muscle pain; heartburn, pain behind the sternum, difficulty or pain with swallowing.

IBREXAFUNGERP

(eye-BREX-a-FUNJ-erp)

Brexafemme

Classification: ANTIFUNGAL; TRITERPENOID

Therapeutic: ANTIFUNGAL

AVAILABILITY Oral tablet

ACTION & *THERAPEUTIC EFFECT* A triterpenoid antifungal that inhibits glucan synthase, an enzyme involved in the formation of an essential component of the fungal cell wall. Used to *treat vaginal fungal infections.*

USES Treatment of vulvovaginal candidiasis.

CONTRAINDICATIONS Hypersensitivity to ibrexafungerp or any component of the formulation; pregnancy (in utero exposure to ibrexafungerp may cause fetal harm; use during pregnancy is contraindicated).

CAUTIOUS USE Lactation.

ROUTE & DOSAGE

Vulvovaginal Candidiasis

Adult: **Oral:** 300 mg twice daily for 1 day

Use with strong CYP3A4 inhibitors

Adult: **Oral:** 150 mg twice daily for 1 day

ADMINISTRATION

Oral

- Administer with or without food.
- Administer doses approximately 12 hours apart.
- Store at 20°–25°C (68°–77°F).

ADVERSE EFFECTS **GU:** Abdominal pain, diarrhea, nausea.

INTERACTIONS **Drug:** Use with strong CYP3A4 inhibitors inhibitors (e.g., **ketoconazole, clarithyromycin**) increases ibrexafungerp exposure; the dose of ibrexafungerp should be decreased. Use with CYP3A4 inducers (e.g., **rifampin, phenobarbital, carbamazepine, phenytoin**) should be avoided.

PHARMACOKINETICS **Peak:** 4–6 h. **Distribution:** 99% protein bound. **Metabolism:** Primarily hydroxylation by CYP3A4. **Half-life:** 20 h. **Elimination:** 90% feces, 1% urine.

NURSING IMPLICATIONS

Assessment & Drug Effects

- Ensure pregnancy testing prior to initiating treatment.

Patient & Family Education

- This drug may be harmful to an unborn baby. A pregnancy test may be done before starting this drug to ensure that you are not pregnant. If you may become pregnant, you must use birth control while taking this drug and for sometime after the last dose. If you get pregnant, call your doctor right away.

IBRUTINIB

(i-brut′i-nib)

Imbruvica

Classification: ANTINEOPLASTIC AGENT; KINASE INHIBITOR

Therapeutic: ANTINEOPLASTIC AGENT

Prototype: Erlotinib

I

AVAILABILITY Capsule

ACTION & *THERAPEUTIC EFFECT* A potent and irreversible inhibitor of Bruton tyrosine kinase (BTK), an enzyme that is an integral component of the B-cell receptor (BCR) and cytokine receptor pathways; activation of B-cell receptor signaling is important for survival of malignant B-cells; *BTK inhibition results in decreased malignant B-cell proliferation and survival.*

USES Treatment of patients with mantle cell lymphoma (MCL) or patients with chronic lymphocytic leukemia (CLL) who have received at least one prior therapy; Waldenström macroglobulinemia; graft-versus-host disease.

CONTRAINDICATIONS Strong CYP3A4 inhibitors; severe renal impairment (CrCl less than 25 mL/min); pregnancy (category D); lactation.

CAUTIOUS USE Neutropenia, thrombocytopenia, anemia; mild to moderate renal impairment; hyperuricemia; mild hepatic impairment; arrhythmias; older adults. Safety and efficacy in children younger than 18 y not established.

ROUTE & DOSAGE

Mantle Cell Lymphoma (MCL)

Adult: **PO** 560 mg once daily at approximately the same time daily

Chronic Lymphocytic Leukemia (CLL)/Waldenström Macroglobulinemia

Adult: **PO** 420 mg once daily at approximately the same time each day until disease progression

Graft-Versus-Host disease (GVHD)

Adult: **PO** 420 mg daily until GVHD progression.

Adverse Reactions Dosage Adjustment

Interrupt therapy for any Grade 3 or greater nonhematological, Grade 3 or greater neutropenia with infection or fever, or Grade 4 hematological toxicities. *After recovery to baseline or Grade 1 toxicity, restart—First occurrence:* 560 mg daily MCL or 420 mg daily CLL; *Second occurrence:* 420 mg daily MCL or 280 mg daily CLL; *Third occurrence:* 280 mg daily MCL or 140 mg daily CLL; *Fourth occurrence:* Discontinue.

Use with CYP3A4 Inhibitors

Strong CYP3A4 inhibitors: Avoid use

Moderate CYP3A4 inhibitors: Decrease dose to 140 mg daily

Hepatic Impairment Dosage Adjustment

Child-Pugh class A: Reduce dose to 140 mg daily
Child-Pugh class B/C: Do not use

ADMINISTRATION

Oral

- Give with water at approximately the same time every day.
- Capsules **must be** swallowed whole; they should not be opened or chewed.
- Store in original container at 15°–30° C (59°–86° F).

ADVERSE EFFECTS **CV:** *Peripheral edema,* hypertension. **Respiratory:** *Upper respiratory infection,* dyspnea, cough, sinusitis, pneumonia, epistaxis, orophayngeal pain, bronchitis. **CNS:** *Fatigue,* dizziness, headache, anxiety, chills. **HEENT:** Dye eye syndrome, increased lacrimation, blurred vision, decreased visual acuity. **Endocrine:** Hyperuricemia, hypoalbuminemia, hypokalemia, dehydration. **Skin:** Skin rash, skin infection, pruritis. **GI:** *Diarrhea, nausea, stomatitis,* constipation, abdominal pain, vomiting, decreased appetite, dyspepsia, gastroesophogeal reflux disease. **GU:** Urinary tract infection. **Musculoskeletal:** Musculoskeletal pain, muscle spasm arthralgia, weakness, arthropathy. **Hematologic:** *Thrombocytopenia, neutropenia,* decreased hemoglobin, *hemorrhage,* petechia. **Other:** Infection, fever, falling.

INTERACTIONS **Drug:** Ibrutinib may enhance the adverse effects of drugs with antiplatelet activity (e.g., P2Y12 INHIBITORS, SSRIS, **aspirin**). Inhibitors of CYP3A4 (e.g., **ketoconazole, itraconazole, voriconazole, posaconazole, clarithromycin, telithromycin**) may increase the levels of ibrutinib. Inducers of CYP3A4 (e.g., **carbamazepine, rifampin, phenytoin**) may decrease the levels of ibrutinib. **Food: Grapefruit** and **grapefruit juice** may increase the levels of ibrutinib. **Herbal: St. John's wort** may decrease the levels of ibrutinib. **Bitter orange** may increase concentration of ibrutinib.

I

PHARMACOKINETICS **Peak:** 1–2 h. **Distribution:** 97% plasma protein bound. **Metabolism:** Extensive hepatic metabolism. **Elimination:** Fecal (80%) and renal (10%). **Half-life:** 4-6 h.

NURSING IMPLICATIONS

Assessment & Drug Effects

- Monitor BP, heart rate, and temperature.
- Monitor ECG, especially with new-onset dyspnea.
- Report irregular heart rate and suspected arrhythmias (e.g., atrial fibrillation or flutter).
- Monitor fluid status and maintain adequate hydration.
- Monitor for and report promptly S&S of bleeding or infection (e.g., UTI, upper respiratory tract infection).
- Monitor lab tests: Baseline and monthly (or as necessary) CBC with differential, platelet count, renal function tests, and LFTs; uric acid clinically indicated.

Patient & Family Education

- Do not consume grapefruit, grapefruit juice or Seville oranges during therapy.
- Report immediately to prescriber any of the following: Temperature 100.5° F or higher, chest pain or

palpitations, unexplained bleeding, or shortness of breath.

- Report GI adverse effects including mouth ulcers, severe reflux or dyspepsia, or severe diarrhea.
- Report excessive weight gain, edema, or numbness or tingling of extremities.
- Women of childbearing potential should use effective means of contraception while taking this drug.
- Do not breast-feed while taking this drug.

I

IBUPROFEN

(eye-byoo'proe-fen)

Advil, Amersol ♣, Caldolor, Children's Motrin, Motrin

Classification: ANALGESIC, NONSTEROIDAL ANTI-INFLAMMATORY DRUG (NSAID) (COX-1 AND COX-2 INHIBITOR); ANTIPYRETIC

Therapeutic: ANALGESIC, NSAID; ANTI-INFLAMMATORY; ANTIPYRETIC

AVAILABILITY Tablet; chewable tablet; suspension; drops; solution for injection

ACTION & *THERAPEUTIC EFFECT* (COX-1 and COX-2) NSAID inhibitor with nonsteroidal anti-inflammatory activity that blocks prostaglandin synthesis. Its activity also includes modulation of T-cell function, inhibition of inflammatory cell chemotaxis, decreased release of superoxide radicals, or increased scavenging of these compounds at inflammatory sites. *Has nonsteroidal anti-inflammatory, analgesic, and antipyretic effects. Inhibits platelet aggregation and prolongs bleeding time.*

USES Chronic, symptomatic rheumatoid arthritis and osteoarthritis; relief of mild to moderate pain; primary dysmenorrhea; reduction of fever.

UNLABELED USES Gout, juvenile rheumatoid arthritis, psoriatic arthritis, ankylosing spondylitis, vascular headache.

CONTRAINDICATIONS Hypersensitivity to ibuprofen; patient in whom urticaria, severe rhinitis, bronchospasm, angioedema, nasal polyps are precipitated by aspirin or other NSAIDs; active peptic ulcer, bleeding abnormalities; perioperative pain related to CABG surgery; signs and symptoms of renal toxicity to ibuprofen; severe hepatic reactions to ibuprofen; development of signs and symptoms of meningitis while taking ibuprofen; salicylate hypersensitivity.

CAUTIOUS USE History of GI ulceration or GI bleeding; intrinsic coagulation defects; DM; impaired hepatic or renal function, chronic renal failure; hypertension, history of CAD; angina, MI, cardiac decompensation; patients with SLE, and related connective tissue disorders; adults older than 60 y; pregnancy (category C). Safe use in children younger than 6 mo not established.

ROUTE & DOSAGE

Inflammatory Disease

Adult: **PO** 400–800 mg tid or qid (max: 3200 mg/day)

Child (weight less than 20 kg): **PO** Up to 400 mg/day in divided doses; *weight 20 kg to less than 30 kg:* Up to 600 mg/day in divided doses; *weight 30–40 kg:* Up to 800 mg/day in divided doses

 Common adverse effects in *italic;* life-threatening effects underlined; generic names in **bold;** classifications in SMALL CAPS; ♣ Canadian drug name; Prototype drug; Alert

Dysmenorrhea

Adult: **PO** 400 mg q4h up to 1200 mg/day

Mild to Moderate Pain

Adult: **PO** 200–800 mg 3–4 × per day **IV** 400 mg q4–6h prn or 100–200 mg q4h prn

Fever

Adult: **PO** 200–400 mg tid or qid (max: 1200 mg/day)
Child (6 mo–12 y): **PO** 5–10 mg/kg q6–8h up to 40 mg/kg/day

ADMINISTRATION

Oral

- Give on an empty stomach, 1 h before or 2 h after meals. May be taken with meals or milk if GI intolerance occurs.
- Ensure that chewable tablets are chewed or crushed before being swallowed.
- Note: Tablet may be crushed if patient is unable to swallow it whole and mixed with food or liquid before swallowing.
- Store in tightly closed, light-resistant container unless otherwise directed by manufacturer.

Intravenous

Patients should be well hydrated before IV infusion to prevent renal damage.
PREPARE: **Infusion:** Dilute required dose with NS, D5W or LR to a final concentration of 4 mg/mL or less.
ADMINISTER: **Infusion:** Infuse over at least 30 min.

ADVERSE EFFECTS **CV:** Edema. **CNS:** Dizziness. **GI:** Epigastric pain, nausea, dyspepsia.

DIAGNOSTIC TEST INTERFERENCE May cause false positive for ***urine phencyclidine.*** May cause false positive **aldosterone/renin ratio.**

INTERACTIONS **Drug:** ORAL ANTICOAGULANTS, **heparin** may prolong bleeding time; avoid other NSAIDs; may increase **lithium** and **methotrexate** toxicity. Do not use **cidofovir** due to toxicity risk. Do not use with **acemetacin, macimorelin, pheylbutazone.** **Herbal: Feverfew, garlic, ginger, ginkgo** may increase bleeding potential.

PHARMACOKINETICS **Absorption:** 85% from GI tract (oral product). **Onset:** 30–60 min. **Peak:** 1–2 h. **Duration:** 6–8 h. **Metabolism:** Hepatic via oxidation. **Elimination:** Primarily in urine; some biliary excretion. **Half-Life:** 2–4 h.

NURSING IMPLICATIONS

Black Box Warning

Ibuprofen has been associated with increased risk of serious, potentially fatal GI bleeding and cardiovascular events (e.g., MI & CVA); risk may increase with duration of use and may be greater in the older adult and those with risk factors for CV disease.

Assessment & Drug Effects

- Monitor for and report promptly S&S of CV thrombotic events (i.e., angina, MI, TIA, or stroke).
- Observe patients with history of cardiac decompensation closely for evidence of fluid retention and edema.
- Monitor for and report promptly S&S of GI ulceration or bleeding. Significant GI bleeding may occur without prior warning.

- Auditory and ophthalmologic examinations are recommended in patients receiving prolonged or high-dose therapy.
- Note: Symptoms of acute toxicity in children include apnea, cyanosis, response only to painful stimuli, dizziness, and nystagmus.
- Monitor lab tests: Baseline and periodic CBC, chemistry profile, renal function tests, and LFTs.

Patient & Family Education

- Stop taking drug and report promptly to prescriber if you experience chest pain, shortness of breath, weakness, slurring of speech, or other signs of a cardiac or neurologic problem.
- Notify prescriber immediately of passage of dark tarry stools, "coffee ground" emesis, frankly bloody emesis, or other GI distress, as well as blood or protein in urine, and onset of skin rash, pruritus, jaundice.
- Do not drive or engage in other potentially hazardous activities until response to the drug is known.
- Do not self-medicate with ibuprofen if taking prescribed drugs or being treated for a serious condition without consulting prescriber.
- Do not give to children younger than 3 mo or for longer than 2 days without consulting pre-scriber.
- Do not take aspirin concurrently with ibuprofen.
- Avoid alcohol and NSAIDs unless otherwise advised by prescriber. Concurrent use may increase risk of GI ulceration and bleeding tendencies.

IBUTILIDE FUMARATE

(i-bu′ti-lide)

Corvert

Classification: CLASS III ANTIARRHYTHMIC

Therapeutic: CLASS III ANTIARRHYTHMIC

Prototype: Amiodarone HCl

AVAILABILITY

Solution for injection

ACTION & THERAPEUTIC EFFECT

Ibutilide is a Class III antiarrhythmic that prolongs cardiac action potential and increases both atrial and ventricular refractoriness without affecting conduction. *Effective in treating recently occurring atrial arrhythmias. It may produce proarrhythmic effects that can be life threatening.*

USES

Rapid conversion of atrial fibrillation or atrial flutter of recent onset.

CONTRAINDICATIONS

Hypersensitivity to ibutilide, hypokalemia, hypomagnesemia.

CAUTIOUS USE

History of CHF, cardiac ejection fraction of 35% or less, recent MI, prolonged QT intervals, ventricular arrhythmias; renal or liver disease, cardiovascular disorder other than atrial arrhythmias; pregnancy (category C); lactation. Safe use in children younger than 18 y not established.

ROUTE & DOSAGE

Atrial Fibrillation or Flutter

Adult (weight less than 60 kg): **IV** 0.01 mg/kg, may repeat in 10 min if inadequate response; *weight 60 kg or greater:* 1 mg, may repeat in 10 min if inadequate response

ADMINISTRATION

- Hypokalemia and hypomagnesemia should be corrected prior to treatment with ibutilide.

Intravenous

PREPARE: **Direct:** Give undiluted. **IV Infusion:** Contents of 1 mg vial may be diluted in 50 mL of D5W or NS to yield 0.017 mg/mL.
ADMINISTER: **Direct/IV Infusion:** Give a single dose by direct injection or infusion over 10 min.
- Stop injection/infusion as soon as presenting arrhythmia is terminated or with appearance of ventricular tachycardia or marked prolongation of QT or QT_c.

- Store diluted solution up to 24 h at 15°–30° C (59°–86° F) or 48 h refrigerated at 2°–8° C (36°–46° F).

ADVERSE EFFECTS **CV:** Proarrhythmic effects (sustained and nonsustained polymorphic ventricular tachycardia), AV block, bundle branch block, ventricular extrasystoles, hypotension, postural hypotension, bradycardia, tachycardia, palpitations, prolonged QT segment. **CNS:** Headache. **GI:** Nausea.

INTERACTIONS **Drug:** Increased potential for proarrhythmic effects when administered with PHENOTHIAZINES, TRICYCLIC ANTIDEPRESSANTS, **amiodarone, disopyramide, procainamide, sotalol** may cause prolonged refractoriness if given within 4 h of ibutilide.

PHARMACOKINETICS **Onset:** 30 min. **Metabolism:** In liver. **Elimination:** 82% in urine, 19% in feces. **Half-Life:** 6 h (range 2–21 h).

NURSING IMPLICATIONS

Black Box Warning

Ibutilide has been associated with potentially fatal arrhythmias usually, but not always, in association of QT prolongation.

Assessment & Drug Effects

- Observe with continuous ECG, BP, and HR monitoring during and for at least 4 h after infusion or until QT_c has returned to baseline. Monitor for longer periods with liver dysfunction or if proarrhythmic activity is observed.
- Hypokalemia and hypomagnesemia should be corrected prior to beginning treatment with ibutilide.
- Monitor for therapeutic effectiveness. Conversion to normal sinus rhythm normally occurs within 30 min of initiation of infusion.
- Monitor lab tests: Baseline serum potassium and magnesium.

Patient & Family Education

- Consult prescriber and understand the potential risks of ibutilide therapy.

IDARUBICIN

(i-da-roo′bi-cin)

Idamycin PFS

Classification: ANTINEOPLASTIC; ANTHRACYCLINE (ANTIBIOTIC)
Therapeutic: ANTINEOPLASTIC
Prototype: Doxorubicin

AVAILABILITY Solution for injection

ACTION & *THERAPEUTIC EFFECT* Cytotoxic anthracycline that exhibits inhibitory effects on DNA topoisomerase II, an enzyme responsible for repairing faulty sections of DNA. It results in breaks in the helix of the DNA, and thus it affects RNA and protein synthesis in rapidly dividing cells. *Has antineoplastic and cytotoxic action on cancer cells that results in cell death.*

USES In combination with other antineoplastic drugs for treatment of AML.

UNLABELED USES Breast cancer, other solid tumors.

CONTRAINDICATIONS Myelosuppression, hypersensitivity to idarubicin or doxorubicin, pregnancy (category D), lactation.

CAUTIOUS USE Impaired renal or hepatic function; patients who have received irradiation or radiotherapy to areas surrounding heart; cardiac disease. Safe use in children younger than 2 y not established.

ROUTE & DOSAGE

I

Acute Myelogenous Leukemia (AML)

Adult: **IV** 12 mg/m² daily for 3 days injected slowly over 10–15 min

Acute Nonlymphocytic Leukemia, Acute Lymphocytic Leukemia

Child: **IV** 10–12 mg/m²/day for 3 days

Renal Impairment Dosage Adjustment

Creatinine greater than 2 mg/dL: Give 75% of dose

Hepatic Impairment Dosage Adjustment

Bilirubin 1.5–5 mg/dL: Give 50% of dose; *if greater than 5 mg/dL:* Do not use drug

ADMINISTRATION

Intravenous

IV administration to infants, children: Verify correct IV concentration and rate of infusion with prescriber.
This drug is a cytotoxic agent and caution should be used to prevent any contact with the drug. Follow institutional or standard guidelines for preparation, handling, and disposal of cytotoxic agents.
PREPARE: **IV Infusion:** Further dilution is not required.
ADMINISTER: **IV Infusion:** Give slowly over 10–15 min into tubing of free flowing IV of NS or D5W. ▪ If extravasation is suspected, immediately stop infusion, elevate the arm, and apply ice pack for 30 min then qid for 30 min × 3 days.
INCOMPATIBILITIES: **Solution/additive:** ALKALINE SOLUTIONS (i.e., **sodium bicarbonate**), **heparin**. **Y-site: Acyclovir, allopurinol, ampicillin/sulbactam, cefazolin, cefepime, ceftazidime, clindamycin, dexamethasone, etoposide, furosemide, gentamicin, heparin, hydrocortisone, imipenem/cilastatin, lorazepam, meperidine, methotrexate, mezlocillin, piperacillin/tazobactam, sargramostim, sodium bicarbonate, teniposide, vancomycin, vincristine.**

- Store reconstituted solutions up to 7 days refrigerated at 2°–8° C (36°–46° F) and 72 h at room temperature 15°–30° C (59°–86° F).

ADVERSE EFFECTS **CV:** CHF, atrial fibrillation, chest pain, MI. **GI:** *Nausea, vomiting, diarrhea, abdominal pain,* mucositis. **Hematologic:** *Anemia, leukopenia,* thrombocytopenia. **Other:** Nephrotoxicity, hepatotoxicity, *alopecia,* rash.

INTERACTIONS **Drug:** IMMUNOSUPPRESSANTS cause additive bone marrow suppression; ANTICOAGULANTS, NSAIDS, SALICYLATES, **aspirin,** THROMBOLYTIC AGENTS increase risk of bleeding; idarubicin may blunt the effects of **filgrastim, sargramostim.**

PHARMACOKINETICS Onset: Median time to remission 28 days. **Peak:** Serum level 4 h. **Duration:** Serum levels 120 h. **Distribution:** Concentrates in nucleated blood and bone marrow cells. **Metabolism:** In liver to idarubicinol, which may be as active as idarubicin. **Elimination:** 16% in urine; 17% in bile. **Half-Life:** Idarubicin 15–45 h, idarubicinol 45 h.

NURSING IMPLICATIONS

Black Box Warning

Idarubicin can cause severe local tissue necrosis if extravasation occurs and it has been associated with severe myelosuppression.

Assessment & Drug Effects

- Monitor infusion site closely, as extravasation can cause severe local tissue necrosis. Notify prescriber if pain, erythema, or edema develops at insertion site.
- Monitor cardiac status closely, especially in older adult patients or those with preexisting cardiac disease.
- Monitor hematologic status carefully; during the period of myelosuppression, patients are at high risk for bleeding and infection.
- Monitor for development of hyperuricemia secondary to lysis of leukemic cells.
- Monitor lab tests: Periodic LFTs and renal function tests, CBC with differential, and coagulation studies.

Patient & Family Education

- Learn all potential adverse reactions to idarubicin.
- Anticipate possible hair loss.
- Discuss interventions to minimize nausea, vomiting, diarrhea, and stomatitis with health care providers.

IDARUCIZUMAB

(i-dare'you-scis-ooh-mab)

Praxbind

Classification: MONOCLONAL ANTIBODY; COAGULATION REVERSAL AGENT

Therapeutic: COAGULATION REVERSAL AGENT

AVAILABILITY Solution for injection

ACTION & THERAPEUTIC EFFECT A humanized monoclonal antibody fragment (Fab) that binds to dabigatran and its acylglucuronide metabolites with higher affinity than dabigatran binds to thrombin. *This action neutralizes dabigatran as well as its active metabolites, thus reversing their anticoagulant effect.*

USES Indicated for the reversal of the anticoagulant effects of dabigatran in patients requiring emergency surgery or other urgent procedures, and in patients with life-threatening or uncontrolled bleeding.

CAUTIOUS USE Hereditary fructose intolerance, thromboembolic disease, pregnancy, lactation.

ROUTE & DOSAGE

Reversal of Dabigatran Effects

Adult: **IV** 5 gram

ADMINISTRATION

Intravenous

PREPARE: **IV Infusion:** Flush the line with 0.9% sodium chloride prior to infusion. Recommended dose provided is 2 vials each containing 2.5 g/50 mL.

ADMINISTER: **IV Infusion:** Administer 5 g dose as either 2 consecutive infusions or inject both vials consecutively via syringe. A preexisting intravenous line may be used for administration.
INCOMPATIBILITIES **Solution/additive:** None listed; however, the solution should not be mixed with other medicinal products or solutions.

- Store refrigerated at 2–8° C (36–46° F).
- Do not freeze; do not shake.
- Prior to use, the unopened vial may be kept at room temperature 25° C (77°F) for up to 48 h if stored in the original package in order to protect from light or up to 6 h when exposed to light.
- Administer within 1 h after solution has been removed from the vial.

ADVERSE EFFECTS **CV:** Thromboembolic events. **CNS:** Delirium, headache. **Endocrine:** Hypokalemia. **GI:** Constipation. **Other:** Hypersensitivity reactions, pneumonia.

PHARMACOKINETICS **Metabolism:** Biodegradation of monoclonal antibody. **Elimination:** Primarily renal. **Half-Life:** 10.3 h.

NURSING IMPLICATIONS

Assessment & Drug Effects

- Obtain baseline aPTT, repeat at 2 h and then every 12 h until aPTT returns to normal.
- Assess for S&S of bleeding and thromboembolism in patients with hereditary fructose intolerance.

Patient & Family Education

- This drug is used to undo the effects of a blood thinner. The chance of blood clots may be raised after using this drug. Follow instructions from your health care provider about prevention of blood clots.
- Report signs or symptoms of a blood clot immediately such as chest pain or pressure; coughing up blood; swelling, warmth, numbness, change of color, or pain in a leg or arm; or trouble breathing or talking.

IDELALISIB

(i-del-a-li′sib)
Zydelig
Classification: ANTINEOPLASTIC; KINASE INHIBITOR
Therapeutic: ANTINEOPLASTIC
Prototype: Erlotinib

AVAILABILITY Tablets

ACTION & *THERAPEUTIC EFFECT* Potent inhibitor of the enzyme, phosphatidylinositol 3-kinase (PI3Kδ), which is highly expressed in malignant lymphoid B-cells. *PI3Kδ inhibition results in apoptosis of malignant tumor cells, thus reducing the number of malignant lymphocytes.*

USES Treatment of patients with relapsed chronic lymphocytic leukemia (CLL), relapsed follicular B-cell non-Hodgkin lymphoma (FL), and relapsed small lymphocytic lymphoma (SLL).

CONTRAINDICATIONS History of serious allergic reactions including anaphylaxis and toxic epidermal necrolysis; intestinal perforation; concurrent CYP3A inducers or substrates; recurrent hepatotoxicity, life-threatening diarrhea, or pneumonitis due to idelalisib; pregnancy (category D); lactation.

CAUTIOUS USE Neutropenia, thrombocytopenia, anemia; preexisting liver impairment; pulmonary toxicity; colitis; older adults. Safety and efficacy in children less than 18 y not established.

ROUTE & DOSAGE

Chronic Lymphocytic Leukemia, B-Cell Non-Hodgkin Lymphoma, Small Lymphocytic Lymphoma

Adult: **PO** 150 mg bid

Hepatic Impairment Dosage Adjustment

ALT/AST greater than 5 to 20 × ULN or bilirubin greater than 3 to 10 × ULN: Interrupt therapy; monitor LFTs at least weekly until ALT/AST and/or bilirubin is ULN or less, then restart therapy at 100 mg bid *ALT/AST greater than 20 × ULN, bilirubin greater than 10 × ULN, or recurrent hepatotoxicity:* Permanently discontinue.

Toxicity Dosage Adjustment

Severe diarrhea or diarrhea requiring hospitalization: Interrupt therapy, monitor at least weekly, restart at 100 mg bid, when diarrhea has resolved. *Life-threatening diarrhea:* Permanently discontinue

Neutropenia ANC less than 500 cells/mm³: Interrupt therapy, monitor ANC at least weekly, then restart at 100 mg bid when ANC 500 cells/mm³ or greater

Thrombocytopenia platelet count less than 25,000 cells/mm³: Interrupt therapy, monitor platelet count at least weekly, then restart at 100 mg bid when platelet count 25,000 cells/mm³ or greater

Symptomatic pneumonitis (any severity): Discontinue

Other severe or life-threatening toxicities: Interrupt therapy until toxicity is resolved; resume treatment at 100 mg bid

Permanently discontinue for any recurrence after re-challenge.

ADMINISTRATION

Oral

- Give without regard to food.
- Tablets **must be** swallowed whole. They must not be crushed or chewed.
- May give a missed dose if within 6 h of usual dosing time. If more than 6 h, skip the missed dose and resume with the next scheduled dose.
- Store at 15°–30° C (59°–86° F).

ADVERSE EFFECTS **Respiratory:** Bronchitis, cough, *dyspnea,* nasal congestion, *pneumonia,* sinusitis, upper respiratory infection. **CNS:** Headache, insomnia. **Endocrine:** Altered glucose level (increase and decrease), altered lymphocyte count (increase and decrease), decreased appetite, decreased hemoglobin, decreased neutrophils, decreased platelets, hypertriglyceridemia, hyponatremia, *increased ALT and AST,* increase gamma glutamyl transpeptidase. **Skin:** Rash. **GI:** *Abdominal pain, diarrhea,* gastroesophageal reflux disease, *nausea,* stomatitis, vomiting. **GU:** Urinary tract infection. **Musculoskeletal:** Arthralgia. **Other:** Asthenia, *chills, fatigue,* night sweats, pain, peripheral edema, *pyrexia,* sepsis *fever.*

INTERACTIONS **Drug:** Coadministration with other drugs that inhibit CYP3A4 (e.g.,

erythromycin, itraconazole, ketoconazole) may increase the levels of idelalisib. Coadministration with other drugs that induce CYP3A4 (e.g., **carbamazepine, phenytoin, rifampin**) may decrease the levels of idelalisib. Idelalisib may increase the levels of other drugs that require CYP3A4 for metabolism. **Food: Grapefruit** and **grapefruit juice** may increase the levels of idelalisib. **Herbal: St. John's wort** may decrease the levels of idelalisib.

PHARMACOKINETICS **Peak:** 1.5 h. **Distribution:** 84% plasma protein bound. **Metabolism:** In liver. **Elimination:** Renal (14%) and fecal (78%). **Half-Life:** 8.2 h.

NURSING IMPLICATIONS

Black Box Warning

Idelalisib has been associated with severe and sometimes fatal cases of hepatotoxicity, diarrhea, colitis, pneumonitis, and intestinal perforation.

Assessment & Drug Effects

- Monitor for and report promptly any of the following: S&S of severe diarrhea/colitis, intestinal perforation, pneumonitis (e.g., cough, dyspnea, hypoxia), dermatologic toxicity (i.e., dermatitis or rash), and hypersensitivity reactions. Withhold drug for any of the foregoing until prescriber is consulted.
- Monitor lab tests: LFTs q2wk first 3 mo, q4wk next 3 mo, then q1–3 mo thereafter, or as necessary; CBC with differential and platelet count q2wk first 3 mo, and at least weekly with neutropenia, or as necessary.

Patient & Family Education

- Report immediately if you develop a fever or any signs of infection.
- Report immediately to prescribed if you experience signs of intestinal toxicity or perforation such as abdominal pain, chills, fever, nausea, vomiting, or severe diarrhea (i.e., six or more bowel movements per day).
- Report signs of skin toxicity including rash with or without itching.
- Report signs of liver damage including jaundice, bruising, abdominal pain, or bleeding.
- Report new or worsening respiratory symptoms including cough or dyspnea.
- Women of childbearing age should use effective means of contraception while taking this drug and for at least 1 mo after ending treatment.
- Do not breast-feed while taking this drug.

IFOSFAMIDE

Ifex

(i-fos'fa-mide)

Classification: ANTINEOPLASTIC; ALKYLATING AGENT

Therapeutic: ANTINEOPLASTIC

Prototype: Cyclophosphamide

AVAILABILITY Solution for injection

ACTION & *THERAPEUTIC EFFECT*

Interacts with DNA as a cell cycle nonspecific agent. Antineoplastic action is primarily due to cross-linking of strands of DNA and RNA as well as inhibition of protein and DNA synthesis. *It has antineoplastic and cytotoxic action on cancer cells that results in cell death.*

USES In combination with other agents in various regimens for germ cell testicular cancer.

CONTRAINDICATIONS Hypersensitivity to ifosfamide; severe bone marrow depression; dehydration; pregnancy (fetal growth retardation and neonatal anemia have been reported with exposure during pregnancy); lactation.

CAUTIOUS USE Impaired renal function, renal failure; hepatic disease; prior radiation or prior therapy with other cytotoxic agents.

ROUTE & DOSAGE

Antineoplastic

Adult: **IV** 1.2 g/m^2/day for 5 consecutive days; repeat q3wk or after recovery from hematologic toxicity (platelets 100,000/mm^3 or greater; WBC 4000/mm^3 or greater)

ADMINISTRATION

Intravenous

This drug is a cytotoxic agent and caution should be used to prevent any contact with the drug. Follow institutional or standard guidelines for preparation, handling, and disposal of cytotoxic agents.

PREPARE: **IV Infusion:** Reconstitute each 1 g or 3 g vial with 20 mL or 60 mL, respectively, of sterile water or bacteriostatic water to yield 50 mg/mL. ▪ Shake well to dissolve. ▪ May be further diluted with D5W, NS, or LR to achieve concentrations of 0.6–20 mg/mL. ▪ Use solution prepared with sterile water within 6 h.

ADMINISTER: **IV Infusion:** Give slowly over 30 min. ▪ Note: Mesna is always given concurrently with ifosfamide; never give ifosfamide alone.

INCOMPATIBILITIES: **Y-site: Cefepime, diazepam, methotrexate, pantoprazole, phenytoin, potassium phosphate.**

▪ Store reconstituted solution prepared with bacteriostatic solution up to a week at 30° C (86° F) or 6 wk at 5° C (41° F).

ADVERSE EFFECTS **CNS:** Brain disease, central nervous system toxicity. **Endocrine:** Metabolic acidosis. **Skin:** *Alopecia.* **GI:** *Nausea, vomiting,* hepatic dysfunction. **GU:** Hematuria, renal insufficiency. **Hematologic:** Thrombocytopenia, leukopenia, anemia. **Other:** Infection.

DIAGNOSTIC TEST INTERFERENCE: May diminish the diagnostic effect of Coccidioides immitis Skin Test.

INTERACTIONS **Drug:** HEPATIC ENZYME INDUCERS (BARBITURATES, **phenytoin**) may increase hepatic conversion of ifosfamide to active metabolite; CORTICOSTEROIDS may inhibit conversion to active metabolites. Do not use with IMMUNOSUPPRESANTS, LIVE VACCINES, MYELEOSUPPRESIVE AGENTS.

PHARMACOKINETICS **Distribution:** Distributed into breast milk. **Metabolism:** In liver via CYP3A4. **Elimination:** in urine. **Half-Life:** 7–15 h.

NURSING IMPLICATIONS

Black Box Warning

Ifosfamide has been associated with hemorrhagic cystitis and CNS toxicities.

Assessment & Drug Effects

- Hold drug and notify prescriber if WBC count is below 2000/mm^3 or platelet count is below 50,000/mm^3.
- Reduce risk of hemorrhagic cystitis by hydrating with 3000 mL of fluid daily prior to therapy and for at least 72 h following treatment to ensure ample urine output.
- Monitor for and report promptly any symptoms of neurotoxicity such as somnolence, confusion, depressive psychosis, and hallucinations.
- Monitor lab tests: CBC with differential prior to each dose and at regular intervals; urinalysis prior to each dose for microscopic hematuria; liver function, renal function.

Patient & Family Education

- Void frequently to lessen contact of irritating chemical with bladder mucosa by keeping well hydrated.
- Note: Susceptibility to infection may increase. Avoid people with infection. Notify prescriber of any infection, fever or chills, cough or hoarseness, lower back or side pain, painful or difficult urination.
- Check with prescriber immediately if there is any unusual bleeding or bruising, black tarry stools, or blood in urine or if pinpoint red spots develop on skin.
- Discuss possible adverse effects (e.g., alopecia, nausea, and vomiting) and measures that can minimize them with health care provider.

ILOPERIDONE

(i-lo-per'i-done)

Fanapt

Classification: ATYPICAL ANTIPSYCHOTIC

Therapeutic: ANTIPSYCHOTIC

Prototype: Clozapine

AVAILABILITY Tablet

ACTION & THERAPEUTIC EFFECT Mechanism of action is unknown, however, thought to be both a dopamine (D_2) and serotonin ($5\text{-}HT_2$) antagonist. *Effective in treating acute schizophrenia uncontrolled by other agents.*

USES Acute treatment of schizophrenia.

CONTRAINDICATIONS Hypersensitivity to iloperidone; older adults with dementia-related psychosis; suicidal ideation; neuroleptic malignant syndrome (NMS); severe hepatic impairment; recent acute MI; ANC less than 100 mm^3; lactation.

CAUTIOUS USE Congenital long QT syndrome; history of cardiac arrhythmias; history of suicidal tendencies; cardiovascular disease; CVA; CHF; cerebrovascular disease; risk for aspiration pneumonia; tardive dyskinesia; DM; history of seizures; history of leukopenia/neutropenia; moderate hepatic impairment; patients at risk for aspiration pneumonia; older adults; pregnancy (antipsychotic use during third trimester of pregnancy has a risk for abnormal muscle movements and/or withdrawal symptoms in newborns). Safety and efficacy in children not established.

ROUTE & DOSAGE

Schizophrenia

Adult: **PO** Initial 1 mg bid, then titrate.

Titration schedule: Increase each dose by 2 mg a day bid (4 mg daily) q24h until desired dose

reached (max: 12 mg bid).
Note: Reduce dose by 50% with concurrent use of a strong CYP2D6 inhibitor (e.g., fluoxetine or paroxetine) or strong CYP3A4 inhibitor (e.g., ketoconazole or clarithromycin).

Pharmacogenetic Dosage Adjustment

Reduce dose 50% for poor CYP2D6 metabolizers

ADMINISTRATION

Oral

- Note that gradual dose titration is recommended initially and whenever patient has been off drug for more than 3 days.
- May administer with or without food.
- Store at 25° C (77° F). Protect from light and moisture.

ADVERSE EFFECTS **CV:** Orthostatic hypotension, *tachycardia*. **Respiratory:** Nasal congestion, nasopharyngitis. **CNS:** *Dizziness,* drowsiness, extrapyramidal reaction, fatigue. **Endocrine:** Increased serum prolactin, weight gain, increased serum triglycerides, increased serum cholesterol. **GI:** Abdominal discomfort, diarrhea, *dry mouth, nausea.*

INTERACTIONS **Drug:** Potential additive QT prolongation if used in combination with drugs with similar effects (e.g., **disopyramide, procainamide, amiodarone**). Inhibitors of CYP3A4 (e.g., **ketoconazole, itraconazole, clarithromycin**) or CYP2D6 (e.g., **fluoxetine, paroxetine**) can increase iloperidone levels. Do not use with **saquinavir** due to risk of torsades de pointes. **Amisulpride** increases the risk of neuroleptic malignant syndrome. May decrease efficacy of ANTIPARINSON AGENTS. Increased risk of adverse effects with CNS DEPRESSANTS.

PHARMACOKINETICS **Peak:** 2–4 h. **Distribution:** 95% plasma protein bound. **Metabolism:** Extensive hepatic metabolism to active and inactive metabolites; CYP2D6 and CYP3A4. **Elimination:** Renal (major) and fecal. **Half-Life:** 18–33 h.

NURSING IMPLICATIONS

Black Box Warning

Iloperidone has been associated with increased mortality in older adults with dementia-related psychosis.

Assessment & Drug Effects

- Monitor for suicidal ideation and report promptly if suspected.
- Monitor BP, HR, and weight. Monitor orthostatic vital signs with concurrent antihypertensive therapy or any condition that predisposes to hypotension (e.g., advanced age, dehydration).
- Monitor for orthostatic hypotension and syncope, especially early in therapy.
- Monitor ECG for prolongation of the QT_c interval.
- Monitor diabetics and those at risk for diabetes for loss of glycemic control.
- Monitor lab tests: Baseline and periodic CBC with differential; electrolytes, liver function, fasting lipid panel.

Patient & Family Education

- Be alert for and report worsening of condition, including ideas of suicide.
- Make position changes slowly, especially from a lying or sitting position to a standing position.

- If diabetic, monitor blood sugar closely for loss of control.
- Stop taking the drug and report immediately any of the following: Feeling faint or fainting, high fever, muscle rigidity, altered mental status, or palpitations.
- Do not drink alcohol while taking this drug.
- Avoid engaging in hazardous activities until response to drug is known.

I

IMATINIB MESYLATE

(i-ma'ti-nib)

Gleevec

Classification: ANTINEOPLASTIC; MONOCLONAL ANTIBODY; EPIDERMAL GROWTH FACTOR RECEPTOR; KINASE INHIBITOR

Therapeutic: ANTINEOPLASTIC

Prototype: Erlotinib

AVAILABILITY Tablet

ACTION & THERAPEUTIC EFFECT Epidermal growth factor receptor-tyrosine kinase inhibitor (EGFR-TKI) that interferes with intracellular signaling pathways that are involved in the development of malignancies. Imatinib inhibits abnormal Bcr-Abl tyrosine kinase created by the Philadelphia chromosome abnormality in chronic myeloid leukemia (CLM). *Inhibits WBC cell proliferation and induces cell death in Bcr-Abl tyrosine kinase positive cells as well as in newly formed leukemic cells. Thus, it interferes with progression of chronic myeloid leukemia (CML). Additionally, imatinib inhibits proliferation and induces cell death in gastrointestinal stomal tumor (GIST) that express a mutation of an activated cKit tyrosine kinase.*

USES Treatment of CML in blast crisis, or in chronic phase after failure of interferon-alpha therapy; unresectable and/or metastatic malignant gastrointestinal stromal tumors (GISTs), acute lymphoblastic leukemia; hypereosinophillic syndrome.

UNLABELED USES Acute lymphocytic leukemia (ALL), soft tissue sarcoma, recurrence of stomach and intestinal tumors.

CONTRAINDICATIONS Pregnancy (category D), lactation.

CAUTIOUS USE History of hypersensitivity to other monoclonal antibodies; hepatic or renal impairment; bleeding, bone marrow suppression; cardiac disease; fungal infections; GI bleeding; history of gastric surgery; heart failure; hepatic disease; infection; jaundice; peripheral edema; renal disease; history of viral infection older adults; females of childbearing age. Safe use in children younger than 3 y not established.

ROUTE & DOSAGE

CML Chronic Phase

Adult: **PO** 400 mg daily
Child (3 y or older): **PO** 340 mg/m^2/day in 1 or 2 divided dose(s) (max dose: 600 mg/day)

CML Accelerated Phase or Blast Crisis

Adult: **PO** 600 mg daily

Philadelphia Chromosome–Positive Acute Lymphoblastic Leukemia

Adult: **PO** 600 mg daily
Child (1 y or older): **PO** 340 mg/m^2/day

Acute Lymphoblastic Leukemia

Adult: **PO** 600 mg/day until disease progression

GISTs/Hyereosinophilic Syndrome

Adult: **PO** 400 mg daily

Renal Impairment Dosage Adjustment

CrCl 20–39 mL/min: Decrease starting dose by 50%;
less than 20 mL/min: Use with caution

Hepatic Impairment Dosage Adjustment

Reduce dose by 25%

Toxicity Dosage Adjustment

Bilirubin greater than 3 × ULN: Withhold therapy until levels have returned to less than 1.5 × ULN
Liver transaminase greater than 5 × ULN: Withhold therapy until levels have returned to less than 2.5 × ULN
Hematologic toxicity: Adjust based on disease state being treated and ANC: See package insert for adjustments

ADMINISTRATION

Oral

- Give with meal and large glass of water (at least 8 oz). Avoid grapefruit juice.
- Store at 15°–30° C (59°–86° F).

ADVERSE EFFECTS **CV:** *Edema,* chest pain, hypotension. **Respiratory:** Nasopharyngitis, *cough,* upper respiratory tract infection, dyspnea, pharyngeal pain, rhinitis, pharyngitis, flu-like symptoms, pneumonia, sinusitis. **CNS:** *Fatigue, headache,* dizziness, insomnia, depression, taste disorder, rigors, anxiety, paresthesia, chills. **HEENT:** *Periorbital edema,* increased lacrimation. **Endo-crine:** *Increased lactate dehydrogenase,* weight gain, decreased serum albumin, hypokalemia. **Skin:** *Skin rash, dermatitis,* pruritis, night sweats, alopecia, diaphoresis. **Hepatic:** *Increased serum AST, increased serum ALT,* increased serum ALP, increased serum bilirubin. **GI:** *Nausea, diarrhea, vomiting, abdominal pain, anorexia,* dyspepsia, flatulence, abdominal distension, constipation, stomatitis, upper abdominal pain. Renal: Increased serum creatinine. **Musculoskeletal:** *Muscle cramps, musculoskeletal pain,* arthralgia, myalgia, weakness, back pain, limb pain, ostealgia. **Hematologic:** *Hemorrhage,* leukopenia, hypoproteinemia, anemia, neutropenia, thrombocytopenia. **Other:** *Fever,* influenza, infection.

INTERACTIONS **Drug:** **Clarithromycin, erythromycin, ketoconazole, itraconazole** may increase imatinib levels and toxicity; **carbamazepine, dexamethasone, phenobarbital, phenytoin, rifampin** may decrease imatinib levels; may increase levels of BENZODIAZEPINES, DIHYDROPYRIDINE, CALCIUM CHANNEL BLOCKERS (e.g., **nifedipine**), **warfarin.** May impact concentration of other medications metabolized via CYP 3A4. **Herbal:** **St. John's wort** may decrease imatinib levels.

PHARMACOKINETICS **Absorption:** Well absorbed, 98% reaches systemic circulation. **Peak:** 2–4 h. **Metabolism:** Primarily by CYP3A4 in liver. **Elimination:** Primarily in feces. **Half-Life:** 18 h imatinib, 40 h active metabolite.

NURSING IMPLICATIONS

Assessment & Drug Effects

- Monitor for S&S of fluid retention. Weigh daily and report rapid weight gain immediately.
- Withhold drug and notify prescriber for any of the following: Bilirubin greater than 3 × ULN, AST/ALT greater than 5 × ULN; treatment may be reinstituted when bilirubin less than 1.5 × ULN and AST/ALT less than 2.5 × ULN.
- Monitor lab tests: CBC with platelet count and differential weekly × 1 mo, biweekly for the 2nd mo, periodically thereafter as clinically indicated; baseline and monthly LFTs; renal function tests; TSH, and electrolytes.

Patient & Family Education

- Do not take any OTC drugs (e.g., acetaminophen, St. John's wort) without consulting prescriber.
- Report any S&S of bleeding immediately to prescriber (e.g., black tarry stool, bright red or cola-colored urine, bleeding from gums).
- Report immediately to prescriber any unexplained change in mental status.
- Use effective means of contraception while taking this drug. Women of childbearing age should avoid becoming pregnant.

IMIPENEM-CILASTATIN SODIUM (Pr)

(i-mi-pen'em sye-la-stat'in)

Primaxin

Classification: BETA-LACTAM ANTIBIOTIC

Therapeutic: ANTIBIOTIC

AVAILABILITY Solution for injection

ACTION & *THERAPEUTIC EFFECT* Fixed combination of imipenem, a beta-lactam antibiotic, and cilastatin. Action of imipenem: Inhibition of mucopeptide synthesis in bacterial cell walls leading to cell death. Cilastatin increases the serum half-life of imipenem. *Effectively used for severe or resistant infections. Acts synergistically with aminoglycoside antibiotics against some isolates of* Pseudomonas aeruginosa.

USES Treatment of serious infections caused by susceptible organisms in the urinary tract, lower respiratory tract, bones and joints, skin and skin structures; also intraabdominal, gynecologic, and mixed infections; bacterial septicemia and endocarditis.

UNLABELED USES Infective endocarditis.

CONTRAINDICATIONS Hypersensitivity to any component of product, multiple allergens; renal impairment with CrCl of less than or equal to 5 mL/min/1.73m^2.

CAUTIOUS USE Hypersensitivity to another carbapenen or penicillin, or cephalosporin; patients with CNS disorders (e.g., seizures, brain lesions, history of recent head injury); renal impairment; older adults; pregnancy (category C); lactation.

ROUTE & DOSAGE

Serious Infections

Adult: **IV:** 250–500 mg q6–8h (max: 4 g/day); **IM:** 500 or 750 mg q12h (max: 4 g/day)
Child (3 mo or older): **IV** 15–25 mg/kg q6h; *1–3 mo:* 25 mg/kg q6–12h
Neonate (weight greater than 1500 g): **IV** 25 mg/kg q8–12h

Renal Impairment Dosage Adjustment

Make adjustments/package insert (based on *CrCl*)

ADMINISTRATION

Caution: IM and IV solutions are **not** interchangeable; **do not** give IM solution by IV, and **do not** give IV solution as IM.

Intramuscular

- Reconstitute powder for IM injection as follows: Add 2 mL or 3 mL of 1% lidocaine HCl solution without epinephrine, respectively, to the 500 mg vial or the 750 mg vial. Agitate to form a suspension then withdraw and inject entire contents of the vial IM.
- Give IM suspension by deep injection into the gluteal muscle or lateral thigh.
- Use reconstituted IM injection within 1 h after preparation.

Intravenous

PREPARE: **Intermittent:** Reconstitute each dose with 10 mL of D5W, NS, or other compatible infusion solution. ▪ Agitate the solution until clear. Color should range from colorless to yellow. ▪ Further dilute with 100 mL of same solution used for initial dilution.

ADMINISTER: **Intermittent:** Give each 500 mg or fraction thereof over 20–30 min. Infuse larger doses over 40–60 min. ▪ **Do not** give as a bolus dose. ▪ Nausea appears to be related to infusion rate, and if it presents during infusion, slow the rate (occurs most frequently with 1-g doses).

INCOMPATIBILITIES: **Solution/additive-:** **Amoxicillin, lactated Ringer's, mannitol,** some **dextrose**-containing solutions, **potassium chloride, sodium bicarbonate, TPN. Y-site: Alemtuzumab, allopurinol, amiodarone, amphotericin B cholesteryl, azathioprine, azithromycin, ceftriaxone, chlorpromazine, dacarbazine, dantrolene, daptomycin, daunorubicin, diazepam, diazoxide, etoposide, fluconazole, gallium, ganciclovir, garenoxacin, gemcitabine, haloperidol, inamrinone, lansoprazole, lorazepam, mannitol, mechlorethamine, metaraminol, meperidine, methyldopa, midazolam, milrinone, minocycline, mycophenolate, nalbuphine, nicardipine, palonosetron, peritoneal dialysis solution, phenytoin, prochlorperazine, pyridoxine, quinpristin/dalfopristin, sargramostim, sodium bicarbonate, SMZ/TMP, temocillin, thiamine, topotecan, vecuronium.**

- Store according to manufacturer's recommendations; stability of IV solutions depends on diluent used for reconstitution. ▪ Most IV solutions retain potency for 4 h at 15°–30° C (59°–86° F) or for 24 h if refrigerated at 4° C (39° F). Avoid freezing.

ADVERSE EFFECTS

Respiratory: Chest discomfort, hyperventilation, dyspnea. **CNS:** Seizures, dizziness, confusion, somnolence, encephalopathy, myoclonus, tremors, paresthesia, headache. **HEENT:** Transient hearing loss. **Endocrine:** Hyponatremia, hyperkalemia alkaline phosphatase, AST, ALT BUN, LDH, creatinine. **Skin:** Rash, pruritus, urticaria, candidiasis, flushing, increased sweating, skin texture

I

change, facial edema. **GI:** *Nausea, vomiting,* diarrhea, pseudomembranous colitis, hemorrhagic colitis, gastroenteritis, abdominal pain, glossitis, heartburn. **Hematologic:** increased WBC, *decreased Hgb, Hct,* eosinophilia, thrombocytopenia. **Other:** Hypersensitivity (rash, fever, chills, dyspnea, pruritus), weakness, oliguria/anuria, polyuria, polyarthralgia; *phlebitis and pain at injection site,* superinfections.

I

INTERACTIONS **Drug: Aztreonam, cephalosporins, penicillins** may antagonize the antibacterial effects. May affect **cyclosporine** levels.

PHARMACOKINETICS **Distribution:** Widely distributed; limited concentrations in CSF; crosses placenta; in breast milk. **Elimination:** 70% in urine within 10 h. **Half-Life:** 1 h.

NURSING IMPLICATIONS

Assessment & Drug Effects

- Determine previous hypersensitivity reaction to beta-lactam antibiotics (penicillins and cephalosporins) or to other allergens.
- Monitor for S&S of hypersensitivity (see Appendix F). Discontinue drug and notify prescriber if S&S occur.
- Monitor closely patients vulnerable to CNS adverse effects.
- Notify prescriber if focal tremors, myoclonus, or seizures occur; dosage adjustment may be needed.
- Monitor for S&S of superinfection (see Appendix F).
- Notify prescriber promptly to rule out pseudomembranous enterocolitis if severe diarrhea accompanied by abdominal pain and fever occurs (see Appendix F).
- Note: Sodium content derived from drug is high; consider in patient on restricted sodium intake.
- Monitor renal, hematologic, and liver function periodically.

Patient & Family Education

- Notify prescriber immediately to report pruritus or symptoms of respiratory distress.
- Report pain or discomfort at IV infusion site.
- Report loose stools or diarrhea promptly.

IMIPRAMINE HYDROCHLORIDE (Pr)

(im-ip′ra-meen)

IMIPRAMINE PAMOATE

Classification: TRICYCLIC ANTIDEPRESSANT (TCA)
Therapeutic: ANTIDEPRESSANT

AVAILABILITY Tablet **Imipramine pamoate:** Capsule

ACTION & *THERAPEUTIC EFFECT* TCAs potentiate both norepinephrine and serotonin in the CNS by blocking their reuptake by presynaptic neurons. Imipramine decreases number of awakenings from sleep, markedly reduces time in REM sleep, and increases stage 4 sleep. Relief of nocturnal enuresis is due to anticholinergic activity and to nervous system stimulation, resulting in earlier arousal to sensation of full bladder. *Effective as an antidepressant. Relieves nocturnal enuresis in children.*

USES Depression, childhood enuresis.

UNLABELED USES ADHD, bulimia nervosa, neuropathic pain, panic disorders, postherpetic

Common adverse effects in *italic;* life-threatening effects underlined; generic names in **bold;** classifications in SMALL CAPS; ♣ Canadian drug name; (P) Prototype drug; ⚠ Alert

neuralgia, overactive bladder, urinary incontinence.

CONTRAINDICATIONS Hypersensitivity to tricyclic drugs; concomitant use of MAOIs within 14 days; suicidal ideation; acute recovery period after MI; initiation in patients receiving linezolid or methylene blue IV; pregnancy (congenital abnormalities have been reported in humans; ACOG recommends that therapy for depression during pregnancy be individualized); lactation.

CAUTIOUS USE History of suicidal thoughts; respiratory difficulties; cardiovascular, hepatic, or GI diseases; blood disorders; increased intraocular pressure, narrow-angle glaucoma; schizophrenia, MDD, bipolar disorder; electroshock therapy; hypomania or manic episodes, patient with suicidal tendencies, seizure disorders; CHF; conductions defects, arrhythmias; strokes, tachycardia; BPH; urinary retention; older adults; adolescents, children younger than 6 y.

ROUTE & DOSAGE

Depression

Adult: **PO** 25–50 mg/day in divided doses; may increase by 25–50 mg/day at greater than 1 week intervals. Usual dose 100–300 mg/day.
Adolescent/Child (over 8 y): **PO** 1.5 mg/kg/day in divided doses; may titrate based on response (max: 5 mg/kg/day)

Enuresis in Childhood

Adolescent/Child (over 6 y): **PO** 10–25 mg at bedtime, may increase by 25 mg/day after 1 week of therapy (max: 50 mg)

Pharmacogenetic Dosage Adjustment

Poor CYP2C19 metabolizers: Start at 30–50% of normal dose

ADMINISTRATION

Oral

- Give with or immediately after food.
- Note: Single doses can be given one hour before bedtime or q AM, respectively, if drowsiness or insomnia results.

ADVERSE EFFECTS **CV:** *Orthostatic hypotension,* tachycardia; *arrhythmias,* hypertension, palpitation, MI, *heart block,* ECG changes, stroke. **CNS:** *Drowsiness,* dizziness, headache, fatigue, numbness, tingling (paresthesias) of extremities; ataxia, tremors, peripheral neuropathy, extrapyramidal symptoms (including parkinsonism effects and tardive dyskinesia); altered EEG patterns, confusion, hallucinations, anxiety, nervousness, insomnia, vivid dreams, restlessness, agitation, hypomania. **HEENT:** Tinnitus; *blurred vision,* disturbances of accommodation, angle-closure glaucoma, *slight mydriasis,* nystagmus. **Endocrine:** Testicular swelling, gynecomastia (men), galactorrhea and breast enlargement (women), increased or decreased libido, increased blood glucose levels. **GI/Hepatic:** *Dry mouth,* constipation, heartburn, weight gain or loss, nausea, vomiting, diarrhea, abdominal cramps, anorexia, stomatitis, black tongue, jaundice, increased serum transaminase. **GU:** *Urinary retention,* hesitency, urinary tract dilation. **Hematologic:** Petechaie, purpura, agranulocytosis, eosinophilia, thrombocytopenia. **Other:**

<u>Angioedema</u> of face, tongue, or generalized.

INTERACTIONS Drug: MAO INHIBITORS may precipitate hyperpyrexic crisis, tachycardia, or seizures; ANTIHYPERTENSIVE AGENTS potentiate orthostatic hypotension; CNS DEPRESSANTS, **alcohol** add to CNS depression; **norepinephrine** and other SYMPATHOMIMETICS may increase cardiac toxicity; **cimetidine** decreases hepatic metabolism, thus increasing imipramine levels; **methylphenidate** inhibits metabolism of imipramine and thus may increase its toxicity. Do not use with other drugs that might prolong the QT interval. Can cause seronotin syndrome if used with other agents that have serotonergic effect. Enhances vasopressor effects of ALPHA/BETA AGONISTS. **Herbal: Ginkgo** may decrease seizure threshold; **St. John's wort** may cause serotonin syndrome.

PHARMACOKINETICS Absorption: Completely absorbed from GI tract. **Peak:** 1–2 h. **Metabolism:** Metabolized to the active metabolite desipramine in liver. (via CYP2D6) **Elimination:** Primarily in urine, small amount in feces; crosses placenta; may be secreted in breast milk. **Half-Life:** 8–16 h.

NURSING IMPLICATIONS

Black Box Warning

Imipramine has been associated with increased risk of suicidal thinking and behavior in children, adolescents, and young adults.

Assessment & Drug Effects

- Monitor children, adolescents, and young adults for increase in suicidality.
- Be alert for and report new or worsening symptoms such as anxiety, agitation, panic attacks, insomnia, irritability, hostility, aggressiveness, impulsivity, hypomania.
- Monitor HR and BP frequently. Orthostatic hypotension may be marked in pretreatment hypertensive or cardiac patients.
- Monitor CV status especially in the older adult and those with preexisting CV disease.
- Monitor older adults for excessive sedation.
- Monitor urinary and bowel elimination, at least until maintenance dosage is stabilized, to detect urinary retention or frequency, constipation, or paralytic ileus.
- Notify prescriber of extrapyramidal symptoms (tremors, twitching, ataxia, incoördination, hyperreflexia, drooling) in patients receiving large doses and especially in older adults.
- Monitor diabetic patients for loss of glycemic control. Hyperglycemia or hypoglycemia (see Appendix F) occurs in some patients.
- Monitor lab tests: CBC in older adults, with high doses, and/or in patients with preexisting cardiovascular disease.

Patient & Family Education

- Report promptly signs of a worsening condition, suicidal ideation, or unusual changes in behavior, especially in children and adolescents.
- Older adults should change position slowly and in stages, especially from lying down to upright posture and dangle legs over bed for a few minutes before walking.
- **Do not** use OTC drugs while on a TCA without prescriber approval.

- Do not drive or engage in other potentially hazardous activities until response to drug is known.
- Avoid exposure to strong sunlight because of potential photosensitivity.

IMIQUIMOD

(i-mi′qui-mod)

Aldara, Zyclara

Classification: KERATOLYTIC; IMMUNOMODULATOR

Therapeutic: IMMUNE RESPONSE MODIFIER; KERATOLYTIC

AVAILABILITY Cream

ACTION & *THERAPEUTIC EFFECT*

An immune response modifier thought to induce cytokine production, which activates immune cells. *Despite destruction of HPV warts, latent or subclinical HPV infection can persist, and recurrence of visible warts is common.*

USES Treatment of external genital and perianal warts *(Condylomata acuminata),* actinic keratosis on the face and scalp of immunocompetent adults, and superficial basal cell carcinoma.

UNLABELED USES Treatment of common warts, herpes simplex virus.

CONTRAINDICATIONS Ocular exposure; excessive sun exposure or sunburn; UV exposure; surgery or drug treatment on affected area.

CAUTIOUS USE Hypersensitivity to benzyl alcohol or paraben; HIV infection; local inflammatory reactions; pregnancy (category C); lactation. Safe use in children younger than 12 y not established.

ROUTE & DOSAGE

Genital and Perianal Warts

Adult/Adolescent (12 y or older): **Topical** Apply a thin layer to the affected areas once daily 3 × wk just before bedtime. Wash off cream after 6–10 h

Actinic Keratosis

Adult: **Topical** Apply a thin layer to the affected areas once daily 2 × wk just before sleep. Wash off cream after 8 h.

Superficial Basal Cell Carcinoma

Adult: **Topical** Apply a thin layer to the affected areas once daily 5 × wk just before sleep for 6 wk. Wash off cream after 8 h.

ADMINISTRATION

Topical

- Handwashing before and after application is recommended.
- Wash treatment area with soap and water and allow to dry thoroughly (at least 10 min).
- Single-use packets contain sufficient cream to cover an area of up to 20 cm^2 (approx. 8 in. by 8 in.).
- Instruct patient to apply a thin layer of cream (avoid using excessive cream), and work into area until no longer visible. Do not occlude the application site.
- After each treatment period, remove the cream by washing the treated area with soap and water.
- Avoid ocular exposure.
- Store below 25° C (77° F).

ADVERSE EFFECTS **Respiratory:** *Upper respiratory tract infection.* **Skin:** *Localized erythema, xeroderma, crusted skin,* skin sclerosis, dermal ulcer, localized vesiculation, excoriation. **Other:** Localized edema, application site discharge, localized pruritis, localized burning, infection.

INTERACTIONS DRUG May enhance adverse effects of other IMMUNO-SUPPRESSANTS. Do not use with LIVE VACCINES.

PHARMACOKINETICS Absorption: Minimal through intact skin.

I

NURSING IMPLICATIONS

Assessment & Drug Effects

- Monitor for and report promptly severe local inflammatory reactions on female external genitalia.

Patient & Family Education

- Uncircumcised males with warts under the foreskin: Pull back the foreskin and clean the area daily to help avoid penile skin reactions.
- Females should not apply cream directly into the vagina. Application to the labia may cause pain or swelling and may cause difficulty in passing urine.
- When being treated for actinic keratosis, avoid or minimize UV light exposure (artificial and sunlight). Wear protective clothing. If sunburn develops, avoid using imiquimod cream until fully recovered.

IMMUNE GLOBULIN INTRAMUSCULAR [IGIM, GAMMA GLOBULIN, IMMUNE SERUM GLOBULIN (ISG)] ⓟ

(im′mune glob′u-lin)

BayGam

IMMUNE GLOBULIN INTRAVENOUS (IGIV)

Flebogamma, Gammagard, Gammar-P IV, IGIV, Iveegam, Octagam

IMMUNE GLOBULIN SUBCUTANEOUS (IGSC, SCIG)

Hizentra, Vivaglobin

Classification: BIOLOGIC RESPONSE MODIFIER; IMMUNOGLOBULIN

Therapeutic: IMMUNOGLOBULIN

AVAILABILITY IGIM: Solution for injection. **IGIV:** Solution for injection; powder for injection. **Subcutaneous:** Solution

ACTION & *THERAPEUTIC EFFECT*

Concentrated solution containing globulin (primarily IgG) from human plasma of either venous or placental origin and processed by a special fractionating technique. *Like hepatitis B immune globulin (H-BIG), contains antibodies specific to hepatitis B surface antigen but in lower concentrations. Therefore, not considered treatment of first choice for postexposure prophylaxis against hepatitis B but usually an acceptable alternative when H-BIG is not available.*

USES IGIM: Provides passive immunity or to modify severity of certain infectious diseases [e.g., rubeola (measles), rubella (German measles), varicella-zoster (chickenpox), type A (infectious) hepatitis], and as replacement therapy in congenital agammaglobulinemia or IgG deficiency diseases. May be used as an alternative to H-BIG to provide passive immunity in hepatitis B infection. Also for postexposure prophylaxis of hepatitis non-A, non-B, and nonspecific hepatitis. **IGIV:** Principally as maintenance therapy in patients unable to manufacture sufficient quantities of IgG antibodies, in patients requiring an immediate increase in immunoglobulin levels, and when IM injections are contraindicated as in patients with bleeding disorders or who have small muscle mass. Also in chronic autoimmune thrombocytopenia and idiopathic thrombocytopenic purpura (ITP). Treatment of primary immunodeficiency disorders associated with defects in humoral immunity. **IGSC:** Primary immune deficiency.

UNLABELED USES Kawasaki syndrome, chronic lymphocytic leukemia, AIDS, premature and low-birth-weight neonates, autoimmune neutropenia, HIV-associated thrombocytopenia, or hemolytic anemia.

CONTRAINDICATIONS History of anaphylaxis or severe reaction to human immune serum globulin (IG) or to any ingredient in the formulations; persons with clinical hepatitis A; IGIV for patients with class-specific anti-IgA deficiencies; IGIM in severe thrombocytopenia or other bleeding disorders.

CAUTIOUS USE Dehydration, diabetes mellitus, children, older adults, hypovolemia, IgA deficiency, infection; renal disease, renal impairment; sepsis; sucrose hypersensitivity; vaccination, viral infection; pregnancy (category C); lactation.

ROUTE & DOSAGE

Hepatitis A Exposure

Adult/Child: **IM** 0.02 mL/kg as soon as possible after exposure; if period of exposure will be 3 mo or longer, give 0.05–0.06 mL/kg once q4–6mo

Hepatitis B Exposure

Adult/Child: **IM** 0.02–0.06 mL/kg as soon as possible after exposure if H-BIG is unavailable

Rubella Exposure

Adult: **IM** 20 mL as single dose in susceptible pregnant women

Rubeola Exposure

Adult/Child: **IM** 0.25 mL/kg within 6 days of exposure

Varicella-Zoster Exposure

Adult/Child: **IM** 0.6–1.2 mL/kg promptly

Immunoglobulin Deficiency

Dosages may vary between brands and formulations; see package insert

Adult/Child: **IV** 200–400 mg/kg monthly; **IM** 1.2 mL/kg followed by 0.6 mL/kg q2–4wk

Idiopathic Thrombocytopenia Purpura

Adult/Child: **IV** 400 mg/kg/day for 5 consecutive days or 1 g/kg × 1–2 days

Obesity Dosage Adjustment

Dose based on IBW or adjusted IBW

ADMINISTRATION

- Note: In hepatitis A (infectious hepatitis), immune globulin is most effective when given before or as soon as possible after exposure but not more than 2 wk after (incubation period for hepatitis A is 15–50 days). ▪ Do not give immune globulin to those presenting clinical manifestations of hepatitis A. ▪ For hepatitis B (serum hepatitis), give immune globulin within 24 h and not more than 7 days after exposure. ▪ Note: IGIM and IGIV formulations are **not** interchangeable.

Intramuscular

- Give adults and older children injections into deltoid or anterolateral aspect of thigh; neonates and small children, into anterolateral aspect of thigh.
- Avoid gluteal injections; however, when large volumes of immune globulin are prescribed or when large doses **must be** divided into several injections, the upper outer quadrant of the gluteus has been used in adults.

Intravenous

PREPARE: **IV Infusion:** Refer to manufacturer's directions for information on the specific product. Allow refrigerated product to come to room temperature.

ADMINISTER: **IV Infusion:** Flow rates vary with product being infused. Refer to manufacturer's directions for the specific product. ▪ Most products may be infused at a rate of 0.5 mg/kg/min for the first 10 min, then increased q20min, if tolerated, by 0.8 mg/kg/min (max rate: 6 mg/kg/min).

INCOMPATIBILITIES: Do not mix other drugs with immunoglobulin.

▪ Store as directed by manufacturer for specific product. Avoid freezing. ▪ Do not use if turbidity has occurred or if product has been frozen.

ADVERSE EFFECTS **Other:** *Pain, tenderness, muscle stiffness at IM site;* local inflammatory reaction, erythema, urticaria, angioedema, headache, malaise, fever, arthralgia, nephrotic syndrome, hypersensitivity (fever, chills, anaphylactic shock), infusion reactions (*nausea, flushing, chills,* headache, chest tightness, wheezing, skeletal pain, back pain, abdominal cramps, anaphylaxis), renal dysfunction, renal failure.

INTERACTIONS **Drug:** May interfere with antibody response to LIVE VIRUS VACCINES (measles/mumps/rubella); give VACCINES 14 days before or 3 mo after IMMUNOGLOBULINS.

PHARMACOKINETICS **Peak:** 2 days. **Distribution:** Rapidly and evenly distributed to intravascular and extravascular fluid compartments. **Half-Life:** 21–23 days.

NURSING IMPLICATIONS

Black Box Warning

IV immune globulin has been associated with renal dysfunction, acute renal failure, osmotic nephropathy, and death.

Assessment & Drug Effects

- Make sure emergency drugs and appropriate emergency facilities are immediately available for treatment of anaphylaxis or sensitization.
- Monitor for S&S adverse reaction to infusion (e.g., nausea, chills, headache, chest tightness); these are indications to slow rate of infusion.
- Note: Hypersensitivity reactions (see Appendix F) are most likely in patients receiving large IM doses, repeated injections, or rapid IV infusion.
- Monitor vital signs and infusion rate closely when patient is receiving IGIV.
- Monitor for and report S&S of renal dysfunction (e.g., decreased urine output, sudden weight gain, fluid retention/edema).

Patient & Family Education

- Report immediately S&S of hypersensitivity (see Appendix F).
- Report promptly to prescriber signs of kidney damage such as decreased

urine output, sudden weight gain, edema, shortness of breath.

INDACATEROL MALEATE

(in′da-ka′ter-ol mal′ee-ate)

Arcapta

Classification: BRONCHODILATOR; RESPIRATORY SMOOTH MUSCLE RELAXANT; BETA-ADRENERGIC AGONIST

Therapeutic: BRONCHODILATOR; RESPIRATORY SMOOTH MUSCLE RELAXANT

Prototype: Albuterol

AVAILABILITY Capsule containing powder for inhalation

ACTION & *THERAPEUTIC EFFECT* Acts primarily on $beta_2$-adrenergic receptors in bronchial smooth muscle with little effect on heart rate. *Causes relaxation of bronchial smooth muscle and bron-chodilation.*

USES Prophylactic, maintenance treatment of chronic obstructive pulmonary disorder (COPD), including chronic bronchitis and emphysema.

CONTRAINDICATIONS Asthma (without concurrent use of a long-term asthma control drug); acutely deteriorating COPD; acute episodes of bronchospasm.

CAUTIOUS USE Paradoxical bronchospasms; cardiovascular disease including hypertension; seizure disorder; thyrotoxicosis; sensitivity to sympathomimetic drugs; concurrent use of other drugs containing long-acting $beta_2$-agonist; pregnancy (category C); lactation. Safety and efficacy in children not established.

ROUTE & DOSAGE

Chronic Obstructive Pulmonary Disorder

Adult: **PO Inhalation** 75 mcg once daily

ADMINISTRATION

Oral Inhalation

- Capsules should be removed from blister immediately before use.
- Capsules should be used only with the neohaler device. Capsules must not be swallowed.
- The Arcapta neohaler should be administered at the same time each day.
- Mouthpiece should be kept dry. Do not rinse mouthpiece.
- Store at 15°–30° C (59°–86° F) in foil package until ready to use.

ADVERSE EFFECTS **Respiratory:** Cough. **CNS:** headache, dizziness.

INTERACTIONS **Drug:** ADRENERGIC AGONISTS and MONOAMINE OXIDASE INHIBITORS may potentiate indacaterol. BETA-BLOCKERS may interfere with the actions of indacaterol. CORTICOSTEROIDS (e.g., **prednisone, dexamethasone), theophylline,** THIAZIDE DIURETICS OR LOOP DIURETICS may increase risk of hypokalemia. CYP3A4 inhibitors and/or P-gp efflux transporters (e.g., **ketoconazole,** HIV PROTEASE INHIBITORS, **erythromycin**) may increase the levels of indacaterol. Indacaterol has been associated with QT prolongation. Drugs that prolong the QT interval (e.g., **disopyramide, procainamide, amiodarone, bretylium, clarithromycin, levofloxacin**) may cause additive effects. TRICYCLIC ANTIDEPRESSANTS (e.g., **amitriptyline**) may potentiate cardiovascular effects of indacaterol.

PHARMACOKINETICS **Absorption:** 43–45% bioavailable. **Peak:** 1–4 h. **Distribution:** 94–96% plasma protein bound. **Metabolism:** In the liver via CYP3A4, CYP2D6, CYP1A1. **Elimination:** Primarily fecal. **Half-Life:** 45.5–126 h.

NURSING IMPLICATIONS

Black Box Warning

Indacaterol has been associated with increased risk of asthma-related death.

Assessment & Drug Effects

- Monitor HR, BP, and respiratory status. Report immediately deterioration in respiratory condition or development of paradoxical bronchospasms following inhalation.
- Periodic ECG monitoring with concurrent use of other drugs associated with QT prolongation.
- Monitor lab tests: Periodic serum potassium; blood glucose in diabetics or prediabetics; periodic pulmonary function tests.

Patient & Family Education

- Do not use for relief of acute symptoms.
- Discontinue drug use and immediately notify prescriber of any of the following: Symptoms of COPD are worsening; indacaterol no longer controls the symptoms of COPD; breathing is worsened following inhalation of indacaterol; the concurrently prescribed short-acting beta$_2$-agonist drug becomes less effective, or more inhalations of the short-acting drug are required.
- Diabetics should monitor blood glucose level more frequently for loss of glycemic control.

INDAPAMIDE

(in-dap'a-mide)

Classification: ELECTROLYTIC AND WATER BALANCE; DIURETIC
Therapeutic: THIAZIDE-LIKE DIURETIC; ANTIHYPERTENSIVE
Prototype: Hydrochlorothiazide

AVAILABILITY Tablet

ACTION & *THERAPEUTIC EFFECT* Sulfonamide derivative that has both diuretic and direct vascular effects. Acts on the proximal portion of the distal renal tubules. Enhances excretion of sodium, chloride, and water by interfering with sodium transfer across renal epithelium of tubules. *Hypotensive activity appears to result from a decrease in plasma and extracellular fluid volume, decreased peripheral vascular resistance, direct arteriolar dilation, and calcium channel blockade.*

USES Hypertension or edema in heart failure.

CONTRAINDICATIONS Hypersensitivity to indapamide or other sulfonamide derivatives, anuria, lactation.

CAUTIOUS USE Electrolyte imbalance, hypokalemia, severe renal impairment; impaired hepatic function or progressive liver disease; prediabetic and type II diabetic patient, history of gout; pregnancy (adverse effects not observed in animal reproduction studies). Safe use in children is not established.

ROUTE & DOSAGE

Edema

Adult: **PO** 1.25 mg once/day, may increase to 5 mg/day if needed

Hypertension

Adult: **PO** 1.25 mg once daily, may increase to 2.5 mg daily after 1 mo (max: 5 mg/day)

ADMINISTRATION

Oral

- Give with food or milk to reduce GI irritation.
- Administer early in day to prevent nocturia.
- Store at 20°C to 25°C (68°F to 77°F). Store in a tight, light-resistant container.

ADVERSE EFFECTS **CV:** Orthostatic hypotension, dysrhythmias. **Respiratory:** Rhinitis. **CNS:** Headache, dizziness, fatigue paresthesia, tension, anxiety, nervousness, agitation. **Endocrine:** Dilutional hyponatremia, *hyperuricemia, hypokalemia,* hyperglycemia, hypochloremia, hypercalcemia. **Skin:** Rash, hives, pruritus, vasculitis, photosensitivity. **GU:** Urinary frequency, nocturia. **Musculoskeletal:** Back pain, muscle cramps, muscle spasm, weakness. **Other:** Infection.

DIAGNOSTIC TEST INTERFERENCE Since indapamide may cause hypercalcemia (and hypophosphatemia), it is generally withheld before tests for ***parathyroid function*** are performed; may lead to false negative aldosterone/renin ratio.

INTERACTIONS **Drug:** Effects of **diazoxide** and indapamide intensified; increased risk of **digoxin** toxicity with hypokalemia; increased risk of nephrotoxicity with **sodium phosphate**; decreased renal **lithium** clearance may increase risk of **lithium** toxicity. BILE ACID SEQUESTRANTS decrease effect. May increase hypotensive effect with ACE INHIBITORS or OTHER ANTIHYPERTENSIVES. Increased risk of adverse effect with other PHOTOSENTITIZING AGENTS. Increased risk of hypokelemia with **topiramate**. Hyponatremic effect may be enhanced by SSRIS.

PHARMACOKINETICS **Absorption:** rapid and complete; 70–79% plasma bound. **Peak:** 2–2.5 h. **Duration:** Up to 36 h. **Metabolism:** In liver. **Elimination:** 60% in urine; 16–23% in feces. **Half-Life:** 14–18 h.

NURSING IMPLICATIONS

Assessment & Drug Effects

- Monitor BP periodically throughout therapy.
- Monitor for digitalis toxicity with concurrent therapy.
- Note: Electrolyte imbalances may be clinically serious with protracted vomiting and diarrhea, excessive sweating, GI drainage, and paracentesis.
- Report promptly signs of hyponatremia or hypokalemia (see Appendix F).
- Monitor diabetics for loss of glycemic control.
- Monitor lab tests: Baseline and periodic renal function, hepatic function, uric acid, and serum electrolytes.

Patient & Family Education

- Notify prescriber of decreased urine output, dizziness, weakness or muscle cramps, nausea, jaundice, or blurred vision.
- Take precautions from sun exposure because of risk of photosensitivity.

- Record weight at least every other day; inspect ankles and legs for edema. Report unexplained, progressive weight gain [e.g., 1–1.5 kg (2–3 lb) in 2–3 days].

INDINAVIR SULFATE

(in-din'a-vir)

Crixivan

Classification: ANTIRETROVIRAL; PRO-TEASE INHIBITOR

Therapeutic: PROTEASE INHIBITOR

Prototype: Saquinavir

I

AVAILABILITY Capsule

ACTION & *THERAPEUTIC EFFECT* Indinavir is an HIV pro-tease inhibitor. HIV protease is an enzyme required to produce the polyprotein precursors of the functional proteins in infectious HIV. Indinavir binds to the protease active site and thus inhibits its activity. *Protease inhibitors prevent cleavage of HIV viral polyproteins, resulting in formation of immature noninfectious virus particles.*

USES Treatment of HIV infection, in combination with other agents.

CONTRAINDICATIONS Hypersensitivity to indinavir; severe leukocyturia of greater than 100 cells/high power field; hemolytic anemia; lactation.

CAUTIOUS USE Hepatic dysfunction, hepatitis; renal impairment, history of nephrolithiasis, diabetes mellitus; hyperglycemia; concurrent HBV infection; history of adverse responses to other protease inhibitors; autoimmune disease; older adults; pregnancy (category C). Optimal dosing regimen for use in children has not been established.

ROUTE & DOSAGE

HIV (dose varies based on concurrent HAART)

Adult: **PO** 800 mg q8h

ADMINISTRATION

Oral

- Give with at least 48 oz of water on an empty stomach 1 h before or 2 h after meal; if needed, may be given with a very light meal or beverage.
- Note: When didanosine and indinavir are ordered concurrently, give each on empty stomach at least 1 h apart.
- Do not administer concurrently with midazolam or triazolam.
- Store tightly closed with desiccant in original bottle.

ADVERSE EFFECTS **Endocrine:** Nephrolithiasis, urolithiasis. **Hepatic/GI:** Hyperbilirubinemia, abdominal pain, nausea.

INTERACTIONS **Drug:** **Rifabutin, rifampin** significantly decrease indinavir levels requiring dose adjustment. **Ketoconazole, itraconazole, delavirdine** significantly increases indinavir levels requiring dose adjustment. Indinavir could inhibit the metabolism and increase the toxicity of **amiodarone, midazolam, sildenafil, tadalafil, trazodone, triazolam, vardenafil.** Indinavir and **didanosine** should be administered at least 1 h apart on empty stomach to permit full absorption of each; increased **ergotamine** toxicity with indinavir. **Rosuvastatin, simvastatin** should not be used concurrently. May impact serum concentrations of other medications metabolized by CYP3A4. **Herbal:** **St. John's wort,** garlic decreases ANTIRETROVIRAL activity of indinavir. **Food:** Avoid taking with high fat food.

PHARMACOKINETICS **Absorption:** Rapidly from GI tract; a meal high in calories, fat, and protein significantly reduces absorption. **Distribution:** 60% protein bound. **Metabolism:** In liver by CYP3A4 and CYP 2D6. **Elimination:** Primarily in feces (greater than 80%), 20% in urine.

NURSING IMPLICATIONS

Assessment & Drug Effects

- Assess for S&S of renal dysfunction, respiratory dysfunction, GI distress, and other common adverse effects.
- Monitor lab tests: Periodic vital load, CD4 count, triglycerides, cholesterol, glucose, LFTs, CBC, urinalysis.

Patient & Family Education

- Learn drug interactions and potential adverse reactions. Drink plenty of liquids to minimize risk of renal stones.
- Notify prescriber of flank pain, hematuria, S&S of jaundice, or other distressing adverse effects.

INDOMETHACIN

(in-doe-meth'a-sin)

Indocin, Tivorbex

Classification:
ANALGESIC, NON-STEROIDAL ANTI-INFLAMMATORY (NSAID)
Therapeutic: ANALGESIC, NSAID; ANTIRHEUMATIC
Prototype: Ibuprofen

AVAILABILITY Capsule; sustained release capsule; oral suspension; rectal suppository; solution for injection

ACTION & *THERAPEUTIC EFFECT* Potent nonsteroidal compound that competes with COX-1 and COX-2 enzymes, thus interfering with formation of prostaglandin. Appears to reduce motility of polymorphonuclear leukocytes, development of cellular exudates, and vascular permeability in injured tissue resulting in its anti-inflammatory effects. Inhibition of prostaglandins is thought to promote closure of the patency of the ductus arteriosus. Antipyretic and anti-inflammatory actions may be related to its ability to inhibit prostaglandin biosynthesis. *It is a potent analgesic, anti-inflammatory, and antipyretic agent. Promotes closure of persistent patent ductus arteriosus.*

USES Palliative treatment in active stages of moderate to severe rheumatoid arthritis, ankylosing rheumatoid spondylitis, acute gouty arthritis, and osteoarthritis of hip in patients intolerant to or unresponsive to adequate trials with salicylates and other therapy. Also used IV to close patent ductus arteriosus in the premature infant. Acute mild to moderate pain (**Tivorbex** only).

UNLABELED USES To relieve biliary pain and dysmenorrhea, Paget's disease, athletic injuries, juvenile arthritis, idiopathic pericarditis.

CONTRAINDICATIONS Allergy to indomethacin, aspirin, or other NSAID; nasal polyps associated with angioedema; history of asthma; history of recurrent GI lesions; perioperative pain with CABG; serious skin reactions to indomethacin; severe hepatic impairment due to indomethecin; pregnancy (D third trimester); lactation; neonates with significant renal failure.

CAUTIOUS USE History of psychiatric illness, epilepsy, parkinsonism; impaired renal or hepatic function; history of ulcer disease or GI bleeding; infection; coagulation disorders; infection, CV disease; CHF, hypertension; fluid retention; preexisting asthma; older adults, persons in hazardous occupations; pregnancy (category C first and second trimester); lactation; children, infants.

ROUTE & DOSAGE

Rheumatoid Arthritis

Adult: **PO** 25–50 mg bid or tid (max: 200 mg/day) or 75 mg sustained release 1–2 × day

Pediatric Arthritis

Child: **PO** 1–2 mg/kg/day in 2–4 divided doses (max: 4 mg/kg/day) or 150–200 mg/day

Acute Gouty Arthritis

Adult: **PO/PR** 50 mg tid until pain is tolerable, then rapidly taper

Bursitis

Adult: **PO** 25–50 mg tid or qid (max: 200 mg/day) or 75 mg sustained release 1–2 × day

Acute Pain (Tivorbex only)

Adult: **PO** 20–40 mg tid or 40 mg bid

ADMINISTRATION

Oral

- Give immediately after meals, or with food, milk, or antacid (if prescribed) to minimize GI side effects.
- Extended-release capsules must be swallowed whole; do not crush.

Rectal

- Indomethacin rectal suppository use is contraindicated with history of proctitis or recent bleeding.

Intravenous

PREPARE: **Direct:** Dilute 1 mg with 1 mL of NS or sterile water for injection without preservatives. Resulting concentration (1 mg/mL) may be further diluted with an additional 1 mL for each 1 mg to yield 0.5 mg/mL.

ADMINISTER: **Direct:** Give by direct IV with a single dose given over 20–30 min.

INCOMPATIBILITIES: **Y-site:** **Amikacin, atracurium, aztreonam, benztropine, buprenorphine, butorphanol, calcium chloride, calcium gluconate, cefoperazone, cefotetan, chlorpromazine, cimetidine, dactinomycin, dantrolene, daunorubicin, diazepam, diazoxide, diphenhydramine, dobutamine, dopamine, doxycycline, epinephrine, erythromycin, esmolol, etoposide, famotidine, gentamicin, glycopyrrolate, haloperidol, hydralazine, iamrinone, isoproterenol, labetalol, levofloxacin, magnesium sulfate, meperidine, metaraminol, midazolam, minocycline, morphine, nalbuphine, netilmicin, norepinephrine, ondansetron, oxytocin, paclitaxel, pantoprazole, papaverine, pentamidine, pentazocine, phenylephrine, phenytoin, polymyxin B sulfate, prochlorperazine, promethazine, propranolol, protamine, pyridoxine, succinylcholine chloride, sufentanil, SMZ/TMP, thiamine, tobramycin, tolazoline, vancomycin, vasopressin, verapamil.**

- Avoid extravasation or leakage; drug can be irritating to tissue.
  - Discard any unused drug, since it contains no preservative.
- Store oral and rectal forms in tight, light-resistant containers unless otherwise directed. Do not freeze.

ADVERSE EFFECTS **CNS:** Headache, dizziness. **GI:** Vomiting, epigastric pain. **Hematologic:** Postoperative hemorrhage.

DIAGNOSTIC TEST INTERFERENCE False-negative ***dexamethasone suppression test;*** may lead to false-positive ***aldosterone/renin ratio.***

INTERACTIONS **Drug:** ORAL ANTICOAGULANTS, **heparin, alcohol** may prolong bleeding time; may increase **lithium** toxicity; effects of ORAL ANTICOAGULANTS, **phenytoin,** SALICYLATES, SULFONAMIDES, SULFONYLUREAS increased because of protein-binding displacement; increased toxicity including GI bleeding with SALICYLATES, NSAIDS; may blunt effects of ANTIHYPERTENSIVES and DIURETICS. May enhance effect of other photo-sensitizing agents. **Herbal:** **Feverfew, garlic, ginger, ginkgo** may increase bleeding potential.

PHARMACOKINETICS **Absorption:** Completely absorbed from GI tract. **Onset:** 1–2 h. **Peak:** 3 h. **Duration:** 4–6 h. **Metabolism:** In liver. **Elimination:** Primarily in urine. **Half-Life:** 2.5–124 h.

NURSING IMPLICATIONS

Black Box Warning

Indomethacin has been associated with increased risk of serious, potentially fatal GI bleeding and cardiovascular events (e.g., MI & CVA); risk may increase with duration of use and may be greater in the older adult and those with risk factors for CV disease.

Assessment & Drug Effects

- Monitor for therapeutic effectiveness: In acute gouty attack, relief of joint tenderness and pain is usually apparent in 24–36 h; swelling generally disappears in 3–5 days. In rheumatoid arthritis: Reduced fever, increased strength, reduced stiffness, and relief of pain, swelling, and tenderness.
- Monitor BP closely throughout therapy.
- Monitor for and report promptly S&S of CV thrombotic events (i.e., angina, MI, TIA, or stroke).
- Monitor for and report promptly S&S of GI ulceration or bleeding. Significant GI bleeding may occur without prior warning.
- Observe patients carefully; instruct to report adverse reactions promptly to prevent serious and sometimes irreversible or fatal effects.
- Monitor weight and observe dependent areas for signs of edema in patients with underlying cardiovascular disease.
- Monitor I&O closely and keep prescriber informed during IV administration for patent ductus arteriosus.
- Monitor lab tests: Periodic renal function tests, LFTs, and CBC with differential.
- Periodic opthalmologic exams with prolonged therapy.

Patient & Family Education

- Stop taking drug and report promptly to prescriber if you experience S&S of GI ulceration: Stomach pain, frequent indigestion and nausea, bloody or tarry stools, vomit with blood or coffee-ground appearance.

- Stop taking drug and report promptly to prescriber if you experience chest pain, shortness of breath, weakness, slurring of speech, or other signs of a cardiac or neurologic problem.
- Do not take aspirin or other NSAIDs; they increase possibility of ulcers.
- Note: Frontal headache is the most frequent CNS adverse effect; if it persists, dosage reduction or drug withdrawal may be indicated. Take drug at bedtime with milk to reduce the incidence of morning headache.
- Do not drive or engage in other potentially hazardous activities until response to drug is known.

INFLIXIMAB

(in-flix'i-mab)

Inflectra, Remicade

Classification: BIOLOGIC RESPONSE MODIFIER; MONOCLONAL ANTIBODY (IgG); TUMOR NECROSIS FACTOR (TNF) MODIFIER

Therapeutic: IMMUNOMODULATOR; ANTI-INFLAMMATORY; DISEASE-MODIFYING ANTIRHEUMATIC DRUG (DMARD)

Prototype: Enteracept

AVAILABILITY Powder for injection

ACTION & *THERAPEUTIC EFFECT*

Inhibits binding of TNF-alpha with its receptors thus preventing the following: Induction of proinflammatory cytokines; enhancement of leukocyte migration out of the vascular system; activation of neutrophil and eosinophil inflammatory activity; and induction of acute inflammatory phase reactants. *Decreases GI inflammation in Crohn's and related diseases. It is also effectively used as a disease-modifying antirheumatic drug (DMARD).*

USES Moderately to severely active Crohn's disease, including fistulizing Crohn's disease, rheumatoid arthritis, psoriatic arthritis, ankylosing spondylitis, ulcerative colitis, plaque psoriasis.

CONTRAINDICATIONS Severe hypersensitivity to infliximab; serious infection, sepsis; heart failure; murine protein hypersensitivity; lactation.

CAUTIOUS USE History of allergic phenomena or untoward responses to monoclonal antibody preparation; chronic infections; previous history of TB infection; history of HBV infection; renal or hepatic impairment; multiple sclerosis (potential exacerbation); fungal infection; human antichimeric antibody (HACA); leukopenia, thrombocytopenia; immunosuppressed patients; autoimmune disorders; neoplastic disease; vasculitis; neurologic disease; neutropenia; seizure disorder; preexisting CNS demyelinating disorders; moderate to severe COPD; history of malignancy; older adults; pregnancy (category B); children.

ROUTE & DOSAGE

Crohn's Disease

Adult: **IV** 5 mg/kg infused over at least 2 h, repeat at 2 and 6 wk for fistulizing disease, then q8wk
Child: **IV** 5 mg/kg at weeks 0, 2, and 6, then 5 mg/kg q8wk

Rheumatoid Arthritis

Adult: **IV** 3 mg/kg at weeks 0, 2, and 6, then q8wk

Ulcerative Colitis

Adult/Adolescent/Child (6 y or older): **IV** 5 mg/kg at weeks 0, 2, and 6, then 5 mg/kg q8wk

Ankylosing Spondylitis

Adult: **IV** 5 mg/kg at weeks 0, 2, and 6, then 5 mg/kg q6wk

Plaque Psoriasis

Adult: **IV** 5 mg/kg at wk 0,2, and 6 and then 5 mg/kg q8wk

ADMINISTRATION

- Note: Do not administer to a patient who has known or suspected sepsis.

Intravenous

PREPARE: **IV Infusion:** Reconstitute each 100 mg vial with 10 mL of sterile water for injection using a 21-gauge or smaller syringe. Inject sterile water against wall of vial, then gently swirl to dissolve but do not shake. ▪ Let stand for 5 min. ▪ Solution should be colorless to light yellow with a few translucent particles. Discard if particles are opaque. ▪ Further dilute by first removing from a 250-mL IV bag of NS a volume of NS equal to the volume of reconstituted infliximab to be added to the IV bag. Slowly add the total volume of reconstituted infliximab solution to the 250-mL infusion bag and gently mix. ▪ Infusion concentration should be 0.4 to 4 mg/mL. ▪ Begin infusion within 3 h of preparation.

ADMINISTER: **IV Infusion:** Give over at least 2 h using a polyethylene-lined infusion set with an in-line, low-protein-binding filter (pore size 1.2 micron or less). ▪ Flush infusion set before and after with NS to ensure delivery of total drug dose. ▪ Discard unused infusion solution.

INCOMPATIBILITIES: **Y-site:** Do not infuse with any other drugs.

- Store unopened vials at 2°–8° C (36°–46° F).

ADVERSE EFFECTS **Respiratory:** *Upper respiratory tract infection,* sinusitis, cough, pharyngitis. **CNS:** Headache. **Hepatic:** *Increased serum ALT.* **GI:** *Abdominal pain,* nausea. **Hematologic:** Anemia. **Other:** *Infection,* infusion-related reaction.

INTERACTIONS **Drug:** May blunt effectiveness of VACCINES given concurrently. Do not give with TUMOR NECROSIS FACTOR MODIFIERS (e.g., **adalimumab, etanercept, infliximab,** or **certolizumab pegol**) or with drugs that block interleukin 1 (**canakinumab, rilonacept**).

PHARMACOKINETICS **Distribution:** Distributed primarily to the vascular compartment. **Half-Life:** 9.5 days.

NURSING IMPLICATIONS

Black Box Warning

Infliximab has been associated with increased risk of serious, potentially fatal, infections and malignancies.

Assessment & Drug Effects

- Discontinue IV infusion and notify prescriber for fever, chills, pruritus, urticaria, chest pain, dyspnea, hypo/hypertension.
- Monitor for up to 2 h post-infusion for an acute infusion reaction

(e.g., chest pain, hypotension, hypertension, dyspnea).
- Monitor for and immediately report S&S of generalized infection.
- Monitor lab tests: Obtain CBC with differential, LFTs, and HBV screen prior to treatment.

Patient & Family Education
- Seek medical evaluation immediately if you suspect an infection.

INGENOL MEBUTATE
(in′ge-nol)
Picato
Classification: DERMATOLOGIC; CELL DEATH INDUCER; ANTIKERATOSIS AGENT
Therapeutic: ANTIKERATOSIS AGENT

AVAILABILITY Gel

ACTION & THERAPEUTIC EFFECT
The mechanism of action is unknown. *Induces cell death in actinic keratosis lesions.*

USES Topical treatment of actinic keratosis.

CONTRAINDICATIONS Healing surgical wound; severe skin reaction beyond the treated area.

CAUTIOUS USE Eye disorders; pregnancy (category C). Safety and efficacy in children younger than 18 y not established.

ROUTE & DOSAGE

Acne Keratosis of Face and Scalp
Adult: **Topical** 0.015% gel once daily to affected area for 3 d

Acne Keratosis of Trunk and Extremities
Adult: **Topical** 0.05% gel once daily to affected area for 2 d

ADMINISTRATION

Topical
- Spread evenly over treatment area and allow to dry for 15 min.
- Patients who self-apply should wash hands immediately after application.
- Store refrigerated.

ADVERSE EFFECTS **Respiratory:** Nasopharyngitis. **Skin:** *Crusting, erosion/ulceration, erythema, flaking/scaling, swelling, vesiculation/postulation.* **Other:** Application-site reactions (infection, irritation, pain, pruritus), headache, periorbital edema.

NURSING IMPLICATIONS

Assessment & Drug Effects
- Monitor for and report severe local skin reactions (e.g., erythema, crusting, swelling, vesiculation, pustulation, erosions, and ulceration).

Patient & Family Education
- Treated area should not be washed or touched for 6 h after application.
- Avoid activities that cause excessive sweating for 6 h after application.
- Avoid sun exposure or use sun protection.

INSULIN ASPART
(in′su-lyn)
NovoLog, NovoLog 70/30
Classification: ANTIDIABETIC; RAPID-ACTING INSULIN
Therapeutic: RAPID-ACTING INSULIN
Prototype: Insulin injection

AVAILABILITY Solution for injection

ACTION & THERAPEUTIC EFFECT
A recombinant insulin analog that is

 Common adverse effects in *italic*; life-threatening effects underlined; generic names in **bold**; classifications in SMALL CAPS; ♣ Canadian drug name; Prototype drug; Alert

more rapidly absorbed than human insulin, with a more rapid onset and shorter duration than regular human insulin. Insulin acts via specific membrane-bound receptors on target tissues to regulate metabolism of carbohydrate, protein, and fats. Target organs for insulin include the liver, skeletal muscle, and adipose tissue. *Provides better blood glucose control than regular human insulin when given before a meal.*

USES Treatment of diabetes mellitus.

CONTRAINDICATIONS Systemic allergic reactions; history of allergic reactions to insulin; hypoglycemia.

CAUTIOUS USE Fever, hyperthyroidism, surgery or trauma; decreased insulin requirements due to diarrhea, nausea, or vomiting, malabsorption; renal or hepatic impairment, hypokalemia; pregnancy [category B **(NovoLog)** and category C **(NovoLog 70/30)**]; lactation. Safe use in children younger than 2 y is not established.

ROUTE & DOSAGE

Diabetes

Adult/Adolescent/Child (older than 2 y): **Subcutaneous** 0.5–1 unit/kg/day; **IV** Dose should be individualized

ADMINISTRATION

- Use only if solution is absolutely clear.

Subcutaneous

- **Must be given no sooner** than 5–10 min before a meal.
- Draw up insulin aspart first when mixing with NPH insulin. Give injection immediately after it is mixed.

Intravenous

Use only under close medical supervision in a clinical setting.

PREPARE: **Infusion:** Dilute with NS or D5W in a polypropylene infusion bag to a final concentration of 0.05–1 unit/mL.

ADMINISTER: **Infusion:** Give at rate ordered by prescriber.

- Store refrigerated at 2°–8° C (36°–46° F); may be stored at room temperature, 15°–30° C (59°–86° F) for up to 28 days. Do not expose to excessive heat or sunlight, and do not freeze.

ADVERSE EFFECTS **Endocrine:** Hypoglycemia, hypokalemia. **Skin:** Injection site reaction, lipodystrophy, pruritus, rash. **Other:** Allergic reactions.

INTERACTIONS **Drug:** ORAL ANTIDIABETIC AGENTS, ACE INHIBITORS, **disopyramide, fluoxetine,** MAO INHIBITORS, **propoxyphene,** SALICYLATES, SULFONAMIDE ANTIBIOTICS, **octreotide** may enhance hypoglycemia; CORTICOSTEROIDS, **niacin, danazol,** DIURETICS, SYMPATHOMIMETIC AGENTS, PHENOTHIAZINES, THYROID HORMONES, ESTROGENS, PROGESTOGENS, **isoniazid, somatropin** may decrease hypoglycemic effects; BETA-BLOCKERS, **clonidine, lithium, alcohol** may either potentiate or weaken effects of insulin; **pentamidine** may cause hypoglycemia followed by hyperglycemia. **Herbal: Garlic, ginseng** may potentiate hypoglycemic effects. See INSULIN INJECTION.

PHARMACOKINETICS **Absorption:** Rapidly absorbed from subcutaneous injection site. **Onset:** 15 min. **Peak:** 1–3 h. **Duration:** 3–5 h. **Distribution:** Low protein binding. **Metabolism:** In liver with some metabolism in the kidneys. **Half-Life:** 81 min.

NURSING IMPLICATIONS

Assessment & Drug Effects

- Monitor for S&S of hypoglycemia (see Appendix F). Initial hypoglycemic response begins within 15 min and peaks 45–90 min after injection.
- Withhold drug and notify prescriber if patient is hypokalemic.
- Monitor lab tests: Periodic postprandial blood glucose and HbA1C.

Patient & Family Education

- Eat immediately after injecting insulin aspart because it has a fast onset and short duration of action.
- Do not inject into areas with redness, swelling, itching, or dimpling.
- Ingest some form of sugar (e.g., orange juice, dissolved table sugar, honey) if symptoms of hypoglycemia develop, and seek medical assistance.
- Check blood sugar as prescribed, especially postprandial values; make note of and notify prescriber of fasting blood glucose less than 80 and greater than 120 mg/dL.
- Notify the prescriber of any of the following: Fever, infection, trauma, diarrhea, nausea or vomiting. Dosage adjustment may be needed.
- Do not take any other medication unless approved by the prescriber.

INSULIN DEGLUDEC

(in′su-lin de-glu′dec)

Tresiba

Classification: ANTIDIABETIC; LONG-ACTING INSULIN

Therapeutic: ANTIDIABETIC

Prototype: Insulin injection

AVAILABILITY Prefilled disposable pens with solution for injection

ACTIONS & THERAPEUTIC EFFECT Slowly absorbed after injection; stimulates peripheral glucose uptake especially in muscle and fat tissue; inhibits hepatic glucose production and stimulates hepatic glycogen synthesis. *Lowers blood glucose levels over an extended period of time and prevents the conversion of glycogen to glucose in the liver.*

USES Treatment of type 1 and type 2 diabetes.

CONTRAINDICATIONS Episodes of severe hypoglycemia; hypersensitivity to insulin degludec or one of its components.

CAUTIOUS USE Changes in meal pattern, level of physical activity, or co-administered drugs; concomitant use of thiazolidinediones (i.e., may cause fluid retention and CHF); regimens designed to achieve tight glycemic control; episodes of mild-to-moderate hypoglycemia; hypokalemia; renal impairment; hepatic impairment; pregnancy; lactation. Safety and efficacy in children and adolescents under 18 y not established.

ROUTE & DOSAGE

Type 1 Diabetes

Adult: **Subcutaneous**
Insulin-naïve patients: Initial dose of 1/3 to 1/2 of total daily insulin dose; use short-acting insulin for remainder of dose
Insulin-experienced patients: Use same unit dose as current long or intermediate-acting insulin unit; adjust according to patient's needs

Type 2 Diabetes

Adult: **Subcutaneous** Initial dose of 10 units once daily; adjust according to patient's needs

ADMINISTRATION

Subcutaneous

- Inject into the thigh, upper arm, or abdomen.
- Rotate injection sites, and do not inject into areas with redness, swelling, itching, or dimpling.
- Do not mix with any other insulin products or solution.
- **Do not** transfer TRESIBA® from the TRESIBA® pen into a syringe for administration.
- Store not-in-use (unopened) disposable prefilled pen in refrigerator. Store in-use pen at room temperature (below 86° F [30° C]) away from direct heat and light). May be used for up to 56 days (8 wk) after being opened, if it is kept at room temperature.

ADVERSE EFFECTS **Respiratory:** Nasopharyngitis, upper respiratory tract infection. **CNS:** Headache. **Endocrine:** Severe hypoglycemia.

INTERACTIONS **Drug:** ANTIDIABETIC AGENTS, ACE INHIBITORS, ANGIOTENSIN II RECEPTOR BLOCKERS, DDP-4 INHIBITORS, **disopyramide,** FIBRATES, **fluoxetine,** GLP-1 RECEPTOR AGONISTS, MONOAMINE OXIDASE INHIBITORS, **pentoxifylline, pramlintide, propoxyphene,** SALICYLATES, SGLT-2 INHIBITORS, SOMATOSTATIN ANALOGS, and SULFONAMIDE ANTIBIOTICS may increase the risk of hypoglycemia. ATYPICAL ANTIPSYCHOTICS (e.g., **clozapine, olanzapine**), CORTICOSTEROIDS, **danazol,** DIURETICS, ESTROGENS, **glucagon, isoniazid, niacin,** ORAL CONTRACEPTIVES, PHENOTHIAZINES, PROGESTINS, PROTEASE INHIBITORS, **somatropin,** SYMPATHOMIMETIC AGENTS (e.g., **albuterol, epinephrine, terbutaline**), and THYROID HORMONES can interfere with the glucose lowering effects of insulin degludec. **Alcohol,** BETA-BLOCKERS, **clonidine, lithium,** and **pentamidine** may either increase or decrease the glucose lowering effects of insulin degludec. BETA-BLOCKERS, **clonidine, guanethidine** may blunt the signs and symptoms of hypoglycemia.

PHARMACOKINETICS **Onset:** 1 h. **Peak:** 3–4 days. **Distribution:** Greater than 99% plasma protein bound. **Metabolism:** Protein degradation to inactive metabolites. **Half-Life:** 25 h.

NURSING IMPLICATIONS

Assessment & Drug Effects

- Monitor for S&S of hypoglycemia (see Appendix F), especially after changes in insulin dose.
- Monitor for S&S of hypokalemia (see Appendix F).
- Withhold drug and notify prescriber if patient is hypoglycemic or hypokalemic (see Appendix F).
- Monitor lab tests: Periodic fasting blood glucose and HbA1C; periodic serum potassium.

Patient & Family Education

- Do not take drug and notify prescriber if experiencing episodes of low blood sugar (hypoglycemia). S&S of hypoglycemia include: Dizziness or light-headedness, sweating, confusion, fast heartbeat, blurred vision, slurred speech, shakiness, anxiety, irritability, or mood changes, and headache.

- Check blood sugar as prescribed; notify prescriber if fasting blood glucose is frequently less than 80 and greater than 120 mg/dL.
- Notify the prescriber of any of the following: Fever, infection, trauma, diarrhea, nausea, or vomiting. Dosage adjustment may be needed.
- Do not take any other medication unless approved by prescriber.
- Women of childbearing age should discuss with prescriber potential risks associated with pregnancy.
- Do not breast-feed while taking this drug without consulting prescriber.

I

INSULIN DETEMIR

(in′su-lyn det′e-mir)

Levemir

Classification: ANTI-DIABETIC; LONG-ACTING INSULIN

Therapeutic: LONG-ACTING INSULIN

Prototype: Insulin injection

AVAILABILITY Solution for injection

ACTION & *THERAPEUTIC EFFECT*

Insulin detemir, a long-acting human insulin, exerts its action by binding to insulin receptors. Receptor-bound insulin lowers blood glucose by facilitating cellular uptake of glucose into skeletal muscle and fat, and inhibiting the output of glucose from the liver. *Insulin detemir is effective as a glucose-lowering agent, with glycemic control equivalent to that of NPH insulin.*

USES Treatment of diabetes mellitus, types 1 and 2.

CONTRAINDICATIONS Hypersensitivity to insulin detemir, or cresol; use in insulin infusion pumps; diabetic ketoacidosis, coma, hyperosmolar hyperglycemic state, hypoglycemia.

CAUTIOUS USE Renal and hepatic impairment; older adults; cardiac disease, CHF, illness, stress; pregnancy (category B); lactation. Safe and effective use in children younger than 2 y has not been established.

ROUTE & DOSAGE

Diabetes

Adult/Child: **Subcutaneous** Insulin-naïve patients: 0.1–0.2 units/kg daily in evening or 10 units daily or bid in evenly spaced doses. For those taking a basal insulin product (i.e., NPH insulin, insulin glargine), a unit-to-unit dose conversion can be used.

ADMINISTRATION

Subcutaneous

- Once-daily injections should be given with the evening meal or at bedtime. With twice-daily dosing, the evening dose may be given with the evening meal, at bedtime, or 12 h after the morning dose.
- Inject into the thigh, upper arm, or abdomen.
- Rotate injection sites, and do not inject into areas with redness, swelling, itching, or dimpling.
- Do not administer IV or IM. With thin patients, inject at a 45-degree angle into a pinched fold of skin to avoid IM injection.
- Do not mix with any other type of insulin. Do not use with an insulin infusion pump.
- Store unopened vials under refrigeration at 2°–8° C (36°–46° F).

Once removed from refrigeration, pens, cartridges, and other delivery devices **must be** kept at room temperature (not to exceed 30° C or 85° F) and either used within 42 days or discarded.

INCOMPATIBILITIES: Solution/additive: Insulin detemir should not be mixed with any other insulin preparations.

ADVERSE EFFECTS Respiratory: Upper respiratory tract infection, pharyngitis, flu-like symptoms. **CNS:** Headache. **Endocrine:** *Hypoglycemia*, severe hypoglycemia. **GI:** Gastroenteritis, abdominal pain. **Other:** Fever.

DIAGNOSTIC TEST INTERFERENCE See INSULIN INJECTION (REGULAR).

INTERACTIONS Drug: See INSULIN INJECTION (REGULAR). **Herbal:** See INSULIN INJECTION (REGULAR).

PHARMACOKINETICS Absorption: Slow, prolonged absorption over 24 h. **Peak:** 3–9 h. **Distribution:** 98–99% protein bound. **Half-Life:** 5–7 h.

NURSING IMPLICATIONS

Assessment & Drug Effects

- Monitor for S&S of hypoglycemia (see Appendix F), especially after changes in insulin dose or type.
- Monitor weight periodically.
- Monitor lab tests: Periodic fasting blood glucose and HbA1C; periodic serum potassium with concurrent potassium-lowering drugs.

Patient & Family Education

- Follow directions for taking the drug (see Administration). Rotate injection sites and never inject into an area with redness, swelling, itching, or dimpling.
- Know parameters for withholding drug. Check blood sugar as prescribed; notify prescriber of fasting blood glucose below 80 or above 120 mg/dL.
- Ingest some form of sugar (e.g., orange juice, dissolved table sugar, honey) if symptoms of hypoglycemia develop; and seek medical assistance.
- Notify the prescriber of any of the following: Fever, infection, trauma, diarrhea, nausea, or vomiting.
- Do not take any other medication unless approved by prescriber.

INSULIN GLARGINE

(in′su-lyn glar′geen)

Basaglar KwikPen, Lantus, Lantus SoloStar, Semglee, Toujeo SoloStar

Classification: ANTIDIABETIC; LONG-ACTING INSULIN

Therapeutic: LONG-ACTING INSULIN

Prototype: Insulin injection

AVAILABILITY Solution for injection

ACTION & *THERAPEUTIC EFFECT* A recombinant human insulin analog with a long duration of action. Lowers blood glucose levels over an extended period of time by stimulating peripheral glucose uptake especially in muscle and fat tissue. In addition, insulin inhibits hepatic glucose production. *Lowers blood glucose levels over an extended period of time. It also prevents the conversion of glucagon to glucose in the liver.*

USES To improve glycemic control in adults with type 1 diabetes mellitus and type 2 diabetes mellitus.

CONTRAINDICATIONS Prior hypersensitivity to insulin glargine; during episodes of hypo-glycemia.

CAUTIOUS USE Renal and hepatic impairment; risks for hypokalemia; older adults; illness; emotional disturbances; stress; pregnancy (may contribute to adverse effects when used during pregnancy); lactation. Safety and efficacy in children younger than 6 y of age not established.

ROUTE & DOSAGE

Type 1 Diabetes

Adult/Child (6 y or older): **Subcutaneous** See package insert; dose is individualized based on multiple patient factors.
Child (6 y or older): **Subcutaneous** See package insert

Type 2 Diabetes

Adult/Child (6 y or older):
Subcutaneous See package insert

ADMINISTRATION

Subcutaneous

- Give subcutaneous only. Do not use if solution is cloudy or viscous.
- Give at same time each day (usually at bedtime) and do not mix with any other insulin product.
- Do not share insulin pens among patients.
- Rotate administration sites.
- Administer at room temperature.
- Store in refrigerator at 2°–8° C (36°–46° F), may store at room temperature, 15°–30° C (59°–86° F). Discard opened refrigerated vials after 28 days and unrefrigerated vials after 14 days. Do not expose to excessive heat or sunlight, and do not freeze.

ADVERSE EFFECTS **CV:** Hypertension, peripheral edema. **Respiratory:** URI, sinusitis, nasopharyngitis, bronchitis, cough. **CNS:** Depression, headache. **HEENT:** Cataract, retinal vascular disease. **Endocrine:** Hypoglycemia. **GI:** Diarrhea. **GU:** Urinary tract infection. **Musculoskeletal:** Arthralgia, back pain, limb pain. **Other:** Influenza, infection, antibody development, accidental injury.

INTERACTIONS **Drug:** ORAL AN-TIDIABETIC AGENTS, ACE INHIBITORS, **disopyramide, fluoxetine,** MAO INHIBITORS, **propoxyphene,** SALICYLATES, SULFONAMIDE ANTIBIOTICS, **octreotide** may enhance hypoglycemia; CORTICOSTEROIDS, **niacin, danazol,** DIURETICS, SYMPATHOMIMETIC AGENTS, PHENOTHIAZINES, THYROID HORMONES, ESTROGENS, PROGESTOGENS, **isoniazid, somatropin** may decrease hypoglycemic effects; BETA-BLOCKERS, **clonidine, lithium, alcohol** may either potentiate or weaken effects of insulin; **pentamidine** may cause hypoglycemia followed by hyperglycemia. **Herbal: Garlic, green tea** may potentiate hypoglycemic effects.

PHARMACOKINETICS **Absorption:** Slowly absorbed from subcutaneous injection site. **Onset:** 1.5 h. **Duration:** 10.4–24 h. **Metabolism:** In liver to active metabolites.

NURSING IMPLICATIONS

Assessment & Drug Effects

- Monitor for S&S of hypoglycemia (see Appendix F), especially after changes in insulin dose or type.
- Withhold drug and notify prescriber if patient is hypokalemic.
- Monitor lab tests: Periodic fasting blood glucose, HbA1C, and potassium; renal function; hepatic function.

Patient & Family Education

- Do not inject into areas with redness, swelling, itching, or dimpling.
- Ingest some form of sugar (e.g., orange juice, dissolved table sugar, honey) if symptoms of hypoglycemia develop and seek medical assistance.
- Instruct patient and caregivers on proper insulin preparation and administration.
- Check blood sugar as prescribed; notify prescriber of fasting blood glucose less than 80 and greater than 120 mg/dL.
- Notify the prescriber of any of the following: Fever, infection, trauma, diarrhea, nausea, or vomiting. Dosage adjustment may be needed.
- Do not take any other medication unless approved by prescriber.

INSULIN GLULISINE

(in′su-lyn glu-li′seen)

Apidra, Apidra SoloSTAR

Classification: ANTIDIABETIC; RAPID-ACTING INSULIN

Therapeutic: RAPID-ACTING INSULIN

Prototype: Insulin injection (Regular)

AVAILABILITY Multidose vials; cartridge system

ACTION & *THERAPEUTIC EFFECT* Insulin glulisine, formed by recombinant DNA, is a rapid-acting insulin. Insulin lowers blood glucose by stimulating peripheral glucose uptake by skeletal muscle and fat and by inhibiting hepatic glucose production. Insulin causes lipolysis in the adipocytes, inhibits proteolysis, and enhances protein synthesis. *Insulin glulisine has a more rapid onset of action and a shorter duration of action than regular human insulin; thus, it provides good postprandial blood glucose control.*

USES Treatment of diabetes mellitus; type I diabetes mellitus in children.

CONTRAINDICATIONS Hypoglycemia; systemic allergy to insulin.

CAUTIOUS USE Renal impairment, hepatic dysfunction; thyroid disease; fever; older adults; pregnancy (category C); lactation, children. Safe use in children younger than 4 y not established.

ROUTE & DOSAGE

Diabetes

Adult/Adolescent/Child (4 y or older): **Subcutaneous** 5–10 units within 15 min before starting a meal or within 20 min after starting a meal. Dose should be individualized.

Adult/Adolescent/Child: **IV** 0.05–1 unit/mL via infusion

ADMINISTRATION

Subcutaneous

- Give within 15 min before or up to 20 min after a meal.
- Store refrigerated at 36°–46° F (2°–8° C). Discard vial if frozen. Protect from light.

Intravenous

Use only under close medical supervision in a clinical setting.

PREPARE: **Infusion:** Dilute with NS or D5W in a polypropylene infusion bag to a final concentration of 0.05–1 unit/mL.

ADMINISTER: **Infusion:** Give at rate ordered by prescriber.

ADVERSE EFFECTS See INSULIN (REGULAR). **Endocrine:**

Hypo-glycemia. **Skin:** Injection site reactions, lipodystrophy, pruritus, rash. **Other:** Allergic reactions.

DIAGNOSTIC TEST INTERFERENCE

See INSULIN INJECTION (REGULAR).

PHARMACOKINETICS

Absorption: 70% bioavailable from injection sites. **Onset:** 15–30 min. **Peak:** 55 min. **Duration:** 3–4 h. **Metabolism:** In liver with some metabolism in the kidney. **Half-Life:** 42 min subcutaneous.

I

NURSING IMPLICATIONS

Assessment & Drug Effects

- Monitor for S&S of hypoglycemia (see Appendix F). Initial hypoglycemic response begins within 15 min and peaks, on average, 40–60 min after injection.
- Monitor lab tests: Periodic fasting and postprandial blood glucose, and HbA1C.

Patient & Family Education

- Follow exactly directions for timing injection in relation to each meal.
- Do not inject into areas with redness, swelling, itching, or dimpling.
- If mixing with NPH human insulin, draw up insulin glulisine first. Inject immediately after mixing.
- Ingest some form of sugar (e.g., orange juice, dissolved table sugar, honey) if symptoms of hypoglycemia develop, and seek medical assistance.
- Check blood sugar as prescribed, especially postprandial values; notify prescriber of fasting blood glucose less than 80 and greater than 140 mg/dL.
- Notify the prescriber of any of the following: Fever, infection, trauma, diarrhea, nausea, or vomiting. Dosage adjustment may be needed.
- Do not take any other medication unless approved by the prescriber.

INSULIN (REGULAR) ✚

(in'su-lyn)

Humulin R, Novolin R

Classification: ANTIDIABETIC; SHORT-ACTING INSULIN

Therapeutic: SHORT-ACTING INSULIN

AVAILABILITY

Solution for injection

ACTION & *THERAPEUTIC EFFECT*

Insulin lowers blood glucose by stimulating peripheral glucose uptake by skeletal muscle and fat and inhibiting hepatic glucose production. Insulin inhibits lipolysis, proteolysis, and gluconeogenesis, and enhance protein synthesis and conversion of excess glucose into fat. *It lowers blood glucose levels by increasing peripheral glucose uptake and by inhibiting the liver from changing glycogen to glucose.*

USES

Treatment of type 1 diabetes mellitus and type 2 diabetes mellitus to improve glycemic control.

CONTRAINDICATIONS

Hypersensitivity to insulin.

CAUTIOUS USE

Renal impairment, renal failure; hepatic impairment, fever, thyroid disease; older adults; pregnancy (category B); children.

ROUTE & DOSAGE

Diabetes Mellitus

Adult: **Subcutaneous** 4–6 units or 0.1 unit/kg or 10% of the basal insulin dose administered before largest meal and as part

of regiment with other agents (dose adjustments based patient response)
Child: **Subcutaneous** 0.2–0.6 units/kg/day in divided doses (adjusted based on response)

ADMINISTRATION

- Note: Insulins should not be mixed unless prescribed by prescriber. In general, regular insulin is drawn up into syringe first. ▪ Any change in the strength (e.g., U-40, U-100), brand (manufacturer), purity, type (regular, etc.), species (pork, human), or sequence of mixing two kinds of insulin is made by the prescriber only, since a simultaneous change in dosage may be necessary.

Subcutaneous

- Use an insulin syringe.
- Give regular insulin 30–60 min before a meal.
- Avoid injection of cold insulin; it can lead to lipodystrophy, reduced rate of absorption, and local reactions.
- Common injection sites: Upper arms, thighs, abdomen [avoid area over urinary bladder and 2 in. (5 cm) around navel], buttocks, and upper back (if fat is loose enough to pick up). Rotate sites.

Intravenous

PREPARE: **Direct:** Give undiluted. **Infusion:** *Humulin R U-100* should be used at a concentration of 0.1 to 1 unit/mL in IV systems with NS in polyvinyl chloride IV bags. *Novolin R* should be used at concentrations of 0.05 to 1 unit/mL in IV systems using propylene IV bags with NS, D5W, or D10W+KCl 40 mmol/L.

ADMINISTER: **Direct:** Give 50 units or a fraction thereof over 1 min. **Infusion:** Rate **must be** ordered by prescriber.

INCOMPATIBILITIES: **Solution/additive:** **Aminophylline, amobarbital, chlorothiazide, cytarabine, dobutamine, octreotide, pentobarbital, phenobarbital, phenytoin, thiopental.** **Y-site:** **Alemtuzumab, butorphanol, cefoperazone, cefoxitin, cefobiprole, chlorpromazine, cisplatin, dantrolene, diazepam, diazoxide, diphenhydramine, gemtuzumab, glycopyrrolate, hydroxyzine, inamrinone, isoproterenol, ketamine, micafungin, minocycline, mitomycin, nestiritide, pentamidine, phentolamine, phenylephrine, phenytoin, piperacillin/tazobactam, polymixin B, prochlorperazine, propranolol, protamine, quinprustin/dalfopristin, rocuronium, SMZ/TMP.**

- Regular insulin may be adsorbed into the container or tubing when added to an IV infusion solution. ▪ Amount lost is variable and depends on concentration of insulin, infusion system, contact duration, and flow rate. ▪ Monitor patient response closely.

- Insulin is stable at room temperature up to 1 mo. Avoid exposure to direct sunlight or to temperature extremes [safe range is wide: 5°–38° C (40°–100° F)]. Refrigerate but do not freeze stock supply. Insulin tolerates temperatures above 38° C with less harm than freezing.

ADVERSE EFFECTS

CNS: With overdose, psychic disturbances (i.e., aphasia, personality changes, maniacal behavior). **Endocrine:**

Posthypoglycemia or rebound hyperglycemia (Somogyi effect), lipoatrophy and lipohyper-trophy of injection sites; insulin resistance. **Skin:** Localized allergic reactions at injection site; generalized urticaria or bullae, lymphade-nopathy. **Other:** Most adverse effects are related to hypoglycemia; anaphylaxis (rare), hyperinsulinemia (*profuse sweating,* hunger, headache, *nausea, tremulousness,* tremors, *palpitation,* tachycardia, weakness, fatigue, nystagmus, circumoral pallor); numb mouth, tongue, and other paresthesias; visual disturbances (diplopia, blurred vision, mydriasis), staring expression, confusion, personality changes, ataxia, incoherent speech, apprehension, irritability, inability to concentrate, personality changes, uncontrolled yawning, loss of consciousness, delirium, hypothermia, convulsions, Babinski reflex, coma. (Urine glucose tests will be negatives.)

INTERACTIONS **Drug: Alcohol,** ANABOLIC STEROIDS, MAO INHIBITORS, **guanethidine,** SALICYLATES, ORAL ANTIDIABETIC agents may potentiate hypoglycemic effects; **dextrothyroxine,** CORTICOSTEROIDS may antagonize hypoglycemic effects; **furosemide,** THIAZIDE DIURETICS increase **serum glucose** levels; **propranolol** and other BETA-BLOCKERS may mask symptoms of hypoglycemic reaction. **Herbal: Garlic, ginseng** may potentiate hypoglycemic effects.

PHARMACOKINETICS **Absorption:** Rapidly absorbed from IM and subcutaneous injections. **Onset:** 0.5–1 h. **Peak:** 2–4 h. **Duration:** 5–7 h. **Distribution:** Throughout extracellular fluids. **Metabolism:** In liver with some metabolism in kidneys. **Elimination:** Less than 2% excreted in urine. **Half-Life:** Biological, up to 13 h.

NURSING IMPLICATIONS

Assessment & Drug Effects

- Note: Frequency of blood glucose monitoring is determined by the insulin regimen and health status of the patient.
- Notify prescriber promptly for markedly elevated blood sugar or presence of acetone with sugar in the urine; may indicate onset of ketoacidosis.
- Monitor for hypoglycemia (see Appendix F) at time of peak action of insulin. Onset of hypoglycemia (blood sugar: 50–40 mg/dL) may be rapid and sudden.
- Check BP, I&O ratio, and blood glucose and ketones every hour during treatment for ketoacidosis with IV insulin.
- Patients with severe hypoglycemia are usually treated with glucagon, epinephrine, or IV glucose 10–50%. As soon as patient is fully conscious, oral carbohydrate (e.g., orange juice with sugar, Gatorade, or Pedialyte) to prevent secondary hypoglycemia may be used.
- Monitor lab tests: Periodic fasting and postprandial blood glucose and HbA1C; urine for ketones in new, unstable, and type 1 diabetes or if patient has lost weight, exercises vigorously, or has an illness and whenever blood glucose is substantially elevated.

Patient & Family Education

- Learn correct injection technique.
- Inject insulin into the abdomen rather than a near muscle that will be heavily taxed, if engaged in active sports.
- Notify prescriber of local reactions at injection site; may develop 1–3 wk after therapy

starts and last several hours to days, usually disappear with continued use.

- Do not change prescription lenses during early period of dosage regulation; vision stabilizes, usually 3–6 wk.
- Check your blood glucose often as directed by the prescriber. Hypoglycemia can result from excess insulin, insufficient food intake, vomiting, diarrhea, unaccustomed exercise, infection, illness, nervous or emotional tension, or overindulgence in alcohol.
- Respond promptly to beginning symptoms of hypoglycemia. Severe hypoglycemia is an emergency situation. Take 4 oz (120 mL) of any fruit juice or regular carbonated beverage [1.5–3 oz (45–90 mL) for child] followed by a meal of longer-acting carbohydrate or protein food. Failure to show signs of recovery within 30 min indicates need for emergency treatment.
- Carry some form of fast-acting carbohydrate (e.g., lump sugar, Life-Savers, or other candy) at all times to treat hypoglycemia.
- Check blood glucose regularly during menstrual period; loss of diabetes control (hyperglycemia or hypoglycemia) is common; adjust insulin dosage accordingly, as prescribed by prescriber.
- Notify prescriber immediately of S&S of diabetic ketoacidosis.
- Continue taking insulin during an illness, go to bed, and drink noncaloric liquids liberally (every hour if possible). Consult prescriber for insulin regulation if unable to eat prescribed diet.
- Avoid OTC medications unless approved by prescriber.

INSULIN, ISOPHANE (NPH)

(in′su-lyn)

Humulin N, Novolin N, ReliOn N

Classification: ANTIDIABETIC; INTERMEDIATE-ACTING INSULIN

Therapeutic: INTERMEDIATE ACTING INSULIN

Prototype: Insulin

AVAILABILITY Solution for injection

ACTION & THERAPEUTIC EFFECT Insulin lowers blood glucose levels by stimulating peripheral glucose uptake, especially by skeletal muscle and fat, and by inhibiting hepatic glucose production. Insulin inhibits lipolysis in the adipocyte, inhibits proteolysis, and enhances protein synthesis. NPH human insulin contains protamine and zinc, providing an intermediate-acting insulin with a slower onset and a longer duration of activity. *Usually without supplemental doses of insulin injection.*

USES Used to control hyperglycemia in the diabetic patient. Mixtard and Novolin 70/30 are fixed combinations of purified regular insulin 30% and NPH 70%.

CONTRAINDICATIONS During episodes of hypoglycemia or in patients sensitive to any ingredient in the formulation; intravenous route; diabetic ketoacidosis; hyperosmolar hyperglycemic state.

CAUTIOUS USE In insulin-resistant patients, hyperthyroidism or hypothyroidism; fever; older adults, renal or hepatic impairment; pregnancy (category B); children.

ROUTE & DOSAGE

Diabetes Mellitus

Adult: **Subcutaneous**
Individualized doses (see INSULIN, REGULAR)

ADMINISTRATION

Subcutaneous

- Give isophane insulin 30 min before first meal of the day. If necessary, a second smaller dose may be prescribed 30 min before supper or at bedtime.
- Ensure complete dispersion by mixing thoroughly by gently rotating vial between palms and inverting it end to end several times. Do not shake.
- **Do not** mix insulins unless prescribed by prescriber. In general, when insulin injection (regular insulin) is to be combined, it is drawn first.
- Store unopened vial at 2°–8° C (36°–46° F). Avoid freezing and exposure to extremes in temperature or to direct sunlight.

ADVERSE EFFECTS See INSULIN (REGULAR).

INTERACTIONS See INSULIN (REGULAR).

PHARMACOKINETICS **Onset:** 1–2 h. **Peak:** 4–12 h NPH. **Duration:** 18–24 h NPH. **Metabolism:** In liver and kidney. **Elimination:** Less than 2% excreted unchanged in urine. **Half-Life:** Up to 13 h.

NURSING IMPLICATIONS

See INSULIN (REGULAR).

Assessment & Drug Effects

- Suspect hypoglycemia if fatigue, weakness, sweating, tremor, or nervousness occur.

Patient & Family Education

- If insulin was given before breakfast, a hypoglycemic episode is most likely to occur between mid-afternoon and dinnertime, when insulin effect is peaking. Advise to eat a snack in mid-afternoon and to carry sugar or candy to treat a reaction. A snack at bedtime will prevent insulin reaction during the night.
- Learn the S&S of hypoglycemia and hyperglycemia (see Appendix F).

INSULIN LISPRO

(in′su-lyn lis′pro)

Humalog

Classification: ANTIDIABETIC; RAPID-ACTING INSULIN
Therapeutic: RAPID-ACTING INSULIN

AVAILABILITY Solution for injection

ACTION & *THERAPEUTIC EFFECT* Insulin lispro of recombinant DNA origin is a human insulin that is a rapid-acting, glucose-lowering agent of shorter duration than human regular insulin. It lowers blood glucose levels by increasing peripheral glucose uptake, especially by skeletal muscle and fat tissue, and by inhibiting the liver from changing glycogen to glucose. *It lowers blood glucose levels and inhibits liver from changing glycogen to glucose.*

USES Treatment of diabetes mellitus.

CONTRAINDICATIONS During episodes of hypoglycemia or in patients sensitive to any ingredient in the formulation.

CAUTIOUS USE In insulin-resistant patients, hyperthyroidism or hypothyroidism; use of alcohol;

- Dust shoes and stockings, as well as feet, with nystatin dusting powder.
- Gently clean infected areas with tepid water before each application of topical preparation.
- Advise patient to avoid sex until treatment is complete, as infection may be spread to sexual partner.
- Continue medication for vulvovaginal candidiasis during menstruation. Do not use tampons, douches, or other vaginal products during therapy. Wear cotton panties and minipad/sanitary napkin, as drug may ooze from vagina and soil clothing.
- Use vaginal tablets up to 6 wk before term to prevent thrush in the newborn.

OBINUTUZUMAB

(o-bi-nu-tu′zu-mab)

Gazyva

Classification: MONOCLONAL ANTIBODY; ANTINEOPLASTIC

Therapeutic: ANTINEOPLASTIC

AVAILABILITY Solution for injection

ACTION & *THERAPEUTIC EFFECT*

Type II anti-CD20 monoclonal antibody that binds to CD20 antigens on the surface of B-lymphocytes and activates complement-dependent cytotoxicity, antibody-dependent cellular cytotoxicity, and antibody-dependent cellular phagocytosis. *Triggers immune responses that result in death of leukemic lymphocytic cells.*

USES Combination use with chlorambucil in the treatment of patients with previously untreated chronic lymphocytic leukemia (CLL); non-Hodgkin's lymphoma.

CONTRAINDICATIONS Grade 4 life-threatening infusion reactions; progressive multifocal leukoencephalopathy (PML); reactivation of latent Hepatitis B; lactation.

CAUTIOUS USE History of Hepatitis B virus infection; infusion reactions; tumor lysis syndrome; bone marrow suppression; pregnancy (category C). Safety and efficacy in children not established.

ROUTE & DOSAGE

Chronic Lymphocytic Leukemia

Adult: IV Six cycles every 28 days *Cycle 1:* 100 mg on day 1; 900 mg on day 2; followed by 1000 weekly for 2 doses on days 8 and 15.
Cycle 2–6: 1000 mg on day 1 of each cycle, then every 28 days for 5 doses

Non-Hodgkin's Lymphoma

Adult: IV 1000 mg on days 1, 8, and 15 on cycle 1; begin the next cycle of therapy on day 29. For cycles 2 to 6, give 1000 mg on day 1 repeated every 28 days

Infusion Reaction Dosage Adjustment

Grade 1–2 (mild or moderate): Slow or interrupt infusion. Upon resolution of symptoms, continue therapy; if no further infusion reactions, rate escalation may resume
Grade 3 (severe): Interrupt infusion and manage symptoms. Upon resolution of symptoms, can restart at no more than ½ the previous rate; if no further infusion symptoms occur, rate escalation may resume. Permanently discontinue if patient experiences another Grade 3 reaction.

Grade 4 (life threatening): Permanently discontinue obinutuzumab

ADMINISTRATION

Intravenous

PREPARE: **Infusion: Cycle 1 (day 1 and day 2):** To prepare 100 mg dose for day 1, withdraw 4 mL (100 mg) of obinutuzumab from vial and inject into a 100 mL NS infusion bag. Use immediately. To prepare 900 mg dose for day 2, withdraw the remaining 36 mL (900 mg) from vial and inject into a 250 mL NS infusion bag. Gently invert to mix; do not shake or freeze. ▪ **Cycle 1 (day 8 and 15) and cycles 2 to 6 (day 1):** To prepare 1000 mg dose, withdraw 40 mL of obinutuzumab from vial and inject into a 250 mL NS infusion bag. Gently invert to mix; do not shake or freeze. ▪ **Note:** Final concentration should be 0.4 to 4 mg/mL. If not used immediately, may store at 2°–8 °C (36°–46° F) for up to 24 h; use immediately after reaching room temperature. Gently invert to mix; do not shake or freeze.

O

ADMINISTER: **Infusion:** Administer only as an infusion through a dedicated line. **Do not** give IV push or bolus. ▪ **Cycle 1 (day 1):** Infuse 100 mg dose at 25 mg/h over 4 h. ▪ **Cycle 1 (day 2):** Infuse 900 mg dose at 50 mg/h; can increase q30 min by 50 mg/min, to max rate of 400 mg/h. ▪ **Cycle 1: (days 8 and 15) and Cycles 2–6 (day 1):** Infuse 1000 mg dose at 100 mg/h; can increase q30 min by 100 mg/h to max rate of 400 mg/h. Note: Patients are usually premedicated with acetaminophen, an antihistamine (e.g., diphenhydramine), and a glucocorticoid (e.g., dexamethasone or methylprednisolone).

INCOMPATIBILITIES: **Solution/additive:** Do not use with diluents other than **0.9% NaCl;** do not mix with other drugs. **Y-site:** Do not mix with any other drug.

ADVERSE EFFECTS

Respiratory: Cough. **Endocrine:** Alkaline phosphatase increased, ALT/AST increased, creatinine increased, hyperkalemia, hypoalbuminemia, hypocalcemia, hypokalemia, hyponatremia. **GI:** Constipation. **Musculoskeletal:** Musculoskeletal pain. **Hematological:** Anemia, leukopenia, *neutropenia, thrombocytopenia*. **Other:** *Infusion related reactions*, infections, pyrexia, tumor lysis syndrome.

PHARMACOKINETICS

Half-Life: 28.4 d.

NURSING IMPLICATIONS

Black Box Warning

Obinutuzumab has been associated with progressive multifocal leukoencephalopathy (PML) including fatal PML, and with Hepatitis B virus (HBV) reactivation, in some cases resulting in fulminant hepatitis, hepatic failure, and death.

Assessment & Drug Effects

- Monitor closely during entire infusion period for S&S of an infusion reaction: Bronchospasm, dyspnea, larynx and throat irritation, wheezing, laryngeal edema, tachycardia, flushing, hypertension, hypotension, fever, nausea, vomiting, diarrhea, headache, and/or chills. Immediately stop infusion if an infusion reaction is suspected and institute supportive measures.

- Monitor for and report promptly S&S of infection. Do not administer this drug if patient has an active infection. Note that infusion reactions are more frequent with first 1000 mg infused and may occur up to 24 h after infusion.
- Monitor for and report promptly signs of tumor lysis syndrome (e.g., nausea, vomiting, diarrhea, lethargy) during 72 h period after first infusion.
- Monitor lab tests: Prior to therapy, HBsAG and anti-HBc; periodic CBC with differential and platelet count, renal function tests, and serum uric acid, serum electrolytes.

Patient & Family Education

- During infusion, immediately report signs of an infusion reaction such as wheezing, chest tightness, fever; itching, bad cough, or swelling of face, lips, tongue, or throat.
- Report promptly signs of tumor lysis syndrome (e.g., nausea, vomiting, diarrhea, lethargy) especially during 72 h period after first infusion.
- Report immediately to prescriber any of the following: Signs of infection, signs of liver toxicity (see Appendix F), tachycardia, severe headache, significant weakness, bruising, or unexplained bleeding.
- Do not accept vaccinations with live viral vaccines.
- Do not breastfeed without consulting prescriber.

OCTREOTIDE ACETATE

(oc-tre′o-tide)

Bynfezia Pen, Mycapssa, Sandostatin, Sandostatin LAR Depot

Classification: SOMATOSTATIN ANALOG

Therapeutic HORMONE SUPPRESSANT; ACROMEGALY AGENT; ANTIDIARRHEAL

AVAILABILITY Solution for injection; depot injection; capsule

ACTION & *THERAPEUTIC EFFECT* A long-acting peptide that mimics natural hormone somatostatin. Suppresses secretion of serotonin, pancreatic peptides, gastrin, vasoactive intestinal peptide, insulin, glucagon, secretin, and motilin. *Stimulates fluid and electrolyte absorption from the GI tract and prolongs intestinal transit time; also inhibits the growth hormone.*

USES Symptomatic treatment of severe diarrhea and flushing episodes associated with metastatic carcinoid tumors. Also watery diarrhea associated with vasoactive intestinal peptide (VIP) tumors, acromegaly.

UNLABELED USES Variceal bleeding, hepatorenal syndrome.

CONTRAINDICATIONS Hypersensitivity to octreotide; pregnancy—fetal risk cannot be ruled out; lactation—infant risk cannot be ruled out.

CAUTIOUS USE Cholelithiasis, renal impairment; dialysis; hepatic disease, liver cirrhosis; cardiac disease, CHF; diabetes, TPN administration; hypothyroidism; older adults.

ROUTE & DOSAGE

Carcinoid Tumors

Adult: **Subcutaneous/IV** 100–600 mcg/day in 2–4 divided doses, titrate to response; **IM** May switch to depot injection after 2 wk of subcutaneous injections, switch to 20 mg q4wk × 2 mo

VIPoma

Adult: **Subcutaneous/IV** 200–300 mcg/day in 2–4 divided

doses, titrate to response; **IM** May switch to depot injection after 2 wk of subcutaneous injections, switch to 20 mg q4wk × 2 mo

Acromegaly

Adult: **Subcutaneous/IV** 50 mcg tid, titrate up to achieve target levels.; **IM(depot)** 20 mg q4 wks × 3 months adjust dose as necessary **PO** 20 mg bid, monitor and adjust dose based on response (max 80 mg daily)

ADMINISTRATION

Oral

- Take capsules orally with a glass of water on an empty stomach, at least 1 hour before a meal or at least 2 hours after a meal.
- Swallow capsules whole. Do not crush or chew capsules.
- Store unopened wallet in a refrigerator between 2 and 8 degrees C (38 and 46 degrees F); do not freeze. After wallet is opened, store between 20 and 25 degrees C (68 and 77 degrees F) for up to 1 month.

Subcutaneous/Intramuscular

- **Sandostatin LAR Depot** should be given IM. Reconstitute according to manufacturer's directions.
- **Sandostatin** may be given subcutaneously or IV.
- Minimize GI side effects by giving injections between meals and at bedtime.
- Avoid multiple injections into the same site. Rotate subcutaneous sites on abdomen, hip, and thigh.
- Give deep IM into a large muscle. To reduce local irritation, allow solution to reach room temperature before injection and administer slowly.
- Store at room temperature for 30–60 minutes prior to drug preparation.

Intravenous

PREPARE: **Direct:** Give **Sandostatin** undiluted. **Intermittent:** Dilute in 50–200 mL D5W.

ADMINISTER: **Direct:** Give a single dose over 3–5 min. In emergency (e.g., carcinoid crisis), give rapid IV bolus over 60 sec. **Intermittent:** Give over 15–30 min.

- Store ampuls and multidose vials in outer carton under refrigeration between 2 and 8 degrees C (36 and 46 degrees F). Protect from light. Open ampuls just prior to administration and discard any unused portion.

INCOMPATIBILITIES: **Solution/additive:** **Fat emulsion, regular insulin.** **Y-site:** **Dantrolene, diazepam, micafungin, phenytoin.**

ADVERSE EFFECTS (≥5%) **CV:** *Bradycardia, cardiac dysrhythmia, peripheral edema (oral).* **Respiratory:** Nasopharyngitis, sinusitis, sinusitis (oral). **CNS:** *Headache, asthenia, fatigue, dizziness,* CVA. **Endocrine:** Hyperglycemia, increased liver transaminases, hypothyroidism (after long-term use), cholelithiasis, pancreatitis. **Skin:** Excessive sweating (oral). **Hepatic:** Cholangiectasis. **GI:** *Nausea, diarrhea, constipation, flatulence, indigestion, abdominal pain, cholelithiasis,* pancreatitis, large intestine polyp, steatorrhea, and discomfort. **GU:** UTI. **Musculoskeletal:** Arthralgia, arthropathy, osteoarthritis. **Hematologic:** Anemia, thrombocytopenia. **Other:** Influenza-like illness, generalized pain.

INTERACTIONS **Drug:** May decrease **cyclosporine** levels;

may alter other drug and nutrient absorption because of alterations in GI motility. May decrease concentration of hormonal contraceptives.

PHARMACOKINETICS **Absorption:** Rapidly from subcutaneous injection. **Peak:** 0.4 h. **Duration:** Up to 12 h. **Metabolism:** In liver. **Elimination:** In urine. **Half-Life:** 1.5 h.

NURSING IMPLICATIONS

Assessment & Drug Effects

- Monitor for hypoglycemia and hyperglycemia (see Appendix F), because octreotide may alter the balance between insulin, glucagon, and growth hormone.
- Monitor fluid and electrolyte balance, as octreotide stimulates fluid and electrolyte absorption from GI tract.
- Monitor vitals signs, especially BP.
- Monitor bowel function, including bowel sounds and stool consistency.
- Monitor lab tests: Baseline and periodic thyroid function tests and vitamin B_{12}. As specific conditions indicate, periodic: Plasma serotonin levels with carcinoid tumors, plasma VIP levels with VIPoma, serum GH, serum IGF-1, and blood glucoses, zinc levels, electrolytes.

Patient & Family Education

- Learn proper technique for subcutaneous injection if self-medication is required.
- Note: Preferred sites for subcutaneous injections of octreotide are the hip, thigh, and abdomen. Multiple injections at the same subcutaneous injection site within short periods of time are not recommended. This is to avoid irritating the area.
- Review adverse effects with patient and/or caregiver.
- Females of reproductive potential use an alternative non-hormonal method of contraception or a backup method when oral form of the drug is uses with combined oral contraceptives.

OFATUMUMAB

(o-fa-tu′mu-mab)

Arzerra

Classification: BIOLOGIC RESPONSE MODIFIER; MONOCLONAL ANTIBODY; CD20 CYTOLYTIC ANTIBODY; ANTINEOPLASTIC

Therapeutic: ANTINEOPLASTIC

AVAILABILITY Solution for injection

ACTION & *THERAPEUTIC EFFECT*

A CD20 cytolytic IgG1 kappa monoclonal antibody. The CD20 molecule is present on normal B lymphocytes, both mature and immature lymphocytes, as well as on B-cells in chronic lymphocytic leukemia (CLL). Ofatumumab causes B-cell lysis possibly by complement-dependent cytotoxicity and by antibody-dependent, cell-mediated cytotoxicity. *Effectiveness in treatment of CLL refractory to the standard drug regimen is based on the clinical improvement in response to ofatumumab.*

USES Chronic lymphocytic leukemia refractory.

CONTRAINDICATIONS Serious infusion reaction; leukoencephalopathy; hepatitis B reactivation; live vaccines; lactation.

CAUTIOUS USE History of hepatitis B; older adults; pregnancy (category C). Safety and efficacy in children not established.

ROUTE & DOSAGE

Chronic Lymphocytic Leukemia (CLL)—First Line or Refractory Dose

Adult: **IV** Initial dose of 300 mg followed 1 wk later by 2000 mg qwk for 7 doses, followed by 2000 mg q4wk for 4 doses

ADMINISTRATION

Intravenous

PREPARE: **Infusion:** Do not shake drug vials. ▪ Determine the volume of the required drug dose and withdraw an equal volume of NS from a 1000 mL polyolefin IV bag. Add ofatumumab to the IV bag and mix by gentle inversion.

ADMINISTER: **Infusion:** Infuse through an in-line filter and PVC administration set supplied with product. ▪ **Do not** give IV push or bolus. ▪ Do not mix or administer with any other drugs or solutions. *For doses 1 and 2:* Initiate infusion at 12 mL/h. If no infusion reaction occurs from 0–30 min, may increase rate q30min as follows: 31–60 min, 25 mL/h; 61–90 min, 50 mL/h; 91–120 min, 100 mL/h; after 120 min, 200 mL/h. ▪ *For doses 3–12:* Initiate infusion at 25 mL/h. If no infusion reaction occurs from 0–30 min, may increase rate q30min as follows: 31–60 min, 50 mL/h; 61–90 min, 100 mL/h; 91–120 min, 200 mL/h; after 120 min, 400 mL/h.

▪ Store diluted solution at 2°–8° C (36°–46° F). ▪ Use within 12 h of preparation. Discard solution after 24 h.

ADVERSE EFFECTS **CV:** Hypertension, hypotension, tachycardia. **Respiratory:** *Bronchitis, cough, dyspnea,* nasopharyngitis, *pneumonia,* sinusitis, *upper respiratory tract infections.* **CNS:** Headache, insomnia. **Skin:** Hyperhidrosis, *rash,* urticaria. **GI:** *Diarrhea, nausea.* **Musculoskeletal:** Back pain, muscle spasms. **Hematologic:** *Anemia, neutropenia.* **Other:** Chills, *fatigue,* herpes zoster infection, *infusion reactions,* peripheral edema, *pyrexia,* sepsis.

PHARMACOKINETICS **Half-Life:** 14 days.

NURSING IMPLICATIONS

Black Box Warning

Ofatumumab has been associated with progressive multifocal leukoencephalopathy (PML) including fatal PML, and with Hepatitis B virus (HBV) reactivation, in some cases resulting in fulminant hepatitis, hepatic failure, and death.

Assessment & Drug Effects

- Monitor for infusion reactions and stop infusion for any of the following: Bronchospasm, dyspnea, angioedema, flushing, significant changes in BP, tachycardia, back or abdominal pain, fever, rash, or urticaria.
- Monitor for and report promptly S&S of changes in neurologic status or suspected intestinal obstruction.
- Monitor lab tests: Baseline HBsAG, anti-HBc, and total anti-HBc (with both IgG and IgM) or anti-HBc IgG tests.

Patient & Family Education

- Report promptly any of the following: New or worsening abdominal pain or nausea, confusion, dizziness, loss of balance, difficulty talking or problems with vision, sore throat, fever, or other signs of infections.

- Avoid live vaccinations and close contact with those who have received live vaccines.

OFLOXACIN

(o-flox'a-cin)

Ocuflox

Classification: QUINOLONE ANTIBIOTIC

Therapeutic: ANTIBIOTIC

Prototype: Ciprofloxacin

AVAILABILITY Tablet; ophthalmic solution; otic solution

ACTION & *THERAPEUTIC EFFECT* Inhibits DNA gyrase, an enzyme necessary for bacterial DNA replication and some aspects of its transcription, repair, recombination, and transposition. *Has a broad spectrum of activity against gram-positive and gram-negative bacteria. Most effective against aerobic and anaerobic gram-negative bacteria.*

USES Uncomplicated gonorrhea, prostatitis, respiratory tract infections, skin and skin structure infections, urinary tract infections, superficial ocular infections, pelvic inflammatory disease. Otic: Otitis externa, otitis media with perforated tympanic membranes.

UNLABELED USES EENT infections, *Helicobacter pylori* infections, *Salmonella* gastroenteritis, anthrax.

CONTRAINDICATIONS Hypersensitivity to ofloxacin or other quinolone antibacterial agents; tendon pain; sunlight (UV) exposure; QT prolongation; viral infection; tendinitis, tendon rupture; history of myasthenia gravis; syphilis.

CAUTIOUS USE Renal disease; patients with a history of epilepsy, psychosis, or increased intracranial pressure, cerebrovascular disease, CNS disorders such as seizures, epilepsy, myasthenia gravis; GI disease, colitis, dehydration; syphilis; atrial fibrillation; acute MI; CVA; pregnancy (category C); lactation; children and adolescents (except for **ophthalmic** and **otic** preparation).

ROUTE & DOSAGE

Uncomplicated Gonorrhea (Not CDC Recommended)

Adult: **PO** 400 mg for 1 dose

Respiratory Tract and Skin and Skin Structure Infections

Adult: **PO** 200–400 mg q12h × 10 days

Urinary Tract Infection

Adult: **PO** 200 mg q12h × 3–10 days

Pelvic Inflammatory Disease

Adult: **PO** 400 mg bid × 14 days

Prostatitis

Adult: **PO** 300 mg bid × 6 wk

Otitis Media with Perforation

Adult: **Otic** 10 drops (0.5 mL) q12h for 14 days

Child (1 y or older): **Otic** 5 drops (0.25 mL) q12h for 14 days

Otitis Externa

Adult: **Otic** 10 drops (0.5 mL) q12h for 7 days

Child (6 mo–13 y): **Otic** 5 drops (0.25 mL) q12h for 7 days

Renal Impairment Dosage Adjustment

CrCl 20–50 mL/min: Dose should be given q24h; *less than 20 mL/min:* ½ the dose q24h

Hepatic Impairment Dosage Adjustment

Severe impairment: 400 mg daily

ADMINISTRATION

Oral

- Administer with or without food.
- Avoid administering mineral supplements or vitamins with iron or zinc within 2 h of drug.
- Do not give antacids with magnesium, aluminum, or sucralfate within 4 h before or 2 h after drug.

Instillation

- **Do not** allow tip of dropper for ocular preparation to contact any surface.

O

ADVERSE EFFECTS **CNS:** *Headache, dizziness, insomnia,* hallucinations. **Skin:** Pruritus, rash. **GI:** Nausea, vomiting, diarrhea, GI discomfort. **GU:** Pruritus, pain, irritation, burning, vaginitis, vaginal discharge, dysmenorrhea, menorrhagia, dysuria, urinary frequency. **Other:** Cartilage erosion.

DIAGNOSTIC TEST INTERFERENCE May cause false positive on ***opiate screening tests.***

INTERACTIONS **Drug:** Ofloxacin absorption decreased when it is administered with MAGNESIUM- or ALUMINUM-CONTAINING ANTACIDS. Other CATIONS, including **calcium, iron,** and **zinc,** also appear to interfere with ofloxacin absorption. May have additive effect with ANTIDIABETICS. Do not use with other agents that prolong QT interval (e.g., **dofetilide, dronedarone, thioridazine, ziprasidone**).

PHARMACOKINETICS **Absorption:** 90–98% from GI tract. **Peak:** 1–2 h. **Distribution:** Distributes to most tissues; 50% crosses into CSF with inflamed meninges; 20–32% protein bound; crosses placenta; distributed into breast milk. **Metabolism:** Slightly in liver. **Elimination:** 72–98% in urine within 48 h. **Half-Life:** 5–7.5 h.

NURSING IMPLICATIONS

Black Box Warning

Ofloxacin has been associated with an increased risk of tendinitis and tendon rupture, and increased muscle weakness in persons with MG.

Assessment & Drug Effects

- Withhold ofloxacin and notify prescriber at first sign of tendon pain, a skin rash, or other allergic reaction.
- Monitor for seizures, especially in patients with known or suspected CNS disorders. Discontinue ofloxacin and notify prescriber immediately if seizure occurs.
- Assess for signs and symptoms of superinfection (see Appendix F).
- Monitor lab tests: C&S tests prior to initial dose.

Patient & Family Education

- Drink fluids liberally unless contraindicated.

- Be aware that dizziness or lightheadedness may occur; use appropriate caution.
- Avoid excessive sunlight or artificial ultraviolet light because of the possibility of phototoxicity.

OLANZAPINE

(olanz-a'peen)

Zyprexa, Zyprexa Relprevv, Zyprexa Zydis

Classification: ATYPICAL ANTIPSYCHOTIC

Therapeutic: ANTIPSYCHOTIC, ANTIMANIC

Prototype: Clozapine

AVAILABILITY Tablet; orally disintegrating tablet; powder for injection

ACTION & *THERAPEUTIC EFFECT* Antipsychotic activity is thought to be due to antagonism for both serotonin 5-$HT_{2A/2C}$ and dopamine D_{1-4} receptors. May inhibit the CNS presynaptic neuronal reuptake of serotonin and dopamine. *Has effective antipsychotic activity.*

USES Management of schizophrenia, treatment of bipolar disorder and bipolar depression, acute agitation (IM); major depressive disorder.

UNLABELED USES Alzheimer dementia, anorexia nervosa, chemotherapy induced nausea/vomiting, hyperactive delirium.

CONTRAINDICATIONS Hypersensitivity to olanzapine; abrupt discontinuation, coma, severe CNS depression; dementia-related psychosis in older adults; lactation.

CAUTIOUS USE Known cardiovascular disease, stroke, MI, HF, CVD, neurologic disease, Parkinson disease; history of seizures, conditions that lower seizure threshold (e.g., Alzheimer dementia); conditions that predispose to hypotension; history of syncope; history of breast cancer; Japanese; DM; BPH; hepatic impairment, jaundice; predisposition to aspiration pneumonia; history of or high risk for suicide; elevated triglyceride levels; hyperlipedemia; older adults; pregnancy (crosses the placenta; may decrease reproductive function in males and females); children. **IM form:** Older adults; debilitated or patients at risk for hypotension. Safety and efficacy in children not established.

ROUTE & DOSAGE

Bipolar Disorders

Adult: **PO** 10–15 mg once/day, may increase by 5 mg until desired response (max: 20 mg/day); **IM Extended release** 150–300 mg q2wk or 405 mg q4wk
Adolescent: 2.5–5 mg daily, may increase in 2.5 or 5 mg increments (max: 20 mg/day)
Geriatric: **PO** Start with 2.5–5 mg once/day; **IM Extended release** varies depending on previous oral dose (see package insert for details)

Major Depressive Disorder

Adult: **PO** 5 mg daily may adjust per response (usual dose 5–20 mg/day)

Acute Agitation

Adult: **IM** 5–10 mg, do not repeat more frequently than q2h (max: 30 mg/24h)
Geriatric: **IM** 2.5–5 mg once daily

ADMINISTRATION

Oral

- Do not push orally disintegrating tablet through blister foil. Peel foil back and remove tablet. Tablet will disintegrate with/without liquid. May be administered with or without food.

Intramuscular

- *Short-acting formulation:* Reconstitute with 2.1 mL of sterile water for injection to yield 5 mg/mL. Use within 1 h of reconstitution.
- *Extended-release formulation:* Reconstitute with supplied syringe and diluent. Use gloves and flush with water if skin contact is made. To produce a 150 mg/mL solution for injection add 1.3 mL of diluent to the 210 mg vial; or add 1.8 mL of diluent to the 300 mg vial; or add 2.3 mL of diluent to the 405 mg vial.
- Give deep IM into the gluteal muscle. Do not inject more than 5 mL into one site.

ADVERSE EFFECTS **CV:** Orthostatic hypotension. **Respiratory:** Rhinitis, cough. **CNS:** *Somnolence, dizziness, headache, insomnia*, akathisia, asthenia, abnormal gait, fatigue, extrapyramidal symptoms (dystonic events, *parkinsonism, akathesia*), tardive dyskinesia. **Endocrine:** *Increased prolactin*, weight gain. **Hepatic/GI:** Abdominal pain, constipation, dyspepsia, dry mouth, increased appetite, decreased serum bilirubin, increased liver enzymes. **Musculoskeletal:** Arthralgia, back pain. **Other:** Accidental injury, bruising, fever.

INTERACTIONS **Drug:** May enhance hypotensive effects of ANTIHYPERTENSIVES; ANTIPARKINSON AGENTS may decrease effect of olanzapine; may enhance effect of ANTICHOLINERGIC AGENTS. May enhance CNS depressant effects of other CNS DEPRESSANTS, **alcohol. Carbamazepine, omeprazole, rifampin** may increase metabolism and clearance of olanzapine. **Fluvoxamine** may inhibit metabolism and clearance of olanzapine. Avoid medications prolong QT interval (e.g., **dofetilide, dronedarone, thioridazine, ziprasidone**). CYP1A2 inhibitors may increase serum concentration of olanzapine, increasing risk of adverse effects; CYP1A2 inducers may decrease serum concentration decreasing efficacy. Do not use with **amisulpride**.

PHARMACOKINETICS **Absorption:** Rapidly from GI tract; 60% reaches systemic circulation. **Onset:** 15 min IM. **Peak:** 6 h. **Distribution:** 93% protein bound, secreted into breast milk of animals (human secretion unknown). **Metabolism:** In liver (CYP1A2). **Elimination:** Approximately 57% in urine, 30% in feces. **Half-Life:** 21–54 h.

NURSING IMPLICATIONS

Black Box Warning

Olanzapine has been associated with increased mortality in older adults with dementia-related psychosis.

Assessment & Drug Effects

- Monitor closely cerebrovascular status in elderly patients with dementia-related psychosis.
- Monitor diabetics for loss of glycemic control.
- Withhold drug and immediately report S&S of neuroleptic malignant syndrome (see Appendix F); assess for and report S&S of tardive dyskinesia (see Appendix F).
- Monitor BP and HR periodically. Monitor temperature, especially with other anticholinergic drugs.

- Monitor for and report orthostatic hypotension, especially during the initial dose-titration period.
- Monitor for seizures, especially in older adults and cognitively impaired persons.
- Monitor weight, BMI, and waist circumference at baseline and again at 4–8–12 wk, then periodically thereafter.
- Taper dosage slowly when discontinuing.
- Monitor lab tests: Periodic CBC, LFTs, lipid profile, serum electrolytes, HbA1C, and blood glucose.

Patient & Family Education

- Report immediately to prescriber behavioral changes, mood changes, or suicidal ideation.
- Report to prescriber difficulty with motor activity, change in balance, severe dizziness, difficulty speaking or swallowing, tremors, difficulty moving, rigidity.
- Carefully monitor blood glucose levels if diabetic.
- Do not drive or engage in potentially hazardous activities until response to drug is known; drug increases risk of orthostatic hypotension and cognitive impairment.
- Avoid alcohol and do not take additional medications without informing prescriber.
- Do not become overheated; avoid conditions leading to dehydration.

OLANZAPINE AND SAMIDORPHAN

(oh-LAN-za-peen & SAM-I-DOR-fan)

Lybalvi

Classifications: OPIOID ANTAGONIST; ATYPICAL ANTIPSYCHOTIC

Therapeutic: ANTIPSYCHOTIC, ANTIMANIC

AVAILABILITY Oral tablet

ACTION & THERAPEUTIC EFFECT A second generation thienobenzodiazepine antipsychotic that displays potent antagonism of serotonin, dopamine, histamine, and alpha1-adrenergic receptors.

USES Treatment of schizophrenia and bipolar I disorder. Used in the acute treatment of bipolar I disorder for mixed or manic episodes as monotherapy and as adjunct to lithium or valproate in adults.

CONTRAINDICATIONS Concomitant use with opioids; patients undergoing opioid withdrawal.

CAUTIOUS USE CNS depression; patients with dementia, esophogeal dysmotility or aspiration risk, hypotension, severe cardiac disease, decreased GI motility, seizure disorder, hepatic impairment, urinary retention, or neuroleptic malignant syndrome; smokers; pregnancy (adverse events were observed in animal reproduction studies; may decrease reproductive function in males and females); lactation.

O

ROUTE & DOSAGE

Bipolar I Disorder

Adult: **Oral** 10–15 mg olanzapine/10 mg samidorpohan once daily

Schizophrenia

Adult: **Oral** 5–10 mg olanzapine/10 mg samidorpohan once daily

Renal Impairment Dosage Adjustment

eGFR 15–29 mL/min: Use caution
eGFR less than 15 mL/min: Not recommended

ADMINISTRATION

Oral

- Administer with or without food. Do not divide tablets or combine strengths.
- Store at 20°–25° C (68°–77° F).

ADVERSE EFFECTS **CNS:** Drowsiness, headache. **Endocrine:** Weight gain, hyperglycemia, increased serum prolactin, increased serum triglycerides. **GI/Hepatic:** Dry mouth, abnormal liver function tests.

INTERACTIONS **Drug:** May enhance hypotensive effects of ANTI-HYPERTENSIVES; ANTIPARKINSON AGENTS may decrease effect of olanzapine; may enhance effect of ANTICHOLINERGIC AGENTS. May enhance CNS depressant effects of other CNS depressants, **alcohol. Carbamazepine, omeprazole, rifampin** may increase metabolism and clearance of olanzapine. Fluvoxamine may inhibit metabolism and clearance of olanzapine. Avoid medications prolong QT interval (e.g., **dofetilide, dronedarone, thioridazine, ziprasidone**). CYP1A2 inhibitors may increase serum concentration of olanzapine, increasing risk of adverse effects; CYP1A2 inducers may decrease serum concentration decreasing efficacy. Do not use with OPIOIDS.

O

PHARMACOKINETICS **Absorption:** Samidorphan: 69% bioavailability. **Peak:** Olanzapine: 4.5–7 h; Samidorphan: 1–2 h. **Distribution:** Olanzapine: 93% protein-bound; Samidorphan: 23–33% protein-bound. **Metabolism:** Olanzapine: Primarily by UGT1A4 and CYP1A2 (major), with CYP2D6 (minor); Samidorphan: Primarily through CYP3A4. Major metabolites do not contribute to drug effect. **Elimination:** Olanzapine: 57% excreted in urine, 30% feces; Samidorphan: 67% excreted in urine, 16% feces. **Half-Life:** Olanzapine: 35–52 h; Samidorphan: 7–11 h

NURSING IMPLICATIONS

Black Box Warning

Increased mortality in elderly patients with dementia-related psychosis.

Assessment & Drug Effects

- Monitor mental status and alertness. Watch and report any abnormal involuntary movements or parkinsonian symptoms.
- Monitor vital signs including Bp at baseline and every 3 months after antipsychotic initiation.
- Monitor weight, height, BMI, waist circumference at baseline and at 4, 8, and 12 weeks after initiating therapy, then quarterly.
- Monitor lab values: CBC, serum electrolytes, LFTs, fasting plasma glucose level, fasting lipid panel.

Patient & Family Education

- Avoid driving and doing other tasks that require alertness until you see how the drug affects you.
- High blood sugar or diabetes, high cholesterol, and weight gain may happen with this drug. This may raise your risk of heart or brain blood vessel disease.
- Do not take opioid drugs while taking this medication. Avoid opioid drugs for at least 5 days after stopping this medication.

OLICERIDINE

(OH li SER I deen)

Olinvyk

Classifications: ANALGESIC; NARCOTIC (OPIATE AGONIST)

Therapeutic: NARCOTIC ANALGESIC

Controlled Substance: Schedule II

AVAILABILITY Solution for injection

ACTION & *THERAPEUTIC EFFECT* A full opioid agonist and is relatively selective for the mu-opioid receptor. The principal therapeutic action is analgesia. The precise mechanism of action is unknown.

USES Management of severe acute pain, where alternative treatments are inadequate.

CONTRAINDICATIONS Acute or severe bronchial asthma in an unmonitored setting or in the absence of resusucitative equipment; Know hypersensitivity to oliceridine; Known or suspected gastrointestinal obstruction; including paralytic ileus; Significant respiratory depression; concomitant use of mixed agonist/antagonist or partial agonist analgesics; impaired consciousness, coma; pregnancy—fetal risk cannot be ruled out; lactation—infant risk cannot be ruled out; safety and efficacy in children have not been established.

CAUTIOUS USE Patients with a personal or family history of substance abuse or mental illness, however, risk should not prevent proper pain management; Patient-controlled analgesia; history of QT prolongation, severe hypotension, orthostatic hypotension, and syncope; history of adrenal insufficiency, patients with biliary tract disease, head trauma, history of seizures, patients with carbon dioxide retention, COPD, cor pulmonale, patients with decreased CYP2D6 function may have increased concentrations of the drug; elderly.

ROUTE & DOSAGE

Acute Pain Management

Adult: **IV** 1.5 mg initial dose, with subsequent hourly titrations. Maximum total daily dose not to exceed 27 mg.

Hepatic Impairment Dosage Adjustment

Child-Pugh class C (Severe impairment): Use with caution

ADMINISTRATION

Intravenous only

- Oliceridien 30 mg/30 mL (1 mg/1 mL) vial is intended for patient-controlled analgesia (PCA) use only. Draw solution directly from the vial into the PCA syringe or IV bag without diluting.
- Store at a controlled room temperature between 20 and 25° C (68 and 77° F), with excursions permitted between 15 and 30° C (59 and 86° F). Protect from freezing and light.

ADVERSE EFFECTS (≥5%) **CNS:** Dizziness, drowsiness, sedation. **Skin:** Itching. **GI:** Constipation, *nausea, vomiting*. **Musculoskeletal:** Back pain.

INTERACTIONS **Drug: Alcohol** and other CNS DEPRESSANTS potentiate effects; Coadministration with potent CYP3A4 or CYP2D6 inhibitors (e.g., **ketoconazole, quinidine, fluoxetine, paroxetine,** etc.) may increase oliceridine levels and toxicity. Use with other serotonergic medications [e.g., SELECTIVE SEROTONIN REUPTAKE INHIBITORS (SSRI), SEROTONIN-NOREPINEPHRINE REUPTAKE INHIBITORS (SNRI), etc.] can increase the risk of serotonin syndrome. Avoid combination with MIXED AGONIST/ANTAGONIST AND PARTIAL AGONIST OPIOID ANALGESICS (e.g., **buprenorphine**).

PHARMACOKINETICS **Distribution:** 77% protein-bound. **Metabolism:** Primarily metabolized by CYP3A4 and CYP2D6 into

O

inactive metabolites. **Elimination:** 70% excreted in urine as inactive metabolites. **Half-Life:** 1.3–3 h.

NURSING IMPLICATIONS

Black Box Warning

Addiction, abuse, misuse; life-threatening respiratory depression, neonatal withdrawal syndrome; and risks from concomitant use with benzodiazepines or other CNS depressants that may be fatal.

Assessment & Drug Effects

- Monitor vital signs
- Monitor for respiratory depression
- Assess pain control
- Be aware that the drug can lead to addiction, abuse, and misuse.

Patient & Family Education

- Report patient confusion, agitation, restlessness, dilated pupils, headache, changes in blood pressure or temperature, nausea, vomiting, diarrhea, rapid heartbeat, tremor, loss of muscle control, shivering, heavy sweating. Symptoms are suggestive of serotonin syndrome.
- Report severe constipation.
- Review adverse effects.

O

OLMESARTAN MEDOXOMIL

(ol-me-sar'tan)

Benicar

Classification: ANGIOTENSIN II RECEPTOR (TYPE AT_1) ANTAGONIST, ANTIHYPERTENSIVE

Therapeutic: ANTIHYPERTENSIVE

Prototype: Losartan

AVAILABILITY Tablet

ACTION & *THERAPEUTIC EFFECT* Angiotensin II receptor (type AT_1) antagonist acts as a potent vasodilator and primary vasoactive hormone of the renin-angiotensin-aldosterone system. Selectively blocks the binding of angiotensin II to the AT_1 receptors found in many tissues (e.g., vascular smooth muscle, adrenal glands). *Antihypertensive effect is due to its potent vasodilation effect.*

USES Treatment of hypertension.

CONTRAINDICATIONS Pregnancy (category D); lactation.

CAUTIOUS USE Renal artery stenosis; severe renal impairment; heart failure; hypovolemia; children younger than 6 y.

ROUTE & DOSAGE

Hypertension

Adult/Child (greater than 35 kg): **PO** 20 mg daily, may increase to 40 mg daily.
Child (6 y or older, weight 20–35 kg): **PO** 10 mg daily; may increase to 20 mg daily

ADMINISTRATION

Oral

- Administer with or without food.
- Store at 20°–25° C (68°–77° F).

ADVERSE EFFECTS **CNS:** Dizziness, headache.

INTERACTIONS **Drug:** May increase hypotensive effect of other ANTIHYPERTENSIVES; may cause hyperkalemia with POTASSIUM-SPARING DIURETICS, POTASSIUM SUPPLEMENTS; increase risk of **lithium** toxicity. Do not use with **colesevelam. Herbal: Ephedra, ma huang** may antagonize antihypertensive effects.

PHARMACOKINETICS **Absorption:** Rapidly absorbed, 26% reaches systemic circulation. **Peak:** 1–2 h. **Distribution:** 99% protein bound. **Metabolism:** Not metabolized by CYP 450 system.

Elimination: 50% in urine, 50% in feces. **Half-Life:** 13 h.

NURSING IMPLICATIONS

Black Box Warning

Olmesartan has been associated with fetal toxicity and death.

Assessment & Drug Effects

- Monitor closely any volumedepleted patient following initial drug doses. If serious hypotension occurs, place patient in supine position and notify prescriber immediately.
- Monitor BP and HR at drug trough (prior to a scheduled dose). Report hypotension or bradycardia.
- Monitor lab tests: Baseline and periodic renal function tests, and serum electrolytes.

Patient & Family Education

- Report immediately to prescriber if a pregnancy is suspected.
- Discontinue drug immediately and notify prescriber if you experience swelling of the face, tongue, or throat, or if you believe you are pregnant.
- Notify prescriber of symptoms of hypotension (e.g., dizziness, fainting).

OLODATEROL HYDROCHLORIDE

(o-lo-da'ter-ol)

Striverdi Respimat

Classification: BRONCHODILATOR RESPIRATORY SMOOTH MUSCLE RELAXANT; BETA-2-ADRENERGIC AGONIST

Therapeutic: BRONCHODILATOR

Prototype: Albuterol

AVAILABILITY Inhaler

ACTION & *THERAPEUTIC EFFECT* Long-acting beta-2-receptor agonist; activates beta-2 airway receptors, resulting in the increase in the synthesis of cyclic-3',5' adenosine monophosphate (cAMP). *Elevated cAMP levels induce bronchodilation by relaxation of airway smooth muscle cells.*

USES Treatment of airflow obstruction in patients with chronic obstructive pulmonary disease (COPD), including chronic bronchitis and/or emphysema.

CONTRAINDICATIONS Asthma without a concomitant long-term asthma control medication; acutely deteriorating COPD; olodaterol-induced bronchospasm; concurrent use of other long-acting beta-2-agonists; severe hypersensitivity reaction.

CAUTIOUS USE Hypersensitivity to other beta-2-agonist; cardiovascular disease; coronary insufficiency, cardiac arrhythmias, hypertrophic obstructive cardiomyopathy, known or suspected prolongation of QT interval, hypertension, hypokalemia; DM; seizure disorders; hyperthyroidism; pregnancy (category C); lactation.

ROUTE & DOSAGE

Chronic Obstructive Pulmonary Disease (COPD)

Adult: **Inhalation** Two inhalations once daily

ADMINISTRATION

Inhalation

- For oral inhalation only.
- Prime inhaler prior to initial use or if not used for longer than 21 days.
- Instruct to breathe in slowly through the mouth, then press the dose release button; patient should continue to breathe in slowly as

long as possible, then hold breath for 10 seconds or for as long as comfortable.

- Store at 15°–30° C (59°–86° F). Protect from freezing. Discard 3 mo after cartridge is inserted into inhaler.

ADVERSE EFFECTS Respiratory: Nasopharyngitis, bronchitis.

INTERACTIONS Drug: Coadministration with other ADRENERGIC AGONISTS may cause a potentiation of sympathetic effects. Concomitant treatment with XANTHINE DERIVATIVES (e.g., **caffeine, theophylline**), LOOP DIURETICS (e.g., **furosemide**), or THIAZIDE DIURETICS (e.g., **hydrochlorothiazide**) may potentiate hypokalemic effects. Olodaterol may have an additive QTc prolongation effect if used in combination with MONOAMINE OXIDASE INHIBITORS, TRICYCLIC ANTIDEPRESSANTS, or other drugs known to cause QTc prolongation. BETA-BLOCKERS (e.g., **atenolol, propranolol**) can interfere with the therapeutic actions of olodaterol.

O

PHARMACOKINETICS Peak: Bioavailability via inhalation is 30%. **Peak:** 10–20 min. **Distribution:** 60% plasma protein bound. **Metabolism:** In liver. **Elimination:** Fecal (53%) and renal (38%) mostly as metabolites. **Half-Life:** 22 h.

NURSING IMPLICATIONS

Black Box Warning

Long-acting beta-2-adrenergic agonists (LABA), such as olodaterol, have been associated with increased risk of asthma-related death.

Assessment & Drug Effects

- Monitor FEV1, FVC, and/or other pulmonary function tests. Report immediately complaints of sudden shortness of breath.
- Monitor BP, HR, and level of CNS stimulation.
- Monitor cardiac status especially in those with preexisting cardiovascular disease.
- Monitor those with seizure disorders for increased seizure activity.
- Monitor for increased use of short-acting beta-2-agonist inhaler; may be marker of a deteriorating condition.
- Diabetics should be monitored for loss of glycemic control.
- Monitor lab tests: Periodic serum potassium and serum glucose.

Patient & Family Education

- Olodaterol should not be used to treat asthma or acute deteriorations of COPD.
- Report promptly to prescriber if you experience sudden shortness of breath, fast or irregular heartbeat or palpitations, or chest pain.
- Monitor blood glucose more frequently if diabetic.
- Persons with seizures disorders should report promptly more frequent seizure activity.
- Do not breastfeed while using this drug.

OLOPATADINE HYDROCHLORIDE

(o-lo-pa′ta-deen)

Patase, Pataday, Patanol

See Appendix A-1.

OLSALAZINE SODIUM

(ol-sal′a-zeen)

Dipentum

Classification: ANTI-INFLAMMATORY

Therapeutic: GI ANTI-INFLAMMATORY

Prototype: Mesalamine

 Common adverse effects in *italic*; life-threatening effects underlined; generic names in **bold**; classifications in SMALL CAPS; ♣ Canadian drug name; ◎ Prototype drug; ⚠ Alert

AVAILABILITY Capsule

ACTION & *THERAPEUTIC EFFECT* Converted to 5-aminosalicylic acid (5-ASA) by colonic bacteria. 5-ASA inhibits prostaglandin production in the colon, thus leading to its anti-inflammatory properties. *5-ASA has anti-inflammatory activity in ulcerative colitis.*

USES Maintenance therapy in patients with ulcerative colitis.

CONTRAINDICATIONS Hypersensitivity to salicylates, aminosalicylates, or olsalazine.

CAUTIOUS USE Patients with preexisting kidney disease; elderly; colitis; pregnancy (animal studies have demonstrated fetal developmental toxicities; use during pregnancy only if clearly indicated); lactation. Safety and efficacy in children not established.

ROUTE & DOSAGE

Ulcerative Colitis Maintenance
Adult: **PO** 500 mg bid

ADMINISTRATION

Oral

- Give with food in evenly divided doses.
- Maintain adequate hydration during therapy.

ADVERSE EFFECTS GI: *Diarrhea*, nausea, abdominal cramping, abdominal pain, anorexia, dyspepsia, indigestion, bloating. **Other:** Arthralgia, URI.

DIAGNOSTIC TEST INTERFERENCE May falsely elevate urinary normetanephrine levels when measured by liquid chromatography with electrochemical detection.

INTERACTIONS Drug: Adverse effects with varicella vaccine including development of Reye's syndrome could occur.

PHARMACOKINETICS Absorption: 1–3% from GI tract; highly protein bound; high colonic concentrations are associated with efficacy. **Metabolism:** Prodrug metabolized to 2 molecules of 5-ASA; **Elimination:** Primarily in feces. **Half-Life:** 2–15 h.

NURSING IMPLICATIONS

Assessment & Drug Effects

- Monitor kidney function in patients with preexisting renal disease.
- Monitor for S&S of a hypersensitivity reaction (see Appendix F). Withhold olsalazine and notify prescriber at first sign of an allergic response.
- Monitor lab tests: Baseline CBC, LFTs, renal function tests and repeat at 6 and 12 months during treatment, then annually.

Patient & Family Education

- Report diarrhea, a possible adverse effect, to the prescriber.

OMACETAXINE MEPESUCCINATE

(o-ma-ce-tax'een)

Synribo

Classification: ANTINEOPLASTIC; INHIBITOR OF ONCOGENIC PROTEINS; PROTEIN SYNTHESIS INHIBITOR

Therapeutic: ANTINEOPLASTIC

AVAILABILITY Lyophilized powder for injection

ACTION & *THERAPEUTIC EFFECT* Mechanism of action not fully understood but believed to include inhibition of protein synthesis with possible reduction in levels of oncoproteins and anti-apoptotic proteins that stimulate CML cell growth. *May slow progression of CML with improvement in disease-related symptoms or increased survival.*

USES Treatment of chronic or accelerated phase chronic myeloid leukemia (CML) in adult patients who have resistance and/or intolerance to two or more tyrosine kinase inhibitors (TKI).

CONTRAINDICATIONS Poorly controlled diabetes (avoid use until controlled); pregnancy (category D); lactation.

CAUTIOUS USE History of GI bleeding; myelosuppression; thrombocytopenia; cerebral hemorrhage; DM or patients with risk factors for DM. Safety and efficacy in children younger than 18 y not established.

ROUTE & DOSAGE

O

Chronic Myeloid Leukemia

Adult: **Subcutaneous** 1.25 mg/m^2 bid for 14 consecutive days in a 28 day cycle; repeat until patient achieves hematological response; follow with 1.25 mg/m^2 bid for 7 consecutive days in a 28-day cycle; can repeat as necessary.

Hematologic Toxicity Dosage Adjustment

Grade 4 neutropenia (ANC less than 0.5 × 10^9/L) or Grade 3 thrombocytopenia (platelet count less than 50 × 10^9/L): Delay next cycle until ANC is greater than or equal to 1.0 × 10^9/L and platelet count is greater than or equal to 50 × 10^9/L; then reduce the number of dosing days to 12 or 5.

ADMINISTRATION

Subcutaneous

- Reconstitute vial with 1 mL of NS for injection; swirl gently until clear. Yields 3.5 mg/mL.
- Avoid contact with the skin. If contact occurs, immediately and thoroughly wash affected area with soap and water.
- Rotate injection sites.
- May store reconstituted solution for 12 h at room temperature or 24 h if refrigerated. Protect from light.

ADVERSE EFFECTS **CV:** <u>Acute coronary syndrome</u>, angina pectoris, <u>arrhythmia</u>, bradycardia, hematoma, hot flush, hypertension, hypotension, palpitations, <u>tachycardia, ventricular extrasystoles</u>. **Respiratory:** Cough, dysphonia, dyspnea, epistaxis, hemoptysis, nasal congestion, pharyngolaryngeal pain, productive cough, rales, rhinorrhea, sinus congestion. **CNS:** Agitation, anxiety, confusional state, depression, headache, insomnia, mental status change. **HEENT:** Blurred vision, cataract, conjunctival hemorrhage, conjunctivitis, diplopia, ear hemorrhage, ear pain, eyelid edema, eye pain, tinnitus. **Endocrine:** Alterations in glucose level, anorexia, decreased appetite, dehydration, increased ALT, increased bilirubin, increased creatinine, *increased uric acid*. **Skin:** Dry skin, ecchymosis, erythema, hyperhidrosis, night sweats, petechiae, pruritus, purpura, rash erythematous, rash papular, skin lesion, skin ulcer, skin exfoliation, skin hyperpigmentation. **GI:** Abdominal distension, anal fissure, aphthous stomatitis, constipation, *diarrhea*, dry mouth, dyspepsia, dysphagia, gastritis, gastroesophageal reflux disease, gastrointestinal hemorrhage, gingival bleeding, gingival pain, gingivitis, hemorrhoids, melena, mouth hemorrhage, mouth ulceration, *nausea*, oral pain, stomatitis, upper abdominal pain, vomiting. **GU:** Dysuria. **Musculoskeletal:** *Arthralgia*, back pain, bone pain, muscle spasms, musculoskeletal pain, stiffness, discomfort and/or weakness, myalgia, musculoskeletal chest pain, pain in extremity. **Hematological:** *Anemia*, bone marrow failure, febrile neutropenia, lymphopenia, *neutropenia*, *thrombocytopenia*. **Other:** *Asthenia*, catheter site pain, chest pain, chills, contusion, *fatigue*, general edema, hypersensitivity reaction, hyperthermia, *infection*, influenza-like illness, *infusion and injection site reactions*, malaise, mucosal inflammation, pain, peripheral edema, *pyrexia*, transfusion reaction.

INTERACTIONS Drug: ANTICOAGULANTS may enhance toxic effects. IMMUNOSUPPRESSANTS may have additive side effects. Do not administer with LIVE VACCINES.

PHARMACOKINETICS Peak: 30 min. **Distribution:** Less than or equal to 50% plasma protein bound. **Metabolism:** Hydrolysis in plasma. **Elimination:** Primary route of elimination not determined. **Half-Life:** 6 h.

NURSING IMPLICATIONS

Assessment & Drug Effects

- Monitor for and report promptly S&S of bleeding and infection.
- Evaluate neurologic status for S&S of cerebral hemorrhage.
- Monitor diabetics and prediabetics for loss of glycemic control.
- Lab test: Weekly CBC with differential during induction and initial maintenance cycles, then q2wk as needed; periodic blood glucose.

Patient & Family Education

- Report promptly any S&S of hemorrhage including easy bruising, blood in urine or stool, slurred speech, confusion, or altered vision.
- Report S&S of infection such as fever of 101° F or greater.
- Report immediately severe or worsening skin rash.
- Monitor blood glucose closely if diabetic. Report immediately if good glycemic control is not maintained.
- Women should use effective means of contraception while taking this drug.
- Do not breast-feed while taking this drug.

OMALIZUMAB

(o-mal-i-zoo′mab)

Xolair

Classification: BIOLOGIC RESPONSE MODIFIER; MONOCLONAL ANTIBODY; RESPIRATORY ANTI-INFLAMMATORY

Therapeutic: ANTIALLERGIC; ANTIASTHMATIC; ANTI-INFLAMMATORY

AVAILABILITY Solution for injection

ACTION & *THERAPEUTIC EFFECT* It inhibits binding of IgE to high-affinity IgE receptors on the surface of mast cells and basophils, limiting the release of inflammatory mediators. *Inhibits release of mediators of the allergic response and has an anti-inflammatory action on the respiratory system.*

USES Control of moderate to severe allergic asthma; chronic idiopathic urticaria; nasal polyps with inadequate response to nasal corticosteroids.

UNLABELED USES
Seasonal allergic rhinitis.

CONTRAINDICATIONS
Severe hypersensitivity to omalizumab; acute asthma, status asthmaticus.

CAUTIOUS USE
Pregnancy (use during pregnancy may be considered when conventional therapies are insufficient); lactation; children younger than 6 y.

ROUTE & DOSAGE

Allergic Asthma/Nasal Polyps

Adult/Adolescent/Child (over 6 y): **Subcutaneous** Dose is based on baseline IgE serum levels and body weight. (see package insert)

Chronic Idiopathic Urticaria

Adult/Adolescent: **Subcutaneous** 150 or 300 mg q4w

ADMINISTRATION

Subcutaneous

- To reconstitute: (1) Draw 1.4 mL of SW into 3-mL syringe with 1-inch, 18-gauge needle. (2) Keep vial upright and inject SW, then gently swirl for about 1 min to wet powder. Do not shake. (3) Gently swirl vial q5min for 5–10 sec to dissolve remaining solids. Discard if not completely dissolved by 40 min. (4) Once dissolved invert vial for 15 sec to allow solution to drain toward stopper. (5) Insert new 3-mL syringe with a 1-inch, 18-gauge needle, into inverted vial with needle tip at the very bottom of solution, then withdraw all solution. (6) Replace 18-gauge with a 25-gauge needle for injection. (7) Expel any excess solution to obtain the 1.2 mL dose.
- Give subcutaneously and rotate injection sites. Doses more than 150 mg should be divided over more than one site. Solution is viscous and takes 5–10 sec to inject.
- Use within 8 h of reconstitution when stored in the vial at 2°–8° C (36°–46° F), or within 4 h of reconstitution when stored at room temperature.

ADVERSE EFFECTS
Respiratory: Upper respiratory tract infections, sinusitis, pharyngitis. **CNS:** Headache, dizziness. **Skin:** Rash, pruritus, urticaria, dermatitis. **GI:** *Abdominal pain.* **Musculoskeletal:** Arthralgia, limb pain. **Other:** Anaphylaxis/anaphylactoid reactions, *injection site reactions (bruising, erythema, warmth, burning, stinging, pruritus, hive formation, pain, induration, inflammation),* fatigue.

INTERACTIONS
Drug: Do not use with inhaled **loxapine**.

PHARMACOKINETICS
Absorption: Slowly absorbed from subcutaneous site; 53–71% reaches systemic circulation. **Peak:** 7–8 days. **Half-Life:** 22 days.

NURSING IMPLICATIONS

Black Box Warning

Omalizumab has been associated with anaphylaxis as early as the first dose and as late as a year following initiation of treatment.

Assessment & Drug Effects

- Monitor closely for S&S of anaphylaxis, presenting as bronchospasm, hypotension, syncope, urticaria, and/or angioedema of the throat or tongue.
- Monitor for injection site reactions including bruising, redness, warmth, burning, stinging, itching, hive formation, pain, indurations, mass, and inflammation.
- Monitor lab tests: Obtain baseline serum total IgE and PFT.

Patient & Family Education

- Do not use this drug for relief of acute bronchospasm or status asthmaticus.
- Promptly report any of the following: Bleeding or unusual bruising, difficulty breathing or shortness of breath, skin rash or hives.
- Do not accept a live virus vaccine without consulting prescriber.

OMEGA-3 FATTY ACIDS (EICOSAPENTAENOIC ACID AND DOCOSAHEXAENOIC ACID) EPA & DHA

(o-me'ga-3)

Dr. Sears OmegaRx, Eskimo-3, Fish Oil, Omega-3 Fatty Acids, ICAR Prenatal Essential Omega-3, Mega Twin EPA, Natrol DHA Neuromins, Natrol Omega-3, Natural Fish Oil, Oleomed Heart, Omacor, Omega-3 Fish Oil Concentrate, Sea Omega, ZonePerfect Omega 3

Classification: NUTRITIONAL SUPPLEMENT; OMEGA-3 FATTY ACIDS

Therapeutic: OMEGA-3 FATTY ACIDS; ANTILIPEMIC

AVAILABILITY Capsule; oil for oral ingestion

ACTION & *THERAPEUTIC EFFECT* Mechanism of action of omega-3-acid ethyl esters is not completely understood. May include inhibition of acetyl-CoA and increased peroxisomal beta-oxidation in the liver. *Triglyceride lowering is the most consistent effect observed.*

USES Adjunct to diet to reduce hypertriglyceridemia.

UNLABELED USES Adjunct nutritional supplementation for hypertriglyceridemia, rheumatoid arthritis, or for the general purpose of maintaining a healthy heart.

CONTRAINDICATIONS Hypersensitivity to any component of the medication.

CAUTIOUS USE Known sensitivity or allergy to fish; pregnancy (category C); lactation; children.

ROUTE & DOSAGE

Hypertriglyceridemia (Lovaza Rx form)

Adult: **PO** 4 g daily (as single or divided dose)

ADMINISTRATION

Oral

- The daily dose may be given as one dose or divided bid
- Store 15°–30° C (59°–86° F).

ADVERSE EFFECTS **HEENT:** Halitosis, taste disturbances. **Metabolic:** Increased total cholesterol and/or LDL levels, weight gain. **Skin:** Rash. **GI:** Diarrhea, dyspepsia, eructation, nausea, vomiting. **Other:** Back pain, flu syndrome, unspecified pain.

INTERACTIONS **Drug:** ANTICOAGULANTS and THROMBOLYTICS are affected by inhibition of platelet aggregation with omega-3 fatty acids.

PHARMACOKINETICS **Metabolism:** Extensive liver metabolism.

NURSING IMPLICATIONS

Assessment & Drug Effects

- Monitor for S&S of hypersensitivity in those with known allergy to fish.
- Monitor diabetics for loss of glycemic control.
- Note: Poor therapeutic response after 2 mo is an indication to discontinue drug.

O

- Monitor blood levels of anticoagulants with concurrent therapy.
- Monitor lab tests: Baseline and periodic lipid profile.

Patient & Family Education

- Do not take omega-3 fatty acids without consulting prescriber if you have a chronic medical disorder.

OMEPRAZOLE

(o-me'pra-zole)

Losec ♣, Prilosec, Prilosec OTC, Zegerid

Classification: PROTON PUMP INHIBITOR; ANTISECRETORY

Therapeutic: ANTIULCER

AVAILABILITY Capsule; powder for oral suspension; delayed release tablet

ACTION & *THERAPEUTIC EFFECT* An antisecretory compound that is a gastric acid pump inhibitor. Suppresses gastric acid secretion by inhibiting the H^+, K^+-ATPase enzyme system [the acid (proton H^+) pump] in the parietal cells. *Suppresses gastric acid secretion relieving gastrointestinal distress and promoting ulcer healing.*

O

USES Duodenal and gastric ulcer. Gastroesophageal reflux disease including severe erosive esophagitis (4 to 8 wk treatment). Long-term treatment of pathologic hypersecretory conditions such as Zollinger-Ellison syndrome, multiple endocrine adenomas, and systemic mastocytosis. In combination with clarithromycin to treat duodenal ulcers associated with *Helicobacter pylori*. Dyspepsia occurring more than twice weekly.

UNLABELED USES Healing or prevention of NSAID-related ulcers; stress gastritis prophylaxis.

CONTRAINDICATIONS Duodenal ulcers; proton pump inhibitors (PPIs), hypersensitivity; concomitant use of **rilpivirine**; lactation; use of **zegerid** in metabolic alkalosis, hypocalcemia, vomiting, GI bleeding.

CAUTIOUS USE Dysphagia; metabolic or respiratory alkalosis; hepatic disease; pregnancy (category C); use in GERD in children younger than 1 y. **OTC form:** Children younger than 18 y.

ROUTE & DOSAGE

Gastroesophageal Reflux, Erosive Esophagitis, Duodenal Ulcer

Adult/Adolescent/Child (weight over 20 kg): **PO** 20–40 mg once/day for 4–8 wk
Child (older than 1 y, weight 10–19 kg): **PO** 10 mg once daily; *weight 5–9 kg:* 5 mg once daily; *weight 3–4 kg:* 2.5 mg once daily

Gastric Ulcer

Adult: **PO** 40 mg daily for 4–8 wk

Hypersecretory Disease

Adult: **PO** 60 mg once/day up to 120 mg tid

***H. pylori* Eradication**

Varies based on regimen

Dyspepsia

Adult: **PO** 20 mg daily × 14 days

ADMINISTRATION

Oral

- Give 30–60 min before meals, preferably breakfast; capsules

must be swallowed whole (do not open, chew, or crush).
- Note: Antacids may be administered with omeprazole.
- *For NG tube administration:* Into a catheter-tipped syringe, empty a 2.5 mg packet of omeprazole spheres into 5 mL of water or a 10 mg packet into 15 mL of water. Immediately shake syringe, then allow to thicken for 2–3 min. Shake syringe again, then inject into NG tube.

ADVERSE EFFECTS **CNS:** Headache. **GI:** Abdominal pain, diarrhea.

DIAGNOSTIC TEST INTERFERENCE Omeprazole has been reported to significantly impair peak cortisol response to exogenous ACTH. May result in false-negative ***13C-urea breath test.*** May falsely elevate serum chromogranin A (CgA) levels.

INTERACTIONS **Drug:** May increase **diazepam, phenytoin, warfarin** levels. May affect levels of ANTIRETROVIRAL AGENTS. Do not use with **acalabrutinib, cefuroxime, dacomitinib, dasatinib, erlotinib, prazopanib, rifampin. Herbal: Ginkgo, St. John's wort** may decrease plasma concentrations. **Food:** Food decreases absorption by up to 35%.

PHARMACOKINETICS **Absorption:** Poorly from GI tract; 30–40% reaches systemic circulation. **Onset:** 0.5–3.5 h. **Peak:** Peak inhibition of gastric acid secretion: 5 days. **Metabolism:** In liver (CYP2C19). **Elimination:** 80% in urine, 20% in feces. **Half-Life:** 0.5–1.5 h.

NURSING IMPLICATIONS

Assessment & Drug Effects

- Monitor for and report lack of improvement or worsening GI symptoms.

Patient & Family Education

- Bone density tests are advised with long-term use.
- Report any changes in urinary elimination such as pain or discomfort associated with urination, or blood in urine.
- Report severe diarrhea; drug may need to be discontinued.

ONABOTULINUMTOXINA A

(oh-nuh-BOT-yoo-lin-num-toks-in-aye)

Botox, Botox Cosmetic

Classification: NEUROMUSCULAR BLOCKER AGENT; ANTISPASMODIC

Therapeutic: MUSCLE RELAXANT; ANTISPASMODIC

AVAILABILITY Powder for injection

ACTION & *THERAPEUTIC EFFECT* Blocks neuromuscular transmission by binding to receptor sites on motor nerve terminals, entering the nerve terminals, and inhibiting the release of acetylcholine and producing a state of denervation. *When injected intramuscularly at therapeutic doses, botulinum toxin type A produces partial chemical denervation of the muscle resulting in a localized reduction in muscle activity.*

USES Treatment of blepharospasm, cervical dystonia, strabismus, facial wrinkles, severe axillary hyperhidrosis, spasticity, urinary incontinence, chronic migraine, overactive bladder.

UNLABELED USES Achalasia, anal fissures, sialorrhea.

CONTRAINDICATIONS Presence of infection at the proposed injection site(s); hypersensitivity to Botox. Patients with dysphagia or respiratory compromise.

O

CAUTIOUS USE Hypersensitivity to botulinum toxin; individuals with peripheral motor neuropathic diseases (e.g., amyotrophic lateral sclerosis, or motor neuropathy), or neuromuscular junctional disorders (e.g., myasthenia gravis or Lambert–Eaton syndrome); neuromuscular disorders; ocular disease; cardiovascular disease; elderly; inflammation at the proposed injection site; weakness in the target muscle(s); pregnancy (use during pregnancy is not recommended); lactation; children.

ROUTE & DOSAGE

Blepharospasm

Adult/Child (12 yr or older): **IM** 1.25–2.5 units injected at each site, may be repeated; cumulative dose should not exceed 200 units in a 30-day period

Cervical Dystonia

Adult/Adolescent (16 yr or older): **IM** 198–300 units divided among affected muscles

Chronic Migraine

Adult: **IM** Administer 5 units/site (recommended total doses 155 once q12w) see package insert for injection locations

Facial Wrinkles

Adult: **IM** 20 units divided among affected muscles in 5 step doses, may repeat in 3–4 mo if needed

Spasticity

Adult/Adolescent/Child: **IM** individualized based on patient size and extent of muscle involvement.

Axillary Hyperhidrosis

Adult: **IM** 50 units/site

Overactive Bladder

Adult: **IM** 100 units/treatment; may repeat dose but no sooner than 12 weeks.

ADMINISTRATION

Intramuscular, Intradermal

- Slowly inject required amount of nonpreserved NS (see dilution calculation) into vial. Discard vial if a vacuum does not pull diluent into vial. Gently rotate to mix. Discard if not clear, colorless, and free of particulate matter. Dilution calculation: Add 1, 2, 4, or 6 mL of NS to yield, respectively, 10 units/0.1 mL, 5 units/0.1 mL, 2.5 units/0.1 mL, 1.25 units/0.1 mL.
- Store at 2°–8°C (36°–46°F) (refrigerated). Administer within 4 h of reconstitution.

INCOMPATIBILITIES: Do not mix with other solutions/additives.

ADVERSE EFFECTS **Respiratory:** Upper respiratory infection. **CNS:** *Headache*, vertical strabismus, dizziness, drowsiness, numbness, speech disturbance. **HEENT:** Dry eyes, ocular irritation, blepharoptosis, diplopia. **GI:** *Dysphagia*, dry mouth, nausea, constipation. **GU:** UTI, bacteriuria, urinary retention, dysuria, increased post void residual volume, hematuria. **Musculoskeletal:** Neck pain, back pain, asthenia. **Hematologic:** Ecchymosis. **Other:** Injection site reactions (localized pain, tenderness, bruising), fever.

INTERACTIONS **Drug:** AMINOGLYCOSIDES, NEUROMUSCULAR BLOCKING AGENTS may potentiate neuromuscular blockade. ANTICHOLINERGIC

AGENTS may have enhanced adverse effects.

NURSING IMPLICATIONS

Black Box Warning

*Distant spread of botulism toxin beyond the site of injection has been reported. Dysphagia and breathing difficulties have occurred and may be **life-threatening**.*

Assessment & Drug Effects

- Evaluate for therapeutic efficacy, maximal at about 1–2 wk (lasting 3–4 mo).
- Monitor post void residual urine volume within 2 weeks posttreatment and periodically thereafter up to 12 weeks in patients not catheterizing.

Patient & Family Education

- Inform prescriber about all prescription, nonprescription, and herbal drugs being taken.
- Report immediately any of the following: Difficulty breathing or swallowing, problem with speech; unusual bleeding, bruising, or swelling around injection site.
- Note: Effects of the injection generally last 3–4 mo and then repeat treatments may be given.

ONDANSETRON HYDROCHLORIDE

(on-dan'si-tron)

Zofran, Zofran ODT, Zuplenz

Classification: 5-HT3 ANTAGONIST; ANTIEMETIC

Therapeutic: ANTIEMETIC

AVAILABILITY Orally disintegrating tablet; oral solution; solution for injection; oral soluble film

ACTION & THERAPEUTIC EFFECT Selective serotonin (5-HT_3) receptor antagonist. Serotonin receptors are located centrally in the chemoreceptor trigger zone (CTZ) and peripherally on the vagal nerve terminals. Serotonin is released from the wall of the small intestine and stimulates the vagal efferent nerves through the serotonin receptors and initiates the vomiting reflex. *Prevents nausea and vomiting associated with cancer chemotherapy and anesthesia.*

USES Prevention of nausea and vomiting associated with chemotherapy or radiation; postoperative nausea and vomiting.

UNLABELED USES Treatment of hyperemesis gravidarum; alcohol dependence; pruritus.

CONTRAINDICATIONS Hypersensitivity to ondansetron; or any component of the formulation; serotonin syndrome reaction to drug.

CAUTIOUS USE Hypersensitivity to other selective 5-HT_3 receptor antagonists; hepatic impairment; QT prolongation; abdominal surgery; PKU; older adults; pregnancy (category B); lactation. **PO:** Children younger than 4 y. **IV:** Infants.

ROUTE & DOSAGE

Prevention of Chemotherapy-Induced Nausea/Vomiting

Adult/Adolescent: **PO** 8–24 mg 30 min before chemotherapy, repeat at 8 h if needed

Adult/Child/Infant (6 mo–18 y): **IV** 0.15 mg/kg infused over 15 min beginning 30 min before chemotherapy, then repeat at 4 and 8 h
Child (older than 4 y): **PO** 4 mg 30 min before chemotherapy, then q8h × 2 more doses

Prevention of Radiation-Induced Nausea/Vomiting

Adult: **PO** 8 mg 1–2 h before each daily fraction of radiotherapy

Nausea and Vomiting with Highly Emetogenic Chemotherapy

Adult: **PO** Single 24 mg dose 30 min before administration of single-day highly emetogenic chemotherapy

Postoperative Nausea and Vomiting

Adult: **PO** 16 mg 1 h preoperatively
Adult/Adolescent/Child (weight greater than 40 kg): **IM/IV** 4 mg injected immediately prior to anesthesia induction or once postoperatively if patient experiences nausea/vomiting shortly after surgery
Child/Infant: (weight less than 40 kg): **IV** 0.05 mg–0.1 mg/kg immediately prior to or following anesthesia induction

Hepatic Impairment Dosage Adjustment

Child-Pugh class C: Max: 8 mg/day

ADMINISTRATION

Oral

- Give tablets 30 min prior to chemotherapy and 1–2 h prior to radiation therapy.
- **Do not** push orally disintegrating tablet through blister foil. Peel foil back and remove tablet. Tablets will disintegrate with/without liquid.

Intramuscular

- Give undiluted into a large muscle.

Intravenous

PREPARE: **Direct for Postoperative Nausea and Vomiting:** May be given undiluted. **IV Infusion for Chemotherapy-Induced Nausea and Vomiting:** Dilute a single dose in 50 mL of D5W or NS. ▪ May be further diluted in selected IV solution.
ADMINISTER: **Direct for Postoperative Nausea and Vomiting:** Give over at least 30 sec, 2–5 min preferred. **IV Infusion for Chemotherapy-Induced Nausea and Vomiting:** Give over 15 min. ▪ When three separate doses are administered, infuse each over 15 min.
INCOMPATIBILITIES: **Solution/additive: Meropenem. Y-site: Acyclovir, allopurinol, aminophylline, amphotericin B, amphotericin B cholesteryl, ampicillin, ampicillin/sulbactam, amsacrine, azathioprine, cefmandole, cefepime, cefoperazone, ceftobiprole, chloramphenicol, dantrolene, diazoxide, ertapenem, foscarnet, fluorouracil, furosemide, ganciclovir, gemtuzumab, indomethacin, lansoprazole, lorazepam, meropenem, methohexital, methylprednisolone, micafungin, milrinone, pantoprazole, pemetrexed, pentobarbital, phenobarbital, phenytoin, rituximab, sargramostim, sodium bicarbonate, SMZ/TMP, thiopental, trastuzumab, TPN.**

ADVERSE EFFECTS CNS: Dizziness, fatigue, light-headedness, *headache, sedation.* **GI:** *Diarrhea,* constipation, dry mouth, transient increases in liver aminotransferases and bilirubin. **Other:** Hypersensitivity reactions.

INTERACTIONS Drug: Do not use with **apomorphine** due to risk of hypotension. Do not use with **hydroxyhloroquine, mifepristone,** and other agents affecting QT interval due to risk of QT prolongation.

PHARMACOKINETICS Peak: 1–1.5 h. **Metabolism:** In liver (CYP3A4). **Elimination:** 44–60% in urine within 24 h; ~25% in feces. **Half-Life:** 3 h.

NURSING IMPLICATIONS

Assessment & Drug Effects

- Monitor fluid and electrolyte status. Diarrhea, which may cause fluid and electrolyte imbalance, is a potential adverse effect of the drug.
- Monitor cardiovascular status, especially in patients with a history of coronary artery disease. Rare cases of tachycardia and angina have been reported.

Patient & Family Education

- Be aware that headache requiring an analgesic for relief is a common adverse effect.

OPICAPONE

(oh-pik'-a-pone)

Ongentys

Classifications: ANTIPARKINSON AGENTS, CATECHOLAMINE O-METHYLTRANSFERASE (COMT) INHIBITOR

Therapeutic: ANTIPARKINSON
Prototype: tolcapone

AVAILABILITY Tablet

ACTION & *THERAPEUTIC EFFECT* A reversible and selective inhibitor of COMT, a major degradation pathway for levodopa resulting in more sustained serum levodopa levels. This provides for increased concentrations available for absorption across the blood–brain barrier thereby providing for increased CNS levels of dopamine, the active metabolite of levodopa. *Provides for increased CNS levels of dopamine.*

USES Adjunctive to levodopa/carbidopa to treat Parkinson's disease

CONTRAINDICATIONS Concomitant use of nonselective monoamine oxidase inhibitors; pheochromocytoma, paraganglioma, or other catecholamine secreting neoplasms.

CAUTIOUS USE Risk for CNS depression, dyskinesia, hallucinations, hypotension, impulse control disorders; hepatic impairment; renal impairment; psychotic disorders; pregnancy (in utero exposure by cause fetal harm); lactation.

ROUTE & DOSAGE

Parkinson's Disease

Adult: **PO** 50 mg once daily

Hepatic Impairment Dosage Adjustment

Child-Pugh class B: 25 mg once daily
Child-Pugh class C: Avoid use

O

ADMINISTRATION

Oral

- Administer at bedtime; do not eat for 1 hour before and at least 1 hour after dose.
- Store at < 30° C (< 86° F).

ADVERSE EFFECTS **CV:** Orthostatic hypotension, hypotension, increased serum CK, syncope. **GI:** Constipation. **Musculoskeletal:** Dyskinesia.

INTERACTIONS **Drug:** Do not combine with nonselective MAO inhibitors (phenelzine, isocarboxazid); **Dobutamine, dopamine, epinephrine, isoetharine, isoproterenol, methyldopa, norepinephrine** may increase heart rates, possible cause arrhythmias, excessive changes in BP. May enhance effects of CNS DEPRESSANTS.

PHARMACOKINETICS **Peak:** 2 h. **Distribution:** 99% protein bound. **Metabolism:** Primarily through sulphation. **Elimination:** 70% excreted in feces **Half-Life:** 1–2 h.

NURSING IMPLICATIONS

Assessment & Drug Effects

- Monitor baseline and periodic BP.
- Monitor lab tests: Liver function tests; renal function tests.

Patient & Family Education

- Avoid driving or doing other tasks that require alertness until you see how this drug affects you.
- To lower the risk of feeling dizzy or passing out, rise slowly from lying or sitting positions. Be careful going up and down stairs.
- Notify your doctor or get medical help right away if you have any of the following signs or symptoms of allergic reaction such as rash, hives, itching; red, swollen, blistered, or peeling skin with or without fever; wheezing; tightness in the chest or throat; trouble breathing, swallowing, or talking; unusual hoarseness; or swelling of the mouth, face, lips, tongue, or throat; or any dizziness or passing out.

OPIUM, POWDERED OPIUM TINCTURE (LAUDANUM) ⚠

(oh′pee-um)

Classification: NARCOTIC (OPIATE AGONIST) ANALGESIC; ANTI-DIARRHEAL

Therapeutic: NARCOTIC ANALGESIC; ANTIDIARRHEAL

Prototype: Morphine

Controlled Substance: Schedule II

AVAILABILITY Tincture

ACTION & *THERAPEUTIC EFFECT* Contains several natural alkaloids including morphine, codeine, papaverine. Antidiarrheal due to inhibition of GI motility and propulsion; leads to prolonged transit of intestinal contents, desiccation of feces, and constipation. *Antidiarrheal activity due to inhibition of GI motility.*

USES Diarrhea.

CONTRAINDICATIONS Diarrhea caused by poisoning (until poison is completely eliminated).

CAUTIOUS USE History of opiate agonist dependence; asthma; severe prostatic hypertrophy; hepatic disease; pregnancy (category C); lactation; children.

ROUTE & DOSAGE

Acute Diarrhea

Adult: **PO** 0.6 mL qid (max: 6 mL/day)

ADMINISTRATION

Oral

- Do not confuse this preparation with camphorated opium tincture (paregoric), which contains only 2 mg anhydrous morphine/5 mL, thus requiring a higher dose volume than that required for therapeutic dose of Deodorized Opium Tincture.
- Give drug diluted with about one third glass of water to ensure passage of entire dose into stomach.
- Store in tight, light-resistant containers.

ADVERSE EFFECTS **CV:** Bradycardia, hypotension. **Respiratory:** Respiratory depression. **CNS:** CNS depression, dizziness, drowsiness. **GI:** Constipation, stomach cramps. **GU:** Decreased urine output. **Musculoskeletal:** Weakness.

INTERACTIONS **Drug: Alcohol** and other CNS DEPRESSANTS add to CNS effects.

PHARMACOKINETICS **Absorption:** Variable absorption from GI tract. **Distribution:** Crosses placenta; distributed into breast milk. **Metabolism:** In liver. **Elimination:** In urine.

NURSING IMPLICATIONS

Assessment & Drug Effects

- Withhold medication and report to prescriber if respirations are 12/min or below or have changed in character and rate.
- Discontinue as soon as diarrhea is controlled; note character and frequency of stools.
- Offer small amounts of fluid frequently but attempt to maintain 3000–4000 mL fluid total in 24 h.
- Monitor body weight, I&O ratio and pattern, and temperature. If patient develops fever of 38.8° C (102° F) or above, electrolyte and hydration levels may need to be evaluated. Consult prescriber.

Patient & Family Education

- Be aware that constipation may be a consequence of antidiarrheal therapy but that normal habit pattern usually is reestablished with resumption of normal dietary intake.
- Note: Addiction is possible with prolonged use or with drug abuse.

OPRELVEKIN

(o-prel've-kin)

Neumega

Classification: BLOOD FORMER; HEMATOPOIETIC GROWTH FACTOR

Therapeutic: HEMATOPOIETIC GROWTH FACTOR

Prototype: Epoetin alfa

AVAILABILITY Solution for injection

ACTION & *THERAPEUTIC EFFECT* The primary hematopoietic activity of oprelvekin is stimulation of production of megakaryocytes (precursors of blood platelets) and thrombocytes by the bone marrow. *Effectiveness indicated by return of postnadir platelet count toward normal (50,000 or higher). Increases platelet count in a dose-dependent manner.*

USES Prevention of severe thrombocytopenia following myelosuppressive chemotherapy (not effective after myeloablative chemotherapy).

CONTRAINDICATIONS Hypersensitivity to oprelvekin; myeloablative chemotherapy; myeloid malignancies; lactation.

CAUTIOUS USE Left ventricular dysfunction, cardiac disease, CHF, history of atrial arrhythmias, or other arrhythmias; electrolyte imbalance, hypokalemia; respiratory disease; papilledema; thromboembolic disorders; older adults; cerebrovascular disease, stroke, TIAs; pleural effusion, pericardial effusion, ascites; ICP, brain tumor, visual disturbances; hepatic or renal dysfunction; pregnancy (category C); children.

ROUTE & DOSAGE

Thrombocytopenia

Adult: **Subcutaneous** 50 mcg/kg once daily starting 6–24 h after completing chemotherapy and continuing until platelet count is 50,000 cells/mcL or higher or up to 21 days

Renal Impairment Dosage Adjustment

CrCl less than 30 mL/min: 25 mcg/kg

ADMINISTRATION

O

- Note: Do not use if solution is discolored or if it contains particulate matter.

Subcutaneous

- Reconstitute solution by gently injecting 1 mL of sterile water for injection (without preservative) toward the sides of the vial. Keep needle in vial and gently swirl to dissolve but do not shake solution. Without removing needle, withdraw specified amount of oprelvekin for injection.
- Give as single dose into the abdomen, thigh, hip, or upper arm.
- Discard any unused portion of the vial. It contains no preservatives.
- Use reconstituted solution within 3 h; store at 2°–8° C (36°–46° F) until used.
- Store unopened vials at 2°–8° C (36°–46° F). Do not freeze.

ADVERSE EFFECTS **CV:** *Tachycardia*, vasodilation, palpitations, syncope, atrial fibrillation/flutter, peripheral edema, capillary leak syndrome. **Respiratory:** *Dyspnea, rhinitis, cough, pharyngitis*, pleural effusion, pulmonary edema, exacerbation of preexisting pleural effusion. **CNS:** *Headache, dizziness, insomnia*, nervousness. **HEENT:** Conjunctival injection, amblyopia. **Skin:** Alopecia, *rash*, skin discoloration, exfoliative dermatitis. **GI:** *Nausea, vomiting, mucositis, diarrhea*, oral moniliasis, anorexia, constipation, dyspepsia. **Hematologic:** Ecchymosis. **Other:** *Edema, neutropenic fever, fever*, asthenia, pain, chills, myalgia, bone pain, dehydration.

INTERACTIONS **Drug:** No clinically significant established.

PHARMACOKINETICS **Absorption:** 80% from subcutaneous injection site. **Onset:** Days 5–9. **Duration:** 7 days after last dose. **Distribution:** Distributes to highly perfused organs. **Elimination:** In urine. **Half-Life:** 6.9 h.

NURSING IMPLICATIONS

Black Box Warning

Oprelvekin has been associated with allergic or hypersensitivity reactions, including anaphylaxis. Oprelvekin should be discontinued if patient develops an allergic or hypersensitivity reaction.

Assessment & Drug Effects

- Monitor carefully for and immediately report S&S of fluid overload, hypokalemia, and cardiac arrhythmias.
- Monitor persons with preexisting fluid retention carefully (e.g., CHF, pleural effusion, ascites) for worsening of symptoms.

- Monitor lab tests: Baseline and periodic CBC; platelet count at nadir and until adequate recovery; periodic serum electrolytes.

Patient & Family Education

- Review patient information leaflet with special attention to administration directions.
- Report any of the following to the prescriber: Shortness of breath, edema of arms and/or legs, chest pain, unusual fatigue or weakness, irregular heartbeat, blurred vision.

ORITAVANCIN

(or-ita-van'sin)

Kimyrsa, Orbactiv

Classification: ANTIBIOTIC; GLYCOPROTEIN

Therapeutic: ANTIBIOTIC

Prototype: Vancomycin

AVAILABILITY Lyophilized powder

ACTION & *THERAPEUTIC EFFECT* Binds to components required for the bacterial cell wall preventing cell wall synthesis. *It is bactericidal against Staphylococcus aureus, Streptococcus pyogenes,* and *Enterococcus faecalis.*

USES Treatment of adult patients with acute bacterial skin and skin structure infections (ABSSSI) caused or suspected to be caused by susceptible isolates of designated gram-positive microorganisms.

CONTRAINDICATIONS Known hypersensitivity to oritavancin; IV unfractionated heparin sodium contraindicated for 48 h after receiving oritavancin; oritavancin induced *Clostridium difficile*–associated diarrhea; oritavanicn induced osteomylitis.

CAUTIOUS USE Hypersensitivity to other antibiotics; concomitant warfarin use; colitis; severe renal or hepatic impairment; pregnancy (adverse effects were not observed in animal reproduction studies); lactation. Safety and efficacy in children younger than 18 y not established.

ROUTE & DOSAGE

Skin and Skin Structure Infections

Adult: **IV** 1200 mg one time dose

ADMINISTRATION

Intravenous

***PREPARE:* IV Infusion:** Three 400 mg vials are need for a single 1200 mg dose. Reconstitute each 400 mg vial with 40 mL of SW for injection to yield 10 mg/mL. Swirl vials gently until completely dissolved. Do not shake. Must be further diluted as follows: Withdraw and discard 120 mL from a 1000 mL bag of D5W; then withdraw 40 mL from each reconstituted vial and add to the D5W bag to bring volume to 1000 mL with a concentration of 1.2 mg/mL.

***ADMINISTER:* IV Infusion:** Kimyrsa: Infuse over 1 hour. Orbactiv: Infuse over 3 h. Flush line before/after with D5W if line used for other drugs or solutions.

***INCOMPATIBILITIES:* Y-site: Aminophylline, amphotericin B, azotreonam, bumetadine, clindamycin, furosemide, heparin, hydrocortisone, meropenem, nitroprusside, phenytoin, sulfamethoxazole/ trimethoprim.**

- Storage: Bag for IV infusion should be used within 6 h when stored at room temperature, or within 12 h when refrigerated at 2–8° C (36–46° F). The combined storage time (reconstituted

O

solution in the vial and diluted solution in the bag) and 3 h infusion time should not exceed 6 h at room temperature or 12 h if refrigerated.

ADVERSE EFFECTS **CV:** Tachycardia. **Respiratory:** Bronchospasm, wheezing. **CNS:** Dizziness, headache. **Endocrine:** Hyperuricemia, hypoglycemia, increased ALT and AST, increased bilirubin. **GI:** Clostridium difficile–associated diarrhea, diarrhea, *nausea*, vomiting. **Hematological:** Positive direct and indirect Coombs test. **Other:** Hypersensitivity reaction, infusion site reaction.

DIAGNOSTIC TEST INTERFERENCE
Drug: Oritavancin has no effect on the coagulation system; however, prolongs ***aPTT*** for 48 h and ***INR*** for up to 24 h.

INTERACTIONS **Drug:** May diminish effect of **heparin**, may decrease the effect of intravesical BCG. Oritavancin may increase the levels of other drugs requiring CYP2C9 or CYP2C19 for metabolism (e.g., **warfarin**).

PHARMACOKINETICS **Distribution:** Widely distributed with 85% plasma protein bound. **Metabolism:** Not significantly metabolized. **Elimination:** Slowly excreted unchanged via renal and fecal elimination. **Half-Life:** 245 h.

NURSING IMPLICATIONS

Assessment & Drug Effects

- Monitor patients for any infusion-related reactions.
- Monitor for S&S of superinfection, including *C. difficile*–associated diarrhea (CDAD) and pseudomembranous colitis, that may develop within days or up to several months after completion of therapy. If superinfection is suspected, withhold drug and contact provider.
- Monitor lab values: Baseline BUN, serum creatinine, and LFTs.

Patient & Family Education

- Report promptly to prescriber if you develop frequent watery or bloody diarrhea.
- Consult with prescriber if you are a female who is or plans to become pregnant.
- Do not breastfeed without consulting prescriber.

ORLISTAT

(or'li-stat)

Alli, Xenical

Classification: ANORECTANT; NONSYSTEMIC LIPASE INHIBITOR
Therapeutic: ANORECTANT
Prototype: Diethylpropion

AVAILABILITY Capsule

ACTION & THERAPEUTIC EFFECT
Nonsystemic inhibitor of gastrointestinal lipase. Reduces intestinal absorption of dietary fat by forming inactive enzymes with pancreatic and gastric lipase in the GI tract. *Indicated by weight loss/decreased body mass index (BMI). Reduces caloric intake in obese individuals.*

USES Weight loss and weight maintenance in conjunction with diet and exercise.

CONTRAINDICATIONS Hypersensitivity to orlistat; malabsorption syndrome; cholestasis; gallbladder disease; hypothyroidism; organic causes of obesity; anorexia nervosa, bulimia nervosa; pregnancy (category X).

CAUTIOUS USE Gastrointestinal diseases including frequent diarrhea; known dietary deficiencies in fat soluble vitamins (i.e., A, D, E); history of calcium oxalate nephrolithiasis or hyperoxaluria; older adults; lactation; children younger than 12 y.

ROUTE & DOSAGE

Weight Loss

Adult/Adolescent (older than 12 y): **PO** 60 or 120 mg tid with each main meal containing fat

ADMINISTRATION

Oral

- Give during or up to 1 h after a meal containing fat.
- Omit dose with nonfat-containing meal or if meal is skipped.
- Store at 15°–30° C (59°–86° F). Keep bottle tightly closed; **do not** use after the printed expiration date.

ADVERSE EFFECTS **CV:** Hypertension, stroke. **CNS:** *Headache*, dizziness, anxiety. **Skin:** Rash. **GI:** *Oily spotting, flatus with discharge, fecal urgency, fatty/oily stool, oily evacuation, increased defecation*, fecal incontinence, *abdominal pain/discomfort*, nausea, infectious diarrhea, rectal pain/discomfort, tooth disorder, gingival disorder, vomiting. **GU:** Menstrual irregularity. **Other:** Fatigue, back pain, infection.

DIAGNOSTIC TEST INTERFERENCE Monitor PT/INR in patients on chronic stable doses of **warfarin.**

INTERACTIONS **Drug:** **Orlistat** may increase absorption of **pravastatin**; may decrease absorption of fat soluble VITAMINS (A, D, E, K), **amiodarone**, THYROID HORMONES, **cyclosporine.** Taking **orlistat** with **atazanavir, ritonavir, tenofovir disoproxil fumarate, emtricitabine, lopinavir; ritonavir**, and **emtricitabine; efavirenz; tenofovir disoproxil fumarate** may decrease HIV control.

PHARMACOKINETICS **Absorption:** Minimal. **Metabolism:** In gastrointestinal wall. **Elimination:** In feces. **Half-Life:** 1–2 h.

NURSING IMPLICATIONS

Assessment & Drug Effects

- Monitor weight and BMI; closely monitor diabetics for hypoglycemia.
- Monitor BP frequently, especially with preexisting hypertension.

Patient & Family Education

- Take a daily multivitamin containing fat-soluble vitamins at least 2 h before/after orlistat.
- Remember common GI adverse effects typically resolve after 4 wk therapy.
- Avoid high-fat meals to minimize adverse GI effects. Distribute fat calories over three main meals daily.
- Monitor weight several times weekly. *Diabetics*: Monitor blood glucose carefully following any weight loss.

O

ORPHENADRINE CITRATE

(or-fen′a-dreen)

Classification: CENTRAL-ACTING SKELETAL MUSCLE RELAXANT

Therapeutic: SKELETAL MUSCLE RELAXANT

Prototype: Cyclobenzaprine

AVAILABILITY Sustained release tablet; solution for injection

ACTION & *THERAPEUTIC EFFECT* Indirect skeletal muscle relaxant thought to work by central atropine-like effects; has some euphorigenic and analgesic properties. *Relieves skeletal muscle spasm.*

USES To relieve muscle spasm discomfort associated with acute musculoskeletal conditions.

CONTRAINDICATIONS Narrow-angle glaucoma; achalasia; pyloric or duodenal obstruction, stenosing peptic ulcers; prostatic hypertrophy or bladder neck obstruction, urinary tract obstruction; myasthenia gravis; cardiospasm.

CAUTIOUS USE History of cardiac disease, arrhythmias, coronary insufficiency; asthma; GERD; hepatic disease; renal disease; renal impairment; older adults; pregnancy (animal reproduction studies have not been conducted); lactation; children.

ROUTE & DOSAGE

Muscle Spasm

Adult: **PO** 100 mg bid; **IM/IV** 60 mg q12h, convert to PO therapy as soon as possible

ADMINISTRATION

Oral

- Ensure that sustained release form is not chewed or crushed. It **must be** swallowed whole.

Intramuscular

- Give undiluted deep into a large muscle.

Intravenous

PREPARE: **Direct:** Give undiluted. Protect from light.
ADMINISTER: **Direct:** Give at a rate of 60 mg (2 mL) over 5 min with patient in supine position. ▪ Keep supine for 5–10 min post-injection.

ADVERSE EFFECTS **CV:** Palpitations, tachycardia. **Respiratory:** Nasal congestion. **CNS:** *Drowsiness*, agitation, confusion, dizziness, euphoria, hallucination, headache. **HEENT:** increased intraocular pressure, mydriasis, nystagmus, blurred vision. **GI:** *Dry mouth*, nausea, vomiting, gastric irritation, constipation. **GU:** *Urinary hesitancy* or *retention*. **Musculoskeletal:** Tremor, weakness. **Other:** Hypersensitivity [pruritus, urticaria, rash, anaphylactic reaction (rare)].

INTERACTIONS **Drug:** May worsen schizophrenic symptoms, or increase risk of tardive dyskinesia with **haloperidol**; additive CNS depressant with ANXIOLYTICS, SEDATIVES, HYPNOTICS, **butorphanol, nalbuphine**, OPIATE AGONISTS, **pentazocine, tramadol, cyclobenzaprine** may increase anticholinergic effects. **Herbal: Valerian, kava** potentiate sedation. **Kratom** may enhance CNS depressant effects.

PHARMACOKINETICS **Absorption:** Readily from GI tract. **Peak:** 2 h. **Duration:** 4–6 h. **Distribution:** Rapidly distributed in tissues; crosses placenta. **Metabolism:** In liver. **Elimination:** In urine. **Half-Life:** 14 h.

NURSING IMPLICATIONS

Assessment & Drug Effects

- Report complaints of mouth dryness, urinary hesitancy or retention, headache, tremors, GI problems, palpitation, or rapid pulse to prescriber. Dosage reduction or drug withdrawal is indicated.

- Monitor elimination patterns. Older adults are particularly sensitive to anticholinergic effects (urinary hesitancy, constipation); closely observe.
- Monitor therapeutic drug effect. In the patient with parkinsonism, orphenadrine reduces muscular rigidity but has little effect on tremors. Some reduction in excessive salivation and perspiration may occur, and patient may appear mildly euphoric.
- Do not discontinue abruptly; taper dosage slowly.

Patient & Family Education

- Relieve mouth dryness by frequent rinsing with clear tepid water, increasing noncaloric fluid intake, sugarless gum, or lemon drops. If these measures fail, a saliva substitute may help.
- Do not drive or engage in potentially hazardous activities until response to drug is known.
- Avoid concomitant use of alcohol and other CNS depressants; these may potentiate depressant effects.

OSELTAMIVIR PHOSPHATE

(o-sel′tam-i-vir)

Tamiflu

Classification: ANTIVIRAL; NEURAMINIDASE INHIBITOR; ANTI-INFLUENZA

Therapeutic: ANTI-INFLUENZA

AVAILABILITY Capsule; oral suspension

ACTION & THERAPEUTIC EFFECT Inhibits influenza A and B viral neuraminidase enzyme, preventing the release of newly formed virus from the surface of the infected cells. Inhibits replication of the influenza A and B virus. *Effectiveness indicated by relief of flu symptoms. Prevents viral spread across the mucous lining of the respiratory tract.*

USES Treatment of uncomplicated acute influenza in adults symptomatic for no more than 2 days; prophylaxis of influenza.

UNLABELED USES H_1N_1 influenza.

CONTRAINDICATIONS Hypersensitivity to oseltamivir; development of allergic-like reaction(s) from drug including anapylaxis and serious skin reactions; severe hepatic impairment or severe hepatic disease; viral infections other than flu. Use within 2 wk of receiving a live vaccine; ESRD. Safety in immunosuppression not established.

CAUTIOUS USE Hereditary fructose intolerance; cardiac disease; COPD, children with asthma; mild or moderate hepatic impairment; psychiatric disorders; renal impairment; pregnancy (category C); lactation; infants younger than 1 y for prophylaxis or neonates younger than 2 wk old for influenza treatment. Safety and efficacy in chronic cardiac/respiratory disease not established.

ROUTE & DOSAGE

Influenza Treatment

Adult/Adolescent/Child (over 40 kg): **PO** 75 mg bid × 5 days
Child (1–12 y, weight 20–40 kg): **PO** 60 mg bid × 5 days; *weight 16–23 kg:* 45 mg bid × 5 days; *weight less than 15 kg:* 30 mg bid × 5 days
Infant: **PO** 3 mg/kg bid × 5 days

O

Influenza Prevention

Adult/Adolescent/Child (1 y or older and weight over 40 kg): **PO** 75 mg daily × 10 days; begin within 2 days of contact with infected person

Child (weight 23–40 kg): **PO** 60 mg daily × 10 days; *weight 15–23 kg:* 45 mg daily × 10 days; *weight less than 15 kg:* 30 mg × 10 days

Renal Impairment Dosage Adjustment

CrCl 10–30 mL/min: **Treatment:** 30 mg daily × 5 days; **Prophylaxis:** 30 mg every other day

ADMINISTRATION

Oral

- Give with food to decrease the risk of GI upset.
- Start within 48 h of onset of flu symptoms.
- Take missed dose as soon as possible unless next dose is due within 2 h.
- Store at 15°–30° C (59°–86° F); protect from moisture, keep dry.

ADVERSE EFFECTS **Respiratory:** Bronchitis, cough. **CNS:** Dizziness, headache, insomnia, vertigo. **GI:** Nausea, vomiting, diarrhea, abdominal pain. **Other:** Fatigue.

PHARMACOKINETICS **Absorption:** Readily absorbed, 75% bioavailable. **Distribution:** 42% protein bound. **Metabolism:** Extensively metabolized to active metabolite oseltamivir carboxylate by liver esterases. **Elimination:** Primarily in urine. **Half-Life:** 1–2 h; oseltamivir carboxylate 6–10 h.

NURSING IMPLICATIONS

Assessment & Drug Effects

- Monitor ambulation in frail and older adult patients due to potential for dizziness and vertigo.
- Monitor children for abnormal behavior such as delirium or self-injury.

Patient & Family Education

- Contact your prescriber regarding the use of this drug in children.

OSIMERTINIB

(oh'si-mer'ti-nib)

Tagrisso

Classification: ANTINEOPLASTIC; KINASE INHIBITOR; EPIDERMAL GROWTH FACTOR RECEPTOR INHIBITOR

Therapeutic: ANTINEOPLASTIC

Prototype: Erlotinib

AVAILABILITY Tablets

ACTION & THERAPEUTIC EFFECT

An irreversible epidermal growth factor receptor (EGFR) tyrosine kinase inhibitor. It preferentially binds to mutant forms of EGFR as compared to the normal wild-type EGFR. It also exhibits anti-tumor activity against cell lines with EGFR-mutations, such as the T790M resistance mutation. *This mutation can cause resistance to other EGFR tyrosine kinase inhibitors.*

USES Treatment of patients with metastatic EGFR T790M mutation-positive non-small-cell lung cancer (NSCLC) who have failed treatment with other EGFR tyrosine kinase inhibitor (TKI) therapy.

CAUTIOUS USE Interstitial pulmonary disease/interstitial lung disease (ILD) or pneumonitis, including fatalities, have been reported. Permanently discontinue use in patients with confirmed, treatment-related ILD or pneumonia. Use cautiously in patients with cardiac disease or other conditions that may increase the risk of QT prolongation including cardiac arrhythmias, congenital long QT syndrome, heart failure, bradycardia, myocardial infarction, hypertension, coronary artery disease, hypomagnesemia, hypokalemia, hypocalcemia or in patients receiving medications for long QT interval. Treatment should be held with an ejection fraction of less than 50% or with more than a 10% decrease from baseline. Geriatric patients (older than 65 y) are at a higher risk of adverse effects. There are no adequate well-controlled studies in pregnant women. It is not known if osimertinib is present in human milk. Recommendations are to discontinue breast-feeding during treatment and for 2 wk after the final dose.

ROUTE & DOSAGE

Non-Small Cell Lung Cancer

Adult: **PO** 80 mg once daily

Adverse Reaction Dosage Adjustment

Interstitial lung disease (ILD)/ pneumonitis: Permanently discontinue

QTc interval greater than 500 msec on at least 2 separate ECGs: Withhold until QTc interval is less than 481 msec; resume at 40 mg

QTc interval prolongation with signs or symptoms of life-threatening arrhythmia: Permanently discontinue

Decrease in LVEF of 10% from baseline and below 50%: Withhold up to 4 wk; resume if improved to baseline; if not, permanently discontinue

Symptomatic congestive heart failure: Permanently discontinue

Other Grade 3 reaction: Withhold for 3 wk; resume at 40–80 mg once daily if resolved to Grade 0–2; if not, permanently

ADMINISTRATION

Oral

- Take without regard to food.

Extemporaneous Compounding Oral

- Disperse tablet in 15 mL of noncarbonated water only.
- Stir until tablet is in small pieces, it will not completely dissolve.
- Administer immediately.
- Rinse the container with 4–8 oz (120 mL–240 mL) of water and immediately drink.
- Store between 15°–30° F (59°–86° F).

ADVERSE EFFECTS **CV:** Prolonged QT interval. **Respiratory:** Cough, dyspnea, upper respiratory infection. **CNS:** Fatigue, headache. **Endocrine:** *Hyperglycemia, hypermagnesemia, hyponatremia*, hypokalemia. **Skin:** *Skin rash, xeroderma, nail disease, pruritus*. **Hepatic/GI:** Increased serum AST, increased serum ALT, hyperbilirubinemia, *diarrhea, stomatitis*, decreased appetite, constipation, nausea, vomiting. **Hematologic:** *Lymphocytopenia, anemia, thrombocytopenia, neutropenia*. **Other:** Fever.

INTERACTIONS **Drug:** Strong CYP3A inhibitors (e.g.,

O

itraconazole, nefazodone, ritonavir, telithromycin) may increase the levels of osimertinib. Strong CYP3A inducers (e.g., **carbamazepine, phenytoin, rifampicin**) may decrease the levels of osimertinib. Do not use with other agents that prolong QT interval. Osimertinib may alter the plasma levels of **carbamazepine, cyclosporine**, ERGOT ALKALOIDS, **fentanyl, quinidine**, and **phenytoin.** Do not use with LIVE VACCINES. May enhance effect of **deferiprone, dipyrone, pazopanib, pimecrolimus, tacrolimus. Herbal: St. John's Wort** may decrease the levels of osimertinib.

PHARMACOKINETICS **Peak:** 6 h. **Metabolism:** Hepatic oxidation by CYP enzymes. **Elimination:** Fecal (68%) and renal (14%). **Half-Life:** 48 h.

NURSING IMPLICATIONS

O

Assessment & Drug Effects

- Hazardous agent (meets NIOSH 2016 criteria for handling and disposing)—double glove, wear a gown if there is a chance of vomit or spit up, eye/face protection for administration of a liquid. Crushed tablets should be prepared in a controlled device.
- Perform respiratory assessments being alert to complaints of shortness of breath and any pain in lower extremities or jugular veins that could be related to thrombosis. Hold drug and notify prescriber if symptoms develop.
- Perform oral exams for inspection of oral mucosa and complaints of pain.
- Monitor daily weight.
- Monitor lab tests: CBC with differential, monitor ECG, ejection fraction, and serum electrolytes.

Patient & Family Education

- Contact medical provider for shortness of breath, new or worsening cough, or pain, edema, or warmth in extremities or neck.
- Women should use effective contraception during therapy and for 6 wk after the last dose. Males with female partners of reproductive potential should also use effective contraception during therapy and for 4 mo after the last dose.
- Report any changes in balance, confusion, weakness, severe dizziness or fainting.

OSPEMIFENE

(os-pem'ih-feen)

Osphena

Classification: ESTROGEN AGONIST/ANTAGONIST; SELECTIVE ESTROGEN RECEPTOR MODIFIER (SERM)

Therapeutic: ESTROGEN AGONIST/ANTAGONIST

Prototype: Tamoxifen

AVAILABILITY Tablet

ACTION & *THERAPEUTIC EFFECT* A selective estrogen receptor agonist/antagonist that activates estrogenic pathways in some tissues (agonist) and blocks the pathways in other tissues (antagonist). *Exerts an estrogen-like effect on the vaginal epithelium thus reversing vulvovaginal atrophy and decreasing dyspareunia.*

USES Treatment of moderate to severe dyspareunia, a symptomatic estrogen-like effect on the vaginal epithelium of vulvar and vaginal atrophy, due to menopause.

CONTRAINDICATIONS Undiagnosed abnormal genital bleeding; known or suspected neoplasia; endometrial cancer; history of breast cancer; history or active VTE, pulmonary embolism (PE), or history of these conditions; active arterial thromboembolic disease (e.g., stroke, MI, or history of these conditions); severe hepatic impairment; known or suspected pregnancy (category X); lactation.

CAUTIOUS USE Risk for DVT, PE, or history of stroke; hypertension; smoking; DM, hypercholesterolemia; obesity, SLE, mild or moderate hepatic impairment.

ROUTE & DOSAGE

Dyspareunia

Adult: PO 60 mg once daily

Hepatic Impairment Dosage Adjustment

Severe hepatic impairment (Child-Pugh class C): Do not administer

ADMINISTRATION

Oral

- Give with food.
- Store at 15°–30° C (59°–86° F).

ADVERSE EFFECTS **Skin:** Hyperhidrosis. **GU:** Genital discharge, vaginal discharge. **Musculoskeletal:** Muscle spasms.

INTERACTIONS **Drug:** Coadministration of CYP2C9 and CYP3A4 Inhibitors (e.g., **fluconazole, ketoconazole**) may increase the levels of ospemifene. Coadministration of CYP2C9 and CYP3A4 inducers (e.g., **rifampin**) may decrease the levels of ospemifene. Coadministration with other drugs that are highly plasma protein bound may cause displacement reactions resulting in increased levels of either ospemifene or other drugs. **Food:** Food increases the bioavailability of ospemifene.

PHARMACOKINETICS **Peak:** 2–2.5 h. **Distribution:** 99% plasma protein bound. **Metabolism:** Hepatic oxidation. **Elimination:** Fecal (75%) and renal (7%). **Half-Life:** 26 h.

NURSING IMPLICATIONS

Black Box Warning

Ospemifene has been associated with increased risk of endometrial cancer in women who are not receiving a progestin, and with increased risk of DVT and CVA.

Assessment & Drug Effects

- Monitor for and report persistent or recurring genital bleeding.
- Monitor closely those with risk factors for cardiovascular disease and thromboembolism (e.g., hypertension, DM, tobacco use, hypercholesterolemia, obesity, history of SLE).

Patient & Family Education

- Notify prescriber immediately if you become pregnant.
- Report promptly all instances of vaginal bleeding.
- This drug may cause or increase the occurrence of hot flashes.

OXACILLIN SODIUM

(ox-a-sill'in)

Classification: PENICILLIN ANTIBIOTIC; PENICILLINASE-RESISTANT PENICILLIN

Therapeutic: ANTIBIOTIC

AVAILABILITY Solution for injection

ACTION & *THERAPEUTIC EFFECT* Oxacillin inhibits final stage of bacterial cell wall synthesis by preferentially binding to specific penicillin-binding proteins (PBPs) located within the bacterial cell wall, leading to destruction of the cell wall of the organism. *It is highly active against most penicillinase-producing staphylococci, and is generally ineffective against gram-negative bacteria and methicillin-resistant staphylococci (MRSA).*

USES Infections caused by staphylococci.

UNLABELED USES Catheter-related infections, skin/soft tissue necrotizing infection.

CONTRAINDICATIONS Hypersensitivity to oxacillin, penicillin, or any component of formulation.

CAUTIOUS USE History of or suspected atopy or allergy (hives, eczema, hay fever, asthma); history of GI disease; hepatic or renal impairment; CHF; older adults; pregnancy (maternal use of penicillins has generally not resulted in an increased risk of adverse fetal effects); lactation (may cause infant diarrhea); premature infants, neonates.

O

ROUTE & DOSAGE

Staphylococcal Infections

Adult: **IV** 2 g q4h
Adolescent/Child: **IV** 100–150 mg/kg/day in divided doses q6h (max: 4000 mg/day)

ADMINISTRATION

Note: The total sodium content (including that contributed by buffer) in each gram of oxacillin is approximately 3.1 mEq or 71 mg.

Intramuscular

- Administer into muscle; avoid sciatic nerve injury.

Intravascular

Note: Verify correct IV concentration and rate of infusion/injection with prescriber before IV administration to neonates, infants, and children.

PREPARE: **Direct:** Reconstitute each 1 g or fraction thereof with 10 mL with sterile water for injection or NS to yield 250 mg/1.5 mL. **Intermittent:** Dilute required dose of reconstituted solution in 50–100 mL of D5W, NS, D5/NS, or LR. **Continuous:** Dilute required dose of reconstituted solution in up to 1000 mL of compatible IV solutions.

ADMINISTER: **Direct:** Give at a rate of 1 g or fraction thereof over 10 min. **Intermittent IVPB:** Give over 30 min.

INCOMPATIBILITIES: **Solution/additive: Cytarabine Y-site: Amphotericin B, calcium, dantrolene, diazepam, diazoxide, diphenhydramine, dobutamine, doxycycline, esmolol, ganciclovir, gentamicin, haloperidol, hydralazine, inamrinone, metaraminol, minocycline, netilmicin, pentazocine, phenytoin, polymixin B, promethazine, protamine, pyridoxine, succinylcholine, SMZ/TMP, tobramycin.**

ADVERSE EFFECTS GI: *C.difficile-associated diarrhea*, hepatotoxicity, elevated liver enzymes. **GU:** Interstitial nephritis, acute renal tubular disease. **Hematologic:** Eosinophilia.

DIAGNOSTIC TEST INTERFERENCE Oxacillin in large doses can cause false-positive ***urine protein tests*** using ***sulfosalicylic acid methods***; may interfere with ***urinary glucose tests***.

INTERACTIONS Do not administer with LIVE VACCINES.

PHARMACOKINETICS **Peak:** 30 min IM; 15 min IV. **Distribution:** Distributes into CNS with inflamed meninges; crosses placenta; distributed into breast milk, 90% protein bound. **Metabolism:** Enters enterohepatic circulation. **Elimination:** Primarily in urine, some in bile. **Half-Life:** 0.5–1 h.

NURSING IMPLICATIONS

Assessment & Drug Effects

- Ask patient prior to first dose about hypersensitivity reactions to penicillins, cephalosporins, and other allergens.
- Hepatic dysfunction (possibly a hypersensitivity reaction) has been associated with IV oxacillin; it is reversible with discontinuation of drug. Symptoms may resemble viral hepatitis or general signs of hypersensitivity and should be reported promptly: Hives, rash, fever, nausea, vomiting, abdominal discomfort, anorexia, malaise, jaundice (with dark yellow to brown urine, light-colored or clay-colored stools, pruritus).
- Withhold next drug dose and report the onset of hypersensitivity reactions and superinfections (see Appendix F).
- Monitor lab tests: Periodic serum LFTs, CBC, BUN, creatinine, and urinalysis.

Patient & Family Education

- Take oral medication around the clock; do not miss a dose. Take all of the medication prescribed even if you feel better, unless otherwise directed by prescriber.

OXALIPLATIN

(ox-a-li-pla′tin)

Classification: ANTINEOPLASTIC; ALKYLATING AGENT

Therapeutic: ANTINEOPLASTIC

Prototype: Cyclophosphamide

AVAILABILITY Solution for injection

ACTION & *THERAPEUTIC EFFECT*
Oxaliplatin forms inter- and intrastrand DNA cross-links that inhibit DNA replication and transcription resulting in cell death. *Antitumor activity of oxaliplatin in combination with 5-fluorouracil (5-FU) has antiproliferative activity against colon carcinoma that is greater than either compound alone.*

USES Metastatic cancer of colon and rectum.

UNLABELED USES Advanced prostate cancer, non-Hodgkin lymphoma, ovarian cancer.

CONTRAINDICATIONS Hypersensitivity to oxaliplatin or other platinum compounds; myelosuppression; pregnancy (may result in fetal harm); lactation.

CAUTIOUS USE Renal impairment, because clearance of ultrafilterable platinum is decreased in mild, moderate, and severe renal impairment; hepatic impairment; older adults; children.

ROUTE & DOSAGE

Metastatic Colon or Rectal Cancer

Adult: **IV** 85 mg/m^2 once every 2 wk until disease progression or unacceptable toxicity; adjust for toxicities (see package insert for adjustments)

Renal Impairment Dosage Adjustment

CrCl less than 30 mL/min: Reduce initial dose to 65 mg/m^2

ADMINISTRATION

Intravenous

Premedication with an antiemetic is recommended.

PREPARE: **IV Infusion:** NEVER reconstitute with NS or any solution containing chloride. ▪ Reconstitute the 50 mg vial or the 100 mg vial by adding 10 mL or 20 mL, respectively, of sterile water for injection or D5W. ▪ MUST further dilute in 250–500 mL of D5W for infusion.

ADMINISTER: **IV Infusion: Do not** use needles or infusion sets containing aluminum parts. ▪ Flush infusion line with D5W before and after administration of any other concomitant medication. ▪ Give over 2 hours with frequent monitoring of the IV insertion site; extend infusion time to 6 hours for acute toxicities. ▪ Discontinue at the first sign of extravasation and restart IV in a different site.

INCOMPATIBILITIES: **Solution/additive: dexamethasone. Y-site: cefepime, cefoperazone, dantrolene, diazepam.**

▪ Store reconstituted solution up to 24 h under refrigeration at 2°–8° C (36°–46° F). ▪ After final dilution, the IV solution may be stored for 6 h at room temperature [20°–25° C (68°–77° F)] or up to 24 h under refrigeration.

O

ADVERSE EFFECTS CV: Chest pain, peripheral edema. **Respiratory:** *Dyspnea, cough,* upper respiratory tract infection. **CNS:** *Fatigue, neuropathy, headache,* insomnia, dizziness, rigors. **Endocrine:** Hypokalemia, dehydration. **Hepatic/GI:** *Diarrhea, nausea, vomiting, anorexia, stomatitis, constipation, abdominal pain,* dyspepsia, dysgeusia, increased liver enzymes. **GU:** Increased serum creatinine. **Hematologic:** *Anemia,* leukopenia, thrombocytopenia, neutropenia. **Musculoskeletal:** Arthralgia. **Other:** *Fever,* back pain, injection site reaction.

INTERACTIONS Drug: MYLEOSUPPRESIVE and IMMUNOSUPRESSIVE AGENTS have increased risk of adverse effects; increases risk of adverse effects with **topotecan**. Do not use with LIVE VACCINES.

PHARMACOKINETICS Distribution: Greater than 90% protein bound. **Metabolism:** Rapid and extensive nonenzymatic biotransformation. **Elimination:** Primarily in urine. **Half-Life:** 391 h.

NURSING IMPLICATIONS

Black Box Warning

Oxaliplatin has been associated with anaphylactic reactions within minutes of administration.

Assessment & Drug Effects

- Monitor for S&S of hypersensitivity (e.g., rash, urticaria, erythema, pruritus; rarely, bronchospasm and hypotension). Discontinue drug and notify prescriber if any of these occur.
- Monitor insertion site. Extravasation may cause local pain and inflammation that may be severe

and lead to complications, including necrosis.
- Monitor for S&S of coagulation disorders including GI bleeding, hematuria, and epistaxis.
- Monitor for S&S of peripheral neuropathy (e.g., paresthesia, dysesthesia, hypoesthesia in the hands, feet, perioral area, or throat, jaw spasm, abnormal tongue sensation, dysarthria, eye pain, and chest pressure). Symptoms may be precipitated or exacerbated by exposure to cold temperature or cold objects.
- Do not apply ice to oral mucous membranes (e.g., mucositis prophylaxis) during the infusion of oxaliplatin as cold temperature can exacerbate acute neurological symptoms.
- Monitor lab tests: Before each administration cycle, CBC with differential, electrolytes, and blood chemistries (including ALT, AST, bilirubin, and creatinine). Baseline and periodic renal function tests. INR and PT in patients on oral anticoagulation therapy. Evaluate pregnancy status.

Patient & Family Education

- Use effective methods of contraception while receiving this drug.
- Avoid cold drinks, use of ice, and cover exposed skin prior to exposure to cold temperature or cold objects.
- Do not drive or engage in potentially hazardous activities until response to drug is known.
- Report any of the following to a health care provider: Difficulty writing, buttoning, swallowing, walking; numbness, tingling or other unusual sensations in extremities; non-productive cough or shortness of breath; fever, particularly if associated with persistent diarrhea or other evidence of infection.
- Report promptly S&S of a bleeding disorder such as black tarry stool, coke-colored or frankly bloody urine, bleeding from the nose or mucous membranes.

OXANDROLONE

(ox-an′dro-lone)

Oxandrin

Classification: ANDROGEN/ANABOLIC STEROID

Therapeutic: ANABOLIC STEROID

Prototype: Testosterone

Controlled Substance: Schedule III

AVAILABILITY

Tablet

ACTION & *THERAPEUTIC EFFECT*

A synthetic derivative of testosterone that promotes weight gain after weight loss following extensive surgery, chronic infections, or severe trauma. It offsets the protein catabolism associated with prolonged administration of corticosteroids, and relieves bone pain frequently accompanying osteoporosis. *Promotes weight gain and relieves bone pain caused by osteoporosis.*

USES

Adjunctive therapy to promote weight gain, offset protein catabolism associated with prolonged administration of corticosteroids, relieve bone pain accompanying osteoporosis.

CONTRAINDICATIONS

Hypersensitivity or toxic reactions to androgens; severe cardiac, hepatic, or renal disease; possibility of virilization of external genitalia of female fetus; polycythemia; hypercalcemia; known or suspected prostatic or breast cancer in males; benign prostatic hypertrophy with obstruction; patients easily stimulated sexually; asthenic males who may react adversely to androgenic overstimulation; conditions

O

aggravated by fluid retention; hypertension; pregnancy (category X); lactation.

CAUTIOUS USE Cardiac, hepatic, and mild to moderate renal disease, hypercholesterolemia, heart failure, peripheral edema, arteriosclerosis, coronary artery disease, MI; cholestasis; DM; BPH; prepubertal males, acute intermittent porphyria; older adults; children.

ROUTE & DOSAGE

Weight Gain

Adult: **PO** 2.5 mg bid to qid (max: 20 mg/day) for 2–4 wk
Child: **PO** 0.1 mg/kg/day

Bone Pain

Adult: **PO** 2.5–20 mg bid to qid for 2–4 wk

ADMINISTRATION

Oral

O

- Individualize doses; great variations in response exist.
- Store at 15°–30° C (59°–86° F).

ADVERSE EFFECTS **CNS:** Habituation, excitation, insomnia, depression, changes in libido. **Endocrine:** Gynecomastia, deepening of voice in females, premature closure of epiphyses in children, edema, decreased glucose tolerance. **Skin:** Hirsutism and male pattern baldness in females, acne. **Hepatic:** Cholestatic jaundice with or without hepatic necrosis and death, hepatocellular neoplasms, peliosis hepatitis (long-term use). **GU:** *Males*: Phallic enlargement, increased frequency or persistence of erections, inhibition of testicular function, testicular atrophy, oligospermia, impotence, chronic priapism, epididymitis, bladder irritability; *Females*: Clitoral enlargement, menstrual irregularities.

DIAGNOSTIC TEST INTERFERENCE May decrease levels of thyroxine-binding globulin (decreased total T_4 and increased T_3 RU and free T_4).

INTERACTIONS **Drug:** May increase INR with **warfarin**. May inhibit metabolism of ORAL HYPOGLYCEMIC AGENTS. Concomitant STEROIDS may increase edema. **Herbal:** **Echinacea** may increase risk of hepatotoxicity.

PHARMACOKINETICS **Half-Life:** 10–13 h (increased in elderly patients).

NURSING IMPLICATIONS

Black Box Warning

Oxandrolone has been associated with hepatic dysfunction, liver failure, liver cell tumors, and increased risk of atherosclerosis from blood lipid changes.

Assessment & Drug Effects

- Monitor weight closely throughout therapy.
- Assess for and report development of edema or S&S of jaundice (see Appendix F).
- Withhold and notify prescriber if hypercalcemia develops in breast cancer patient.
- Monitor growth in children closely.
- Monitor lab tests: Periodic LFTs, lipid profile, Hct, and Hgb.

Patient & Family Education

- Women: Report signs of virilization, including acne and changes in menstrual periods.

- Men: Report too frequent or prolonged erections or appearance/worsening of acne.
- Report S&S of jaundice (see Appendix F) or edema.
- Monitor blood glucose for loss of glycemic control if diabetic.

OXAPROZIN

(ox-a-pro′zin)

Daypro

Classification: ANALGESIC, NON-STEROIDAL ANTI-INFLAMMATORY DRUG (NSAID)

Therapeutic: NONNARCOTIC ANALGESIC, NSAID; ANTIRHEUMATIC; ANTIPYRETIC

Prototype: Ibuprofen

AVAILABILITY Tablet

ACTION & *THERAPEUTIC EFFECT*

Long-acting NSAID agent, which is an effective prostaglandin synthetase inhibitor. It inhibits COX-1 and COX-2 enzymes needed for prostaglandin synthesis at the site of inflammation. *Has anti-inflammatory, antipyretic, and analgesic properties.*

USES Treatment of osteoarthritis and rheumatoid arthritis, juvenile rheumatoid arthritis.

UNLABELED USES Ankylosing spondylitis, chronic pain, gout, oral surgery pain, temporal arteritis, tendinitis.

CONTRAINDICATIONS Hypersensitivity to oxaprozin, salicylates, or any other NSAID; UGI bleeding; complete or partial syndrome of nasal polyps; angioedema; CABG perioperative pain; pregnancy (category D third trimester); lactation.

CAUTIOUS USE History of GI bleeding, alcoholism, smoking; history of severe hepatic dysfunction, renal insufficiency; cardiac disease; coagulopathy; photosensitivity; older adults; pregnancy (category C first and second trimester). Safety and efficacy in children younger than 6 y not established.

ROUTE & DOSAGE

Osteoarthritis, Rheumatoid Arthritis

Adult: **PO** 1200 mg daily (max: 1800 mg/day or 26 mg/kg, whichever is lower)

Juvenile Rheumatoid Arthritis

Adolescent/Child (6 y or older, weight over 55 kg): **PO** 1200 mg qd; *weight 32–54 kg:* 900 mg qd; *weight 22–31 kg:* 600 mg qd

ADMINISTRATION

Oral

- Give with meals or milk to decrease GI distress.
- Divide doses in those unable to tolerate once-daily dosing.
- Use lower starting doses for those with renal or hepatic dysfunction, advanced age, low body weight, or a predisposition to GI ulceration.

ADVERSE EFFECTS CV: Edema. **CNS:** Confusion, depression, disturbed sleep, dizziness, drowsiness, headache, sedation. **HEENT:** Tinnitus. **Skin:** Pruritis, skin rash. **Hepatic/GI:** Increased liver enzymes, abdominal pain, anorexia, constipation, dyspepsia, flatulence. **GU:** Dysuria, urinary frequency. **Hematologic:** Anemia, prolonged bleeding time.

DIAGNOSTIC TEST INTERFERENCE May cause false-positive reactions for BENZODIAZEPINES with ***urine drug-screening*** tests. May lead to false-positive aldosterone/renin ratio.

INTERACTIONS Drug: May attenuate the antihypertensive response to DIURETICS. NSAIDS increase the risk of **methotrexate** or **lithium** toxicity. Use caution with ANTICOAGULANTS, PLATELET INHIBITORS. May increase **aspirin** toxicity. Do not use with **cidofovir** or **ketorolac. Herbal: Feverfew, garlic, ginger, ginkgo** may increase risk of bleeding.

O

PHARMACOKINETICS Absorption: Readily from GI tract. **Peak:** 125 min. **Onset:** 1–6 wk for maximum therapeutic effect. **Distribution:** 99% protein bound. Distributes into synovial fluid, crosses placenta. Distributed into breast milk. **Metabolism:** In the liver. **Elimination:** 60% in urine, 30–35% in feces. **Half-Life:** 40 h.

NURSING IMPLICATIONS

Black Box Warning

Oxaprozin has been associated with increased risk of serious, potentially fatal, GI bleeding and cardiovascular events (e.g., MI & CVA); risk may increase with duration of use and may be greater in the older adult and those with risk factors for CV disease.

Assessment & Drug Effects

- Monitor for S&S of GI bleeding, especially in patients with a history of inflammation or ulceration of upper GI tract, or those treated chronically with NSAIDs.
- Monitor patients with CHF for increased fluid retention and edema. Report rapid weight increases accompanied by edema.
- Auditory and ophthalmologic exams are recommended with prolonged or high-dose therapy.
- Monitor lab tests: Baseline and periodic CBC, LFTs, and renal function tests.

Patient & Family Education

- Report immediately dark tarry stools, "coffee ground" or bloody emesis, or other GI distress.
- Avoid aspirin or other NSAIDs without explicit permission of prescriber.
- Stop taking drug and report promptly to prescriber if you experience chest pain, shortness of breath, weakness, slurring of speech, or other signs of a cardiac or neurologic problem.
- Be aware of the possibility of photosensitivity, which results in a rash on sun-exposed skin.
- Report immediately to prescriber ringing in ears, decreased hearing, or blurred vision.
- Do not exceed ordered dose. The goal of therapy is lowest effective dose.

OXAZEPAM

(ox-a′ze-pam)

Ox-Pam ♦

Classification: ANXIOLYTIC; SEDATIVE-HYPNOTIC; BENZODIAZEPINE

Therapeutic: ANTIANXIETY; SEDATIVE-HYPNOTIC

Prototype: Lorazepam

Controlled Substance: Schedule IV

AVAILABILITY Capsule

ACTION & *THERAPEUTIC EFFECT* Benzodiazepine derivative related to lorazepam. Effects are mediated by the inhibitory neurotransmitter GABA, and acts on the thalamic, hypothalamic, and limbic levels of CNS. *Has anxiolytic, sedative, hypnotic, and skeletal muscle relaxant effects.*

USES Management of anxiety; control acute withdrawal symptoms in chronic alcoholism.

CONTRAINDICATIONS Hypersensitivity to oxazepam and other benzodiazepines; respiratory depression; psychoses, suicidal ideation; acute alcohol intoxication; acute-angle glaucoma; pregnancy (teratogenic effects have been observed with some benzodiazepines); lactation.

CAUTIOUS USE Impaired kidney and liver function; alcoholism; addiction-prone patients; COPD; history of seizures; history of suicide; mental depression; bipolar disorder; older adults and debilitated patients; children younger than 6 y.

ROUTE & DOSAGE

Anxiety

Adult/Adolescent/Child (6 y or older): **PO** 10–15 mg tid or qid

Acute Alcohol Withdrawal

Adult: **PO** 10–30 mg PRN (based on institution protocol)

ADMINISTRATION

Oral

- Give with food if GI upset occurs.
- Store in a tightly closed container at 15°–30° C (59°–86° F) unless otherwise specified.

ADVERSE EFFECTS **CV:** Hypotension, edema. **CNS:** *Drowsiness*, dizziness, mental confusion, vertigo, ataxia, headache, lethargy, syncope, tremor, slurred speech, paradoxic reaction (euphoria, excitement). **Skin:** Skin rash, edema. **GI:** Nausea, xerostomia, jaundice. **GU:** Altered libido. **Hematologic:** <u>Leukopenia</u>.

INTERACTIONS **Drug: Alcohol**, CNS DEPRESSANTS, ANTICONVULSANTS potentiate CNS depression; **cimetidine** increases oxazepam plasma levels, increasing its toxicity; may decrease antiparkinsonism effects of **levodopa**; may increase **phenytoin** levels; smoking decreases sedative and antianxiety effects. **Herbal: Kava, kratom, valerian** may potentiate sedation.

PHARMACOKINETICS **Absorption:** Readily absorbed from GI tract. **Peak:** 2–3 h. **Distribution:** Crosses placenta; distributed into breast milk. **Metabolism:** In liver. **Elimination:** Primarily in urine, some in feces. **Half-Life:** 2–8 h.

NURSING IMPLICATIONS

Black Box Warning

Concomitant use of benzodiazepines and opioids may result in profound sedation, respiratory depression, coma, and death. The use of benzodiazepines exposes users to abuse, misuse, physical dependence, and addiction which can lead to overdose and death.

Assessment & Drug Effects

- Observe older adult patients closely for signs of overdosage. Report to prescriber if daytime psychomotor function is depressed.
- Monitor for increased signs and symptoms of suicidality.
- Note: Excessive and prolonged use may cause physical dependence.
- Monitor lab tests: Periodic LFTs and CBC count.

Patient & Family Education

- Report promptly any mild paradoxic stimulation of affect and excitement with sleep disturbances that may occur within the first 2 wk of therapy. Dosage reduction is indicated.
- Consult prescriber before self-medicating with OTC drugs.
- Do not drive or engage in potentially hazardous activities until response to drug is known.
- Do not drink alcoholic beverages while taking oxazepam. The CNS depressant effects of each agent may be intensified.
- Contact prescriber if you intend to or do become pregnant during therapy about discontinuing the drug.
- Withdraw drug slowly following prolonged therapy to avoid precipitating withdrawal symptoms (seizures, mental confusion, nausea, vomiting, muscle and abdominal cramps, tremulousness, sleep disturbances, unusual irritability, hyperhidrosis).

O

OXCARBAZEPINE

(ox-car'ba-ze-peen)

Oxtellar XR, Trileptal

Classification: ANTICONVULSANT

Therapeutic: ANTICONVULSANT

Prototype: Carbamazepine

AVAILABILITY Tablet; extended release tablet; oral suspension

ACTION & *THERAPEUTIC EFFECT* Anticonvulsant properties may result from blockage of voltage-sensitive sodium channels, which results in stabilization of hyperexcited neural membranes. *Inhibits repetitive neuronal firing, and decreased propagation of neuronal impulses.*

USES Focal (partial) onset seizures.

UNLABELED USES Trigeminal neuralgia.

CONTRAINDICATIONS Hypersensitivity to oxcarbazepine including skin reactions; suicidal ideation or behavior; drug induced agranulocytosis, pancytopenia, leukopenia; pregnancy—fetal risk cannot be ruled out; lactation—infant risk cannot be ruled out.

CAUTIOUS USE Renal impairment; renal failure; severe hepatic impairment; patients at risk for hyponatremia; history of hypothyroidism; suicidal tendencies; history of poor coordination or gait disturbances; pregnancy; older adults; children younger than 2 y. **Extended Release:** Use in children less than 6 y.

ROUTE & DOSAGE

Focal Onset Seizures

Adult: **PO** Immediate release 300–600 mg/day in divided doses (max: 2.4 g/day) *Extended release:* 600 mg daily, may increase at weekly intervals (max: 2.4 g/day)

Child (4–16 y): **PO** Initiate with 8–10 mg/kg/day divided bid, gradually increase weekly to target dose (divided bid) based on weight: *Weight 20–35 kg:* 600–1200 mg/day; *weight 35.1–50 kg:* 900–1500 mg/day; *weight 30.1–70 kg:* 1200–2100 mg/day; *weight greater than 70 kg:* 1500–2100 mg/day

Renal Impairment Dosage Adjustment

CrCl less than 30 mL/min: Initiate at ½ usual starting dose

ADMINISTRATION

Oral

- NIOSH recommends use of single gloves by anyone handling intact tablets or capsules or administering from a unit-dose package. If cutting, crushing, or manipulating, or handling of uncoated tablets, use double gloves and protective gown. During administration, eye/face protection is needed if the patient may resist or if there is a potential to vomit or spit up.
- Ensure that extended release tablet is swallowed whole. It should not be crushed or chewed.
- Extended release: Take a single daily dose on an empty stomach, at least 1 hour before or 2 hours after a meal.
- Immediate release: Can be taken with or without food.
- Immediate release suspension: Shake well and prepare dose immediately using the oral dosing syringe. Can be mixed in a small glass of water just prior to administration or may be swallowed directly from the syringe.
- Do not abruptly stop this medication; withdraw drug gradually when discontinued to minimize seizure potential.
- Store at controlled room temperature of 25° C (77° F), with excursions permitted between 15 and 30 degrees C (59 and 86 degrees F). Protect extended-release tablets from moisture and light. Use suspension within 7 weeks of first opening the bottle.

ADVERSE EFFECTS (≥ 5%) **CNS:** *Headache, dizziness, somnolence, ataxia, nystagmus, abnormal gait, drowsiness,* tremor, abnormal coordination. **HEENT:** *Diplopia, abnormal vision,* nystagmus. **Endocrine:** Hyponatremia, weight gain. **GI:** *Nausea, vomiting, abdominal pain,* dyspepsia. **Other:** *Fatigue.*

DIAGNOSTIC TEST INTERFERENCE

May decrease serum T4.

INTERACTIONS **Drug: Carbamazepine, phenobarbital, phenytoin, valproic acid, verapamil;** CALCIUM CHANNEL BLOCKERS may decrease oxcarbazepine levels; may increase levels of **phenobarbital, phenytoin;** may decrease levels of **felodipine,** ORAL CONTRACEPTIVES. Do not use with transdermal **selegiline, cobicistat, dolutegravir, doravirine, elvitegravir, eslicarbazepine, ledipasvir, selegiline, simeprevir, sofosbuvir, tendofovir, dasabuvir/ombitasvir/**

paritaprevir/ritonavir. Herbal: Ginkgo may decrease anticonvulsant effectiveness. **Evening primrose oil** may decrease the seizure threshold.

PHARMACOKINETICS Absorption: Rapidly and completely from GI tract. **Peak:** Steady-state levels reached in 2–3 days. **Distribution:** 40% protein bound. **Metabolism:** Extensively metabolized in liver to active 10-monohydroxy metabolite (MHD). **Elimination:** 95% in kidneys. **Half-Life:** 2 h, MHD 9 h.

NURSING IMPLICATIONS

Assessment & Drug Effects

- Monitor for and report S&S of: Hyponatremia (e.g., nausea, malaise, headache, lethargy, confusion); CNS impairment (e.g., somnolence, excessive fatigue, cognitive deficits, speech or language problems, incoordination, gait disturbances).
- Monitor for worsening of depression or suicidal thoughts, changes in mood or behavior.
- Monitor phenytoin levels when administered concurrently.
- Monitor lab tests: Periodic serum sodium; plasma level of the concomitant antiepileptic drug during titration of the oxcarbazepine dose.

Patient & Family Education

- Notify prescriber of the following: Dizziness, excess drowsiness, frequent headaches, malaise, double vision, lack of coordination, or persistent nausea.
- Report any worsening depression, suicidal ideation, or unusual changes in behavior.
- Exercise special caution with concurrent use of alcohol or CNS depressants.
- Use caution with potentially hazardous activities and driving until response to drug is known.
- Advise against sudden discontinuation as this may lead to seizures.
- Use or add barrier contraceptive since drug may render hormonal methods ineffective.

O

OXICONAZOLE NITRATE

(ox-i-con′a-zole)

Oxistat

Classification: AZOLE ANTIFUNGAL

Therapeutic: ANTIFUNGAL

Prototype: Fluconazole

AVAILABILITY Cream; lotion

ACTION & *THERAPEUTIC EFFECT* Topical synthetic antifungal agent that presumably works by altering the cellular membrane of the fungi, resulting in increased membrane permeability, secondary metabolic effects, and growth inhibition. *Prevents growth of fungi that cause tinea pedis, tinea cruris, and tinea corporis.*

USES Topical treatment of tinea pedis, tinea cruris, and tinea corporis due to *Trichophyton rubrum* and *Trichophyton mentagrophytes;* also used for cutaneous candidiasis caused by *Candida albicans* and *Candida tropicalis.*

CONTRAINDICATIONS Hypersensitivity to oxiconazole.

CAUTIOUS USE Hypersensitivity to other azole antifungals; pregnancy (category B); lactation.

ROUTE & DOSAGE

Tinea and Other Dermal Infections

Adult: **Topical** Apply to affected area once daily in the evening

ADMINISTRATION

Topical

- Apply cream to cover the affected areas once daily (in the evening).
- Treat tinea corporis and tinea cruris for 2 wk; tinea pedis for 1 mo to reduce the possibility of recurrence.
- Store at 15°–30° C (59°–86° F).

ADVERSE EFFECTS **Skin:** Transient burning and stinging, dryness, erythema, pruritus, and local irritation.

PHARMACOKINETICS **Absorption:** Less than 0.3% is absorbed systemically.

NURSING IMPLICATIONS

Patient & Family Education

- Use only externally. Do not use intravaginally.
- Discontinue drug and contact prescriber if irritation or sensitivity develops.
- Avoid contact with eyes.
- Contact prescriber if no improvement is noted after the prescribed treatment period.

OXYBUTYNIN CHLORIDE

(ox-i-byoo′ti-nin)

Ditropan XL, Gelnique, Oxytrol

Classification: ANTICHOLINERGIC; ANTIMUSCARINIC; GU ANTISPASMODIC
Therapeutic: GU ANTISPASMODIC

AVAILABILITY Tablet; extended release tablet; oral solution; transdermal patch; topical gel

ACTION & *THERAPEUTIC EFFECT* Exerts a direct antispasmodic effect on smooth muscle and inhibits the muscarinic action of acetylcholine on smooth muscle. *Relaxes bladder smooth muscle and increases bladder capacity.*

USES To relieve symptoms associated with overactive bladder.

CONTRAINDICATIONS Hypersensitivity of oxybutynin; narrow-angle glaucoma, myasthenia gravis, partial or complete GI obstruction, gastric retention, paralytic ileus, intestinal atony (especially older adult or debilitated patients), megacolon, pyloric stenosis, severe colitis, GU obstruction, urinary retention, unstable cardiovascular status; pregnancy—fetal risk cannot be ruled out; lactation—infant risk cannot be ruled out. **Extended Release:** With renal impairment or pediatric patients that cannot swallow a tablet whole.

CAUTIOUS USE Autonomic neuropathy, hiatal hernia with reflex esophagitis; gastric obstructive disorders due to risk of gastric retention; gastric motility problems, hepatic or renal dysfunction; urinary infection; hyperthyroidism; CHF, coronary artery disease, hypertension; myasthenia gravis, Parkinson disease; prostatic hypertrophy; older adults; children 5y and older.

O

ROUTE & DOSAGE

Overactive Bladder

Adult/Adolescent: **PO Immediate release** 5 mg 2–3 × day (max: 20 mg/day) **Sustained release** 5–10 mg daily, may adjust as needed (max 30 mg/day); **Topical** Apply 1 patch twice weekly; or apply contents of 1 10% gel package once daily

Geriatric: **PO Immediate release** 2.5–5 mg bid (max: 15 mg/day); use adult dosing for topical or sustained release products

Child (5 y or older): **PO** 5 mg bid; increase as necessary (max: 5 mg qid)

ADMINISTRATION

Oral

- Ensure that sustained release form is not chewed or crushed. It **must be** swallowed whole. May be given without regard to meals and should be given at the same time each day with plenty of fluids.
- Store syrup, tablet, extended release tablet, at controlled room temperature between 15 and 30 degrees C (59 and 86 degrees F). Protect from light. Store extended release tablets at controlled room temperature at 25 degrees C (77 degrees F), excursions permitted to 15 to 30 degrees C (59 to 86 degrees F). Protect from light.

Topical

- Ensure that old patch is removed prior to application of new patch.
- Gel may be applied to abdomen, upper arms/shoulder, and thigh. Rotate site application and avoid using the same site on 2 consecutive days. Squeeze entire contents of the gel packet onto application site. Wear gloves and gently rub into skin until dried.
- Avoid exposure to open fire or smoking until gel has dried.
- Avoid contact with eyes, nose, open sores, recently shaved skin, and skin with rashes.
- Do not shower or immerse area in water for 1 hour after gel application.
- Cover application site with clothing if skin-to-skin contact is anticipated.
- Storage variances for each trade drug. All can be stored at controlled room temperature at 25 degrees for other variances see package insert. Protect from moisture.

O

ADVERSE EFFECTS (≥ 5%) CNS: *Drowsiness,* dizziness headache. **HEENT:** *Blurred vision.* **GI:** *Dry mouth,* nausea, *constipation,* diarrhea, indigestion, bloated feeling.

DIAGNOSTIC TEST INTERFERENCE

May suppress the wheal and flare reactions to skin test antigen.

INTERACTIONS: Drugs: Do not use with, ANTICHOLINERGIC AGENTS. CYP3A4 inhibitors may increase serum concentrations.

PHARMACOKINETICS Absorption: Diffuses across intact skin. **Onset:** 0.5–1 h. (oral immediate release) **Peak:** 3–6 h. (PO Immediate); 3 days (PO Extended) **Duration:** 6–10 h (PO immediate). 96 h transdermal. **Metabolism:** In liver (CYP 3A4). **Elimination:** Primarily in urine. **Half-Life:** 2–5 h.

NURSING IMPLICATIONS

Assessment & Drug Effects

- Periodic interruptions of therapy are recommended to determine patient's need for continued treatment. Tolerance has occurred in some patients.
- Keep prescriber informed of expected responses to drug therapy (e.g., effect on urinary frequency, urgency, urge incontinence, nocturia, completeness of bladder emptying).
- Monitor patients with colostomy or ileostomy closely; abdominal distention and the onset of diarrhea in these patients may be early signs of intestinal obstruction or of toxic megacolon.

Patient & Family Education

- Do not drive or engage in potentially hazardous activities until response to drug is known.
- Exercise caution in hot environments. By suppressing sweating, oxybutynin can cause fever and heat stroke.
- Review adverse effects with patient and/or caregiver.
- Report hallucinations, agitation, and confusion especially during the first few months of therapy and with dose increase.
- Avoid alcohol as it will increase drowsiness.

OXYCODONE HYDROCHLORIDE

(ox-i-koe′done)

Oxaydo, OxyContin, Roxicodone, Roxybond, Xtampza

Classification: NARCOTIC (OPIATE AGONIST); ANALGESIC

Therapeutic: NARCOTIC ANALGESIC

Prototype: Morphine

Controlled Substance: Schedule II

AVAILABILITY Tablet. **OxyContin:** Sustained release tablet; oral solution

ACTION & THERAPEUTIC EFFECT Semisynthetic derivative of an opium agonist that binds with stereospecific receptors in various sites of CNS to alter both perception of pain and emotional response to pain. *Active against moderate to moderately severe pain. Appears to be more effective in relief of acute than longstanding pain.*

USES Relief of moderate to moderately severe pain, neuralgia. Relieves postoperative, postextractional, postpartum pain.

CONTRAINDICATIONS Hypersensitivity to oxycodone and principle drugs with which it is combined; bronchial asthma; known gastrointestinal obstruction; significant respiratory depression. pregnancy (category D for prolonged use or high doses at term); lactation.

CAUTIOUS USE Alcoholism; renal or hepatic disease; viral infections; Addison's disease; cardiac arrhythmias; chronic ulcerative colitis; history of drug abuse or dependency; gallbladder disease, acute abdominal conditions; head injury, intracranial lesions; history of seizures, hypothyroidism; BPH; respiratory disease; urethral stricture; peptic ulcer or coagulation abnormalities (combination products containing aspirin); older adult or debilitated patients; children.

ROUTE & DOSAGE

Moderate to Severe Pain

(Dose individualized per opioid tolerance and patient response)

O

Adult: **PO** 5–15 mg q4–6h prn; **Controlled release** 10 mg q12h (reserved for opioid tolerant patients)

Hepatic Impairment Dosage Adjustment

Start initial therapy at ⅓ to ½ normal dose and titrate carefully

ADMINISTRATION

Oral

- Ensure that sustained release form is not chewed or crushed. It **must be** swallowed whole.
- Administer with approximately the same amount of food to ensure consistent plasma levels.
- May be administered via gastrostomy or nasogastric tube. Flush the tube with water, pour capsule contents into the tube with 15 mL of water; flush tube 2 more times with 10 mL of water per flush; milk or nutritional supplements may be used for flushing instead of water.
- Store at 15°–30° C (59°–86° F). Protect from light and moisture.

ADVERSE EFFECTS **CV:** Bradycardia, flushing, edema, orthostatic hypotension. **Respiratory:** Shortness of breath, cough, <u>respiratory depression</u>. **CNS:** Euphoria, dysphoria, abnormal dreaming, agitation, abnormal thinking, anxiety, lightheadedness, *headache, dizziness, sedation*. **Endocrine:** Hyperglycemia, hyponatremia. **Skin:** Pruritus, skin rash. **GI:** Anorexia, nausea, abdominal pain, vomiting, *constipation,* jaundice, <u>hepatotoxicity</u> (combinations containing acetaminophen). **GU:** Dysuria, frequency of urination, urinary retention. **Ocular:** Miosis. **Other:** Unusual bleeding or bruising, arthralgia, back pain, fever, blurred vision.

DIAGNOSTIC TEST INTERFERENCE ***Serum amylase*** levels may be elevated because oxycodone causes spasm of sphincter of Oddi. ***Blood glucose determinations:*** False decrease (measured by ***glucose oxidase-peroxidase method***). ***5-HIAA determination:*** False positive with use of ***nitrosonaphthol reagent*** (quantitative test is unaffected).

INTERACTIONS **Drug: Alcohol** and other CNS DEPRESSANTS add to CNS depressant activity. Monitor closely if used with **amiodarone.** Use caution with CYP3A4 INHIBITORS due to increased risk of toxicities. Serotonin syndrome could occur when used with TRIPTANS. Do not use with BENZODIAZEPINES due to increased risk of sedation. **Herbal: St. John's wort** may increase sedation. **Food:** Grapefruit juice can increase adverse effects.

PHARMACOKINETICS **Absorption:** Readily from GI tract. **Onset:** 10–15 min. **Peak:** 30–60 min. **Duration:** 4–5 h. **Distribution:** Crosses placenta; distributed into breast milk. **Metabolism:** In liver by CYP3A4, CYP2D6. **Elimination:** Primarily in urine. **Half-Life:** 3–5 h.

NURSING IMPLICATIONS

Black Box Warning

Oxycodone has been associated with high abuse potential, and life-threatening respiratory depression, neonatal opioid withdrawal, Cytochrome P450 3A4 interaction.

Assessment & Drug Effects

- Monitor respiratory status. Withhold drug and notify prescriber if respiratory depression occurs.
- Monitor patient's response closely, especially to sustained-release preparations.
- Consult prescriber if nausea continues after first few days of therapy.
- Note: Lightheadedness, dizziness, sedation, or fainting appears to be more prominent in ambulatory than in nonambulatory patients and may be alleviated if patient lies down. Monitor blood pressure.
- Evaluate patient's continued need for oxycodone preparations. Monitor effectiveness of pain relief. Psychic and physical dependence and tolerance may develop with repeated use. The potential for drug abuse is high.
- Be aware that serious overdosage of any oxycodone preparation presents problems associated with a narcotic overdose (respiratory depression, circulatory collapse, extreme somnolence progressing to stupor, coma, or death.) After long term use, discontinuation should be tapered. Monitor for signs of opioid withdrawal.

Patient & Family Education

- Do not alter dosage regimen by increasing, decreasing, or shortening intervals between doses. Habit formation and liver damage may result.
- Avoid potentially hazardous activities such as driving a car or operating machinery while using oxycodone preparation.
- Do not drink large amounts of alcoholic beverages while using oxycodone preparations; risk of liver damage is increased.
- Check with prescriber before taking OTC drugs for colds, stomach distress, allergies, insomnia, or pain.
- Inform surgeon or dentist that you are taking an oxycodone preparation before any surgical procedure is undertaken.

OXYMETAZOLINE HYDROCHLORIDE

(ox-i-met-az′oh-leen)

Afrin, Nafrine ♣, Neo-Synephrine 12 Hour, Rhofade

Classification: NASAL PREPARATION; DECONGESTANT

Therapeutic: DECONGESTANT

Prototype: Naphazoline

AVAILABILITY Intranasal solution; cream; ophthalmic drop

ACTION & *THERAPEUTIC EFFECT* Sympathomimetic agent that acts directly on alpha receptors of sympathetic nervous system resulting in relief of nasal congestion. *Constricts smaller arterioles in nasal passages and has prolonged decongestant effect.*

USES Relief of nasal congestion in a variety of allergic and infectious disorders of the upper respiratory tract; ocular pruritis (ophthalmic drops); acne rosacea (cream).

CONTRAINDICATIONS Specific contraindications have not been determined; pregnancy—fetal risk cannot be ruled out; lactation—infant risk cannot be ruled out.

CAUTIOUS USE CAD, hypertension, history of narrow-angle glaucoma; children younger than 6 y.

O

ROUTE & DOSAGE

Nasal Congestion

Adult/Adolescent/Child (6 y and older): **Intranasal** 2–3 drops or 2–3 sprays of 0.05% solution into each nostril bid for up to 3 days

Acne Rosacea (cream only)

Adult: Topical Apply thin layer once daily

ADMINISTRATION

Topical

- Prime the pump. Apply a smooth and even layer across entire face (forehead, each cheek, nose, and chin). Avoid eyes and lips. Do not apply to open wounds or irritated skin. Wash hands after application.

Instillation of Nasal Spray

- Shake well before use and place spray nozzle in nostril without occluding it and do not tilt head; instruct patient to sniff briskly during administration.
- Rinse dropper or spray tip in hot water after each use to prevent contamination of solution by nasal secretions.
- Wash hands after administration.

O

ADVERSE EFFECTS (≥5%) HEENT: *Burning,* stinging, dryness of nasal mucosa, *sneezing.* **Other:** Headache, *rebound congestion.*

INTERACTIONS Drug: Do not use nasal preparation with ERGOT DERIVATIVES.

PHARMACOKINETICS Onset: 5–10 min. **Duration:** 6–10 h.

NURSING IMPLICATIONS

Assessment & Drug Effects

- Monitor for S&S of excess use. If noted, discuss possibility of rebound congestion (nasal).
- Monitor for improvement of facial erythema due to rosacea (topical).

Patient & Family Education

- Do not to exceed recommended dosage. Rebound congestion (chemical rhinitis) may occur with prolonged or excessive use (nasal administration).
- Systemic effects can result from swallowing excessive medication (nasal administration).
- Report any development of facial acne.

OXYMETHOLONE

(ox-i-meth′oh-lone)

Anadrol-50

Classification: ANDROGEN/ ANABOLIC STEROID

Therapeutic: ANABOLIC STEROID

Prototype: Testosterone

Controlled Substance: Schedule III

AVAILABILITY Tablet

ACTION & *THERAPEUTIC EFFECT* Mechanism of action in refractory anemias is unclear but may be due to direct stimulation of bone marrow, protein anabolic activity, or to androgenic stimulation of erythropoiesis. *Stimulates formation of red blood cells in the bone marrow. Stimulates bone growth, aids in bone matrix reconstitution.*

USES Aplastic anemia.

CONTRAINDICATIONS Hypersensitivity to oxymetholone;

prostatic hypertrophy with obstruction; prostatic or male breast cancer; carcinoma of the breast in women with hypercalcemia; hepatic decompensation; hepatic carcinoma; nephrosis or nephrotic stage of nephritis; females of childbearing age; pregnancy (category X); lactation.

CAUTIOUS USE Prepubertal males; older males; DM; history of cardiac, renal, or hepatic impairment; CAD; atherosclerosis; children.

ROUTE & DOSAGE

Aplastic Anemia

Adult/Adolescent/Child: **PO** 1–2 mg/kg/day (may require doses up to 5 mg/kg/day)

ADMINISTRATION

Oral

- For treatment of anemias, a minimum trial period of 3–6 mo is recommended, since response tends to be slow.
- Store at 15°–30° C (59°–86° F). Protect from heat and light.

ADVERSE EFFECTS **CV:** *Edema,* skin flush. **Endocrine:** Androgenic in women: Suppression of ovulation, lactation, or menstruation; *hoarseness or deepening of voice* (often irreversible); *hirsutism; oily skin; acne;* clitoral enlargement; regression of breasts; male-pattern baldness. Hypoestrogenic effects in women: Flushing, sweating; vaginitis with pruritus, drying, bleeding; menstrual irregularities. Hypercalcemia. **GI:** *Nausea, vomiting, anorexia,* diarrhea, jaundice, <u>hepatotoxicity</u>. **GU:** Bladder irritability. **Hematologic:** Bleeding (with concurrent anticoagulant therapy), iron deficiency anemia, leukemia. **Other:** Premature epiphyseal closure, phallic enlargement, priapism. Postpubertal: Testicular atrophy, decreased ejaculatory volume, azoospermia, oligospermia (after prolonged administration or excessive dosage), impotence, epididymitis, gynecomastia; increased risk of atherosclerosis.

INTERACTIONS **Drug:** May enhance hypoprothrombinemic effects of **warfarin. Herbal: Echinacea** may increase risk of hepatotoxicity.

PHARMACOKINETICS **Absorption:** Readily from GI tract. **Metabolism:** In liver. **Elimination:** In urine. **Half-Life:** 9 h.

NURSING IMPLICATIONS

Black Box Warning

Oxymetholone has been associated with hepatic dysfunction, liver failure, liver cell tumors, and increased risk of atherosclerosis from blood lipid changes.

Assessment & Drug Effects

- Monitor patient with a history of seizures closely because an increase in their frequency may be noted.
- Monitor periodically for edema that may develop with or without CHF.
- Monitor for and report jaundice or other S&S of hepatotoxicity (see Appendix F). Withhold drug at first sign of liver toxicity.
- Monitor for hypercalcemia (see Appendix F), especially in women with breast cancer.
- Monitor lab tests: Periodic Hgb and Hct, serum iron and iron binding capacity, and LFTs.

O

Patient & Family Education

- Monitor blood glucose for loss of glycemic control if diabetic.
- Stop taking drug and notify prescriber if jaundice appears.
- Women: Notify prescriber of signs of virilization.

OXYMORPHONE HYDROCHLORIDE

(ox-i-mor′fone)

Numorphan, Opana, Opana ER

Classification: NARCOTIC (OPIATE AGONIST); ANALGESIC
Therapeutic: NARCOTIC ANALGESIC
Prototype: Morphine
Controlled Substance: Schedule II

AVAILABILITY Solution for injection; suppository; extended release tablet; tablet

ACTION & *THERAPEUTIC EFFECT* The precise mechanism of the action is unknown; however, specific CNS opioid receptors for endogenous compounds with opioid-like activity have been identified throughout the CNS and play a role in the analgesic effects of this drug. *Effective in relief of moderate to severe pain.*

O

USES Relief of moderate to severe pain, preoperative medication, support of anesthesia.

CONTRAINDICATIONS Hypersensitivity to oxymorphone; pulmonary edema resulting from chemical respiratory irritants; ileus; respiratory depression without appropriate monitoring; acute or severe bronchial asthma; upper airway obstruction; hypercapnia; moderate and severe hepatic function impairment; status asthmaticus.

CAUTIOUS USE Alcoholism; biliary tract disease; bladder obstruction; severe pulmonary disease, respiratory insufficiency, COPD; head injury; circulatory shock; history of seizures; renal impairment; depression; older adults and debilitated patients; pregnancy (category C); lactation; children younger than 18 y.

ROUTE & DOSAGE

Moderate to Severe Pain

Adult: **PO** 10–20 mg q4–6h prn; **Extended release** 5–10 mg q12h; **Subcutaneous/IM** 1–1.5 mg q4–6h prn **IV** 0.5 mg q4–6h then switch to alternate route **PR** 5 mg q4–6h prn

ADMINISTRATION

Oral

- Give on an empty stomach at least 1 h before or 2 h after eating.
- Extended-release tablets must be swallowed whole with enough water to ensure immediate, complete swallowing. Tablets must not be crushed or chewed.

Subcutaneous/Intramuscular

- Give undiluted.

Intravenous

PREPARE: **Direct:** May be given undiluted or diluted in 5 mL of sterile water or NS.
ADMINISTER: **Direct:** Give at a rate of 0.5 mg over 2–5 min.

- Protect drug from light. Store suppositories in refrigerator 2°–15° C (36°–59° F).

ADVERSE EFFECTS **CV:** Cardiac arrest, circulatory depression. **Respiratory:** Respiratory depression (see morphine), apnea, respiratory arrest. **CNS:** *Dizziness,* lightheadedness, sedation. **GI:** *Nausea, vomiting, euphoria.* **Other:** Sweating, coma, shock.

INTERACTIONS **Drug: Alcohol** and other CNS DEPRESSANTS add to CNS depression; **propofol** increases risk of bradycardia.

PHARMACOKINETICS **Onset:** 5–10 min IV; 10–15 min IM; 15–30 min PR. **Peak:** 1–1.5 h. **Duration:** 3–6 h. **Distribution:** Crosses placenta. **Metabolism:** In liver. **Elimination:** In urine. **Half-Life:** PO 7–9 h; extended release 9–11 h.

NURSING IMPLICATIONS

Black Box Warning

Oxymorphone has been associated with high abuse potential, respiratory depression, accidental overdose (especially in children), and death with co-ingestion of alcohol.

Assessment & Drug Effects

- Monitor respiratory rate. Withhold drug and notify prescriber if rate falls below 12 breaths/min.
- Supervise ambulation and advise patient of possible lightheadedness. Older adult and debilitated patients are most susceptible to CNS depressant effects of drug.
- Evaluate patient's continued need for narcotic analgesic. Prolonged use can lead to dependence of morphine type.
- Medication contains sulfite and may precipitate a hypersensitivity reaction in susceptible patient.

Patient & Family Education

- Use caution when walking because of potential for injury from dizziness.
- Do not consume alcohol while taking oxymorphone.

OXYTOCIN INJECTION

(ox-i-toe′sin)

Pitocin

Classification: OXYTOCIC

Therapeutic: OXYTOCIC

AVAILABILITY Solution for injection

ACTION & *THERAPEUTIC EFFECT* Synthetic polypeptide identical pharmacologically to natural oxytocin released by posterior pituitary. By direct action on myofibrils, produces phasic contractions characteristic of normal delivery. Uterine sensitivity to oxytocin increases during gestational period and peaks sharply before parturition. *Effective in initiating or improving uterine contractions at term.*

USES To initiate or improve uterine contraction at term, management of inevitable, incomplete, or missed abortion; stimulation of uterine contractions during third stage of labor; stimulation to overcome uterine inertia; control of postpartum hemorrhage and promotion of postpartum uterine involution. Also used to induce labor in cases of maternal diabetes, preeclampsia, eclampsia, and erythroblastosis fetalis.

CONTRAINDICATIONS Hypersensitivity to oxytocin; significant cephalopelvic disproportion, unfavorable fetal position or presentations that are undeliverable without conversion before delivery, obstetric emergencies that favor surgical intervention, fetal distress in which delivery is not imminent, prematurity, placenta previa, prolonged use in severe toxemia or uterine inertia, hypertonic uterine patterns, conditions predisposing to thromboplastin or amniotic fluid embolism (dead fetus, abruptio placentae), grand multiparity, invasive cervical carcinoma, primipara older than 35 y, past history of uterine sepsis or of traumatic delivery; pregnancy (category C).

CAUTIOUS USE Preeclampsia; history of seizures; history of mental hypertension.

ROUTE & DOSAGE

Labor Induction

Adult: **IV** 0.5–2 milliunits/min, may increase by 1–2 milliunits/min q15–60 min (max: 20 milliunits/min); dose is decreased when labor is established; **High dose regimen** 6 milliunits/min, may increase by 6 milliunits/min q15–60 min until contraction pattern established.

Postpartum Bleeding

Adult: **IM** 10 units total dose; **IV** Infuse a total of 10–40 units at a rate of 20–40 milliunits/min after delivery

Incomplete Abortion

Adult: **IV** 10–20 milliunits/min

ADMINISTRATION

Intramuscular

- NIOSH recommends the use of double gloves and protective gown. During administration, if there is a potential that the substance could splash or if the patient may resist, use eye/face protection.
- Give 10 units IM after delivery of the placenta.

Intravenous

PREPARE: **IV Infusion:** When diluting oxytocin for IV infusion, rotate bottle gently to distribute medicine throughout solution. **IV Infusion for Inducing Labor:** Add 10 units (1 mL) to 1 L of D5W, NS, LR, or D5NS to yield 10 milliunits/mL. **IV Infusion for Postpartum Bleeding/Incomplete Abortion:** Add 10–40 units (1–4 mL) to 1 L of D5W, NS, LR, or D5NS to yield 10–40 milliunits/mL.

ADMINISTER: **IV Infusion:** Use an infusion pump for accurate control of infusion rate. **IV Infusion for Inducing Labor:** Initially infuse 0.5–2 milliunits/min; increase by 1–2 milliunits/min at 30–60 min intervals. **IV Infusion for Postpartum Bleeding:** Initially infuse 10–40 milliunits/min, then adjust to control uterine atony. **IV Infusion for Incomplete Abortion:** Infuse 10–20 milliunits/min. Do not exceed 30 units in 12 h.

INCOMPATIBILITIES: **Y-site: Amphotericin B, ampicillin, chlorpromazine, dantrolene, diazepam, diazoxide, dimenhydrinate, haloperidol, hydralazine, inamrinone lactate, indomethacin, insulin, methohexital, pantoprazole, phenytoin, sulfamethoxazole/trimethoprim.**

ADVERSE EFFECTS **CV:** Dysrhythmia, fetal bradycardia, hypertensive episodes. **CNS:** Brain injury, central nervous system deficit, coma, convulsion. **Endocrine:** Water intoxication. **GI:** Nausea, vomiting. **GU:** Pelvic hematoma. **Hematologic:** Afibrinogenemia.

INTERACTIONS **Drug:** VASOCONSTRICTORS cause severe hypertension; **cyclopropane anesthesia** causes hypotension, maternal bradycardia, arrhythmias. **Herbal: Ephedra, ma huang** may cause hypertension.

PHARMACOKINETICS **Duration:** 1 h. **Distribution:** Distributed throughout extracellular fluid; small amount may cross placenta. **Metabolism:** Rapidly destroyed in liver and kidneys. **Elimination:** Small amounts excreted unchanged in urine. **Half-Life:** 3–5 min.

NURSING IMPLICATIONS

Assessment & Drug Effects

- Start flow charts to record maternal BP and other vital signs, I&O ratio, weight, strength, duration, and frequency of contractions, as well as fetal heart tone and rate, before instituting treatment.
- Monitor fetal heart rate and maternal BP and pulse at least q15min during infusion period; evaluate tonus of myometrium during and between contractions and record on flow chart. Report change in rate and rhythm immediately.
- Stop infusion to prevent fetal anoxia, turn patient on her side, and notify prescriber if contractions are prolonged (occurring at less than 2-min intervals) and if monitor records contractions about 50 mm Hg or if contractions last 90 sec or longer. Stimulation will wane rapidly within 2–3 min. Oxygen administration may be necessary.
- If local or regional (caudal, spinal) anesthesia is being given to the patient receiving oxytocin, be alert to the possibility of hypertensive crisis (sudden intense occipital headache, palpitation, marked hypertension, stiff neck, nausea, vomiting, sweating, fever, photophobia, dilated pupils, bradycardia or tachycardia, constricting chest pain).
- Monitor I&O during labor. If patient is receiving drug by prolonged IV infusion, watch for symptoms of water intoxication (drowsiness, listlessness, headache, confusion, anuria, weight gain). Report changes in alertness and orientation and changes in I&O ratio (i.e., marked decrease in output with excessive intake).
- Check fundus frequently during the first few postpartum hours and several times daily thereafter.

Patient & Family Education

- Be aware of purpose and anticipated effect of oxytocin.
- Report sudden, severe headache immediately to health care providers.

OZENOXACIN

(oz-en-ox'a sin)

Xepi

Classification: QUINOLONE ANTIBIOTIC

Therapeutic: ANTIBIOTIC

Prototype: Ciprofloxacin

AVAILABILITY Topical 1% external cream

ACTION & *THERAPEUTIC EFFECT* Similar to other quinolone antibiotics, inhibits DNA gyrase A and topoisomerase IV, enzymes responsible for bacterial DNA replication. *Bactericidal against S. aureus and S. pyogenes which treats common impetigo infections.*

USES Treatment of impetigo.

CAUTIOUS USE Prolonged use may result in overgrowth of resistant bacteria or fungi; only for external topical use.

ROUTE & DOSAGE

Impetigo

Adult and Child: **Topical** Apply a thin film 2 × day for five days to the affected areas

ADMINISTRATION

Topical

- Apply a thin film of cream 2 × day to the affected area.
- Wash hands after application. Treated area may be covered with a sterile bandage or gauze dressing.
- Store at 20°–25° C (68°–77° F).

ADVERSE EFFECTS **Skin:** Rosacea, seborrheic dermatitis.

PHARMACOKINETICS **Absorption:** Due to topical application, negligible systemic absorption. **Elimination:** Not metabolized.

P

NURSING IMPLICATIONS

Assessment & Drug Effects

- Assess for effective use and severe skin irritation.

Patient & Family Education

- Apply medication topically only.
- Report any skin irritation to your provider.

PACLITAXEL

(pac-li-tax′el)

Abraxane, Taxol

Classification: ANTINEOPLASTIC TAXANE

Therapeutic: ANTINEOPLASTIC; ANTIMICROTUBULE

AVAILABILITY Solution for injection; powder for injection (with 900 mg human albumin)

ACTION & *THERAPEUTIC EFFECT* During cell division paclitaxel acts as an antimicrotubular agent that interferes with the microtubule network essential for interphase and mitosis. This results in abnormal spindle formation during mitosis. *Interferes with growth of rapidly dividing cells including cancer cells, and eventually causes cell death. Additionally, the breakup of the cytoskeleton within non-dividing cells interrupts intracellular transport and communications.*

USES Ovarian cancer, breast cancer, Kaposi's sarcoma, non–small-cell lung cancer (NSCLC).

UNLABELED USES Squamous cell head and neck cancer, small-cell lung cancer, endometrial cancer, esophageal cancer, gastric cancer, testicular cancer, germ cell tumors, and other solid tumors, leukemia, melanoma.

CONTRAINDICATIONS **Taxol:** Hypersensitivity to paclitaxel, or taxanes; baseline neutrophil count less than 1500 cells/mm^3; thrombocytopenia; with AIDS-related Kaposi's sarcoma baseline neutrophil count less than 1000 cells/mm^3; pregnancy (category D); lactation (infant risk cannot be ruled out). For **Abraxane:** Baseline neutrophil count less than 1500 cells/mm^3.

CAUTIOUS USE Cardiac arrhythmias, cardiac disease; impaired liver function; alcoholism; older adults; peripheral neuropathy. Safety and efficacy in children not established.

ROUTE & DOSAGE

Ovarian Cancer, NSCLC

Adult: **IV** 135 mg/m^2 over 24 h infusion repeated q3wk

Breast Cancer

Adult: **IV** 175 mg/m^2 over 3 h q3wk
Abraxane: **IV** 260 mg/m^2 over 30 min q3wk

Kaposi's Sarcoma

Adult: **IV** 135 mg/m^2 infused over 3 h q3wk or 100 mg/m^2 infused over 3 h q2wk

ADMINISTRATION

Intravenous

▪ NIOSH recommends double gloves and a protective gown when handling. If there is a potential for a splash or the patient may resist, use eye/face protection. Note: Premedication is required (except with **Abraxane**) to avoid severe hypersensitivity. ▪ Follow institutional or standard guidelines for preparation, handling, and disposal of cytotoxic agents.

PREPARE: **IV Infusion: Dilution of Conventional Paclitaxel:** Do not use equipment or devices containing polyvinyl chloride (PVC) in preparation of infusion. ▪ Dilute to a final concentration of 0.3–1.2 mg/mL in any of the following: D5W, NS, D5/NS, or D5W in Ringer's injection. The prepared solution may be hazy, but this does not indicate a loss of potency. **Abraxane Vial Reconstitution:** Slowly inject 20 mL NS over at least 1 min onto the inside wall of the vial to yield 5 mg/mL. ▪ **Do not** inject directly into the cake powder. Allow vial to sit for at least 5 min, then gently swirl for at least 2 min to completely dissolve. If foaming occurs, let stand for at least 15 min until foam subsides. ▪ If particulates or settling are visible, gently invert vial to ensure complete resuspension prior to use. ▪ Remove the required dose and inject into an empty sterile, PVC or non-PVC type IV bag.

ADMINISTER: **IV Infusion:** Because tissue necrosis occurs with extravasation, frequently assess patency of a peripheral IV site. ▪ **Conventional Paclitaxel:** Infuse over 1–24 h through IV tubing containing an in-line (0.22 -micron or less) filter. Do not use equipment containing PVC. ▪ **Abraxane: Do not** use an in-line filter. Infuse over 30 min.

INCOMPATIBILITIES: **Solution/additive: PVC bags** and **infusion sets** should be avoided (except with Abraxane) due to leaching of DEHP (plasticizer). ▪ Do not mix with any other medications. **Y-site: Amiodarone hydrochloride, amphotericin B, amphotericin B cholesteryl sulfate complex, chlorpromazine, diazepam, digoxin, doxorubicin liposome, gemtuzumab, hydroxyzine, idarubicin, indomethacin, labetalol, methylprednisolone, mitoxantrone, phenytoin, propranolol.**

▪ **Conventional paclitaxel** solutions diluted for infusion are stable at room temperature (approximately 25° C/77° F) for up to 27 h. ▪ Reconstituted **Abraxane** should be used immediately but may be kept refrigerated for up to 8 h if needed.

ADVERSE EFFECTS

CV: *Flushing, edema,* hypotension.

CNS: *Peripheral neuropathy.* **Skin:** *Alopecia,* rash. **Hepatic:** Increased serum alkaline phosphatase, increased serum AST. **GI:** *Diarrhea, inflammation of mucous membrane, nausea, vomiting.* **Musculoskeletal:** Weakness. **Hematologic:** *Anemia, lekopenia, neutropenia, thrombocytopenia.*

INTERACTIONS Drug: Increased myelosuppression if **cisplatin, doxorubicin** is given before paclitaxel; **ketoconazole** can inhibit metabolism of paclitaxel; additive bradycardia with BETA-BLOCKERS, **digoxin, verapamil;** additive risk of bleeding with ANTICOAGULANTS, NSAIDS, PLATELET INHIBITORS (including **aspirin**), THROMBOLYTIC AGENTS. Do not use with LIVE VACCINES, **conivaptan, deferiprone, dipyrone, natalizumab, pimecrolimus, tacrolimus.**

PHARMACOKINETICS Distribution: Greater than 90% protein bound; does not cross CSF. **Metabolism:** In liver (CYP3A4, 2C8). **Elimination:** Feces 70%, urine 14%. **Half-Life:** 1–9 h.

P

NURSING IMPLICATIONS

Black Box Warning

Paclitaxel has been associated with severe hypersensitivity, anaphylaxis, and neutropenia.

Assessment & Drug Effects

- Monitor for hypersensitivity reactions, especially during first and second administrations of the paclitaxel. S&S requiring treatment, but not necessarily discontinuation of the drug, include dyspnea, hypotension, and chest pain. Discontinue immediately and manage symptoms aggressively if angioedema and generalized urticaria develop.
- Monitor vital signs frequently, especially during the first hour of infusion. Bradycardia occurs in approximately 12% of patients, usually during infusion. It does not normally require treatment. Cardiac monitoring is indicated for those with severe conduction abnormalities.
- Monitor for anemia, neutropenia, and thrombocytopenia.
- Monitor for peripheral neuropathy, the severity of which is dose dependent. Severe symptoms occur primarily with higher than recommended doses.
- Monitor lab tests: Periodic CBC with differential and platelet count, and Hct & Hgb throughout course of treatment.

Patient & Family Education

- Immediately report to prescriber S&S of paclitaxel hypersensitivity: Difficulty breathing, chest pain, palpitations, angioedema (subcutaneous swelling usually around face and neck), and skin rashes or itching.
- Be sure to have periodic blood work as prescribed.
- Avoid aspirin, NSAIDS, and alcohol to minimize GI distress.
- Be aware of high probability of developing hair loss (greater than 80%).

PALBOCICLIB

(pal-bo-cyc′lib)

Ibrance

Classification: ANTINEOPLASTIC; KINASE INHIBITOR; CYCLIN-DEPENDENT KINASE (CDK) INHIBITOR

Therapeutic: ANTINEOPLASTIC

 Common adverse effects in *italic;* life-threatening effects underlined; generic names in **bold;** classifications in SMALL CAPS; ♣ Canadian drug name; ⊙ Prototype drug; ⚠ Alert

AVAILABILITY Capsules

ACTION & THERAPEUTIC EFFECT Inhibits an enzyme (cyclin-dependent kinase) that is essential for cancer cells to progress through the cell cycle at the G1/S phase. *Reduces proliferation of breast cancer cells by preventing progression through the cell cycle.*

USES Treatment of postmenopausal women with estrogen receptor (ER) positive, human epidermal growth factor receptor 2 (HER2) negative advanced breast cancer in combination with letrozole.

CONTRAINDICATIONS Pregnancy; lactation.

CAUTIOUS USE Concomitant use of moderate or strong CYP3A4 inhibitor; grapefruit products; bone marrow suppression; infection; thromboembolic events including pulmonary embolism.

ROUTE & DOSAGE

Breast Cancer

Adult: **PO** 125 mg once daily in combination with letrozole for 21 days, followed by 7 days with letrozole only; repeat cycle until progressive disease or unacceptable toxicity occur

Hematologic Toxicity Dosage Adjustment

Grade 3: Withhold initiation of next cycle until recovery to Grade 2 or less
Grade 3 with ANC (less than 1000 to 500/mm³) and Fever 38.5° C (101.3° F) or greater and/or infection: Withhold until recovery to Grade 2 or less (at least 1000/mm³); resume at 100 mg once daily if first occurrence or 75 mg once daily if second occurrence
Grade 4: Withhold until recovery to Grade 2 or less; resume at 100 mg once daily if first occurrence or 75 mg once daily if second occurrence

Non-Hematologic Toxicity Dosage Adjustment

Grade 3 or higher: Withhold until recovery to Grade 2 or less depending on toxicity; resume at 100 mg once daily if first occurrence or 75 mg once daily if second occurrence

Co-Administered Strong CYP3A Inhibitor Dosage Adjustment

Decrease dose to 75 mg once daily

ADMINISTRATION

Oral

- Give with food at approximately the same time each day.
- Capsules must be swallowed whole. They must not be crushed, chewed, or opened prior to swallowing (do not administer if capsules are broken, cracked, or not fully intact).
- Do not administer with grapefruit juice.
- Store at 20°–25° C (68°–77° F).

ADVERSE EFFECTS Respiratory: Epistaxis, pulmonary embolism, *upper respiratory infection*. **Endocrine:** Decreased appetite. **Skin:** *Alopecia*. **GI:** *Diarrhea, nausea, stomatitis*, vomiting. **Hematologic:** *Anemia, leukopenia, neutropenia*, thrombocytopenia. **Other:** Asthenia, *fatigue*, peripheral neuropathy.

INTERACTIONS **Drug:** Concomitant use of strong CYP3A inhibitors (e.g., **clarithromycin, indinavir, itraconazole, ketoconazole, lopinavir/ritonavir, nefazodone, nelfinavir, posaconazole, ritonavir, saquinavir, telaprevir, telithromycin, verapamil,** and **voriconazole**) increases the levels of palbociclib. Concomitant use of strong CYP3A inducers (e.g., **phenytoin, rifampin, carbamazepine**) decreases the levels of palbociclib. Concomitant use of moderate CYP3A inducers (e.g., **bosentan, efavirenz, etravirine, modafinil, nafcillin**) may decrease the levels of palbociclib. Palbociclib increases the levels of midazolam. Palbociclib may increase the levels of other drugs requiring CYP3A isozymes (e.g., **alfentanil, cyclosporine, dihydroergotamine, ergotamine, everolimus, fentanyl, pimozide, quinidine, sirolimus, tacrolimus**). **Food: Grapefruit** or **grapefruit juice** may increase the levels of palbociclib. **Herbal: St John's wort** decreases the levels of palbociclib.

P

PHARMACOKINETICS **Absorption:** 46% bioavailable. **Peak:** 6–12 h. **Distribution:** 85% plasma protein bound. **Metabolism:** In liver. **Elimination:** Fecal (74.1%) and renal (17.5%). **Half-Life:** 29 h.

NURSING IMPLICATIONS

Assessment & Drug Effects

- Monitor for and report promptly S&S of infection; report fever of 101° F or greater.
- Monitor for S&S of pulmonary embolism (e.g., shortness of breath, anxiety, chest pain, hemoptysis, fainting, irregular or rapid HR).
- Monitor lab tests: Baseline CBC with differential, repeat q2wk for first 2 cycles, then prior to each cycle or more often if indicated.

Patient & Family Education

- Report immediately to prescriber any of the following S&S: Fever, chills, dizziness, weakness, increased tendency to bleed and/or bruise, shortness of breath or rapid breathing, chest pain, or rapid heart rate.
- Do not consume grapefruit or grapefruit juice while taking this drug.
- Women should use effective contraception during treatment and for at least 2 wk after the last dose.
- Do not breast-feed while taking this drug.

PALIFERMIN

(pal-i-fur′men)

Kepivance

Classification: BIOLOGIC RESPONSE MODIFIER; KERATINOCYTE GROWTH FACTOR; CYTOKINE

Therapeutic: KERATINOCYTE GROWTH FACTOR (KGF)

AVAILABILITY Powder for injection

ACTION & *THERAPEUTIC EFFECT*

Naturally occurring keratinocyte growth factor (KGF) is produced and regulated in response to epithelial tissue injury. Binding of KGF to its receptors in epithelial cells results in proliferation, differentiation, and repair of injury to epithelial cells. Palifermin is a synthetic form of KGF; thus it enhances replacement of injured cells. *Reduces the incidence of severe oral mucositis that interferes with food consumption in the cancer patient.*

USES Reduction of the incidence and duration of severe oral mucositis in patients with hematologic malignancies who are receiving myelotoxic therapy requiring hematopoietic stem cell support.

CONTRAINDICATIONS Hypersensitivity to *Escherichia coli*-derived protein, palifermin; nonhematologic malignancies; within 24 h of chemotherapy; lactation.

CAUTIOUS USE Use contraception for females of childbearing age; pregnancy (category C); children.

ROUTE & DOSAGE

Mucositis Prophylaxis

Adult: **IV** 60 mcg/kg/day for 3 days before and 3 days after myelotoxic therapy (total: 6 doses)

ADMINISTRATION

Intravenous

Do not give within 24 h before/after or during myelotoxic chemotherapy.

PREPARE: **Direct:** Use double gloves and protective gown while preparing and administering. If there is any chance that the patient may resist, wear eye/face protection. Reconstitute powder with 1.2 mL sterile water **only** to yield 5 mg/mL. Gently swirl to dissolve but do not shake. ▪ Powder will dissolve in about 3 min. Should be used immediately.

ADMINISTER: **Direct:** Give as a bolus dose. ▪ If heparin is used to maintain the IV line, flush before/after with NS. ▪ If diluted solution was refrigerated (max refrigeration time: 24 h), may warm to room temperature for up to 1 h but protect from light.

INCOMPATIBILITIES: **Y-site: Heparin.**

▪ Store powder vial at 2°–8° C (36°–46° F). Protect from light. ▪ If needed, may store reconstituted solution refrigerated for up to 24 h. ▪ Discard any reconstituted solution left at room temperature for longer than 1 h.

ADVERSE EFFECTS **CNS:** *Dysesthesia.* **Endocrine:** *Elevated serum amylase, elevated serum lipase.* **Skin:** *Erythema, pruritus, rash.* **GI:** *Mouth/tongue thickness or discoloration, taste alterations, abdominal pain, anorexia, vomiting.* **GU:** Proteinuria. **Musculoskeletal:** *Arthralgia.* **Other:** *Edema, arthralgia, fever, pain.*

INTERACTIONS **Drug:** Should not be administered within 24 h before, during infusion of or within 24 h after administration of ANTINEOPLASTIC agents.

PHARMACOKINETICS **Distribution:** Extravascular distribution. **Half-Life:** 4.5 h.

NURSING IMPLICATIONS

Assessment & Drug Effects

- Monitor for improvement in mucositis.
- Monitor for S&S of oral toxicities and skin toxicities.

Patient & Family Education

- Report any of the following to a health care provider: Alteration of taste, discoloration or enlargement of the tongue, lack of sensation around the mouth, skin rash, itching, or edema.

P

PALIPERIDONE

(pa-li′per-i-done)

Invega

PALIPERIDONE PALMITATE

Invega Sustenna, Invega Trinza

Classification: ATYPICAL ANTI-PSYCHOTIC

Therapeutic: ANTIPSYCHOTIC

Prototype: Clozapine

AVAILABILITY Extended release tablet; solution for injection

ACTION & *THERAPEUTIC EFFECT* While the mechanism is unknown, its proposed action interferes with binding of dopamine to dopamine type 2 (D2) receptors, serotonin (5-HT2A) receptors, and alpha-adrenergic receptors. *Effective in controlling symptoms of schizophrenia as well as other psychotic symptoms.*

USES Treatment of schizophrenia, schizoaffective disorder.

P

UNLABELED USES Agitation associated with dementia, bipolar disorder.

CONTRAINDICATIONS Hypersensitivity to paliperidone, risperidone; concurrent administration with drugs that produce QT_c prolongation; severe GI narrowing (pathologic or iatrogenic); drug induced NMS; older adults with dementia-related psychosis; pregnancy—fetal risk cannot be ruled out; lactation—infant risk cannot be ruled out.

CAUTIOUS USE History of cerebrovascular events; hypovolemia, dehydration; cardiovascular disease; QT prolongation; history of cardiac arrhythmias; risk factors for hypotension; renal impairment; CNS pathology; history of seizures; systemic infection; DM; hyperglycemia; obesity; Parkinson's disease; Lewy bodies dementia; older adults; children younger than 12 y.

ROUTE & DOSAGE

Schizophrenia

Adult: **PO** Initially 6 mg/day; may adjust up/down in 3 mg increments; at least 5 day intervals needed for dosage increments (max: 12 mg/day); **IM** 234 mg on day 1, then 156 mg on day 8, then monthly dose of 117 mg (dose may vary based on patient response)
Adolescent: **PO** 3 mg daily

Schizoaffective Disorder

Adult: **PO** 6 mg daily, dose adjusted at intervals of more than 4 days (max: 12 mg/day); **IM** 234 mg on day 1, then 156 mg on day 8, then monthly dose of 117 mg (dose may vary based on patient response)

Renal Impairment Dosage Adjustment

CrCl 50–79 mL/min: Max: **PO** 6 mg/day; **IM** 156 mg on day 1 and 117 mg 1 wk later, then monthly 78 mg injections; *CrCl 10–49 mL/min:* Max: **PO** 3 mg/day; **IM** not recommended

ADMINISTRATION

Oral

- Extended release tablets **must be** swallowed whole. They should not be chewed or crushed.
- Give in the morning with or without food.
- Store extended release tablets at 25 degrees C (77 degrees F), with excursion permitted to 15 to

30 degrees C (59 to 86 degrees F). Protect from moisture.

Intramuscular

- Give as a single injection; do not administer in divided doses. Must be administered by a healthcare provider.
- First 2 doses on day 1 and 1 wk later: Inject slowly, deep into the deltoid muscle.
- Monthly maintenance dose: Inject slowly, deep into the deltoid or gluteal muscle.
- Store extended release tablets at 25 degrees C (77 degrees F), with excursion permitted to 15 to 30 degrees C (59 to 86 degrees F).

ADVERSE EFFECTS (≥ 5%) CV: *tachycardia*. **Respiratory:** Nasopharyngitis. **CNS:** *Akathisia, anxiety,* dystonia, dyskinesia, extrapyramidal disorder, Parkinsonism, *somnolence,* tremor. **Endocrine:** Hyperprolactinemia, weight gain. **GI:** Dyspepsia, constipation.

INTERACTIONS Drug: Enhanced CNS depression with **alcohol** or CNS DEPRESSANTS. Paliperidone may enhance the effects of ANTIHYPERTENSIVE AGENTS. Paliperidone can diminish the effects of DOPAMINE AGONISTS **(levodopa, cabergoline, pergolide, pramipexole, ropinirole);** ANTIPARKINSON AGENTS. **Carbamazepine** decreases effectiveness. Avoid with agents that increase QT interval (e.g., **bepridil, ziprasidone**). Avoid CYP3A4 inhibitors (e.g., AZOLE ANTIFUNGALS). **Amisulpride** may increase risk of adverse effects. **Food:** High-fat/high-caloric meal increases paliperidone levels.

PHARMACOKINETICS Absorption: Bioavailability is 28%. **Peak:** 24 h. **Distribution:** 74% protein bound. **Metabolism:** In liver (26–41%). **Elimination:** Urine (major, 50–70% unchanged) and stool (minor). **Half-Life:** 23 h.

NURSING IMPLICATIONS

Black Box Warning

Paliperidone has been associated with increased mortality in older adults with dementia-related psychosis.

Assessment & Drug Effects

- Baseline ECG recommended to rule out congenital, long-QT syndrome.
- Prior to initiating therapy, hypokalemia and hypo-magnesemia should be corrected.
- Monitor weight.
- Monitor CV status and monitor orthostatic BP especially in those prone to hypotension.
- Reassess patient periodically in order to maintain on the lowest effective drug dose.
- Monitor closely neurologic status of older adults.
- Supervise closely those with suicidal ideation.
- Monitor closely those at risk for seizures.
- Assess degree of cognitive and motor impairment, and assess for environmental hazards.
- Monitor diabetics for loss of glycemic control.
- Monitor lab tests: Baseline and periodic serum electrolytes; periodic renal function tests, LFTs, lipid profile, thyroid function tests, blood glucose, and CBC.

Patient & Family Education

- Exercise caution with hazardous activities until response to drug is known.
- The capsule should be swallowed whole.

P

- Risk of orthostatic hypotension. Encourage rising slowly from sitting/supine position.
- Use caution when participating in activities leading to an increased core temperature such as strenuous exercise, exposure to extreme heat or dehydration.
- Do not be surprised by seeing the tablet shell and core components in the stool because they are insoluble.
- Avoid alcohol while taking this medication.
- Carefully monitor blood glucose levels if diabetic.
- Be aware of the risk of orthostatic hypotension.
- Monitor for signs and symptoms of suicidal ideation.
- Be aware of the possibility of seizure activity.

PALIVIZUMAB

(pal-i-viz′u-mab)

Synagis

Classification:
IMMUNOMODULATOR; MONOCLONAL ANTIBODY; IMMUNOGLOBULIN
Therapeutic: IMMUNOGLOBULIN (IGG)

P

AVAILABILITY Solution for injection

ACTION & *THERAPEUTIC EFFECT*
Exhibits neutralizing and fusion-inhibitory activity against the respiratory syncytial virus (RSV). *Provides passive immunity against respiratory syncytial virus. Indicated by prevention of lower respiratory tract infection.*

USES Prevention of serious lower respiratory tract infections in children susceptible to RSV.

CONTRAINDICATIONS Hypersensitivity to palivizumab.

CAUTIOUS USE Hypersensitivity to other immunoglobulin preparations, blood products, or other medications; kidney or liver dysfunction; acute RSV infection; pregnancy (category C).

ROUTE & DOSAGE

RSV

Child: **IM** 15 mg/kg qmo during RSV season

ADMINISTRATION

Intramuscular

- Give IM only into the anterolateral aspect of the thigh. Volumes greater than 1 mL should be divided and given in different sites.

ADVERSE EFFECTS **Respiratory:** *URI, rhinitis,* pharyngitis, cough, wheeze, bronchiolitis, asthma, croup, dyspnea, sinusitis, apnea. **Skin:** *Rash*. **GI:** Increased AST, diarrhea, nausea, vomiting, gastroenteritis. **Other:** *Otitis media,* pain, hernia.

PHARMACOKINETICS **Half-Life:** 20 days.

NURSING IMPLICATIONS

Assessment & Drug Effects

- Monitor carefully for and immediately report S&S of respiratory illness including fever, cough, wheezing, and chest retractions.
- Assess for and report erythema or indurations at injection site.

Patient & Family Education

- Contact prescriber for S&S of respiratory illness, vomiting, diarrhea, or if redness develops at injection site.

PALONOSETRON

(pal-o-no′si-tron)

Aloxi

Classification: SEROTONIN 5-HT_3 RECEPTOR ANTAGONIST; ANTIEMETIC

Therapeutic: ANTIEMETIC

Prototype: Ondansetron

AVAILABILITY Solution for injection

ACTION & *THERAPEUTIC EFFECT* Selectively blocks serotonin 5-HT_3 receptors found centrally in the chemoreceptor trigger zone (CTZ) of the hypothalamus, and peripherally at vagal nerve endings in the intestines. *Prevents acute chemotherapy-induced nausea and vomiting associated with initial and repeat courses of moderately or highly emetogenic chemotherapy.*

USES Prevention of acute and delayed nausea and vomiting associated with highly emetogenic cancer chemotherapy; post-operative nausea/vomiting.

CONTRAINDICATIONS Hypersensitivity to palonosetron.

CAUTIOUS USE Dehydration; cardiac arrhythmias, QT prolongation; electrolyte imbalance; pregnancy (category B); lactation; children younger than 18 y.

ROUTE & DOSAGE

Prevention of Chemotherapy-Induced Nausea and Vomiting

Adult: **IV** 0.25 mg infused over 30 sec 30 min prior to chemotherapy; do not repeat for at least 7 days

Child: **IV** 20 mcg/kg Infused over 15 min prior to chemotherapy

Post-Operative Nausea/Vomiting

Adult: **IV** 0.075 mg single dose administered over 10 sec immediately before anesthesia

ADMINISTRATION

Intravenous

PREPARE: **Direct:** Do not dilute and do not mix with other drugs. ***ADMINISTER:*** Prevention of chemotherapy-induced nausea and vomiting. **Direct:** Give 30 min prior to start of chemotherapy. Adults: Give over 30 sec. Children: Give over 15 min. Flush IV line with NS before and after administration. Prevention of nausea and vomiting; infuse over 10 sec prior to anesthesia induction.
INCOMPATIBILITIES: Do not mix with other drugs.

- Store at room temperature of 15°–30° C (59°–86° F). Protect from light.

ADVERSE EFFECTS **CNS:** Headache, anxiety, dizziness. **GI:** Constipation, diarrhea, abdominal pain. **Cardiac:** Prolonged QT interval. **Dermatologic:** Pruritus.

INTERACTIONS **Drug:** Can cause profound hypotension with **apomorphine**. May cause serotonin syndrome with other serotonergic drugs (e.g., SSRI).

PHARMACOKINETICS **Metabolism:** In liver (CYP2D6, 1A2, 3A4). **Elimination:** Primarily renal. **Half-Life:** 40 h.

P

NURSING IMPLICATIONS

Assessment & Drug Effects

- Monitor closely cardiac status especially in those taking diuretics or otherwise at risk for hypokalemia or hypomagnesemia, with congenital QT syndrome, or patients taking antiarrhythmic or other drugs that lead to QT prolongation.

Patient & Family Education

- Report promptly any of the following: Difficulty breathing, wheezing, or shortness of breath; palpitations or chest tightness; skin rash or itching; swelling of the face, tongue, throat, hands, or feet.

PAMIDRONATE DISODIUM

(pa-mi'dro-nate)

Classification: BISPHOSPHONATE
Therapeutic: BONE METABOLISM REGULATORY
Prototype: Etidronate

AVAILABILITY Powder for injection; solution for injection

ACTION & *THERAPEUTIC EFFECT* A bone-resorption inhibitor thought to absorb calcium phosphate crystals into bone. May also inhibit osteoclast activity, thus contributing to inhibition of bone resorption. *Reduces bone turnover and, when used in combination with adequate hydration, it increases renal excretion of calcium, thus reducing serum calcium concentrations.*

USES Hypercalcemia of malignancy and Paget's disease, bone metastases in multiple myeloma or breast cancer.

UNLABELED USES Primary hyperparathyroidism, osteoporosis prophylaxis.

CONTRAINDICATIONS Hypersensitivity to pamidronate; breast cancer, severe renal disease, hypercalcemia, hypercholesterolemia, polycythemia, prostatic cancer; pregnancy (category D); lactation (infant risk cannot be ruled out).

CAUTIOUS USE Hypersensitivity to pamidronate or other bisphosphonates; heart failure, nephrosis or nephrotic syndrome, moderate renal disease, chronic kidney failure; hepatic disease, cholestasis; peripheral edema, prostate hypertrophy; cancer patients with stomatitis; older adults. Safe use in children not established.

ROUTE & DOSAGE

Moderate Hypercalcemia of Malignancy (corrected calcium 12–13.5 mg/dL)

Adult: **IV** 60–90 mg may repeat in 7 days

Severe Hypercalcemia of Malignancy (corrected calcium greater than 13.5 mg/dL)

Adult: **IV** 90 may repeat in 7 days

Paget's Disease

Adult: **IV** 30 mg once daily for 3 days (90 mg total)

Osteolytic Metastases

Adult: **IV** 90 mg once/mo

ADMINISTRATION

Intravenous

PREPARE: NIOSH recommends the use of double gloves and protective gown. During administration, if there is potential that the substance could splash or if the patient may resist, use eye/face protection. **IV Infusion:** Add 10 mL sterile water for injection to reconstitute the 30 or 90 mg vial to yield 3 or 9 mg/mL, respectively. Allow to completely dissolve. **IV Infusion for Hypercalcemia of Malignancy:** Withdraw the required dose and dilute in D5W, NS, or 1/2NS as follows: Use 1000 mL. **IV Infusion for Paget's Disease and Multiple Myeloma:** Withdraw the required dose and dilute in D5W, NS, or 1/2NS as follows: Use 500 mL. **IV Infusion for Breast Cancer Bone Metastases:** Withdraw the required dose and dilute in D5W, NS, or 1/2NS as follows: Use 250 mL.

ADMINISTER: **IV Infusion:** Regulate infusion rate carefully. Rapid infusion may cause renal damage. **IV Infusion for Hypercalcemia of Malignancy:** Infuse over 2–24 h. **IV Infusion for Paget's Disease and Multiple Myeloma:** Infuse over 4 h. **IV Infusion for Breast Cancer Bone Metastases:** Infuse over 2 h.

INCOMPATIBILITIES: **Solution/additive:** **Hetastarch,** CALCIUM-CONTAINING SOLUTIONS (including **lactated Ringer's**). **Y-site:** **Amphotericin B, caspofungin, dantrolene, diazepam, gemtuzumab, leucovorin, phenytoin.**

- Refrigerate reconstituted pamidronate solution at 2°–8° C (36°–46° F); the IV solution may be stored at room temperature. Both are stable for 24 h.

ADVERSE EFFECTS

CV: Hypertension. **Respiratory:** *Dyspnea, cough.* **CNS:** *Fatigue,* hypercalcemia, *headache, insomnia,* anxiety, pain. **Endocrine:** Hypophosphatemia, hypokalemia, hypocalcemia, hypomagnesemia. **GI:** *Nausea, vomiting, anorexia,* abdominal pain. **GU:** UTI, increased creatinine. **Musculoskeletal:** Muscle pain, weakness, joint pain. **Hematologic:** Anemia. **Other:** Fever.

DIAGNOSTIC TEST INTERFERENCE

May interfere with diagnostic imaging agents such as technetium-99m-diphosphonate in bone scans.

INTERACTIONS

Drug: Concurrent use of **foscarnet** may further decrease serum levels of ionized calcium.

PHARMACOKINETICS

Absorption: 50% of dose is retained in body. **Onset:** 24–48 h. **Peak:** 6 days. **Duration:** 2 wk–3 mo. **Distribution:** Accumulates in bone; once deposited, remains bound until bone is remodeled. **Metabolism:** Not metabolized. **Elimination:** 50% excreted in urine unchanged. **Half-Life:** 28 h.

NURSING IMPLICATIONS

Assessment & Drug Effects

- Assess IV injection site for thrombophlebitis.
- Monitor for S&S of hypocalcemia, hypokalemia, hypomagnesemia, and hypophosphatemia. Continue monitoring for hypocalcemia at least 2 wk after treatment completed.
- Monitor for seizures especially in those with a preexisting seizure disorder.
- Monitor vital signs. Be aware that drug fever, which may occur with pamidronate use, is self-limiting, usually subsiding in 48 h even with continued therapy.

- Monitor I&O and hydration status. Patient should be adequately hydrated, without fluid overload.
- Monitor lab tests: Baseline and prior to each treatment serum creatinine; frequent serum electrolytes; periodic CBC with differential.

Patient & Family Education

- Be aware that transient, self-limiting fever with/without chills may develop.
- Generalized malaise, which may last for several weeks following treatment, is an anticipated adverse effect.
- Report to prescriber immediately perioral tingling, numbness, and paresthesia. These are signs of hypocalcemia.

PANCRELIPASE

(pan-kre-li'pase)

Creon, Pancreaze, Pertzye, Ultresa, Viokace, Zenpep

Classification: ENZYME REPLACEMENT THERAPY

Therapeutic: PANCREATIC ENZYME REPLACEMENT THERAPY

P

AVAILABILITY Tablet or capsule containing lipase, protease, and amylase

ACTION & *THERAPEUTIC EFFECT* Pancreatic enzyme concentrate similar to natural pancreatin but on a weight basis has 12 times the lipolytic activity and at least 4 × the trypsin and amylase content of pancreatin. *Facilitates hydrolysis of fats into glycerol and fatty acids, starches into dextrins and sugars, and proteins into peptides for easier absorption.*

USES Replacement therapy in symptomatic treatment of malabsorption syndrome due to cystic fibrosis; management of exocrine pancreatic insufficiency due to pancreatectomy.

CONTRAINDICATIONS None listed in the manufacturer's labeling.

CAUTIOUS USE Hypersensitivity to pancrelipase or porcine; GI disease, gout; hyperuricemia; renal impairment; Crohn's disease, short bowel syndrome; pregnancy (category C); lactation.

ROUTE & DOSAGE

Pancreatic Insufficiency

Various brands are not interchangeable, see package insert for interchangeability

Adult/Adolescent/Child (4 y or older): **PO** 500 lipase units/kg/meal; titrate based on symptoms

Child (1–3 y): **PO** 1000 lipase units/kg/meal; titrate based on symptoms

Neonate/Infant (younger than 12 mo): **PO** varies per brand, see package insert

ADMINISTRATION

Oral

- Give capsules with food and sufficient liquid. Do not crush or chew capsules or capsule contents; capsules should be swallowed whole.
- May open capsule and sprinkle contents on soft acidic food, which should be swallowed without chewing. Follow with a full glass of water or juice.
- Determine dosage in relation to fat content in diet (suggested ratio: 300 mg pancrelipase for each 17 g dietary fat).

ADVERSE EFFECTS **CV:** Peripheral edema. **Respiratory:** Nasal congestion, cough. **CNS:** Dizziness, headache, otalgia. **HEENT:** *Ear pain.* **Endocrine:** Hyperuricosuria. hyperglycemia. **GI:** Anorexia, *abdominal pain,* nausea, vomiting, abdominal pain, dyspepsia diarrhea. **Hematologic:** Lymphadenopathy.

INTERACTIONS **Drug:** Effectiveness can be decreased by concurrent ANTACID use.

PHARMACOKINETICS **Distribution:** Acts locally in GI tract. **Elimination:** Feces.

NURSING IMPLICATIONS

Assessment & Drug Effects

- Monitor I&O and weight. Note appetite and quality of stools, weight loss, abdominal bloating, polyuria, thirst, hunger, itching. Pancreatic insufficiency is frequently associated with steatorrhea, bulky stools, and insulin dependent diabetes.
- Monitor uric acid levels in patients with hyperuricemia, gout or renal impairment.
- S&S of colon stricture (cramping, abdominal pain, constipation, vomiting, inability to pass gas or stool).

Patient & Family Education

- Notify prescriber if breast-feeding or intending to breast-feed during treatment.

PANCURONIUM BROMIDE

(pan-kyoo-roe'nee-um)

Classification: NONDEPOLARIZING SKELETAL MUSCLE RELAXANT

Therapeutic: SKELETAL MUSCLE RELAXANT

Prototype: Atracurium

AVAILABILITY Solution for injection

ACTION & THERAPEUTIC EFFECT Produces skeletal muscle relaxation or paralysis by competing with acetylcholine at cholinergic receptor sites on the skeletal muscle endplate and thus blocks nerve impulse transmission. *Induces skeletal muscle relaxation or paralysis.*

USES Adjunct to anesthesia to induce skeletal muscle relaxation. Also to facilitate management of patients undergoing mechanical ventilation.

CONTRAINDICATIONS Hypersensitivity to the drug or bromides.

CAUTIOUS USE History of severe anaphylactic reactions to other neuromuscular blocking agents requires appropriate emergency treatment. Debilitated patients; dehydration; MG; neuromuscular disease; pulmonary, liver, or kidney disease; fluid or electrolyte imbalance; pregnancy (category C); lactation; neonate less than 1 mo.

ROUTE & DOSAGE

Skeletal Muscle Relaxation

Adult/Child/Infant: **IV** 0.04–0.1 mg/kg initial dose, may give additional doses of 0.01 mg/kg at 30–60 min intervals

Neonate: **IV** 0.02 mg/kg test dose

ADMINISTRATION

Intravenous

Plastic syringe may be used for administration, but drug may adsorb to plastic with prolonged storage.

PREPARE: **Direct:** Give undiluted.

ADMINISTER: **Direct:** Give over 30–90 sec.

INCOMPATIBILITIES: **Solution/ additive: Allopurinol, amphotericin B (conventional and lipid), caspofungin, dantrolene, diazepam, furosemide, gemtuzumab, lansoprazole, mitomycin, pantoprazole, phenytoin.**

- Refrigerate at 2°–8° C (36°–46° F). Do not freeze.

ADVERSE EFFECTS **CV:** *Increased pulse rate and BP,* ventricular extrasystoles. **Skin:** Transient acneiform rash, burning sensation along course of vein. **Other:** Salivation, skeletal muscle weakness, respiratory depression.

DIAGNOSTIC TEST INTERFERENCE Pancuronium may decrease ***serum cholinesterase*** concentrations.

INTERACTIONS **Drug:** GENERAL ANESTHETICS increase neuromuscular blocking and duration of action; AMINOGLYCOSIDES, **polymyxin B, clindamycin, lidocaine,** parenteral **magnesium, quinidine, quinine, trimethaphan, verapamil** increase neuromuscular blockade; DIURETICS may increase or decrease neuromuscular blockade; **lithium** prolongs duration of neuromuscular blockade; NARCOTIC ANALGESICS possibly add to respiratory depression; **succinylcholine** increases onset and depth of neuromuscular blockade; **phenytoin** may cause resistance to or reversal of neuromuscular blockade.

PHARMACOKINETICS **Onset:** 30–45 sec. **Peak:** 2–3 min. **Duration:** 60 min. **Distribution:** Well distributed to tissues and extracellular fluids; crosses placenta in small amounts. **Metabolism:** Small amount in liver. **Elimination:** Primarily in urine. **Half-Life:** 2 h.

NURSING IMPLICATIONS

Assessment & Drug Effects

- Assess cardiovascular and respiratory status continuously.
- Observe patient closely for residual muscle weakness and signs of respiratory distress during recovery period. Monitor BP and vital signs. Peripheral nerve stimulator may be used to assess the effects of pancuronium and to monitor restoration of neuromuscular function.
- Note: Consciousness is not affected by pancuronium. Patient will be awake and alert but unable to speak.

PANITUMUMAB

(pan-i-tu-mu′mab)

Vectibix

Classification: ANTINEOPLASTIC TYROSINE KINASE INHIBITOR

Therapeutic: ANTINEOPLASTIC

Prototype: Erlotinib

AVAILABILITY Solution for injection

ACTION & *THERAPEUTIC EFFECT* Epidermal growth factor receptors (EGFRs) are overexpressed in many human cancers, including those of the colon and rectum. EGFRs control the activity of intra-cellular tyrosine kinases that regulate transcription of DNA molecules involved in cancer cell growth, survival, and proliferation. *Panitumumab inhibits overexpression of EGFRs in cancer cells, decreasing their proliferation, survival, and decreasing their invasive capacity and metastases.*

USES Treatment of EGFR-expressing metastatic colorectal carcinoma in patients with disease progression on or following fluoropyrimidine-, oxaliplatin-, and irinotecan-containing chemotherapy regimens.

CONTRAINDICATIONS Pulmonary fibrosis; interstitial lung disease; pregnancy (fetal risk cannot be ruled out); lactation (infant risk cannot be ruled out).

CAUTIOUS USE Photosensitivity with drug use; electrolyte imbalances, especially hypomagnesemia, and hypocalcemia; lung disorders; older patients. Safe use in children not established.

ROUTE & DOSAGE

Metastatic Colorectal Carcinoma

Adult: **IV** 6 mg/kg q14days

Dosage Adjustments for Infusion Reactions and Dermatologic Reactions

Mild or moderate infusion reactions (Grade 1 or 2): Reduce infusion rate by 50%

Severe infusion reactions (Grade 3 or 4): Discontinue permanently

Intolerable or severe dermatologic toxicity (greater than Grade 3): Withhold drug. If toxicity does not improve to at least Grade 2 within 1 mo, permanently discontinue. If toxicity improves to at least Grade 2 and patient is symptomatically improved after withholding no more than 2 doses, resume at 50% of original dose. If toxicities recur, discontinue permanently. If toxicities do not recur, subsequent doses may be increased by increments of 25% of original dose until 6 mg/kg is reached.

ADMINISTRATION

Intravenous

PREPARE: **IV Infusion:** Dilute doses up to 1000 mg with NS to a total volume of 100 mL. ▪ Dilute higher doses with NS to a total volume of 150 mL. ▪ Final concentration should not exceed 10 mg/mL. ▪ Mix by gentle inversion and do not shake. Solution will contain small translucent particles that will be removed by filtration during infusion.

ADMINISTER: **IV Infusion:** Infuse doses less than 1000 mg over 60 min. ▪ Infuse doses greater than 1000 mg over 90 min. ▪ Use an infusion pump and a 0.2 or 0.22 micron in-line filter. ▪ Flush the line before/after infusion with NS. ▪ Discontinue infusion immediately if an anaphylactic reaction is suspected (i.e., bronchospasm, fever, chills, hypotension).

▪ Store unopened vials at 2°–8° C (36°–46° F). Protect vials from direct sunlight. ▪ Use diluted infusion solution within 6 h if stored at room temperature, or within 24 h if stored at 2°–8° C (36°–46° F).

P

ADVERSE EFFECTS **CV:** Peripheral edema. **Respiratory:** Cough, dyspnea. **HEENT:** Eye irritation, abnormal eyelash growth. **Endocrine:** hypomagnesemia. **Skin:** *Acne,* fissures, dermatitis, *nail changes, pruritis, rash.* **GI:** *Abdominal pain,* constipation, *diarrhea,* nausea, mucositis, stomatitis, vomiting. **Other:** *Fatigue.*

INTERACTIONS **Drugs:** Do not use with **aminolevulinic acid.**

PHARMACOKINETICS **Half-Life:** 7.5 days.

NURSING IMPLICATIONS

Black Box Warning

Panitumumab has been associated with frequent, sometimes severe, dermatologic toxicities, and severe infusion reactions.

Assessment & Drug Effects

- Monitor for S&S of a severe infusion reaction; check vital signs q30min during infusion and 30 min post infusion.
- Monitor for and report S&S of dermatologic toxicity such as acne-like dermatitis, pruritus, erythema, rash, skin exfoliation, dry skin, and skin fissures; inflammatory or infectious sequelae in those who experience severe dermatologic toxicities.
- Withhold drug and notify prescriber for any signs of drug toxicity.
- Monitor lab tests: Periodic serum electrolytes during and for 8 wk following completion of therapy.

Patient & Family Education

- Immediately report any discomfort experienced during and shortly after drug infusion.
- Wear sunscreen and limit sun exposure while receiving panitumumab.
- Report any of the following to a health care provider: Any signs of irritation, inflammation, or infection of the skin, nails, or eyes; shortness of breath or any other breathing difficulty.
- Women of childbearing age should use reliable means of contraception during and for 6 mo after the last dose of panitumumab.

P

PANTOPRAZOLE SODIUM

(pan-to′pra-zole)

Protonix

Classification: PROTON PUMP INHIBITOR; ANTISECRETORY

Therapeutic: ANTIULCER

Prototype: Omeprazole

AVAILABILITY Delayed release tablet; solution for injection; delayed release oral suspension

ACTION & THERAPEUTIC EFFECT Gastric acid secretion is decreased by inhibiting the H^+, K^+-ATPase enzyme system responsible for acid production. *Suppresses gastric acid secretion by inhibiting the acid (proton H^+) pump in the parietal cells.*

USES Short-term treatment of erosive esophagitis associated with gastroesophageal reflux disease (GERD), hypersecretory disease.

UNLABELED USES Peptic ulcer disease, dyspepsia, stress ulcer prophylaxis, heartburn, duodenal ulcer.

CONTRAINDICATIONS Hypersensitivity to pantoprazole or other proton pump inhibitors (PPIs).

CAUTIOUS USE Mild to severe hepatic insufficiency, cirrhosis; concurrent administration of EDTA-containing products; elderly (avoid after 8 wk); history of lupus erythematosus, history of osteoporosis; pregnancy (category B); lactation (infant risk cannot be ruled out). Safety and efficacy in children younger than 5 y not established for uses other than erosive esophagitis.

There is no commercially available dosage formulation appropriate for children younger than 5 y.

ROUTE & DOSAGE

Erosive Esophagitis

Adult: **PO** 40 mg daily × 8 wks
IV 40 mg daily × 7–10 days
Adolescent/Child (5 y and older, weight 40 kg or more): **PO** 40 mg daily × 8 wk; *weight 15–39 kg:* 20 mg daily × 8 wk

Hypersecretory Disease

Adult: **PO** 40 mg bid (doses up to 240 mg/day have been used)
IV 80 mg bid; adjust based on acid output

ADMINISTRATION

Oral

- Do not crush or break in half. **Must be** swallowed whole with or without food.
- Granules for oral suspension should be given 30 min before meals. Granules should be put into apple juice or applesauce, not water and given within 10 min of preparation.
- *NG tube administration:* Add granules for suspension to a catheter tip syringe inserted into a 16 French catheter (or larger). Add 40 mL of apple juice in 10 mL increments to fully suspend granules and ensure that all of the drug is washed into the stomach.
- Store tablet and oral suspension at 20°–25° C (66°–77° F), but room temperature permitted. Excursions permitted to 15°–30° C (59°–86° F).

Intravenous

PREPARE: **IV 15 Min Infusion:** Reconstitute each 40 mg vial with 10 mL NS to yield 4 mg/mL. ▪ The required dose of 40 or 80 mg may be further diluted to a **total volume** of 100 mL in D5W, NS, or LR to yield 0.4 mg/mL or 0.8 mg/mL, respectively.

ADMINISTER: **IV Infusion:** Give through a dedicated line or flushed IV line before and after each dose with D5W, NS, or LR. ▪ Give the 4 mg/mL concentration over at least 2 min. ▪ Infuse the 0.4 or 0.8 mg/mL concentration over 15 min.

INCOMPATIBILITIES: **Solution/additive:** **Nefopam,** solutions containing **zinc, nefopam hydrochloride. Y-site: Acyclovir sodium, alemtuzumab, alfentanil, amikacin, amiodarone hydrochloride, amphotericin b, atenolol, atracurium, atropine, aztreonam, blinatumomab, bretylium, buprenorphine, butorphanol, caffeine, calcium salts, caspofungin, acetate, cefazolin sodium, cefepime, cefoperazone, cefotaxime, cefotetan disodium, cefoxitin, ceftazidime, ceftobiprole medocaril, cefuroxime, chloramphenicol, chlorpromazine, cimetidine, ciprofloxacin, cisatracurium, cisplatin, clindamycin phosphate, cloxacillin sodium, cyclosporine, dacarbazine, dactinomycin, dantrolene, daptomycin, daunorubicin, dexamethasone sodium phosphate, dexmedetomidine hydrochloride, dexrazoxane, diazepam, digoxin,**

P

diltiazem, dimenhydrinate, diphenhydramine, dobutamine, dolasetron, dopamine hydrochloride, doxacurium chloride doxorubicin, droperidol, enalaprilat, ephedrine, epinephrine hydrochloride, epirubicin, esmolol, estrogens, etoposide, famotidine, fenoldopam, fentanyl, fluconazole, fludarabine, furosemide, gatifloxacin, gemcitabine, gemtuzumab, gentamicin sulfate, glycopyrrolate, haloperidol, heparin, hydralazine, hydrocortisone, hydromorphone, hydroxyzine, idarubicin, ifosfamide, indomethacin, insulin, isoproterenol hydrochloride, isavuconazonium, ketorolac, labetalol, leucovorin, levofloxacin, levorphanol, lidocaine, linezolid, lorazepam, magnesium sulfate, mannitol, mechlorethamine, melphalan, meperidine, meropenem, methotrexate, methylprednisolone, metoclopramide hydrochloride, metoprolol, metronidazole, midazolam hydrochloride, milrinone, minocycline, mitomycin, mitoxantrone hydrochloride, mivacurium chloride, morphine sulfate, moxifloxacin, multiple vitamin injections, mycophenolate, nalbuphine, naloxone, nicardipine, nitroglycerin, nitroprusside sodium, norepinephrine bitartrate, octreotide acetate, ondansetron, oxytocin, palonosetron, pancuronium, pemetrexed, pentamidine isethionate, phenobarbital sodium, phenytoin, piperacillin sodium–tazobactam sodium, polymyxin B, potassium acetate, potassium phosphate, prochlorperazine, promethazine, propofol, propranolol, quinupristin/dalfopristin, remifentanil, rocuronium, salbutamol, sodium acetate, sodium bicarbonate, sodium phosphate, streptozocin, sulfamethoxazole-trimethoprim, tacrolimus, thiopental sodium, thiotepa, tobramycin sulfate, tolazoline hydrochloride, topotecan, trimethobenzamide hydrochloride, vancomycin, vecuronium, verapamil, vinblastine, vincristine, vinorelbine, voriconazole.

▪ Reconstituted IV solutions may be stored for up to 6 h at 15°–30° C (59°–86° F) before further dilution. ▪ The diluted 100 mL solution should be infused within 24 h or infused within 24 h of reconstitution.

ADVERSE EFFECTS CNS: *Headache.* **GI:** Diarrhea.

DIAGNOSTIC TEST INTERFERENCE May cause false–positive ***urine tetrahydrocannabinol (THC) test;*** may increase CgA levels, which may interfere with neuroendocrine tumor detection.

INTERACTIONS Drug: Contraindicated with **atazanavir** or **rilpivirine.** Do not use with **acalabrutinib, dacomitinib, dasatinib, delavirdine, erlotinib, nelfinavir, neratinib, pazopanib, rilpivirine, risedronate, velpatasvir.** May decrease absorption of **ampicillin,** IRON SALTS, **itraconazole, ketoconazole;** increases INR with **warfarin.** May decrease concentration of CEPHALOSPORINS. **Herbal: Ginkgo** may decrease plasma levels.

PHARMACOKINETICS **Absorption:** Well absorbed with 77% bioavailability. **Peak:** 2.4 h. **Distribution:** 98% protein bound. **Metabolism:** In liver (CYP2C19). **Elimination:** 71% in urine, 18% in feces. **Half-Life:** 1 h.

NURSING IMPLICATIONS

Assessment & Drug Effects

- Monitor for and immediately report S&S of angioedema or a severe skin reaction.
- Monitor for improvement in gastroesophageal comfort.
- Monitor lab tests: Vitamin B_{12} and magnesium with long-term therapy.

Patient & Family Education

- Contact prescriber promptly if any of the following occur: Peeling, blistering, or loosening of skin; skin rash, hives, or itching; swelling of the face, tongue, or lips; difficulty breathing or swallowing.

PAPAVERINE HYDROCHLORIDE

(pa-pav'er-een)

Classification: NONNITRATE VASODILATOR
Therapeutic: VASODILATOR; SMOOTH MUSCLE RELAXANT
Prototype: Hydralazine

AVAILABILITY Solution for injection

ACTION & *THERAPEUTIC EFFECT* Exerts nonspecific direct spasmolytic effect on smooth muscles unrelated to innervation. Acts directly on myocardium, depresses conduction and irritability, and prolongs refractory period. *Relaxes the smooth muscle of the heart as well as produces relaxation of vascular smooth muscles.*

USES Smooth muscle spasms.

UNLABELED USES Impotence, cardiac bypass surgery.

CONTRAINDICATIONS Parenteral use in complete AV block.

CAUTIOUS USE Glaucoma; myocardial depression; QT prolongation, angina pectoris; recent stroke; pregnancy (category C); lactation.

ROUTE & DOSAGE

Smooth Muscle Spasm
Adult: **IM/IV** 30–120 mg q3h as needed

ADMINISTRATION

Intramuscular

- Aspirate carefully before injecting IM to avoid inadvertent entry into blood vessel, and administer slowly.

Intravenous

- IV administration to children: Verify correct IV concentration and rate of infusion with prescriber.

PREPARE: **Direct:** Give undiluted or diluted in an equal volume of sterile water for injection.
ADMINISTER: **Direct:** Give slowly over 1–2 min. Avoid rapid injection.
INCOMPATIBILITIES: **Solution/additive:** **Aminophylline, heparin, lactated Ringer's.** **Y-site:** **aminophylline, amphotericin B, ampicillin, bumetanide,** CEPHALOSPORINS, **clindamycin, dantrolene, diazepam, diazoxide, furosemide, heparin, indomethacin, ketorolac, methylprednisolone, phenobarbital, phenytoin, piperacillin.**

ADVERSE EFFECTS **CV:** Slight rise in BP, paroxysmal tachycardia, transient ventricular ectopic rhythms, AV block, arrhythmias. **Respiratory:** Increased depth of respiration, <u>respiratory depression, fatal apnea</u>. **CNS:** Dizziness, drowsiness, headache, sedation. **HEENT:** Diplopia, nystagmus. **Skin:** Pruritus, skin rash. **GI:** Nausea, anorexia, constipation, diarrhea, abdominal distress, dry mouth and throat, <u>hepatotoxicity</u> (jaundice, eosinophilia, abnormal liver function tests); with rapid IV administration. **GU:** Priapism. **Other:** General discomfort, facial flushing, sweating, weakness, coma.

INTERACTIONS

Drug: May decrease **levodopa** effectiveness; **morphine** may antagonize smooth muscle relaxation effect of papaverine.

PHARMACOKINETICS

Absorption: Readily from GI tract. **Peak:** 1–2 h. **Duration:** 12 h sustained release. **Metabolism:** In liver. **Elimination:** In urine chiefly as metabolites. **Half-Life:** 90 min.

P

NURSING IMPLICATIONS

Assessment & Drug Effects

- Monitor pulse, respiration, and BP in patients receiving drug parenterally. If significant changes are noted, withhold medication and report promptly to prescriber.

Patient & Family Education

- Notify prescriber if any adverse effect persists or if GI symptoms, jaundice, or skin rash appears. Liver function tests may be indicated.
- Do not drive or engage in potentially hazardous activities until response to drug is known. Alcohol may increase drowsiness and dizziness.

PAREGORIC

(par-e-gor′ik)

Classification: ANTIDIARRHEAL; NARCOTIC (OPIATE AGONIST) ANALGESIC

Therapeutic: ANTIDIARRHEAL

Prototype: Loperamide

Controlled Substance: Schedule III

AVAILABILITY

Liquid

ACTION & *THERAPEUTIC EFFECT*

Decreases GI motility and effective propulsive peristalsis while diminishing digestive secretions. *Delayed transit of intestinal contents results in desiccation of feces and constipation.*

USES

Short-term treatment for symptomatic relief of acute diarrhea.

CONTRAINDICATIONS

Hypersensitivity to opium alkaloids; diarrhea caused by poisons (until eliminated); COPD; children; pregnancy—fetal risk cannot be ruled out; lactation—infant risk cannot be ruled out.

CAUTIOUS USE

Asthma; liver disease; severely impaired renal function; GI disease or hemorrhage; history of opiate agonist dependence; severe prostatic hypertrophy; Addison's disease; hypothyroidism; atrial flutter and other supraventricular tachycardias; low blood volume; history of respiratory depression or emphysema; elderly.

ROUTE & DOSAGE

Acute Diarrhea

Adult: **PO** 5–10 mL after loose bowel movement, 1–4 × daily if needed

Child: **PO** 0.25–0.5 mL/kg 1–4 × day

ADMINISTRATION

Oral

- Give paregoric in sufficient water (2 or 3 swallows) to ensure its passage into the stomach (mixture will appear milky).
- Extra precaution in double-checking dose and administering. A 25 fold difference in morphine content exists between paregoric an opium tincture.
- Store tincture at controlled room temperature between 15 and 30 degrees C (59 and 86 degrees F.)

ADVERSE EFFECTS **CNS:** *Dizziness, lightheadedness, sedated.* **GI:** *Nausea, vomiting, constipation.*

INTERACTIONS **Drug: Alcohol** and other CNS DEPRESSANTS add to CNS effects.

PHARMACOKINETICS **Distribution:** Crosses placenta; distributed into breast milk. **Metabolism:** In liver. **Elimination:** In urine.

NURSING IMPLICATIONS

Assessment & Drug Effects

- Paregoric may worsen the course of infection-associated diarrhea by delaying the elimination of pathogens.
- Be aware that adverse effects are primarily due to morphine content. Paregoric abuse results because of the narcotic content of the drug.
- Assess for fluid and electrolyte imbalance until diarrhea has stopped.

Patient & Family Education

- Adhere strictly to prescribed dosage schedule.
- Avoid activities requiring mental alertness or coordination until the drug effects are realized.
- Review adverse effects with patient and/or caregiver.
- Maintain bed rest if diarrhea is severe with a high level of fluid loss.
- Replace fluids and electrolytes as needed for diarrhea. Drink warm clear liquids and avoid dairy products, concentrated sweets, and cold drinks until diarrhea stops.
- Observe character and frequency of stools. Discontinue drug as soon as diarrhea is controlled. Report promptly to prescriber if diarrhea persists more than 3 days, if fever is higher than 38.8° C (102° F), abdominal pain develops, or if mucus or blood is passed.
- Understand that constipation is often a consequence of antidiarrheal treatment and a normal elimination pattern is usually established as dietary intake increases.
- There are many drugs that paregoric interacts with. Consult healthcare professional prior to new drug use (including over-the-counter drugs).

P

PARICALCITOL

(par-i-cal′ci-tol)

Zemplar

Classification: VITAMIN D ANALOG

Therapeutic: VITAMIN D ANALOG

Prototype: Calcitriol

AVAILABILITY Vial; capsule

ACTION & *THERAPEUTIC EFFECT* Synthetic vitamin D analog that reduces parathyroid hormone (PTH) activity levels in chronic kidney failure (CRF). Lowers serum levels of calcium and phosphate. Decreases parathyroid hormone release as well as bone resorption in some patients. *Effectiveness indicated by iPTH levels less than 1.5–3 × the upper limit of normal.*

USES Prevention and treatment of secondary hyperparathyroidism associated with CRF.

CONTRAINDICATIONS Hypersensitivity to paricalcitol; hypercalcemia; evidence of vitamin D toxicity; concurrent administration of phosphate preparations and vitamin D.

CAUTIOUS USE Severe liver disease; abnormally low levels of PTH; pregnancy (fetal risk cannot be ruled out); lactation (infant risk cannot be ruled out). Safety and efficacy in children younger than 5 y not established.

ROUTE & DOSAGE

Secondary Hyperparathyroidism

Adult: **IV** 0.04 mcg/kg–0.1 mcg/kg (max: 0.24 mcg/kg), no more than every other day during dialysis; adjust based on serum iPTH **PO** based on baseline iPTH level divided by 80 and administered 3 × weekly, no more than every other day

Renal Impairment Dosage Adjustment

Stage 5 Chronic Kidney Disease (CKD): See package insert

ADMINISTRATION

Oral

- Give no more frequently than every other day when dosing 3 × wk.
- Store at 15°–30° C (59°–86° F).

Intravenous

PREPARE: **Direct:** Give undiluted.
ADMINISTER: **Direct:** Give IV bolus dose anytime during dialysis.

- Store at 25° C (77° F). Discard unused portion of a single dose vial.

ADVERSE EFFECTS **CV:** Edema, hypertension, hypotension. **Respiratory:** Rhinitis. **CNS:** Dizziness, insomnia, headache. **Endocrine:** hypervolemia. **Skin:** Rash. **GI:** Diarrhea, *nausea*, vomiting, gastrointestinal hemorrhage, peritonitis, constipation. **GU:** Urinary urgency. **Other:** Sepsis.

INTERACTIONS **Drug:** Hypercalcemia may increase risk of **digoxin** toxicity; may increase **magnesium** absorption and toxicity in renal failure. Do not use with **vitamin D analogs. Herbal:** Be cautious of **vitamin D** content in herbal and OTC products.

PHARMACOKINETICS **Distribution:** Greater than 99% protein bound. **Metabolism:** Via CYP3A4. **Elimination:** In feces. **Half-Life:** 15 h.

NURSING IMPLICATIONS

Assessment & Drug Effects

- Monitor for S&S of hypercalcemia (see Appendix F).
- Withhold drug and notify prescriber if hypercalcemia occurs.
- Coadministered drugs: Monitor for digoxin toxicity if serum calcium level is elevated.
- Monitor lab tests: Serum calcium, serum phosphorus, and serum or plasma intact PTH at least every 2 wk for 3 mo, then monthly for 3 mo, and every 3 mo thereafter. Increase frequency of lab tests with coadministration of strong CYP3A inhibitors.

Patient & Family Education

- Report immediately any of the following to the prescriber: Weakness, anorexia, nausea, vomiting, abdominal cramps, diarrhea, muscle or bone pain, or excessive thirst.
- Adhere strictly to dietary regimen of calcium supplementation and phosphorus restriction to ensure successful therapy.
- Avoid excessive use of aluminum-containing compounds such as antacids/vitamins.

PAROMOMYCIN SULFATE

(par-oh-moe-mye′sin)

Classification: AMINOGLYCOSIDE ANTIBIOTIC; AMEBICIDE

Therapeutic: AMEBICIDE

AVAILABILITY Capsule

ACTION & *THERAPEUTIC EFFECT* Aminoglycoside antibiotic with broad-spectrum antibacterial activity. *Exerts direct bactericidal and amebicidal action, primarily in lumen of GI tract. Ineffective against extraintestinal amebiasis.*

USES Acute and chronic intestinal amebiasis; adjunctive therapy for hepatic coma/encephalopathy.

CONTRAINDICATIONS Aminoglycoside hypersensitivity; intestinal obstruction; impaired kidney function.

CAUTIOUS USE GI ulceration; renal failure, renal impairment; older adults; myasthenia gravis; parkinsonism; pregnancy (category C); children.

ROUTE & DOSAGE

Intestinal Amebiasis

Adult/Child: **PO** 25–35 mg/kg divided in 3 doses for 7–10 days

Hepatic Coma

Adult: **PO** 4 g/day in divided doses for 5–10 days

ADMINISTRATION

Oral

- Administer with meals.

ADVERSE EFFECTS CNS: Headache, vertigo. **HEENT:** Ototoxicity. **Skin:** Exanthema, rash, pruritus. **GI:** *Diarrhea, abdominal cramps,* steatorrhea, *nausea, vomiting, heartburn,* secondary enterocolitis. **GU:** Nephrotoxicity (in patients with GI inflammation or ulcerations) oliguria, proteinuria, pyuria. **Other:** Eosinophilia, overgrowth of nonsusceptible organisms.

DIAGNOSTIC TEST INTERFERENCE Prolonged use of paromomycin may cause reduction in ***serum cholesterol.***

INTERACTIONS Drug: May decrease absorption of **cyanocobalamin.** Do not use with **cidofovir** or **gallium.** Use caution with other AMINOGLYCOSIDES or agents that may increase risk of nephrotoxicity.

PHARMACOKINETICS Absorption: Poorly from intact GI tract. **Elimination:** In feces. **Half-Life:** 2–3 h.

NURSING IMPLICATIONS

Assessment & Drug Effects

- Monitor therapeutic effectiveness. Criterion of cure is absence

P

of amoebae in stool specimens examined at weekly intervals for 6 wk after completion of treatment, and thereafter at monthly intervals for 2 y.

- Monitor for appearance of a superinfection during therapy (see Appendix F).
- Monitor closely patients with history of GI ulceration for nephrotoxicity and ototoxicity (see Appendix F). Drug absorption can take place through diseased mucosa.

Patient & Family Education

- Do not prepare, process, or serve food until treatment is complete when receiving drug for intestinal amebiasis. Isolation is not required.
- Practice strict personal hygiene, particularly hand washing after defecation and before eating food.

PAROXETINE

(par-ox′e-teen)

Brisdelle, Pexeva, Paxil, Paxil CR

Classification: ANTIDEPRESSANT; SELECTIVE SEROTONIN 5-HT REUPTAKE INHIBITOR (SSRI)

Therapeutic: ANTIDEPRESSANT; SSRI; ANTIANXIETY

Prototype: Fluoxetine

AVAILABILITY Tablet; sustained release tablet; suspension; capsule

ACTION & *THERAPEUTIC EFFECT* Antidepressant that is a serotonin 5-HT reuptake inhibitor. It is highly potent and a highly selective inhibitor of serotonin reuptake by neurons in CNS. *Efficacious in depression resistant to other antidepressants and in depression complicated by anxiety.*

USES Depression, obsessive-compulsive disorders, panic attacks, excessive social anxiety, generalized anxiety, post traumatic stress disorder (PTSD), premenstrual dysphoric disorder (PMDD), vasomotor symptoms.

UNLABELED USES Diabetic neuropathy, myoclonus, bipolar depression in conjunction with lithium, chronic headache, premature ejaculation, fibromyalgia.

CONTRAINDICATIONS Hypersensitivity to paroxetine; suicidal ideation; concomitant use of MAO inhibitors, pimozide, or thioridazine; alcohol abuse; pregnancy—known to cause fetal harm; lactation—infant risk cannot be ruled out.

CAUTIOUS USE History of mania, suicidal tendencies, bipolar disorder; seizure disorder; renal/hepatic impairment; history of metabolic disorders; volume-depleted patients; abrupt discontinuation; older adults. Not FDA approved for children and adolescents.

ROUTE & DOSAGE

Major Depressive Disorder

Adult: **PO** Immediate release: 20 mg/day may increase by 10 mg weekly (max: 50 mg/day); sustained release 25 mg daily in morning, may increase by 12.5 mg (max: 62.5 mg/day); use lower starting doses for patients with renal or hepatic insufficiency
Geriatric: **PO** Start with 10 mg/day immediate release (12.5 mg/day sustained release), [max: 40 mg/day (50 mg/day sustained release)]

Panic Disorder

Adult: **PO** Immediate Release 10 mg daily then increase to 40 mg/day; **Sustained release** 12.5 mg daily, may increase (max: 75 mg/day)

Social Anxiety Disorder

Adult: **PO** Immediate Release 10 mg/day may increase based on response (max: 60 mg/day). Extended Release 12.5 mg/day may increase based on response (max: 37.5 mg/day)

PTSD, OCD

Adult: **PO** Start with 20 mg once daily, may increase by 10 mg/day at weekly intervals if needed to target dose of 40 mg once daily (max: 60 mg/day)
Geriatric: **PO** Start with 10 mg once daily, may increase by 10 mg/day at weekly intervals if needed (max: 40 mg/day)

Generalized Anxiety

Adult: **PO** Immediate Release Start 10 mg daily, may increase based on response to 50 mg/day

Premenstrual Dysphoric Disorder

Adult: **PO** Extended Release 12.5 mg once daily (up to 25 mg once daily) throughout the month

Hot Flashes

Adult: **PO** 7.5 mg daily (Brisdelle formulation); **Extended release** 12.5 mg daily may titrate up to 25 mg daily

Pharmacogenetic Dosage Adjustment

Poor CYP2D6 metabolizers: Start with 50% of dose and titrate to response

ADMINISTRATION

Oral

- NIOSH guidelines warn drug has risk to men and women actively trying to conceive, women who are pregnant or lactating. Use single gloves when handling intact tablets or capsules or when administering from unit-doses packaging. If cutting, crushing, manipulating or handling uncoated tablets, use double gloves and a protective gown. Wear single gloves for administration and eye/face protection if the formulation is hard to swallow or if the patient may resist, vomit or spit up.
- Ensure that sustained release form is not chewed or crushed. **Must be** swallowed whole.
- Usually administered every morning. Administering with food will decrease GI adverse effects. Do not administer concomitantly with antacids.
- Suspension should be shaken well before administration.
- Be aware that at least 14 days should elapse when switching a patient from/to an MAO inhibitor to/from paroxetine.
- Store extended release tablets and suspension at or below 25° C (77° F). Immediate release tablets should be stored between 15 and 30° C (59 and 86° F).

ADVERSE EFFECTS (≥5%) **CV:** Vasodilation. **CNS:** *Headache*, tremor, asthenia, dizziness, insomnia, *sedation*. **HEENT:** Blurred vision. **Endocrine:** Hyponatremia in older adults. **Skin:** Diaphoresis. **GI:** *Nausea*, constipation, anorexia, diarrhea, *dry mouth*. **GU:** Abnormal ejaculation, erectile dysfunction, orgasm disorder, decrease in libido.

INTERACTIONS Drug: Use with other serotonergic agents (e.g. SSRIs) or MAOIs can cause serotonin syndrome. Do not use with **pimozide. Activated charcoal** reduces absorption of paroxetine. **Cimetidine** increases paroxetine levels. MAO INHIBITORS, **selegiline** may cause an increased vasopressor response leading to hypertensive crisis or death. **Phenytoin** can cause liver enzyme induction resulting in lower paroxetine levels and shorter half-life. **Warfarin** may increase risk of bleeding and **thioridazine** levels, and prolong QT_c interval leading to heart block; increase **ergotamine** toxicity with **dihydroergotamine, ergotamine.** May reduce the efficacy of **tamoxifen. Herbal: St. John's wort** may cause serotonin syndrome (headache, dizziness, sweating, agitation).

PHARMACOKINETICS Absorption: 99% from GI tract. **Onset:** 2 wk. **Peak:** 5–8 h. **Distribution:** Very lipophilic. 95% protein bound. Distributes into breast milk. **Metabolism:** Extensively in the liver to inactive metabolites via CYP2D6. **Elimination:** Less than 2% is excreted unchanged in urine. 65% of dose appears in urine as metabolites. Metabolites of paroxetine are also excreted in feces, presumably via bile. **Half-Life:** 24 h.

P

NURSING IMPLICATIONS

Black Box Warning

Paroxetine has been associated with suicidal ideation and behavior in children, adolescents, and young adults.

Assessment & Drug Effects

- Monitor for worsening of depression or emergence of suicidal ideation. Closely monitor those younger than 18 y for suicidal thinking and behavior.
- Monitor for adverse effects, which include headache, weakness, sedation, dizziness, insomnia; nausea, constipation, or diarrhea; dry mouth; sweating; male ejaculatory disturbance. These occur in more than 10% of all patients and may result in poor compliance with drug regimen.
- Monitor older adults for fluid and sodium imbalances.
- Monitor weight.
- Monitor patients with history of mania for reactivation of condition.
- Monitor patients with preexisting cardiovascular disease carefully because paroxetine may adversely affect hemodynamic status.

Patient & Family Education

- For off-label use; monitor children, adolescents, and young adults for changes in behavior that may indicate suicidal ideation.
- Use caution when operating hazardous machinery or equipment until response to drug is known.
- Avoid use of alcohol, aspirin, NSAIDS or St. Johns Wort while taking this drug.
- Adaptation to some adverse effects (especially dizziness and nausea) may occur over a period of 4–6 wk.
- Do not stop drug therapy after improvement in emotional status occurs.
- Notify prescriber of any distressing adverse effects.

PATIROMER

(pa-tir'oh-mer)

Veltassa

Classification: CATIONIC EXCHANGE POLYMER; POTASSIUM BINDER

Therapeutic: POTASSIUM BINDER

AVAILABILITY Powder for oral suspension

ACTION & *THERAPEUTIC EFFECT* A nonabsorbed, cation exchange polymer that binds to potassium in the lumen of the gastrointestinal tract and increases its fecal elimination. *The binding of potassium reduces the concentration of free potassium in the gastrointestinal lumen, resulting in a reduction of serum potassium levels.*

USES Treatment of hyperkalemia. Due to its delayed onset of action, it should not be used in the emergency treatment of life-threatening hyperkalemia.

CONTRAINDICATIONS Hypersensitivity to patiromer. Avoid use in patients with severe constipation, GI obstruction, fecal impaction, including post-operative bowel motility disorders.

CAUTIOUS USE Use cautiously in patients with a history of hypomagnesemia. Maternal use during pregnancy is not expected to result in fetal risk. According to the manufacturer, breast-feeding is not expected to result in risk to the infant. If an infant does experience adverse effects, it should be reported to the FDA.

ROUTE & DOSAGE

Hyperkalemia

Adult: **PO** 8.4 grams once daily; may increase to 25.2 grams once daily

ADMINISTRATION

Oral

- Administer patiromer 6 h before or 6 h after other orally administered medications to prevent patiromer from binding to other oral medications.
- Administer with food.
- Do not administer in its dry form.
- Do not heat or add to heated food or liquids.

Oral Liquid Formulation

- Prepare each dose immediately before administration.
- Measure 1/3 cup of water. Pour half into the cup and then empty the entire contents of the packet into the glass. Stir thoroughly and add the remaining water. Stir again, the particles will not completely dissolve. The mixture will look cloudy. Add more water if needed for desired consistency.
- Drink immediately, rinse the glass with more water and drink again. Repeat as needed to ensure that the entire dose has been given.
- Store at 2°–8° C (36°–46° F). If stored at room temperature 25° C (77° F), use within 3 mo of being taken out of refrigeration. Avoid exposure to excessive heat above 40° C (104° F).

ADVERSE EFFECTS **CNS:** Nausea. **Endocrine:** Hypokalemia, hypomagnesemia. **GI:** Abdominal

P

discomfort, constipation, diarrhea, flatulence.

INTERACTIONS Drug: Patiromer can bind to other coadministered oral drugs and reduce their absorption. Oral drugs should be taken at least 6 h before or 6 h after patiromer.

PHARMACOKINETICS Absorption: Not orally absorbed.

NURSING IMPLICATIONS

Assessment & Drug Effects

- Older adults may experience more gastrointestinal adverse reactions.
- Monitor lab tests: Serum magnesium and potassium levels.

Patient & Family Education

- Immediately report to prescriber for any of the following: Mood changes, muscle pain, weakness, muscle cramps or spasms, seizures, lack of appetite, severe nausea or vomiting, or an abnormal heart beat.
- Report signs of a significant reaction: Wheezing, chest tightness, itching, swelling of face, lips, tongue, or throat.

P

PAZOPANIB

(pas-o′pa-nib)

Votrient

Classification: ANTINEOPLASTIC; KINASE INHIBITOR

Therapeutic: ANTINEOPLASTIC

Prototype: Erlotinib

AVAILABILITY Tablet

ACTION & THERAPEUTIC EFFECT A multityrosine kinase (i.e., multikinase) inhibitor that limits tumor growth by inhibiting cell surface vascular endothelial growth factor receptors and other receptors needed for tumor angiogenesis and growth. *Pazopanib inhibits growth of advanced renal cell carcinoma.*

USES Treatment of advanced renal cell carcinoma; soft tissue sarcoma.

CONTRAINDICATIONS Hepatotoxicity; severe hepatic impairment; ALT elevation greater than 3 × ULN concurrently with bilirubin elevation of greater than 2 × ULN; cerebral or GI bleeding within last 6 mo; GI perforation or fistula; uncontrolled hypertension; drug induced left ventricular ejection fraction (LVEF); wound dehiscence; stop drug 7 days before surgical procedures; patients who have had an arterial thrombotic event within 6 mo; reversible posterior leukoencephalopathy syndrome; nephrotic syndrome; pregnancy—fetal risk cannot be ruled out; lactation—infant risk cannot be ruled out.

CAUTIOUS USE Risk for QT prolongation or history of QT prolongation; electrolyte imbalance; CHF; cardiac dysfunction; risk for or history of thrombotic event; risk for or history of GI perforation or fistula; moderate hepatic impairment; history of hypothyroidism; infection; older adults; children younger than 18 y.

ROUTE & DOSAGE

Renal Cell Carcinoma/Soft Tissue Sarcoma

Adult: **PO** 800 mg once daily reduce until disease progression or unacceptable toxicity

Hepatic Impairment Dosage Adjustment

See package insert for details

ADMINISTRATION

Oral

- NIOSH guidelines recommend single gloves by anyone handling intact tablets or capsules or administering from a unit-dose package.
- Give without food at least 1 h before or 2 h after a meal.
- Ensure that the tablets are swallowed whole. They should not be crushed or chewed.

ADVERSE EFFECTS (≥ 5%) CV: *Hypertension,* **Respiratory:** *Dyspnea.* **CNS:** *Headache.* **Endocrine:** *Alterations- in glucose, anorexia, AST and ALT elevation, decreased magnesium, decreased phosphorus, decreased sodium,* decreased weight, *elevated bilirubin,* hypothyroidism, lipase enzyme elevation, proteinuria. **Skin:** Hair color change. **Hepatic:** Increase alkaline phosphatase. **GI:** *Abdominal pain, diarrhea, nausea, vomiting.* **Musculoskeletal:** Myalgia, pain, weakness. **Hematologic:** *Leukopenia, lymphocytopenia, neutropenia,* thrombocytopenia. **Other:** *Soft tissue sarcoma, cancer pain.*

INTERACTIONS Drug: Multiple significant interactions exist, consult a drug interaction database for most complete information. Strong INHIBITORS OF CYP3A4 (e.g., **ketoconazole, ritonavir, clarithromycin**) may increase pazopanib levels. INDUCERS OF CYP3A4 (e.g., **rifampin**) may decrease pazopanib levels. Pazopanib may increase the levels of other drugs that require CYP3A4, CYP2D6, or CYP2C8 for their metabolism. Do not use with agents that prolong QT interval (e.g., **bepridil, cisapride, dofetilide, quinidine, ziprasidone**). Do not use with LIVE VACCINES. **Food: Grapefruit juice** may increase pazopanib levels.

PHARMACOKINETICS Peak: 2–4 h. **Distribution:** Greater than 99% plasma protein bound. **Metabolism:** Hepatic oxidation by CYP3A4, minor metabolism via CYP1A2 and CYP2C8. **Elimination:** Primarily fecal. **Half-Life:** 31 h.

NURSING IMPLICATIONS

Black Box Warning

Pazopanib has been associated with severe, sometimes fatal, hepatotoxicity.

Assessment & Drug Effects

- Monitor BP closely. Consult prescriber for desired parameters and report promptly BP elevations above desired levels.
- Monitor cardiac status, especially in those at higher risk for QT interval prolongation. ECG monitoring as warranted.
- Withhold drug and notify prescriber immediately if ALT exceeds 3 × ULN and bilirubin exceeds 2 × ULN.
- Monitor lab tests: CBC with differential. Baseline LFTs, then q4wk for 4 mo, and periodically thereafter; periodic thyroid function tests, urinalysis for proteinuria; baseline and periodic serum electrolytes, pregnancy test before starting therapy.

Patient & Family Education

- Report promptly any of the following: Unexplained signs of bleeding, jaundice, unusually dark urine, unusual tiredness, or pain in the right upper abdomen.
- Do not take OTC drugs, herbs, vitamins or dietary supplements without consulting prescriber.

- Women of childbearing age should use adequate means of contraception to avoid pregnancy while on this drug and for at least 2 weeks after discontinuing the drug.
- Take a missed dose as soon as possible, but if the next dose is less than 12 hours skip the missed dose.

PEGFILGRASTIM

(peg-fil-gras'tim)

Neulasta, Fulphila, Udenyca

Classification: HEMATOPOIETIC GROWTH FACTOR; GRANULOCYTE COLONY-STIMULATING FACTOR (G-CSF)

Therapeutic: HEMATOPOIETIC GROWTH FACTOR; G-CSF

Prototype: Filgrastim

AVAILABILITY Solution for injection

ACTION & *THERAPEUTIC EFFECT* Endogenous G-CSF regulates the production of neutrophils within the bone marrow; primarily affects neutrophil proliferation, differentiation, and selected end-cell functional activity (including enhanced phagocytic activity, antibody-dependent killing, and increased expression of some functions associated with cell-surface antigens). *Increases neutrophil proliferation and differentiation within the bone marrow.*

USES To decrease the incidence of infection, as manifested by febrile neutropenia, in patients with non-myeloid malignancies receiving myelosuppressive anticancer drugs associated with a significant incidence of severe neutropenia with fever.

CONTRAINDICATIONS Severe hypersensitivity to perfilgrastim, filgrastin, or any component of the formulation; myeloid cancers; splenomegaly; ARDS from drug.

CAUTIOUS USE Sickle cell disorders; neutropenic patients with sepsis; leukemia; pregnancy (category C); lactation. Safety and efficacy in children not established.

ROUTE & DOSAGE

Neutropenia

Adult (weight greater than 45 kg): **Subcutaneous** 6 mg once/chemotherapy cycle at least 24 h after chemotherapy

ADMINISTRATION

Subcutaneous

- Do not administer pegfilgrastim in the period 14 days before or 24 h after cytotoxic chemotherapy.
- Use only one dose/vial; do not reenter the vial.
- Prior to injection, pegfilgrastim may be allowed to reach room temperature for a maximum of 6 h. Discard any vial left at room temperature for longer than 6 h.
- Aspirate prior to injection to avoid injection into a blood vessel. Inject subcutaneously; do not inject intradermally. Recommended injection sites include outer area of upper arms, abdomen (excluding 2-in. area around navel), front of middle thighs, and upper outer areas of the buttocks.
- Store refrigerated at 2°–8° C (36°–46° F). Do not freeze. Avoid shaking.

ADVERSE EFFECTS **Musculoskeletal:** *Bone pain*, limb pain.

DIAGNOSTIC TEST INTERFERENCE May interfere with ***bone imaging studies.***

INTERACTIONS Drug: Can interfere with activity of CYTOTOXIC AGENTS; do not use 14 days before or less than 24 h after CYTOTOXIC AGENTS; **lithium** may increase release of neutrophils. Do not use with **tisagenlecleucel.**

PHARMACOKINETICS Absorption: Readily absorbed from subcutaneous site. **Half-Life:** 15–80 h.

NURSING IMPLICATIONS

Assessment & Drug Effects

- Discontinue pegfilgrastim if absolute neutrophil count exceeds 10,000/mm^3 after the chemotherapy-induced nadir. Neutrophil counts should then return to normal.
- Monitor patients with preexisting cardiac conditions closely. MI and arrhythmias have been associated with a small percent of patients receiving pegfilgrastim.
- Monitor temperature q4h. Incidence of infection should be reduced after administration of pegfilgrastim.
- Assess degree of bone pain if present. Consult prescriber if nonnarcotic analgesics do not provide relief.
- Monitor lab tests: Baseline CBC with differential and platelet count; then CBC twice weekly during therapy; regular Hct and Hgb, and platelet count.

Patient & Family Education

- Report bone pain and, if necessary, request analgesics to control pain.
- Note: Proper drug administration and disposal is important. A puncture-resistant container for the disposal of used syringes and needles should be utilized.

PEGINTERFERON ALFA-2A

(peg-in-ter-fer′on)

Pegasys

Classification: BIOLOGIC RESPONSE MODIFIER; IMMUNOMODULATOR; ALPHA INTERFERON

Therapeutic: ANTIVIRAL; ANTIHEPATITIS

AVAILABILITY Solution for injection

ACTION & *THERAPEUTIC EFFECT* Interferon-stimulated genes modulate processes leading to inhibition of viral replication in infected cells, inhibition of cell proliferation, and immunomodulation. *Induces antiviral effects by activation of macrophages, natural killer cells, and T-cells, thus boosting cellular immunity and suppressing hepatic inflammation and replication of hepatitis C virus.*

USES Chronic hepatitis B.

CONTRAINDICATIONS Hypersensitivity to peginterferon alfa-2a or any of its components; drug induced life-threatening neuromuscular, autoimmune, ischemic or infectious disorder(s); severe immunosuppression; autoimmune thyroid diseases (e.g., Graves' disease, thyroiditis); autoimmune hepatitis; encephalopathy; history of significant or uncontrolled cardiac disease; pancreatitis; dental work; sepsis; *E. coli* hypersensitivity, neonates and infants because it contains benzyl alcohol; pregnancy—fetal risk cannot be ruled out; lactation—infant risk cannot be ruled out.

CAUTIOUS USE History of neuropsychiatric disorder; alcoholism, substance abuse; risk of pulmonary failure; bipolar disorder, mania, psychosis, history of suicides; bone marrow suppression; cardiac arrhythmias, history of MI, cardiac disease, heart failure, uncontrolled hypertension; pulmonary disease, including COPD; thyroid dysfunction; DM; autoimmune disorders; ulcerative and hemorrhagic colitis; pancreatitis; pulmonary disorders; liver impairment; HBV or HIV coinfection; retinal disease; history of depression, renal impairment with creatinine clearance less than 50 mL/min; organ transplant recipients; older adults;. Safe use in children younger than 3 y not established.

ROUTE & DOSAGE

Chronic Hepatitis B

Adult: **Subcutaneous** 180 mcg once weekly × 48 wk

Hematologic Parameters, Adverse Effects, Renal Impairment, and Hepatic Impairment Dosage Adjustments

See package insert

ADMINISTRATION

Subcutaneous

- Give dose on the same day of each week. Consider night time administration to increase patient's tolerance. Administer subcutaneously in the abdomen or thigh and rotate injection sites.
- Warm refrigerated vial by rolling in hands for about 1 min. Do not use if particulate matter is visible in the vial or product is discolored. Discard any unused portion.
- Withhold drug and notify prescriber for any of the following: ANC less than 750/mm^3 or platelet count less than 50,000/mm^3.
- Store in the refrigerator at 36°–46° F (2°–8° C), do not freeze or shake. Protect from light. Vials, prefilled syringes and autoinjectors are for single use only. Discard unused portions. Do not leave out of the refrigerator longer than 24 hours.

ADVERSE EFFECTS **Respiratory:** *Cough, dyspnea.* **CNS:** *Headache, irritability, insomnia, dizziness, impaired concentration.* **Endocrine:** Increased serum triglycerides, decreased weight. **Skin:** *Alopecia, pruritus, dermatitis, rash, injection site inflammation.* **Hepatic:** Elevated ALT/SGPT. **GI:** *Nausea, diarrhea, abdominal pain, anorexia.* **Musculoskeletal:** *Arthralgia, myalgia.* **Hematologic:** Thrombocytopenia, *neutropenia.* **Other:** *Fatigue, flu-like symptoms, rigors, fever.*

INTERACTIONS **Drug:** additive myelosuppression with ANTINEOPLASTICS. Do not administer LIVE VACCINES.

PHARMACOKINETICS **Peak:** 72–96 h. **Half-Life:** 50–160 h.

NURSING IMPLICATIONS

Black Box Warning

Peginterferon Alfa-2A has been associated with fatal or life-threatening neuropsychiatric, autoimmune, ischemic, and infectious disorders.

Assessment & Drug Effects

- Monitor for S&S of hypersensitivity (e.g., angioedema, bronchoconstriction) and, if noted, institute appropriate medical action immediately. Note that transient rashes are not an indication to discontinue treatment.

P

- Withhold drug and notify prescriber for any of the following: Severe neuropsychiatric events (e.g., psychosis, hallucinations, suicidal ideation, depression, bipolar disorders, and mania), severe neutropenia or thrombocytopenia, abdominal pain accompanied by bloody diarrhea and fever, S&S of pancreatitis, new or worsening ophthalmologic disorders, or any other severe adverse event (see CAUTIOUS USE).
- Monitor respiratory and cardiovascular status; report dyspnea, chest pain, and hypotension immediately; perform baseline and periodic ECG and chest x-ray.
- Baseline and periodic ophthalmology exams are recommended.
- Monitor lab tests: Baseline creatinine clearance, uric acid, CBC with differential, platelet count, Hct and Hgb, TSH, ALT, AST, bilirubin, blood glucose; CBC with differential, platelet count, Hct and Hgb after 2 wk and other blood chemistries after 4 wk. Serum HCV RNA level after 24 wk of treatment.

Patient & Family Education

- If you miss a drug dose and remember within 2 days of the scheduled dose, take the dose and continue with your regular schedule. If more than 2 days have passed, contact prescriber for instructions.
- Instruct and provide opportunity for return demonstration of proper subcutaneous injection technique and placement of injections.
- Notify prescriber immediately for any of the following: Severe depression or suicidal thoughts, severe chest pain, difficulty breathing, changes in vision, unusual bleeding or bruising, bloody diarrhea, high fever, severe stomach or lower back pain, severe chest pain, development of a new or worsening of a preexisting skin condition.
- Follow up with lab tests; compliance with lab testing is extremely important while taking this drug.
- Review adverse effects with patient and/or caregiver.
- Do not drive or engage in other potentially hazardous activities until reaction to drug is known.
- Report any visual disturbances.
- Avoid drinking alcohol.
- Women should use reliable means of contraception while taking this drug and up to 6 months after therapy ends. Notify prescriber immediately if they become pregnant. Adverse effects to the fetus may be caused by either male of female patients receiving this drug in combination with ribavirin.

PEGINTERFERON ALFA-2B

(peg-in-ter-fer′on)

PegIntron, Sylatron

Classification: BIOLOGIC RESPONSE MODIFIER; IMMUNOMODULATOR; ALPHA INTERFERON

Therapeutic: ANTIVIRAL; ANTIHEPATITIS

Prototype: Peginterferon alfa-2a

AVAILABILITY
Powder for injection

ACTION & *THERAPEUTIC EFFECT*

Binds to specific membrane receptors on the cell surface, thereby initiating suppression of cell proliferation, enhanced phagocytic activity of macrophages, augmentation of specific cytotoxic lymphocytes for target cells, and inhibition of viral replication in virus-infected cells. *Induces antiviral effects by activation of macrophages, natural killer cells, and T-cells, thus boosting cellular immunity and suppressing hepatic inflammation and replication of hepatitis C virus.*

USES Adjuvant therapy of melanoma.

CONTRAINDICATIONS Hypersensitivity to peginterferon or interferon alfa; autoimmune hepatitis; decompensated liver disease {Child-Pugh (class B and C)} in cirrhotic chronic hepatitis C patients before or during treatment; pancreatitis; persistently severe or worsening S&S of life-threatening neuropsychiatric, autoimmune, ischemic, or infectious disorders; history of significant or unstable cardiac disease; uncontrollable DM or hypo- or hyperthyroidism; pregnancy—fetal risk cannot be ruled out; lactation—infant risk cannot be ruled out. **Sylatron:** Hepatic decompensation. {Child-Pugh (class B and C)}.

CAUTIOUS USE History of neuropsychiatric disorder; suicidal tendencies; substance abuse disorders; bone marrow suppression; ulcerative and hemorrhagic colitis; pulmonary disorders; HBV or HIV coinfection; thyroid dysfunction; DM; cardiovascular disease; autoimmune disorders; pulmonary disease, COPD; retinal disease; renal impairment with creatinine clearance less than 50 mL/min; older adults; Safety and efficacy in children younger than 3 y not established.

ROUTE & DOSAGE

Melanoma (Sylatron only)

Adult: **Subcutaneous** 6 mcg/kg/wk × 8 doses then 3 mcg/kg/wk for up to 5 y

Renal Impairment Dosage Adjustment

CrCl 30–50 mL/min: reduce initial dose to 4.5 mcg/kg/week; then 2.25 mcg/kg/week; CrCl less than 30 mL/min: reduce initial dose to 3 mcg/kg/week; then 1.5 mcg/kg/week

ADMINISTRATION

Subcutaneous

- Give dose on the same day of each week.
- *Vial reconstitution:* Be aware that two Safety Lok™ syringes are provided in the drug package: One for reconstitution and one for injection. Reconstitute with only 0.7 mL of supplied diluent and discard remaining diluent. Enter the vial only once as it does not contain a preservative. Swirl gently to produce a clear, colorless solution. Use solution immediately.
- Store dry vial at 15°–30° C (59°–86° F). If necessary, store reconstituted solution up to 24 h at 2°–8° C (36°–46° F).

ADVERSE EFFECTS (≥ 5%) **CNS:** *Headache, dizziness.* **Skin:** *Alopecia.* **Hepatic:** *Increased liver enzymes.* **GI:** *Nausea, anorexia, diarrhea,* vomiting. **Musculoskeletal:** *Arthralgia, myalgia.* **Hematologic:** Thrombocytopenia, neutropenia. **Other:** *Fatigue, inflammation at injection site, rigors, fever.*

INTERACTIONS **Drug:** additive myelosuppression with ANTINEOPLASTICS; **zidovudine** may increase hematologic toxicity; i increase neurotoxicity with **telbivudine; aldesleukin (IL-2)** may potentiate

P

the risk of kidney failure. Do not administer LIVE VACCINES.

PHARMACOKINETICS

Peak: 15–44 h. **Elimination:** 30% in urine. **Half-Life:** 40-50 h.

NURSING IMPLICATIONS

Black Box Warning

PegIntron has been associated with fatal or life-threatening neuropsychiatric, autoimmune, ischemic, and infectious disorders. Sylatron has been associated with serious depression with suicidal ideation, completed suicides, and other serious neuropsychiatric disorders.

Assessment & Drug Effects

- Monitor for S&S of hypersensitivity (e.g., angioedema, bronchoconstriction) and, if noted, institute appropriate medical action immediately. Note that transient rashes are not an indication to discontinue treatment.
- Monitor for and report immediately S&S of neuropsychiatric disorders (e.g., psychosis, hallucinations, suicidal ideation, depression). Every 3 weeks during the initial 8 weeks of treatment, every 6 months thereafter while on therapy, and for at least 6 months after discontinuing therapy.
- Regular dental exams.
- Monitor respiratory and cardiovascular status; report dyspnea, chest pain, and hypotension immediately; baseline and periodic ECG and chest x-ray.
- Withhold drug and notify prescriber for any of the following: Severe neuropsychiatric events, severe neutropenia or thrombocytopenia, abdominal pain accompanied by bloody diarrhea and fever, S&S of pancreatitis, or any other severe adverse event (see CAUTIOUS USE).
- Baseline and periodic ophthalmology exams are recommended.
- Monitor lab tests: Baseline and periodic creatinine clearance, serum uric acid, CBC with differential, platelet count, Hct and Hgb, TSH, ALT, AST, bilirubin, blood glucose; triglycerides, serum HCV RNA level after 24 wk of treatment, pregnancy test immediately prior to initiation of therapy and monthly during therapy and for 6 months after therapy.

Patient & Family Education

- Drink fluids liberally while taking this drug, especially during the initial stages of therapy.
- Instruct, and provide opportunity for return demonstration of subcutaneous injections.
- Learn reasons for withholding drug (see ASSESSMENT & DRUG EFFECTS).
- Use effective means of contraception while taking this drug. Women should not become pregnant. Use 2 forms of birth control during therapy and for 6 months after the last dose.
- Review adverse effects with patient and/or caregiver.
- Immediately report chest pain, lightheadedness, fainting episode, or racing heartbeat.
- Follow up with lab tests; compliance with lab testing is extremely important while taking this drug.

PEGINTERFERON BETA-1A

(peg-in-ter-fer'on)

Plegridy

Classification: BIOLOGIC RESPONSE MODIFIER; IMMUNOMODULATOR; BETA INTERFERON

Therapeutic: IMMUNOMODULATOR

Prototype: Peginterferon alfa-2A

AVAILABILITY Prefilled solution for injection

ACTION & *THERAPEUTIC EFFECT* Exact mechanism of action in the treatment of multiple sclerosis is unknown. Interferon beta-1A alters the expression and response to surface antigens and enhances immune cell activities. *Improves symptoms and functionality in patients with relapsing MS.*

USES Treatment of patients with relapsing forms of multiple sclerosis.

CONTRAINDICATIONS History of hypersensitivity to natural or recombinant interferon beta or peginterferon, or any other component of the formulation; suicidal ideation or other severe psychiatric symptoms.

CAUTIOUS USE Severe renal impairment; seizure disorder; hepatic impairment; depression, history of suicidal thoughts; seizure disorder; myelosuppression; CHF; cardiomyopathy; serious injections site reactions; older adults; pregnancy (category C); lactation. Safety and efficacy in children younger than 18 y not established.

P

ROUTE & DOSAGE

Multiple Sclerosis

Adult: **Subcutaneous** 63 mcg on day 1; 94 mcg on day 15; 125 mcg on day 29 and 125 mcg every 14 days thereafter

ADMINISTRATION

Subcutaneous

- Allow prefilled syringe or pen to warm to room temperature (approx. 30 min) prior to injection; do not use external heat sources (e.g., hot water) to warm.
- Inject into the abdomen, back of the upper arm, or thigh; rotate injection sites; do not inject into area where skin is red, irritated, bruised, or scarred.
- Store in the closed original carton to protect from light, at 2°–8° C (36°–46° F). Do not freeze; discard if frozen.

ADVERSE EFFECTS **CNS:** *Headache.* **Endocrine:** Increased ALT and AST, increased gamma glutamyl transferase. **Skin:** Pruritus. **GI:** Nausea, vomiting. **Musculoskeletal:** Arthralgia, *myalgia.* **Hematologic:** Decreased white cell counts. **Other:** *Asthenia, chills,* hyperthermia, *influenza-like illness,* injection site edema, *injection site erythema,* injection site hematoma, *injection site illness, injection site pain, injection site pruritus,* injection site rash, injection site hematoma, pain, *pyrexia.*

INTERACTIONS **Drugs:** Use with NRTIS should be done with caution as it may impact antiviral clearance. Avoid use with **vigabatrin.**

PHARMACOKINETICS **Peak:** 1–1.5 days. **Distribution:** Well distributed to tissues. **Metabolism:** Not extensive. **Elimination:** Primarily renal. **Half-Life:** 78 h.

NURSING IMPLICATIONS

Assessment & Drug Effects

- Monitor for injection site reactions (e.g., erythema, pain, pruritus, edema, necrosis).
- Monitor for and report promptly any of the following: S&S of hypersensitivity or hepatic injury; S&S of myelosuppression (e.g., infections, bleeding, anemia); new onset or worsening signs of CV disease (i.e., CHF); mental status changes.
- Monitor for increased seizure activity with a preexisting seizure disorder.
- Monitor lab tests: Baseline and periodic CBC with differential and platelet count, LFTs, renal function tests; periodic thyroid function tests.

Patient & Family Education

- Report promptly to prescriber if you develop signs of infection or bleeding.
- Consult your prescriber if you experience mental status changes (e.g., depression, suicidal ideation, anxiety, emotional instability, illogical thinking).
- Notify prescriber immediately if you experience worsening symptoms of heart failure such as shortness of breath, swelling of your lower legs, or excessive weight gain.
- Notify your prescriber if you are pregnant or plan to become pregnant.
- Do not breast-feed without first consulting your prescriber.

PEGLOTICASE

(peg-lo′ti-case)

Krystexxa

Classification: ANTIGOUT; URIC ACID METABOLIZING ENZYME

Therapeutic: ANTIGOUT

AVAILABILITY Solution for injection

ACTION & *THERAPEUTIC EFFECT* Pegloticase is a recombinant uric acid specific enzyme that catalyzes the conversion of uric acid to a water soluble, inert metabolite readily eliminated by the kidney. *It lowers the serum uric acid, thus reducing uric acid induced inflammation.*

USES Treatment of chronic gout.

CONTRAINDICATIONS Established G6PD deficiency; lactation.

CAUTIOUS USE African or Mediterranean ancestry; consider discontinuing if uric acid level above 6 mg/mL; retreatment with pegloticase following discontinuation of therapy for longer than 6 wk; CHF; pregnancy (category C); children younger than 18 y.

ROUTE & DOSAGE

Chronic Gout

Adult: **IV** 8 mg over 2 hrs q2wk

ADMINISTRATION

Intravenous

- Note: Premedication with antihistamines and corticosteroids is required to minimize the risk of anaphylaxis and infusion reactions. ▪ Pegloticase should only be administered in a health care setting and by health care providers trained to manage anaphylaxis and infusion reactions.

PREPARE: **IV Infusion:** Do not shake vial. ▪ Withdraw 1 mL of pegloticase from the 2 mL vial and inject into 250 mL of NS. Do not mix or dilute with other drugs. ▪ Invert IV bag to mix but do not shake. ▪ Discard unused pegloticase remaining in vial.

ADMINISTER: **IV Infusion:** If refrigerated, bring to room temperature prior to infusion. **Do not** give IV push or bolus. Infuse over NO LESS THAN 120 min. ▪ Monitor closely throughout infusion and for 2 h post-infusion for S&S of anaphylaxis or an infusion reaction (e.g., urticarial, erythema, dyspnea, flushing, chest discomfort, chest pain, and rash). ▪ If S&S of anaphylaxis or an infusion reaction occur, stop infusion and immediately notify prescriber. ▪ If anaphylaxis is ruled out and infusion is restarted, it should be run at a slower rate. ▪ Infusion bags may be stored refrigerated for 4 h after dilution.

INCOMPATIBILITIES: **Solution/additive:** Do not mix with another drug. **Y-site:** Do not mix with another drug.

▪ Store unopened vials in refrigerator at (2°–8° C or 36°–46° F) and protect from light. Do not shake or freeze.

▪ Diluted solution may be stored up to 4 h at 2°–8° C (36°–46° F). Warm to room temperature before administration. Diluted solution is also stable at room temperature for up to 4 h, but should be protected from light.

ADVERSE EFFECTS **CV:** Chest pain. **Respiratory:** Dyspnea, nasopharyngitis. **CNS:** Headache. **Endocrine:** Anemia. **Skin:** Erythema, urticaria. **GI:** *Nausea* vomiting, constipation **Other:** Anaphylaxis, contusion, ecchymosis, arthralgia, gout flare, infusion reaction, pruritus.

INTERACTIONS **Drug:** Potential interaction with other pegylated products (**pegfilgrastim, peginterferon alfa-2a**). Do not use with **allopurinol, febuxostat, probenecid, sulfinpyrazone.**

NURSING IMPLICATIONS

Black Box Warning

Pegloticase has been associated with anaphylaxis and infusion reactions during and after administration. G6PD deficiency-associated hemolysis and methemoglobinemia.

Assessment & Drug Effects

- Monitor closely during infusion and for 2 h post-infusion for S&S of anaphylaxis (see Appendix F) or an infusion reaction (see IV ADMINISTRATION).
- Assess vital signs frequently during and for 2 h post-infusion.
- Monitor cardiac status, especially with preexisting congestive heart failure.
- Notify prescriber if uric acid level is 6 mg/mL or above. Two consecutive readings above 6 mm/mL may indicate need to discontinue treatment.
- Monitor lab tests: Baseline and periodic serum uric acid level.

Patient & Family Education

- Report promptly any discomfort (e.g., wheezing, facial swelling, skin rash, redness of the skin, difficulty breathing, flushing, chest discomfort, chest pain, rash) during or following IV infusion.

- Gout flares may increase during the first 3 mo of therapy and are not a reason to discontinue pegloticase.

PEMBROLIZUMAB

(pem-bro-li′zu-mab)

Keytruda

Classification: IMMUNOMODULATOR; MONOCLONAL ANTIBODY; PROGRAMMED DEATH RECEPTOR-1 BLOCKER

Therapeutic: IMMUNOSUPPRESSANT

Prototype: Basiliximab

AVAILABILITY Lyophilized powder

ACTION & THERAPEUTIC EFFECT A monoclonal antibody that acts as an immune checkpoint inhibitor. Activation of programmed cell death (PD-1) receptors found on T cells inhibits T cell proliferation and cytokine production. Increased activation of PD-1 receptors occurs in some tumors and can contribute to inhibition of active T-cell immune response to tumors. Pembrolizumab binds to the PD-1 receptor and blocks its activation thus removing inhibition of the immune response, including the antitumor immune response. *Blocking PD-1 activity results in decreased tumor growth.*

USES Treatment of patients with unresectable or metastatic melanoma and disease progression following ipilimumab and a BRAF inhibitor (for those patients who have a BRAF V600 mutation), metastatic non–small-cell lung cancer; head/neck cancer; colorectal cancer; cervical cancer; Hodgkin lymphoma; urothelial cancer.

CONTRAINDICATIONS Any life-threatening adverse reaction; drug induced Grade 3–4 renal failure, hepatitis, or infusion-related reactions; drug induced life-threatening immune-mediated colitis; pregnancy—fetal risk cannot be ruled out; lactation—infant risk cannot be ruled out.

CAUTIOUS USE Renal or hepatic impairment; drug induced pneumonitis; asthma; COPD; prior thoracic radiation; inflammation of the pituitary (hypophysitis); DM; thyroid disorders; colitis; organ donor recipients; women of childbearing age. Safety and efficacy in children younger than 18 y not established.

ROUTE & DOSAGE

Metastatic Melanoma/Hodgkin Lymphoma

Adult: **IV** 200 mg every 3 wk or 400 mg every 6 wk until disease progression or unacceptable toxicity

Breast Cancer

Adult: IV 200 mg every 3wk or 400 mg every 6 wk; duration varies based on concurrent medications.

Non–Small-Cell Lung Cancer/Head/Neck Cancer

Adult: **IV** 200 mg q3w for up to 24 mo until disease progression or unacceptable toxicity

Toxicity Dosage Adjustment

See package insert

ADMINISTRATION

Intravenous

PREPARE: **IV Infusion:** Dilute prior to administration in NS or D5W to a final concentration of 1 to 10 mg/mL. Slowly swirl vial; do

P

not shake. Allow up to 5 min for bubbles to dissipate. Mix by gently inverting bag. Discard unused portion of the vial.
ADMINISTER: **IV Infusion:** Infuse over 30 min through a 0.2–0.5 micron sterile, nonpyrogenic, low-protein-binding in-line or add-on filter.
INCOMPATIBILITIES: Do not mix or infuse with any other medications.

- Store intact vials at 2°–8° C (36°–46° F). Reconstituted and solutions diluted for infusion may be stored at room temperature for up to 6 h (infusion must be completed within 6 h of reconstitution) or refrigerated at 2°–8° C (36°–46° F) for no more than 96 h from the time of reconstitution.

ADVERSE EFFECTS (≥5%) **CV:** *Hypertension.* **Respiratory:** *Cough,* dyspnea. **CNS:** Neuropathy. **Endocrine:** Hyperglycemia, hypercholesterolemia, hypertriglyceridemia, hypoalbuminemia, hyponatremia. **Skin:** Pruritus, *rash, alopecia.* **Hepatic:** Aspartate aminotransferase serum elevations. **GI:** *Constipation, anorexia, diarrhea, nausea.* **GU:** *Proteinuria.* **Musculoskeletal:** *Arthralgia.* **Hematologic:** Anemia. **Other:** *Fatigue.*

INTERACTIONS **Drug:** May enhance toxicity of **thalidomide**. CORTICOSTEROIDS may decrease efficacy of pembrolizumab. If used with **clozapine** monitor ANC.

PHARMACOKINETICS **Half-Life:** 26 days.

NURSING IMPLICATIONS

Assessment & Drug Effects

- Monitor for S&S of hypersensitivity or infusion-related reactions.
- Monitor for tumor response.
- Monitor for S&S of drug toxicity including pneumonitis, colitis, hepatitis, pituitary disorders, nephritis, thyroid dysfunction.
- Monitor lab tests: Baseline and periodic LFTs, renal function tests, thyroid function tests; periodic lipid profile and serum electrolytes, blood glucose levels, pregnancy test prior to drug treatment for women with reproductive potential.

Patient & Family Education

- Report promptly to prescriber if you experience signs of pulmonary toxicity such as new or worsening cough, chest pain, or shortness of breath.
- Report signs of colitis or liver damage such as diarrhea, severe abdominal pain, jaundice, severe nausea or vomiting, or easy bruising or bleeding.
- Report signs of endocrine dysfunction including persistent or unusual headache, extreme weakness, dizziness or fainting, or vision changes.
- Women of childbearing potential should use highly effective contraception during and for 4 mo after the last dose of this drug.
- Do not breastfeed while taking this drug.

PEMETREXED

(pe-me-trex′ed)
Alimta
Classification: ANTINEOPLASTIC; ANTIMETABOLITE, ANTIFOLATE
Therapeutic: ANTINEOPLASTIC
Prototype: Methotrexate

AVAILABILITY Powder for injection

ACTION & *THERAPEUTIC EFFECT* Suppresses tumor growth by inhibiting both DNA synthesis and folate metabolism at multiple target enzymes. *Appears to arrest the cell cycle, thus inhibiting tumor growth.*

USES Treatment of malignant pleural mesothelioma that is unresectable or in patients that are not surgery candidates in combination with cisplatin; treatment of locally advanced or metastatic non–small-cell lung cancer (NSCLC).

UNLABELED USES Solid tumors, including bladder, breast, colorectal, gastric, head and neck, pancreatic, and renal cell cancers.

CONTRAINDICATIONS Mannitol hypersensitivity; creatinine clearance is less than 45 mL/min, renal failure, active infection; vaccines; pregnancy (category D); lactation.

CAUTIOUS USE Anemia, thrombocytopenia, neutropenia, dental disease; older adults; hepatic disease, renal impairment; hypoalbuminemia, hypovolemia, dehydration, ascites, pleural effusion; children younger than 18 y.

ROUTE & DOSAGE

Malignant Mesothelioma, Non–Small-Cell Lung Cancer

Adult: IV 500 mg/m^2 on day 1 of each 21-day cycle

Renal Impairment Dosage Adjustment

CrCl less than 45 mL/min: Not recommended

ADMINISTRATION

Intravenous

Pre/posttreatment with folic acid, vitamin B_{12}, and dexamethasone are needed to reduce hematologic and gastrointestinal toxicity, and the possibility of severe cutaneous reactions from pemetrexed.

This drug is a cytotoxic agent and caution should be used to prevent any contact with the drug. Follow institutional or standard guidelines for preparation, handling, and disposal of cytotoxic agents.

***PREPARE:* IV Infusion:** Reconstitute each 100 mg or 500 mg vial with 4.2 mL or 20 mL, respectively, of preservative-free NS. ▪ Do not use any other diluent. Swirl gently to dissolve. Each vial will contain 25 mg/mL. ▪ Withdraw the needed amount of reconstituted solution and add to 100 mL of preservative-free NS. ▪ Discard any unused portion.

***ADMINISTER:* IV Infusion: Do not** give a bolus dose. ▪ Infuse over 10 min.

***INCOMPATIBILITIES:* Solution/additive:** Solutions containing **calcium, lactated Ringer's. Y-site: Amphotericin B, calcium, cefazolin, cefotaxime, cefotetan, cefoxitin, ceftazidime, chlorpromazine, ciprofloxacin, dobutamine, doxorubicin, doxycycline, droperidol, gemcitabine, gentamicin, irinotecan, metronidazole, minocycline, mitoxantrone, nalbuphine, ondansetron, prochlorperazine, tobramycin, topotecan.**

▪ Store unopened single-use vials at room temperature at 15°–30° C (59°–86° F). ▪ The reconstituted drug is stable for up to 24 h at 2°–8° C (36°–46° F) or at 25° C (77° F).

ADVERSE EFFECTS **CV:** Chest pain, thromboembolism. **Respiratory:** *Dyspnea.* **CNS:** Neuropathy, *mood alteration, depression.* **Skin:** *Rash, desquamation,* alopecia. **GI:** *Nausea, vomiting, constipation, anorexia, stomatitis, diarrhea,* dehydration, dysphagia, esophagitis, odynophagia, increased LFTs. **GU:** *Increases serum creatinine,* renal failure. **Hematologic:** *Neutropenia,* leukopenia, anemia, thrombocytopenia. **Other:** *Fatigue, fever,* hypersensitivity reaction, edema, myalgia, arthralgia.

INTERACTIONS Drug: Increased risk of renal toxicity with other nephrotoxic drugs (**acyclovir, adefovir, amphotericin B,** AMINOGLYCOSIDES, **carboplatin, cidofovir, cisplatin, cyclosporine, foscarnet, ganciclovir, sirolimus, tacrolimus, vancomycin**); NSAIDS may increase risk of renal toxicity in patients with preexisting renal insufficiency; may cause additive risk of bleeding with ANTICOAGULANTS, PLATELET INHIBITORS, **aspirin,** THROMBOLYTIC AGENTS.

PHARMACOKINETICS Metabolism: Not extensively. **Elimination:** Primarily in urine. **Half-Life:** 3.5 h.

P

NURSING IMPLICATIONS

Assessment & Drug Effects

- Withhold drug and notify prescriber if the absolute neutrophil count (ANC) is less than 1500 cells/mm^3 or the platelet count is less than at least 100,000 cells/mm^3, or if the CrCl is less than 45 mL/min.
- Notify prescriber for S&S of neuropathy (paresthesia) or thromboembolism.
- Monitor lab tests: Baseline and periodic CBC with differential; monitor for nadir and recovery before each dose (on days 8 and 15, respectively, of each cycle); periodic LFTs, serum creatinine, and BUN.

Patient & Family Education

- Report promptly any of the following to prescriber: Symptoms of anemia (e.g., chest pain, unusual weakness or tiredness, fainting spells, lightheadedness, shortness of breath); symptoms of poor blood clotting (e.g., bruising; red spots on skin; black, tarry stools; blood in urine); symptoms of infection (e.g., fever or chills, cough, sore throat, pain or difficulty passing urine); symptoms of liver problems (e.g., yellowing of skin).
- Do not take nonsteroidal antiinflammatory drugs (NSAIDS) without first consulting the prescriber.

PENBUTOLOL

(pen-bu'tol-ol)

Levatol

Classification: BETA-ADRENERGIC ANTAGONIST; ANTIHYPERTENSIVE
Therapeutic: ANTIHYPERTENSIVE
Prototype: Propranolol

AVAILABILITY Tablet

ACTION & *THERAPEUTIC EFFECT* Synthetic beta-1- and beta-2-adrenergic blocking agent that competes with epinephrine and norepinephrine for available beta receptor sites. Lowers both supine and standing BP in hypertensive patients. Hypotensive effect is associated with decreased cardiac output, suppressed renin activity as well as beta blockage. *Effective in lowering mild to moderate blood pressure.*

USES Mild to moderate hypertension.

CONTRAINDICATIONS Hypersensitivity to penbutolol; cardiogenic shock, acute CHF, sinus bradycardia, second and third degree AV block; bronchial asthma, acute bronchospasm; Raynaund's disease; COPD; abrupt withdrawal.

CAUTIOUS USE Cardiac failure; PVD; chronic bronchitis; diabetes; mental depression; myasthenia gravis, cerebrovascular insufficiency, stroke; renal disease; major surgery; hyperthyroid; older adults; pregnancy (category C); lactation. Safety and efficacy in children not established.

ROUTE & DOSAGE

Hypertension

Adult: **PO** 20 mg daily, may increase to 40–80 mg/day

ADMINISTRATION

Oral

- Discontinue by reducing the dose gradually over 1 to 2 wk.

ADVERSE EFFECTS **CV:** AV block, bradycardia. **Respiratory:** Cough, dyspnea. **CNS:** Dizziness, fatigue, *headache,* insomnia. **GI:** Nausea, diarrhea, dyspepsia. **GU:** Impotence.

INTERACTIONS **Drug:** DIURETICS and other HYPOTENSIVE AGENTS increase hypotensive effect; effects of **albuterol, metaproterenol, terbutaline, pirbuterol,** and **penbutolol** are antagonized; NSAIDS blunt hypotensive effect; decreases hypoglycemic effect of **glyburide; amiodarone** increases risk of bradycardia and sinus arrest.

PHARMACOKINETICS **Absorption:** Readily from GI tract. **Peak:** 2–3 h. **Duration:** 20 h. **Metabolism:** In liver. **Elimination:** In urine. **Half-Life:** 5 h.

NURSING IMPLICATIONS

Assessment & Drug Effects

- Take apical pulse before administering drug. If pulse is below 60, or other established parameter, hold the drug and contact prescriber.
- Take a BP reading before giving drug, if BP is not stabilized. If systolic pressure is 90 mm Hg or less, hold drug and contact prescriber.
- Check BP near end of dosage interval or before administration of next dose to evaluate effectiveness.
- Monitor therapeutic effectiveness. Full effectiveness of the drug may not be seen for 4–6 wk.
- Watch for S&S of bronchial constriction. Report promptly and withhold drug.
- Monitor diabetics for loss of glycemic control. Drug suppresses clinical signs of hypoglycemia (e.g., BP changes, increased pulse rate) and may prolong hypoglycemic state.
- Monitor carefully for exacerbation of angina during drug withdrawal.

Patient & Family Education

- Do not discontinue the drug without prescriber's advice because of the possible exacerbation of ischemic heart disease.
- If diabetic, report persistent S&S of hypoglycemia (see Appendix F) to prescriber (diabetics).
- Avoid driving or other potentially hazardous activities until response to drug is known.
- Make position changes slowly and avoid prolonged standing. Notify prescriber if dizziness and lightheadedness persist.
- Comply with and do not alter established regimen (i.e., do not

omit, increase, or decrease dosage or change dosage interval).

- Avoid prolonged exposure of extremities to cold.
- Avoid excesses of alcohol. Heavy alcohol consumption [i.e., greater than 60 mL (2 oz)/day] may elevate arterial pressure; therefore, to maintain treatment effectiveness, either avoid alcohol or drink moderately (less than 60 mL/day). Consult prescriber.

PENCICLOVIR

(pen-cy'clo-vir)

Denavir

Classification: ANTIVIRAL

Therapeutic: TOPICAL ANTIVIRAL

Prototype: Acyclovir

AVAILABILITY Cream

ACTION & *THERAPEUTIC EFFECT* Antiviral agent active against herpes simplex virus type 1 (HSV-1) and type 2 (HSV-2). HSV-1 and HSV-2 infected cells phosphorylate penciclovir utilizing viral thymidine kinase. Competes with viral DNA, thus inhibiting both viral DNA synthesis and replication. *Effectiveness is measured in decreased viral load.*

USES Treatment of recurrent herpes labialis (cold sores).

CONTRAINDICATIONS Hypersensitivity to penciclovir or famciclovir.

CAUTIOUS USE Acyclovir, or related antiviral hypersensitivity; pregnancy—fetal risk minimal; lactation—infant risk minimal. Safety and efficacy in children younger than 12 y not established. Safety in immunocompromised patients not established.

ROUTE & DOSAGE

Cold Sores

Adult: **Topical** Apply q2h while awake × 4 days

ADVMINISTRATION

Topical

- Apply as soon as possible after developing lesion.
- Do not apply to mucous membranes or near the eyes.
- Store at 20 to 25 degrees C (68 to 77 degrees F).

ADVERSE EFFECTS No adverse effects with occurrence of 1% or greater.

PHARMACOKINETICS **Absorption:** Minimally absorbed from cold sore.

NURSING IMPLICATIONS

Assessment & Drug Effects

- Monitor the extent of lesions and treatment effectiveness.

Patient & Family Education

- Wash hands before and after application. Avoid contact of drug with eyes.
- Start using treatment at the earliest sign of a cold sore.
- Apply sunscreen to lips; may minimize recurrence of lesions.

PENICILLAMINE

(pen-i-sill'a-meen)

Cuprimine, Depen

Classification: DISEASE-MODIFYING ANTIRHEUMATIC DRUG (DMARD)

Therapeutic: CHELATING AGENT; ANTIRHEUMATIC (DMARD)

AVAILABILITY Capsule; tablet

ACTION & *THERAPEUTIC EFFECT*

Combines chemically with cystine to form a soluble disulfide complex that prevents stone formation and may even dissolve existing cystic stones. Forms stable soluble chelate with copper, zinc, iron, lead, mercury, and possibly other heavy metals and promotes their excretion in urine. Mechanism of action in rheumatoid arthritis appears to be related to inhibition of collagen formation. *With Wilson's disease, therapeutic effectiveness is indicated by improvement in psychiatric and neurologic symptoms, visual symptoms, and liver function. With rheumatoid arthritis, therapeutic effectiveness is indicated by improvement in grip strength, decrease in stiffness following immobility, reduction of pain, decrease in sedimentation rate and rheumatoid factor.*

USES To promote renal excretion of excess copper in Wilson's disease (hepatolenticular degeneration); cystinuria.

UNLABELED USES Scleroderma, primary biliary cirrhosis, porphyria cutanea tarda, lead poisoning.

CONTRAINDICATIONS Hypersensitivity to penicillamine or to any penicillin; history of penicillamine-related aplastic anemia or agranulocytosis; rheumatoid arthritis patients with renal insufficiency or who are pregnant; renal failure; concomitant administration with drugs that can cause severe hematologic or renal reactions (e.g., antimalarials, gold salts); pregnancy; lactation.

CAUTIOUS USE Allergy-prone individuals; DM; renal disease, renal impairment; hepatic impairment, hepatic disease; history of hematologic disease; children.

ROUTE & DOSAGE

Wilson's Disease

Adult: **PO** 750–1,500 mg/day in divided doses (max: 2000 mg/day)

Cystinuria

Adult: **PO** 250–500 mg qid, with doses adjusted to limit urinary excretion of cystine to 100–200 mg/day
Child: **PO** 20–40 mg/kg/day in 4 divided doses with doses adjusted to limit urinary excretion of cystine to 100–200 mg/day

Renal Impairment Dosage Adjustment

CrCl less than 50 mL/min: Avoid use

ADMINISTRATION

Oral

- Give on empty stomach (60 min before or 2 h after meals) to avoid absorption of metals in foods by penicillamine.
- Give contents in 15–30 mL of chilled fruit juice or pureed fruit (e.g., applesauce) if patient cannot swallow capsules or tablets.
- Drink copious amounts of water, about 1 pint at bedtime and another pint once during the night.
- Store in tight, well-closed containers.

ADVERSE EFFECTS **Skin:** Rash. **GI:** Diarrhea, loss of appetite, loss of taste, nausea, vomiting, ulcers in the mouth. **GU:** Proteinuria.

INTERACTIONS **Drug:** ANTIMALARIALS, CYTOTOXICS, **gold** therapy may potentiate hematologic and renal adverse effects; **iron** may decrease penicillamine absorption.

PHARMACOKINETICS Absorption: Readily from GI tract. **Peak:** 1 h. **Distribution:** Crosses placenta. **Metabolism:** In liver. **Elimination:** In urine. **Half-Life:** 1–7 h.

NURSING IMPLICATIONS

Black Box Warning

Penicillamine has been associated with serious hematological and renal adverse reactions.

Assessment & Drug Effects

- Monitor for and report promptly S&S of granulocytopenia and/or thrombocytopenia such as fever, sore throat, chills, bruising, or bleeding.
- Monitor skin, lymph nodes, and body temperature, during the first month of therapy, every 2 wk for the next 5 mo, and monthly thereafter.
- Withhold drug and contact prescriber if the patient with rheumatoid arthritis develops proteinuria greater than 1 g (some clinicians accept greater than 2 g) or if platelet count drops to less than 100,000/mm^3, or platelet count falls below 3500–4000/mm^3, or neutropenia occurs.
- Monitor lab tests: Baseline WBC with differential, direct platelet count, Hgb, LFTs (every 6 months), and urinalyses prior to initiation of therapy and twice weekly during the first month of therapy, then every 2 wk for the next 5 mo, and monthly thereafter.

Patient & Family Education

- Note: Clinical evidence of therapeutic effectiveness may not be apparent until 1–3 mo of drug therapy.
- Take exactly as prescribed. Allergic reactions occur in about one third of patients receiving penicillamine. Temporary interruptions of therapy increase possibility of sensitivity reactions.
- Take temperature nightly during first few months of therapy. Fever is a possible early sign of allergy.
- Observe skin over pressure sites: Knees, elbows, shoulder blades, toes, buttocks. Penicillamine increases risk of skin breakdown.
- Report unusual bruising or bleeding, sore mouth or throat, fever, skin rash, or any other unusual symptoms to prescriber.

PENICILLIN G BENZATHINE

(pen-i-sill′in)

Bicillin, Bicillin L-A, Permapen

Classification: BETA-LACTAM ANTIBIOTIC; NATURAL PENICILLIN

Therapeutic: ANTIBIOTIC

Prototype: Penicillin G potassium

AVAILABILITY Solution for injection

ACTION & *THERAPEUTIC EFFECT* Acts by interfering with synthesis of mucopeptides essential to formation and integrity of the bacterial cell wall. *Effective against many strains of* Staphylococcus aureus, *gram-positive cocci, gram-negative cocci. Also effective against gram-positive bacilli and gram-negative bacilli as well as some strains of* Salmonella, Shigella, *and spirochetes.*

USES Infections highly susceptible to penicillin G, such as streptococcal, pneumococcal, and staphylococcal infections, venereal disease such as syphilis (including early, late, and congenital forms), and nonvenereal diseases. Also used in prophylaxis of rheumatic fever.

CONTRAINDICATIONS Hypersensitivity to penicillins; IV administration.

CAUTIOUS USE History of or suspected allergy (eczema, hives, hay fever, asthma); hypersensitivity to cephalosporins or carbapenems; history of colitis; IBD; renal disease, renal impairment; GI disease; pregnancy (category B); lactation; infants, neonates.

ROUTE & DOSAGE

Mild to Moderate Infections

Adult: **IM** 1,200,000 units once/day
Child (weight greater than 27 kg): **IM** 900,000 units once/day; *weight less than 27 kg:* 300,000–600,000 units once/day

Syphilis

Adult: **IM** Less than 1 y duration: 2,400,000 units as single dose; greater than 1 y duration: 2,400,000 units/wk for 3 wk
Child (younger than 2 y): **IM** 50,000 units/kg as single dose

Prophylaxis for Rheumatic Fever

Adult: **IM** 1.2 million units q4wk
Child: **IM** 1.2 million units q3–4wk

ADMINISTRATION

Intramuscular

- Do not confuse penicillin G benzathine with preparations containing procaine penicillin G (e.g., Bicillin C-R).
- Make IM injection deep into upper outer quadrant of buttock. In infants and small children, the preferred site is the midlateral aspect of the thigh.
- Shake multiple-dose vial vigorously before withdrawing desired IM dose. Shake prepared cartridge unit vigorously before injecting drug.
- Select IM site with care. Injection into or near a major peripheral nerve can result in nerve damage.
- Inadvertent IV administration has resulted in arterial occlusion and cardiac arrest.
- Make injections at a slow steady rate to prevent needle blockage.
- Store at 15°–30° C (59°–86° F).

ADVERSE EFFECTS **Skin:** Pruritus, urticaria, and other skin eruptions. **Hematologic:** Eosinophilia, hemolytic anemia, and other blood abnormalities. Also see PENICILLIN G POTASSIUM. **Other:** *Local pain,* tenderness, and fever associated with IM injection, chills, fever, wheezing, anaphylaxis, neuropathy, nephrotoxicity; superinfections, Jarisch-Herxheimer reaction in patients with syphilis.

INTERACTIONS **Drug: Probenecid** decreases renal elimination; may decrease efficacy of ORAL CONTRACEPTIVES.

PHARMACOKINETICS **Absorption:** Slowly absorbed from IM site. **Peak:** 12–24 h. **Duration:** 26 days. **Distribution:** Crosses placenta; distributed into breast milk. **Metabolism:** Hydrolyzed to penicillin in body. **Elimination:** Excreted slowly by kidneys.

NURSING IMPLICATIONS

Black Box Warning

Penicillin G has been associated with serious adverse reaction due to inadvertent IV administration.

P

Note: See penicillin G potassium for numerous additional clinical implications.

Assessment & Drug Effects

- Determine history of hypersensitivity reactions to penicillins, cephalosporins, or other allergens prior to initiation of drug therapy.
- Monitor lab tests: Baseline C&S and repeat at completion of therapy.

Patient & Family Education

- Report immediately to prescriber the onset of an allergic reaction. There is great risk of severe and prolonged reactions because drug is absorbed so slowly.

PENICILLIN G POTASSIUM (Pr)

(pen-i-sill'in)

Megacillin ♣

PENICILLIN G SODIUM

Classification: BETA-LACTAM ANTIBIOTIC; NATURAL PENICILLIN
Therapeutic: ANTIBIOTIC

AVAILABILITY Vial; solution for injection

ACTION & *THERAPEUTIC EFFECT* Acid labile, penicillinase-sensitive, natural penicillin that acts by interfering with synthesis of mucopeptides essential to formation and integrity of bacterial cell wall. Antimicrobial spectrum is narrow compared to that of semisynthetic penicillins. *Highly active against gram-positive cocci (e.g., non-penicillinase-producing* Staphylococcus, Streptococcus *groups) and gram-negative cocci. Also effective against gram-positive bacilli and gram-negative bacilli as well as some strains of* Salmonella, Shigella, *and spirochetes.*

USES Moderate to severe systemic infections caused by penicillin-sensitive microorganisms. Certain staphylococcal infections; streptococcal infections. Also used as prophylaxis in patients with rheumatic or congenital heart disease. Since oral preparations are absorbed erratically and thus **must be** given in comparatively high doses, this route is generally used only for mild or stabilized infections or long-term prophylaxis.

UNLABELED USES Skin/soft tissue infection.

CONTRAINDICATIONS Hypersensitivity to any of the penicillins or corn for dextrose solution prep; cardiospasm; viral infections; patients on sodium restriction.

CAUTIOUS USE History of or suspected allergy (asthma, eczema, hay fever, hives); history of allergy to cephalosporins; GI disorders; kidney or liver dysfunction, cardiac or vascular conditions; electrolyte imbalance; renal disease or renal impairment; MG; older adults; pregnancy (category B); lactation; young infants; neonates.

ROUTE & DOSAGE

Moderate to Severe Infections

Adult: **IV/IM** 2–24 million units divided q4h
Child: **IV/IM** 250,000–400,000 units/kg divided q4h

ADMINISTRATION

Note: Check whether prescriber has prescribed penicillin G potassium or sodium.

Intramuscular

- Do not use the 20,000,000 unit dosage form for IM injection.
- Reconstitute for IM: Loosen powder by shaking bottle before adding diluent (sterile water for injection or sterile NS). Keep the total volume to be injected small. Solutions containing up to 100,000 units/mL cause the least discomfort. Adding 10 mL diluent to the 1,000,000 unit vial = 100,000 units/mL. Shake well to dissolve.
- Select IM site carefully. IM injection is made deep into a large muscle mass. Inject slowly. Rotate injection sites.

Intravenous

PREPARE: **Intermittent/Continuous:** Reconstitute as for IM injection then withdraw the required dose and add to 100–1000 mL of D5W or NS IV solution, depending on length of each infusion.
ADMINISTER: **Intermittent:** *Adults:* Give over at least 1 h; *Infants and Children:* Give over 15–30 min. **Continuous:** Give at a rate required to infuse the daily dose in 24 h. ▪ With high doses, IV penicillin G should be administered slowly (usually over 24 h) to prevent electrolyte imbalance from potassium or sodium content. ▪ Prescriber will often prescribe specific flow rate.
INCOMPATIBILITIES: **Solution/additive:** **Dextran 40, fat emulsion, aminophylline, amphotericin B, cephalothin, chlorpromazine, dopamine, hydroxyzine, metaraminol, metoclopramide, pentobarbital, prochlorperazine, promazine, sodium bicarbonate,** TETRACYCLINES.

- Store dry powder (for parenteral use) at room temperature. After reconstitution (initial dilution), store solutions for 1 wk under refrigeration. ▪ Intravenous infusion solutions containing penicillin G are stable at room temperature for at least 24 h.

ADVERSE EFFECTS **CV:** Hypotension, circulatory collapse, cardiac arrhythmias, cardiac arrest. **Respiratory:** Bronchospasm, asthma. **Endocrine:** Hyperkalemia (penicillin G potassium); hypokalemia, alkalosis, hypernatremia, CHF (penicillin G sodium). **Skin:** Itchy palms or axilla, pruritus, *urticaria,* flushed skin, *delayed skin rashes* ranging from urticaria to exfoliative dermatitis, Stevens–Johnson syndrome, fixed-drug eruptions, contact dermatitis. **GI:** Vomiting, diarrhea, severe abdominal cramps, nausea, epigastric distress, diarrhea, flatulence, dark discoloration of tongue, sore mouth or tongue. **GU:** Interstitial nephritis, Loeffler's syndrome, vasculitis. **Hematologic:** Hemolytic anemia, thrombocytopenia. **Other:** Coughing, sneezing, feeling of uneasiness; systemic anaphylaxis, fever, widespread increase in capillary permeability and vasodilation with resulting edema (mouth, tongue, pharynx, larynx), laryngospasm, malaise, serum sickness (fever, malaise, pruritus, urticaria, lymphadenopathy, arthralgia, angioedema of face and extremities, neuritis prostration, eosinophilia), SLE-like syndrome, injection site reactions (pain, inflammation, abscess, phlebitis), superinfections (especially with *Candida* and gram-negative bacteria), neuromuscular irritability (twitching, lethargy, confusion, stupor, hyperreflexia, multi-focal myoclonus, localized or generalized seizures, coma).

DIAGNOSTIC TEST INTERFERENCE

Blood grouping and compatibility tests: Possible interference associated with penicillin doses greater than 20 million units daily. ***Urine glucose:*** Massive doses of penicillin may cause false-positive test results with ***Benedict's solution*** and possibly ***Clinitest*** but not with ***glucose oxidase methods*** (e.g., ***Clinistix, Diastix, TesTape***). ***Urine protein:*** Massive doses of penicillin can produce false-positive results when turbidity measures are used (e.g., ***acetic acid*** and ***heat, sulfosalicylic acid***); ***Ames reagent*** reportedly not affected. ***Urinary PSP excretion tests:*** False decrease in urinary excretion of PSP. ***Urinary steroids:*** Large IV doses of penicillin may interfere with accurate measurement of ***urinary 17-OHCS*** (***Glenn–Nelson technique*** not affected).

P

INTERACTIONS

Drug: Probenecid decreases renal elimination; penicillin G may decrease efficacy of ORAL CONTRACEPTIVES; **colestipol** decreases penicillin absorption; POTASSIUM-SPARING DIURETICS may cause hyperkalemia with penicillin G potassium. **Food:** Food increases breakdown in stomach.

PHARMACOKINETICS

Peak: 15–30 min IM. **Distribution:** Widely distributed; good CSF concentrations with inflamed meninges; crosses placenta; distributed in breast milk. **Metabolism:** 16–30% metabolized. **Elimination:** 60% in urine within 6 h. **Half-Life:** 0.4–0.9 h.

NURSING IMPLICATIONS

Assessment & Drug Effects

- Obtain an exact history of patient's previous exposure and sensitivity to penicillins and cephalosporins and other allergic reactions of any kind prior to treatment with penicillin.
- Hypersensitivity reactions are more likely to occur with parenteral penicillin than with the oral drug. Skin rash is the most common type allergic reaction and should be reported promptly to prescriber.
- Observe all patients closely for at least 30 min following administration of parenteral penicillin. The rapid appearance of a red flare or wheal at the IM or IV injection site is a possible sign of sensitivity. Also suspect an allergic reaction if patient becomes irritable, has nausea and vomiting, breathing difficulty, or sudden fever. Report any of the foregoing to prescriber immediately.
- Be aware that reactions to penicillin may be rapid in onset or may not appear for days or weeks. Symptoms usually disappear fairly quickly once drug is stopped, but in some patients may persist for 5 days or more.
- Allergy to penicillin is unpredictable. It has occurred in patients with a negative history of penicillin allergy and also in patients with no known prior contact with penicillin (sensitization may have occurred from penicillin used commercially in foods and beverages).
- Be alert for neuromuscular irritability in patients receiving parenteral penicillin in excess of 20 million units/day who have

renal insufficiency, hyponatremia, or underlying CNS disease, notably myasthenia gravis or epilepsy. Seizure precautions are indicated. Symptoms usually begin with twitching, especially of face and extremities.

- Monitor I&O, particularly in patients receiving high parenteral doses. Report oliguria, hematuria, and changes in I&O ratio. Consult prescriber regarding optimum fluid intake. Dehydration increases the concentration of drug in kidneys and can cause renal irritation and damage.
- Observe closely for signs of toxicity, especially in neonates, young infants, older adults, and patients with impaired kidney function receiving high-dose penicillin therapy. Urinary excretion of penicillin is significantly delayed in these patients.
- Observe patients on high-dose therapy closely for evidence of bleeding, and bleeding time should be monitored. (In high doses, penicillin interferes with platelet aggregation.)
- Monitor lab tests: Baseline C&S; periodic LFTs, kidney function tests, and serum electrolytes with high-dose therapy.

Patient & Family Education

- Understand that hypersensitivity reaction may be delayed. Report skin rashes, itching, fever, malaise, and other signs of a delayed reaction to prescriber immediately (see ADVERSE EFFECTS).
- Notify prescriber if following symptoms appear when taking penicillin for treatment of syphilis: Headache, chills, fever, myalgia, arthralgia, malaise, and worsening of syphilitic skin lesions. Reaction is usually self-limiting. Check with prescriber if symptoms do not improve within a few days or get worse.
- Report S&S of superinfection (see Appendix F).

PENICILLIN G PROCAINE

(pen-i-sill'in)

Classification: BETA-LACTAM ANTIBIOTIC; NATURAL PENICILLIN

Therapeutic: ANTIBIOTIC

Prototype: Penicillin G potassium

AVAILABILITY Solution for injection

ACTION & *THERAPEUTIC EFFECT* Long-acting form of penicillin G. The procaine salt has low solubility and thus creates a tissue depot from which penicillin is slowly absorbed. Slower onset of action than penicillin G potassium, but longer duration of action. It inhibits the final stage of bacterial cell wall synthesis by binding to specific penicillin-binding proteins (PBPs) located in the bacterial cell wall. This results in cell death of bacteria. *Same actions and antibacterial activity as for penicillin G potassium and is similarly inactivated by penicillinase and gastric acid.*

USES Moderately severe infections due to penicillin G-sensitive microorganisms that are susceptible to low but prolonged serum penicillin concentrations. Commonly, uncomplicated pneumococcal pneumonia, uncomplicated gonorrheal infections, and all stages of syphilis. May be used concomitantly with penicillin G or probenecid when more rapid action and higher blood levels are indicated.

CONTRAINDICATIONS History of hypersensitivity to any of the penicillins.

P

CAUTIOUS USE History of or suspected allergy, hypersensitivity to cephalosporins, carbapenem; asthmatics; procaine; history of seizures; asthmatics; GI disease, renal disease; severe renal impairment; pregnancy (category B); lactation; children.

ROUTE & DOSAGE

Moderate to Severe Infections

Adult: **IM** 600,000–1,200,000 units once/day
Child: **IM** 300,000 units once/day

Pneumococcal Pneumonia

Adult: **IM** 600,000 units q12h

Uncomplicated Gonorrhea

Adult: **IM** 4,800,000 units divided between 2 different injection sites at one visit preceded by 1 g of probenecid 30 min before injections

Syphilis

Adult: **IM** Primary, secondary, latent: 600,000 units/day for 8 days; late latent, tertiary, neurosyphilis: 600,000 units/day for 10–15 days
Child: **IM** 500,000–1,000,000 units/m^2 once/day

ADMINISTRATION

Intramuscular

- Shake multiple-dose vial thoroughly before withdrawing medication to ensure uniform suspension of drug.
- Use 20-gauge needle to avoid clogging.
- Give IM deep into upper outer quadrant of gluteus muscle; in infants and small children midlateral aspect of thigh is generally preferred. Select IM site carefully. Accidental injection into or near major peripheral nerves and blood vessels can cause neurovascular damage.
- Aspirate carefully before injecting drug to avoid entry into a blood vessel. Inadvertent IV administration reportedly has resulted in pulmonary infarcts and death.
- Inject drug at a slow, but steady rate to prevent needle blockage. Give in two sites if the dose is very large. Rotate injection sites.

ADVERSE EFFECTS **Other:** Procaine toxicity [e.g., mental disturbances (anxiety, confusion, depression, combativeness, hallucinations), expressed fear of impending death, weakness, dizziness, headache, tinnitus, unusual tastes, palpitation, changes in pulse rate and BP, seizures. Also see PENICILLIN G POTASSIUM.

INTERACTIONS **Drug: Probenecid** decreases renal elimination; may decrease efficacy of ORAL CONTRACEPTIVES.

PHARMACOKINETICS **Absorption:** Slowly from IM site. **Peak:** 1–3 h. **Duration:** 15–20 h. **Distribution:** Crosses placenta; distributed into breast milk. **Metabolism:** Hydrolyzed to penicillin in body. **Elimination:** By kidneys within 24–36 h.

NURSING IMPLICATIONS

Assessment & Drug Effects

- Obtain an exact history of patient's previous exposure and sensitivity to penicillins, cephalosporins, and to procaine, and other allergic reactions of any kind prior to treatment.
- Test patient by injecting 0.1 mL of 1–2% procaine hydrochloride intradermally if sensitivity is suspected. Appearance of a wheal,

P

flare, or eruption indicates procaine sensitivity.

- Be alert to the possibility of a transient toxic reaction to procaine, particularly when large single doses are administered. The reaction manifested by mental disturbance and other symptoms (see ADVERSE EFFECTS) occurs almost immediately and usually subsides after 15–30 min.

Patient & Family Education

- Report any skin reaction at the site of injection.
- Report onset of rash, itching, fever, chills, or other symptoms of an allergic reaction to prescriber.

PENICILLIN V

PENICILLIN V POTASSIUM

(pen-i-sill'in)

Apo-Pen-VK ♣, Nadopen-V ♣, Novopen-VK ♣

Classification: BETA-LACTAM ANTIBIOTIC; NATURAL PENICILLIN

Therapeutic: ANTIBIOTIC

Prototype: Penicillin G potassium

AVAILABILITY Tablet; suspension

ACTION & *THERAPEUTIC EFFECT* Acid stable analog of penicillin G with which it shares actions. It binds with the necessary penicillin-binding proteins (PBP) in cell wall of bacteria interfering with cell wall synthesis and resulting in cell lysis. *Penicillin V is bactericidal and is inactivated by penicillinase. Less active than penicillin G against gonococci and other gram-negative microorganisms.*

USES Mild to moderate infections caused by susceptible *Streptococci*, *Pneumococci*, and *Staphylococci*. Also Vincent's infection and as prophylaxis in rheumatic fever.

UNLABELED USES Bite wounds, cutaneous anthrax, pharyngitis.

CONTRAINDICATIONS Hypersensitivity to any penicillin.

CAUTIOUS USE History of or suspected allergy (hay fever, asthma, hives, eczema) reactions; hypersensitivity to cephalosporins, beta-lactamase inhibitors, or carbapenem; GI disease; cystic fibrosis; renal impairment, hepatic impairment; pregnancy (category B); lactation; children.

ROUTE & DOSAGE

Mild to Moderate Infections

Adult: **PO** 250–500 mg q6h
Child (younger than 12 y): **PO** 15–50 mg/kg/day in 3–6 divided doses

Rheumatic Fever Prophylaxis

Adult: **PO** 125–250 mg bid

Endocarditis Prophylaxis

Adult: **PO** 2 g 30–60 min before procedure, then 500 mg q6h for 8 doses
Child (weight less than 30 kg): **PO** 1 g 30–60 min before procedure, then 250 mg q6h for 8 doses

ADMINISTRATION

Oral

- Give after a meal rather than on an empty stomach; drug may be better absorbed and result in higher blood levels.
- Shake well before pouring. Following reconstitution, oral solution is stable for 14 days under refrigeration.

ADVERSE EFFECTS Other: Nausea, vomiting, *diarrhea*, epigastric

P

distress. *Hypersensitivity reactions* (e.g., flushing, pruritus, urticaria, or other skin eruptions, eosinophilia, anaphylaxis; hemolytic anemia, leukopenia, thrombocytopenia, neuropathy, superinfections).

INTERACTIONS **Drug: Probenecid** decreases renal elimination; may decrease efficacy of ORAL CONTRACEPTIVES; **colestipol** decreases absorption. **Food:** Food increases breakdown in stomach.

PHARMACOKINETICS **Absorption:** 60–73% absorbed from GI tract. **Peak:** 30–60 min. **Duration:** 6 h. **Distribution:** Highest levels in kidneys; crosses placenta; distributed into breast milk. **Elimination:** In urine. **Half-Life:** 30 min.

NURSING IMPLICATIONS

Note: See penicillin G potassium for numerous additional nursing implications.

Assessment & Drug Effects

- Obtain careful history concerning hypersensitivity reactions to penicillins, cephalosporins, and other allergens before therapy begins.
- Monitor lab tests: Baseline C&S; LFTs, and hematologic studies at regular intervals in patients receiving prolonged therapy.

Patient & Family Education

- Take penicillin V around the clock at specific intervals to maintain a constant blood level.
- Do not miss any doses and continue taking medication until it is all gone unless otherwise directed by the prescriber.
- Discontinue medication and promptly report to prescriber the onset of hypersensitivity reactions and superinfections (see Appendix F).
- Use specially marked measuring device to ensure accurate doses of oral liquid preparation.

PENTAMIDINE ISETHIONATE

(pen-tam′i-deen)

Nebupent, Pentacarinat ♣, Pentam

Classification: ANTIPROTOZOAL

Therapeutic: ANTIPROTOZOAL

AVAILABILITY Solution for injection; aerosol

ACTION & *THERAPEUTIC EFFECT* Blocks parasite reproduction by interfering with nucleotide (DNA, RNA), phospholipid, and protein synthesis. *Effective against the protozoan parasite* Pneumocystis carinii *in AIDS patients.*

USES *Pneumocystis jirovecii* pneumonia (PCP).

UNLABELED USES African trypanosomiasis and visceral leishmaniasis. (Drug supplied for latter uses is through the Centers for Disease Control and Prevention, Atlanta, GA.)

CONTRAINDICATIONS QT prolongation, history of torsades de pointes; lactation (infant risk cannot be ruled out).

CAUTIOUS USE Hypertension, hypotension; hyperglycemia; pancreatitis; hypoglycemia; hypocalcemia; blood dyscrasias; liver or kidney dysfunction; diabetes mellitus; pancreatitis; asthma; history of smoking, cardiac arrhythmias; pregnancy (category C); children.

ROUTE & DOSAGE

Treatment of *Pneumocystis jirovecii* Pneumonia

Adult/Child: **IM/IV** 4 mg/kg/day for 21 days

Prophylaxis of *Pneumocystis jirovecii* Pneumonia

Adult: **Inhaled** 300 mg/nebulizer q4wk
Child: **Inhaled** 300 mg/nebulizer monthly

ADMINISTRATION

Inhaled

- Reconstitute contents of one vial in 6 mL sterile water (not saline) and administer using nebulizer.
- Do not mix with any other drug.

Intramuscular

- Dissolve contents of 1 vial (300 mg) in 3 mL sterile water for injection.
- Give deep IM into a large muscle.
- The IM injection is painful and frequently causes local reactions (pain, indurations, swelling). Select alternate sites for daily doses and institute local treatment if indicated.

Intravenous

PREPARE: **IV Infusion:** Dissolve contents of 1 vial in 3–5 mL sterile water for injection or D5W. ▪ Further dilute in 50–250 mL of D5W.

ADMINISTER: **IV Infusion:** Give over 60–120 min.

INCOMPATIBILITIES: **Y-site:** Extensive list of incompatibilities, do not administer with other medications.

- Note: IV solutions are stable at room temperature for up to 48 h. Protect solution from light.

ADVERSE EFFECTS

Respiratory: Bronchospasm, *cough, dyspnea, wheezing*. **CNS:** *Fatigue dizziness*. **Endocrine:** Hypoglycemia. **GI:** *Decreased appetite*. **GU:** *Nephrotoxicity, renal impairment,* increased serum creatinine. **Hematologic:** Leukopenia.

INTERACTIONS

Drug: AMINOGLYCOSIDES, **amphotericin B, cidofovir, cisplatin, ganciclovir, cyclosporine, vancomycin,** other nephrotoxic drugs increase risk of nephrotoxicity.

PHARMACOKINETICS

Absorption: Readily after IM injection. **Distribution:** Leaves bloodstream rapidly to bind extensively to body tissues. **Elimination:** 50–66% in urine within 6 h; small amounts found in urine for as long as 6–8 wk. **Half-Life:** 6.5–13.2 h.

P

NURSING IMPLICATIONS

Assessment & Drug Effects

- Monitor BP and HR continuously during the infusion, every half hour for 2 h thereafter, and then every 4 h until BP stabilizes. Sudden severe hypotension may develop after a single dose. Place patient in supine position while receiving the drug.
- Measure and record I&O ratio and pattern.
- Be alert and report promptly S&S of impending kidney dysfunction

(e.g., changed I&O ratio, oliguria, edema).
- Characteristics of pneumonia in the immunocompromised patient include constant fever, scanty (if any) sputum, dyspnea, tachypnea, and cyanosis.
- Monitor temperature changes and institute measures to lower the temperature as indicated. Fever is a constant symptom in *P. carinii* pneumonia, but may be rapidly elevated [as high as 40° C (104° F)] shortly after drug infusion.
- Monitor lab tests: Periodic serum electrolytes, renal function tests, LFTs, CBC with differential, platelet count, BUN, creatinine, and blood glucose.

Patient & Family Education

- Report promptly to prescriber increasing respiratory difficulty.
- Monitor blood glucose for loss of glycemic control if diabetic.
- Report any unusual bruising or bleeding. Avoid using aspirin or other NSAIDS.
- Increase fluid intake (if not contraindicated) to 2–3 qt (L)/day.

P

PENTAZOCINE HYDROCHLORIDE

(pen-taz'oh-seen)

Talwin

Classification: NARCOTIC (OPIATE AGONIST-ANTAGONIST); ANALGESIC
Therapeutic: NARCOTIC ANALGESIC
Controlled Substance: Schedule IV

AVAILABILITY Solution for injection

ACTION & *THERAPEUTIC EFFECT* Synthetic analgesic with potency approximately one-third that of morphine. Opiates exert their effects by stimulating specific opiate receptors that produce analgesia, respiratory depression, and euphoria as well as physical dependence. *Effective for moderate to severe pain relief. Acts as weak narcotic antagonist and has sedative properties.*

USES Relief of moderate to severe pain; also used for preoperative analgesia or sedation, and as supplement to surgical anesthesia.

CONTRAINDICATIONS Hypersensitivity to sulfite; head injury, increased intracranial pressure; seizures; emotionally unstable patients, respiratory depression, or history of drug abuse.

CAUTIOUS USE Impaired kidney or liver function; cardiac disease; COPD, asthmas, GI obstruction; biliary surgery; patients with MI who have nausea and vomiting; pregnancy (category C); lactation; children younger than 12 y.

ROUTE & DOSAGE

Moderate to Severe Pain (Excluding Patients in Labor)

Adult: **IM/IV/Subcutaneous** 30 mg q3–4h (max: 360 mg/day)

Anesthesia

Adult: **IM/IV/Subcutaneous** 30 mg dose; may repeat q3–4h as needed (max: 360 mg daily)
Adolescent/Child: **IM** 0.5 mg/kg single dose (max: 30 mg)

Pain during Labor

Adult: **IM** 30 mg dose; **IV** 20 mg dose may repeat q2–3h (total: 2–3 doses)

Renal Impairment Dosage Adjustment

CrCl 10–50 mL/min: Give 75% of dose; *less than 10 mL/min:* Give 50% of dose

ADMINISTRATION

Subcutaneous/Intramuscular

- IM is preferred to subcutaneous route when frequent injections over an extended period are required.
- Observe injection sites daily for signs of irritation or inflammation.

Intravenous

PREPARE: **Direct:** Give undiluted or diluted with 1 mL sterile water for injection for each 5 mg.
ADMINISTER: **Direct:** Give slowly at a rate of 5 mg over 60 sec.
INCOMPATIBILITIES: **Solution/additive:** **Alemtuzumab, aminophylline,** BARBITURATES, **sodium bicarbonate, glycopyrrolate, heparin, nafcillin. Y-site: Alemtuzumab, aminophylline, amphotericin B, ampicillin, atenolol, azathioprine, aztreonam, bivalirudin, cefamandole, cefazolin, cefoperazone, cefotaxime, cefotetan, cefoxitin, ceftizoxime, ceftriaxone, cefuroxime, chloramphenicol, dantrolene, daptomycin, diazepam, diazoxide, foscarnet, furosemide, gallium, ganciclovir, gemtuzumab, indomethacin, ketorolac, methylprednisolone, mitomycin, nafcillin, nitroprusside, oxacillin, pemetrexed, penicillin G, pentobarbital, phenobarbital, phenytoin, piperacillin, SMZ/TMP, ticarcillin, nafcillin.**

ADVERSE EFFECTS **CV:** Hypertension, palpitation, tachycardia. **Respiratory:** Respiratory depression. **CNS:** *Drowsiness,* sweating, *dizziness, light-headedness, euphoria,* psychotomimetic effects, confusion, anxiety, hallucinations, disturbed dreams, bizarre thoughts, euphoria, and other mood alterations. **HEENT:** Visual disturbances. **Skin:** Injection site reactions (induration, nodule formation, sloughing, sclerosis, cutaneous depression), rash, pruritus. **GI:** *Nausea, vomiting,* constipation, dry mouth, alterations of taste. **GU:** Urinary retention. **Other:** Flushing, allergic reactions, shock.

INTERACTIONS **Drug: Alcohol** and other CNS DEPRESSANTS add to CNS depression; NARCOTIC ANALGESICS may precipitate narcotic withdrawal syndrome.

P

PHARMACOKINETICS **Onset:** 15 min IM, Subcutaneous; 2–3 min IV. **Peak:** 1 h IM, 15 min IV. **Duration:** 3 h IM, 1 h IV. **Distribution:** Crosses placenta. **Metabolism:** Extensively in liver. **Elimination:** Primarily in urine; small amount in feces. **Half-Life:** 2–3 h.

NURSING IMPLICATIONS

Assessment & Drug Effects

- Monitor therapeutic effect. Tolerance to analgesic effect sometimes occurs. Psychologic and physical dependence have been reported in patients with history of drug abuse, but rarely in patients without such history. Addiction liability matches that of codeine.

- Monitor vital signs and assess for respiratory depression. Keep supine to minimize adverse effects.
- Monitor drug-induced CNS depression.
- Be aware that pentazocine may produce acute withdrawal symptoms in some patients who have been receiving opioids on a regular basis.
- Monitor I&O as drug may cause urinary retention.

Patient & Family Education

- Avoid driving and other potentially hazardous activities until response to drug is known.
- Do not discontinue drug abruptly following extended use; may result in chills, abdominal and muscle cramps, yawning, runny nose, tearing, itching, restlessness, anxiety, drug-seeking behavior.

P

PENTOBARBITAL

(pen-toe-bar'bi-tal)

PENTOBARBITAL SODIUM

Nembutal, Novopentobarb ♣

Classification: ANXIOLYTIC; SEDATIVE-HYPNOTIC; BARBITURATE; ANTICONVULSANT

Therapeutic: ANTIANXIETY; SEDATIVE-HYPNOTIC; ANTI-CONVULSANT

Prototype: Secobarbital

Controlled Substance: Schedule II

AVAILABILITY Solution for injection

ACTION & *THERAPEUTIC EFFECT* Short-acting barbiturate with anticonvulsant properties. Potent respiratory depressant. Initially, barbiturates suppress REM sleep, but with chronic therapy REM sleep returns to normal. *Effective as a sedative and hypnotic and anticonvulsant.*

USES Sedative or hypnotic for preanesthetic medication, induction of general anesthesia, adjunct in manipulative or diagnostic procedures, and emergency control of acute convulsions.

CONTRAINDICATIONS History of sensitivity to barbiturates; parturition, fetal immaturity, uncontrolled pain; ethanol intoxication; hepatic encephalopathy; porphyria; suicidal ideation; pregnancy (category D); lactation.

CAUTIOUS USE COPD, sleep apnea; heart failure; hypertension, hypotension, pulmonary disease; alcoholism; mental status changes, suicidality, major depression; neonates; renal impairment, renal failure; children.

ROUTE & DOSAGE

Preoperative Sedation

Adult: **IM** 150–200 mg in 2 divided doses

Child: **IV** 2–6 mg/kg (max: 100 mg)

Hypnotic/Insomnia

Adult: **IM** 150–200 mg

Child: **IM** 2–6 mg/kg (max: 100 mg)

Status Epilepticus

Adult: **IV** 5–15 mg/kg loading, then 0.5–3 mg/kg/h
Child: **IM** 5–15 mg/kg loading, then 0.5–5 mg/kg/h

ADMINISTRATION

Note: Do not give within 14 days of starting/stopping an MAO inhibitor.

Intramuscular

- Do not use parenteral solutions that appear cloudy or in which a precipitate has formed.
- Make IM injections deep into large muscle mass, preferably upper outer quadrant of buttock. Aspirate needle carefully before injecting it to prevent inadvertent entry into blood vessel. Inject no more than 5 mL (250 mg) in any one site because of possible tissue irritation.

Intravenous

PREPARE: **Direct:** Give undiluted or diluted (preferred) with sterile water, D5W, NS, or other compatible IV solutions.
ADMINISTER: **Direct:** Give slowly. Do not exceed rate of 50 mg/min.
INCOMPATIBILITIES: **Solution/additive: Atropine, butorphanol, chlorpheniramine, chlorpromazine, cimetidine, codeine, dimenhydrinate, diphenhydramine, droperidol, ephedrine, fentanyl, glycopyrrolate, hydrocortisone, hydroxyzine, inulin, levorphanol, meperidine, methadone, midazolam, morphine, nalbuphine, norepinephrine,** TETRACYCLINES, **penicillin G, pentazocine, perphenazine, phenytoin, promazine, prochlorperazine, promethazine, sodium bicarbonate, streptomycin, succinylcholine, triflupromazine, vancomycin. Y-site: Amphotericin B cholesteryl, fenoldopam, TPN.**

- Take extreme care to avoid extravasation. Necrosis may result because parenteral solution is highly alkaline. ▪ Do not use cloudy or precipitated solution.

ADVERSE EFFECTS **CV:** Hypotension with rapid IV. **Respiratory:** With rapid IV (respiratory depression, laryngospasm, bronchospasm, apnea). **Other:** Drowsiness, lethargy, hang-over, paradoxical excitement in the older adult patient.

INTERACTIONS **Drug: Phenmetrazine** antagonizes effects of pentobarbital; CNS DEPRESSANTS, **alcohol,** SEDATIVES add to CNS depression; MAO INHIBITORS cause excessive CNS depression; **methoxyflurane** creates risk of nephrotoxicity. **Herbal: Kava, valerian** may potentiate sedation.

PHARMACOKINETICS **Onset:** 10–15 min IM; 1 min IV. **Duration:** 15 min IV. **Distribution:** Crosses placenta. **Metabolism:** Primarily in liver. **Elimination:** In urine. **Half-Life:** 4–50 h.

P

NURSING IMPLICATIONS

Assessment & Drug Effects

- Monitor BP, pulse, and respiration q3–5min during IV administration. Observe patient closely; maintain airway. Have equipment for artificial respiration immediately available.
- Observe patient closely for adverse effects for at least 30 min after IM administration of hypnotic dose.
- Monitor for hypersensitivity reactions (see Appendix E) especially with a history of asthma or angioedema.
- Monitor for adverse CNS effects including exacerbation of depression and suicidal ideation.
- Monitor those in acute pain, children, the elderly, and debilitated patients for paradoxical excitement restlessness.
- Concurrent drug: Monitor warfarin and phenytoin levels frequently to ensure therapeutic range.
- Monitor lab tests: Periodic pentobarbital level. Note: Plasma level greater than 30 mcg/mL may be toxic and 65 mcg/mL and above may be lethal.

P

Patient & Family Education

- Exercise caution when driving or operating machinery for the remainder of day after taking drug.
- Avoid alcohol and other CNS depressants for 24 h after receiving this drug.
- Women using oral contraceptives should use an additional, alternative form of contraception.

PENTOXIFYLLINE

(pen-tox-i′fi-leen)

Classification: HEMATOLOGIC; RED BLOOD CELL MODIFIER; BLOOD VISCOSITY REDUCER

Therapeutic: RED BLOOD CELL MODIFIER; BLOOD VISCOSITY IMPROVER

AVAILABILITY Sustained release tablet

ACTION & *THERAPEUTIC EFFECT* Maintains the flexibility of RBCs, increasing erythrocyte cAMP activity, thus allowing erythrocyte membranes to maintain their integrity and become more resistant to deformity. Improvement in blood viscosity results in increased blood flow to the microcirculation and enhanced tissue oxygenation. *Results in increased blood flow to the extremities, reduced pain and paresthesia of intermittent claudication.*

USES Intermittent claudication associated with occlusive peripheral vascular disease; diabetic angiopathies.

UNLABELED USES To improve psychopathologic symptoms in patient with cerebrovascular insufficiency and to reduce incidence of stroke in the patient with recurrent TIAs.

CONTRAINDICATIONS Intolerance to pentoxifylline or to methylxanthines (caffeine and theophylline); intracranial bleeding; retinal bleeding; lactation.

CAUTIOUS USE Angina, hypotension, arrhythmias, cerebrovascular disease; peptic ulcer disease; renal failure; renal impairment; risk of bleeding; pregnancy (category C); children younger than 18 y.

ROUTE & DOSAGE

Intermittent Claudication

Adult: **PO** 400 mg tid with meals

 Common adverse effects in *italic;* life-threatening effects underlined; generic names in **bold;** classifications in SMALL CAPS; ♣ Canadian drug name; ⊙ Prototype drug; ⚠ Alert

ADMINISTRATION

Oral

- Give on an empty stomach or with food; be consistent with time of day and relationship to food in establishing the daily regimen.
- Store tablets at 15°–30° C (59°–86° F).

ADVERSE EFFECTS CV: Angina, chest pain, dyspnea, arrhythmias, palpitations, hypotension, edema, flushing. **CNS:** Agitation, nervousness, *dizziness,* drowsiness, headache, insomnia, tremor, confusion. **Skin:** Brittle fingernails, pruritus, rash, urticaria. **GI:** Abdominal discomfort, belching, flatus, bloating, diarrhea, *dyspepsia, nausea, vomiting.* **Eye:** Blurred vision, conjunctivitis, scotomas. **Other:** Fever, flushing, convulsions, somnolence, loss of consciousness. Earache, unpleasant taste, excessive salivation, leukopenia, malaise, sore throat, swollen neck glands, weight change.

INTERACTIONS Drug: Ciprofloxacin, cimetidine may increase levels and toxicity, **warfarin** may have additive effects. Do not use with **ketorolac**. **Herbal: Evening primrose oil, ginseng, ginkgo** may increase bleeding risk.

PHARMACOKINETICS Absorption: Readily from GI tract; 10–50% reaches systemic circulation (first pass metabolism). **Peak:** 2–4 h. **Distribution:** Distributed into breast milk. **Metabolism:** In liver and erythrocytes. **Elimination:** Primarily in urine. **Half-Life:** 0.4–0.8 h.

NURSING IMPLICATIONS

Assessment & Drug Effects

- Monitor therapeutic effectiveness which is indicated by relief from pain and cramping in calf muscles, buttocks, thighs, and feet during exercise and improves walking performance (time and duration).
- Monitor BP if patient is also on antihypertensive treatment. Drug may slightly decrease an already stabilized BP, necessitating a reduced dose of the hypotensive drug.

Patient & Family Education

- Consult prescriber to determine CV status and capacity before reestablishing walking as exercise.
- Pay particular attention to care of the feet because of arterial insufficiency (diminished perfusion to feet).
- Be aware that bleeding and prolonged PT/INR associated with this treatment have been reported. Report promptly unexplained bleeding, easy bruising, nose bleed, pinpoint rash to prescriber.
- Avoid driving or working with hazardous machinery until drug response has stabilized because of potential for tiredness, blurred vision, dizziness.

PERAMIVIR

(per-a-mi'vir)

Rapivab

Classification: ANTIVIRAL; NEURAMINIDASE INHIBITOR

Therapeutic: ANTI-INFLUENZA

Prototype: Oseltamivir

AVAILABILITY Solution for injection

ACTION & *THERAPEUTIC EFFECT*
Inhibits influenza A and B viral neuraminidase enzyme, preventing the release of newly formed viruses from the surface of the infected cells. Inhibits replication of the

influenza A and B virus. *Relieves flu symptoms and prevents viral spread across the mucous lining of the respiratory tract.*

USES Treatment of acute uncomplicated influenza in patients 18 y or older who have been symptomatic for no more than 2 days.

CAUTIOUS USE Serious skin reactions; abnormal behavior including hallucinations and delirium; renal impairment; pregnancy (category C); lactation. Safety and efficacy in patients younger than 18 y not established.

ROUTE & DOSAGE

Influenza

Adult: **IV** Single 600 mg dose within 48 h of symptoms

Renal Impairment Dosage Adjustment

CrCL 30–49 mL/min: Reduce to 200 mg
CrCL 10–29 mL/min: Reduce To Whom It May Concern: 100 mg

P

ADMINISTRATION

Intravenous

PREPARE: **IV Infusion:** Dilute required dose in NS, 0.45% NaCl, D5W, or LR to a max volume of 100 mL.
ADMINISTER: **IV Infusion:** Give over 15–30 min.
INCOMPATIBILITIES: **Solution/additive:** Do not mix with other IV medications. **Y-site:** Do not co-infuse with other IV medications

- Store refrigerated at 2°–8° C (36°–46° F) for up to 24 h if not administered immediately. If refrigerated, allow solution to reach room temperature then administer immediately.

ADVERSE EFFECTS CV: Hypertension. **CNS:** Insomnia. **Endocrine:** Hyperglycemia, increased ALT/AST, increased creatine phosphokinase. **Skin:** Exfoliative dermatitis, rash, Stevens–Johnson syndrome. **GI:** Constipation, *diarrhea*. **Hematological:** Neutropenia.

PHARMACOKINETICS Distribution: 30% plasma protein bound. **Metabolism:** Minimal. **Elimination:** Primarily renal (90%). **Half-Life:** 20 h.

NURSING IMPLICATIONS

Assessment and Drug Effects

- Monitor for and report promptly skin rash, dermatitis, erythema.
- Monitor for neuropsychiatric events, especially in children.
- Monitor lab tests: Baseline serum urea nitrogen and serum creatinine.

Patient & Family Education

- Seek immediate medical attention if a skin reaction occurs.
- Contact prescriber for any signs of abnormal behavior including illogical thinking, altered speech, hallucinations, or delusions.

PERINDOPRIL ERBUMINE

(per-in'do-pril)

Classification: ANGIOTENSIN-CONVERTING ENZYME (ACE) INHIBITOR; ANTIHYPERTENSIVE
Therapeutic: ANTIHYPERTENSIVE
Prototype: Captopril

AVAILABILITY Tablet

ACTION & *THERAPEUTIC EFFECT* Inhibits the renin angiotensin-converting enzyme (ACE) that catalyzes the conversion of angiotensin I to angiotensin II, a potent vasoconstrictor substance. Also reduces aldosterone production causing a potassium-sparing effect. In addition, it decreases systemic vascular resistance (afterload) and pulmonary capillary wedge pressure (PCWP), a measure of preload, and improves cardiac output as well as activity tolerance. *Effective in lowering blood pressure by vasodilatation resulting from inhibition of ACE. Improves cardiac output as well as activity tolerance in CAD.*

USES Hypertension, reduce the risk of myocardial infarction in patients with stable CAD.

UNLABELED USES Heart failure, ST elevation acute coronary syndrome.

CONTRAINDICATIONS Hypersensitivity to perindopril or any other ACE inhibitors; history of angioedema induced by an ACE inhibitor, patients with hypertrophic cardiomyopathy, hepatoxicity; renal artery stenosis; concomitant use with aliskiren in patients with diabetes mellitus; concomitant use or within 36 hours of switching to or from a neprilysin inhibitor; pregnancy (exposure to an ACE inhibitor during the first trimester of pregnancy may be associated with an increased risk of fetal malformation); lactation.

CAUTIOUS USE Renal insufficiency, volume-depleted patients, severe liver dysfunction; autoimmune diseases, immunosuppressant drug therapy; hyperkalemia or potassiumsparing diuretics; surgery; neutropenia; febrile illness; older adults. Safety and efficacy in children not established.

ROUTE & DOSAGE

Hypertension

Adult: **PO** 4 mg once daily, may be titrated to 16 mg daily

Stable Coronary Artery Disease

Adult: **PO** 4 mg daily × 2 wk, then 8 mg daily

Renal Impairment Dosage Adjustment

CrCl 30–79 mL/min: Start at 2 mg daily; *CrCl less than mL/min:* not recommended

ADMINISTRATION

Oral

- Manufacturer recommends an initial dose of 2–4 mg in 1 or 2 divided doses if concurrently ordered diuretic cannot be discontinued 2–3 days before beginning perinodopril. Consult prescriber.
- Give on an empty stomach 1 h before meals.
- Dosage adjustments are generally made at intervals of at least 1 wk.
- Store at 20°–25° C (68°–77° F) and protect from moisture.

ADVERSE EFFECTS **CV:** Edema, *angioedema*. **Respiratory:** Cough, upper respiratory infection, sinusitis, rhinitis. **CNS:** Headache. **GI:** Diarrhea. **GU:** Urinary tract infection. **Musculoskeletal**: Weakness, back pain, leg pain. **Other:** Infection.

DIAGNOSTIC TEST INTERFERENCE May lead to false negative aldosterone/renin ratio.

INTERACTIONS **Drug:** POTASSIUM SPARING DIURETICS (**amiloride, spironolactone, triamterene**)

P

may increase the risk of hyperkalemia. POTASSIUM SUPPLEMENTS increase the risk of hyperkalemia; **lithium** levels can be increased; ANTIHYPERTENSIVES may increase risk of hypotension; use with **azathioprine** may cause anemia and leukopenia; may increase adverse effects of **iron**; may increase risk of nephrotoxicity with **sodium phosphate**. **Pregabalin** may increase risk of angioedema. **Food:** Food can decrease drug absorption 35%.

PHARMACOKINETICS **Absorption:** Readily from GI tract, absorption significantly decreased when taken with food. **Peak:** 1–2 h. **Metabolism:** Hydrolyzed in the liver to its active form, perindoprilat. **Elimination:** Primarily in urine. **Half-Life: Perindopril:** 0.8–1 h, **perindoprilat:** 30–120 h.

NURSING IMPLICATIONS

Black Box Warning

Perindropril has been associated with fetal injury and death.

Assessment & Drug Effects

- Monitor BR and HR carefully following initial dose for several hours until stable, especially in patients using concurrent diuretics, on salt restriction, or volume depleted.
- Place patient immediately in a supine position if excess hypotension develops.
- Monitor closely kidney function in patients with CHF.
- Monitor serum lithium levels and assess for S&S of lithium toxicity when used concurrently; increased caution is needed when diuretic therapy is also used.
- Monitor lab tests: Periodic serum potassium, BUN, and creatinine; periodic CBC with differential.

Patient & Family Education

- Discontinue drug and immediately report S&S of angioedema (i.e., swelling) of face or extremities to prescriber. Seek emergency help for swelling of the tongue or any other signs of potential airway obstruction.
- Contact prescriber immediately if you become pregnant.
- Be aware that light-headedness can occur, especially during early therapy; excess fluid loss of any kind (e.g., vomiting, diarrhea) will increase risk of hypotension and fainting.
- Avoid using potassium supplements unless specifically directed to do so by prescriber.
- Report S&S of infection (e.g., sore throat, fever) promptly to prescriber.

PERMETHRIN (Pr)

(per-meth'rin)

Nix, Elimite, Acticin

Classification: SCABICIDE; PEDICULICIDE

Therapeutic: SCABICIDE; PEDICULICIDE

AVAILABILITY Cream; liquid

ACTION & *THERAPEUTIC EFFECT* Inhibits sodium ion influx through nerve cell membrane channels, resulting in delayed repolarization of the action potential and paralysis of the pest. *It prevents burrowing into host's skin. Since lice are completely dependent on blood for survival, they die within 24–48 h. Also active against ticks, mites, and fleas.*

USES Pediculosis capitis.

CONTRAINDICATIONS Hypersensitivity to pyrethrins, chrysanthemums, sulfites, or other preservatives or dyes; acute inflammation of the scalp; lactation.

CAUTIOUS USE Children younger than 2 y **(liquid),** and less than 2 mo **(lotion);** asthma; pregnancy (category B).

ROUTE & DOSAGE

Head Lice

Adult/Child (2 y or older):
Topical Apply sufficient volume to clean wet hair to saturate the hair and scalp; leave on 10 min, then rinse hair thoroughly

ADMINISTRATION

Topical

- Saturate scalp as well as hair with the lotion; this is not a shampoo. Shake lotion well before application.
- Hair should be washed with regular shampoo before treatment with permethrin, thoroughly rinsed and dried.
- Rinse hair and scalp thoroughly and dry with a clean towel following 10 min exposure to the medication. Head lice are usually eliminated with one treatment.
- Store drug away from heat at 15°–25° C (59°–77° F) and direct light. Avoid freezing.

ADVERSE EFFECTS **Skin:** *Pruritus, transient tingling,* burning, stinging, numbness; erythema, edema, rash.

PHARMACOKINETICS **Absorption:** Less than 2% of amount applied is absorbed through intact skin. **Metabolism:** Rapidly hydrolyzed to inactive metabolites. **Elimination:** Primarily in urine.

NURSING IMPLICATIONS

Assessment & Drug Effects

- Do not attempt therapy if patient is known to be sensitive to any pyrethrin or pyrethroid. Stop treatment if a reaction occurs.

Patient & Family Education

- When hair is dry, comb with a fine-tooth comb (furnished with medication) to remove dead lice and remaining nits or nit shells.
- Be aware that drug remains on hair shaft up to 14 days; therefore, recurrence of infestation rarely occurs (less than 1%).
- Inspect hair shafts daily for at least 1 wk to determine drug effectiveness. Contact prescriber if live lice are observed after 7 days. Signs of inadequate treatment: Itching, redness of skin, skin abrasion, infected scalp areas.
- Resume regular shampooing after treatment; residual deposit of drug on hair is not reduced.
- Be aware that drug is usually irritating to the eyes and mucosa. Flush well with water if medicine accidentally gets into eyes.

P

PERPHENAZINE

(per-fen′a-zeen)

Classification: PHENOTHIAZINE ANTIPSYCHOTIC; ANTIEMETIC
Therapeutic: ANTIPSYCHOTIC; ANTIEMETIC
Prototype: Chlorpromazine

AVAILABILITY Tablet

ACTION & *THERAPEUTIC EFFECT* Affects all parts of CNS, particularly the hypothalamus. Antipsychotic effect is due to its ability to antagonize neurotransmitter dopamine by acting on its receptors in the brain. Antiemetic action results from direct blockade of dopamine in the chemoreceptor trigger zone (CTZ) in the medulla. *Has antipsychotic and antiemetic properties.*

USES Schizophrenia, symptomatic control of severe nausea and vomiting.

CONTRAINDICATIONS Hypersensitivity to perphenazine and other phenothiazines; preexisting liver damage; suspected or established subcortical brain damage, comatose states, CNS depression; dementia-related psychosis; hepatic encephalopathy; QT prolongation; bone marrow depression; hematological disease; pregnancy (jaundice has been observed in newborns following maternal use of phenothiazines); lactation.

CAUTIOUS USE Previously diagnosed breast cancer; liver or kidney dysfunction; renal impairment; cardiovascular disorders; drug or alcohol abuse; epilepsy; psychic depression, patients with suicidal tendency; cardiac and pulmonary disease; glaucoma; history of intestinal or GU obstruction; older adults or debilitated patients; children younger than 12 y.

ROUTE & DOSAGE

Schizophrenia

Adult/Adolescent: **PO** 8–16 mg/day in divided doses; titrate to response (max: 64 mg/day)

Nausea

Adult: **PO** 8–16 mg daily in divided doses (max: 24 mg/day)

ADMINISTRATION

Oral

- May be taken with or without food. Administer with food, milk, or full glass of water to minimize gastric irritation.
- Storage: Store at 20°C to 25°C (68°F to 77°F).

ADVERSE EFFECTS **CV:** *Orthostatic hypotension,* bradycardia, ECG changes. **CNS:** *Extrapyramidal effects (dystonic reactions, akathisia, parkinsonian syndrome, tardive dyskinesia), sedation,* convulsions, bizarre dreams, catatonic-like state, cerebral edema. **HEENT:** Mydriasis, blurred vision, corneal and lenticular deposits. **Endocrine:** Hyperprolactinemia, galactorrhea, weight gain. **GI:** Constipation, *dry mouth,* increased appetite, adynamic ileus, abnormal liver function tests, cholestatic jaundice. **GU:** *Urinary retention,* gynecomastia, menstrual irregularities, inhibited ejaculation. **Hematologic:** Agranulocytosis, thrombocytopenic purpura, aplastic or hemolytic anemia. **Other:** Photosensitivity, itching, erythema, urticaria, angioneurotic edema, drug fever, anaphylactoid reaction, sterile abscess. Nasal congestion, decreased sweating.

INTERACTIONS **Drug:** **Alcohol** and other CNS DEPRESSANTS enhance CNS depression; ANTICHOLINERGIC AGENTS add to anticholinergic effects including fecal impaction and paralytic ileus; BARBITURATES, ANESTHETICS increase hypotension, excitation and may increase risk of QT prolongation; PHOTOSENSITIZING AGENTS may have additive effect; ANTIPARKINSON AGENTS may decrease efficacy of perphenazine; may increase ulcerogenic effect of **potassium**. **Herbal:** **Kava** increased risk and severity of dystonic reactions.

PHARMACOKINETICS Absorption: Poorly absorbed from GI tract; 20% reaches systemic circulation. **Onset of action:** 2–4 weeks. **Duration:** 6–12 h. **Distribution:** Crosses placenta. **Metabolism:** In liver (CYP2D6). **Elimination:** In urine and feces. **Half-Life:** 9–12 h.

NURSING IMPLICATIONS

Black Box Warning

Perphenazine has been associated with increased mortality in older adults with dementia-related psychosis.

Assessment & Drug Effects

- Monitor mental status and report promptly suicidal ideation, significant changes in mood, behavior, or functional ability.
- Monitor vital signs periodically and report significant changes in HR or BP (especially with marked dosage increases).
- Report restlessness, weakness of extremities, dystonic reactions (spasms of neck and shoulder muscles, rigidity of back, difficulty swallowing or talking); motor restlessness (akathisia: inability to be still); and parkinsonian syndrome (tremors, shuffling gait, drooling, slow speech).
- Withhold medication and report immediately to prescriber S&S of tardive dyskinesia (i.e., fine, wormlike movements or rapid protrusions of the tongue, chewing motions, lip smacking).
- ECG and ophthalmologic examination are recommended prior to initiation and periodically during therapy.
- Suspect hypersensitivity, withhold drug, and report to prescriber if jaundice appears between weeks 2 and 4.
- Monitor urine and bowel elimination pattern especially with daily doses greater than 24 mg.
- Monitor ophthalmic screening at onset of therapy and periodically throughout.
- Monitor lab tests: Periodic CBC with differential, LFTs, renal function tests, serum electrolytes, fasting blood glucose, HgA1C, and lipid panel.

Patient & Family Education

- Make all position changes slowly and in stages, particularly from recumbent to upright posture, and to lie down or sit down if lightheadedness or dizziness occurs.
- Do not drive or engage in potentially hazardous activities until response to drug is known.
- Discontinue drug and report to prescriber immediately if jaundice appears between weeks 2 and 4.
- Avoid long exposure to sunlight and to sunlamps. Photosensitivity results in skin color changes from brown to blue-gray.
- Adhere strictly to dosage regimen. Contact prescriber before changing it for any reason.
- Drug should be discontinued gradually over a period of several weeks following prolonged therapy.
- Avoid OTC drugs unless prescriber prescribes them.
- Be aware that perphenazine may discolor urine reddish brown.

PERTUZUMAB

(per-tu′zu-mab)

Perjeta

Classification: MONOCLONAL ANTIBODY; HUMAN EPIDERAL GROWTH FACTOR RECEPTOR 2 PROTEIN (HER2) ANTAGONIST; ANTINEOPLASTIC

Therapeutic: ANTINEOPLASTIC; HER2 ANTAGONIST

Prototype: Trastuzumab

AVAILABILITY Solution for injection

ACTION & *THERAPEUTIC EFFECT* Inhibits kinase-mediated intracellular signaling pathways by blocking HER2 receptors which results in cancer cell growth arrest and apoptosis; stimulates antibody-dependent cell-mediated cytotoxicity (ADCC) of cancer cells. *Inhibits proliferation of tumor cells with HER2 receptors.*

USES Indicated for the treatment of patients with HER2-positive metastatic breast cancer (with trastuzumab and docetaxel).

CONTRAINDICATIONS Hyersensitivity to pertuzumab; severe infusion reaction; clinical significant decrease in left ventricular function due to drug; pregnancy (category D); lactation.

CAUTIOUS USE Hepatic impairment; severe renal impairment; prior use of anthracycline or radiation; uncontrolled hypertension; recent MI, serious cardiac arrhythmias; CHF. Safety and efficacy in children younger than 18 y not established.

P

ROUTE & DOSAGE

Metastatic Breast Cancer

Adult: **IV** Initial dose of 840 mg; follow q3wk with 420 mg in combination with trastuzumab and docetaxel. Withhold or discontinue if trastuzumab is withheld or discontinued.

Dosing Interruption Due to Decreased Left Ventricular Ejection Fraction (LVEF)

Decreased LVEF to less than 45% or LVEF between 45%–49% with a 10% or greater absolute decrease below pretreatment values: Withhold pertuzumab and trastuzumab for at least 3 wk. *If the LVEF recovers to greater than 49% or to 45%–49% with less than 10% absolute decrease from baseline:* Resume pertuzumab therapy. *If the LVEF does not improve or declines further within approximately 3 wk:* Discontinue pertuzumab and trastuzumab.

ADMINISTRATION

Intravenous

This drug is a cytotoxic agent and caution should be used to prevent any contact with the drug. Follow institutional or standard guidelines for preparation, handling, and disposal of cytotoxic agents.

PREPARE: **IV Infusion:** Dilute required dose in 250 mL NS in a PVC or non-PVC polyolefin bag. Invert to mix but do not shake. Prepare just before use.
ADMINISTER: **IV Infusion:** Infuse initial dose of pertuzumab over 60 min; infuse subsequent doses of pertuzumab over 30–60 min. If trastuzumab is given concurrently with initial dose of pertuzumab, infuse trastuzumab over 90 min; give subsequent doses of trastuzumab over 30–90 min.
INCOMPATIBILITIES: **Solution/additive:** Do not mix with other drugs. Do not mix/dilute with dextrose (5%) solution. **Y-site:** Do not mix with other drugs.

- Observe closely during first 60 min after initial infusion and for 30 min after subsequent infusions. Slow or stop infusion for significant infusion-related reactions.

Monitor vital signs and other parameters frequently until complete return to baseline. ▪ Store vials at 2°–8° C (36°–46° F). Store IV infusion refrigerated for up to 24 h.

ADVERSE EFFECTS **Respiratory:** Dyspnea, cough, nasopharyngitis, URI, epistaxis. **CNS:** Asthenia, dizziness, *fatigue*, headache, insomnia, *peripheral neuropathy*. **Skin:** *Alopecia*, dry skin, nail disorder, pruritus, *rash*. **GI:** Constipation, decreased appetite, *diarrhea*, dyspepsia, dysgeusia, *nausea*, stomatitis, vomiting. **Musculoskeletal:** Arthralgia, myalgia, weakness. **Hematological:** Anemia, febrile neutropenia, leukopenia, neutropenia. **Cardiac:** Decreased left ventricular ejection fraction. **Other:** Hypersensitivity, increased lacrimation, mucosal inflammation, peripheral edema, pyrexia.

PHARMACOKINETICS **Half-Life:** 18 d.

NURSING IMPLICATIONS

Black Box Warning

Pertuzumab has been associated with a significant decrease in left ventricular function, and with fetal death and birth defects.

Assessment & Drug Effects

- Monitor vital signs and cardiac status closely during drug administration and for 60 min after initial infusion and 30 min after subsequent infusions.
- Assess frequently for infusion-related reactions. Slow or stop infusion for significant infusion-related reactions. Institute appropriate support therapies.
- Assess for and report S&S of peripheral neuropathy and infection.
- Monitor lab tests: Baseline and periodic CBC with differential.

Patient & Family Education

- Report promptly S&S of infection.
- Use effective means of contraception during and for 6 mo following end of therapy.
- Report promptly to prescriber if you become pregnant.
- Do not breast-feed while taking this drug.
- Monitor weight daily and report greater than 2 lb weight gain in a day, swelling in the lower extremities, or shortness of breath.

PHENAZOPYRIDINE HYDROCHLORIDE

(fen-az-oh-peer′i-deen)

Azo-Standard, Baridium, Geridium, Phenazo ♣, Phenazodine, Pyridiate, Pyridium, Pyronium ♣, Urodine, Urogesic

Classification: URINARY TRACT ANALGESIC

Therapeutic: URINARY TRACT ANALGESIC

AVAILABILITY Tablet

ACTION & *THERAPEUTIC EFFECT* Azo dye that has local anesthetic action on urinary tract mucosa, which imparts little or no antibacterial activity. *Effective as a urinary tract analgesic*.

USES Symptomatic relief of pain, burning, frequency, and urgency arising from irritation of urinary tract mucosa, as from infection, trauma, surgery, or instrumentation.

CONTRAINDICATIONS Renal insufficiency, renal disease including glomerulonephritis, pyelonephritis, renal failure, uremia; hepatic disease; glucose-6-phosphate dehydrogenase deficiency, severe hepatitis.

CAUTIOUS USE GI disturbances; older adults; pregnancy (category B); lactation; children.

ROUTE & DOSAGE

Cystitis

Adult: **PO** 200 mg tid
Child: **PO** 12 mg/kg/day in 3 divided doses

ADMINISTRATION

Oral

- Give with or after meals.

ADVERSE EFFECTS **Endocrine:** Methemoglobinemia, hemolytic anemia. **Skin:** Skin pigmentation. **GI:** Mild GI disturbances. **GU:** Kidney stones, transient acute kidney failure. **Special Senses:** May stain soft contact lenses. **Other:** Headache, vertigo.

P

DIAGNOSTIC TEST INTERFERENCE Phenazopyridine may interfere with any urinary test that is based on color reactions or spectrometry: ***Bromsulphalein*** and ***phenolsulfonphthalein*** excretion tests; urinary ***glucose*** test using ***Clinistix*** or ***Tes-Tape*** (***copper-reduction methods*** such as ***Clinitest*** and ***Benedict's test*** reportedly not affected); ***bilirubin*** using "foam test" or ***Ictotest; ketones*** using ***nitroprusside*** (e.g., ***Acetest, Ketostix,*** or ***Gerhardt ferric chloride***); ***urinary protein*** using ***Albustix, Albutest,*** or ***nitric acid ring test;*** urinary ***steroids; urobilinogen; assays*** for ***porphyrins.***

PHARMACOKINETICS **Absorption:** Readily absorbed from GI tract. **Distribution:** Crosses placenta in trace amounts. **Metabolism:** In liver and other tissues. **Elimination:** Primarily in urine.

NURSING IMPLICATIONS

Assessment & Drug Effects

- Monitor for therapeutic effectiveness as indicated by relief from pain and burning upon urination.

Patient & Family Education

- Drug will impart an orange to red color to urine and may stain clothing.

PHENELZINE SULFATE

(fen'el-zeen)

Classification: ANTIDEPRESSANT; MONOAMINE OXIDASE (MAO) INHIBITOR
Therapeutic: ANTIDEPRESSANT; MAO INHIBITOR

AVAILABILITY Tablet

ACTION & *THERAPEUTIC EFFECT* Antidepressant action believed to be due to irreversible inhibition of MAO, thereby permitting increased concentrations of endogenous epinephrine, norepinephrine, serotonin, and dopamine within presynaptic neurons and at receptor sites. *Antidepressant utilization is limited to individuals who do not respond well to other classes of antidepressants.*

USES Atypical or nonendogenous depression.

CONTRAINDICATIONS Hypersensitivity to MAO inhibitors; suicidal ideation; pheochromocytoma; untreated hyperthyroidism; cardiac arrhythmias, uncontrolled hypertension; increased intracranial pressure; intracranial bleeding; atonic colitis; glaucoma; frequent headaches; bipolar depression; accompanying alcoholism or drug addiction; paranoid schizophrenia; older adults or debilitated patients; lactation.

CAUTIOUS USE Epilepsy; pyloric stenosis; DM; manic-depressive states; agitated patients; schizophrenia or psychosis; seizures; suicidal tendencies; chronic brain syndromes; pregnancy (category C); children and adolescents.

ROUTE & DOSAGE

Depression

Adult: **PO** 15 mg tid, rapidly increase to at least 60 mg/day, may need up to 90 mg/day

ADMINISTRATION

Oral

- Avoid rapid discontinuation, particularly after high dosage, since a rebound effect may occur (e.g., headache, excitability, hallucinations, and possibly depression).
- Store in tightly covered containers away from heat and light.

ADVERSE EFFECTS **CV:** Hypertensive crisis (intense occipital headache, palpitation, marked hypertension, stiff neck, nausea, vomiting, sweating, fever, photophobia, dilated pupils, bradycardia or tachycardia, constricting chest pain, intracranial bleeding), hypotension or hypertension, circulatory collapse. **CNS:** Mania, hypomania, confusion, memory impairment, delirium, hallucinations, euphoria, acute anxiety reaction, toxic precipitation of schizophrenia, convulsions, peripheral neuropathy. **HEENT:** Blurred vision. **Skin:** Hyperhidrosis, skin rash, photosensitivity. **GI:** *Constipation, dry mouth, nausea,* vomiting, *anorexia,* weight gain. **Hematologic:** Normocytic and normochromic anemia, leukopenia. **Other:** Dizziness or vertigo, headache, *orthostatic hypotension,* drowsiness or *insomnia,* weakness, fatigue, edema, tremors, twitching, akathisia, ataxia, hyperreflexia, faintness, hyperactivity, marked agitation, anxiety, seizures, trismus, opisthotonos, respiratory depression, coma.

DIAGNOSTIC TEST INTERFERENCE

Phenelzine may cause a slight false increase in ***serum bilirubin.***

INTERACTIONS **Drug:** TRICYCLIC ANTIDEPRESSANTS may cause hyperpyrexia, seizures; **fluoxetine, sertraline, paroxetine** may cause serotonin syndrome (see Appendix E); SYMPATHOMIMETIC AGENTS (e.g., **amphetamine, phenylephrine, phenylpropanolamine**), **guanethidine** may cause hypertensive crisis; CNS DEPRESSANTS have additive CNS depressive effects; OPIATE ANALGESICS (especially **meperidine**) may cause hypertensive crisis and circulatory collapse; **buspirone,** hypertension; GENERAL ANESTHETICS, prolonged hypotensive and CNS depressant effects; hypertension, headache, hyperexcitability reported with **dopamine, methyldopa, levodopa, tryptophan; metrizamide** may increase risk of seizures; HYPOTENSIVE AGENTS and DIURETICS have additive hypotensive effects. **Food:** Aged meats or aged cheeses, protein extracts, sour cream, alcohol, anchovies, liver, sausages, overripe figs, bananas, avocados, chocolate, soy

P

sauce, bean curd, natural yogurt, fava beans—**tyramine**-containing foods—may precipitate hypertensive crisis. Avoid **chocolate** or **caffeine. Herbal: Ginseng, ephedra, ma huang, St. John's wort** may cause hypertensive crisis.

PHARMACOKINETICS **Absorption:** Readily absorbed from GI tract. **Onset:** 2 wk. **Metabolism:** Rapidly metabolized. **Elimination:** 79% of metabolites excreted in urine in 96 h.

NURSING IMPLICATIONS

Black Box Warning

Phenelzine has been associated with increased risk of suicidal thinking and behavior (suicidality) in children, adolescents, and young adults.

Assessment & Drug Effects

- Monitor children, adolescents, and adults for changes in behavior that may indicate suicidality.
- Prior to initiation of treatment, evaluate patient's BP in standing and recumbent positions.
- Monitor BP and pulse between doses when titrating initial dosages. Observe closely for evidence of adverse drug effects. Thereafter, monitor at regular intervals throughout therapy.
- Report immediately if hypomania (exaggeration of motility, feelings, and ideas) occurs as depression improves. This reaction may also appear at higher than recommended doses or with long-term therapy.
- Observe for and report therapeutic effectiveness of drug: Improvement in sleep pattern, appetite, physical activity, interest in self and surroundings, as well as lessening of anxiety and bodily complaints.
- Observe patient with diabetes closely for S&S of hypoglycemia (see Appendix E).
- Patients on prolonged therapy should be checked periodically for altered color perception, changes in fundi or visual fields. Changes in red-green vision may be the first indication of eye damage.

Patient & Family Education

- Maximum antidepressant effects generally appear in 2–6 wk and persist several weeks after drug withdrawal.
- Avoid self-medication. OTC preparations (e.g., cough, cold, hay fever remedies, and appetite suppressants) can precipitate severe hypertensive reactions if taken during therapy or within 2–3 wk after discontinuation of an MAO inhibitor.
- Report immediately to prescriber the onset of headache and palpitation, or any other unusual effects which may indicate need to discontinue therapy.
- Do not consume foods and beverages containing tyramine or tryptophan or drugs containing pressor agent. These can cause severe hypertensive reactions. Get a list from your care provider.
- Avoid drinking excessive caffeine and chocolate beverages (e.g., coffee, tea, cocoa, or cola).
- Make position changes slowly, especially from recumbent to upright posture, and dangle legs over bed a few minutes before rising to walk. Avoid standing still for prolonged periods. Also avoid hot showers and baths (resulting vasodilatation may potentiate hypotension); lie down immediately if feeling light-headed or faint.

- Check weight 2 or 3 × wk and report unusual gain.
- Report jaundice. Hepatotoxicity is believed to be a hypersensitivity reaction unrelated to dosage or duration of therapy.

PHENOBARBITAL

(fee-noe-bar'bi-tal)

Solfoton

PHENOBARBITAL SODIUM

Luminal

Classification: ANTICONVULSANT; SEDATIVE-HYPNOTIC; BARBITURATE

Therapeutic: ANTICONVULSANT; SEDATIVE-HYPNOTIC

Controlled Substance: Schedule IV

AVAILABILITY Tablet; capsule; liquid; solution for injection

ACTION & *THERAPEUTIC EFFECT* Sedative and hypnotic effects appear to be due primarily to interference with impulse transmission of cerebral cortex by inhibition of reticular activating system. Limiting spread of seizure activity results by increasing the threshold for motor cortex stimulation. *Effective as a sedative, hypnotic, and an anticonvulsant with no analgesic effect.*

USES Long-term management of tonic-clonic (grand mal) seizures and partial seizures; status epilepticus, eclampsia, febrile convulsions in young children. Also used as a sedative in anxiety or tension states; in pediatrics as preoperative and postoperative sedation and to treat pylorospasm in infants.

UNLABELED USES Treatment and prevention of hyperbilirubinemia in neonates and in the management of chronic cholestasis; benzodiazepine withdrawal.

CONTRAINDICATIONS Hypersensitivity to barbiturates; manifest hepatic or familial history of porphyria; severe respiratory or kidney disease; history of previous addiction to sedative hypnotics; alcohol intoxication; uncontrolled pain; renal failure, anuria; pregnancy (category D).

CAUTIOUS USE Impaired liver, kidney, cardiac, or respiratory function; sleep apnea; COPD; history of allergies; patients with fever; hyperthyroidism; diabetes mellitus or severe anemia; seizure disorders; during labor and delivery; patient with borderline hypoadrenal function; older adult or debilitated patients; lactation; young children and neonates.

ROUTE & DOSAGE

Anticonvulsant

Adult: **PO/IV** 1–3 mg/kg/day in divided doses
Child: **PO/IV** 4–8 mg/kg/day in divided doses

Status Epilepticus

Adult: **IV** 300–800 mg, then 120–240 mg q20min (total max: 1–2 g)
Child: **IV** 10–20 mg/kg in single or divided doses, then 5 mg/kg/dose q15–30min (total max: 40 mg/kg)
Neonate: **IV** 15–20 mg/kg in single or divided doses

Sedative/Hypnotic

Adult: **PO** 30–120 mg/day; **IV/IM** 100–320 mg/day
Child: **PO** 2 mg/kg/day in 3 divided doses **IV/IM** 3–5 mg/kg

P

Renal Impairment Dosage Adjustment

CrCl less than 10 mL/min: Dose q12–16h

Hemodialysis Dosage Adjustment

20–50% dialyzed

ADMINISTRATION

Oral

- Give crushed and mixed with a fluid or with food if patient cannot swallow pill. Do not permit patient to swallow dry crushed drug.

Intramuscular

- Give IM deep into large muscle mass; do not exceed 5 mL at any one site.

Intravenous

Note: Verify correct IV concentration and rate of infusion for neonates, infants, children with prescriber. Use IV route ONLY if other routes are not feasible.

P

PREPARE: **Direct:** May be given undiluted or diluted in 10 mL of sterile water for injection.

ADMINISTER: **Direct:** Give no faster than 60 mg/min in adults and 30 mg/min in children. Give within 30 min after preparation.

INCOMPATIBILITIES: **Solution/additive:** **Ampicillin, cephalothin, chlorpromazine, cimetidine, clindamycin, dexamethasone, diphenhydramine, erythromycin, ephedrine, hydralazine, hydrocortisone sodium succinate, hydroxyzine, insulin, kanamycin, levorphanol, meperidine, methadone, methylphenidate, morphine, nitrofurantoin, norepinephrine, pentazocine, pentobarbital, phytonadione, procaine, prochlorperazine, promazine, promethazine, sodium bicarbonate, streptomycin,** TETRACYCLINES, **vancomycin, warfarin.** **Y-site:** **Amphotericin B cholesteryl complex, hydromorphone, TPN with albumin.**

- Be aware that extravasation of IV phenobarbital may cause necrotic tissue changes that necessitate skin grafting. Check injection site frequently.

ADVERSE EFFECTS

CV: Bradycardia, syncope, hypotension. **Respiratory:** Respiratory depression. **CNS:** *Somnolence,* nightmares, insomnia, "hangover," headache, anxiety, thinking abnormalities, dizziness, nystagmus, irritability, paradoxic excitement and exacerbation of hyperkinetic behavior (in children); confusion or depression or marked excitement (older adult or debilitated patients); ataxia. **Endocrine:** Hypocalcemia, osteomalacia, rickets. **Skin:** Mild maculopapular, morbilliform rash; erythema multiforme, Stevens–Johnson syndrome, exfoliative dermatitis (rare). **GI:** Nausea, vomiting, constipation, diarrhea, epigastric pain, liver damage. **Musculoskeletal:** Folic acid deficiency, vitamin D deficiency. **Hematologic:** Megaloblastic anemia, agranulocytosis, thrombocytopenia. **Other:** Myalgia, neuralgia, CNS depression, coma, and death.

DIAGNOSTIC TEST INTERFERENCE

BARBITURATES may affect ***bromsulphalein*** retention tests (by enhancing liver uptake and excretion of dye) and increase ***serum phosphatase.***

INTERACTIONS

Drug: Alcohol, CNS DEPRESSANTS compound CNS depression; phenobarbital may decrease absorption and increase metabolism of ORAL ANTICOAGULANTS; increases metabolism of CORTICOSTEROIDS, ORAL CONTRACEPTIVES, ANTICONVULSANTS, **digitoxin,** possibly decreasing their effects; ANTIDEPRESSANTS potentiate adverse effects of phenobarbital; **griseofulvin** decreases absorption of phenobarbital; **quinine** increases plasma levels. **Herbal: Kava, valerian** may potentiate sedation.

PHARMACOKINETICS **Absorption:** 70–90% slowly from GI tract. **Peak:** 8–12 h PO; 30 min IV. **Duration:** 4–6 h IV. **Distribution:** 20–45% protein bound; crosses placenta; enters breast milk. **Metabolism:** In liver (CYP2C19). **Elimination:** In urine. **Half-Life:** 2–6 days.

NURSING IMPLICATIONS

Assessment & Drug Effects

- Observe patients receiving large doses for at least 30 min to ensure that sedation is not excessive.
- Chronic use in children or infants requires continuous assessment related to normal cognitive and behavioral functioning.
- Keep patient under constant observation when drug is administered IV, and record vital signs at least every hour or more often if indicated.
- Check IV injection site very frequently to prevent extravasation of phenobarbital. It could result in tissue damage requiring skin grafting.
- Monitor serum drug levels. Serum concentrations greater than 50 mcg/mL may cause coma. Therapeutic serum concentrations of 15–40 mcg/mL produce anticonvulsant activity in most patients. These values are usually attained after 2 or 3 wk of therapy with a dose of 100–200 mg/day.
- Expect barbiturates to produce restlessness when given to patients in pain because these drugs do not have analgesic action.
- Be prepared for paradoxical responses and report promptly in older adult or debilitated patient and children [i.e., irritability, marked excitement (inappropriate tearfulness and aggression in children), depression, and confusion].
- Monitor for drug interactions. Barbiturates increase the metabolism of many drugs, leading to decreased pharmacologic effects of those drugs.
- Monitor for and report chronic toxicity symptoms (e.g., ataxia, slurred speech, irritability, poor judgment, slight dysarthria, nystagmus on vertical gaze, confusion, insomnia, somatic complaints).
- Monitor lab tests: Periodic LFTs, CBC with differential, Hct and Hgb, and renal function tests.

Patient & Family Education

- Be aware that anticonvulsant therapy may cause drowsiness during first few weeks of treatment, but this usually diminishes with continued use.
- Avoid potentially hazardous activities requiring mental alertness until response to drug is known.
- Do not consume alcohol in any amount when taking a barbiturate; it may severely impair judgment and abilities.
- Increase vitamin D-fortified foods (e.g., milk products) because drug increases vitamin D metabolism. A vitamin D supplement may be prescribed.
- Maintain adequate dietary folate intake: Fresh vegetables (especially green leafy), fresh fruits, whole grains, liver. Long-term therapy may result in nutritional

folate (B_9) deficiency. A supplement of folic acid may be prescribed.

- Adhere to drug regimen (i.e., do not change intervals between doses or increase or decrease doses) without contacting prescriber.
- Do not stop taking drug abruptly because of danger of withdrawal symptoms (8–12 h after last dose), which can be fatal.
- Report to prescriber the onset of fever, sore throat or mouth, malaise, easy bruising or bleeding, petechiae, jaundice, rash when on prolonged therapy.
- Avoid pregnancy when receiving barbiturates. Use or add barrier device to hormonal contraceptive when taking prolonged therapy.

PHENTERMINE HYDROCHLORIDE

(phen-ter′meen)

Adipex-P, Lomaira

Classification: ANOREXIANT
Therapeutic: APPETITE SUPPRESSANT
Prototype: Diethylpropion
Controlled Substance: Schedule IV

P

AVAILABILITY Tablet; capsule

ACTION & *THERAPEUTIC EFFECT* Sympathetic amine with actions lead to CNS stimulation including stimulation of the hypothalamus to release norepinephrine. *Appetite suppression or metabolic effects along with diet adjustment result in weight loss in obese individuals.*

USES Short-term (8–12 wk) adjunct for weight loss.

CONTRAINDICATIONS Known hypersensitivity to sympathetic amines; glaucoma; moderate to severe uncontrolled hypertension, history of cardiovascular disease, cardiac arrhythmias, stroke; hyperthyroidism; agitated states; history of drug abuse; during or within 14 days of administration of MAO inhibitor; glaucoma; pregnancy (use of phentermine is contraindicated during pregnancy due to potential fetal harm); lactation.

CAUTIOUS USE Hypertension, DM; seizures; renal impairment; older adults; children younger than 16 y.

ROUTE & DOSAGE

Obesity

Adult/Adolescent: **PO** 15–37.5 mg each morning; 8 mg tid (Lomaira)

Renal Impairment Dosage Adjustment

eGFR 15–29 mL/min: Max dose: 15 mg/day

ADMINISTRATION

Oral

- Ensure that at least 14 days have elapsed between the first dose of phentermine and the last dose of an MAO inhibitor.
- Give 30 min before meals or 1 to 2 hours after meals.
- Do not administer if an SSRI is currently prescribed.
- Avoid late evening administration. Most effective when combined with a low-calorie diet and behavior modification counseling.
- Store in a tight container.

ADVERSE EFFECTS **CV:** Palpitations, tachycardia, hypertension ischemia. **CNS:** Overstimulation, restlessness, dizziness, insomnia, euphoria, dysphoria, tremor, headache, psychosis. **Endocrine:** Change in libido. **Skin:** Urticaria. **GI:** Dry mouth, altered taste, diarrhea, constipation, stomach pain. **GU:** Impotence.

DIAGNOSTIC TEST INTERFERENCE May cause false positive with urine detection of amphetamines/ methamphetamine.

INTERACTIONS **Drug:** MAO INHIBITORS may increase pressor response resulting in hypertensive crisis. TRICYCLIC ANTIDEPRESSANTS may enhance cardiovascular side effects. May have increased arrhythmia risk when used with of **guanethidine.** **Herbal:** Kratom will increase risk of adverse effects.

PHARMACOKINETICS **Absorption:** Absorbed from the small intestine. **Duration:** 4–14 h. **Elimination:** Primarily in urine. **Half-Life:** 19–24 h.

NURSING IMPLICATIONS

Assessment & Drug Effects

- Monitor periodic cardiovascular status, including BP.
- Monitor weight and waist circumference every month for the first 3 months, then at 3-month intervals.

Patient & Family Education

- Do not take this drug late in the evening because it could cause insomnia.
- Report immediately any of the following: Shortness of breath, chest pains, dizziness or fainting, swelling of the extremities.
- Tolerance to the appetite suppression effects of the drug usually develops in a few weeks. Notify prescriber, but do not increase the drug dose.
- Weigh yourself at least 3 × wk at the same time of day with the same amount of clothing.

PHENTOLAMINE MESYLATE

(fen-tole′a-meen)

OraVerse

Classification: ALPHA-ADRENERGIC RECEPTOR ANTAGONIST; VASODILATOR

Therapeutic: VASODILATOR; ANTIHYPERTENSIVE

Prototype: Prazosin

AVAILABILITY Solution for injection

ACTION & *THERAPEUTIC EFFECT* Alpha-adrenergic blocking agent that competitively blocks alpha-adrenergic receptors, but action is transient and incomplete. Causes vasodilation and decreases general vascular resistance as well as pulmonary arterial pressure, primarily by direct action on vascular smooth muscle. *Prevents hypertension resulting from elevated levels of circulating epinephrine or norepinephrine.*

USES Diagnosis of pheochromocytoma and to prevent or control hypertensive episodes associated with pheochromocytoma; management of extravasation of norepinephrine.

UNLABELED USES Extravasation of sympathomimetic vasopressors

CONTRAINDICATIONS Hypersensitivity to phentolamine; MI (or history of MI), CAD; coronary insufficiency; angina; peptic ulcer disease.

CAUTIOUS USE Gastritis; pregnancy (adverse effects have been observed in some animal reproduction studies); lactation; children.

ROUTE & DOSAGE

Diagnosis of Pheochromocytoma

Adult: **IV/IM** 5 mg
Child: **IM** 3 mg; **IV** 1 mg

To Treat Extravasation

Adult: **Intradermal** 5–10 mg diluted in 10 mL of normal saline injected into affected area within 12 h of extravasation
Child: **Intradermal** small amount of a 0.5 to 1 mg/mL solution injected into affected area within 12 h of extravasation

ADMINISTRATION

Note: Place patient in supine position when receiving drug parenterally. ▪ Monitor BP and pulse q5min until stabilized.

Intramuscular

- Reconstitute 5 mg vial with 1 mL of sterile water for injection.

Intravenous

PREPARE: **Direct:** Reconstitute as for IM. May be further diluted with up to 10 mL of sterile water. ▪ Use immediately.

ADMINISTER: **Direct:** Inject rapidly. Monitor BP immediately after injection, every 30 seconds for 3 minutes, then every minute for 7 minutes.

INCOMPATIBILITIES: **Y-site: Amphotericin B (conventional), carmustine, cefamandole, cefazolin, cefoperazone, cefotaxime, cefotetan, cefoxitin, cefuroxime, clindamycin, dantrolene, diazepam, diazoxide, ganciclovir, gemtuzumab, insulin, ketorolac, phenobarbital, phenytoin, sulfamethoxazole/trimethoprim.**

ADVERSE EFFECTS **CV:** *Orthostatic hypotension, bradycardia, flushing.* **Respiratory:** Nasal congestion. **CNS:** Mouth pain, headache, weakness, dizziness. **Other:** Pain at injection site.

INTERACTIONS **Drug:** May antagonize BP raising effects of **epinephrine, ephedrine;** may increase antihypertensive effects of other ANTIHYPERTENSIVES.

PHARMACOKINETICS **Peak:** 2 min IV; 15–20 min IM. **Duration:** 10–30 min IV; 30-45 min IM. **Elimination:** In urine. **Half-Life:** 19 min.

NURSING IMPLICATIONS

Assessment & Drug Effects

Test for pheochromocytoma:

- *IV administration:* Keep patient at rest in supine position throughout test, preferably in quiet darkened room. ▪ Prior to drug administration, take BP q10min for at least 30 min to establish that BP has stabilized before IV injection. ▪ Record BP immediately after injection and at 30-sec intervals for first 3 min; then at 1-min intervals for next 7 min.
- *IM administration:* Post-injection, BP determinations at 5-min intervals for 30–45 min.

Patient & Family Education

- Avoid sudden changes in position, particularly from reclining to upright posture and dangle legs and exercise ankles and toes for a few minutes before standing to walk.
- Lie down or sit down in head-low position immediately if lightheaded or dizzy.

PHENYLEPHRINE HYDROCHLORIDE

(fen-ill-ef′rin)

AK-Dilate Ophthalmic, Altafrin
Classification: EYE AND NOSE PREPARATION; ALPHA-ADRENERGIC AGONIST; MYDRIATIC; VASOPRESSOR; DECONGESTANT
Therapeutic: VASOCONSTRICTOR; DECONGESTANT; MYDRIATIC
Prototype: Dexmedetomide

AVAILABILITY Tablet; nasal solution; ophthalmic solution; solution for injection; suppository

ACTION & *THERAPEUTIC EFFECT*
Potent, synthetic, direct-acting sympathomimetic with strong alpha-adrenergic cardiac stimulant actions. Elevates systolic and diastolic pressures through arteriolar constriction. Reduces intraocular pressure by increasing outflow and decreasing rate of aqueous humor secretion. *Effective antihypotensive agent. Topical applications to eye produce vasoconstriction and prompt mydriasis of short duration, usually without causing cycloplegia. Nasal decongestant action qualitatively similar to that of epinephrine but more potent.*

USES Parenterally for hypotension or shock. Used topically for rhinitis of common cold, allergic rhinitis, and sinusitis; in selected patients with wide-angle glaucoma; as mydriatic for ophthalmoscopic examination or surgery, and for relief of uveitis; used orally for nasal congestion.

CONTRAINDICATIONS Severe CAD, hypertension, atrial fibrillation, atrial flutter, cardiac disease, cardiomyopathy; uncontrolled hypertension; ventricular arrhythmias; thyrotoxicosis; cerebral arteriosclerosis, MAOI; labor, delivery, infants, neonates. **Ophthalmic preparations:** Narrow-angle glaucoma.

CAUTIOUS USE Hyperthyroidism; DM; heart failure; thyroid disease; BPH; 21 days before or following termination of MAO inhibitor therapy; older adults; pregnancy (no study data available; when administered intravenously, phenylephrine crosses the placenta); children younger than 6 y. **Ophthalmic:** Lactation.

ROUTE & DOSAGE

Hypotension during Anesthesia
Adult: **IV** Bolus 40–100 mcg/dose every 1–2 min as needed (total dose not to exceed 200 mcg)

Vasoconstrictor
Adult: **Ophthalmic** See Appendix A-1; **Intranasal** 2–3 sprays of 0.25–0.5% solution 4h as needed
Child (6–12 y): **Intranasal** 2–3 drops or sprays of 0.25% solution 4h as needed

ADMINISTRATION
Instillation
- Nasal preparations: Instruct patient to blow nose gently (with both nostrils open) to clear nasal passages before administration of medication.
- Instillation (drops): Tilt head back while sitting or standing up, or lie on bed and hang head over side. Stay in position a few minutes to permit medication to spread through nose. (Spray): With head upright, squeeze bottle quickly and firmly to produce 1 or 2 sprays into each nostril; wait 3–5 min, blow nose, and repeat dose. (Jelly): Place in each nostril and sniff it well back into nose.
- Clean tips and droppers of nasal solution dispensers with hot

P

water after use to prevent contamination of solution. Droppers of ophthalmic solution bottles should not touch any surface including the eye.

- Ophthalmic preparations: To avoid excessive systemic absorption, apply pressure to lacrimal sac during and for 1–2 min after instillation of drops. Patient should remove contacts prior to instillation and wait at least 15 minutes before reinsertion.

Subcutaneous/Intramuscular

- Give undiluted.

Intravenous

Note: Ensure patency of IV site prior to administration.

PREPARE: **Direct:** Dilute each 10 mg (1 mL) of 1% solution in 9 mL of sterile water. **IV Infusion:** Dilute each 10 mg in 500 mL D5W or NS (concentration: 0.02 mg/mL).
ADMINISTER: **Direct:** Give a single dose over 30 sec. **IV Infusion:** Titrate to maintain BP.
INCOMPATIBILITIES: **Y-site:** **Acyclovir, amphotericin B (conventional and lipid), azathioprine, dantrolene, diazepam, diazoxide, ganciclovir, indomethacin, insulin, lansoprazole, minocycline, mitomycin, pentamidine, phenytoin, SMZ/TMP, thiopental.**

P

- Protect from exposure to air, strong light, or heat, any of which can cause solutions to change color to brown, form a precipitate, and lose potency.

ADVERSE EFFECTS **CV:** Palpitation, tachycardia, bradycardia, arrhythmia, hypertension, peripheral vasoconstriction. **Respiratory:** Dyspnea, respiratory distress. **HEENT:** Blurred vision, increased sensitivity to light. *Rebound nasal congestion* (hyperemia and edema of mucosa), *nasal burning,* stinging, dryness, *sneezing*. **Endocrine:** Metabolic acidosis. **Skin:** Pallor, piloerection, pruritis. **GI:** Nausea, vomiting, epigastric pain, gastric irritation. **GU:** Decreased renal blood flow, decreased urine output. **Other:** Neck pain, weakness, restlessness, anxiety, *tremor,* severe visceral or peripheral vasoconstriction, necrosis if IV infiltrates.

INTERACTIONS **Drug:** ERGOT ALKALOIDS, **guanethidine,** TRICYCLIC ANTIDEPRESSANTS increase pressor effects of phenylephrine; **halothane, digoxin** increase risk of arrhythmias; MAO INHIBITORS cause hypertensive crisis; **oxytocin** causes persistent hypertension; ALPHA-BLOCKERS, BETA-BLOCKERS antagonize effects of phenylephrine.

PHARMACOKINETICS **Onset:** Immediate IV; 10–15 min IM/Subcutaneous; 15–30 min Nasal. **Duration:** 15–20 min IV; 30–120 min IM/Subcutaneous; 3–6 h topical. **Metabolism:** In liver and tissues by monoamine oxidase.

NURSING IMPLICATIONS

Assessment & Drug Effects

- Monitor infusion site closely as extravasation may cause tissue necrosis and gangrene. If extravasation does occur, area should be immediately injected with 5–10 mg of phentolamine (Regitine) diluted in 10–15 mL of NS.
- Monitor pulse, BP, and cardiac output, pulmonary wedge pressure (q2–5min) during IV administration.
- Control flow rate and dosage to prevent excessive dosage. IV overdoses can induce ventricular dysrhythmias.

- Observe for congestion or rebound miosis after topical administration to eye.

Patient & Family Education

- Be aware that instillation of 2.5–10% strength ophthalmic solution can cause burning and stinging.
- Do not exceed recommended dosage regardless of formulation.
- Inform the prescriber if no relief is experienced from preparation in 5 days.
- Wear sunglasses in bright light because after instillation of ophthalmic drops, pupils will be large and eyes may be more sensitive to light than usual. Stop medication and notify prescriber if sensitivity persists beyond 12 h after drug has been discontinued.
- Be aware that some ophthalmic solutions may stain contact lenses.

PHENYTOIN (Prototype)

(fen′i-toy-in)

Dilantin-125, Dilantin

PHENYTOIN SODIUM EXTENDED

Dilantin, Phentek

PHENYTOIN SODIUM PROMPT

Dilantin

Classification: ANTICONVULSANT; HYDANTOIN

Therapeutic: ANTICONVULSANT

AVAILABILITY Capsule; sustained release capsule; chewable tablet; suspension; solution for injection

ACTION & THERAPEUTIC EFFECT Stabilizes neuronal membranes and decreases seizure activity by increasing efflux or decreasing influx of sodium ions across cell membranes in the motor cortex during generation of nerve impulses; prolongs refractory period and suppresses ventricular pacemaker automaticity; shortens action potential in the heart. *Inhibits seizure activity. Effective in treating arrhythmias associated with QT prolongation.*

USES To treat focal (partial onset) seizures and generalized onset seizures; treatment of status epilepticus.

UNLABELED USES Treatment of trigeminal neuralgia (tic douloureux).

CONTRAINDICATIONS Hypersensitivity to phenytoin; concurrent use of delavirdine; rash; sinus bradycardia, complete or incomplete heart block; Adams-Stokes syndrome; pregnancy (increased risk of congenital malformations and adverse outcomes may occur following in utero phenytoin exposure).

CAUTIOUS USE Impaired liver or kidney function; alcoholism; blood dyscrasias; hypotension, severe myocardial insufficiency, impending or frank heart failure; pancreatic adenoma; DM, hyperglycemia; respiratory depression; acute intermittent porphyria; older adult, debilitated, or gravely ill patients.

ROUTE & DOSAGE

Status Epilepticus

Adult: **IV** 20 mg/kg at a max rate of 50 mg/minute; if necessary, may give an additional

P

dose of 5–10 mg/kg 10 min after the loading dose *Adolescent/Child/Infant:* **IV** 20 mg/kg (max dose: 1000 mg/dose)

Focal and generalized onset Seizures

Adult: **PO Extended release** 1 g divided into 3 doses administrated at 2 hour intervals then start maintenance dosing 24 hours after first dose *Maintenance dose:* 100 mg 3–4 times/day. Adjust dose based on response.
Adolescent/Child: **PO/IV** 15–20 mg/kg/day in divided doses then 5 mg/kg/day in divided doses (max: 300 mg/day)

ADMINISTRATION

Oral

- Ensure that sustained release form is not chewed or crushed. **Must be** swallowed whole.
- Do not give within 2–3 h of antacid ingestion.
- Shake suspension vigorously before pouring to ensure uniform distribution of drug.
- Note: Chewable tablets are not intended for once-a-day dosage since drug is too quickly bioavailable and can therefore lead to toxic serum levels.
- Use sustained release capsules ONLY for once-a-day dosage regimens.

Intravenous

Note: Verify correct rate of IV injection for administration to infants or children with prescriber.
- Inspect solution prior to use. May use a slightly yellowed injectable solution safely. Precipitation may be caused by refrigeration, but slow warming to room temperature restores clarity.

PREPARE: **Direct:** Give undiluted. Use only when clear without precipitate.
ADMINISTER: **Direct for Adult** Give at a max rate of 50 mg/minute. (20 mg/min in older adult or when used as antiarrhythmic). **Do not** give more rapidly. ▪ Follow with an injection of sterile saline through the same in-place catheter or needle. **Do not** use solutions containing dextrose.
Direct for Child/Neonate: Give 1 mg/kg/min. **Do not** give more rapidly. ▪ Follow with an injection of sterile saline through the same in-place catheter or needle. **Do not** use solutions containing dextrose.
INCOMPATIBILITIES: **Solution/additive: Do not administer with other medications. Y-site:** Extensive incompatibilities; **Do not administer with other medications.**
- Observe injection site frequently during administration to prevent infiltration. Local soft tissue irritation may be serious, leading to erosion of tissues.

ADVERSE EFFECTS **CV:** Atrial conduction depression, <u>cardiac arrhythmia, ventricular fibrillation,</u> hypotension. **CNS:** Ataxia, confusion, dizziness, drowsiness, headache, insomnia, nervousness, paresthesia, slurred speech, twitching, vertigo, suicidal ideation. **HEENT:** Nystagmus. **Endocrine:** Decreased T4, vitamin D deficiency. **Skin:** Dermatitis, rash, Stevens–Johnson syndrome, injection site reaction, local tissue necrosis/reaction. **Hepatic/GI:** Acute hepatic injury, increased ALP, constipation, gingival hyperplasia, nausea, vomiting, swelling of lips, dysgeusia. **GU:** Peyronie disease. **Hematologic:** Macrocytosis, megaloblastic anemia, pseudolymphoma, purpuric dermatitis. **Musculoskeletal:** Osteomalacia.

DIAGNOSTIC TEST INTERFERENCE

Phenytoin (HYDANTOINS) may produce lower than normal values for T4 and T3, ***dexamethasone*** or ***metyrapone*** tests; may increase serum levels of ***TSH, glucose, BSP,*** and ***alkaline phosphatase*** and may decrease ***PBI*** and ***urinary steroid*** levels.

INTERACTIONS

Drug: May impact serum concentrations of other medications metabolized by CYP3A4. **Alcohol** decreases phenytoin effects; OTHER ANTICONVULSANTS may increase or decrease phenytoin levels; phenytoin may decrease absorption and increase metabolism of ORAL ANTICOAGULANTS; phenytoin increases metabolism of CORTICOSTEROIDS, ORAL CONTRACEPTIVES, and **nisoldipine,** decreasing their effectiveness; **amiodarone, chloramphenicol, omeprazole,** and **ticlopidine** increase phenytoin levels; ANTITUBERCULOSIS AGENTS decrease phenytoin levels. Closely monitor if used with ANTIRETROVIRALS. Avoid use of P-glycoprotein inducers. **Food: Folic acid, calcium,** and **vitamin D** absorption may be decreased by phenytoin; phenytoin absorption may be decreased by enteral nutrition supplements. **Herbal: Ginkgo** may decrease anticonvulsant effectiveness.

PHARMACOKINETICS

Absorption: Completely from GI tract. **Peak:** 1.5–3 h prompt release; 4–12 h sustained release. **Distribution:** 95% protein bound; crosses placenta; small amount in breast milk. **Metabolism:** Oxidized in liver to inactive metabolites; induces CYP 3A4. **Elimination:** By kidneys. **Half-Life:** 22 h.

NURSING IMPLICATIONS

Black Box Warning

Phenytoin has been associated with severe adverse cardiovascular effects when administered too rapidly.

Assessment & Drug Effects

- Monitor infusion site closely as extravasation may cause tissue necrosis.
- Continuously monitor vital signs and symptoms during IV infusion and for an hour afterward. Watch for respiratory depression. Constant observation and a cardiac monitor are necessary with older adults or patients with cardiac disease. Margin between toxic and therapeutic IV doses is relatively small.
- Be aware of therapeutic serum concentration: 10–20 mcg/mL; toxic level: 30–50 mcg/mL; lethal level: 100 mcg/mL. Steady-state therapeutic levels are not achieved for at least 7–10 days.
- Observe patient closely for neurologic adverse effects following IV administration. Monitor patient for suicidal tendencies.
- Monitor for gingival hyperplasia, which appears most commonly in children and adolescents and never occurs in patients without teeth.
- Make sure patients on prolonged therapy have adequate intake of vitamin D-containing foods and sufficient exposure to sunlight.
- Monitor diabetics for loss of glycemic control.

P

- Monitor for S&S of hypocalcemia (see Appendix E), especially in patients receiving other anticonvulsants concurrently, as well as those who are inactive, have limited exposure to sun, or whose dietary intake is inadequate.
- Observe for symptoms of folic acid deficiency: Neuropathy, mental dysfunction.
- Be alert to symptoms of hypomagnesemia (see Appendix E); neuromuscular symptoms: Tetany, positive Chvostek's and Trousseau's signs, seizures, tremors, ataxia, vertigo, nystagmus, muscular fasciculations.
- Monitor lab tests: Periodic serum phenytoin concentration, CBC, LFTs, comprehensive metabolic profile.

Patient & Family Education

- Be aware that drug may make urine pink or red to red-brown.
- Report symptoms of fatigue, dry skin, deepening voice when receiving long-term therapy because phenytoin can unmask a low thyroid reserve.
- Do not alter prescribed drug regimen. Stopping drug abruptly may precipitate seizures and status epilepticus.
- Do not request/accept change in drug brand when refilling prescription without consulting prescriber.
- Understand the effects of alcohol: Alcohol intake may increase phenytoin serum levels, leading to phenytoin toxicity.
- Discontinue drug immediately if a measles-like skin rash or jaundice appears and notify prescriber.
- Be aware that influenza vaccine during phenytoin treatment may increase seizure activity. Consult prescriber.

P

PHYSOSTIGMINE SALICYLATE

(fi-zoe-stig'meen)

Classification: CHOLINESTERASE INHIBITOR
Therapeutic: ANTICHOLINERGIC ANTIDOTE, CHOLINESTERASE INHIBITOR
Prototype: Neostigmine

AVAILABILITY Solution for injection

ACTION & *THERAPEUTIC EFFECT*

Inhibits the destructive action of acetylcholinesterase and thereby prolongs and exaggerates the effect of the acetylcholine on the skeletal muscle, GI tract and within the CNS. *Effective in reversing anticholingeric toxicity.*

USES To reverse anticholinergic toxicity.

CONTRAINDICATIONS Asthma; DM; gangrene, cardiovascular disease; mechanical obstruction of intestinal or urogenital tract; peptic ulcer disease; asthma; any vagotonic state; closed-angle glaucoma; secondary glaucoma; inflammatory disease of iris or ciliary body; lactation.

CAUTIOUS USE Epilepsy; parkinsonism; bradycardia; hyperthyroidism; seizure disorders; hypotension; pregnancy (category C); children.

ROUTE & DOSAGE

Reversal of Anticholinergic Effects

Adult: **IM/IV** 0.5–2 mg (IV not faster than 1 mg/min), repeat as needed
Child: **IV** 0.02 mg/kg/dose, may repeat q5–10min (max total dose: 2 mg)

ADMINISTRATION

- Use only clear, colorless solutions. Redtinted solution indicates oxidation, and such solutions should be discarded.

Intramuscular

- Give undiluted.

Intravenous

Note: Verify correct rate of IV injection for infants or children with prescriber.

PREPARE: **Direct:** Give undiluted. ***ADMINISTER:*** **Direct for Adult:** Give slowly at a rate of no more than 1 mg/min. ▪ Rapid administration and overdosage can cause a cholinergic crisis. **Direct for Child:** Give 0.5 mg or fraction thereof over at least 1 min. ▪ Rapid administration and overdosage can cause a cholinergic crisis.

INCOMPATIBILITIES: **Solution/additive:** **Phenytoin.** **Y-site:** **Dobutamine.**

ADVERSE EFFECTS **CV:** Irregular pulse, palpitations, bradycardia, rise in BP. **Respiratory:** Dyspnea, bronchospasm, respiratory paralysis, pulmonary edema. **CNS:** Restlessness, hallucinations, twitching, tremors, *sweating,* weakness, ataxia, convulsions, collapse. **HEENT:** Miosis, *lacrimation,* rhinorrhea. **GI:** *Nausea, vomiting, epigastric pain, diarrhea, salivation.* **GU:** Involuntary urination or defecation. **Other:** *Sweating,* cholinergic crisis (acute toxicity), hyperactivity, respiratory distress, convulsions.

INTERACTIONS **Drug:** Antagonizes effects of **isofluorphate.**

PHARMACOKINETICS **Absorption:** Readily from mucous membranes, muscle, subcutaneous tissue; 10–12% absorbed from GI tract. **Onset:** 3–8 min IM/IV. **Duration:** 0.5–5 h IM/IV. **Distribution:** Crosses blood–brain barrier. **Metabolism:** In plasma by cholinesterase. **Elimination:** Small amounts in urine. **Half-Life:** 15–40 min.

NURSING IMPLICATIONS

Assessment & Drug Effects

- Monitor vital signs and state of consciousness closely in patients receiving drug for atropine poisoning. Since physostigmine is usually rapidly eliminated, patient can lapse into delirium and coma within 1 to 2 h; repeat doses may be required.
- Monitor closely for adverse effects related to CNS and for signs of sensitivity to physostigmine. Have atropine sulfate readily available for clinical emergency.
- Discontinue parenteral or oral drug if following symptoms arise: Excessive salivation, emesis, frequent urination, or diarrhea.
- Eliminate excessive sweating or nausea with dose reduction.

P

PHYTONADIONE (VITAMIN K_1)

(fye-toe-na-dye′one)

Mephyton

Classification: VITAMIN K; ANTIDOTE

Therapeutic: VITAMIN K; ANTIDOTE

AVAILABILITY Tablet; solution for injection

ACTION & *THERAPEUTIC EFFECT* Fat-soluble substance chemically identical to and with similar activity as naturally occurring vitamin K. Vitamin K is essential for hepatic biosynthesis of blood clotting Factors II, VII, IX, and X. *Promotes liver synthesis of clotting factors.*

USES Reversal of anticoagulation due to warfarin, treatment of vitamin K deficiency, prophylaxis and treatment of vitamin K deficiency bleeding of the newborn.

CONTRAINDICATIONS Hypersensitivity to phytonadione, benzyl alcohol, or castor oil; severe liver disease.

CAUTIOUS USE Biliary tract disease, obstructive jaundice, pregnancy (phytonadione crosses the placenta in limited concentrations). **IV:** Older adults.

ROUTE & DOSAGE

Anticoagulant Overdose

Adult: Dose based on INR and severity of bleeding. Typical range **PO/IV** 2.5–10 mg as single dose. See institution protocol.

Prophylaxis for Hemorrhagic Disease of Newborns

Infant: **Subcutaneous** 0.5–1 mg immediately after delivery

Vitamin K deficiency

Adult: **PO/IM/IV** 10 mg, may repeat in 48–72 hours
Child/Infant: **IM/Subcutaneous/ IV** 0.5–5 mg

ADMINISTRATION

Oral

- May administer diluted or undiluted in a beverage.
- Store in tightly closed container and protect from light. Vitamin K is rapidly degraded by light.

Intramuscular/Subcutaneous

- Subcutaneous route is generally not preferred due to unpredictable absorption. IM route should be avoided due to the risk of hematoma formation.
- Apply gentle pressure to site following injection. Swelling (internal bleeding) and pain sometimes occur with injection.

Intravenous

Note: Reserve IV route only for emergencies.

PREPARE: **Direct:** Dilute a single dose in 10 mL D5W, NS, or D5/NS. ▪ Protect infusion solution from light.
ADMINISTER: **Direct:** Give solution immediately after dilution at a rate not to exceed 1 mg/min.
INCOMPATIBILITIES: **Solution/additive: Ranitidine. Y-site: Dantrolene, diazepam, diazoxide, magnesium sulfate, phenytoin, sulfamethoxazole/trimethoprim, temocillin.**

- Protect infusion solution from light by wrapping container with aluminum foil or other opaque material. ▪ Discard unused solution and contents in open ampule.

ADVERSE EFFECTS **CV:** Chest pain, flushing, hypotension, tachycardia, weak pulse. **Respiratory:** Cyanosis, dyspnea. **CNS:** Dizziness. **HEENT:** Peculiar taste sensation. **Endocrine:** Hyperbilirubinemia, kernicterus. **Skin:** Diaphoresis, eczematous rash, erythema, erythematous rash, pruritic patches of the skin, urticaria. **GI/Hepatic:** Dysgeusia, hyperbilirubinemia. **Hematologic:** Paradoxic hypoprothrombinemia (patients with severe liver disease), severe hemolytic anemia. **Other:** Hypersensitivity or anaphylaxis-like reaction: Facial flushing, cramp-like pains, convulsive movements, chills, fever, diaphoresis, weakness, dizziness, shock, cardiac arrest.

DIAGNOSTIC TEST INTERFERENCE Falsely elevated ***urine steroids*** (by modifications of ***Reddy, Jenkins, Thorn procedure***).

INTERACTIONS Drug: Antagonizes effects of **warfarin; cholestyramine, colestipol, mineral oil** decrease absorption of oral phytonadione.

PHARMACOKINETICS Absorption: Readily from intestinal lymph if bile is present. **Onset:** 6–12 h PO; 1–2 h IM/Subcutaneous; 15 min IV. **Peak:** Hemorrhage usually controlled within 3–8 h; normal prothrombin time may be obtained in 12–14 h after administration. **Distribution:** Concentrates briefly in liver after absorption; crosses placenta; distributed into breast milk. **Metabolism:** Rapidly in liver. **Elimination:** In urine and bile.

NURSING IMPLICATIONS

Black Box Warning

Phytonadione has been associated with severe reactions (resembling hypersensitivity or anaphylaxis) during and immediately after IV and IM administration.

Assessment & Drug Effects

- Monitor patient constantly. Severe reactions, including fatalities, have occurred during and immediately after IV and IM injection (see ADVERSE EFFECTS).
- Frequency, dose, and therapy duration are guided by PT/INR clinical response.
- Monitor therapeutic effectiveness which is indicated by shortened PT, INR, bleeding, and clotting times, as well as decreased hemorrhagic tendencies.
- Be aware that patients on large doses may develop temporary resistance to coumarin-type anticoagulants. If oral anticoagulant is reinstituted, larger than former doses may be needed. Some patients may require change to heparin.
- Monitor lab tests: Baseline and frequent PT, INR.

Patient & Family Education

- Maintain consistency in diet and avoid significant increases in daily intake of vitamin K-rich foods when drug regimen is stabilized. Know sources rich in vitamin K: Asparagus, broccoli, cabbage, lettuce, turnip greens, pork or beef liver, green tea, spinach, watercress, and tomatoes.

PILOCARPINE HYDROCHLORIDE (Pr)

PILOCARPINE NITRATE

(pye-loe-kar′peen)

Adsorbocarpine, Isopto Carpine, Minims Pilocarpine ♣, Miocarpine ♣, Ocusert, Pilo, Pilocar, Salagen

Classification: EYE PREPARATION; MIOTIC (ANTIGLAUCOMA); DIRECT-ACTING CHOLINERGIC

Therapeutic: ANTIGLAUCOMA

AVAILABILITY Ophthalmic solution; ophthalmic gel; ocular insert; tablet

ACTION & *THERAPEUTIC EFFECT* In open-angle glaucoma, pilocarpine causes contraction of the ciliary muscle, increasing the outflow of aqueous humor, which reduces intraocular pressure (IOP). In closed-angle glaucoma, it induces miosis by opening the angle of the anterior chamber of the eye, through which aqueous humor exits. *Decrease in IOP results from stimulation of ciliary and papillary sphincter muscles, thus facilitating outflow of aqueous humor.*

P

USES Open-angle and angle-closure glaucomas; to reduce IOP and to protect the lens during surgery and laser iridotomy; to counteract effects of mydriatics and cycloplegics following surgery or ophthalmoscopic examination; to treat xerostomia.

CONTRAINDICATIONS Secondary glaucoma, acute iritis, acute inflammatory disease of anterior segment of eye; uncontrolled asthma; lactation. **Ocular therapeutic system:** Not used in acute infectious conjunctivitis, keratitis, retinal detachment, or when intense miosis is required, or with contact lens use.

CAUTIOUS USE Bronchial asthma; biliary tract disease; COPD; hypertension; pregnancy (category C).

ROUTE & DOSAGE

Acute Glaucoma

Adult/Child: **Ophthalmic** 1 drop of 1–2% solution in affected eye q5–10min for 3–6 doses, then 1 drop q1–3h until IOP is reduced

Chronic Glaucoma

Adult/Child: **Ophthalmic** 1 drop of 0.5–4% solution in affected eye q4–12h or 1 ocular system (Ocusert) q7days

Miotic

Adult/Child: **Ophthalmic** 1 drop of 1% solution in affected eye

Xerostomia

Adult: **PO** 5 mg tid, may increase up to 10 mg tid

ADMINISTRATION

Oral

- Give with a full glass of water, if not contraindicated.

Instillation

- Note: During acute phase, prescriber may prescribe instillation of drug into unaffected eye to prevent bilateral attack of acute glaucoma.
- Apply gentle digital pressure to periphery of nasolacrimal drainage system for 1–2 min immediately after instillation of drops to prevent delivery of drug to nasal mucosa and general circulation.

ADVERSE EFFECTS CV: Tachycardia. **Respiratory:** Bronchospasm, rhinitis. **CNS:** Oral (asthenia, headaches, dizziness, chills). **HEENT:** Ciliary spasm with brow ache, twitching of eyelids, eye pain with change in eye focus, miosis, *diminished vision in poorly illuminated areas,* blurred vision, reduced visual acuity, sensitivity, contact allergy, lacrimation, follicular conjunctivitis, conjunctival irritation, cataract, <u>retinal detachment</u>. **GI:** *Nausea,* vomiting, abdominal cramps, diarrhea, epigastric distress, *salivation.* **Other:** Tremors, *increased sweating,* urinary frequency.

INTERACTIONS Drug: The actions of pilocarpine and **carbachol** are additive when used concomitantly. Oral form may cause conduction disturbances with BETA-BLOCKERS. Antagonizes the effects of concurrent ANTICHOLINERGIC DRUGS (e.g., **atropine, ipratropium**). **Food:** High-fat meal decreases absorption of pilocarpine.

PHARMACOKINETICS Absorption: Topical penetrates cornea rapidly; readily absorbed from GI tract. **Onset:** Miosis 10–30 min; IOP reduction 60 min; salivary stimulation 20 min. **Peak:** Miosis 30 min; IOP reduction 75 min; salivary stimulation 60 min. **Duration:** Miosis 4–8 h; IOP reduction 4–14 h (7 days with Ocusert); salivary stimulation 3–5 h. **Metabolism:** Inactivated at neuronal synapses and in plasma. **Elimination:** In urine. **Half-Life:** 0.76–1.35 h.

NURSING IMPLICATIONS

Assessment & Drug Effects

- Be aware that hourly tonometric tests may be done during early treatment because drug may cause an initial transitory increase in IOP.
- Monitor changes in visual acuity.
- Monitor for adverse effects. Brow pain and myopia tend to be more prominent in younger patients and generally disappear with continued use of drug.

Patient & Family Education

- Understand that therapy for glaucoma is prolonged and that adherence to established regimen is crucial to prevent blindness.
- Do not drive or engage in potentially hazardous activities until vision clears. Drug causes blurred vision and difficulty in focusing.
- Discontinue medication if symptoms of irritation or sensitization persist and report to prescriber.

PIMAVANSERIN

(pim-a-van′ser-in)

Nuplazid

Classification: ATYPICAL ANTIPSYCHOTIC

Therapeutic: ANTIPSYCHOTIC

Prototype: Clozapine

AVAILABILITY Tablets

ACTION & *THERAPEUTIC EFFECT* An inverse agonist and antagonist with a high binding affinity for the serotonin 5-HT_{2A} receptor and a lower binding affinity for the 5-HT_{2C} receptor.

USES Treatment of hallucinations and delusions associated with Parkinson disease.

CONTRAINDICATIONS Avoid use in patients with cardiac disease or other risk factors for prolonged QT intervals, torsade de pointes, and/or sudden death such as cardiac arrhythmias, congenital long QT syndrome, heart failure, bradycardia, myocardial infarction, hypertension, coronary artery disease, hypomagnesemia, hypokalemia, hypocalcemia, or in patients receiving medications known to prolong the QT interval. Females and elderly patients are also at risk for QT prolongation. Pimavanserin is not recommended for patients with severe renal impairment (CrCl less than 30 mL/min), including renal failure. Not recommended for patients with mild, moderate or severe hepatic disease or impairment. Drug has not been evaluated in this population. Not approved for patients with dementia, related psychosis and delusions associated with Parkinson's disease.

CAUTIOUS USE Cautious use for older adults. No data on use in pregnant or lactating women.

ROUTE & DOSAGE

Hallucinations and Delusions

Adult: **PO** 34 mg once daily

Hepatic Impairment Dosage Adjustment

Not recommended in patients with hepatic impairment

P

Renal Impairment Dosage Adjustment

CrCl less than 30 mL/min: Not recommended

Concomitant Use with CYP3A4 Inhibitors Dosage Adjustment

Decrease dose to 17 mg once daily if used with a strong CYP3A4 inhibitor

ADMINISTRATION

Oral

- May be administered without regard to food.
- Store at 15°–30° C (59°–86° F).

ADVERSE EFFECTS CV: QT interval prolongation. **CNS:** Confusional state, hallucinations. **GI:** Constipation, nausea. **Other:** Gait disturbance, peripheral edema.

INTERACTIONS Drug: Concomitant use of drugs that prolong the QT interval (e.g., **amiodarone, chlorpromazine, disopyramide, gatifloxacin, moxifloxacin, procainamide, quinidine, sotalol, thioridazine, ziprasidone**) may be additive to the QT effects of pimavanserin and increase the risk of cardiac arrhythmia. Concomitant use with a strong CYP3A4 inhibitor (e.g., **clarithromycin, indinavir, itraconazole, ketoconazole**) increases the levels of primavanserin. Concomitant use with a strong CYP3A4 inducer (e.g., **carbamazepine, phenytoin, rifampin**) may decrease the levels of primavanserin. **Herbal: St. John's wort** may decrease the levels of primavanserin.

PHARMACOKINETICS Peak: 6 h. **Distribution:** 95% plasma protein bound. **Metabolism:** Hepatic oxidation to active and inactive metabolites. **Elimination:** Renal and fecal. **Half-Life:** 57 h.

NURSING IMPLICATIONS

Assessment & Drug Effects

- Monitor ECG: Prolonged QT interval has been reported.
- Monitor vital signs.
- Assess for peripheral edema and perform daily weights.
- Assess cognition and gait, patient at risk for confusion, hallucinations, and altered gait that impact safety.
- Monitor lab tests: LFTs, serum creatinine, and electrolytes.

Patient & Family Education

- No data on use in pregnant women; contraceptive measures should be taken.
- Check with provider before taking any over the counter medication and make sure to tell healthcare providers the patient is currently taking this medication.
- Avoid drinking alcohol while taking this medication.
- Report any swelling noted in hands or feet.
- Report a fast or pounding heartbeat, chest pain, confusion, or severe dizziness.

PIMECROLIMUS

(pim-e-cro-lim'us)

Elidel

Classification: BIOLOGIC RESPONSE MODIFIER; IMMUNOMODULATOR
Therapeutic: IMMUNOSUPPRESSANT; ANTI-INFLAMMATORY
Prototype: Cyclosporine

AVAILABILITY Cream

ACTION & *THERAPEUTIC EFFECT*

Selectively inhibits inflammatory

action of skin cells by blocking T-cell activation and cytokine release. It appears to inhibit the production of IL-2, IL-4, IL-10, and interferon gamma in T-cells. *Produces significant anti-inflammatory activity without evidence of skin atrophy.*

USES Short-term intermittent treatment of mild to moderate atopic dermatitis, eczema.

CONTRAINDICATIONS Hypersensitivity to pimecrolimus or components in the cream; Netherton's syndrome; immunocompromised individuals; application to active cutaneous viral infection; occlusive dressing; artificial or natural sunlight (UV) exposure; continuous long-term use; lactation; children younger than 2 y.

CAUTIOUS USE Infection at topical treatment sites; history of untoward effects with topical cyclosporine or tacrolimus; skin papillomas; immunocompromised patients; pregnancy (category C).

ROUTE & DOSAGE

Atopic Dermatitis

Adult/Adolescent/Child (older than 2 y): **Topical** Apply thin layer to affected skin bid (avoid continuous long-term use)

ADMINISTRATION

Topical

- Do not apply to any skin surface that appears to be infected.
- Limit application to areas of involvement with atopic dermatitis.

ADVERSE EFFECTS **Respiratory:** Sore throat, *upper respiratory infection, cough,* nasal congestion, asthma exacerbation, rhinitis, epistaxis. **CNS:** Headache. **HEENT:** Ear infection, earache, conjunctivitis. **Skin:** *Burning,* irritation, pruritus, skin infection, impetigo, folliculitis, skin papilloma, herpes simplex dermatitis, urticaria, acne. **GI:** Gastroenteritis, abdominal pain, nausea, vomiting, diarrhea, constipation. **Other:** Flu-like symptoms, infections, fever, increased risk of cancer.

PHARMACOKINETICS **Absorption:** Minimal through intact skin. **Metabolism:** No evidence of skin-mediated metabolism, metabolized in liver by CYP3A4. **Elimination:** Primarily in feces.

NURSING IMPLICATIONS

Assessment & Drug Effects

- Assess for and report persistent skin irritation that develops following application of the cream and lasts for more than 1 wk.

Patient & Family Education

- Minimize exposure of treated area to natural or artificial sunlight.
- Immediately report a new or changed skin lesion to the prescriber.
- Stop topical application once signs of dermatitis have disappeared. Resume application at the first sign of recurrence.
- Continuous, long-term use of this cream is not recommended.
- Wash hands thoroughly after application if hands are not the treatment sites.
- Report any significant skin irritation that results from application of the cream.

PIMOZIDE

(pi'moe-zide)

Classification: ANTIPSYCHOTIC

Therapeutic: ANTIPSYCHOTIC; CNS DOPAMINERGIC RECEPTOR ANTAGONIST

Prototype: Haloperidol

AVAILABILITY Tablet

ACTION & THERAPEUTIC EFFECT Potent central dopamine antagonist that alters release and turnover of central dopamine stores. Blockade of CNS dopaminergic receptors results in suppression of the motor and phonic tics that characterize Tourette's disorder. *Effective in suppressing motor and phonic tics associated with Tourette's disorder.*

USES Tourette's syndrome resistant to standard therapy.

UNLABELED USES Delusional parasitosis.

CONTRAINDICATIONS Hypersensitivity to pimozide or any component of the formulation; treatment of simple tics other than those associated with Tourette's disorder; drug-induced tics; history of cardiac dysrhythmias and conditions marked by prolonged QT syndrome, patient taking drugs that may prolong QT interval (e.g., quinidine); congenital heart defects, cardiac arrhythmias; torsade de pointes; electrolyte imbalance; Parkinson's disease; NMS; severe toxic CNS depression or coma states; lactation.

CAUTIOUS USE Kidney and liver dysfunction; cardiac disease; glaucoma; BPH; renal or hepatic impairment; urinary retention; low WBC; seizure disorders; older adults; pregnancy (adverse effects observed in some animal reproduction studies). Safe use in children younger than 12 y is not known.

ROUTE & DOSAGE

Tourette's Disorder

Adult: **PO** 1–2 mg/day in divided doses, gradually increase dose every other day up to 0.2 mg/kg/day or 10 mg/day in divided doses (max: 0.2 mg/kg/day or 10 mg/day)

Adolescent: **PO** 0.05 mg/kg/day at bedtime, gradually increase as needed (max: 0.2 mg/kg/day or 10 mg, whichever is less)

Pharmacogenetic dosage adjustment

CYP2D6 poor metabolizers should be dose titrated in ≥14-day increments; max dose 4 mg/day

ADMINISTRATION

Oral

- May be taken with or without food; preferable to administer dose at bedtime.
- Increase drug dose gradually, usually over 1–3 wk, until maintenance dose is reached.
- Follow regimen prescribed by prescriber for withdrawal: Usually slow, gradual changes over a period of days or weeks (drug has a long half-life). Sudden withdrawal may cause reemergence of original symptoms (motor and phonic tics) and of neuromuscular adverse effects of the drug.

ADVERSE EFFECTS CNS: Headache, *sedation, drowsiness,* insomnia, depression, akathisia, behavioral changes, rigidity, nervousness. **HEENT:** Visual disturbances, photophobia, decreased accommodation, blurred vision, cataracts. **Skin:** Rash. **GI:** Increased thirst, increased salivation, diarrhea, dysgeusia, increased appetite, anorexia, *dry mouth, constipation*. **GU:** Impotence, nocturia. **Musculoskeletal:** Akinesia, weakness, muscle rigidity, stooped posture. **Other:** Speech disorder, handwriting changes, tardive dyskinesia.

INTERACTIONS **Drug:** **Alcohol** and other CNS DEPRESSANTS increase CNS depression; CYP2D6 INHIBITORS increase concentration of pimozide; CYP3A4 INHIBITORS increase concentration of pimozide; ANTICHOLINERGIC AGENTS (e.g., TRICYCLIC ANTIDEPRESSANTS, **atropine**) increase anticholinergic effects; medications that increase QT interval, PHENOTHIAZINES, TRICYCLIC ANTIDEPRESSANTS, ANTIARRHYTHMICS, MACROLIDE ANTIBIOTICS, AZOLE ANTIFUNGALS, PROTEASE INHIBITORS, **nefazodone, sertraline, zileuton** increase risk of arrhythmias and heart block; pimozide antagonizes effects of ANTICONVULSANTS—there is loss of seizure control; increases risk of ulcer formation with potassium; SSRIS increase the risk of adverse effects. **Food: Grapefruit juice** (greater than 1 qt/day) may increase plasma concentrations and adverse effects.

PHARMACOKINETICS **Absorption:** Slowly and variably from GI tract (40–50% absorbed). **Peak:** 6–8 h. **Metabolism:** In liver (by CYP3A4, CYP2D6, CYP1A2). **Elimination:** 80–85% in urine, 15–20% in feces.

NURSING IMPLICATIONS

Note: See haloperidol for additional nursing implications.

Assessment & Drug Effects

- Obtain ECG baseline data at beginning of therapy and check periodically, especially during dosage adjustments.
- Notify prescriber immediately for widening or prolongation of the QT interval, which suggests developing cardiotoxicity.
- Risk of tardive dyskinesia appears to be greatest in women, older adults, and those on high-dose therapy.
- Be aware that extrapyramidal reactions often appear within the first few days of therapy, are dose-related, and usually occur when dose is high.
- Be aware that anticholinergic effects (dry mouth, constipation) may increase as dose is increased.
- Monitor mental status, vital signs, weight, height, BMI, waist circumference.
- Annual ocular examination.
- Monitor lab values: Baseline and periodic CBC, electrolytes, liver function fasting plasma glucose level/HbA1c, fasting lipid panel.

Patient & Family Education

- Adhere to established drug regimen (i.e., do not change dose or intervals and discontinue only with prescriber's guidance).
- Use measures to relieve dry mouth (frequent rinsing with water, saliva substitute, increased fluid intake) and constipation (increased dietary fiber, drink 6–8 glasses of water daily).
- Do not drive or engage in potentially hazardous activities because drug-caused hand tremors, drowsiness, and blurred vision may impair alertness and abilities.
- Pseudoparkinsonism symptoms are usually mild and reversible with dose adjustment.

- Be alert to the earliest symptom of tardive dyskinesia ("flycatching"—an involuntary movement of the tongue), and report promptly to the prescriber.
- Return to prescriber for periodic assessments of therapy benefit and cardiac status.
- Understand dangers of ingesting alcohol to prevent augmenting CNS depressant effects of pimozide.

PINDOLOL

(pin'doe-lole)

Classification: BETA-ADRENERGIC RECEPTOR ANTAGONIST; ANTIHYPERTENSIVE
Therapeutic: ANTIHYPERTENSIVE; ANTIANGINAL
Prototype: Propranolol

AVAILABILITY Tablet

ACTION & *THERAPEUTIC EFFECT* Competitively blocks beta-adrenergic receptors primarily in myocardium, and beta receptors within smooth muscle. *Lowers blood pressure by decreasing peripheral vascular resistance. Exerts vasodilation as well as hypotensive effects.*

USES Management of hypertension.

UNLABELED USES Angina, traumatic brain injury.

CONTRAINDICATIONS Bronchospastic diseases, asthma; cardiogenic shock, AV block, second and third degree heart block; severe bradycardia; overt cardiac failure; pulmonary failure; abrupt withdrawal; lactation.

CAUTIOUS USE Nonallergic bronchospasm; COPD; CHF; angina; history of cardiac failure that is well controlled; major surgery; DM; hyperthyroidism; MG; impaired liver and kidney function; pregnancy (category B). Safety and efficacy in children not established.

ROUTE & DOSAGE

Hypertension

Adult: **PO** 5 mg bid, may increase by 10 mg/day q3–4wk if needed up (max: 60 mg/day in 2–3 divided doses)
Geriatric: **PO** Start with 5 mg daily

ADMINISTRATION

Oral

- Give drug at same time of day each day with respect to time of food intake for most predictable results.
- Withdraw or discontinue treatment gradually over a period of 1–2 wk.

ADVERSE EFFECTS **CV:** *Bradycardia,* hypotension, CHF. **Respiratory:** Bronchospasm, pulmonary edema, dyspnea. **CNS:** *Fatigue,* dizziness, insomnia, drowsiness, confusion, fainting, decreased libido. **Endocrine:** Hypoglycemia (may mask symptoms of a hypoglycemic reaction). **GI:** Nausea, *diarrhea, constipation,* flatulence. **GU:** Impotence. **Hematologic:** Agranulocytosis. **Other:** Back or joint pain. Sensitivity reactions seen as antinuclear antibodies (ANA) (10–30% of patients).

INTERACTIONS **Drug:** DIURETICS and other HYPOTENSIVE AGENTS increase hypotensive effect; effects of **albuterol, metaproterenol, terbutaline, pirbuterol,** and **pindolol** antagonized; NSAIDS blunt hypotensive effect; decreases hypoglycemic effect of **glyburide; amiodarone** increases risk of bradycardia and sinus arrest.

PHARMACOKINETICS Absorption: Rapidly from GI tract; 50–95% reaches systemic circulation (first pass metabolism). **Onset:** 3 h. **Peak:** 1–2 h. **Duration:** 24 h. **Distribution:** Distributed into breast milk. **Metabolism:** 40–60% in liver. **Elimination:** In urine. **Half-Life:** 3–4 h.

NURSING IMPLICATIONS

Assessment & Drug Effects

- Monitor HR and BP. Report bradycardia and hypotension. Dosage adjustment may be indicated.
- Note: Hypotensive effect may begin within 7 days but is not at maximum therapeutically until about 2 wk after beginning of treatment.

Patient & Family Education

- Pindolol masks the dizziness and sweating symptoms of hypoglycemia. Monitor blood glucose for loss of glycemic control.
- Adhere to the prescribed drug regimen; if a change is desired, consult prescriber first. Abrupt withdrawal of drug might precipitate a thyroid crisis in a patient with hyperthyroidism, and angina in the patient with ischemic heart disease, leading to an MI.

PIOGLITAZONE HYDROCHLORIDE

(pi-o-glit'a-zone)

Actos

Classification: ANTIDIABETIC; THIAZOLIDINEDIONE (GLITAZONE)

Therapeutic: ANTIDIABETIC; INSULIN SENSITIZER

Prototype: Rosiglitazone maleate

AVAILABILITY Tablet

ACTION & *THERAPEUTIC EFFECT* Decreases hepatic glucose output and increases insulin-dependent muscle glucose uptake in skeletal muscle and adipose tissue. Improves glycemic control in non-insulin-dependent diabetics (type 2) by enhancing insulin sensitivity of cells without stimulating pancreatic insulin secretion. *Improves glycemic control as indicated by improved blood glucose levels and decreased HbA1C.*

USES Adjunct to diet in the treatment of type 2 diabetes mellitus.

CONTRAINDICATIONS Hypersensitivity to pioglitazone, rosiglitazone; type 1 diabetes, or treatment of DKA; New York Heart Association (NYHA) Class III or IV heart failure; active liver disease or ALT levels greater than 2.5 × NL; jaundice; fracture risk factors; lactation.

CAUTIOUS USE Liver dysfunction; cardiovascular disease; hypertension, CHF, anemia, edema; osteoporosis; history of bladder cancer; older adults; pregnancy (category C). Safety and efficacy in children younger than 18 y not recommended.

ROUTE & DOSAGE

Type 2 Diabetes Mellitus

Adult: **PO** 15–30 mg once daily (max: 45 mg daily)

Disease State Dosage Adjustment

Patients with NHYA Class I or II heart failure: 15 mg once daily

Drug Interaction Dosage Adjustment

If used with gemfibrozil (max: 15 mg)

ADMINISTRATION

Oral

- Give without regard to food.
- Do not initiate therapy if baseline serum ALT greater than 2.5 × normal.
- Store at 15°–30° C (59°–86° F) in tightly closed container; protect from humidity and moisture.

ADVERSE EFFECTS **CV:** *Edema.* **Respiratory:** Upper respiratory infection. **CNS:** Headache. **Endocrine:** Hypoglycemia.

INTERACTIONS **Drug:** **Pioglitazone** may decrease serum levels of ORAL CONTRACEPTIVES; **ketoconazole, gemfibrozil, mifepristone** may increase serum levels of **pioglitazone.** Increased risk of hypoglycemia when used with insulin or ANTIDIABETIC medications. BILE ACID SEQUESTRANTS, **bosentan** may decrease effect. Serum concentrations may be increased by CYP2C8 inhibitors. **Herbal: Garlic, ginseng** may potentiate hypoglycemic effects.

P

PHARMACOKINETICS **Absorption:** Rapidly absorbed. **Peak:** 2 h; steady state concentrations within 7 days. **Duration:** 24 h. **Distribution:** Greater than 99% protein bound. **Metabolism:** In liver to active metabolites. **Elimination:** Primarily in bile and feces. **Half-Life:** 16–24 h.

NURSING IMPLICATIONS

Black Box Warning

Pioglitazone has been associated with exacerbation of CHF.

Assessment & Drug Effects

- Monitor for S&S hypoglycemia (possible when insulin/sulfonylureas are coadministered).
- Monitor closely for S&S of CHF or exacerbation of symptoms with preexisting CHF.
- Withhold drug and notify prescriber if ALT greater than 3 × ULN or patient has jaundice.
- Monitor weight and notify prescriber of development of edema.
- Monitor lab tests: Baseline and periodic LFTs; periodic fasting plasma glucose and HbA1C.

Patient & Family Education

- Be aware that resumed ovulation is possible in nonovulating premenopausal women.
- Use or add barrier contraceptive if using hormonal contraception.
- Report immediately to prescriber: Unexplained anorexia, nausea, vomiting, abdominal pain, fatigue, dark urine; or S&S of fluid retention such as weight gain, edema, or activity intolerance.
- Combination therapy: May need adjustment of other antidiabetic drugs to avoid hypoglycemia.
- Learn of and adhere strictly to guidelines for liver function tests. Be sure to have blood tests for liver function periodically.

PIPERACILLIN/TAZOBACTAM

(pi-per'a-cil-lin/taz-o-bac'tam)

Zosyn

Classification: ANTIBIOTIC; EXTENDED SPECTRUM PENICILLIN

Therapeutic: ANTIBIOTIC

AVAILABILITY Solution for injection

ACTION & *THERAPEUTIC EFFECT* Tazobactam has little antibacterial activity itself; however, in combination with piperacillin, it extends the spectrum of bacteria that are susceptible to piperacillin. *Two-drug combination has antibiotic*

activity against an extremely broad spectrum of gram-positive, gram-negative, and anaerobic bacteria.

USES Treatment of moderate to severe appendicitis, uncomplicated and complicated skin and skin structure infections, endometritis, pelvic inflammatory disease, or nosocomial- or community-acquired pneumonia caused by beta-lactamase-producing bacteria.

CONTRAINDICATIONS Hypersensitivity to piperacillin, tazobactam, penicillins; coagulopathy.

CAUTIOUS USE Hypersensitivity to cephalosporins, carbapenem, or betalactamase inhibitors such as clavulanic acid and sulbactam; GI disease, colitis; CF; eczema; kidney failure; complicated urinary tract infections; pregnancy (category B); lactation.

ROUTE & DOSAGE

Moderate to Severe Infections

Adult: **IV** 3.375 g q6h, infused over 30 min, for 7–10 days
Child (younger than 6 mo): **IV** 150–300 mg piperacillin/kg/day divided q6–8h; *6 mo or older:* 240 mg piperacillin component/kg/day divided q8h

Nosocomial Pneumonia

Adult: **IV** 4.5 g q6h, infused over 30 min, for 7–10 days

Renal Insufficiency Dosage Adjustment

CrCl 20–40 mL/min: 2.25 g q6h; *less than 20 mL/min:* 2.25 g q8h

Hemodialysis Dosage Adjustment

2.25 g q12h (for nosocomial pneumonia dose q8h); give additional 0.75 g after dialysis session

ADMINISTRATION

Note: Verify correct IV concentration and rate of infusion for administration to infants or children with prescriber.

Intravenous

PREPARE: **Intermittent:** Reconstitute powder with 5 mL of diluent (e.g., D5W, NS) for each 1 g or fraction thereof; shake well until dissolved. ▪ Further dilute to a total of 50 to 150 mL in selected diluent (e.g., NS, sterile water for injection, D5W, dextran 6% in NS, and LR only with solution containing EDTA).

ADMINISTER: **Intermittent:** Give over at least 30 min. ▪ **Do not** administer through a line with another infusion.

INCOMPATIBILITIES: **Solution/additive:** **Aminoglycosides, lactated Ringer's, albumin, blood products, solutions containing sodium bicarbonate.** **Y-site:** **Acyclovir, aminoglycosides, amiodarone, amphotericin B, amphotericin B cholesteryl complex, azithromycin, chlorpromazine, cisatracurium, cisplatin, dacarbazine, daunorubicin, dobutamine, doxorubicin, doxorubicin liposome, doxycycline, droperidol, famotidine, ganciclovir, gatifloxacin, gemcitabine, haloperidol, hydroxyzine, idarubicin, miconazole, minocycline, mitomycin, mitoxantrone, nalbuphine, prochlorperazine, promethazine, streptozocin, vancomycin.**

ADVERSE EFFECTS **CNS:** Headache, insomnia, fever. **Skin:** Rash, pruritus, hypersensitivity reactions. **GI:** Diarrhea, constipation, nausea, vomiting, dyspepsia, pseudomembranous colitis.

P

INTERACTIONS **Drug:** May increase risk of bleeding with ANTICOAGULANTS; **probenecid** decreases elimination of piperacillin.

PHARMACOKINETICS **Distribution:** Distributes into many tissues, including lung, blister fluid, and bile; crosses placenta; distributed into breast milk. **Metabolism:** In liver. **Elimination:** In urine. **Half-Life:** 0.7–1.2 h.

NURSING IMPLICATIONS

Assessment & Drug Effects

- Obtain history of hypersensitivity to penicillins, cephalosporins, or other drugs prior to administration.
- Monitor patient carefully during the first 30 min after initiation of the infusion for signs of hypersensitivity (see Appendix E).
- Monitor lab tests: Baseline C&S; periodic renal function tests, CBC with differential, PT and PTT, serum electrolytes, and LFTs.

Patient & Family Education

- Report rash, itching, or other signs of hypersensitivity immediately.
- Report loose stools or diarrhea as these may indicate pseudomembranous colitis.

P

PIROXICAM

(peer-ox′i-kam)

Feldene

Classification: NONNARCOTIC ANALGESIC; NONSTEROIDAL ANTI-INFLAMMATORY DRUG (NSAID)
Therapeutic: ANALGESIC; NSAID; ANTIPYRETIC
Prototype: Ibuprofen

AVAILABILITY Capsule

ACTION & THERAPEUTIC EFFECT Nonsteroidal anti-inflammatory agent that strongly inhibits enzyme cyclooxygenase, both COX1 and COX2, the catalyst of prostaglandin synthesis. Decreased prostaglandin results in anti-inflammatory properties, analgesic and antipyretic effects. *Decreases inflammatory processes in bone-joint disease as well as has analgesic and antipyretic effects.*

USES Acute and long-term relief of mild to moderate pain and for symptomatic treatment of osteoarthritis and rheumatoid arthritis; headache.

CONTRAINDICATIONS Hypersensitivity to NSAIDS or salicylates; hemophilia; active peptic ulcer, GI bleeding; CABG perioperative pain; ST-elevated MI; lactation.

CAUTIOUS USE History of upper GI disease including ulcerative colitis; SLE; kidney dysfunction; hepatic disease; CHF; acute MI; compromised cardiac function; hypertension or other conditions predisposing to fluid retention; renal disease; alcoholism; coagulation disorders; older adults; pregnancy (category C). Safe use in children not established.

ROUTE & DOSAGE

Arthritis, Pain
Adult: **PO** 20 mg daily

ADMINISTRATION

Oral

- Give at the same time every day.
- Give capsule with food or fluid to help reduce GI irritation.
- Dose adjustments should be made on basis of clinical response at

intervals of weeks rather than days in order to prevent over dosage.

- Store in tightly closed container at 15°–30° C (59°–86° F) unless otherwise directed.

ADVERSE EFFECTS **CV:** Edema. **CNS:** Dizziness, headache. **HEENT:** Tinnitus. **Skin:** Pruritis, skin rash. **Hepatic/GI:** Increased liver enzymes, abdominal pain, anorexia, constipation, diarrhea, dyspepsia, gastrointestinal bleeding. **Hematologic:** Anemia, prolonged bleeding time.

DIAGNOSTIC TEST INTERFERENCE May lead to false-positive ***aldosterone/renin ratio.***

INTERACTIONS **Drug:** ORAL ANTICOAGULANTS, **heparin** may prolong bleeding time; may increase **lithium** toxicity; **alcohol,** NONSTEROIDAL ANTIINFLAMMATORIES increase risk of GI hemorrhage; enhances nephrotoxic effects of **cylcosporine**. Do not use with **cidofovir.** **Herbal: Feverfew, garlic, ginger, ginkgo** may increase bleeding potential.

PHARMACOKINETICS **Absorption:** Extensively from GI tract. **Onset:** 1 h analgesia; 7 days for rheumatoid arthritis. **Peak:** 3–5 h analgesia; 2–4 wk antirheumatic. **Duration:** 48–72 h analgesia. **Distribution:** Small amount distributed into breast milk. **Metabolism:** Extensively in liver by (CYP2C9). **Elimination:** Primarily in urine, some in bile (less than 5%). **Half-Life:** 50 h.

NURSING IMPLICATIONS

Black Box Warning

Piroxican has been associated with increased risk of serious, potentially fatal, GI bleeding and cardiovascular events (e.g., MI and CVA); risk may increase with duration of use and may be greater in the older adult and those with risk factors for CV disease.

Assessment & Drug Effects

- Clinical evidence of benefits from drug therapy include pain relief in motion and in rest, reduction in night pain, stiffness, and swelling; increased ROM (range of motion) in all joints.
- Monitor for and report promptly S&S of GI ulceration or bleeding. Significant GI bleeding may occur without prior warning.
- Monitor for and report promptly S&S of CV thrombotic events (i.e., angina, MI, TIA, or stroke).
- Monitor lab tests: Periodic renal function tests, LFTs, CBC, and electrolytes in the older adult and during long-term therapy.

Patient & Family Education

- Do not self-dose with aspirin or other OTC drug without prescriber's advice.
- Do not increase dosage beyond prescribed regimen. Higher than recommended doses are associated with increased incidence of GI irritation and peptic ulcer.
- Incidence of GI bleeding with this drug is relatively high. Report symptoms of GI bleeding (e.g., dark, tarry stools, coffee-colored emesis) or severe gastric pain promptly to prescriber.
- Stop taking drug and report promptly to prescriber if you experience chest pain, shortness of breath, weakness, slurring of speech, or other signs of a cardiac or neurologic problem.
- Be alert to symptoms of drug-induced anemia: Profound fatigue, skin and mucous membrane pallor, lethargy.

- Avoid alcohol since it may increase the risk of GI bleeding.
- Be alert to signs of hypoprothrombinemia including bruises, pinpoint rash, unexplained bleeding, nose bleed, blood in urine, when piroxicam is taken concomitantly with an anticoagulant.
- Do not drive or engage in potentially hazardous activities until response to drug is known.
- Drink at least 6–8 full glasses of water daily and report signs of renal insufficiency (see Appendix E) to prescriber because most of drug is excreted by kidneys and impaired kidney function increases danger of toxicity.

PITAVASTATIN CALCIUM

(pit-a-vah-stat′in)

Livalo, Zypitamag

Classification: ANTIHYPERLIPIDEMIC; LIPID-LOWERING AGENT; HMG-COA REDUCTASE INHIBITOR (STATIN)
Therapeutic: ANTILIPEMIC; LIPID-LOWERING AGENT; STATIN
Prototype: Lovastatin

P

AVAILABILITY Tablet

ACTION & *THERAPEUTIC EFFECT* Pitavastatin is a HMG-CoA reductase inhibitor that reduces plasma cholesterol levels by interfering with the production of cholesterol in the liver. It also promotes removal of LDL and VLDL from plasma. *Effectiveness is measured by decrease in blood level of total cholesterol, LDL cholesterol, and triglycerides and an increase in HDL cholesterol.*

USES Treatment of primary hyperlipidemia and mixed dyslipidemia.

UNLABELED USES Regression of coronary atherosclerosis in patients with acute coronary syndrome (ACS).

CONTRAINDICATIONS Hypersensitivity to pitavastatin; myopathy and rhabdomyolysis; acute renal failure; ESRD not on hemodialysis; active liver disease; large amounts of alcohol; coadministration with cyclosporine; pregnancy (category X); lactation.

CAUTIOUS USE Renal impairment; hepatic impairment; DM; older adults. Safety and efficacy in children not established.

ROUTE & DOSAGE

Hypercholesterolemia, Hyperlipoproteinemia, and/or Hypertriglyceridemia

Adult: **PO** Initially 2 mg once daily; can be adjusted to 1–4 mg once daily

Renal Impairment Dosage Adjustment

CrCl 15 to less than 60 mL/min: Initially, 1 mg once daily; do not exceed 2 mg once daily

ADMINISTRATION

Oral

- May give without regard to meals any time of day.
- Store at 15°–30° C (59°–86° F).

ADVERSE EFFECTS **Respiratory:** Nasopharyngitis. **CNS:** Headache. **Hepatic/GI:** Increased liver enzymes, constipation. **Musculoskeletal:** Back pain.

INTERACTIONS **Drug: Cyclosporine, erythromycin,** HIV PROTEASE INHIBITORS, and **rifampin** increase pitavastatin levels. FIBRATES may increase the risk of myopathy and rhabdomyolysis. Combination use with **niacin** may increase the risk of skeletal muscle effects. Do not use with **fusidic acid**.

PHARMACOKINETICS **Absorption:** 51% bioavailable. **Peak:** 1 h. **Distribution:** Greater than 99% plasma protein bound. **Metabolism:** In liver. **Elimination:** Primarily fecal (79%) with minor renal (15%) elimination. **Half-Life:** 12 h.

NURSING IMPLICATIONS

Assessment & Drug Effects

- Monitor for and report muscle pain, tenderness, or weakness.
- Withhold drug and notify prescriber for ALT/AST greater than 3 × ULN.
- Monitor lab tests: Lipid profile at baseline, at 4 wk, and periodically thereafter; LFTs at baseline, at 12 wk after initiation or elevation of dose, and periodically thereafter; creatine kinase levels if patient experiences muscle pain.

Patient & Family Education

- Report promptly unexplained muscle pain, tenderness, or weakness.
- Avoid or minimize alcohol consumption while on this drug.
- Use effective contraceptive measures to avoid pregnancy while taking this drug.

PLASMA PROTEIN FRACTION

(plas′ma)

Plasmanate

Classification: PLASMA VOLUME EXPANDER

Therapeutic: PLASMA VOLUME EXPANDER; ALBUMIN

Prototype: Normal serum albumin, human

AVAILABILITY Solution for injection

ACTION & *THERAPEUTIC EFFECT* Provides plasma proteins that increase colloidal osmotic pressure within the intravascular compartment equal to human plasma. It shifts water from the extravascular tissues back into the intravascular space, thus expanding plasma volume. *Used to maintain cardiac output by expanding plasma volume in the treatment of shock due to various causes.*

USES Emergency treatment of hypovolemic shock; temporary measure in treatment of blood loss when whole blood is not available.

CONTRAINDICATIONS Hypersensitivity to albumin; severe anemia; cardiac failure; patients undergoing cardiopulmonary bypass surgery.

CAUTIOUS USE Patients with low cardiac reserve; absence of albumin deficiency; liver or kidney failure; pregnancy (category C); children.

ROUTE & DOSAGE

Plasma Volume Expansion

Adult: **IV** 250–500 mL at a maximum rate of 10 mL/min

ADMINISTRATION

Intravenous

Do not use solutions that show a sediment or appear turbid. Do not use solutions that have been frozen.

PREPARE: **IV Infusion:** Give undiluted. ▪ Once container is opened, solution should be used within 4 h because it contains no preservatives. ▪ Discard unused portions.

ADMINISTER: **IV Infusion:** Rate of infusion and volume of total dose will depend on patient's age, diagnosis, degree of venous and pulmonary congestion, Hct, and Hgb determinations. As with any oncotically active solution, infusion rate should be relatively slow. Range may vary from 1–10 mL/min.

INCOMPATIBILITIES: PROTEIN HYDROLYSATES or solutions containing alcohol.

ADVERSE EFFECTS **GI:** Nausea, vomiting, hypersalivation, headache. **Other:** Tingling, chills, fever, cyanosis, chest tightness, backache, urticaria, erythema, shock (systemic anaphylaxis), circulatory overload, pulmonary edema.

NURSING IMPLICATIONS

Assessment & Drug Effects

- Monitor vital signs (BP and pulse). Frequency depends on patient's condition. Flow rate adjustments are made according to clinical response and BP. Slow or stop infusion if patient suddenly becomes hypotensive.
- Report a widening pulse pressure (difference between systolic and diastolic); it correlates with increase in cardiac output.
- Report changes in I&O ratio and pattern.
- Observe patient closely during and after infusion for signs of hypervolemia or circulatory overload (see Appendix E). Report these symptoms immediately to prescriber.
- Make careful observations of patient who has had either injury or surgery in order to detect bleeding points that failed to bleed at lower BP.

P

PLAZOMICIN

(pla-zoe-mye′sin)

Zemdri

Classification: ANTIBIOTIC; AMINOGLYCOSIDE

Therapeutic: ANTIBIOTIC

Prototype: Gentamycin

AVAILABILITY Solution for injection

ACTION & THERAPEUTIC EFFECT Broad-spectrum aminoglycoside antibiotic that binds to 30S subunit of bacterial ribosomes, resulting in cell death. *Active against microorganisms, specifically gram-negative bacilli and gram-positive cocci, which may be resistant to other treatment options.*

USES Treatment of complicated urinary tract infections including pyelonephritis.

CONTRAINDICATIONS History of hypersensitivity to other aminoglycosides; pregnancy.

CAUTIOUS USE Only to be used with proven or strongly suspected bacterial infection to prevent drug-resistance.

ROUTE & DOSAGE

Complicated Urinary Tract Infection

Adult: **IV** 15 mg/kg once a day for 4–7 days

Renal Impairment Dosage Adjustment

CrCL greater than or equal to 60 mL/min: No dosage adjustment; *30 to less than 60 mL/min:* 10 mg/kg every 24 h; *15 to less than 30 mL/min:* 10 mg/kg every 48 h

Obese Patient Dosage Adjustment

TBW greater than IBW by more than 25%: Utilize ABW for dosing weight

ADMINISTRATION

Intravenous

PREPARE: Dilute to volume of 50 mL with NS or LR; solution is stable for 24 h.
ADMINISTER: **IV Infusion:** Infuse over 30 min.
INCOMPATIBILITIES: Incompatibilities have yet to be established; the manufacturer recommends against simultaneous infusion with other medications

- Store solution at refrigerated temperatures 2°–8° C (35°–46° F).

ADVERSE EFFECTS CV: Hypotension or hypertension. **CNS:** Headache, dizziness. **HEENT:** Ototoxicity. **GU:** Diarrhea, nausea, vomiting, nephrotoxicity, increased serum creatinine. **Other:** Hypokalemia, hypersensitivity, (rash, pruritus, drug fever, anaphylaxis).

INTERACTIONS Drug: Amphotericin B, capreomycin, cisplatin, methoxylurane, polymyxin B, vancomycin, ethacrynic acid and **furosemide** increase risk of adverse effects. PENICILLINS may decrease effect of plazomicin. NEUROMUSCULAR BLOCKING AGENTS (e.g., **succinylcholine**) potentiate neuromuscular blockade.

PHARMACOKINETICS Absorption: Administered intravenously. **Peak:** Peaks quickly after infusion. **Distribution:** Distributed widely in body fluids; 20% protein bound. **Metabolism:** Not metabolized. **Elimination:** Excreted primarily in the urine. **Half-Life:** 3.5 h.

NURSING IMPLICATIONS

Black Box Warning

Associated with nephrotoxicity, ototoxicity, and increased risk of adverse effect with neuromuscular blockade.

Assessment & Drug Effects

- Monitor urine output.
- Monitor for symptoms of ototoxicity or neuromuscular blockade.
- Monitor lab tests: Urinalysis, BUN, serum creatinine, plasma plazomicin trough.

Patient & Family Education

- Notify prescriber if experiencing any of the following symptoms: Unable to pass urine, change in urine amount, blood in the urine, or a significant weight gain.
- Notify prescriber of S&S of an allergic reaction such as hives; rash; itching; red, swollen, blistered, or peeling skin with or without fever; wheezing; tightness in the chest or throat; trouble breathing, swallowing, or talking; unusual hoarseness; or swelling of the mouth, face, lips, tongue, or throat.

PLECANATIDE

(ple-kan′a-tide)

Trulance

Classification: GUANYLATE CYCLASE-C AGONIST; ACCELERANT OF GI TRANSIT
Therapeutic: ACCELERANT OF GI TRANSIT

AVAILABILITY Tablet

P

ACTION & *THERAPEUTIC EFFECT*

Plecanatide increases the cyclic guanosine monophosphate (cGMP) levels by acting as an agonist of guanylate cyclase-C. This results in an increase of intestinal fluid and transit by stimulating chloride and bicarbonate excretion into the intestinal lumen. *Gastrointestinal time is accelerated which is helpful in combatting constipation.*

USES Treatment of chronic idiopathic constipation.

CONTRAINDICATIONS Known or suspected mechanical gastrointestinal obstruction. Patient currently has diarrhea; pediatric patients younger than 6 y.

CAUTIOUS USE There are no adequate well-controlled studies of plecanatide used in pregnancy. Risk of birth defect or miscarriage cannot be determined. There are no data on the presence of plecanatide in animal or human milk, the effects on breast-feeding infants, or the effects of the milk production.

P

ROUTE & DOSAGE

Chronic Idiopathic Constipation

Adult: **PO** 3 mg daily

ADMINISTRATION

Gastric or Nasogastric

- Tablets may be mixed with water and administered through a gastric feeding tube.
- Mix 30 mL of room temperature water into a cup with the tablet and swirl for at least 15 sec, flush the feeding tube with 30 mL of water, draw up the mixture with a syringe and administer the mixture via the feeding tube immediately.
- Add additional 30 mL of water to the cup if any part of the tablet remains, swirl for at least 15 sec, and use the same syringe to administer via the feeding tube.
- Flush the feeding tube with at least 10 mL of water after administration.

Oral

- Swallow tablets whole.
- Take with or without food.
- If patient has difficulty swallowing, tablets may be crushed and administered orally with water or applesauce.
- For administration with water, mix 30 mL of room temperature water into a cup with the tablet, swirl for at least 10 sec, and swallow entire amount immediately; add an additional 30 mL of water if any part of the tablet remains, swirl again, swallow immediately; do not store for later use.
- For administration with applesauce, crush the tablet into a powder and mix with 1 teaspoonful of applesauce at room temperature, consume the entire mixture immediately, do not store for later use.
- Store at 20°–25° C (68°–77° F); excursions permitted to 15°–30° C (59°–86° F). Do not subdivide or repackage; protect from moisture.

ADVERSE EFFECTS **GI:** Diarrhea.

PHARMACOKINETICS **Absorption:** Minimal systemic absorption. **Metabolism:** Metabolized within GI tract to active metabolite; degraded in intestinal lumen to small peptides and amino acids.

NURSING IMPLICATIONS

Black Box Warning

Safety and efficacy of plecanaide not established in patients younger than 18 y. Diarrhea, sometimes severe, has been reported and dose interruption was required. Risk of serious dehydration in pediatric patients.

Assessment & Drug Effects

- Monitor the frequency and consistency of bowel movements.
- Monitor for S&S of dehydration.
- Improvement of constipation is indicative of efficacy.

Patient & Family Education

- Notify all health care providers that this drug is being taken. This includes doctors, nurses, pharmacists and dentists.
- If this drug is taken by accident, get help right away.
- Notify prescriber if you become pregnant or plan on getting pregnant while taking this drug.
- Notify prescriber if you are breast-feeding.
- Notify prescriber right away if very loose stools persist.
- If a dose is missed, skip the dose and go back to normal administration time. Do not take 2 doses at the same time or extra doses.
- Consult with prescriber before taking any other prescription drugs, over the counter drugs, natural products or vitamins.

PLERIXAFOR

(ple-rix′a-for)

Mozobil

Classification: BIOLOGICAL RESPONSE MODIFIER; INHIBITOR OF CXCR4 CHEMOKINE RECEPTOR

Therapeutic: CXCR4 CHEMOKINE RECEPTOR INHIBITOR; STEM CELL MOBILIZER

AVAILABILITY Solution for injection

ACTION & THERAPEUTIC EFFECT A hematopoietic stem cell mobilizer that induces leukocytosis and increases the number of circulating hematopoietic progenitor cells. *Plerixafor enables collection of peripheral blood stem cell (PBSC) for autologous transplantation.*

USES In combination with granulocyte colony-stimulating factor (G-CSF), used to mobilize peripheral blood stem cell (PBSC) for collection and subsequent autologous transplantation in patients with non-Hodgkin's lymphoma and multiple myeloma.

CONTRAINDICATIONS Leukemia; pregnancy (category D); lactation.

CAUTIOUS USE Neutrophil count greater than 50,000/mm^3; thrombocytopenia; splenomegaly; moderate-to-severe renal impairment; concurrent drugs that reduce renal function. Safety and efficacy in children not established.

ROUTE & DOSAGE

Peripheral Blood Stem Cell Mobilization

Adult: **Subcutaneous** 0.24 mg/kg once daily (max: 0.40 mg/day), 11 h prior to initiation of apheresis; administer with filgrastim for up to 4 consecutive days.

Renal Impairment Dosage Adjustment

CrCl less than or equal to 50 mL/min: Reduce dose to 0.16 mg/kg (max: 27 mg/day)

Obesity Dosage Adjustment

Dose based on actual body weight up to 175% of IBW

ADMINISTRATION

Subcutaneous

- Give undiluted approximately 11 h prior to apheresis.
- Calculate the required dose as follows: 0.012 × actual weight in kg = mL to administer. Note that each vial contains 1.2 mL of 20 mg/mL solution. Discard unused solution.
- Store single-use vials at 15°–30° C (59°–86° F).

ADVERSE EFFECTS **CNS:** *Dizziness, fatigue, headache,* insomnia. **GI:** *Diarrhea,* flatulence, *nausea, vomiting.* **Other:** *Arthralgia, injection-site reactions.*

PHARMACOKINETICS **Peak:** 30–60 min. **Distribution:** 58% plasma protein bound. **Metabolism:** Not significantly metabolized. **Elimination:** Primarily in urine. **Half-Life:** 3–5 h.

NURSING IMPLICATIONS

Assessment & Drug Effects

- Monitor (during and for 1 h after administration) for and promptly report: Signs of a systemic reaction (e.g., urticaria, periorbital swelling, dyspnea, or hypoxia); signs of splenic enlargement (e.g., upper abdominal pain and/or scapular or shoulder pain).
- Monitor for orthostatic hypotension and syncope during or within 1 h of drug injection. Monitor ambulation or take other precautions as warranted.
- Monitor injection sites for skin reactions.
- Monitor lab tests: Baseline and periodic WBC with differential.

Patient & Family Education

- Report promptly any discomfort experienced during or shortly after drug injection.
- Exercise caution when changing position from lying or sitting to standing as rapid movement shortly after injection may trigger fainting.
- Report skin reactions at the injection site (e.g., itching, rash swelling, or pain).
- Females should use effective contraception while taking this drug.

P

PNEUMOCOCCAL 13-VALENT VACCINE, DIPHTHERIA

(noo-moe′KOK-al)

Prevnar 13

See Appendix J.

PODOPHYLLUM RESIN (PODOPHYLLIN)

(pode-oh-fill′um)

Podoben, Podofin

PODOFILOX

Condylox

Classification: KERATOLYTIC

Therapeutic: CYTOTOXIC; KERATOLYTIC

AVAILABILITY **Podophyllum:** Liquid. **Podofilox:** Gel; solution

ACTION & *THERAPEUTIC EFFECT* Directly affects epithelial cell metabolism by arresting mitosis through binding to protein subunits of microtubules; causes necrosis of visible wart tissue. *Slow disruption of cells and tissue erosion as a result of its caustic action. Selectively affects embryonic and tumor cells more than adult cells.*

USES Benign growths including external genital and perianal warts, papillomas, fibroids.

CONTRAINDICATIONS Birthmarks, moles, or warts with hair

growth from them; cervical, urethral, oral warts; normal skin and mucous membranes peripheral to treated areas; DM; patient with poor circulation; concurrent use of steroids; irritated, or bleeding skin; application of drug over large area.

CAUTIOUS USE Pregnancy (category C); lactation. Safe use in children is not known.

ROUTE & DOSAGE

Condylomata Acuminata

Adult: **Topical** Use 10% solution and repeat 1–2 × wk for up to 4 applications

Verruca Vulgaris (Common Wart)

Adult: **Topical** Apply 0.5% solution q12h for up to 4 wk

Genital/Perianal Warts

Adult: **Topical** Apply bid × 3 days then withhold treatment × 4 days, may repeat cycle up to 4 ×

ADMINISTRATION

Note: Use 10–25% solution for areas less than 10 cm^2 or 5% solution for areas of 10–20 cm^2, anal, or genital warts; apply drug to dry surface, allowing area to dry between drops, wash off after 1–4 h.

Topical

- Avoid podophyllum resin contact with eyes or similar mucosal surfaces; if it occurs, flush thoroughly with lukewarm water for 15 min and remove film precipitated by the water.
- Avoid application of drug to normal tissue. If it occurs, remove with alcohol. Protect surfaces surrounding area to be treated with a layer of petrolatum or flexible collodion.
- Remove drug thoroughly with soap and water after each treatment of accessible tissue surface.
- Apply a protective coat of talcum powder after treatment and drying of anogenital area.
- Remove drug with alcohol, if application causes extreme pain, pruritus, or swelling.
- Store in a tight, light-resistant container; avoid exposure to excessive heat.

ADVERSE EFFECTS **CNS:** Localized burning, localized pain. **Skin:** *Skin erosion*, localized inflammation, localized pruritis. **Hematologic:** Localized hemorrhage.

NURSING IMPLICATIONS

Assessment & Drug Effects

- Warts become blanched, then necrotic within 24–48 h. Sloughing begins after about 72 h with no scarring. Frequently, a mild topical anti-infective agent, with or without a dressing, is applied until the healing is complete.
- Monitor neurologic status. Sensorimotor polyneuropathy, if it occurs, appears about 2 wk after application of drug, worsens for 3 mo, and may persist for up to 9 mo. Cerebral effects may persist for 7–10 days; ataxia, hypotonia, and areflexia improve more slowly than effects on sensorium.

Patient & Family Education

- Learn proper technique of treatment if self-administered as treatment of verruca vulgaris (common wart). Also be fully aware of the need to report treatment failure to prescriber.
- Be aware that as with any STD, the patient's sex partner should be examined.

P

- Systemic toxicity may be severe and serious and is associated with application of drug to large areas, to tissue that is friable, bleeding, or recently biopsied, or for prolonged time. Toxicity may occur within hours of application. There are significant dangers from overuse or misuse of this drug.
- Learn symptoms of toxicity and report any that appear promptly to prescriber (see ADVERSE EFFECTS).

POLYCARBOPHIL

(pol-i-kar'boe-fil)

FiberNorm, Fiber-LAX

Classification: BULK-PRODUCING LAXATIVE; ANTIDIARRHEAL

Therapeutic: BULK LAXATIVE; ANTI-DIARRHEAL

Prototype: Psyllium

AVAILABILITY Tablet; chewable tablet

ACTION & *THERAPEUTIC EFFECT* Hydrophilic agent that absorbs free water in intestinal tract and opposes dehydrating forces of bowel by forming a gelatinous mass. *Restores more normal moisture level and motility in the lower GI tract; produces well-formed stool and reduces diarrhea.*

USES Constipation or diarrhea associated with acute bowel syndrome, diverticulosis, irritable bowel and in patients who should not strain during defecation. Also choleretic diarrhea, diarrhea caused by small-bowel surgery or vagotomy, and disease of terminal ileum.

CONTRAINDICATIONS Partial or complete GI obstruction; fecal impaction; dysphagia; acute abdominal pain; rectal bleeding; undiagnosed abdominal pain, or other symptoms symptomatic of appendicitis; poisonings; before radiologic bowel examination; bowel surgery.

CAUTIOUS USE Renal failure, renal impairment; pregnancy (category C); children younger than 3 y.

ROUTE & DOSAGE

Constipation or Diarrhea

Adult/Adolescent/Child (older than 6 y): **PO** 625 mg calcium polycarbophil 1–4 × day

ADMINISTRATION

Oral

- Chewable tablets should be chewed well before swallowing.
- Give each dose with a full glass [240 mL (8 oz)] of water or other liquid.
- Store at 15°–30° C (59°–86° F) in tightly closed container unless otherwise directed.

ADVERSE EFFECTS GI: Abdominal fullness.

INTERACTIONS Drug: May decrease absorption and clinical effects of ANTIBIOTICS, **warfarin, digoxin, nitrofurantoin,** SALICYLATES. Do not use with CALCIUM SALTS.

PHARMACOKINETICS Absorption: Not absorbed from GI tract. **Onset:** 12–24 h. **Peak:** 1–3 days.

NURSING IMPLICATIONS

Assessment & Drug Effects

- Determine duration and severity of diarrhea in order to anticipate signs of fluid-electrolyte losses.

- Monitor and record number and consistency of stools/day, presence and location of abdominal discomfort (i.e., tenderness, distention), and bowel sounds.
- Monitor and record I&O ratio and pattern. Dehydration is indicated if output is less than 30 mL/h.

Patient & Family Education

- Consult prescriber if sudden changes in bowel habit persist more than 1 wk, action is minimal or ineffective for 1 wk, or if there is no antidiarrheal action within 2 days.
- Be aware that extended use of this drug may cause dependence for normal bowel function.
- Do not discontinue polycarbophil unless prescriber advises if also taking an oral anticoagulant, digoxin, salicylates, or nitrofurantoin.

POLYMYXIN B SULFATE

(pol-i-mix′in)

Classification: ANTIBIOTIC; POLYMYXIN

Therapeutic: ANTIBIOTIC

AVAILABILITY Solution for injection

ACTION & *THERAPEUTIC EFFECT* Binds to lipid phosphates in bacterial membranes and changes permeability to permit leakage of cytoplasm from bacterial cells, resulting in cell death. *Bactericidal against susceptible gram-negative but not gram-positive organisms.*

USES Topically and in combination with other anti-infectives or corticosteroids for various superficial infections of eye, ear, mucous membrane, and skin. Concurrent systemic anti-infective therapy may be required for treatment of intraocular infection and severe progressive corneal ulcer. Used parenterally only in hospitalized patients for treatment of severe acute infections of urinary tract, bloodstream, and meninges; and in combination with Neosporin for continuous bladder irrigation to prevent bacteremia associated with use of indwelling catheter.

CONTRAINDICATIONS Hypersensitivity to polymyxin antibiotics; respiratory insufficiency; concurrent use of products that inhibit peristalsis, skeletal muscle relaxants, ether, or sodium citrate.

CAUTIOUS USE Impaired kidney function, renal failure; inflammatory bowel disease; myasthenia gravis; pulmonary disease. **IV/IM form:** Pregnancy (category C); lactation. **Topical form:** Pregnancy (category B). Safety and efficacy in children younger than 1 mo not established.

ROUTE & DOSAGE

Infections

Adult/Child: **IV** 15,000–25,000 units/kg/day divided q12h; **IM** 25,000–30,000 units/kg/day divided q4–6h; **Intrathecal** 50,000 units × 3–4 days then every other day × 2 wk; *younger than 2 y:* 20,000 units × 3–4 days, then 25,000 units every other day
Infant: **IV** Up to 40,000 units/kg/day

Renal Impairment Dosage Adjustment

Reduce, specific dose unknown

ADMINISTRATION

Intramuscular

- Routine administration by IM routes not recommended because it causes intense discomfort, along the peripheral nerve distribution, 40–60 min after IM injection.
- Make IM injection in adults deep into upper outer quadrant of buttock. Select IM site carefully to avoid injection into nerves or blood vessels. Rotate injection sites. Follow agency policy for IM site used in children.

Intravenous

PREPARE: **Intermittent:** Reconstitute by dissolving 500,000 units in 5 mL sterile water for injection or NS to yield 100,000 units/mL. Withdraw a single dose and then further dilute in 300–500 mL of D5W.

ADMINISTER: **Intermittent:** Infuse over period of 60–90 min. ▪ Inspect injection site for signs of phlebitis and irritation.

INCOMPATIBILITIES: **Solution/additive:** **Amphotericin B, cefazolin, cephalothin, cephapirin, chloramphenicol, heparin, nitrofurantoin, prednisolone, tetracycline.**

- Protect unreconstituted product and reconstituted solution from light and freezing. Store in refrigerator at 2°–8° C (36°–46° F). ▪ Parenteral solutions are stable for 1 wk when refrigerated. Discard unused portion after 72 h.

ADVERSE EFFECTS

CNS: Drowsiness, dizziness, vertigo, convulsions, coma; neuromuscular blockade (generalized muscle weakness, respiratory depression or arrest); meningeal irritation, increased protein and cell count in cerebrospinal fluid, fever, headache, stiff neck (intrathecal use). **HEENT:** Blurred vision, nystagmus, slurred speech, dysphagia, ototoxicity (vestibular and auditory) with high doses. **GI:** GI disturbances. **GU:** Albuminuria, cylindruria, azotemia, hematuria; nephrotoxicity. **Other:** Irritability, facial flushing, ataxia, circumoral, lingual, and peripheral paresthesias (stocking-glove distribution); severe pain (IM site), thrombophlebitis (IV site), superinfections, electrolyte disturbances (prolonged use; also reported in patients with acute leukemia); local irritation and burning (topical use), anaphylactoid reactions (rare).

INTERACTIONS

Drug: ANESTHETICS and NEUROMUSCULAR BLOCKING AGENTS may prolong skeletal muscle relaxation. AMINOGLYCOSIDES, LOOP DIURETICS, and **amphotericin B** have additive nephrotoxic potential.

PHARMACOKINETICS

Peak: 2 h IM. **Distribution:** Widely distributed except to CSF, synovial fluid, and eye; does not cross placenta. **Metabolism:** Unknown. **Elimination:** 60% excreted unchanged in urine. **Half-Life:** 4.3–6 h.

NURSING IMPLICATIONS

Black Box Warning

Polymixin B has been associated with nephrotoxicity and neurotoxicity.

Assessment & Drug Effects

- Review electrolyte results. Patients with low serum calcium are particularly prone to develop neuromuscular blockade.
- Inspect tongue every day. Assess for S&S of superinfection (see Appendix E). Polymyxin therapy

supports growth of opportunistic organisms. Report symptoms promptly.

- Monitor I&O. Maintain fluid intake sufficient to maintain daily urinary output of at least 1500 mL. Some degree of renal toxicity usually occurs within first 3 or 4 days of therapy even with therapeutic doses. Consult prescriber.
- Withhold drug and report findings to prescriber for any of the following: Decreases in urine output (change in I&O ratio), proteinuria, cellular casts, rising BUN, serum creatinine, or serum drug levels (not associated with dosage increase). All can be interpreted as signs of nephrotoxicity.
- Nephrotoxicity is generally reversible, but it may progress even after drug is discontinued. Therefore, close monitoring of kidney function is essential, even following termination of therapy.
- Be alert for respiratory arrest after the first dose and also as long as 45 days after initiation of therapy. It occurs most commonly in patients with kidney failure and high plasma drug levels and is often preceded by dyspnea and restlessness.
- Monitor lab tests: Baseline C&S and renal function tests; frequent serum drug levels during therapy.

Patient & Family Education

- Report to prescriber immediately any muscle weakness, shortness of breath, dyspnea, depressed respiration. These symptoms are rapidly reversible if drug is withdrawn.
- Report promptly to prescriber transient neurologic disturbances (burning or prickling sensations, numbness, dizziness). All occur commonly and usually respond to dosage reduction.
- Report promptly to prescriber the onset of stiff neck and headache (possible symptoms of neurotoxic reactions, including neuromuscular blockade). This response is usually associated with high serum drug levels or nephrotoxicity.
- Report promptly S&S of superinfection (see Appendix E).
- Report any S&S of colitis for up to 2 mo following discontinuation of drug.

PONATINIB

(poe-na'ti-nib)

Iclusig

Classification: ANTINEOPLASTIC; KINASE INHIBITOR

Therapeutic: ANTINEOPLASTIC

Prototype: Erlotinib

AVAILABILITY Tablet

ACTION & THERAPEUTIC EFFECT Inhibits the action of certain tyrosine kinases (a family of enzymes needed for viability of leukemia cells). *Inhibits the growth and replication of mutant leukemic cells.*

USES Treatment of chronic phase, accelerated phase, or blast phase chronic myeloid leukemia (CML) and Philadelphia chromosome-positive acute lymphocytic leukemia (Ph+ALL) that is resistant or intolerant to prior tyrosine kinase inhibitor therapy.

CONTRAINDICATIONS Arterial thrombosis; stroke or MI, severe CHF, serious or severe hemorrhage induced by ponatinib; hepatotoxicity; tumor lysis syndrome; severe myelosuppression; compromised wound healing; GI perforation; pregnancy (category D); lactation.

CAUTIOUS USE CHF, hypertension, cardiac arrhythmias, myelosuppression, DVT; pancreatitis; fluid retention; moderate to severe hepatic impairment.

ROUTE & DOSAGE

Chronic Myeloid Leukemia (CML)/Acute Lymphocyte Leukemia (ALL)

Adult: PO 45 mg once daily

Toxicity Dosage Adjustment

See package insert

Strong CYP3A4 Inhibitors Dosage Adjustment

30 mg once daily

ADMINISTRATION

Oral

- May give without regard to food.
- Tablets must be swallowed whole. They must not be crushed or chewed.
- Avoid intake of grapefruit juice.
- Store at 15°–30° C (59°–86° F).

P

ADVERSE EFFECTS **CV:** *Hypertension, arterial ischemia, peripheral vascular disease, arterial embolism, cerebral ischemia, cerebrovascular accident, myocardial infarction*, peripheral edema, coronary occlusive disease, cardiac arrhythmia, cardiac failure, hypertensive crisis. **Respiratory:** Cough, dyspnea, pleural effusion, nasopharyngitis, pneumonia, upper respiratory tract infection. **CNS:** *Fatigue, headache*, peripheral neuropathy, pain, dizziness, insomnia, chills. **HEENT:** Conjunctival edema, conjunctival hemorrhage, conjunctivitis, dry eye syndrome, eye pain. **Endocrine:** *Hyperglycemia, hypophosphatemia, fluid retention, hypocalcemia, hypoalbuminemia, hyponatremia*, decreased serum bicarbonate, hyperkalemia. **Skin:** *Skin rash, xeroderma*, pruritus, cellulitis, alopecia. **Hepatic/GI:** *Increased liver enzymes, hepatotoxicity, increased serum bilirubin, constipation, abdominal pain, increased serum lipase, nausea, decreased appetite*, vomiting, diarrhea, stomatitis, increased serum amylase. **GU:** UTI, increased serum creatinine. **Musculoskeletal:** *Arthralgia*, myalgia, limb pain, back pain, ostealgia, muscle spasm, muscle pain. **Hematologic:** *Leukopenia, bone marrow depression, neutropenia, anemia, thrombocytopenia, lymphocytopenia, hemorrhage*, febrile neutropenia.

INTERACTIONS **Drug:** Coadministration with strong CYP3A4 inducers (e.g., **carbamazepine, phenytoin, rifampin**) may decrease the levels of ponatinib. Coadministration with strong CYP3A4 inhibitors (e.g. **clarithromycin, conivaptan, indinavir, itraconazole, ketoconazole, lopinavir, nefazodone, nelfinavir, posaconazole, ritonavir, saquinavir, telaprenavir, telithromycin, voriconazole**) may increase the levels of ponatinib. Coadministration with drugs that elevate gastric pH (e.g., ANTACIDS, H_2 BLOCKERS, PROTON PUMP INHIBITORS) may decrease the levels of ponatinib. Studies have yet been done; however, since ponatinib inhibits the ABCG2 and P-gp transporter systems, it may alter the transport of drugs requiring either of these transporters. **Food:** Grapefruit juice may increase the levels of ponatinib. **Herbal:** **St. John's wort** may decrease the levels of ponatinib.

PHARMACOKINETICS **Peak:** 6 h. **Distribution:** Greater than 99% plasma protein bound. **Metabolism:** Hepatic oxidation and hydrolysis. **Elimination:** Fecal (87%) and renal (5%). **Half-Life:** 24 h.

NURSING IMPLICATIONS

Black Box Warning

Ponatinib has been associated with cardiovascular, cerebrovascular, and peripheral vascular thrombosis, including fatal MI and stroke; and with hepatotoxicity and liver failure.

Assessment & Drug Effects

- Monitor cardiovascular status closely.
- Report bradycardia, development of edema, and S&S of CHF.
- Monitor I&O and daily weight. Report rapid weight gain.
- Monitor BP frequently. Be alert for S&S of hypertensive crisis (e.g., confusion, headache, chest pain, or shortness of breath).
- Monitor for and promptly report S&S of hepatotoxicity or pancreatitis.
- Monitor lab tests: Baseline and monthly LFTs; serum lipase q2wk for first month, and monthly thereafter or more often as indicated; CBC with differential and platelet count q2wk for the first 3 mo; periodic serum electrolytes and uric acid.

Patient & Family Education

- Do not drink grapefruit juice while taking this drug.
- Report promptly signs of thrombosis (e.g., chest pain, shortness of breath, one-sided weakness, speech problems, leg pain or swelling).
- Report promptly signs of liver toxicity (e.g., jaundice, dark urine, clay-colored stool).
- Report promptly signs of heart failure (e.g., shortness of breath, chest pain, palpitations, dizziness, fainting, rapid weight gain, abdominal swelling).
- Women should use effective means of contraception to avoid pregnancy as ponatinib can cause severe fetal harm.

PORACTANT ALFA

(por-ac'tant)

Curosurf

Classification: LUNG SURFACTANT

Therapeutic: LUNG SURFACTANT

AVAILABILITY Suspension

ACTION & *THERAPEUTIC EFFECT* Endogenous pulmonary surfactant lowers the surface tension on alveoli surfaces during respiration, and stabilizes the alveoli against collapse at resting pressures. *Alleviates respiratory distress syndrome (RDS) in premature infants caused by deficiency of surfactant.*

USES Treatment (rescue) of respiratory distress syndrome in premature infants.

CONTRAINDICATIONS Hypersensitivity to porcine products or poractant alpha.

CAUTIOUS USE Infants born more than 3 wk after ruptured membranes; intraventricular hemorrhage of grade III or IV; major congenital malformations; nosocomial infection; pretreatment of hypothermia or acidosis due to increased risk of intracranial hemorrhage.

P

ROUTE & DOSAGE

Respiratory Distress Syndrome

Neonate: **Intratracheal** 2.5 mL/kg birth weight, may repeat with 1.25 mL/kg q12h × 2 more doses if needed (max: 5 mL/kg)

ADMINISTRATION

Note: Correction of acidosis, hypotension, anemia, hypoglycemia, and hypothermia is recommended prior to administration of poractant alfa.

Intratracheal

- Warm vial slowly to room temperature; gently turn upside down to form uniform suspension, but do NOT shake.
- Withdraw slowly the entire contents of a vial (concentration equals 80 mg/mL) into a 3 or 5 mL syringe through a large gauge (greater than 20 gauge) needle.
- Attach a 5 French catheter, precut to 8 cm, to the syringe.
- Fill the catheter with poractant alfa and discard excess through the catheter so that only the total dose to be given remains in the syringe.
- Refer to specific instruction provided by manufacturer for proper dosing technique. Follow instructions carefully regarding installation of drug and ventilation of infant. Note that catheter tip should not extend beyond distal tip of endotracheal tube.
- Store refrigerated at 2°–8° C (36°–46° F) and protect from light. Do not shake vials. Do not warm to room temperature and return to refrigeration more than once.

ADVERSE EFFECTS **CV:** Bradycardia, hypotension. **Respiratory:** Intratracheal tube blockage, oxygen desaturation; pulmonary hemorrhage.

PHARMACOKINETICS Not studied.

NURSING IMPLICATIONS

Assessment & Drug Effects

- Stop administration of poractant alfa and take appropriate measures if any of the following occur: Transient episodes of bradycardia, decreased oxygen saturation, reflux of poractant alfa into endotracheal tube, or airway obstruction. Dosing may resume after stabilization.
- Do not suction airway for 1 h after poractant alfa instillation unless there is significant airway obstruction.

POSACONAZOLE

(pos-a-con′a-zole)

Noxafil

Classification: AZOLE ANTIFUNGAL

Therapeutic: ANTIFUNGAL

Prototype: Fluconazole

AVAILABILITY Oral suspension; delayed release tablets

ACTION & *THERAPEUTIC EFFECT*

Inhibits ergosterol synthesis, the principal sterol in the fungal cell membrane, thus interfering with the functions of fungal cell membrane. This results in increased membrane permeability causing leakage of cellular contents. *Has a broad spectrum of antifungal activity against common fungal pathogens.*

USES Prophylactic treatment of invasive *Aspergillus* and *Candida*, oropharyngeal candidiasis.

UNLABELED USES Treatment of febrile neutropenia or refractory invasive fungal infection; treatment of periorbital cellulitis due to *Rhizopus* sp.; treatment of refractory histoplasmosis; treatment of refractory coccidioidomycosis; treatment of fungal necrotizing fasciitis.

CONTRAINDICATIONS Hypersensitivity to posaconazole or other azole antifungals; coadministration with sirolimus, ergot alkaloids, or CYP3A4 substrates; history of QT prolongation; abnormal levels of potassium, magnesium, or calcium; liver disease caused by posaconazole; lactation.

CAUTIOUS USE Hypersensitivity to other azole antifungal antibiotics; hepatic disease or hepatitis; cardiac arrhythmias, hypokalemia; history of proarrhythmic conditions; CHF, myocardial ischemia, atrial fibrillation; AIDS; obesity; severe renal impairment; pregnancy (category C); children younger than 13 y.

ROUTE & DOSAGE

Prophylactic Treatment of Invasive *Aspergillus* and *Candida* Infections

Adult/Adolescent: **PO** 200 mg tid

Thrush

Adult/Adolescent: **PO Oral Suspension** 100 mg bid × 1 day then 100 mg qd × 13 days;
PO Tablet 300 mg bid for one day then 300 mg daily until recovery

ADMINISTRATION

Oral Suspension

- Shake well before use. Give with a full meal or liquid nutritional supplement.

Oral Tablet

- Swallow whole, do not crush. Administer with food.
- Store at 15°–30° C (59°–86° F).

ADVERSE EFFECTS **CV:** *Hypertension, hypotension, tachycardia.* **Respiratory:** *Cough, dyspnea, epistaxis, pharyngitis,* upper respiratory tract infection. **CNS:** QT/QT_C prolongation, tremor. **HEENT:** Blurred vision, taste disturbances. **Endocrine:** *Bilirubinemia,* creatinine levels increased, elevated liver enzymes, hypocalcemia, *hyperglycemia, hypokalemia, hypomagnesemia.* **Skin:** *Pruritus, rash.* **GI:** *Abdominal pain, anorexia constipation, diarrhea, dyspepsia, mucositis, nausea,* vomiting. **GU:** *Vaginal hemorrhage.* **Musculoskeletal:** *Arthralgia, back pain, musculoskeletal pain.* **Hematologic:** *Anemia, febrile neutropenia, neutropenia, petechiae,* <u>thrombocytopenia</u>. **Other:** Anxiety, *bacteremia, dizziness, edema, fatigue, fever, headache, infection, insomnia, rigors,* weakness.

INTERACTIONS **Drug:** Posaconazole is known to increase the plasma levels of **cyclosporine, tacrolimus, rifabutin, midazolam,** and **phenytoin.** Coadministration with other drugs that cause QT prolongation (e.g., **quinidine**) can result in torsades de pointes. Posaconazole may increase the plasma levels of ERGOT ALKALOIDS, VINCA ALKALOIDS, HMG COA REDUCTASE INHIBITORS, and CALCIUM CHANNEL BLOCKERS. Avoid use with cimetidine, efavirenz, esomeprazole, phenytoin, due to decreases in efficacy. **Food:** Administration with food increases absorption of posaconazole.

PHARMACOKINETICS **Peak:** 3–5 h. **Distribution:** 98% protein bound.

Metabolism: Conjugated to inactive metabolites. **Elimination:** Primarily fecal elimination (71%) with minor renal elimination. **Half-Life:** 35 h.

NURSING IMPLICATIONS

Assessment & Drug Effects

- Monitor for and report S&S of breakthrough fungal infections, especially in those with severe renal impairment, or experiencing vomiting and diarrhea, or who cannot tolerate a full meal or supplement along with posaconazole.
- Monitor and report degree of improvement of oropharyngeal candidiasis.
- Monitor those with proarrhythmic conditions for development of arrhythmias.
- Withhold drug and notify prescriber of abnormal serum potassium, magnesium, or calcium levels.
- Monitor blood levels of phenytoin, cyclosporine, tacrolimus, and sirolimus with concurrent therapy. Monitor for adverse effects of concurrently administered statins or calcium channel blockers.
- Monitor lab tests: Baseline and periodic LFTs; periodic renal function tests, serum electrolytes, and CBC.

Patient & Family Education

- Do not take any prescription or nonprescription drugs without informing your prescriber.
- Know parameters for withholding drug (i.e., inability to take with a full meal or nutritional supplement).
- Report immediately any of the following to your health care provider: Vomiting, diarrhea, inability to eat, jaundice of skin, yellowing of eyes, itching, or skin rash.

P

POTASSIUM CHLORIDE ⚠

(poe-tass′ee-um)

Apo-K ♣, K-Dur, K-Long ♣, KCl 5% and 20%, Klor, Klor-10%, Klor-Con, Micro-K Extentabs, Slo-Pot ♣

POTASSIUM GLUCONATE

Classification: ELECTROLYTIC REPLACEMENT SOLUTION

Therapeutic: ELECTROLYTE REPLACEMENT

AVAILABILITY **Chloride:** Sustained release tablet; tablet; effervescent tablet; liquid; powder; solution for injection; vial. **Gluconate:** Liquid

ACTION & *THERAPEUTIC EFFECT* Principal intracellular cation that is essential for maintenance of intracellular isotonicity, transmission of nerve impulses, contraction of cardiac, skeletal, and smooth muscles, maintenance of normal kidney function, and for enzyme activity. *Effectiveness in hypokalemia is measured by serum potassium concentration greater than 3.5 mEq/L.*

USES To prevent and treat potassium deficit; effective in the treatment of hypokalemic alkalosis (chloride, not the gluconate).

CONTRAINDICATIONS Severe renal impairment; severe hemolytic reactions; untreated Addison's disease; crush syndrome; early postoperative oliguria (except during GI drainage); adynamic ileus; acute dehydration; heat cramps, hyperkalemia, patients receiving potassium-sparing diuretics, digitalis intoxication with AV conduction disturbance.

CAUTIOUS USE Cardiac or kidney disease; systemic acidosis;

 Common adverse effects in *italic;* life-threatening effects underlined; generic names in **bold;** classifications in SMALL CAPS; ♣ Canadian drug name; ⊙ Prototype drug; ⚠ Alert

risk for hypokalemia; renal or hepatic impairment; older adults; pregnancy (category B); lactation; children.

ROUTE & DOSAGE

Diabetes Mellitus (type 1)

Adult/Adolescent/Child (older than 3 y): **Subcutaneous** 05.–1 unit/kg/day (dose adjustments based on blood glucose determinations)
Humalog Mix Formulation: Individualize dosage

Renal Impairment Dosage Adjustment

CrCl 10–50 mL/min: Administer at 75% of normal dose
CrCl less than 10 mL/min: Administer at 50% of dose and monitor closely

ADMINISTRATION

Subcutaneous

- Give within 15 min before or immediately after a meal. Give only if solution is clear and colorless.
- Note: May be given in same syringe with longer-acting insulins but absorption may be delayed.

ADVERSE EFFECTS See INSULIN INJECTION (REGULAR).

INTERACTIONS See INSULIN INJECTION (REGULAR).

PHARMACOKINETICS **Absorption:** Rapidly absorbed from IM and subcutaneous injection sites. **Onset:** Less than 15 min. **Peak:** 0.5–1 h. **Duration:** 3–4 h. **Distribution:** Throughout extracellular fluids. **Metabolism:** Metabolized in liver with some metabolism in kidneys. **Elimination:** Less than 2% excreted in urine. **Half-Life:** 1 h.

NURSING IMPLICATIONS

See INSULIN INJECTION (REGULAR).

Assessment & Drug Effects

- Assess for hypoglycemia from 1 to 3 h after injection.
- Assess highly insulin-dependent patients for need for increases in intermediate/long-acting insulins.

Patient & Family Education

- Note: Risk of hypoglycemia is greatest 1–3 h after injection.

INTERFERON ALFA-2B

(in-ter-feer'on)

Intron A

Classification: BIOLOGICAL RESPONSE MODIFIER; IMMUNOMODULATOR; INTERFERON; ANTINEOPLASTIC
Therapeutic: ANTINEOPLASTIC; IMMUNOMODULATOR; INTERFERON; ANTIVIRAL
Prototype: Peginterferon alfa-2a

AVAILABILITY Solution for injection

ACTION & THERAPEUTIC EFFECT Interferon (IFN) alfa-2b, one of 4 types of alpha interferons, is a highly purified protein and natural product of human leukocytes within 4–6 h after viral stimulation. Produced by recombinant DNA technology. **Antiviral action:** Reprograms virus-infected cells to inhibit various stages of virus replication. **Antitumor action:** Suppresses cell proliferation. **Immunomodulating action:** Enhances phagocytic activity of macrophages and augments specific cytotoxicity of lymphocytes for target cells. The immune system and the interferon system of defense are complementary. *Has a broad spectrum of antiviral, cytotoxic, and immunomodulating activity (i.e., favorably adjusts immune system to better combat foreign invasion of antigens, cancers, and viruses).*

I

USES Hairy cell leukemia, chronic hepatitis B, malignant melanoma, condylomata acuminata, follicular lymphoma, AIDS-related Kaposi sarcoma.

UNLABELED USES Chronic myeloid leukemia.

CONTRAINDICATIONS Hypersensitivity to interferon alfa-2b or to any components of the product; patients with or development of decompensated liver disease; autoimmune hepatitis; development of hemorrhagic or ischemic cerebrovascular event; patients with visceral AIDS-related Kaposi sarcoma. Coadministration with ribavirin in pregnant women, in men with pregnant partners, thalassemia major, sickle-cell anemia, CrCl less than 50 mL/min or hypersensitivity to ribavirin; pancreatitis; suicidal ideation; lactation; neonates.

CAUTIOUS USE Severe, preexisting cardiac, renal, or hepatic disease; pulmonary disease (e.g., COPD); DM; preexisting thyroid disorders; patients prone to ketoacidosis; coagulation disorders; preexisting myelosuppression; previous dysrhythmias; history of pulmonary disease; autoimmune disorders; hypertriglyceridemia; history of depression or suicidal tendencies; or other neuropsychiatric disorders; substance abuse disorders; debilitating conditions; ocular disorders; pregnancy (may cause increased risk during pregnancy; use with caution); lactation. Safety and efficacy in children younger than 18 y not established for indications other than chronic hepatitis B. Safety for chronic hepatitis B in children younger than 1 y not established.

ROUTE & DOSAGE

Hairy Cell Leukemia

Adult: **IM/Subcutaneous** 2 million units/m^2 three times per week for up to 6 mo

Kaposi Sarcoma

Adult: **IM/Subcutaneous** 30 million units/m^2 three times per week

Condylomata Acuminata

Adult: **Subcutaneous** 1 million units/lesion three times per week x3w

Chronic Hepatitis B

Adult: **Subcutaneous** 5 million units daily or 10 million units 3 times per week x16w

Malignant Melanoma

Adult: **IV** 20 million international units/m^2 daily for 5 days/wk × 4 wk; maintenance dose is 10 million international units/m^2 given **subcutaneously** weekly × 48 wk

Follicular Lymphoma

Adult: **Subcutaneous** 5 million units three times per week for up to 18 mo

ADMINISTRATION

Subcutaneous/Intramuscular

- Reconstitution: The final concentration with the amount of required diluent is determined by the condition being treated (see manufacturer's directions). Inject diluent (bacteriostatic water for injection) into interferon alfa-2b vial; gently agitate solution before withdrawing dose with a sterile syringe.
- Make sure reconstituted solution is clear and colorless to light yellow and free of particulate

material; discard if there are particles or solution is discolored.

- Administer dose in the evening to enhance tolerability.
- Store vials and reconstituted solutions at 2°–8° C (36°–46° F); remains stable for 1 mo. Discard any remaining drug in reconstituted vials.

Intravenous

PREPARE: **IV Infusion:** Prepare **immediately** before use. Select the appropriate number of vials (i.e., 10, 18, or 50 million international units) of recombinant powder for injection and add to each the 1 mL of supplied diluent. Swirl gently to dissolve but do not shake. ▪ Further dilute by adding the required dose to 100 mL of NS. ▪ The final concentration should not be less than 10 million international units/100 mL.

ADMINISTER: **IV Infusion:** Infuse over 20 min.

INCOMPATIBILITIES: **Solution/additive: Dextrose**-containing solutions; sterile water for injection.

ADVERSE EFFECTS **CV:** Hypertension, chest pain, peripheral edema. **Respiratory:** Bronchitis. **CNS:** Depression, nervousness, anxiety, confusion, *dizziness, fatigue,* somnolence, insomnia, altered mental states, ataxia, tremor, paresthesias, *headache*. **Skin:** Pruritus, alopecia, rash, diaphoresis, injection site reaction. **Hepatic/GI:** Increased liver enzymes, *anorexia,* weight loss, *nausea,* vomiting, xerostomia, abdominal pain, *diarrhea, dyspepsia*. **GU:** Amenorrhea, increased BUN, polyuria. **Hematologic:** Mild thrombocytopenia, transient granulocytopenia, anemia, *neutropenia,* leukopenia, decreased platelet count. **Musculoskeletal:** Myalgia, asthenia, musculoskeletal pain, arthralgia, back pain. **Other:** Chills, flu-like symptoms, fever, flushing, infection.

INTERACTIONS **Drug:** May increase **theophylline** levels; additive myelosuppression with ANTINEOPLASTICS, **zidovudine** may increase hematologic toxicity, do not use with **telbivudine, tizanidine** due to increased risk of adverse reactions. Use with **ribavirin** increases risk of hemolytic anemia; do not use in combination with **ribavirin** if CrCl less than 50 mL/min.

PHARMACOKINETICS **Peak:** 3-12 h. **Metabolism:** In kidneys. **Half-Life:** 2–3 h.

NURSING IMPLICATIONS

Black Box Warnings

Interferon alfa-2b has been associated with fatal or life-threatening neuropsychiatric, autoimmune, ischemic, and infectious disorders.

Assessment & Drug Effects

- Monitor for and report any of the following S&S immediately: Depression, suicidal ideation, suicide attempt, or other indications of psychiatric disturbance.
- Assess hydration status; patient should be well hydrated, especially during initial stage of treatment and if vomiting or diarrhea occurs.
- Monitor for and promptly report any of the following: Chest pain, dyspnea, ecchymoses, petechiae, fever, severe abdominal pain, or psychic disturbances.
- Assess for flu-like symptoms, which may be relieved by acetaminophen (if prescribed).
- Monitor level of GI distress and ability to consume fluids and food.

- Monitor mental status and alertness; implement safety precautions if needed.
- Monitor lab tests: Baseline and periodic CBC with differential, platelet count, serum electrolytes, LFTs, and TSH; chest x-ray, ophthalmic exam, ECG

Patient & Family Education

- Seek medical attention promptly for any of the following: Chest pain, shortness of breath, easy bruising, persistent fever, decrease or loss of vision, severe abdominal pain, depression or suicidal ideation.
- Note: If flu-like symptoms develop, take acetaminophen as advised by prescriber and take interferon at bedtime.
- Use caution with hazardous activities until response to drug is known.
- Learn about adverse effects and notify prescriber about those that cause significant discomfort.

INTERFERON BETA-1A

(in-ter-fer′on)

Avonex, Rebif

Classification: BIOLOGIC RESPONSE MODIFIER; IMMUNOMODULATOR; INTERFERON

Therapeutic: IMMUNOMODULATOR; INTERFERON

Prototype: Peginterferon alfa-2a

AVAILABILITY **Avonex:** Solution for injection; prefilled syringe. **Rebif:** Solution for injection

ACTION & *THERAPEUTIC EFFECT* Interferon beta-1a is produced by recombinant DNA technology. Interferon beta-1a inhibits expression of pro-inflammatory cytokines including INF-G, thought to be a major factor in triggering the autoimmune reaction that leads to multiple sclerosis. It is believed that INF-G stimulates cytotoxic T-cells and causes degradation by macrophages' enzymes on the myelin sheath of neurons in the spinal cord. *Effective in improving time of onset of progression in disability; it was significantly longer in patients treated with interferon beta-1a.*

USES Relapsing-remitting multiple sclerosis.

CONTRAINDICATIONS Previous hypersensitivity to interferon-beta or human albumin, albumin hypersensitivity, hamster protein hypersensitivity; lactation (using **Rebif**).

CAUTIOUS USE Suicidal tendencies, depression, preexisting psychiatric disorders; bone marrow depression; cardiac disease; seizure disorders; thyroid disease; hepatic impairment; pregnancy (category C); lactation (using **Avonex**). Safety and efficacy in children younger than 18 y not established.

ROUTE & DOSAGE

Multiple Sclerosis

Adult: **IM Avonex** 30 mcg qwk; **Subcutaneous Rebif** 22 or 44 mcg 3 × wk

ADMINISTRATION

Intramuscular

- **Avonex:** Reconstitute single use Avonex vial (33 mcg of lyophilized powder) with 1.1 mL of supplied diluent and swirl gently to dissolve.
- Withdraw 1 mL for administration.

- Discard any residual drug as the product contains no preservatives.
- Use within 6 h of reconstitution.

Subcutaneous

- **Rebif:** Give at the same time each day (preferably in the late afternoon or evening) on the same three days of the week at least 48 h apart each week.
- Inject subcutaneously using either a 22 or 44 mcg prefilled syringe. Discard any residual drug as the product contains no preservatives.
- Store unreconstituted vials or prefilled syringes at 2°–8° C (36°–46° F).
- May store for up to 30 days at room temperature up to 25° C (77° F). Do not use beyond expiration date.

ADVERSE EFFECTS CV: Tachycardia, CHF (rare). **CNS:** Headache, *fever,* fatigue, lethargy, depression, somnolence, weakness, agitation, malaise, confusion or reduced ability to concentrate, anxiety, dementia, emotional lability, depersonalization, suicide attempts, worsening of psychiatric disorders. **Endocrine:** Hypocalcemia, elevated serum creatinine, elevated liver transaminases. **Skin:** Local skin necrosis at injection site, *pain at injection site.* **GI:** Nausea, vomiting, *diarrhea, hepatic injury.* **Hematologic:** Leukopenia, anemia, pancytopenia (rare), thrombocytopenia (rare). **Other:** Alopecia, myalgias, *flu-like syndrome,* anaphylaxis.

PHARMACOKINETICS Peak: **Avonex** 7.8–9.8 h; **Rebif** 16 h. **Metabolism:** Rapidly inactivated in body fluids and tissue. **Half-Life:** **Avonex** 8.6–10 h; **Rebif** 69 h.

NURSING IMPLICATIONS

Assessment & Drug Effects

- Withhold drug and notify prescriber if depression or suicidal ideation develops or if there is a worsening of psychiatric symptoms.
- Monitor patients with cardiac disease carefully for worsening cardiac function.
- Monitor lab tests: Periodic LFTs, renal function tests, routine blood chemistry, and CBC with differential, and platelet count; thyroid function tests q6mo with preexisting thyroid dysfunction or when clinically indicated.

Patient & Family Education

- Take a missed dose as soon as possible but not within 48 h of next scheduled dose.
- Learn about common adverse effects, especially flu-like syndrome (headache, fatigue, fever, rigors, chest pain, back pain, myalgia).
- Withhold drug and notify prescriber of depression or suicidal ideation or exacerbation of a preexisting seizure disorder.
- Women who become pregnant should notify prescriber promptly.

INTERFERON BETA-1B

(in-ter-fer'on)

Betaseron, Extavia

Classification: BIOLOGIC RESPONSE MODIFIER; IMMUNOMODULATOR; INTERFERON

Therapeutic: IMMUNOMODULATOR; INTERFERON

Prototype: Peginterferon alfa-2a

AVAILABILITY Solution for injection

ACTION & THERAPEUTIC EFFECT
Interferon beta-1b is a glycoprotein produced by recombinant DNA technique. It is thought to inhibit expression of pro-inflammatory cytokines including INF-G, thought to be a major factor in triggering

the autoimmune reaction. It is believed that INF-G stimulates cytotoxic T-cells and causes degradation by macrophages' enzymes on the myelin sheath of neurons in the spinal cord. *Possess antiviral, antiproliferative, antitumor, and immunomodulatory activity. The effectiveness of interferon beta-1b for multiple sclerosis (MS) is based on the assumption that MS is an immunologically mediated illness.*

USES Relapsing and relapsing-remitting multiple sclerosis.

CONTRAINDICATIONS Previous hypersensitivity to interferon beta-1b or human albumin, mannitol hypersensitivity; suicidal ideation; jaundice due to hepatic injury; worsening of CHF.

CAUTIOUS USE History of suicidal tendencies or mental disorders especially chronic depression; seizures; cardiac disease; hepatic impairment; pregnancy (category C) but may cause a spontaneous abortion; lactation. Safety and efficacy in children younger than 18 y not established.

ROUTE & DOSAGE

Multiple Sclerosis

Adult: **Subcutaneous** 62.5 mcg every other day during wk 1 and 2; 125 mcg every other day during wk 3 and 4; 187.5 mcg every other day during wk 5 and 6; then 250 mcg every other day

ADMINISTRATION

Subcutaneous

- Reconstitute by adding 1.2 mL of the supplied diluent (0.54% NaCl) to vial and gently swirl. **Do not** shake. The resultant solution contains 0.25 mg (8 million units)/mL.
- Discard reconstituted solution if it contains particulate matter or is discolored. Also discard unused solution.
- Rotate injection sites; use 27-gauge needle to administer drug.
- Store vials under refrigeration, 2°–8° C (36°–46° F) or at room temperature.

ADVERSE EFFECTS **CV:** Tachycardia, peripheral edema, CHF (rare). **CNS:** Headache, *fever,* fatigue, dizziness, lethargy, depression, somnolence, weakness, agitation, malaise, confusion or reduced ability to concentrate, anxiety, dementia, emotional lability, depersonalization, suicide attempts, hypertonia, chills. **Endocrine:** Hypocalcemia, elevated serum creatinine, elevated liver transaminases, autoimmune hepatitis, hepatic failure. **Skin:** Local skin necrosis at injection site, rash, *pain at injection site.* **GI:** Nausea, vomiting, *diarrhea,* abdominal pain. **Hematologic:** Leukopenia, thrombocytopenia, anemia. **Other:** Alopecia, myalgias, *flu-like syndrome.*

INTERACTIONS **Drug:** Use with NRTIS or PROTEASE INHIBITORS should be done with caution.

PHARMACOKINETICS **Absorption:** About 50% absorbed from subcutaneous sites. **Distribution:** Penetrates intact blood–brain barrier poorly; crosses placenta; distributed into breast milk. **Metabolism:** Rapidly inactivated in body fluids and tissue.

NURSING IMPLICATIONS

Assessment & Drug Effects

- Monitor vital signs, neurologic status, and neuropsychiatric status frequently during therapy.
- Assess for and promptly treat flu-like symptom complex (fever, chills, myalgia, etc.).
- Assess injection sites; pain and redness are common reactions. Report tissue ulceration promptly.
- Monitor lab tests: LFTs at 1, 3, and 6 mo after initiation of therapy and as clinically warranted thereafter; periodic renal function tests, CBC, thyroid function, and serum electrolytes.

Patient & Family Education

- Learn and understand potential adverse drug reactions.
- Learn proper technique for solution preparation and injection.
- Self-medicate with acetaminophen (if not contraindicated) if flu-like symptom complex develops.
- Avoid prolonged exposure to sunlight.
- Use caution when performing hazardous activities until response to drug is known.

IODOQUINOL

(eye-oh-do-kwin'ole)

Yodoxin

Classification: AMEBICIDE
Therapeutic: AMEBICIDE
Prototype: Emetine

AVAILABILITY Tablet

ACTION & THERAPEUTIC EFFECT Direct-acting (contact) amebicide. *Effective against both trophozoites and cyst forms of* Entamoeba histolytica *in intestinal lumen.*

USES Intestinal amebiasis and for asymptomatic passers of cysts. Commonly used either concurrently or in alternating courses with another intestinal amebicide.

CONTRAINDICATIONS Hypersensitivity to any 8-hydroxyquinoline or to iodine-containing preparations or foods; hepatic or renal damage; lactation.

CAUTIOUS USE Severe thyroid disease; minor self-limiting problems; prolonged high-dosage therapy; preexisting optic neuropathy; pregnancy (category C).

ROUTE & DOSAGE

Intestinal Amebiasis

Adult: **PO** 650 mg tid for 20 days (max: 2 g/day); may repeat after a 2–3 wk drug-free interval

Child: **PO** 30–40 mg/kg/day in 2–3 divided doses for 20 days (max: 1.95 g/day); may repeat after a 2–3 wk drug-free interval

ADMINISTRATION

Oral

- Give drug after meals. If patient has difficulty swallowing tablet, crush and mix with applesauce.

ADVERSE EFFECTS CNS: Headache, agitation, retrograde amnesia, vertigo, ataxia, peripheral neuropathy (especially in children); muscle pain, weakness usually below T12 vertebrae, dysesthesias especially of lower limbs, paresthesias, increased sense of warmth. **HEENT:** Blurred vision, optic atrophy, optic neuritis, permanent loss of vision.

Endocrine: Thyroid hypertrophy, iodism [generalized furunculosis (iodine toxiderma), skin eruptions, fever, chills, weakness]. **Skin:** Discoloration of hair and nails, acne, hair loss, urticaria, various forms of skin eruptions. **GI:** Nausea, vomiting, anorexia, abdominal cramps, diarrhea, constipation, rectal irritation and itching. **Hematologic:** Agranulocytosis (rare). **Other:** Hypersensitivity (urticaria, pruritus).

DIAGNOSTIC TEST INTERFERENCE Iodoquinol can cause elevations of ***PBI*** and decrease of ***I-131 uptake*** (effects may last for several weeks to 6 mo even after discontinuation of therapy). ***Ferric chloride test for PKU*** (phenylketonuria) may yield false-positive results if iodoquinol is present in urine.

PHARMACOKINETICS **Absorption:** Small amount from GI tract. **Elimination:** In feces.

NURSING IMPLICATIONS

Assessment & Drug Effects

- Monitor I&O ratio. Record characteristics of stools: Color, consistency, frequency, presence of blood, mucus, or other material.
- Note: Ophthalmologic examinations are recommended at regular intervals during prolonged therapy.
- Monitor and report immediately the onset of blurred or decreased vision or eye pain. Also report symptoms of peripheral neuropathy: Pain, numbness, tingling, or weakness of extremities.

Patient & Family Education

- Report any of the following: Skin rash, blurred vision, fever or other signs of infection.
- Complete full course of treatment. Stool needs to be examined again 1, 3, and 6 mo after termination of treatment.
- Note: Intestinal amebiasis is spread mainly by contaminated water, raw fruits or vegetables, flies, roaches, and hand-to-mouth transfer of infected feces. It is very important to wash hands after defecation and before eating.

IPILIMUMAB

(ip'i-lim'ue-mab)

Yervoy

Classification: MONOCLONAL ANTIBODY; ANTINEOPLASTIC

Therapeutic: ANTINEOPLASTIC

AVAILABILITY Solution for injection

ACTION & THERAPEUTIC EFFECT A recombinant, human monoclonal antibody thought to augment T-cell activation and proliferation thus enhancing T-cell mediated antitumor immune responses. *Enhances the immune system's ability to seek out and destroy metastatic melanoma cells.*

USES Treatment of unresectable or metastatic malignant melanoma.

CAUTIOUS USE Immune-mediated hepatitis, dermatitis, neuropathies, endocrinopathies, nephritis, pneumonitis, meningitis, pericarditis, uveitis, iritis, and hemolytic anemia; pregnancy (category C); lactation. Safety and efficacy in children not established.

ROUTE & DOSAGE

Malignant Melanoma

Adult: **IV** 3 mg/kg q3wks for a total of 4 doses

Adverse Reaction Dosage Adjustment

Moderate immune-mediated adverse reaction or for symptomatic endocrinopathy: Withhold dose

If the adverse reaction completely or partial resolves (Grade 0–1) and if patient is receiving less than 7.5 mg prednisone or equivalent/day: Resume at 3 mg/kg q3wks until all 4 doses are given or 16 wks from first dose, whichever comes first.

If treatment course not completed within 16 wk; or if moderate adverse reactions are persistent; or if corticosteroid dose cannot be reduced to 7.5 mg prednisone; or if severe or life-threatening adverse reactions occur: Permanently discontinue ipilimumab

ADMINISTRATION

Intravenous

PREPARE: **IV Infusion:** Place vials at room temperature for 5 min. Do not shake. Withdraw required volume and add to an IV bag with enough NS or D5W to yield a final concentration of 1–2 mg/mL. Gently invert IV bag to mix.

ADMINISTER: **IV Infusion:** Give over 90 min through an IV line containing a low-protein-binding in-line filter. Flush line with NS or D5W after each dose.

INCOMPATIBILITIES: **Solution/additive:** Do not mix ipilimumab, or administer as an infusion with other drugs or compounds.

- Store at 2°–8°C (36°–46° F). Protect from light. May store diluted solution for up to 24 h under refrigeration or at 20°–25°C (68°–77°F). Discard partially used vials.

ADVERSE EFFECTS **Skin:** *Pruritus, rash;* Stevens–Johnson syndrome, toxic epidermal necrolysis. **Hepatic:** AST or ALT greater 5 × the ULN or total bilirubin greater than 3 × the ULN. **GI:** *Diarrhea*; enterocolitis; GI hemorrhage; GI perforation. **Other:** *Fatigue*.

PHARMACOKINETICS **Half-Life:** 14.7 d.

NURSING IMPLICATIONS

Black Box Warning

Ipilimumab has been associated with severe immune-mediated adverse reactions including enterocolitis, hepatitis, dermatitis, neuropathy, and endocrinopathy.

Assessment & Drug Effects

- Use the *Nursing Immune-Mediated Adverse Reaction Symptom Checklist* (found on the product web site) to assess the patient.
- Monitor closely for and report immediately severe adverse reactions that may occur during or after (weeks to months) infusing. These include but are not limited to: Severe motor or sensory neuropathy; severe skin reactions; colitis with abdominal pain, fever, ileus, peritoneal signs, increased stool frequency (7 or more over baseline) or stool incontinence, need for intravenous hydration for more than 24 h, and GI hemorrhage.
- Report immediately ALT elevations of more than 5 × the ULN or total bilirubin elevations more than 3 × the ULN.
- Monitor lab tests: Baseline and before each dose: LFTs and

thyroid function tests; periodic renal function tests.

Patient & Family Education

- Read the *Medication Guide* for ipilimumab prior to each infusion.
- Report immediately to prescribe any adverse reaction experienced during or after (weeks to months) infusion.
- Women should inform prescriber if they become pregnant.

IPRATROPIUM BROMIDE

(i-pra-troe′pee-um)

Atrovent, Atrovent HFA

Classification: ANTICHOLINERGIC; ANTIMUSCARINIC; BRONCHODILATOR

Therapeutic: BRONCHODILATOR

Prototype: Atropine

AVAILABILITY Solution for inhalation; inhaler; nasal spray

ACTION & *THERAPEUTIC EFFECT* Local application to nasal mucosa inhibits serous and seromucous gland secretions. Blocks action of acetylcholine at parasympathetic sites in bronchial smooth muscle causing bronchodilation. *Produces local, site-specific effects on the larger central airways including bronchodilation and prevention of bronchospasms.*

USES Maintenance therapy in COPD including chronic bronchitis and emphysema; nasal spray for perennial rhinitis and symptomatic relief of rhinorrhea associated with the common cold.

UNLABELED USES Perennial nonallergic rhinitis.

CONTRAINDICATIONS Hypersensitivity to atropine, bromides, peanut oils, soy lecithin; paradoxical bronchospasm.

CAUTIOUS USE Narrow-angle glaucoma; BPH; bladder neck obstruction; pregnancy (category B). lactation; children.

ROUTE & DOSAGE

COPD

Adult: **Inhalation** 2 inhalations of MDI qid (max: 12 inhalations in 24 h) **Nebulizer** 500 mcg (1 unit dose vial) q6–8h

Rhinitis

Adult/Adolescent/Child (6 y or older): **Intranasal** 2 sprays of 0.03% each nostril bid or tid

ADMINISTRATION

Intranasal/Inhalation/Nebulizer

- Demonstrate aerosol use and check return demonstration.
- Wait 3 min between inhalations if more than one inhalation/dose is ordered.
- Avoid contact with eyes.
- Instruct patient to rinse mouth with water to minimize dry mouth.

ADVERSE EFFECTS **Respiratory:** Bronchitis, exacerbation of COPD, sinusitis, dyspnea. **CNS:** Headache.

INTERACTIONS DRUG May enhance anticholinergic effects of other ANTICHOLINERGIC agents.

PHARMACOKINETICS **Absorption:** 10% of inhaled dose reaches lower airway; approximately 0.5% of dose is systemically absorbed. **Peak:** 1.5–2 h. **Duration:** 4–6 h. **Elimination:** 48% of dose excreted in feces; less than 5% excreted in urine. **Half-Life:** 1.5–2 h.

NURSING IMPLICATIONS

Assessment & Drug Effects

- Monitor respiratory status; auscultate lungs before and after inhalation.
- Report treatment failure (exacerbation of respiratory symptoms) to prescriber.
- Monitor pulmonary function tests.

Patient & Family Education

- Note: This medication is not an emergency agent because of its delayed onset and the time required to reach peak bronchodilation.
- Review patient information sheet on proper use of nasal spray.
- Allow 30–60 sec between puffs for optimum results. Do not let medication contact your eyes.
- Wait 5 min between this and other inhaled medications. Check with prescriber about sequence of administration.
- Take medication only as directed, noting some leniency in number of puffs within 24 h. Supervise child's administration until certain all of dose is being administered.
- Rinse mouth after medication puffs to reduce bitter taste.
- Discuss changes in normal urinary pattern with the prescriber (more common in older adults).
- Call prescriber if you note changes in sputum color or amount, ankle edema, or significant weight gain.

IRBESARTAN

(ir-be-sar′tan)

Avapro

Classification: ANGIOTENSIN II RECEPTOR ANTAGONIST; ANTIHYPERTENSIVE

Therapeutic: ANTIHYPERTENSIVE

Prototype: Losartan

AVAILABILITY Tablet

ACTION & *THERAPEUTIC EFFECT* Irbesartan is an angiotensin II receptor (type AT_1) antagonist. Irbesartan selectively blocks the binding of angiotensin II to the AT_1 receptors found in many tissues (e.g., vascular smooth muscle, adrenal glands), resulting in vasodilation of vascular smooth muscle. *This blocks vasoconstricting and aldosterone-secreting effects of angiotensin II, thus resulting in an antihypertensive effect.*

USES Hypertension, treatment of diabetic nephropathy in patients with hypertension and type 2 diabetes.

UNLABELED USES CHF, acute coronary syndrome.

CONTRAINDICATIONS Hypersensitivity to irbesartan, losartan, or valsartan; hypovolemia; pregnancy (category D second and third trimester); lactation.

CAUTIOUS USE Arterial stenosis of the renal artery, hepatic disease; severe CHF, African American patients; pregnancy (category C first trimester). Safe use in children not established.

ROUTE & DOSAGE

Hypertension

Adult: **PO** Start with 150 mg once daily, may increase to 300 mg/day

Diabetic Nephropathy

Adult: **PO** 300 mg daily

ADMINISTRATION

Oral

- Give without regard to food.
- Store at 15°–30° C (59°–86° F).

ADVERSE EFFECTS CV: Orthostatic dizziness, orthostatic hypotension. **CNS:** Dizziness. **Endocrine:** Hyperkalemia.

INTERACTIONS Drug: May increase risk of hypotension with other ANTIHYPERTENSIVE agents.

DIAGNOSTIC TEST INTERFERENCE May lead to false-negative ***aldosterone/renin ratio.***

PHARMACOKINETICS Absorption: Rapidly absorbed from GI tract, 60–80% bioavailability. **Distribution:** 90% protein bound. **Metabolism:** In the liver primarily by CYP2C9. **Elimination:** Primarily in feces. **Half-Life:** 11–15 h.

NURSING IMPLICATIONS

Black Box Warning

Irbesartan has been associated with fetal injury and death.

Assessment & Drug Effects

- Monitor for therapeutic effectiveness: Maximum pressure-lowering effect may not be evident for 6–12 wk; indicated by decreases in systolic and diastolic BP.
- Monitor BP periodically; trough readings, just prior to the next scheduled dose, should be made when possible.
- Monitor lab tests: Periodic BUN and creatinine, serum potassium.

Patient & Family Education

- Inform prescriber immediately if you become pregnant.
- Notify prescriber of episodes of dizziness, especially when making position changes.

IRINOTECAN HYDROCHLORIDE

(eye-ri-no′te-can)

Camptosar

Classification: ANTINEOPLASTIC; CAMPTOTHECIN ANALOG

Therapeutic: ANTINEOPLASTIC

Prototype: Topotecan

AVAILABILITY Solution for injection

ACTION & *THERAPEUTIC EFFECT*

Antitumor activity due to inhibition of the intranuclear enzyme topoisomerase I (DNA-gyrase). By inhibiting topoisomerase I, irinotecan and its active metabolite, SN-38, cause double-stranded DNA damage during the synthesis (S) phase of DNA synthesis. *Irinotecan inhibits both DNA and RNA synthesis.*

USES Metastatic carcinoma of colon or rectum.

UNLABELED USES Gastric cancer, malignant glioma, non-small cell lung cancer, pancreatic cancer.

CONTRAINDICATIONS Previous hypersensitivity to irinotecan, topotecan, or other camptothecin analogs; hereditary fructose intolerance; interstitial pulmonary disease; previous pelvic/abdominal radiation recipients; acute infection, severe diarrhea, bowel obstruction; pregnancy (category D); lactation.

CAUTIOUS USE Gastrointestinal disorders, myelosuppression, renal or hepatic impairment, history of bleeding disorders, previous cytotoxic or radiation therapy; older adults. Safe use in children not established.

 Common adverse effects in *italic*; life-threatening effects underlined; generic names in **bold**; classifications in SMALL CAPS; ♣ Canadian drug name; ● Prototype drug; ⚠ Alert

ROUTE & DOSAGE

Metastatic Carcinoma

Adult: **IV** 125 mg/m^2 once weekly for 4 wk, then a 2-wk rest period (future courses may be adjusted to range from 50 to 150 mg/m^2 depending on tolerance; see complete prescribing information for specific dosage adjustment recommendations based on toxic effects)

Pharmacogenetic Dosage Adjustment

Patients with UGT1A1*28 allele have increased risk of side effects, start with decreased dose

ADMINISTRATION

Intravenous

Administer only after premedication (at least 30 min prior) with an antiemetic.
- Wash immediately with soap and water if skin contacts drug during preparation.

PREPARE: **IV Infusion:** Dilute the ordered dose in enough D5W (preferred) or NS to yield a concentration of 0.12–2.8 mg/mL. ▪ Typical amount of diluent used is 250–500 mL.

ADMINISTER: **IV Infusion:** Infuse over 90 min. ▪ Closely monitor IV site; if extravasation occurs, immediately flush with sterile water and apply ice.

INCOMPATIBILITIES: **Y-site: Acyclover, allopurinol, amphotericin B, cefepime, cefotaxime, ceftriaxone, chloramphenicol, chlorpromazine, dantrolene, dexmedetomidine, diazepam, droperidol, fluorouracil, fosphenytoin, furosemide, ganciclovir, gemcitabine, glycopyrrolate, methothexital, methylprenisolone, mitomycin, nafcillin, nitroprusside, premetrexed, phenytoin, piperacillin/tazobactam, trastuzumab.**

- Store undiluted at 15°–30° C (59°–86° F) and protect from light. Use reconstituted solutions within 24 h.

ADVERSE EFFECTS

CV: Vasodilation/flushing. **Respiratory:** *Dyspnea,* cough, rhinitis. **CNS:** Headache, *insomnia, dizziness.* **Skin:** *Alopecia,* sweating, rash. **GI:** *Diarrhea (early and late onset), dehydration, nausea, vomiting, anorexia, weight loss, constipation, abdominal cramping and pain,* flatulence, stomatitis, dyspepsia, increased alkaline phosphatase and AST. **Hematologic:** Leukopenia, neutropenia, *anemia.* **Other:** *Asthenia, fever, pain,* chills, edema, abdominal enlargement, back pain.

INTERACTIONS

Drug: ANTICOAGULANTS, ANTIPLATELET AGENTS, NSAIDS may increase risk of bleeding; **carbamazepine, phenytoin, phenobarbital** may decrease irinotecan levels. **Herbal: St. John's wort** may decrease irinotecan levels.

PHARMACOKINETICS

Peak: 1 h. **Distribution:** Irinotecan is 30% protein bound; active metabolite SN-38 is 95% protein bound. **Metabolism:** In liver by carboxylesterase enzyme to active metabolite SN-38. **Elimination:** 10 h for SN-38; 20% excreted in urine. **Half-Life:** 10–20 h.

NURSING IMPLICATIONS

Black Box Warning

Irinotecan has been associated with severe, potentially life-threatening diarrhea that may occur during or shortly after infusion, or more than 24 h after infusion.

Assessment & Drug Effects

- Monitor closely for fluid and electrolyte imbalance. If severe diarrhea occurs during infusion, stop infusion and notify prescriber.
- Monitor for acute GI distress, especially early diarrhea (within 24 h of infusion), which may be preceded by diaphoresis and cramping, and late diarrhea (more than 24 h after infusion).
- Monitor lab tests. Prior to each dose, WBC with differential, Hgb, platelet count, and serum electrolytes especially during periods of diarrhea.

Patient & Family Education

- Learn about common adverse effects and measures to control or minimize when possible.
- Notify prescriber immediately when you experience diarrhea, vomiting, and S&S of infection. Diarrhea requires prompt treatment to prevent serious fluid and electrolyte imbalances.

IRON DEXTRAN

(i′ern dek′stran)

INFeD

Classification: BLOOD FORMER; IRON SUPPLEMENT; ANTIANEMIC

Therapeutic: ANTIANEMIC; IRON SUPPLEMENT

Prototype: Ferrous sulfate

AVAILABILITY Solution for injection

ACTION & *THERAPEUTIC EFFECT*

A complex of ferric hydroxide with dextran in solution for injection. Reticuloendothelial cells of liver, spleen, and bone marrow dissociate iron (ferric ion) from iron dextran complex. The released ferric ion combines with transferrin and is transported to bone marrow, where it is incorporated into hemoglobin. *Effective in replacement of iron needed in iron deficiency anemia, thus replenishing hemoglobin and depleted iron stores.*

USES Only in patients with clearly established iron deficiency anemia when oral administration of iron is unsatisfactory or impossible.

CONTRAINDICATIONS Hypersensitivity to the product; all anemias except iron-deficiency anemia; acute phase of infectious renal disease.

CAUTIOUS USE Rheumatoid arthritis, ankylosing spondylitis; renal disease; SLE; impaired hepatic function; cardiac disease; history of allergies or asthma; pregnancy (risk of adverse maternal reactions following the use of parenteral iron that may result in fetal bradycardia especially during second and third trimesters); lactation. Use not recommended in infants younger than 4 mo old.

ROUTE & DOSAGE

Iron Deficiency

Adult: **IM/IV** Total dose (mL) = 0.0442 (desired hemoglobin [g/dL] − observed hemoglobin [g/dL]) × IBW (kg) + (0.26 × IBW [kg]) dose administered as multiple daily doses of less than 100 mg

Child: **IM/IV**
Dose is based on age, weight, and current hemoglobin. See package insert for dosing table.

 Common adverse effects in *italic;* life-threatening effects underlined; generic names in **bold;** classifications in SMALL CAPS; ♣ Canadian drug name; ⊙ Prototype drug; ⚠ Alert

ADMINISTRATION

May be administered IV or IM.

Test Dose

- Prior to the first *INFeD* IM dose, administer an IM test dose of 0.5 mL.
- Prior to the first IV dose, administer a 0.5 mL test dose at a gradual rate over at least 30 seconds (**INFeD**).
- Note: Although anaphylactic reactions (see Appendix F) usually occur within a few minutes after injection, it is recommended that 1 h or more elapse before remainder of initial dose is given following test dose.

Intramuscular

- Give injection only into the muscle mass in upper outer quadrant of buttock (never in the upper arm). In small child, use the lateral thigh. Use a 2- or 3-inch, 19- or 20-gauge needle. The Z-track technique is recommended. Use one needle to withdraw drug from container and another needle for injection.
- Note: If patient is receiving IM in standing position, patient should be bearing weight on the leg opposite the injection site; if in bed, patient should be in the lateral position with injection site uppermost.

Intravenous

PREPARE: **Direct:** Give undiluted. **IV Infusion:** Dilute in 250–1000 mL of NS.

ADMINISTER: **Direct** *Test Dose:* A test dose is given before the first IV therapeutic dose. ▪ *DexFerrum:* Give test dose of 25 mg (0.5 mL) slowly over 30 seconds to 5 min. ▪ *INFeD:* Give test dose over 30 sec. Wait 1–2 h and if no adverse reaction occurs, give the remainder of the first dose by IV infusion.

IV Infusion: Infuse at a rate not to exceed 50 mg (1 mL) or fraction thereof over 60 sec. Avoid rapid infusion.

INCOMPATIBILITIES: **Solution/additive: TPN. Y-site: Dopamine** After infusion is completed, flush vein with 10 mL of NS. ▪ Have patient remain in bed for at least 30 min after IV administration to prevent orthostatic hypotension. Monitor BP and pulse.

- Store below 20°–25°C (68°–77°F) unless otherwise directed.

ADVERSE EFFECTS

CV: *Peripheral vascular flushing (rapid IV), hypotension,* precordial pain or pressure sensation, bradycardia, tachycardia, <u>fatal cardiac arrhythmias, circulatory collapse</u>. **CNS:** Headache, shivering, transient paresthesias, syncope, dizziness, <u>coma</u>, seizures. **Endocrine:** Hemosiderosis, metabolic acidosis, hyperglycemia, reactivation of quiescent rheumatoid arthritis, exogenous hemosiderosis. **Skin:** Sterile abscess and brown skin discoloration (IM site), local phlebitis (IV site), lymphadenopathy, *pain at IM injection site.* **GI:** Nausea, vomiting, transient loss of taste perception, metallic taste, diarrhea, melena, abdominal pain, hemorrhagic gastritis, intestinal necrosis, hepatic damage. **Hematologic:** Bleeding disorder with severe toxicity. **Other:** Hypersensitivity (urticaria, skin rash, allergic purpura, pruritus, fever, chills, dyspnea, arthralgia, myalgia; <u>anaphylaxis</u>).

DIAGNOSTIC TEST INTERFERENCE

Falsely elevated ***serum bilirubin*** and falsely decreased ***serum calcium*** values may occur. Large doses of iron dextran may impart a brown color to serum drawn 4 h after iron administration. ***Bone scans*** involving Tc-99m diphosphonate have shown dense areas of activity along contour of iliac crest 1–6 days after IM injections of iron dextran.

INTERACTIONS A toxic complex may form with **dimercaprol.** ACE INHIBITORS may increase adverse effects.

PHARMACOKINETICS **Absorption:** 60% from IM site by 3 days; 90% absorbed by 1–3 wk. **Distribution:** Crosses placenta; distributed into breast milk. **Metabolism:** In reticuloendothelial system. **Half-Life:** 6 h.

I

NURSING IMPLICATIONS

Black Box Warning Pr

Iron dextran has been associated with anaphylactic-type reactions.

Assessment & Drug Effects

- Monitor closely for hypersensitivity-type reaction. Report immediately urticaria, rash, pruitus, chills, dyspnea or other S&S of hypersensitivity.
- Systemic reactions may occur over 24 h after parenteral iron has been administered. Large IV doses are associated with increased frequency of adverse effects.
- Monitor lab tests: Periodic Hgb, Hct, reticulocyte count, serum ferritin, serum iron, TIBC, transferrin saturation.

Patient & Family Education

- Do not take oral iron preparations when receiving iron injections.
- Eat foods high in iron and vitamin C.
- Notify prescriber of any of the following: Backache or muscle ache, chills, dizziness, fever, headache, nausea or vomiting, paresthesias, pain or redness at injection site, skin rash or hives, or difficulty breathing.

IRON SUCROSE

(i′ron su′crose)

Venofer, Velphoro

Classification: BLOOD FORMER; IRON REPLACEMENT; ANTIANEMIC

Therapeutic: ANTIANEMIC; IRON DEFICIENCY REPLACEMENT

Prototype: Ferrous sulfate

AVAILABILITY Solution for injection; chewable tablet

ACTION & *THERAPEUTIC EFFECT* A complex of iron (ferric) (III) hydroxide in sucrose. It is dissociated by the reticuloendothelial system (RES) into iron and sucrose. Normal erythropoiesis depends on the concentration of iron and erythropoietin available in the plasma; both are decreased in renal failure. *Increases serum iron level in chronic renal failure patients, and results in increased hemoglobin level.*

USES Treatment of iron deficiency anemia in chronic kidney disease.

CONTRAINDICATIONS Patients with iron overload, hypersensitivity to Venofer, or for anemia not caused by iron deficiency; hemochromatosis.

CAUTIOUS USE Patients with a history of hypotension; older adults, decreased renal, hepatic, or cardiac function; pregnancy (risk of adverse maternal reactions following use of parenteral iron that may result in fetal bradycardia, especially during the second and third trimester); lactation. Safety and efficacy in children or infants not established.

ROUTE & DOSAGE

Iron Deficiency Anemia

Adult: **IV Hemodialysis dependent (HDD-CKD):** 100 mg elemental iron given at least 15 min/hemodialysis session (cumulative dose: 1000 mg); **Nonhemodialysis dependent (NDD-CKD):** 200 mg elemental iron on 5 different occasions within the 14-day period; **Peritoneal dialysis dependent (PDD-CKD):** 300 mg on days 1 and 15, then 400 mg 14 days later

ADMINISTRATION

Intravenous

PREPARE: **Direct/Infusion: HDD-CKD:** Give direct IV undiluted or diluted immediately prior to infusion in a maximum of 100 mL NS. ▪ **NDD-CKD:** Give direct IV undiluted. ▪ **PDD-CKD:** Dilute 300–400 mg in a maximum of 250 mL of NS for infusion.

ADMINISTER: **Direct:** Give the undiluted solution slowly by direct IV over 2–5 min. **IV Infusion** ▪ Infusion diluted solution for **HDD-CKD patient** over at least 15 min and for **PDD-CKD patient** over 90 min. ▪ Avoid rapid infusion.

INCOMPATIBILITIES: **Solution/additive:** Do not mix with other medications or parenteral nutrition solutions. **Y-site:** **Cefiderocol, dopamine, tacrolimus.**

- Store unopened vials preferably at 25° C (77° F), but room temperature permitted. Discard unused portion in opened vial.

ADVERSE EFFECTS **CV:** *Hypotension,* peripheral edema, hypertension. **Respiratory:** Nasopharyngitis, pharyngitis, sinusitis, URI, dyspnea. **CNS:** Headache, dizziness. **Skin:** Injection site reaction. **GI:** Nausea, vomiting, diarrhea. **Musculoskeletal:** Muscle cramps. **Other:** Graft complications, anaphylactoid reactions.

INTERACTIONS **Drug:** May reduce absorption of ORAL IRON PREPARATIONS. May decrease absorption of **levothyroxine**. A toxic complex may form with **dimercaprol**. Monitor closely if used with **obinutuzumab** or **amifostine**.

PHARMACOKINETICS **Peak:** 4 wk. **Distribution:** Primarily to blood with some distribution to liver, spleen, bone marrow. **Metabolism:** Dissociated to iron and sucrose in reticuloendothelial system. **Elimination:** Sucrose is eliminated in urine, 5% of iron excreted in urine. **Half-Life:** 6 h.

NURSING IMPLICATIONS

Assessment & Drug Effects

- Withhold drug and notify prescriber when serum ferritin level equals or exceeds established guidelines.
- Stop infusion and notify prescriber for S&S overdosage or infusing too rapidly: Hypotension, edema; headache, dizziness, nausea, vomiting, abdominal pain, joint or muscle pain, and paresthesia.
- Monitor patient carefully during the first 30 min after initiation of IV therapy for signs of hypersensitivity and anaphylactoid reaction (see Appendix F).
- Monitor lab tests: Periodic serum ferritin, serum iron, TIBC, transferrin saturation, Hct, and Hgb.

Patient & Family Education

- Report any of the following promptly: Itching, rash, chest pain, headache, dizziness, nausea, vomiting, abdominal pain, joint or

I

muscle pain, and numbness and tingling.

ISAVUCONAZONIUM SULFATE

(i-sa-vu-con'a-zo-ni-um)

Cresemba

Classification: AZOLE ANTIFUNGAL

Therapeutic: ANTIFUNGAL

Prototype: Fluconazole

AVAILABILITY Capsules; solution for injection

I

ACTION & *THERAPEUTIC EFFECT* Inhibits the synthesis of ergosterol, a key component of the fungal cell membrane, through the inhibition of a cytochrome P-450 dependentenzyme (lanosterol 14-alpha-demethylase). *Depletion of ergosterol within the fungal cell membrane weakens the membrane structure and impairs its function, inhibiting fungal growth*.

USES Treatment of invasive aspergillosis and invasive mucormycosis in patients 18 y or older.

UNLABELED USES Treatment of esophageal candidiasis.

CONTRAINDICATIONS Known hypersensitivity to isavuconazole; coadministration of strong CYP3A4 inhibitors; coadministration with strong CYP3A4 inhibitors (e.g., ketoconazole or high-dose ritonavir); coadministration with strong CYP3A4 inducers (e.g., rifampin, carbamazepine, St. John's wort, or long acting barbiturates); patients with familial short QT syndrome; lactation.

CAUTIOUS USE Severe hepatic impairment; infusion-related reactions; concurrent immunosuppressants; concurrent drugs with narrow therapeutic window that are P-gp substrates (e.g., digoxin); pregnancy. Safety and efficacy in patients younger than 18 y not established.

ROUTE & DOSAGE

Invasive Aspergillosis or Mumormycosis

Adult: **PO/IV** Loading dose of 372 mg q8h for 6 doses; then 372 mg; **PO** once daily

ADMINISTRATION

Oral

- May be given without regard to food.
- Capsules must be swallowed whole; do not crush, dissolve, or open.
- Store at 15°–30° C (59°–86°F).

Intravenous

PREPARE: **IV Infusion:** Reconstitute by adding 5 mL of SW to vial to yield 1.5 mg/mL; shake gently to dissolve. Remove solution from vial and add to 250 mL of NS or D5W. Mix gently and do not shake bag.

ADMINISTER: **IV Infusion:** Infuse over at least 1 h using an infusion set with an in-line filter (pore size 0.2 to 1.2 micron).

INCOMPATIBILITIES: **Solution/additive:** Do not mix with any other medication. Should only be administered with NS or D5W.

- Storage: Reconstituted solution may be stored below 25° C (77° F) for maximum 1 h prior to preparation of infusion solution. Infusion should be completed within 6 h of dilution at room temperature. If this is not possible, immediately refrigerate at 2°–8° C (36°–46°F) the infusion solution after dilution and complete the infusion within 24 h.

ADVERSE EFFECTS **CV:** Atrial fibrillation, atrial flutter, bradycardia, cardiac arrest, hypotension, palpitations, reduced QT interval, supraventricular extrasystoles, supraventricular tachycardia, thrombophlebitis, ventricular extrasystoles. **Respiratory:** Acute respiratory failure, bronchospasm, *cough*, *dyspnea*, tachypnea. **CNS:** Anxiety, confusion, convulsion, depression, dysgeusia, encephalopathy, hallucination, *headache*, hypoesthesia, insomnia, migraine, peripheral neuropathy, paresthesia, somnolence, stupor, syncope, tremor delirium. **HEENT:** Optic neuropathy, tinnitus, vertigo. **Endocrine:** Hypoalbuminemia, hypoglycemia, *hypokalemia*, hypomagnesemia, hyponatremia, increased ALT/AST, increased blood alkaline phosphatase, increased blood bilirubin, increased gamma-glutamyltransferase. **Skin:** Alopecia, dermatitis, exfoliative dermatitis, erythema, petechiae, pruritus, rash, urticaria. **GI:** Abdominal distension, abdominal pain, *constipation*, *diarrhea*, dyspepsia, gastritis, gingivitis, *nausea*, stomatitis, *vomiting*. **GU:** Hematuria, proteinuria, renal failure. **Musculoskeletal:** *Back pain*, bone pain, neck pain. **Hematological:** Agranulocytosis, leukopenia, pancytopenia. **Other:** Chest pain, chills, decreased appetite, fatigue, hypersensitivity, injection site reactions, malaise, *peripheral edema*.

INTERACTIONS **Drug:** Coadministration with CYP3A4 inhibitors (e.g., **ketoconazole, lopinavir, ritonavir**) increases the levels of isavuconazole. Coadministration with CYP3A4 inducers (e.g., **rifampin**) decreases the levels of isavuconazole. Isavuconazole decreases the levels of **bupropion,** and **lopinavir/ritonavir,** and increases the levels of **atorvastatin, cyclosporine, digoxin, midazolam, mycophenolate mofetil, sirolimus,** and **tacrolimus.**

PHARMACOKINETICS **Absorption:** 98% bioavailable. **Peak:** 2–3 h. **Distribution:** Greater than 99% plasma protein bound. **Metabolism:** In liver after conversion to isavuconazole (active drug). **Elimination:** Renal (45.5%) and fecal (46.1%) **Half-Life:** 130 h.

I

NURSING IMPLICATIONS

Assessment & Drug Effects

- Monitor baseline ECG and frequently monitor BP during IV infusion.
- Monitor closely for infusion-related reactions (e.g., hypotension, dyspnea, chills, dizziness, paresthesia) or hypersensitivity reactions (e.g., severe skin reactions, Stevens–Johnson syndrome). Discontinue the infusion and notify prescriber if these reactions occur.
- Monitor lab tests: Baseline and periodic LFTs; serum electrolytes as indicated.

Patient & Family Education

- Report immediately if experiencing any of the following during IV infusion: Difficulty breathing, chills, dizziness, numbness and tingling, changes in sense of touch, skin rash.
- Report to prescriber if signs of liver injury develop (e.g., itchy skin, nausea or vomiting, yellowing of eyes, extreme fatigue, flu-like symptoms).

- Women who are or plan to become pregnant should consult prescriber regarding potential risks to fetus.
- Use effective means of contraception while taking this drug.
- Do not breastfeed while taking this drug.

ISOCARBOXAZID

(eye-soe-kar-box'a-zid)

Marplan

Classification: ANTIDEPRESSANT; MONOAMINE OXIDASE INHIBITOR (MAOI)

Therapeutic: ANTIDEPRESSANT

Prototype: Phenelzine

AVAILABILITY Tablet

ACTION & *THERAPEUTIC EFFECT* Inhibits monoamine oxidase, the enzyme involved in the catabolism of catecholamine neurotransmitters and serotonin. *Effectiveness as an antidepressant is due to its inhibition of MAO.*

USES Symptomatic treatment of depressed patients refractory to or intolerant of TCAs or electroconvulsive therapy.

CONTRAINDICATIONS Hypersensitivity to MAO inhibitors; pheochromocytoma; children (younger than 16 y); older adults (over 60 y) or debilitated patients; cardiac arrhythmias, hypertension, CVA; severe renal or hepatic impairment; history of headache; increased intracranial pressure, surgery; stroke, head trauma; suicidal ideation; lactation.

CAUTIOUS USE Hyperthyroidism, parkinsonism, epilepsy, schizophrenia; bipolar disorder; psychosis; suicidal risks; dental work; pregnancy (category C). Safety and efficacy in children not established.

ROUTE & DOSAGE

Refractory Depression

Adult: **PO** 10–30 mg/day in 1–3 divided doses (max: 30 mg/day)

ADMINISTRATION

Oral

- Note: Dosage is individualized on the basis of patient response. Lowest effective dosage should be used.
- Store in a tight, light-resistant container.

ADVERSE EFFECTS **CV:** *Orthostatic hypotension,* paradoxical hypertension, palpitation, tachycardia, other arrhythmias. **CNS:** Dizziness, light-headedness, tiredness, weakness, *drowsiness,* vertigo, headache, *overactivity,* hyperreflexia, muscle twitching, tremors, mania hypomania, *insomnia,* confusion, memory impairment. **HEENT:** *Blurred vision,* nystagmus, glaucoma. **GI:** Increased appetite, weight gain, *nausea,* diarrhea, *constipation, anorexia,* black tongue, *dry mouth,* abdominal pain. **GU:** Dysuria, *urinary retention,* incontinence, sexual disturbances. **Other:** Peripheral edema, excessive sweating, chills, skin rash, hepatitis, jaundice.

INTERACTIONS **Drug:** TRICYCLIC ANTIDEPRESSANTS, **fluoxetine,** AMPHETAMINES, **ephedrine, guanethidine, buspirone, methyldopa, dopamine, levodopa, tryptophan** may precipitate hypertensive crisis, headache, or hyperexcitability; **alcohol** and other CNS DEPRESSANTS compound CNS depressant effects; **meperidine** can cause fatal cardiovascular collapse; ANESTHETICS exaggerate hypotensive and CNS depressant effects; **metrizamide**

increases risk of seizures; compounds hypotensive effects of DIURETICS and other ANTIHYPERTENSIVE AGENTS. **Food:** All **tyramine**-containing foods (aged cheeses, processed cheeses, sour cream, wine, champagne, beer, pickled herring, anchovies, caviar, shrimp, liver, dry sausage, figs, raisins, overripe bananas or avocados, chocolate, soy sauce, bean curd, yeast extracts, yogurt, papaya products, meat tenderizers, broad beans) may precipitate hypertensive crisis. **Herbal: Ginseng, ephedra, ma huang, St. John's wort** may precipitate hypertensive crisis.

PHARMACOKINETICS Duration: Up to 2 wk. **Metabolism:** In liver.

NURSING IMPLICATIONS

Black Box Warning

Isocarboxazid has been associated with suicidal thinking and behavior in children, adolescents, and young adults.

Assessment & Drug Effects

- Monitor for and report promptly signs of clinical deterioration or suicidal ideation. Children, adolescents and young adults are at particular risk.
- Monitor for therapeutic effectiveness: May be apparent within 1 wk or less, but in some patients there may be a time lag of 3–4 wk before improvement occurs.
- Monitor BP. Monitor for orthostatic hypotension by evaluating BP with patient recumbent and standing.
- Check for peripheral edema daily and monitor weight several times weekly.
- Note: Toxic symptoms from over-dosage or from ingestion of contraindicated substances (e.g., foods high in tyramine) may occur within hours.
- Monitor I&O and bowel elimination patterns.

Patient & Family Education

- Monitor closely behavior of children, adolescents and young adults; report immediately unusual changes in behavior or suicidal ideation.
- Make position changes slowly and in stages; lie down or sit down if faintness occurs.
- Use caution when performing potentially hazardous activities.
- Consult prescriber before self-medicating with OTC agents (e.g., cough, cold, hay fever, or diet medications).
- Avoid alcohol and excessive caffeine-containing beverages and tryptophan and tyramine-containing foods including cheeses, yeast, meat extracts, smoked or pickled meat, poultry, or fish, fermented sausages, and overripe fruit.

ISOMETHEPTENE/ DICHLORALPHENAZONE/ ACETAMINOPHEN

(i-so-meth'ep-tene/di-chlor-al-phen'a-zone/a-cet'a-min-o-phen)

Duradrin, Nodolor, Migragesic IDA

Classification: SYMPATHOMIMETIC; NONNARCOTIC ANALGESIC

Therapeutic: ANTIMIGRAINE; NON-NARCOTIC ANALGESIC

Controlled Substance: Schedule C-IV

AVAILABILITY Capsule

ACTION & *THERAPEUTIC EFFECT*

Isometheptene is a sympathomimetic amine that acts by constricting cranial and cerebral arterioles. Isometheptene relieves vascular headaches. Dichloralphenazone is a mild sedative that helps reduce headache pain. Acetaminophen is a mild analgesic. *Effective as a mild sedative, reduces headache pain as well as being a mild analgesic.*

USES Relief for tension, vascular, and migraine headaches.

CONTRAINDICATIONS Patients with glaucoma; severe renal disease, organic heart disease; hepatic disease; concurrent MAO inhibitors.

I

CAUTIOUS USE Hypertension; peripheral vascular disease, and recent cardiovascular attacks; older adults; pulmonary disease; pregnancy (category C); lactation; children.

ROUTE & DOSAGE

Tension Headache

Adult: **PO** 1–2 capsules q4h up to 8 capsules/24 h

Migraine Headache

Adult: **PO** 2 capsules at onset, then 1 capsule qh until relief (max: 5 capsules/12 h)

ADMINISTRATION

Oral

- Do not give this drug to anyone who is concurrently using an MAOI. Allow 14 days to elapse between discontinuation of the MAOI and administration of this drug.
- Do not give more than 8 capsules in a 24 h period.
- Store at 15°–30° C (59°–86° F) in a dry place.

ADVERSE EFFECTS **CNS:** Transient dizziness. **GI:** Acetaminophen hepatotoxicity. **Skin:** Rash.

INTERACTIONS **Drug:** MAOIS may cause hypertensive crisis; other **acetaminophen**-containing drugs (including OTC) may increase risk of hepatotoxicity.

PHARMACOKINETICS **Absorption:** Rapidly absorbed. **Metabolism:** Dichloralphenazone is metabolized to an antipyrine. See ACETAMINOPHEN and for more detail. **Elimination:** Renal and hepatic. **Half-Life:** 12 h.

NURSING IMPLICATIONS

Assessment & Drug Effects

- Monitor BP closely with preexisting hypertension.
- Monitor lower extremity perfusion with a history of PVD.

Patient & Family Education

- Avoid, or moderate, alcohol use while taking this drug.
- Do not drive or engage in other potentially hazardous activities until response to drug is known.
- Report any decrease in tolerance to walking if you have a history of PVD.

ISONIAZID (ISONICOTINIC ACID HYDRAZIDE)

(eye-soe-nye′a-zid)

Isotamine ♣

Classification: ANTI-INFECTIVE; ANTITUBERCULOSIS

Therapeutic: ANTITUBERCULOSIS

AVAILABILITY Tablet; syrup; solution for injection

ACTION & *THERAPEUTIC EFFECT* Inhibits the synthesis of mycolic acids, an essential component of the bacterial cell wall. At therapeutic levels, isoniazid is bactericidal against actively growing intracellular and extracellular *Mycobacterium tuberculosis* organisms. *Exerts bacteriostatic action against actively growing tubercle bacilli; may be bactericidal in higher concentrations.*

USES Treatment of all forms of active tuberculosis caused by susceptible organisms; treatment of latent tuberculosis infection.

UNLABELED USES Treatment of nontuberculous mycobacterium.

CONTRAINDICATIONS Hypersensitivity to isoniazid or any component of the formulation; hepatic injury; acute liver disease; drug-induced hepatitis; lactation.

CAUTIOUS USE Chronic liver disease; HIV infection; hepatitis; severe renal dysfunction; history of convulsive disorders; chronic alcoholism; persons older than 50 y; pregnancy. (Benefits may outweigh the risks; use with caution during pregnancy.)

ROUTE & DOSAGE

Treatment of Active Tuberculosis

Adult/Adolescent/Child (over 40kg): **PO/IM** 5 mg/kg/dose daily(usual dose: 300 mg/day)
Child (less than 40 kg): **PO/IM** 10–15 mg/kg/dose daily (max: 300mg/day)

Latent Tuberculosis

Adult/Child: varies based on concurrent disease state and other agents; see package insert

ADMINISTRATION

Oral

- Give on an empty stomach at least 1 h before or 2 h after meals.

Intramuscular

- Note: Isoniazid solution for IM injection tends to crystallize at low temperatures; if this occurs, solution should be allowed to warm to room temperature to redissolve crystals before use.
- Give deep into a large muscle and rotate injection sites; local transient pain may follow IM injections.
- Store in tightly closed, light-resistant containers.

ADVERSE EFFECTS **CV:** Vasculitis. **CNS:** *Paresthesias, peripheral neuropathy,* hallucinations. **HEENT:** Optic neuritis, optic atrophy. **Endocrine:** Pyridoxine (vitamin B_6) deficiency, pellagra, gynecomastia, hyperglycemia, metabolic acidosis. **Skin:** Rash. **GI:** Nausea, vomiting, epigastric distress, pancreatitis; hepatotoxicity (*elevated AST, ALT;* bilirubinemia, jaundice, hepatitis). **Hematologic:** Agranulocytosis, hemolytic or aplastic anemia, thrombocytopenia, eosinophilia. **Other:** Drug-related fever, rheumatic and lupus erythematosus-like syndromes, irritation at injection site.

DIAGNOSTIC TEST INTERFERENCE Isoniazid may produce false-positive results using ***copper sulfate tests*** (e.g., ***Clinitest***)

INTERACTIONS **Drug:** **Cycloserine, ethionamide** enhance CNS toxicity; may increase **phenytoin, fosphenytoin** levels, resulting in toxicity; **methoxyflurane** increases risk of nephrotoxic metabolites; increases concentration of **lemborexant, lomitapide**. Do not use with LIVE VACCINES. **Food:** Food decreases rate and extent of isoniazid absorption; should be taken 1 h before meals.

PHARMACOKINETICS Absorption: Readily from GI tract; food may reduce rate and extent of absorption. **Peak:** 1–2 h. **Distribution:** Distributed to all body tissues and fluids including the CNS; crosses placenta. **Metabolism:** Inactivated by acetylation in liver. **Elimination:** 75–96% in urine in 24 h; excreted in breast milk. **Half-Life:** 1–4 h.

NURSING IMPLICATIONS

Black Box Warning

Isoniazid has been associated with severe, potentially fatal hepatitis.

Assessment & Drug Effects

- Withhold drug and notify prescriber immediately of a hypersensitivity reaction; generally occurs within 3–7 wk after initiation of therapy.
- Monitor for and report promptly signs of hepatic toxicity (see Appendix F).
- Monitor for and report promptly signs of peripheral neuritis (e.g., paresthesias of feet and hands with numbness, tingling, burning).
- Monitor BP during period of dosage adjustment. Some experience orthostatic hypotension; therefore, caution against rapid positional changes.
- Monitor diabetics for loss of glycemic control.
- Check weight at least twice weekly under standard conditions.
- Monitor lab tests: Baseline and periodic LFTs; sputum cultures monthly until 2 consecutive negative cultures reported.

Patient & Family Education

- Report promptly any of the following signs of liver toxicity: Unexplained weakness, nausea/vomiting, loss of appetite, dark urine, jaundice, clay-colored stools.
- Avoid or at least reduce alcohol intake while on isoniazid therapy because of increased risk of hepatotoxicity.

ISOPROTERENOL HYDROCHLORIDE (Pr)

(eye-soe-proe-ter′e-nole)

Isuprel

Classification: BETA-ADRENERGIC AGONIST; BRONCHODILATOR; CARDIAC STIMULATOR

Therapeutic: BRONCHODILATOR; ANTIARRHYTHMIC; CARDIAC STIMULATOR

AVAILABILITY Solution for injection

ACTION & THERAPEUTIC EFFECT Stimulates beta1-and beta2-receptors resulting in relaxation of bronchial, GI, and uterine smooth muscle, increased heart rate, and contractility, vasodilation of peripheral vasculature. *Reverses bronchospasm and facilitates removal of bronchial secretion. Increases cardiac output and cardiac workload. Also has antiarrhythmic properties by affecting AV node conduction.*

USES Reversible bronchospasm induced by anesthesia. As cardiac stimulant in cardiac arrest, carotid sinus hypersensitivity, cardiogenic and bacteremic shock, Adams-Stokes syndrome, or ventricular arrhythmias. Used in treatment of shock that persists after replacement of blood volume.

UNLABELED USES Treatment of status asthmaticus in children.

CONTRAINDICATIONS Preexisting cardiac arrhythmias associated with tachycardia; tachycardia caused by digitalis intoxication, central hyperexcitability, cardiogenic shock secondary to coronary artery occlusion and MI; ventricular fibrillation; angina.

CAUTIOUS USE Sensitivity to sympathomimetic amines; older adult and debilitated patients, hypertension, coronary insufficiency and other cardiovascular disorders, angina; renal dysfunction, hyper-thyroidism, diabetes, prostatic hypertrophy, glaucoma, tuberculosis; pregnancy (category C); lactation.

ROUTE & DOSAGE

Cardiac Arrhythmias/Cardiac Resuscitation

Adult: **IV** varies based on rhythm, range usually 2–10 mcg/min

ADMINISTRATION

Intravenous

Note: Maximum concentration on IV solution for both adults and children: 20 mcg/mL (0.02 mg/mL)

PREPARE: **Direct IV Injection for Adult with AV Block/Arrhythmia/Bradycardia/Cardiac Arrest:** Dilute 1 mL (0.2) of 1:5000 solution with 9 mL NS or D5W to produce a 1:50,000 (0.02 mg/mL) solution or use 1:50,000 solution undiluted. **Continuous Infusion for Adult with AV Block/Arrhythmia/Bradycardia/Cardiac Arrest:** Dilute 10 mL (2 mg) of 1:5000 solution in 500 mL D5W to produce a 1:250,000 (4 mcg/mL) solution. **IV Infusion for Adult with Shock Hypoperfusion:** Dilute 5 mL (1 mg) of 1:5000 solution in 500 mL D5W to produce a 1:500,000 (2 mcg/mL) solution. **Direct IV Injection for Adult with Bronchospasm:** Dilute 1 mL (0.2 mg) of 1:5000 solution with 9 mL NS or D5W to produce a 1:50,000 solution undiluted. **Continuous Infusion for Child with AV Block/Bradycardia:** Dilute to a range of 4–12 mcg/mL in 100 mL of D5W or NS.

ADMINISTER: **Direct IV for Adult/Child:** Give at a rate of 0.2 mg or fraction thereof over 1 min. ▪ Flush with 15–20 mL NS. **Continuous IV Infusion for Adult/Child:** Rate is adjusted according to patient response. Infusion rate is generally decreased or infusion may be temporarily discontinued if heart rate exceeds 110 bpm, because of the danger of precipitating arrhythmias. ▪ Microdrip or constant-infusion pump is recommended to prevent sudden influx of large amounts of drug. ▪ IV administration is regulated by continuous ECG monitoring. ▪ Patient **must be** observed and response to therapy **must be** monitored continuously.

INCOMPATIBILITIES: **Solution/additive: Aminophylline, furosemide, sodium bicarbonate. Y-site: Amphotericin B, azathioprine, dantrolene, diazepam, diazoxide, ganciclovir, gemtuzumab, ibuprofen, indomethacin, insulin, mitomycin, pentobarbital, phenytoin, sodium bicarbonate, SMZ/TMP.**

- Isoproterenol solutions lose potency with standing. ▪ Discard if precipitate or discoloration is present.

ADVERSE EFFECTS **CV:** Flushing, palpitations, tachycardia, unstable BP, anginal pain, ventricular arrhythmias. **CNS:** Headache, mild tremors, nervousness, anxiety, insomnia, excitement, fatigue. **GI:** Swelling of parotids (prolonged use), bad taste, buccal ulcerations (sublingual administration), nausea. **Acute Poisoning:** Overdosage, especially after excessive use of aerosols (*tachycardia,* palpitations, nervousness, nausea, vomiting). **Other:** Severe prolonged asthma attack, sweating, bronchial irritation and edema.

INTERACTIONS Drug: Epinephrine and other SYMPATHOMIMETIC AMINES, TRICYCLIC ANTIDEPRESSANTS increase effects and cause cardiac toxicity. HALOGENATED GENERAL ANESTHETICS exacerbate arrhythmias; while BETA-BLOCKERS antagonize effects.

I

PHARMACOKINETICS Absorption: Rapidly from parenteral administration. **Onset:** Immediate. **Metabolism:** Metabolized by COMT in liver, lungs, and other tissues. **Elimination:** 40–50% unchanged in urine.

NURSING IMPLICATIONS

Assessment & Drug Effects

- Check pulse before and during IV administration. Rate greater than 110 usually indicates need to slow infusion rate or discontinue infusion. Consult prescriber for guidelines.
- Incidence of arrhythmias is high, particularly when drug is administered IV to patients with cardiogenic shock or ischemic heart disease, digitalized patients, or to those with electrolyte imbalance.
- Note: Tolerance to bronchodilating effect and cardiac stimulant effect may develop with prolonged use.
- Note: Once tolerance has developed, continued use can result in serious adverse effects including rebound bronchospasm.

ISOSORBIDE DINITRATE

(eye-soe-sor'bide)

Coronex ♣, Dilatrate-SR, Iso-Bid, Isordil, Novosorbide ♣

Classification: NITRATE VASODILATOR

Therapeutic: VASODILATOR; ANTIANGINAL

Prototype: Nitroglycerin

AVAILABILITY Sublingual tablet; chewable tablet; tablet; capsule

ACTION & *THERAPEUTIC EFFECT* Relaxes vascular smooth muscle with resulting vasodilation. Dilation of peripheral blood vessels tends to cause peripheral pooling of blood, decreased venous return to heart, and decreased left ventricular end-diastolic pressure, with consequent reduction in myocardial oxygen consumption. *Has an antianginal effect as a result of vasodilation of the coronary arteries.*

USES Relief of acute anginal attacks and for management of long-term angina pectoris.

UNLABELED USES Alone or in combination with a cardiac glycoside or with other vasodilators (e.g., hydralazine, prazosin, for refractory CHF; diffuse esophageal spasm without gastro-esophageal reflux and heart failure).

CONTRAINDICATIONS Hypersensitivity to nitrates or nitrites.

CAUTIOUS USE Glaucoma, hypotension, hypovolemia; hypertrophic cardiomyopathy; older adults;

pregnancy (category C), lactation. Safety and efficacy in children not established.

ROUTE & DOSAGE

Angina Prophylaxis

Adult: **PO** 2.5–30 mg qid a.c. and at bedtime; **Sublingual tablet** 2.5–10 mg q4–6h; **Chewable tablet** 5–30 mg chewed q2–3h

Acute Anginal Attack

Adult: **PO Sublingual tablet** 2.5–10 mg q2–3h prn; **Chewable tablet** 5–30 mg chewed prn for relief

ADMINISTRATION

Oral

- Do not confuse with isosorbide, an oral osmotic diuretic.
- Give regular oral forms on an empty stomach (1 h a.c. or 2 h p.c.). If patient complains of vascular headache, however, it may be taken with meals.
- Advise patient not to eat, drink, talk, or smoke while sublingual tablet is under tongue.
- Instruct patient to place sublingual tablet under tongue at first sign of an anginal attack. If pain is not relieved, repeat dose at 5–10 min intervals to a maximum of 3 doses. If pain continues, notify prescriber or go to nearest hospital emergency room.
- Chewable tablet **must be** thoroughly chewed before swallowing.
- Have patient sit when taking rapid-acting forms of isosorbide dinitrate (sublingual and chewable tablets) because of the possibility of faintness.
- Store in a tightly closed container in a cool, dry place. Do not expose to extremes of temperature.

ADVERSE EFFECTS **CV:** Palpitation, postural hypotension, tachycardia. **CNS:** Headache, dizziness, weakness, *light-headedness*, restlessness. **Skin:** *Flushing*, pallor, perspiration, rash, exfoliative dermatitis. **GI:** Nausea, vomiting. **Other:** Hypersensitivity reaction, paradoxical increase in anginal pain, methemoglobinemia (overdose).

INTERACTIONS **Drug: Alcohol** may enhance hypotensive effects and lead to cardiovascular collapse; ANTIHYPERTENSIVE AGENTS, PHENOTHIAZINES add to hypotensive effects.

PHARMACOKINETICS **Absorption:** Significant first-pass metabolism with PO absorption, with 10–90% reaching systemic circulation. **Onset:** 2–5 min SL; within 1 h regular tabs; within 3 min chewable tabs; 30 min sustained release tabs. **Duration:** 1–2 h SL; 4–6 h regular tabs; 0.5–2 h chewable tabs; 6–8 h sustained release tabs. **Metabolism:** In liver. **Elimination:** 80–100% in urine within 24 h.

NURSING IMPLICATIONS

Assessment & Drug Effects

- Monitor effectiveness of drug in relieving angina.
- Note: Headaches tend to decrease in intensity and frequency with continued therapy but may require administration of analgesic and reduction in dosage.
- Note: Chronic administration of large doses may produce tolerance and thus decrease effectiveness of nitrate preparations.

Patient & Family Education

- Make position changes slowly, particularly from recumbent to upright posture, and dangle feet and ankles before walking.

- Lie down at the first indication of light-headedness or faintness.
- Keep a record of anginal attacks and the number of sublingual tablets required to provide relief.
- Do not drink alcohol because it may increase possibility of light-headedness and faintness.

ISOSORBIDE MONONITRATE

(eye-soe-sor′bide)

Ismo, Imdur, Monoket

Classification: NITRATE VASODILATOR

Therapeutic: ANTIANGINAL

Prototype: Nitroglycerin

AVAILABILITY Tablet; sustained release tablet

ACTION & *THERAPEUTIC EFFECT* Isosorbide mononitrate is a long-acting metabolite of the coronary vasodilator isosorbide dinitrate. It decreases preload as measured by pulmonary capillary wedge pressure (PCWP), and left ventricular end volume and diastolic pressure (LVEDV), with a consequent reduction in myocardial oxygen consumption. *It is equally or more effective than isosorbide dinitrate in the treatment of chronic, stable angina. It is a potent vasodilator with antianginal and antiischemic effects.*

USES Prevention of angina. Not indicated for acute attacks.

CONTRAINDICATIONS Hypersensitivity to nitrates.

CAUTIOUS USE Hypotension; hypertrophic cardiomyopathy; older adults; pregnancy (category B, C) depends on manufacturer; lactation. **Extended release form:** Should not be used in patients with GI disease (e.g., GI motility, malabsorption).

ROUTE & DOSAGE

Prevention of Angina

Adult: **PO Regular release (ISMO, Monoket)** 20 mg bid 7 h apart; **Sustained release (Imdur)** 30–60 mg every morning, may increase up to 120 mg once daily after several days if needed (max: 240 mg)

ADMINISTRATION

Oral

- Give first dose in morning on arising and second dose 7 h later with twice daily dosing regimen. Give in morning on arising with once daily dosing.
- Store sustained release tablets in a tight container.

ADVERSE EFFECTS **CV:** Aggravation of angina, abnormal heart sounds, murmurs, <u>MI</u>, transient hypotension, palpitations. **Respiratory:** Bronchitis, pneumonia, upper respiratory tract infection, nasal congestion, bronchospasm, coughing, dyspnea, rales, rhinitis. **CNS:** Headache, agitation, anxiety, confusion, loss of coordination, hypoesthesia, hypokinesia, insomnia or somnolence, nervousness, migraine headache, paresthesia, vertigo, ptosis, tremor. **HEENT:** Diplopia, blurred vision, photophobia, conjunctivitis. **Endocrine:** Hyperuricemia, hypokalemia. **Skin:** Rash, pruritus, hot flashes, acne, abnormal texture. **GI:** Nausea, vomiting, dry mouth, abdominal pain, constipation, diarrhea, dyspepsia, flatulence, tenesmus, gastric ulcer, hemorrhoids, gastritis, glossitis.

GU: Renal calculus, UTI, atrophic vaginitis, dysuria, polyuria, urinary frequency, decreased libido, impotence. **Hematologic:** Hypochromic anemia, purpura, thrombocytopenia, methemoglobinemia (high doses).

INTERACTIONS Drug: Alcohol may cause severe hypotension and cardiovascular collapse. **Aspirin** may increase nitrate serum levels. CALCIUM CHANNEL BLOCKERS may cause orthostatic hypotension.

PHARMACOKINETICS Absorption: Completely and rapidly absorbed from GI tract; 93% reaches systemic circulation. **Onset:** 1 h. **Peak:** Regular release 30–60 min; sustained release 3–4 h. **Duration:** Regular release 5–12 h; sustained release 12 h. **Metabolism:** In liver by denitration and conjugation to inactive metabolites. **Elimination:** Primarily by kidneys. **Half-Life:** 4–5 h.

NURSING IMPLICATIONS

Assessment & Drug Effects

- Monitor cardiac status, frequency and severity of angina, and BP.
- Assess for and report possible S&S of toxicity, including orthostatic hypotension, syncope, dizziness, palpitations, light-headedness, severe headache, blurred vision, and difficulty breathing.
- Monitor lab tests: Periodic serum electrolytes.

Patient & Family Education

- Do not crush or chew sustained release tablets. May break tablets in two and take with adequate fluid (4–8 oz).
- Do not withdraw drug abruptly; doing so may precipitate acute angina.
- Maintain correct dosing interval with twice daily dosing.
- Note: Geriatric patients are more susceptible to the possibility of developing postural hypotension.
- Avoid alcohol ingestion and aspirin unless specifically permitted by prescriber.

ISOTRETINOIN (13-*cis*-RETINOIC ACID)

(eye-soe-tret′i-noyn)

Amnesteem, Claravis, Sotret

Classification: ANTIACNE (RETINOID)

Therapeutic: ANTIACNE; ANTI-NEOPLASTIC

AVAILABILITY Capsule

ACTION & THERAPEUTIC EFFECT Decreases sebum secretion by reducing sebaceous gland size; inhibits gland cell differentiation; blocks follicular keratinization. *Has antiacne properties and may be used as a chemotherapeutic agent for epithelial carcinomas.*

USES Treatment of severe recalcitrant cystic or conglobate acne in patient unresponsive to conventional treatment, including systemic antibiotics.

UNLABELED USES Lamellar ichthyosis, oral leukoplakia, hyperkeratosis, acne rosacea, scarring gram-negative folliculitis; adjuvant therapy of basal cell carcinoma of lung and cutaneous T-cell lymphoma (mycosis fungoides); psoriasis; chemoprevention for prostate cancer.

CONTRAINDICATIONS Tinnitus; hypersensitivity to parabens (preservatives in the formulation), retinoid hypersensitivity, leukopenia,

I

neutropenia; UV exposure; pregnancy (category X), females of childbearing age; lactation.

CAUTIOUS USE Coronary artery disease; major depression, psychosis, history of suicides, alcoholism; hepatitis, hepatic disease; visual disturbance; rheumatologic disorders, osteoporosis; history of pancreatitis, inflammatory bowel disease; diabetes mellitus; obesity; retinal disease; elevated triglycerides, hyperlipidemia.

I

ROUTE & DOSAGE

Cystic Acne

Adult: **PO** 0.5–1 mg/kg/day in 2 divided doses (max recommended dose: 2 mg/kg/day) for 15–20 wk

Disorders of Keratinization

Adult: **PO** Up to 4 mg/kg/day in divided doses

ADMINISTRATION

Oral

- Give with or shortly after meals.
- Note: A single course of therapy provides adequate control in many patients. If a second course is necessary, it is delayed at least 8 wk because improvement may continue without the drug.
- Store in a tight, light-resistant container. Capsules remain stable for 2 y.

ADVERSE EFFECTS **Respiratory:** Epistaxis, *dry nose*. **CNS:** Lethargy, headache, fatigue, visual disturbances, pseudotumor cerebri, paresthesias, dizziness, depression, psychosis, suicide (rare). **HEENT:** Reduced night vision, dry eyes, papilledema, eye irritation, *conjunctivitis*, corneal opacities. **Endocrine:** Hyperuricemia, *increased serum concentrations of triglycerides by 50–70%*, serum cholesterol by 15–20%, VLDL cholesterol by 50–60%, LDL cholesterol by 15–20%. **Skin:** *Cheilitis*, skin fragility, dry skin, pruritus, peeling of face, palms, and soles; photosensitivity (photoallergic and phototoxic), erythema, skin infections, petechiae, rash, urticaria, exaggerated healing response (painful exuberant granulation tissue with crusting), brittle nails, alopecia. **GI:** *Dry mouth*, anorexia, nausea, vomiting, abdominal pain, nonspecific GI symptoms, acute hepatotoxic reactions (rare), inflammation and bleeding of gums, increased AST, ALT, acute pancreatitis. **Musculoskeletal:** Arthralgia; bone, joint, and muscle pain and stiffness; chest pain, skeletal hyperostosis (especially in athletic people and with prolonged therapy), mild bruising, decreased bone mineral density. **Hematologic:** Decreased Hct, Hgb, elevated sedimentation rate. **Other:** Most are dose-related (i.e., occurring at doses greater than 1 mg/kg/day), reversible with termination of therapy.

INTERACTIONS **Drug:** VITAMIN A SUPPLEMENTS increase toxicity; decreases effectiveness of ESTROGEN hormonal contraceptives in oral form as well as topical/injectable/implantable/insertable ESTROGEN hormonal birth control. Use with systemic CORTICOSTEROIDS or **phenytoin** may increase bone loss.

PHARMACOKINETICS Absorption: Rapid absorption after slow dissolution in GI tract; 25% of administered drug reaches systemic circulation. **Peak:** 3.2 h. **Distribution:** Not fully understood; appears in liver, ureters, adrenals, ovaries, and lacrimal glands. **Metabolism:** In liver; enterohepatically cycled. **Elimination:** In urine and feces in equal amounts. **Half-Life:** 10–20 h.

NURSING IMPLICATIONS

Black Box Warning

Isotretinoin has been associated with an extremely high risk of severe birth defects if pregnancy occurs while taking isotretinoin; it must not be used by women who are pregnant or who could become pregnant.

Assessment & Drug Effects

- Report signs of liver dysfunction (jaundice, pruritus, dark urine) promptly.
- Monitor closely for loss of glycemic control in diabetic and diabetic-prone patients.
- Monitor for development of depression and suicidal ideation.
- Note: Persistence of hypertriglyceridemia (levels above 500–800 mg/dL) despite a reduced dose indicates necessity to stop drug to prevent onset of acute pancreatitis.
- Monitor lab tests: Baseline lipid profile and repeat at 2 wk, 1 mo, and every month thereafter throughout course of therapy; LFTs at 2- or 3-wk intervals for 6 mo and once a month thereafter during treatment.

Patient & Family Education

- Rule out pregnancy within 2 wk of starting treatment. Use a reliable contraceptive 1 mo before, throughout, and 1 mo after therapy is discontinued.
- Maintain drug regimen even if during the first few weeks transient exacerbations of acne occur. Recurring symptoms may signify response of deep unseen lesions.
- Discontinue medication at once and notify prescriber if visual disturbances occur along with nausea, vomiting, and headache.
- Do not self-medicate with multivitamins, which usually contain vitamin A. Toxicity of isotretinoin is enhanced by vitamin A supplements.
- Avoid or minimize exposure of the treated skin to sun or sunlamps. Photosensitivity (photoallergic and phototoxic) potential is high.
- Notify prescriber immediately of abdominal pain, rectal bleeding, or severe diarrhea, which are possible symptoms of drug-induced inflammatory bowel disease.
- Keep lips moist and softened (use thin layer of lubricant such as petroleum jelly); dry mouth and cheilitis (inflamed, chapped lips), frequent adverse effects of isotretinoin.
- Notify prescriber of joint pain, such as pain in the great toe (symptom of gout and hyperuricemia).

ISOXSUPRINE HYDROCHLORIDE

(eye-sox'syoo-preen)

Classification: BETA-ADRENERGIC AGONIST; ALPHA-ADRENERGIC RECEPTOR INHIBITOR; VASODILATOR

Therapeutic: VASODILATOR

AVAILABILITY Tablet

ACTION & *THERAPEUTIC EFFECT* Sympathomimetic with beta-adrenergic stimulant activity and with an inhibitory effect on alpha receptors. Vasodilating action on arteries within skeletal muscles is greater than on cutaneous vessels. *Has both cerebral and peripheral vasodilatory properties.*

USES Treatment of cerebral vascular insufficiency and peripheral vascular disease, such as Raynaud's disease.

CONTRAINDICATIONS Immediately postpartum; presence of arterial bleeding; parenteral use in presence of hypotension, fetal distress; intrauterine fetal death; vaginal bleeding; tachycardia; presence of rash.

CAUTIOUS USE Bleeding disorders; severe cerebrovascular disease, severe obliterative coronary artery disease, recent MI; pregnancy (crosses the placenta; adverse effects observed in infants born to mothers who received isoxsuprine during pregnancy); lactation.

ROUTE & DOSAGE

Cerebral Vascular Insufficiency, Peripheral Vascular Disease

Adult: **PO** 10–20 mg tid or qid

ADMINISTRATION

Oral

- May give without regard to meals.
- Store at room temperature.

ADVERSE EFFECTS **CV:** Hypotension, tachycardia, chest pain. **CNS:** Dizziness. **GI:** Nausea, vomiting, abdominal distress. **Skin:** Skin rash.

INTERACTIONS Do not use with **tranylcypromine.**

PHARMACOKINETICS **Absorption:** Readily from GI tract. **Peak:** 1 h. **Duration:** 3 h. **Distribution:** Crosses placenta. **Elimination:** In urine. **Half-Life:** 1.25 h.

NURSING IMPLICATIONS

Assessment & Drug Effects

- Monitor for therapeutic effectiveness: Response to treatment of peripheral vascular disorders may take several weeks. Evaluate clinical manifestations of arterial insufficiency.
- Monitor BP and pulse; may cause hypotension and tachycardia. Supervise ambulation.
- Observe both mother and baby for hypotension and irregular and rapid heartbeat if isoxsuprine is used to delay premature labor.

Hypocalcemia, hypoglycemia, and ileus have been observed in babies born of mothers taking isoxsuprine.

Patient & Family Education

- Notify prescriber of adverse reactions (skin rash, palpitation, flushing) promptly; symptoms are usually effectively controlled by dosage reduction or discontinuation of drug.
- Prevent orthostatic hypotension by making position changes slowly and in stages, particularly from lying down to sitting upright and avoid standing still.
- Note: For treatment of menstrual cramps, isoxsuprine is usually started 1–3 days before onset of menstruation and continued until pain is relieved or menstrual flow stops.

ISRADIPINE

(is-ra′di-peen)

Classification: CALCIUM CHANNEL ANTAGONIST; ANTIHYPERTENSIVE

Therapeutic: ANTIHYPERTENSIVE; ANTIANGINAL

Prototype: Nifedipine

AVAILABILITY Capsule

ACTION & *THERAPEUTIC EFFECT* Inhibits calcium ion influx into cardiac muscle and smooth muscle without changing calcium concentrations, thus affecting contractility. Isradipine relaxes coronary vascular smooth muscle. It significantly decreases systemic vascular resistance. *Reduces BP at rest and during isometric and dynamic exercise. Reduces BP and has an antianginal effect.*

USES Mild to moderate hypertension.

UNLABELED USES Angina.

CONTRAINDICATIONS Hypersensitivity to isradipine.

CAUTIOUS USE CHF, heart failure; hypertrophic cardiomyopathy with outflow tract obstruction; aortic stenosis; acute MI, severe bradycardia, cardiogenic shock, ventricular dysfunction; mild renal impairment, hepatic impairment; GERD, hiatal hernia with esophageal reflux; older adult; pregnancy (category C); lactation. Safety and efficacy in children not established.

ROUTE & DOSAGE

Hypertension

Adult: **PO** 2.5 mg bid (max: 20 mg/day)

ADMINISTRATION

Oral

- Note: After the first 2–4 wk of therapy, dose may be increased for improved BP control in increments of 5 mg/day at 2–4 wk intervals up to a maximum dose of 20 mg/day.
- Store in a tight, light-resistant container.

ADVERSE EFFECTS CV: Flushing, ankle edema, palpitations, tachycardia, hypotension, chest pain, CHF.

Respiratory: Dyspnea. **CNS:** Headache, dizziness, fainting, fatigue, sleep disturbances, vertigo. **Skin:** Rash, decreased skin sensation. **GI:** Nausea, vomiting, abdominal discomfort, constipation, increased liver enzymes.

INTERACTIONS **Drug: Adenosine** may prolong bradycardia. May increase **cyclosporine** levels and toxicity. **Rifampin, phenytoin, carbamazepine** and other CYP3A4 inducers may decrease effect. **Food: Grapefruit juice** may increase side effects.

PHARMACOKINETICS **Absorption:** Rapidly and completely absorbed from GI tract, 95% protein bound, but only 15–24% reaches systemic circulation because of first-pass metabolism. **Onset:** 1 h. **Peak:** 2–3 h. **Duration:** 12 h. **Metabolism:** Extensive first-pass metabolism in liver. **Elimination:** 70% in urine as inactive metabolites; 30% in feces. **Half-Life:** 8 h.

NURSING IMPLICATIONS

Assessment & Drug Effects

- Monitor BP throughout course of therapy.
- Monitor patients with a history of CHF carefully, especially with concurrent beta-blocker use. Promptly report S&S of worsening heart failure.
- Monitor ambulation, especially with older adult patients, until response to drug is known.

Patient & Family Education

- Notify prescriber promptly of shortness of breath, palpitations, or other signs of adverse cardiovascular effects.
- Do not drive or engage in other potentially hazardous activities until response to drug is known.

ISTRADEFYLLINE

(is-tra-def-i-lin)

Nourianz

Classifications: ADENOSINE RECEPTOR ANTAGONIST

Therapeutic: ANTIPARKINSON

AVAILABILITY Oral tablet

ACTION & THERAPEUTIC EFFECT
Exact action is unknown, but studies suggest activity as an adenosine antagonist. *Works as an adjunctive treatment to levodopa/carbidopa in patients with Parkinson disease experiencing "off" episodes.*

USES Adjunctive treatment for patients with Parkinson disease experiencing "off" episodes.

CONTRAINDICATIONS Not recommended for patient with a major psychotic disorder; pregnancy—fetal risk cannot be ruled out; lactation—infant risk cannot be ruled out.

CAUTIOUS USE Patients with a history of compulsive behaviors.

ROUTE & DOSAGE

Parkinson's Disease, "off" Episodes

Adult: **PO** 20 mg once a day

Hepatic Impairment Dosage Adjustment

Child-Pugh class B: Maximum dose 20 mg/day
Child-Pugh class C: Avoid use

ADMINISTRATION

Oral

- May be given with or without food.

- Store at controlled room temperature between 20 and 25 degrees C (68 and 77 degrees F), with excursions permitted between 15 and 30 degrees C (59 and 86 degrees F).

ADVERSE EFFECTS **CNS:** *Dizziness, dyskinesia.* **GI:** *Nausea, constipation.* **Other:** Abnormal behavior, disturbance in thinking, *hallucinations.*

INTERACTIONS **Drug:** Strong CYP3A4 inducers (e.g. **rifampin, phenytoin, carbamazepine, efavirenz**, and **phenobarbital**) can decrease istradefylline levels. Strong CYP3A4 inhibitors (e.g., **ketoconazole, clarithromycin**) can increase istradefylline levels—in this case max dose of istradefylline should be 20 mg **Herbal: St. John's wort** may decrease the levels of istradefylline.

PHARMACOKINETICS **Peak:** 3–4h. **Distribution:** 557 L; 98% protein bound. **Metabolism:** Primarily by CYP1A1 and CYP3A4 (major). **Elimination:** 48% excreted in feces; 39% in urine. **Half-Life:** 83 h.

NURSING IMPLICATIONS

Assessment & Drug Effects

- Monitor for improvement of tremor, sluggish movements, and gait disturbance.
- Monitor for new or exacerbation of dyskinesia.
- Monitor for behavioral changes, hallucinations and impulse control disorders.

Patient & Family Education

- Review adverse effects.
- Report any hallucinations or abnormal behaviors.
- Report any impulse control disorders such as pathological gambling, hypersexuality, or compulsive spending or eating.
- Female patients of childbearing potential to use contraception during therapy.
- Avoid the use of St. John's Wort during therapy.

ITRACONAZOLE

(i-tra-con'a-zole)

Onmel, Sporanox

Classification: ANTIBIOTIC; AZOLE ANTIFUNGAL

Therapeutic: AZOLE ANTIFUNGAL

Prototype: Fluconazole

I

AVAILABILITY Capsule; tablet; oral solution; solution for injection

ACTION & *THERAPEUTIC EFFECT* Interferes with formation of ergosterol, the principal sterol in the fungal cell membrane that, when depleted, interrupts fungal membrane functioning. *Antifungal properties affect the fungal cell membrane functioning.*

USES Treatment of systemic fungal infections caused by blastomycosis, histoplasmosis, aspergillosis, onychomycosis due to dermatophytes of the toenail with or without fingernail involvement; oropharyngeal and esophageal candidiasis; orally to treat superficial mycoses (*Candida*, pityriasis versicolor).

UNLABELED USES Systemic and vaginal candidiasis; meningitis.

CONTRAINDICATIONS Hypersensitivity to itraconazole; hypotension; CrCl less than 30 mL/min; ventricular dysfunction as in CHF; or history of CHF when treating onychomycosis; neuropathy; systemic candidiasis; lactation.

CAUTIOUS USE Hypersensitivity to other azole antifungals, achlorhydria; GERD; COPD, cystic fibrosis; dialysis; older adults, females of childbearing age; hepatic disease, hepatitis, HIV infection; hypochlorhydria; pulmonary disease; renal disease, renal impairment; valvular heart disease, ventricular dysfunction; angina, cardiac disease; pregnancy (category C). Safe use in children has not been established.

ROUTE & DOSAGE

Blastomycosis, Aspergillosis

Adult: **PO** 200–400 mg daily mg once daily and continue for at least 3 mo

Oropharyngeal Candidiasis (solution)

Adult: **PO** 200 mg daily for 1–2 wk

Esophageal Candidiasis

Adult: **PO** 100 mg daily for at least 3 wk (max: 200 mg/day)

Onychomycosis

Adult: **PO** 200 mg daily × 3 mo

Histoplasmosis

Adult: **PO** 200 mg daily then increase to max dose of 400 mg daily × 3 mo

ADMINISTRATION

Oral

- Give capsules with a full meal.
- Give oral solution without food. Liquid should be vigorously swished for several seconds and swallowed.
- Do not interchange oral solution and capsules.
- Do not give with proton pump inhibitors, H2-blockers, or antacids.
- Divide dosages greater than 200 mg/day into two doses.
- Store capsules at room temperature of 15°–25° C (59°–77° F). Protect from light and moisture.
- Store liquid at or below 25° C (77° F).

ADVERSE EFFECTS **CV:** Hypertension with higher doses, chest pain. **CNS:** Headache, dizziness, fatigue, somnolence, abnormal dreams, hearing loss (euphoria, drowsiness less than 1%). **Endocrine:** Gynecomastia, hypokalemia (especially with higher doses), hypertriglyceridemia. **Skin:** Rash, pruritus. **GI:** *Nausea, vomiting, dyspepsia, abdominal pain, diarrhea, anorexia, flatulence, gastritis*; elevations of serum transaminases, alkaline phosphatase, and bilirubin. **GU:** Decreased libido, impotence. **Other:** Severe toxicity (doses exceeding 400 mg daily have been associated with higher risk of hypokalemia, hypertension, adrenal insufficiency).

INTERACTIONS **Drug:** Use with **alfuzosin, alprazolam, buprenorphine,** ERGOT ALKALOIDS, **dofetilide, donepezil, doxorubicin, dronedarone, efavirenz, flibanserin, haloperidol, isavuconazonium, ivabradine, lomitapide, loperamide, lovastatin, lurasidone, methadone,** oral **midazolam, naloxegol, nisoldipine, pimavanserin, pimozide, quinidine, ranolazine, silodosin, simvastatin, thioridazine, ticagrelor triazolam, venetoclax, ziprasidone** is contraindicated. Itraconazole may increase levels and toxicity of **alprazolam, ergotamine,**

dihydroergotamine, ORAL HYPOGLYCEMIC AGENTS, **warfarin, ritonavir, indinavir, vinca alkaloids, busulfan, methylergonovine, midazolam, triazolam, diazepam, nifedipine, nicardipine, amlodipine, felodipine, lovastatin, simvastatin, cyclosporine, tacrolimus, methylprednisolone, digoxin.** Combination with **dofetilide, levomethadyl, oral midazolam, pimozide, quinidine, triazolam** may cause severe cardiac events including cardiac arrest or sudden death. Itraconazole levels are decreased by **carbamazepine, phenytoin, phenobarbital, isoniazid, rifabutin, rifampin. Herbal: St. John's wort** and **garlic** may decrease itraconazole levels.

PHARMACOKINETICS Absorption: Best when taken with food. **Onset:** 2 wk–3 mo. **Peak:** Peak levels at 1.5–5 h. Steady-state concentrations reached in 10–14 days. **Distribution:** Highly protein bound (greater than 99%), minimal concentrations in CSF. Higher concentrations in tissues than in plasma. **Metabolism:** Extensively in liver by CYP3A4, may undergo enterohepatic recirculation. **Elimination:** 35% in urine, 55% in feces. **Half-Life:** 34–42 h.

NURSING IMPLICATIONS

Black Box Warning

Itraconazole has been associated with worsening CHF in those with ventricular dysfunction and with serious adverse cardiac effects when coadministered with other drugs metabolized by the CYP450-3A4 pathway.

Assessment & Drug Effects

- Monitor cardiac status and liver function throughout therapy. Withhold drug and notify prescriber immediately if S&S of CHF, other cardiac dysfunction, or signs of liver dysfunction appear.
- Monitor for digoxin toxicity when given concurrently with digoxin.
- Monitor PT and INR carefully when given concurrently with warfarin.
- Monitor for S&S of hypersensitivity (see Appendix F); discontinue drug and notify prescriber if noted.
- Monitor lab tests: Baseline C&S and periodic LFTs especially in those with preexisting hepatic abnormalities.

Patient & Family Education

- Discontinue drug and report promptly to prescriber S&S of CHF (see Appendix F).
- Notify prescriber promptly for S&S of liver dysfunction, including anorexia, nausea, and vomiting; weakness and fatigue; dark urine and clay-colored stool.
- Note: Risk of hypoglycemia may increase in diabetics on oral hypoglycemic agents.
- Women should use effective means of contraception during and for 2 mo following termination of treatment.

IVABRADINE

(i-va-bra′deen)

Corlanor

Classification: ANTIARRHYTHMIC; HYPERPOLARIZATION-ACTIVATED CYCLIC NUCLEOTIDE-GATED (HCN) CHANNEL BLOCKER

Therapeutic: ANTIARRHYTHMIC

AVAILABILITY Tablets

I

ACTION & *THERAPEUTIC EFFECT*

Blocks the hyperpolarization-activated cyclic nucleotide-gated (HCN) channel responsible for the cardiac pacemaker current which regulates heart rate. *Reduces the resting heart rate.*

USES Reduction of the risk of hospitalization for worsening heart failure in patients with stable, symptomatic chronic heart failure with left ventricular ejection fraction 35% or less, who are in sinus rhythm with resting heart rate of 70 or more beats per minute and either are on maximally tolerated doses of beta-blockers or have a contraindication to beta-blocker use.

CONTRAINDICATIONS Acute decompensated heart failure; BP less than 90/50 mm Hg; sick sinus syndrome, sinoatrial block or 3rd degree AV block, unless a functioning demand pacemaker is present; resting HR less than 60 bpm prior to treatment; severe hepatic impairment (Child-Pugh class C); pacemaker dependence; concurrent strong CYP3A4 inhibitors; pregnancy; lactation.

CAUTIOUS USE Atrial fibrillation; decreases in HR; bradycardia symptoms; 2nd degree AV block; concurrent moderate CYP3A4 inhibitors or CYP3A4 inducers. Safety and efficacy in children younger than 18 y not established.

ROUTE & DOSAGE

Heart Failure

Adult: **PO** 5 mg bid; adjust depending on heart rate and tolerability; with conduction defects, start with 2.5 mg bid

Heart Rate Dosage Adjustments

Greater than 60 bpm: Increase dose by 2.5 mg up to max of 7.5 mg bid
Less than 50 bpm or S&S of bradycardia: Decrease dose by 2.5 mg; discontinue if patient is taking 2.5 mg bid

ADMINISTRATION

Oral

- Give with meals.
- Dose may be adjusted based on HR after 2 wk of treatment.
- Store at 15°–30° C (59°–86° F).

ADVERSE EFFECTS **CV:** Atrial fibrillation, *bradycardia, hypertension.* **HEENT:** Phosphenes, visual brightness.

INTERACTIONS **Drug:** Concomitant use of strong CYP3A4 inhibitors (e.g., AZOLE ANTIFUNGALS, MACROLIDE ANTIBIOTICS, HIV PROTEASE INHIBITORS, **nefazodone**) and moderate CYP3A4 inhibitors (e.g., **diltiazem, verapamil**) increases the levels of ivabradine. Concomitant use of CYP3A4 inducers (e.g., BARBITURATES, **phenytoin, rifampicin**) decreases the levels of ivabradine. **Food: Grapefruit** and grapefruit juice increase the levels of ivabradine. **Herbal: St. John's wort** decreases the levels of ivabradine.

PHARMACOKINETICS **Absorption:** 40% bioavailable. **Peak:** 1 h. **Distribution:** 70% plasma protein bound. **Metabolism:** Extensive first-pass metabolism in liver. **Elimination:** Renal and fecal. **Half-Life:** 6 h.

NURSING IMPLICATIONS

Assessment & Drug Effects

- Monitor ECG regularly for atrial fibrillation.
- Report promptly symptoms of atrial fibrillation, such as heart palpitations or racing, chest pressure, or worsening shortness of breath.
- Monitor HR and BP regularly. Report promptly HR outside the range of 50–60 bpm and BP less than 90/50 mm Hg.
- Monitor HR more frequently if dosage increased or decreased, or if receiving other negative chronotropes (e.g., amiodarone, beta-blockers, digoxin).
- Monitor for and promptly report S&S of worsening heart failure.

Patient & Family Education

- Notify prescriber promptly of any of the following: Symptoms of heart failure worsening; BP less than 90/50 mm Hg; resting HR less than 60; heart palpitations or racing; excessive fatigue or dizziness.
- Avoid drinking grapefruit juice and taking St. John's wort during treatment.
- Luminous phenomena may occur while taking this drug; experienced as temporary brightness in field of vision, or halos, or colored bright lights, usually triggered by sudden variations in light intensity, primarily during the first 2 mo of therapy.
- Use caution when driving or using machinery in situations where sudden changes in light intensity may occur (e.g., driving at night).
- Women should use effective means of contraception and notify prescriber of a known or suspected pregnancy.
- Do not breastfeed while taking this drug without consulting prescriber.

IVERMECTIN

(i-ver-mec'tin)

Stromectol

Classification: ANTHELMINTIC

Therapeutic: ANTHELMINTIC; ANTIPARASITIC

Prototype: Praziquantel

AVAILABILITY Tablet; skin lotion

ACTION & *THERAPEUTIC EFFECT*

A semisynthetic anthelmintic agent which is a broad-spectrum antiparasitic agent that causes an increase in permeability to chloride ions of the parasitic cell membrane, resulting in hyperpolarization of nerve or muscle cells of parasites. This results in their paralysis and cell death. *Causes cell death of parasites.*

USES Treatment of strongyloidiasis of the intestinal tract, onchocerciasis.

CONTRAINDICATIONS Hypersensitivity to ivermectin.

CAUTIOUS USE Asthma; moderate or severe hepatic disease; hyperreactive onchodermatitis; older adults; pregnancy (category C); lactation (infant risk cannot be ruled out); (**oral tablet**) children less than 15 kg of weight. (**Topical**) safety and efficacy not established in patients younger that 6 mo.

ROUTE & DOSAGE

Strongyloides

Adult/Child (weight 15 kg or greater): **PO** 200 mcg/kg × 1 dose

Onchocerciasis

Adult/Child (weight 15 kg or greater): **PO** 150 mcg/kg × 1 dose, may repeat q3–12mo prn

I

ADMINISTRATION

Oral

- Give tablets with water rather than any other type of liquid on an empty stomach.
- Store tablets below 30° C (86° F).

Topical

- **Lotion:** Apply to dry hair and scalp, leave on for 10 min, rinse with water. Wait 24 h then shampoo hair and scalp. Discard unused portion.
- **Cream:** Apply pea-sized amount to each affected area and apply as a thin film.
- Store topical cream or lotion between 15°–30° C (59°–86° F).

ADVERSE EFFECTS **Skin:** Pruritis, rash. **Musculoskeletal:** Joint pain, synovitis. **Hematologic:** Lymphadenitis. **Other:** Fever

INTERACTIONS **Drug:** May increase effect of **warfarin.** Avoid LIVE VACCINES.

PHARMACOKINETICS **Peak:** 4 h. **Distribution:** Distributed into breast milk. **Metabolism:** In the liver. **Elimination:** In feces over 12 days. **Half-Life:** 16 h.

NURSING IMPLICATIONS

Assessment & Drug Effects

- Monitor for therapeutic effectiveness: Indicated by negative stool samples.
- Monitor for cardiovascular effects such as orthostatic hypotension and tachycardia.
- Monitor for and report inflammatory conditions of the eyes.
- Monitor lab tests: Stool culture per mo then 3 mo following therapy.

Patient & Family Education

- Get a follow-up stool examination to determine effectiveness of treatment. Treatment for worms does not kill adult parasites; repeated follow-up and retreatment are usually needed.
- Notify prescriber if eye discomfort develops.

IXABEPILONE

(ix-a-be-pi′lone)

Ixempra

Classification: ANTINEOPLASTIC; EPOTHILONE

Therapeutic: ANTINEOPLASTIC; ANTIMITOTIC

AVAILABILITY Lyophilized powder for injection

ACTION & *THERAPEUTIC EFFECT* Binds directly to microtubules needed to form the spindles required in mitosis of dividing cells. *Blocks new cell formation during the mitotic phase of their cell division cycle, thus leading to cancer cell death.*

USES Metastatic or locally advanced breast cancer alone or in combination with capecitabine in patients who have failed therapy with an anthracycline and a taxane.

CONTRAINDICATIONS Polyoxyethylated castor oil hypersensitivity; hepatic impairment in patients with AST or ALT greater than 10 × ULN, and/or bilirubin greater than 3 × ULN; neutrophil count less than 1,500/mm^3 or platelet count less than 100,000/mm^3; concomitant use of capecitabine and bilirubin greater than 1 × ULN, or AST or ALT greater than 2.5 × ULN; grade 4 neuropathy or any other grade 4 toxicity; pregnancy—fetal risk cannot be ruled out; lactation—infant risk cannot be ruled out.

CAUTIOUS USE Hypersensitivity to ixabepilone; monotherapy of patients with hepatic impairment baseline values of AST or ALT greater than 5 × ULN; patients with preexisting cardiac history, myelosuppression.

ROUTE & DOSAGE

Breast Cancer

Adult: **IV** 40 mg/m^2 q3wk

Obesity Dosage Adjustment

BSA greater than 2.2 m^2: Dosage should be calculated based on 2.2 m^2 instead of actual m^2

Dosage Adjustments

- *Grade 2 neuropathy 7 days or more, or grade 3 neuropathy less than 7 days, or grade 3 toxicity other than neuropathy:* reduce dose by 20%
- *Neutrophil less than 500 cells/mm^3 7 days or more, or febrile neutropenia, or platelets less than 25,000/mm^3 or platelets less than 50,000/mm^3 with bleeding:* Reduce dose by 20%
- *Grade 3 neuropathy 7 days or more or disabling neuropathy, or any grade 4 toxicity:* Do not administer

Hepatic Impairment Dosage Adjustment in Monotherapy

- *AST and ALT 2.5–10 × ULN o and bilirubin 1–1.5 × ULN:* 32 mg/m^2
- *AST and ALT 10 time or more ULN and bilirubin greater than 1.5 × ULN but less than 3 × ULN:* 20–30 mg/m^2
- *AST and ALT greater than 10 × ULN or bilirubin greater than 3 × ULN:* Do not administer

ADMINISTRATION

Intravenous

This drug is a cytotoxic agent and caution should be used to prevent any contact with the drug. Follow institutional or standard guidelines for preparation, handling, and disposal of cytotoxic agents. Wear double gloves and protective gown. During administration, if there is a potential that the substance could splash or if the patient may resist, use eye/face protection.

PREPARE: **IV Infusion:** Supplied in a kit containing a powder vial and diluent vial. Allow kit to come to room temperature for 30 min before reconstitution. ▪ Slowly inject diluent into the powder vial to yield 2 mg/mL. Swirl gently and invert vial to dissolve. ▪ Further dilute in LR solution in DEHP-free bags. Select a volume of LR to produce a final concentration of 0.2–0.6 mg/mL. Mix thoroughly.

ADMINISTER: **IV Infusion:** Use DEHP-free infusion line with a 0.2–1.2-micron in-line filter. ▪ Infuse at a rate appropriate to the total volume of solution. Complete infusion within 6 h of preparation.

INCOMPATIBILITIES: **Solution/additive:** Diluents other than **lactated Ringer's injection** should not be combined with ixabepilone. **Y-site:** Do not use a Y-site connection with this drug.

- Store drug kit refrigerated at 2°–8° C (36°–46° F) in original packaging.
- Reconstituted solution may be stored in the vial for a maximum of only 1 h at room temperature/light.
- Once further diluted with lactated Ringer's injection, solution is stable at room temperature/light for 6 h.

ADVERSE EFFECTS (≥5%) **CNS:** Aesthenia, peripheral neuropathy. **Skin:** *Alopecia*, nail disorder, palmar-plantar erythrodysesthesia syndrome. **GI:** *Abdominal pain, anorexia, constipation, diarrhea, mucositis, nausea, stomatitis, vomiting*, taste disorder. **Musculoskeletal:** *Arthralgia, myalgia, musculoskeletal pain.* **Hematologic:** Anemia, leukopenia, *neutropenia.* **Other:** *Fatigue.*

INTERACTIONS **Drug:** Inhibitors of CYP3A4 (e.g., HIV PROTEASE INHIBITORS, MACROLIDE ANTIBIOTICS, AZOLE ANTIFUNGAL AGENTS) increase the plasma level of ixabepilone. Strong CYP3A4 inducers (e.g., **dexamethasone, phenytoin, carbamazepine, rifampin, rifabutin, phenobarbital**) decrease the plasma level of ixabepilone. Do not administer with LIVE VACCINES. Avoid **metronidazole** or **disulfram.** May enhance adverse effects with MYLEOSUPPRESSIVE AGENTS. **Food: Grapefruit** and **grapefruit juice** increase the plasma level of ixabepilone. **Herbal: St. John's wort** decreases the plasma level of ixabepilone.

PHARMACOKINETICS **Distribution:** 67–77% protein bound. **Metabolism:** In liver (CYP3A4). **Elimination:** Stool (major) and urine (minor). **Half-Life:** 52 h.

NURSING IMPLICATIONS

Black Box Warning

Ixabepilone in combination with capecitabine is contraindicated in patients with AST or ALT greater than 2.5 × ULN or bilirubin greater than 1 × ULN because of an increased risk of toxicity and neutropenia-related death.

Actions & Drug Effects

- Monitor for signs of an infusion-related hypersensitivity reaction.
- Monitor for and promptly report signs of peripheral neuropathy.
- Monitor lab tests: Baseline and periodic CBC with differential, platelet count, LFTs; periodic serum electrolytes.

Patient & Family Education

- Report promptly any of the following: Numbness and tingling of the hands or feet, S&S of infection (e.g., fever of 100.5° F or greater, chills, cough, burning, or pain on urination), hives, itching, rash, flushing, swelling, shortness of breath, difficulty breathing, chest tightness or pain, palpitations or unusual weight gain.
- Patient should avoid driving and other activities requiring mental alertness or coordination until drug effects are realized, as the medication may cause dizziness or somnolence.
- Avoid grapefruit or grapefruit juice while receiving this drug.
- Use effective contraceptive measures to prevent pregnancy.

IXEKIZUMAB

(ix′e′kiz-ue-mab)

Taltz

Classification: INTERLEUKIN-17A ANTAGONIST; IMMUNOSUPPRESSANT; MONOCLONAL ANTIBODY

Therapeutic: IMMUNOSUPPRESSANT

Prototype: Basiliximab

AVAILABILITY Solution for injection

ACTION & *THERAPEUTIC EFFECT* A humanized IgG4 monoclonal antibody that selectively binds with the interleukin 17A (IL-17A) cytokine and inhibits its interaction with the IL-17 receptor. *This action inhibits the release of proinflammatory cytokines and chemokines that are involved in the normal inflammatory and immune responses.*

USES Treatment of adults with moderate-to-severe plaque psoriasis who are candidates for systemic therapy or phototherapy.

CONTRAINDICATIONS Hypersensitivity to ixekizumab.

CAUTIOUS USE Immunosuppression, Crohn's disease, infection, inflammatory bowel disease, tuberculosis, vaccination, pregnancy, lactation, children.

ROUTE & DOSAGE

Psoriasis

Adult: **Subcutaneous** 160 mg at wk 0; then 80 mg q2wk for 6 doses; then 80 mg q4wk

ADMINISTRATION

Subcutaneous

- Available as a pre-filled syringe containing 80 mg ixekizumab. Each 160 mg dose is administered as 2 subcutaneous injections.
- Remove from refrigerator and allow to warm to room temperature for 30 min.
- Do not administer where skin is tender, bruised, erythematous, indurated, or affected by psoriasis.
- Rotate sites of injection.
- Discard syringe after each use.
- Store unopened pre-filled syringes in refrigerator at 2°–8° C (36°–46° F).

ADVERSE EFFECTS **Respiratory:** Upper respiratory tract infections. **Endocrine:** Neutropenia, thrombocytopenia. **GI:** Nausea. **Other:** Hypersensitivity, injection site reactions, tinea infections.

INTERACTIONS **Drug:** Ixekizumab can alter the formation of CYP450 enzymes and could possibly cause interactions with other drugs requiring these enzymes for metabolism.

PHARMACOKINETICS **Absorption:** Bioavailability is 60–81%. **Peak:** 4 days. **Metabolism:** Peptide degradation. **Half-Life:** 13 days.

NURSING IMPLICATIONS

Assessment & Drug Effects

- Assess for signs or symptoms of hypersensitivity, infection, active tuberculosis, and inflammatory bowel disease.

Patient & Family Education

- Notify healthcare provider if you have active tuberculosis or inflammatory bowel disease such as Crohn's disease or ulcerative colitis.
- You may have a greater chance of getting an infection. Wash hands often. Avoid people with colds or infections. Stay current on all of your vaccinations.
- Tell your healthcare provider if you are breastfeeding or if you are pregnant or planning to get pregnant.

KETOCONAZOLE

(ke-to-con'a-zol)

Extina, Nizoral, Xolegel

Classification: AZOLE ANTIFUNGAL

Therapeutic: AZOLE ANTIFUNGAL

Prototype: Fluconazole

AVAILABILITY Tablet; cream; shampoo; foam; gel

K

ACTION & THERAPEUTIC EFFECT

Interferes with formation of ergosterol, the principal sterol in the fungal cell membrane that, when depleted, interrupts membrane function by increasing its permeability. *Antifungal properties are related to the drug effect on the fungal cell membrane functioning.*

USES **Oral:** Severe systemic fungal infections. **Topical:** Tinea corporis and tinea cruris and in treatment of tinea versicolor (pityriasis), seborrheic dermatitis.

UNLABELED USES **Oral:** Onychomycosis, vaginal candidiasis, Cushing's syndrome associated with adrenal or pituitary adenoma; precocious puberty, and candidiasis prophylaxis.

K

CONTRAINDICATIONS Hypersensitivity to ketoconazole or any component in the formulation; chronic alcoholism, fungal meningitis; onychomycosis; ocular exposure, ophthalmic administration, acute or chronic liver disease; coadministration of dofetilide, quinidine, pimozide, methadone, disopyramide, dronedarone, and ranolazine.

CAUTIOUS USE Azole antifungal hypersensitivity; achlorhydria, hypochlorhydria; hypovolemia, asthma; alcoholism; older adult; HIV infection; hyperactive onchodermatitis; pregnancy (category C); lactation. Safe use in children younger than 2 y is not established.

ROUTE & DOSAGE

Fungal Infections

Adult: **PO** 200–400 mg once/day; **Topical** Apply 1–2 × day to affected area and surrounding skin
Child (2 y or older): **PO** 3.3–6.6 mg/kg/day as single dose (do not exceed adult doses)

Dandruff

Adult/Child: **Topical** Shampoo twice a week for 4 wk with at least 3 days between shampoos; **Topical (Extina)** Apply bid × 4 wk; **(Xolegel)** Apply daily × 2 wk

ADMINISTRATION

Oral

- Give with water, fruit juice, coffee, or tea; drug requires an acid medium for dissolution and absorption.
- Relieve nausea and vomiting during early therapy by taking drug with food and dividing into 2 daily doses.
- Do not give with antacids.
- Store in tightly covered container at 15°–30° C (59°–86° F) unless otherwise directed.

Topical

- Apply sufficient shampoo to produce lather to wash scalp and hair and gently massage over entire scalp area for 5 min, rinse hair thoroughly and repeat, leaving shampoo on scalp for 3 min. Rinse thoroughly.

ADVERSE EFFECTS **CV:** Cardiac dysrhythmia, prolonged QT interval, Torsades de pointes, ventricular arrhythmia. **Skin:** Mild transient erythema, severe irritation, pruritus, stinging. **GI:** *Nausea, vomiting,* anorexia, dry mouth, epigastric or abdominal pain, constipation, diarrhea, transient elevation in serum liver enzymes, <u>fatal hepatic necrosis</u> (rare). **GU:** Gynecomastia (males), breast pain; uterine bleeding, loss of libido, impotence, oligospermia, hair loss. **Hematologic:** With high doses, lowers serum testosterone and ACTH-induced corticosteroid serum levels, transient decreases in serum cholesterol and triglycerides; hyponatremia (rare). **Oral: Other:** Skin rash, erythema, urticaria, pruritus, angioedema, anaphylaxis. **Other:** Acute hypoadrenalism (reduction of adrenal stress syndrome), renal hypofunction.

INTERACTIONS **Drug: Alcohol** may cause sunburn-like reaction; ANTACIDS, ANTICHOLINERGICS, H_2-RECEPTOR ANTAGONISTS decrease ketoconazole absorption; **isoniazid, rifampin** increase ketoconazole metabolism, thus decreasing its activity; levels of **phenytoin** and ketoconazole decreased; do not use with BENZODIAZEPINEs; may increase levels of **cyclosporine** or **carbamazepine,** increasing the risk of toxicity; **warfarin** may potentiate hypoprothrombinemia; may increase ergotamine toxicity of **dihydroergotamine, ergotamine;** may increase concentration and toxicity of **trazodone.** Contraindicated with medications that prolong the QT interval (i.e., **dofetilide, dolansetron, donepezil,** etc.). Do not use with agents extensively metabolized by CYP 3A4 (e.g., **lovastatin, quinidine,** etc.). **Herbal: Echinacea** may increase risk of hepatotoxicity.

PHARMACOKINETICS **Absorption:** Erratically from GI tract (needs an acid pH); minimal absorption topically. **Peak:** 1–2 h. **Distribution:** Distributed to saliva, urine, sebum, and cerumen; CSF levels unpredictable; distributed into breast milk. **Metabolism:** In liver (CYP3A4). **Elimination:** Primarily in feces, 13% in urine. **Half-Life:** 8 h.

NURSING IMPLICATIONS

Black Box Warning

Ketoconazole has been associated with serious, potentially fatal, hepatotoxocity and QT prolongation when coadministered with dofetilide, quinidine, pimozide, methadone, disopyramide, dronedarone, and ranolazine.

Assessment & Drug Effects

- Monitor for S&S of hepatotoxicity (see Appendix F). Discontinue drug immediately to prevent irreversible liver damage and report to prescriber.
- Monitor lab tests: Baseline LFTs and repeat at least monthly throughout therapy. INR, adrenal function.

Patient & Family Education

- Report S&S of hepatotoxicity promptly to prescriber (see Appendix F).
- Do not drive or engage in potentially hazardous activities until response to drug is known.
- Avoid OTC drugs for gastric distress, such as Rolaids, Tums, Alka-Seltzer and check with prescriber before taking any other nonprescription medicines.
- Notify prescriber if skin condition fails to respond to topical therapy or worsens or if signs of irritation or sensitivity occur.

KETOPROFEN

(kee-toe-proe′fen)

Classification: NONSTEROIDAL ANTI-INFLAMMATORY DRUG (NSAID); ANTIPYRETIC
Therapeutic: ANALGESIC, NSAID
Prototype: Ibuprofen

AVAILABILITY Capsule; sustained release capsule

K

ACTION & *THERAPEUTIC EFFECT*

Nonsteroidal anti-inflammatory drug (NSAID) that inhibits both COX-1 and COX-2 enzymes; thus it also inhibits prostaglandin synthesis, and therefore interferes with the inflammatory process. It inhibits platelet aggregation and prolongs bleeding time. *Has analgesic, anti-inflammatory, antiarthritic, and antiplatelet properties.*

USES Acute or long-term treatment of rheumatoid arthritis and osteoarthritis; primary dysmenorrhea; symptomatic relief of postoperative, dental, and postpartum pain.

K

UNLABELED USES Reiter's syndrome, juvenile arthritis, acute gouty arthritis, biliary pain, renal colic.

CONTRAINDICATIONS Patient in whom aspirin, salicylate, or another NSAID induces asthma, urticaria, bronchospasm, severe rhinitis, shock; perioperatively for CABG surgery; renal nephritis, nephritic syndrome; pregnancy; lactation (infant risk cannot be ruled out).

CAUTIOUS USE History of GI disease, GI bleeding, active ulcer; renal or hepatic impairment, patient who may be adversely affected by prolongation of bleeding time; heart failure, fluid retention; hypertension; patient receiving diuretics; geriatric patient; anemia; dental work; myasthenia gravis. Safe use in children younger than 16 y not established.

ROUTE & DOSAGE

Arthritis

Adult: **PO** 75 mg tid or 50 mg qid (max: 300 mg/day) or **Sustained release** 200 mg daily

Geriatric: **PO** Start with 75 mg bid, or 50 mg tid; **Sustained release** 100–150 mg once daily

Mild to Moderate Pain, Dysmenorrhea

Adult: **PO** 25–50 mg q6–8h (max: 300 mg/day)

ADMINISTRATION

Oral

- Ensure that extended release capsule is swallowed whole. It should not be crushed or chewed.
- Give with food, milk, or prescribed antacid to reduce GI irritation.
- Store tablets at 15°–30° C (59°–86° F) in a tightly closed, light-resistant container unless otherwise directed.
- Store capsules and suppositories at 20°–25° C (68°–77° F). Protect from light and excessive heat and humidity.

ADVERSE EFFECTS **CNS:** CNS depression, CNS stimulation, headache. **Hepatic:** Increased LFTs. **GI:** Abdominal pain, constipation, diarrhea, flatulence, indigestion, nausea. **GU:** Renal impairment.

INTERACTIONS **Drug:** ORAL ANTICOAGULANTS, **heparin** may prolong bleeding time; may increase **lithium** toxicity; may increase **methotrexate** toxicity. Avoid use of other NSAIDS. Do not use with **cidofovir** or **ketorolac.** **Herbal:** **Feverfew, garlic, ginger, ginkgo** increase bleeding potential.

PHARMACOKINETICS **Absorption:** Readily from GI tract. **Onset:** 1–2 h. **Peak:** 1–2 h. **Duration:** 4–6 h. **Metabolism:** In liver. **Elimination:** Primarily in urine, some biliary excretion. **Half-Life:** 1.1–4 h.

NURSING IMPLICATIONS

Black Box Warning

Ketoprofen has been associated with increased risk of serious, potentially fatal, GI bleeding and cardiovascular thrombolytic events (e.g., MI and CVA); risk may increase with duration of use and may be greater in the older adult and those with risk factors for CV disease.

Assessment & Drug Effects

- Monitor for hypertension and report promptly S&S of CV thrombotic events (i.e., angina, MI, TIA, or stroke).
- Monitor for and report tinnitus, hearing impairment, and visual disturbance, especially during prolonged or high-dose therapy.
- Monitor for S&S of GI ulceration (e.g., stool for occult blood, persistent indigestion).
- Monitor lab tests: Baseline and periodic hemoglobin, renal function tests, CBC, and LFTs.

Patient & Family Education

- Report promptly signs of jaundice (see Appendix F) as well as the following: Blurred vision, tinnitus, urinary urgency or frequency, unexplained bleeding, weight gain with edema.
- Stop taking drug and report promptly to prescriber if you experience chest pain, shortness of breath, weakness, slurring of speech, or other signs of a cardiac or neurologic problem.
- Note: Alcohol, aspirin, or other NSAIDs may increase risk of GI ulceration and bleeding tendencies and therefore should be avoided.
- Do not drive or engage in potentially hazardous activities until response to drug is known.

KETOROLAC TROMETHAMINE

(ke-tor′o-lac)

Acular, Acular LS, Acuvail, SPRIX

Classification: ANALGESIC, NONSTEROIDAL ANTI-INFLAMMATORY DRUG (NSAID); ANTIPYRETIC

Therapeutic: NONNARCOTIC ANALGESIC; NSAID

Prototype: Ibuprofen

AVAILABILITY Tablet; solution for injection; ophthalmic solution; nasal spray

ACTION & *THERAPEUTIC EFFECT* It inhibits synthesis of prostaglandins by inhibiting both COX-1 and COX-2 enzymes. Is a peripherally acting analgesic. It inhibits platelet aggregation and prolongs bleeding time. *Exhibits analgesic, anti-inflammatory, and antipyretic activity. Effective in controlling acute postoperative pain.*

USES *Short-term* management of pain; ocular itching due to seasonal allergic conjunctivitis, reduction of postoperative pain and photophobia after refractive surgery.

CONTRAINDICATIONS Hypersensitivity to ketorolac; hypersensitivity reaction to aspirin, salicylates, or other NSAIDs; major surgery; severe renal impairment or at risk for renal failure due to volume depletion; perioperative use in CABG surgery for 10–14 days after; suspected or confirmed CV bleeding, hemorrhagic diathesis, incomplete hemostasis; patients with risk of bleeding; active or recent GI bleeding; history of GI bleeding or peptic ulcer; pre-op or intraoperatively; exfoliative dermatitis; in combination with other NSAIDs; during labor and delivery; lactation.

K

CAUTIOUS USE Impaired renal or hepatic function; liver disease; Crohn's disease or IBD; bleeding disorders; myelosuppressive chemotherapy; debilitated patients; DM; preexisting asthma; lactase deficiency; coagulation disorders; SLE; CHF; history of hypertension; older adults; pregnancy (category C); lactation. Safe use in children younger than 17 y for all other forms not established.

ROUTE & DOSAGE

Pain

Adult: **IV Loading Dose** 30 mg (15 mg if less than 50 kg); **IM** 30–60 mg loading dose, then 15–30 mg q6h [max: 150 mg/day on first day, then 120 mg subsequent days (30 mg load, then 15 mg q6h if less than 50 kg)]; **PO** (continuation of IV/IM therapy) 20 mg initial dose then 10 mg q6h prn (max: 40 mg/day) max duration all routes 5 days **Nasal Spray** 1 spray q6–8h (max: 8/day)
Geriatric: **IV Loading Dose** 15 mg; **IM** 30 mg loading dose, then 15 mg q6h; **PO** 5–10 mg q6h prn (max: 40 mg/day) max duration all routes 5 days
Child: **IM** 1 mg/kg (max: 30 mg); **IV** 0.5 mg/kg (max: 15 mg)

ADMINISTRATION

WARNING: Do not administer IV, IM, or PO ketorolac longer than 5 days.

Oral

- Give with food to reduce GI effects.

Instillation Ophthalmic

- Do not touch container to the eye when applying ophthalmic drops.

Intramuscular

- Inject IM drug slowly and deeply into a large muscle.
- Rotate injection sites to avoid injection site pain in patients receiving multiple doses.

Intravenous

PREPARE: **Direct:** Give undiluted.
ADMINISTER: **Direct:** Give IV bolus dose over at least 15 sec. Preferred method is to give through a Y-tube in a free-flowing IV.
INCOMPATIBILITIES: **Solution/additive:** **Haloperidol, hydroxyzine, meperidine, morphine, prochlorperazine, promethazine.** **Y-site:** **Acyclovir, amphotericin B, azathioprine, azithromycin, calcium chloride, capsofungin, chlorpromazine, dantrolene, diazepam, diazoxide, diltiazem, diphenhydramine, dobutamine, doxycycline, epirubicin, erythromycin, esmolol, fenoldopam, gemcitabine, gemtuzumab, haloperidol, hydroxyzine, idarubicin, labetalol, levofloxacin, metaraminol, midazolam, milrinone acetate, minocycline, nalbuphine, pantoprazole, papaverine, pentamidine, pentazocine, phentolamine, phenytoin, prochlorperazine, promethazine, protamine, pyridoxine, quinupristin/dalfopristin, rocuronium, sulfamethoxazole/trimethoprim, tolazoline, vancomycin, vecuronium, vinorelbine.**

- Store injection at 15°–30° C (59°–86° F).
- Store tablet at 20°–25° C (68°–77° F). Protect from light and humidity.

ADVERSE EFFECTS **CNS:** *Drowsiness*, dizziness, headache. **HEENT:**

Tinnitus. **GI:** *Nausea*, dyspepsia, GI pain, hemorrhage. **Other:** Edema, sweating, pain at injection site.

INTERACTIONS **Drug:** Do not use with other NSAIDs. Do not use with **cidofovir.** May increase **methotrexate** levels and toxicity; do not use with **pentoxifylline.** **Herbal: Feverfew, garlic, ginger, ginkgo** increase bleeding potential.

PHARMACOKINETICS **Peak:** 45–60 min. **Distribution:** Into breast milk. **Metabolism:** In liver. **Elimination:** In urine. **Half-Life:** 4–6 h.

NURSING IMPLICATIONS

Black Box Warning

Ketorolac has been associated with increased risk of serious, potentially fatal GI bleeding and cardiovascular events (e.g., MI & CVA); risk may be greater in the older adult and those with risk factors for CV disease. Ketorolac has also been associated with increased risk of bleeding.

Assessment & Drug Effects

- Correct hypovolemia prior to administration of ketorolac.
- Monitor urine output in older adults and patients with a history of cardiac decompensation, renal impairment, heart failure, or liver dysfunction as well as those taking diuretics. Discontinuation of drug will return urine output to pretreatment level.
- Monitor for S&S of GI distress or bleeding including nausea, GI pain, diarrhea, melena, or hematemesis. GI ulceration with perforation can occur anytime during treatment. Drug decreases platelet aggregation and thus may prolong bleeding time.
- Monitor for and report promptly S&S of CV thrombotic events (i.e., angina, MI, TIA, or stroke).
- Monitor for fluid retention and edema in patients with a history of CHF.
- Monitor lab tests: CBC, periodic serum electrolytes and LFTs; urinalysis (for hematuria and proteinuria) with long-term use.

Patient & Family Education

- Watch for S&S of GI ulceration and bleeding (e.g., bloody emesis, black tarry stools) during long-term therapy.
- Stop taking drug and report promptly to prescriber if you experience chest pain, shortness of breath, weakness, slurring of speech, or other signs of a cardiac or neurologic problem.
- Note: Possible CNS adverse effects (e.g., light-headedness, dizziness, drowsiness).
- Do not drive or engage in potentially hazardous activities until response to drug is known.
- Do not use other NSAIDs while taking this drug.

KETOTIFEN FUMARATE

(kee-toe-tye'fen)

Zaditor

See Appendix A-1.

LABETALOL HYDROCHLORIDE

(la-bet'a-lole)

Classification: ALPHA- and BETA-ADRENERGIC ANTAGONIST; ANTIHYPERTENSIVE

Therapeutic: ANTIHYPERTENSIVE

Prototype: Propranolol

AVAILABILITY Tablet; solution for injection

ACTION & *THERAPEUTIC EFFECT*

Acts as an adrenergic receptor blocking agent that combines selective alpha activity and nonselective beta-adrenergic blocking actions. The alpha blockade results in vasodilation, decreased peripheral resistance, and orthostatic hypotension. It has beta-blocking effects on the sinus node, AV node, and ventricular muscle, which lead to bradycardia, delay in AV conduction, and depression of cardiac contractility. *Effective in reducing blood pressure by vasodilation as well as depression of cardiac contractility.*

USES Hypertension, hypertensive emergency.

CONTRAINDICATIONS Bronchial asthma or obstructive airway disease; uncontrolled cardiac failure, heart block (greater than first degree), cardiogenic shock, severe bradycardia; systolic blood pressure less than 100 mm Hg; perioperative CABG pain; abrupt withdrawal; pregnancy—fetal risk cannot be ruled out.

CAUTIOUS USE Renal disease, renal failure, hepatic disease; well-compensated patients with history of heart failure; CHF; acute MI; coronary artery disease; pheochromocytoma; DM; major surgery; liver dysfunction, jaundice; diabetes mellitus; SLE; myasthenia gravis; PVD; older adults; lactation—infant risk is minimal. Safety and efficacy in children not established.

ROUTE & DOSAGE

Hypertension

Adult: **PO** 100 mg bid, may gradually increase to 200–400 mg bid (max: 1200–2400 mg/day); **IV** 5–20 mg slowly over 2 min, repeat q10min if needed (max: 300 mg total dose)

ADMINISTRATION

Oral

- Give with or immediately after food consistently. Food increases drug bioavailability.

Intravenous

Note: Amount of IV solution may be changed depending on patient status.

PREPARE: **Direct:** Give undiluted. **Continuous:** Dilute 200 mg in 160 mL of D5W, NS, D5/NS, LR, or other compatible IV solution to yield 1 mg/mL; or dilute 200 mg in 250 mL compatible IV fluid to yield approximately 2 mg/3mL.

ADMINISTER: **Direct:** Give a 20-mg dose slowly over 2 min. ▪ Maximum hypotensive effect occurs 5–15 min after each administration. **Continuous:** Normal rate is 2 mg/min. ▪ Controlled infusion pump device is recommended for maintaining accurate flow rate during IV infusion. ▪ Keep patient supine when receiving labetalol IV. ▪ Take BP immediately before administration. Rate is adjusted according to BP response. ▪ Discontinue drug once the desired BP is attained.

INCOMPATIBILITIES: **Solution/additive:** **sodium bicarbonate.** **Y-site:** **Acyclovir, albumin, amphotericin B cholesteryl, azathioprine, cangrelor, cefmandole, cefepime, cefoperazone, cefotaxime, cefoxitin, ceftaroline, ceftobiprole, ceftriaxone, cefuroxime, cloxacillin, dantrolene, diazepam, diazoxide, esomeprazole, foscarnet,**

fosfomycin, gemtuzumab, hydrocortisone, ibuprofen, ketorolac, lansoprazole, micafungin, mitomycin, paclitaxel, pantoprazole, penicillin, phenytoin, piperacillin/tazobactam, thiopental.

▪ Store at 2°–30° C (36°–86° F) unless otherwise advised. Do not freeze. ▪ Protect tablets from moisture.

ADVERSE EFFECTS (≥5%)

CNS: Dizziness. **Skin:** Tingling of skin. **GI:** Nausea. **Other:** Fatigue.

DIAGNOSTIC TEST INTERFERENCE

False increases in ***urinary catecholamines*** when measured by ***nonspecific trihydroxyindole (THI) reaction*** (due to labetalol metabolites); false positive ***urine amphetamine*** if measured by thin-layer chromatography or radioenzymatic assay; false positive aldosterone/renin ratio.

INTERACTIONS

Drug: Cimetidine may increase effects of labetalol; **glutethimide** decreases effects of labetalol; **halothane** adds to hypotensive effects; may mask symptoms of hypoglycemia caused by ORAL SULFONYLUREAS, **insulin;** BETA AGONISTS antagonize effects of labetalol. ANTIHYPERTENSIVES can increase risk of hypotension. ALPHA2 AGONISTS increase AV blocking effects. **Dronedarone, rivastigmine** increase risk of bradycardia.

PHARMACOKINETICS

Absorption: Readily from GI tract, only 25% reaches systemic circulation due to first pass metabolism. **Onset:** 20 min–2 h PO; 2–5 min IV. **Peak:** 2–4 h PO; 5–15 min IV. **Duration:** 8–24 h PO; 16–18 h IV. **Distribution:** Crosses placenta; distributed into breast milk. **Metabolism:** In liver (CYP2D6). **Elimination:** 60% in urine, 40% in bile. **Half-Life:** 3–8 h.

NURSING IMPLICATIONS

Assessment & Drug Effects

- Monitor BP and pulse during dosage adjustment period. Use standing BP as indicator for making dosage adjustments for oral drugs and assessing patient's tolerance of dosage increases. Take after patient stands for 10 min. Clarify with prescriber.
- Monitor BP at 5 min intervals for 30 min after IV administration; then at 30 min intervals for 2 h; then hourly for about 6 h; and as indicated thereafter.
- Monitor diabetic patients closely; drug may mask usual cardiovascular response to acute hypoglycemia (e.g., tachycardia).
- Maintain patient in supine position for at least 3 h after IV administration. Then determine patient's ability to tolerate elevated and upright positions before allowing ambulation. Manage this slowly.
- Monitor lab tests: Periodic LFTs and renal function tests.

Patient & Family Education

- Note: Postural hypotension is most likely to occur during peak plasma levels (i.e., 2–4 h after drug administration).
- Make all position changes slowly and in stages, particularly from lying to upright position. Older adult patients are especially sensitive to hypotensive effects.
- Do not drive or engage in other potentially hazardous activities until response to drug is known.
- Diabetics should closely monitor blood sugar for loss of glycemic control.

- Do not abruptly stop taking this drug. It is usually discontinued gradually.

LACOSAMIDE

(lac-os′a-mide)

Vimpat

Classification: ANTICONVULSANT

Therapeutic: ANTICONVULSANT

Controlled Substance: Schedule V

AVAILABILITY Tablet; oral solution; solution for injection

ACTION & *THERAPEUTIC EFFECT* Lacosamide selectively enhances slow inactivation of voltage-gated sodium channels, thus stabilizing hyperexcitable membranes and inhibiting repetitive neuronal firing. *Decreases frequency of partial-onset seizures in those treated with multiple antiepileptic drugs.*

L

USES Treatment of focal (partial) onset seizures; primary generalized tonic-clonic seizures.

UNLABELED USES Refractory status epilepticus.

CONTRAINDICATIONS Specific contraindications have not been determined; pregnancy—fetal risk cannot be ruled out; lactation—infant risk cannot be ruled out.

CAUTIOUS USE History of multiorgan hypersensitivity reactions; CrCl 30 mL/min or less; renal disease; hepatic impairment; history of suicidal tendencies, history of chronic depression; cardiovascular disease, cardiac conduction problems (e.g., second-degree AV block); myocardial ischemia, heart failure; seizure disorders; diabetic neuropathy; older adults. Safety and efficacy in children younger than 4 y not established.

ROUTE & DOSAGE

Focal (Partial) Onset Seizures

Adult: **PO/IV** 50–100 mg bid; may increase by 50 mg bid qwk to 100–200 mg bid. Note: Patients may be switched from PO to IV (or vice versa) using equivalent doses and administration frequency.

Generalized Tonic-Clonic Seizure

Adult: **PO/IV** 50 mg bid; may be increased at weekly intervals by 50 mg bid.

Hepatic Impairment Dosage Adjustment

Mild to moderate impairment: Reduce dose to 75% of dose

Severe impairment: Not recommended

Renal Impairment Dosage Adjustment

CrCl less than 30 mL/min: Reduce dose to 75%

ADMINISTRATION

Oral

- Do not abruptly stop medication; it should be withdrawn gradually, over a minimum of 1 wk.
- Tablets and oral solution may be given with or without food.
- Tablets should be given whole and not divided.
- For oral solution, use calibrated measuring device.
- Discard any unused oral solution 7 weeks after opening the bottle.
- Store tablets and solution at 20°–25° C (68°–77° F).

Intravenous

PREPARE: **IV Infusion:** May give undiluted or diluted in NS, D5W, LR.
ADMINISTER: **IV Infusion:** Preferably infuse over 30–60 min. For adults, may infuse over 15 minutes if needed.
INCOMPATIBILITIES: **Solution/additive:** Do not mix with other drugs.

- May be stored diluted for up to 26 h at 20°–25° C (68°–77° F). Excursions permitted between 15 and 30° C (59–86° F). Do not freeze. Once diluted, do not store for more than 4 hours at room temperature and discard any unused portion.

ADVERSE EFFECTS (≥5%) **CNS:** *Dizziness, headache.* **HEENT:** *Diplopia.* **Skin:** Pruritus. **GI:** *Nausea.*

INTERACTIONS **Drug:** May prolong QT interval when given with other drugs known to affect QT interval (e.g., ANTIARRYTHMICS, **astemizole, bepridil, droperidol**). **Mefloquine** decreases therapeutic effect.

PHARMACOKINETICS **Absorption:** Approximately 100% oral absorption. **Peak:** 1–4 h. **Distribution:** Less than 15% protein bound. **Metabolism:** Hepatic oxidation to less active metabolite (via CYP3A4, CYP2C9, CYP2C19). **Elimination:** Primarily fecal (95%). **Half-Life:** 13 h.

NURSING IMPLICATIONS

Assessment & Drug Effects

- Monitor for and record all seizure activity.
- Monitor for and report promptly suicidal behavior and ideation.
- Monitor closely patients with known cardiac conduction abnormalities. Baseline and periodic ECGs are recommended.
- Monitor older adults for adverse reactions after each upward dose titration. Institute safety precautions as needed to avoid injury from falls.
- Monitor lab tests: Periodic CBC with differential, especially with long-term therapy, lacosamide serum level, saliva level.

Patient & Family Education

- Exercise caution with hazardous activities until reaction to drug is known.
- Report promptly feelings of depression, unusual changes in mood or behavior, or thoughts of inflicting harm to self.
- Report any signs of liver toxicity: yellowing of the skin and the whites of the eyes, itching, abdominal pain, fatigue, loss of appetite, nausea, vomiting, rash, or fever.
- Report bothersome neurologic symptoms such as dizziness, loss of balance, and changes in vision.
- Do not abruptly stop taking this drug. It **must be** tapered off. Stopping abruptly can lead to a seizure.

LACTITOL

(lak-ti-tol)

Pizensy

Classifications: HYPEROSMOTIC LAXATIVE
Therapeutic: LAXATIVE; AMMONIUM DETOXICANT
Prototype: Mannitol

AVAILABILITY Oral solution

ACTION & THERAPEUTIC EFFECT
Lactitol is a sugar compound that exerts an osmotic effect, causing an influx of water into the intestine. *Works to produce a laxative effect.*

USES Treatment of chronic idiopathic constipation.

UNLABELED USES Prevention and treatment of hepatic encephalopathy.

CONTRAINDICATIONS Known or suspected mechanical gastrointestinal obstruction, galactosemia; pregnancy—fetal risk cannot be ruled out; lactation—infant risk cannot be ruled out.

CAUTIOUS USE Specific precautions have not been determined.

ROUTE & DOSAGE

Treatment of Chronic Idiopathic Constipation

Adult: **PO** 20 g once daily

Treatment of Hepatic Encephalopathy

Adult: **PO** Initially, 0.5g/kg/day in 2 divided doses

ADMINISTRATION

Oral

- Measure the 1-g or 20-g dose (from multidose bottle or unit-dose packets) and pour into an 8-ounce glass of water, juice, or other beverage (e.g., coffee, tea, soda) and stir thoroughly to dissolve.
- Drink entire contents of the glass.
- Administer with a meal.
- Administer other oral medications at least 2 hours before or 2 hours after lactitol administration.
- Store powder for solution at room temperature between 20 and 25 degrees C (68 and 77 degrees F), with excursions permitted between 15 and 30 degrees C (59 and 86 degrees F).

ADVERSE EFFECTS **Respiratory:** *Upper respiratory infection.* **GI:** *Flatulence.*

INTERACTIONS **Drugs:** May reduce absorption of other oral medications; separate from other medications by 2 hours.

PHARMACOKINETICS **Absorption:** Minimally absorbed. **Elimination:** Degraded into organic acids in colon. **Half-Life:** 2.4 h

NURSING IMPLICATIONS

Assessment & Drug Effects

- Monitor for regular bowel movements

Patient & Family Education

- Report persistent loose stools.
- Review adverse effects with patient and/or caregivers.
- Make sure to add to 8 ounces of water or other beverage and drink entire contents.
- Make sure to space out other oral medications at least 2 hours before or 2 hours after taking the drug.

LACTULOSE

(lak′tyoo-lose)

Cephulac, Chronulac

Classification: HYPEROSMOTIC LAXATIVE; NEUROLOGIC

Therapeutic: LAXATIVE; AMMONIUM DETOXICANT

AVAILABILITY Oral and rectal solution; syrup

ACTION & *THERAPEUTIC EFFECT* Reduces blood ammonia by acidifying colon contents, thus retarding diffusion of nonionic ammonia (NH_3) from colon to blood while promoting its migration from blood to colon. In the acidic colon, NH_3 is converted to nonabsorbable ammoniumions (NH_4^+) and is then expelled in feces. *Osmotic effect of* *lactulose moves water from plasma to intestines, softening stools, and stimulates peristalsis by pressure from water content of stool. Decreases blood ammonia in a patient with hepatic encephalopathy. Effectiveness is marked by improved EEG patterns and mental state (clearing of confusion, apathy, and irritation).*

USES Prevention and treatment of portal-systemic encephalopathy (PSE), including stages of hepatic precoma and coma, and by prescription for relief of chronic constipation.

UNLABELED USES To restore regular bowel habit posthemorrhoidectomy; to evacuate bowel in older adult patients with severe constipation after barium studies; and for treatment of chronic constipation in children.

CONTRAINDICATIONS Low galactose diet.

CAUTIOUS USE Diabetes mellitus; concomitant use with electrocautery procedures (proctoscopy, colonoscopy); older adult and debilitated patients; pregnancy (category B); lactation; children.

ROUTE & DOSAGE

Prevention and Treatment of Portal-Systemic Encephalopathy

Adult: **PO** 30–45 mL tid or qid adjusted to produce 2–3 soft stools/day
Adolescent/Child: **PO** 40–90 mL/day in divided doses adjusted to produce 2–3 soft stools/day
Infant: **PO** 2.5–10 mL/day in 3–4 divided doses adjusted to produce 2–3 soft stools/day

Management of Acute Portal-Systemic Encephalopathy

Adult: **PO** 30–45 mL q1–2h until laxation is achieved, then adjusted to produce 2–3 soft stools/day; **Rectal** 300 mL diluted with 700 mL water given via rectal balloon catheter, and retained for 30–60 min, may repeat in 4–6 h if necessary or until patient can take PO

Chronic Constipation

Adult: **PO** 30–60 mL/day prn
Child: **PO** 7.5 mL/day after breakfast

ADMINISTRATION

Oral

- Give with fruit juice, water, or milk (if not contraindicated) to increase palatability. Laxative effect is enhanced by taking with ample liquids. Avoid meal times.

Rectal

- Administer as a retention enema via a rectal balloon catheter. If solution is evacuated too soon, instillation may be promptly repeated.
- Do not freeze. Avoid prolonged exposure to temperatures above 30° C (86° F) or to direct light. Normal darkening does not affect action, but discard solution that is very dark or cloudy.

ADVERSE EFFECTS GI: Flatulence, borborygmi, belching, abdominal cramps, pain, and distention (initial dose); *diarrhea* (excessive dose); nausea, vomiting, colon accumulation of hydrogen gas; hypernatremia.

INTERACTIONS Drug: LAXATIVES may incorrectly suggest therapeutic action of lactulose.

PHARMACOKINETICS Absorption: Poorly absorbed from GI tract. **Metabolism:** In gut by intestinal bacteria.

NURSING IMPLICATIONS

Assessment & Drug Effects

- In children if the initial dose causes diarrhea, dosage is reduced immediately. Discontinue if diarrhea persists.
- Promote fluid intake (1500–2000 mL/day or greater) during drug therapy for constipation; older adults often self-limit liquids. Lactulose-induced osmotic changes in the bowel support intestinal water loss and potential hypernatremia. Discuss strategy with prescriber.

Patient & Family Education

- Laxative action is not instituted until drug reaches the colon; therefore, about 24–48 h is needed.
- Do not self-medicate with another laxative due to slow onset of drug action.
- Notify prescriber if diarrhea (i.e., more than 2 or 3 soft stools/day) persists more than 24–48 h. Diarrhea is a sign of overdosage. Dose adjustment may be indicated.

LAMIVUDINE

(lam-i-vu′deen)

Epivir, Epivir-HBV, Heptovir ♣

Classification: ANTIRETROVIRAL; NUCLEOSIDE REVERSE TRANSCRIPTASE INHIBITOR (NRTI)

Therapeutic: ANTIRETROVIRAL; NRTI

AVAILABILITY Tablet; oral solution

ACTION & *THERAPEUTIC EFFECT* Lamivudine is a synthetic nucleoside analog reverse transcriptase inhibitor. It inhibits the transcription of the HIV viral RNA chain as well as the hepatitis B viral RNA chain. *Antiviral action is effective against HIV viruses and hepatitis B (HBV) viral infections.*

USES HIV infection in combination with other retroviral agents; treatment of chronic hepatitis B.

CONTRAINDICATIONS Hypersensitivity to lamivudine; lactic acidosis; severe hepatomegaly; exacerbation of hepatitis B; immune reconstitution syndrome; pregnancy—fetal risk cannot be ruled out; lactation—infant risk cannot be ruled out.

CAUTIOUS USE Renal impairment, renal failure; diabetes mellitus; autoimmune disorders; obesity.

ROUTE & DOSAGE

HIV Infection

Adult/Adolescent/Child (25 kg or more): **Epivir PO** 150 mg bid or 300 mg daily
Child (over 3 y and 20–24 kg): **PO** 75 mg in morning and 150 mg in evening
Infant/Child (3 mo to 3 y): **Epivir PO** 4 mg/kg bid (max: 150 mg bid)

Renal Impairment Dosage Adjustment (Adult)

CrCl 30–49 mL/min: 150 mg daily; *15–29 mL/min:* 150 mg first dose, then 100 mg daily; *5–14 mL/min:* 150 mg first dose, then 50 mg daily; *less than 5 mL/min:* 50 mg first dose, then 25 mg daily

Chronic Hepatitis B

Adult: **Epivir-HBV PO** 100 mg daily

Adolescent/Child (2–16 y): **PO** 4 mg/kg bid (max: 150 mg)

Renal Impairment Dosage Adjustment (Adult)

CrCl 30–49 mL/min: 100 mg first dose, then 50 mg daily; *15–29 mL/min:* 100 mg first dose, then 25 mg daily; *5–14 mL/min:* 35 mg first dose, then 15 mg daily; *less than 5 mL/min:* 35 mg first dose, then 10 mg daily

ADMINISTRATION

Oral

- May be administered without regard to meals.
- Give Epivir bid in combination with AZT. The recommended dose for adults who weigh less than 50 kg (110 lb) is 2 mg/kg. Give Epivir-HBV daily; **do not** give in combination with AZT.
- Store solution at 20°–25° C (68°–77° F) tightly closed.

ADVERSE EFFECTS (≥5%) **Respiratory:** *Nasal symptoms, cough.* **CNS:** *Headache.* **Endocrine:** Lactic acidosis. **Hepatic:** Hepatomegaly. **GI:** *Nausea, diarrhea.* **Other:** Fever, malaise, fatigue.

INTERACTIONS **Drug:** Do not use with **emtricitabine** or **cladribine. Trimethoprim-sulfamethoxazole** increases serum levels of lamivudine. **Sorbitol** decreases concentration of lamivudine. **Herbal:** Do not use with **echinacea**.

PHARMACOKINETICS **Absorption:** Rapidly absorbed from GI tract (86% reaches systemic circulation). **Distribution:** Low binding to plasma proteins. **Metabolism:** Minimal. **Elimination:** Excreted primarily unchanged in urine. **Half-Life:** 2–4 h.

NURSING IMPLICATIONS

Black Box Warning

Lamivudine has been associated with severe, potentially fatal, lactic acidosis, hepatomegaly with steatosis, and exacerbations of hepatitis B.

Assessment & Drug Effects

- Monitor children closely for S&S of hepatic dysfunction, lactic acidosis (see metabolic acidosis Appendix F), and pancreatitis; if they occur, immediately stop drug and notify prescriber.
- Monitor for and report all significant adverse reactions.
- Monitor lab tests: Periodic CBC with differential, renal function tests, hepatitis B screening (baseline and at modification), Hepatitis C antibody testing prior to initiation or modification, LFTs, and serum amylase throughout therapy.

Patient & Family Education

- Report any of the following immediately: Nausea, vomiting, anorexia, abdominal pain, jaundice.
- Report any signs of infection (fever, pain, inflammation).
- Review adverse effects.
- Do not discontinue the drug unless directed by a healthcare professional.
- Note: The drug may cause redistribution or accumulation of body fat and the long-term effect of these conditions are unknown.

LAMOTRIGINE

(la-mo′tri-geen)

Lamictal, Lamictal CD, Lamictal ODT, Lamictal XR

Classification: ANTICONVULSANT

Therapeutic: ANTICONVULSANT

AVAILABILITY Tablet; chewable tablet; orally disintegrating tablet; extended release tablet

ACTION & *THERAPEUTIC EFFECT* May act by inhibiting the release of glutamate and aspartate, excitatory neurotransmitters at voltage-sensitive sodium channels, resulting in decreased seizure activity in the brain. This stabilizes neuronal membranes. *Effectiveness is measured by decreasing seizure activity.*

USES Treatment of focal (partial) onset seizures and generalized onset seizures, treatment of bipolar disorder (immediate release only).

UNLABELED USES Prevention of migraines.

CONTRAINDICATIONS Hypersensitivity to lamotrigine, development of any skin rash unless it is clearly not related to the drug; multiorganic hypersensitivity reactions; acute mania; suicidal ideation especially if severe or abrupt in onset; aseptic meningitis; pregnancy—fetal risk cannot be ruled out; lactation—infant risk cannot be ruled out. **Extended release:** not approved for children younger than 13 y. **Immediate release:** tablet not approved for children younger than 2 y.

CAUTIOUS USE Renal insufficiency, blood dyscrasias, bipolar disorder, history of suicidal tendencies; CHF, cardiac or liver function impairment; severe renal impairment; moderate to severe hepatic impairment; older adults. Safety and efficacy in acute treatment of a mood episode not established.

ROUTE & DOSAGE

Focal (Partial) Onset/Generalized Onset Seizures (Not Taking Interacting Medication)

Adult/Adolescent: **PO** 25 mg/day × 2 w then may increase to 50 mg/day × 2w, may increase by 50 mg/day q1–2w based on response.

Partial Seizures, Patients Receiving Drugs that Induce Metabolism

Adult: **PO** 50 mg/day for 2 wk, then 100 mg/day for 2 wk, may titrate by 100mg/day q1–2 w
Child (2–6 y): **PO** Dose individualized based on age and concurrent medications, see package insert.

Focal (Partial) Onset/Generalized Onset Seizures Taking Valproate

Adult: **PO** 25 mg every other day for 2 wk, then 25 mg daily for 2 wk, may increase by 25–50 mg q1–2w based on response.
Child (2–16 y): **PO** Dose individualized based on age and concurrent medications, see package insert.

Bipolar Disorder, Patients Not Receiving Valproate or Carbamazepine

Adult: **PO** 25 mg daily for 2 wk, then 50 mg daily for 2 wk, then 100 mg/day for 1 wk, then 200 mg daily

Bipolar Disorder, Patients Receiving Valproic Acid

Adult/Adolescent (16 y or older): **PO** 25 mg every other day for 2 wk, then 25 mg daily for 2 wk, then 50 mg daily for 1 wk, then 100 mg daily

Bipolar Disorder, Patients Receiving Drugs that Induce Metabolism

Adult/Adolescent (16 y or older): **PO** Start with 50 mg daily for 2 wk, then 100 mg/day for 2 wk, then 200 mg/day for 1 wk, then 300 mg/day

Hepatic Impairment Dosage Adjustment

Moderate: Reduce dose by 25%
Severe with Ascites Reduce dose by 50%

ADMINISTRATION

Oral

- *Orally disintegrating tablet (ODT)* should be placed on the tongue and moved around the mouth. It will rapidly disintegrate. It may be swallowed with/without water or food.
- Ensure that *chewable tablets* are chewed or crushed before being swallowed with a liquid.
- *Chewable dispersible tablets* may be swallowed whole, chewed, or mixed in water or diluted juice.
- When discontinued, drug should be tapered off gradually over a 2-wk period, unless patient safety is at risk.
- Storage of chewable, disintegrating and extended release tablets between 20–25° C (68–77° F) with excursions between 15–30° C (59–86° F). Store in a dry place and protect from light.

ADVERSE EFFECTS (≥5%) **Respiratory:** *Rhinitis*, pharyngitis. **CNS:** *Dizziness, ataxia, somnolence, headache*, aphasia, vertigo, confusion, weakness, tremor. **HEENT:** *Diplopia, blurred vision.* **Skin:** Rash (including Stevens–Johnson syndrome, toxic epidermal necrolysis), urticaria, pruritus, alopecia, acne. **GI:** *Nausea*, vomiting, anorexia, abdominal pain, diarrhea, dyspepsia. **GU:** Hematuria, dysmenorrhea. **Musculoskeletal:** Backache. **Other:** Fever.

DIAGNOSTIC TEST INTERFERENCE May cause false-positive in rapid urine drug screens (phencyclidine).

INTERACTIONS **Drug: Carbamazepine, phenobarbital, primidone, phenytoin, fosphenytoin, rifampin**, ORAL CONTRACEPTIVES induce lamotrigine metabolism and may decrease lamotrigine levels (dosage needs adjusted). CNS DEPRESSANT may have increased sedation. **Valproic acid** may increase risk of serious rash. Lamotrigine may decrease serum levels of **valproic acid**. May affect efficacy of ORAL CONTRACEPTIVES. Chronic **acetaminophen** use may affect serum concentrations of lamotrigine. Do not use with **mefloquine** or **topiramate**. **Herbal: Ginkgo** may decrease anticonvulsant effectiveness. **Evening primrose** oil may affect seizure threshold.

PHARMACOKINETICS **Absorption:** Readily from GI tract; 98% reaches systemic circulation. **Onset:** 12 wk. **Peak:** 1–4 h. **Distribution:** 55% protein bound; crosses placenta; distributed into breast milk. **Metabolism:** In liver to inactive metabolite. **Elimination:** Can induce own metabolism; excreted in urine. **Half-Life:** 25–30 h.

NURSING IMPLICATIONS

Black Box Warning

Lamotrigine has been associated with severe, potentially fatal, rashes especially during wk 2–8 of therapy.

Assessment & Drug Effects

- Withhold drug if rash develops and immediately report to prescriber.
- Monitor the plasma levels of lamotrigine and other anticonvulsants when given concomitantly.
- Monitor patients with bipolar disorder for worsening of their symptoms and suicidal ideation. Withhold the drug and immediately report to prescriber.
- Monitor for adverse reactions when lamotrigine is used with other anticonvulsants, especially valproic acid.
- Monitor for signs of an unexpected infection, bleeding, nuchal rigidity.
- Be aware of drug interactions and closely monitor when interacting drugs are added or discontinued.

Patient & Family Education

- Do not take drug if a skin rash develops. Contact your prescriber immediately.
- Notify prescriber for any of the following: Worsening seizure control, skin rash, ataxia, blurred vision or double vision, fever or flu-like symptoms.
- Report symptoms of depression, suicidal ideation, or behavioral or psychiatric adverse reactions.
- Do not drive or engage in other potentially hazardous activities until response to the drug is known.
- Women using oral contraceptives to avoid pregnancy should add a barrier contraceptive.
- Schedule periodic ophthalmologic exams with long-term use.
- Do not discontinue abruptly. It could lead to a seizure.

LANSOPRAZOLE

(lan′so-pra-zole)

Prevacid, Prevacid 24 HR

DEXLANSOPRAZOLE

DexiLant

Classification: PROTON PUMP INHIBITOR

Therapeutic: ANTIULCER; ANTISECRETORY

Prototype: Omeprazole

AVAILABILITY Sustained release capsule; orally disintegrating tablet; **Dexlansoprazole:** delayed release capsule

ACTION & *THERAPEUTIC EFFECT* Suppresses gastric acid secretion by inhibiting the H^+, K^+-ATPase enzyme [the acid (proton H^+) pump] in the parietal cells. *Suppresses gastric acid formation in the stomach.*

USES Short-term treatment of duodenal ulcer (up to 4 wk) and erosive esophagitis (up to 8 wk), pathologic hypersecretory disorders, gastric ulcers; in combination with antibiotics for *Helicobacter pylori*. Gastroesophageal reflux disease (GERD).

UNLABELED USES Stress gastritis prophylaxis.

CONTRAINDICATIONS Hypersensitivity to lansoprazole or dexlansoprazole; proton pump inhibitors (PPIs) hypersensitivity;

lactation (infant risk cannot be ruled out).

CAUTIOUS USE Hepatic impairment; gastric malignancy; older adults; history of phenylketonuria; history of lupus erythematosus; renal impairment; pregnancy (category B), infants.

ROUTE & DOSAGE

Duodenal Ulcer

Adult: **PO** 15 mg once daily

Erosive Esophagitis

Adult: **PO** 30 mg once daily × 8 wk, then decrease to 15 mg once daily; **(dexlansoprazole)** 60 mg daily

GERD

Adult/Adolescent: **PO** 15 mg once daily for up to 8 wk
Child (1–11 y, weight 30 kg or greater): **PO** 30 mg daily; *weight less than 30 kg:* 15 mg daily (max: 30 mg/day)

Hypersecretory Disorder

Adult: **PO** 60 mg once daily (max: 120 mg/day in divided doses), may need to be adjusted for hepatic impairment; **(dexlansoprazole)** 30 mg daily

NSAID-Associated Gastric Ulcer

Adult: **PO** 30 mg daily for up to 8 wk

H. pylori

Adult: **PO** 30 mg bid × 2 wk, in combination with antibiotics

Healing Erosive Esophagitis (Dexlansoprazole)

Adult: **PO** 60 mg daily for up to 8 wk

Maintenance of Healed Erosive Esophagitis (Dexlansoprazole)

Adult: **PO** 30 mg daily

Non-Erosive GERD (Dexlansoprazole)
Adult: **PO** 30 mg daily for 4 wk

Hepatic Impairment Dosage Adjustment

Severe hepatic disease (Child-Pugh class C): Reduce dose (max: 30 mg/day **dexlansoprazole**)

ADMINISTRATION

Oral

- *All forms:* Administer dosage 30 min a.c. Give once daily dose before breakfast.
- Give at least 30 min prior to any concurrent sucralfate therapy.
- Do not crush or chew capsules. Capsules can be opened and granules sprinkled on food or mixed with 40 mL of apple juice and administered through an NG tube. Do not crush or chew granules.
- Note: Disintegrating tablets contain phenylalanine and should not be used for patients with PKU. Capsule and syrup formulations do not contain phenylalanine.

ADVERSE EFFECTS **CNS:** Headache. **GI:** Abdominal pain, constipation, diarrhea.

INTERACTIONS **Drug:** May decrease **theophylline** levels. **Sucralfate** decreases lansoprazole bioavailability. May interfere with absorption of **ketoconazole, digoxin, ampicillin,** or IRON SALTS. Use with **warfarin** may increase INR. May alter **tacrolimus, bosutinib** concentration. May decrease absorption of **cefuroxime. Food:** Food reduces peak lansoprazole levels by 50%.

L

PHARMACOKINETICS **Absorption:** Rapidly from GI tract after leaving stomach. **Onset:** Acid reduction within 2 h; ulcer relief within 1 wk. **Peak:** 1.5–3 h. Dexlansoprazole has 2 peaks, at 1–2 h then at 4–5 h. **Duration:** 24 h. **Distribution:** 97% bound to plasma proteins. **Metabolism:** In liver via CYP2C19 and 3A4. **Elimination:** 14–25% in urine; part of dose eliminated in bile and feces. **Half-Life:** 1.5 h.

NURSING IMPLICATIONS

Assessment & Drug Effects

- Monitor for therapeutic effectiveness of concurrently used drugs that require an acid medium for absorption (e.g., digoxin, ampicillin, ketoconazole).
- Monitor lab tests: Periodic CBC, renal function tests, LFTs, and serum gastric levels, serum magnesium levels, serum vitamin B_{12}.

Patient & Family Education

- Inform prescriber of significant diarrhea.
- Inform prescriber of S&S of hypomagnesemia: Muscle spasms, or cramps, muscle weakness, abnormal eye movement.

LANTHANUM CARBONATE

(lan-tha′num)

Fosrenol

Classification: ELECTROLYTE AND WATER BALANCE AGENT; PHOSPHATE BINDER
Therapeutic: PHOSPHATE BINDER
Prototype: Sevelamer hydrochloride

AVAILABILITY Chewable tablet

ACTION & *THERAPEUTIC EFFECT* Lanthanum is used for the management of hyperphosphatemia in end-stage renal disease; it is a calcium/aluminum-free phosphate binding agent. It has a higher affinity for binding to phosphate than calcium or aluminum. Low systemic absorption minimizes the risk of aluminum intoxication and hypercalcemia. Lanthanum decreases phosphate absorption from the diet. *Lowers serum phosphate.*

USES Reduce serum phosphate levels in patients with end-stage renal disease.

CONTRAINDICATIONS Prior hypersensitivity to lanthanum carbonate, lactation.

CAUTIOUS USE Bowel obstruction, Crohn's disease, acute peptic ulcer, ulcerative colitis; pregnancy (category B); children younger than 18 y.

ROUTE & DOSAGE

Hyperphosphatemia

Adult: **PO** 1500 mg daily in divided doses then titrate to serum phosphate less than 6 mg/dL

ADMINISTRATION

Oral

- Give with or immediately after a meal.
- Tablets **must be** chewed completely before swallowing. Whole tablets should not be swallowed.
- Store at 15°–30° C (59°–86° F).

ADVERSE EFFECTS **CV:** Hypotension. **Respiratory:** Bronchitis, rhinitis. **CNS:** Headache. **GI:** *Nausea, vomiting, diarrhea,* abdominal pain, constipation. **Other:** Dialysis graft occlusion.

PHARMACOKINETICS **Absorption:** Minimal from GI tract. **Metabolism:** Not metabolized. **Elimination:** In feces. **Half-Life:** 53 h.

NURSING IMPLICATIONS

Assessment & Drug Effects

- Monitor for dialysis graft occlusion, as lanthanum therapy may increase occlusion risk.
- Monitor lab tests: Serum phosphate levels during dosage titration and regularly throughout treatment; periodic serum calcium, bicarbonate, and chloride.

Patient & Family Education

- Chew chewable tablets completely, then swallow.
- Report promptly any of the following: Headache, drowsiness, dizziness, fainting, confusion, irritability, nausea, vomiting, or loss of appetite.

LAPATINIB DITOSYLATE

(la-pa′ti-nib di-toe′si-late)

Tykerb

Classification: ANTINEOPLASTIC TYROSINE KINASE INHIBITOR

Therapeutic: ANTINEOPLASTIC

Prototype: Erlotinib

AVAILABILITY Tablet

ACTION & *THERAPEUTIC EFFECT*

An inhibitor of intracellular tyrosine kinase domains of both epidermal growth factor receptors [EGFR (ErbB1) and HER2 (ErbB2)] required for cell proliferation of certain breast cancers. *Inhibits ErbB-driven tumor cell growth in those who are positive for the HER2 receptor.*

USES Treatment of advanced or metastatic breast cancer in patients whose tumor overexpresses the human epidermal receptor type 2 (HER2) protein and who have received prior therapy.

CONTRAINDICATIONS Hypersensitivity to lapatinib, capecitabine, doxifluridine, 5-FU; decreased left ventricular ejection fraction (LVEF) of grade 1, that is below lower limits of normal (LLN); jaundice; severe hepatotoxicity to drug; development of interstitial lung disease or pneumonitis of at least Grade 3; hypokalemia, hypomagnesemia; females of childbearing age; pregnancy (category D); lactation.

CAUTIOUS USE Moderate to severe hepatic impairment; coronary artery disease; angina, cardiac arrhythmias, congenital QT_c prolongation syndrome. Safe use in children younger than 18 y not established.

L

ROUTE & DOSAGE

Breast Cancer (HER2-Positive Metastatic)

Adult: **PO** 1250 mg daily (in combination with capecitabine) until disease progression or unacceptable toxicity.

Hepatic Impairment Dosage Adjustment

Severe hepatic impairment (Child-Pugh class C): Reduce dose

Toxicity Dosage Adjustment

Grade 2 or more (excluding cardiac): Discontinue and restart at standard dose when toxicity improves to Grade 1

Decreased left ventricular ejection fraction: Discontinue treatment for at least 2 wk

Diarrhea: Interrupt therapy; reintroduce at lower rate.

ADMINISTRATION

Oral

- Give lapatinib at least 1 h before/after a meal.
- Give capecitabine with food or within 30 min after food.
- Note that concurrent use with strong CYP3A4 inhibitors/inducers should be avoided (see Drug Interactions). If concurrent use is necessary, dosage adjustments are required.
- Store at 15°–30° C (59°–86° F) in a tightly closed container.

ADVERSE EFFECTS **Respiratory:** Dyspnea. **CNS:** Headache, insomnia. **Skin:** Hand-foot syndrome, rash. **GI:** *Diarrhea,* indigestion, *nausea, vomiting.* **Musculoskeletal:** Backache, limb pain. **Other:** Fatigue.

L

INTERACTIONS **Drug:** INHIBITORS OF CYP3A4 (**ketoconazole, clarithromycin, atazanavir, indinavir, nefazodone, nelfinavir, ritonavir, saquinavir, telithromycin, voriconazole**) will increase lapatinib plasma level. INDUCERS OF CYP3A4 (**dexamethasone, phenytoin, carbamazepine, rifampin, rifabutin, rifapentine, phenobarbital**) will decrease lapatinib plasma level. Lapatinib can increase plasma levels of **theophylline** and **warfarin. Food: Grapefruit juice** may increase the plasma level of lapatinib; co-administration with food increases lapatinib plasma levels. **Herbal: St. John's wort** will decrease plasma levels of lapatinib.

PHARMACOKINETICS **Peak:** 4 h. **Distribution:** 9% plasma protein bound. **Metabolism:** Extensive hepatic metabolism. **Elimination:** Fecal (major) and renal (minor). **Half-Life:** 24 h.

NURSING IMPLICATIONS

Black Box Warning

Lapatinib has been associated with severe, potentially fatal, hepatotoxocity.

Assessment & Drug Effects

- Prior to initiating therapy, hypokalemia and hypomagnesemia should be corrected.
- Monitor cardiac status (i.e., LV ejection fraction, ECG with QT measurement) throughout therapy.
- Monitor for and report severe diarrhea as it may cause dehydration and serious electrolyte imbalances.
- Withhold drug and notify prescriber if changes in LFTs parameters are significant and/or S&S of hepatotoxicity appear (see Appendix F).
- Monitor for theophylline and warfarin toxicity with concurrent use.
- Monitor lab tests: Baseline and periodic serum electrolytes; baseline and q4–6 wk LFTs; periodic CBC with differential and platelet count, Hgb, Hct.

Patient & Family Education

- Adhere to directions regarding medication and food.
- Report promptly any of the following: Palpitations, shortness of breath, severe diarrhea.
- Do not take a double dose if the dose is missed.
- Do not eat grapefruit or drink grapefruit juice while taking lapatinib.
- Do not take St. John's wort or OTC medications for stomach ulcers while taking lapatinib unless approved by the prescriber.
- Women are advised to use effective means of contraception while taking lapatinib.

LATANOPROST

(la-tan'o-prost)

Xalatan

Classification: EYE PREPARATION; PROSTAGLANDIN

Therapeutic: PROSTAGLANDIN

AVAILABILITY Ophthalmic solution

ACTION & THERAPEUTIC EFFECT Prostaglandin analog that is thought to reduce intraocular pressure (IOP) by increasing the outflow of aqueous humor. *Reduces elevated intraocular pressure in patients with open-angle glaucoma.*

USES Treatment of open-angle glaucoma, ocular hypertension, and elevated intraocular pressure (IOP).

CONTRAINDICATIONS Hypersensitivity to latanoprost, benzalkonium chloride, or another component in the solution.

CAUTIOUS USE Active intraocular inflammation such as iritis or uveitis; ocular disease; patients at risk for macular edema; history of or active herpes simplex keratitis; hepatic or renal impairment; contact lens wearers; pregnancy (category C); lactation. Safety and efficacy in children not established.

ROUTE & DOSAGE

Glaucoma

Adult: **Ophthalmic** 1 drop in affected eye(s) daily in evening

ADMINISTRATION

Installation

- Ensure that contact lenses are removed prior to installation and not reinserted for 15 min after installation.
- Apply only to affected eye(s). Ensure that only one drop is instilled.
- Do not allow tip of dropper to touch eye.
- Wait at least 5 min before/after instillation of other eyedrops.
- Refrigerate at 2°–8° C (36°–46° F). Protect from light. Once opened, the container may be stored at room temperature up to 25° C (77° F) for 6 wk.

ADVERSE EFFECTS **HEENT:** *Conjunctival hyperemia, growth of eyelashes, ocular pruritus*, ocular dryness, visual disturbance, ocular burning, *foreign body sensation*, eye pain, pigmentation of the periocular skin, blepharitis, cataract, superficial punctate keratitis, eyelid erythema, ocular irritation, eyelash darkening, eye discharge, tearing, photophobia, allergic conjunctivitis, increases in iris pigmentation (brown pigment), conjunctival edema. **Skin:** Rash. **GI:** Abnormal liver function tests. **Other:** Headache, asthenia, flu-like symptoms.

INTERACTIONS **Drug:** Precipitation may occur if mixed with eyedrops containing **thimerosal**; space other EYE PREPARATIONS at least 5 min apart.

PHARMACOKINETICS **Absorption:** Absorbed through the cornea. **On-set:** 3–4 h. **Peak IOP Reduction:** 8–12 h. **Distribution:** Minimal systemic distribution. **Metabolism:** Hydrolyzed in aqueous humor to active form. **Elimination:** Renally excreted. **Half-Life:** 17 min.

NURSING IMPLICATIONS

Assessment & Drug Effects

- Withhold eyedrops and notify prescriber if acute intraocular inflammation (iritis or uveitis) or external eye inflammation are noted.

- Note that increased pigmentation of the iris and eyelid, and additional growth of eyelashes on the treated eye are adverse effects that may develop gradually over months to years.

Patient & Family Education

- Contact prescriber immediately if any ocular reaction occurs, especially conjunctivitis and lid reactions.
- Note: Increased pigmentation of the iris and eyelid, and additional growth of eyelashes on the treated eye, are possible adverse effects of this drug. Persons with light colored eyes receiving treatment to one eye may develop a darker eye.

L

LATANOPROSTENE BUNOD

(la-tan-oh-pros′teen-bu′nod)

Vyzulta

Classification: EYE PREPERATION; PROSTAGLANDIN

Therapeutic: PROSTAGLANDIN

Prototype: Latanoprost

AVAILABILITY Ophthalmic solution

ACTION & *THERAPEUTIC EFFECT* Prostaglandin analog that is thought to reduce intraocular pressure (IOP) by increasing the outflow of aqueous humor. *Reduces elevated intraocular pressure in patients with open-angle glaucoma or ocular hypertension.*

USES Treatment of open-angle glaucoma, ocular hypertension, and elevated intraocular pressure (IOP).

CAUTIOUS USE Active intraocular inflammation such as iritis or uveitis; patients at risk for macular edema; ocular disease; history of active herpes simplex keratitis; use with contact lens; safety in pregnancy has not been established (category C); use in patients 16 y or younger is not recommended due to pigmentation risk.

ROUTE & DOSAGE

Glaucoma

Adult: **Ophthalmic** 1 drop in affected eye(s) daily in evening

ADMINISTRATION

Installation

- Ensure that contact lenses are removed prior to installation and not reinserted for 15 min after installation.
- Appy only to affected eye(s). Ensure that only one drop is instilled.
- Do not allow tip of dropper to touch eye.
- Wait at least 5 min before/after use of other eyedrops.
- Store unopened bottles refrigerated at 2°–8° C (36°–46° F). Once opened, bottle may be stored at 2°–25° C (36°–77° F) for 8 wk.

ADVERSE EFFECTS **HEENT:** *Conjunctival hyperemia, growth of eyelashes, ocular pruritus*, application site pain, conjunctival hyperemia, eye irritation and pain, blurred vision. **Skin:** Increase in iris pigmentation (brown pigment).

INTERACTIONS **Drug:** NSAIDs may enhance or diminish therapeutic effect of prostaglandins, use with bimatoprost may increase intraocular pressure.

PHARMACOKINETICS **Absorption:** Minimal systemic absorption. **Peak:** 5 min (plasma). **Metabolism:** Latanoprostene bunod is metabolized to latanoprost acid (active agent) and butanediol mononitrate. **Elimination:** Occurs within 15 min of administration.

NURSING IMPLICATIONS

Assessment & Drug Effects

- Monitor IOP at baseline and periodically.

Patient & Family Education

- Notify prescriber of signs of an allergic reaction such as rash, hives, itching, or swelling of the eyes; wheezing, tightness in the chest or throat; trouble breathing, swallowing, or talking; unusual hoarseness; or swelling of the mouth, face, lips, tongue, or throat.

LEDIPASVIR AND SOFOSBUVIR

(le-di-pas′vir and so-fos′bu-vir)

Harvoni

Classification: ANTIVIRAL; DIRECT-ACTING ANTIVIRAL; VIRAL PROTEIN INHIBITOR; ANTIHEPATITIS

Therapeutic: ANTIHEPATITIS

AVAILABILITY Tablet

ACTION & *THERAPEUTIC EFFECT* Ledipasvir inhibits a protein (HCV NS5A) necessary for viral replication. Sofosbuvir is a prodrug converted to its active form (GS-461203) which inhibits an enzyme (S5B RNA-dependent RNA polymerase), essential for viral replication. *Inhibits replication of the HCV virus.*

USES Treatment of chronic hepatitis C (CHC) genotype 1 infection in adults.

CAUTIOUS USE Concurrent use of potent P-gp inducers (e.g., rifampin, St. John's wort) or amiodarone in combination with an additional direct-acting antihepaciviral agent.

ROUTE & DOSAGE

Chronic Hepatitis C Infection

Adult: 1 tablet (90 mg ledipasvir/400 mg sofosbuvir) once daily for 12–24 wk

ADMINISTRATION

Oral

- May be given without regard to food.
- Store below 30° C (86° F).

ADVERSE EFFECTS **CNS:** *Fatigue, headache,* insomnia. **Endocrine:** Elevated lipase, increased bilirubin. **GI:** Diarrhea, nausea.

INTERACTIONS **Drug:** Ledipasvir may increase the levels of other drugs that require P-gp or breast cancer resistance protein (BCRP). P-gp inducers (e.g., rifampin) may decrease the levels of ledipasvir and sofosbuvir. ANTACIDS, H_2-RECEPTOR ANTAGONISTS, and PROTON PUMP INHIBITORS may decrease the levels of ledipasvir. **Carbamazepine, oxcarbazepine, phenobarbital, phenytoin**, RIFAMYCINS, **ritonavir**, and **tipranavir** may decrease the levels of ledipasvir and sofosbuvir. **Simeprevir** may increase the levels of ledipasvir and sofosbuvir. Ledipasvir and sofosbuvir may increase the levels of **digoxin, rosuvastatin**, and **tenofovir. Herbal: St. John's wort** may decrease the levels of ledipasvir and sofosbuvir.

PHARMACOKINETICS **Peak:** Ledipasvir: 4–4.5 h. sofosbuvir: 0.8–1 h. **Distribution:** Ledipasvir greater than 99.8% plasma protein bound; sofosbuvir is 61–65% plasma protein bound. **Metabolism:** Minimal for ledipasvir; extensive for sofosbuvir (required for formation

L

of active metabolite). **Elimination:** Primarily fecal (86%) for ledipasvir; primarily renal (80%) for sofosbuvir. **Half-Life:** Ledipasvir, 47 h.; sofosbuvir, 27 h (active metabolite).

NURSING IMPLICATIONS

Assessment & Drug Effects

- Monitor ECG during first 48 h of treatment when used in combination with amiodarone and another hepatitis C direct-acting antiviral or in patients who discontinued amiodarone just prior to initiating sofosbuvir in combination with a direct-acting antihepaciviral.
- Monitor lab tests: Baseline and periodic LFTs and serum creatinine; baseline and periodic serum HCV-RNA, and repeat at end of treatment and during follow-up.

L

Patient & Family Education

- Do not take OTC drugs without consulting prescriber.
- Check heart rate daily during the first 2 wk of treatment. Report promptly if outside of the parameters set by prescriber.
- Do not breastfeed without consulting prescriber.

LEFLUNOMIDE

(le-flu′no-mide)

Arava

Classification: DISEASE-MODIFYING ANTIRHEUMATIC DRUG (DMARD)

Therapeutic: DISEASE-MODIFYING ANTIRHEUMATIC DRUG (DMARD)

AVAILABILITY Tablet

ACTION & *THERAPEUTIC EFFECT* An immunomodulator that demonstrates anti-inflammatory effects. Suppression of pyrimidine synthesis in T and B lymphocytes interferes with RNA and protein synthesis in cells that are involved in the inflammatory process within affected joints. This reduces cytokine and antibody-mediated destruction of the synovial joints by decreasing the inflammatory process. *Reduces the S&S of rheumatoid arthritis (RA), retards structural joint damage, and improves physical function.*

USES Active RA.

UNLABELED USES Juvenile idiopathic arthritis, psoriasis.

CONTRAINDICATIONS Hepatic disease; jaundice; lactase deficiency; hypersensitivity to leflunomide; patients with positive hepatitis B or C serology; malignancy, particularly lymphoproliferative disorders; severe immunosuppression; live vaccination, infants; uncontrolled infection; pregnancy; lactation.

CAUTIOUS USE Renal insufficiency; renal failure; hepatic impairment; alcoholism; immunosuppression; lactase deficiency; infection. Use in children younger than 18 y has not been fully studied.

ROUTE & DOSAGE

Rheumatoid Arthritis

Adult: **PO** Initiate with a loading dose of 100 mg/day × 3 days, then maintenance dose of 20 mg daily, may decrease to 10 mg/day if higher dose is not tolerated

ADMINISTRATION

Oral

- NIOSH recommends the use of single gloves by anyone handling intact tablets, capsules, or administering from a unit-dose package.

Double glove if cutting or crushing or manipulating or handling uncoated tablets. Wear eye/face protection if the formulation is hard to swallow or if the patient may resist, vomit, or spit up.
- Initiate with a 3-day loading dose followed by a lower maintenance dose.
- Store between 15°–30° C (59°–86° F) and protect from light.

ADVERSE EFFECTS **CV:** Hypertension. **Respiratory:** Respiratory tract infection, bronchitis, rhinitis. **CNS:** Dizziness, headache. **Skin:** Alopecia, rash. **Hepatic:** Abnormal hepatic function tests. **GI:** *Diarrhea*, abdominal pain, ulcers in the mouth, nausea, vomiting. **Musculoskeletal:** Back pain, weakness, inflammation of tendons.

INTERACTIONS **Drug: Rifampin** may significantly increase leflunomide levels; **cholestyramine, charcoal** decrease absorption; caution should be used with other hepatotoxic drugs. Do not use with LIVE VACCINES. Do not use with **teriflunomide**.

PHARMACOKINETICS **Absorption:** Approximately 80% reaches systemic circulation. **Peak:** 6–12 h for active metabolite. **Distribution:** Greater than 99% protein bound. **Metabolism:** Metabolized primarily to M1 (active metabolite). **Elimination:** 43% in urine, 48% in feces. **Half-Life:** 19 days for active metabolite.

NURSING IMPLICATIONS

Black Box Warning

Leflunomide has been associated with severe, potentially fatal, hepatotoxicity and embryo-fetal toxicity.

Assessment & Drug Effects
- Monitor carefully for and report immediately S&S of infection; withhold leflunomide if infection is suspected.
- Withhold drug and notify prescriber if S&S of hepatotoxicty appear (see Appendix F).
- Monitor BP and weight periodically. Doses greater than 25 mg/day are associated with a greater incidence of side effects such as alopecia, weight loss, and elevated liver enzymes.
- Monitor lab tests: Baseline screening to rule out hepatitis B or C; baseline then monthly × 6 WBC, platelet count, H&H, then q6–8 wk thereafter; baseline and monthly LFTs × 6 mo, then every 6–8 wks thereafter.

Patient & Family Education
- Use reliable contraception while taking leflunomide.
- Note: Both women and men need to discontinue leflunomide and undergo a drug elimination procedure prescribed by the prescriber BEFORE conception.
- Withhold drug if you develop an infection and notify the prescriber before resuming the drug.
- Notify prescriber about any of the following: Hair loss, weight loss, GI distress, bruising, bleeding, paleness, fatigue, fever, rash, or itching.
- Avoid live vaccines.

LENVATINIB
(len-va′ti-nib)

Lenvima

Classification: ANTINEOPLASTIC TYROSINE KINASE INHIBITOR
Therapeutic: ANTINEOPLASTIC
Prototype: Erlotinib

AVAILABILITY Capsules

ACTION & THERAPEUTIC EFFECT

A tyrosine kinase inhibitor of multiple receptors including vascular endothelial growth factor receptors, fibroblast growth factor receptors, and platelet derived growth factor receptors which are implicated in tumor angiogenesis, tumor growth, and cancer progression. *Interferes with development of blood vessels and essential cell components needed for thyroid tumor growth.*

USES Treatment of patients with locally recurrent or metastatic, progressive, radioactive iodine-refractory differentiated thyroid cancer (DTC).

CONTRAINDICATIONS Life-threatening hypertension; arterial thrombotic event; hepatic failure; nephrotic syndrome; GI perforation or life-threatening fistula; pregnancy; lactation.

CAUTIOUS USE QT prolongation; hypertension; mild-to-moderate liver or renal impairment. Safety and efficacy in children younger than 18 y not established.

ROUTE & DOSAGE

Thyroid Cancer

Adult: **PO** 24 mg once daily

Advanced Renal Cell Cancer

Adult: **PO** 18 mg once daily

Hepatocellular Carcinoma

Adult: **PO** 12 mg once daily

Hepatic Impairment Dosage Adjustment

Severe impairment (Child-Pugh class C): Decrease to 14 mg once daily

Renal Impairment Dosage Adjustment

Severe impairment (CrCL less than 30 mL/min): Decrease to 14 mg once daily (thyroid cancer) or 10 mg once daily (renal cell cancer)

Dose Adjustments for Persistent and Intolerable Grade 2 or Grade 3 Adverse Reactions or Grade 4 Laboratory Abnormalities

See package insert

ADMINISTRATION

Oral

- May give without regard to food at the same time each day.
- Swallow capsules whole or dissolve capsules in 1 tbsp of water or apple juice. Do not break or crush capsules and allow to sit for more than 10 min. Stir for at least 3 min. After drinking, add another 1 tbsp of water or apple juice to the glass and swirl a few times and swallow.
- Store at room temperature 15°–30° C (59°–86° F).

ADVERSE EFFECTS **CV:** *Hypertension, peripheral edema,* hypotension, prolonged QT interval. **Respiratory:** *Cough,* bloody nose, pulmonary edema. **CNS:** *Headache,* dizziness, insomnia. **Endocrine:** *Increased TSH level,* dehydration, hypokalemia, hypercalcemia, hypercholesterolemia, hypoalbuminemia, hypoglycemia, hypomagnesemia. **Skin:** *Hand-foot syndrome, impaired wound healing,* rash, alopecia, thickening of skin. **Hepatic:** Increased serum alkaline phosphate, hyperbilirubinemia, increased serum AST. **GI:** *Abdominal pain, anorexia,* *nausea, stomatitis, diarrhea, vomiting, constipation, weight loss,* indigestion, dry mouth, increased serum lipase. **GU:** *Proteinuria,* UTI. **Musculoskeletal:** Joint and muscle pain. **Hematologic:** Hemorrhage. **Other:** *Difficulty speaking, fatigue.*

INTERACTIONS **Drug:** Avoid use with other agents that impact QT prolongation.

PHARMACOKINETICS **Peak:** 1–4 h. **Distribution:** 98–99% plasma protein bound. **Metabolism:** In liver. **Elimination:** Fecal (64%) and renal (25%). **Half-Life:** 28 h.

NURSING IMPLICATIONS

Assessment & Drug Effects

- Monitor ECG at baseline and periodically thereafter; withhold drug and notify prescriber for QT prolongation or other arrhythmias.
- Monitor HR and BP and report promptly irregular heart rate and significant BP elevation.
- Withhold drug and notify prescriber for S&S of any of the following: Hepatic impairment, proteinuria, bleeding, arterial thrombotic events, cardiac dysfunction, or GI perforation or fistula formation.
- Monitor lab tests: Baseline and periodic thyroid function tests, renal function tests, LFTs, Hct & Hgb, serum electrolytes, and serum lipase.

Patient & Family Education

- If a dose is missed and cannot be taken within 12 h, skip that dose and take the next dose at the usual time.
- Monitor HR and BP regularly.
- Contact prescriber immediately for any of the following: S&S of cardiac impairment (e.g., shortness of breath, swelling of ankles, chest pain, or irregular heart beat); S&S of a stroke (e.g., numbness or weakness on one side of body, trouble speaking, sudden severe headache, sudden vision change); S&S of liver damage (e.g., jaundice, dark "tea colored" urine, light-colored stool); S&S of bleeding.
- Women should use an effective method of birth control during treatment and for at least 2 wk after the last dose of this drug.
- Do not breastfeed while taking this drug.

LESINURAD

(le-sin′-ure-ad)

Zurampic

Classification: ANTIGOUT; URIC ACID TRANSPORTER 1 (URAT 1) INHIBITOR

Therapeutic: ANTIGOUT

AVAILABILITY Tablets

ACTION & *THERAPEUTIC EFFECT* Decreases uric acid levels by inhibiting the function of uric acid transporter 1 (URAT1) and organic anion transporter 4 (OAT4). *These two transporter proteins are involved in the renal reabsorption of uric acid. URAT1 is responsible for the majority of the reabsorption of filtered uric acid from the renal tubular lumen, while OAT4 is a uric acid transporter associated with diuretic-induced hyperuricemia.*

USES Treatment of hyperuricemia associated with gout in patients who have not achieved target serum uric acid levels with a xanthine oxidase inhibitor alone. Lesinurad should be used in combination with a xanthine oxidase inhibitor.

CONTRAINDICATIONS Severe renal impairment (CrCL less than 30 mL/min), end stage renal disease, kidney transplant recipients, or patients on dialysis; tumor lysis syndrome or Lesch-Nyhan syndrome.

CAUTIOUS USE Hepatic disease, organ transplant, cardiac disease, renal impairment, secondary hyperuricemia, pregnancy, lactation.

ROUTE & DOSAGE

Hyperuricemia

Adult: **PO** 200 mg once daily

Hepatic Impairment Dosage Adjustment

Severe hepatic impairment (Child-Pugh class C): Not recommended

Renal Impairment Dosage Adjustment

CrCL less than 45 mL/min: Not recommended

ADMINISTRATION

Oral

- **Must be** coadministered with a xanthine oxidase inhibitor such as allopurinol or febuxostat.
- Administer in the morning with food and water at the same time as the morning dose of xanthine oxidase inhibitor
- If treatment with xanthine oxidase inhibitor is interrupted, lesinurad should also be interrupted. Failure to follow these instructions may increase risk of adverse renal events.
- Instruct patient to stay well-hydrated.

ADVERSE EFFECTS **CV:** Cardiovascular death, nonfatal myocardial infarction, nonfatal stroke. **CNS:** Headache. **GI:** Gastroesophageal reflux disease. **GU:** Nephrolithiasis, renal failure. **Hematological:** Increased serum creatinine. **Other:** Influenza.

INTERACTIONS **Drug:** Inhibitors of CYP2C9 (e.g., **fluconazole, amiodarone**) may increase the levels of lesinurad. Lesinurad can reduce the levels of **sildenafil** and **amlodipine** and may interfere with the actions of HORMONAL CONTRACEPTIVES. **Aspirin** at doses higher than 325 mg per day may decrease the efficacy of lesinurad in combination with allopurinol.

PHARMACOKINETICS **Absorption:** Bioavailability is 100%. **Peak:** 1–4 h. **Distribution:** 98% plasma protein bound. **Metabolism:** Hepatic oxidation by CYP enzymes. **Elimination:** Renal (63%) and fecal (32%). **Half-Life:** 5 h.

NURSING IMPLICATIONS

Black Box Warning

Lesinurad has lead to acute renal failure when given alone. It should only be used in combination with a xanthine oxidase inhibitor.

Assessment & Drug Effects

- Monitor serum creatinine and creatinine clearance levels. Report any signs or symptoms of nephrotoxicity.
- Monitor baseline and periodic uric acid levels.

Patient & Family Education

- Notify healthcare provider if you have kidney disease or a history of kidney transplant.
- Report any signs or symptoms of kidney problems such as difficulty

urinating, a change in the amount of urine, blood in the urine, or a significant weight gain.
- Report any signs or symptoms of an allergic reaction such as rash; hives; wheezing; tightness in the chest or throat; trouble breathing or talking; unusual hoarseness; or swelling of the face, lips, mouth, tongue, or throat.
- All forms of hormonal contraceptives may be less effective during therapy with lesinurad. Additional methods of contraception are recommended during therapy.
- Take this medication with a full glass of water; drink lots of non-caffeinated liquids each day unless told otherwise by your health care provider.

LETERMOVIR
(le-term′-oh-vir)
Prevymis
Classification: ANTIVIRAL
Therapeutic: ANTIVIRAL

AVAILABILITY Tablet; solution for injection

ACTION & THERAPEUTIC EFFECT
Interferes with DNA synthesis of CMV thereby inhibiting replication. *It reduces formation of new lesions and speeds healing time.*

USES Prophylaxis of CMV infection.

CONTRAINDICATIONS Co-administration with pimozide, ergot alkaloids, or cyclosprine and pitavastatin/simvastatin.

CAUTIOUS USE Not recommended in severe hepatic impairment, renal impairment (CrCl less than 50 mL/min), pregnancy, lactation.

ROUTE & DOSAGE

CMV Prophylaxis
Adult: **PO** 480 mg daily started between day 0–28 post transplant, continue through day 100 post transplant; **IV** Same as PO dose

ADMINISTRATION
Oral
- Swallow tablet whole. May give without regard to food.

Intravenous

PREPARE: **IV Infusion:** Vials are for single use only; do not shake the vials. Dilute contents of a single-use vial with 250 mL of NS or D5W only. Diluted solution may be colorless to yellow. ▪ Diluted solution is stable for up to 24 h at room temperature or up to 48 h if refrigerated at 2°–8° C (36°–46°F); time includes storage of the diluted solution through the duration of the infusion. ▪ Do not give as an IV bolus; give only as an IV infusion. ▪ Only use infusion sets made from PVC, polyethylene (PE), polybutadiene (PBD), silicone rubber (SR), styrene-butadiene copolymer (SBC) styrene-butadiene-styrene (SBS) or polystyrene (PS). ▪ Only use catheters made from radiopaque polyurethane.
ADMINISTER: **IV** Use only in patients unable to tolerate oral therapy. Administer infusion over 1 h via peripheral or central venous catheter. Do not administer with poly-urethane containing IV administration sets.
INCOMPATIBILITIES: **New medication.** Drug incompatibilities have not been tested. Do not use with polyurethane containing tubing.

ADVERSE EFFECTS CV: Peripheral edema, tachycardia, atrial fibrillation. **Respiratory:** Cough. **CNS:** Headache, fatigue. **GI:** *nausea*, vomiting diarrhea, abdominal pain. **Hematology:** Decreased platelet count.

INTERACTIONS Drug: Letermovir is a substrate and inhibitor of OATP1B1/3 transporters. Avoid use with other inhibitors/substrates of the OATP1B1/3 transporters. Letermovir acts as a CYP3A4 inhibitor; monitor use with CYP3A substrates (e.g., **fentanyl, midazolam**). Letermovir may increase plasma concentrations of **amiodarone**, ANTIDIABETIC AGENTS, **ergotamine**, HMG-CoA REDUCTASE INHIBITORS, IMMUNOSUPPRESSANTS. Letermovir may decrease plasma concentrations of PROTON PUMP INHIBITORS, **phenytoin**, and **warfarin**.

PHARMACOKINETICS Absorption: Oral dose has 94% bioavailability. **Distribution:** 99% protein bound. **Metabolism:** Primarily eliminated unchanged. **Elimination:** 93% in feces, 2% in urine. **Half-Life:** 12 h.

NURSING IMPLICATIONS

Assessment & Drug Effects

- Monitor for CMV reactivation.
- Closely monitor in patients with CrCl less than 50mL/min receiving IV formulation.
- Monitor lab tests: Serum creatinine/BUN.

Patient & Family Education

- This drug interacts with many other drugs. Report any new medications to your pharmacist/prescriber.
- If patient misses a dose, take as soon as they remember. If patient does not remember until the next dose is due, skip the missed dose and go back to the regular schedule; do not double the next dose or take more than prescribed.
- Notify prescriber if pregnant or planning a pregnancy.
- Notify prescriber if breast-feeding.
- Report promptly any of the following to prescriber: Swelling in arms/legs, signs of allergic reaction.

LETROZOLE

(le′tro-zole)

Femara

Classification: ANTINEOPLASTIC; AROMATASE INHIBITOR

Therapeutic: ANTINEOPLASTIC

Prototype: Anastrozole

AVAILABILITY Tablet

ACTION & *THERAPEUTIC EFFECT* Nonsteroid competitive inhibitor of aromatase, the enzyme that converts androgens to estrogens. It does not inhibit adrenal steroid synthesis. *Results in the regression of estrogen-dependent tumors.*

USES Treatment of breast cancer in postmenopausal women.

CONTRAINDICATIONS Hypersensitivity to letrozole; pregnant women, women of childbearing age, premenopausal females, hormone replacement therapy (HRT); pregnancy, lactation (infant risk cannot be ruled out).

CAUTIOUS USE Moderate to severe hepatic impairment; older adults. Safety and efficacy in children not established.

ROUTE & DOSAGE

Breast Cancer

Adult: **PO** 2.5 mg daily

Hepatic Impairment Dosage Adjustment

Severe hepatic impairment (Child-Pugh class C): Reduce the dose by 50%

ADMINISTRATION

Oral

- NIOSH recommends the use of single gloves by anyone handling tablets or capsules or administering from a unit-dose package. In the preparation of tablets, capsules including cutting, crushing, manipulating, or handling of uncoated tablets, use double gloves and protective gown. During administration wear single gloves and wear eye/face protection if formulation is hard to swallow or if the patient may resist, vomit, or spit up.
- Give without regard to food.

ADVERSE EFFECTS **CV:** Edema, chest pain, hypertension. **Respiratory:** Dyspnea, cough. **CNS:** *Fatigue*, dizziness, headache, insomnia, pain. **Endocrine:** *Hypercholesterolemia*, weight gain, weight loss. **Skin:** *Hot sweats*, sweating, rash, alopecia. **GI:** Constipation, diarrhea, anorexia, nausea, vomiting. **GU:** UTI, vaginal dryness, breast pain, vaginal hemorrhage, vaginal irritation. **Musculoskeletal:** *Joint pain, arthritis*, backache, bone pain, muscle pain, osteoporosis, bone fracture. **Other:** Infection, influenza, viral infection.

INTERACTIONS **Drug:** ESTROGENS, ORAL CONTRACEPTIVES could interfere with the pharmacologic action of letrozole.

PHARMACOKINETICS **Absorption:** Rapidly from GI tract. **Metabolism:** In liver (CYP3A4 and 2A6). **Elimination:** 90% in urine. **Half-Life:** 2 days.

NURSING IMPLICATIONS

Assessment & Drug Effects

- Pregnancy test in women with reproductive potential prior to therapy.
- Monitor carefully for S&S of thrombophlebitis or thromboembolism; report immediately.
- X-rays and DXA scans baseline and routinely.
- Monitor lab tests: Periodic serum calcium and CBC with differential.

Patient & Family Education

- Notify prescriber immediately if S&S of thrombophlebitis develop (see Appendix F).
- Report osteoporosis and bone fractures.

LEUCOVORIN CALCIUM

(loo-koe-vor′in)

LEVOLEUCOVORIN

(levo-loo-koe-vor′in)

Fusilev

Classification: BLOOD FORMER; ANTIANEMIC

Therapeutic: ANTIANEMIC; CHEMOTHERAPEUTIC PROTECTANT

AVAILABILITY Tablet; solution for injection

ACTION & *THERAPEUTIC EFFECT*

Both leucovorin and levoleucovorin are reduced forms of folic acid. Unlike folic acid, they do not require enzymatic reduction by dihydrofolate reductase. Thus, they are readily available as an essential cell growth factor. During antineoplastic therapy, both forms of the drug prevent serious toxicity by

L

protecting cells from the action of folic acid antagonists. *Antidote against folic acid antagonists such as methotrexate.*

USES Methotrexate toxicity, megalobalstic anemia, colorectal cancer.

UNLABELED USES Treatment of non-Hodgkin's lymphoma, esophageal cancer, gastric cancer.

CONTRAINDICATIONS Pernicious anemia, or other megaloblastic anemias secondary to vitamin B_{12} deficiency. Pregnancy—fetal risk cannot be ruled out. Lactation—infant risk cannot be ruled out. **Oral form:** Stomatitis.

CAUTIOUS USE Inadequate hydration; history of seizures; debilitated patients; older adults; HIV patients; patients with renal insufficiency; children.

ROUTE & DOSAGE

Note: Levoleucovorin is dosed at half the normal dose of leucovorin

Megaloblastic Anemia

Adult/Child: **IV/IM** Up to 1 mg/day

Methotrexate-Rescue

Adult/Child: **PO/IM/IV** 15 mg q6h until serum methotrexate levels are reduced

Folic Acid Antagonist Overdose

Adult/Child: **PO** 5–15 mg/day

Advanced Colorectal Cancer

Adult: **IV** 200 mg/m^2 × 5 days q4w for 2 cycles (in combination with fluorouracil)

ADMINISTRATION

Oral

- Note: Oral route is **not** recommended for doses higher than 25 mg or if patient is likely to vomit.
- Store tablets at 15–25° C. Protect from light and moisture.

Intravenous

PREPARE: **Leucovorin Direct/IV Infusion:** For doses less than 10 mg/m^2, reconstitute each 50 mg in 5 mL of bacteriostatic water for injection with benzyl alcohol as a preservative to yield 10 mg/mL. ▪ For doses greater than 10 mg/m^2 reconstitute, as above, but with sterile water for injection without a preservative. Final concentration is 10 mg/mL. ▪ Further dilute in 100–500 mL of IV solutions (e.g., D5W, NS, LR) to yield a concentration of 10–20 mg/mL of IV solution. **Levoleucovorin Direct:** Reconstitute the 50-mg vial with 5.3 mL NS injection to yield 10 mg/mL. ▪ May further dilute, immediately, in NS or D5W to 0.5–5 mg/mL. ▪ Do not mix with other solutions or additives.

ADMINISTER: **Leucovorin/Levoleucovorin Direct:** Give 160 mg or fraction thereof over 1 min. **Leucovorin/Levoleucovorin IV Infusion:** Do not exceed direct IV rate. ▪ Give more slowly if the volume of IV solution to be infused is large.

INCOMPATIBILITIES: **Leucovorin only: Solution/additive: Fluorouracil. Y-site: Amiodarone, Amphotericin B cholesteryl complex, carboplatin, ceftriazone, chlorpromazine, dantrolene, diazepam, droperidol, epirubicin, foscarnet, gemtuzumab, lansoprazole, methylprednisolone, naloxone,**

pamidronate, pantoprazole, pentamidine, phenytoin, potassium phosphate, quinupristin/dalfopristin, sodium bicarbonate, thiopental, vancomycin.

▪ **Leucovorin:** Use solution reconstituted with bacteriostatic water within 7 days. ▪ Use solution reconstituted with sterile water for injection immediately. **Levoleucovorin:** Solutions with NS may be held at 15°–30° C (59°–86° F) for up to 12 h. Solutions with D5W may be held at 15°–30° C (59°–86° F) for up to 4 h. ▪ Protect from light.

ADVERSE EFFECTS **GI:** Diarrhea, nausea, vomiting, stomatitis. **Other:** Allergic sensitization (urticaria, pruritus, rash, wheezing) and fatigue.

INTERACTIONS **Drug:** May enhance adverse effects of **fluorouracil**; may reverse therapeutic effects of **trimethoprim-sulfamethoxazole**. Do not use with **raltitrexed**.

PHARMACOKINETICS **Onset:** Within 30 min. **Peak:** 0.9 h (levoleucovorin). **Duration:** 3–6 h. **Distribution:** Crosses placenta; distributed into breast milk. **Metabolism:** In liver and intestinal mucosa to tetrahydrofolic acid derivatives. **Elimination:** 80–90% in urine, 5–8% in feces. **Half-Life:** 6 h; 0.77 h (levoleucovorin).

NURSING IMPLICATIONS

Assessment & Drug Effects

- Monitor neurologic status. Use of leucovorin alone in treatment of pernicious anemia or other megaloblastic anemias associated with vitamin B_{12} deficiency can result in an apparent hematological remission while allowing already present neurologic damage to progress.
- Monitor lab tests: Baseline and daily serum creatinine and methotrexate level when treated for methotrexate toxicity; CBC with differential and platelets prior to each treatment and weekly during the first two courses and then one each cycle.

Patient & Family Education

- Notify prescriber of S&S of a hypersensitivity reaction immediately (see Appendix F).
- Report nausea, vomiting diarrhea or sores in the mouth.
- Notify healthcare provider if dose is missed or if vomiting occurs after taking the medication.

LEUPROLIDE ACETATE (Prototype drug)

(loo-proe'lide)

Eligard, Lupron, Lupron Depot, Lupron Depot-Ped

Classification: GONADOTROPIN-RELEASING HORMONE (GnRH) ANALOG

Therapeutic: GnRH ANALOG; ANTINEOPLASTIC

AVAILABILITY Solution for injection; microspheres for injection (depot formulations)

ACTION & *THERAPEUTIC EFFECT* A luteinizing hormone-releasing hormone (LH-RH) and GnRH agonist; acts as a potent inhibitor of gonadotropin secretion when given continuously in therapeutic doses. **Antitumor effect:** *May inhibit growth of hormone-dependent tumors as indicated by reduction in concentrations of PSA and serum testosterone to levels equal to or less than pretreatment levels.* **Contraceptive effect:** *By inhibiting gonadotropin release, ovulation or spermatogenesis is suppressed.*

USES Palliative treatment of advanced prostatic carcinoma; endometriosis; anemia caused by leiomyomata; precocious puberty.

UNLABELED USES Breast cancer; BPH, PMS; infertility.

CONTRAINDICATIONS Known hypersensitivity to benzyl alcohol, GnRH analog hypersensitivity; following orchiectomy or estrogen therapy; metastatic cerebral lesions; menstruation, abnormal vaginal bleeding, pregnancy (category X); lactation.

CAUTIOUS USE Life-threatening carcinoma in which rapid symptomatic relief is necessary; osteoporosis; older adults.

L

ROUTE & DOSAGE

Palliative Treatment for Prostate Cancer

Adult: **Subcutaneous** 1 mg/day; **IM** 7.5 mg/mo or 22.5 mg q3mo or 30 mg q4mo or 45 mg q6mo (depends on specific depot preparation)

Endometriosis

Adult: **IM** 3.75 mg qmo or 11.25 mg q3mo (max: 6 mo)

Precocious Puberty

Child (weight greater than 37.5 kg): **IM** 15 mg q4wk; *weight 25–37.5 kg:* 11.25 mg q4wk; *weight less than 25 kg:* 7.5 mg q4wk

Precocious Puberty (Depot Form)

Child (2–11 y): **IM** 11.25 or 30 mg q3mo

ADMINISTRATION

Subcutaneous

- Use double gloves and protective gown for all preparation and administration of subcutaneous and intramuscular injection. Use eye protection if there is any chance of splash or if the patient may resist.
- Do not use Depot form for subcutaneous injection.
- Assemble two-syringe mixing system. Mix as directed and allow to reach room temperature and administer within 30 min of mixing. Also available as a subcutaneous implant.
- Rotate injection sites.

Intramuscular

- Prepare solution for Depot-Ped injection. Screw plunger into the end stopper until stopper begins to turn; hold syringe upright; slowly push (6–8 sec) until first stopper is at the blue line in the middle of the barrel to combine the diluent with microspheres; keep syringe upright while mixing suspension gently until all of the powder is completely dissolved into suspension; expel air from the syringe; use within 2 h; do not use if the powder has not dissolved into a suspension. Inject at 90° angle and inject intramuscularly immediately because suspension settles quickly.
- Do not administer parenteral drug formulation if particulate matter or discoloration is present.
- Storage directions are different for different brands. Follow package insert for each brand.

ADVERSE EFFECTS **CV:** *Peripheral edema*, cardiac arrhythmias, <u>MI</u>. **Respiratory:** Pleural rub, pulmonary fibrosis flare, cough, <u>pulmonary embolism</u>. **CNS:** Dizziness, pain, headache, fatigue, insomnia, paresthesia. **Endocrine:** *Hot flushes, impotence, decreased libido,* gynecomastia, breast tenderness, amenorrhea, vaginal bleeding, thyroid enlargement, hypoglycemia. Increased hematuria, dysuria, flank pain. **Skin:** Pruritus, rash, hair loss, acne. **GI:** Nausea, vomiting, constipation, anorexia, sour taste, GI bleeding, diarrhea. **Musculoskeletal:** Increased bone pain, *myalgia, fractures of vertebral column.* **Hematologic:** Decreased Hct, Hgb. **Other:** *Disease flare (worsening of S&S of carcinoma), injection site irritation,* asthenia, fatigue, depression, fever, facial swelling.

INTERACTIONS Drug: ANDROGENS, ESTROGENS counteract therapeutic effects. Avoid using QT prolonging agents (e.g., **bretylium, dofetilide**, etc.).

PHARMACOKINETICS Absorption: Readily absorbed from subcutaneous or IM sites. **Metabolism:** By enzymes in hypothalamus and anterior pituitary. **Half-Life:** 3 h.

NURSING IMPLICATIONS

Assessment & Drug Effects

- Monitor PSA and testosterone levels in males with prostate cancer. A gradual rise in values after their decrease may signify treatment failure.
- Inspect injection site. If local hypersensitivity reactions occur (erythema, induration), suspect sensitivity to benzyl alcohol. Report to prescriber.
- Monitor I&O ratio and pattern. Report hematuria and decreased output. Carefully monitor voiding problems, monitor Hgb and Hct, and hemoglobin A1C within 3–6 mo of beginning therapy.

Patient & Family Education

- When used for prostate cancer, bone pain and voiding problems (i.e., symptoms of tumor obstruction) usually increase during first several weeks of continuous treatment but are transient. Hot flushes also may be experienced.
- Notify prescriber of neurologic S&S (paresthesia and weakness in lower limbs). Exercise caution when walking without assistance.
- When used for endometriosis, continuous treatment may cause amenorrhea and other menstrual irregularities.

LEVALBUTEROL HYDROCHLORIDE

(lev-al-bu′ter-ole)

Xopenex, Xopenex HFA

Classification: BETA-ADRENERGIC RECEPTOR AGONIST

Therapeutic: BRONCHODILATOR

Prototype: Albuterol

AVAILABILITY Inhalation solution, inhaler.

ACTION & *THERAPEUTIC EFFECT* An isomer of albuterol with beta$_2$-adrenergic agonist properties; acts on the beta$_2$ receptors of the smooth muscles of the bronchial tree, thus resulting in bronchodilation. *Effective bronchodilator that decreases airway resistance, facilitates mucous drainage, and increases vital capacity.*

USES Treatment or prevention of bronchospasm in patients with reversible obstructive airway disease.

CONTRAINDICATIONS Hypersensitivity to levalbuterol or albuterol; angioedema; pregnancy (fetal risk cannot be ruled out); lactation (infant risk cannot be ruled out).

CAUTIOUS USE Cardiovascular disorders especially coronary insufficiency, cardiac arrhythmias, hypertension, QT elongation, convulsive disorders; diabetes mellitus, diabetic ketoacidosis; hyperthyroidism, hypokalemia, older adults; seizures, status asthmaticus, tachycardia; hypersensitivity to sympathetic amines; hyperthyroidism, thyrotoxicosis; children.

ROUTE & DOSAGE

Bronchospasm

Adult: **Inhalation** 2 inhalations q4–6h prn; nebulized solution; 0.63 mg by nebulization q6–8h, may increase to 1.25 mg tid if needed

Child (6–11 y): **Inhalation** 2 inhalations q4–6h prn; nebulized solution 0.31 mg by nebulization tid q6–8h (max: 0.63 mg tid)

ADMINISTRATION

Inhalation

- Use vials within 2 wk of opening pouch. Protect vial from light and use within 1 wk after removal from pouch. Use only if solution in vial is colorless.

INCOMPATIBILITIES: **Solution/additive:** Compatibility when mixed with other drugs in a nebulizer has not been established.

- Store at 15°–25° C (59°–77° F) in protective foil pouch.

ADVERSE EFFECTS **Respiratory:** Asthma, rhinitis, viral disease, pharyngitis. **CNS:** Feeling nervous, tremor. **Skin:** rash. **GI:** Diarrhea. **Other:** Accidental injury, fever

INTERACTIONS **Drug:** BETA-ADRENERGIC BLOCKERS may antagonize levalbuterol effects; MAOI, TRICYCLIC ANTIDEPRESSANTS may potentiate levalbuterol effects on vascular system; ECG changes or hypokalemia may be exacerbated by LOOP OR THIAZIDE DIURETICS.

PHARMACOKINETICS **Onset:** 5–15 min. **Duration:** 3–6 h. **Half-Life:** 3.3 h.

NURSING IMPLICATIONS

Assessment & Drug Effects

- Monitor for S&S of CNS or cardiovascular stimulation (e.g., BP, HR, respiratory status).
- Monitor diabetics for loss of glycemic control.
- Monitor lab tests: Periodic serum potassium especially with coadministered loop or thiazide diuretics, BUN, creatinine levels.

Patient & Family Education

- Seek medical advice immediately if a previously effective dose becomes ineffective.
- Report immediately to prescriber: Chest pain or palpitations, swelling of the eyelids, tongue, lips, or face; increased wheezing or difficulty breathing.
- Do not use drug more frequently than prescribed.
- Exercise caution with hazardous activities; dizziness and vertigo are possible side effects.
- Check with prescriber before taking OTC cold medication.

LEVETIRACETAM

(lev-e-tir′a-ce-tam)

Elepsia XR, Keppra, Keppra XR, Spritam

Classification: ANTICONVULSANT

Therapeutic: ANTICONVULSANT

AVAILABILITY Tablet; extended release tablets; oral solution;

 Common adverse effects in *italic;* life-threatening effects underlined; generic names in **bold;** classifications in SMALL CAPS; ♣ Canadian drug name; ➲ Prototype drug; ⚠ Alert

solution for injection; oral disintegrating tablet

ACTION & THERAPEUTIC EFFECT

The precise mechanism of antiepileptic effects is unknown. It is a broad spectrum antiepileptic agent that does not involve GABA inhibition. It prevents epileptiform burst firing and propagation of seizure activity. *Inhibits complex partial seizures and prevents epileptic and seizure activity.*

USES Adjunctive therapy for focal (partial) onset, and generalized onset myoclonic, tonic clonic seizures.

UNLABELED USES Status epilepticus, short-term seizure prophylaxis in subarachnoid hemorrhage.

CONTRAINDICATIONS Hypersensitivity to levetiracetam; suicidal ideation; labor; pregnancy—fetal risk cannot be ruled out; lactation—infant risk cannot be ruled out. Avoid use in older adults with a history of falls or fractures (unless used for seizure or mood disorders). **Extended release tablets:** Children younger than 12.

CAUTIOUS USE Renal impairment; renal disease; renal failure; older adults; history of psychosis or depression, suicidal tendencies. **Immediate release tablet** for children younger than 4 y.

ROUTE & DOSAGE

Focal (Partial) Onset Seizures

Adult/Adolescent (16 y or older): **PO/IV** 500 mg bid, may increase by 500 mg bid q2wk (max: 3000 mg/day) OR **Extended release** 1 gram/day may increase q2wk by 1 g/day

Child (4–15 y): **PO Solution form/IV** 10 mg/kg bid; may increase by 10 mg/kg bid q2wk up to 30 mg/kg bid

Child/Infant (older than 6 mo): **PO** 10 mg/kg bid may increase q2wk by 10 mg/kg/dose to 25 mg/kg bid; **IV** 7 mg/kg bid may increase to dose of 21 mg/kg bid

Infant (1–6 mo): **PO** 7 mg/kg bid may increase by 7 mg/kg bid up to dose of 21 mg/kg bid

Tonic Clonic; Primary Generalized Seizures

Adult/Adolescent (16 y or older): **PO/IV** 500 mg bid, increase by 1000 mg q2wk to dose of 3000 mg/day

Child (6 y or older): **PO Immediate release** or **Solution form** 10 mg/kg bid, increase by 10 mg/kg bid q2wk to dose of 30 mg/kg/day bid

Adolescent/Child (6 y or older 20–40 kg): **PO Fast melt tablet** 250 mg bid then increase dose by 250 bid q2wk to 750 mg bid

Adolescent/Child (6 y or older over 40 kg): **PO Fast melt tablet** 500 mg bid then increase dose by 500 mg bid q2w to max dose of 1500 mg bid

Renal Impairment Dosage Adjustment

CrCl 50–80 mL/min: **Immediate release or IV** 500–1000 mg q12h; **Extended release** 1000–2000 mg q24;

CrCl 30–49 mL/min: **Immediate release or IV** 250–750 mg q12h; **Extended release** 500–1500 mg q24h

L

CrCl 15–30 mL/min: **Immediate release or IV** 250–500 mg q12h; Extended release 500 mg–1g q24

ADMINISTRATION

Oral

- Ensure that extended release tablets are swallowed whole. They should not be cut or chewed.
- May be given with our without food.
- Dose increment changes should be made no more often than at 2-wk intervals.
- Taper dose if discontinued.
- Give supplemental doses to dialysis patients after dialysis.
- Store at 15°–30° C (59°–86° F).

L

Intravenous

PREPARE: **Intermittent:** Levetiracetam supplied in NS needs no further dilution. If using the concentrated solution, dilute required dose in 100 mL of D5W, NS or LR.
ADMINISTER: **Intermittent:** Give over 15 min.
INCOMPATIBILITIES: **Solution/additives: Dobutamine, dopamine. Y Site: Posaconazole.**

- Diluted solution may be stored up to 4 h at 15°–30° C (59°–86° F).

ADVERSE EFFECTS (≥5%) Respiratory: Cough, pharyngitis. **CNS:** Headache, lack of energy, dizziness. **GI:** Anorexia, *vomiting*. **Musculoskeletal:** Decreased bone mineral density, neck pain. **Other:** Risk for infectious disease, abnormal behavior, irritability.

INTERACTIONS Drug: AMPHETAMINES may decrease seizure threshold. CNS DEPRESSANTS have additive sedation. **Herbal:** Avoid use of **kava**.

PHARMACOKINETICS Absorption: Rapidly and almost completely absorbed. **Peak:** 1 h; steady-state 2 days. **Distribution:** Less than 10% protein bound. **Metabolism:** Minimal hepatic metabolism. **Elimination:** Renally eliminated. **Half-Life:** 7.1 h (9.6 h in older adults).

NURSING IMPLICATIONS

Assessment & Drug Effects

- Monitor individuals with a history of psychosis or depression for signs and symptoms of suicidal tendencies, suicidal ideation, and suicidality. Report any of these symptoms to the prescriber.
- Monitor blood pressure.
- Monitor and notify prescriber of difficulty with gait or coordination.
- Monitor lab tests: Periodic CBC with differential, levetiracetam plasma or saliva levels, serum creatinine/BUN, Hct and Hgb, and LFTs.

Patient & Family Education

- Monitor for signs and symptoms of suicidality, especially in children with a history of depression or psychosis.
- Do not drive or engage in potentially hazardous activities until response to drug is known.
- Watch for serious skin reactions.
- Do not abruptly discontinue drug. MUST use gradual dose reduction/taper.

LEVOBUNOLOL

(lee-voe-byoo′noe-lole)

Betagan

See Appendix A-1.

LEVOCETIRIZINE

(lev-o-ce-tir'i-zeen)

Xyzal

See Cetirizine.

LEVODOPA (L-DOPA)

(lee-voe-doe'pa)

Classification: DOPAMINE RECEPTOR AGONIST; ANTIPARKINSON

Therapeutic: ANTIPARKINSON

AVAILABILITY Capsule for inhalation

ACTION & *THERAPEUTIC EFFECT* Levodopa readily crosses the blood–brain barrier; it is believed that the dopamine level is severely reduced in parkinsonism. Levodopa restores dopamine levels in extrapyramidal centers of the brain. *Effective in controlling the involuntary muscle movement such as tremors and rigidity associated with Parkinson disease.*

USES Intermittent treatment of off episodes in Parkinson disease.

CONTRAINDICATIONS Known hypersensitivity to levodopa; narrow-angle glaucoma patients with suspicious pigmented lesion or history of melanoma; acute psychoses, within 2 wk of use of MAOIs, suicidal ideation; pregnancy—fetal risk cannot be ruled out; lactation—infant risk is established.

CAUTIOUS USE Cardiovascular, kidney, liver, or endocrine disease, history of MI with residual arrhythmias; peptic ulcer; convulsions; history of suicidal tendencies; depression; bipolar disorder; psychiatric disorders; chronic wide-angle glaucoma; diabetes; pulmonary diseases, bronchial asthma. Safe use in children not established.

ROUTE & DOSAGE

Parkinson Disease

Adult: **Inhalation** 84 mg up to 5 times daily prn

ADMINISTRATION

Oral

- Capsules are for oral inhalation only; do not swallow.
- Remove capsule for insertion into inhaler immediately prior to use. Do not load more than one capsule.
- Do not open capsules or use capsules that look crushed or damaged or wet.
- Only push the handle and mouthpiece together 1 time.
- Inhale orally and hold breath for 5 seconds; reload the inhaler with a second capsule and repeat.
- Store in a dry place between 20 and 25 degrees C (69 to 77 degrees F), with excursions permitted between 15 and 30 degrees C (59 and 86 degrees F). Store in original blister package and only remove immediately before use.

ADVERSE EFFECTS **Respiratory:** *Cough, discolored sputum, upper respiratory infection.* **GI:** *Nausea.* **Other:** Impulse control disorder.

DIAGNOSTIC TEST INTERFERENCE False diagnosis for pheochromocytoma.

INTERACTIONS **Drug:** MAO INHIBITORS may precipitate hypertensive crisis; increased risk of hypotension with ANTIHYPERTENSIVES, **pyridoxine** can reverse effects of levodopa; ANTICHOLINERGICS may exacerbate abnormal involuntary movements; may decrease the effect of ANTIPSYCHOTIC AGENTS; HALOGENATED GENERAL ANESTHETICS increase risk

L

of arrhythmias. Do not use with **alizapride, amisulpride, bromperidol, macimorelin, metoclopramide, sulpride.** MULTIVITAMINS **with fluoride, folate, iron** may decrease effect of levodopa. **Food:** Food decreases the rate and extent of levodopa absorption. Vitamin B supplements can decrease therapeutic effect. **Herbal: Kava** may worsen parkinsonian symptoms.

PHARMACOKINETICS Absorption: Rapidly and well absorbed from GI tract; lower absorption if taken with food. **Peak:** 1–3 h. **Distribution:** Widely distributed in body. **Metabolism:** Most of drug is decarboxylated to dopamine in lumen of GI tract, liver, and serum. **Elimination:** 80–85% of dose excreted in urine in 24 h. **Half-Life:** 2 h.

L

NURSING IMPLICATIONS

Assessment & Drug Effects

- Monitor vital signs, particularly during period of dosage adjustment. Report alterations in BP, pulse, and respiratory rate and rhythm.
- Supervise ambulation as indicated. Orthostatic hypotension is usually asymptomatic, but some patients experience dizziness and syncope. Tolerance to this effect usually develops within a few months of therapy.
- Make accurate observations and report adverse reactions and therapeutic effects promptly. Rate of dosage increase is determined primarily by patient's tolerance and response to drug.
- Monitor all patients closely for compulsive behavior changes; increased gambling urges, sexual urges, uncontrolled spending or other urges.
- Report promptly muscle twitching and spasmodic winking (blepharospasm); these are early signs of overdosage. Patients on full therapeutic doses for longer than 1 y may develop such abnormal involuntary movements as well as jerky arm and leg movements. Symptoms tend to increase if dosage is not reduced.
- Report to prescriber any S&S of the on–off phenomenon sometimes associated with chronic management: Rapid unpredictable swings in intensity of motor symptoms of parkinsonism evidenced by increase in bradykinesia (attacks of "leg freezing" or slow body movement).
- Monitor for changes in intraocular pressure.

Patient & Family Education

- Make positional changes slowly, particularly from lying to upright position, and dangle legs a few minutes before standing.
- Resume activities gradually, observing safety precautions to avoid injury. Elevation of mood and sense of well-being may precede objective improvement. Significant improvement usually occurs during second or third wk of therapy, but may not occur for 6 mo or more in some patients.
- Review adverse effects with patient and/or caregiver.
- Report any symptoms of impulsive control disorders.

LEVOFLOXACIN

(lev-o-flox′a-sin)

Levaquin

Classification: QUINOLONE ANTIBIOTIC

Therapeutic: ANTIBIOTIC

Prototype: Ciprofloxacin

AVAILABILITY Tablet; oral solution; solution for injection; ophthalmic solution

ACTION & *THERAPEUTIC EFFECT*

A broad-spectrum fluoroquinolone antibiotic that inhibits DNA-gyrase, an enzyme necessary for bacterial replication, transcription, repair, and recombination. *Effective against many aerobic gram-positive and aerobic gram-negative organisms.*

USES Treatment of maxillary sinusitis, acute exacerbations of bacterial bronchitis, community-acquired pneumonia, uncomplicated skin/skin structure infections, UTI, acute pyelonephritis caused by susceptible bacteria; acute bacterial sinusitis; chronic bacterial prostatitis; bacterial conjunctivitis; treatment of pneumonic and septicemic plague.

UNLABELED USES Epididymitis, infective carditis, tuberculosis.

CONTRAINDICATIONS Hypersensitivity to levofloxacin and quinolone antibiotics; tendon pain, inflammation or rupture; syphilis; viral infections; photosensitivity/phototoxicity from drug; suicidal ideation; psychotic manifestations; manifestations of peripheral neuropathy; S&S of hepatitis; hypoglycemic reaction or peripheral neuropathy to drug; MG; QT prolongation.

CAUTIOUS USE History of suicidal ideation; psychosis; anxiety, confusion, depression; known or suspected CNS disorders; predisposed to seizure activity; risk factors associated with potential seizures (e.g., some drug therapy, renal insufficiency), dehydration, renal impairment (CrCl less than 50 mL/min); colitis; cardiac arrhythmias; DM; older adults; pregnancy (category C); lactation. Safe use in children younger than 6 mo not established.

ROUTE & DOSAGE

Infections

Adult: **PO** 500 mg q24h × 10 days; **IV** 500 mg infused over 60 min q24h × 7–14 days

Community-Acquired Pneumonia

Adult: **PO/IV** 750 mg q24h × 5 days

Uncomplicated UTI

Adult: **PO/IV** 250 mg q24h × 14 days

Complicated UTI, Pyelonephritis

Adult: **PO/IV** 250 mg q24h × 10 days

Acute Bacterial Sinusitis

Adult: **PO/IV** 750 mg daily × 5 days

Chronic Bacterial Prostatitis

Adult: **PO/IV** 500 mg q24h × 28 days

Skin & Skin Structure Infections

Adult: **PO** 750 mg q24h × 14 days

Inhaled Anthrax

Adult/Adolescent/Child (weight at least 50 kg): **IV** 500 mg daily × 60 days

Infant/Child (6 mo or older and weight less than 50 kg): **IV** 8 mg/kg q12h (no more than 250 mg/dose)

Plague

Adult: **PO** 500 mg daily for 10–14 days

Renal Impairment Dosage Adjustment

For initial dose of 500 mg, adjust as follows: *CrCl 20–50 mL/min:* 250 mg q24h; *less than 20 mL/min:* 250 mg q48h

L

For initial dose of 750 mg, adjust as follows: *CrCl 20–50 mL/min:* 750 mg q48h; *10–19 mL/min:* 500 mg q48h; *less than 20 mL/min:* 250 mg q48h

ADMINISTRATION

Oral

- Do not give oral drug within 2 h of drugs containing aluminum or magnesium (antacids), iron, zinc, or sucralfate.

Intravenous

PREPARE: **Intermittent:** Withdraw the desired dose from 500 or 750 mg (25 mg/mL) single-use vial. ▪ Add to enough D5W, NS, D5/NS, D5/LR, or other compatible solutions to produce a concentration of 5 mg/mL [e.g., 500 mg (or 20 mL) added to 80 mL]. ▪ Discard any unused drug remaining in the vial.

ADMINISTER: **Intermittent:** Infuse 500 mg or less over 60 min. ▪ Infuse 750 mg over at least 90 min. ▪ **Do not** give a bolus dose or infuse too rapidly.

INCOMPATIBILITIES: **Y-site:** Do not add any drugs to levofloxacin solution or infuse simultaneously through the same line (manufacturer recommendation).

- Store tablets in a tightly closed container. IV solution is stable for 72 h at 25° C (77° F).

ADVERSE EFFECTS **CNS:** Headache, insomnia, dizziness. **HEENT:** Decreased vision, foreign body sensation, transient ocular burning, ocular pain, photophobia. **Skin:** Rash, pruritus. **GI:** Nausea, diarrhea, constipation, vomiting, abdominal pain, dyspepsia. **GU:** Vaginitis. **Other:** Cartilage erosion. Injection site pain or inflammation, chest or back pain, fever, pharyngitis.

DIAGNOSTIC TEST INTERFERENCE

May cause false positive on opiate screening tests.

INTERACTIONS **Drug: Magnesium**- or **aluminum**-containing antacids, **sucralfate, iron, zinc** may decrease levofloxacin absorption; NSAIDS may increase risk of CNS reactions, including seizures; may cause hyper- or hypoglycemia in patients on ORAL HYPOGLYCEMIC AGENTS. Do not use with agents known to prolong QT interval (**bepridil, doeftilide, dronedarone, halofantrine, levomethadyl, pimozide, thioridazine, ziprasidone**).

PHARMACOKINETICS **Absorption:** Rapidly from GI tract. **Peak:** PO 1–2 h. **Distribution:** Penetrates lung tissue, 24–38% protein bound. **Metabolism:** Minimally in the liver. **Elimination:** Primarily unchanged in urine. **Half-Life:** 6–8 h.

NURSING IMPLICATIONS

Black Box Warning

Levofloxacin has been associated with tendinitis and tendon rupture; drug may exacerbate muscle weakness in those with MG.

Assessment & Drug Effects

- Withhold therapy and report to prescriber immediately any of the following: Skin rash or other signs of a hypersensitivity reaction (see Appendix F); CNS symptoms such as seizures, restlessness, confusion, hallucinations, depression; skin eruption following sun exposure; symptoms of colitis such as persistent diarrhea; joint pain, inflammation, or rupture of a tendon.
- Monitor diabetics on oral hypolgycemic agents for loss of glycemic control.

- Monitor lab tests: C&S test prior to beginning therapy, serum creatinine/BUN, and LFTs.

Patient & Family Education

- Discontinue drug and notify prescriber if S&S of hypersensitivity occur (e.g., skin rash, hives, rapid heartbeat, difficulty swallowing or breathing).
- If tendon pain occurs, discontinue the drug and notify the prescriber.
- Consume fluids liberally while taking levofloxacin. Failure to do so can lead to crystallization of urine.
- Allow a minimum of 2 h between drug dosage and taking any of the following: Aluminum or magnesium antacids, iron supplements, multivitamins with zinc, or sucralfate.
- Avoid exposure to excess sunlight or artificial UV light.
- Closely monitor blood glucose if taking oral hypoglycemic agents for diabetic control.

LEVOLEUCOVORIN

(levo-loo-koe-vor′in)

Fusilev

See Leucovorin.

LEVONORGESTREL-RELEASING INTRAUTERINE SYSTEM

(lee′vo-nor-jes-trel)

Kyleena, Liletta, Mirena, Skyla

Classification: PROGESTIN HORMONE

Therapeutic: PROGESTIN

Prototype: Norgestrel

AVAILABILITY IUD, tablet

ACTION & *THERAPEUTIC EFFECT* A progestogen that induces morphological changes in the endometrium including glandular atrophy, leukocytic infiltration, and decrease in glandular and stromal mitoses. Contraceptive effect may result by preventing follicular maturation and ovulation, thickening of the cervical mucus of the uterus, thus preventing passage of sperm into the uterus, or decreasing ability of sperm to survive in an environment of altered endometrium. *Effective contraceptive.*

USES Hormonal contraception, menorrhagia, postcoital contraception.

CONTRAINDICATIONS Hypersensitivity to any component of the product; previously inserted IUD which has not been removed; suspicion of pregnancy; history of ectopic pregnancy; history of uterine anomalies which distort the uterine cavity; acute PID; vaginal bleeding of unknown etiology; septic abortion in past 3 mo; abnormal Pap or suspected/known cervical neoplasm; known or suspected carcinoma of the breast; thrombophlebitis or thromboembolic disorders, pregnancy (category X).

CAUTIOUS USE Women at risk for or have a venereal disease; anemia; history of migraines; presence or history of salpingitis; genital bleeding of unknown etiology; severe arterial disease; coagulopathy; previous pelvic surgery.

ROUTE & DOSAGE

Contraception

Adult: **Intrauterine** Insert device at any point in menstrual cycle; may leave in place up to 3 y (**Skyla**), 4y (**Liletta**) or 5 y (**Mirena** or **Kyleena**)

Post Coital Contraception

Adult/Adolescent: **Oral** 1 tablet as soon as possible after intercourse

L

ADMINISTRATION

Intrauterine

- Inserted only by prescriber or other person qualified by special training in the intrauterine system.

ADVERSE EFFECTS **CV:** Hypertension. **CNS:** Depression, emotional lability, headache (including migraine), nervousness, *fatigue*. **Endocrine:** Breast tenderness/pain. Weight gain. **Skin:** *Acne*, alopecia, eczema. **GI:** *Abdominal pain*, nausea. **GU:** *Amenorrhea*, *intermenstrual bleeding*, dysmenorrhea, leukorrhea, decreased libido, vaginal moniliasis, vulvovaginal disorders, cervicitis, dyspareunia. **Hematologic:** Anemia.

INTERACTIONS **Drug:** Do not use with **bosentan**.

L

PHARMACOKINETICS **Peak:** Few weeks. **Duration:** 5 y. **Distribution:** 86% protein bound. **Metabolism:** In liver. **Elimination:** In both urine and feces. **Half-Life:** 37 h.

NURSING IMPLICATIONS

Assessment & Drug Effects

- Monitor for decreased pulse, perspiration, or pallor during insertion. Keep patient supine until these signs have disappeared.
- Monitor BP especially with preexisting hypertension.

Patient & Family Education

- Report S&S of PID immediately: (e.g., prolonged or heavy bleeding, unusual vaginal discharge, abdominal or pelvic pain or tenderness, painful sexual intercourse, chills, fever, and flu-like symptoms).
- Report S & S of depression.
- Report any of the following to prescriber immediately: Migraine (if not experienced before) or exceptionally severe headache, or jaundice.

LEVORPHANOL TARTRATE

(lee-vor′fa-nole)

Classification: ANALGESIC; NARCOTIC (OPIATE AGONIST)
Therapeutic: NARCOTIC ANALGESIC
Prototype: Morphine sulfate
Controlled Substance: Schedule II

AVAILABILITY Tablet

ACTION & *THERAPEUTIC EFFECT*

A potent synthetic morphine derivative with agonist activity only. Reported to cause less nausea, vomiting, and constipation than equivalent doses of morphine but may produce more sedation, smooth-muscle relaxation, and respiratory depression. *More potent as an analgesic and has somewhat longer duration of action than morphine.*

USES To relieve moderate to severe pain.

CONTRAINDICATIONS Hypersensitivity to levorphanol; labor and delivery, pregnancy (category D with long time use or high doses); lactation.

CAUTIOUS USE Patients with impaired respiratory reserve, or depressed respirations from another cause (e.g., severe infection, obstructive respiratory conditions, chronic bronchial asthma); head injury or increased intracranial pressure; acute MI, cardiac dysfunction; liver disease, biliary surgery, alcohol or delirium tremens; liver or kidney dysfunction, hypothyroidism, Addison's disease, toxic psychosis, prostatic hypertrophy, or urethral stricture; older adults, other vulnerable populations; pregnancy (category B, short-term use of low doses); children.

ROUTE & DOSAGE

Moderate to Severe Pain

Adult: **PO** 2 mg q6–8h prn

ADMINISTRATION

Oral

- Give in the smallest effective dose to minimize the possibility of tolerance and physical dependence.

ADVERSE EFFECTS **CV:** Hypotension, arrhythmias. **Respiratory:** Respiratory depression. **CNS:** Euphoria, *sedation, drowsiness,* nervousness, confusion. **HEENT:** Blurred vision. **GI:** *Nausea*, vomiting, dry mouth, cramps, *constipation*. **GU:** Urinary frequency, urinary retention, sedation. **Other:** Physical dependence.

INTERACTIONS **Drug: Alcohol** and other CNS DEPRESSANTS compound sedation and CNS depression. **Herbal: St. John's wort** may increase sedation.

PHARMACOKINETICS **Peak:** 60–90 min. **Duration:** 6–8 h. **Distribution:** Crosses placenta; distributed into breast milk. **Metabolism:** In liver. **Elimination:** In urine. **Half-Life:** 11–16 h.

NURSING IMPLICATIONS

Assessment & Drug Effects

- Assess degree of pain relief. Drug is most effective when peaks and valleys of pain relief are avoided.
- Monitor bowel function.
- Monitor ambulation, especially in older adult patients.

Patient & Family Education

- Do not drive or engage in other potentially hazardous activities.
- Avoid alcohol and other CNS depressants unless approved by prescriber.
- Note: Ambulation may increase frequency of nausea and vomiting.
- Increase fluid and fiber intake to offset constipating effects of the drug.

LEVOTHYROXINE SODIUM (T_4) Pr

(lee-voe-thye-rox′een)

Eltroxin ♣, Levoxyl, Synthroid, Unithroid

Classification: THYROID REPLACEMENT

Therapeutic: THYROID HORMONE REPLACEMENT

AVAILABILITY Tablet; solution for injection

ACTION & *THERAPEUTIC EFFECT* Synthetically prepared levo-isomer of thyroxine (T_4, principal component of thyroid gland secretions, determines normal thyroid function). Principal effects include diuresis, loss of weight and puffiness, increased sense of well-being and activity tolerance, plus rise of T_3 and T_4 serum levels toward normal. *By replacing decreased or absent thyroid hormone, it restores metabolic rate of a hypothyroid individual.*

USES Administered orally: Replacement or supplemental therapy in congenital or acquired hypothyroidism of any etiology. Administered IV for treatment of myxedema coma.

CONTRAINDICATIONS Hypersensitivity to levothyroxine or glycerol; thyrotoxicosis; severe cardiovascular conditions, acute MI; obesity treatment; uncorrected adrenal insufficiency.

CAUTIOUS USE Cardiac disease, angina pectoris, cardiac arrhythmias, hypertension; diabetes mellitus;

older adult; impaired kidney function; pregnancy (fetal risk minimal); lactation (infant risk is minimal).

ROUTE & DOSAGE

Thyroid Replacement

Adult: **PO** 1.6 mcg/kg/day; adjust dose by 12.5–25 mcg/day q4–6wk prn **IV** 75% of established oral dose

Child (3–6 mo): **PO** 8–10 mcg/kg/day or 25–50 mcg/day; *6–12 mo:* 6–8 mcg/kg/day *1–5 y:* 5-6 mcg/kg/day *6–12 y:* 4–5 mcg/kg/day *12 y or older:* 2–3 mcg/kg/day

Myxedematous Coma

Adult: **IV** 200–400 mcg day 1, then 1.2 mcg/kg/day if needed

L

ADMINISTRATION

Oral

- Give as a single dose, preferably 30 min–1 h before breakfast. Give consistently with respect to meals. Administer 4 h apart from antacids, iron, and calcium supplements.
- Maintenance dosage for older adults may be 25% lower than for heavier and younger adults.
- Store in a tight, light-resistant container.

Intravenous

PREPARE: **Direct:** Reconstitute vial by adding 5 mL of NS for injection to each 100 mcg. Shake well to dissolve. Use immediately.

ADMINISTER: **Direct:** Give bolus dose over 1 min not to exceed 100 mcg per min.

INCOMPATIBILITIES: **Y-site: Tacrolimus.**

- Store capsules and tablets between 15°–30° C (59°–77° F).
- Store dry powder at 20°–25° C (68°–77° F).

ADVERSE EFFECTS

CV: Palpitations, angina, cardiac arrest, hypertension, myocardial infarction. **Respiratory:** Dyspnea. **CNS:** Insomnia, anxiety, feeling nervous. **Endocrine:** Weight loss, menstrual disease. **Skin:** Alopecia, sweating. **Hepatic:** Increased liver enzymes. **GI:** Diarrhea, abdominal cramps, gag reflex, increased appetite, vomiting. **GU:** Infertility. **Other:** Fever.

INTERACTIONS

Drug: Cholestyramine, colestipol decrease absorption of levothyroxine; **epinephrine, norepinephrine** increase risk of cardiac insufficiency; ORAL ANTICOAGULANTS may potentiate hypoprothrombinemia. **Food:** Food can inhibit absorption so should be taken on an empty stomach.

PHARMACOKINETICS

Absorption: Variable and incompletely absorbed from GI tract (50–80%). **Peak:** 3–4 wk. **Duration:** 1–3 wk. **Distribution:** Gradually released into tissue cells; 99% protein bound. **Half-Life:** 6–7 days.

NURSING IMPLICATIONS

Black Box Warning

In euthyroid patients, levothyroxine doses within the range of daily hormonal requirements are ineffective for weight reduction. Larger doses may produce serious or even life-threatening manifestations of toxicity, particularly when given in association with sympathomimetic amines such as those used for their anorectic effects.

Assessment & Drug Effects

- Monitor HR and BP. Report promptly tachycardia or suspected arrhythmias.
- Monitor for adverse effects during early adjustment. If metabolism increases too rapidly, especially in older adults and heart disease patients, symptoms of angina or cardiac failure may appear.
- Monitor bone age, growth, and psychomotor function in children.
- Some children have partial hair loss after a few months; it returns even with continued therapy.
- Synthroid 100 and 300 mcg tablets contain tartrazine, which may cause an allergic-type reaction in certain patients; particularly those who are hypersensitive to aspirin.
- Monitor lab tests: Baseline and periodic tests of thyroid function. Frequent PT/INR with concurrent anticoagulant therapy, renal function tests.

Patient & Family Education

- Thyroid replacement therapy is usually lifelong.
- Notify prescriber immediately of signs of toxicity (e.g., chest pain, palpitations, nervousness).
- Avoid OTC medications unless approved by prescriber.

LIDOCAINE HYDROCHLORIDE

(lye'doe-kane)

Lidoderm, Xylocaine, ZTlido, Xylocard ♣

Classification: CLASS IB ANTIARRHYTHMIC; LOCAL ANESTHETIC (AMIDE TYPE)

Therapeutic: CLASS IB ANTIARRHYTHMIC; LOCAL ANESTHETIC; ANTICONVULSANT

AVAILABILITY Injection; solution; ointment; cream; gel; spray; jelly; patch; intradermal patch

ACTION & *THERAPEUTIC EFFECT* Exerts antiarrhythmic action (Class IB) by suppressing automaticity in His-Purkinje system. Combines with fast sodium channels in myocardial cell membranes, thus inhibiting sodium influx into myocardial cells. Thus it decreases ventricular depolarization, automaticity, and excitability during diastole. As a local anesthetic, it decreases pain through a reversible nerve conduction blockade. *Suppresses automaticity in His-Purkinje system of the heart and elevates electrical stimulation threshold of ventricle during diastole. Prompt, intense, and longer-lasting local anesthetic than procaine.*

USES Local and regional anesthesia and to relieve local discomfort of skin and mucous membranes. **Patch** for relief of pain associated with post-herpetic neuralgia.

UNLABELED USES Sudden cardiac arrest due to ventricular fibrillation or pulseless ventricular tachycardia, interstitial cystitis.

CONTRAINDICATIONS History of hypersensitivity to amide-type local anesthetics; application or injection of lidocaine anesthetic in presence of severe trauma or sepsis; pregnancy—fetal risk cannot be ruled out.

CAUTIOUS USE Liver or kidney disease, CHF, marked hypoxia, respiratory depression, hypovolemia, shock; myasthenia gravis; debilitated patients, older adults; family history of malignant hyperthermia (fulminant hypermetabolism); lactation—infant risk is minimal. **Topical use:** In eyes, over large body areas, over prolonged periods, in severe or extensive trauma or skin disorders.

ROUTE & DOSAGE

Ventricular Arrhythmias

Adult: **IV** 50–100 mg bolus at a rate of 20–50 mg/min, may repeat in 5 min, then start infusion of 1–4 mg/min immediately after first bolus, not more than 300 mg/h; IM 200–300 mg, may repeat once after 60–90 min
Child: IV 1 mg/kg bolus dose, then 20–50 mcg/kg/min infusion

Anesthetic Uses

Adult: Varies based on procedure, degree of anesthesia needed, tissue vascularity and patient condition. See institutional protocols.

Post-Herpetic Neuralgia

Adult: **Topical** Apply up to 3 patches over intact skin in most painful areas once for up to 12 h per 24 h period

L

ADMINISTRATION

Subcutaneous and Intradermal

- Give in abdomen as preferred site.
- Slowly and steadily inject small volumes while withdrawing the needle.
- Store intradermal powder at controlled room temperature between 15 and 25° C (59–86° F).

Topical

- Do not apply topical lidocaine to large areas of skin or to broken or abraded surfaces. Consult prescriber about covering area with a dressing.
- Avoid topical preparation contact with eyes.
- Store Gel/Jelly at controlled room temperature between 20 and 25° C (68–77° F). Store solution between 15–30° C (59–86° F). Protect from freezing.

Intravenous

- Note: Do not use lidocaine solutions containing preservatives for spinal or epidural (including caudal) block. Use ONLY lidocaine HCl injection without preservatives or epinephrine that is specifically labeled for IV injection or infusion.

PREPARE: **Direct:** Give undiluted. **IV Infusion:** Use D5W for infusion. For adults, add 1 g to 250 or 500 mL to yield 2 or 4 mg/mL, respectively; for children, add 120 mg to 100 m to yield 1.2 mg/mL. ▪ Do not use solutions with particulate matter or discoloration.

ADMINISTER: **Direct:** Give at a rate of 50 mg or fraction thereof over 1 min. **IV Infusion:** Use microdrip and infusion pump. *Adult:* Rate of flow is usually 1–4 mg/min or less. *Child:* Infuse at 20–50 mcg/kg/min.

INCOMPATIBILITIES: Solution/additive: **Methohexital, phenytoin.** Y-site: **Acyclovir, amphotericin B cholesteryl complex, azathioprine, caspofungin, ceftobiprole, dantrolene, diazepam, diazoxide, ganciclovir, gemtuzumab, lansoprazole, milrone, pantoprazole, phenytoin, sulfamethoxazole, thiopental.**

- Discard partially used solutions of lidocaine without preservatives.

ADVERSE EFFECTS (≥5%) **CV:** Edema. **CNS:** Headache. **HEENT:** Burning sensation in eye, conjunctival hyperemia, corneal epithelial defect. **Skin:** Site of topical application may develop erythema, edema, bruising, itching. **GI:** Anorexia, nausea, vomiting.

INTERACTIONS **Drug:** Lidocaine patch may increase toxic effects of **tocainide, mexiletine**; BARBITURATES decrease lidocaine activity; **cimetidine**, BETA-BLOCKERS,

quinidine increase pharmacologic effects of lidocaine; **phenytoin** increases cardiac depressant effects; **procainamide** compounds neurologic and cardiac effects. Do not use with **saquinavir**, may increase arrhythmogenic effects.

PHARMACOKINETICS **Absorption:** Topical application is 3% absorbed through intact skin. **Onset:** 45–90 sec IV; 5–15 min IM; 2–5 min topical. **Duration:** 10–20 min IV; 60–90 min IM; 30–60 min topical; greater than 100 min injected for anesthesia. **Distribution:** Crosses blood–brain barrier and placenta; distributed into breast milk. **Metabolism:** In liver via CYP3A4 and 2D6. **Elimination:** In urine. **Half-Life:** 1.5–2 h.

NURSING IMPLICATIONS

Assessment & Drug Effects

- Stop infusion immediately if ECG indicates excessive cardiac depression (e.g., prolongation of PR interval or QRS complex and the appearance or aggravation of arrhythmias).
- Monitor BP and ECG constantly; assess respiratory and neurologic status frequently to avoid potential overdosage and toxicity.
- Auscultate lungs for basilar rales, especially in patients who tend to metabolize the drug slowly (e.g., CHF, cardiogenic shock, hepatic dysfunction).
- Watch for neurotoxic effects (e.g., drowsiness, dizziness, confusion, paresthesias, visual disturbances, excitement, behavioral changes) in patients receiving IV infusions or with high lidocaine blood levels.
- Signs of methemoglobinemia: cyanotic skin color, abnormal color of the blood.

Patient & Family Education

- Swish and spit out when using lidocaine solution for relief of mouth discomfort; gargle for use in pharynx, may be swallowed (as prescribed).
- Oral topical anesthetics (e.g., Xylocaine Viscous) may interfere with swallowing reflex. **Do not** ingest food within 60 min after drug application; especially pediatric, geriatric, or debilitated patients.
- Topical do not apply to broken skin and avoid occlusive dressing and heat to site.
- Report signs of lidocaine toxicity: restlessness, anxiety, tinnitus, dizziness, blurred vision, tremors, depression, and drowsiness.

LIFITEGRAST

(lif-i-teg′-rast)

Xiidra

Classification: IMMUNOMODULATOR; LYMPHOCYTE FUNCTION-ASSOCIATED ANTIGEN-1 (LFA-1) ANTAGONIST

Therapeutic: IMMUNOMODULATOR

AVAILABILITY Ophthalmic solution

ACTION & THERAPEUTIC EFFECT The exact mechanism of action is unknown; however, lifitegrast binds to the integrin lymphocyte function-associated antigen-1 (LFA-1) and blocks the interaction of LFA-1 with intercellular adhesion molecule-1 (ICAM-1). *ICAM-1 may be overexpressed in corneal and conjunctival tissues in dry eye disease.*

USES Treatment of the signs and symptoms of dry eye disease (DED).

CAUTIOUS USE Use of contact lenses, lactation, pregnancy.

ROUTE & DOSAGE

Dry Eye Disease

Adult: **Ophthalmic** 1 drop bid

ADMINISTRATION

Ophthalmic

- Remove contact lenses before instilling drops. Wait 15 min before re-inserting lenses.
- Avoid touching tip of dropper to the eye or any surface.
- Gently instill one drop onto lower eyelid. Repeat for second eye.
- Discard single-use container after instilling in each eye.

ADVERSE EFFECTS **Respiratory:** Sinusitis. **CNS:** Headache. **HEENT:** Blurred vision, conjunctival hyperemia, eye discharge, eye discomfort, eye irritation, eye pruritus, increased lacrimation, instillation site irritation, reduced visual acuity. **Other:** Dysgeusia.

PHARMACOKINETICS Due to ophthalmic administration, pharmacokinetic data is limited.

NURSING IMPLICATIONS

Assessment & Drug Effects

- Monitor patient for signs or symptoms of an allergic reaction such as rash; hives; itching; shortness of breath; wheezing; cough; or swelling of the face, lips, tongue, or throat.

Patient & Family Education

- Use caution when driving or performing other tasks that require clear eyesight.
- Tell your doctor if you are breastfeeding or pregnant.
- Wash hands before instilling eye drops.
- Avoid touching tip of eyedropper to eye or any other surface.

L

LINACLOTIDE

(lin′a-clo-tide)

Linzess

Classification: ACCELERANT OF GI TRANSIT; GUANYLATE CYCLASE-C AGONIST

Therapeutic: ACCELERANT OF GI TRANSIT

AVAILABILITY Capsule

ACTION & *THERAPEUTIC EFFECT* Acts on the inner surface of the intestinal epithelium to increase concentrations of cGMP. Increased intracellular cGMP results in increased intestinal fluid and accelerated transit. Increased extracellular cGMP decreases the activity of pain-sensing nerves. *Improves bowel function by decreasing constipation and associated pain due to bowel irritation.*

USES Treatment of irritable bowel syndrome with constipation and chronic idiopathic constipation.

CONTRAINDICATIONS Severe diarrhea; known or suspected mechanical GI obstruction; children younger than 6 y.

CAUTIOUS USE Pregnancy (category C); lactation. Safety and efficacy in children younger than 18 y not established.

ROUTE & DOSAGE

Irritable Bowel Syndrome with Constipation

Adult: **PO** 290 mcg once daily

Chronic Idiopathic Constipation

Adult: **PO** 145 mcg once daily

ADMINISTRATION

Oral

- Give on an empty stomach at least 30 min prior to first meal of day.
- Ensure that capsules are swallowed whole. They should not be opened or chewed.
- Store at 20°–25° C (68°–77° F).

ADVERSE EFFECTS Respiratory: Sinusitis, upper respiratory tract infection. **GI:** Abdominal distension, abdominal pain, *diarrhea*, dyspepsia, fecal incontinence, flatulence, gastroesophageal reflux disease, viral gastroenteritis, vomiting. **Other:** Headache, fatigue.

PHARMACOKINETICS Absorption: Minimally absorbed. **Metabolism:** In the GI tract to active metabolite. **Elimination:** Fecal.

NURSING IMPLICATIONS

Assessment & Drug Effects

- Monitor bowel pattern. Report severe abdominal pain, severe diarrhea, or passage of bloody stools.

Patient & Family Education

- Stop taking drug and seek immediate medical attention if you develop unusual or severe abdominal pain, and /or severe diarrhea, especially if in combination with red blood in the stool or passage of black, tarry stool.

LINAGLIPTIN

(lin'a glip'tin)

Tradjenta

Classification: DIPEPTIDYL PEPTIDASE-4 (DPP-4) INHIBITOR

Therapeutic: ANTIDIABETIC; DDP-4 INHIBITOR

Prototype: Sitagliptin

AVAILABILITY Tablet

ACTION & *THERAPEUTIC EFFECT* Slows inactivation of incretin hormones released by the intestine. When the blood glucose begins to rise, incretin hormones stimulate insulin secretion and reduce glucagon secretion, resulting in decreased hepatic glucose production. *Sitagliptin lowers both fasting and postprandial plasma glucose levels.*

USES Treatment of type 2 diabetes mellitus in combination with diet and exercise.

CONTRAINDICATIONS History of hypersensitivity to linagliptin (e.g., urticaria, angioedema, or bronchial hyperreactivity); acute pancreatitis.

CAUTIOUS USE Previous history of angioedema with another DPP-4 inhibitor; concurrent use with an insulin secretagogue (e.g., sulfonylurea); history of pancreatitis; pregnancy (category B); lactation. Safety and efficacy in children not established.

ROUTE & DOSAGE

Type 2 Diabetes Mellitus

Adult: **PO** 5 mg once daily

ADMINISTRATION

Oral

- May be given with or without food.
- Store at 15°–30° C (59°–86° F).

ADVERSE EFFECTS Respiratory: Nasopharyngitis. **Endocrine:** Hypoglycemia. **GI:** Increased serum lipase.

INTERACTIONS Drug: Strong inducers of CYP3A4 (e.g., **rifampin, dexamethasone, phenytoin, phenobarbital**) or P-glycoprotein (e.g., **rifampin**) may decrease the therapeutic effect of linagliptin. Combination use with a SULFONYLUREA (e.g., **glyburide**) may increase the risk of hypoglycemia. **Herbal:** St John's wort may affect efficacy.

PHARMACOKINETICS **Absorption:** 30% bioavailable. **Peak:** 1.5 h. **Metabolism:** Primarily excreted unchanged via CYP 3A4. **Elimination:** Enterohepatic system (80%) and renal elimination (5%). **Half-Life:** 12 h.

NURSING IMPLICATIONS

Assessment & Drug Effects

- Monitor for S&S of hypoglycemia when used in combination with a sulfonylurea drug or insulin.
- Monitor blood pressure.
- Monitor for serious hypersensitivity reactions (e.g., angioedema, exfoliative skin conditions). Onset may occur any time during the first 3 mo of treatment.
- Monitor lab tests: Baseline and periodic HbA1C, blood glucose, serum creatinine/BUN.

Patient & Family Education

- Seek medical attention during periods of stress or illness as dosage adjustments may be required.
- Monitor both fasting and postprandial blood glucose levels as directed.
- Report promptly for medical evaluation if you experience any of the following: Wheezing; chest tightness; fever; itching; bad cough; blue skin color; seizures; or swelling of face, lips, tongue, or throat.
- Note that when taken alone to control diabetes, linagliptin is unlikely to cause hypoglycemia because it only works when the blood sugar is rising.

LINCOMYCIN HYDROCHLORIDE

(lin-koe-mye′sin)

Lincocin

Classification: LINCOSAMIDE ANTIBIOTIC

Therapeutic: ANTIBIOTIC

Prototype: Clindamycin

AVAILABILITY Solution for injection

ACTION & THERAPEUTIC EFFECT Derived from *Streptomyces lincolnensis* and binds to the 50S ribosomal subunits of the bacteria inhibiting protein synthesis, eventually resulting in inhibition of bacterial cell growth or bacterial cell death. *Effective against most common gram-positive pathogens. Also effective against many anaerobic bacteria.*

USES Reserved for treatment of serious infections caused by susceptible bacteria in penicillin-allergic patients or patients for whom penicillin is inappropriate.

CONTRAINDICATIONS Previous hypersensitivity to lincomycin and clindamycin; impaired liver function, known monilial infections (unless treated concurrently); lactation.

CAUTIOUS USE Impaired kidney function; history of GI disease, particularly colitis; history of liver, endocrine, or metabolic diseases; history of asthma, hay fever, eczema, drug or other allergies; older adult patients, pregnancy (category B); infants younger than 1 mo.

ROUTE & DOSAGE

Infections

Adult: **IM** 600 mg q12–24 h **IV** 600 mg–1 g q8–12h (max: 8 g/day)

Adolescent/Child/Infant (older than 1 mo): **IM** 10 mg/kg q12–24h; **IV** 10–20 mg/kg/day divided q8–12h

ADMINISTRATION

Intramuscular

- Give injection deep into large muscle mass; inject slowly to minimize pain. Rotate injection sites.

Intravenous

PREPARE: **Intermittent:** Dilute each 1 g of lincomycin in at least 100 mL of D5W, NS, or other compatible solution.
ADMINISTER: **Intermittent:** Give at a rate of 1 g/h.
INCOMPATIBILITIES: **Solution/additive:** **Colistimethate, kanamycin, methicillin, penicillin G, phenytoin.**

- Follow manufacturer's directions for further information on reconstitution, storage time, compatible IV fluids, and IV administration rates.

ADVERSE EFFECTS **CV:** Hypotension, syncope, cardiopulmonary arrest (particularly after rapid IV). **HEENT:** Tinnitus. **GI:** Glossitis, stomatitis, *nausea, vomiting*, anorexia, decreased taste acuity, unpleasant or altered taste, abdominal cramps, *diarrhea*, acute enterocolitis, pseudomembranous colitis (potentially fatal). **Hematologic:** Neutropenia, leukopenia, agranulocytosis, thrombocytopenic purpura, aplastic anemia. **Other:** Hypersensitivity [pruritus, urticaria, skin rashes, exfoliative and vesiculobullous dermatitis, erythema multiforme (rare), angioedema, photosensitivity, anaphylactoid reaction, serum sickness]; superinfections (proctitis, pruritus ani, vaginitis); vertigo, dizziness, headache, generalized myalgia, thrombophlebitis following IV use; pain at IM injection site.

INTERACTIONS **Drug: Kaolin and pectin** decrease lincomycin absorption; **tubocurarine, pancuronium** may enhance neuromuscular blockade.

PHARMACOKINETICS **Peak:** 30 min IM. **Duration:** 12–14 h IM; 14 h IV. **Distribution:** High concentrations in bone, aqueous humor, bile, and peritoneal, pleural, and synovial fluids; crosses placenta; distributed into breast milk. **Metabolism:** Partially in liver. **Elimination:** In urine and feces. **Half-Life:** 5 h.

NURSING IMPLICATIONS

Black Box Warning

Lincomycin has been associated with severe, potentially fatal, C. difficile pseudomembranous colitis.

Assessment & Drug Effects

- Monitor BP and pulse. Have patient remain recumbent following drug administration until BP stabilizes.
- Monitor closely and report changes in bowel frequency. Discontinue drug if significant diarrhea occurs.
- Diarrhea, acute colitis, or pseudomembranous colitis (see Appendix F) may occur up to several weeks after cessation of therapy.
- Examine IM/IV injection sites daily for signs of inflammation.
- Monitor serum drug levels closely in patients with severe impairment of kidney function.
- Monitor for S&S of superinfections that are most likely to occur when therapy exceeds 10 days (see Appendix F).
- Monitor lab tests: C&S prior to initiating therapy; periodic LFTs, renal function tests, and CBC during prolonged drug therapy.

L

Patient & Family Education

- Notify prescriber immediately of symptoms of hypersensitivity (see Appendix F). Drug should be discontinued.
- Notify prescriber promptly of the onset of perianal irritation, diarrhea, or blood and mucus in stools.

LINDANE

(lin'dane)

Classification: SCABICIDE; PEDICULICIDE
Therapeutic: ANTIPARASITIC; PEDIC-ULICIDE

AVAILABILITY Shampoo

ACTION & *THERAPEUTIC EFFECT* Action related to its direct absorption by parasites and ova (nits). Drug absorption through the parasite exoskeleton results in death of parasites and their ova. *Has ectoparasitic and ovicidal activity against the two variants of* Pediculus humanus, Pediculus capitis *(head louse) and* Pediculus pubis *(crab louse), and the arthropod* Sarcoptes scabiei *(scabies).*

USES To treat head and crab lice and scabies infestations and to eradicate their ova.

CONTRAINDICATIONS Premature neonates, patient with known seizure disorders; application to eyes, face, mucous membranes, urethral meatus, open cuts or raw, weeping surfaces; prolonged or excessive applications or simultaneous application of creams, ointments, oils; extensive dermatitis; uncontrolled seizures; lactation.

CAUTIOUS USE History of seizures; HIV infection; history of head trauma; elderly, individuals weighing less than 50 kg (110 lbs); alcoholism; pregnancy (category C); infants, children younger than 10 y, or individuals weighing less than 110 lb.

ROUTE & DOSAGE

Lice and Scabies Infestation

Adult/Child: **Topical** Apply to all body areas except the face, leave lotion on 8–12 h, then rinse off; leave shampoo on 4 min, then rinse thoroughly; **do not** repeat in less than 1 wk

ADMINISTRATION

Note: Caregiver needs to wear plastic disposable or rubber gloves when applying lindane (nitrile, latex with neoprene or sheer vinyl). Thoroughly clean hands after application, especially if pregnant or applying medication to more than one patient to avoid prolonged skin contact.

Topical

- Remove all skin lotions, creams, and oil-based hair dressings completely and allow skin to dry and cool before applying lindane; this will reduce percutaneous absorption.
- Shake cream or lotion container well. Apply thin film over the affected areas. Leave in place 8–12 h and follow with bath or shower.
- Shampoo: Hair should be dry before application. Apply to dry hair without adding water. Work drug thoroughly onto hair shafts and scalp and allow to remain in place 4 min. Immediately rinse all lather away and avoid unnecessary contact with other body surfaces. Towel dry briskly and then remove nits with nit comb or tweezers.
- Store in a tight container away from direct light and heat. Protect from freezing. Store at 20°–25° C (68°–77° F).

ADVERSE EFFECTS CNS: CNS stimulation (usually after accidental ingestion or misuse of product): Restlessness, anxiety, dizziness, tremors, convulsions; seizures; death. **Skin:** Eczematous eruptions. **Other:** Inhalation (headache, nausea, vomiting, myelosuppression, irritation of ENT).

INTERACTIONS Drug: No clinically significant interactions established.

PHARMACOKINETICS Absorption: Slowly and incompletely absorbed through intact skin; maximum absorption from face, scalp, axillae. **Distribution:** Stored in body fat. **Metabolism:** In liver. **Elimination:** In urine and feces.

NURSING IMPLICATIONS

Black Box Warning

Lindane has been associated with seizures and death with repeated or prolonged application.

Assessment & Drug Effects

- Monitor for seizure activity in individuals with a history of seizures. Withhold drug and report to prescriber immediately.
- Exercise caution when using lindane on infants, children, the elderly, and individuals with other skin conditions (e.g., atopic dermatitis, psoriasis) and in those who weigh less than 110 lbs (50 kg) as they may be at risk of serious neurotoxicity.

Patient & Family Education

- Lindane is highly toxic drug if topical applications are excessive or if swallowed or inhaled. Keep out of reach of children. **Do not** use more often than prescribed.
- Discontinue medication and notify prescriber if skin eruptions appear.
- Do not apply medication to face, mouth, open skin lesions, or to eyelashes; avoid contact with eyes. If accidental eye contact occurs, flush with water.

LINEZOLID

(lin-e-zo′lid)

Zyvox, Zyvoxam ♣

Classification: OXAZOLIDINONE ANTIBIOTIC

Therapeutic: ANTIBIOTIC

AVAILABILITY Tablet; suspension; solution for injection

ACTION & *THERAPEUTIC EFFECT* Synthetic antibiotic that binds to a site on the 23S ribosomal RNA of bacteria, which prevents the bacterial RNA translation process, thus preventing further growth. *Is bactericidal against gram-positive, gram-negative, and anaerobic bacteria. Bacteriostatic against enterococci and staphylococci, and bactericidal against streptococci.*

USES Treatment of vancomycin-resistant *Enterococcus faecium* (VREF), nosocomial pneumonia, bacteremia, complicated and uncomplicated skin and skin structure infections, community-acquired pneumonia.

CONTRAINDICATIONS Hypersensitivity to linezolid; concurrent or within 2 weeks of MAOI therapy.

CAUTIOUS USE History of thrombocytopenia, thrombocytopenia; patients on serotonin reuptake inhibitors, or adrenergic agents, active alcoholism, anemia, bleeding, bone marrow suppression, history of seizures; chemotherapy, coagulopathy, colitis, diarrhea, hypertension, hyperthyroidism,

L

leukopenia, hypertension; diabetes mellitus; pheochromocytoma; carcinoid syndrome.

ROUTE & DOSAGE

Vancomycin-Resistant *Enterococci*

Adult/Adolescent (12 y or older): **PO/IV** 600 mg q12h × 7–14 days
Infant/Child: **PO/IV** 10 mg/kg q8h × 10–28 days

Nosocomial or Community-Acquired Pneumonia, Complicated Skin Infections

Adult/Adolescent (12 y or older): **PO/IV** 600 mg q12h × duration varies based on disease severity and patient response
Infant/Child: **PO/IV** 10 mg/kg (Max: 600 mg) q8h × 10–14 days

L

ADMINISTRATION

Note: No dosage adjustment is necessary when switching from IV to oral administration.

Oral

- Reconstitute suspension by adding 123 mL distilled water in two portions; after adding first half, shake to wet all of the powder, then add second half of water and shake vigorously to produce a uniform suspension with a concentration of 100 mg/5 mL.
- Before each use, mix suspension by inverting bottle 3–5 × but **do not shake**. Discard unused suspension after 21 days.

Intravenous

PREPARE: **Intermittent:** IV solution is supplied in a single-use, ready-to-use infusion bag. Remove from protective wrap immediately prior to use. ▪ Check for minute leaks by firmly squeezing bag. Discard if leaks are detected.

ADMINISTER: **Intermittent:** Do not use infusion bag in a series connection. ▪ Give over 30–120 min. If IV line is used to infuse other drugs, flush before and after with D5W, NS, or LR.

INCOMPATIBILITIES: **Solution/additive:** **Amikacin, ceftriaxone, erythromycin, hydrocortisone, methylprednisolone, trimethoprim-sulfamethoxazole.** **Y-site:** **Amphotericin B, chlorpromazine, dantrolene, daunorubicin, diazepam, garenoxacin, letermovir, pantoprazole, pentamidine, phenytoin, thiopental.**

- Store at 25° C (77° F). Protect from light and keep bottles tightly closed.

ADVERSE EFFECTS (≥5%) **CNS:** Headache. **Skin:** Rash. **GI:** Diarrhea, nausea.

INTERACTIONS **Drug:** MAO INHIBITORS may cause hypertensive crisis; **pseudoephedrine** may cause elevated BP; may cause **serotonin** syndrome with agents that effect serotonin like SELECTIVE SEROTONIN REUPTAKE INHIBITORS. AMPHETAMINES may have increase hypertensive effects. Do not administer with LIVE VACCINES. Use caution with MYLEOSUPPRESIVE AGENTS. **Food:** Tyramine-containing food may cause elevated BP. **Herbal:** **Ginseng, ephedra, ma huang** may lead to elevated BP, headache, nervousness.

PHARMACOKINETICS **Absorption:** Rapidly absorbed, 100% bioavailable. **Peak:** 1–2 h PO. **Distribution:** 31% protein bound. **Metabolism:** By oxidation. **Elimination:** Primarily in urine. **Half-Life:** 6–7 h.

NURSING IMPLICATIONS

Assessment & Drug Effects

- Monitor for S&S of: Bleeding; hypertension; or pseudomembranous colitis that begins with diarrhea.
- Monitor blood pressure.
- Visual function assessment for patients taking 3 months or longer.
- Monitor lab tests: C&S before initiating therapy; periodic CBC, platelet count, Hgb and Hct, in those at risk for bleeding or with longer than 2 wk of linezolid therapy.

Patient & Family Education

- Report any of the following to prescriber promptly: Onset of diarrhea; easy bruising or bleeding of any type; or S&S of superinfection (see Appendix F), S&S of seizure activity.
- Report any vision changes that may include seeing flashing or flickering lights or any numbness or tingling in hands or feet.
- Avoid foods and beverages high in tyramine (e.g., aged, fermented, pickled, or smoked foods, and beverages). Limit tyramine intake to less than 100 mg per meal (see *Information for Patients* provided by the manufacturer).
- Do not take OTC cold remedies or decongestants without consulting prescriber.
- Note for phenylketonurics: Each 5 mL oral suspension contains 20 mg phenylalanine.

LIOTHYRONINE SODIUM (T_3)

(lye-oh-thye′roe-neen)

Cytomel, Triostat

Classification: THYROID REPLACEMENT

Therapeutic: THYROID HORMONE REPLACEMENT

Prototype: Levothyroxine sodium

AVAILABILITY Tablet; solution for injection

ACTION & *THERAPEUTIC EFFECT* Synthetic form of natural thyroid hormone (T_3). Shares actions and uses of thyroid but has more rapid action and more rapid disappearance of effect, permitting quick dosage adjustment, if necessary. *Replacement therapy for absent or decreased thyroid hormone. Principal effect is an increase in the metabolic rate of all body tissues.*

USES Replacement or supplemental therapy for cretinism, myxedema, goiter, secondary (pituitary) or tertiary (hypothalamic) hypothyroidism, and T_3 suppression test.

CONTRAINDICATIONS Hypersensitivity to liothyronine; thyrotoxicosis; obesity treatment; severe cardiovascular conditions, acute MI, uncontrolled hypertension; adrenal insufficiency.

CAUTIOUS USE Angina pectoris, hypertension; diabetes mellitus; impaired kidney function, renal failure; severe and prolonged hypothyroidism; older adult; pregnancy (category A); lactation (infant risk cannot be ruled out); children.

ROUTE & DOSAGE

Thyroid Replacement

Adult: **PO** 25–75 mcg/day
Geriatric: **PO** 5 mcg/day, increase by 5 mcg/day every 2 wk

Myxedema

Adult: **IV** 5–20 mcg loading dose, maintenance 2.5–10 mcg q8h

Geriatric: **PO** Start at 5 mcg/day

T_3 Suppression Test

Adult: **PO** 75–100 mcg/day × 7 days

ADMINISTRATION

Oral

- Give daily before breakfast.

Intravenous

PREPARE: **Direct:** Give undiluted.
ADMINISTER: **Direct:** Give each 10 mcg or fraction thereof over 1 min.

- Store tablets in a heat-, light-, and moisture-proof container.
- Store tablets between 15°–30° C (59°–86° F). Store solution between 2°–8° C (36°–46° F).

L

ADVERSE EFFECTS CV: Cardiac arrhythmia.

INTERACTIONS Drug: Cholestyramine, colestipol decrease absorption; **epinephrine, norepinephrine** increase risk of cardiac insufficiency; ORAL ANTICOAGULANTS may potentiate hypoprothrombinemia. CALCIUM salts may decrease effect of product, separate does by 4 h.

PHARMACOKINETICS Absorption: Completely absorbed from GI tract. **Peak:** 24–72 h. **Duration:** Up to 72 h. **Distribution:** Gradually released into tissue cells. **Half-Life:** 6–7 days.

NURSING IMPLICATIONS

Black Box Warning

In euthyroid patients, levothyroxine doses within the range of daily hormonal requirements are ineffective for weight reduction. Larger doses may produce serious or even life-threatening manifestations of toxicity, particularly when given in association with sympathomimetic amines such as those used for their anorectic effects.

Assessment & Drug Effects

- Watch for possible additive effects during the early period of liothyronine substitution for another preparation, particularly in older adults, children, and patients with cardiovascular disease. Residual actions of other thyroid preparations may persist for weeks.
- Metabolic effects of liothyronine persist a few days after drug withdrawal.
- Withhold drug and notify prescriber at onset of overdosage symptoms (hyperthyroidism, see Appendix F); usually therapy can be resumed with lower dosage.
- Monitor lab tests: Serum T3 and TSH levels.

Patient & Family Education

- Take medication exactly as ordered.
- Learn S&S of hyperthyroidism (see Appendix F); notify prescriber promptly if they appear.

LIOTRIX (T_3–T_4)

(lye′oh-trix)

Classification: THYROID REPLACEMENT

Therapeutic: THYROID HORMONE REPLACEMENT

Prototype: Levothyroxine sodium

AVAILABILITY Tablet

ACTION & *THERAPEUTIC EFFECT*

Synthetic levothyroxine (T_4) and liothyronine (T_3) that influence growth and maturation of tissues, increase energy expenditure, and affect turnover of essentially all substrates. These hormones play an integral role in metabolic processes, and are important to development of the CNS in newborns. *Increases metabolic rate of all body tissues.*

USES Replacement or supplemental therapy for cretinism, myxedema, goiter, and secondary (pituitary) or tertiary (hypothalamic) hypothyroidism. Also with antithyroid agents in thyrotoxicosis and to prevent goitrogenesis and hypothyroidism.

CONTRAINDICATIONS Untreated thyrotoxicosis, acute MI, morphologic hypogonadism, nephrosis, adrenal deficiency due to hypopituitarism; tartrazine dye hypersensitivity, obesity treatment.

CAUTIOUS USE Myxedema; hypertension, angina, cardiac arrhythmias, cardiac disease, coronary artery disease; chronic hypothyroidism; diabetes mellitus, diabetes insipidus older adults; hypertension; arteriosclerosis; kidney dysfunction, pregnancy (category A); lactation; neonates, infants, children.

ROUTE & DOSAGE

Thyroid Replacement

Adult/Child: **PO** 12.5–25 mcg/day, gradually increase to desired response

ADMINISTRATION

Oral

- Give as a single daily dose, preferably before breakfast.
- Make dose increases at 1- to 2-wk intervals.
- Store in a heat-, light-, and moisture-proof container. Shelf-life: 2 y.
- Store at 2°–8° C (36°–46° F).

ADVERSE EFFECTS CV: Cardiac arrhythmia, chest pain, increased blood pressure, palpitations, tachycardia. **Respiratory:** Dyspnea. **CNS:** Anxiety, ataxia, headache, insomnia, nervousness. **Endocrine:** Weight loss, menstrual disease. **Skin:** Alopecia, sweating, itching. **GI:** Abdominal cramps, constipation, diarrhea, increased appetite, nausea, vomiting. **Other:** Fever.

INTERACTIONS Drug: Cholestyramine, colestipol decrease absorption; **epinephrine, norepinephrine** increase risk of cardiac insufficiency; ORAL ANTICOAGULANTS may potentiate hypoprothrombinemia. CALCIUM SALTS decrease effect of thyroid supplement.

L

NURSING IMPLICATIONS

Black Box Warning

In euthyroid patients, levothyroxine doses within the range of daily hormonal requirements are ineffective for weight reduction. Larger doses may produce serious or even life-threatening manifestations of toxicity, particularly when given in association with sympathomimetic amines such as those used for their anorectic effects.

Assessment & Drug Effects

- Watch for possible additive effects during the early period of liothyronine substitution for another preparation, particularly in older adults, children, and patients with cardiovascular disease. Residual actions of other thyroid preparations may persist for weeks.
- Note: Metabolic effects of liotrix persist a few days after drug withdrawal.

- Withhold drug and notify prescriber at onset of overdosage symptoms (hyperthyroidism, see Appendix F); usually therapy can be resumed with lower dosage.
- Monitor diabetics for glycemic control; an increase in insulin or oral hypoglycemic may be required.
- Monitor lab tests: T3, T4, unbound T4 and TSH levels.

Patient & Family Education

- Notify prescriber of headache (euthyroid patients); may indicate need for dosage adjustment or change to another thyroid preparation.
- Take medication exactly as ordered.
- Learn S&S of hyperthyroidism (see Appendix F); notify prescriber if they appear.

L

LIRAGLUTIDE

(lir-a-glu′tide)

Saxenda, Victoza

Classification: ANTIDIABETIC; GLUCAGON-LIKE PEPTIDE-1 RECEPTOR AGONIST; INCRETIN MIMETICS

Therapeutic: ANTIDIABETIC

Prototype: Exenatide

AVAILABILITY Solution for injection

ACTION & *THERAPEUTIC EFFECT* Liraglutide is a glucagon-like peptide-1 (GLP-1) receptor agonist that causes increased insulin release and decreased glucagon release in the presence of elevated blood glucose, and delays the rate of gastric emptying. *Liraglutide lowers postprandial blood glucose levels and helps normalize HbA1C.*

USES Treatment of type 2 diabetes mellitus in combination with diet and exercise; reduction of cardiovascular mortality **(Victoza)**; chronic weight management **(Saxenda)**.

CONTRAINDICATIONS Family or personal history of medullary thyroid carcinoma (MTC); history of multiple endocrine neoplasia syndrome type 2 (MEN 2); serious hypersensitive reaction to liraglutide; treatment with insulin; diabetic ketoacidosis; pancreatitis; history of suicidal attempts or active suicidal ideation; pregnancy—fetal risk has been demonstrated; lactation—infant risk cannot be ruled out.

CAUTIOUS USE History of pancreatitis; alcohol abuse; history of cholelithiasis; history of severe hypoglycemia; gastroparesis; type 2 diabetes; history of angioedema; renal or hepatic impairment; history of thyroid nodules concurrent use with insulin secretagogues (e.g., sulfonylurea); obesity; older adults. Safe use in children younger than 10 y not established.

ROUTE & DOSAGE

Type 2 Diabetes Mellitus (Victoza)

Adult/Adolescent/Child (over 10 y): **Subcutaneous** Initial dose of 0.6 mg once daily for 1 wk. Then increase dose to 1.2–1.8 mg once daily to achieve glycemic control.

Chronic Weight Management (Saxenda only)

Adult/Adolescent: **Subcutaneous** 0.6 mg daily for 1 wk then increase by 0.6 mg/day at weekly intervals to target dose of 3 mg daily

ADMINISTRATION

Subcutaneous

- NIOSH guidelines recommend double gloves and a protective gown for preparation and administration. If there is any chance that the patient may resist, use eye/face protection.
- Inject into abdomen, thigh, or upper arm without regard to meals.
- Injection timing can be changed without dose adjustment (i.e., injection may be given any time of day).
- Store refrigerated between 2 and 8° C (36 and 46° F). After first use, then may be stored refrigerated at 15°–30° C (59°–86° F) for up to 30 days. Do not freeze. Discard pen 30 days after first use. Protect from excessive heat and sunlight. Do not store in the freezer.

ADVERSE EFFECTS (≥5%)

Respiratory: *Upper respiratory tract infection.* **CNS:** *Headache.* **Endocrine:** *Hypoglycemia.* **GI:** *Constipation, diarrhea, nausea, vomiting, decreased appetite, dyspepsia.*

INTERACTIONS

Drug: Due to its ability to slow gastric emptying, liraglutide can decrease absorption rate and plasma levels of oral medications; increases risk of hypoglycemia with INSULIN and SULFONYLUREAS

PHARMACOKINETICS

Peak: 8–12 h. **Distribution:** 98% plasma protein bound. **Metabolism:** Peptide hydrolysis/degradation. **Elimination:** Urine and feces as inactive metabolites. **Half-Life:** 12–13 h.

NURSING IMPLICATIONS

Black Box Warning

Liraglutide has been associated with thyroid tumors in animal studies; relevance to humans has not been established.

Assessment & Drug Effects

- Monitor for S&S of hypoglycemia. Note that the initial week of dosing (0.6 mg/d) is not effective for glycemic control but is designed to reduce GI distress.
- Monitor weight.
- Monitor for emergence or worsening of depression, suicidal thoughts or behavior, or changes in mood or behavior.
- Monitor for and report S&S of significant GI distress, including nausea, vomiting, and diarrhea.
- Monitor for and promptly report S&S of acute pancreatitis (acute abdominal pain with/without vomiting). If pancreatitis is suspected, withhold drug and notify prescriber immediately.
- Monitor lab tests: Frequent fasting and postprandial plasma glucose and periodic HbA1C; calcitonin levels, periodic renal function tests and LFTs.

Patient & Family Education

- Monitor blood glucose daily as directed. Report to prescriber significant hypoglycemia.
- Report worsening or development of depression, suicidal ideation, or unusual changes in behavior.
- Review adverse effects with patient and/or caregiver.
- Administered daily, at any time independent of meals.
- Demonstration of correct subcutaneous administration.
- If a dose is missed, instruct the patient to skip the missed dose

L

and resume the normal schedule. Contact provider if more than 3 days are missed.
- Report promptly any of the following: A lump in the neck; hoarseness; difficulty swallowing or difficulty breathing; significant GI distress such as persistent, severe abdominal pain that may be accompanied by vomiting.
- Discard any pen that has been in use for greater than 30 days. Do not share the injection pen.
- Liraglutide may cause decreased appetite and some weight loss.

LISDEXAMFETAMINE DIMESYLATE

(lis-dex-am-fet′a-meen)

Vyvanse

Classification: CEREBRAL STIMULANT; AMPHETAMINE; ANOREXIGENIC

Therapeutic: STIMULANT; ANOREXIGENIC; ATTENTION DEFICIT AGENT

Prototype: Amphetamine

Controlled Substance: Schedule II

AVAILABILITY Capsule; chewable tablet

ACTION & *THERAPEUTIC EFFECT* An isomer of amphetamine that has anorexigenic action; this is thought to result from CNS stimulation and possibly from loss of acuity of smell and taste. *In hyperkinetic children, amphetamines reduce motor restlessness by an unknown mechanism.*

USES Treatment of attention-deficit hyperactivity disorder (ADHD); binge eating disorder.

CONTRAINDICATIONS Hypersensitivity to sympathomimetic amines, dextroamphetamine, or amphetamine; advanced arteriosclerosis; serious structural cardiac abnormalities, cardiomyopathy, cardiac arrhythmias, or symptomatic cardiovascular disease; uncontrollable hypertension; glaucoma; agitated states; during or within 14 days of administering MAOIs; emergence of new psychotic or manic symptoms caused by amphetamine use; suicidal ideation; lactation.

CAUTIOUS USE Controlled hypertension, heart failure, recent MI, or recent ventricular arrhythmia; preexisting psychotic disorder; suicidal tendencies; bipolar disorder, depression; history of aggressive or hostile behavior; renal impairment; Tourette syndrome/tics; history of drug abuse or alcoholism; older adults; pregnancy (category C); children younger than 6 y.

ROUTE & DOSAGE

Attention-Deficit Hyperactivity Disorder

Adult/Child (6–12 y): **PO** 30 mg daily in a.m.; may increase to 50–70 mg daily at weekly intervals (max: 70 mg daily)

Binge Eating Disorder

Adult: 30 mg daily in a.m. then titrate up by 20 mg at weekly interval to target dose of 50–70 mg/day

ADMINISTRATION

Oral
- Give daily dose in the morning.
- Capsule may be taken whole or opened and dissolved in a glass of water, yogurt, or orange juice.
- Store at 15°–30° C (59°–86° F) and protect from light.

ADVERSE EFFECTS **CV:** Increased blood pressure, increased heart rate. **Respiratory:** Dyspnea **CNS:** Affect lability, dizziness, *headache, insomnia, irritability*, somnolence, tic. **Endocrine:** Decreased appetite, weight loss. **Skin:** Rash. **GI:** *Abdominal pain, dry mouth*, nausea, xerostomia, vomiting, *decreased appetite*. **GU:** Erectile dysfunction. **Other:** Pyrexia.

DIAGNOSTIC TEST INTERFERENCE Can cause a significant elevation in plasma CORTICOSTEROID levels and may interfere with ***urinary steroid determinations***.

INTERACTIONS **Drug:** **Chlorpromazine** and **haloperidol** inhibit the CNS stimulant effects of amphetamines. **Furazolidone** and MAO INHIBITORS can increase adverse effects. **Lithium** may inhibit the effects of lisdexamfetamine. Compounds that acidify the urine lower the plasma levels of lisdexamfetamine. Lisdexamfetamine inhibits the actions of **adrenergic blockers**. Coadministration of ANTIHISTAMINES with lisdexamfetamine can counteract desired sedative effects. Lisdexamfetamine may antagonize the hypotensive effects of ANTIHYPERTENSIVE AGENTS. Lisdexamfetamine may delay the absorption of **ethosuximide** and **phenytoin**. Lisdexamfetamine may potentiate the actions of TRICYCLIC ANTIDEPRESSANTS, **meperidine** and **norepinephrine**. **Albuterol** can cause increased cardiovascular effects.

PHARMACOKINETICS **Absorption:** Rapidly from GI tract. **Peak:** 1 h. **Distribution:** Extensive throughout body. **Metabolism:** Prodrug converted in liver to dextroamphetamine. **Elimination:** Urine (96%). **Half-Life:** 1 h (lisdexamfetamine) 6–8 h (dextroamphetamine).

NURSING IMPLICATIONS

Black Box Warning

Lisdexamfetamine has been associated with high potential for abuse and dependence.

Assessment & Drug Effects

- Monitor children, adolescents, and adults for signs and symptoms of adverse cardiac reactions (e.g., hypertension, arrhythmias). Report promptly exertional chest pain or syncope.
- Monitor closely growth rate in children.
- Typically therapy is interrupted or dosage reduced periodically to assess effectiveness in behavior disorders.
- Monitor children and adolescents for development of aggressive or abnormal behaviors.

Patient & Family Education

- Do not drive or engage in other potentially hazardous activities until response to drug is known.
- Report promptly any of the following: Chest pain with activity, new or worse behavior or thought problems, psychotic symptoms (e.g., hearing voices, believing things that are not true).
- Taper drug gradually following long-term use to avoid extreme fatigue, mental depression, and prolonged abnormal sleep pattern.

LISINOPRIL

(ly-sin′o-pril)

Prinivil, Qbrelis, Zestril

Classification: ANTIHYPERTENSIVE; ANGIOTENSIN-CONVERTING ENZYME (ACE) INHIBITOR

Therapeutic: ANTIHYPERTENSIVE

Prototype: Enalapril

AVAILABILITY Tablet; oral solution

ACTION & *THERAPEUTIC EFFECT* Lowers BP by specific inhibition of the angiotensin-converting enzyme (ACE). This interrupts conversion sequences initiated by renin that form angiotensin II, a potent vasoconstrictor. ACE inhibition alters hemodynamics without compensatory reflex tachycardia or changes in cardiac output (except in patients with CHF). *Improves cardiac output and exercise tolerance. Aldosterone is also reduced, thus permitting a potassium-sparing effect. Migraine prophylaxis.*

USES Hypertension; heart failure with reduced ejection fraction, ST elevation MI.

L

CONTRAINDICATIONS History of angioedema related to treatment with an ACE inhibitor, ACE inhibitor hypersensitivity; history of idiopathic or hereditary angioedema; hypotension; pregnancy—fetal risk has been demonstrated; lactation—infant risk cannot be ruled out.

CAUTIOUS USE Impaired kidney function, renal artery stenosis, renal disease, renal failure, hyperkalemia, aortic stenosis, cardiomyopathy; cerebrovascular disease; collagen vascular disease; CAD; dialysis; heart failure, hyperkalemia, hyponatremia, hypotension, hypovolemia; major surgery; African Americans; autoimmune diseases, especially systemic lupus erythematosus (SLE); women of reproductive age; use during anesthesia; older adults; children younger than 6 y or if child's GFR is greater than 30 mL/min/1.73 m(2).

ROUTE & DOSAGE

Hypertension

Adult/Adolescent: **PO** 5–10 mg once/day, after 4 weeks may titrate up to 40 mg/day
Child (6–16 y): **PO** Start at 0.07 mg/kg (max: 5 mg) once/day (max: 40 mg/day)

Heart Failure

Adult: **PO** 2.5–5 mg daily may increase weekly to highest tolerated dose (usually 5–40 mg daily)

Acute MI

Adult: **PO** 2.5–5 mg daily then titrate up to 10 mg/day as tolerated

Renal Impairment Dosage Adjustment

CrCl 10–30 mL/min: initial dose of 5 mg daily (max 40 mg/day); *CrCl less than 10 mL/min:* initial dose of 2.5 mg daily (max 40 mg/day)

ADMINISTRATION

Oral

- Monitor drug effect for several hours or until the BP is stabilized for at least 1 additional hour. Concurrent administration with a diuretic may compound hypotensive effect.
- Store solutions and tablets in controlled room temperature between 20 and 25 degrees C (68 and 77 degrees F); protect from freezing and excessive heat.

ADVERSE EFFECTS (≥5%) **CV:** Hypotension, *chest pain*. **Respiratory:** *Cough*. **CNS:** *Headache, dizziness.*

DIAGNOSTIC TEST INTERFERENCE: May lead to false-negative aldosterone/renin ratio.

INTERACTIONS Drug: NSAIDS may decrease antihypertensive activity; POTASSIUM SUPPLEMENTS, POTASSIUM-SPARING DIURETICS, **aliskiren** may cause hyperkalemia; may increase **lithium** levels and toxicity; may increase risk of adverse effects if used with ANTGIOTENSIN II BLOCKERS or **iron dextran, sodium pho**; **lanthanum** decreases concentration of lisinopril. Do not use with **sacubitril** due to risk of angioedema.

PHARMACOKINETICS Absorption: 25% absorbed from GI tract. **Onset:** 1 h. **Peak:** 5–7 h. **Duration:** 24 h. **Distribution:** Limited amount crosses blood–brain barrier; crosses placenta; small amount distributed in breast milk. **Metabolism:** Is not metabolized. **Elimination:** Primarily in urine. **Half-Life:** 12 h.

NURSING IMPLICATIONS

Black Box Warning

Lisinopril has been associated with fetal injury and death.

Assessment & Drug Effects

- Place patient in supine position and notify prescriber if sudden and severe hypotension occurs within the first 1–5 h after initial drug dose; greatest risk for hypotension is in patients who are sodium- or volume-depleted because of diuretic therapy.
- Measure BP just prior to dosing to determine whether satisfactory control is being maintained for 24 h. If the antihypertensive effect is diminished in less than 24 h, an increase in dosage may be necessary.
- Monitor closely for angioedema of extremities, face, lips, tongue, glottis, and larynx. Discontinue drug promptly and notify prescriber if such symptoms appear; carefully monitor for airway obstruction until swelling is relieved.
- Monitor serum sodium and serum potassium levels for hyponatremia and hyperkalemia.
- Withhold therapy and notify prescriber if neutropenia (neutrophil count less than 1000/mm^3) develops; kidney function tests at periodic intervals, especially in patients with severe volume or sodium replacement or those with severe CHF.
- Monitor lab tests: Baseline WBC count, then every month for the first 3–6 mo of therapy, and at periodic intervals for 1 y; electrolytes 2–4 weeks after initiation, serum creatinine/BUN, serum potassium, serum sodium, LFTs.

Patient & Family Education

- Discontinue drug and contact prescriber immediately for severe hypersensitivity reaction (e.g., hoarseness, swelling of the face, mouth, hands, or feet, or sudden trouble breathing).
- Women should use reliable means of contraception throughout therapy.
- Report immediately to prescriber if a pregnancy occurs.
- Be aware of importance of proper diet, including sodium and potassium restrictions. **Do not** use salt substitute containing potassium.
- Continued compliance with high BP medication is very important. If a dose is missed, take it as soon as possible but not too close to next dose.

- Review adverse effects with patient and/or caregivers.
- Do not drive or engage in other potentially hazardous activities until response to the drug is known.
- With concomitant therapy, lisinopril increases the risk of lithium toxicity.
- Notify prescriber promptly of any indication of infection (e.g., sore throat, fever).
- Do not suddenly discontinue the drug.
- Do not store drug in a moist area. Heat and moisture may cause the medicine to break down. Do not freeze.

LITHIUM CARBONATE

(li'thee-um)

Lithobid

LITHIUM CITRATE

Classification: ANTIPSYCHOTIC; MOOD STABILIZER

Therapeutic: ANTIPSYCHOTIC; ANTI-MANIC; ANTIDEPRESSANT

AVAILABILITY **Lithium Carbonate:** Capsule; tablet; sustained release tablet. **Lithium Citrate:** oral solution.

ACTION & *THERAPEUTIC EFFECT* Lithium competes with various physiologically important cations: Na^+, K^+, Ca^{2+}, Mg^{2+}; therefore, it affects cell membranes, body water, and neurotransmitters. At the synapse, it accelerates catecholamine destruction, inhibits the release of neurotransmitters and decreases sensitivity of postsynaptic receptors. Decreases overactivity of receptors involved in stimulating manic states. *Effective response evidenced by changed facial affect, improved posture, assumption of self-care, improved ability to concentrate, improved sleep pattern. Treatment for bipolar disorder and mania.*

USES Treatment of manic and mixed episodes of bipolar disorder.

UNLABELED USES Bipolar major depression.

CONTRAINDICATIONS Hypersensitivity to lithium or any component of formulation; history of ACE inhibitor induced angioedema; severe cardiovascular or kidney disease, severe debilitation, sodium depletion; manifestations of hypercalcemia; pregnancy—fetal risk cannot be ruled out; lactation—infant risk cannot be ruled out.

CAUTIOUS USE Thyroid disease; hypothyroidism; epilepsy; mild to moderate cardiac disease, cardiac arrhythmias, dehydration, diarrhea; mental status changes, risk of suicidal thoughts or behavior; renal disease, renal impairment; sodium restriction, urinary retention; DM: debilitative patients; older adults; children younger than 7 y for immediate release tablet or capsule; children younger than 12 y for extended release tablet.

ROUTE & DOSAGE

Mania

Adult/Adolescent: **PO Loading Dose** 600–900 mg in 2–3 divided doses then increase based on response to usual dose of 900 mg/day

Child (over 30 kg): **PO** 8 mEq tid, increase q3days to clinical response; *(under 30 kg):*8 mEq bid, increase at weekly intervals to clinical response.

ADMINISTRATION

Oral

- Ensure that sustained release tablets are not chewed or crushed; **must be** swallowed whole.
- Store capsules and tablets at a controlled room temperature of 25 degrees C (77 degrees F), with excursions permitted between 15 and 30 degrees C (59 and 86 degrees F). Protect from moisture.

ADVERSE EFFECTS (≥5%) **CNS:** *Dizziness*, deep tendon hyperreflexia. **HEENT:** Blurred vision. **Endocrine:** *Hypothyroidism, weight gain, hyperparathyroidism*. **Skin:** *Acne* (lithium citrate). **GI:** *Nausea, gastritis, dry mouth*. **GU:** *Nephrotoxicity polyuria* (lithium citrate). **Hematologic:** *Reversible leukocytosis* (14,000 to 18,000/mm^3). **Other:** Fatigue, increased thirst.

INTERACTIONS **Drug:** **Carbamazepine**, increase risk of adverse effects DIURETICS, NSAIDS, **methyldopa**, TETRACYCLINES decrease renal clearance of lithium, increasing pharmacologic and toxic effects; THEOPHYLLINES, **urea, sodium bicarbonate, sodium** or **potassium citrate** increase renal clearance of lithium, decreasing its pharmacologic effects; **calcium polystyrene sulfonate** decreases concentration of lithium; **dapoxetine, linezolid**, MAOI INHIBITORS may cause serotonin syndrome. ACE INHIBITORS and ANGIOTENSION II RECEPTOR BLOCKERS increase concentration of **lithium.** Do not use with agents known to prolong QT interval (i.e., **bepridil, dofetilide, dronedarone, halofantrine, haloperidol, levomethadyl, pimozide, thioridazine, ziprasidone**).

PHARMACOKINETICS **Absorption:** Readily absorbed from GI tract. **Peak:** 0.5–3 h carbonate; 15–60 min citrate. **Distribution:** Crosses blood–brain barrier and placenta; distributed into breast milk. **Metabolism:** Not metabolized. **Elimination:** 95% in urine, 1% in feces, 4–5% in sweat. **Half-Life:** 20–27 h.

NURSING IMPLICATIONS

Black Box Warning

Lithium toxicity can occur at doses close to therapeutic levels.

Assessment & Drug Effects

- Monitor for S&S of lithium toxicity (e.g., vomiting, diarrhea, lack of coordination, drowsiness, muscular weakness, slurred speech when level is 1.5–2 mEq/L; ataxia, blurred vision, giddiness, tinnitus, muscle twitching, coarse tremors, polyuria when greater than 2 mEq/L). Withhold one dose and call prescriber. Drug should not be stopped abruptly.
- Monitor older adults carefully to prevent toxicity, which may occur at serum levels ordinarily tolerated by other patients.
- Be alert to and report symptoms of hypothyroidism (see Appendix F).
- Weigh patient daily; check for edema. Report changes in I&O ratio, sudden weight gain, or edema.
- Report early signs of extrapyramidal reactions promptly to prescriber.
- Monitor lab tests: Periodic lithium levels (draw blood sample prior to next dose or 8–12 h after last dose) at least every 6 mo; periodic thyroid function tests, CBC with differential, serum electrolytes, renal function tests, thyroid function tests.

L

Patient & Family Education

- Be alert to increased output of dilute urine and persistent thirst. Dose reduction may be indicated.
- Contact prescriber if diarrhea or fever develops. Avoid practices that may encourage dehydration: Hot environment, excessive caffeine beverages (diuresis).
- Drink plenty of liquids (2–3 L/day) during stabilization period and at least 1–1.5 L/day during ongoing therapy.
- Do not drive or engage in other potentially hazardous activities until response to drug is known. Lithium may impair both physical and mental ability.
- Use effective contraceptive measures during lithium therapy.

L

LIXISENATIDE

(lix-i-sen′-a-tide)

Adlyxin

Classification: ANTIDIABETIC; GLUCAGON-LIKE PEPTIDE-1 RECEPTOR AGONIST; INCRETIN MIMETIC

Therapeutic: ANTIDIABETIC

Prototype: Exenatide

AVAILABILITY Solution for injection

ACTION & *THERAPEUTIC EFFECT* An agonist of glucagon-like peptide-1 (GLP-1) that increases glucose-dependent insulin release, decreases glucagon secretion, and slows gastric emptying. *It improves glycemic control by reducing fasting and postprandial glucose concentrations in patients with type 2 diabetes.*

USES Type 2 diabetes mellitus in combination with diet and exercise.

CONTRAINDICATIONS Hypersensitivity to lixisenatide; angioedema; end-stage renal disease; severe gastroparesis; pregnancy—fetal risk cannot be ruled out; lactation—infant risk cannot be ruled out.

CAUTIOUS USE Children.

ROUTE & DOSAGE

Type 2 Diabetes Mellitus

Adult: **Subcutaneous** Initial dose of 10 mcg once daily for 14 days; increase to 20 mcg on day 15

Renal Impairment Dosage Adjustment

Close monitoring required with renal impairment

ADMINISTRATION

Subcutaneous Injection

- Administer subcutaneously in thigh, abdomen, or upper arm; do not give IM or IV.
- Rotate injection sites.
- Available as a pre-filled pen. Activate before using the first time. Do not share injection pens between patients.
- Administer once daily 1 h before first meal of the day.
- Store unopened pen in original packaging under refrigerated conditions between 2 and 8 degrees C (36 and 46 degrees F); protect from light and freezing. After first use, store opened pen below 30 degrees C (85 degrees F). Replace pen cap after each use to protect from light. Discard pen 14 days after the first use.

ADVERSE EFFECTS (≥5%) **CNS:** *Dizziness, headache.* **Endocrine:** *Hypoglycemia.* **GI:** *Diarrhea, nausea, vomiting.*

INTERACTIONS **Drug:** Lixisenatide delays gastric emptying and may reduce the rate of absorption of orally administered medications. Lixisenatide increases the potential risk of hypoglycemia when used in combination with a SULFONYLUREA or **basal insulin.**

PHARMACOKINETICS **Peak:** 1–3.5 h. **Metabolism:** Peptide degradation. **Elimination:** Primarily renal. **Half-Life:** 3 h.

NURSING IMPLICATIONS

Assessment & Drug Effects

- Monitor HbA1c levels at least twice annually.
- Monitor renal function.
- Monitor patient for S&S of GI effects.
- Monitor patient for S&S of hypersensitivity.

Patient & Family Education

- Check blood sugar levels as ordered by your healthcare provider.
- Watch for S&S of hypoglycemia such as feeling cold, sweaty, irritable, or confused.
- Avoid driving if blood sugar is low.
- Follow diet and exercise plan as ordered by your healthcare provider.
- Report S&S of injection site reaction, stomach pain, difficulty urinating, blood in the urine, or significant weight gain.
- Birth control taken by mouth should be taken at least 1 h before or 11 h after taking this drug.

LODOXAMIDE

(lo-dox'a-mide)

Alomide

See Appendix A-1.

LOFEXIDINE

(loe-fex'i-deen)

Lucemyra

Classification: ANTIADRENERGIC; CENTRAL ALPHA-2 AGONIST

Therapeutic: CENTRAL ALPHA-2 AGONIST

AVAILABILITY Tablet

ACTION & *THERAPEUTIC EFFECT*

Lofexidine is a central alpha-2 adrenergic agonist which binds to adrenergic neurons, decreasing the release of norepinephrine and overall sympathetic tone. *This decreases the overall severity of opioid withdrawal symptoms in patients with abrupt opioid discontinuation.*

USES Opioid withdrawal.

CAUTIOUS USE Use may potentiate CNS depressive effects of other medications, including alcohol. Vital signs should be monitored for sudden orthostasis, hypotension, or bradycardia. May cause QT prolongation, which is more pronounced in hepatic or renal impairment. Abrupt discontinuation is not advised; medication should slowly be tapered to discontinuation.

ROUTE & DOSAGE

Opioid Withdrawal Symptoms

Adult: **PO** 0.54 mg (3 tablets) 4 × day with and titrated to withdrawal symptoms [max: 2.88 mg in one day, or 0.72 mg (4 tablets) in one dose]; discontinuation requires tapering discussed in the package label

Renal Impairment Dosage Adjustment

eGFR 30–89.9 mL/min/m²: 2 tablets, 4 × day (1.44 mg/day)
eGFR less than 30 mL/min/m²: 1 tablet, 4 × day (0.72 mg/day)

Hepatic Impairment Dosage Adjustment

Moderate hepatic impairment (Child-Pugh class B): 2 tablets, 4 × day (1.44 mg/day)
Severe hepatic impairment (Child-Pugh class C): 1 tablet, 4 × day (0.72 mg/day)

ADMINISTRATION

Oral/Intranasal/Inhalation/Nebulizer

- Given with or without food.
- Store in original container at 25° C (77° F) away from heat and moisture; excursions permitted between 15°–30° C (59°–86° F).

ADVERSE EFFECTS **CV:** Hypotension, syncope, QT prolongation. **CNS:** Insomnia, dizziness, somnolence, sedation. **HEENT:** Dry mouth, tinnitus.

INTERACTIONS **Drug:** Coadministration with QT prolongating medications (e.g., **methadone**) may further prolong the QT interval. Coadministration with oral **naltrexone** may significantly change the efficacy of naltrexone. Use with other CNS depressant medications may potentiate CNS depressant effects. Coadministration with strong CYP2D6 inhibitor (e.g., **paroxetine**) increases the risk of "hypotension" and bradycardia.

PHARMACOKINETICS **Absorption:** 72% bioavailability. **Peak:** 3-5 h. **Distribution:** 55% protein bound. **Metabolism:** Primarily hepatic through CYP2D6; additional metabolism through CYP1A2 and CYP2C19. **Elimination:** 30% inactivated through first-pass absorption; 94% urine, 1% feces. **Half-Life:** 12 h.

NURSING IMPLICATIONS

Assessment & Drug Effects

- Monitor vital signs prior to dosing and with changes in dose.
- Baseline ECG in patients with history of cardiac dysfunction, hepatic impairment, renal impairment, or patients taking other medications that can cause QT prolongation (methadone).
- Monitor for reduction of S&S of opioid withdrawal and compliance of therapy.
- Monitor lab tests: Electrolytes at initiation of therapy.

Patient & Family Education

- Drink plenty of fluids and avoid overheating.
- Avoid driving or operating heavy machinery until the effects of the drug are realized.
- Notify prescriber if you feel light headed or faint. Be cautious when going from lying to standing or sitting to standing.
- Notify prescriber if unable to carry out activities of daily living because of fatigue.
- Do not use alcohol or other sedating drugs.
- Do not discontinue drug without contacting prescriber. Abrupt stoppage of the drug can lead to a marked rise in blood pressure.

LOMUSTINE

(loe-mus'teen)

CeeNU ♣, Gleostine

Classification: ANTINEOPLASTIC; ALKYLATING AGENT; NITROSOUREA

Therapeutic: ANTINEOPLASTIC

Prototype: Cyclophosphamide

AVAILABILITY Capsule

ACTION & *THERAPEUTIC EFFECT* Has cell cycle-nonspecific activity against rapidly proliferating cell populations. Inhibits synthesis of both DNA and RNA. *Has antineoplastic and myelosuppressive effect.*

USES Palliative therapy in addition to other modalities or with other chemotherapeutic agents in malignant glioma and as secondary therapy in Hodgkin lymphoma.

CONTRAINDICATIONS Immunization with live virus vaccines, viral infections; severe bone marrow suppression; active infection; pregnancy—fetal risk cannot be ruled out; lactation—infant risk cannot be ruled out.

CAUTIOUS USE Patients with decreased circulating platelets, leukocytes, or erythrocytes; kidney or liver function impairment; previous cytotoxic or radiation therapy; secondary malignancies; pulmonary disease.

ROUTE & DOSAGE

Brain Tumor

Adult/Adolescent: **PO** 130 mg/m^2 as single dose, repeated in 6 wk; subsequent doses based on hematologic response (WBC greater than $4000/mm^3$, platelets greater than $100,000/mm^3$)

Child: **PO** 75–150 mg/m^2 q6wk

Hodgkin lymphoma

Adult: **PO** 130 mg/m^2 as single dose, repeated in 6 wk; reduce dose to 100 mg/m^2 in patients with compromised bone marrow function

Renal Impairment Dosage Adjustment

CrCl 10–50 mL/min: reduce dose to 75% of normal dose; *CrCl less than 10 mL/min* reduce dose to 25–50% of normal dose

ADMINISTRATION

Oral

- NIOSH guideline recommend wearing single gloves when handling intact capsules or tablets from unit-dosed packaging. Avoid exposure with inadvertently broken capsules. If dermal contact occurs, wash areas of skin immediately and thoroughly with soap and water.
- Give on an empty stomach to reduce possibility of nausea, may also give an antiemetic before drug to prevent nausea.
- Store capsules at controlled room temperature of 25 degrees C (77 degrees F), with excursions permitted between 15 and 30 degrees C (59 and 86 degrees F). Protect from excessive heat over 40° C (104 degrees F).

ADVERSE EFFECTS **Respiratory:** Pulmonary toxicity (rare). **HEENT:** Optic atrophy, visual disturbances. **Hepatic:** hepatotoxicity. **GU:** Nephrotoxicity. **Hematologic:** Delayed (cumulative) myelosuppression: (Thrombocytopenia, leukopenia).

INTERACTIONS Drug: MYLEOSUPPRESSIVE AGENTS can increase bone marrow toxicity; ANTICOAGULANTS, NSAIDS, SALICYLATES increase risk of bleeding; can reduce the effect of some IMMUNOSUPPRESSANTS. Some ANTINEOPLASTIC AGENTS may decrease therapeutic effect of **lomustine**. Do not use with LIVE VACCINES; use caution with inactivated VACCINES. **Herbal: Echinacea** may decrease therapeutic effect.

PHARMACOKINETICS Absorption: Readily absorbed from GI tract. **Peak:** 3 h. **Distribution:** Readily crosses blood–brain barrier; crosses placenta; distributed into breast milk. **Metabolism:** In liver to several active metabolites. **Elimination:** In urine. **Half-Life:** 16–48 h.

L

NURSING IMPLICATIONS

Black Box Warning

Lomustine has been associated with bone marrow suppression resulting in bleeding and severe infection.

Assessment & Drug Effects

- A repeat course is not given until platelets have returned to above 100,000/mm^3 and leukocytes to above 4000/mm^3.
- Avoid invasive procedures during nadir of platelets.
- Thrombocytopenia occurs about 4 wk and leukopenia about 6 wk after a dose, persisting 1–2 wk.
- Pulmonary function tests prior to initiation and frequently during treatment.
- Inspect oral cavity daily for S&S of superinfections (see Appendix F) and stomatitis or xerostomia.
- Monitor lab tests: Blood counts weekly and for at least 6 wk after last dose. Periodic LFTs and renal function tests, electrolytes during treatment.

Patient & Family Education

- Nausea and vomiting may occur 3–5 h after drug administration, usually lasting less than 24 h.
- Report any difficulty with breathing.
- Review adverse effects with patient and/or caregiver.
- Anorexia may persist for 2 or 3 days after a dose.
- Notify prescriber of signs of sore throat, cough, fever. Also report unexplained bleeding or easy bruising.
- Use reliable contraceptive measures during therapy. Females should prevent pregnancy for at least 2 weeks after the last dose. Male patients should prevent pregnancy in their partners for at least 3.5 months after the last dose.
- Be aware of the possibility of hair loss while taking this drug.
- A given dose may include capsules of different colors; the pharmacist prepares prescribed dose by combining various capsule strengths.

LOPERAMIDE

(loe-per′a-mide)

Imodium, Imodium AD

Classification: ANTIDIARRHEAL

Therapeutic: ANTIDIARRHEAL

AVAILABILITY Tablet; capsule; oral liquid

ACTION & *THERAPEUTIC EFFECT* Inhibits GI peristaltic activity by direct action on circular and longitudinal intestinal muscles. Prolongs transit time of intestinal contents, increases consistency of stools, and reduces fluid and electrolyte loss. *Effectiveness as an antidiarrheal agent is due to prolonging transit time in the colon.*

USES Acute nonspecific diarrhea, chronic diarrhea associated with inflammatory bowel disease, and to reduce fecal volume from ileostomies.

CONTRAINDICATIONS Conditions in which constipation should be avoided, ileus, severe colitis, abdominal pain; bacterial gastroenteritis; acute diarrhea caused by broad-spectrum antibiotics (pseudomembranous colitis) or associated with microorganisms that penetrate intestinal mucosa (e.g., toxigenic *Escherichia coli, Salmonella*, or *Shigella*); hypersensitivity to loperamide; GI bleeding; infants less than 24 months of age; pregnancy—fetal risk cannot be ruled out; lactation—infant risk cannot be ruled out.

CAUTIOUS USE Dehydration; diarrhea caused by invasive bacteria; ulcerative colitis; impaired liver function; prostatic hypertrophy; history of narcotic dependence; patients with AIDS.

ROUTE & DOSAGE

Acute Diarrhea

Adult: **PO** 4 mg followed by 2 mg after each loose stool (max: 16 mg/day)
Child (2 to 5 y; weight 13–21 kg): **PO** 1 mg followed by 1 mg/dose after each loose stool (max 3 mg/day); *6 to 8y; weight 21–27 kg:* 2 mg followed by 1 mg/dose after each loose stool (max 4 mg/day); *9–12 y; weight 27–43 kg:* 2 mg followed by 1 mg/dose after each loose stool (max 6 mg/day).

Chronic Diarrhea

Adult: **PO** 4 mg followed by 2 mg after each loose stool until diarrhea is controlled (max: 16 mg/day)

ADMINISTRATION

Oral

- Do not give prn doses to a child with acute diarrhea.
- Provide appropriate fluid and electrolyte replacement and monitor I and O.
- Store at 15 to 25 degrees C (59 to 77 degrees F).

ADVERSE EFFECTS **CNS:** *Drowsiness, dizziness.* **GI:** *Abdominal discomfort or pain, nausea, vomiting, dry mouth.* **Other:** Fatigue.

INTERACTIONS **Drug:** No clinically significant interactions established.

PHARMACOKINETICS **Absorption:** Poorly absorbed from GI tract. **Onset:** 30–60 min. **Peak:** 2.5 h solution; 4–5 h capsules. **Duration:** 4–5 h. **Elimination:** Primarily in feces, less than 2% in urine. **Half-Life:** 11 h.

NURSING IMPLICATIONS

Assessment & Drug Effects

- Monitor therapeutic effectiveness. Chronic diarrhea usually responds within 10 days. If improvement does not occur within this time, it is unlikely that symptoms will be controlled by further administration.
- Discontinue if there is no improvement after 48 h of therapy for acute diarrhea.
- Monitor fluid and electrolyte balance.
- Notify prescriber promptly if the patient with ulcerative colitis develops abdominal distention or other GI symptoms (possible signs of potentially fatal toxic megacolon).

Patient & Family Education

- Notify prescriber if diarrhea does not stop in a few days or if abdominal pain, distention, or fever develops.

- Record number and consistency of stools.
- Do not drive or engage in other potentially hazardous activities until response to drug is known.
- Review adverse effects with patient and/or caregiver.
- Do not take alcohol and other CNS depressants concomitantly unless otherwise advised by prescriber; may enhance drowsiness.
- Do not take more than 16 mg in a 24-hour period.
- Learn measures to relieve dry mouth; rinse mouth frequently with water, suck hard candy.

LOPINAVIR/RITONAVIR

(lop-i-na'ver/rit-o-na'ver)

Kaletra

Classification: PROTEASE INHIBITOR

Therapeutic: PROTEASE INHIBITOR

Prototype: Saquinavir mesylate

AVAILABILITY Tablet; oral suspension

ACTION & *THERAPEUTIC EFFECT* Inhibits the activity of HIV protease and prevents the cleavage of viral polyproteins essential for the maturation of HIV. Ritonavir inhibits the CYP3A metabolism of lopinavir, thereby, increasing the blood level of lopinavir. *Decreases plasma HIV RNA level; reduces viral load as a result of the combined therapy of the two drugs in HIV infected patients.*

USES Treatment of HIV infection in combination with other antiretroviral agents.

CONTRAINDICATIONS Hypersensitivity to lopinavir or ritonavir; lactation.

CAUTIOUS USE Hepatic impairment, patients with hepatitis B or C, cirrhosis; history of elevated transaminase; older adults; DM; history of pancreatitis; cardiac disease; potential for PR prolongation and QT prolongation; congenital prolongation, hypokalemia; conduction abnormalities, ischemic heart disease, and cardiomyopathy; history of triglyceride elevation; autoimmune disorders (e.g., Graves' disease, polymyositis, Guillain-Barre syndrome); elevated total cholesterol and triglycerides; hemophilia; older adults; pregnancy (fetal risk cannot be ruled out); infants less than 14 days old.

ROUTE & DOSAGE

HIV Infection (without Efavirenz, Nelfinavir, or Nevirapine)

Adult: **PO** 800/200 mg daily or 400/100 mg bid

HIV Infection (with Efavirenz, Nelfinavir, or Nevirapine)

Adult: **PO** 500/125 mg bid or 6.5 mL of solution bid
Child: Dose varies based on weight, concurrent medication and previous antiretroviral exposure, see package insert.

ADMINISTRATION

Oral

- Give with a meal or light snack.
- Note: If didanosine is concurrently ordered, give didanosine 1 h before or 2 h after lopinavir/ritonavir.
- Store oral solution refrigerated at 2°–8° C (36°–46° F). If stored at room temperature 25° C (77° F) or below, discard after 2 mo.
- Store tablets at 15°–30° C (59°–86° F) in tightly sealed container.

ADVERSE EFFECTS **Respiratory:** URI. **CNS:** Fatigue, headache, migraine. **Endocrine:** *Hypercholesterolemia, increased triglycerides, increased gamma-glutamyl transferase*, hyperglycemia. **Skin:** Rash. **Hepatic:** Increased serum ALT. **GI:** *Diarrhea*, nausea, vomiting, abdominal pain, increased serum lipase. **Hematologic:** Abnormal neutrophil count.

INTERACTIONS **Drug:** **Flecainide, propafenone, pimozide** may lead to life-threatening arrhythmias; **rifampin** may decrease antiretroviral response; **dihydroergotamine, ergotamine, methylergonovine** may lead to acute ergot toxicity; HMG-COA REDUCTASE INHIBITORS may increase risk of myopathy and rhabdomyolysis; BENZODIAZEPINES may have prolonged sedation or respiratory depression; **efavirenz, nevirapine**, ANTICONVULSANTS, STEROIDS may decrease lopinavir levels; **delavirdine, ritonavir** may increase lopinavir levels; may increase levels of **amprenavir, indinavir, saquinavir, ketoconazole, itraconazole, midazolam, triazolam, rifabutin, sildenafil, atorvastatin, cerivastatin**, IMMUNOSUPPRESSANTS; may decrease levels of **atovaquone, methadone**, may increase trazodone toxicity; decrease efficacy of hormonal contraceptives, increases midazolam concentration and toxicity. Also see INTERACTIONS in **ritonavir** monograph. **Herbal:** **St. John's wort, garlic** may decrease effect.

PHARMACOKINETICS **Absorption:** Increased absorption when taken with food. **Peak:** 4 h. **Distribution:** 98–99% protein bound. **Metabolism:** Extensively metabolized by CYP3A. **Elimination:** Primarily in feces. **Half-Life:** 5–6 h lopinavir.

NURSING IMPLICATIONS

Assessment & Drug Effects

- Monitor for S&S of: Pancreatitis, especially with marked triglyceride elevations; new onset diabetes or loss of glycemic control; hypothyroidism or Cushing's syndrome.
- Monitor lab tests: Periodic fasting blood glucose, LFTs, lipid profile, serum amylase, baseline and periodic screening for hepatitis C, renal function tests, serum electrolytes, inorganic phosphorus, CBC with differential, and thyroid function tests.

Patient & Family Education

- Report all prescription and nonprescription drugs being taken. Do not use herbal products, especially St. John's wort, without first consulting the prescriber.
- Become familiar with the potential adverse effects of this drug; report those that are bothersome to prescriber.
- Concurrent use of sildenafil (Viagra) increases risk for adverse effects such as hypotension, changes in vision, and sustained erection; promptly report any of these to the prescriber.
- Use additional or alternative contraceptive measures if estrogen-based hormonal contraceptives are being used.
- Notify provider right away if pregnant.

LORATADINE

(lor′a-ta-deen)

Alavert, Claritin, Claritin Reditabs

Classification: NONSEDATING ANTIHISTAMINE; H_1-RECEPTOR ANTAGONIST

Therapeutic: NONSEDATING ANTIHISTAMINE

AVAILABILITY Tablet; syrup

ACTION & *THERAPEUTIC EFFECT*

Long-acting nonsedating antihistamine with selective peripheral H_1-receptor antagonism, thus blocking histamine release. Loratadine diminishes capillary permeability, edema formation, and constriction of respiratory, GI, and vascular smooth muscle. *Effective in relieving allergic reactions related to histamine release.*

L

USES Relief of symptoms of seasonal allergic rhinitis; idiopathic chronic urticaria.

CONTRAINDICATIONS Hypersensitivity to loratadine, or structurally related antihistamines.

CAUTIOUS USE Hepatic and renal impairment, renal disease, renal failure; emphysema, chronic bronchitis; asthma; pregnancy (category B); lactation. **Syrup and chewable tablets:** Children 2 y and older. **Orally disintegrating tablets:** Children 6 y and older.

ROUTE & DOSAGE

Allergic Rhinitis

Adult/Adolescent/Child (6 y or older): **PO** 10 mg once/day or 5 mg q12h

Child (2 to less than 6 y): **PO** 5 mg daily

ADMINISTRATION

Oral

- Give on an empty stomach, 1 h before or 2 h after a meal.
- Store in a tightly closed container.

ADVERSE EFFECTS **CV:** Hypotension, hypertension, palpitations, syncope, tachycardia. **CNS:** Dizziness, dry mouth, fatigue, headache, somnolence, altered salivation and lacrimation, thirst, flushing, anxiety, depression, impaired concentration. **HEENT:** Blurred vision, earache, eye pain, tinnitus. **Skin:** Rash, pruritus, photosensitivity. **GI:** Nausea, vomiting, flatulence, abdominal distress, constipation, diarrhea, weight gain, dyspepsia. **Other:** Arthralgia, myalgia.

PHARMACOKINETICS **Absorption:** Readily from GI tract. **Onset:** 1–3 h. **Peak:** 8–12 h; reaches steady state levels in 3–5 days. **Duration:** 24 h. **Distribution:** Distributed into breast milk. **Metabolism:** In liver to active metabolite, descarboethoxyloratidine. **Elimination:** In urine and feces. **Half-Life:** 12–15 h.

NURSING IMPLICATIONS

Assessment & Drug Effects

- Assess carefully for and report distressing or dangerous S&S that occur after initiation of the drug. A variety of adverse effects, although not common, are possible. Some are an indication to discontinue the drug.
- Monitor cardiovascular status and report significant changes in BP and palpitations or tachycardia.

Patient & Family Education

- Drug may cause significant drowsiness in older adult patients and those with liver or kidney impairment.
- Note: Concurrent use of alcohol and other CNS depressants may have an additive effect.

LORAZEPAM

(lor-a′ze-pam)

Ativan, Loreev XR

Classification: ANXIOLYTIC; SEDATIVE-HYPNOTIC; BENZODIAZEPINE

Therapeutic: ANTIANXIETY; SEDATIVE-HYPNOTIC

Controlled Substance: Schedule IV

AVAILABILITY Tablet; oral solution; solution for injection; extended release capsule; oral concentrate.

ACTION & *THERAPEUTIC EFFECT*

Effects (antianxiety, sedative, hypnotic, and skeletal muscle relaxant) are mediated by the inhibitory neurotransmitter GABA. Action sites are thalamic, hypothalamic, and limbic levels of CNS. *Antianxiety agent that also causes mild suppression of REM sleep, while increasing total sleep time.*

USES Management of anxiety disorders and for short-term relief of symptoms of anxiety. Also used for preanesthetic medication to produce sedation and to reduce anxiety and recall of events related to day of surgery; for management of status epilepticus.

UNLABELED USES Chemotherapy-induced nausea and vomiting, antipsychotic-induced akathisia, alcohol withdrawal syndrome, catatonia, acute vertigo episodes.

CONTRAINDICATIONS Known sensitivity to benzodiazepines; acute narrow-angle glaucoma; primary depressive disorders or psychosis; COPD; coma, shock, sleep apnea; acute alcohol intoxication; dementia; intraarterial administration; respiratory depression; sleep apnea syndrome; pregnancy—fetal risk cannot be ruled out.

CAUTIOUS USE Renal or hepatic impairment; renal failure; organic brain syndrome; myasthenia gravis; narrow-angle glaucoma; pulmonary disease; mania; psychosis; suicidal tendency; history of seizure disorders; GI disorders; adults over 50 y and debilitated patients; lactation—infant risk is minimal; children younger than 12 y.

ROUTE & DOSAGE

Anxiety

Adult: **PO/IM/IV** 0.5–2 mg q4–6h (max: 10 mg/day)

Geriatric: **PO** 1–2 mg/day (max: 2 mg/day)

Preoperative Sedation Induction

Adult: **IV** 1 to 4 mg or 0.02 to 0.04 mg/kg (max single dose 4 mg) 5–20 min before procedure

Status Epilepticus

Adult: **IV** 4 mg injected slowly at 2 mg/min, may repeat dose once if inadequate response after 10 min

ADMINISTRATION

Oral

- Increase the evening dose when higher oral dosage is required, before increasing daytime doses.
- Use only the calibrated dropper for dosing. Concentrated solution can be mixed with liquid or semi-solid food (water, juices, soda or soda-like beverages, applesauce, or puddings)
- Store capsules and tablets at 25° C (77° F). Excursions permitted between 15 and 30° C (59 and 86° F).

Intramuscular

- Injected undiluted, deep into a large muscle mass.
- Store original carton under refrigeration and protect from light.

Intravenous

▪ IV administration to neonates, infants, children: Verify correct IV concentration and rate of infusion with prescriber. ▪ Patients older than 50 y may have more profound and prolonged sedation with IV lorazepam (usual max initial dose: 2 mg).

PREPARE: **Direct:** Prepare lorazepam immediately before use. Dilute with an equal volume of sterile water, D5W, or NS.

ADMINISTER: **Direct:** Inject directly into vein or into IV infusion tubing at rate not to exceed 2 mg/min and with repeated aspiration to confirm IV entry. ▪ Take extreme precautions to PREVENT intra-arterial injection and perivascular extravasation.

INCOMPATIBILITIES: **Solution/additive: Dexamethasone, metoclopramide. Y-site: Aldesleukin, liposomal amphotericin B, ampicillin, aztreonam, cefiderocol, cloxacillin, codeine, dantrolene, daunorubicin, fluconazole, foscarnet, gallium, gemtuzumab, hydralazine, idarubicin, imipenem/cilastatin, lansoprazole, letermovir, meperidine, mitomycin, omeprazole, ondansetron, pantoprazole, phenytoin, potassium phosphate, rocuronium, sargramostim, sufentanil.**

▪ Keep parenteral preparation in refrigerator; do not freeze. ▪ Do not use a discolored solution or one with a precipitate.

ADVERSE EFFECTS (≥5%)

CNS: *Sedation*, dizziness. **Other:** Psychiatric depression.

INTERACTIONS

Drug: Alcohol, CNS DEPRESSANTS, ANTICONVULSANTS potentiate CNS depression; **cimetidine** increases lorazepam plasma levels, increases toxicity;

lorazepam may decrease antiparkinsonism effects of **levodopa;** may increase **phenytoin** levels; smoking decreases sedative and antianxiety effects. **Herbal: Kava, valerian** may potentiate sedation.

PHARMACOKINETICS Absorption: Readily absorbed from GI tract. **Onset:** 1–5 min IV; 15–30 min IM. **Peak:** 60–90 min IM; 2 h PO. **Duration:** 12–24 h. **Distribution:** Crosses placenta; distributed into breast milk. **Metabolism:** Not metabolized in liver. **Elimination:** In urine. **Half-Life:** 10–20 h.

NURSING IMPLICATIONS

Assessment & Drug Effects

- IM or IV lorazepam injection of 2–4 mg is usually followed by a depth of drowsiness or sleepiness that permits patient to respond to simple instructions whether patient appears to be asleep or awake.
- Monitor vital signs, CNS status, and ability to void following administration.
- Supervise ambulation of older adult patients for at least 8 h after lorazepam injection to prevent falling and injury.
- Supervise patient who exhibits depression with anxiety closely; the possibility of suicide exists, particularly when there is apparent improvement in mood.
- Monitor lab tests: Periodic CBC and LFTs with long-term therapy.

Patient & Family Education

- Do not drive or engage in other hazardous activities for at least 24–48 h after receiving an injection of lorazepam.
- Do not consume alcoholic beverages for at least 24–48 h after an injection and avoid when taking an oral regimen.
- Notify prescriber if daytime psychomotor function is impaired; a change in regimen or drug may be needed.
- Terminate regimen gradually over a period of several days. Do not stop long-term therapy abruptly; withdrawal may be induced with feelings of panic, tonic-clonic seizures, tremors, abdominal and muscle cramps, sweating, vomiting.
- Discuss discontinuation of drug with prescriber if you wish to become pregnant.

LOSARTAN POTASSIUM

(lo-sar′tan)

Cozaar

Classification: ANGIOTENSIN II RECEPTOR ANTAGONIST; ANTIHYPERTENSIVE

Therapeutic: ANTIHYPERTENSIVE

AVAILABILITY Tablet

ACTION & *THERAPEUTIC EFFECT*

Angiotensin II receptor (type AT_1) antagonist acts as a potent vasoconstrictor and primary vasoactive hormone of the renin–angiotensin–aldosterone system. Selectively blocks the binding of angiotensin II to the AT_1 receptors found in many tissues (e.g., vascular smooth muscle, adrenal glands). *Antihypertensive effect is due to vasodilation and inhibition of aldosterone effects on sodium and water retention.*

USES Hypertension, diabetic nephropathy.

CONTRAINDICATIONS Hypersensitivity to losartan, pregnancy (category D second and third trimester), lactation.

CAUTIOUS USE Patients on diuretics, heart failure; hyperkalemia;

hypo-volemia; renal or hepatic impairment, pregnancy (category C discontinue use as soon as detected); children younger than 6 y.

ROUTE & DOSAGE

Hypertension, Diabetic Nephropathy

Adult: **PO** 50 mg daily, titrate as needed (max: 100 mg/day); *Adolescent/Child (older than 6 y and weight over 20 kg):* **PO** 0.7 mg/kg daily

ADMINISTRATION

Oral

- Administer without regard to meals. Administer at approximately the same time every day.

L

ADVERSE EFFECTS CV: Chest pain, hypotension, orthostatic hypo-tension. **CNS:** Fatigue. **Endocrine:** Hyperkalemia.

INTERACTIONS Drug: Phenobarbital decreases serum levels of losartan and its metabolite. **Aliskiren** and other ANTIHYPERTENSIVES may increase hypotensive effects. Medications that affect CYP3A4 or CYP2C9 may affect serum concentrations.

PHARMACOKINETICS Absorption: Rapidly absorbed from GI tract; approximately 25–33% reaches systemic circulation. **Peak:** 6 h. **Duration:** 24 h. **Distribution:** Highly bound to plasma proteins; does not appear to cross blood–brain barrier. **Metabolism:** Extensively metabolized in liver by CYP 2C9 and CYP 3A4. **Elimination:** 35% in urine, 60% in feces. **Half-Life:** Losartan 1.5–2 h; metabolite 6–9 h.

NURSING IMPLICATIONS

Black Box Warning

Losartan has been associated with fetal injury and death when used during the second and third trimesters.

Assessment & Drug Effects

- Monitor BP at drug trough (prior to a scheduled dose).
- Inadequate response may be improved by splitting the daily dose into twice-daily dose.
- Monitor lab tests: Periodic electrolytes, and renal function tests with long-term therapy.

Patient & Family Education

- Do not use potassium supplements or salt substitutes without consulting prescriber.
- Notify prescriber of symptoms of hypotension (e.g., dizziness, fainting).
- Notify prescriber immediately of pregnancy.
- Teach patient to change positions slowly to minimize risk of orthostatic hypotension.

LOTEPREDNOL ETABONATE

(lo-te'pred-nol e-ta-bo'nate)

Alrex, Lotemax

See Appendix A-1.

LOVASTATIN Pr

(loe-vah-stat'in)

Altoprev

Classification: ANTILIPEMIC; LIPID-LOWERING; HMG-COA REDUCTASE INHIBITOR (STATIN)

Therapeutic LIPID-LOWERING; STATIN

AVAILABILITY Tablet; extended release tablet

ACTION & *THERAPEUTIC EFFECT*

Reduces plasma cholesterol levels by interfering with body's ability to produce its own cholesterol. This cholesterol-lowering effect triggers induction of LDL receptors, which promote removal of LDL and VLDL remnants (precursors of LDL) from plasma. Also results in an increase in plasma HDL concentrations (HDL collects excess cholesterol from body cells and transports it to liver for excretion). *Reduces plasma cholesterol levels by interfering with body's ability to produce its own cholesterol, and it also lowers LDL and VLDL cholesterol.*

USES Hypercholesterolemia, coronary heart disease, heterozygous familial hypercholesterolemia in adolescents, primary/secondary prevention of atherosclerotic cardiovascular disease.

CONTRAINDICATIONS Hypersensitivity to lovastatin; active liver disease, unexplained persistent elevations of serum transaminases; cholestasis, hepatic encephalopathy, hepatitis, jaundice; rhabdomyolysis, or myopathy; surgery, trauma; hypotension, renal failure; homozygous familial hypercholesterolemia; pregnancy (category X); lactation.

CAUTIOUS USE Patient who consumes substantial quantities of alcohol; history of liver disease; electrolyte imbalance, endocrine disease; infection, severe renal impairment, seizure disorder; DM; patient with risk factors predisposing to development of kidney failure secondary to rhabdomyolysis; older adults; females of childbearing age; children younger than 10 y. **Extended release tablets:** Safety and efficacy in children not established.

ROUTE & DOSAGE

Hypercholesterolemia/Coronary Heart Disease

Adult: **PO Extended release** 20–60 mg daily; **Immediate release** 20 mg daily

Adolescent: **PO Immediate release** 10–40 mg once/day

Prevention of Cardiovascular Disease (Moderate-Intensity Therapy)

Adult: **PO Immediate release** 40 mg daily

ADMINISTRATION

Oral

- Give with the evening meal if daily. Give the first of 2 daily doses with breakfast.
- Ensure that extended release tablets are not crushed or chewed. They **must be** swallowed whole.
- Store tablets at 5°–30° C (41°–86° F) in light-resistant, tightly closed container.

ADVERSE EFFECTS **Hepatic:** Impaired hepatic function. **Musculoskeletal:** Increased creatine phosphokinase (CPK).

INTERACTIONS **Drug: Clarithromycin, clofibrate, cyclosporine, danazol, erythromycin, fenofibrate, fluconazole, gemfibrozil, itraconazole, ketoconazole, miconazole, niacin,** and PROTEASE INHIBITORS increase risk of myopathy and rhabdomyolysis; potentiate hypoprothrombinemia with **warfarin**. Do not use with **conivaptan, idelalisib, mifepristone, telaprevir, telithromycin. Food: Grapefruit juice** (greater than 1 qt/day) may increase risk of myopathy and rhabdomyolysis.

PHARMACOKINETICS **Absorption:** 30% from GI tract; extensive first-pass metabolism. **Onset:** 2 wk. **Peak:** 4–6 wk. **Distribution:** Crosses blood–brain barrier and placenta; distributed into breast milk. **Metabolism:** In liver to active metabolites. **Elimination:** 83% in feces; 10% in urine. **Half-Life:** 1.1–1.7 h.

NURSING IMPLICATIONS

Assessment & Drug Effects

- Drug-induced increases in serum transaminases, usually not associated with jaundice or other clinical S&S, return to normal when drug is discontinued. If these values rise and remain at 3 × upper level of normal, drug will be discontinued and liver biopsy considered.
- Monitor diabetics for loss of glycemic control.
- Monitor lab tests: LFTs at 6 and 12 wk after initiation of therapy and periodically thereafter; periodic HbA1C, and lipid profile.

Patient & Family Education

- Notify prescriber promptly of muscle tenderness or pain, especially if accompanied by fever or malaise. If CPK is elevated or if myositis is diagnosed, drug will be discontinued.
- Avoid or at least reduce alcohol consumption.
- Understand that lovastatin is not a substitute for, but an addition to, diet therapy.
- Diabetics should monitor blood glucose frequently for loss of glycemic control.

LOXAPINE SUCCINATE

(lox′a-peen)

Adasuve

Classification: ANTIPSYCHOTIC

Therapeutic: ANTIPSYCHOTIC

Prototype: Clozapine

AVAILABILITY Capsule; powder for inhalation

ACTION & THERAPEUTIC EFFECT Blocks postsynaptic dopamine receptors in the brain; Also possesses serotonin-blocking activity. *Stabilizes emotional component of schizophrenia.*

USES Schizophrenia, agitation associated with bipolar disorder.

CONTRAINDICATIONS Hypersensitivity to loxapine and amoxapine; severe drug-induced CNS depression; coma; dementia-related psychosis in older adults; NMS; severe neutropenia; history of/current diagnosis of asthma, COPD, or other lung disease associated with bronchospasm, acute respiratory signs or symptoms; lactation.

CAUTIOUS USE Tardive dyskinesia; cardiovascular disease; seizure disorder; glaucoma, prostatic hypertrophy, urinary retention, history of convulsive disorders, cardiovascular disease; transient hypotensive episodes; alcoholism; brain tumor; hematologic disease; hepatic disease; renal impairment; decreased GI motility; thyroid disease; older adults; pregnancy (adverse effects observed in animal reproduction studies); children younger than 16 y.

ROUTE & DOSAGE

Schizophrenia

Adult: **PO** Start with 10 mg bid and rapidly increase to maintenance dose of 60–100 mg/day in divided doses (max: 250 mg/day)

Agitation with Schizophrenia/ Bipolar Disorder

Adult: **Inhalation** 10 mg daily (max: 10 mg/24 hours)

ADMINISTRATION

Oral

- Mix prior to administration.
- Cadasuve Inhaler: Refer to manufacturer's information for specific instructions for administration of the oral inhalation powder using the Cadasuve inhaler.

ADVERSE EFFECTS **CV:** *Orthostatic hypotension,* hypertension, tachycardia. **Respiratory:** Respiratory distress. **CNS:** *Drowsiness, sedation,* dizziness, syncope, EEG changes, paresthesias, staggering gait, muscle weakness, *extrapyramidal effects,* akathisia, tardive dyskinesia, neuroleptic malignant syndrome. **HEENT:** Nasal congestion, tinnitus; blurred vision, ptosis. **Skin:** Dermatitis, facial edema, pruritus, photosensitivity. **GI:** Constipation, dry mouth, *dysgeusia*. **GU:** Urinary retention, menstrual irregularities. **Other:** Polydipsia, weight gain or loss, hyperpyrexia, hypersensitivity, transient leukopenia.

DIAGNOSTIC TEST INTERFERENCE False positives for phenylketonuria, amylase, uroporphyrins, urobilinogen.

INTERACTIONS **Drug:** **Alcohol** and other CNS DEPRESSANTS potentiate CNS depression. Use caution with other ANTIPSYCHOTICS; use with other ANTICHOLINERGIC AGENTS increases risk of adverse effects. Do not use with **metoclopramide** due to increased risk of extrapyramidal effects; **iohexol** increases seizure risk. Do not use with **amilsulpride, bromopride, caberolgine, clozapine**.

PHARMACOKINETICS **Absorption:** Readily absorbed from GI tract. **Onset:** 20–30 min (PO) 2 min (inhalation). **Peak:** 1.5–3 h. **Duration:** 12 h (PO). **Distribution:** Widely distributed; crosses placenta; distributed into breast milk; 97% protein bound. **Metabolism:** In liver. **Elimination:** 50% in urine, 50% in feces. **Half-Life:** 19 h.

NURSING IMPLICATIONS

Black Box Warning

Loxapine has been associated with increased mortality in the older adult with dementia-related psychosis. Loxapine inhalation can cause bronchospasm that has the potential to lead to respiratory distress and respiratory arrest.

Assessment & Drug Effects

- Monitor baseline BP pattern prior and during therapy; both hypotension and hypertension have been reported as adverse reactions.
- Observe carefully for mental status changes, seizure activity, and extrapyramidal effects such as acute dystonia (see Appendix F) during early therapy. Most symptoms disappear with dose adjustment or with antiparkinsonism drug therapy.
- Discontinue therapy and report promptly to prescriber the first signs of impending tardive dyskinesia (fine vermicular movements of the tongue) when patient is on long-term treatment.
- Monitor height, weight, and periodic waist circumference.
- Baseline and annual ocular examination for visual changes.
- Monitor lab studies: Baseline and periodic CBC, electrolytes, liver function, lipid panel, and fasting HbA_{1C}

Patient & Family Education

- **Do not** change dosage regimen in any way without prescriber approval.

- Avoid self-dosing with OTC drugs unless approved by the prescriber.
- Drowsiness usually decreases with continued therapy. If it persists and interferes with daily activities, consult prescriber. A change in time of administration or dose may help.
- Avoid potentially hazardous activity until response to drug is known.
- Learn measures to relieve dry mouth; rinse mouth frequently with water, suck hard candy. Avoid commercial products that may contain alcohol and enhance drying and irritation.
- Notify prescriber of blurred or colored vision.
- Do not take drug dose and notify prescriber of following: Light-colored stools, bruising, unexplained bleeding, prolonged constipation, tremor, restlessness and excitement, sore throat and fever, rash.
- Stay out of bright sun; cover exposed skin with sunscreen.

LUBIPROSTONE

(lu-bi-pros′tone)

Amitiza

Classification: LAXATIVE AND STOOL SOFTENER; CHLORIDE CHANNEL ACTIVATOR

Therapeutic: LAXATIVE AND STOOL SOFTENER

AVAILABILITY Capsule

ACTION & *THERAPEUTIC EFFECT*

A chloride channel activator that acts locally on the apical membrane of the gastrointestinal tract to increase intestinal fluid secretion and improve fecal transit. This action bypasses the antisecretory effects of opiates which suppress secretomotor neuron excitability. *The increase in intestinal fluid secretion enhances intestinal motility, thereby increasing the passage of stool and alleviating symptoms associated with chronic idiopathic constipation.*

USES Treatment of chronic idiopathic constipation; constipation-predominant irritable bowel syndrome (IBS-C); opioid-induced constipation.

CONTRAINDICATIONS Hypersensitivity to lubiprostone; history of mechanical GI obstruction: Crohn's disease, volvulus, diverticulitis, etc.; severe diarrhea; lactation.

CAUTIOUS USE GI disease, hepatic impairment; pregnancy (category C); children.

ROUTE & DOSAGE

Chronic Idiopathic/Opioid-Induced Constipation

Adult: PO 24 mcg bid

IBS-C

Adult: PO 8 mcg bid

Hepatic Dose Adjustment (for Chronic Constipation)

Child-Pugh class B: Start with 16 mcg bid

Child-Pugh class C: Start with 8 mcg bid

(for IBS)

Child-Pugh class C: Start with 8 mcg daily

ADMINISTRATION

Oral

- Administer with food and water to minimize nausea.
- Capsule should be swallowed whole.
- Do not administer to a patient with severe diarrhea or suspected bowel obstruction.
- Store at 15°–30° C (59°–86° F).

ADVERSE EFFECTS **CNS:** Headache. **GI:** *Nausea*, diarrhea, abdominal pain.

PHARMACOKINETICS **Absorption:** Very low. **Peak:** 1.1 h (M3). **Distribution:** 94% protein bound. **Metabolism:** Extensive nonhepatic metabolism. **Elimination:** Urine (major) and feces. **Half-Life:** 0.9–1.4 h.

NURSING IMPLICATIONS

Assessment & Drug Effects

- Monitor for and report S&S of bowel obstruction.
- Monitor lab tests: Baseline and periodic LFTs.

Patient & Family Education

- Report to prescriber if you experience severe or prolonged diarrhea, or new or worsening abdominal pain or dyspnea following dosing.
- Do not drive or engage in potentially hazardous activities until response to drug is known.

LULICONAZOLE

(lu-li-con′a-zole)

Luzu

Classification: AZOLE ANTIFUNGAL

Therapeutic: AZOLE ANTIFUNGAL

Prototype: Fluconazole

AVAILABILITY Cream

ACTION & *THERAPEUTIC EFFECT* An azole antifungal that appears to inhibit an enzyme required for formation of fungal cell membranes. *Inhibits fungal cell formation and fungal growth.*

USES Topical treatment of interdigital *tinea pedis, tinea cruris,* and *tinea corporis* caused by the organisms *Trichophyton rubrum* and *Epidermophyton floccosum*, in patients 18 y and older.

CAUTIOUS USE Pregnancy (category C); lactation. Safety and efficacy in children younger than 18 y not established.

ROUTE & DOSAGE

Fungal Infection

Adult: Topical Apply once daily to affected and immediately surrounding areas for 1 or 2 wk

ADMINISTRATION

Topical

- Apply to affected area out to about 1 inch of surrounding healthy skin.
- Store at 15°–30° C (59°–86° F).

ADVERSE EFFECTS **Skin:** Application site reactions, cellulitis, dermatitis.

INTERACTIONS **Drug:** Luliconazole may increase the levels of other drugs that require CYP2C19 and CYP3A4 for oxidative metabolism.

PHARMACOKINETICS **Peak:** 5.8–16.9 h. **Distribution:** Greater than 99% plasma protein bound.

NURSING IMPLICATIONS

Assessment & Drug Effects

- Monitor affected area for clearance of fungal infection.

Patient & Family Education

- Wash your hands after application to affected areas.
- Avoid contacting mucous membranes (e.g., mouth, vagina, eyes) with this cream.
- Report to prescriber if you are pregnant or plan to become pregnant.

LURASIDONE

(lu-ra′si-done)

Latuda

Classification: ATYPICAL ANTIPSYCHOTIC

Therapeutic: ANTIPSYCHOTIC

Prototype: Clozapine

AVAILABILITY Tablet

ACTION & THERAPEUTIC EFFECT

A benzoisothiazol-derivative atypical antipsychotic with mixed serotonin-dopamine antagonist activity thought to improve negative symptoms of psychoses and reduce the incidence of extrapyramidal side effects. *Controls schizophrenic ideation and behavior.*

L

USES Bipolar disorder and schizophrenia.

CONTRAINDICATIONS Hypersensitivity to lurasidone; older adults with dementia-related psychosis; suicidal ideation; severe neutropenia or leukopenia; agranulocytosis; severe suicidality; neuroleptic malignant syndrome (NMS); patients at risk for aspiration pneumonia; lactation.

CAUTIOUS USE Moderate and severe renal impairment; Child-Pugh class B and C hepatic impairment; cardiovascular disease; dyslipidemia; orthostatic hypotension; history of suicide; disorders that lower seizure threshold (e.g., Alzheimer dementia; Parkinson disease; dementia with Lewy bodies; history of drug abuse or dependence); history of seizures or NMS; tardive dyskinesia; hyperglycemia; diabetes mellitus or with family history of DM; history of breast cancer; infection; older adults; pregnancy (antipsychotic use during the third trimester of pregnancy has a risk of abnormal muscle movements and/or withdrawal symptoms in newborns following delivery). Safety and efficacy in children not established.

ROUTE & DOSAGE

Schizophrenia

Adult: **PO** 40 mg daily then increase as needed (max: 160 mg)

Bipolar Disorder

Adult: **PO** 20 mg daily then increase (normal range 20–120 mg/day)

Hepatic Impairment Dosage Adjustment

Child-Pugh class B Reduce dose (max: 80 mg once daily;) *Child-Pugh class B and C:* Reduce dose (max: 40 mg once daily)

Renal Impairment Dosage Adjustment

CrCl less than 50 mL/min: Reduce dose (max: 80 mg once daily)

ADMINISTRATION

Oral

- Administer consistently at the same time every day with food (at least 350 calories). Evening administration may help reduce adverse effects.
- Store at 25°C (77°F).

ADVERSE EFFECTS **CV:** Tachycardia. **Respiratory:** Rhinitis, **CNS:** *Akathisia*, agitation, anxiety, dizziness, dystonia, *Parkinsonian-like syndrome, drowsiness,* insomnia, extrapyramidal reaction. **Endocrine:** Elevated serum creatinine, elevated serum triglycerides, increased serum cholesterol, increased serum glucose, increased serum prolactin, weight gain. **GI:** Diarrhea, dyspepsia, *nausea*, vomiting, xerostomia. **Musculoskeletal:** Back pain. **Other:** Viral infection.

INTERACTIONS **Drug:** Do not use with strong inhibitors of CYP3A4 (e.g., **ketoconazole, ritonavir, voriconazole**); with moderate CYP3A4 inhibitors (e.g., **carbamazepine, diltiazem, erythromycin, fluconazole**) start with half dose. Inducers of CYP3A4 (e.g., **rifampin**) decrease the levels of lurasidone. **Amisulpride, metoclopramide** or CNS DEPRESSANTS increases risk of adverse effects; may increase QT prolongation when used with **disopyramide**; **dopamine, ephedrine** increases hypotensive effects. ANTIPARKSINON AGENTS may decrease therapeutic effect. **Food:** Avoid **Grapefruit juice. Herbal: St. John's wort** can decrease the levels of lurasidone.

PHARMACOKINETICS **Absorption:** increases with food, 9-19% bioavailable. **Peak:** 1–3 h. **Distribution:** 99% plasma protein bound. **Metabolism:** Hepatic via CYP3A4. **Elimination:** Fecal (80%) and renal (9%). **Half-Life:** 18 h.

NURSING IMPLICATIONS

Black Box Warning

Lurasidone has been associated with increased mortality in older adults with dementia-related psychosis and with increased risk of suicidal thoughts and behavior in children, adolescents, and young adults.

Assessment & Drug Effects

- Monitor for and report promptly suicidal ideation.
- Monitor orthostatic vital signs, especially in those at risk for hypotension. Risk is highest at time of dose initiation or escalation. Monitor fall risk.
- Monitor closely patients with neutropenia. Report promptly development of fever or other signs of infection.
- Monitor weight and report significant weight gain.
- Monitor diabetics closely for loss of glycemic control.
- Monitor for and report promptly any mental status changes, seizure activity, or S&S tardive dyskinesia (see Appendix F).
- Taper dosage slowly when discontinuing.
- Baseline and annual ocular examination.
- Monitor lab tests: Baseline and periodic blood glucose, HbA_{1C}, lipid profile, LFTs, electrolytes, renal and liver function, and CBC with differential.

Patient & Family Education

- Do not engage in hazardous activities until response to drug is known.
- Rise slowly from a lying or sitting position to avoid dizziness and fainting.
- Report immediately any of the following: Suicidal thoughts, fever, muscle rigidity, palpitations, signs of infection, dizziness or fainting upon standing.
- Avoid situations that may cause overheating or dehydration.
- Avoid alcohol while taking lurasidone.
- Monitor blood glucose levels frequently if diabetic.

MAFENIDE ACETATE

(ma′fe-nide)

Sulfamylon

Classification: SULFONAMIDE ANTIBIOTIC

Therapeutic: ANTIBIOTIC

Prototype: Sulfisoxazole

AVAILABILITY Powder, cream

ACTION & THERAPEUTIC EFFECT Produces marked reduction of bacterial growth in vascular tissue. Active in presence of purulent matter and serum. *Bacteriostatic against many gram-positive and gram-negative organisms, including Pseudomonas aeruginosa, and certain strains of anaerobes.*

USES Treatment of second- and third-degree burns.

M

CONTRAINDICATIONS History of hypersensitivity to mafenide or sulfonamides; respiratory (inhalation) injury, pulmonary infection; lactation.

CAUTIOUS USE Impaired kidney or pulmonary function, G6PD deficiency and hemolytic anemia with DIC; burn patients with acute kidney failure; pregnancy (category C); children younger than 3 mo.

ROUTE & DOSAGE

Burns

Adult/Adolescent/Child: **Topical** Apply aseptically to burn areas to a thickness of approximately 15 mm (1/16 in.) once or twice daily

ADMINISTRATION

Topical

- Apply cream or solution aseptically to cleansed, debrided burn areas with sterile gloved hand.
- Cover burn areas with cream at all times. Make reapplications to areas from which cream has been removed as necessary.
- Store in tight, light-resistant containers. Avoid extremes of temperature.

ADVERSE EFFECTS **Skin:** *Intense pain, burning, or stinging at application sites,* bleeding of skin, excessive body water loss, excoriation of new skin, superinfections. **Hypersensitivity:** Pruritus, rash, urticaria, blisters, eosinophilia. **Other:** Metabolic acidosis.

PHARMACOKINETICS **Absorption:** Rapidly from burn surface. **Peak:** 2–4 h. **Metabolism:** Rapidly inactivated in blood to a weak carbonic anhydrase inhibitor. **Elimination:** Via kidneys.

NURSING IMPLICATIONS

Assessment & Drug Effects

- Monitor vital signs. Report immediately changes in BP, pulse, and respiratory rate and volume.
- Monitor I&O. Report oliguria or changes in I&O ratio and pattern.
- Be alert to S&S of metabolic acidosis (see Appendix F).
- Be alert to evidence of superinfections (see Appendix F), particularly in and below burn eschar.
- Observe carefully; accuracy is critical. It is frequently difficult to distinguish between adverse reactions to mafenide and the effects of severe burns.

- Note: Allergic reactions have reportedly occurred 10–14 days after initiation of mafenide therapy. Temporary discontinuation of drug may be necessary.
- Report intense local pain to prescriber; pain caused by drug may require administration of analgesic.
- Monitor lab tests: Periodic serum electrolytes and tests for acid-base balance.

Patient & Family Education

- Apply only a thin dressing over burns unless otherwise directed.
- Therapy is usually continued until healing is progressing well (usually 60 days) or site is ready for grafting (after about 35–40 days). It is not withdrawn while there is a possibility of infection unless adverse reactions intervene.
- Report any of the following to the prescriber immediately: Foul-smelling drainage from wounds, bleeding at wound site, unexplained fever.

MAGNESIUM CITRATE

(mag-nes'i-um)

Citrate of Magnesia, Citroma

Classification: SALINE CATHARTIC

Therapeutic: LAXATIVE

Prototype: Magnesium hydroxide

AVAILABILITY Solution

ACTION & *THERAPEUTIC EFFECT* Hyperosmotic laxative that promotes bowel evacuation by causing osmotic retention of fluid; this distends colon and stimulates peristaltic activity. *Evacuates bowels.*

USES To evacuate bowel prior to certain surgical and diagnostic procedures; intermittently as laxative to treat acute constipation.

CONTRAINDICATIONS Severe renal impairment, renal failure; gastrointestinal bleeding; nausea, vomiting, diarrhea, abdominal pain, acute surgical abdomen; intestinal impaction, obstruction or perforation; rectal bleeding; use of solutions containing sodium bicarbonate in patients on sodium-restricted diets.

CAUTIOUS USE Mild or moderate renal impairment; cardiac disease; older adults; pregnancy (category A); lactation; children younger than 2 y.

ROUTE & DOSAGE

Acute Constipation

Adult/Adolescent: **PO** 150–300 mL

Child (6–12 y): **PO** 100–150 mL; *2–5 y:* 60–120 mL

Bowel Prep

Adult/Adolescent: **PO** 150–300 mL once

Child (2 to younger than 6 y): **PO** 0.5 mL/kg (max: 200 mL) under supervision of physician; *6–12 y:* 75–150 mL one time

ADMINISTRATION

Oral

- Give on an empty stomach with a full (240 mL) glass of water. Time dosing so that it does not interfere with sleep. Drug produces a watery or semifluid evacuation in 2–6 h.
- Chill solution by pouring it over ice or refrigerate it until ready to use to increase palatability.
- Be aware that once container is opened, effervescence will decrease. This does not affect the quality of preparation.
- Store at 2°–30° C (36°–86° F) in tightly covered containers.

ADVERSE EFFECTS GI: Abdominal cramps, nausea, flatulence, fluid and electrolyte imbalance, hypermag-nesemia (prolonged use).

INTERACTIONS Drug: May decrease effectiveness of **digoxin,** ORAL AN-TICOAGULANTS, PHENOTHIAZINES; will decrease absorption of **ciprofloxacin,** TETRACYCLINES; **sodium polystyrene sulfonate** will bind magnesium, decreasing its effectiveness.

PHARMACOKINETICS Onset: 3–6 h.

NURSING IMPLICATIONS

Assessment & Drug Effects

- Monitor for dehydration, hypo-kalemia, and hyponatremia (see Appendix F) since drug may cause intense bowel evacuation.

Patient & Family Education

- Do not use for routine treatment of constipation (especially in older adult).
- Expect some degree of abdominal cramping.

M

MAGNESIUM HYDROXIDE

(mag-nes'i-um)

Magnesia, Magnesia Magma, Milk of Magnesia, M.O.M.

Classification: SALINE CATHARTIC; ANTACID

Therapeutic: LAXATIVE; ANTACID

AVAILABILITY Tablet; suspension

ACTION & THERAPEUTIC EFFECT Aqueous suspension of magnesium hydroxide with rapid and long-acting neutralizing action. Causes osmotic retention of fluid, which distends colon, resulting in mechanical stimulation of peristaltic activity. *Acts as antacid in low doses and as mild saline laxative at higher doses.*

USES Short-term treatment of occasional constipation, for relief of GI symptoms associated with hyperacidity, and as adjunct in treatment of peptic ulcer. Also has been used in treatment of poisoning by mineral acids and arsenic, and as mouthwash to neutralize acidity.

CONTRAINDICATIONS Abdominal pain, nausea, vomiting, chronic diarrhea, severe kidney dysfunction, fecal impaction, intestinal obstruction or perforation, rectal bleeding, colostomy, ileostomy.

CAUTIOUS USE Renal impairment, renal disease; older adults; pregnancy (category A); lactation; children younger than 2 y.

ROUTE & DOSAGE

Laxative

Adult: **PO** 2.4–4.8 g (30–60 mL)/day in 1 or more divided doses
Child (2 to less than 6 y): **PO** 0.4–1.2 g (5–15 mL)/day in 1 or more divided doses; *6–11 y:* 1.2–2.4 g (15–30 mL)/day in 1 or more divided doses

ADMINISTRATION

Oral

- Shake bottle well before pouring to assure mixing of suspension.
- Follow drug with at least a full glass of water to enhance drug action for laxative effect. Administer in the morning or at bedtime. Most effective when taken on an empty stomach.

- Store at 15°–30° C (59°–86° F) in tightly covered container. Slowly absorbs carbon dioxide on exposure to air. Avoid freezing.

ADVERSE EFFECTS **CV:** Hypotension, bradycardia, complete heart block and other ECG abnormalities. **Respiratory:** Respiratory depression. **Endocrine:** Electrolyte imbalance with prolonged use. **GI:** Nausea, vomiting, abdominal cramps, *diarrhea*. **GU:** Alkalinization of urine. **Other:** Weakness, lethargy, mental depression, hyporeflexia, dehydration, coma.

INTERACTIONS **Drug:** Milk of Magnesia decreases absorption of **chlordiazepoxide, dicumarol, digoxin, isoniazid,** QUINOLONES, TETRACYCLINES.

PHARMACOKINETICS **Absorption:** 15–30% of magnesium is absorbed. **Onset:** 3–6 h. **Distribution:** Small amounts distributed in saliva and breast milk. **Elimination:** In feces; some renal excretion.

NURSING IMPLICATIONS

Assessment & Drug Effects

- Evaluate the patient's continued need for drug. Prolonged and frequent use of laxative doses may lead to dependence. Additionally, even therapeutic doses can raise urinary pH and thereby predispose susceptible patients to urinary infection and urolithiasis.

Patient & Family Education

- Investigate the cause of persistent or recurrent constipation or gastric distress with prescriber.

MAGNESIUM OXIDE

(mag-nes'i-um)

Mag-Ox, Maox, Par-Mag, Uro-Mag

Classification: ANTACID; SALINE CATHARTIC

Therapeutic: ANTACID; MAGNESIUM SUPPLEMENT; LAXATIVE

Prototype: Magnesium hydroxide

AVAILABILITY Tablet; capsule

ACTION & *THERAPEUTIC EFFECT* Nonsystemic antacid with high neutralizing capacity and relatively long duration of action. *Acts as an antacid in low doses and a mild saline laxative at higher doses. Also effective as a magnesium supplement.*

USES Essentially the same as magnesium hydroxide. May also be used as magnesium supplement.

CONTRAINDICATIONS Abdominal pain, nausea, vomiting, diarrhea, severe kidney dysfunction, fecal impaction, intestinal obstruction or perforation, ileus; rectal bleeding, colostomy, ileostomy; AV block; hypermagnesia.

CAUTIOUS USE Cardiac disease, renal disease, renal impairment; electrolyte imbalance; pregnancy (category A); lactation.

ROUTE & DOSAGE

Antacid

Adult: **PO** 280–1500 mg with water or milk qid, p.c. and at bedtime

Laxative

Adult: **PO** 2–4 g with water or milk at bedtime

M

Magnesium Supplement

Adult: **PO** 400–1200 mg/day in divided doses

ADMINISTRATION

Oral

- Separate administration of this drug from other oral drugs by 1–2 h.
- Store at 15°–30° C (59°–86° F) in airtight containers. On exposure to air, magnesium oxide rapidly absorbs moisture and carbon dioxide.

ADVERSE EFFECTS GI: *Diarrhea,* abdominal cramps, nausea; hypermagnesemia, kidney stones (chronic use).

INTERACTIONS Drug: See magnesium hydroxide.

PHARMACOKINETICS Absorption: 30–50% from GI tract. **Elimination:** In urine.

M

NURSING IMPLICATIONS

Assessment & Drug Effects

- Monitor for dehydration, hypokalemia, and hyponatremia (see Appendix F) since drug may cause intense bowel evacuation.
- Monitor lab tests: Periodic serum magnesium.

Patient & Family Education

- Liquid preparation is reportedly more effective than the tablet form, as with other antacids.

MAGNESIUM SALICYLATE

(mag-nes′i-um)

Doan's Pills

Classification: ANALGESIC; NONSTEROIDAL ANTI-INFLAMMATORY DRUG (NSAID)

Therapeutic: NONNARCOTIC ANALGESIC, NSAID; ANTIPYRETIC

Prototype: Aspirin

AVAILABILITY Caplet

ACTION & THERAPEUTIC EFFECT Sodium-free salicylate derivative that is a nonsteroidal anti-inflammatory drug (NSAID). It inhibits prostaglandin synthesis. *In equal doses, less potent than aspirin as an analgesic and antipyretic. Has anti-inflammatory effects.*

USES Relief of pain and inflammation.

CONTRAINDICATIONS Hypersensitivity to salicylates; erosive gastritis, peptic ulcer; advanced renal insufficiency, liver damage; thrombolytic therapy; bleeding disorders; before surgery; pregnancy (category D third trimester).

CAUTIOUS USE Serious acid-base imbalances; renal disease, history of GI bleeding, or peptic ulcers; SLE; history of acute bronchospasm; pregnancy (category C first and second trimester); lactation; children younger than 12 y.

ROUTE & DOSAGE

Analgesic/Antipyretic

Adult: **PO** 1–2 caplets q4–6h prn

ADMINISTRATION

Oral

- Give with a full glass of water to minimize gastric irritation.

ADVERSE EFFECTS Other: Salicylism [dizziness, drowsiness, tinnitus, hearing loss, nausea, vomiting, hypermagnesemia (with high doses in patients with renal insufficiency)].

INTERACTIONS Drug: Aminosalicylic acid increases risk of SALICYLATE toxicity; ACIDIFYING

AGENTS decrease renal elimination and increase risk of SALICYLATE toxicity; anticoagulants—added risk of bleeding with ANTICOAGULANTS; CARBONIC ANHYDRASE INHIBITORS enhance SALICYLATE toxicity; CORTICOSTEROIDS compound ulcerogenic effects; increases **methotrexate** toxicity; low doses of SALICYLATES may antagonize uricosuric effects of **probenecid, sulfinpyrazone.** May increase the risk of CNS depression with **gabapentin.**

PHARMACOKINETICS **Absorption:** Well absorbed from the GI tract. **Peak:** 20 min. **Distribution:** Widely distributed with high levels of salicylic acid in liver and kidney, crosses placenta, excreted in breast milk. **Metabolism:** Salicylic acid is metabolized in liver. **Elimination:** In kidneys. **Half-Life:** 2–3 h with single dose, 15–30 h with chronic dosing.

NURSING IMPLICATIONS

Assessment & Drug Effects

- Monitor lab tests: Periodic serum magnesium if used in high dosages or with renal impairment.

Patient & Family Education

- Report to prescriber promptly tinnitus, hearing loss, or dizziness.
- Do not take aspirin-containing drugs without consent of prescriber.
- Check ingredients. Doan's pills may contain acetaminophen plus salicylamide.

MAGNESIUM SULFATE

(mag-nes′i-um)

Classification: SALINE CATHARTIC; ELECTROLYTE REPLACEMENT; ANTICONVULSANT
Therapeutic: ELECTROLYTE REPLACEMENT; ANTICONVULSANT
Prototype: Magnesium hydroxide

AVAILABILITY Solution for injection; oral capsules

ACTION & *THERAPEUTIC EFFECT* **Oral:** Acts as a laxative by osmotic retention of fluid, which distends colon, increases water content of feces, and causes mechanical stimulation of bowel activity. **Parenteral:** Acts as a depressant of smooth, skeletal, and cardiac muscle function. Decreases acetylcholine liberated from motor nerve terminals, producing peripheral neuromuscular blockade and slowing rate of S-A node impulse formation in the myocardium prolonging conduction time. *Effective parenterally as a smooth muscle relaxant in labor and delivery, and cardiac disorders caused by hypomagnesemia. When taken orally, it is a laxative.*

USES Parenterally to control seizures in severe preeclampsia and treatment of hypomagnesemia. Orally for relief of constipation.

UNLABELED USES To inhibit premature labor (tocolytic action) and as adjunct in hyperalimentation, to alleviate bronchospasm of acute asthma; torsades de pointes.

CONTRAINDICATIONS Myocardial damage; AV heart block; cardiac arrest except for certain arrhythmias; hypermagnesemia; GI obstruction; pregnancy (continuous maternal use can lead to fetal hypocalcemia and bone abnormalities). **IV:** For toxemia during the 2 h preceding delivery. **Oral:** In patients with abdominal pain, nausea, vomiting or other signs of appendicitis; fecal impaction, or intestinal irritation, obstruction, or perforation; magnesium-restricted diet.

CAUTIOUS USE Renal disease; renal failure; renal impairment; acute MI; digitalized patients; older adults. **IV:** Children.

ROUTE & DOSAGE

Preeclampsia, Eclampsia

Adult: **IV** 4–6 g slowly; then 1–2g/hour for at least 24 hours after delivery. **IM** 5g in each in buttock (10 g total) then 5g q4h for at least 24 hours after delivery; monitor closely

Hypomagnesemia

Adult: **IM** *Mild:* 1 g q6h for 4 doses; **IV** 1–2 g over 1–2 hours *Severe:* **IV** 4–8 g infused over 24 h

Total Parenteral Nutrition

Adult: **IV** 8–20 mEq elemental magnesium/day

Constipation

Adult/Adolescent: **PO** 10–20 g dissolved in 8 ounces of water, may repeat in 4 hours (max: 2 doses/day)

Renal Impairment Dosage Adjustment

Monitor closely to avoid adverse effects

ADMINISTRATION

- Magnesium 1%, 2%, 4%, and 8% solutions are for IV route only. Both IV and IM routes are appropriate for magnesium 20% and 50%; 50% solution must be diluted prior to IV administration.

Intramuscular

- IM injection is painful and should be reserved for patients with limited IV access and severe hypomagnesemia.
- Give deep using the 50% concentration for adults and the 20% concentration for children.

Intravenous

Note: Verify correct IV concentration and rate of infusion for administration to infants, children with prescriber.

PREPARE: **Direct/IV Infusion:** Give solutions with concentrations of 20% or less undiluted. ▪ Dilute more concentrated solutions to 20% (200 mg/mL) or less with D5W or NS.

ADMINISTER: **Direct:** Give at a rate of 150 mg over at least 1 min. Note: 20% solution contains 200 mg/mL, 10% solution contains 100 mg/mL. **IV Infusion:** Must be diluted to a <20% solution for IV infusion and may be administered IVP, IVPB, or as a continuous IV infusion.

INCOMPATIBILITIES: **Solution/additive:** **amphotericin B, ampicillin, cyclosporine, dobutamine, polymyxin B, procaine.** **Y-site:** **Aminophylline, amphotericin B, anidulafungin, azathioprine, calcium chloride, cefepime, ceftobiprole, ceftriaxone, cefuroxime, dantrolene, dexamethasome, diazepam, diazoxide, dicoloxacillin, doxorubicin, epirubicin, ganciclovir, garenoxacin, haloperidol, inamrinone, indomethacin, lansoprazole, methylprednisolone, pentamidine, phenytoin, phytonadione, tedizolid.**

ADVERSE EFFECTS **CV:** Flushing, hypotension, vasodilation. **Endocrine:** Hypermagnesemia.

INTERACTIONS **Drug:** NEUROMUSCULAR BLOCKING AGENTS, CNS DEPRESSANTS add to respiratory depression and apnea. Oral administration with CALCIUM SALTS will impact efficacy.

Magnesium will decrease concentration of QUINOLONES. Do not use with calcium polystyrene or sodium polystyrene, it may result in metabolic acidosis.

PHARMACOKINETICS **Onset:** 1–2 h PO; 1 h IM. **Duration:** 30 min IV; 3–4 h PO. **Distribution:** Crosses placenta; distributed into breast milk. **Elimination:** In kidneys.

NURSING IMPLICATIONS

Assessment & Drug Effects

- Observe constantly when given IV. Check BP and pulse q10–15 min or more often if indicated.
- Early indicators of magnesium toxicity (hypermagnesemia) include cathartic effect, profound thirst, feeling of warmth, sedation, confusion, depressed deep tendon reflexes, and muscle weakness.
- Monitor respiratory rate closely. Report immediately if rate falls below 12.
- Check urinary output, especially in patients with impaired kidney function. Therapy is generally not continued if urinary output is less than 100 mL during the 4 h preceding each dose.
- Observe newborns of mothers who received parenteral magnesium sulfate within a few hours of delivery for signs of toxicity, including respiratory and neuromuscular depression.
- Observe patients receiving drug for hypomagnesemia for improvement in the following signs of deficiency: Irritability, choreiform movements, tremors, tetany, twitching, muscle cramps, tachycardia, hypertension, psychotic behavior.
- Have calcium gluconate readily available in case of magnesium sulfate toxicity.
- Monitor lab tests: Periodic serum magnesium, calcium, and potassium.

Patient & Family Education

- Drink sufficient water during the day when drug is administered orally to prevent net loss of body water.

MANNITOL ⓟ

(man′ni-tole)

Osmitrol

Classification: ELECTROLYTIC AND WATER BALANCE AGENT; OSMOTIC DIURETIC

Therapeutic: OSMOTIC DIURETIC

AVAILABILITY Solution for injection

ACTION & THERAPEUTIC EFFECT

Increases rate of electrolyte excretion by the kidney, particularly sodium, chloride, and potassium. Induces diuresis by raising osmotic pressure of glomerular filtrate, thereby inhibiting tubular reabsorption of water and solutes. Reduces elevated intraocular and cerebrospinal pressures by increasing plasma osmolality, thus inducing diffusion of water from these fluids back into plasma and extravascular space. *Osmotic diuretic that reduces intracranial pressure, cerebral edema, intraocular pressure, and promotes diuresis, thus preventing or treating oliguria.*

USES To promote diuresis in prevention and treatment of oliguric phase of acute kidney failure following cardiovascular surgery, severe traumatic injury, surgery in presence of severe jaundice, hemolytic transfusion reaction. Also used to reduce elevated intraocular (IOP) and intracranial pressure (ICP), to measure glomerular filtration rate (GFR), to promote excretion of toxic substances, to relieve symptoms of pulmonary

M

edema, and as irrigating solution in transurethral prostatic reaction to minimize hemolytic effects of water. Commercially available in combination with sorbitol for urogenital irrigation.

CONTRAINDICATIONS Anuria; severe renal failure with azotemia or increasing oliguria; marked pulmonary congestion or edema; severe CHF; metabolic edema; hypovolemia; organic CNS disease, intracranial bleeding; shock, severe dehydration; progressive heart failure; concomitantly with blood.

CAUTIOUS USE Electrolyte imbalance; older adult; pregnancy (category B); lactation; children.

ROUTE & DOSAGE

M

Edema, Ascites

Adult: **IV** 100 g as a 10–20% solution over 2–6 h

Elevated IOP or ICP

Adult: **IV** 1.5–2 g/kg as a 15–25% solution over 30–60 min

Acute Chemical Toxicity

Adult: **IV** 100–200 g depending on urine output

ADMINISTRATION

Intravenous

Note: Verify correct IV concentration and rate of infusion for administration to infants, children with prescriber.

PREPARE: **IV Infusion:** Give undiluted.

ADMINISTER: **IV Infusion:** Give a single dose over 30–60 min. ***Oliguria:*** A test dose is given to patients with marked oliguria to check adequacy of kidney function. Response is considered satisfactory if urine flow of at least 30–50 mL/h is produced over 2–3 h after drug administration; then rate is adjusted to maintain urine flow at 30–50 mL/h with a single dose usually being infused over 90 min or longer. ▪ Concentrations higher than 15% have a greater tendency to crystallize. ▪ Use an administration set with a 5 micron in-line IV filter when infusing concentrations of 15% or above.

INCOMPATIBILITIES: **Solution/additive:** **Cephapirin, ertapenem, imipenem-cilastatin, meropenem.** **Y-site:** **Amphotericin B, cefepime, codeine, dantrolene, diazepam, diazoxide, doxorubicin liposome, filgrastim, imipenemcilastin, phenytoin, SMZ/TMP.**

▪ Store at 15°–30° C (59°–86° F) unless otherwise directed. Avoid freezing.

ADVERSE EFFECTS **CV:** Chest pain, cardiac failure, hypertension, local thrombophlebitis, peripheral edema, tachycardia. **Respiratory:** Pulmonary edema, rhinitis. **CNS:** Chills, dizziness, headache, seizure. **HEENT:** Blurred vision. **Endocrine:** Dehydration, dilutional hyponatremia, fluid and electrolyte imbalance, hypovolemia, hyperglycemia, hyperkalemia. **Skin:** Rash, urticaria. **GI:** Nausea, vomiting, xerostomia. **GU:** Dysuria, acute renal failure, tubular necrosis, polyuria. **Other:** Fever, tissue necrosis, local pain.

INTERACTIONS **Drug:** Increases urinary excretion of **lithium,** SALICYLATES, BARBITURATES, **imipramine, potassium.** May increase nephrotoxic effect of AMINOGLYCOSIDES.

PHARMACOKINETICS Onset: 1–3 h diuresis; 30–60 min IOP; 15 min ICP. **Duration:** 4–6 h IOP; 3–8 h ICP. **Distribution:** Confined to extracellular space; does not cross blood–brain barrier except with very high plasma levels in the presence of acidosis. **Metabolism:** Small quantity metabolized to glycogen in liver. **Elimination:** Rapidly excreted by kidneys. **Half-Life:** 100 min.

NURSING IMPLICATIONS

Assessment & Drug Effects

- Take care to avoid extravasation. Observe injection site for signs of inflammation or edema.
- Measure I&O accurately and record to achieve proper fluid balance.
- Monitor vital signs closely. Report significant changes in BP and signs of CHF.
- Monitor for possible indications of fluid and electrolyte imbalance (e.g., thirst, muscle cramps or weakness, paresthesias, and signs of CHF).
- Be alert to the possibility that a rebound increase in ICP sometimes occurs about 12 h after drug administration. Patient may complain of headache or confusion.
- Take accurate daily weight.
- Monitor lab tests: Periodic serum electrolytes and renal function tests. Monitor serum and urine osmolality.

Patient & Family Education

- Report any of the following: Thirst, muscle cramps or weakness, paresthesia, dyspnea, or headache.
- Family members should immediately report any evidence of confusion.

MAPROTILINE HYDROCHLORIDE

(ma-proe′ti-leen)

Classification: TETRACYCLIC ANTIDEPRESSANT

Therapeutic: ANTIDEPRESSANT

AVAILABILITY Tablet

ACTION & *THERAPEUTIC EFFECT* Increases the synaptic concentration of norepinephrine in the CNS by inhibition of its reuptake by the presynaptic neuronal membrane. *Useful in depression associated with anxiety and sleep disturbances.*

USES Treatment of major depressive disorder and anxiety associated with depression.

CONTRAINDICATIONS Hypersensitivity to maprotiline or any component of the formulation; seizure disorder; Acute MI; MAOI therapy within 14 days.

CAUTIOUS USE History of seizure activity; psychotic disorders; history of suicidal tendencies; DM; hepatic disease; GI disease; GERD; BPH; respiratory depression; labor and delivery; pregnancy (limited information regarding use during pregnancy); lactation; children younger than 18 y.

ROUTE & DOSAGE

Mild to Moderate Depression

Adult: **PO** 25–75 mg/day may increase in 25 mg increments q2wk up to 150–225 mg/day in single or divided doses

Geriatric: **PO** 25 mg daily, increase in 25 mg increments after 2w to typical dose of 50–75 mg daily.

M

ADMINISTRATION

Oral

- Give as single dose or in divided doses.
- Store at 20°–25° C (68°–77° F) unless otherwise specified.

ADVERSE EFFECTS **CNS:** Nervousness, dizziness, suicidal ideation, *drowsiness*. **HEENT:** Blurred vision. **GI:** *Constipation, dry mouth*.

INTERACTIONS **Drug:** May decrease some response to ANTIHYPERTENSIVES; CNS DEPRESSANTS, **alcohol,** HYPNOTICS, BARBITURATES, SEDATIVES potentiate CNS depression; with **levodopa,** SYMPATHOMIMETICS (e.g., **epinephrine, norepinephrine**) there is possibility of sympathetic hyperactivity with hypertension and **hyperpyrexia;** with MAO INHIBITORS or **linezolid** there is possibility of severe reactions, toxic psychosis, cardiovascular instability; THYROID DRUGS increase possibility of arrhythmias; **cimetidine** may increase plasma TCA levels. ANTICHOLENERGIC AGENTS have increased risk of adverse effects. Do not use with **potassium salts** due to increased risk of adverse effects.

PHARMACOKINETICS **Absorption:** Slowly absorbed from GI tract. **Peak:** 12 h. **Distribution:** Distributed chiefly to brain, lungs, liver, and kidneys. **Metabolism:** In liver. **Elimination:** 70% in urine, 30% in feces. **Half-Life:** 28–105 h.

NURSING IMPLICATIONS

Black Box Warning

Maprotiline has been associated with suicidal thinking and behavior in children, adolescents, and young adults.

Assessment & Drug Effects

- Monitor for increased suicidality, unusual changes in behavior, or suicide attempt. Inform the prescriber immediately.
- Assess level of sedative effect. If recovering patient becomes too lethargic to care for personal hygiene or to maintain food intake and interactions with others, report to prescriber.
- Monitor bowel elimination pattern. Baseline and periodic BMI and weight monitoring.
- Observe seizure precautions; risk of seizures appears to be high in heavy drinkers.
- Monitor ECG, heart rate, blood pressure in patients with preexisting cardiac disease or at an increased risk for QT-prolonging effects.
- Monitor lab results: Serum electrolytes and blood glucose at baseline and periodically during therapy.

Patient & Family Education

- Report immediately to prescriber signs of worsening mental status such as suicidal ideation, aggressiveness, agitation, anxiety, hostility, impulsivity, insomnia, irritability, panic attacks, and worsening of depression.
- Use caution with tasks that require alertness and skill; ability may be impaired during early therapy.
- Do not use OTC drugs unless approved by prescriber.
- Avoid alcohol; the effects of maprotiline are potentiated when both are used together and for 2 wk after maprotiline is discontinued.

MARAVIROC

(mar-a-vir'ok)

Selzentry

Classification: ANTIRETROVIRAL; FUSION INHIBITOR; CELLULAR CHEMOKINE RECEPTOR (CCR5) ANTAGONIST

Therapeutic: ANTIRETROVIRAL

AVAILABILITY
Tablet

ACTION & THERAPEUTIC EFFECT
Selectively binds to human chemokine coreceptor-5 (CCR-5) on cell membranes of helper T cell lymphocytes preventing interaction with the HIV-1 protein necessary for the HIV virus to enter helper T cells. *Prevents infection of helper T cells by HIV-1 viruses with CCR-5 tropism.*

USES
Treatment of human immunodeficiency virus (HIV-1) infection in combination with other antiretroviral agents.

CONTRAINDICATIONS
Patients with severe renal impairment (CrCl < 30 mL/minute) or end-stage renal disease (ESRD) who are taking concomitant potent CYP3A inhibitors or inducers.

CAUTIOUS USE
Hepatic impairment; renal impairment cardiovascular disease; older adults; postural hypotension; pregnancy (insufficient data to evaluate human teratogenic risk); children younger than 16 y; lactation.

ROUTE & DOSAGE

Regimen without CYP3A Inducers or Inhibitors

Adult/Adolescent: **PO** 300 mg bid

Regimen with CYP3A Inhibitor with/without CYP3A Inducer

Adult/Adolescent: **PO** 150 mg bid

Regimen with CYP3A Inducers without a Strong CYP3A Inhibitor

Adult/Adolescent: **PO** 600 mg bid

Renal/Hepatic Dosage Adjustment

See package insert.

ADMINISTRATION

Oral

- May be administered with or without food.
- **Must be** given in combination with other antiretroviral drugs.
- Store at 20°–25° C (68°–77° F).

ADVERSE EFFECTS
Respiratory: Bronchitis, *cough*, sinusitis, *upper respiratory tract infection*. **CNS:** Insomnia, *dizziness*. **Skin:** Nail and nailbed disorders, folliculitis, *rash*. **Hepatic/GI:** *Increased AST, abdominal distension*, bloating, flatulence, decreased GI motility, change in appetite, constipation. **Musculoskeletal:** Arthropathy, myalgia. **Hematologic:** Neutropenia, anemia. **Other:** *Infection*, fever, herpes viral infection, bacterial infection.

INTERACTIONS
Drug: Extensive drug interactions, confirm with a drug interaction database. STRONG CYP3A4 INHIBITORS (HIV PROTEASE INHIBITORS with the exception of **tipranavir/ritonavir, delavirdine, ketoconazole, itrazonazole, clarithromycin**) increase maraviroc plasma level. CYP3A4 INDUCERS (**efavirenz, rifampin, carbamazepine, phenobarbital, phenytoin**) decrease maraviroc plasma level. **Herbal: St. John's wort** may decrease the plasma levels of maraviroc.

PHARMACOKINETICS **Absorption:** Bioavailability is 23–33%. **Peak:** 0.5–4 h (dose-dependent). **Distribution:** 75% protein bound. **Metabolism:** In liver via CYP3A4. **Elimination:** Primarily in feces. **Half-Life:** 14–18 h.

NURSING IMPLICATIONS

Black Box Warning

Maraviroc has been associated with severe hepatotoxicity. Severe rash or evidence of a systemic allergic reaction may occur prior to the development of hepatotoxicity.

Assessment & Drug Effects

- Monitor for and report promptly S&S of hepatotoxicity, hepatitis or infection.
- Report promptly rash, fever, or other signs of an allergic reaction.
- Monitor BP especially in those on antihypertensive drugs and with a history of postural hypotension.
- Monitor CV status especially in those with preexisting conditions that cause myocardial ischemia.
- Monitor lab tests: Baseline and periodic CD4+ cell count and HIV RNA viral load; periodic LFTs, transaminase, bilirubin, and WBC with differential.

Patient & Family Education

- Report promptly any of the following: Itchy rash, yellow skin or eyes, nausea or vomiting, upper abdominal pain, flu-like symptoms, unexplained fatigue.
- Exercise caution when arising from a lying or sitting position. Dizziness is a common adverse effect.
- Do not engage in dangerous activities until response to drug is known.

MECHLORETHAMINE HYDROCHLORIDE

(me-klor-eth′a-meen)

Classification: ANTINEOPLASTIC; ALKYLATING AGENT; NITROGEN MUSTARD
Therapeutic: ANTINEOPLASTIC
Prototype: Cyclophosphamide

AVAILABILITY Powder for injection; gel

ACTION & *THERAPEUTIC EFFECT* Bifunctional alkylating agent which inhibits DNA and RNA synthesis via formation of carbonium ions resulting in cross-links in DNA causing miscoding, breakage, and failure to replicate. *Antineoplastic agent that simulates actions of x-ray therapy, but nitrogen mustards produce more acute tissue damage and more rapid recovery.*

USES Hodgkin lymphoma; cutaneous T cell lymphoma.

CONTRAINDICATIONS Hypersensitivity to mechlorethamine or any component of the formulation; myelosuppression; infectious granuloma; known infectious diseases, acute herpes zoster; intracavitary use with other systemic bone marrow suppressants; pregnancy (may cause fetal harm if administered during pregnancy); lactation.

CAUTIOUS USE Bone marrow infiltration with malignant cells, chronic lymphocytic leukemia; men or women in childbearing age.

ROUTE & DOSAGE

Advanced Hodgkin Disease

Adult: **IV** 6 mg/m^2 on day 1 of every 4 weeks (in combination with other agents)

Cutaneous T-cell lymphoma

Adult: **Topical** Thin film daily to affected area of skin

Obesity Dosage Adjustment

Dose based on IBW

ADMINISTRATION

Topical

- Apply a thin film topically to affected area. Apply within 30 minutes after removal from refrigerator and return to refrigerator promptly after each use.
- Apply to completely dry skin at least 4 hours before or 30 minutes after showering/washing. Allow treated areas to dry for 5 to10 minutes after application before covering with clothing.
- Apply emollients to treated area 2 hours before or 2 hours after mechlorethamine application. Avoid fire, flame, or smoking until medication has dried.
- Caregivers should wear gloves when applying to patients. Wash hands thoroughly with soap and water after handling medication. If accidental skin exposure occurs, wash thoroughly for at least 15 minutes with soap and water and remove contaminated clothing.

Intravenous

Wear surgical gloves during preparation and administration of solution. ▪ Avoid inhalation of vapors and dust and contact of drug with eyes and skin. ▪ Flush contaminated area immediately if drug contacts the skin. Use copious amounts of water for at least 15 min, followed by 2% sodium thiosulfate solution. Irritation may appear after a latent period. ▪ Irrigate immediately if eye contact occurs. Use copious amounts of NS followed by ophthalmologic examination as soon as possible.

PREPARE: **Direct:** Reconstitute immediately before use by adding 10 mL sterile water for injection or NS injection to vial to yield 1 mg/mL. With needle still in stopper, shake vial several times to dissolve. ▪ Discard colored solution or contents of any vial with drops of moisture.

ADMINISTER: **Direct:** To reduce risk of severe local reactions from extravasation or high concentration of the drug, inject slowly over 3–5 min into tubing or sidearm of freely flowing IV infusion. ▪ Flush vein with running IV solution for 2–5 min to clear tubing of any remaining drug. ▪ Be alert for extravasation. Treat promptly with subcutaneous or intradermal injection with isotonic sodium thiosulfate solution (1/6 molar) and application of ice compresses intermittently for a 6–12 h period to reduce local tissue damage and discomfort. ▪ Tissue induration and tenderness may persist 4–6 wk, and tissue may slough.

INCOMPATIBILITIES: **Solution/additive: D5W, methohexital, methotrexate, normal saline. Y-site: Allopurinol, amiodarone, amphotericin B, ampicillin/sulbactam, cefepime, dantrolene, diazepam, garenoxacin, imipenem/cilastin, methohexital, methotrexate, pantoprazole, pentobarbital, phenytoin, sulfamethoxazole/trimethoprim, thiopental.**

M

ADVERSE EFFECTS CNS: Neurotoxicity: Vertigo, tinnitus, headache, drowsiness, light-headedness, sedation, cerebral deterioration, coma. **HEENT:** Tinnitus, deafness. **Skin:** Pruritus, alopecia, rash, diaphoresis. **Hepatic/GI:** Stomatitis, xerostomia, anorexia, *nausea, vomiting,* diarrhea, metallic taste, jaundice. **GU:** Amenorrhea, azoospermia, chromosomal abnormalities, hyperuricemia. **Hematologic:** Leukopenia, *thrombocytopenia,* lymphocytopenia, petechiae, agranulocytosis, *anemia.* **Other:** Weakness, hypersensitivity reactions, anaphylaxis. *With extravasation: Painful inflammatory reaction, tissue necrosis, sloughing, thrombosis, localized thrombophlebitis.*

INTERACTIONS Drug: May reduce effectiveness of ANTIGOUT AGENTS by raising serum **uric acid** levels; dosage adjustments may be necessary; may prolong neuromuscular blocking effects of **succinylcholine;** may potentiate bleeding effects of ANTICOAGULANTS, SALICYLATES, NSAIDS, PLATELET INHIBITORS; OTHER IMMUNOSUPPRESSANTS or MYELOSUPPRESSIVE AGENTS may increase effects. Do not use with LIVE VACCINES. **Herbal:** Do not use with **Echinacea**.

PHARMACOKINETICS Metabolism: Rapid hydrolysis. **Half-Life:** 15–20 min.

NURSING IMPLICATIONS

Black Box Warning

This drug is highly toxic and must be handled and administered with care. Inhalation of dust or vapors and contact with skin or mucous membranes, especially those of the eyes, must be avoided. Avoid exposure during pregnancy. Mechlorethamine extravasation has been associated with painful tissue inflammation and sloughing.

Assessment & Drug Effects

- Monitor infusion site closely. If infiltration is suspected, immediately DC infusion (see ADMINISTRATION).
- Monitor and record patient's fluid losses. Prolonged vomiting and diarrhea can produce volume depletion.
- Report immediately petechiae, ecchymoses, or abnormal bleeding from intestinal and buccal membranes. Keep injections and other invasive procedures to a minimum during period of thrombocytopenia.
- Report symptoms of agranulocytosis (e.g., unexplained fever, chills, sore throat, tachycardia, and mucosal ulceration).
- Monitor lab tests: Periodic CBC with differential and platelet count; renal and hepatic function.

Patient & Family Education

- Report any signs of bleeding immediately.
- Avoid exposure to people with infection, especially upper respiratory tract infections.
- Use caution to prevent falls or other traumatic injuries, especially during periods of low platelet counts.
- Increase fluid intake up to 3000 mL/day if allowed to minimize risk of kidney stones. Report promptly all symptoms, including flank or joint pain, swelling of lower legs and feet, changes in voiding pattern.
- If you are pregnant or get pregnant while taking this drug, call your doctor right away. Use birth control that you can trust to prevent pregnancy while taking this drug.

MECLIZINE HYDROCHLORIDE

(mek'li-zeen)

Antivert, Antrizine, Bonamine ♣, Bonine, Dizmiss, RuVert-M

Classification: ANTIHISTAMINE; H_1-RECEPTOR ANTAGONIST; ANTIVERTIGO

Therapeutic: ANTIHISTAMINE, ANTIVERTIGO

AVAILABILITY Tablet; capsule

ACTION & *THERAPEUTIC EFFECT* An H_1 receptor antagonist with anticholinergic, CNS depressant, and local anesthetic effects. Its antiemetic and antivertigo effects are not fully understood. It depresses inner ear labyrinth excitability and vestibular stimulation, and it may affect chemoreceptor trigger zone in the CNS. *Exhibits antivertigo, and antiemetic effects.*

USES Management of nausea, vomiting, and dizziness associated with motion sickness and in vertigo associated with diseases affecting vestibular system.

CONTRAINDICATIONS Hypersensitivity to meclizine; GI obstruction, ileus.

CAUTIOUS USE Angle-closure glaucoma, older adults, asthma, prostatic hypertrophy, pregnancy (category B), lactation. Use in children younger than 12 y not recommended.

ROUTE & DOSAGE

Motion Sickness

Adult/Adolescent: **PO** 25–50 mg 1 h before travel, may repeat q24h if necessary for duration of journey

Vertigo

Adult/Adolescent: **PO** 25–100 mg/day in divided doses

ADMINISTRATION

Oral

- Give without regard to meals.
- Ensure that chewable tablets are chewed or crushed before being swallowed with a liquid.

ADVERSE EFFECTS **CNS:** *Drowsiness.* **HEENT:** Blurred vision. **GI:** Dry mouth. **Other:** Fatigue.

INTERACTIONS **Drug: Alcohol,** CNS DEPRESSANTS may potentiate sedative effects of meclizine.

PHARMACOKINETICS **Absorption:** Readily absorbed from GI tract. **Onset:** 1 h. **Duration:** 8–24 h. **Distribution:** Crosses placenta. **Elimination:** Primarily in feces. **Half-Life:** 6 h.

NURSING IMPLICATIONS

Assessment & Drug Effects

- Supervision of ambulation, particularly with the older adult, since drug may cause drowsiness.
- Assess effectiveness of drug and inform prescriber when prescribed for vertigo; dosage adjustment may be required.

Patient & Family Education

- Do not drive or engage in potentially hazardous activities until response to drug is known.
- Be aware that sedative action may add to that of alcohol, barbiturates, narcotic analgesics, or other CNS depressants.
- Take 1 h before departure when prescribed for motion sickness.

MECLOFENAMATE SODIUM

(me-kloe-fen-am′ate)

Classification: ANALGESIC, NONSTEROIDAL ANTI-INFLAMMATORY DRUG (NSAID)

Therapeutic: ANALGESIC, NSAID; ANTIPYRETIC; ANTIRHEUMATIC

Prototype: Ibuprofen

AVAILABILITY Capsule

ACTION & *THERAPEUTIC EFFECT* Inhibits prostaglandin synthesis by inhibiting both the COX-1 and COX-2 enzymes necessary for its synthesis and competes for binding at prostaglandin receptor sites. Does not appear to alter course of arthritis. *Palliative anti-inflammatory and analgesic activity.*

USES Symptomatic treatment of acute or chronic rheumatoid arthritis and osteoarthritis; treatment of dysmenorrhea; treatment of bursitis/tendinitis; fever, ankylosing spondylitis.

M

UNLABELED USES Management of psoriatic arthritis, mild to moderate postoperative pain.

CONTRAINDICATIONS Hypersensitivity to aspirin or other NSAIDS; active peptic ulcer, ulcerative colitis; perioperative pain related to CABG surgery; renal disease; pregnancy (category D third trimester), patient designated as functional class IV rheumatoid arthritis (incapacitated, bedridden, etc.).

CAUTIOUS USE History of upper GI tract disease; coronary artery disease; acute MI, cardiac arrhythmias; CVA; diabetes mellitus; SLE; compromised cardiac and kidney function, or other conditions predisposing to fluid retention; pregnancy (category C first and second trimester); lactation; children younger than 14 y.

ROUTE & DOSAGE

Inflammatory Disease

Adult: **PO** 200–400 mg/day in 3–4 divided doses (max: 400 mg/day)

Dysmenorrhea

Adult: **PO** 100 mg tid starting at onset of menstrual flow (for up to 6 days)

ADMINISTRATION

Oral

- Give with food or milk if patient complains of GI distress.
- Withhold dose and report to prescriber if significant diarrhea occurs.
- Store at 15°–30° C (59°–86° F) in airtight, light-resistant container.

ADVERSE EFFECTS **CNS:** Dizziness. **Skin:** Skin rash. **GI:** Abdominal cramps, diarrhea, dyspepsia, nausea.

INTERACTIONS **Drug:** ORAL ANTICOAGULANTS, **heparin,** ANTIPLATELETS may prolong bleeding time; may increase **lithium** toxicity; do not use with other NSAIDS, increases pharmacologic and toxic activity of SULFONYLUREAS, SULFONAMIDES, **warfarin** through protein-binding displacement. **Herbal: Feverfew, garlic, ginger, ginkgo** increase bleeding potential.

DIAGNOSTIC TEST INTERFERENCE May lead to false-positive ***aldosterone/renin ratio.***

PHARMACOKINETICS **Absorption:** Rapidly and completely from GI tract. **Peak:** 1–2 h. **Duration:** 2–4 h. **Distribution:** Crosses placenta.

Metabolism: In liver. **Elimination:** 60% in urine, 30% in feces. **Half-Life:** 2–3.3 h.

NURSING IMPLICATIONS

Black Box Warning

Meclofenamate has been associated with increased risk of serious, potentially fatal, GI bleeding and cardiovascular events (e.g., MI & CVA); risk may increase with duration of use and may be greater in the older adult and those with risk factors for CV disease.

Assessment & Drug Effects

- Report diarrhea promptly. It is the most frequent adverse effect and usually dose related.
- Monitor I&O ratio. Encourage fluid intake of at least 8 glasses of liquid a day.
- Monitor for and report promptly S&S of CV thrombotic events (i.e., angina, MI, TIA, or stroke).
- Monitor for and report promptly S&S of GI ulceration or bleeding. Significant GI bleeding may occur without prior warning.
- Monitor lab tests: CBC, chemistry profile, occult blood loss, and periodic LFTs and renal function tests.

Patient & Family Education

- Report immediately to prescriber any sign of bleeding (e.g., melena, epistaxis, ecchymosis) when taking concomitant oral anticoagulant.
- Stop taking drug and promptly notify the prescriber if nausea, vomiting, severe diarrhea, and abdominal pain occur.
- Report to prescriber without delay: Blurred vision, tinnitus, or taste disturbances.
- Dizziness, a troublesome early side effect, frequently disappears in time. Avoid driving or potentially hazardous activities until response to drug is known.

MEDROXYPROGESTERONE ACETATE

(me-drox′ee-proe-jess′te-rone)

Depo-Provera, Depo-subQ Provera 104, Provera

Classification: PROGESTIN

Therapeutic: PROGESTIN

Prototype: Progesterone

AVAILABILITY Tablet; suspension for injection

ACTION & *THERAPEUTIC EFFECT* Induces and maintains endometrium, preventing uterine bleeding; inhibits production of pituitary gonadotropin, thus preventing ovulation and producing thick cervical mucus resistant to passage of sperm. *Slows release of luteinizing hormone (LH) preventing follicular maturation and ovulation.*

USES Dysfunctional uterine bleeding; secondary amenorrhea; endometrial hyperplasia, parenteral form **(Depo-Provera)** used in adjunctive, palliative treatment of inoperable, recurrent, and metastatic endometrial or renal carcinoma; contraception; endometriosis-associated pain.

UNLABELED USES Obstructive sleep apnea, treatment of hot flashes.

CONTRAINDICATIONS Hypersensitivity to medroxyprogesterone or any component of drug; history of arterial thromboembolic disorders; active DVT; breast cancer, vaginal cancer, uterine cancer, undiagnosed abnormal genital bleeding; hepatic impairment or disease; incomplete abortion; pregnancy (category X); lactation.

CAUTIOUS USE Asthma, seizure disorders, CVA; history of DVT; DM, hypercholesterolemia, hypertension, SLE, obesity, tobacco use; migraine, cardiac or kidney dysfunction. **IM:** Owing to potential for irreversible bone loss, long-term birth control use should be avoided or used in adolescents and early adulthood.

ROUTE & DOSAGE

Secondary Amenorrhea

Adult: **PO** 5–10 mg/day for 5–10 days beginning any time if endometrium is adequately estrogen primed (withdrawal bleeding occurs in 3–7 days after discontinuing therapy)

Abnormal Bleeding due to Hormonal Imbalance

Adult: **PO** 5–10 mg/day for 5–10 days beginning on the assumed or calculated 16th or 21st day of menstrual cycle; if bleeding is controlled, administer 2 subsequent cycles

Endometrial Hyperplasia

Adult: **PO** 5–10 mg daily for 12–14 days/mo beginning on day 1 or 16 of cycle

Carcinoma

Adult: **IM** 400–1000 mg/wk; continue at 400 mg/mo if improvement occurs and disease stabilizes

Contraceptive

Adult: **IM** 150 mg q3mo
Subcutaneous 104 mg q3mo

M

ADMINISTRATION

Oral

- Oral drug may be given with food to minimize GI distress.

Intramuscular

- Shake vial vigorously for at least 1 min prior to drawing up dose.
- Administer IM deep into a large muscle.
- Shake vial vigorously for at least 1 min prior to drawing up dose.
- Inject into anterior thigh or abdomen.
- Store all formulations at 15°–30° C (59°–86° F); protect from freezing.

ADVERSE EFFECTS **CV:** Hypertension, pulmonary embolism, edema. **CNS:** Cerebral thrombosis or hemorrhage, depression. **Skin:** Angioneurotic edema. **GI:** Vomiting, nausea, cholestatic jaundice, abdominal cramps. **GU:** *Breakthrough bleeding,* changes in menstrual flow, dysmenorrhea, vaginal candidiasis. **Musculoskeletal:** Loss of bone mineral density. **Other:** Weight changes; *breast tenderness,* enlargement or secretion.

INTERACTIONS **Drug:** **Amino-glu-tethimide** decreases serum concentrations of medroxyprogesterone; BARBITURATES, **carbamazepine, oxcarbazepine, phenytoin, primidone, rifampin, modafinil, rifabutin, topiramate** can increase metabolism and decrease serum levels of medroxyprogesterone. **Herbal:** Intermenstrual bleeding and loss of contraceptive efficacy may occur with **St. John's wort.**

PHARMACOKINETICS **Peak:** 2–4 h PO, 3 wk IM. **Distribution:** Greater than 90% protein bound. **Metabolism:** In liver. **Elimination:** Primarily in feces. **Half-Life:** 30 days PO, 50 days IM.

NURSING IMPLICATIONS

Black Box Warning

Compounds with estrogen plus progestin have been associated with increased risk of DVT, PE, CVA, MI, dementia, and invasive breast cancer in postmenopausal women.

Assessment & Drug Effects

- See progesterone for numerous additional nursing implications.
- Be aware that IM injection may be painful. Monitor sites for evidence of sterile abscess. A residual lump and discoloration of tissue may develop.
- Monitor for S&S of thrombophlebitis (see Appendix F).

Patient & Family Education

- Initially menstrual cycle may be irregular with unpredictable bleeding or spotting. Over time amenorrhea develops. Be aware that after repeated IM injections, infertility and amenorrhea may persist as long as 18 mo.

MEFENAMIC ACID

(me-fe-nam'ik)

Classification: ANALGESIC, NONSTEROIDAL ANTI-INFLAMMATORY DRUG (NSAID)
Therapeutic: ANALGESIC, NSAID; ANTIPYRETIC
Prototype: Ibuprofen

AVAILABILITY Tablet

ACTION & THERAPEUTIC EFFECT NSAID that inhibits COX-1 and COX-2 enzymes necessary for prostaglandin synthesis affecting platelet function. *Analgesic, anti-pyretic, and anti-inflammatory actions.*

USES Short-term relief of mild to moderate pain including primary dysmenorrhea.

CONTRAINDICATIONS Angiodema, anaphylactic reaction or hypersensitivity to mefenamic; undiagnosed abnormal genital bleeding, breast cancer (known or suspected); DVT or PE (current or history of); active or history of arterial thromboembolic disease (e.g., stroke, MI); hepatic impairment or disease; pancreatitis; pregnancy; lactation.

CAUTIOUS USE Hypersensitivity to aspirin, history of UGI bleeding; blood dyscrasias; asthma; seizure disorders; hepatic hemangioma; migraines; porphyria; hypoparathyroidism; prior history of cholestatic jaundice; cardiac arrhythmias; hypertriglyceridemia; CHF; edema; history of DVT; DM; SLE; older adults. Long-term use increases risk of serious adverse events (see DRUG ADVERSE EFFECTS). Safety and efficacy in children younger than 14 y not established.

ROUTE & DOSAGE

ADMINISTRATION

Dysmenorrhea

Adult/Adolescent: **PO** 500 mg tid for up to 5 days

Oral

- Give with food, milk, or antacids to minimize GI adverse effects.
- Duration of therapy should not exceed 1 wk (manufacturer's warning).

ADVERSE EFFECTS CNS: Dizziness, headache, nervousness. **GI:** Abdominal cramps, abdominal pain, constipation, diarrhea, dyspepsia, gastric ulcer, gastritis, nausea, vomiting.

DIAGNOSTIC TEST INTERFERENCE False-positive reactions for ***urinary bilirubin*** (using ***diazo tablet test***); may lead to false-positive ***aldosterone/renin ratio.***

INTERACTIONS Drug: Mefenamic acid may prolong bleeding time with ORAL ANTICOAGULANTS, ORAL ANTI-PLATLETS, **heparin;** may increase **lithium** toxicity; increases pharmacologic and toxic activity of SULFONYL-UREAS, SULFONAMIDES, **warfarin** because of protein-binding displacement. Do not use with other NSAIDS. **Herbal: Feverfew, garlic, ginger, ginkgo** increase bleeding potential.

M

PHARMACOKINETICS Absorption: Rapidly and completely from GI tract. **Peak:** 2–4 h. **Duration:** 6 h. **Distribution:** Distributed in breast milk. **Metabolism:** Partially in liver. **Elimination:** 50% in urine, 50% in feces. **Half-Life:** 2 h.

NURSING IMPLICATIONS

Black Box Warning

Mefenamic acid has been associated with increased risk of serious, potentially fatal, GI bleeding and cardiovascular events (e.g., MI & CVA); risk may increase with duration of use and may be greater in the older adult and those with risk factors for CV disease.

Assessment & Drug Effects

- Monitor for and report promptly S&S of GI ulceration or bleeding. Significant GI bleeding may occur without prior warning.
- Monitor for and report promptly S&S of CV thrombotic events (i.e., angina, MI, TIA, or stroke).
- Assess patients who develop severe diarrhea and vomiting for dehydration and electrolyte imbalance.
- Monitor lab tests: Periodic CBC, chemistry profile, occult blood loss, LFTs, and renal function tests.

Patient & Family Education

- Discontinue drug promptly if diarrhea, dark stools, hematemesis, ecchymoses, epistaxis, or rash occur and do not use again. Contact prescriber.
- Notify prescriber if persistent GI discomfort, sore throat, fever, or malaise occur.
- Stop taking drug and report promptly to prescriber if you experience chest pain, shortness of breath, weakness, slurring of speech, or other signs of a cardiac or neurologic problem.
- Do not drive or engage in potentially hazardous activities until response to drug is known. It may cause dizziness and drowsiness.
- Monitor blood glucose for loss of glycemic control if diabetic.

MEFLOQUINE HYDROCHLORIDE

(me-flo′quine)

Classification: ANTIPROTOZOAL; ANTIMALARIAL
Therapeutic: ANTIMALARIAL
Prototype: Chloroquine

AVAILABILITY Tablet

ACTION & *THERAPEUTIC EFFECT* Antimalarial agent that inhibits replication of parasites. *Effective against all types of malaria, including chloroquine-resistant malaria.*

USES Treatment and prophylaxis of malaria.

CONTRAINDICATIONS Hypersensitivity to mefloquine or a related compound; aggressive behavior; active depression, or history of depression, suicidal ideation; generalized anxiety disorder, psychosis, schizophrenia, or other major psychiatric disorders; seizure disorders; lactation.

CAUTIOUS USE Persons piloting aircraft or operating heavy machinery; persons using a calcium channel blocking agent or with severe heart arrhythmias, history of QT_C prolongation; pregnancy (mefloquine crosses the placenta but has not shown an increased risk of adverse effects in pregnant women).

ROUTE & DOSAGE

Note: The U.S. Public Health Service does **not** recommend its use in children less than 15 kg or in pregnant women

Treatment of Malaria

Adult: **PO** 750 mg as initial dose; then 500 mg 6–12 hours later
Child: **PO** 15 mg/kg once then 6–12 h later a 10mg/kg dose

Prophylaxis for Malaria

Adult: **PO** 250 mg once/wk (beginning 2 wk before travel), then 250 mg weekly during travel and for 4 weeks after leaving area
Child: **PO** 5 mg/kg/dose once weekly starting 2 wk before travel and then weekly through travel and for 4 wk after leaving area

ADMINISTRATION

Oral

- Give with food and at least 8 oz water.
- When used for malaria prophylaxis, dose should be taken once weekly on the same day each week.
- Tablets may be crushed or suspended in small amount of water, milk, or other beverage if unable to swallow tablets.
- Do not give concurrently with quinine or quinidine; wait at least 12 h beyond last dose of either drug before administering mefloquine.
- Store at 20°–25° C (68°–77° F).

ADVERSE EFFECTS **CNS:** Abnormal dreams, insomnia. **GI:** Vomiting.

INTERACTIONS **Drug:** Strong CYP3A4 inducers may decrease efficacy. Mefloquine can prolong cardiac conduction in patients taking BETA-BLOCKERS, CALCIUM CHANNEL BLOCKERS, other agents impacting QT interval. ANTIMALARIALS may increase adverse effects. Increased risk of cardiac arrest and seizures with **quinidine.**

PHARMACOKINETICS **Absorption:** 85% absorbed, concentrates in red blood cells. **Distribution:** Concentrated in red blood cells due to high-affinity binding to red blood cell membranes; 98% protein bound; distributed minimally into breast milk. **Metabolism:** In liver by CYP 3A4. **Elimination:** Primarily in bile and feces. **Half-Life:** 10–21 days (shorter in patients with acute malaria and in children).

NURSING IMPLICATIONS

Black Box Warning

Mefloquine has been associated with neuropsychiatric reactions that can persist after drug has been discontinued.

Assessment & Drug Effects

- Monitor carefully during prophylactic use for development of unexplained anxiety, depression, restlessness, or confusion; such manifestations may indicate a need to discontinue the drug.
- Monitor blood levels of anticonvulsants with concomitant therapy closely.
- Baseline and periodic ocular examinations.
- Monitor lab tests: Periodic LFTs during prolonged use.

M

Patient & Family Education

- Take drug on the same day each week when used for malaria prophylaxis.
- Do not perform potentially hazardous activities until response to drug is known.
- Report any of the following immediately: Fever, sore throat, muscle aches, visual problems, anxiety, confusion, mental depression, hallucinations.

MEGESTROL ACETATE

(me-jess'trole)

Megace, Megace ES

Classification: ANTINEOPLASTIC; PROGESTIN

Therapeutic: ANTINEOPLASTIC; APPETITE ENHANCER

Prototype: Progesterone

AVAILABILITY Suspension; tablet

ACTION & THERAPEUTIC EFFECT

Progestational hormone with antineoplastic properties for which an antiluteinizing effect mediated via the pituitary has been postulated. *Effective for treating breast, renal cell, or endometrial carcinoma. Also effective as an appetite enhancer. Has a local effect when instilled directly into the endometrial cavity.*

USES Palliative agent for treatment of advanced carcinoma of breast or endometrium, AIDS-related wasting or cachexia.

CONTRAINDICATIONS Diagnostic test for pregnancy; pregnancy (category X oral suspension, category D tablet); lactation.

CAUTIOUS USE Older adults; severe hepatic disease; diabetes mellitus; renal impairment; thromboembolic disease.

ROUTE & DOSAGE

Palliative Treatment for Advanced Breast Cancer

Adult: **PO** 40 mg qid

Palliative Treatment for Advanced Endometrial Cancer

Adult: **PO** 40–320 mg/day in divided doses

HIV-Related Cachexia/Anorexia

Adult: **PO (suspension)** 800 mg daily or 625 mg of **Megace ES**

ADMINISTRATION

Oral

- Give with meals or food if GI distress occurs.
- Shake oral suspension well before use.

- Use appropriate handling and disposal precautions.
- Store at 15°–30° C (59°–86° F) in tightly closed container.

ADVERSE EFFECTS **GI:** Abdominal pain, nausea, vomiting, diarrhea. **GU:** Vaginal bleeding, impotence. **Hematologic:** DVT. **Other:** Breast tenderness, headache, increased appetite, weight gain, allergic-type reactions (including bronchial asthma), rash.

INTERACTIONS **Drug:** May increase levels of **warfarin;** may decrease renal clearance of **dofetilide.** Do not use with **bosentan.**

PHARMACOKINETICS **Absorption:** Appears to be well absorbed from GI tract. **Peak:** 1–3 h. **Duration:** 3–12 mo. **Metabolism:** Completely metabolized in liver. **Elimination:** 57–78% of dose excreted in urine within 10 days.

NURSING IMPLICATIONS

Assessment & Drug Effects

- Monitor weight periodically.
- Notify prescriber if abdominal pain, headache, nausea, vomiting, or breast tenderness become pronounced.
- Monitor for allergic reactions, including breathing distress characteristic of asthma, rash, urticaria, anaphylaxis, tachypnea, anxiety. Stop medication if they appear and notify prescriber.

Patient & Family Education

- Use contraception measures to prevent pregnancy while taking this medication.
- Learn breast self-examination.
- Learn S&S of thrombophlebitis (see Appendix F).
- Review package insert to ensure understanding of megestrol therapy.
- Maintain adequate hydration while taking medication.

MELOXICAM

(mel-ox′i-cam)

Anjeso, Mobic, Qmizz ODT, Vivlodex

Classification: ANALGESIC, NONSTEROIDAL ANTI-INFLAMMATORY DRUG (NSAID)

Therapeutic: ANALGESIC, NSAID; ANTIPYRETIC; ANTIRHEUMATIC

Prototype: Ibuprofen

AVAILABILITY Tablet; capsule; oral disintegrating tablet; solution for injection

ACTION & *THERAPEUTIC EFFECT* A nonsteroidal anti-inflammatory drug (NSAID) that inhibits both COX-1 and COX-2 enzymes necessary for synthesis of prostaglandin, which is part of the inflammatory response. *Exhibits analgesic and anti-inflammatory actions. It improves the S&S of RA.*

USES Relief of the signs and symptoms of osteoarthritis, rheumatoid arthritis; moderate to severe pain in adults.

CONTRAINDICATIONS Hypersensitivity to meloxicam, aspirin, salicylates, or NSAIDs; GI bleeding; moderate to severe renal insufficiency (injection only); severe hepatic disease; history of asthma, urticarial, or other allergic-type reactions after taking aspirin or other nonsteroidal anti-inflammatory drugs; perioperative pain with CABG surgery; lactation.

CAUTIOUS USE History of coagulation defects, liver dysfunction, gastrointestinal disease, anemia; bone marrow suppression;

dehydration, edema, history of UGI bleeding; CV disease; jaundice; hepatic or renal impairment; hypertension, hypovolemia, immunosuppression; asthma; lactase deficiency, advanced renal dysfunction; hypertension or cardiac conditions aggravated by fluid retention and edema; older adults; females of childbearing age; pregnancy (birth defects have been observed following in utero NSAID exposure); children.

ROUTE & DOSAGE

Osteoarthritis/Rheumatoid Arthritis

Adult: **PO** 5 mg once daily; can increase up to 10 mg daily; ODT form 7.5 mg daily can increase up to 15 mg daily

Moderate to Severe Pain

Adult: **IV** 30 mg once daily

ADMINISTRATION

Oral

- Use the lowest effective dose for the shortest duration to minimize risk of serious adverse effects.
- May be taken with food to minimize gastrointestinal irritation.
- Oral: Store at 25° C (77° F).

Intravenous

- Administer undiluted as an IV bolus over 15 seconds.
- Injection: Store at 15°C–25°C (59°F–77° F).

ADVERSE EFFECTS GI: Abdominal pain, diarrhea, dyspepsia, flatulence, nausea, constipation, ulceration, GI bleed. **Other:** Edema, accidental injury, flu-like syndrome.

DIAGNOSTIC TEST INTERERENCE

May lead to false positive aldosterone/renin ratio.

INTERACTIONS Drug: Do not use with **ketorolac.** May decrease effectiveness of ACE INHIBITORS, DIURETICS; **aspirin, warfarin**, ANTICOAGULANTS may increase risk of bleed; may increase **lithium** levels and toxicity; may increase photosensitizing effect with other agents; may increase nephrotoxic effect of **cyclosporine;** increases serum concentration of **methotrexate**. **Herbal: Feverfew, garlic, ginger, ginkgo** may increase bleeding potential.

PHARMACOKINETICS Absorption: 89% bioavailable. **Peak:** 4–5 h. **Distribution:** Greater than 99% protein bound, distributes into synovial fluid. **Metabolism:** In liver (CYP2C9, CYP3A4). **Elimination:** Equally in urine and feces. **Half-Life:** 15–20 h (PO); 24 hr (IV).

NURSING IMPLICATIONS

Black Box Warning

Meloxicam has been associated with increased risk of serious, potentially fatal, GI bleeding and cardiovascular events (e.g., MI & CVA); risk may increase with duration of use and may be greater in the older adult and those with risk factors for CV disease.

Assessment & Drug Effects

- Monitor for and immediately report S&S of GI ulceration or bleeding, including black, tarry stool, abdominal or stomach pain; hepatotoxicity, including fatigue, lethargy, pruritus, jaundice, flu-like symptoms; skin rash; weight gain and edema.
- Withhold drug and notify prescriber if hepatotoxicity or GI bleeding is suspected.

- Monitor carefully patients with a history of CHF, HTN, or edema for fluid retention.
- Monitor for and report promptly S&S of CV thrombotic events (i.e., angina, MI, TIA, or stroke). Monitor BP.
- Coadministered drugs: With warfarin, closely monitor INR when meloxicam is initiated or dose changed; monitor for lithium toxicity, especially during addition, withdrawal, or change in dose of meloxicam.
- Periodic ophthalmologic exam with long term therapy.
- Monitor lab tests: Baseline and periodic CBC with differential, chemistry profile, renal function.

Patient & Family Education

- Report any of the following to the prescriber immediately: Nausea, black tarry stool, abdominal or stomach pain, unexplained fatigue or lethargy, itching, jaundice, flu-like symptoms, skin rash, weight gain, or edema.
- Discontinue drug if hepatotoxicity or GI bleeding is suspected. Note that GI bleeding may occur without forewarning and is more likely in older adults, in those with a history of ulcers or GI bleeding, and with alcohol consumption and cigarette smoking.
- Stop taking drug and report promptly to prescriber if you experience chest pain, shortness of breath, weakness, slurring of speech, or other signs of a cardiac or neurologic problem.

MELPHALAN

(mel′fa-lan)

Alkeran, Evomela

Classification: ANTINEOPLASTIC; ALKYLATING AGENT

Therapeutic: ANTINEOPLASTIC

Prototype: Cyclophosphamide

AVAILABILITY Tablet; solution for injection

ACTION & THERAPEUTIC EFFECT Forms a highly reactive carbonium ion that causes cross-linking in DNA, thereby interfering with DNA and RNA replication as well as protein synthesis. *Antineoplastic effects result from its activity against both resting and rapidly dividing tumor cells.*

USES treatment of multiple myeloma and ovarian cancer.

UNLABELED USES Hodgkin lymphoma, light chain amyloidosis.

CONTRAINDICATIONS Hypersensitivity to melphalan or any component of the formulation; severe bone marrow suppression; pregnancy (may cause fetal harm if administered during pregnancy); lactation.

CAUTIOUS USE Recent treatment with other chemotherapeutic agents; moderate to severe anemia, neutropenia, or thrombocytopenia; renal or hepatic impairment; men and women of child bearing age; older adults.

ROUTE & DOSAGE

Multiple Myeloma

Adult: **PO** 6 mg/day for 2–3 wk, drug then 4 weeks rest, restart at 2 mg/day when WBC and platelet counts start to rise; or 10 mg/day for 7–10 days then reduce to 2 mg daily dose **IV (Evomela or Alkeran)** 16 mg/m^2 q2wk for 4 doses then at 4 week intervals.

Multiple Myeloma conditioning regimen

IV(Evomela) 100 mg/m^2 daily × 2 days on day −3 and −2 prior to stem cell transplant (day 0)

Epithelial Ovarian Cancer

Adult: **PO** 0.2 mg/kg/day for 5 days as single course, may repeat course q4–5wk

ADMINISTRATION

Oral

- Administer on an empty stomach.

Intravenous

This drug is a cytotoxic agent and caution should be used to prevent any contact with the drug. Follow institutional or standard guidelines for preparation, handling, and disposal of cytotoxic agents.

PREPARE: **IV Infusion:** Reconstitute melphalan powder by **rapidly** injecting 10 mL of the provided diluent into the vial to yield 5 mg/mL. Shake vigorously until clear. ▪ Immediately dilute further with NS to a concentration of 0.45 mg/mL or less. ▪ Note: 45 mg in 100 mL yields 0.45 mg/mL. ▪ Do not refrigerate reconstituted solution prior to infusion.

ADMINISTER: **IV Infusion:** Infuse over 15 to 20 minutes. Administration **must be** completed within 60 min of reconstitution of drug because both reconstituted and diluted solutions are unstable. ▪ Ensure patency of IV site prior to infusion.

INCOMPATIBILITIES: **Solution/additive: D5W, lactated Ringer's. Y-site: Amiodoarone, Amphotericin B, chlorpromazine, garenoxacin, pantoprazole.**

- Store at 15°–30° C (59°–86° F) in light-resistant, airtight containers.

ADVERSE EFFECTS

Cardiovascular: Peripheral edema. **CNS:** Fatigue, dizziness. **Endocrine:** Hypokalemia, hypophosphatemia. **GI:** Nausea, vomiting, diarrhea, decreased appetite, constipation, stomatitis, abdominal pain, dysgeusia, dyspepsia. **Hematologic:** Leukopenia, agranulocytosis, thrombocytopenia, anemia, febrile neutropenia. **Other:** Amenorrhea, fever.

DIAGNOSTIC TEST INTERFERENCE

May cause false positive ***Coombs' test***.

INTERACTIONS

Drug: Increases risk of nephrotoxicity with **cyclosporine, cimetidine** may decrease efficacy. Do not use with LIVE VACCINES; MYLEOSUPPRESSIVE or IMMUNOSUPPRESIVE AGENTS due to increased risk of adverse effects. **Food:** Food decreases absorption.

PHARMACOKINETICS

Absorption: Incompletely and variably absorbed from GI tract. **Peak:** 2 h. **Distribution:** Widely distributed to all tissues; low penetration in CSF (Alkeran). **Metabolism:** By spontaneous hydrolysis in plasma. **Elimination:** 25–50% in feces; 10% in urine. **Half-Life:** 1.5 h.

NURSING IMPLICATIONS

Black Box Warning

Melphalan has been associated with severe bone marrow suppression (with resulting infection and bleeding), development of leukemia, and with production of chromosomal aberrations thus making it potentially mutagenic in humans.

Assessment & Drug Effects

- Monitor laboratory reports to anticipate leukopenic and thrombocytopenic periods.

- A degree of myelosuppression is maintained during therapy so as to keep leukocyte count in range of 3000–3500/mm^3.
- Assess for flank and joint pains that may signal onset of hyperuricemia.
- Monitor for extravasation at infusion site.
- Monitor lab tests: CBC with differential, platelet count, serum electrolytes, renal/liver function tests, and serum uric acid before each treatment and periodically as needed.

Patient & Family Education

- Be alert to onset of fever, profound weakness, chills, tachycardia, cough, sore throat, changes in kidney function, or prolonged infections and report to prescriber.
- If you get pregnant while taking this drug or within several months after lase dose, call your provider right away. Use a reliable form of birth control to prevent pregnancy during treatment and for some time after taking last dose.

MEMANTINE

(me-man'teen)

Namenda, Namenda XR

Classification: N-METHYL-D-ASPARTATE (NMDA) RECEPTOR ANTAGONIST; ANTIDEMENTIA

Therapeutic: ANTIDEMENTIA; ANTI-ALZHEIMER

AVAILABILITY Tablet; oral solution; extended release capsule

ACTION & *THERAPEUTIC EFFECT* Excess glutamate may play a role in Alzheimer disease by overstimulating NMDA receptors. Blockade of NMDA receptors may slow intracellular calcium accumulation, preventing nerve damage without interfering with actions of glutamate that are required for memory and learning. *Improves cognitive functioning in moderate to severe Alzheimer disease (AD) and in mild to moderate vascular dementia.*

USES Treatment of symptoms of moderate to severe Alzheimer disease.

UNLABELED USES Treatment of moderate to severe vascular dementia

CONTRAINDICATIONS Known memantine hypersensitivity.

CAUTIOUS USE Severe renal impairment; severe hepatic impairment; cardiovascular disease; history of seizure disorder; older adults; pregnancy (adverse effects have been observed in animal reproduction studies); lactation; children.

ROUTE & DOSAGE

Alzheimer Disease

Adult: **PO Immediate release** Initiate with 5 mg once daily, increase dose by 5 mg/wk over a 3-wk period to target dose of 10 mg bid; **PO Extended release** 7 mg daily, increase at weekly intervals to 28 mg daily

Severe Renal Impairment Dosage Adjustment

Decrease to 5 mg daily

ADMINISTRATION

Oral

- Ensure that extended-release capsule is swallowed whole. It should not be opened or chewed.

- Withdraw and administer oral solution with provided dosing device; dose should be slowly squirted into corner of patient's mouth. Do not mix oral solution with any other liquid.
- Administer with or without food.
- Note: The recommended interval between dose increases is 1 wk.
- Dose reductions should be considered with moderate renal impairment.
- Store at 20°–25° C (68°–77° F).

ADVERSE EFFECTS **CV:** Hypertension. **Respiratory:** Cough. **CNS:** Dizziness, headache, confusion anxiety. **GI:** Constipation, diarrhea. **Musculoskeletal:** Back pain. **Other:** Flu-like symptoms.

INTERACTIONS **Drug:** Drugs that increase the pH of the urine (CARBONIC ANHYDRASE INHIBITORS, **sodium bicarbonate**) may increase levels of memantine; **tafenoquine** may increase concentration of memantine.

PHARMACOKINETICS **Absorption:** 100% from GI tract. **Duration:** 4–6 h. **Distribution:** Easily crosses the blood–brain barrier. **Metabolism:** Minimal. **Elimination:** Primarily excreted unchanged in urine. **Half-Life:** 60–80 h.

NURSING IMPLICATIONS

Assessment & Drug Effects

- Monitor respiratory and CV status including BP, especially with preexisting heart disease.
- Monitor cognitive function; report S&S of focal neurologic deficits (e.g., TIA, ataxia, vertigo).
- Periodic ophthalmic exam.

Patient & Family Education

- Report any of the following to the prescriber: Problems with vision, skin rash, shortness of breath, swelling in throat or tongue, agitation or restlessness, confusion, dizziness, or incontinence.
- Do not drive or engage in other hazardous activities until reaction to drug is known.

MENINGOCOCCAL DIPHTHERIA TOXOID CONJUGATE

(me-nin'joe-kok-al)

Menactra, Menveo

See Appendix J.

MEPERIDINE HYDROCHLORIDE

(me-per'i-deen)

Demerol

Classification: NARCOTIC (OPIATE AGONIST) ANALGESIC

Therapeutic: NARCOTIC ANALGESIC

Prototype: Morphine

AVAILABILITY Tablet; syrup; solution for injection

ACTION & *THERAPEUTIC EFFECT* Analgesia occurs through inhibition of ascending pain pathways, altering the perception of and response to pain; produces generalized CNS depression. *Control of moderate to severe pain. Does not alter pain threshold.*

USES Relief of moderate to severe acute pain, for preoperative medication, for support of anesthesia, and for obstetric analgesia.

CONTRAINDICATIONS Hypersensitivity to meperidine; convulsive disorders; acute abdominal conditions prior to diagnosis; chronic pain; MAOI therapy; pregnancy (category D at term).

CAUTIOUS USE Head injuries, increased intracranial pressure;

asthma and other respiratory conditions; supraventricular tachycardia; prostatic hypertrophy; urethral stricture; glaucoma; older adult or debilitated patients; impaired kidney or liver function, hypothyroidism, Addison's disease; pregnancy (category B); children.

ROUTE & DOSAGE

Moderate to Severe Pain

Note: Should be titrated to pain response

Adult: **PO/Subcutaneous/IM/IV** 50–150 mg q3–4h prn

Child: **PO/Subcutaneous/IM/IV** 1–1.8 mg/kg q3–4h (max: 100 mg q4h) prn

Preoperative

Adult: **IM/Subcutaneous** 50–100 mg 30–90 min before surgery

Child: **IM/Subcutaneous** 1.1–2.2 mg/kg 30–90 min before surgery

Obstetric Analgesia during Labor/Delivery

Adult: **IM/Subcutaneous** 50–100 mg when pains become regular, may be repeated q1–3h

Hepatic/Renal Impairment Dosage Adjustment

Metabolite accumulation can occur, adjust based on patient response

ADMINISTRATION

Oral

- Give syrup formulation in half a glass of water. Undiluted syrup may cause topical anesthesia of mucous membranes.
- May be administered with food or milk to minimize GI irritation.

Subcutaneous/Intramuscular

- Be aware that subcutaneous route is painful and can cause local irritation. IM route is generally preferred when repeated doses are required.
- Aspirate carefully before giving IM injection to avoid inadvertent IV administration. IV injection of undiluted drug can cause a marked increase in heart rate and syncope.

Intravenous

Note: Verify correct IV concentration and rate of infusion/injection for administration to infants or children with prescriber.

PREPARE: **Direct:** Dilute 50 mg in at least 5 mL of NS or sterile water to yield 10 mg/mL. **IV Infusion:** Dilute to a concentration of 1–10 mg/mL in NS, D5W, or other compatible solution.

ADMINISTER: **Direct:** Give slowly over 3–5 min at a rate not to exceed 25 mg/min. Slower injection preferred. **IV Infusion:** Usually given through a controlled infusion device at a rate not to exceed 25 mg/min.

INCOMPATIBILITIES: **Solution/additive:** **Aminophylline,** BARBITURATES, **furosemide, heparin, methicillin, morphine, phenytoin, sodium bicarbonate.** **Y-site:** **Allopurinol, amphotericin B cholesteryl complex, cefepime, doxorubicin liposome, furosemide, idarubicin, imipenem/cilastatin, lansoprazole, mezlocillin, minocycline, tetracycline.**

- Store at 15°–30° C (59°–86° F) in tightly closed, light-resistant containers unless otherwise directed by manufacturer.

ADVERSE EFFECTS **CV:** Facial flushing, light-headedness, hypotension, syncope, palpitation, bradycardia, tachycardia, cardiovascular collapse, cardiac arrest (toxic doses). **Respiratory:** Respiratory

M

depression in newborn, bronchoconstriction (large doses). **CNS:** *Dizziness,* drowsiness, weakness, euphoria, dysphoria, *sedation,* headache, uncoordinated muscle movements, disorientation, decreased cough reflex, miosis, corneal anesthesia, respiratory depression. Toxic doses: Muscle twitching, tremors, hyperactive reflexes, excitement, hypersensitivity to external stimuli, agitation, confusion, hallucinations, dilated pupils, convulsions. **Endocrine:** Increased levels of serum amylase, BSP retention, bilirubin, AST, ALT. **Skin:** Phlebitis (following IV use), pain, tissue irritation and induration, particularly following subcutaneous injection. **GI:** Dry mouth, *nausea,* vomiting, *constipation,* biliary tract spasm. **GU:** Oliguria, urinary retention. **Other:** Allergic (*Pruritus,* urticaria, skin rashes, wheal and flare over IV site), profuse perspiration, physical dependence, psychological dependence.

M

DIAGNOSTIC TEST INTERFERENCE

High doses of meperidine may interfere with ***gastric emptying studies*** by causing delay in gastric emptying.

INTERACTIONS

Drug: Alcohol and other CNS DEPRESSANTS, **cimetidine** cause additive sedation and CNS depression; AMPHETAMINES may potentiate CNS stimulation; MAO INHIBITORS, **selegiline** may cause excessive and prolonged CNS depression, convulsions, cardiovascular collapse; **phenytoin** may increase toxic meperidine metabolites. Do not use with **ritonavir. Herbal: St. John's wort** may increase sedation.

PHARMACOKINETICS

Absorption: 50–60% from GI tract. **Onset:** 15 min PO; 10 min IM, Subcutaneous; 5 min IV. **Peak:** 1 h PO, IM, Subcutaneous. **Duration:** 2–4 h PO, IM, Subcutaneous; 2 h IV. **Distribution:** Crosses placenta; distributed into breast milk. **Metabolism:** In liver. **Elimination:** In urine. **Half-Life:** 3–5 h.

NURSING IMPLICATIONS

Assessment & Drug Effects

- Give narcotic analgesics in the smallest effective dose and for the least period of time compatible with patient's needs.
- Assess patient's need for prn medication. Record time of onset, duration, and quality of pain.
- Note respiratory rate, depth, and rhythm and size of pupils in patients receiving repeated doses. If respirations are 12/min or below and pupils are constricted or dilated (see ACTION and USES) or breathing is shallow, or if signs of CNS hyperactivity are present, consult prescriber before administering drug.
- Monitor vital signs closely. Heart rate may increase markedly, and hypotension may occur. Meperidine may cause severe hypotension in postoperative patients and those with depleted blood volume.
- Schedule deep breathing, coughing (unless contraindicated), and changes in position at intervals to help to overcome respiratory depressant effects.
- Chart patient's response to drug and evaluate continued need.
- Repeated use can lead to tolerance as well as psychic and physical dependence of the morphine type.
- Be aware that abrupt discontinuation following repeated use results in morphine-like withdrawal symptoms. Symptoms develop

more rapidly (within 3 h, peaking in 8–12 h) and are of shorter duration than with morphine. Nausea, vomiting, diarrhea, and pupillary dilatation are less prominent, but muscle twitching, restlessness, and nervousness are greater than produced by morphine.

Patient & Family Education

- Exercise caution with ambulation and moving from a lying/sitting position to a standing position.
- Be aware that nausea, vomiting, dizziness, and faintness associated with fall in BP are more pronounced when walking than when lying down (these symptoms may also occur in patients without pain who are given meperidine). Symptoms are aggravated by the head-up position.
- Do not drive or engage in potentially hazardous activities until any drowsiness and dizziness have passed.
- Do not take other CNS depressants or drink alcohol because of their additive effects.

MEPOLIZUMAB

(me-poe-liz′ue-mab)

Nucala

Classification: MONOCLONAL ANTIBODY; INTERLEUKIN-5 ANTAGONIST; ANTIASTHMATIC

Therapeutic: ANTIASTHMATIC

AVAILABILITY Lyophilized powder for reconstitution and injection

ACTION & *THERAPEUTIC EFFECT* An antibody that acts as an interleukin-5 antagonist (IgG1 kappa). IL-5 is the major cytokine responsible for the growth and differentiation, recruitment, activation, and survival of eosinophils. Eosinophils are involved in the inflammation associated with the pathogenesis of asthma. *The inhibition of IL-5 signaling by mepolizumab, reduces the production and survival of eosinophils.*

USES Treatment of patients with severe asthma who are 6 y or older, and who exhibit an eosinophilic phenotype; eosinophilic granulomatosis with polyangiitis, hypereosinoophilic syndrome, rhinosinusitis with nasal polyps.

CONTRAINDICATIONS Hypersensitivity to mepolizumab.

CAUTIOUS USE Treat patients with a pre-existing helminth infection prior to starting therapy with mepolizumab. Clinical trials show no dosing differences with geriatric patients, but greater sensitivity cannot be ruled out and hepatic, renal, and cardiac function need to be considered. Pregnancy exposure data is insufficient to inform risk. Potential fetal effects are likely to be greater in the second and third trimesters. There is no information regarding transfer of mepolizumab to human milk and the effects on the breast-fed infant. The FDA approved product label recommends considering developmental and health benefits of breast-feeding and the mother's need for therapy.

ROUTE & DOSAGE

Asthma

Adult/Adolescent/Child over 12y: **Subcutaneous** 100 mg q4wk

Child 6–11: **Subcutaneous** 40 mg q4w

Hypereosinophilic syndrome
Adult/Adolescent: Subcutaneous 300 mg q4w

ADMINISTRATION

Subcutaneous ONLY

- Visually inspect parenteral products for particulate matter. Solution can appear colorless, pale yellow, or pale brown and should be free of particles.
- Reconstitute mepolizumab in the vial with 1.2 mL sterile water for injection preferably using a 2–3 mL syringe and a 21- to 27-gauge, 1/2-inch needle, to result in a final concentration of 100mg/mL and should not be mixed with other medication.
- Direct the sterile water into the vial and then gently swirl the medication until the powder is dissolved (usually taking 5 min). Do not shake.
- If not used immediately, store below 25° C (77° F), but do not freeze. Discard if not used within 8 h of reconstitution.
- Remove 1 mL of the reconstitute from the vial and administer subcutaneously into the upper arm, thigh or abdomen.

ADVERSE EFFECTS Respiratory: Oropharyngeal pain. **CNS:** Fatigue, *headache.* **Other:** Hypersensitivity reactions, antibody development, *injection site reaction.*

INTERACTIONS Drug: No significant interactions noted.

PHARMACOKINETICS Absorption: 80% bioavailability. **Metabolism:** Degraded by proteolytic enzymes. **Half-Life:** 16–22 days.

NURSING IMPLICATIONS

Assessment & Drug Effects

- Patient may experience dizziness, headache, back pain, loss of strength and energy. Patient may need assistance when ambulating.
- Assess respiratory status and report any shortness of breath or abnormally low pulse oximetry readings.

Patient & Family Education

- Notify prescriber if dizziness or fainting occurs.
- Seek out medical assistance with any signs of a significant drug reaction: Fever, itching, chest tightness, swelling of face, lips, tongue, or throat.
- This is not a rescue medication for an asthma attack, it is a maintenance drug.
- Check with provider before taking additional prescription or over the counter medications.

MEPROBAMATE Pr

(me-proe-ba′mate)

Classification: CARBAMATE; ANXIOLYTIC; SEDATIVE-HYPNOTIC
Therapeutic: ANTIANXIETY; SEDATIVE-HYPNOTIC
Controlled Substance: Schedule IV

AVAILABILITY Tablet

ACTION & *THERAPEUTIC EFFECT* Affects the thalamus and limbic system; inhibits multineuronal spinal reflexes. *Antianxiety agent. Hypnotic doses suppress REM sleep.*

USES Management of anxiety disorders.

CONTRAINDICATIONS History of hypersensitivity to meprobamate or related carbamates; history of acute intermittent

porphyria; pregnancy (maternal use associated with congential malformations; avoid use during pregnancy); lactation.

CAUTIOUS USE Impaired kidney or liver function; convulsive disorders; history of alcoholism or drug abuse; patients with suicidal tendencies; children younger than 6 y.

ROUTE & DOSAGE

Anxiety

Adult: **PO** 1.2–1.6 g/day in 3–4 divided doses (max: 2.4 g/day)
Child (6 y or older): **PO** 100–200 mg bid or tid

Renal Impairment Dosage Adjustment

CrCl 10–50 mL/min: Extend dosing interval to q9–12h
CrCl less than 10 mL/min: Extend dosing interval to q12–18h

ADMINISTRATION

Oral

- Give with food to minimize gastric distress.
- Treat physical dependence by gradual drug withdrawal over 1–2 wk to prevent onset of withdrawal symptoms.
- Store at 15°–30° C (59°–86° F) unless otherwise specified by manufacturer.

ADVERSE EFFECTS **CV:** Cardiac arrhythmia, peripheral edema, palpitations, severe hypotension, syncope, tachycardia. **Respiratory:** Bronchospasm. **CNS:** *Drowsiness, ataxia,* dizziness, vertigo, slurred speech, headache, weakness, paresthesias, impaired visual accommodation, euphoria, paradoxical excitation, abnormal EEG. **Integumentary:** Dermatitis, erythema multiforme, skin rash, Stevens–Johnson syndrome. **GI:** Stomatitis, nausea, vomiting, diarrhea, proctitis. **Hematologic:** Aplastic anemia (rare); Leukopenia, agranulocytosis, thrombocytopenia, exacerbation of porphyria. **Other:** Allergy or idiosyncratic reactions (itchy, urticarial, or erythematous maculopapular rash); exfoliative dermatitis, fever, anaphylaxis.

INTERACTIONS **Drug:** **Alcohol, entacapone,** TRICYCLIC ANTIDEPRESSANTS, ANTIPSYCHOTICS, OPIATES, SEDATING ANTIHISTAMINES, **pentazocine, tramadol,** MAOIS, SEDATIVE-HYPNOTICS, ANXIOLYTICS may potentiate CNS depression. Do not use with **perampanel** or **sodium oxybate.** **Herbal:** **Kava, valerian** may potentiate sedation.

PHARMACOKINETICS **Absorption:** Well absorbed from GI tract. **Peak:** 1–3 h. **Onset:** 1 h. **Distribution:** Uniformly throughout body; crosses placenta. **Metabolism:** Rapidly in liver. **Elimination:** Renally excreted; excreted in breast milk. **Half-Life:** 10–11 h.

NURSING IMPLICATIONS

Assessment & Drug Effects

- Supervise ambulation, if necessary. Older adults and debilitated patients are prone to oversedation and to hypotensive effects, especially during early therapy.
- Utilize safety precautions for hospitalized patients. Hypnotic doses may cause increased motor activity during sleep.
- Consult prescriber if daytime psychomotor function is impaired.

M

A change in regimen or drug may be indicated.

- Withdraw gradually in physically dependent patients to prevent preexisting symptoms or withdrawal reactions within 12–48 h: Vomiting, ataxia, muscle twitching, mental confusion, hallucinations, convulsions, trembling, sleep disturbances, increased dreaming, nightmares, insomnia. Symptoms usually subside within 12–48 h.

Patient & Family Education

- Take drug as prescribed. Psychic or physical dependence may occur with long-term use of high doses.
- Be aware that tolerance to alcohol will be lowered.
- Make position changes slowly, especially from lying down to upright; dangle legs for a few minutes before standing.
- Avoid driving or engaging in hazardous activities until response to drug is known.
- Report immediately onset of skin rash, sore throat, fever, bruising, unexplained bleeding.

MEQUINOL/TRETINOIN

(me-qui′nol/tre-ti′noyn)

Solagé

Classification: RETINOID

Therapeutic: DEPIGMENTING AGENT; RETINOID

Prototype: Isotretinoin

AVAILABILITY Solution

ACTION & *THERAPEUTIC EFFECT*

Mequinol is a depigmenting agent and tretinoin is a retinoid used to improve dermatologic changes (e.g., fine wrinkling, mottled hyperpigmentation, roughness) associated with photo-damage and aging. Mequinol's mechanism of depigmentation is probably due to oxidation by tyrosine to cytotoxic products in melanocytes, and/or inhibition of melanin formation. Tretinoin, a retinoid, is used to improve photo-damage to the skin by acting via retinoic acid receptors (RARs). *Mequinol has depigmenting properties; tretinoin improves sun-damaged skin.*

USES Treatment of solar lentigines (age spots).

UNLABELED USES Facial wrinkles.

CONTRAINDICATIONS Hypersensitivity to mequinol or tretinoin; pregnancy (category X); lactation.

CAUTIOUS USE History of hypersensitivity to acitretin, isotretinoin, etretinate, or other vitamin A derivatives, or hydroquinone; patients with eczema, moderate to severe skin pigmentation, vitiligo; cold weather; children.

ROUTE & DOSAGE

Solar Lentigines

Adult: **Topical** Apply to solar lentigines bid at least 8 h apart

ADMINISTRATION

Topical

- Apply doses at least 8 h apart; avoid application to unaffected areas.
- Avoid contact with eyes, lips, mucous membranes, or paranasal creases.
- Protect from light.

ADVERSE EFFECTS **Skin:** *Erythema, burning, stinging, tingling, desquamation, pruritus,* skin irritation, temporary hypopigmentation, rash, dry skin, crusting, application site reaction.

INTERACTIONS Drug: THIAZIDE DIURETICS, TETRACYCLINES, FLUOROQUINOLONES, PHENOTHIAZINES, SULFONAMIDES may augment phototoxicity.

PHARMACOKINETICS Absorption: 4.4% through skin. **Peak:** 1–2 h.

NURSING IMPLICATIONS

Assessment & Drug Effects

- Monitor for and report peeling, erythema, or hypopigmentation.
- Monitor for signs of tretinoin toxicity: Headache, fever, weakness, and fatigue.

Patient & Family Education

- Do not apply larger than recommended amounts.
- Do not wash affected area for at least 6 h after drug application; do not apply cosmetics to affected area for at least 30 min after drug application.
- Minimize exposure to sunlight or sunlamps. Use extra caution if also taking concurrently other drugs that are photosensitizing (e.g., thiazide diuretics, phenothiazines).
- Notify prescriber if vitiligo (hypopigmentation of skin) or S&S of tretinoin toxicity develop (see ASSESSMENT & DRUG EFFECTS).

MERCAPTOPURINE (6-MP, 6-MERCAPTOPURINE)

(mer-kap-toe-pyoor′een)

Purixan

Classification: ANTINEOPLASTIC; ANTIMETABOLITE, PURINE ANTAGONIST

Therapeutic: ANTINEOPLASTIC; IMMUNOSUPPRESSANT

AVAILABILITY Tablet

ACTION & *THERAPEUTIC EFFECT* Purine antagonist which inhibits DNA and RNA synthesis; acts as false metabolite and is incorporated into DNA and RNA eventually inhibiting their synthesis; specific for the S phase of the cell cycle. *Has delayed immunosuppressive properties and carcinogenic potential.*

USES Treatment of acute lymphoblastic leukemia (ALL), as part of a combination chemotherapy regimen.

UNLABELED USES Prevention of transplant graft rejection; SLE; rheumatoid arthritis; Crohn's disease.

CONTRAINDICATIONS Prior resistance to mercaptopurine; infections; pregnancy (category D); lactation.

CAUTIOUS USE Impaired kidney or liver function.

ROUTE & DOSAGE

Leukemias

Adult/Child: 1.5–2.5 mg/kg once daily then continue based on patient response

ADMINISTRATION

Oral

- Give total daily dose at one time at same time every day.
- Administer on empty stomach; avoid concomitant intake of milk products.
- Reduce dose of mercaptopurine usually by ⅓–¼ when given concurrently with allopurinol.
- Store tablets in light- and air-resistant container.

ADVERSE EFFECTS Respiratory: Pulmonary fibrosis. **CNS:** Malaise. Hyperuricemia. **Skin:** Skin rash. **GI:** Anorexia, diarrhea, nausea, vomiting. **GU:** Renal toxicity. **Hematologic:** *Bone marrow depression*, anemia, leukopenia, immunosuppression. **Other:** Infection.

INTERACTIONS **Drug: Allopurinol** may inhibit metabolism and thus increase toxicity of mercaptopurine; may potentiate or antagonize anticoagulant effects of **warfarin.** Do not use with **azathioprine, deferiprone, febuxostat, pimecrolimus, tacrolimus.**

PHARMACOKINETICS **Absorption:** Approximately 50% absorbed from GI tract. **Peak:** 2 h. **Distribution:** Distributes into total body water. **Metabolism:** Rapidly by xanthine oxidase in liver. **Elimination:** 11% in urine within 6 h. **Half-Life:** 20–50 min.

NURSING IMPLICATIONS

Assessment & Drug Effects

- Monitor for S&S of liver damage. Hepatic toxicity occurs most often when dose exceeds 2.5 mg/kg/day. Jaundice signals onset of hepatic toxicity and may necessitate terminating use.
- Withhold drug and notify prescriber at the first sign of an abnormally large or rapid fall in platelet and leukocyte counts.
- Record baseline data related to I&O ratio and pattern and body weight.
- Check vital signs daily. Report febrile states promptly.
- Protect patient from exposure to trauma, infections, or other stresses (restrict visitors and personnel who have colds) during periods of leukopenia.
- Report nausea, vomiting, or diarrhea. These may signal excessive dosage, especially in adults.
- Watch for signs of abnormal bleeding (ecchymoses, petechiae, melena, bleeding gums) if thrombocytopenia develops; report immediately.
- Monitor lab tests: Periodic CBC with differential, platelet count, bone marrow exam, and LFTs.

Patient & Family Education

- Report any signs of bleeding (e.g., hematuria, bruising, bleeding gums).
- Report signs of hepatic toxicity (see Appendix F).
- Increase hydration (10–12 glasses of fluid daily) to reduce risk of hyperuricemia. Consult prescriber about desirable volume.
- Notify prescriber of onset of chills, nausea, vomiting, flank or joint pain, swelling of legs or feet, or symptoms of anemia.

MEROPENEM

(mer-o′pe-nem)

Merrem

Classification: CARBAPENEM ANTIBIOTIC

Therapeutic: ANTIBIOTIC

Prototype: Imipenem

AVAILABILITY Solution for injection

ACTION & *THERAPEUTIC EFFECT* Broad-spectrum antibiotic that inhibits cell wall synthesis of bacteria by its strong affinity for penicillin-binding proteins of bacterial cell wall. *Effective against both gram-positive and gram-negative bacteria.*

USES Complicated appendicitis and peritonitis, bacterial meningitis caused by susceptible bacteria, complicated skin infections, intra-abdominal infections, skin/soft tissue infections.

UNLABELED USES Febrile neutropenia.

CONTRAINDICATIONS Hypersensitivity to meropenem, other carbapenem antibiotics or history of anaphylactic reactions to beta-lactams.

CAUTIOUS USE History of asthma or allergies, renal impairment, renal disease; epileptics, history of neurologic disorders, older adults, pregnancy (category B), lacatation; children younger than 3 mo.

ROUTE & DOSAGE

Intra-Abdominal Infections

Adult/Child (weight greater than 50 kg): **IV** 1 g q8h
Child (3 mo or older, weight less than 50 kg): **IV** 20 mg/kg q8h (max: 1 g q8h)

Bacterial Meningitis

Adult/Child (weight greater than 50 kg): **IV** 2 g q8h
Child (3 mo or older, weight less than 50 kg): **IV** 40 mg/kg q8h (max: 2 g q8h)

Complicated Skin Infection

Adult/Child (weight greater than 50 kg): **IV** 500 mg –1g q8h
Child (3 mo or older, weight less than 50 kg): **IV** 10 mg/kg q8h (max: 500 mg q8h)

Renal Impairment Dosage Adjustment

CrCl 26–50 mL/min: q12h; *10–25 mL/min:* ½ dose q12h; *less than 10 mL/min:* ½ dose q24h

ADMINISTRATION

Intravenous

Note: Dosage reduction is recommended for older adults.

PREPARE: **Direct:** Reconstitute the 500-mg or 1-g vial, respectively, by adding 10 or 20 mL sterile water for injection to yield approximately 50 mg/mL. ▪ Shake to dissolve and let stand until clear. **IV Infusion:** Further dilute reconstituted solution in 50–250 mL of D5W, NS, or D5/NS.

ADMINISTER: **Direct:** Give doses of 5–20 mL over 3–5 min. **IV Infusion:** Give over 15–30 min.

INCOMPATIBILITIES: **Solution/additive:** **D5W, lactated Ringer's, amphotericin B, mannitol, multivitamins, potassium chloride, sodium bicarbonate.** **Y-site:** **Amiodarone, amphotericin B, ciprofloxacin, dacarbazine, daunorubicin, diazepam, dolasetron, doxorubicin, doxycycline, epirubicin, fenoldopam, garenoxacin, idarubicin, ketamine, metronidazole, mycophenolate, nicardapine, ondansetron, oritavancin, pantoprazole, quinupristin/dalfopristin, temocillin, topotecan, zidovudine.**

▪ Store undiluted at 15°–30° C (59°–86° F), diluted IV solutions should generally be used within 1 h of preparation.

ADVERSE EFFECTS **CNS:** Headache. **Endocrine:** Hyperbilirubinemia. **Skin:** Rash, pruritus, diaper rash. **GI:** Diarrhea, nausea, vomiting, constipation. **Hematologic:** Anemia. **Other:** Inflammation at injection site, phlebitis, thrombophlebitis. Apnea, oral moniliasis, sepsis, shock.

INTERACTIONS **Drug:** **Probenecid** delays meropenem excretion; may decrease **valproic acid** serum levels.

PHARMACOKINETICS Distribution: Attains high concentrations in bile, bronchial secretions, cerebrospinal fluid. **Metabolism:** Renal and extrarenal metabolism via dipeptidases or nonspecific degradation. **Elimination:** In urine. **Half-Life:** 0.8–1 h.

NURSING IMPLICATIONS

Assessment & Drug Effects

- Determine history of hypersensitivity reactions to other betalactams, cephalosporins, penicillins, or other drugs.
- Discontinue drug and immediately report S&S of hypersensitivity (see Appendix F).
- Report S&S of superinfection or pseudomembranous colitis (see Appendix F).
- Monitor for seizures especially in older adults and those with renal insufficiency.
- Monitor lab tests: Baseline C&S; periodic LFTs and renal function tests.

Patient & Family Education

- Learn S&S of hypersensitivity, superinfection, and pseudomembranous colitis; report any of these to prescriber promptly.

M

MESALAMINE

(me-sal′a-meen)

Apriso, Asacol, Canasa, Delzicol, Lialda, Pentasa, Rowasa, Salofalk ♣

Classification:
ANTI-INFLAMMATORY;
5-AMINOSALICYLIC ACID DERIVATIVE INHIBITOR
Therapeutic: GI;
ANTI-INFLAMMATORY

AVAILABILITY Controlled release capsule; delayed release tablet; suppository; rectal suspension

ACTION & *THERAPEUTIC EFFECT* Modulates local chemical mediators of the inflammatory response, especially leukotrienes, and is a free radical scavenger; inhibits tumor necrosis factor (TNF). *Provides topical anti-inflammatory action in the colon of patients with ulcerative colitis.*

USES Indicated in active mild to moderate distal ulcerative colitis, proctosigmoiditis, or proctitis; maintenance of remission of ulcerative colitis.

UNLABELED USES Crohn's disease.

CONTRAINDICATIONS Hypersensitivity to mesalamine, salicylates (including aspirin); colitis exacerbation.

CAUTIOUS USE Sulfite hyper-sensitivity; predisposition to myocarditis or pericarditis; sensitivity to sulfasalazine; renal disease, renal impairment; asthmatic patients; older adults; pregnancy (an increased rate of congenital malformations has not been observed in humans; when treatment for IBD is needed in pregnant patients, mesalamine can be continued without interruption); lactation; children younger than 12 y.

ROUTE & DOSAGE

Ulcerative Colitis

Adult: **Rectal (Rowasa)** 4 g once/day at bedtime, enema should be retained for about 8 h if possible or 1 suppository (500 mg) bid; **(Canasa)** 500 mg bid, may increase up to 500 mg tid **PO (Asacol)** 800 mg tid × 6 wk; **(Pentasa)** 1 g four times daily × 6 wk; **(Lialda)** 2.4 g–4.8 g daily **Maintenance Dose (Asacol)** 800 mg bid or 400 mg qid

Adolescent/Child (weight 54–90 kg): **PO** (Dezlicol) 1.2 g bid; *weight 33 to less than 54 kg:* 1.2 g QAM and 800 mg QPM *weight 17 less than 33 kg:* 800 mg QAM and 400 mg QPM

ADMINISTRATION

Oral

- Ensure that controlled-release and enteric forms of the drug are not crushed or chewed.
- Shake the bottle well to make sure the suspension is mixed.
- Administer with or without food.

Rectal

- Use rectal suspension at bedtime with the objective of retaining it all night.
- Rectal enema: Shake bottle well. Instill full contents of bottle. Have patient retain enema for 8 hours or as long as practical.
- Rectal foam: Warm canister to room temperature. Attach applicator and shake for 20 seconds. Insert applicator tip into rectum. Press pump once and slowly release to administer dose; hold in rectum for 10–15 seconds. For the second spray, press dome again and release slowly. Wait 10–15 seconds then remove applicator.
- Suppository: Remove foil wrapper; insert into rectum. Retain suppository for 1–3 hours or longer.
- Store at 15°–30° C (59°–86° F) away from heat and light.

ADVERSE EFFECTS **Respiratory:** Nasopharyngitis, cough, sinusitis, URI. **CNS:** *Headache,* dizziness. **Skin:** Rash. **GI:** *Abdominal pain,* flatulence, nausea, eructation, constipation. **GU:** Urinary frequency. **Other:** Influenza.

INTERACTIONS **Drug:** Do not administer within 6 weeks of varicella vaccination due to risk of Reye's syndrome.

PHARMACOKINETICS **Absorption:** Rectal 5–35% absorbed from colon depending on retention time of enema or suppository. **PO Asacol,** approximately 28% absorbed; 80% of drug is released in colon 12 h after ingestion. **PO Pentasa,** 50% of drug is released in colon at a pH less than 6. **Peak:** 3–6 h. **Distribution:** Rectal administration may reach as high as the ascending colon. **Asacol** is released in the ileum and colon; **Pentasa** is released in the jejunum, ileum, and colon. Low concentrations of mesalamine and higher concentrations of its metabolites are excreted in breast milk. **Metabolism:** Rapidly acetylated in the liver and colon wall. **Elimination:** Primarily in feces; absorbed drug excreted in urine. **Half-Life:** 2–15 h (depending on formulation).

NURSING IMPLICATIONS

Assessment & Drug Effects

- Assess for S&S of allergic-type reactions (e.g., hives, itching, wheezing, anaphylaxis). Suspension contains a sulfite that may cause reactions in asthmatics and some nonasthmatic persons.
- Expect response to therapy within 3–21 days; however, the usual course of therapy is from 3–6 wk depending on symptoms and sigmoidoscopic examinations.
- Monitor lab tests: Periodic renal function, liver function, CBC.

Patient & Family Education

- Report to prescriber promptly: Cramping, abdominal pain, bloody diarrhea, or other signs of rectal irritation.

- Check with prescriber before using any new medicine (prescription or OTC).
- Continue medication for full time of treatment even if you are feeling better.

MESNA

(mes'na)

Mesnex

Classification: CHEMOPROTECTANT; DETOXIFYING AGENT

Therapeutic: DETOXIFYING AGENT

AVAILABILITY Solution for injection; tablet

ACTION & *THERAPEUTIC EFFECT* Detoxifying agent used to inhibit hemorrhagic cystitis induced by ifosfamide. *Reacts chemically with urotoxic ifosfamide metabolites, resulting in their detoxification, and thus significantly decreases the incidence of hematuria.*

M

USES Prophylaxis for ifosfamide-induced hemorrhagic cystitis. Not effective in preventing hematuria due to other pathologic conditions such as thrombocytopenia.

UNLABELED USES Reduces the incidence of cyclophosphamide-induced hemorrhagic cystitis.

CONTRAINDICATIONS Hypersensitivity to mesna or other thiol compounds.

CAUTIOUS USE Autoimmune diseases; infants (injection); pregnancy (category B); lactation; neonates.

ROUTE & DOSAGE

Ifosfamide-Induced Hemorrhagic Cystitis

Adult: **IV** Dose = 20% of ifosfamide dose given 15 min before ifosfamide administration and 4 and 8 h after ifosfamide dose; **PO** 40% of ifosfamide dose 2 and 6 h after each ifosfamide dose

ADMINISTRATION

Oral

- Give at 2 and 6 h after each dose of ifosfamide.

Intravenous

PREPARE: **Direct:** Add 4 mL of D5W, NS, or LR for each 100 mg of mesna to yield 20 mg/mL.

ADMINISTER: **Direct:** Give a single dose by direct IV over 60 sec.

INCOMPATIBILITIES: **Solution/additive:** **Carboplatin, cisplatin, ifosfamide with epirubicin.** **Y-site:** **Amphotericin B cholesteryl complex, lansoprazole.**

- Inspect parenteral drug products visually for particulate matter and discoloration prior to administration. ▪ Discard any unused portion of the ampul because drug oxidizes on contact with air.

- Refrigerate diluted solutions or use within 6 h of mixing even though diluted solutions are chemically and physically stable for 24 h at 25° C (77° F). ▪ Store unopened ampul at 15°–30° C (59°–86° F) unless otherwise specified.

ADVERSE EFFECTS **GI:** *Bad taste in mouth, soft stools,* nausea, vomiting.

DIAGNOSTIC TEST INTERFERENCE May produce a false-positive result in test for ***urinary ketones.***

INTERACTIONS **Drug:** May decrease the effect of **warfarin.**

PHARMACOKINETICS **Bioavailability:** 45%–79% **Metabolism:** Rapidly oxidized in liver to active metabolite dimesna; dimesna is further metabolized in kidney. **Elimination:** 65% in urine within 24 h. **Half-Life:** Mesna 0.36 h, dimesna 1.17 h.

NURSING IMPLICATIONS

Assessment & Drug Effects

- Monitor urine for hematuria.
- About 6% of patients treated with mesna along with ifosfamide still develop hematuria.

Patient & Family Education

- Mesna prevents ifosfamide-induced hemorrhagic cystitis; it will not prevent or alleviate other adverse reactions or toxicities associated with ifosfamide therapy.
- Report any unusual or allergic reactions to prescriber.
- Drink at least a quart of liquid a day when taking mesna.

METAPROTERENOL SULFATE

(met-a-proe-ter′e-nole)

Classification: BETA-ADRENERGIC AGONIST; BRONCHODILATOR

Therapeutic: BRONCHODILATOR

Prototype: Albuterol

AVAILABILITY Tablet; solution for inhalation

ACTION & *THERAPEUTIC EFFECT* Potent synthetic beta-adrenergic agonist that acts selectively on beta$_2$-adrenergic receptors resulting in bronchial smooth muscle relaxation. *Effective as a bronchodilator; additionally, it controls bronchospasm in asthmatics.*

USES Bronchodilator in symptomatic relief of asthma and reversible bronchospasm associated with bronchitis and emphysema.

UNLABELED USES Treatment and prophylaxis of heart block and to avert progress of premature labor (tocolytic action).

CONTRAINDICATIONS Sensitivity to metaproterenol or other sympathomimetic agents; seizure disorders; DM; hyperthyroidism.

CAUTIOUS USE Older adults; hypertension, cardiovascular disorders including coronary artery disease, cardiac arrhythmias, QT prolongation; MAOI therapy; pregnancy (category C); lactation; children. Not recommended for children younger than 6 y **(tablets).**

ROUTE & DOSAGE

Bronchospasm

Adult: **PO** 20 mg tid–qid; **Nebulizer** 1 vial of inhaled solution not more than q4h.

ADMINISTRATION

- Note: Patient may use tablets and aerosol concomitantly.

Oral

- Give with food to reduce GI distress.

Inhalation

- Instruct patient to shake metered dose aerosol container, exhale through nose as completely as possible, administer aerosol while inhaling deeply through mouth, and to hold breath about 10 sec before exhaling slowly. Administer second inhalation 10 min after first.
- Store all forms at 15°–30° C (59°–86° F); protect from light and heat.

ADVERSE EFFECTS **CV:** Tachycardia. **CNS:** Nervousness. **Musculoskeletal:** Tremor.

INTERACTIONS **Drug: Epinephrine,** other SYMPATHOMIMETIC BRONCHODILATORS may compound effects of metaproterenol; MAO INHIBITORS, TRICYCLIC ANTIDEPRESSANTS potentiate action of metaproterenol on vascular system; the effects of both metaproterenol and BETA ADRENERGIC BLOCKERS are antagonized.

PHARMACOKINETICS **Absorption:** 40% of PO doses reach systemic circulation. **Onset:** Inhaled: 1 min; PO 15 min. **Peak:** 1 h all routes. **Duration:** Inhaled: 1–5 h; PO 4 h. **Metabolism:** In liver. **Elimination:** In urine.

NURSING IMPLICATIONS

Assessment & Drug Effects

- Monitor respiratory status. Auscultate lungs before and after inhalation to determine efficacy of drug in decreasing airway resistance.
- Monitor cardiac status. Report tachycardia and hypotension.
- Monitor pulmonary function tests.

Patient & Family Education

- Report failure to respond to usual dose. Drug may have shorter duration of action after long-term use.
- Do not increase dose or frequency unless ordered by prescriber; there is the possibility of serious adverse effects.

METFORMIN (Pr)

(met-for′min)

Fortamet, Glucophage, Glucophage XR, Glumetza, Riomet

Classification: ANTIDIABETIC; BIGUANIDE

Therapeutic: ANTIHYPERGLYCEMIC

AVAILABILITY Tablet; sustained release tablet; oral solution

ACTION & *THERAPEUTIC EFFECT* Thought to both increase the binding of insulin to its receptors and potentiate insulin action. Improves tissue sensitivity to insulin, increases glucose transport into skeletal muscles and fat, and suppresses gluconeogenesis and hepatic production of glucose. *Effective in lowering serum glucose level and, ultimately, the HbA1C value.*

USES Treatment of type 2 diabetes mellitus as adjunct to diet and exercise.

UNLABELED USES Antipsychotic-induced weight gain, polycystic ovary syndrome.

CONTRAINDICATIONS Hypersensitivity to metformin; acute MI, cardiogenic shock; Type I DM; diabetic ketoacidosis; metabolic acidosis with or without coma; lactic acidosis; radiographic contrast administration; renal disease, renal failure, renal impairment with CrCl of 1.5 md/dL in men and 1.4 md/dL in women; sepsis; surgery.

CAUTIOUS USE Previous hypersensitivity to phenformin or buformin; anemia; coma; dehydration, diarrhea; impaired liver function; renal impairment; ethanol use; fever; gastroparesis, GI obstruction; CHF: hyperthyroidism, pituitary insufficiency; polycystic ovary syndrome; trauma, emesis; debilitated patients; older adults; pregnancy (category B); children younger than 10 y.

ROUTE & DOSAGE

Type 2 Diabetes Mellitus

Adult: **PO** Start with 500 mg daily to tid or 850 mg daily to bid with meals, may increase by 500–850 mg/day q1–3wk (max: 2550 mg/day); or start with 500 mg sustained release with p.m. meal, may increase by 500 mg/day at p.m. meal qwk (max: 2000 mg/day)
Adolescent/Child (10 y or older): **PO Glucophage** only: 500 mg bid, may increase by 500 mg/day qwk (max: 2000 mg/day)

ADMINISTRATION

Oral

- Ensure that extended release tablets are not crushed or chewed. They **must be** swallowed whole.
- Use a calibrated oral syringe or container to measure the oral solution for accurate dosing.
- Give with or shortly after main meals.
- Withhold metformin 48 h before and 48 h after receiving IV contrast dye.
- Dose increments are usually made at 2- to 3-wk intervals.
- Store at 15°–30° C (59°–86° F).

ADVERSE EFFECTS **CNS:** Headache, dizziness, agitation, fatigue. **Endocrine:** Lactic acidosis. **Skin:** Flushing, increased sweating. **GI:** *Nausea, vomiting, abdominal pain, bitter or metallic taste, diarrhea, bloatedness, anorexia;* malabsorption of amino acids, vitamin B_{12}, and folic acid possible.

INTERACTIONS **Drug: Captopril, furosemide, nifedipine** may increase risk of hypoglycemia. **Cimetidine** reduces clearance of metformin. Concomitant therapy with AZOLE ANTIFUNGAL AGENTS (**fluconazole, ketoconazole, itraconazole**) and ORAL HYPOGLYCEMIC DRUGS has been reported in severe hypoglycemia. IODINATED RADIOCONTRAST DYES can cause lactic acidosis and acute kidney failure. **Amiloride, cimetidine digoxin, dofetilide, midodrine, morphine, procainamide, quinidine, quinine, triamterene, trimethoprim,** or **vancomycin** may decrease metformin elimination by competing for common renal tubular transport systems. **Acarbose** may decrease metformin levels. **Iodinated contrast dyes** may cause lactic acidosis or acute kidney failure. **Herbal: Garlic, ginseng, glucomannan** may increase hypoglycemic effects. **Guar gum** decreases absorption.

M

PHARMACOKINETICS **Absorption:** 50–60% of dose reaches systemic circulation. **Peak:** 1–3 h. **Distribution:** Not bound to plasma proteins. **Metabolism:** Not metabolized. **Elimination:** In urine. **Half-Life:** 6.2–17.6 h.

NURSING IMPLICATIONS

Black Box Warning

Metformin has been associated with potentially fatal lactic acidosis.

Assessment & Drug Effects

- Monitor vital signs and fasting and postprandial blood glucose values.
- Report promptly any of the following signs of lactic acidosis: Malaise, myalgia, somnolence, respiratory depression, abdominal distress.

- Monitor known or suspected alcoholics carefully for decreased liver function.
- Monitor cardiopulmonary status throughout course of therapy; cardiopulmonary insufficiency may predispose to lactic acidosis.
- Monitor lab tests: Periodic urine for glucose and ketones, fasting blood glucose, and HbA1C; baseline and periodic Hct & Hgb and RBC indices for anemia.

Patient & Family Education

- Be aware that hypoglycemia is not a risk when drug is taken in recommended therapeutic doses unless combined with other drugs which lower blood glucose.
- Report to prescriber immediately S&S of infection, which increase the risk of lactic acidosis (e.g., abdominal pains, nausea, and vomiting, anorexia).
- Report promptly severe vomiting, diarrhea, fever, or any illness that causes limited fluid intake.
- Avoid drinking alcohol while taking this drug.

M

METHADONE HYDROCHLORIDE

(meth′a-done)

Dolophine, Methadose

Classification: NARCOTIC (OPIATE AGONIST); ANALGESIC

Therapeutic: NARCOTIC ANALGESIC; TOXICOLOGY AGENT

Prototype: Morphine

Controlled Substance: Schedule II

AVAILABILITY Tablet; oral solution; injection

ACTION & *THERAPEUTIC EFFECT* Synthetic narcotic that is a CNS depressant, which causes sedation and respiratory depression. Highly addictive, with abuse potential; abstinence syndrome develops more slowly, and withdrawal symptoms are less intense but more prolonged. *Relieves severe pain and manages withdrawal therapy from narcotics, especially heroin.*

USES To relieve severe pain; for detoxification and temporary maintenance treatment in hospital and in federally controlled maintenance programs for ambulatory patients with narcotic abstinence syndrome.

CONTRAINDICATIONS Hypersensitivity to methadone; significant respiratory depression; severe pulmonary disease; acute or severe bronchial asthma in absence of resuscitative equipment; hypercarpnia; known or suspected paralytic ileus; obstetric analgesia.

CAUTIOUS USE History of QT prolongation; liver, kidney, or cardiac dysfunction; COPD, acute or chronic asthma; preexisting respiratory depression, hypoxia, or hypercapnia; head injuries; severe hepatic or renal impairment; hypothyroidism; adrenal insufficiency; Addison's disease; patients at risk for hypotension; BPH; urethral stricture; older adults; pregnancy (category C); lactation. Safety and efficacy in children not established.

ROUTE & DOSAGE

Pain

Adult: **PO/Subcutaneous/IM** 2.5–10 mg q3–4h prn **IV** 2.5–10 mg q8–12h prn (opiate naïve patient)

Child: **PO/IV/Subcutaneous/IM** 0.1–0.2 mg/kg q4h × 2–3 doses, then q6–12h prn (max: 5–10 mg/dose)

Detoxification Treatment

Adult: **PO/Subcutaneous/IM** (Doses are very patient specific and these are general ranges) 15–40 mg once/day, usually maintained at 20–120 mg/day

Renal Impairment Dosage Adjustment

CrCl less than 10 mL/min: Use 50–75% of dose

ADMINISTRATION

Oral

- Give for analgesic effect in the smallest effective dose to minimize the possible tolerance and physical and psychic dependence.
- Dilute dispersible tablets in 120 mL of water or fruit juice and allow at least 1 min for dispersion.

Subcutaneous/Intramuscular

- Note: IM route is preferred over subcutaneous when repeated parenteral administration is required (subcutaneous injections may cause local irritation and induration). Rotate injection sites.

Intravenous

PREPARE: **Direct/IV Infusion:** May be given undiluted or diluted with 1–5 mL of NS.

ADMINISTER: **Direct/IV Infusion:** Give over 5 or more minutes.

INCOMPATIBILITIES: **Y-site: Acyclovir, allopurinol, amphotericin B, dantrolene, daunorubicin, fluorouracil, ganciclovir, lansoprazole, lethohexital, pentobarbital, phenytoin pipercillin/tazobacatam, SMZ/TMP, thiopental.**

- Store at 15°–30° C (59°–86° F) in tight, light-resistant containers.

ADVERSE EFFECTS **Respiratory:** Respiratory depression. **CNS:** *Drowsiness,* light-headedness, dizziness, hallucinations. **GI:** Nausea, vomiting, dry mouth, *constipation.* **GU:** Impotence. **Other:** Transient fall in BP, bone and muscle pain.

INTERACTIONS **Drug: Alcohol** and other CNS DEPRESSANTS, **cimetidine** add to sedation and CNS depression; AMPHETAMINES may potentiate CNS stimulation; with MAO INHIBITORS, **selegiline, furazolidone** causes excessive and prolonged CNS depression, convulsions, cardiovascular collapse. **Food: Grapefruit juice** may increase serum levels and adverse effects. **Herbal: St. John's wort** decreases plasma levels.

PHARMACOKINETICS **Absorption:** Well absorbed from GI tract, variable IM absorption. **Onset:** 30–60 min PO; 10–20 min IM/Subcutaneous. **Peak:** 1–2 h. **Duration:** 6–8 h PO, IM, Subcutaneous; may last 22–48 h with chronic dosing. **Distribution:** Crosses placenta; distributed into breast milk. **Metabolism:** In liver (CYP3A4). **Elimination:** In urine. **Half-Life:** 15–25 h.

NURSING IMPLICATIONS

Black Box Warning

Methadone has been associated with abuse potential, respiratory depression, and QT prolongation.

Assessment & Drug Effects

- Evaluate patient's continued need for methadone for pain. Adjustment of dosage and lengthening of between-dose intervals may be possible.
- Monitor respiratory status. Principal danger of overdosage, as with morphine, is extreme respiratory depression.

- Monitor closely for changes in cardiac status (e.g., QT interval prolongation) especially during drug initiation and titration.
- Be aware that because of the cumulative effects of methadone, abstinence symptoms may not appear for 36–72 h after last dose and may last 10–14 days. Symptoms are usually of mild intensity (e.g., anorexia, insomnia, anxiety, abdominal discomfort, weakness, headache, sweating, hot and cold flashes).
- Observe closely for recurrence of respiratory depression during use of narcotic antagonists such as naloxone.

Patient & Family Education

- Be aware that orthostatic hypotension, sweating, constipation, drowsiness, GI symptoms, and other transient adverse effects of therapeutic doses appear to be more prominent in ambulatory patients. Most adverse effects disappear over a period of several weeks.
- Make position changes slowly, particularly from lying down to upright position; sit or lie down if you feel dizzy or faint.
- Do not drive or engage in potentially hazardous activities until response to drug is known.

METHAMPHETAMINE HYDROCHLORIDE

(meth-am-fet′a-meen)

Desoxyn

Classification: ADRENERGIC AGONIST; CEREBRAL STIMULANT; AMPHETAMINE

Therapeutic: CEREBRAL STIMULANT; ANOREXIANT

Prototype: Amphetamine sulfate

Controlled Substance: Schedule II

AVAILABILITY Tablet; long-acting tablet

ACTION & *THERAPEUTIC EFFECT* CNS stimulant actions approximately equal to those of amphetamine, but accompanied by less peripheral activity. *CNS stimulation results in increased motor activity, diminished sense of fatigue, alertness, increased focus, and mood elevation. Anorexigenic effect is due to direct inhibition of hypothalamic appetite center.*

USES Short-term adjunct in management of exogenous obesity, as adjunctive therapy in attention deficit disorder (ADD), narcolepsy, epilepsy, and postencephalitic parkinsonism, and in treatment of certain depressive reactions, especially when characterized by apathy and psychomotor retardation.

CONTRAINDICATIONS Hypersensitivity or idiosyncracy to sympathomimetic amines; children with structural cardiac abnormalities; glaucoma; advanced arteriosclerosis; symptomatic cardiovascular disease; moderate to severe hypertension; hyperthyroidism; patients in agitated state or history of drug abuse; lactation.

CAUTIOUS USE Mild hypertension; psychopathic personalities; hyperexcitability states; history of suicide attempts; older adult or debilitated patients; pregnancy (category C); ADHD treatment in children younger than 6 y or for obesity treatment in children younger than 12 y; longer-term use in children.

ROUTE & DOSAGE

Attention Deficit Disorder

Child (6 y or older): **PO** 2.5–5 mg 1–2 × day, may increase by 5 mg at weekly intervals up to 20–25 mg/day

Obesity

Adult: **PO** 5 mg 1–3 × day 30 min before meals or 5–15 mg of long-acting form once/day

ADMINISTRATION

Oral

- Give early in the day, if possible, to avoid insomnia.
- Ensure that long-acting tablets are not chewed or crushed; these need to be swallowed whole.
- Give 30 min before each meal when used for treatment of obesity. If insomnia results, advise patient to inform prescriber.
- Preserve in tight, light-resistant containers.

ADVERSE EFFECTS **CV:** Palpitation, arrhythmias, hypertension, hypotension, circulatory collapse. **CNS:** Restlessness, tremor, hyperreflexia, insomnia, headache, nervousness, anxiety, dizziness, euphoria, or dysphoria. **HEENT:** Increased intraocular pressure. **GI:** Dry mouth, unpleasant taste, nausea, vomiting, diarrhea, constipation.

INTERACTIONS **Drug: Acetazolamide, sodium bicarbonate** decreases methamphetamine elimination; **ammonium chloride, ascorbic acid** increases methamphetamine elimination; effects of both methamphetamine and BARBITURATES may be antagonized; **furazolidone** may increase BP effects of AMPHETAMINES—interaction may persist for several weeks after discontinuing **furazolidone;** antagonizes antihypertensive effects of **guanethidine;** MAO INHIBITORS, **selegiline** can cause hypertensive crisis (fatalities reported)—do not administer AMPHETAMINES during or within 14 days of administration of these drugs; PHENOTHIAZINES may inhibit mood elevating effects of AMPHETAMINES; TRICYCLIC ANTIDEPRESSANTS enhance methamphetamine effects because they increase norepinephrine release; BETA-ADRENERGIC AGONISTS increase adverse cardiovascular effects of AMPHETAMINES.

PHARMACOKINETICS **Absorption:** Readily absorbed from the GI tract. **Duration:** 6–12 h. **Distribution:** All tissues especially the CNS; excreted in breast milk. **Metabolism:** In liver. **Elimination:** Renal elimination.

M

NURSING IMPLICATIONS

Black Box Warning

Methamphetamine has been associated with a high potential for abuse.

Assessment & Drug Effects

- Monitor weight throughout period of therapy.
- Be alert for a paradoxical increase in depression or agitation in depressed patients. Report immediately; drug should be withdrawn.

Patient & Family Education

- Be alert for development of tolerance; happens readily, and prolonged use may lead to drug dependence. Abuse potential is high.

- Withdrawal after prolonged use is frequently followed by lethargy that may persist for several weeks.
- Weigh every other day under standard conditions and maintain a record of weight loss.

METHAZOLAMIDE

(meth-a-zoe'la-mide)

Classification: EYE PREPARATION; CARBONIC ANHYDRASE INHIBITOR; ANTIGLAUCOMA

Therapeutic: ANTIGLAUCOMA

Prototype: Acetazolamide

AVAILABILITY Tablet

ACTION & *THERAPEUTIC EFFECT* Inhibits carbonic anhydrase activity in eye by reducing rate of aqueous humor formation with consequent lowering of intraocular pressure. *Effective in lowering intraocular pressure in glaucoma patients.*

USES Treatment of chronic open-angle glaucoma or secondary glaucoma.

CONTRAINDICATIONS Long term treatment of angle-closure glaucoma; hypokalemia, hyponatremia; dialysis; hepatic disease; renal disease; adrenal gland failure; cirrhosis.

CAUTIOUS USE Pulmonary disease, COPD; diabetes mellitus; renal impairment; pregnancy (adverse effects have been observed in animal reproduction studies); lactation.

ROUTE & DOSAGE

Glaucoma

Adult: **PO** 50–100 mg bid or tid

ADMINISTRATION

Oral

- Give with meals to minimize GI distress.
- Storage: Store at 20°C to 25°C (68°F to 77°F).

ADVERSE EFFECTS **CNS:** Seizure, paresthesia, confusion, drowsiness, fatigue, flaccid paralysis, malaise. **HEENT:** Myopia, tinnitus, auditory disturbance. **Endocrine:** Electrolyte disturbance, glycosuria, metabolic acidosis. **Skin:** Erythema multiforme, skin photosensitivity, skin rash, Stevens–Johnson syndrome, toxic epidermal necrolysis, urticarial. **GI:** Decreased appetite, diarrhea, dysgeusia, melena, nausea, vomiting. **GU:** Crystalluria, hematuria, nephrolithiasis, polyuria. **Other:** Anaphylaxis, hypersensitivity reaction, fever.

DIAGNOSTIC TEST INTERFERENCE May lead to false negative aldosterone/renin ratio.

INTERACTIONS **Drug:** Do not use with CARBONIC ANHYDRASE INHIBITORS; patients on high doses of SALICYLATES are at higher risk for SALICYLATE toxicity.

PHARMACOKINETICS **Absorption:** Slowly from GI tract. **Onset:** 2–4 h. **Peak:** 6–8 h. **Duration:** 10–18 h. **Distribution:** Throughout body, concentrating in RBCs, plasma, and kidneys; crosses placenta. **Metabolism:** Partially in liver. **Elimination:** Primarily in urine.

NURSING IMPLICATIONS

Assessment & Drug Effects

- Supervise ambulation in older adult, since drug may cause vertigo.
- Assess patient's ability to perform ADL since drug may cause fatigue and lethargy.

- Monitor lab tests: Baseline and periodic CBC with platelet count; periodic serum electrolytes.

Patient & Family Education

- Be aware that drug may cause drowsiness. Advise caution with hazardous activities until response to drug is known.

METHENAMINE HIPPURATE

(meth-en′a-meen hip′yoo-rate)

Hiprex, Urex

METHENAMINE MANDELATE

Classification: URINARY TRACT ANTI-INFECTIVE

Therapeutic: URINARY TRACT ANTI-INFECTIVE

Prototype: Trimethoprim

AVAILABILITY **Methenamine Hippurate:** Tablet. **Methenamine Mandelate:** Tablet; suspension

ACTION & THERAPEUTIC EFFECT Tertiary amine that liberates formaldehyde in an acid medium, which is a nonspecific antibiotic agent with bactericidal activity. *Currently used only for suppression and prophylaxis of frequently recurring urinary tract infections such as in patients with neurogenic bladder or in those who require intermittent catheterization routinely.*

USES Prophylactic treatment of recurrent urinary tract infections (UTIs). Also long-term prophylaxis when residual urine is present (e.g., neurogenic bladder).

CONTRAINDICATIONS Renal insufficiency; liver disease; gout; severe dehydration; lactation.

CAUTIOUS USE Oral suspension for patients susceptible to lipoid pneumonia (e.g., older adults, debilitated patients); gout; pregnancy (category C); children.

ROUTE & DOSAGE

UTI Prophylaxis

Adult: **PO (Hippurate)** 1 g bid; **(Mandelate)** 1 g qid

Child (6 y or younger): **PO (Mandelate)** 18.4 mg/kg qid; *6–12 y:* **(Hippurate)** 0.5–1 g bid; **(Mandelate)** 500 mg qid or 50 mg/kg/day in 3 divided doses

ADMINISTRATION

Oral

- Give after meals and at bedtime to minimize gastric distress.
- Give oral suspension with caution to older adult or debilitated patients because of the possibility of lipid (aspiration) pneumonia; it contains a vegetable oil base.
- Store at 15°–30° C (59°–86° F) in tightly closed container; protect from excessive heat.

ADVERSE EFFECTS **Endocrine:** Bladder irritation, dysuria, frequency, albuminuria, hematuria, crystalluria. **GI:** Nausea, vomiting, diarrhea, abdominal cramps, anorexia.

DIAGNOSTIC TEST INTERFERENCE Methenamine (formaldehyde) may produce falsely elevated values for ***urinary catecholamines*** and ***urinary steroids (17-hydroxycorticosteroids)*** (by ***Reddy method***). Possibility of false ***urine glucose determinations*** with ***Benedict's*** test. Methenamine interferes with ***urobilinogen*** and possibly ***urinary VMA*** determinations.

INTERACTIONS Drug: Sulfamethoxazole forms insoluble precipitate in acid urine; **acetazolamide, sodium bicarbonate** may prevent hydrolysis to formaldehyde.

PHARMACOKINETICS Absorption: Readily from GI tract, although 10–30% of dose is hydrolyzed to formaldehyde in stomach. **Peak:** 2 h. **Duration:** Up to 6 h or until patient voids. **Distribution:** Crosses placenta; distributed into breast milk. **Metabolism:** Hydrolyzed in acid pH to formaldehyde. **Elimination:** In urine. **Half-Life:** 4 h.

NURSING IMPLICATIONS

Assessment & Drug Effects

- Monitor urine pH; value of 5.5 or less is required for optimum drug action.
- Monitor I&O ratio and pattern; drug most effective when fluid intake is maintained at 1500 or 2000 mL/day.
- Consult prescriber about changing to enteric-coated tablet if patient complains of gastric distress.
- Supplemental acidification to maintain pH of 5.5 or below required for drug action may be necessary. Accomplish by drugs (ascorbic acid, ammonium chloride) or by foods.

Patient & Family Education

- Do not self-medicate with OTC antacids containing sodium bicarbonate or sodium carbonate (to prevent raising urine pH).
- Achieve supplementary acidification by limiting intake of foods that can increase urine pH [e.g., vegetables, fruits, and fruit juice (except cranberry, plum, prune)] and increasing intake of foods that can decrease urine pH (e.g., proteins, cranberry juice, plums, prunes).

METHIMAZOLE

(meth-im′a-zole)

Tapazole

Classification: ANTITHYROID HORMONE

Therapeutic: ANTITHYROID

Prototype: Propylthiouracil

AVAILABILITY Tablet

ACTION & *THERAPEUTIC EFFECT* Inhibits synthesis of thyroid hormones as the drug accumulates in the thyroid gland. Does not affect existing T_3 or T_4 levels. *Corrects hyperthyroidism by inhibiting synthesis of the thyroid hormone.*

USES Hyperthyroidism and prior to surgery or radiotherapy of the thyroid; may be used cautiously to treat hyperthyroidism in pregnancy.

CONTRAINDICATIONS Pregnancy (category D).

CAUTIOUS USE Bone marrow suppression; older adults; hepatic disease.

ROUTE & DOSAGE

Hyperthyroidism

Adult: **PO** 5–15 mg q8h
Child: **PO** 0.2–0.4 mg/kg/day divided q8h

ADMINISTRATION

Oral

- Give at same time each day relative to meals.
- Store at 15°–30° C (59°–86° F) in light-resistant container.

ADVERSE EFFECTS CNS: Peripheral neuropathy, drowsiness, neuritis, paresthesias, vertigo.

Endocrine: Hypothyroidism. **Skin:** Rash, alopecia, skin hyperpigmentation, urticaria, and pruritus. **GI:** Hepatotoxicity (rare). **GU:** Nephrotic syndrome. **Musculoskeletal:** Arthralgia. **Hematologic:** Leukopenia, agranulocytosis, granulocytopenia, thrombocytopenia, pancytopenia, and aplastic anemia.

INTERACTIONS Drug: Can reduce anticoagulant effects of **warfarin;** may increase serum levels of **digoxin;** may alter **theophylline** levels; may need to decrease dose of BETA-BLOCKERS.

PHARMACOKINETICS Absorption: Readily absorbed from GI tract. **Onset:** 30–40 min. **Peak:** 1 h. **Duration:** 2–4 h. **Distribution:** Crosses placenta; distributed into breast milk. **Elimination:** 12% in urine within 24 h. **Half-Life:** 5–13 h.

NURSING IMPLICATIONS

Assessment & Drug Effects

- Closely monitor PT and INR in patients on oral anticoagulants. Anticoagulant activity may be potentiated.
- Monitor lab tests: Baseline and periodic thyroid function tests; periodic CBC with differential, prothrombin time, and LFTs.

Patient & Family Education

- Be aware that skin rash or swelling of cervical lymph nodes may indicate need to discontinue drug and change to another antithyroid agent. Consult prescriber.
- Notify prescriber promptly if the following symptoms appear: Bruising, unexplained bleeding, sore throat, fever, jaundice.
- Methimazole does not induce hypothyroiditis.

METHOCARBAMOL

(meth-oh-kar′ba-mole)

Robaxin

Classification: CENTRALLY ACTING SKELETAL MUSCLE RELAXANT; CARBAMATE

Therapeutic: SKELETAL MUSCLE RELAXANT

Prototype: Cyclobenzaprine

AVAILABILITY Solution for injection; tablet

ACTION & *THERAPEUTIC EFFECT* Exerts skeletal muscle relaxant action by general CNS depression. *Acts on multisynaptic pathways in spinal cord that control muscular spasms.*

USES Adjunct treatment of muscle spasm. Also used intravenously as adjunct in management of neuromuscular manifestations of tetanus.

CONTRAINDICATIONS Comatose states; CNS depression; acidosis; older adults; renal impairment.

CAUTIOUS USE Epilepsy; renal disease, renal failure, renal impairment, seizure disorder; females of childbearing age; pregnancy (fetal and congenital abnormalities have been reported following in utero exposure in animal reproduction studies); lactation; children.

ROUTE & DOSAGE

Acute Musculoskeletal Disorders

Adult: **PO** 1.5 g tid or qid for 2–3 days, then 4–4.5 g/day in 3–4 divided doses; **IV/IM** 1 g q8h for up to 3 days

Tetanus

Adult: **IV** 1–2 g may be repeated q6h

M

Child: **PO** 15 mg/kg may repeat q6h as needed up to 1.8 g/m^2/day for 3 consecutive days if necessary

ADMINISTRATION

Oral

- Tablets may be crushed and mixed with food or liquid if needed.

Intramuscular

- Do not exceed IM dose of 5 mL (0.5 g) into each gluteal region. Insert needle deep and carefully aspirate. Inject drug slowly. Rotate injection sites and observe for evidence of irritation.

Intravenous

PREPARE: **Direct:** May be given undiluted or diluted. **IV Infusion:** May dilute in up to 250 mL of NS or D5W.

ADMINISTER: **Direct:** Give at a maximum rate of 3 mL/minute. May be administered diluted or undiluted. **IV Infusion:** Infuse at a rate consistent with amount of fluid, but do not exceed direct rate. ▪ Keep patient recumbent during and for 10–15 min after IV injection in order to reduce possibility of orthostatic hypotension and other adverse reactions. ▪ Monitor vital signs and IV flow rate. ▪ Take care to avoid extravasation of IV solution, which may result in thrombophlebitis and sloughing.

- Store at 20°–25° C (68°–77° F).

ADVERSE EFFECTS **CV:** Hypotension, bradycardia, flushing, syncope, thrombophlebitis, angioedema. **Respiratory:** Nasal congestion. **CNS:** *Drowsiness, dizziness,* headache, amnesia, ataxia, confusion, insomnia, sedation, seizure. **HEENT:** Conjunctivitis, blurred vision, diplopia, nystagmus. **Skin:** Urticaria, pruritus, rash, sloughing (with extravasation). **GI/Hepatic:** Nausea, metallic taste, vomiting, dyspepsia, jaundice. **Hematologic:** Leukopenia. **Other:** Hypersensitivity reaction, anaphylactic reaction.

DIAGNOSTIC TEST INTERFERENCE Methocarbamol may cause false increases in ***urinary 5-HIAA*** (with ***nitrosonaphthol reagent***) and ***VMA (Gitlow method).***

INTERACTIONS **Drug: Alcohol** and other CNS DEPRESSANTS enhance CNS depression.

PHARMACOKINETICS **Absorption:** Readily absorbed from GI tract; 46–50% protein bound. **Onset:** 30 min. **Peak:** 1–2 h. **Metabolism:** In liver. **Elimination:** In urine. **Half-Life:** 1–2 h.

NURSING IMPLICATIONS

Assessment & Drug Effects

- Monitor vital signs closely during IV infusion.
- Supervise ambulation following parenteral administration.
- Monitor IV site closely to prevent extravasation.

Patient & Family Education

- Make position changes slowly, particularly from lying down to upright position; dangle legs before standing.
- Be aware that adverse reactions after oral administration are usually mild and transient and subside with dosage reduction. Use caution regarding drowsiness and dizziness. Avoid activities requiring mental alertness and physical coordination until response to drug is known.

METHOTREXATE SODIUM

(meth-oh-trex'ate)

MTX, Otrexup, Rasuvo, Trexall, Xatmep

Classification: ANTINEOPLASTIC; ANTIMETABOLITE; IMMUNOSUPPRESSANT; DISEASE-MODIFYING ANTIRHEUMATIC DRUG (DMARD)

Therapeutic: ANTINEOPLASTIC; ANTIFOLATE; ANTIRHEUMATIC; ANTI-PSORIATIC

AVAILABILITY Tablet; solution for injection; oral solution

ACTION & *THERAPEUTIC EFFECT* Antimetabolite and folic acid antagonist that blocks folic acid participation in nucleic acid synthesis, thereby interfering with mitotic cell process. Rapidly proliferating tissues (malignant cells, bone marrow, and psoriasis) are sensitive to interference of the mitotic process by this drug. *Induces remission slowly; use often preceded by other antineoplastic therapies. Additionally has immunosuppressant effects, antipsoriatic, and antirheumatic effects.*

USES In combination regimens to maintain induced remissions in neoplastic diseases. Effective in treatment of gestational choriocarcinoma and hydatidiform mole and as immunosuppressant in kidney transplantation, for acute and subacute leukemias and leukemic meningitis, especially in children. Used in lymphosarcoma, in certain inoperable tumors of head, neck, and pelvis, and in mycosis fungoides. Also used to treat severe psoriasis nonresponsive to other forms of therapy, rheumatoid arthritis, active polyarticular-course juvenile idiopathic arthritis.

UNLABELED USES Psoriatic arthritis, SLE, polymyositis.

CONTRAINDICATIONS Hypersensitivity to methotrexate; chronic liver disease; alcoholism or alcoholic liver disease; vaccination; ultraviolet exposure to psoriatic lesions; preexisting blood dyscrasias; rheumatoid arthritis; men and women of childbearing age; pregnancy (category X); lactation.

CAUTIOUS USE Infections; peptic ulcer, ulcerative colitis; renal impairment; very young or old patients; cancer patients with preexisting bone marrow impairment; poor nutritional status; children.

ROUTE & DOSAGE

Oncology Uses

Varies based on concurrent antineoplastic agents and patient specific factors; see package insert

Psoriasis

Adult: **PO** 2.5 mg q12h for 3 doses each wk or 10–25 mg weekly, adjust dose gradually

Rheumatoid Arthritis

Adult: **PO** 10–15 mg weekly, increase by 5 mg q2–4 wk (max: 20–30 mg weekly): **Subcutaneous/IM** 7.5 mg weekly, adjust dose to response

ADMINISTRATION

Oral

- May be taken without respect to meals.
- Avoid skin exposure and inhalation of drug particles.

Intramuscular

- Inject deeply into a large muscle.

Intravenous

Note: Verify correct IV concentration and rate of infusion for administration to children with prescriber.
PREPARE: **Direct:** Reconstitute powder vial by adding 2 mL of NS or D5W without preservatives to each 5 mg to yield 2.5 mg/mL. Reconstitute 1 g high-dose vial with 19.4 mL D5W or NS to yield 50 mg/mL. **IV Infusion:** Further dilute contents of the reconstituted 1 g high-dose vial in D5W or NS to a 25 mg/mL or less.
ADMINISTER: **Direct:** Give at rate of 10 mg or fraction thereof over 60 sec. **IV Infusion:** Give over 1–4 h or as prescribed.
INCOMPATIBILITIES: **Solution/additive:** **Bleomycin, metoclopramide.** **Y-site:** **Amiodarone, amphotericin B, capsofungin, chlorpromazine, codeine, dacarbazine, daptomycin, dexrazone, diazepam, diltiazem, dobutamine, dopamine, doxycycline, gemcitabine, gentamicin, idarubicin, ifosfamide, levofloxacin, mechlorethamine, midazolam, mycphenolate, nalbuphine, nicardipine, pantoprazole, phenytoin, propacetamil, propofol quinupristin/dalfopristin, ranacuronium.**

- Preserve drug in tight, light-resistant container.

ADVERSE EFFECTS **CV:** Arterial thrombosis, cerebral thrombosis, chest pain, deep vein thrombosis, hypotension, pericardial effusion, pericarditis, pulmonary embolism, retinal thrombosis, thrombophlebitis, vasculitis. **Respiratory:** Interstitial pneumonitis, cough, epistaxis, pharyngitis, pneumonia, upper respiratory tract infection. **CNS:** Drowsiness, fatigue, malaise, mood changes, neurological signs and symptoms. **HEENT:** Blurred vision, conjunctivitis, eye pain, visual disturbance, tinnitus. **Endocrine:** Decreased libido, decreased serum albumin, diabetes mellitus, gynecomastia, menstrual disease. **Skin:** Alopecia, burning sensation of the skin, skin photosensitivity. **Hepatic/GI:** Increased liver enzymes, hepatotoxicity, diarrhea, nausea, vomiting, stomatitis. **GU:** Azotemia, cystitis, renal failure. **Musculoskeletal:** Arthralgia, myalgia. **Hematologic:** Thrombocytopenia, leukopenia. **Other:** Infection, fever.

INTERACTIONS **Drug: Acitretin, alcohol, azathioprine, sulfasalazine** increase risk of hepatotoxicity; **chloramphenicol, etretinate,** SALICYLATES, NSAIDS, SULFONAMIDES, SULFONYLUREAS, **phenylbutazone, phenytoin,** TETRACYCLINES, **PABA, penicillin, probenecid**, PROTON PUMP INHIBITORS may increase methotrexate levels with increased toxicity; **folic acid** may alter response to methotrexate. May increase **theophylline** levels; **cholestyramine** enhances methotrexate clearance. Avoid use with **deferiprone, foscarnet, pimecrolimus, tacrolimus,** SALICYLATES. Do not use with LIVE VACCINES. **Herbal: Echinacea** may increase risk of hepatotoxicity. **Food: Caffeine** greater than 180 mg/day (3–4 cups) may decrease effectiveness for rheumatoid arthritis.

PHARMACOKINETICS **Absorption:** Readily absorbed from GI tract. **Peak:** 0.5–2 h IM/IV; 1–4 h PO. **Distribution:** Widely distributed with highest concentrations in kidneys, gallbladder, spleen, liver,

M

and skin; minimal passage across blood–brain barrier; crosses placenta; distributed into breast milk. **Metabolism:** In liver. **Elimination:** Primarily in urine. **Half-Life:** 2–4 h.

NURSING IMPLICATIONS

Black Box Warning

Methotrexate has been associated with hepatotoxicity, lung damage, severe skin reactions, tumor lysis syndrome, and potentially fatal infections.

Assessment & Drug Effects

- Prolonged treatment with small frequent doses may lead to hepatotoxicity, which is best diagnosed by liver biopsy.
- Monitor for and report ulcerative stomatitis with glossitis and gingivitis, often the first signs of toxicity. Inspect mouth daily; report patchy necrotic areas, bleeding and discomfort, or overgrowth (black, furry tongue).
- Monitor I&O ratio and pattern. Keep patient well hydrated (about 2000 mL/24 h).
- Prevent exposure to infections or colds during periods of leukopenia. Be alert to onset of agranulocytosis (cough, extreme fatigue, sore throat, chills, fever) and report symptoms promptly.
- Be alert for and report symptoms of thrombocytopenia (e.g., ecchymoses, petechiae, epistaxis, melena, hematuria, vaginal bleeding, slow and protracted oozing following trauma).
- Monitor lab tests: Baseline and periodic LFTs, renal function tests, CBC with differential, and platelet count. Monitor methotrexate levels and urine pH.

Patient & Family Education

- Report promptly any of the following: Diarrhea, mouth sores, fever, dehydration, cough, bleeding, shortness of breath, any signs of infection, or a skin rash.
- Use contraceptive measures during and for at least 3 mo (males) or 1 ovulatory cycle (females) after cessation of therapy.
- Avoid or moderate alcohol ingestion, which increases the incidence and severity of methotrexate hepatotoxicity.
- Do not use OTC proton pump inhibitors (e.g., omeprazole) without consulting prescriber.
- Practice fastidious mouth care to prevent infection, provide comfort, and maintain adequate nutritional status.
- Do not self-medicate with vitamins. Some OTC compounds may include folic acid (or its derivatives), which alters methotrexate response.
- Use contraceptive measures during and for at least 3 mo following therapy.
- Avoid exposure to sunlight and ultraviolet light. Wear sunglasses and sunscreen.

METHOXSALEN (Pr)

(meth-ox′a-len)

Uvadex

Classification: PSORALEN; PIGMENTING AGENT

Therapeutic: PIGMENTING AGENT; ANTIPSORIATIC

AVAILABILITY

Capsule; solution for injection; lotion

ACTION & *THERAPEUTIC EFFECT*

Plant derivative with strong photosensitizing effects: Used with ultraviolet-A light (UVA) in therapeutic regimens called PUVA (P-psoralen). After photoactivation by long wavelength, UVA, methoxsalen combines with epidermal cell DNA causing photo-damage (cytotoxic action). *Photo-damage inhibits rapid and uncontrolled epidermal cell turn-over characteristic of psoriasis. Results in an inflammatory reaction with erythema. Strongly melanogenic.*

USES Repigmentation of idiopathic vitiligo; control of severe, recalcitrant disabling psoriasis; cutaneous T cell lymphoma.

CONTRAINDICATIONS Hypersensitivity to methoxsalen or any component of the formulation; sunburn, sensitivity (or its history) to psoralens, diseases associated with photosensitivity (e.g., SLE, albinism, melanoma or its history); invasive squamous cell cancer; cataract; aphakia; previous exposure to arsenic or ionizing radiation.

CAUTIOUS USE Hepatic insufficiency; GI disease; chronic infection; treatment with known photosensitizing agents; immunosuppressed patient; cardiovascular disease; pregnancy (adverse effects were observed in animal reproduction studies); lactation. Safety **(lotion)** in children younger than 12 y not established. Safety **(oral)** in children not established.

ROUTE & DOSAGE

Idiopathic Vitiligo

Adult: **Topical** Apply lotion 1–2 h before exposure to UV light once/wk **PO** 20 mg 2–4 hours prior to UVA exposure

Psoriasis

Adult: **PO** 10–70 mg 1.5–2 h before exposure to UV light 2–3 × wk: (specific dose based on patient weight and skin type; see package insert)

Cutaneous T cell lymphoma

Adult: **IV** see package insert for treatment calculations

ADMINISTRATION

- Note: Methoxsalen therapy with UV light (PUVA therapy) should be done under the complete control of a prescriber with special competence and experience in photochemotherapy.

Oral

- Oxsoralen-Ultra soft gelatin capsules are **not** interchangeable with 8-MOP hard gelatin capsules.
- Give with milk or food to prevent GI distress.
- Maintain consistent time relationship between food–drug ingestion. Food digestion and absorption appear to affect drug serum levels.

Topical

- Only small (less than 10 cm^2), well-defined areas are treated with lotion. Systemic treatment is used for large areas.
- Apply lotion with cotton swabs, allow to dry 1–2 min, then reapply. Protect borders of the lesion with petrolatum and sunscreen lotion to prevent hyperpigmentation.
- Use finger cots or gloves to apply lotion and prevent photosensitization and burned skin.
- Apply sunscreen lotion to the skin for about one third of the initial exposure time during PUVA therapy until there is sufficient tanning. Do not apply to psoriatic areas before treatment.
- Store lotion and capsules at 15°–30° C (59°–86° F) in light-resistant containers unless otherwise directed by manufacturer.

ADVERSE EFFECTS **CNS:** Nervousness, dizziness, headache, mental depression or excitation, vertigo, insomnia. **HEENT:** Cataract formation, ocular damage. **Skin:** Phototoxic effects: Severe edema and erythema, *pruritus,* painful blisters; burning, peeling, thinning, freckling, and accelerated aging of skin; hyper- or hypopigmentation; severe skin pain (lasting 1–2 mo), photoallergic contact dermatitis (with topical use), exacerbation of latent photosensitive dermatoses. **GI:** Cheilitis, *nausea* and other GI disturbances, toxic hepatitis. **Other:** Transient loss of muscular coordination, edema, leg cramps, systemic immune effects, drug fever.

INTERACTIONS

Drug: May increase concentration of CYP1A2 substrates (eg **alosetron, bendamustine, rasagiline, tizanidine**) **Food:** Food will increase peak and extent of absorption.

PHARMACOKINETICS

Absorption: Variably from GI tract. **Peak:** 2 h. **Duration:** 8–10 h. **Distribution:** Preferentially taken up by epidermal cells; reversibly protein bound. **Elimination:** 80–90% in urine within 8 h. **Half-Life:** 0.75–2.4 h.

NURSING IMPLICATIONS

Assessment & Drug Effects

- Schedule a pretreatment ophthalmologic exam to rule out cataracts; repeat periodically during treatment and at yearly intervals thereafter.
- Fair-skinned patients appear to be at greatest risk for phototoxicity from PUVA therapy (see ADVERSE EFFECTS).
- Be aware that repigmentation is more rapid on fleshy areas (i.e., face, abdomen, buttocks) than on hands or feet.
- Monitor lab tests: Baseline and every 6-12 months CBC with differential, LFT, renal function tests, and antinuclear antibody tests.

Patient & Family Education

- Expect that effective repigmentation may require 6–9 mo of treatment; periodic treatment usually is necessary to retain pigmentation. If, after 3 mo of treatment, there is no apparent response, drug is discontinued.
- Avoid additional exposure to UV light (direct or indirect) for at least 8 h after oral drug ingestion and UVA exposure.
- Understand intended treatment schedule: After topical application, the initial sunlight exposure is limited to 1 min, with subsequent gradual and incremental exposures by prescription.
- Avoid additional UV light for 24–48 h after topical application and UVA exposure.
- Wear sunscreen lotion (with SPF 15 or higher) and protective clothing (hat, gloves) to cover all exposed areas including lips, to prevent burning or blistering if sunlight cannot be avoided after the treatment.
- Do not sunbathe for at least 48 h after PUVA treatment. Sunburn and photochemotherapy are additive in the production of burning and erythema.
- Wear wraparound sunglasses with UVA-absorbing properties both indoors and outdoors during daylight hours for 24 h. Do not substitute prescription sunglasses or photosensitive darkening glasses; they may actually increase danger of cataract formation.
- Alert prescriber to appearance of new psoriatic areas, flares, or regressed cleared skin areas during treatment and maintenance periods.

M

METHYCLOTHIAZIDE

(meth-i-kloe-thye′a-zide)

Classification: THIAZIDE DIURETIC; ANTIHYPERTENSIVE

Therapeutic: THIAZIDE DIURETIC; ANTIHYPERTENSIVE

Prototype: Hydrochlorothiazide

AVAILABILITY Tablet

ACTION & *THERAPEUTIC EFFECT* Inhibits sodium reabsorption in the distal tubules causing increased excretion of sodium and water, as well as, potassium and hydrogen ions. *Antihypertensive effect as well as enhanced excretion of sodium and water.*

USES Treatment of edema and hypertension.

M

CONTRAINDICATIONS Hypersensitivity to thiazides, and sulfonamide derivatives; anuria; hypokalemia; lactation.

CAUTIOUS USE Renal disease; impaired kidney or liver function; older adults; gout; SLE; hypercalcemia; DM; moderate to high cholesterol, elevated triglyceride level; pregnancy (category B); children.

ROUTE & DOSAGE

Edema

Adult: **PO** 2.5–10 mg daily

Hypertension

Adult: **PO** 2.5–5 mg/day

ADMINISTRATION

Oral

- Give early in the morning to reduce sleep interruption because of diuresis. If 2 doses are ordered, administer second dose no later than 6 p.m.
- May be taken with food or milk.
- Store at 15°–30° C (59°–86° F) unless otherwise instructed.

ADVERSE EFFECTS **CV:** Necrotizing angiitis, orthostatic hypotension. **Respiratory:** Pneumonitis, pulmonary edema, respiratory distress. **CNS:** Dizziness, headache, paresthesia, restlessness, vertigo. **HEENT:** Transient blurred vision. **Endocrine:** Electrolyte disturbance, glycosuria, hypercalcemia, hyperglycemia, hyperuricemia, *hypokalemia*. **Skin:** Skin photosensitivity, skin rash, Stevens–Johnson syndrome, urticaria. **Hepatic/GI:** Jaundice, anorexia, constipation, diarrhea, epigastric distress, nausea. **Musculoskeletal:** Muscle cramps, muscle spasm, weakness. **Hematologic:** Agranulocytosis, aplastic anemia, hemolytic anemia, leukopenia, purpura, thrombocytopenia. **Other:** Fever, anaphylaxis.

INTERACTIONS **Drug:** **Amphotericin B,** CORTICOSTEROIDS increase hypokalemic effects; may antagonize hypoglycemic effects of **insulin,** SULFONYLUREAS; **cholestyramine, colestipol** decrease thiazide absorption; intensifies hypoglycemic and hypotensive effects of **diazoxide;** increased potassium and magnesium loss may cause **digoxin** toxicity; decreases **lithium** excretion, increasing its toxicity; NSAIDS may attenuate diuresis, and risk of NSAID-induced kidney failure increased. Do not use with **levosulpride, bromperidol, promazine**.

PHARMACOKINETICS **Absorption:** Incompletely absorbed. **Onset:** 2 h. **Peak:** 6 h. **Duration:** Greater than 24 h. **Distribution:** Distributed throughout extracellular tissue; concentrates in kidney; crosses placenta; distributed in breast milk. **Metabolism:** Does not appear to be metabolized. **Elimination:** In urine.

NURSING IMPLICATIONS

Assessment & Drug Effects

- Expect antihypertensive effects in 3–4 days; maximal effects may require 3–4 wk.
- Monitor BP and I&O ratio during first phase of antihypertensive therapy. Report a sudden fall in BP, which may initiate severe postural hypotension and potentially dangerous perfusion problems, especially in the extremities.
- Monitor patient for S&S of hypokalemia (see Appendix F). Report promptly. Prescriber may change dose and institute replacement therapy.
- Monitor lab tests: Periodic serum electrolytes, BUN and creatinine, and CBC with differential.

Patient & Family Education

- Eat a balanced diet to protect against hypokalemia; generally not severe even with long-term therapy. Prevent onset by eating potassium-rich foods including a banana (about 370 mg potassium) and at least 180 mL (6 oz) orange juice (about 330 mg potassium) every day.
- Watch carefully for loss of glycemic control (diabetics) and early signs of hyperglycemia (see Appendix F). Symptoms are slow to develop.
- Avoid OTC drugs unless the prescriber approves them. Many preparations contain both potassium and sodium, and may induce electrolyte imbalance adverse effects.
- Older adults are more responsive to excessive diuresis; orthostatic hypotension may be a problem.
- Change positions slowly and in stages from lying down to upright positions; avoid hot baths or showers, extended exposure to sunlight, and standing still. Accept assistance as necessary to prevent falling.
- Do not drive or engage in potentially hazardous activities until adjustment to the hypotensive effects of drug has been made.

METHYLDOPA (Pr)

(meth-ill-doe′pa)

Classification: CENTRALLY ACTING ANTIHYPERTENSIVE; ALPHA-ADRENERGIC AGONIST

Therapeutic: CENTRALLY ACTING ANTIHYPERTENSIVE

AVAILABILITY Tablet; solution for injection

ACTION & *THERAPEUTIC EFFECT* Structurally related to catecholamines and their precursors. Inhibits decarboxylation of dopa, thereby reducing concentration of dopamine, a precursor of norepinephrine. It also inhibits the precursor of serotonin. Reduces renal vascular resistance; maintains cardiac output without acceleration, but may slow heart rate; tends to support sodium and water retention. *Lowers standing and supine BP.*

USES Hypertension, hypertensive urgency or emergency.

CONTRAINDICATIONS Hypersensitivity to methyldopa; active liver disease (hepatitis, cirrhosis); pheochromocytoma; coadministration with MAOIs; blood dyscrasias.

CAUTIOUS USE History of impaired liver or kidney function or disease; renal failure; autoimmune disease; cardiac disease; angina pectoris; history of mental depression; Parkinson's disease;

M

blood transfusion type and cross matching; young or older adults; pregnancy (category B); lactation; children.

ROUTE & DOSAGE

Hypertension

Adult/Adolescent: **PO** 250 mg bid or tid, may be increased up to 3 g/day in divided doses, usual range 250–1000 mg total/day
Geriatric: **PO** lower doses may be needed
Child: **PO** 10 mg/kg/day in 2–4 divided doses (max: 3 g/day)

Hypertensive Emergency/ Urgency

Adult: **IV** 250–500 mg q6h
Child: **IV** 20–40 mg/kg/day

Renal Impairment Dosage Adjustment

CrCl 10–50 mL/min: Dose q8–12h; *less than 10 mL/min:* Dose q12–24h

M

ADMINISTRATION

Oral

- Make dosage increases in evening to minimize daytime sedation.

Intravenous

PREPARE: **Intermittent:** Dilute in 100 mL of D5W, as needed, to yield 10 mg/mL.
ADMINISTER: **Intermittent:** Give over 30–60 min.
INCOMPATIBILITIES: **Solution/additive:** **Amphotericin B, hydrocortisone, methohexital, tetracycline.** **Y-site:** **Acyclovir, amphotericin B, ampicillin, azathioprine, cefoperazone, dantrolene, diazepam, diazoxide, ganciclovir, gemtuzumab, haloperidol, hydralazine, imipenem, indomethacin, ketorolac, mitomycin, pentobarbital, phenytoin, piperacillin/tazobacam.**

ADVERSE EFFECTS **CV:** Orthostatic hypotension, syncope, bradycardia, myocarditis, edema, weight gain *(sodium and water retention),* paradoxic hypertensive reaction (especially with IV administration). **CNS:** *Sedation, drowsiness,* sluggishness, headache, weakness, fatigue, dizziness, vertigo, *decrease in mental acuity,* inability to concentrate, amnesia-like syndrome, parkinsonism, mild psychoses, depression, nightmares. **HEENT:** *Nasal stuffiness.* **Endocrine:** Gynecomastia, lactation, *decreased libido, impotence,* hypothermia (large doses), positive tests for lupus and rheumatoid factors. **Skin:** Granulomatous skin lesions. **GI:** Diarrhea, constipation, abdominal distention, malabsorption syndrome, nausea, vomiting, dry mouth, sore or black tongue, sialadenitis, abnormal liver function tests, jaundice, hepatitis, hepatic necrosis (rare). **Hematologic:** *Positive direct Coombs' test* (common especially in African-Americans), granulocytopenia. **Other:** Hypersensitivity (*fever,* skin eruptions, ulcerations of soles of feet, flu-like symptoms, lymph-adenopathy, eosinophilia).

DIAGNOSTIC TEST INTERFERENCE

Methyldopa may interfere with ***serum creatinine*** measurements using ***alkaline picrate method, AST*** by ***colorimetric methods,*** and ***uric acid*** measurements by ***phosphotungstate method*** (with high methyldopa blood levels); it may produce false elevations of ***urinary catecholamines*** and increase in ***serum amylase*** in methyldopa-induced sialadenitis.

INTERACTIONS

Drug: AMPHETAMINES, TRICYCLIC ANTIDEPRESSANTS, PHENOTHIAZINES, BARBITURATES may attenuate antihypertensive response; methyldopa may inhibit effectiveness of **ephedrine; haloperidol** may exacerbate psychiatric symptoms; with **levodopa** additive hypotension, increased CNS toxicity, especially psychosis; increases risk of **lithium** toxicity; **methotrimeprazine** causes excessive hypotension; MAO INHIBITORS may cause hallucinations; **phenoxybenzamine** may cause urinary incontinence. **Herbal: Licorice** may affect electrolyte levels; **ephedra, yohimbe, ginseng** may decrease efficacy.

PHARMACOKINETICS

Absorption: About 50% absorbed from GI tract. **Peak:** 4–6 h. **Duration:** 24 h PO; 10–16 h IV. **Distribution:** Crosses placenta, distributed into breast milk. **Metabolism:** In liver and GI tract. **Elimination:** Primarily in urine. **Half-Life:** 1.7 h.

NURSING IMPLICATIONS

Assessment & Drug Effects

- Check BP and pulse at least q30min until stabilized during IV infusion and observe for adequacy of urinary output.
- Take BP at regular intervals in lying, sitting, and standing positions during period of dosage adjustment.
- Supervision of ambulation in older adults and patients with impaired kidney function; both are particularly likely to manifest orthostatic hypotension with dizziness and light-headedness during period of dosage adjustment.
- Monitor fluid and electrolyte balance and I&O. Weigh patient daily, and check for edema because methyldopa favors sodium and water retention.
- Be alert that rising BP indicating tolerance to drug effect may occur during week 2 or 3 of therapy.
- Monitor lab tests: Baseline and periodic blood counts and LFTs especially during first 6–12 wk of therapy or if patient develops unexplained fever; periodic serum electrolytes.

Patient & Family Education

- Exercise caution with hot baths and showers, prolonged standing in one position, and strenuous exercise that may enhance orthostatic hypotension. Make position changes slowly, particularly from lying down to upright posture; dangle legs a few minutes before standing.
- Be aware that transient sedation, drowsiness, mental depression, weakness, and headache commonly occur during first 24–72 h of therapy or whenever dosage is increased. Symptoms tend to disappear with continuation of therapy or dosage reduction.
- Avoid potentially hazardous tasks such as driving until response to drug is known; drug may affect ability to perform activities requiring concentrated mental effort, especially during first few days of therapy or whenever dosage is increased.
- Do not to take OTC medications unless approved by prescriber.

METHYLERGONOVINE MALEATE

(meth-ill-er-goe-noe′veen)

Methergine

Classification: ERGOT ALKALOID; OXYTOCIC

Therapeutic: OXYTOCIC

Prototype: oxytocin

AVAILABILITY Tablet; solution for injection

ACTION & *THERAPEUTIC EFFECT* Increases the tone, rate, and amplitude of contractions on the smooth muscles of the uterus, producing sustained contractions which shortens the third stage of labor and reduces blood loss. *Administered after delivery of the placenta to minimize the risk of postpartal hemorrhage.*

M

USES Routine management after delivery of placenta and for postpartum atony, subinvolution, and hemorrhage. With full obstetric supervision, may be used during second stage of labor.

CONTRAINDICATIONS Hypersensitivity to ergot preparations; induction of labor; use prior to delivery of placenta; threatened spontaneous abortion; prolonged use; uterine sepsis; hypertension; toxemia; angina; arteriosclerosis; CAD; dysfunctional uterine bleeding; eclampsia; hypertension; MI; neonates; PVD; preeclampsia; Raynaud's disease; sepsis; stroke; thromboangiitis obliterans; thrombophlebitis.

CAUTIOUS USE DM; hepatic disease; migraine headaches; renal impairment; pulmonary disease; pregnancy (category C); lactation.

ROUTE & DOSAGE

Postpartum Hemorrhage

Adult: **PO** 0.2 q6–8h × 2–7 days; **IM** 0.2 mg q2–4h

ADMINISTRATION

- Use parenteral routes only in emergencies.

Oral

- Note: Dosing should not exceed 1 wk.

Intramuscular

- Inject undiluted deep into a large muscle.

Intravenous

PREPARE: **Direct:** Give undiluted or diluted in 5 mL of NS.
ADMINISTER: **Direct:** Administer slowly over at least 60 sec. ▪ Do not use ampules containing discolored solution or visible particles.

- Store at 15°–30° C (59°–86° F) unless otherwise directed. Protect from light.

ADVERSE EFFECTS **CV:** Angina pectoris, AV block, bradycardia, hypertension. **Respiratory:** Dyspnea, nasal congestion. **CNS:** Dizziness, hallucination, headache, seizure. **HEENT:** Tinnitus. **Skin:** Diaphoresis, skin rash. **GI:** Abdominal pain, diarrhea, nausea, unpleasant taste, vomiting. **GU:** Hematuria. **Musculoskeletal:** Leg cramps. **Other:** Anaphylaxis.

INTERACTIONS **Drug:** PARENTERAL SYMPATHOMIMETICS, other ERGOT ALKALOIDS, TRIPTANS add to pressor effects and carry risk of hypertension; PROTEASE INHIBITORS, **itraconazole** may increase the risk of toxicity. Can affect other agents metabolized by CYP3A4.

PHARMACOKINETICS **Absorption:** Readily from GI tract. **Onset:** 5–15 min PO; 2–5 min IM; immediate IV. **Duration:** 3 or more h PO; 3 h IM; 45 min IV. **Distribution:** Distributed into breast milk. **Metabolism:** Slowly in liver. **Elimination:** Mainly in feces, small amount in urine. **Half-Life:** 3 h.

NURSING IMPLICATIONS

Assessment & Drug Effects

- Monitor vital signs (particularly BP) and uterine response during and after parenteral administration of methylergonovine until partum period is stabilized (about 1–2 h).
- Notify prescriber if BP suddenly increases or if there are frequent periods of uterine relaxation.

Patient & Family Education

- Report severe cramping or increased bleeding.
- Report any of the following: Cold or numb fingers or toes, nausea or vomiting, chest or muscle pain.

METHYLNALTREXONE BROMIDE

(meth-yl-nal-trex′own bro′mide)

Relistor

Classification: NARCOTIC (OPIATE ANTAGONIST)

Therapeutic: GI STIMULANT (OPIOID INDUCED)

AVAILABILITY Solution for injection

ACTION & *THERAPEUTIC EFFECT* A selective, peripherally acting antagonist of opioid binding to mu opioid receptors in tissues such as the GI tract. *Decreases constipating effects of opioids without interfering with analgesic effect of opioids in the CNS.*

USES Treatment of opioid-induced constipation in patients with advanced illness who are receiving palliative care when response to laxative therapy has not been sufficient.

UNLABELED USES Management of nausea and vomiting related to morphine. Treatment of pruritus related to morphine. Management of urinary retention caused by opioids.

CONTRAINDICATIONS Known or suspected mechanical GI obstruction; severe or persistent diarrhea.

CAUTIOUS USE Renal impairment; history of GI tract lesions; pregnancy (category B); older adults; lactation. Safety and efficacy in children not established.

ROUTE & DOSAGE

Opioid-Induced Constipation

Adult (weight less than 38 kg): **Subcutaneous** Administer every other day *weight less than 38 kg:* 0.15 mg/kg; *weight 38 to less than 62 kg:* 8 mg; *weight 62 to less than 114 kg:* 12 mg; *weight greater than 114 kg:* 0.15 mg/kg

Renal Impairment Dosage Adjustment

CrCl less than 30 mL/min: Reduce normal adult dose by 50%

ADMINISTRATION

Subcutaneous

- An 8 mg dose equals 0.4 mL and a 12 mg dose equals 0.6 mL.
- Insert needle at a 45-degree angle into a pinched fold of skin on the abdomen, thigh, or upper arm. Release skin and inject. Rotate injection sites.

- Store at 20°–25° C (68°–77° F) away from light. May store drawn up into syringe for 24 h at room temperature with ambient light.

ADVERSE EFFECTS CNS: Dizziness. **GI:** *Abdominal pain*, diarrhea, *flatulence, nausea*.

PHARMACOKINETICS Peak: 0.5 h. **Distribution:** 11–15% protein bound. **Metabolism:** Hepatic. **Elimination:** Primarily eliminated unchanged (85%) in urine and feces. **Half-Life:** 8 h.

NURSING IMPLICATIONS

Assessment & Drug Effects

- Monitor bowel pattern.
- Withhold drug and report promptly severe or persistent diarrhea.

Patient & Family Education

- Ensure that patient/caregiver knows how to correctly inject subcutaneous medication.
- Stop methylnaltrexone and notify prescriber if severe or persistent diarrhea develops.

M

METHYLPHENIDATE HYDROCHLORIDE

(meth-ill-fen′i-date)

Aptensio XR, Concerta, Cotempla, Daytrana, Focalin XR, Metadate CD, Metadate ER, Methylin, Methylin ER, Quilivant XR, QuiliChew Ritalin, Ritalin LA, Ritalin SR

Classification: CEREBRAL STIMULANT

Therapeutic: CEREBRAL STIMULANT

Prototype: Amphetamine

Controlled Substance: Schedule II

AVAILABILITY Tablet; chewable tablet; oral solution; sustained release capsule/tablet; transdermal patch; oral disintegrating tablet

ACTION & *THERAPEUTIC EFFECT* Acts mainly on cerebral cortex exerting a stimulant effect. Results in mild CNS and respiratory stimulation with potency intermediate between amphetamine and caffeine. *Effects are more prominent on mental rather than on motor activities. Also believed to have an anorexiant effect.*

USES Treatment of ADHD, narcolepsy.

UNLABELED USES Depression.

CONTRAINDICATIONS Hypersensitivity to drug; history of marked anxiety, tension, agitation; aortic stenosis; glaucoma; motor tics; family history or diagnosis of Tourette syndrome; glaucoma; concurrent use of MAOIs or within 14 days of their use; substance abuse; suicidal ideation. **Metadate CD, Metadate ER,** and **Methylin ER:** Patients with severe hypertension; angina pectoris, cardiac arrhythmias, heart failure; recent MI, hyperthyroidism or thyrotoxicosis.

CAUTIOUS USE History of drug dependency; alcoholism; emotionally unstable individual; personality disturbances; aggressive behavior or hostility; bipolar disorder, psychosis; abrupt discontinuation; anxiety, cardiac arrhythmias, cardiac disease, hypertension; dysphagia, esophageal stricture, GI obstruction, heart failure, hepatic disease, hyperthyroidism, history of paralytic ileus, CF; peripheral vasculopathy; mania; radiographic contrast administration; history of seizures; older adults; pregnancy (category C); lactation; children younger than 6 y of age.

ROUTE & DOSAGE

Narcolepsy

Adult: **PO** 10 mg bid or tid 30–45 min p.c. (range: 10–60 mg/day)
Adolescent/Child (6 y or older): **PO** 5 mg bid, may increase weekly (max dose: 60 mg/day)

Attention Deficit Disorder

Adult: **PO Immediate release products:** 20–30 mg daily in divided doses; **Concerta extended release product:** 18–36 mg daily; (dose varies per previous methylphenidate use, see package insert for table) **Aptensio Extended release** 10 mg daily; **other extended release capsules:** corresponds to the previously titrated 8-h dosage of the IR tablets; in treatment naive patients initial dose of 20 mg each morning is appropriate.
Adolescent/Child (6 y or older): **PO** 5 mg before breakfast and lunch, with a gradual increase of 5–10 mg/wk as needed (max: 60 mg/day) or 20–40 mg sustained release daily before breakfast (max dose: 72 mg daily);. **Concerta Extended release** 18 mg daily (max: 54 mg/day); (dose varies per previous methylphenidate use, see package insert for table) **Transdermal patch** 10 mg patch worn for 9 hours × 1 wk then taper as needed. Increase no more than once weekly. Apply 2 h before desired effect. **Cotempla disintegrating tablet** 17.3 mg daily

ADMINISTRATION

Oral

- Give 30–45 min before meals. To avoid insomnia, give last dose before 6 p.m.
- Ensure that sustained release form is not chewed or crushed. It **must be** swallowed whole.
- May open Metadate CD capsules and sprinkle on food
- Store at 15°–30° C (59°–86° F).

Transdermal

- Apply patch to hip area 2 h before desired effect and remove not later than 9 h after application. Patch may be removed earlier than 9 h if a shorter duration of effect is desired.
- Alternate application site daily. Do not apply under tight clothing.

ADVERSE EFFECTS **CV:** Palpitations, changes in BP and pulse rate, angina, cardiac arrhythmias, exacerbation of underlying CV conditions. **Respiratory:** Nasopharyngitis, cough, URI. **CNS:** Dizziness, drowsiness, *nervousness, insomnia,* irritability, headache, emotional lability, anxiety, tremor. **HEENT:** Difficulty with accommodation, blurred vision. **GI:** Dry throat, anorexia, nausea, vomiting, xerostomia, hepatotoxicity, abdominal pain, decreased appetite, xerostomia, weight loss. **Other:** Hypersensitivity reactions (rash, fever, arthralgia, urticaria, exfoliative dermatitis, erythema multiforme), decreased libido; long-term growth suppression.

INTERACTIONS **Drug:** MAO INHIBITORS may cause hypertensive crisis; antagonizes effects of ANTIHYPERTENSIVES, potentiates action of CNS STIMULANTS (e.g., **amphetamine, caffeine**); may inhibit metabolism and increase serum levels of **fosphenytoin, phenytoin, phenobarbital,** and **primidone, warfarin,** TRICYCLIC ANTIDEPRESSANTS. Could cause serotonin syndrome with other serotenergic drugs (e.g., SSRIs).

PHARMACOKINETICS **Absorption:** Readily from GI tract. Transdermal absorption increased with heat or inflamed skin. **Peak:** 1.9 h; 4–7 h sustained release, 2 h transdermal. **Duration:** 3–6 h; 8 h sustained release. **Elimination:** In urine.

NURSING IMPLICATIONS

Black Box Warning

Methylphenidate has been associated with development of marked tolerance, dependence, abnormal behavior, and psychotic episodes; and with severe depression following withdrawal from abusive use.

M

Assessment & Drug Effects

- Monitor BP and pulse at appropriate intervals.
- Monitor closely patient with a history of drug dependence or alcoholism. Chronic abusive use can lead to tolerance, psychic dependence, and psychoses.
- Supervise drug withdrawal carefully following prolonged use. Abrupt withdrawal may result in severe depression and psychotic behavior.
- Monitor lab tests: Periodic CBC with differential and platelet count; periodic LFTs during first 6–12 wk of therapy.

Patient & Family Education

- Report adverse effects to prescriber, particularly nervousness and insomnia. These effects may diminish with time or require reduction of dosage or omission of afternoon or evening dose.
- Check weight at least 2 or 3 × weekly and report weight loss. Check height and weight in children; failure to gain in either should be reported to prescriber.
- Withhold patch from an ADHD child who exhibits anxiety, tension or agitation. Consult prescriber.
- Do not apply heat or heating pad over area where patch is located.

METHYLPREDNISOLONE

(meth-ill-pred-niss′oh-lone)

Medrol

METHYLPREDNISOLONE ACETATE

Depo-Medrol

METHYLPREDNISOLONE SODIUM SUCCINATE

Solu-Medrol

Classification: BIOLOGICAL RESPONSE MODIFIER; ADRENAL CORTICOSTE-ROID; GLUCOCORTICOID
Therapeutic: GLUCOCORTICOID; ANTI-INFLAMMATORY
Prototype: Prednisone

AVAILABILITY **Methylprednisolone:** Tablet. **Methylprednis-olone Acetate:** Solution for injection. **Methylprednisolone Sodium Succinate:** Powder for injection

ACTION & *THERAPEUTIC EFFECT* Corticosteroids modulate carbohydrate, protein, and lipid metabolism and maintenance of fluid and electrolyte homeostasis. It influences cardiovascular, immunologic, musculoskeletal, endocrine, and neurologic physiology. It decreases inflammation by suppression of migration of leukocytes and reversal of increased capillary permeability. *Has anti-inflammatory and immunosuppressive properties.*

USES An anti-inflammatory or immunosuppresive agent in the management of acute and chronic inflammatory diseases, for palliative management of neoplastic diseases, and for control of severe acute and chronic allergic processes.

UNLABELED USES Acute respiratory distress syndrome, transplant rejection, COPD, COVID-19, refractory nausea/vomiting of pregnancy, pneumocystis pneumonia.

CONTRAINDICATIONS Hypersensitivity to corticosteroid drugs; Kaposi sarcoma; systemic fungal infections; live or attenuated virus vaccines; immune thrombocytopenia; use of solutions with benzyl alcohol preservative for premature infants or neonates.

CAUTIOUS USE Cushing's syndrome; GI disease, GI ulceration; hepatic disease; renal disease; hypertension; varicella, vaccinia; CHF; diabetes mellitus; ocular herpes simplex; glaucoma; coagulopathy; emotional instability or psychotic tendencies; pregnancy (some evidence of an association between first trimester systemic corticosteroid use and oral clefts; methylprednisolone is a preferred oral corticosteroid for the treatment of maternal conditions during pregnancy); lactation.

ROUTE & DOSAGE

Usual Dosing Range for Inflammation

Adult: **PO** 16–64 mg/day at once or in divided doses; **IM** (Acetate or succinate) 40–60 mg as single dose; **IV** (succinate) 40–125 mg/day in single or divided doses

Child: **PO/IM/IV** Individualize for disease state and patient response.

Acute Asthma Exacerbation

Adult/Child (over 12 year): **PO/IV** 40–60 mg/day in 1–2 doses × 3–10 days

Child: **PO** 1–2 mg/kg/day in divided doses × 3–10 days (Max: 60 mg/day)

Obesity Dosage Adjustment

Dose based on IBW if lower than actual weight

ADMINISTRATION

Oral

- If prescribed once daily, administer in the morning.
- Note: Preparation less irritating if given with food.

Intramuscular

- Use methylprednisolone acetate for IM injection.
- Give injection deep into large muscle (not deltoid).

Intravenous

Use methylprednisolone sodium succinate for IV administration.

PREPARE: **Direct/Intermittent:** Available in ACT-O-Vial from which the desired dose may be withdrawn after initial dilution with supplied diluent. ▪ May be further diluted according to prescriber's orders.

ADMINISTER: **Direct:** Administer as a slow IV injection over several minutes. **Intermittent:** Give over 15–60 min.

INCOMPATIBILITIES: **Solution/additive:** **Calcium gluconate, glycopyrrolate, linezolid, metaraminol, nafcillin, penicillin G sodium.**

Y-site: **Alemtuzumab, allopurinol, amophotericin B, ampicillin, amsacrine, blinatumomab, calcium chloride, calcium gluconate, caspofungin, cefiderocol, cefotaxime, cefoxitin, ciprofloxacin, dacarbazine, dantrolene, daunorubicin, dexrazoxane, diazepam, diazoxide, diphenhydramine, docetaxel, dolasetron, doxycycline, epirubicin, etoposide, fenoldopam, filgrastim, foscarnet, ganciclovir, garenoxacin, gemcitabine, gemtuzumab, haloperidol, hydralazine, idarubicin, irinotecan, isavuconazonium, lansoprazole, leucovorin, magnesium sulfate, minocycline, mitoxantrone, mycophenolate, nalbuphine, netilmicin, paclitaxel, palonosetron, pantoprazole, papaverine, pentamidine, pentazocine, phenytoin, plazomicin, posaconazole, promethazine, propofol, protamine, pyridoxine, rocuronium, sargramostim, thiamine, vercuronium, vinorelbine.**

- Store at 20°–25° C (68°–77° F). Do not freeze.

M

ADVERSE EFFECTS **CV:** Bradycardia, cardiac arrest, cardiac arrhythmia, edema, thrombophlebitis, vasculitis. **CNS:** Euphoria, headache, insomnia, emotional lability, psychosis. **HEENT:** Cataracts, exophthalmoses, glaucoma. **Endocrine:** Cushingoid state, growth suppression in children, carbohydrate intolerance, hyperglycemia, hypokalemia, hyperlipidemia, hypokalemic acidosis. **Hematologic:** Leukocytosis, petechia. **GI/Hepatic:** Nausea, abdominal distension, peptic ulcer, increased liver enzymes. **Musculoskeletal:** Athropathy, delayed wound healing, osteoporosis, aseptic necrosis of bone, spontaneous fractures.

DIAGNOSTIC TEST INTERFERENCE May decrease response to skin tests.

INTERACTIONS **Drug:** **Amphotericin B, furosemide,** THIAZIDE DIURETICS increase potassium loss; with ATTENUATED VIRUS VACCINES, may enhance virus replication or increase vaccine adverse effects; **isoniazid, phenytoin, phenobarbital, rifampin** decrease effectiveness of methylprednisolone because they increase metabolism of STEROIDS. May decrease therapeutic effects of **aldesleukin, mifamurtide.** ANTACIDS may decrease the bioavailability of steroids.

PHARMACOKINETICS **Absorption:** Readily absorbed from GI tract. **Peak:** 1–2 h PO; 1 h IV. **Duration:** 1.25–1.5 days PO; 1–5 wk IM. **Metabolism:** In liver. **Half-Life:** 2.5 h; HPA suppression: 18–36 h.

NURSING IMPLICATIONS

Assessment & Drug Effects

- Monitor diabetics for loss of glycemic control.
- Monitor serum potassium and report S&S of hypokalemia (see Appendix F).
- Monitor for and report S&S of Cushing's syndrome (see Appendix F).
- Monitor lab tests: Periodic blood glucose, electrolytes.

Patient & Family Education

- Consult prescriber for any of the following: Slow wound healing, significant insomnia or confusion, or unexplained bone pain.

- Do not alter established dosage regimen (i.e., not to increase, decrease, or omit doses or change dose intervals). Withdrawal symptoms (rebound inflammation, fever) can be induced with sudden discontinuation of therapy.
- Report onset of signs of hypocorticism adrenal insufficiency immediately: Fatigue, nausea, anorexia, joint pain, muscular weakness, dizziness, fever.

METHYLTESTOSTERONE

(meth-ill-tess-toss′te-rone)

Android, Metandren ♣, Testred, Virilon

Classification: ANDROGEN/ANABOLIC STEROID

Therapeutic: ANABOLIC STEROID

Prototype: Testosterone

Controlled Substance: Schedule III

AVAILABILITY Tablet

ACTION & *THERAPEUTIC EFFECT* Stimulates receptors in organs and tissues to promote growth and development of male sex organs and maintains secondary sex characteristics in androgen-deficient males. *Androgen activity is similar to testosterone; used in replacement therapy, and palliative treatment of postmenopausal female hormone responsive breast cancer.*

USES Androgen replacement therapy, delayed puberty (male), palliation of female mammary cancer (1–5 y postmenopausal), postpartum breast engorgement.

CONTRAINDICATIONS Liver dysfunction; prostate cancer; severe cardiac, renal, or hepatic disease; pregnancy (category X); lactation.

CAUTIOUS USE Mild or moderate liver, kidney, or cardiac dysfunction; heart failure, diabetes mellitus; prostatic hypertrophy.

ROUTE & DOSAGE

Replacement

Adult: **PO** 10–50 mg/day in divided doses

Breast Cancer

Adult: **PO** 50–200 mg/day in divided doses for duration of therapeutic response or no longer than 3 mo if no remission

Postpartum Breast Engorgement

Adult: **PO** 80 mg/day for 3–5 days

ADMINISTRATION

Oral

- Place buccal tablets between cheek and gum. Ensure that tablet is absorbed, not chewed or swallowed; and eating or drinking avoided until absorption is complete.
- Store at 15°–30° C (59°–86° F). Avoid freezing.

ADVERSE EFFECTS **Endocrine:** *Acne, gynecomastia, edema,* oligospermia, menstrual irregularities. **GI:** Cholestatic hepatitis with jaundice, irritation of oral mucosa with buccal administration. **GU:** Renal calculi (especially in immobilized patient), priapism.

INTERACTIONS **Drug:** Increases risk of bleeding associated with ORAL ANTICOAGULANTS; possibly increases risk of **cyclosporine** toxicity; may decrease glucose level, making adjustment of doses of **insulin,** SULFONYLUREAS necessary. **Herbal:** **Echinacea** may increase risk of hepatotoxicity.

PHARMACOKINETICS **Absorption:** Readily from GI tract. **Metabolism:** In liver. **Elimination:** In urine.

NURSING IMPLICATIONS

Assessment & Drug Effects

- Report signs of hepatic toxicity (see Appendix F).
- Monitor for flank pain, abdominal pain radiating to groin, or other symptoms of renal calculi.
- Monitor lab tests: Periodic LFTs.

Patient & Family Education

- Be prepared for distressing and undesirable adverse effects of virilization (women) since dosage sufficient to produce remission in breast cancer is quantitatively similar to that used for androgen replacement in the male.
- Report signs of virilism promptly. Voice change and hirsutism may be irreversible, even after drug is withdrawn.
- Report priapism (men) or other signs of excess sexual stimulation. The prescriber will terminate therapy.
- Report symptoms of jaundice with or without pruritus to prescriber; appears to be dose related. If liver function tests are altered at the same time, this drug will be withdrawn.

M

METIPRANOLOL HYDROCHLORIDE

(me-ti-pran′ol-ol)

OptiPranolol

See Appendix A-1.

METOCLOPRAMIDE HYDROCHLORIDE

(met-oh-kloe-pra′mide)

Gimoti, Maxolon ♣, Reglan

Classification: GI STIMULANT; PROKINETIC AGENT

Therapeutic: GI STIMULANT; ANTIEMETIC

AVAILABILITY Tablet; oral solution; injection; orally disintegrating tablet; nasal spray

ACTION & THERAPEUTIC EFFECT Potent central dopamine receptor antagonist that increases lower esophageal sphincter tone and enhances GI motility and gastric emptying without stimulating gastric, biliary, or pancreatic secretions. *Effective as an antiemetic agent as part of a chemotherapy regimen. In diabetic gastroparesis, it relieves anorexia, nausea, vomiting, or persistent fullness after meals.*

USES Management of diabetic gastric stasis (gastroparesis); to prevent nausea and vomiting associated with emetogenic cancer chemotherapy; symptomatic treatment of refractory gastroesophageal reflux.

UNLABELED USES Radiation induced nausea/vomiting, hiccups, partial bowel obstruction.

CONTRAINDICATIONS Sensitivity or intolerance to metoclopramide; uncontrolled seizures; pheochromocytoma; mechanical GI obstruction, haemorrhage, or perforation; ileus; symptomatic control of tardive dyskinesia; concomitant use with other agents likely to increase extrapyramidal reactions; lactation.

CAUTIOUS USE CHF, cardiac disease; sulfite hypersensitivity, asthma, hypokalemia, hypertension; history of depression; hepatic disease, infertility, methemoglobin reductase deficiency, Parkinson's disease, kidney dysfunction; GI hemorrhage; G6PD deficiency, procainamide hypersensitivity, seizure disorder, seizures, tardive dyskinesia; history of intermittent porphyria; older adults; pregnancy (may increase prolactin levels; extrapyramidal symptoms may occur in the neonate); no longer than 12 wk; children.

ROUTE & DOSAGE

Gastroesophageal Reflux

Adult: **PO** 10–15 mg qid a.c. and at bedtime (max 60 mg/day)
Child: **PO** 0.1–0.2 mg/kg qid

Diabetic Gastroparesis

Adult: **PO/IV/IM** 5–10 mg 2–3 times daily before meals; titrate to lowest effective dose (max 40 mg/day in divided dose)
Nasal 15 mg in one nostril 4 times daily x2–8w (max 60 mg/day)
Geriatric: **PO** 5 mg a.c and at bedtime

Chemotherapy-Induced Emesis

Adult: **PO** 10–20 mg 4 times daily on post-chemotherapy days 2–4

Postoperative Nausea/Vomiting

Adult: **IM** 10–20 mg near end of surgery

Renal Impairment Dosage adjustment

CrCl 10–60 mL/min: Administer 50% of normal dose;
CrCl less than 10 mL/min: Administer 33% of normal dose

Hepatic Impairment Dosage Adjustment

Child Pugh class B or C: max dose 20 mg/day

ADMINISTRATION

Oral

- Give 30 min before meals and at bedtime.
- Remove orally disintegrating tablet (ODT) from blister immediately before use. Place on tongue. ODT will melt and should then be swallowed.

Intranasal

- Prime pump (press 10 times until spray appears) prior to first use or if spray is unused > 2 weeks. Insert applicator into nostril, tilt head slightly forward keeping bottle upright, and close off the other nostril. Have patient breathe in through nose. While inhaling, press pump to release spray; exhale through mouth. Avoid spraying directly into nasal septum, eyes, or mouth.
- After each use, wipe the spray tip with a clean tissue and replace cap. If spray nozzle gets clogged, clean by removing nozzle and soaking in warm water; do not insert a pin or other sharp object into the nozzle.
- Discard after 4 months, even if bottle is not completely empty.

Intramuscular

- Give deep IM into a large muscle.

Intravenous

Note: Verify correct IV concentration and rate of infusion for administration to infants or children with prescriber.
PREPARE: **Direct:** Doses of 10 mg or less may be given undiluted. **IV Infusion:** Doses greater than 10 mg IV should be diluted in at least 50 mL of D5W, NS, D5/0.45% NaCl, LR or other compatible solution.

M

ADMINISTER: **Direct:** Give over 1–2 min (or longer in pediatric patients). **IV Infusion:** Give over not less than 15 min.

INCOMPATIBILITIES: **Solution/additive:** **erythromycin, floxacillin, furosemide, lorazepam.** **Y-site:** **amphotericin B cholesteryl complex, amsacrine, carmustine, cefepime, ceftobiprole, dantrolene, diazepam, diazoxide, doxorubicin liposome, ganciclovir, garenoxacin, gemtuzumab, inamrinone, lansoprazole, phenytoin, propofol, sulfamethoxazole/trimethoprim.**

- Discard open ampules; do not store for future use. ▪ Store at 15°–30° C (59°–86° F) in light-resistant bottle. Tablets are stable for 3 y; solutions and injections, for 5 y.

M

ADVERSE EFFECTS

CV: Atrioventricular block, bradycardia, flushing, hypertension. **CNS:** *Mild sedation, fatigue, restlessness,* agitation, headache, insomnia, disorientation, *extrapyramidal symptoms* (acute dystonic type), tardive dyskinesia, dizziness, neurologic malignant syndrome with injection. **HEENT:** Visual disturbance. **Skin:** Urticarial or maculopapular rash. **Endocrine:** Galactorrhea, gynecomastia, amenorrhea, impotence. **GI:** Nausea, *diarrhea,* vomiting. **GU:** Urinary frequency, urinary incontinence. **Hematologic:** Methemoglobinemia. **Other:** Glossal or periorbital edema.

DIAGNOSTIC TEST INTERFERENCE

Metoclopramide may interfere with gonadorelin test by increasing ***serum prolactin*** levels.

INTERACTIONS

Drug: Alcohol and other CNS DEPRESSANTS add to sedation; ANTICHOLINERGICS, OPIATE ANALGESICS may antagonize effect on GI motility; PHENOTHIAZINES may potentiate extra-pyramidal symptoms; may increase hypertensive effect of MAO INHIBITORS; may diminish the effects of **amantadine, bromocriptine, levodopa, pergolide, ropinirole, pramipexole;** may cause increase in extrapyramidal and dystonic reactions with PHENOTHIAZINES, THIOANTHENES, **droperidol, haloperidol, loxapine, metyrosine;** strong CYP2D6 inhibitors may increase concentration of **metoclopramide**; may enhance adverse effects of ANTIPSYCHOTIC AGENTS; may prolong neuromuscular blocking effects of **succinylcholine.**

PHARMACOKINETICS

Absorption: Readily from GI tract. **Onset:** 30–60 min PO; 10–15 min IM; 1–3 min IV. **Peak:** 1–2 h. **Duration:** 1–3 h. **Distribution:** To most body tissues including CNS; crosses placenta; distributed into breast milk. **Metabolism:** Minimally in liver via CYP2D6. **Elimination:** 95% in urine, 5% in feces. **Half-Life:** 2.5–6 h.

NURSING IMPLICATIONS

Black Box Warning

Metoclopramide has been associated with tardive dyskinesia. Discontinue metoclopramide in patients who develop S&S of tardive dyskinesia.

Assessment & Drug Effects

- Report immediately the onset of restlessness, involuntary movements, facial grimacing, rigidity, or tremors. Extrapyramidal symptoms are most likely to occur in children, young adults, and the older adult and with high-dose treatment of vomiting associated with cancer chemotherapy.

Symptoms can take months to regress.

- Monitor for possible hypernatremia and hypokalemia (see Appendix F), especially if patient has HF or cirrhosis.
- Monitor lab tests: Periodic serum electrolytes.

Patient & Family Education

- Report S&S of acute dystonia, such as trembling hands and facial grimacing (see Appendix F), immediately.
- Avoid driving and other potentially hazardous activities for a few hours after drug administration.
- Avoid alcohol and other CNS depressants.
- Adverse reactions associated with increased serum prolactin concentration (galactorrhea, menstrual disorders, gynecomastia) usually disappear within a few weeks or months after drug treatment is stopped.

METOLAZONE

(me-tole′a-zone)

Zaroxolyn ♣

Classification: THIAZIDE DIURETIC; ANTIHYPERTENSIVE

Therapeutic: DIURETIC; ANTI-HYPERTENSIVE

Prototype: Hydrochlorothiazide

AVAILABILITY Tablet

ACTION & *THERAPEUTIC EFFECT* Causes diuretic action by inhibiting sodium reabsorption in the distal tubules causing increased excretion of sodium, water, potassium, and hydrogen ions. *Produces a decrease in the systolic and diastolic BPs, and reduces edema in CHF and kidney failure patients.*

USES Edema associated with HF and kidney disease.

CONTRAINDICATIONS Hypersensitivity to metolazone and sulfonamides; anuria, hypokalemia; hepatic coma or precoma; SLE; pregnancy (hypoglycemia, hypokalemia, hyponatremia, jaundice, and thrombocytopenia reported as complications to the fetus or newborn following maternal use of thiazide diuretics); lactation.

CAUTIOUS USE History of gout; allergies; kidney and liver dysfunction; older adults; children.

ROUTE & DOSAGE

Edema

Adult: **PO** 5–20 mg/day

ADMINISTRATION

Oral

- Schedule doses to avoid nocturia and interrupted sleep. Give early in a.m. after eating to prevent gastric irritation (if given in 2 doses, schedule second dose no later than 3 p.m.). May be taken with or without food.
- Store at 25° C (77° F) in tightly closed container.

ADVERSE EFFECTS Cardiovascular: Orthostatic hypotension, palpitations, syncope. **Endocrine:** Dehydration, *hypokalemia, hyperuricemia, hyperglycemia*. **GI:** Cholestatic jaundice. **Hematologic:** Venous thrombosis, <u>leukopenia</u>.

DIAGNOSTIC TEST INTERFERENCE May lead to false negative aldosterone/renin ratio.

INTERACTIONS Drug: CORTICOSTEROIDS increase hypokalemic effects; may antagonize hypoglycemic effects of SULFONYLUREAS, **insulin; cholestyramine, colestipol**

decrease thiazide absorption; intensifies hypoglycemic and hypotensive effects of **diazoxide;** do not use with **levosulpiride**; decreases **lithium** excretion, increasing its toxicity; NSAIDS may attenuate diuresis; increased risk of NSAID-induced kidney failure; may cause increased risk of QT prolongation with **promazine**; may have additive effect with other ANTIHYPERTENSIVE AGENTS.

PHARMACOKINETICS **Absorption:** Incomplete. **Onset:** 1 h. **Peak:** 2–8 h. **Duration:** 12–24 h. **Distribution:** Distributed throughout extracellular tissue; concentrates in kidney; crosses placenta; distributed in breast milk. **Metabolism:** Does not appear to be metabolized. **Elimination:** In urine. **Half-Life:** 14 h.

M

NURSING IMPLICATIONS

Assessment & Drug Effects

- Anticipate overdosage and adverse reactions in geriatric patients; may be more sensitive to effects of usual adult dose.
- Terminate therapy when adverse reactions are moderate to severe.
- Expect possible antihypertensive effects in 3 or 4 days, but 3–4 wk are required for maximum effect.
- Monitor BP (orthostatic) and fluid balance.
- Monitor lab tests: Periodic serum electrolytes, uric acid, renal function.

Patient & Family Education

- Do not drink alcohol; it potentiates orthostatic hypotension.
- Antihypertensive therapy may require as adjunct a high-potassium, low-sodium, and low-calorie diet.
- Include potassium-rich foods in the diet.
- Be aware that if hypokalemia develops, dietary potassium supplement of 1000–2000 mg (25–50 mEq) is usually adequate treatment.

METOPROLOL TARTRATE

(me-toe′proe-lole)

Betaloc ♣, Kapspargo Sprinkle, Lopressor, Toprol XL

Classification: CARDIOSELECTIVE; BETA-ADRENERGIC ANTAGONIST; ANTIHYPERTENSIVE

Therapeutic: ANTIHYPERTENSIVE; ANTIANGINAL

Prototype: Propranolol

AVAILABILITY Tablet; sustained release tablet; solution for injection

ACTION & *THERAPEUTIC EFFECT* Beta-adrenergic antagonist with preferential effect on $beta_1$ receptors located primarily on cardiac muscle. Antihypertensive action may be due to competitive antagonism of catecholamines at cardiac adrenergic neuron sites, drug-induced reduction of sympathetic outflow to the periphery, and to suppression of renin activity. *Reduces heart rate and cardiac output at rest and during exercise; lowers both supine and standing BP, slows sinus rate, and decreases myocardial automaticity. Antianginal effect is like that of propranolol.*

USES Management of mild to severe hypertension, treatment of heart failure, long-term treatment of angina pectoris and prophylactic management of stable angina pectoris reduce the risk of mortality after an MI.

UNLABELED USES CHF, migraine prophylaxis, arrhythmias.

CONTRAINDICATIONS Hypersensitivity to metoprolol or other beta blockers; cardiogenic shock, severe bradycardia, advanced AV block without a pacemaker, bradycardia, sick sinus syndrome; pheochromocytoma, moderate to severe cardiac failure, right ventricular failure secondary to pulmonary hypertension; abrupt discontinuation; lactation.

CAUTIOUS USE Severe impairment of liver function; cardiomegaly, CHF controlled by digitalis and diuretics; major surgery; mental illness; bronchial asthma and other bronchospastic diseases; thyrotoxicosis, hyperthyroidism; moderate to severe cholesterol concentrations; elevated triglycerides; DM; PVD; MG; cerebrovascular insufficiency; pregnancy (category C), children younger than 6 y.

ROUTE & DOSAGE

Hypertension

Adult: **PO Immediate release** 50 mg bid then titrate based on response; **Extended release** 25–100 mg daily then titrate based on response up to 100–450 mg/day

Angina Pectoris

Adult: **PO Immediate release** 50 mg bid; **Extended release** 100 mg daily, may increase weekly up to 100–400 mg/day

Heart Failure

Adult: **PO Extended release** 12.5–25 mg/day × 2 wk, then adjust dose

Myocardial Infarction

Adult: **IV** 5 mg q2min for 3 doses, followed by PO therapy; **PO** 25–50 mg q6–12h for 48 h, then titrate dose; **Extended release** 25–50 mg daily then titrate dose

ADMINISTRATION

Oral

- Ensure that sustained-release form is not chewed or crushed. It **must be** swallowed whole.
- Give with food to slightly enhance absorption; however, administration with food not essential. It is important to give with or without food consistently to minimize possible variations in bioavailability.

Intravenous

PREPARE: **Direct:** Give undiluted.
ADMINISTER: **Direct:** Give at a rate of 5 mg over 60 sec. ▪ Note conditions which are contraindications to drug administration.
INCOMPATIBILITIES: **Y-site: Allopurinol, amphotericin B cholesteryl complex, amphotericine B lipid, dantrolene, diazepam, diazoxide, gemtuzumab, lepirudin, pantoprazole, phenytoin, SMZ/TMP.**

- Store at 15°–30° C (59°–86° F). Protect from heat, light, and moisture.

ADVERSE EFFECTS **CV:** *Bradycardia,* palpitation, cold extremities, Raynaud's phenomenon, intermittent claudication, angina pectoris, CHF, intensification of AV block, AV dissociation, complete heart block, cardiac arrest. **Respiratory:** Bronchospasm (with high doses), *shortness of breath.* **CNS:** *Dizziness, fatigue, insomnia,* increased dreaming, mental depression. **HEENT:** Dry mouth and mucous membranes. **Endocrine:** Hypoglycemia. **Skin:** Dry skin, pruritus, skin eruptions.

GI: Nausea, *heartburn,* gastric pain, diarrhea or constipation, flatulence. **Hematologic:** Eosinophilia, thrombocytopenic and nonthrombocytopenic purpura, agranulocytosis (rare). **Other:** Hypersensitivity (erythematous rash, fever, headache, muscle aches, sore throat, laryngospasm, respiratory distress).

DIAGNOSTIC TEST INTERFERENCE

In common with other beta-blockers, metoprolol may cause elevated ***BUN*** and ***serum creatinine levels*** (patients with severe heart disease), elevated ***serum transaminase, alkaline phosphatase, lactate dehydrogenase,*** and ***serum uric acid.***

INTERACTIONS

Drug: BARBITURATES, **rifampin** may decrease effects of metoprolol; **cimetidine, methimazole, propylthiouracil,** ORAL CONTRACEPTIVES may increase effects of metoprolol; additive bradycardia with **digoxin;** effects of both metoprolol and **hydralazine** may be increased; **indomethacin** may attenuate hypotensive response; BETA AGONISTS and metoprolol mutually antagonistic; **verapamil** may increase risk of heart block and bradycardia; increases **terbutaline** serum levels. Do not use with **bromperidol, floctafenine, methacholine, rivastigmine.**

PHARMACOKINETICS

Absorption: Readily from GI tract; 50% of dose reaches systemic circulation. **Onset:** 15 min. **Peak:** 1.5 h; 20 min (IV). **Duration:** 13–19 h. **Distribution:** Crosses blood–brain barrier and placenta; distributed into breast milk. **Metabolism:** Extensively in liver (CYP2D6). **Elimination:** In urine. **Half-Life:** 3–4 h.

NURSING IMPLICATIONS

Black Box Warning

Metoprolol has been associated with exacerbations of ischemic heart disease when stopped abruptly.

Assessment & Drug Effects

- Take apical pulse and BP before administering drug. Report to prescriber significant changes in rate, rhythm, or quality of pulse or variations in BP prior to administration.
- Monitor BP, HR, and ECG carefully during IV administration.
- Expect maximal effect on BP after 1 wk of therapy.
- Observe hypertensive patients with CHF closely for impending heart failure: Dyspnea on exertion, orthopnea, night cough, edema, distended neck veins.
- Monitor I&O, daily weight; auscultate daily for pulmonary rales.
- Reduce dosage gradually over a period of 1–2 wk when drug is discontinued.
- Monitor lab tests: Baseline and periodic blood cell count, blood glucose, LFTs and renal function tests.

Patient & Family Education

- Do not abruptly stop taking this drug. Sudden withdrawal can result in increase in anginal attacks and MI in patients with angina pectoris and thyroid storm in patients with hyperthyroidism.
- Learn how to take radial pulse before each dose. Report to prescriber if pulse is slower than base rate (e.g., 60 bpm) or becomes irregular. Consult prescriber for parameters.
- Reduce insomnia or increased dreaming by avoiding late evening doses.

- Monitor blood glucose (diabetics) for loss of glycemic control. Drug may mask some symptoms of hypoglycemia (e.g., BP and HR changes) and prolong hypoglycemia. Be alert to other possible signs of hypoglycemia not affected by metoprolol and report to prescriber if present: Sweating, fatigue, hunger, inability to concentrate.
- Report immediately to prescriber the onset of problems with vision.
- Relieve eye dryness by using sterile artificial tears available OTC.
- Do not drive or engage in potentially hazardous activities until response to drug is known.

METRONIDAZOLE

(me-troe-ni′da-zole)

Flagyl, Flagyl ER, MetroCream, MetroGel, MetroLotion, Nuvessa, Rosadan, Vandazole

Classification: ANTITRICHOMONAL; AMEBICIDE

Therapeutic: AMEBICIDE; ANTIBACTERIAL

AVAILABILITY Tablet; capsule; sustained release tablet; vial; lotion, emulsion; cream; gel

ACTION & *THERAPEUTIC EFFECT* Interacts with DNA to cause loss of DNA structure and strand breakage resulting in inhibition of protein synthesis and cell death in susceptible organisms. *Has direct trichomonacidal and amebicidal activity; exhibits antibacterial activity against obligate anaerobic bacteria, gram-negative anaerobic bacilli, and* Clostridia.

USES Asymptomatic and symptomatic trichomoniasis in females and males; acute intestinal amebiasis and amebic liver abscess; preoperative prophylaxis in colorectal surgery, elective hysterectomy or vaginal repair, and emergency appendectomy. **IV:** Serious infections caused by susceptible anaerobic bacteria in intra-abdominal infections, skin infections, gynecologic infections, septicemia, and for both pre- and postoperative prophylaxis, bacterial vaginosis. **Topical:** Rosacea.

UNLABELED USES Treatment of pseudomembranous colitis, Crohn's disease, *H. pylori* eradication, bacterial vaginosis prophylaxis, gastric ulcer, pelvic inflammatory disease.

CONTRAINDICATIONS Hypersensitivity to metronidazole or other nitroimidazole drugs; use of disulfiram within 2 wk; use of alcohol within 24 h; development of abnormal neurologic signs; first trimester of pregnancy; lactation.

CAUTIOUS USE Coexistent candidiasis; CNS disorders; seizure disorders; heart failure; severe hepatic impairment; QT prolongation; severe renal impairment/failure; alcoholism; liver disease; older adults.

ROUTE & DOSAGE

Trichomoniasis

Adult: **PO** 2 g once or 500 mg bid × 7 days

Giardiasis, *Gardnerella*

Adult: **PO** 500 mg bid × 7 days or 750 ER tablet daily × 7 days **Vaginal** Once or twice daily × 5 days

M

Pelvic Inflammatory Disease (with other antibiotics)

Adult: **PO** 500 mg bid × 14 days

Amebiasis

Adult: **PO** 500–750 mg tid × 5–10 days
Child: **PO** 35–50 mg/kg/day in 3 divided doses × 10 days

Anaerobic Infections

Adult: **PO** 7.5 mg/kg q6h (max: 4 g/day); **IV** 15 mg/kg; then 7.5 mg/kg q6h (max: 4 g/day)
Child: **PO** 30–50 mg/kg/day divided q6–8h (max: 4 g/day); **IV** 22.5–40 mg/kg/day divided q8h
Neonate (weight less than 1.2 kg): **IV**

Rosacea

Adult: **Topical** Apply 0.75% gel as a thin film to affected area bid; apply 1% gel as a thin film to affected area daily

ADMINISTRATION

Oral

- Crush tablets before ingestion if patient cannot swallow whole.
- Ensure that Flagyl ER (extended release form) is not chewed or crushed. It **must be** swallowed whole. Give on an empty stomach, 1 h before or 2 h after meals.
- Give immediately before, with, or immediately after meals or with food or milk to reduce GI distress.
- Give lower than normal doses in presence of liver disease.

Topical

- Apply a thin film to affected area only.

Intravenous

Note: Verify correct IV concentration and rate of infusion for administration to neonates, infants, or children with prescriber.

PREPARE: **Intermittent:** Single-dose flexible containers (500 mg/100 mL) are ready for use without further dilution.

ADMINISTER: **Intermittent:** Give IV solution slowly over 30–60 min.

INCOMPATIBILITIES: **Solution/additive: TPN, aztreonam. Y-site: Amphotericin B cholesteryl complex, aztreonam, dantrolene, daptomycin, diazepam, drotecogin, filgrastim, ganciclovir, garenoxacin, lansoprazole, minocycline, pantoprazole, pemetrexed, phenytoin, procainamide, propofol, quinupristin/dalfopristin.**

- Note: Precipitation occurs if neutralized solution is refrigerated. ▪ Note: Use diluted and neutralized solution within 24 h of preparation.

- Store at 15°–30° C (59°–86° F); protect from light. ▪ Reconstituted Flagyl IV is chemically stable for 96 h when stored below 30° C (86° F) in room light. ▪ Diluted and neutralized IV solutions containing Flagyl IV should be used within 24 h of mixing.

ADVERSE EFFECTS **CV:** ECG changes (flattening of T wave). **CNS:** Vertigo, headache, ataxia, confusion, irritability, depression, restlessness, weakness, fatigue, drowsiness, insomnia, paresthesias, sensory neuropathy (rare). **HEENT:** Nasal congestion. **GI:** *Nausea,* vomiting, anorexia, epigastric distress, abdominal cramps, diarrhea, constipation, dry mouth, metallic taste, proctitis. **GU:** Polyuria, dysuria, pyuria, incontinence, cystitis, decreased libido, dysmenorrhea, dryness of vagina and vulva, sense of pelvic pressure, vaginitis. **Other:** Hypersensitivity (rash, urticaria, pruritus, flushing), fever, fleeting joint pains, bacterial infection, overgrowth of *Candida*.

DIAGNOSTIC TEST INTERFERENCE

Metronidazole may interfere with certain chemical analyses for ***AST,*** resulting in decreased values.

INTERACTIONS

Drug: ORAL ANTICOAGULANTS potentiate hypoprothrombinemia; **alcohol** may elicit disulfiram reaction; oral solutions of **citalopram, ritonavir; lopinavir/ritonavir,** and IV formulations of **sulfamethoxazole; trimethoprim, nitroglycerin** may elicit disulfiram reaction due to the alcohol content of the dosage form; **disulfiram** causes acute psychosis; **phenobarbital** increases metronidazole metabolism; may increase **lithium** levels; **fluorouracil, azathioprine** may cause transient neutropenia. Use with **ziprasidone** could increase QT prolongation. **Warfarin** effects can be increased.

PHARMACOKINETICS

Absorption: 80% absorbed from GI tract. **Peak:** 1–3 h. **Distribution:** Widely distributed to most body tissues, including CSF, bone, cerebral and hepatic abscesses; crosses placenta; distributed in breast milk. **Metabolism:** 30–60% in liver. **Elimination:** 77% in urine; 14% in feces within 24 h. **Half-Life:** 6–8 h.

NURSING IMPLICATIONS

Assessment & Drug Effects

- Discontinue therapy immediately if symptoms of CNS toxicity (see Appendix F) develop. Monitor especially for seizures and peripheral neuropathy (e.g., numbness and paresthesia of extremities).
- Monitor for S&S of sodium retention, especially in patients on corticosteroid therapy or with a history of CHF.
- Monitor patients on lithium for elevated lithium levels.
- Report appearance of candidiasis or its becoming more prominent with therapy to prescriber promptly.
- Repeat feces examinations, usually up to 3 mo, to ensure that amebae have been eliminated.
- Monitor lab tests: Total and differential WBC counts before, during, and after therapy, especially if a second course is necessary.

Patient & Family Education

- Adhere closely to the established regimen without schedule interruption or changing the dose.
- Refrain from intercourse during therapy for trichomoniasis unless male partner wears a condom to prevent reinfection.
- Have sexual partners receive concurrent treatment. Asymptomatic trichomoniasis in the male is a frequent source of reinfection of the female.
- Do not drink alcohol during therapy; may induce a disulfiram-type reaction (see Appendix F). Avoid alcohol or alcohol-containing medications for at least 48 h after treatment is completed.
- Urine may appear dark or reddish brown (especially with higher than recommended doses). This appears to have no clinical significance.
- Report symptoms of candidal overgrowth: Furry tongue, color changes of tongue, glossitis, stomatitis; vaginitis, curd-like, milky vaginal discharge; proctitis.

M

Treatment with a candidacidal agent may be indicated.

MEXILETINE

(mex-il′e-teen)

Mexitil

Classification: CLASS IB ANTI-ARRHYTHMIC

Therapeutic: CLASS IB ANTIARRHYTHMIC

Prototype: Lidocaine

AVAILABILITY Capsule

ACTION & *THERAPEUTIC EFFECT* Analog of lidocaine with class IB antiarrhythmic properties. Shortens action potential refractory period duration and improves resting potential. Produces modest suppression of sinus node automatically and AV nodal conduction. Prolongs the his-to-ventricular interval only if patient has preexisting conduction disturbance. *Has antiarrhythmic properties for ventricular disturbances.*

USES Acute and chronic ventricular arrhythmias; prevention of recurrent cardiac arrests; suppression of PVCs due to ventricular tachyarrhythmias.

UNLABELED USES Wolff-Parkinson-White syndrome and supraventricular arrhythmias.

CONTRAINDICATIONS Severe left ventricular failure, cardiogenic shock, severe bradyarrhythmias. Preexisting second- or third-degree heart block without pacemaker; cardiogenic shock; lactation.

CAUTIOUS USE Patients with sinus node conduction irregularities, intraventricular conduction abnormalities; hypotension; severe congestive heart failure; renal failure; liver dysfunction; pregnancy (category C).

ROUTE & DOSAGE

Ventricular Arrhythmias

Adult: **PO** 200–300 mg q8h (max: 1200 mg/day)
Adult: **PO** 1.4–5 mg/kg q8h

ADMINISTRATION

Oral

- Give with food or milk to reduce gastric distress.

ADVERSE EFFECTS **CV:** <u>Exacerbated arrhythmias</u>, palpitations, chest pain, syncope, hypotension. **CNS:** *Dizziness, tremor, nervousness, incoordination,* headache, blurred vision, paresthesias, numbness. **Skin:** Rash. **GI:** *Nausea, vomiting, heartburn,* diarrhea, constipation, dry mouth, abdominal pain. **GU:** Impotence, urinary retention. **Other:** Dyspnea, edema, arthralgia, fever, malaise, hiccups.

INTERACTIONS **Drug:** **Phenytoin, phenobarbital, rifampin** may decrease mexiletine levels; **cimetidine, fluvoxamine** may increase mexiletine levels; may increase **theophylline** levels; may increase proarrhythmic effects of **dofetilide** (separate administration by at least 1 wk).

PHARMACOKINETICS **Absorption:** Readily from GI tract. **Peak:** 2–3 h. **Distribution:** Distributed into breast milk. **Metabolism:** In liver. **Elimination:** In urine; renal elimination increases with urinary acidification. **Half-Life:** 10–12 h.

NURSING IMPLICATIONS

Black Box Warning

Mexiletine has been associated with excessive mortality and non-fatal cardiac arrest; therefore, its use should be reserved for patients with life-threatening ventricular arrhythmias.

Assessment & Drug Effects

- Check pulse and BP before administration; make sure both are stabilized.
- Effective serum concentration range is 0.5–2 mcg/mL.
- Supervise ambulation in the weak, debilitated patient or the older adult during drug stabilization period. CNS adverse reactions predominate (e.g., intention tremors, nystagmus, blurred vision, dizziness, ataxia, confusion, nausea).
- Encourage drug compliance; affected particularly by the distressing adverse effects of tremor, ataxia, and eye symptoms.
- Check frequently with patient about adherence to drug regimen. If adverse effects are increasing, consult prescriber. Dose adjustment or discontinuation may be needed.
- Monitor lab tests: Baseline and periodic LFTs.

Patient & Family Education

- Learn about pulse parameters to be reported: Changes in rhythm and rate (bradycardia = pulse below 60); symptomatic bradycardia (light-headedness, syncope, dizziness), and postural hypotension.

MICAFUNGIN

(my-ca-fun'gin)

Mycamine

Classification: ANTIFUNGAL; ECHINOCANDIN

Therapeutic: ANTIFUNGAL

Prototype: Caspofungin

AVAILABILITY Intravenous solution

ACTION & *THERAPEUTIC EFFECT* Micafungin is an antifungal agent that inhibits the synthesis of glucan, an essential component of fungal cell walls. Micafungin does not allow *Candida* fungi to replicate. *Has antifungal effects against various species of Candida.*

USES Treatment of patients with esophageal candidiasis, and for prophylaxis of *Candida* infections in patients undergoing hematopoietic stem cell transplantation. Susceptible organisms include *C. albicans, C. glabrata, C. krusei, C. parapsilosis,* and *C. tropicalis.*

UNLABELED USES Treatment of pulmonary *Aspergillus* infection.

CONTRAINDICATIONS Hypersensitivity to any component in micafungin.

CAUTIOUS USE Hepatic and renal dysfunction; older adult; pregnancy (category C); lactation; children younger than 4 mo.

ROUTE & DOSAGE

Esophageal Candidiasis

Adult: **IV** 150 mg/day over 1 h

Candidiasis Prophylaxis in Hematopoietic Stem Cell Transplantation Patients

Adult: **IV** 50 mg/day over 1 h

Disseminated Candidiasis

Child/Infant (older than 4 mo): **IV** 2 mg/kg once daily

ADMINISTRATION

Intravenous

PREPARE: **IV Infusion:** Reconstitute the 50 or 100 mg vial with 5 mL NS (without a bacteriostatic agent) to yield 10 mg/mL or 20 mg/mL, respectively. ▪ Gently swirl, but do not shake, to dissolve. Solution should be clear. ▪ Add required dose to 100 mL NS.

ADMINISTER: **IV Infusion:** Give slowly over 1 h. ▪ Flush existing IV line with NS before/after infusion. ▪ Protect IV solution from light.

INCOMPATIBILITIES: **Y-site: Albumin, amiodarone, cisatracurium, diltiazem, dobutamine, ephine-phrine, insulin, isavuconazonium, labetaoll, levofloxacin, meperidine, midazolam, morphine, mycophenolate, nicardipine, octreotide, ondansetron, phenytoin, plazomicin, rocuronium, telvancin, vecuronium.**

▪ Store reconstituted vial and IV solution for up to 24 h at 25° C (77° F).

ADVERSE EFFECTS **CV:** Phlebitis. **GI:** Vomiting, diarrhea. **GU:** Renal failure. **Hematologic:** Anemia. **Other:** Fever.

INTERACTIONS **Drug:** Micafungin increases levels of **sirolimus** and **nifedipine.**

PHARMACOKINETICS **Distribution:** 99% protein bound. **Metabolism:** Biotransformation primarily in the liver. **Elimination:** Fecal (major) and renal. **Half-Life:** 14–17 h.

NURSING IMPLICATIONS

Assessment & Drug Effects

- Monitor for S&S of hypersensitivity during IV infusion; frequently monitor IV site for thrombophlebitis.
- Monitor for S&S of hemolytic anemia (i.e., jaundice).
- Monitor lab tests: Periodic LFTs, renal function tests, serum electrolytes, and CBC.

Patient & Family Education

- Report immediately any of the following: Facial swelling, wheezing, difficulty breathing or swallowing, tightness in chest, rash, hives, itching, or sensation of warmth.

MICONAZOLE NITRATE

(mi-kon′a-zole)

Desenex, Femizol-M, Fungoid, Lotrimin AF, Micatin, Monistat 3, Monistat 7, Monistat-Derm, M-Zole, Tetterine

Classification: AZOLE ANTIFUNGAL

Therapeutic: ANTIFUNGAL

Prototype: Fluconazole

AVAILABILITY Vaginal suppository; cream; ointment; powder; spray; solution

ACTION & *THERAPEUTIC EFFECT* Broad-spectrum agent with fungicidal activity. Appears to inhibit uptake of components essential for cell reproduction and growth as well as cell wall structure, thus promoting cell death of fungi. *Effective against* Candida albicans *and other species of this genus. Inhibits growth of common dermatophytes, and the organism responsible for tinea versicolor.*

USES Vulvovaginal candidiasis, tinea pedis (athlete's foot), tinea cruris, tinea corporis, and tinea versicolor caused by dermatophytes.

CONTRAINDICATIONS Hypersensitivity to miconazole.

CAUTIOUS USE Hypersensitivity to azole antifungals; diabetes mellitus; bone marrow suppression; pregnancy (category C); lactation; children younger than 2 y **(topical)** and children younger than 12 y **(vaginal)**.

ROUTE & DOSAGE

Fungal Infection

Adult: **Topical** Apply cream sparingly to affected areas twice a day, and once daily for tinea versicolor, for 2 wk (improvement expected in 2–3 days, tinea pedis is treated for 1 mo to prevent recurrence); **Intravaginal** Insert suppository or vaginal cream each night × 7 days (100 mg) or 3 days (200 mg)

ADMINISTRATION

Topical

- Apply cream sparingly to intertriginous areas (between skin folds) to avoid maceration of skin.
- Massage affected area gently until cream disappears.
- Store at 15°–30° C (59°–86° F) unless otherwise directed.

ADVERSE EFFECTS **GU:** Vulvovaginal burning, itching, or irritation; maceration, allergic contact dermatitis.

INTERACTIONS **Drug:** May increase INR with **warfarin;** may inactivate **nonoxynol-9** spermicides.

PHARMACOKINETICS **Absorption:** Small amount absorbed from vagina. **Metabolism:** Rapidly metabolized in liver. **Elimination:** In urine and feces. **Half-Life:** 2.1–24 h.

NURSING IMPLICATIONS

Assessment & Drug Effects

- Expect clinical improvement from topical application in 1 or 2 wk. If no improvement in 4 wk, diagnosis is reevaluated. Treat tinea pedis infection for 1 mo to assure permanent recovery.

Patient & Family Education

- Complete full course of treatment to ensure recovery.
- Do not interrupt vaginal application during menstrual period.
- Avoid contact of drug with eyes.

MIDAZOLAM HYDROCHLORIDE

(mid'az-zoe-lam)

Nayzilam

Classification: ANESTHETIC; BENZODIAZEPINE; ANXIOLYTIC; SEDATIVE-HYPNOTIC

Therapeutic: ANESTHETIC; ANTIANXIETY; SEDATIVE-HYPNOTIC

Prototype: Lorazepam

Controlled Substance: Schedule IV

AVAILABILITY Syrup; solution for injection

ACTION & THERAPEUTIC EFFECT Short-acting benzodiazepine that intensifies activity of gammaaminobenzoic acid (GABA), a major inhibitory neurotransmitter of the brain, interfering with its reuptake and promoting its accumulation at neuronal synapses. Calms the patient, relaxes skeletal muscles, and in high doses produces sleep. *A CNS depressant with muscle relaxant,* *sedative-hypnotic, anticonvulsant, and amnestic properties.*

USES Sedation before general anesthesia, induction of general anesthesia; to impair memory of perioperative events (anterograde amnesia); for conscious sedation prior to short diagnostic and endoscopic procedures; and as the hypnotic supplement to nitrous oxide and oxygen (balanced anesthesia) for short surgical procedures; acute treatment of intermittent seizure activity different than usual pattern.

UNLABELED USES Treatment of acute agitation, cocaine intoxication, refractory status epilepticus.

CONTRAINDICATIONS Intolerance to benzodiazepines; acute narrow-angle glaucoma; shock; coma; acute alcohol intoxication; intra-arterial injection; status asthmaticus; pregnancy (teratogenic effects have been observed with some benzodiazepines however more studies are needed; the incidence of premature birth and low birth weight may be increased following maternal use of benzodiazepines), obstetric delivery; lactation.

CAUTIOUS USE COPD; chronic kidney failure; cardiac disease; pulmonary insufficiency; dementia; electrolyte imbalance; neuromuscular disease; Parkinson's disease; psychosis; CHF; bipolar disorder; older adults.

ROUTE & DOSAGE

General Anesthesia

Adult: **IV** Premedication: usual dosing range 0.5–2 mg administered in 0.5–1 mg increments based on effect.

Sedation, Amnesia Prior to Procedure

Adolescent/Child/Infant: **IM** 0.1–0.15 mg/kg 30–60 min before procedure (max dose: 10 mg)
Child (over 6y): **IV** 0.025–0.05 mg/kg titrate to effect (max dose: 10 mg)

Intermittent Seizures

Adult/Adolescent: **Nasal** 5mg (1 spray) as single dose may repeat in 10 min in alternate nostril based on response (max: 2 sprays/episode)

ADMINISTRATION

Oral

- Oral route is reserved for children.Use supplied oral dispenser to dispense directly into mouth.
- Do not mix with any liquid prior to administering.

Intramuscular

- Inject IM drug undiluted, deep into a large muscle mass.

Intravenous

PREPARE: **Direct:** For procedural sedation, administer by slow IV injection over at least 2 minutes using a concentration of 1 mg/mL. **IV Infusion:** Add 5 mL of the 5 mg/mL concentration to 45 mL of D5W or NS to yield 0.5 mg/mL.

ADMINISTER: **Direct for Conscious Sedation:** Give over 2 min or longer. **Direct for Induction of Anesthesia:** Give over 20–30 sec. **Direct for Neonate: Do not** give bolus dose; give over at least 2 min. **IV Infusion:** Give at a rate based on weight.

INCOMPATIBILITIES: Solution/additive: **Fospropofol.** Y-site: **Acyclovir, albumin, aminophylline, amoxicillin, amphotericin B cholesteryl complex, ampicillin, ascorbic acid, atenolol, azathioprine, blinatumomab, cefepime, cefoperazone, ceftazidime, ceftobiprole, cefuroxime, chloramphenicol, cloxacillin, dantrolene, dexamethasone, diazepam, diazoxide, ertapenem, esomeprazole, floxacillin, foscarnet, fosfomycin, fosphenytoin, fosproprol, ganciclovir, gemtuzumab, indomethacin, ketorolac, lansoprazole, letermovir, meropenem, methotrexate, micafungin, mitomycin, omeprazole, pentobarbial, phenobarbital, piperacillin/tazobactam, potassium acetate, prochlorperazine, sodium bicarbonate, trimethoprim/sulfamethoxazole, temocillin, thiopental.**

- Store at 20°–25° C (68°–77° F), therapeutic activity is retained for 2 y from date of manufacture.

ADVERSE EFFECTS **CV:** Hypotension. **Respiratory:** Airway obstruction, respiratory arrest, apnea *bradypnea*, decreased tidal volume, nasal discomfort, throat irritation, oxygen *desaturation*. **CNS:** *Retrograde amnesia,* headache, euphoria, drowsiness, excessive sedation, confusion. **Skin:** Injection site discomfort. **GI:** Nausea, vomiting.

INTERACTIONS **Drug: Alcohol,** CNS DEPRESSANTS, ANTICONVULSANTS potentiate CNS depression; **cimetidine** increases midazolam plasma levels, increasing its toxicity; may decrease antiparkinsonism effects of **levodopa;** may increase **phenytoin** levels; **smoking** decreases sedative and antianxiety effects. Do not use with **lonafarnib, delviridine,** or **abametapir**. Oral midazolam is contraindicated with ANTIHEPAVIRAL combination products and with PROTEASE INHIBITORS. **Food: Grapefruit juice** (greater than 1 qt/day) may increase risk of myopathy and rhabdomyolysis. **Herbal: Kava, valerian, kratom** may potentiate sedation. **Echinacea, St. John's wort** may reduce efficacy.

PHARMACOKINETICS **Onset:** 1–5 min IV; 5–15 min IM, 20–30 min PO. **Peak:** 20–60 min. **Duration:** Less than 2 h IV; 1–6 h IM. **Distribution:** Crosses blood–brain barrier and placenta. **Metabolism:** In liver (CYP3A4). **Elimination:** In urine. **Half-Life:** 1–4 h.

M

NURSING IMPLICATIONS

Black Box Warning

IV midazolam has been associated with respiratory depression and respiratory arrest. Rapid injection (less than 2 min) has been associated with seizures, and with severe hypotension in neonates, particularly when the patient has received fentanyl.

Assessment & Drug Effects

- Inspect insertion site for redness, pain, swelling, and other signs of extravasation during IV infusion.
- Monitor closely for indications of impending respiratory arrest. Resuscitative drugs and equipment should be immediately available.
- Monitor for hypotension, especially if the patient is premedicated with a narcotic agonist analgesic.

- Monitor vital signs for entire recovery period. In obese patient, half-life is prolonged during IV in-fusion; therefore, duration of effects is prolonged (i.e., amnesia, postoperative recovery).
- Be aware that overdose symptoms include somnolence, confusion, sedation, diminished reflexes, coma, and untoward effects on vital signs.

Patient & Family Education

- Do not drive or engage in potentially hazardous activities until response to drug is known. You may feel drowsy, weak, or tired for 1–2 days after drug has been given.

MIDODRINE HYDROCHLORIDE

(mid'o-dreen)

Classification: VASOPRESSOR
Therapeutic: ANTIHYPOTENSIVE
Prototype: Dexmedetomide

AVAILABILITY Tablet

ACTION & *THERAPEUTIC EFFECT* Vasopressor and $alpha_1$ agonist that activates the alpha-adrenergic receptors of the arteries and veins, resulting in increased vascular tone and elevation in blood pressure. *Affects standing, sitting, and supine systolic and diastolic blood pressures. Effectiveness indicated by an increase in 1-min standing systolic BP and subjective feelings of clinical improvement.*

USES Orthostatic hypotension.

CONTRAINDICATIONS Severe organic heart disease; heart failure; kidney disease, renal failure; urinary retention; pheochromocytoma; thyrotoxicosis; MAOI therapy; persistent and excessive supine hypertension.

CAUTIOUS USE Renal impairment, hepatic impairment; history of visual problems; diabetes with hypotension or visual disorders; pregnancy (category C); lactation. Safety and efficacy in children not established.

ROUTE & DOSAGE

Orthostatic Hypotension

Adult: **PO** 10 mg tid during the daytime hours, dosed not less than 3 h apart with last dose at least 4 h before bedtime (max: 20 mg/dose)

ADMINISTRATION

Oral

- Do not give at bedtime or before napping (within 4 h of lying supine for any length of time).
- Give with caution in persons with pretreatment, supine systolic BP 170 mm Hg or higher.
- Store at 15°–30° C (59°–86° F).

ADVERSE EFFECTS CV: *Hypertension.* **CNS:** Confusion, nervousness, anxiety. **Skin:** *Pruritus, piloerection,* rash. **GI:** Dry mouth. **GU:** *Dysuria, urinary retention, urinary frequency.* **Other:** *Paresthesia,* chills, pain, facial flushing.

INTERACTIONS Drug: May antagonize effects of **doxazosin, prazosin, terazosin;** may potentiate vasoconstrictive effects of **ephedrine, phenylephrine, pseudoephedrine;** may cause hypertensive crisis with MAOIS.

PHARMACOKINETICS Absorption: Rapidly from GI tract. **Peak:** Midodrine 0.5 h; desglymidodrine 1–2 h. **Metabolism:** Rapidly metabolized to the active metabolite.

Elimination: In urine. **Half-Life:** 25 min.

NURSING IMPLICATIONS

Assessment & Drug Effects

- Monitor supine and standing BP regularly. Withhold drug and notify prescriber if supine BP increases excessively; determine acceptable parameters.
- Monitor carefully effect of the drug in diabetics with orthostatic hypotension and those taking fludrocortisone acetate, which may increase intraocular pressure.
- Monitor lab tests: Baseline LFTs and renal function tests.

Patient & Family Education

- Take last daily dose 4 h before bedtime.
- Report immediately to prescriber sensations associated with supine hypertension (e.g., pounding in ears, headache, blurred vision, awareness of heart beating).
- Discontinue drug and report to prescriber if S&S of bradycardia develop (e.g., dizziness, pulse slowing, fainting).
- Do not take allergy drugs, cold preparations, or diet pills without consulting prescriber.

MIDOSTAURIN

(mye-doe-staw′rin)

Rydapt

Classification: ANTINEOPLASTIC; TYROSINE KINASE INHIBITOR; FLT3 INHIBITOR

Therapeutic: ANTINEOPLASTIC

AVAILABILITY Capsule

ACTION & *THERAPEUTIC EFFECT* Inhibits multiple receptor tyrosine kinases. *Induces cell death in leukemic cells, resulting in decreased cell proliferation and cell survival.*

USES Treatment of mast cell leukemia; also used for the treatment of systemic mastocytosis and treatment of acute myeloid leukemia, if FLT3-positive, in combination with cytarabine and daunorubicin.

CONTRAINDICATIONS Pregnancy; lactation. Hypersensitivity to midostaurin or any components.

CAUTIOUS USE History of lung or gastrointestinal disease or hematological abnormalities. Concurrent use of products that impact QT interval. Safety and efficacy in children not established.

ROUTE & DOSAGE

Mast Cell Leukemia

Adult: **PO** 100 mg bid

Aggressive Systemic Mastocytosis (ASM)

Adult: **PO** 100 mg bid

Acute Myeloid Leukemia

Adult: **PO** 50 mg bid on days 8–21 of each induction cycle (with cytarabine and daunorubicin), and on days 8–21 of each consolidation cycle (high-dose cytarabine)

Hepatic and Renal Impairment Dosage Adjustment

Unstudied in this population

Toxicity Dosage Adjustment

Specific adjustments available in the package insert

M

ADMINISTRATION

Oral

- Administer with food every 12 h.
- Do not crush/open capsules.
- Administer prophylactic antiemetics before therapy.
- Store at 25° C (77° F); excursions permitted to 15°–30° C (59°–86° F). Store in original package to protect from moisture.

ADVERSE EFFECTS **CV:** *Edema*, QT changes, heart failure, myocardial infarction hypotension. **Respiratory:** URTI, epistaxis, dyspnea, cough. **CNS:** *Headache, fatigue*, dizziness, insomnia, arthralgia, musculoskeletal pain. **Endocrine:** *Hyperglycemia, hypocalemia, hyperuricemia*, hyponatremia, hypoalbuminemia, hypokalemia, hyperkalemia, hypophosphatemia. **Skin:** Hyperhidrosis, rash. **GI:** Gastrointestinal hemorrhage, *nausea, vomiting, mucositis*, diarrhea, increased serum lipase, abdominal pain, constipation, hemorrhoids. **GU:** Urinary tract infection, renal failure. **Hematologic:** *Febrile neutropenia, lymphocytopenia*, leukopenia, anemia, thromobocytopenia, neutropenia, petechia. **OTHER:** Sepsis, mycosis.

INTERACTIONS Major substrate of CYP3A4. Avoid combination with strong CYP3A4 inducers (e.g., **carbamazepine, phenytoin, rifampin**). Avoid use with other medications which may increase risk for QT_C-prolongation (e.g., **hydroxychloroquine, ketoconazole, ziprasidone**).

PHARMACOKINETICS **Absorption:** C_{max} decreased if administered with food. **Distribution:** 99% protein bound. **Onset:** Peak in 1–3 h. **Metabolism:** Hepatic, primarily through CYP3A4, to active metabolites **Elimination:** 95% in feces, 5% in urine. **Half-Life:** 21 h.

NURSING IMPLICATIONS

Assessment & Drug Effects

- Monitor for potential pulmonary toxicity or signs of bone marrow suppression.
- Verify pregnancy status within 7 days of initiating therapy in women with reproductive potential.
- Respiratory assessments for signs and symptoms of pulmonary toxicity.
- Assess EKG for QT interval if patient is on concurrent medication that may prolong the QT interval.
- Weekly CBC for the first 4 wk of treatment, every other week for the next 8 wk, and monthly thereafter during therapy.

Patient and Family Education

- Report immediately to prescriber any signs of infection, high blood sugar, signs of bleeding, signs of kidney problems blood in the urine, difficulty urinating, prolonged nausea, vomiting and diarrhea, coffee ground emesis.
- May impair male fertility.
- Women and men should use effective means to avoid pregnancy while taking this drug for at least 4 mo after the last dose. Do not breast-feed for at least 4 mo after the last dose.

MIGLITOL

(mig′li-toll)

Glyset

Classification: ANTIDIABETIC; ALPHA-GLUCOSIDASE INHIBITOR

Therapeutic: ANTIDIABETIC; GLYCEMIC CONTROL ENHANCER

Prototype: Acarbose

 Common adverse effects in *italic*; life-threatening effects underlined; generic names in **bold**; classifications in SMALL CAPS; ♣ Canadian drug name; Prototype drug; Alert

AVAILABILITY Tablet

ACTION & *THERAPEUTIC EFFECT* Enzyme inhibits intestinal glucosidases thus delaying the formation of glucose from saccharides in the small intestine resulting in a smaller rise in postprandial blood glucose concentration. *Helps control postprandial hyperglycemia, and reduces the levels of glysylated hemoglobin (HbA1C) in type 2 diabetics.*

USES Adjunct to diet for control of type 2 diabetes.

UNLABELED USES Type 1 diabetes.

CONTRAINDICATIONS Hypersensitivity to miglitol; diabetic ketoacidosis; digestive or absorptive disorders; history of or partial intestinal obstruction, IBD; lactation.

CAUTIOUS USE Hypersensitivity to acarbose; creatinine clearance greater than 2 mg/dL; high stress conditions (i.e., surgery, trauma); pregnancy (category B). Safety and efficacy in children younger than 18 y not established.

ROUTE & DOSAGE

Type 2 Diabetes Mellitis

Adult: **PO** 25 mg tid at the start of each meal, may increase after 4–8 wk to 50 mg tid (max: 100 mg tid)

ADMINISTRATION

Oral

- Give drug with first bite of each of the three main meals.
- Store at 15°–30° C (59°–86° F).

ADVERSE EFFECTS **GI:** *Flatulence, diarrhea,* abdominal pain.

INTERACTIONS **Drug:** Miglitol may reduce bioavailability of **propranolol; charcoal, pancreatin, amylase, pancrelipase** may decrease effectiveness of miglitol. **Herbal: Garlic, ginseng** may potentiate hypoglycemic effects.

PHARMACOKINETICS **Absorption:** 25 mg dose is completely absorbed, amount absorbed decreases with increasing dose to where 100 mg dose is 50–70% absorbed. **Peak:** 2–3 h. **Distribution:** Minimal protein binding (less than 4%). **Metabolism:** Not metabolized. **Elimination:** Half-life 2 h; 95% excreted unchanged in urine, lower doses should be used in patients with renal impairment.

NURSING IMPLICATIONS

Assessment & Drug Effects

- Monitor for therapeutic effectiveness: Indicated by improved blood glucose levels and decreased HbA1C.
- Monitor for S&S of hypoglycemia when used in combination with sulfonylureas, insulin, other hypoglycemia agents.
- Treat hypolgycemia with oral glucose (dextrose); miglitol interferes with the breakdown of sucrose (table sugar).
- Monitor lab tests: Daily postprandial blood glucose and HbA1C q3mo.

Patient & Family Education

- Keep a source of oral glucose available to treat low blood sugar; miglitol prevents digestive breakdown of table sugar.
- Abdominal discomfort, flatulence, and diarrhea tend to diminish with continued therapy.

M

MILNACIPRAN

(mil-na-see′pran)

Savella

Classification: ANTIDEPRESSANT; SEROTONIN NOREPINEPHRINE REUPTAKE INHIBITOR (SNRI); ANALGESIC

Therapeutic: ANALGESIC; SNRI

Prototype: Venlafaxine

AVAILABILITY Tablet

ACTION & *THERAPEUTIC EFFECT*

A potent inhibitor of norepinephrine and serotonin reuptake without affecting uptake of other neurotransmitters. *Effective in reducing the pain associated with fibromyalgia.*

USES Management of fibromyalgia.

M

UNLABELED USES Treatment of depression.

CONTRAINDICATIONS Within 14 days discontinued use of MAOIs; abrupt discontinuation of milnacipran; suicidal ideation; major depressive disorder; uncontrolled narrow-angle glaucoma; substantial alcohol use; chronic liver disease; ESRD; lactation.

CAUTIOUS USE Suicidal tendencies; history of seizures or depression; history of cardiac disease or preexisting tachyarrhythmias; male obstructive uropathies; history of GI bleeding; moderate and severe renal impairment; hepatic impairment; older adults; pregnancy (adverse events have been observed in animal reproduction studies); children younger than 18 y.

ROUTE & DOSAGE

Fibromyalgia

Adults/Adolescents (17 y or older): **PO** Initial dose of 12.5 mg once daily on day 1, increase to 12.5 mg bid on days 2 and 3, 25 mg bid on days 4–7, and then 50 mg bid; Dose can be increased to 100 mg bid if needed.

Renal Impairment Dosage Adjustment

CrCl less than 29 mL/min: Decrease dose by 50% (i.e., 25–50 mg bid)

ADMINISTRATION

Oral

- Dose titration should occur over a period of 1 wk to the recommended dose.
- Give with food, if needed, to improve tolerability of drug.
- Do not give within 14 days of an MAOI.
- Store at 15°–30° C (59°–86° F).

ADVERSE EFFECTS **CV:** Hypertension, palpitations, <u>tachycardia</u>. **CNS:** *Dizziness, headache, insomnia,* migraine. **Endocrine:** Hot flash. **Skin:** Hyperhidrosis. **GI:** *Constipation,* dry mouth, *nausea,* vomiting.

INTERACTIONS **Drug:** Concurrent use with SELECTIVE SEROTONIN REUPTAKE INHIBITORS, SELECTIVE NOREPINEPHRINE REUPTAKE INHIBITORS, MAOIS, **tramadol**, OR 5-HT-2B/2D AGONISTS (TRIPTANS) may cause additive serotonergic effects, hypertension, and coronary vasoconstriction. Lithium may increase risk of serotonin syndrome. **Milnacipran** may inhibit antihypertensive effect of **clonidine** and other ALPHA$_2$ AGONISTS. **IV digoxin** may increase the risk of postural hypotension and tachycardia. Milnacipran may increase bleeding ANTIPLATELET agents; concurrent use with **epinephrine** or **norepinephrine** may cause paroxysmal hypertension and arrhythmia.

PHARMACOKINETICS **Absorption:** 85–90% bioavailability. **Distribution:** Minimal (13%) plasma protein binding. **Metabolism:** Less than 50% metabolized by liver. **Elimination:** Primarily renal. **Half-Life:** 6–8 h.

NURSING IMPLICATIONS

Black Box Warning

Milnacipan has been associated with suicidal thinking and behavior in children, adolescents, and young adults.

Assessment & Drug Effects

- Monitor for and report promptly unusual changes in behavior (e.g., depression, anxiety, panic attack, insomnia, aggressiveness, mania) or suicidal ideation. Monitor closely during initial few months of therapy and during periods of dosage adjustment.
- Monitor HR and BP closely and report promptly sustained BP elevations. Pre-existing hypertension should be controlled before initiating this drug.
- Monitor for orthostatic hypotension and tachycardia with concurrent digoxin use.
- Intraocular pressure should be monitored in those with baseline elevation or a history of glaucoma.
- Monitor lab tests: Periodic renal function.

Patient & Family Education

- Do not abruptly stop taking this drug. It should be tapered off gradually after extended use.
- Report prompt unusual changes in behavior or suicidal ideas.
- Do not engage in potentially hazardous activities until reaction to drug is known.
- Exercise care to take prescribed BP medications exactly as ordered.
- Concurrent use of aspirin or NSAIDs is not recommended due to increased risk of bleeding. Consult prescriber.
- Avoid consuming alcohol while taking this drug.

MILRINONE LACTATE

(mil′ri-none)

Classification: INOTROPIC AGENT; VASODILATOR

Therapeutic: INOTROPIC AGENT

Prototype: Milrinone acetate

AVAILABILITY Solution for injection

ACTION & *THERAPEUTIC EFFECT* Has a positive inotropic action and is a vasodilator with little chronotropic activity. Inhibitory action against cyclic-AMP phosphodiesterase in cardiac and smooth vascular muscle. Increases cardiac contractility and myocardial contractility. *Therefore, increases cardiac output and decreases pulmonary wedge pressure and vascular resistance, without increasing myocardial oxygen demand or significantly increasing heart rate.*

USES Short-term management of CHF.

UNLABELED USES Short-term use to increase the cardiac index in patients with low cardiac output after surgery. To increase

M

cardiac function prior to heart transplantation.

CONTRAINDICATIONS
Hypersensitivity to milrinone; valvular heart disease; acute MI.

CAUTIOUS USE
Atrial fibrillation, atrial flutter; renal disease; renal impairment, renal failure; older adults; pregnancy (category C); lactation; children.

ROUTE & DOSAGE

Heart Failure

Adult: **IV Loading Dose** 50 mcg/kg IV over 10 min; **IV Maintenance Dose** 0.375–0.75 mcg/kg/min

ADMINISTRATION

Intravenous

Note: Correct preexisting hypokalemia before administering milrinone. ▪ See manufacturer's information for dosage reduction in the presence of renal impairment.

PREPARE: **IV Infusion Loading Dose:** Give undiluted or dilute each 1 mg in 1 mL NS or 0.45% NaCl. **IV Infusion Maintenance Dose:** Dilute 20 mg of milrinone in D5W, NS, or 0.45% NaCl to yield: 100 mcg/mL with 180 mL diluent; 150 mcg/mL with 113 mL diluent; 200 mcg/mL with 80 mL diluent.

ADMINISTER: **IV Infusion Loading Dose:** Give 50 mcg/kg over 10 min. **IV Infusion Maintenance Dose:** Give at a rate based on weight. Use a microdrip set and infusion pump.

INCOMPATIBILITIES: **Solution/additive:** **Furosemide, procainamide.** **Y-site:** **Furosemide, imipenem/cilastatin, procainamide.**

▪ Store according to manufacturer's directions.

ADVERSE EFFECTS
CV: Increased ectopic activity, PVCs, ventricular tachycardia, ventricular fibrillation, supraventricular arrhythmias; possible increase in angina symptoms, hypotension. **CNS:** Headache. **Other:** Hypokalemia.

INTERACTIONS
Drug: Disopyramide may cause excessive hypotension.

PHARMACOKINETICS
Peak: 2 min. **Duration:** 2 h. **Distribution:** 70% protein bound. **Elimination:** 80–85% excreted unchanged in urine within 24 h. Active renal tubular secretion is primary elimination pathway. **Half-Life:** 1.7–2.7 h.

NURSING IMPLICATIONS

Assessment & Drug Effects

- Monitor cardiac status closely during and for several hours following infusion. Supraventricular and ventricular arrhythmias have occurred.
- Monitor BP and promptly slow or stop infusion in presence of significant hypotension. Closely monitor those with recent aggressive diuretic therapy for decreasing blood pressure.
- Monitor fluid and electrolyte status. Hypokalemia should be corrected whenever it occurs during administration.
- Monitor lab tests: Periodic serum electrolytes.

Patient & Family Education

- Report immediately angina that occurs during infusion to prescriber.
- Be aware that drug may cause a headache, which can be treated with analgesics.

MINOCYCLINE HYDROCHLORIDE

(mi-noe-sye′kleen)

Arestin, Minocin, Minolira, Solodyn, Ximino

Classification: TETRACYCLINE ANTIBIOTIC

Therapeutic: ANTIBIOTIC

Prototype: Tetracycline

AVAILABILITY Capsule; tablet; sustained release microsphere; solution for injection

ACTION & *THERAPEUTIC EFFECT* Bacteriostatic action that appears to be a result of reversible binding to ribosomal units of susceptible bacteria and inhibition of bacterial protein synthesis. *Effective against gram-positive and gram-negative bacteria, but usually used against gram-negative bacteria.*

USES Treatment of mucopurulent cervicitis, granuloma inguinale, lymphogranuloma venereum, proctitis, bronchitis, lower respiratory tract infections caused by *Mycoplasma pneumoniae,* Rickettsial infections, chlamydial infections, non-gonococcal urethritis, chlamydial conjunctivitis, plague, brucellosis, bartonellosis, tularemia, UTI, and prostatitis; acne vulgaris, gonorrhea, cholera, meningococcal carrier state, amebiasis, anthrax.

CONTRAINDICATIONS Hypersensitivity to minocyline or other tetracyclines; pregnancy (category D); lactation.

CAUTIOUS USE Renal and hepatic impairment; older adults; children younger than 8 y.

ROUTE & DOSAGE

Anti-Infective

Adult: **PO/IV** 200 mg followed by 100 mg q12h
Child (8 y or older): **PO/IV** 4 mg/kg (max: 200 mg) followed by 2 mg/kg q12h (max: 100 mg)

Syphilis (when penicillin is contraindicated)

Adult: **PO/IV** 200 mg then 100 mg q12h × 10–15 days

Acne

Adult: **PO** 200 mg × 1 then 100 mg q12h

Moderate to Severe Acne (Solodyn, Minolira, Ximino only)

Adult/Adolescent/Child (older than 12 y): **PO** 1 mg/kg daily × 12 wk

Meningococcal Infection Prophylaxis

Adult: **PO** 100 mg q12h × 5 days
Child (8 y or older): **PO** 4 mg/kg followed by 2 mg/kg q12h × 5 days (max: 100 mg/dose)

Renal Impairment Dosage Adjustment

Do not exceed 200 mg/day in patients with renal impairment

ADMINISTRATION

Oral

- Shake suspension well before administration.
- Ensure that sustained release tablets are swallowed whole.
- Administer with adequate fluid to decrease the risk of esophageal irritation.

- Check expiration date. Outdated tetracycline can cause severe adverse effects.

Intravenous

PREPARE: **IV Infusion:** Reconstitute with 5 mL of sterile water for injection and immediately further dilute in 100 to 1,000 mL of NS, D5W, D5NS, or 250 mL to 1,000 mL of LR.

ADMINISTER: Infuse over 60 min; avoid rapid administration. The injectable route should be used only if the oral route is not feasible or adequate. Prolonged intravenous therapy may be associated with thrombophlebitis.

INCOMPATIBILITIES: **Solution/Additive:** LR, TPN, TNA, **Doxapram hydrochloride, Rifampin**.

- Store intact vials at 20°–25° C (68°–77° F). Diluted solution in NS, D5W, D5NS, or LR is stable at room temperature for up to 4 h or at 2°–8° C (36°–46° F) for up to 24 h.

M

ADVERSE EFFECTS **CNS:** *Weakness, light-headedness, ataxia, dizziness, headache, fatigue, drowsiness, vertigo, tinnitus.* **Skin:** Pruritus. **Hepatic:** Hepatitis, increased liver enzyme, hepatotoxicity. **GI:** *Nausea, vomiting,* anorexia, cramps, diarrhea, flatulence. **Other:** Dental caries, dental pain.

INTERACTIONS **Drug:** ANTACIDS, **iron, calcium, magnesium, zinc, kaolin and pectin, sodium bicarbonate, bismuth subsalicylate** can significantly decrease minocycline absorption; effects of both **desmopressin** and minocycline antagonized; increases **digoxin** absorption, increasing risk of **digoxin** toxicity; **methoxyflurane** increases risk of kidney failure. Do not use with **acitretin** or **isotretinoin**. **Food:** Dairy products significantly decrease minocycline absorption; food may also decrease its absorption.

PHARMACOKINETICS **Absorption:** 90–100% from GI tract. **Peak:** 2–3 h. **Distribution:** Tends to accumulate in adipose tissue; crosses placenta; distributed into breast milk. **Metabolism:** Partially metabolized. **Elimination:** 20–30% in feces; ~12% in urine. **Half-Life:** 11–26 h.

NURSING IMPLICATIONS

Assessment & Drug Effects

- Obtain history of hypersensitivity reactions prior to administration; drug is contraindicated with known tetracycline hypersensitivity.
- Monitor carefully for signs of hypersensitivity response (see Appendix F), particularly in patients with history of allergies, especially to drugs.
- Monitor at-risk patients for S&S of superinfection (see Appendix F).
- Assess risk of toxic effects carefully; increases with renal and hepatic impairment.
- Supervise ambulation, since light-headedness, dizziness, and vertigo occur frequently.
- Monitor lab tests: Baseline C&S, LFTs, BUN, renal function, serum magnesium with periodic testing for long-term therapy.

Patient & Family Education

- Avoid hazardous activities or those requiring alertness while taking minocycline.
- Use sunscreen when outdoors and otherwise protect yourself from direct sunlight since

photosensitivity reaction may occur.

- Report vestibular adverse effects (e.g., dizziness), which usually occur during first week of therapy. Effects are reversible if drug is withdrawn.
- Report loose stools or diarrhea or other signs of superinfection promptly to prescriber.
- Use or add barrier contraceptive while taking this drug if using hormonal contraceptive.
- Maintain adequate hydration while taking this drug.

MINOXIDIL

(mi-nox'i-dill)

Rogaine

Classification: NONNITRATE VASODILATOR; ANTIHYPERTENSIVE

Therapeutic: ANTIHYPERTENSIVE

Prototype: Hydralazine

AVAILABILITY Tablet; solution

ACTION & *THERAPEUTIC EFFECT* Direct-acting vasodilator that appears to act by blocking calcium uptake through cell membranes. Reduces elevated systolic and diastolic blood pressures in supine and standing positions, by decreasing peripheral vascular resistance. *Effective as an antihypertensive. It increases heart rate and cardiac output.* **Topical:** *Reverses balding to some degree.*

USES Treat severe hypertension that is symptomatic or associated with damage to target organs and is not manageable with maximum therapeutic doses of a diuretic plus two other antihypertensive drugs. **Topical:** Treats alopecia areata and male pattern alopecia.

CONTRAINDICATIONS Hypersensitivity to minoxidil; pheochromocytoma; mild hypertension; recent acute MI, dissecting aortic aneurysm, valvular dysfunction; pulmonary hypertension; pericardial effusion; lactation.

CAUTIOUS USE Severe renal impairment; malignant hypertension; recent MI (within preceding month); CAD, chronic CHF; tachycardia; worsening of angina; older adults; pregnancy (category C); children younger than 12 y.

ROUTE & DOSAGE

Hypertension

Adult: **PO** 5–10 mg daily, titrate up as needed (max: 100 mg)
Adolescent: **PO** 5 mg/day titrate carefully (max: 100 mg/day)

Alopecia

Adult: **Topical** Apply 1 mL of 2% solution to affected area bid

ADMINISTRATION

Oral

- Dose increments are usually made at 3–5 days intervals. If more rapid adjustment is necessary, adjustments can be made q6h with careful monitoring.

Topical

- Do not apply topical product to an irritated scalp (e.g., sunburn, psoriasis).
- Store at 15°–30° C (59°–86° F) in tightly covered container unless otherwise directed.

ADVERSE EFFECTS **CV:** *Tachycardia*, angina pectoris, *ECG changes*, pericardial effusion and tamponade, rebound hypertension (following drug withdrawal); *edema*, including

M

pulmonary edema; *CHF (salt and water retention)*. **Skin:** *Hypertrichosis,* transient pruritus, darkening of skin, hypersensitivity rash, Stevens–Johnson syndrome. With topical use: Itching, flushing, scaling, dermatitis, folliculitis. **Other:** Fatigue.

INTERACTIONS Drug: Epinephrine, norepinephrine cause excessive cardiac stimulation; **guan-ethidine** causes profound ortho-static hypotension.

PHARMACOKINETICS Absorption: Readily absorbed from GI tract. **Onset:** 30 min PO; at least 4 mo topical. **Peak:** 2–8 h PO. **Duration:** 2–5 days PO; new hair growth will remain 3–4 mo after withdrawal of topical. **Distribution:** Widely distributed including into breast milk. **Metabolism:** In liver. **Elimination:** 97% in urine and feces. **Half-Life:** 4.2 h.

M

NURSING IMPLICATIONS

Black Box Warning

Minoxidil has been associated with pericardial effusion, occasionally progressing to tamponade, and it can exacerbate angina pectoris.

Assessment & Drug Effects

- Take BP and apical pulse before administering medication and report significant changes. Consult prescriber for parameters.
- Do not stop drug abruptly. Abrupt reduction in BP can result in CVA and MI. Keep prescriber informed.
- Monitor fluid and electrolyte balance closely throughout therapy. Sodium and water retention commonly occur. Monitor potassium intake and serum potassium levels in patient on diuretic therapy.
- Monitor I&O and daily weight. Report unusual changes in I&O ratio or daily weight gain, greater than 1 kg (2 lb).
- Observe patient daily for edema and auscultate lungs for rales. Be alert to signs and symptoms of CHF (see Appendix F).
- Observe for symptoms of pericardial effusion or tamponade. Symptoms are similar to those of CHF, but additionally patient may have paradoxical pulse (normal inspiratory reduction in systolic BP may fall as much as 10–20 mm Hg).
- Monitor lab tests: Periodic serum electrolytes.

Patient & Family Education

- Learn about usual pulse rate and count radial pulse for one full minute before taking drug. Report an increase of 20 or more bpm.
- Notify prescriber promptly if the following S&S appear: Increase of 20 or more bpm in resting pulse; breathing difficulty; dizziness; light-headedness; fainting; edema (tight shoes or rings, puffiness, pitting); weight gain, chest pain, arm or shoulder pain; easy bruising or bleeding.
- Develops 3–9 wk after start of therapy and occurs in approximately 80% of patients; reversible within 1–6 mo after drug withdrawal.

MIRABEGRON

(mir-a-be'gron)

Myrbetriq

Classification: GENITOURINARY AGENT; BETA-3 ADRENERGIC AGONIST, ANTISPASMOTIC

Therapeutic: ANTISPASMOTIC

AVAILABILITY Extended release tablet; oral suspension

ACTION & THERAPEUTIC EFFECT A beta adrenergic receptor agonist that relaxes the detrusor smooth muscle during the storage phase of the urinary bladder fill–void cycle thus increasing bladder capacity and tone. *Decreases episodes of urge incontinence and reduces urinary frequency.*

USES Treatment of overactive bladder; treatment neurogenic detursor overactivity in pediatric patients.

CONTRAINDICATIONS Uncontrolled hypertension; ESRD; severe hepatic and renal impairment; lactation; hypersensitivity to mirabegron.

CAUTIOUS USE Hypertension; significant bladder outlet obstruction; moderate hepatic impairment; moderate renal impairment; pregnancy (adverse effects have been observed in animal reproduction studies). Safety and efficacy in children younger than 18 y not established.

ROUTE & DOSAGE

Overactive Bladder

Adult: **PO** 25 mg once daily; can be increased to 50 mg once daily after 4–8w

Neurogenic detrusor overactivity

Child (over 3y and over 35 kg): **PO** 25 mg tablet or 48 mg granules daily. *(over 3y and 22–35 kg)* 32 mg granules daily. *(over 3y and 11–22 kg)* 24 mg granules daily

Hepatic Impairment Dosage Adjustment

Moderate hepatic impairment (Child Pugh class B): Max: 25 mg once daily (adult)
Severe hepatic impairment (Child Pugh class C): Not recommended

Renal Impairment Dosage Adjustment

eGFR 15–29 mL/min: Max: 25 mg once daily (adult) *eGFR less than 15 mL/min:* Not recommended

ADMINISTRATION

Oral

- May be given without regard to food.
- Ensure that tablet is swallowed whole. It should not be crushed, divided, or chewed.
- Store at 25° C (77° F).

ADVERSE EFFECTS **CV:** *Hypertension*, tachycardia. **Respiratory:** *Nasopharyngitis*, sinusitis. **CNS:** Dizziness, *headache*. **GI:** Xerostomia. **GU:** *Urinary tract infection*. **Musculoskeletal:** Back pain. **Other:** Influenza.

INTERACTIONS **Drug:** Mirabegron may increase the levels of other drugs requiring CYP2D6 for metabolism (e.g., **clozapine, doxorubicin, eliglustat, metoprolol, desipramine**). Mirabegron increases the levels of **digoxin**. Reduce dose of **mirabegron** if used with propafenone or **solifenacin.**

PHARMACOKINETICS **Absorption:** 29–35% bioavailable. **Peak:** 3.5 h. **Distribution:** 71% plasma protein bound. **Metabolism:** Extensive hepatic metabolism (CYP2D6, CYP3A4). **Elimination:** Renal (55%) and fecal (34%). **Half-Life:** 50 h.

NURSING IMPLICATIONS

Assessment & Drug Effects

- Monitor baseline and periodic BP, especially in those with a history of hypertension.
- Monitor for signs and symptoms of urinary retention.
- Monitor lab tests: Baseline and periodic renal function tests.

Patient & Family Education

- Report promptly signs of urinary tract infection, difficulty passing urine or urinary retention.
- Report to your prescriber if you are or plan to become pregnant.
- Do not breast-feed without consulting prescriber.

M

MIRTAZAPINE

(mir-taz'a-peen)

Remeron, Remeron SolTab

Classification: TETRACYCLIC ANTIDEPRESSANT; ANXIOLYTIC

Therapeutic: ANTIDEPRESSANT; ANTIANXIETY

AVAILABILITY Tablet; orally disintegrating tablet

ACTION & *THERAPEUTIC EFFECT* Tetracyclic antidepressant pharmacologically and therapeutically similar to tricyclic antidepressants. Tetracyclics enhance central nonadrenergic and serotonergic activity; mechanism of action thought to be due to normalization of neurotransmission efficacy. Mirtazapine is a potent antagonist of 5-HT_2 and 5-HT_3 serotonin receptors. *Acts as antidepressant. Effectiveness is indicated by mood elevation.*

USES Treatment of depression.

UNLABELED USES Prophylaxis of chronic tension-type headache, panic disorder.

CONTRAINDICATIONS Hypersensitivity to mirtazapine or mianserin; hypersensitivity to other antidepressants (e.g., tricyclic antidepressants and MAOI depressants), acute MI; fever, infection; agranulocytosis, suicidal ideation; jaundice, ethanol intoxication; lactation.

CAUTIOUS USE History of cardiovascular or GI disorders; BPH, urinary retention; preexisting hematological disease; thrombocytopenia; narrow-angle glaucoma, increased intraocular pressure; renal impairment, renal failure; moderate to severe hepatic impairment; hypercholesterolemia, hypertriglyceridem-ia, cardiac disease; angina, cardiac arrhythmias; bipolar disorder, mania, bone marrow suppression, PKU, history of MI; CVD; seizure disorder, seizures; depression; history of suicidal tendencies; hypovolemia, surgery; closed-angle glaucoma; ileus, GI obstruction, dehydration; diabetes mellitus, diabetic ketoacidosis; older adults; pregnancy (a significant increase in major teratogenic effects has not been observed following in utero exposure). Safety and efficacy in children not established.

ROUTE & DOSAGE

Depression

Adult: **PO** 15 mg/day in single dose at bedtime, may increase q1–2wk (max: 45 mg/day)
Geriatric: **PO** 7.5 mg in single dose at bedtime

Renal Impairment Dosage Adjustment

eGFR less than 30 mL/min: Initiate with 50% of typical dose

ADMINISTRATION

Oral

- Give preferably prior to sleep to minimize injury potential.
- Begin drug no sooner than 14 days after discontinuation of an MAO inhibitor.
- Reduce dosage as warranted with severe renal or hepatic impairment and in older adults.
- Store at 20°–25° C (68°–77° F) in tight, light-resistant container.

ADVERSE EFFECTS

Respiratory: Flu-like symptoms. **CNS:** *Drowsiness,* dizziness, abnormal dreams, abnormal thinking, tremor. **Endocrine:** Increased serum cholesterol, weight gain, increased serum triglycerides. **GI/Hepatic:** *Increased appetite*/weight gain, *dry mouth, constipation,* increased liver enzymes. **Other:** Asthenia, flu syndrome.

INTERACTIONS

Drug: Additive cognitive and motor impairment with **alcohol** or BENZODIAZEPINES or CNS DEPRESSANTS; increase risk of hypertensive crisis with MAOIS. **Herbal: Kava, kratom, valerian** may potentiate sedative effects.

PHARMACOKINETICS

Absorption: Rapidly absorbed from GI tract, 50% reaches systemic circulation. **Peak:** 2 h. **Distribution:** 85% protein bound. **Metabolism:** In liver by cytochrome P450 system (CYP2D6, CYP1A2, CYP3A4). **Elimination:** 75% in urine, 15% in feces. **Half-Life:** 20–40 h.

NURSING IMPLICATIONS

Black Box Warning

Mirtazapine has been associated with suicidal thinking and behavior in children, adolescents, and young adults

Assessment & Drug Effects

- Monitor for worsening of depression or suicidal ideation.
- Assess for weight gain and excessive somnolence or dizziness.
- Monitor for orthostatic hypotension with a history of cardiovascular or cerebrovascular disease. Periodically monitor ECG especially in those with known cardiovascular disease.
- Monitor those with history of seizures for lowering of the seizure threshold.
- Monitor lab tests: Periodic WBC with differential, lipid profile, renal function, and LFTs.

Patient & Family Education

- Report immediately to prescriber signs of worsening mental status such as suicidal ideation, aggressiveness, agitation, anxiety, hostility, impulsivity, insomnia, irritability, panic attacks, and worsening of depression.
- Do not drive or engage in potentially hazardous activities until response to drug is known.

M

- Do not use alcohol while taking drug.
- Report immediately unexplained fever or S&S of infection, especially flu-like symptoms, to prescriber.
- Do not take other prescription or OTC drugs without consulting prescriber.
- Make position changes slowly especially from lying or sitting to standing. Report dizziness, palpitations, and fainting.
- Monitor weight periodically and report significant weight gains.

MISOPROSTOL

(my-so-prost'ole)

Cytotec

Classification: PROSTAGLANDIN

Therapeutic: PROSTAGLANDIN

AVAILABILITY Tablet

ACTION & *THERAPEUTIC EFFECT* Synthetic prostaglandin E_1 analog, with both antisecretory (inhibiting gastric acid secretion) and mucosal protective properties. Increases bicarbonate and mucosal protective properties. Inhibits basal and nocturnal gastric acid secretion and acid secretion in response to a variety of stimuli, including meals, histamine, pentagastrin, and coffee. Produces uterine contractions that may endanger pregnancy and cause a miscarriage. *Inhibits basal and nocturnal gastric acid secretion.*

USES Prevention of NSAID (including aspirin-induced) gastric ulcers in patients at high risk of complications from a gastric ulcer (e.g., the older adult and patients with a concomitant debilitating disease or a history of ulcers). Drug is taken for the duration of NSAID therapy and does not interfere with the efficacy of the NSAID.

UNLABELED USES Short-term treatment of duodenal ulcers; cervical ripening and induction of labor.

CONTRAINDICATIONS History of allergies to prostaglandins. **Topical:** Abnormal fetal position, caesarean section, ectopic pregnancy; fetal disease, incomplete abortion; multiparity, placenta previa, vaginal bleeding; pregnancy (category X).

CAUTIOUS USE Renal impairment; cardiovascular disease; IBD; lactation. Safety and efficacy in children not established.

ROUTE & DOSAGE

Prevention of NSAID-Induced Ulcers

Adult: **PO** 100–200 mcg qid p.c. and at bedtime

ADMINISTRATION

Oral

- Give with food to minimize GI adverse effects (manufacturer recommendation).
- Store away from heat, light, and moisture.

ADVERSE EFFECTS **CNS:** Headache. **GI:** *Diarrhea, abdominal pain,* nausea, flatulence, dyspepsia, vomiting, constipation. **GU:** Spotting, cramps, dysmenorrhea, uterine contractions.

INTERACTIONS **Drug:** MAGNESIUM-CONTAINING ANTACIDS may increase diarrhea.

PHARMACOKINETICS **Absorption:** Readily from GI tract; extensive first pass metabolism. **Onset:** 30 min. **Peak:** 60–90 min. **Duration:** At least 3 h. **Metabolism:** In liver.

Elimination: Primarily in urine; small amount in feces. **Half-Life:** 20–40 min.

NURSING IMPLICATIONS

Black Box Warning

Misoprostol can cause abortion, premature birth, or birth defects.

Assessment & Drug Effects

- Monitor for diarrhea; may be minimized by giving drug after meals and at bedtime. Diarrhea is a common adverse effect that is dose related and usually self-limiting (often resolving in 8 days).

Patient & Family Education

- Avoid pregnancy during misoprostol therapy; use an effective contraception method while taking drug.
- Avoid using concurrent magnesium-containing antacids because of increased incidence of diarrhea.
- Report postmenopausal bleeding to prescriber; it may be drug related.
- Drug has abortifacient property. Contact prescriber and immediately discontinue drug if you become pregnant.

MITOMYCIN

(mye-toe-mye'sin)

Mutamycin, Mytozytrex

Classification: ANTINEOPLASTIC (ANTIBIOTIC); ANTHRACYCLINE

Therapeutic: ANTINEOPLASTIC

Prototype: Doxorubicin

AVAILABILITY Solution for injection

ACTION & *THERAPEUTIC EFFECT* Potent antibiotic antineoplastic effective in certain tumors unresponsive to surgery, radiation, or other agents. It selectively inhibits synthesis of DNA. At high concentrations, cellular and enzymatic RNA as well as protein synthesis are suppressed. *Highly destructive to rapidly proliferating cells and slowly developing carcinomas.*

USES In combination with other chemotherapeutic agents in palliative, adjunctive treatment of disseminated adenocarcinoma of breast, pancreas, or stomach, squamous cell carcinoma of head, neck, lung, and cervix. Not recommended to replace surgery or radiotherapy or as a single primary therapeutic agent.

CONTRAINDICATIONS Hypersensitivity or idiosyncratic reaction; severe bone marrow suppression; coagulation disorders or bleeding tendencies; over-hydration; pregnancy (category D); lactation.

CAUTIOUS USE Renal impairment; myelosuppression; pulmonary disease or respiratory insufficiency; older adults; children.

ROUTE & DOSAGE

Cancer

Adult/Child: **IV** 10–20 mg/m^2/day as a single dose q6–8wk, additional doses based on hematologic response

Renal Impairment Dosage Adjustment

CrCl less than 10 mL/min: Use 75% of dose

M

ADMINISTRATION

Intravenous

Note: Verify correct IV concentration and rate of infusion/injection for administration to children with prescriber.

PREPARE: **Direct:** Reconstitute each 5 mg vial with 10 mL sterile water for injection. Shake to dissolve. If product does not clear immediately, allow to stand at room temperature until solution is obtained. Reconstituted solution is purple. **IV Infusion:** Reconstituted solution may be further diluted to concentrations of 20–40 mcg in D5W, NS, or LR.

ADMINISTER: **Direct:** Give reconstituted solution over 5–10 min or longer. **IV Infusion:** Give over 10 min or longer as determined by total volume of solution. ▪ D5W IV solutions **must be** infused within 3 h of preparation (see storage, below). ▪ Monitor IV site closely. Avoid extravasation to prevent extreme tissue reaction (cellulitis) to the toxic drug.

INCOMPATIBILITIES: **Solution/additive:** DEXTROSE-CONTAINING SOLUTIONS, **bleomycin. Y-site: Aztreonam, cefepime, etoposide, filgrastim, gemcitabine, piperacillin/tazobactam, sargramo-stim, topotecan, vinorelbine.**

▪ Store drug reconstituted with sterile water for injection (0.5 mg/mL) for 14 days refrigerated or 7 days at room temperature. ▪ Drug diluted in D5W (20–40 mcg/mL) is stable at room temperature for 3 h.

ADVERSE EFFECTS

Respiratory: Acute bronchospasm, hemoptysis, dyspnea, nonproductive cough, pneumonia, interstitial pneumonitis. **CNS:** Paresthesias. **Skin:** Desquamation; induration, pain, necrosis, cellulitis at injection site; reversible alopecia, purple discoloration of nail beds. **GI:** Stomatitis, *nausea, vomiting,* anorexia, hematemesis, diarrhea. **GU:** Hemolytic uremic syndrome, renal toxicity. **Hematologic:** Bone marrow toxicity (*thrombocytopenia, leukopenia* occurring 4–8 wk after treatment onset), thrombophlebitis, anemia. **Other:** Pain, headache, fatigue, edema.

PHARMACOKINETICS

Metabolism: Metabolized rapidly in liver. **Elimination:** In urine. **Half-Life:** 23–78 min.

NURSING IMPLICATIONS

Black Box Warning

Mitomycin has been associated with severe bone marrow suppression, serious infections, hemorrhage, and irreversible renal failure.

Assessment & Drug Effects

- Withhold drug and notify prescriber if serum creatinine is greater than 1.7 mg/dL or if platelet count falls below 150,000/mm^3 and WBC is down to 4000/mm^3 or if prothrombin or bleeding times are prolonged.
- Monitor I&O ratio and pattern. Report any sign of impaired kidney function: Change in ratio, dysuria, hematuria, oliguria, frequency, urgency. Keep patient well hydrated (at least 2000–2500 mL orally daily if tolerated). Drug is nephrotoxic.
- Observe closely for signs of infection. Monitor body temperature frequently.

- Inspect oral cavity daily for signs of stomatitis or superinfection (see Appendix F).
- Monitor lab tests: Frequent CBC with differential, platelet count, Hgb, Hct, and serum creatinine during and for at least 7 wk after treatment.

Patient & Family Education

- Report to prescriber immediately if you have respiratory distress.
- Report signs of common cold to prescriber immediately.
- Understand that hair loss is reversible after cessation of treatment.

MITOTANE

(mye'toe-tane)

Lysodren

Classification: ANTINEOPLASTIC
Therapeutic: ANTINEOPLASTIC

AVAILABILITY Tablet

ACTION & *THERAPEUTIC EFFECT* Cytotoxic agent with suppressant action on the adrenal cortex. Modifies peripheral metabolism of steroids and reduces production of adrenal steroids. Extra-adrenal metabolism of cortisol is altered, leading to reduction in 17-hydroxycorticosteroids (17-OHCS); however, plasma levels of corticosteroids do not fall. *Cytotoxic agent with suppressant action on the adrenal cortex.*

USES Inoperable adrenal cortical carcinoma (functional and nonfunctional).

UNLABELED USES Cushing's syndrome.

CONTRAINDICATIONS Shock, severe trauma; lactation.

CAUTIOUS USE Liver disease; infection; preexisting neurologic disease; pregnancy (category C); children.

ROUTE & DOSAGE

Adrenocortical Carcinoma

Adult: **PO** Initially 1–6 g/day in divided doses tid or qid then increased to 9–10 g/day in divided doses (tolerated dose range: 2–16 g/day)

ADMINISTRATION

Oral

- Alert: Withhold temporarily and consult prescriber if shock or trauma occurs, since adrenal suppression is its prime action. Exogenous steroids may be required until the already depressed adrenal starts secreting steroids.
- Store at 15°–30° C (59°–86° F) in tight, light-resistant containers.

ADVERSE EFFECTS **CV:** Hypertension, hypotension, flushing **CNS:** Vertigo, dizziness, drowsiness, tiredness, depression, *lethargy, sedation,* headache, confusion, tremors. **HEENT:** Blurred vision, diplopia, lens opacity, toxic retinopathy. **Endocrine:** Adrenocortical insufficiency. *Hypouricemia, hypercholesterolemia.* **Skin:** *Rash,* cutaneous eruptions and pigmentation. **GI:** *Anorexia, nausea, vomiting, diarrhea.* **GU:** Hematuria, hemorrhagic cystitis, albuminuria. **Other:** Generalized aching, fever, muscle twitching, hypersensitivity reactions, hyperpyrexia.

DIAGNOSTIC TEST INTERFERENCE

Mitotane decreases ***protein-bound iodine (PBI)*** and ***urinary 17-OHCS levels.***

INTERACTIONS

Drug: Potentiates sedative effects of **alcohol** and other CNS DEPRESSANTS; may increase the metabolism of **phenytoin, phenobarbital, warfarin,** decreasing their effectiveness. POTASSIUM SPARING DIURETICS may decrease the effect.

PHARMACOKINETICS

Absorption: Approximately 40% absorbed from GI tract. **Onset:** 2–4 wk. **Peak:** 3–5 h. **Distribution:** Deposits in most body tissues, especially adipose tissue. **Metabolism:** In liver. **Elimination:** 10% in urine, 1–17% in feces. **Half-Life:** 18–159 days.

M

NURSING IMPLICATIONS

Assessment & Drug Effects

- Monitor pulse and BP for early signs of shock (adrenal insufficiency).
- Observe for symptoms of hepatotoxicity (see Appendix F). Report them promptly, since reduced hepatic capacity can increase toxicity of mitotane and because dose may have to be decreased.
- Notify prescriber if following persist and become more severe: Aching muscles, fever, flushing, and muscle twitching.
- Monitor obese patient for symptoms of adrenal hypofunction. Because a large portion of the drug deposits in fatty tissue, the obese are particularly susceptible to prolonged adverse effects.
- Make neurologic and behavioral assessments at regular intervals throughout therapy.

Patient & Family Education

- Be aware that mitotane does not cure but does reduce tumor mass, pain, weakness, anorexia, and steroid symptoms.
- Report symptoms of adrenal insufficiency (weakness, fatigue, orthostatic hypotension, pigmentation, weight loss, dehydration, anorexia, nausea, vomiting, and diarrhea) to prescriber.
- Exercise caution when driving or performing potentially hazardous tasks requiring alertness because of drug-induced drowsiness, tiredness, dizziness. Symptoms tend to recede with continuation in therapy.

MITOXANTRONE HYDROCHLORIDE

(mi-tox'an-trone)

Novantrone

Classification: ANTINEOPLASTIC
Therapeutic: ANTINEOPLASTIC; IMMUNOSUPPRESSANT
Prototype: Doxorubicin

AVAILABILITY

Solution for injection

ACTION & *THERAPEUTIC EFFECT*

Non-cell-cycle specific antitumor agent with less cardiotoxicity than doxorubicin. Interferes with DNA synthesis by intercalating with the DNA double helix, blocking effective DNA and RNA transcription. *Highly destructive to rapidly proliferating cells in all stages of cell division.*

USES

In combination with other drugs for the treatment of acute nonlymphocytic leukemia (ANLL) in adults, bone pain in advanced prostate cancer. Reducing neurologic disability and/or frequency of clinical relapses in multiple sclerosis.

UNLABELED USES Breast cancer, non-Hodgkin's lymphomas, autologous bone marrow transplant.

CONTRAINDICATIONS Hypersensitivity to mitoxantrone; myelosuppression; baseline LVEF less than 50%; multiple sclerosis; pregnancy (category D); lactation.

CAUTIOUS USE Impaired cardiac function; impaired liver and kidney function; systemic infections; previous treatment with daunorubicin or doxorubicin due to increased possibility of decreased cardiac function; children.

ROUTE & DOSAGE

Combination Therapy (with Cytarabine) for ANLL

Adult: **IV Induction Therapy** 12 mg/m^2/day on days 1–3, may need to repeat induction course; **IV Consolidation Therapy** 12 mg/m^2 on days 1 and 2 (max lifetime dose: 80–120 mg/m^2)

Prostate Cancer

Adult: **IV** 12–14 mg/m^2 q21days

Multiple Sclerosis

Adult: **IV** 12 mg/m^2 q3mo (max lifetime dose: 140 mg/m^2) Discontinue drug in MS patients if LVEF drops below 50% or if there is a clinically significant reduction in LVEF.

ADMINISTRATION

Intravenous

If mitoxantrone touches skin, wash immediately with copious amounts of warm water.

PREPARE: **IV Infusion: Must be** diluted prior to use. Withdraw contents of vial and add to at least 50 mL of D5W or NS. ▪ May be diluted to larger volumes to extend infusion time. ▪ Use goggles, gloves, and protective gown during drug preparation and administration.

ADMINISTER: **IV Infusion:** Administer into the tubing of a freely running IV of D5W or NS and infused over at least 3 min or longer (i.e., 30–60 min) depending on the total volume of IV solution. ▪ If extravasation occurs, stop infusion and immediately restart in another vein.

INCOMPATIBILITIES: Solution/additive: **Heparin, hydrocortisone, paclitaxel.** Y-site: **Amphotericin B cholesteryl complex, ampicillin, ampicillin/sulbactam, atenolol, azithromycin, aztreonam, cefazolin, cefoperazone, ceftaxime, cefoxitin, ceftazidime, ceftriaxone, cefuroxime, clindamycin, dantrolene, dexamethasone, diazepam, digoxin, cefepime, doxorubicin liposome, ertapenem, foscarnet, fosphenytion, furosemide, gemtuzumab, heparin, idarubicin, lansoprazole, methylprednisolone, nafcillin, nitroprusside, paclitaxel, pantoprazole, pemetrexed, phenytoin, piperacillin/tazobactam, propofol, ticarcillin, voriconazole, TPN.**

M

▪ Discard unused portions of diluted solution. ▪ Once opened, multiple-use vials may be stored refrigerated at 2°–8° C (35°–46° F) for 14 days.

ADVERSE EFFECTS **CV:** Arrhythmias, decreased left ventricular function, *CHF*, tachycardia, ECG changes, MI (occurs with cumulative doses of greater than 80–100 mg/m^2), edema, increased risk of cardiotoxicity. **GI:** *Nausea, vomiting,* constipation, diarrhea, hepatotoxicity. **Hematologic:** Leukopenia, thrombocytopenia. **Other:** Discolors urine and sclera a blue-green color. **Skin:** Mild phlebitis, blue skin discoloration, alopecia.

INTERACTIONS **Drug:** May impair immune response to VACCINES such as influenza and pneumococcal infections. May have increased risk of infection with **yellow fever vaccine.**

PHARMACOKINETICS **Distribution:** Rapidly taken up by tissues and slowly released into plasma, 95% protein bound. **Metabolism:** In liver. **Elimination:** Primarily in bile. **Half-Life:** 37 h.

NURSING IMPLICATIONS

Black Box Warning

Mitoxantrone has been associated with potentially fatal CHF that may occur during therapy or months to years after end of therapy; extravasation has been associated with severe, local tissue damage.

Assessment & Drug Effects

- Monitor IV insertion site. Transient blue skin discoloration may occur at site if extravasation has occurred.
- Monitor cardiac functioning throughout course of therapy including LVEF; report signs and symptoms of CHF or cardiac arrhythmias.
- Monitor lab tests: Baseline and periodic LFTs and CBC with differential.

Patient & Family Education

- Understand potential adverse effects of mitoxantrone therapy.
- Expect urine to turn blue-green for 24 h after drug administration; sclera may also take on a bluish color.
- Be aware that stomatitis/mucositis may occur within 1 wk of therapy.
- Do not risk exposure to those with known infections during the periods of myelosuppression.

MODAFINIL

(mod-a′fi-nil)

Provigil, Alertec ♣

ARMODAFINIL

Nuvigil

Classification: CNS STIMULANT, ANALEPTIC

Therapeutic: CNS STIMULANT; ANTINARCOLEPTIC

Controlled Substance: Schedule IV

AVAILABILITY Tablet

ACTION & THERAPEUTIC EFFECT

Primary sites of CNS stimulant activity of modafinil appear to be in the hippocampus, the centrolateral nucleus of the thalamus, and the central nucleus of the amygdala. Modafinil may increase excitatory transmission in the thalamus and hippocampus. *Modafinil causes wakefulness, increased locomotor activity, and psychoactive and euphoric effects.*

USES Improve wakefulness in patients with narcolepsy or excessive sleepiness associated with shift work sleep disorder, obstructive sleep apnea/hypopnea syndrome.

UNLABELED USES Fatigue related to organic brain syndrome or multiple sclerosis, ADHD.

CONTRAINDICATIONS Hypersensitivity to modafinil.

CAUTIOUS USE Cardiovascular disease including left ventricular hypertrophy; cardiac disease, ischemic ECG changes, chest pain, arrhythmias, mitral valve prolapse, recent MI, unstable angina; history of drug or alcohol abuse; psychosis or emotional instability, depression, mania; neurologic disease, Tourette syndrome; severe hepatic impairment; renal impairment; sleep apnea; older adults; pregnancy (category C); lactation (infant risk cannot be ruled out); Safety and efficacy in children under 18 y not established.

ROUTE & DOSAGE

Narcolepsy, Fatigue

Adult: **PO (Provigil)** 200 mg/each morning; **(Nuvigil)** 150 or 250 mg each morning

Shift Work Sleep Disorder

Adult: **PO (Provigil)** 200 mg 1 h prior to shift; **(Nuvigil)** 150 mg 1 h prior to shift

Obstructive Sleep Apnea

Adult: **PO (Nuvigil)** 150 mg each morning

Hepatic Impairment Dosage Adjustment

Reduce dose by 50%

ADMINISTRATION

Oral

- Give in the morning shortly after awakening.
- Store at 20°–25° C (68°–77° F).

ADVERSE EFFECTS **Respiratory:** Rhinitis. **CNS:** Dizziness, *headache*, insomnia, anxiety, feeling nervous. **GI:** Nausea. **Musculoskeletal:** Back pain.

INTERACTIONS **Drug: Methylphenidate** may delay absorption of modafinil; modafinil may decrease levels of **cyclosporine,** ORAL CONTRACEPTIVES; modafinil may increase levels of **clomipramine, phenytoin, warfarin,** TRICYCLIC ANTIDEPRESSANTS. Do not take with **ritonavir.** Do not take with other CNS STIMULANTS. May decrease concentration of other medications metabolized by CYP3A4.

PHARMACOKINETICS **Absorption:** Rapidly absorbed. **Peak:** 2–4 h. **Distribution:** Approximately 60% protein bound. **Metabolism:** In liver to inactive metabolites via CYP 3A4. **Elimination:** In urine. **Half-Life:** 15 h.

NURSING IMPLICATIONS

Assessment & Drug Effects

- Therapeutic effectiveness: Indicated by improved daytime wakefulness.
- Monitor BP and cardiovascular status, especially with preexisting hypertension and mitral valve prolapse or other CV condition.
- Monitor for S&S of psychosis, especially when history of psychotic episodes exists.
- Coadministered drugs: Monitor INR with warfarin for first several months and when dosage is changed; monitor for toxicity with phenytoin.
- Monitor lab tests: CBC, periodic LFTs.

Patient & Family Education

- Use barrier contraceptive instead of/in addition to hormonal contraceptive.
- Inform prescriber of all prescription or OTC drugs in/added to your regimen.
- Notify prescriber if any S&S of an allergic reaction appear.

M

MOEXIPRIL HYDROCHLORIDE

(mo-ex'i-pril)

Classification: ANGIOTENSIN-CONVERTING ENZYME (ACE) INHIBITOR; ANTIHYPERTENSIVE
Therapeutic: ANTIHYPERTENSIVE
Prototype: Enalapril

AVAILABILITY Tablet

ACTION & *THERAPEUTIC EFFECT* ACE inhibitor that results in decreased conversion of angiotensin I to angiotensin II. Results in decreased vasopressor activity and aldosterone secretion. Lowering angiotensin II plasma levels results in blood pressure decreases and plasma renin activity increases. *ACE inhibition and decreased aldosterone secretion are responsible for its antihypertensive effect.*

USES Hypertension.

UNLABELED USES Stable coronary artery disease, non-ST-elevation acute coronary syndrome.

CONTRAINDICATIONS Hypersensitivity to moexipril; history of angioedema related to an ACE inhibitor; pregnancy—fetal injury has been reported; lactation—infant risk cannot be ruled out.

CAUTIOUS USE Hypersensitivity to any other ACE inhibitor; ischemic heart disease, aortic stenosis, or cerebrovascular disease; renal impairment, renal artery stenosis, volume-depleted patients; hypertensive patient with CHF; history of autoimmune disease; severe liver dysfunction; immunosuppressed patients; hyperkalemia; patients undergoing surgery/anesthesia; preexisting neutropenia; black patients; safety and efficacy in children not established.

ROUTE & DOSAGE

Hypertension

Adult: **PO** 3.75–7.5 mg once/day, may increase up to 30 mg/day in divided doses

Renal Impairment Dosage Adjustment

CrCl 40 mL/min or less: Start with 3.75 mg daily (max: Titrate up to 15 mg daily)

ADMINISTRATION

Oral

- Give 1 h before meals. Food greatly reduces absorption of moexipril.

- May need to reduce starting dose 50% in patients with possible volume depletion or a history of renal insufficiency.
- Store in a tightly closed container at 15°–30° C (59°–86° F). Protect from moisture.

ADVERSE EFFECTS (≥5%) Respiratory: *Cough* Other: *Influenza-like symptoms.*

DIAGNOSTIC TEST INFERENCE: May increase BUN, creatinine, potassium, positive Coomb'; may cause false-positive results in urine acetone determinations; may lead to false-negative aldosterone/renin ratio.

INTERACTIONS Drug: NSAIDS may reduce antihypertensive effects. May increase **lithium** levels and toxicity. ANTIHYPERTENSIVE AGENTS may increase hypotensive effects. POTASSIUM SUPPLEMENTS and POTASSIUM SPARING DIURETICS may increase risk of hyperkalemia. Enhance toxic effects of **iron dextran**. **Food:** Food greatly reduces absorption of moexipril.

PHARMACOKINETICS Absorption: Readily absorbed from GI tract; approximately 13% of active metabolite reaches systemic circulation; absorption greatly reduced by food. **Onset:** 1 h. **Duration:** 24 h. **Distribution:** Approximately 50% protein bound. **Metabolism:** In liver to moexiprilat (active metabolite). **Elimination:** 13% in urine, 53% in feces. **Half-Life:** 2–9 h.

NURSING IMPLICATIONS

Black Box Warning

Moexipril has been associated with fetal injury and death.

Assessment & Drug Effects

- Monitor closely for systematic hypotension that may occur within 1–3 h of first dose, especially in those with high blood pressure, on a diuretic or restricted salt intake, or otherwise volume depleted.
- Monitor BP and HR frequently during initiation of therapy, whenever a diuretic is added, and periodically throughout therapy.
- Determine trough BP (just before next dose) before dose adjustments are made.
- Monitor for and report promptly significant behavioral changes and/or neuropsychiatric events.
- Monitor lab tests: Periodic serum electrolytes, uric acid, calcium levels, WBC with differential, Hct and Hgb, fasting blood glucose, urinalysis, LFTs, and renal function tests.

Patient & Family Education

- Report to prescriber immediately if you suspect you are pregnant.
- Review adverse effects with patient and/or caregiver.
- Report to prescriber immediately swelling around face or neck or in extremities.
- Report S&S of hypotension (e.g., dizziness, weakness, syncope); nonproductive cough; skin rash; flu-like symptoms; jaundice; irregular heartbeat or chest pains; and dehydration from vomiting, diarrhea, or diaphoresis.
- Report promptly behavioral changes (e.g., aggression, anxiety, hostility, mood changes, insomnia, memory impairment).

MOMETASONE FUROATE

(mo-met'a-sone)

Asmanex, Elocon, Nasonex

See Appendix A-3.

MONTELUKAST
(mon-te-lu′cast)
Singulair
Classification: LEUKOTRIENE INHIBITOR
Therapeutic: BRONCHODILATOR
Prototype: Zafirlukast

AVAILABILITY Tablet; chewable tablet; oral granules

ACTION & *THERAPEUTIC EFFECT* Selective receptor antagonist of leukotriene, thus inhibiting bronchoconstriction. Leukotrienes (inflammatory agents) induce bronchoconstriction and mucus production. Elevated sputum and blood levels of leukotrienes are present during acute asthma attacks. Montelukast controls asthmatic attacks by inhibiting leukotriene release as well as inflammatory action associated with the attack. *Effectiveness is indicated by improved pulmonary functions and better controlled asthmatic symptoms.*

USES Prophylaxis and chronic treatment of asthma or allergic rhinitis; exercise induced bronchoconstriction (EIB).

UNLABELED USES Refractory urticaria, atopic dermatitis.

CONTRAINDICATIONS Hypersensitivity to montelukast; acute asthma attacks; bronchoconstriction due to acute asthma; status asthmaticus; suicidal ideation.

CAUTIOUS USE Hypersensitivity to other leukotriene receptor antagonists (e.g., zafirlukast, zileuton); history of mental illness; history of suicidal thoughts or behavior; severe liver disease; jaundice, PKU; severe asthma; pregnancy (category B); lactation; (infant risk cannot be ruled out). Children younger than 6 mo.

ROUTE & DOSAGE

Asthma
Adult/Adolescent: **PO** 10 mg daily in evening
Child (12 mo–5 y): **PO** 4 mg daily in evening; *6–14 y:* 5 mg chewable tablet daily in evening

EIB
Adult/Adolescent (15 y or older): **PO** 10 mg 2 h before exercise (not more than 1/day)
Child (6–14 y): **PO** 5 mg 2 h before exercise

Allergic Rhinitis
Adult/Adolescent: **PO** 10 mg daily
Child (6–14 y): **PO** 5 mg daily; *6 mo–5 y:* 4 mg daily

ADMINISTRATION

Oral
- Give in the evening for maximum effectiveness.
- Ensure chewable tablets for children are not swallowed whole.
- Store at 15°–30° C (59°–86° F) in a tightly closed container and protect from light.

ADVERSE EFFECTS **CNS:** Headache.

INTERACTIONS **Drugs:** Do not use with **loxapine**.

PHARMACOKINETICS **Absorption:** Rapidly absorbed from GI tract, bioavailability 64%. **Peak:** 3–4 h for oral tablet, 2–2.5 h for chewable tablet. **Distribution:** Greater than 99% protein bound.

M

Metabolism: Extensively metabolized by CYP3A4 and 2C9. **Elimination:** In feces. **Half-Life:** 2.7–5.5 h.

NURSING IMPLICATIONS

Assessment & Drug Effects

- Monitor effectiveness carefully when used in combination with phenobarbital or other potent cytochrome P450 enzyme inducers.
- Lab test: Periodic liver function tests.

Patient & Family Education

- Do not use for reversal of an acute asthmatic attack.
- Inform prescriber if short-acting inhaled bronchodilators are needed more often than usual with montelukast.
- Use chewable tablets (contain phenylalanine) with caution with PKU.
- Report changes in mood, suicidal ideation, depression or sleep problems.

MORPHINE SULFATE

(mor′feen)

Arymo, Astramorph, DepoDur, Duramorph, Infumorph, Kadian, MS Contin, MorphaBond ER, Statex ♣

Classification: ANALGESIC; NARCOTIC (OPIATE AGONIST)

Therapeutic: NARCOTIC ANALGESIC

Controlled Substance: Schedule II

AVAILABILITY Tablet; controlled release tablet/capsule; oral solution; injection; extended release lysosomal injection; suppository

ACTION & *THERAPEUTIC EFFECT* Natural opium alkaloid with agonist activity that binds with the same receptors as endogenous opioid peptides. Narcotic agonist effects are identified with different locations of receptors: Analgesia at supraspinal level, euphoria, respiratory depression and physical dependence; analgesia at spinal level, sedation and miosis; and dysphoric, hallucinogenic, and cardiac stimulant effects. *Controls severe pain; also used as an adjunct to anesthesia.*

USES Symptomatic relief of severe acute and chronic pain.

CONTRAINDICATIONS Hypersensitivity to morphine or opiate agonists; convulsive disorders; acute or severe bronchial asthma with resuscitative equipment; severe respiratory depression; head injury; heart failure secondary to chronic lung disease; chemical-irritant-induced pulmonary edema; hypovolemia; undiagnosed acute abdominal conditions; following biliary tract surgery and surgical anastomosis; pancreatitis, known or suspected GI ileus; severe liver insufficiency; concomitant use of alcohol; hypothyroidism; within 14 days of use of MAOI; during labor for delivery of a premature infant, premature infants; pregnancy (category C all trimesters). **Release Oral Solution:** Hypersensitivity to morphine, respiratory insufficiency or depression; severe CNS depression; attack of bronchial asthma; heart failure secondary to chronic lung disease; cardiac arrhythmias; increased intracranial or cerebrospinal pressure; head injuries; brain tumor; acute alcoholism, DT; convulsive disorders; after biliary tract surgery; suspected surgical abdomen; surgical anastomosis; concomitantly with MAOIs or within 14 days of use. **ER:** Lactation.

CAUTIOUS USE Head trauma; increased cranial pressure; toxic psychosis; renal impairment; mild or moderate hepatic impairment; circulatory shock; CNS depression or coma; seizure disorders; elevated ICP; GI obstruction; mild or moderate hepatic impairment; Addison's disease; hypothyroidism; BPH; urethra stricture; psychosis; history of orthostatic hypotension in ambulatory patients; cardiac arrhythmias, CVD; ulcerative colitis; constipation; emphysema; history of acute asthma attacks, COPD; pancreatic or biliary tract disease; kyphoscoliosis; cor pulmonale; severe obesity; reduced blood volume; BPH; renal disease; history of substance abuse or alcoholism; older adults, young, or debilitated patients; children; labor, pregnancy (category C for low doses, short-term use, and not close to term); lactation.

ROUTE & DOSAGE

Pain Relief

There is substantial interpatient variability in the relative potency of different opioid products. Opioid tolerance will impact dosing.

Adult: **PO** 10–30 mg q4h prn or 15–30 mg sustained release q8–12h; **(Kadian)** dose q12–24h, increase dose prn for pain relief; **IV/IM/Subcutaneous** 2–10 mg/70 kg q3–4h; **Epidural** 5 mg given epidurally, may administer incremental doses of 1–2 mg with time between (max 10 mg q24h) **(DepoDur** only) 15 mg as single dose 30 min before surgery (max: 20 mg); **PR** 10–20 mg q4h prn

Child: **IV/IM/Subcutaneous** 0.05–0.2 mg/kg q2–4h or 0.025–2.6 mg/kg/h by continuous infusion (max: 10 mg/dose)

Renal Impairment Dosage Adjustment

Dose may need adjustment to prevent metabolite accumulation

ADMINISTRATION

Oral

- A fixed, individualized schedule is recommended when narcotic analgesic therapy is started to provide effective management; blood levels can be maintained and peaks of pain can be prevented (usually a 4-h interval is adequate).
- Lower dosages are recommended for older adult or debilitated patients.
- Do not break in half, crush, or allow sustained release tablet to be chewed.
- Do not give patient sustained release tablet within 24 h of surgery.
- Dilute oral solution in approximately 30 mL or more of fluid or semisolid food. A calibrated dropper comes with the bottle. Read labels carefully when using liquid preparation; available solutions: 20 mg/mL; 100 mg/mL.

Intramuscular/Subcutaneous

- Give undiluted.

Intravenous

Note: Verify correct IV concentration and rate of infusion/injection for administration to neonates, infants, or children with prescriber.

PREPARE: **Direct:** Dilute 2–10 mg in at least 5 mL of sterile water for injection. **Continuous:** Typically diluted to a range of 0.1–1 mg/mL. ▪ More concentrated

solutions may be required with fluid restriction.
ADMINISTER: **Direct:** Give a single dose over 4–5 min. Avoid rapid administration. **Continuous:** Infuse via a controlled infusion device at a rate determined by patient response as ordered.
INCOMPATIBILITIES: **Solution/ additive:** **Aminophylline, amobarbital, chlorothiazide, floxacillin, fluorouracil, haloperidol, heparin, meperidine, phenobarbital, phenytoin, sodium bicarbonate, thiopental sodium.** **Y-site:** **Alatrofloxacin mesylate, Alemtuzumab, amphotericin B cholesteryl complex, azathioprine, ceftobiprole, cloxacillin sodium dantrolene, diazoxide, daunorubicin citrate liposome, folic acid, ganciclovir sodium, garenoxacin mesylate, gemtuzumab, inamrinone lactate indomethacin, lansoprazole, micafungin, mitomycin, pentamidine, pentobarbital, phenytoin, sargramostim, trastuzumab.**

- Store oral and parenteral medication at 15°–30° C (59°–86° F). Avoid freezing. Refrigerate suppositories. Protect all formulations from light.

ADVERSE EFFECTS

CV: Bradycardia, palpitations, syncope; flushing of face, neck, and upper thorax; orthostatic hypotension, peripheral edema, hypertension, tachycardia, cardiac arrest. **Respiratory:** Severe respiratory depression (as low as 2–4/min) or arrest; pulmonary edema. **CNS:** Euphoria, insomnia, disorientation, visual disturbances, dysphoria, paradoxic CNS stimulation (restlessness, tremor, delirium, insomnia), convulsions (infants and children); decreased cough reflex, drowsiness, dizziness, deep sleep, coma, continuous intrathecal infusion may cause granulomas leading to paralysis, withdrawal syndrome. **HEENT:** Miosis, visual disturbances, nystagmus. **GI:** *Constipation,* anorexia, flatulence, dry mouth, biliary colic, *nausea,* vomiting, elevated transaminase levels. **GU:** Urinary retention or urgency, dysuria, oliguria, reduced libido or potency (prolonged use), amenorrhea, impotence. **Hematologic:** Precipitation of porphyria. **Other:** Hypersensitivity [*pruritus,* rash, urticaria, edema, hemorrhagic urticaria (rare), anaphylactoid reaction (rare)], sweating, skeletal muscle flaccidity; cold, clammy skin, hypothermia. Prolonged labor and respiratory depression of newborn.

DIAGNOSTIC TEST INTERFERENCE

False positive ***urine glucose*** determinations may occur using ***Benedict's solution. Plasma amylase*** and ***lipase*** determinations may be falsely positive for 24 h after use of morphine; ***transaminase levels*** may be elevated.

INTERACTIONS

Drug: CNS DEPRESSANTS, SEDATIVES, BARBITURATES, BENZODIAZEPINES, and TRICYCLIC ANTIDEPRESSANTS potentiate CNS depressant effects. Contraindicated with MAO INHIBITORS use in previous 14 days; they may precipitate hypertensive crisis. PHENOTHIAZINES may antagonize analgesia. Use with SSRIs can increase risk of serotonin syndrome. Use with **alcohol** may lead to potentially fatal overdoses (contraindicated with **Avinza**). **Herbal: Kava, valerian, St. John's wort** may increase sedation.

PHARMACOKINETICS

Absorption: Variably from GI tract. **Peak:** 60 min PO; 20–60 min PR; 50–90 min subcutaneous; 30–60 min IM; 20 minIV. **Duration:** Up to 7 h. **Distribution:** Crosses blood–brain barrier and placenta; distributed in breast milk. **Metabolism:** In liver. **Elimination:** 90% in urine in 24 h; 7–10% in bile.

NURSING IMPLICATIONS

Black Box Warning

Morphine has been associated with potentially fatal respiratory depression, high abuse potential, risk with neuraxial administration.

Assessment & Drug Effects

- Obtain baseline respiratory rate, depth, and rhythm and size of pupils before administering the drug. Respirations of 12/min or below and miosis are signs of toxicity. Withhold drug and report to prescriber.
- Observe patient closely to be certain pain relief is achieved. Record relief of pain and duration of analgesia.
- Monitor carefully those at risk for severe respiratory depression after epidural or intrathecal injection: Older adult or debilitated patients or those with decreased respiratory reserve (e.g., emphysema, severe obesity, kyphoscoliosis).
- Continue monitoring for respiratory depression for at least 24 h after each epidural or intrathecal dose.
- Assess vital signs at regular intervals. Morphine induced respiratory depression may occur even with small doses, and it increases progressively with higher doses (generally max: 90 min after subcutaneous, 30 min after IM, and 7 min after IV).
- Encourage changes in position, deep breathing, and coughing (unless contraindicated) at regularly scheduled intervals. Narcotic analgesics also depress cough and sigh reflexes and thus may induce atelectasis, especially in postoperative patients.
- Be alert for nausea and orthostatic hypotension (with light-headedness and dizziness) in ambulatory patients or when a supine patient assumes the head-up position or in patients not experiencing severe pain.
- Monitor I&O ratio and pattern. Report oliguria or urinary retention. Morphine may dull perception of bladder stimuli; therefore, encourage the patient to void at least q4h. Palpate lower abdomen to detect bladder distention.
- Monitor bowel patterns; promote oral fluids and ambulation when able to aid in prevention of constipation. May need to contact provider for stool softeners and/or laxatives as needed.

Patient & Family Education

- Avoid alcohol and other CNS depressants while receiving morphine.
- Do not use of any OTC drug unless approved by prescriber.
- Do not ambulate without assistance after receiving drug.
- Use caution or avoid tasks requiring alertness (e.g., driving a car) until response to drug is known since morphine may cause drowsiness, dizziness, or blurred vision.

MOXIFLOXACIN HYDROCHLORIDE

(mox-i-flox′a-sin)

Avelox, Moxeza, Vigamox

Classification: QUINOLONE ANTIBIOTIC

Therapeutic: ANTIBIOTIC

Prototype: Ciprofloxacin

AVAILABILITY Tablet; ophthalmic solution; solution for injection

ACTION & *THERAPEUTIC EFFECT* It inhibits DNA gyrase, an enzyme required for DNA replication, transcription, repair, and recombination of bacterial DNA. *Broad spectrum antibiotic that is bactericidal against gram-positive and gram-negative organisms.*

USES Treatment of acute bacterial sinusitis, acute bacterial exacerbation of chronic bronchitis, community-acquired pneumonia, skin and skin structure infections, plague, bacterial conjunctivitis, complicated skin infections.

UNLABELED USES Hospital acquired pneumonia, infective endocarditis, tuberculosis, plague prophylaxis.

CONTRAINDICATIONS Hypersensitivity to moxifloxacin or other quinolones; moderate to severe hepatic insufficiency; syphilis; MG; tendon pain; viral infection; history of torsades de pointes; lactation.

CAUTIOUS USE CNS disorders; history of seizures; severe cerebral arteriosclerosis; peripheral neuropathy; cerebrovascular disease, history of ventricular arrhythmias, atrial fibrillation; hypokalemia; bradycardia, acute myocardial ischemia, acute MI; colitis, diarrhea, GI disease; DM; mild or moderate heart insufficiency; QT prolongation; seizure disorder; sunlight (UV) exposure; hepatic impairment; older adults; pregnancy (category C). Safety and efficacy in children younger than 18 y not established. **Ocular preparation:** Use in children younger than 4 mo.

ROUTE & DOSAGE

Acute Bacterial Sinusitis, Acute Bacterial Exacerbation of Chronic Bronchitis, Community-Acquired Pneumonia, Skin Infections, Plague

Adult: **PO/IV** 400 mg daily × 5–14 days

Complicated Skin Infection

Adult: **PO/IV** 400 mg daily × 7–21 days

ADMINISTRATION

Oral

- Administer 4 h before or 8 h after multivitamins (containing iron or zinc), antacids (containing magnesium, calcium, or aluminum), sucralfate, or didanosine.

Intravenous

PREPARE: **IV Infusion:** Avelox (400 mg) is supplied in ready-to-use 250 mL IV bags. No further dilution is necessary.
ADMINISTER: **IV Infusion:** Give over 60 min. AVOID RAPID OR BOLUS DOSE.
INCOMPATIBILITIES: **Allopurinol, aminophylline, amphotericin B (Abelcet), ceftobiprole, dantrolene, fluorouracil, fosphenytoin, furosemide, nitroprusside, pantoprazole, phenytoin, vancomycin, voriconazole.**

- Store at 15°–30° C (59°–86° F); protect from high humidity.

ADVERSE EFFECTS CV: Arrhythmia, heart failure, QT prolongation. **CNS:** Dizziness, headache, insomnia, peripheral neuropathy. **HEENT:** Visual impairment, ocular __hemorrhage.__ **Endocrine:** Decreased amylase, decreased glucose, increased albumin, hyperchloremia. **GI:** Nausea, diarrhea, abdominal pain, vomiting, taste perversion, abnormal liver function tests, dyspepsia. **Musculoskeletal:** Tendon rupture, cartilage erosion.

DIAGNOSTIC TEST INTERFERENCE

May cause false-positive on ***opiate screening tests.***

INTERACTIONS **Drug: Iron, zinc,** ANTACIDS, **aluminum, magnesium, calcium, sucralfate** decrease absorption; use cautiously with other agents that can prolong QT interval (e.g., **erythromycin, amiodarone, bepridil, cisapride, dofetilide, procainamide, ziprasidone**).

M

PHARMACOKINETICS **Absorption:** 90% bioavailable. **Steady State:** 3 d. **Distribution:** 50% protein bound. **Metabolism:** In liver. **Elimination:** Unchanged drug: 20% in urine, 25% in feces; metabolites: 38% in feces, 14% in urine. **Half-Life:** 12 h.

NURSING IMPLICATIONS

Black Box Warning

Moxifloxacin has been associated with increased risk of tendinitis and tendon rupture.

Assessment & Drug Effects

- Monitor for and notify prescriber immediately of adverse CNS effects.
- Notify prescriber immediately for S&S of hypersensitivity (see Appendix F).
- Monitor lab tests: Baseline C&S and serum potassium with history of hypokalemia, LFTs, serum creatinine/BUN.

Patient & Family Education

- Notify prescriber immediately if you experience pain, swelling, or inflammation of a tendon, or weakness or inability to use one of your joints.
- Drink fluids liberally, unless directed otherwise.
- Increased seizure potential is possible, especially when history of seizure exists.
- Stop taking drug and notify prescriber if experiencing palpitations, fainting, skin rash, severe diarrhea, dizziness, light-headedness, vision disorders, agitation, insomnia.
- Avoid engaging in hazardous activities until reaction to drug is known.

MUPIROCIN

(mu-pi-ro'sin)

Bactroban, Bactroban Nasal, Centany

Classification: PSEUDOMONIC ACID ANTIBIOTIC

Therapeutic: ANTIBIOTIC

AVAILABILITY Ointment; cream

ACTION & *THERAPEUTIC EFFECT*

Inhibits bacterial protein synthesis by binding with the bacterial transfer RNA. *Susceptible bacteria are* Staphylococcus aureus *[including methicillin-resistant (MRSA) and beta-lactamase-producing strains] and other* Staphylococcus *and* Streptococcus pyogenes.

USES Impetigo due to *Staphylococcus aureus*, beta-hemolytic *Streptococci*, and *Streptococcus pyogenes;* nasal carriage of *S. aureus.*

UNLABELED USES Superficial skin infections; burns.

 Common adverse effects in *italic;* life-threatening effects __underlined;__ generic names in **bold;** classifications in SMALL CAPS; ♣ Canadian drug name; ● Prototype drug; ⚠ Alert

CONTRAINDICATIONS Hypersensitivity to any of its components and for ophthalmic use; lactation. **Topical:** Do not apply to breast.

CAUTIOUS USE Renal impairment; pregnancy (category B); lactation; children.

ROUTE & DOSAGE

Impetigo

Adult/Child (2 mo or older): **Topical** Apply to affected area tid, if no response in 3–5 days, reevaluate (usually continue for 1–2 wk)

Elimination of Staphylococcal Nasal Carriage

Adult/Child: **Intranasal** Apply intranasally bid for 5 days

ADMINISTRATION

Topical

- Apply thin layer of medication to affected area. Wash hands before and after application.
- Cover area being treated with a gauze dressing if desired.

ADVERSE EFFECTS **CNS:** Headache. **HEENT:** Intranasal, local stinging, soreness, dry skin, pruritus. **Skin:** Burning, stinging, pain, pruritus, rash, erythema, dry skin, tenderness, swelling.

INTERACTIONS **Drug:** Incompatible with **salicylic acid 2%**; do not mix in HYDROPHILIC VEHICLES (e.g., **Aquaphor**) or COAL TAR SOLUTIONS; **chloramphenicol** may interfere with bactericidal action of mupirocin.

PHARMACOKINETICS **Absorption:** Not systemically absorbed.

NURSING IMPLICATIONS

Assessment & Drug Effects

- Watch for signs and symptoms of superinfection (see Appendix F). Prolonged or repeated therapy may result in superinfection by nonsusceptible organisms.
- Reevaluate drug use if patient does not show clinical response within 3–5 days.
- Discontinue the drug and notify prescriber if signs of contact dermatitis develop or if exudate production increases.

Patient & Family Education

- Discontinue drug and contact prescriber if a sensitivity reaction or chemical irritation occurs (e.g., increased redness, itching, burning).

NABILONE

(nab'i-lone)

Classification: SYNTHETIC CANNABINOID; ANTIEMETIC
Therapeutic: ANTIEMETIC
Prototype: Aprepitant
Controlled Substance: Schedule II

AVAILABILITY Capsule

ACTION & *THERAPEUTIC EFFECT* Nabilone is a synthetic cannabinoid with multiple effects on the CNS. It is thought that the antiemetic effect results from its interaction with the cannabinoid receptor system (CB1-receptor) in neural tissues. In therapeutic doses, it produces relaxation, drowsiness, and euphoria. *It effectively controls emesis in patients receiving chemotherapy when other drugs have failed.*

USES Refractory nausea and vomiting.

CONTRAINDICATIONS Hypersensitivity to any cannabinoid; hypovolemia; safety and efficacy not established in children younger than 18 y; pregnancy—fetal risk cannot be ruled out; lactation—infant risk cannot be ruled out.

CAUTIOUS USE History of psychiatric disorders; history of heart disease; hepatic dysfunction; history of substance abuse; older adults.

ROUTE & DOSAGE

Nausea and Vomiting

Adult: **PO** Initial dose of 1 or 2 mg bid. May increase (max: 2 mg tid)

ADMINISTRATION

Oral

- Give 1–3 h before chemotherapy is begun. A dose of 1–2 mg the night before chemotherapy may be helpful in relieving nausea.
- Store at 25 degrees C (77 degrees F), excursions permitted between 15°–30° C (59°–86° F).

ADVERSE EFFECTS **CV:** *Hypotension*. **CNS:** Asthenia, *ataxia, confusion difficulties, drowsiness, headache, sedation, vertigo*. **HEENT:** *Visual disturbances*. **GI:** *Dry mouth*. **Other:** *Dysmorphic mood, euphoria*.

INTERACTIONS **Drug:** SEDATIVES, HYPNOTICS, and other psychoactive substances can potentiate the CNS effects of nabilone. Coadministration of cannabinoids with **amphetamine**, TRICYCLIC ANTIDEPRESSANTS, and/or SYMPATHOMIMETIC AGENTS can produce additive hypertension and tachycardia. **Obinutuzumab** may increase hypotensive effects. **Food: Alcohol** can potentiate the CNS effects of nabilone.

PHARMACOKINETICS **Absorption:** Complete absorption from GI tract. **Peak:** 2 h. **Metabolism:** Extensive hepatic metabolism. **Elimination:** Fecal (major) and urine. **Half-Life:** 2 h.

NURSING IMPLICATIONS

Assessment & Drug Effects

- Monitor for and report S&S of adverse psychiatric reactions (e.g., disorientation, hallucinations, psychosis) for 48–72 h after last dose of nabilone.
- Monitor for S&S of tachycardia and postural hypotension, especially in the older adult and those with a history of heart disease or hypertension.

Patient & Family Education

- Do not use alcohol or other CNS depressants while using this medication.
- Do not drive or engage in potentially hazardous activities until response to drug is known.
- Instruct patient to rise slowly from sitting/supine position.
- Report any of the following to a health care provider: Confusion, disorientation, hallucinations, or other bizarre behavior.

NABUMETONE

(na-bu-me'tone)

Classification: NON-STEROIDAL ANTI-INFLAMMATORY DRUG (NSAID)
Therapeutic: ANALGESIC, NSAID; ANTIRHEUMATIC; ANTIPYRETIC
Prototype: Ibuprofen

AVAILABILITY Tablet

ACTION & *THERAPEUTIC EFFECT* Blocks prostaglandin synthesis by inhibiting cyclooxygenase, an enzyme that converts arachidonic acid to precursors of prostaglandins. *Anti-inflammatory, analgesic, and antipyretic effects. Effective antirheumatic agent. Inhibits platelet aggregation and prolongs bleeding time.*

USES Rheumatoid arthritis and osteoarthritis.

CONTRAINDICATIONS Patients in whom urticaria, severe rhinitis, bronchospasm, angioedema, or nasal polyps are precipitated by aspirin or other NSAIDS; salicylate hypersensitivity; active peptic ulcer; bleeding abnormalities; CABG perioperative pain; lactation (infant risk cannot be ruled out).

CAUTIOUS USE Hypertension, fluid retention, heart failure; first MI, history of GI ulceration, impaired liver or kidney function, chronic kidney failure, cardiac decompensation, history of preexisting asthma, bone marrow suppression; patients with SLE; elderly; pregnancy (category C). Safety and efficacy in children not established.

ROUTE & DOSAGE

Rheumatoid & Osteoarthritis

Adult: **PO** 1000 mg/day or 500 mg bid may increase (max: 2000 mg/day)

Renal Impairment Dosage Adjustment

CrCl 30–49 mL/min: max daily dose: 1500 mg/day; *less than 30 mL/min:* max daily dose: 1000 mg/day

ADMINISTRATION

Oral

- Give with food, milk, or antacid (if prescribed) to reduce the possibility of GI upset.
- Store at 20° C–25° C (68° F–77° F). Protect from light.

ADVERSE EFFECTS **CV:** Edema. **CNS:** Dizziness, headache. **HEENT:** Tinnitus. **Skin:** Pruritis, rash. **Hepatic:** Increased LFTs. **GI:** Abdominal pain, constipation, diarrhea, flatulence, indigestion, nausea, occult blood in stools.

INTERACTIONS **Drug:** May attenuate the antihypertensive response to DIURETICS. Has additive bleeding risk with ANTICOAGULANTS. NSAIDS increase the risk of **methotrexate** toxicity. Do not use with **cidofovir** or **ketorolac.** Do not use with photosensitizing agents. **Food:** Food may increase the peak but not the overall absorption of nabumetone. Alcohol usage can increase risk of gastric irritation. **Herbal:** **Feverfew, garlic, ginger, ginkgo** may increase bleeding potential.

PHARMACOKINETICS **Absorption:** Readily absorbed from GI tract; approximately 35% is converted to its active metabolite on first pass through the liver. **Onset:** 1–3 wk for antirheumatic action. **Peak:** 3–6 h. **Distribution:** 99% protein bound; distributes into synovial fluid. **Metabolism:** In liver to its active metabolite, 6-methoxy-2-naphthylacetic acid (6MNA). **Elimination:** 80% of dose is excreted in urine as 6MNA; 10% excreted in feces. **Half-Life:** 24 h (6MNA).

NURSING IMPLICATIONS

Black Box Warning

Nabumetone has been associated with increased risk of serious, potentially fatal, GI bleeding and cardiovascular events (e.g., MI & CVA); risk may increase with duration of use and may be greater in the older adult and those with risk factors for CV disease.

Assessment & Drug Effects

- Monitor for signs and symptoms of GI bleeding.
- Monitor for and report promptly S&S of CV thrombotic events (i.e., angina, MI, TIA, or stroke).
- Monitor lab tests: Baseline and periodic Hgb and Hct with prolonged or high-dose therapy; CBC, LFTs, serum creatinine/BUN, stool guaiac.

Patient & Family Education

- Use caution with hazardous activities since nabumetone may cause dizziness, drowsiness, and blurred vision.
- Report abdominal pain, nausea, dyspepsia, or black tarry stools.
- Stop taking drug and report promptly to prescriber if you experience chest pain, shortness of breath, weakness, slurring of speech, or other signs of a cardiac or neurologic problem.
- Be aware that alcohol and aspirin will increase the risk of GI ulceration and bleeding.
- Notify your prescriber if any of the following occur: Persistent headache, skin rash or itching, visual disturbances, weight gain, or edema.

NADOLOL

(nay-doe'lole)

Corgard

Classification: BETA-ADRENERGIC ANTAGONIST; ANTIHYPERTENSIVE

Therapeutic: ANTIHYPERTENSIVE

Prototype: Propranolol

AVAILABILITY Tablet

ACTION & *THERAPEUTIC EFFECT*

Nonselective beta-adrenergic blocking agent that inhibits response to adrenergic stimuli by competitively blocking these receptors within the heart. Reduces heart rate and cardiac output at rest and during exercise, and also decreases conduction velocity through AV node and myocardial automaticity. *Decreases both systolic and diastolic BP at rest and during exercise.*

USES Hypertension, either alone or in combination with a diuretic. Also long-term prophylactic management of angina pectoris.

CONTRAINDICATIONS Bronchial asthma, severe COPD, inadequate myocardial function, sinus bradycardia, greater than first-degree conduction block, overt cardiac failure, cardiogenic shock; abrupt withdrawal; lactation.

CAUTIOUS USE CHF; DM; ischemic heart disease; hyperthyroidism; renal failure, renal impairment; pregnancy (category C); children younger than 18 y.

ROUTE & DOSAGE

Hypertension, Angina

Adult: **PO** 40 mg once/day, may increase up to 240–320 mg/day in 1–2 divided doses

 Common adverse effects in *italic*; life-threatening effects underlined; generic names in **bold**; classifications in SMALL CAPS; ♣ Canadian drug name; Prototype drug; Alert

ADMINISTRATION

Oral

- Do not discontinue abruptly; reduce dosage over a 1–2-wk period. Abrupt withdrawal can precipitate MI or thyroid storm in susceptible patients.
- Store at 15°–30° C (59°–86° F); protect drug from light.

ADVERSE EFFECTS **CV:** *Bradycardia, peripheral vascular insufficiency (Raynaud's type),* palpitation, postural hypotension, conduction or rhythm disturbances, CHF. **CNS:** *Dizziness, fatigue,* sedation, headache, paresthesias, behavioral changes. **HEENT:** Blurred vision, dry eyes. **Skin:** Dry skin. **GI:** Dry mouth, anorexia, flatulence. **GU:** Impotence. **Other:** Hypersensitivity (rash, pruritus, laryngospasm, respiratory disturbances).

INTERACTIONS **Drug:** NSAIDS may decrease hypotensive effects; may mask symptoms of a hypoglycemic reaction to **insulin**, SULFONYLUREAS; **prazosin, terazosin** may increase severe hypotensive response to first dose. **Amiodarone** causes additive effects.

PHARMACOKINETICS **Absorption:** 30–40% of PO dose absorbed. **Peak:** 2–4 h. **Duration:** 17–24 h. **Distribution:** Widely distributed; crosses placenta; distributed in breast milk. **Elimination:** 70% in urine; also in feces. **Half-Life:** 10–24 h.

NURSING IMPLICATIONS

Black Box Warning

Nadolol has been associated with exacerbations of ischemic heart disease following abrupt withdrawal.

Assessment & Drug Effects

- Assess heart rate and BP before administration of each dose. Withhold drug and notify prescriber if apical pulse drops below 60 bpm or systolic BP below 90 mm Hg.
- Do not abruptly stop this medication. It should be tapered off over 1–2 wk to prevent exacerbation of angina.
- Monitor for signs of CHF (e.g., cough, fatigue, dyspnea, rapid pulse, edema).
- Monitor patients with diabetes mellitus closely. Nadolol may prevent clinical manifestations of hypoglycemia (e.g., tachycardia, BP changes).
- Monitor I&O ratio and creatinine clearance in patients with impaired kidney function or with cardiac problems.

Patient & Family Education

- Check pulse before taking each dose. Do not take your medication if pulse rate drops below 60 (or other parameter set by prescriber) or becomes irregular. Consult your prescriber right away.
- Do not stop taking your medication or alter dosage without consulting your prescriber. Monitor weight. Report weight gain of 1–1.5 kg (2–3 lb) in a day and any other possible signs of CHF (e.g., cough, fatigue, dyspnea, rapid pulse, edema).
- Do not drive or engage in potentially hazardous activities until response to drug is known.

NAFARELIN ACETATE

(na-fa're-lin)

Synarel

Classification: GONADOTROPIN-RELEASING HORMONE (GnRH) ANA-LOG

Therapeutic: GnRH ANALOG

Prototype: Leuprolide

AVAILABILITY Spray solution

ACTION & THERAPEUTIC EFFECT Inhibits pituitary gonadotropin secretion of LH and FSH resulting a temporary increase in ovarian steroid hormone production. *Decrease in serum estradiol concentrations results in the quiescence of tissues and functions that depend on LH and FSH.*

USES Endometriosis and precocious puberty.

UNLABELED USES Uterine leiomyomas, benign prostatic hyperplasia.

CONTRAINDICATIONS Hypersensitivity to GnRH or GnRH agonist analog; undiagnosed abnormal vaginal bleeding; women who may become pregnant; pregnancy (category X); lactation.

CAUTIOUS USE Polycystic ovarian disease; menstruation; osteoporosis; pituitary insufficiency; children.

ROUTE & DOSAGE

Endometriosis

Adult: **Inhalation** 400 mcg in one nostril in morning and 200 mcg in other nostril in evening beginning between days 2 and 4 of menstrual cycle; if patient doesn't achieve amenorrhea after 2 mo of therapy, may increase to 200 mcg in each nostril bid; do not exceed 6 mo of treatment

Precocious Puberty

Child: **Inhalation** 400 mcg into each nostril every morning and evening. (total: 8 sprays)

ADMINISTRATION

Inhalation

- Withhold any topical nasal decongestant, if being used, until at least 2 h after nafarelin administration.
- Store at 15°–30° C (59°–86° F); protect from light.

ADVERSE EFFECTS **Respiratory:** Nasal irritation. **CNS:** Transient headache, inertia, mild depression, *moodiness,* fatigue. **Endocrine:** *Hot flashes, anovulation, decreased libido, hypocalcemia, hyperphosphatemia, hypertriglyceridemia, amenorrhea, vaginal dryness,* galactorrhea. Decreased bone mineral content (reversible). **Skin:** Acne. **GI:** *Bloating, abdominal cramps,* weight gain, nausea. **GU:** *Impotence, decreased libido,* dyspareunia.

DIAGNOSTIC TEST INTERFERENCE Increased ***alkaline phosphatase***; marked increase in ***estradiol*** in first 2 wk, then decrease to below baseline; decreased ***FSH*** and ***LH*** levels; decreased ***testosterone*** levels.

INTERACTIONS **Drugs:** Do not use with ESTROGENS or ANDROGENS. **Herbal:** Do not use with black cohosh.

PHARMACOKINETICS **Absorption:** 21% absorbed from nasal mucosa. **Onset:** 4 wk. **Peak:** 12 wk. **Duration:** 30–50 days after discontinuing drug. **Distribution:** 78–84% bound to plasma proteins; crosses placenta. **Metabolism:** Hydrolyzed in kidney. **Elimination:** 44–55% in urine over 7 days, 19–44% in feces. **Half-Life:** 2.7 h.

NURSING IMPLICATIONS

Assessment & Drug Effects

- Make appropriate inquiries about breakthrough bleeding, which may indicate that patient has missed successive drug doses.
- Monitor for and report immediately S&S of thromboembolism, including signs of TIA, CVA, or MI.
- Monitor lab tests: Blood glucose, glycosylated hemoglobin A1C, prostate-specific antigen, serum estradiol concentrations, serum gonadotropin concentrations, serum testosterone concentrations.

Patient & Family Education

- Read the information pamphlet provided with nafarelin.
- Inform prescriber if breakthrough bleeding occurs or menstruation persists.
- Use or add barrier contraceptive during treatment.

NAFCILLIN SODIUM

(naf-sill′in)

Classification: PENICILLIN ANTI-BIOTIC; PENICILLINASE-RESISTANT PENICILLIN

Therapeutic: PENICILLIN ANTIBIOTIC

Prototype: Oxacillin sodium

AVAILABILITY Solution for injection

ACTION & *THERAPEUTIC EFFECT* Interferes with synthesis of mucopeptides essential to formation and integrity of bacterial cell wall leading to bacterial cell lysis. *Effective against both penicillin-sensitive and penicillin-resistant strains of Staphylococcus aureus. Also active against pneumococci and group A beta-hemolytic streptococci.*

USES Primarily, infections caused by penicillinase-producing staphylococci.

CONTRAINDICATIONS Hypersensitivity to penicillins, cephalosporins, and other allergens; use of oral drug in severe infections, gastric dilatation, cardiospasm, or intestinal hypermotility; pregnancy—fetal risk cannot be ruled out.

CAUTIOUS USE History of or suspected atopy or allergy (eczema, hives, hay fever, asthma); GI disease; hepatic disease or impairment; renal disease; lactation—infant risk is minimal.

ROUTE & DOSAGE

Staphylococcal Infections

Adult: **IV** 1–2 g q4h × 7–10 days
Child: **IV** 50–200 mg/kg/day divided q4–6h (max: 12 g/day)
Child (weight greater than 40 kg):
Neonate: **IV** 50–100 mg/kg/day divided q6–12h

ADMINISTRATION

Intramuscular

- Reconstitute each 500 mg with 1.7 mL of sterile water for injection or NaCl injection to yield 250 mg/mL. Shake vigorously to dissolve.
- In adults: Make certain solution is clear. Select site carefully. Inject deeply into gluteal muscle. Rotate injection sites.
- In children: The preferred IM site in children younger than 3 y is the midlateral or anterolateral thigh. Check agency policy.
- Label and date vials of reconstituted solution. Remains stable for 7 days under refrigeration and for 3 days at 15°–30° C (59°–86° F).

Intravenous

Note: Vials in the *ADD-Vantage Drug Delivery System* are to be used with *ADD-Vantage* diluent containers of NS 50 and 100 mL. See the manufacturer's instructions for reconstitution and administration.

PREPARE: **Intermittent:** Reconstitute powder as for IM injection. Dilute the required dose of reconstituted solution in 100–150 mL of compatible IV solution.

ADMINISTER: **Intermittent:** Give over 30–60 min.

INCOMPATIBILITIES: **Solution/additive:** **ascorbic acid, aztreonam, bleomycin, cytarabine, gentamicin, hydrocortisone, methylprednisolone, promazine.** **Y-site:** **Alemtuzumab, amphotericin B, azathioprine, capreomycin, caspofungin, chloramphenicol, dacarbazine, dantrolene, daunorubicin, dexrazoxane, diazoxide, doxycycline, droperidol, epirubicin, fentanyl, garenoxacin, gemcitabine, haloperidol, hydroxyzine, idarubicin, inamrinone, irinotecan, meperidine, metaraminol, minocycline, mitoxantrone, mycophenolate, netilmicin, palonosetron, pentazocine, phenytoin, promethazine, protamine, pyridoxine, succinylcholine, sulfamethoxazole/trimethoprim, topotecan, vecuronium, vincristine, vinorelbine.**

- Note: Usually, limit IV therapy to 24–48 h because of the possibility of thrombophlebitis (see Appendix F), particularly in older adults.
- Discard unused portions 24 h after reconstitution.

ADVERSE EFFECTS

Endocrine: Hypokalemia (with high IV doses). **Skin:** Injection site extravasation. **GI:** *Diarrhea.* **GU:** Allergic interstitial nephritis. **Hematologic:** Eosinophilia, thrombophlebitis following IV; neutropenia (long-term therapy). **Other:** Anaphylaxis (particularly following parenteral therapy).

DIAGNOSTIC TEST INTERFERENCE

Can cause false-positive ***urine protein*** tests using *sulfosalicylic acid method* or serum protein tests, positive Coombs'-test.

INTERACTIONS

Drug: May diminish effects of **warfarin;** may decrease concentration of **CYP3A4** substrates; may increase metabolism of ESTROGENS; decreases serum concentration of **letermovir, nifedipine. Probenecid** increases serum concentrations.

PHARMACOKINETICS

Peak: 30–120 min IM; 15 min IV. **Duration:** 4–6 h IM. **Distribution:** Distributes into CNS with inflamed meninges; crosses placenta; distributed into breast milk, 90% protein bound. **Metabolism:** Enters enterohepatic circulation. **Elimination:** Primarily in feces; 10–30% in urine. **Half-Life:** 1 h.

NURSING IMPLICATIONS

Assessment & Drug Effects

- Obtain a careful history before therapy to determine any prior allergic reactions to penicillins, cephalosporins, and other allergens.
- Inspect IV site for inflammatory reaction. Also check IV site for leakage; in the older adult patient especially, loss of tissue elasticity with aging may promote extravasation around the needle.
- Monitor for fever.
- Note: Allergic reactions, principally rash, occur most commonly.
- Monitor neutrophil count. Nafcillin-induced neutropenia

(agranulocytosis) occurs commonly during third week of therapy. It may be associated with malaise, fever, sore mouth, or throat. Perform periodic assessments of liver and kidney functions during prolonged therapy.

- Be alert for signs of bacterial or fungal superinfections (see Appendix F) in patients on prolonged therapy.
- Determine IV sodium intake for patients with sodium restriction. Nafcillin sodium contains approximately 3 mEq of sodium per gram; periodic WBC with differential, renal function tests, LFTs.
- Monitor lab tests: Baseline and periodic CBC with differential; periodic LFTs, and renal function tests with nafcillin therapy longer than 2 wk.

Patient & Family Education

- Report promptly S&S of neutropenia (see Assessment & Drug Effects), superinfection, or hypokalemia (see Appendix F).
- Report severe diarrhea.
- Demonstrate competency in administering injections and remind to rotate injection sites.
- Call healthcare provider if a treatment is missed.

NAFTIFINE

(naf′ti-feen)

Naftin

Classification: ANTIBIOTIC; ANTIFUNGAL

Therapeutic: ANTIFUNGAL

Prototype: Terbinafine

AVAILABILITY Cream; gel

ACTION & *THERAPEUTIC EFFECT* Synthetic broad-spectrum antifungal agent that may be fungicidal depending on the organism. Interferes in the synthesis of ergosterol, the principal sterol in the fungus cell membrane. Ergosterol becomes depleted and membrane function is affected. *Effective against topical infections caused by fungal organisms.*

USES Tinea pedis, tinea cruris, and tinea corporis.

CONTRAINDICATIONS Hypersensitivity to naftifine; occlusive dressing.

CAUTIOUS USE Pregnancy (category B); lactation. Safety and efficacy in children not established.

ROUTE & DOSAGE

Tinea Infections

Adult: **Topical** Apply cream daily, or apply gel twice daily, up to 4 wk

ADMINISTRATION

Topical

- Gently massage into affected area and surrounding skin. Wash hands before and after application.
- Do not apply occlusive dressing unless specifically directed to do so.
- Store at 15°–30° C (59°–86° F).

ADVERSE EFFECTS **Skin:** Burning or stinging, dryness, erythema, itching, local irritation.

PHARMACOKINETICS **Absorption:** 2.5–6% absorbed through intact skin. **Onset:** 7 days. **Metabolism:** In liver. **Elimination:** In urine and feces. **Half-Life:** 2–3 days.

NURSING IMPLICATIONS

Assessment & Drug Effects

- Assess for irritation or sensitivity to cream; these are indications to discontinue use.

- Reevaluate use of drug if no improvement is noted after 4 wk.

Patient & Family Education

- Learn correct application technique.
- Avoid contact with eyes or mucous membranes.

NALBUPHINE HYDROCHLORIDE

(nal′byoo-feen)

Nubain

Classification: ANALGESIC; NARCOTIC (OPIATE AGONIST-ANTAGONIST)

Therapeutic: NARCOTIC ANALGESIC

Prototype: Pentazocine

AVAILABILITY Solution for injection

ACTION & *THERAPEUTIC EFFECT* Synthetic narcotic analgesic with agonist and weak antagonist properties that is a potent analgesic. *Analgesic action that relieves moderate to severe pain with apparently low potential for dependence.*

USES Symptomatic relief of moderate to severe pain. Also preoperative sedation analgesia and as a supplement to surgical anesthesia.

CONTRAINDICATIONS History of hypersensitivity to nalbuphine, opiate agonists; pregnancy (category D in prolonged use or in high doses at term).

CAUTIOUS USE History of emotional instability or drug abuse; head injury, increased intracranial pressure; cardiac disease; impaired respirations, COPD; GI disorders; impaired kidney or liver function; MI; biliary tract surgery; pregnancy (category B; see CONTRAINDICATIONS); lactation.

ROUTE & DOSAGE

Moderate to Severe Pain

Adult: **IV/IM/Subcutaneous** 10 mg/70 kg q3–6h prn (max: 160 mg/day)

Surgery Anesthesia Supplement

Adult: **IV** 0.3–3 mg/kg, then 0.25–0.5 mg/kg as required

ADMINISTRATION

Intramuscular/Subcutaneous

- Inject undiluted.

Intravenous

PREPARE: **Direct:** Give undiluted.
ADMINISTER: **Direct:** Give at a rate of 10 mg or fraction thereof over 3–5 min.
INCOMPATIBILITIES: **Solution/additive:** **Diazepam, dimenhydrinate, ketorolac, pentobarbital, promethazine, thiethylperazine.** **Y-site:** **Allopurinol, amphotericin B cholesteryl, cefepime, docetaxel, methotrexate, nafcillin, pemetrexed, piperacillin/tazobactam, sargramostim, sodium bicarbonate.**

- Store at 15°–30° C (59°–86° F), avoid freezing.

ADVERSE EFFECTS **CV:** Hypertension, hypotension, bradycardia, tachycardia, flushing. **Respiratory:** Dyspnea, asthma, respiratory depression. **CNS:** *Sedation, dizziness,* nervousness, depression, restlessness, crying, euphoria, dysphoria, distortion of body image, unusual dreams, confusion, hallucinations; numbness and tingling sensations, headache, vertigo. **HEENT:** Miosis, blurred vision, speech difficulty.

Skin: Pruritus, urticaria, burning sensation, *sweaty, clammy skin.* **GI:** Abdominal cramps, bitter taste, *nausea, vomiting,* dry mouth. **GU:** Urinary urgency.

INTERACTIONS **Drug: Alcohol** and other CNS DEPRESSANTS add to CNS depression.

PHARMACOKINETICS **Onset:** 2–3 min IV; 15 min IM. **Peak:** 30 min IV. **Duration:** 3–6 h. **Distribution:** Crosses placenta. **Metabolism:** In liver. **Elimination:** In urine. **Half-Life:** 5 h.

NURSING IMPLICATIONS

Assessment & Drug Effects

- Assess respiratory rate before drug administration. Withhold drug and notify prescriber if respiratory rate falls below 12.
- Watch for allergic response in persons with sulfite sensitivity.
- Administer with caution to patients with hepatic or renal impairment.
- Monitor ambulatory patients; nalbuphine may produce drowsiness.
- Watch for respiratory depression of newborn if drug is used during labor and delivery.
- Avoid abrupt termination of nalbuphine following prolonged use, which may result in symptoms similar to narcotic withdrawal: Nausea, vomiting, abdominal cramps, lacrimation, nasal congestion, piloerection, fever, restlessness, anxiety.

Patient & Family Education

- Do not drive or engage in potentially hazardous activities until response to drug is known.
- Avoid alcohol and other CNS depressants.

NALDEMEDINE

(nal-dem′e-deen)

Symproic

Classification: GI AGENT; PERIPHERALLY ACTING OPIOID ANTAGONIST

Therapeutic: GI AGENTS

AVAILABILITY Tablet

ACTION & *THERAPEUTIC EFFECT* Blocks opioid binding at mu, delta, and kappa receptors; peripherally blocks actions in GI tract. *It competitively blocks the effect of opioids on the GI tract, decreasing the constipating effects of opioids.*

USES Treatment of opioid-induced constipation in patients with chronic noncancer pain.

CONTRAINDICATIONS Severe hepatic impairment; known or suspected GI obstruction, or risk of recurrent obstruction. No well-controlled studies have been done on pregnant women. Naldemedine does cross the placenta and can cause opioid withdrawal in the fetus.

CAUTIOUS USE History of peptic ulcer disease, diverticular disease, peritoneal metasteses; disruption to blood–brain barrier; not known if safe in hepatic impairment; pregnancy; lactation (breastfeeding can resume 3 days after last dose). Efficacy has only been established in patients that have had 4 or more wk of opioid use; patients taking opioids for less than 4 wk may be less responsive. Safety and efficacy in children not established.

ROUTE & DOSAGE

Opioid-Induced Constipation

Adult: **PO** 0.2 mg daily

ADMINISTRATION

Oral

- Administer without regard to meals.
- Discontinue if treatment with the opioid pain medication is also discontinued.
- Store at 20°–25° C (68°–77° F). Protect from light.

ADVERSE EFFECTS GI: *Abdominal pain, diarrhea,* nausea, vomiting, gastroenteritis, gastrointestinal perforation. **Other:** Opioid withdrawal.

INTERACTIONS Drug: Substrate of P-glycoprotein/ABCB1, CYP3A4, and UGT1A3. Avoid use with strong CYP3A4 inducers (e.g., **carbamazepine, phenytoin, rifampin**). Avoid use with OPIOID ANTAGONISTS. **Herbal:** Avoid use with **St. John's wort**.

N

PHARMACOKINETICS Distribution: 93–94% protein bound. **Onset:** Peak concentration in 0.75 h. **Metabolism:** Primarily hepatic via CYP3A. **Elimination:** 35% in feces, 57% in urine. **Half-Life:** 11 h.

NURSING IMPLICATIONS

Assessment & Drug Effects

- Assess for symptoms of GI obstruction.
- Monitor for S&S of opioid withdrawal.
- Monitor for signs of GI perforation.

Patient & Family Education

- Report to prescriber immediately any swelling or pain in stomach, persistent diarrhea, signs of allergic reaction.
- Report to prescriber any signs of withdrawal: Muscle aches, restlessness, anxiety that may progress to nausea, vomiting, abdominal cramping, goose bumps, and excessive yawning.
- Do not take with the following drugs: **Carbamazepine, phenytoin, rifampin,** or **St. John's wort.**
- Notify prescriber if discontinuing the opioid pain medication; naldemedine is only to be taken when a person is taking opioids.
- Notify prescriber if planning to get pregnant. If taken during pregnancy, it may cause withdrawal in the unborn baby.

NALOXEGOL

(na-lox'i-gol)

Movantik

Classification: NARCOTIC (OPIATE ANTAGONIST)

Therapeutic: NARCOTIC ANTAGONIST

Prototype: Naloxone

Controlled Substance: Schedule II

AVAILABILITY Tablets

ACTION & THERAPEUTIC EFFECT A mu-opioid receptor antagonist with limited ability to cross the blood–brain barrier. *Functions peripherally in tissues such as the GI tract thereby decreasing the constipation associated with opioids.*

USES Treatment of opioid-induced constipation (OIC) in adult patients with chronic non-cancer pain.

CONTRAINDICATIONS Severe hypersensitivity to naloxegol; known or suspected GI obstruction;

severe hepatic impairment; concurrent use of strong CYP3A4 inhibitors or inducers.

CAUTIOUS USE Concurrent use of moderate CYP3A4 inhibitors; renal impairment; mild to moderate hepatic impairment; pregnancy (category C); lactation. Safety and efficacy in pediatric patients not established.

ROUTE & DOSAGE

Opioid-Induced Constipation

Adult: **PO** 25 mg once daily in the a.m.; if unable to tolerate, reduce to 12.5 mg

Renal Impairment Dosage Adjustment

CrCL less than 60 mL/min: Initial dose is 12.5 mg once daily; may increase to 25 mg once daily if well tolerated

Co-Administered Drugs Dosage Adjustment

Strong CYP3A4 inhibitors or inducers: Not recommended

Moderate CYP 3A4 inhibitors: Reduce dose to 12.5 mg once daily

ADMINISTRATION

Oral

- Give on an empty stomach at least 1 h before or 2 h after the first meal of the day.
- Tablets **must be** swallowed whole, do not crush or chew.
- Laxative should be discontinued prior to administering this drug and may be resumed after 3 days if response to naloxegol is suboptimal.
- Drug should be discontinued if opioid pain medication is also discontinued.
- Store at 15°–30° C (59°–86°F).

ADVERSE EFFECTS **CNS:** Headache. **GI:** *Abdominal pain*, diarrhea, flatulence, nausea, vomiting. **Other:** Hyperhidrosis.

INTERACTIONS **Drug:** Strong CYP3A4 inhibitors (e.g., **clarithromycin, itraconazole, ketoconazole**) and moderate CYP3A4 inhibitors (e.g., **diltiazem, erythromycin, verapamil**) will increase the levels of naloxegol and may increase the risk of adverse effects. Strong CYP3A4 inducers (e.g., **carbamazepine, rifampin**) may significantly decrease plasma levels of naloxegol. **Food: Grapefruit** or **grapefruit juice** may increase the levels of naloxegol. **Herbal: St. John's Wort** may significantly decrease plasma levels of naloxegol.

PHARMACOKINETICS **Peak:** Less than 2h. **Distribution:** Readily distributed in peripheral tissue; not plasma protein bound. **Metabolism:** In liver to inactive metabolites. **Elimination:** Fecal (68%) and renal (16%). **Half-Life:** 6–11 h.

NURSING IMPLICATIONS

Assessment & Drug Effects

- Monitor for symptoms of GI obstruction (e.g., severe, persistent, or worsening abdominal pain).
- Monitor closely for GI perforation especially in those at risk (e.g., peptic ulcer disease, diverticular disease, GI tract malignancies, peritoneal metastases).
- Monitor vital signs and report symptoms of opioid withdrawal (e.g., chills, diaphoresis, anxiety, irritability, changes in BP or HR).

Patient & Family Education

- Avoid consumption of grapefruit or grapefruit juice during treatment.

- Discontinue all maintenance laxative therapy prior to taking this drug. Laxative(s) can be used as needed if there is a poor response to naloxegol after 3 days.
- Do not breast-feed while taking this drug.

NALOXONE HYDROCHLORIDE

(nal-ox'one)

Narcan

Classification: NARCOTIC (OPIATE ANTAGONIST)

Therapeutic: NARCOTIC ANTAGONIST

AVAILABILITY Solution for injection

ACTION & *THERAPEUTIC EFFECT* A potent narcotic antagonist, essentially free of agonistic (morphine-like) properties. *Reverses the effects of opiates, including respiratory depression, sedation, and hypotension.*

USES Narcotic overdosage; complete or partial reversal of narcotic depression. Drug of choice when nature of depressant drug is not known and for diagnosis of suspected acute opioid overdosage. Challenge for opioid dependence.

UNLABELED USES Shock and to reverse alcohol-induced or clonidine-induced coma or respiratory depression.

CONTRAINDICATIONS Hypersensitivity to naloxone, naltrexone, nalmefene; respiratory depression due to nonopioid drugs; substance abuse.

CAUTIOUS USE Known or suspected narcotic dependence; brain tumor, head trauma, increased ICP; history of substance abuse; cardiac irritability; seizure disorders; pregnancy (category B); lactation.

ROUTE & DOSAGE

Opiate Overdose

Adult: **IV** 0.4–2 mg, may repeat q2–3min up to 10 mg if necessary
Child (5 y or older and weight at least 20 kg): **IV** 2 mg, may repeat q2–3min if needed
Child/Infant (weight less than 20 kg): **IV** 0.01–0.1 mg/kg, may repeat q2–3min up to 10 mg if necessary
Neonate: **IV/Subcutaneous/IM** 0.01 mg/kg, may repeat q2–3min

Postoperative Opiate Depression

Adult: **IV** 0.1–0.2 mg, may repeat q2–3min for up to 3 doses if necessary
Child: **IV** 0.005–0.01 mg/kg, may repeat q2–3min up to 3 doses if necessary

Challenge for Opioid Dependence

Adult: **IM** 0.2 mg, observe for 30 sec for signs/symptoms of withdrawal, if no signs/symptoms then 0.6 mg and observe for 20 min

ADMINISTRATION

Intramuscular/Subcutaneous

- Inject undiluted.

Intravenous

PREPARE: **Direct:** May be given undiluted. **IV Infusion:** Dilute 2 mg in 500 mL of D5W or NS to yield 4 mcg/mL (0.004 mg/mL).

ADMINISTER: **Direct:** Give bolus dose over 30 sec. **IV Infusion:** Adjust rate according to patient response.
INCOMPATIBILITIES: **Y-site: Amphotericin B cholesteryl complex, lansoprazole.**

- Use IV solutions within 24 h.
- Store at 15°–30° C (59°–86° F), protect from excessive light.

ADVERSE EFFECTS CV: Increased BP, tachycardia. **GI:** Nausea, vomiting. **Hematologic:** Elevated partial thromboplastin time. **Other:** Reversal of analgesia, tremors, hyperventilation, slight drowsiness, sweating.

INTERACTIONS Drug: Reverses analgesic effects of NARCOTIC (OPIATE) AGONISTS and NARCOTIC (OPIATE) AGONIST-ANTAGONISTS.

PHARMACOKINETICS Onset: 2 min. **Duration:** 45 min. **Distribution:** Crosses placenta. **Metabolism:** In liver. **Elimination:** In urine. **Half-Life:** 60–90 min.

NURSING IMPLICATIONS

Assessment & Drug Effects

- Observe patient closely; duration of action of some narcotics may exceed that of naloxone. Keep prescriber informed; repeat naloxone dose may be necessary.
- May precipitate opiate withdrawal if administered to a patient who is opiate dependent.
- Note: Effects of naloxone generally start to diminish 20–40 min after administration and usually disappear within 90 min.
- Monitor respirations and other vital signs.
- Monitor surgical and obstetric patients closely for bleeding. Naloxone has been associated with abnormal coagulation test results. Also observe for reversal of analgesia, which may be manifested by nausea, vomiting, sweating, tachycardia.

Patient & Family Education

- Report postoperative pain that emerges after administration of this drug to prescriber.

NALTREXONE HYDROCHLORIDE

(nal-trex′one)
Vivitrol, ReVia

BROMIDE METHYLNALTREXONE

Relistor
Classification: NARCOTIC (OPIATE ANTAGONIST)
Therapeutic: NARCOTIC ANTAGONIST
Prototype: Naloxone HCl

N

AVAILABILITY Tablet; intramuscular injection. **Bromide Methylnaltrexone:** Solution for injection

ACTION & *THERAPEUTIC EFFECT* Opioid antagonist with a mechanism of action that appears to result from competitive binding at opioid receptor sites, thus it reduces euphoria and drug craving without supporting addiction. *Weakens or completely and reversibly blocks the subjective effects (the "high") of IV opioids and analgesics possessing both agonist and antagonist activity.*

USES Alcoholism, opiate agonist dependence. Opioid-related constipation in patients nonresponsive to laxatives (**Relistor**).

UNLABELED USES Pruritus.

CONTRAINDICATIONS Hypersensitivity to naltrexone; patients receiving opioid analgesics; opiate agonist use within 7–10 days; acute opioid agonist withdrawal; opioid-dependent patient; acute hepatitis, liver failure, hepatic encephalopathy; suicidal ideation; any individual who (1) fails naloxone challenge, (2) has a positive urine screen for opioids, or (3) has a history of sensitivity to naltrexone; lactation.

CAUTIOUS USE Mild to moderate hepatic impairment (Child-Pugh class A or B); history of suicidal tendencies; renal impairment; pregnancy (category C). **IM form:** Special at-risk patients: Thrombocytopenia, coagulopathy (e.g., hemophilia), severe hepatic impairment; children younger than 18 y.

ROUTE & DOSAGE

Opioid Dependence

Adult: **PO** 25 mg qd, if no response increase to 50 mg/day
Adult: **IM** 380 mg q4w

Alcohol Dependence

Adult: **PO** 50 mg once/day **IM** 380 mg q 4 wk

Opioid-Related Constipation (Relistor)

Adult (weight less than 38 kg or greater than 114 kg): **Subcutaneous** 0.15 mg/kg every other day (max: 0.15 mg/kg in 24 h); *weight 38–62 kg:* 8 mg every other day (max: 8 mg/24 h); *weight 62–114 kg:* 12 mg every other day (max: 12 mg/24 h)

Renal Impairment Dosage Adjustment (Relistor)

CrCl less than 30 mL/min: Reduce dose by 50%

ADMINISTRATION

Oral

- Give with food to decrease nausea.

Intramuscular

- Give IM into the gluteal muscle, alternating buttocks per injection. Aspirate before injection to ensure that drug is not injected IV.

Subcutaneous (Methylnaltrexone Only)

- Give subcutaneously into upper arm, abdomen, or thigh.

ADVERSE EFFECTS **CNS:** *Difficulty sleeping, anxiety, headache, nervousness,* reduced or increased energy, irritability, dizziness, depression. **Skin:** Skin rash. **GI:** Dry mouth, anorexia, *nausea, vomiting,* constipation, *abdominal cramps/pain,* <u>hepatotoxicity</u>. **Musculoskeletal:** *Muscle and joint pains.* **Hematologic: IM extended release form:** Hematoma formation at injection site. **Other:** Chills.

INTERACTIONS **Drug:** Increased somnolence and lethargy with PHENOTHIAZINES; reverses analgesic effects of NARCOTIC (OPIATE) AGONISTS and NARCOTIC (OPIATE) AGONIST-ANTAGONISTS.

PHARMACOKINETICS **Absorption:** Rapidly from GI tract; 20% reaches systemic circulation (first-pass effect). **Onset:** 15–30 min. **Peak:** 1 h; 30 min (Relistor). **Duration:** 24–72 h PO; 4 wk IM. **Metabolism:** In liver to active metabolite. **Elimination:** In urine. **Half-Life:** 10–13 h PO, 5–10 days IM.

NURSING IMPLICATIONS

Assessment & Drug Effects

- Monitor for development of depression or suicidal thinking.

- Monitor for and report promptly S&S of hepatotoxicity (see Appendix F).
- Monitor lab tests: LFTs before the treatment is started, at monthly intervals for 6 mo, and then periodically.

Patient & Family Education

- Note: Naltrexone therapy may put you in danger of overdosing if you use opiates. Small doses even at frequent intervals will give no desired effects; however, a dose large enough to produce a high is dangerous and may be -fatal.
- Do not self-dose with OTC drugs for treatment of cough, colds, diarrhea, or analgesia. Many available preparations contain small doses of an opioid. Consult prescriber for safe drugs if they are needed.

NAPHAZOLINE HYDROCHLORIDE

(naf-az'oh-leen)

Classification: EYE AND EAR PREPARATION; VASOCONSTRICTOR; ALPHA-ADRENERGIC AGONIST; DECONGESTANT

Therapeutic: DECONGESTANT

AVAILABILITY Ophthalmic solution

ACTION & *THERAPEUTIC EFFECT* Direct-acting alpha-adrenergic agonist that produces rapid and prolonged vasoconstriction of arterioles. *It decreases fluid exudation and mucosal engorgement.*

USES Ocular vasoconstrictor. Nasal congestion.

CONTRAINDICATIONS Narrow-angle glaucoma; hypersensitivity to adrenergic agents; pregnancy—fetal risk cannot be ruled out; lactation—infant risk cannot be ruled out.

CAUTIOUS USE Hypertension, cardiac disease, advanced arteriosclerosis; diabetes; hyperthyroidism; ocular infection or ocular trauma; children; safety and efficacy not established in children under 12 y.

ROUTE & DOSAGE

Eye Redness

Adult: **Topical** 1–2 drops of a 0.012–0.03% solution up to 4 times daily

ADMINISTRATION

Optic

- Remove contact lenses before instilling ophthalmic drops.
- Do not touch the tip of the dropper to the eye, fingertips, or other surface to prevent contamination.
- Wash hands before and after use.
- Tilt the head back slightly and pull the lower eyelid down with the index finger to form a pouch. Squeeze the number of ordered drops in the pouch. Close eyes to spread drops.
- To avoid contamination or the spread of infection, do not use dropper for more than one person.
- Store ophthalmic solutions at controlled room temperature between 8 and 27° C (36 and 80° F).

Nasal

- Wash hands before and after use.
- To avoid contamination, do not use for more than one person.
- Close the nostril that is not receiving the medication, insert the bottle tip in the open nostril. Breathe deeply as you squeeze the bottle.

- Store nasal solutions and sprays between 15 and 30° C (59 and 86° F).

ADVERSE EFFECTS (Common)

HEENT: Transient nasal stinging or burning, nasal discharge, sneezing, pupillary dilation, increased intraocular pressure.

INTERACTIONS

Drug: ERGOT DERIVATIVES may enhance vasoconstrictive effects.

PHARMACOKINETICS

Onset: Within 5 min. **Duration:** 6–8 h.

NURSING IMPLICATIONS

Assessment & Drug Effects

- Watch for rebound congestion and chemical rhinitis with frequent and continued use.
- Monitor BP periodically for development or worsening of hypertension, especially with ophthalmic route.
- Overdose: Bradycardia and hypotension can result. Report promptly.

Patient & Family Education

- Do not exceed prescribed regimen. Systemic effects can result from swallowing excessive medication.
- Discontinue medication and contact prescriber if nasal congestion is not relieved after 3 days.
- Contact healthcare provider if eye symptoms are not relieved after 48 hours of therapy.
- Prevent contamination of eye solution by taking care not to touch eyelid or surrounding area with dropper tip.

N

NAPROXEN

(na-prox'en)

EC-Naprosyn, Naprosyn

NAPROXEN SODIUM

Aleve, Anaprox, Anaprox DS

Classification: NON-STEROIDAL ANTI-INFLAMMATORY DRUG (NSAID)

Therapeutic: NONNARCOTIC ANALGESIC, NSAID

Prototype: Ibuprofen

AVAILABILITY

Tablet; sustained release tablet

ACTION & THERAPEUTIC EFFECT

Propionic acid derivative that is an NSAID. Mechanism of action is related to inhibition of prostaglandin synthesis by inhibiting COX-1 and COX-2 isoenzymes. *Analgesic, anti-inflammatory, and antipyretic effects; also inhibits platelet aggregation and prolongs bleeding time.*

USES

Anti-inflammatory and analgesic effects in symptomatic treatment of acute and chronic rheumatoid arthritis, juvenile arthritis (naproxen only), and for treatment of primary dysmenorrhea. Also management of ankylosing spondylitis, osteoarthritis, and gout.

UNLABELED USES

Paget's disease of bone, Bartter's syndrome.

CONTRAINDICATIONS

Hypersensitivity to naproxen or any other NSAIDs; active peptic ulcer; patients in whom asthma, rhinitis, urticaria, bronchospasm, or shock is precipitated by aspirin or other NSAIDs; perioperative pain associated with CABG; pregnancy (fetal risk cannot be ruled out); lactation (infant risk cannot be ruled out).

CAUTIOUS USE

History of upper GI tract disorders; history of GI bleeding; impaired kidney, liver, or cardiac function; patients on sodium restriction **(naproxen sodium);** low pretreatment Hgb concentration; fluid retention, hypertension, heart failure; coagulopathy; SLE; children younger than 2 y. **OTC:** Children younger than 12 y.

ROUTE & DOSAGE

Note: 200 mg naproxen = 220 naproxen sodium

Inflammatory Disease

Adult: **PO** 250–500 mg bid
Child (12 y or older): **PO** 5 mg/kg bid (max: 1000 mg/day)

Mild to Moderate Pain, Dysmenorrhea

Adult: **PO** 500 mg followed by 250 mg q6–8h prn up to 1000 mg
Child (12 y or older): **PO** 250 to 375 mg twice daily (max: 1000 mg/day)

ADMINISTRATION

Oral

- Ensure that extended release or enteric-coated form is not chewed or crushed. It **must be** swallowed whole. Administer with a full glass of water or other liquid.
- Give with food or an antacid (if prescribed) to reduce incidence of GI upset.
- Store at 15°–30° C (59°–86° F) in tightly closed container; protect from freezing and excessive heat.

ADVERSE EFFECTS

CV: Edema. **Respiratory:** Dyspnea. **CNS:** Dizziness, headache, somnolence. **HEENT:** Ototoxicity, tinnitus. **Skin:** Bruising, pruritis, rash. **GI:** Abdominal pain, constipation, heartburn, nausea. **Hematologic:** Hemolysis.

DIAGNOSTIC TEST INTERFERENCE

Transient elevations in ***BUN*** and serum ***alkaline phosphatase*** may occur. Naproxen may interfere with some urinary assays of ***5-HIAA*** and may cause falsely high ***urinary 17-KGS*** levels (using ***m-dinitrobenzene reagent***). Naproxen should be withdrawn 72 h before adrenal function tests. May lead to false positive ***aldosterone/renin ratio.***

INTERACTIONS

Drug: Bleeding time effects of ORAL ANTICOAGULANTS, **heparin** may be prolonged; may increase **lithium** toxicity. Do not use with **floctafenine, macimorelin, mifamurtide, mornflumate, phenylbutazone, alniflmate, tenoxicam,** or with NSAIDS. Do not use with photo-sensitizing agents. **Herbal: Feverfew, garlic, ginger, ginkgo, evening primrose oil, glucosamine** may increase bleeding potential.

PHARMACOKINETICS

Absorption: Almost completely from GI tract when taken on empty stomach. **Peak:** 2 h naproxen; 1 h naproxen sodium. **Duration:** 7 h. **Metabolism:** In liver. **Elimination:** Primarily in urine; some biliary excretion (less than 1%). **Half-Life:** 12–15 h.

NURSING IMPLICATIONS

Black Box Warning

Naproxen has been associated with increased risk of serious, potentially fatal, GI bleeding and cardiovascular events (e.g., MI & CVA); risk may increase with duration of use and may be greater in the older adult and those with risk factors for CV disease.

Assessment & Drug Effects

- Monitor for and report promptly S&S of GI ulceration or bleeding. Significant GI bleeding may occur without prior warning.
- Baseline blood pressure and during therapy.
- Monitor for and report promptly S&S of CV thrombotic events (i.e., angina, MI, TIA, or stroke).
- Take detailed drug history prior to initiation of therapy. Observe for signs of allergic response in those with aspirin or other NSAID sensitivity.
- Baseline and periodic auditory and ophthalmic examinations are recommended in patients receiving prolonged or high dose therapy.
- Monitor lab tests: Baseline and periodic CBC, LFTs, stool guaiac, and renal function tests with prolonged or high dose therapy.

Patient & Family Education

- Be aware that the therapeutic effect of naproxen may not be experienced for 3–4 wk.
- Stop taking drug and report promptly to prescriber if you experience S&S of GI ulceration: Stomach pain, frequent indigestion and nausea, bloody or tarry stools, vomit with blood or coffee-ground appearance.
- Avoid alcohol and aspirin (as well as other NSAIDs) unless otherwise advised by a prescriber. Potential to increase risk of GI ulceration and bleeding.
- Stop taking drug and report promptly to prescriber if you experience chest pain, shortness of breath, weakness, slurring of speech, or other signs of a cardiac or neurologic problem.

NARATRIPTAN

(nar-a-trip′tan)

Amerge

Classification: 5-HT$_1$ RECEPTOR AGONIST

Therapeutic: ANTIMIGRAINE

Prototype: Sumatriptan

AVAILABILITY Tablet

ACTION & THERAPEUTIC EFFECT Binds to the serotonin receptors (5-HT$_{1D}$ and 5-HT$_{1B}$) on intracranial blood vessels, resulting in selective vasoconstriction of dilated vessels in the carotid circulation. It also inhibits the release of inflammatory neuropeptides associated with a migraine attack. *Inhibits vasoconstriction of dilated vessels selectively. This results in the relief of acute migraine headache attacks.*

USES Acute migraine headaches with or without aura.

CONTRAINDICATIONS Hypersensitivity to naratriptan; severe renal impairment (creatinine clearance less than 15 mL/min); severe hepatic impairment; history of ischemic heart disease (i.e., angina pectoris, MI), arteriosclerosis, cardiac arrhythmias; cardiac disease, CAD, peripheral vascular disease; cerebrovascular syndromes (i.e., strokes or TIA); uncontrolled hypertension; patients with hemiplegic or basilar migraine; ischemic bowel disease; older adults.

CAUTIOUS USE Cardiovascular disease; renal or hepatic insufficiency; elderly; pregnancy (category C); lactation pregnancy (fetal risk cannot be ruled out); lactation (infant risk cannot be ruled out).

Safety and efficacy in children younger than 18 y not established.

ROUTE & DOSAGE

Acute Migraine

Adult: **PO** 1–2.5 mg; may repeat in 4 h if necessary (max: 5 mg/24 h)

Renal Impairment Dosage Adjustment

Patients with mild or moderate renal or hepatic impairment should not exceed 2.5 mg/24 h

ADMINISTRATION

Oral

- Administer as soon as symptoms appear. If the first tablet was effective but symptoms return, a second tablet may be given, but no sooner than 4 h after the first. Do not exceed 5 mg in 24 h.
- If there is no response to the first tablet, contact prescriber before administering a second tablet.
- Do not give within 24 h of an ergot-containing drug or other 5-HT_1 agonist.
- Store at 20°–25° C (68°–77° F); protect from light.

ADVERSE EFFECTS

GI: Nausea.

INTERACTIONS

Drug: Dihydroergotamine, methysergide, ERGOT derivatives and other 5-HT_1 AGONISTS may cause prolonged vasospastic reactions; SSRIS have rarely caused weakness, hyperreflexia, and incoordination; MAOIS should not be used with 5-HT_1 AGONISTS. Do not use with **dapoxetine. Herbal: Gingko, ginseng, echinacea, St. John's wort** may increase triptan toxicity.

PHARMACOKINETICS

Absorption: Rapidly absorbed, 70% bioavailability. **Peak:** 2–4 h. **Distribution:** 28–31% protein bound. **Metabolism:** In liver. **Elimination:** Primarily in urine. **Half-Life:** 6 h.

NURSING IMPLICATIONS

Assessment & Drug Effects

- Monitor blood pressure during therapy.
- Monitor carefully cardiovascular status following first dose in patients at risk for CAD (e.g., postmenopausal women, men older than 40 y, persons with known CAD risk factors) or coronary artery vasospasms.
- Be aware that ECG is recommended following first administration of naratriptan to someone with known CAD risk factors and periodically with long-term use.
- Report immediately to the prescriber: Chest pain, nausea, or tightness in chest or throat that is severe or does not quickly resolve.
- Obtain periodic cardiovascular evaluation with continued use.

Patient & Family Education

- Carefully review patient information leaflet and guidelines for administration.
- Contact prescriber immediately for any of the following: Symptoms of angina (e.g., severe and/or persistent pain or tightness in chest or throat, severe nausea); hypersensitivity (e.g., wheezing, facial swelling, skin rash, or hives); or abdominal pain.
- Report any other adverse effects (e.g., tingling, flushing, dizziness) at next prescriber visit.
- Avoid activities requiring mental alertness or coordination until drug effects are realized.

N

- Report worsening headaches as overuse may result in medication overuses headaches.
- Report confusion, hallucinations, sudden or severe abdominal pain, bloody diarrhea.

NATALIZUMAB

(na-tal′-i-zu-mab)

Tysabri

Classification: INTEGRIN INHIBITOR

Therapeutic: IMMUNOMODULATOR; MONOCLONAL ANTIBODY (IgG)

Prototype: Basiliximab

AVAILABILITY Solution for injection

ACTION & *THERAPEUTIC EFFECT* Natalizumab binds to integrins expressed on the surface of all leukocytes (except neutrophils) and inhibits adhesion of leukocytes to their counter-receptor(s) on activated vascular endothelial cells of the GI tract. Disruption of these interactions prevents transmigration of leukocytes across the endothelium into inflamed tissue. *Inhibition of T-cell infiltration into the brain is thought to impede the demyelinating process of MS. It reduces relapses and occurrence of brain lesions. Natalizumab is also thought to attenuate T-lymphocyte–mediated intestinal inflammation in Crohn's disease and possibly ulcerative colitis.*

USES Treatment of relapsing forms of multiple sclerosis, treatment of Crohn's disease.

CONTRAINDICATIONS Prior hypersensitivity to natalizumab; murine protein hypersensitivity; have or have had progressive multifocal leukoencephalopathy (PML); active infection; S&S of PML; females of childbearing age; pregnancy (fetal risk cannot be ruled out); lactation (infant risk cannot be ruled out).

CAUTIOUS USE Diabetes mellitus, immunocompromised patients; exposure to infection or tuberculosis; hepatic dysfunction; children younger than 18 y.

ROUTE & DOSAGE

Multiple Sclerosis/Moderate to Severe Crohn's Disease

Adult: **IV** 300 mg infused over 1 h every 4 wk

ADMINISTRATION

Intravenous

PREPARE: **IV Infusion:** Before and after dilution, solution should be colorless and clear to slightly opaque. Do not use if the solution has visible particles, flakes, color, or is cloudy. ▪ Withdraw 300 mg (15 mL) from the vial and add to an IV bag with 100 mL of NS. Do not use with any other diluent. ▪ Gently invert the bag to mix; do not shake. ▪ The IV solution **must be** used immediately or stored at 2°–8° C (36°–46° F) and used within 8 h.

ADMINISTER: **IV Infusion:** Flush IV line before/after with NS. Infuse over 1 h. ▪ Do not give a bolus dose. ▪ Stop infusion immediately if S&S of hypersensitivity appear.

INCOMPATIBILITIES: **Solution/additive/Y-site:** Do not mix or infuse with other drugs.

- Store IV solution for up to 8 h at 2°–8° C (36°–46° F). ▪ Allow solution to warm to room temperature before administration. Protect from light.

ADVERSE EFFECTS **Respiratory:** Upper or lower respiratory infection. **CNS:** *Headache*. **Skin:** Rash. **GI:** Abdominal pain, diarrhea, gastroenteritis, nausea. **GU:** UTI. **Musculoskeletal:** Joint pain, limb pain. **Other:** Depression, *fatigue*.

INTERACTIONS **Drug:** May reduce the effectiveness of VACCINES and TOXOIDS; may increase risk of infection with IMMUNOSUPPRESSANTS.

PHARMACOKINETICS **Half-Life:** 11 days.

NURSING IMPLICATIONS

Black Box Warning

Natalizumab has been associated with increased risk of progressive multifocal leukoencephalopathy (PML), an opportunistic viral infection of the brain that usually leads to death or severe disability.

Assessment & Drug Effects

- During IV infusion and for 1–2 h after, monitor closely for S&S of hypersensitivity (e.g., urticaria, dizziness, fever, rash, chills, pruritus, nausea, flushing, hypotension, dyspnea, and chest pain).
- Monitor neurologic status frequently. Report promptly any emerging S&S of dysfunction.
- Monitor lab tests: Baseline and periodic CBC with differential; periodic LFTs.

Patient & Family Education

- Report immediately any of the following during/after IV infusion: Difficulty breathing, wheezing or shortness of breath, swelling or tightness about the neck and throat, chest pain, skin rash or hives.
- Report promptly S&S of infection (e.g., cough, fever, chills, or sore throat).
- Report yellowing of skin or whites of the eyes.

NATAMYCIN

(na-ta-mye′sin)

Natacyn

Classification: ANTIFUNGAL ANTIBIOTIC

Therapeutic: ANTIFUNGAL

Prototype: Amphotericin B

AVAILABILITY Opthalmic suspension

ACTION & *THERAPEUTIC EFFECT* Mechanism of action is by binding to sterols in the fungal cell membrane resulting in cell death of fungi. *Effective against many yeasts and filamentous fungi including* Candida, Aspergillus, Cephalosporium, Fusarium, *and* Penicillium.

USES Ocular fungal infections.

CONTRAINDICATIONS Hypersensitivity to natamycin or any of its components; pregnancy—fetal risk cannot be ruled out; lactation—infant risk cannot be ruled out.

CAUTIOUS USE Safety and efficacy in children not established.

ROUTE & DOSAGE

Fungal Keratitis

Adult: **Ophthalmic** 1 drop in conjunctival sac of infected eye q1–2h for 3–4 days, then decrease to 1 drop q6–8h, then gradually decrease to 1 drop q4–7days

Fungal Conjuctivitis

Adult: **Ophthalmic** 1 drop in conjunctival sac of infected eye 4–6 times daily

ADMINISTRATION

Instillation

- Wash hands thoroughly before and after treatment. Infection is easily transferred from infected to noninfected eye and to other individuals.
- Shake well before using.
- Store at 2°–24° C (36°–75° F). Do not freeze. Protect from light and heat.

ADVERSE EFFECTS **HEENT:** Eye irritation.

PHARMACOKINETICS **Absorption:** Drug adheres to ulcerated surface of the cornea and is retained in conjunctival fornices. Does not appear to be systemically absorbed.

N

NURSING IMPLICATIONS

Assessment & Drug Effects

- Inspect eye for response and tolerance at least twice weekly.
- Note: Lack of improvement in keratitis within 7–10 days suggests that causative organisms may not be susceptible to natamycin. Reevaluation is indicated and possibly a change in therapy.

Patient & Family Education

- Learn appropriate technique for application of eye drops.
- Expect temporary light sensitivity. Be prepared to wear sunglasses outdoors after drug administration and perhaps for a few hours indoors.
- Return to ophthalmologist for reevaluation of eye problem if you experience symptoms of conjunctivitis: Pain, discharge, itching, scratching "foreign body sensation," changes in vision.
- Do not share facecloths and hand towels; this will help prevent transmission of the fungal infection.

NATEGLINIDE

(nat-e-gli′nide)

Starlix

Classification: ANTIDIABETIC; MEGLITINIDE

Therapeutic: ANTIDIABETIC

Prototype: Repaglinide

AVAILABILITY Tablet

ACTION & *THERAPEUTIC EFFECT*

Lowers blood glucose levels by stimulating the release of insulin from the pancreatic cells of a type 2 diabetic. Significantly reduces postprandial blood glucose in type 2 diabetics and improves glycemic control when given before meals. *Effectiveness is indicated by preprandial blood glucose between 80 and 120 mg/dL and HbA1C 6.5% or less.*

USES Alone or in combination with metformin for the treatment of non-insulin-dependent diabetes mellitus.

CONTRAINDICATIONS Prior hypersensitivity to nateglinide. Type 1 (insulin-dependent) diabetes mellitus, diabetic ketoacidosis; hypoglycemia.

CAUTIOUS USE Renal impairment; liver dysfunction; adrenal or pituitary insufficiency; malnutrition; infection, trauma, surgery or unusual stress; surgery; trauma; pregnancy (category C); lactation.

ROUTE & DOSAGE

Diabetes Mellitus

Adult: **PO** 60–120 mg tid 1–30 min prior to meals

ADMINISTRATION

Oral

- Give, preferably, 1–30 min before meals. Omit the dose if the meal is skipped. Add a dose if an extra meal is eaten. Never double the dose.
- Store at 15°–30° C (59°–86° F).

ADVERSE EFFECTS **CV:** Dizziness. **Respiratory:** Upper respiratory infection, bronchitis, cough. **Endocrine:** Hypoglycemia. **GI:** Diarrhea. **Musculoskeletal:** Arthropathy. **Other:** Back pain, flu-like symptoms.

INTERACTIONS **Drug:** NSAIDS, SALICYLATES, MAO INHIBITORS, BETA-ADRENERGIC BLOCKERS, may potentiate hypoglycemic effects; THIAZIDE DIURETICS, CORTICOSTEROIDS, THYROID PREPARATIONS, SYMPATHOMIMETIC AGENTS may attenuate hypoglycemic effects. **Herbal: Garlic, ginseng** may potentiate hypoglycemic effects.

PHARMACOKINETICS **Absorption:** Rapidly absorbed, 73% bioavailability. **Peak:** 1 h. **Distribution:** 98% protein bound. **Metabolism:** In liver by CYP2C9 (70%) and CYP3A4 (30%). **Elimination:** Primarily in urine. **Half-Life:** 1.5 h.

NURSING IMPLICATIONS

Assessment & Drug Effects

- Monitor carefully for S&S of hypoglycemia especially during the 1-wk period following transfer from a longer acting sulfonylurea.
- Monitor lab tests: Frequent 2 h postprandial blood glucose and FBS, and HbA1C q3mo.

Patient & Family Education

- Take only before a meal to lessen the chance of hypoglycemia.
- When transferred to nateglinide from another oral hypoglycemia drug, start nateglinide the morning after the other agent is stopped, unless directed otherwise by prescriber.
- Watch for S&S of hyperglycemia or hypoglycemia (see Appendix F); report poor blood glucose control to prescriber.
- Report gastric upset or other bothersome GI symptoms to prescriber.

NEBIVOLOL HYDROCHLORIDE

(ne-bi-vol′ol)

Bystolic

Classification: BETA-BLOCKER
Therapeutic: ANTIHYPERTENSIVE
Prototype: Propranolol

AVAILABILITY Tablet

ACTION & *THERAPEUTIC EFFECT* A beta-adrenergic receptor blocker that is a beta-1 selective antagonist in majority of individuals and a nonselective beta-blocker in poor metabolizers. At higher doses nebivolol blocks both beta-1 and beta-2 receptors. *Effectiveness is measured by decreasing both systolic and diastolic pressures associated with hypertension.*

USES Management of hypertension either alone or in combination with other antihypertensive agents.

UNLABELED USES Management of heart failure.

CONTRAINDICATIONS Hypersensitivity to nebivolol; severe bradycardia; greater than first degree heart block; sick sinus syndrome without pacemaker; severe hepatic impairment (Child-Pugh greater than class C); decompensated HF; bronchospastic disease; abrupt discontinuation; pregnancy (fetal risk cannot be ruled out); lactation (infant risk cannot be ruled out).

CAUTIOUS USE Hypersensitivity to nebivolol or other beta-blockers; compensated CHF; history of angina or recent MI; PVD; bronchospastic disease; major surgery, anesthesia; moderate hepatic and moderate to severe renal impairment; pheochromocytoma; spontaneous hypoglycemia or DM; hyperthyroidism; history of peripheral vascular disease. Safety and efficacy in children not established.

ROUTE & DOSAGE

Hypertension

Adult: **PO** 5 mg daily; can increase q2wk up to 40 mg daily

Hepatic Impairment Dosage Adjustment

Moderate hepatic impairment (Child-Pugh class B): 2.5 mg daily and increase cautiously as needed; *severe hepatic impairment:* Use is contraindicated

Renal Impairment Dosage Adjustment

CrCl less than 30 mL/min: 2.5 mg daily and cautiously increase as needed

ADMINISTRATION

Oral

- May give without regard to meals.
- Store at 20°–25° C (68°–77° F) in a tight, light-resistant container.

ADVERSE EFFECTS CNS: Headache, fatigue.

INTERACTIONS Drug: Catecholamine-depleting agents **(guanethidine)** may produce excessive reduction in sympathetic activity if used with nebivolol. Compounds that inhibit CYP2D6 **(fluoxetine, paroxetine, propafenone, quinidine)** may increase nebivolol levels. If used in combination with **clonidine**, simultaneous discontinuation of both drugs may cause life threatening increases in blood pressure. Combination use with **digoxin** may increase the risk of bradycardia. **Cimetidine** increases the levels of nebivolol metabolites. **Verapamil** and **diltiazem** may increase the pharmacologic effects of nebivolol. Nebivolol may decrease the clearance of **disopyramide.** Nebivolol may decrease the AUC and C_{max} of **sildenafil.** Do not use with **sotalol** or **tranylcypromine.**

PHARMACOKINETICS Peak: 1.5–4 h. **Distribution:** 98% plasma protein bound. **Metabolism:** Hepatic (via CYP2D6); extent depends on genetic profile. **Elimination:** In urine (38–67%) and feces (13–44%). **Half-Life:** 12–19 h depending on genetic differences in metabolism.

NURSING IMPLICATIONS

Assessment & Drug Effects

- Monitor closely BP and HR. Report promptly significant bradycardia or S&S of heart failure.
- Monitor closely during the perioperative period for depressed cardiac functioning.
- Monitor diabetics for loss of glycemia control.
- Monitor respiratory status in those at risk for bronchospasm.
- Monitor lab tests: LFTs, blood glucose (in diabetics), and serum creatinine.

Patient & Family Education

- Use caution with dangerous activities until reaction to drug is known.
- Report promptly any of the following: Sudden weight gain, increasing shortness of breath, swelling in lower legs and feet; heart rate less than 60 beats per minute or other value established by prescriber.
- Diabetics may experience hypoglycemia without the usual signs and symptoms while on this drug.
- Avoid activities requiring mental alertness or coordination until drug effects are realized.
- Do not abruptly stop taking this medication. It should be tapered off over 1–2 wk.

NECITUMUMAB

(ne-si-toom'oo-mab)

Portrazza

Classification: IMMUNOMODULATOR; MONOCLONAL ANTIBODY; ANTINEOPLASTIC; EPIDERMAL GROWTH FACTOR RECEPTOR (EGFR) ANTAGONIST

Therapeutic: ANTINEOPLASTIC; EPIDERMAL GROWTH FACTOR RECEPTOR (EGFR) ANTAGONIST

Prototype: Trastuzumab

AVAILABILITY Solution for injection

ACTION & *THERAPEUTIC EFFECT*

A recombinant human IgG1 monoclonal antibody that binds to the human epidermal growth factor receptor (EGFR) and blocks the binding of EGFR to its biological targets. *Expression and activation of EGFR has been correlated with malignant progression, induction of angiogenesis, and inhibition of apoptosis. The binding of necitumumab to EGFR induces its internalization and degradation.*

USES First-line treatment of patients with metastatic squamous non-small-cell lung cancer in combination with gemcitabine and cisplatin.

CAUTIOUS USE Cardiac arrest, cardiopulmonary arrest, venous and arterial thromboembolism (VTE and ATE), serious rash, and/or sudden death have occurred in patients treated with necitumumab in combination with gemcitabine and cisplatin. There are no adequate well-controlled studies in pregnant women; in animal data, it does cause fetal harm. It is not known whether necitumumab is present in human milk and the safest course is to advise women to discontinue breast-feeding during treatment and for 3 mo after the last dose.

ROUTE & DOSAGE

Non-Small-Cell Lung Cancer

Adult: **IV** 800 mg over 60 m on days 1 and 8 of 3wk cycle
Previous Grade 1 or 2 infusion-related reaction: Pre-medicate with diphenhydramine
Additional Grade 1 or 2 infusion-related reaction: Pre-medicated with diphenhydramine, acetaminophen, and dexamethasone

Infusion-Related Reactions (IRR) Dosage Adjustment

Grade 1: Decrease infusion rate by 50%
Grade 2: Stop infusion until resolution to Grade 0 or decrease infusion rate by 50%
Grade 3 or 4: Permanently discontinue

Dermatologic Toxicity Dosage Adjustment

Grade 3 or acneiform rash: Withhold until symptoms resolve to less than or equal to Grade 2; resume at reduced dose of 400 mg for 1 cycle; may increase to 600 mg and 800 mg in subsequent cycles if symptom free. Permanently discontinue if rash does not resolve to less than or equal to Grade 2 within 6 wk or if symptoms worsen.

N

ADMINISTRATION

Intravenous

PREPARE: **IV Infusion:** Withdraw the required volume of the drug and dilute with 0.9% sodium chloride injection in an IV infusion container to a final volume of 250 mL. Do not use solutions containing dextrose. Mix by gently inverting. Do not infuse with other electrolytes or medications.

ADMINISTER: **IV Infusion:** Administer via an infusion pump over 60 min through a separate infusion line. Flush the line with 0.9% sodium chloride injection at the end of the infusion.

INCOMPATIBILITIES **Solution/additive:** Do not mix with dextrose. **Y-site:** Administer through separate line.

- Store diluted solution at room temperature up to 25° C (77° F) for no more than 4 h, or under refrigeration 2°–8° C (36°–46° F) for no more than 24 h. Discard partially used or empty vials of necitumumab.

ADVERSE EFFECTS **CV:** Cardiopulmonary arrest. **Respiratory:** *Hemoptysis*, oropharyngeal pain, pulmonary embolism. **CNS:** *Headache*. **HEENT:** Conjunctivitis. **Endocrine:** Weight loss. **Skin:** Acne, *dermatitis acneiform*, dry skin, erythema, *generalized rash, maculopapular rash*, pruritus, skin fissures. **GI:** *Diarrhea*, stomatitis, *vomiting*. **Musculoskeletal:** Muscle spasm. **Hematological:** *Hypocalcemia, hypokalemia, hypomagnesemia, hypophosphatemia*. **Other:** Dysphagia, paronychia, phlebitis.

INTERACTIONS **Drug:** Necitumumab increases the levels of **gemcitabine.**

PHARMACOKINETICS **Half-Life:** 14 days.

NURSING IMPLICATIONS

Assessment & Drug Effects

- Monitor electrolytes prior to administration of each dose and for 8 wk after the last dose.
- Most infusion-related reactions have been reported after the first or second administration.
- Monitor respiratory status and pulse oximetry in case of pulmonary embolism.
- Assess oral mucosa for sores and pain.
- Monitor daily weight.

Patient & Family Education

- Use contraceptive measures during treatment.
- Report any shortness of breath, coughing up of blood, muscle spasms, or any eye infections.

- Encourage family members to become CPR certified.

NEFAZODONE

(nef-a-zo'done)

Classification:
ANTIDEPRESSANT; SEROTONIN RE-UPTAKE INHIBITOR/ ANTAGONIST
Therapeutic: ANTIDEPRESSANT; SNRI

AVAILABILITY Tablet

ACTION & *THERAPEUTIC EFFECT*
Antidepressant with a dual mechanism of action. Inhibits neuronal serotonin (5-HT_2) and norepinephrine reuptake. *Effective in treating major depression without major cardiovascular adverse effects.*

USES Treatment of depression.

CONTRAINDICATIONS Hypersensitivity to nefazodone or alcohol; active hepatic disease, hepatitis, jaundice; elevated hepatic transaminase levels; MAOI therapy; mania; severe restlessness, suicidal ideation; surgery; pregnancy—fetal risk cannot be ruled out; lactation—infant risk has been demonstrated.

CAUTIOUS USE History of seizure disorders, seizures; narrow angle glaucoma; renal impairment; recent MI, unstable cardiac disease; hypotension; angina, stroke, hypovolemia, dehydration, bipolar disorder; history of mania; Safety and efficacy in children younger than 18 y not established.

ROUTE & DOSAGE

Depression
Adult: **PO** 50–100 mg daily, may increase based on response 150–600 mg/day in 2 divided doses
Geriatric: **PO** Start with 50 mg bid, gradually increase based on response.

ADMINISTRATION

Oral
- Do not give within 14 days of discontinuation of an MAO inhibitor.
- Can be given without regard to food.
- Store at room temperature below 40° C (104° F).

ADVERSE EFFECTS (≥5%) **CNS:** *Headache, dizziness, drowsiness,* confusion, asthenia. **HEENT:** Blurred vision. **GI:** Dry mouth, constipation, nausea.

INTERACTIONS **Drug:** May cause serotonin syndrome (see Appendix F) with MAOIS or SSRIS; may increase plasma levels of some BENZODIAZEPINES, including **alprazolam** and **triazolam.** May decrease plasma levels and effects of **propranolol.** May increase levels and toxicity of **buspirone, carbamazepine, cilostazol, digoxin;** reports of QT_c prolongation and ventricular arrhythmias with **pimozide;** increased risk of rhabdomyolysis with **lovastatin, simvastatin;** increased risk of **ergotamine** toxicity with **dihydroergotamine, ergotamine**, or ERGOT ALKALOIDS. Nefazodone inhibits CYP 3A4 and increases risk of adverse effects of other medications metabolized via this pathway, so do not use concurrently. **Herbal: St. John's wort** may cause **serotonin** syndrome. Do not take **red yeast rice.**

PHARMACOKINETICS **Onset:** 1 wk. **Distribution:** 99% protein bound. **Peak:** 3–5 wk. **Metabolism:** In liver via CYP3A4, CYP1A2, CYP2D6, CYP2C to at least two active metabolites. **Half-Life:** Nefazodone 3.5 h, metabolites 2–8 h.

NURSING IMPLICATIONS

Black Box Warning

Nefazodone has been associated with suicidal thinking and behavior in children, adolescents, and young adults, and with potentially fatal hepatotoxicity.

Assessment & Drug Effects

- Monitor for worsening of depression or emergence of suicidal ideation.
- Monitor patients with a history of seizures for increased activity.
- Monitor for and report promptly S&S of hepatotoxicity (see Appendix F).
- ECG for high-risk patients prior to starting therapy.
- Assess safety, as dizziness and drowsiness are common adverse effects.
- Monitor lab tests: Periodic LFTs and CBC during long-term therapy.

Patient & Family Education

- Report immediately to prescriber signs of worsening mental status such as suicidal ideation, aggressiveness, agitation, anxiety, hostility, impulsivity, insomnia, irritability, panic attacks, and worsening of depression.
- Be aware that significant improvement in mood may not occur for several weeks following initiation of therapy.
- Do not drive or engage in potentially hazardous activities until response to the drug is known.
- Report changes in visual acuity.
- Report signs of jaundice such as yellow coloration of the cornea of the eye or other S&S of liver dysfunction (anorexia, GI complaints, malaise, etc.).
- Report prolonged penile erection.
- Avoid alcohol.
- Notify healthcare provider before taking any over the counter medication.

NELARABINE

Arranon

Classification: PYRIMIDINE ANTIMETABOLITE

Therapeutic: ANTINEOPLASTIC

Prototype: 5-Fluorouracil

AVAILABILITY Solution

ACTION & *THERAPEUTIC EFFECT* Nelarabine inhibits DNA synthesis in lymphoblastic T-cells of acute leukemia and lymphoma. *The incorporation of a nelarabine metabolite in the leukemic blast cells halts DNA synthesis and causes cell death.*

USES Treatment of patients with T-cell acute lymphoblastic leukemia lymphoma.

CONTRAINDICATIONS Hypersensitivity to nelarabine; severe bone marrow suppression; older adults; pregnancy (infant risk cannot be ruled out); lactation (infant risk cannot be ruled out).

CAUTIOUS USE Severe renal impairment, severe renal failure;

hepatic impairment; risk of infection, bleeding.

ROUTE & DOSAGE

Adult T-Cell Leukemia/ Lymphoma

Adult: **IV** 1500 mg/m^2 on days 1, 3, and 5, repeated every 21 days
Child: **IV** 650 mg/m^2 /dose for 5 days, repeat cycle every 21 days

Toxicity Dosage Adjustment

Grade 2 or higher neurologic toxicity: Discontinue therapy; *hematologic toxicities:* Delay therapy

ADMINISTRATION

- NIOSH recommends the use of double gloves and protective gown. If there is potential during administration for splash or if the patient could resist, use eye/face protection.

Intravenous

This drug is a cytotoxic agent and caution should be used to prevent any contact with the drug. Follow institutional or standard guidelines for preparation, handling, and disposal of cytotoxic agents.

PREPARE: **IV Infusion:** Do not dilute. Transfer the required dose to a PVC or glass container for infusion.
ADMINISTER: **IV Infusion for Adult:** Give over 2 h. **IV Infusion for Child:** Give over 1 h.

- Store vials at 15°–30° C (59°–86° F). Nelarabine is stable in PVC bags or glass infusion containers for 8 h up to 30° C.

ADVERSE EFFECTS

CV: Peripheral edema. **Respiratory:** *Cough,* dyspnea. **CNS:** Weakness, dizziness, headache, reduced sense of touch, prickly sensation, peripheral neuropathy, somnolence. **Skin:** Bruising. **GI:** Constipation, diarrhea, *nausea,* vomiting. **Musculoskeletal:** Muscle pain. **Hematologic:** *Anemia, leukopenia, neutropenia, thrombocytopenia*. **Other:** *Fatigue,* fever.

INTERACTIONS

Drugs: Do not use with LIVE VACCINES. Avoid use with **deferiprone, dipyrone, lenograstim, natalizumab, pentostatin, pimecrolimus, tacrolimus**. **Herbal:** Use echinacea with caution.

PHARMACOKINETICS

Distribution: Extensive. **Metabolism:** Bioactivation to ara-GTP, oxidized to uric acid. **Elimination:** Renal. **Half-Life:** 3 h (active metabolite).

NURSING IMPLICATIONS

Black Box Warning

Nelarabine has been associated with severe neurologic reactions.

Assessment & Drug Effects

- Monitor for and report immediately S&S of adverse CNS effects, including altered mental status (e.g., confusion, severe somnolence), seizures, and peripheral neuropathy (e.g., numbness, paresthesias, motor weakness, ataxia, paralysis). Note: Previous or concurrent treatment with intra-thecal chemotherapy or previous craniospinal irradiation may increase risk of CNS toxicity.
- Discontinue IV and notify prescriber for neurologic adverse events of NCI Common Toxicity Criteria grade 2 or greater.

N

- Monitor for S&S of bleeding, especially with platelet counts less than 50,000/mm^3.
- Monitor diabetics for loss of glycemic control.
- Monitor lab tests: Baseline and periodic CBC with differential and platelet count; periodic serum electrolytes, serum uric acid, LFTs, and renal function test.

Patient & Family Education

- Do not drive or engage in potentially hazardous activities until response to drug is known.
- Report any of the following to a health care provider: Seizures; tingling or numbness in hands and feet; problems with fine motor coordination; unsteady gait and increased weakness with ambulating; fever or other signs of infections; black tarry stools, blood tinged urine, or other signs of bleeding.
- Use effective contraceptive measures to avoid pregnancy (males with partners of child-bearing potential) and female patients while taking this drug.

NELFINAVIR MESYLATE

(nel-fin′a-vir)

Viracept

Classification: PROTEASE INHIBITOR

Therapeutic: PROTEASE INHIBITOR

Prototype: Saquinavir

AVAILABILITY Tablet; powder for oral suspension

ACTION & *THERAPEUTIC EFFECT* Inhibits HIV-1 protease, which is responsible for the production of HIV-1 viral particles in an infected individual. This prevents the cleavage of viral polypeptide, resulting in the production of an immature, noninfectious virus. *Effectiveness is indicated by decreased viral load.*

USES Treatment of HIV infection in combination with other agents.

CONTRAINDICATIONS Hypersensitivity to nelfinavir; pancreatitis; Grade 2 or higher neurologic toxicity to drug; lactation (infant risk cannot be ruled out).

CAUTIOUS USE Liver function impairment, hemophilia; diabetes mellitus, hyperglycemia; pregnancy (category B); children younger than 2 y.

ROUTE & DOSAGE

HIV Infection

Adult/Adolescent: **PO** 750 mg tid or 1250 mg bid with food
Child (2–13 y): **PO** 45–55 mg/kg/dose bid (max dose: 1250 mg/dose) or 25–35 mg/kg/dose tid (max dose: 750 mg/dose)

ADMINISTRATION

Oral

- Give with a meal or light snack.
- Oral powder may be mixed with a small amount of water, milk, soy milk, or dietary supplements; liquid should be consumed immediately. Do not mix oral powder in original container nor with acid food or juice (e.g., orange or apple juice, or apple sauce).
- Store at 15°–30° C (59°–86° F).

ADVERSE EFFECTS **GI:** *Diarrhea*, nausea, flatulence. **Hematologic:** Lymphocytopenia, decreased neutrophils. **Other:** Fatigue.

INTERACTIONS **Drug:** Other PROTEASE INHIBITORS, **ketoconazole** may increase nelfinavir levels;

rifabutin, rifampin, PROTON PUMP INHIBITORS may decrease nelfinavir levels; nelfinavir will decrease ORAL CONTRACEPTIVE levels; may increase levels of **amiodarone, atorvastatin, simvastatin, sildenafil,** PDE 5 INHIBITORS; increase risk of **ergotamine** toxicity with **dihydroergotamine, ergotamine,** HMG-COA REDUCTASE INHIBITORS may have increased risk of rhabdomyolysis. BENZODIAZEPINES may increase risk of sedation. **Herbal: St. John's wort, garlic** may decrease antiretroviral activity. Use with **red yeast rice** may increase risk of rhabdomyolysis.

PHARMACOKINETICS **Absorption:** Food increases the amount of drug absorbed. **Distribution:** Greater than 98% protein bound. **Metabolism:** In the liver (CYP3A). **Elimination:** Primarily in feces. **Half-Life:** 3.5–5 h.

NURSING IMPLICATIONS

Assessment & Drug Effects

- Monitor hemophiliacs (type A or B) closely for spontaneous bleeding.
- Monitor carefully patients with hepatic impairment for toxic drug effects.
- Monitor labs at baseline and with modification: Viral load, Hepatitis B screening, Hepatitis C antibody testing, LFTs, CBC with differential, BUN, creatinine, pregnancy test in women prior to therapy, blood glucose or HbA1c.

Patient & Family Education

- Drug **must be** taken exactly as prescribed. Do not alter dose or discontinue drug without consulting prescriber.
- Use a barrier contraceptive even if using hormonal contraceptives.
- Be aware that diarrhea is a common adverse effect.
- Contact health care provider prior to taking any OTC or herbal medications.

NEOMYCIN SULFATE

(nee-oh-mye'sin)

Mycifradin, Myciguent, Neo-Tabs, Neo-Fradin

Classification: AMINOGLYCOSIDE ANTIBIOTIC

Therapeutic: ANTIBIOTIC

Prototype: Gentamicin

AVAILABILITY Tablet; oral solution; ointment, cream

ACTION & *THERAPEUTIC EFFECT*

Inhibits bacterial protein synthesis through irreversible binding to the 30S ribosomal subunit within susceptible bacteria, thus causing bacteria not to replicate. *Active against a wide variety of gram-negative bacteria. Effective against certain gram-positive organisms, particularly penicillin-sensitive and some methicillin-resistant strains of Staphylococcus aureus (MRSA).*

USES Severe diarrhea caused by enteropathogenic *Escherichia coli;* preoperative intestinal antisepsis; to inhibit nitrogen-forming bacteria of GI tract in patients with cirrhosis or hepatic coma and for urinary tract infections caused by susceptible organisms. Also topically for short-term treatment of eye, ear, and skin infections.

CONTRAINDICATIONS Hypersensitivity to aminoglycosides; use of oral drug in patients with intestinal obstruction; ulcerative bowel lesions; IBD; topical applications

N

over large skin areas; aminoglycosides; drug induced loss of hearing.

CAUTIOUS USE Dehydration; renal disease, renal impairment; hearing impairment; myasthenia gravis, parkinsonism; pregnancy (category C); lactation; children. **Topical otic applications:** Patients with perforated eardrum.

ROUTE & DOSAGE

Intestinal Antisepsis

Adult: **PO** 1 g q1h × 4 doses, then 1 g q4h × 5 doses
Child: **PO** 10.3 mg/kg q4–6h for 3 days

Hepatic Coma

Adult: **PO** 4–12 g/day in 4 divided doses for 5–6 days
Child: **PO** 437.5–1225 mg/m^2 q6h for 5–6 days

Diarrhea

Adult: **PO** 50 mg/kg in 4 divided doses for 2–3 days
Child: **PO** 8.75 mg/kg q6h for 2–3 days

Cutaneous Infections

Adult: **Topical** Apply 1–3 × day

ADMINISTRATION

Oral

- Preoperative bowel preparation: Saline laxative is generally given immediately before neomycin therapy is initiated.

Topical

- Consult prescriber about what to use for cleansing skin before each application.
- Make sure ear canal is clean and dry prior to instillation for topical therapy of external ear.

ADVERSE EFFECTS **HEENT:** Ototoxicity. **Skin:** *Redness,* scaling, pruritus, dermatitis. **GI:** Mild laxative effect, diarrhea, nausea, vomiting; prolonged therapy: malabsorption-like syndrome including cyanocobalamin (vitamin B_{12}) deficiency, low serum cholesterol. **GU:** Nephrotoxicity. **Other:** Neuromuscular blockade with muscular and respiratory paralysis; hypersensitivity reactions.

INTERACTIONS **Drug:** May decrease absorption of **cyanocobalamin.**

PHARMACOKINETICS **Absorption:** 3% absorbed from GI tract in adults; up to 10% absorbed in neonates. **Peak:** 1–4 h. **Elimination:** 97% excreted unchanged in feces. **Half-Life:** 3 h.

NURSING IMPLICATIONS

Black Box Warning

Neomycin has been associated with neurotoxicity (including ototoxicity) and nephrotoxicity.

Assessment & Drug Effects

- Monitor closely for ototoxicity and nephrotoxicity. Risk is greatest in those with impaired renal function.
- Monitor I&O in patients receiving drug orally. Report oliguria or changes in I&O ratio. Inadequate neomycin excretion results in high serum drug levels and risk of nephrotoxicity.
- Monitor lab tests: Baseline and periodic serum renal function tests.

Patient & Family Education

- Stop treatment and consult your prescriber if irritation occurs when you are using topical neomycin. Allergic dermatitis is common.

- Report any unusual symptom related to ears or hearing (e.g., tinnitus, roaring sounds, loss of hearing acuity, dizziness).
- Do not exceed prescribed dosage or duration of therapy.

NEOSTIGMINE METHYLSULFATE

(nee-oh-stig′meen)

Bloxiverz

Classification: CHOLINERGIC MUSCLE STIMULANT; CHOLINESTERASE INHIBITOR

Therapeutic: MUSCLE NERVE STIMULANT

AVAILABILITY Solution for injection

ACTION & THERAPEUTIC EFFECT Produces reversible cholinesterase inhibition or inactivation with direct stimulant action on voluntary muscle fibers and possibly on autonomic ganglia and CNS neurons. Allows intensified and prolonged effect of acetylcholine at cholinergic synapses (basis for use in myasthenia gravis). *Produces generalized cholinergic response including miosis, increased tonus of intestinal and skeletal muscles, constriction of bronchi and ureters, slower pulse rate, and stimulation of salivary and sweat glands.*

USES To prevent and treat postoperative abdominal distention and urinary retention; for symptomatic control of and sometimes for differential diagnosis of myasthenia gravis; and to reverse the effects of nondepolarizing muscle relaxants (e.g., tubocurarine).

CONTRAINDICATIONS Hypersensitivity to neostigmine, cholinergics; bromides; ileus; mechanical obstruction of intestinal or urinary tract; peritonitis.

CAUTIOUS USE Recent ileorectal anastomoses; epilepsy; asthma; hepatic disease; bradycardia, CAD, recent coronary occlusion; vagotonia; cardiac arrhythmias; renal failure; renal impairment; renal disease; hyperthyroidism; MG; peptic ulcer; seizure disorder; older adults; pregnancy (category C); children; lactation.

ROUTE & DOSAGE

Diagnosis of Myasthenia Gravis

Adult: **IM** 0.02 mg/kg
Child: **IM** 0.04 mg/kg

Treatment of Myasthenia Gravis

Adult: **IM/Subcutaneous** 0.5–2.5 mg q1–3h (max: 10 mg/day)
Child: **IM/Subcutaneous** 0.01–0.04 mg/kg q2–4h

Reversal of Nondepolarizing Neuromuscular Blockade

Adult: **IV** 0.5–2.5 mg slowly (max dose: 5 mg); may repeat
Child: **IV** 0.025–0.08 mg/kg
Infant: **IV** 0.025–0.1 mg/kg

Postoperative Abdominal Distention and Urinary Retention

Adult: **IM/Subcutaneous** 0.25 mg q4–6h for 2–3 days

Myasthenia Gravis

Adult: **IV** 0.5–2 mg q1–3h
Child: **IV** 0.01–0.04 mg/kg q2–4h

Renal Impairment Dosage Adjustment

CrCl 10–50 mL/min: Use 50% of dose; *less than 10 mL/min:* Use 25% of dose

ADMINISTRATION

Intramuscular/Subcutaneous

- Give undiluted.

Intravenous

PREPARE: **Direct:** Give undiluted.
ADMINISTER: **Direct:** Give at a rate of 0.5 mg or a fraction thereof over 1 min.
INCOMPATIBILITIES: **Fluorescein.**

ADVERSE EFFECTS **CV:** Tightness in chest, bradycardia, hypotension, elevated BP. **Respiratory:** *Increased salivation* and bronchial secretions, sneezing, cough, dyspnea, diaphoresis, respiratory depression. **CNS:** CNS stimulation. **HEENT:** Lacrimation, miosis, blurred vision. **GI:** *Nausea,* vomiting, eructation, epigastric discomfort, abdominal cramps, diarrhea, involuntary or difficult defecation. **GU:** Difficult micturition. **Other:** Muscle cramps, *fasciculations,* twitching, pallor, fatigability, generalized weakness, paralysis, agitation, fear, death.

INTERACTIONS **Drug: Succinylcholine decamethonium** may prolong phase I block or reverse phase II block; neostigmine antagonizes effects of **tubocurarine; atracurium, vecuronium, pancuronium; procainamide, quinidine, atropine** antagonize effects of neostigmine.

PHARMACOKINETICS **Onset:** 10–30 min IM or IV. **Peak:** 20–30 min IM or IV. **Distribution:** Not reported to cross placenta or appear in breast milk. **Metabolism:** In liver. **Elimination:** 80% of drug and metabolites excreted in urine within 24 h. **Half-Life:** 50–90 min.

NURSING IMPLICATIONS

Assessment & Drug Effects

- Check pulse before giving drug to bradycardic patients. If below 60/min or other established parameter, consult prescriber. Atropine will be ordered to restore heart rate.
- Monitor respiration, maintain airway or assisted ventilation, and give oxygen as indicated when used as antidote for tubocurarine or other nondepolarizing neuromuscular blocking agents (usually preceded by atropine).
- Monitor pulse, respiration, and BP during period of dosage adjustment in treatment of myasthenia gravis.
- Report promptly and record accurately the onset of myasthenic symptoms and drug adverse effects in relation to last dose.
- Note carefully time of muscular weakness onset. It may indicate whether patient is in cholinergic or myasthenic crisis: Weakness that appears approximately 1 h after drug administration suggests cholinergic crisis (overdose) and is treated by prompt withdrawal of neostigmine and immediate administration of atropine. Weakness that occurs 3 h or more after drug administration is more likely due to myasthenic crisis (underdose or drug resistance) and is treated by more intensive anticholinesterase therapy.
- Record drug effect and duration of action. S&S of myasthenia gravis relieved by neostigmine include lid ptosis; diplopia; drooping facies; difficulty in chewing, swallowing, breathing, or coughing; and weakness of neck, limbs, and trunk muscles.
- Manifestations of neostigmine overdosage often appear first in muscles of neck and those

involved in chewing and swallowing, with muscles of shoulder girdle and upper extremities affected next.

- Report to prescriber if patient does not urinate within 1 h after first dose when used to relieve urinary retention.

Patient & Family Education

- Keep a diary of "peaks and valleys" of muscle strength.
- Keep an accurate record for prescriber of your response to drug. Learn how to recognize adverse effects, how to modify dosage regimen according to your changing needs, or how to administer atropine if necessary.
- Be aware that certain factors may require an increase in size or frequency of dose (e.g., physical or emotional stress, infection, menstruation, surgery), whereas remission requires a decrease in dosage.

NEPAFENAC

(nep'a-fe-nac)

Nevanac

See Appendix A-1.

NERATINIB MALEATE

(neh-ra'tih-nib may'lee-ayt')

Nerlynx

Classification: ANTINEOPLASTIC; ANTI-HER2 AGENT; EGFR INHIBITOR; TYROSINE KINASE INHIBITOR

Therapeutic: ANTINEOPLASTIC

AVAILABILITY Tablet

ACTION & *THERAPEUTIC EFFECT* Neratinib is an irreversible inhibitor of epidermal growth factor receptor (EGFR), human epidermal growth factor receptor 2 (HER2), and HER4. *Approved as adjuvant treatment of breast cancer to help maintain remission.*

USES Treatment of early stage HER2-Positive breast cancer, post-trastuzumab treatment.

CONTRAINDICATIONS Pregnancy, lactation.

CAUTIOUS USE History of hepatic disease, geriatric patients.

ROUTE & DOSAGE

Breast Cancer

Adult: **PO** 240 mg daily for 1 year

Toxicity Dosage Adjustment

First dose reduction: 200 mg once daily
Second dose reduction: 160 mg once daily
First dose reduction: 120 mg once daily
Specific toxicity and dose reduction strategies available in the package insert

ADMINISTRATION

Oral

- Take dose with food at approximately the same time every day.
- Swallow tablets whole; do not chew, crush, or spit.
- Separate neratinib from antacids; may give 3 h after the antacid.
- Store at 20°–25° C (68°–77° F); excursions permitted at 15°–30° C (59°–86° F).

ADVERSE EFFECTS **Endocrine:** Weight loss, elevated liver enzymes. UTI. **Skin:** Dry skin, rash, nail changes. **GI:** *Abdominal pain,* anorexia, *diarrhea, nausea,* vomiting, stomatitis, swollen abdomen. **Musculoskeletal:** Spasm. **Other:** *Fatigue.*

INTERACTIONS Drug: Major substrate of CYP3A4, avoid use with CYP3A4 inducers (e.g., **carbamazepine, phenytoin, rifampin**) and inhibitors (e.g., **amiodarone, clarithromycin, erythromycin, itraconazole, verapamil**). Inhibits P-glycoprotein/ABCB1, avoid use with substrates of that glycoprotein (e.g., **topotecan, vincristine**). Avoid use with medications that reduce gastric acid, such as PROTON PUMP INHIBITORS and H_2-receptor ANTAGONISTS. **Herbal:** Avoid use with **St. John's wort.**

PHARMACOKINETICS Distribution: 99% protein bound (primarily albumin). **Onset:** Peak in 2–8. **Metabolism:** Hepatic, primarily through CYP3A4. **Elimination:** 97% in feces, 1% in urine. **Half-Life:** 7–17 h.

NURSING IMPLICATIONS

Assessment & Drug Effects

- Antidiarrheal prophylaxis is recommended for the first 2 cycles.
- Monitor intake and output. Risk for fluid deficit related to diarrhea.
- Monitor lab tests: LFTs and pregnancy test prior to treatment.

Patient & Family Education

- Many drugs and over the counter medications interact with this drug. Notify all prescribers that you are on this medication and check with prescriber before taking any other over the counter or natural products.
- Do not breast-feed while taking this medication. Resume breast- feeding 1 mo after taking the final dose.
- Call prescriber if diarrhea persists.
- Avoid grapefruit and grapefruit juice.
- If older than 65 y, more side effects may occur.
- Patients and spouses with reproductive potential should use effective birth control while taking this medication and 3 mo after the last dose.
- If pregnancy occurs while taking this drug or within 1 mo of the final dose, call your prescriber right away.
- Report any confusion, mood changes, muscle pain/weakness, inability to pass urine, pass blood in the urine, if the urine is dark, loss of appetite, urinary urgency, more than 2 bowel movements in a day, or swelling of the belly.
- If a dose is missed, skip the dose and go back to the usual time. Do not take 2 doses at the same time or extra doses.

NETARSUDIL

(ne-tar'soo-dil)

Rhopressa

Classification: EYE PREPARATION; RHO KINASE INHIBITOR

Therapeutic: RHO KINASE INHIBITOR

AVAILABILITY Ophthalmic solution

ACTION & *THERAPEUTIC EFFECT* As a rhokniase inhibitor, exact mechanism is unknown; thought to increase outflow of aqueous humor. *Reduces elevated intraocular pressure in patients with open-angle glaucoma.*

USES Treatment of open-angle glaucoma, ocular hypertension, and elevated intraocular pressure (IOP).

CAUTIOUS USE Bacterial keratitis is associated with multiple-dose containers of topical ophthalmic products; the medication should not be used with contact lenses.

ROUTE & DOSAGE

Glaucoma

Adult: **Ophthalmic** 1 drop in affected eye(s) once daily in the evening

ADMINISTRATION

Ocular

- Ensure that contact lenses are removed prior to installation and not reinserted for 15 min after installation.
- Apply only to affected eye(s). Ensure that only one drop is instilled.
- Do not allow tip of dropper to touch eye.
- Wait at least 5 min before/after instillation of other eyedrops.
- Store at 2°–8° C (35°–46° F) until opened, after which it may be stored at 2°–25° C (35°–77° F) for up to 6 wk.

ADVERSE EFFECTS **HEENT:** Conjunctival *hyperemia*, corneal verticillata, instillation site pain, conjunctival hemorrhage, blurred vision, increased lacrimation, reduced visual acuity. **Skin:** Erythema of the eyelid.

PHARMACOKINETICS **Absorption:** No clinically relevant systemic absorption occurs. **Metabolism:** Eye enzyme esterases metabolize netarsudil to its active metabolite, AR-13503.

NURSING IMPLICATIONS

Assessment & Drug Effects

- Obtain baseline intraocular pressure and monitor periodically.

Patient & Family Education

- Teach patient importance of proper administration and proper timing of multiple eye medications.
- Report any changes in vision.

NEVIRAPINE

(ne-vir'a-peen)

Viramune, Viramune XR

Classification: NONNUCLEOSIDE REVERSE TRANSCRIPTASE INHIBITOR (NNRTI)

Therapeutic: ANTIRETROVIRAL; NNRTI

Prototype: Efavirenz

AVAILABILITY Tablet; oral suspension; extended release tablet

ACTION & *THERAPEUTIC EFFECT* Nonnucleoside reverse transcriptase inhibitor (NNRTI) of HIV-1. Binds directly to reverse transcriptase and blocks RNA- and DNA-dependent polymerase activities, thus preventing replication of the virus. Does not inhibit HIV-2 RT. *Prevents replication of the HIV-1 virus. Resistant strains appear rapidly.*

USES Treatment of HIV with other agents.

UNLABELED USES Prevention of maternal-fetal HIV transmission.

CONTRAINDICATIONS Hypersensitivity to nevirapine; development of rash; severe skin reactions to the drug; hepatitis B or C; or early possible S&S of hepatitis; increased transaminases combined with rash or sign of hepatotoxicity; hepatic impairment of Child-Pugh class B or C use in post-exposure to HIV prophylaxis treatment; immune reconstitution complex; hormonal contraception; lactation (infant risk cannot be ruled out).

CAUTIOUS USE Renal disease; hemodialysis; mild hepatic impairment, CNS disorders; pregnant women with CD4+ lymphocyte

N

counts greater than 250/mm^3; patients with autoimmune disorders; older adults; pregnancy (category B) (fetal risk cannot be ruled out); neonates children.

ROUTE & DOSAGE

HIV

Adult/Adolescent: **PO Immediate release** 200 mg once daily for 14 days, then increase to 200 mg bid; or **Extended release** 400 mg daily
Infant/Child (8 y and younger): **PO** 200 mg/m^2/dose daily × 14 d then 200 mg/m^2/dose bid (max: 200 mg bid)
Child (older than 8 y): **PO Immediate release** 120–150 mg/m^2 daily × 14 days, then 120–150 mg/m^2 bid (max: 400 mg) (max: 200 mg/dose)

Hepatic Impairment Dosage Adjustment

Do not use in Child-Pugh class B or C

N

ADMINISTRATION

Oral

- NIOSH recommends the use of single gloves by anyone handling intact tablets or capsules or administering from a unit-dose package. Use double gloves if cutting or manipulating uncoated tablets. During administration, wear single gloves, eye/face protection if the formulation is hard to swallow or if the patient may resist, vomit, or spit up. Use double gloves and protective gown if administering an oral liquid via a feeding tube.
- Reinitiate with 200 mg/day for 14 days, then increase to bid dosing, when dosing is interrupted for more than 7 days.
- Ensure that extended release tablet is swallowed whole. It must not be crushed or chewed.
- Store at 15°–30° C (59°–86° F) in a tightly closed container.

ADVERSE EFFECTS **Endocrine:** Increased cholesterol, increased LDL, increased amylase. **Skin:** Rash. **Hepatic:** Increased ALT, **GI:** *Diarrhea, nausea.* **Hematologic:** Neutropenia.

INTERACTIONS **Drug:** May decrease plasma concentrations of PROTEASE INHIBITORS, ORAL CONTRACEPTIVES; may decrease **methadone, dronedarone** levels. **Fluconazole** may increase adverse effects. Do not take with **carbamazepine, ergonovine, itraconazole.** Herbal: **St. John's wort, garlic** may decrease antiretroviral activity.

PHARMACOKINETICS **Absorption:** Rapidly from GI tract. **Peak:** 4h. **Distribution:** 60% protein bound, crosses placenta, distributed into breast milk. **Metabolism:** In liver (CYP3A). **Elimination:** Primarily in urine. **Half-Life:** 25–40 h.

NURSING IMPLICATIONS

Black Box Warning

Nevirapine has been associated with severe, potentially fatal, hepatotoxicity and skin reactions.

Assessment & Drug Effects

- Monitor carefully, especially during first 18 wk of therapy, for severe rash (with or without fever, blistering, oral lesions, conjunctivitis, swelling, joint aches, or general malaise) and for S&S of hepatotoxicity (see Appendix F).

- Withhold drug and notify prescriber if rash develops or liver function tests are abnormal.
- Monitor lab tests at baseline and with modification: LFTs, CBC with differential, CD4 cell counts, Hepatitis B screening, Hepatitis A antibody testing, BUN, creatinine, electrolytes, urinalysis.

Patient & Family Education

- Withhold drug and notify prescriber if severe rash appears or if you develop S&S of hepatitis.
- Do not drive or engage in potentially hazardous activities until response to drug is known. There is a high potential for drowsiness and fatigue.
- Use or add barrier contraceptive if using hormonal contraceptive.
- It is normal for part of the extended release tablet to be seen in the stool.
- Do not take St. John's wort while taking this medication.

NIACIN (VITAMIN B_3, NICOTINIC ACID)

(nye'a-sin)

Niacor, Niaspan, Novoniacin ♣, Slo-Niacin, Tri-B3 ♣

NIACINAMIDE (NICOTINAMIDE)

Classification: VITAMIN B_3; ANTILIPEMIC

Therapeutic: ANTILIPEMIC; LIPID-LOWERING AGENT

AVAILABILITY Tablet; sustained release tablet; capsule

ACTION & THERAPEUTIC EFFECT Water-soluble, heat-stable, B-complex vitamin (B_3) that functions with riboflavin as a control agent in coenzyme system that converts protein, carbohydrate, and fat to energy through oxidation-reduction. Niacinamide, an amide of niacin, is used as an alternative in the prevention and treatment of pellagra. *Produces vasodilation by direct action on vascular smooth muscles. Inhibits hepatic synthesis of VLDL, cholesterol, and triglyceride, and, indirectly, LDL. Large doses effectively reduce elevated serum cholesterol and total lipid levels in hypercholesterolemia and hyperlipidemic states.*

USES In prophylaxis and treatment of niacin deficiency. Also in adjuvant treatment of hyperlipidemia (elevated cholesterol or triglycerides) in patients who do not respond adequately to diet or weight loss (not considered a primary or secondary agent for this use).

CONTRAINDICATIONS Hypersensitivity to niacin or niacinamide; hepatic impairment; active hepatic disease, significant or unexplained elevations of hepatic transaminses two or three times ULN; hepatotoxicity; hemorrhaging or arterial bleeding; active peptic ulcer; persistent cutaneous reactions to niacin use; pregnancy—fetal risk cannot be ruled out; lactation—infant risk cannot be ruled out.

CAUTIOUS USE History of gallbladder disease, liver disease, and peptic ulcer; excessive alcohol consumption; renal impairment; glaucoma; unstable angina or MI; new onset atrial fibrillation; coronary artery disease; diabetes mellitus; CAD; poorly controlled DM; predisposition to gout; allergy; thrombocytopenia; patients at risk for hypophosphatemia; Safety and effectiveness of immediate-release tablets have not been established in pediatric patients; safety and

N

efficacy of extended-release tablets not established in pediatric patients 16 y or younger.

ROUTE & DOSAGE

Dietary Supplementation

Adult: **PO** 50 mg bid or 100 mg daily

Hyperlipidemia

Adult: **PO** Not typically recommended, dose varies based on specific product

ADMINISTRATION

Oral

- Give with meals to decrease GI distress. Give with cold water (not hot beverage) to facilitate swallowing.
- May take at bedtime with a low-fat snack.
- May pretreat with aspirin or ibuprofen 30 minutes before dose to reduce severity and frequency of flushing, itching, and GI distress.
- Ensure that sustained release form is not chewed or crushed. It **must be** swallowed whole.
- Store at 15°–30° C (59°–86° F) in a light and moisture proof container.

ADVERSE EFFECTS (≥5%) **Skin:** *Flushing* **GI:** *Nausea,* vomiting.

DIAGNOSTIC TEST INTERFERENCE

Decreases ***serum cholesterol*** 15–30% and may cause false elevations with certain ***fluorometric methods*** of determining ***urinary catecholamines.*** Niacin may cause false-positive ***urine glucose*** tests using ***copper sulfate reagents*** (e.g., ***Benedict's*** solution).

INTERACTIONS **Drug:** BILE ACID SEQUESTRANTS may decrease absorption of niacin. May increase risk of myopathy with **simvastatin**.

PHARMACOKINETICS **Absorption:** Readily from GI tract. **Peak:** 20–70 min. **Distribution:** Into breast milk. **Metabolism:** In liver. **Elimination:** Primarily in urine. **Half-Life:** 45 min.

NURSING IMPLICATIONS

Assessment & Drug Effects

- Monitor therapeutic effectiveness and record effect of therapy on clinical manifestations of deficiency (fiery red tongue, excessive saliva secretion and infection of oral membranes, nausea, vomiting, diarrhea, confusion). Therapeutic response usually begins within 24 h.
- Monitor patients with DM and patients on high doses for decreased glucose tolerance and loss of glycemic control.
- Observe patients closely for evidence of liver dysfunction (jaundice, dark urine, light-colored stools, pruritus) and hyperuricemia in patients predisposed to gout (flank, joint, or stomach pain; altered urine excretion pattern).
- Monitor lab tests: Baseline and periodic blood glucose, LFTs with prolonged high dose therapy, serum creatine phosphokinase (CPK) and potassium, periodic phosphorus (patients at risk for hypophosphatemia), prothombin time in patients going to surgery.

Patient & Family Education

- Be aware that you may feel warm and flushed in face, neck, and ears within first 2 h after oral ingestion and it may last several hours. Effects are usually transient and subside as therapy continues.
- Sit or lie down and avoid sudden posture changes if you feel weak

or dizzy. Report these symptoms and persistent flushing to your prescriber.
- Be aware that alcohol and large doses of niacin cause increased flushing and sensation of warmth.
- Avoid exposure to direct sunlight until lesions have entirely cleared if you have skin manifestations.
- Notify healthcare provider if dose is missed for several days, the dose may need to be adjusted before the medication can be resumed.

NICARDIPINE HYDROCHLORIDE

(ni-car′di-peen)

Cardene

Classification: CALCIUM CHANNEL BLOCKER; ANTIHYPERTENSIVE
Therapeutic: ANTIHYPERTENSIVE; ANTIANGINAL
Prototype: Nifedipine

AVAILABILITY Capsule; sustained release capsule; solution for injection

ACTION & *THERAPEUTIC EFFECT*

Calcium channel entry blocker that inhibits the transmembrane influx of calcium ions into cardiac muscle and smooth muscle, thus affecting contractility. Selectively affects vascular smooth muscle more than cardiac muscle. *Significantly decreases systemic vascular resistance. It reduces BP at rest and during isometric and dynamic exercise.*

USES Either alone or with beta-blockers for chronic, stable (effort-associated) angina; either alone or with other antihypertensives for essential hypertension.

UNLABELED USES CHF, cerebral ischemia, migraine.

CONTRAINDICATIONS Hypersensitivity to nicardipine; advanced aortic stenosis; cardiogenic shock; hypotension.

CAUTIOUS USE CHF; renal and hepatic impairment; severe bradycardia; older adult; GERD; hiatal hernia; renal disease; renal impairment; acute stroke; angina; CHF; acute myocardial infarction; older adults; pregnancy (category C); lactation. Safety and efficacy in children not established.

ROUTE & DOSAGE

Hypertension, Angina

Adult: **PO** 20–40 mg tid or 30–60 mg SR bid; *Initiation of therapy in a drug-free patient:* **IV** 5 mg/h initially, increase dose by 2.5 mg/h q15min (or faster) (max: 15 mg/h); *for severe hypertension:* 4–7.5 mg/h; *for postop hypertension:* 10–15 mg/h initially, then 1–3 mg/h

ADMINISTRATION

Note: To prevent symptoms of withdrawal, do not abruptly discontinue drug.

Oral

- Give on empty stomach. High-fat meals may decrease blood levels.
- Ensure that sustained release form is not chewed or crushed. It **must be** swallowed whole.
- When converting from IV to oral dose, give first dose of tid regimen 1 h before discontinuing infusion.

Intravenous

PREPARE: **IV Infusion:** Dilute each 25 mg with 240 mL of D5W or NS to yield 0.1 mg/mL.

ADMINISTER: **IV Infusion:** Usually initiated at 50 mL/h (5 mg/h) with rate increases of 25 mL/h (2.5 mg/h) q5–15min up to a maximum of 150 mL/h. ▪ Infusion is usually slowed to 30 mL/h once the target BP is reached. *Substitute for oral doses:* Oral 20 mg q8h, IV equivalent is 0.5 mg/h; oral 30 mg q8h, IV equivalent is 1.2 mg/h; oral 40 mg q8h, IV equivalent is 2.2 mg/h.

INCOMPATIBILITIES: **Solution/additive:** **Sodium bicarbonate.** **Y-site:** **Acyclovir, aminocaproic acid, aminophylline, amphotericin B, ampicillin, ampicillin/sulbactam, atenolol, azithromycin, cefoperazone, ceftazidime, cefuroxime, clindamycin, dexamethasone, diazepam, ertapenem, fludarabine, fluorouracil, foscarnet, fosphenytoin, furosemide, ganciclovir, gemtuzumab, hydrocortisone, heparin, imipenem/cilastatin, ketorolac, lansoprazole, meropenem, mesna, methohexital, methotrexate, micafungin, pantoprazole, pemetrexed, pentobarbital, phenobarbital, phenytoin, piperacillin, potassium acetate, potassium phosphates.**

ADVERSE EFFECTS **CV:** Pedal edema, hypotension, flushing, palpitations, tachycardia, increased angina. **CNS:** Dizziness or headache, fatigue, anxiety, depression, paresthesias, insomnia, somnolence, nervousness. **Skin:** Rash, pruritus. **GI:** Anorexia, nausea, vomiting, dry mouth, constipation, dyspepsia. **Other:** Arthralgia or arthritis.

INTERACTIONS **Drug:** **Adenosine** prolongs bradycardia. **Amiodarone** may cause sinus arrest and AV block. **Benazepril** blunts increase in heart rate and increase in plasma **norepinephrine** and **aldosterone** seen with nicardipine. BETA-BLOCKERS cause hypotension and bradycardia. **Cimetidine** increases levels of nicardipine, resulting in hypotension. Concomitant nicardipine and **cyclosporine** result in significant increase in **cyclosporine** serum concentrations 1–30 days after initiation of nicardipine therapy; following withdrawal of nicardipine, **cyclosporine** levels decrease. **Magnesium,** when used to retard premature labor, may cause severe hypotension and neuromuscular blockade. **Food:** **Grapefruit juice** (greater than 1 qt/day) may increase plasma concentrations and adverse effects.

PHARMACOKINETICS **Absorption:** Immediately 35% of oral dose reaches systemic circulation. **Onset:** 1 min IV; 20 min PO. **Peak:** 0.5–2 h. **Duration:** 3 h IV. **Distribution:** 95% protein bound; distributed in breast milk. **Metabolism:** Rapidly and extensively in liver (CYP3A4); active metabolite has less than 1% activity of parent compound. **Elimination:** 35% in feces, 60% in urine; not affected by hemodialysis. **Half-Life:** 8.6 h.

NURSING IMPLICATIONS

Assessment & Drug Effects

- Establish baseline data before treatment is started including BP and pulse.
- Monitor closely BP values during initiation and titration of dosage. Hypotension with or without an increase in heart rate may occur.

- Avoid too rapid reduction in either systolic or diastolic pressure during parenteral administration.
- Discontinue IV infusion if hypotension or tachycardia develop.
- Observe for large peak and trough differences in BP. Initially, measure BP at peak effect (1–2 h after dosing) and at trough effect (8 h after dosing).

Patient & Family Education

- Record and report any increase in frequency, duration, and severity of angina when initiating or increasing dosage. Keep a record of nitroglycerin use and promptly report any changes in previous anginal pattern.
- Do not change dosage regimen without consulting prescriber.
- Be aware that abrupt withdrawal may cause an increased frequency and duration of chest pain. This drug **must be** gradually tapered under medical supervision.
- Rise slowly from a recumbent position; avoid driving or operating potentially dangerous equipment until response to nicardipine is known.
- Notify prescriber if any of the following occur: Irregular heartbeat, shortness of breath, swelling of the feet, pronounced dizziness, nausea, or drop in BP.

NICOTINE

(nik′o-teen)

Nicotrol NS, Nicotrol Inhaler, Commit

NICOTINE POLACRILEX

Nicorette Gum, Nicorette DS, Thrive

NICOTINE TRANSDERMAL SYSTEM

Habitrol, Nicoderm, Nicotrol

Classification: SMOKING DETERRENT; CHOLINERGIC RECEPTOR ANTAGONIST
Therapeutic: SMOKING DETERRENT

AVAILABILITY Gum; lozenges; nasal spray; inhaler; transdermal patch

ACTION & *THERAPEUTIC EFFECT* Ganglionic cholinergic receptor antagonist that has both adrenergic and cholinergic effects. Includes stimulant and depressant effects on the peripheral nervous system and CNS; respiratory stimulation; peripheral vasoconstriction; increased heart rate, cardiac output, and stroke volume; increased tone and motor activity of GI smooth muscles; increased bronchial secretions (initially); antidiuretic activity. Heavy smokers are tolerant of these effects. *Rationale for use is to reduce withdrawal symptoms accompanying cessation of smoking. Success rate appears to be greatest in smokers with high "physical" type of nicotine dependence.*

USES Treatment to aid smoking cessation.

CONTRAINDICATIONS Nonsmokers, immediate post-MI period; life-threatening arrhythmias; active temporomandibular joint disease; severe angina pectoris; women with childbearing potential (unless effective contraception is used); pregnancy—fetal risk cannot be ruled out; lactation—infant risk has been demonstrated.

CAUTIOUS USE Vasospastic disease (e.g., Buerger's disease, Prinzmetal's variant angina), cardiac arrhythmias, hyperthyroidism, type 1 diabetes, pheochromocytoma, esophagitis, oral and pharyngeal inflammation; renal impairment, hepatic impairment, chronic nasal disorders, asthma, denture use, denture caps, or partial bridges; hypertension and peptic ulcer disease (active or inactive); GERD. Children younger than 18 y.

ROUTE & DOSAGE

Smoking Cessation

Adult: **PO** Chew 1 piece of gum whenever having an urge to smoke, may be repeated as needed (max: 24 pieces of gum/day); continue to extend the time between doses after the first 6 weeks **Intranasal** 1 spray in each nostril, start with 1–2 doses (2–4 sprays) each hour (max: 5 doses or 10 sprays/hour to max of 80 sprays/day), may continue for 3 mo
Topical Patients smoking greater than 10 cigarettes/day begin with Step 1 (21 mg/day) × 6w then Step 2 (14 mg/day) × 2w then Step 3 (7 mg/day) × 2w. Patients smoking less than 10 cigarettes/day begin with Step 2 (14 mg/day) × 6w then Step 3 (7 mg/day) × 2w.

ADMINISTRATION

Oral

- Note: Most adverse local effects (irritation of tongue, mouth, and throat, jaw-muscle aches, dislike of taste) are transient and subside in a few days. Modification of the chewing technique may help.
- Store gum/lozenges/troche between 20 and 25° C (68–77° F). Protect from light.

Nasal

- Tilt head back slightly when spray is administered. Do not sniff, swallow, or inhale through the nose during administration.
- Rinse exposed skin, lips, mouth, eyes or ears immediately with water only.
- Store at controlled room temperature of 25° C (77° F), excursions permitted between 15 and 30° C (59 and 86° F).

Inhalation

- Use regularly during the first week to help adapt to the irritant effects of the inhaler.
- After using the inhaler, separate the mouthpiece and remove and discard the used cartridge. Clean mouthpiece with soap and water and store in the plastic case.
- Store at room temperature not to exceed 25° C (77° F). Protect cartridges from light.

Transdermal

- Remove the old patch before applying the next new patch.
- Apply patch to nonhairy, clean, dry skin site; immediately remove from protective container.
- Store between 20 and 25° C (68 and 77° F).

ADVERSE EFFECTS (≥5%) **Respiratory:** *Sore mouth or throat, nasal irritation,* (nasal spray) **CNS:** *Headache, dizziness, light-headedness,* insomnia, irritability, dependence on nicotine *nose, nasal irritation, throat irritation, watering eyes,* minor epistaxis, nasal ulceration. **Skin:** *Erythema, pruritus, local edema, rash;* skin reactions may be delayed, occurring after 3 wk of patch use. **Other:** Acute overdose/nicotine intoxication (perspiration; severe headache; dizziness; disturbed hearing and vision; mental confusion; severe weakness;

fainting; hypotension; dyspnea; weak, rapid, irregular pulse; seizures); death (from respiratory failure secondary to drug-induced respiratory muscle paralysis).

INTERACTIONS **Drug:** May increase tachycardic effect of **adenosine**. **Varenicline** may increase adverse effects of nicotine replacement therapy. May increase metabolism of **caffeine, theophylline, acetaminophen, insulin, oxazepam, pentazocine propranolol. Food:** Coffee, cola may decrease nicotine absorption from nicotine lozenge.

PHARMACOKINETICS **Absorption:** Approximately 90% of the nicotine in a piece of gum is released slowly over 15–30 min; rate of release is controlled by vigor and duration of chewing; readily absorbed from buccal mucosa; transdermal 75–90% absorbed through skin; 53–58% of nasal spray is absorbed. **Peak:** Transdermal 8–9 h; nasal spray 4–15 min. **Distribution:** Crosses placenta; distributed into breast milk. **Metabolism:** In liver, primarily to cotinine. **Elimination:** In urine. **Half-Life:** 30–120 min. (depending on dosage form)

NURSING IMPLICATIONS

Assessment & Drug Effects

- Be aware that transient erythema, pruritus, or burning is common with transdermal patch and usually disappears 24 h after patch removal.
- Monitor pulse and blood pressure.
- Differentiate cutaneous hypersensitivity (contact sensitization) that does not resolve in 24 h from a transient local reaction. The former is an indication to discontinue the transdermal patch.

Patient & Family Education

- Chew a piece of gum for approximately 30 min to get the full dose of nicotine.
- Chew only one piece of gum at a time. Chewing gum too rapidly can cause excessive buccal absorption and lead to adverse effects: Nausea, hiccups, throat irritation.
- Gradually decrease number of pieces of gum chewed in 24 h. Usually, a period of 3 mo is allowed before tapering use of gum.
- Do not use nasal and inhalation forms of the drug beyond 6 months.
- Promptly discontinue use of transdermal patch and notify prescriber if a severe or persistent local or generalized skin reaction occurs.
- Remove transdermal patch before having magnetic resonance imaging (MRI), exposure may lead to skin burns.
- Smoking while using the transdermal nicotine patch increases the risk of adverse reactions.
- Report any episodes of tachycardia and palpitations.
- Immediately report to healthcare provider any symptoms of nicotine overdose (severe headache, dizziness, upset stomach, vomiting, blurred vision).

NIFEDIPINE

(nye-fed′i-peen)

Adalat CC, Afeditab CR, Nifedical XL, Procardia, Procardia XL

Classification: CALCIUM CHANNEL BLOCKER; ANTIANGINAL, ANTIHYPERTENSIVE

Therapeutic: ANTIHYPERTENSIVE, ANTIANGINAL

AVAILABILITY Capsule; sustained release tablet

ACTION & *THERAPEUTIC EFFECT* Blocks calcium ion influx across cell membranes of cardiac muscle and vascular smooth muscle. Reduces myocardial oxygen utilization and supply and relaxes and prevents coronary artery spasm. Decreases peripheral vascular resistance and increases cardiac output. *The rise in peripheral blood flow is the basis for use in treatment of Raynaud's phenomenon as well as hypertension. Effective antianginal agent.*

USES Vasospastic "variant" or Prinzmetal's angina and chronic stable angina without vasospasm. Mild to moderate hypertension.

UNLABELED USES Vascular headaches; Raynaud's phenomenon; asthma; cardiomyopathy; primary pulmonary hypertension.

CONTRAINDICATIONS Known hypersensitivity to nifedipine; unstable angina; acute MI; cardiogenic shock; aortic stenosis; GI obstruction.

CAUTIOUS USE GERD; CHF; pregnancy (category C); lactation; children.

ROUTE & DOSAGE

Variant Angina

Adult: **PO** 10 mg tid may titrate up to 180 mg/day; **Extended release** 30–60 mg daily; titrate up if necessary (max: 90 mg/day)

Hypertension

Adult: **PO Extended release** 30–60 mg once/day; titrate up if necessary (max: 90 mg/day)

ADMINISTRATION

Oral

- Do not give within the first 1–2 wk following an MI.
- Do not give with grapefruit juice.
- Use only the sustained release form to treat chronic hypertension. Ensure that sustained release form is not chewed or crushed. It **must be** swallowed whole.
- Discontinue drug gradually, with close medical supervision to prevent severe hypertension and other adverse effects.
- Store intermediate release capsules at 15°–25° C (59°–77° F); protect from light and moisture.

ADVERSE EFFECTS **CV:** Hypotension, *facial flushing, heat sensation,* palpitations, *peripheral edema,* MI (rare), prolonged systemic hypotension with overdose. **Respiratory:** Nasal congestion, dyspnea, cough, wheezing. **CNS:** *Dizziness, light-headedness,* nervousness, mood changes, weakness, jitteriness, sleep disturbances, blurred vision, retinal ischemia, difficulty in balance, *headache.* **Skin:** Dermatitis, pruritus, urticaria. **GI:** Nausea, heartburn, *diarrhea,* constipation, cramps, flatulence, gingival hyperplasia, hepatotoxicity. **GU:** Sexual difficulties, possible male infertility. **Musculoskeletal:** Inflammation, joint stiffness, muscle cramps. **Other:** Sore throat, weakness, fever, sweating, chills, febrile reaction.

DIAGNOSTIC TEST INTERFERENCE Nifedipine may cause mild to moderate increases of ***alkaline phosphatase, CPK, LDH, AST, ALT.***

INTERACTIONS **Drug:** BETA-BLOCKERS may increase likelihood of CHF; may increase risk of

phenytoin toxicity. Do not use with strong CYP3A4 inducers (e.g., BARBITURATES, **carbamazepine, phenobarbital, rifabutin, rifampin**). **Herbal: Melatonin** may increase blood pressure and heart rate. **Ginkgo, ginseng** may increase plasma concentrations. **St. John's wort** may decrease plasma concentrations. **Food: Grapefruit juice** (greater than 1 qt/day) may increase plasma concentrations and adverse effects.

PHARMACOKINETICS Absorption: Readily from GI tract; 45–75% reaches systemic circulation. **Onset:** 10–30 min. **Peak:** 30 min. **Distribution:** Distributed into breast milk; 92–98% protein bound. **Metabolism:** In liver via CYP3A4, P-glycoprotein. **Elimination:** 75–80% in urine, 15% in feces. **Half-Life:** 2–5 h.

NURSING IMPLICATIONS

Assessment & Drug Effects

- Monitor BP carefully during titration period. Patient may become severely hypotensive, especially if also taking other drugs known to lower BP. Withhold drug and notify prescriber if systolic BP less than 90.
- Monitor blood sugar in diabetic patients. Nifedipine has diabetogenic properties.
- Monitor for gingival hyperplasia and report promptly. This is a rare but serious adverse effect (similar to phenytoin-induced hyperplasia).

Patient & Family Education

- Keep a record of nitroglycerin use and promptly report any changes in previous pattern. Occasionally, people develop increased frequency, duration, and severity of angina when they start treatment with this drug or when dosage is increased.
- Be aware that withdrawal symptoms may occur with abrupt discontinuation of the drug (chest pain, increase in anginal episodes, MI, dysrhythmias).
- Inspect gums visually every day. Changes in gingivae may be gradual, and bleeding may be exhibited only with probing.
- Seek prompt treatment for symptoms of gingival hyperplasia (easy bleeding of gingivae and gradual enlarging of gingival mass, especially on buccal side of lower anterior teeth). Drug will be discontinued if gingival hyperplasia occurs.
- Research shows that smoking decreases the efficacy of nifedipine and has direct and adverse effects on the heart in the patient on nifedipine treatment.

NILOTINIB HYDROCHLORIDE

(ni-lot′i-nib hy-dro-chlor′ide)

Tasigna

Classification: ANTINEOPLASTIC TYROSINE KINASE INHIBITOR

Therapeutic: ANTINEOPLASTIC

Prototype: Erlotinib

AVAILABILITY Capsule

ACTION & *THERAPEUTIC EFFECT*

Nilotinib is a tyrosine kinase inhibitor designed to selectively inhibit the BCR-ABL tyrosine kinase on the Philadelphia chromosome found in chronic myelogenous leukemia (CML). It prevents tyrosine kinase enzyme from converting to its active conformation. Thus, it prevents proliferation of BCR-ABL cells and ultimately induces cell death in CML. Nilotinib enhances binding site affinity by offering alternate binding pathways for the ABL tyrosine kinases. *Increased kinase selectivity and binding site affinity makes nilotinib more potent than other similar drugs (imatinib) in preventing the proliferation of CML.*

USES Treatment of Philadelphia chromosome positive (Ph^+) chronic myelogenous leukemia (CML) in patients resistant to or intolerant to prior therapy that included imatinib.

CONTRAINDICATIONS Hypoglycemia; hypomagnesemia; hypokalemia; long QT syndrome; drug-induced QT prolongation; severe galactose or lactose intolerance; glucose-galactose malabsorption syndromes; pregnancy (fetal risk cannot be ruled out); lactation (infant risk cannot be ruled out).

CAUTIOUS USE History of pancreatitis; history of cardiac disease, recent MI, CHF, unstable angina; myelosuppression; total gastrectomy; hepatic impairment. Safety and efficacy in children younger than 18 y not established.

N

ROUTE & DOSAGE

Chronic Myelogenous Leukemia

Adult: **PO** 300 or 400 mg bid

QT Prolongation Dosage Adjustment

See package insert.

Myelosuppression Dosage Adjustment

- If ANC less than 1×10^9/L or platelet count less than 50×10^9/L, discontinue nilotinib.
- If ANC greater than 1×10^9/L and platelet count greater than 50×10^9/L within 2 wk, resume previous dose.
- If ANC less than 1×10^9/L or platelet count less than 50×10^9/L for more than 2 wk, reduce to 400 mg PO daily

Nonhematologic Abnormalities Dosage Adjustment

For grade 3 or higher serum lipase, amylase, bilirubin, or hepatic transaminases: Withhold nilotinib and monitor abnormal level(s).
Resume nilotinib at 400 mg PO daily if toxicity resolves to grade 1 or lower.
Other moderate/severe nonhematologic toxicities: Withhold nilotinib until toxicity resolves, then resume at 400 mg PO daily. May increase to 400 mg bid

ADMINISTRATION

Oral

- Give on an empty stomach, at least 1 h before or 2 h after eating.
- Ensure that capsules are swallowed whole with water.
- For those unable to swallow, contents of capsule may be added to 1 tsp of applesauce immediately before administration.
- Note: Hypokalemia and hypomagnesemia should be corrected prior to drug administration.
- Store at 15°–30° C (59°–86° F)

ADVERSE EFFECTS **CV:** Peripheral edema, hypertension, ischemic heart disease. **Respiratory:** *Cough, nasopharyngitis,* URI, dyspnea, oropharyngeal pain, flu-like symptoms. **CNS:** *Fatigue, headache,* insomnia, dizziness. **Endocrine:** Hypertriglyceridemia, hyponatremia, hypophosphatemia, *increased serum cholesterol, increased blood glucose,* increased serum triglycerides. **Skin:** *Rash,* alopecia, *night sweats, pruritis.*

Hepatic: *Increased serum ALT, increased serum AST,* hyperbilirubinemia. **GI:** Abdominal pain, *constipation, diarrhea,* increased serum lipase, *nausea, vomiting.* **Musculoskeletal:** *Joint pain,* back pain, limb pain, muscle weakness, muscle pain, muscle spasm. **Hematologic:** Neutropenia, thrombocytopenia, anemia. **Other:** *Fever.*

INTERACTIONS Drug: CYP3A4 Inducers (**carbamazepine, dexamethasone, phenobarbital, phenytoin, rifabutin, rifampin, rifapentine**) decrease nilotinib levels. Inhibitors of CYP3A4 (**clarithromycin, indinavir, itraconazole, ketoconazole, nefazodone, nelfinavir, ritonavir, saquinavir, telithromycin, voriconazole**) increase nilotinib levels. Nilotinib increases the levels of **midazolam, warfarin. Food:** Food increases bioavailability. **Grapefruit** juice may increase nilotinib levels. **Herbal: St. John's wort** decreases nilotinib levels.

PHARMACOKINETICS Peak: 3 h. **Distribution:** 98% plasma protein bound. **Metabolism:** Hepatic to in active metabolites CYP 3A4. **Elimination:** 93% fecal. **Half-Life:** 17 h.

NURSING IMPLICATIONS

Black Box Warning

Nilotinib has been associated with prolongation of the QT interval and sudden death.

Assessment & Drug Effects

- Obtain a baseline ECG, then again 7 days after first drug dose, and periodically thereafter. Withhold drug and report immediately QT prolongation.
- Monitor closely patients with hepatic impairment for QT interval prolongation.
- Monitor diabetics for loss of glycemic control.
- Monitor signs and symptoms of bleeding, fluid retention and respiratory compromise during treatment.
- Monitor lab tests: Baseline and periodic serum electrolytes, lipid profile, serum glucose, LFTs, serum lipase/amylase; CBC q2wk first 2 mo then monthly thereafter.

Patient & Family Education

- Women of childbearing age should use reliable forms of contraception, including a barrier type.
- Report any bright red bleeding noted in the stool, black tarry stools, or coffee ground or obvious blood in emesis.
- Report any yellowing of the skin or the whites of the eyes.
- Avoid grapefruit products while on nilotinib.

N

NILUTAMIDE

(ni-lu′ta-mide)

Nilandron

Classification: ANTINEOPLASTIC; ANTIANDROGEN

Therapeutic: ANTINEOPLASTIC; ANTI ANDROGEN

Prototype: Flutamide

AVAILABILITY Tablet

ACTION & *THERAPEUTIC EFFECT* Blocks the effects of testosterone at the androgen receptor sites, thus preventing the normal androgenic response. *Effective in blocking testosterone in treatment of metastatic prostate carcinoma.*

USES Use with surgical castration for metastatic prostate cancer.

CONTRAINDICATIONS

CONTRAINDICATIONS Hypersensitivity to nalutamide; females, severe hepatic impairment, hepatitis; severe respiratory insufficiency; drug-induced interstitial pneumonitis; pregnancy—fetal risk cannot be ruled out; lactation—infant risk cannot be ruled out.

CAUTIOUS USE Asian patients relative to causing interstitial pneumonitis; alcoholics. Safety and efficacy in children not established.

ROUTE & DOSAGE

Metastatic Prostate Cancer

Adult: **PO** 300 mg daily × 30 days, then 150 mg daily

ADMINISTRATION

Oral

- Give first dose on the day of or day after surgical castration.
- Give without regard to food.
- Store at 25 degrees C (77 degrees F), excursions permitted between 15°–30° C (59°–86° F) and protect from light.

ADVERSE EFFECTS **Respiratory:** *Dyspnea.* **CNS:** *Headache, insomnia.* **HEENT:** Poor adaptation to darkened environments. **Endocrine:** *Hot sweats.* **Skin:** Pruritus. **GU:** Atrophy of testis, reduced libido.

INTERACTIONS **Drug:** Use caution in low therapeutic margin drugs. **Herbal:** **St. John's wort** may decrease levels. **Food:** Avoid alcohol (increased risk of ethanol intolerance).

PHARMACOKINETICS **Absorption:** Rapidly from GI tract. **Metabolism:** In the liver (CYP2C19). **Elimination:** In urine. **Half-Life:** 38–50 h.

NURSING IMPLICATIONS

Black Box Warning

Nilutamide has been associated with development of interstitial pneumonitis.

Assessment & Drug Effects

- Obtain baseline chest x-ray before treatment and periodically thereafter.
- Closely monitor for S&S of pneumonitis; at the first sign of adverse pulmonary effects, withhold drug and notify prescriber. Abnormal ABGs may indicate need to discontinue drug.
- Monitor patients taking phenytoin, theophylline, or warfarin closely for toxic levels of these drugs.
- Monitor lab tests: Baseline LFTs, then regularly during first 4 mo, and periodically thereafter; LFTs with first sign of liver dysfunction; serum prostate specific antigen and serum alkaline phosphatase; serum transaminase at baseline and at regular intervals for the first 4 months of therapy and periodically thereafter.

Patient & Family Education

- Report to prescriber immediately the following S&S of adverse effects on lungs: Development of chest pain, dyspnea, and cough with fever.
- Review adverse effect with patient and/or caregiver.
- Avoid drinking alcohol while taking this drug.
- Report S&S of liver injury to prescriber: Jaundice, dark urine, fatigue, or signs of GI distress including nausea, vomiting, abdominal pain.
- Use caution when moving from lighted to dark areas because the

drug may slow visual adaptation to darkness. Tinted glasses may partially alleviate the problem.

- Avoid an abrupt discontinuation of the drug.
- Contact healthcare provider if a dose is missed.

NIMODIPINE

(ni-mod′i-peen)

Nymalize

Classification: CALCIUM CHANNEL BLOCKER; CEREBRAL ANTISPASMODIC

Therapeutic: CEREBRAL ANTISPASMODIC

Prototype: Nifedipine

AVAILABILITY Capsule; oral solution

ACTION & *THERAPEUTIC EFFECT* Calcium channel blocking agent that is relatively selective for cerebral arteries compared with arteries elsewhere in the body. *Reduces vascular spasms in cerebral arteries during a stroke.*

USES To improve neurologic deficits due to spasm following subarachnoid hemorrhage.

CONTRAINDICATIONS Hypotension; cardiogenic shock; pregnancy—fetal risk cannot be ruled out; lactation—infant risk cannot be ruled out.

CAUTIOUS USE Hepatic impairment or cirrhosis; acute MI; bradycardia, heart failure, ventricular dysfunction; older adults. Safety and efficacy in children not established.

ROUTE & DOSAGE

Subarachnoid Hemorrhage

Adult: **PO** 60 mg q4h for 21 days, start therapy within 96 h of subarachnoid hemorrhage

Hepatic Impairment Dosage Adjustment

Decrease dose to 30 mg q4h

ADMINISTRATION

Oral

- Administer 1 h before or 2 h after a meal. Do not eat grapefruit or drink grapefruit juice while taking this drug.
- Oral solution: Use the supplied oral syringe labeled “Oral Use Only.” Following drug administration via enteral tube, fill syringe with 20 mL NS and flush the enteral tube.
- Capsule: If capsule cannot be swallowed whole, make a hole in both ends of the capsule with an 18-gauge needle and extract the contents into a syringe. Remove needle and administer contents of syringe orally or via an enteral tube. NEVER administer capsule contents parenterally.
- Store capsule at controlled room temperature between 20 and 25 degrees C (68 and 77 degrees F); protect from light. Store solutions at controlled room temperature at 25 degrees C (77 degrees F), with excursions allowed between 15 and 30 degrees C (59 and 86 degrees F); do not refrigerate. Protect from light.

ADVERSE EFFECTS (>5%) CV: *Hypotension.* **CNS:** Headache.

DIAGNOSTIC TEST INTERFERENCE May lead to false negative aldosterone/renin ratio.

INTERACTIONS Drug: Hypotensive effects increased when combined with other CALCIUM CHANNEL BLOCKERS, ALPHA-1 BLOCKERS or OTHER ANTIHYPERTENSIVES. Effects could be decreased when used with CYP 3A4 inducers and can be increased when used with CYP3A4 inhibitors. **Rifamycin** may decrease concentration of nimodipine; **cimetidine** may increase concentration of nimodipine. **Food: Grapefruit juice** (greater than 1 qt/day) may increase plasma concentrations and adverse effects. **Herbal:** Avoid use of **St. John's wort.**

PHARMACOKINETICS Absorption: Readily from GI tract; approximately 13% reaches systemic circulation (first pass metabolism). **Peak:** 1 h. **Distribution:** Crosses blood–brain barrier; possibly crosses placenta; distributed into breast milk; 95% protein bound. **Metabolism:** extensively hepatic via CYP3A4. **Elimination:** Greater than 50% in urine, 32% in feces. **Half-Life:** 1–2 h.

NURSING IMPLICATIONS

Black Box Warning

Do not administer nimodipine intravenously or by other parenteral routes. Deaths and serious, life threatening adverse events have occurred when the contents of nimodipine capsules have been injected parenterally.

Assessment & Drug Effects

- Take apical pulse prior to administering drug and hold it if pulse is below 60. Notify the prescriber.
- Establish baseline data before treatment is started: BP, pulse, and laboratory evaluations of liver and kidney function.
- Monitor frequently for adverse drug effects, including hypotension, peripheral edema, tachycardia, or skin rash.
- Monitor frequently for dizziness or light-headedness in older adult patients; risk of hypotension is increased.

Patient & Family Education

- Report gradual weight gain and evidence of edema (e.g., tight rings on fingers, ankle swelling).
- Review adverse effects with patient and/or caregiver.
- Notify provider before taking any other medication (including over the counter and herbal drugs).
- Keep follow-up appointments for monitoring of progress during therapy.

NISOLDIPINE

(ni-sol′di-peen)

Sular

Classification: CALCIUM CHANNEL BLOCKER; ANTIHYPERTENSIVE

Therapeutic: ANTIHYPERTENSIVE; ANTIANGINAL

Prototype: Nifedipine

AVAILABILITY Extended release tablet

ACTION & *THERAPEUTIC EFFECT* Inhibits calcium ion influx across cell membranes of cardiac muscle and vascular smooth muscle, which results in vasodilation, inotropism, and negative chronotropism. Inhibits vasoconstriction in the peripheral vasculature. *Significantly reduces total peripheral resistance, decreases blood pressure, and increases cardiac output. It is also a potent coronary vasodilator.*

USES Hypertension.

UNLABELED USES CHF, angina.

CONTRAINDICATIONS Hypersensitivity to nisoldipine or other calcium blockers; systolic BP less than 90 mm Hg, cardiogenic shock, severe hypotension, acute MI, sick sinus syndrome.

CAUTIOUS USE Severe hepatic impairment; severe obstructive coronary artery disease; class II to IV heart failure, especially with concurrent administration of a beta-blocker; severe aortic stenosis; hypertrophic cardiomyopathy with outflow tract obstruction; paroxysmal atrial fibrillation; GERD; CHF; digital ischemia, ulceration, or gangrene; nonobstructive hypertrophic cardiomyopathy; Duchenne muscular dystrophy; older adults; pregnancy (category C); lactation, children.

ROUTE & DOSAGE

Hypertension

Adult: **PO** 17 mg daily may increase by 8.5 mg weekly as needed
Geriatric: **PO** 8.5 mg daily, may increase weekly as needed

ADMINISTRATION

Oral

- Give drug with food to decrease GI distress, but do not give with grapefruit juice or a high-fat meal.
- Ensure that extended release form is not chewed or crushed. It **must be** swallowed whole.
- Drug is usually discontinued gradually to prevent adverse effects.
- Store at 15°–30° C (59°–86° F).

ADVERSE EFFECTS **CV:** Hypotension, *peripheral edema*, palpitations, orthostatic hypotension. **Respiratory:** Pulmonary edema (patients with CHF), wheezing, dyspnea, sinusitis. **CNS:** Dizziness, anxiety, tremor, weakness, fatigue, *headache*. **Skin:** *Flushing*, rash, erythema, urticaria. **GI:** Abdominal pain, cramps, constipation, dry mouth, diarrhea, nausea. **GU:** Urinary frequency. **Other:** Myalgia.

INTERACTIONS **Drug:** May cause significant increase in **digoxin** level in patients with CHF. BETA-BLOCKERS may cause hypotension and bradycardia. **Phenytoin, carbamazepine, phenobarbital** may significantly decrease levels. Azole antifungals may affect metabolism; avoid combination. **Food:** High-fat food increases availability.

PHARMACOKINETICS **Absorption:** Rapidly from GI tract; 4–8% reaches systemic circulation. **Peak Effect:** 1–3 h. **Duration:** 8–12 h for hypertension, 7–8 h for angina. **Distribution:** 99% protein bound. **Metabolism:** Extensively in liver. **Elimination:** 70–75% in urine as metabolites. **Half-Life:** 2–14 h.

NURSING IMPLICATIONS

Assessment & Drug Effects

- Monitor blood pressure carefully during period of drug initiation and with dosage increments.
- Monitor cardiovascular status especially heart rate, frequency of angina attacks, or worsening heart failure.
- Assess for and report edematous weight gain.
- Monitor lab tests: Frequent digoxin levels with concurrent use.

Patient & Family Education

- Do not discontinue the drug abruptly.
- Report symptoms of orthostatic hypotension or other bothersome adverse effects to prescriber.
- Do not drive or engage in potentially hazardous activities until response to drug is known.

NITAZOXANIDE

(nit-a-zox′a-nide)

Alinia

Classification: ANTIPROTOZOAL

Therapeutic: ANTIPROTOZOAL

Prototype: Metronidazole

AVAILABILITY Oral suspension; tablet

ACTION & *THERAPEUTIC EFFECT* Antiprotozoal activity believed to be due to interference with an essential enzyme needed for anaerobic energy metabolism in protozoa. *Inhibits growth of sporozoites and oocysts of* Cryptosporidium parvum *and trophozoites of* Giardia lamblia.

N

USES Diarrhea caused by *Cryptosporidium parvum* and *Giardia lamblia.*

UNLABELED USES Rotavirus infection.

CONTRAINDICATIONS Prior hypersensitivity to nitazoxanide.

CAUTIOUS USE Hepatic and biliary disease, renal disease, renal impairment, renal failure, and combined renal and hepatic disease; HIV patients, pregnancy (fetal risk cannot be ruled out); lactation (infant risk cannot be ruled out). Safety and efficacy in children younger than 1 y not studied.

ROUTE & DOSAGE

Infectious Diarrhea

Adult/Adolescent: **PO** 500 mg q12h × 3 days
Child (1–3 y): **PO** 100 mg q12h × 3 days; *4–11 y:* 200 mg q12h × 3 days

ADMINISTRATION

Oral

- Take tablets or suspension with food.
- Prepare suspension as follows: Tap bottle until powder loosens. Draw up 48 mL of water, add half to bottle, shake to suspend powder, then add remaining 24 mL of water and shake vigorously.
- Give required dose (5 or 10 mL) with food.
- Keep container tightly closed, and shake well before each administration.
- Suspension may be stored for 7 days at 15°–30° C (59°–86° F), after which any unused portion **must be** discarded.

INTERACTIONS Food: Increases levels.

PHARMACOKINETICS Peak: 1–4 h. **Distribution:** 99% protein bound. **Metabolism:** Rapidly hydrolyzed in liver to an active metabolite, tizoxanide (desacetyl-nitazoxanide). **Elimination:** In urine, bile, and feces.

NURSING IMPLICATIONS

Assessment & Drug Effects

- Monitor for therapeutic effectiveness: No watery stools and 2 or less soft stools with no hematochezia within the past 24 h or no symptoms and no unformed stools within the past 48 h.

- Monitor closely patients with preexisting hepatic or biliary disease for adverse reactions.
- Assess appetite, level of abdominal discomfort and extent of bloating.
- Assess frequency and quantity of diarrhea and monitor total hydration status.
- Weigh daily to aid in assessment of possible fluid loss from diarrhea.

Patient & Family Education

- Note that 5 mL of the oral suspension contains approximately 1.5 g of sucrose.
- Report either no improvement in or worsening of diarrhea and abdominal discomfort.

NITROFURANTOIN

(nye-troe-fyoor'an-toyn)

Furadantin, Novo-Furan ♣

NITROFURANTOIN MACROCRYSTALS

Macrobid, Macrodantin

Classification: URINARY TRACT ANTI-INFECTIVE; NITROFURAN

Therapeutic: URINARY TRACT ANTIBIOTIC

AVAILABILITY Suspension; capsule

ACTION & THERAPEUTIC EFFECT Synthetic nitrofuran derivative presumed to act by interfering with several bacterial enzyme systems. Highly soluble in urine and reportedly most active in acid urine. Antimicrobial concentrations in urine exceed those in blood. *Active against wide variety of gram-negative and gram positive microorganisms.*

USES Uncomplicated urinary tract infection, including cystitis.

CONTRAINDICATIONS Hypersensitivity to nitrofurantoin including hepatic dysfunction; anuria, oliguria, significant impairment of kidney function (CrCl less than 60 mL/min); G6PD deficiency; history of cholestatic jaundice; pregnancy at term (38–42 wk), labor, or obstetric delivery; lactation.

CAUTIOUS USE History of asthma, anemia, diabetes, vitamin B deficiency, hepatic disease; pulmonary disease; mild to moderate renal disease; electrolyte imbalance, debilitating disease; B_{12} deficiency; pregnancy (category B); infants younger than 1 mo.

ROUTE & DOSAGE

UTI, Cystitis

Adult: **PO** 50–100 mg qid × 7 days, or 3 days after sterile urine sample
Child/Infant (1 mo–12 y): **PO** 1.25–1.75 mg/kg q6h (max: 400 mg/day)
Adult/Adolescent (Macrobid only): **PO** 100 mg q12h × 7 days

Chronic Suppressive Therapy for UTI

Adult: **PO** 50–100 mg at bedtime
Child (1 mo–12 y): **PO** 1 mg/kg/day in 1–2 divided doses (max: 100 mg/day)

Renal Impairment Dosage Adjustment

Avoid if CrCl less than 60 mL/min

ADMINISTRATION

Oral

- Give with food or milk to minimize gastric irritation.
- Avoid crushing tablets because of the possibility of tooth staining; dilute oral suspension in milk,

water, or fruit juice, and rinse mouth thoroughly after taking drug.

ADVERSE EFFECTS **Respiratory:** Allergic pneumonitis, asthmatic attack (patients with history of asthma), pulmonary sensitivity reactions (interstitial pneumonitis or fibrosis). **CNS:** Peripheral neuropathy, headache, nystagmus, drowsiness, vertigo. **Skin:** Skin eruptions, pruritus, urticaria, exfoliative dermatitis, transient alopecia. **GI:** *Anorexia, nausea, vomiting,* abdominal pain, diarrhea, cholestatic jaundice, hepatic necrosis. **GU:** Genitourinary superinfections (especially with *Pseudomonas*), crystalluria (older adult patients), dark yellow or brown urine. **Hematologic (rare):** Hemolytic or megaloblastic anemia (especially in patients with G6PD deficiency), granulocytosis, eosinophilia. **Other:** Angioedema, anaphylaxis, drug fever, arthralgia. Tooth staining from direct contact with oral suspension and crushed tablets (infants).

N

DIAGNOSTIC TEST INTERFERENCE Nitrofurantoin metabolite may produce false-positive ***urine glucose*** test results with ***Benedict's reagent.***

INTERACTIONS **Drug:** ANTACIDS may decrease absorption of nitrofurantoin; **nalidixic acid,** other QUINOLONES may antagonize antimicrobial effects; **probenecid, sulfinpyrazone** increase risk of nitrofurantoin toxicity.

PHARMACOKINETICS **Absorption:** Readily from GI tract. **Peak:** Urine: 30 min. **Distribution:** Crosses placenta; distributed into breast milk. **Metabolism:** Partially in liver. **Elimination:** Primarily in urine. **Half-Life:** 20 min.

NURSING IMPLICATIONS

Assessment & Drug Effects

- Monitor I&O. Report oliguria and any change in I&O ratio.
- Be alert to signs of urinary tract superinfections (e.g., milky urine, foul-smelling urine, perineal irritation, dysuria).
- Assess for nausea (which occurs fairly frequently). May be relieved by using macrocrystalline preparation (Macrodantin).
- Watch for acute pulmonary sensitivity reaction, usually within first week of therapy and apparently more common in older adults. May be manifested by mild to severe flu-like syndrome.
- With prolonged therapy, monitor for subacute or chronic pulmonary sensitivity reaction, commonly manifested by insidious onset of malaise, cough, dyspnea on exertion, altered ABGs.
- Monitor for S&S of peripheral neuropathy, which can be severe and irreversible. Withhold drug and notify prescriber immediately.
- Monitor lab tests: Baseline C&S, LFTs, PFTs, serum creatinine/BUN.

Patient & Family Education

- Report promptly muscle weakness, tingling, numbness.
- Nitrofurantoin may impart a harmless brown color to urine.
- Consult prescriber regarding fluid intake. Generally, fluids are not forced; however, intake should be adequate.

NITROGLYCERIN

(nye-troe-gli'ser-in)

Minitran, Nitrocap, Nitrodisc, Nitro-Dur, Nitrogard, Nitrogard-SR, Nitrong SR, Nitrospan, Nitro-stat, Nitrostat I.V., ProStakan

 Common adverse effects in *italic;* life-threatening effects underlined; generic names in **bold;** classifications in SMALL CAPS; ♣ Canadian drug name; ⊙ Prototype drug; ⚠ Alert

Classification: NITRATE VASODILATOR
Therapeutic: ANTIANGINAL; VASODILATOR

AVAILABILITY Solution for injection; sublingual tablet; sustained release tablet; capsule; transdermal patch; ointment.

ACTION & *THERAPEUTIC EFFECT* Organic nitrate and potent vasodilator that relaxes vascular smooth muscle. After conversion to nitric oxide, it leads to dose-related dilation of both venous and arterial blood vessels. Promotes peripheral pooling of blood, reduction of peripheral resistance, and decreased venous return to the heart. Both left ventricular preload and afterload are reduced and myocardial oxygen consumption or demand is decreased. *Produces antianginal, antiischemic, and antihypertensive effects.*

USES Prophylaxis, treatment, and management of angina pectoris. IV nitroglycerin is used to control BP in perioperative hypertension, CHF associated with acute MI; to produce controlled hypotension during surgical procedures, and to treat angina pectoris in patients who have not responded to nitrate or beta-blocker therapy. Treatment of pain associated with chronic anal fissure.

UNLABELED USES Sublingual and topical to reduce cardiac workload in patients with acute MI and in CHF. Ointment for adjunctive treatment of Raynaud's disease.

CONTRAINDICATIONS Hypersensitivity, idiosyncrasy, or tolerance to nitrates; severe anemia; head trauma, increased ICP. **Sublingual:** Early MI; severe anemia, increased ICP; hypersensitivity to nitroglycerin. **Sustained release form:** Glaucoma. **IV form:** Hypotension, uncorrected hypovolemia, constrictive pericarditis, pericardial tamponade; restrictive cardiomyopathy.

CAUTIOUS USE Severe liver or kidney disease, conditions that cause dry mouth, pregnancy (category C), lactation.

ROUTE & DOSAGE

Angina

Adult: **Sublingual** 1–2 sprays (0.4–0.8 mg) or a 0.3–0.6-mg tablet q3–5 min as needed (max: 3 doses in 15 min); **PO** 1.3–9 mg q8–12h **IV** Start with 5 mcg/min and titrate q3–5 min until desired response (up to 200 mcg/min);
Transdermal Unit Apply once q24h or leave on for 10–12 h, then remove and have a 10–12 h nitrate free interval;
Topical Apply 1.5–5 cm (½–2 in) of ointment q4–6h
Child: **IV** 0.25–0.5 mcg/kg/min, titrate by 0.5–1 mcg/kg/min q3–5min (max: 5 mg/kg/min)

Anal Fissure

Adult: **Topical** 1 inch every 12 h for up to 3 wk

ADMINISTRATION

Sublingual Tablet

- Give 1 tablet and if pain is not relieved, give additional tablets at 5-min intervals, but not more than 3 tablets in a 15-min period.
- Typically available for self-administration in their original container.

N

Instruct in correct use. Request patient to report all attacks.

- Instruct to sit or lie down upon first indication of oncoming anginal pain and to place tablet under tongue or in buccal pouch (hypotensive effect of drug is intensified in the upright position).

Sustained Release Tablet or Capsule

- Give on an empty stomach (1 h before or 2 h after meals), with a full glass of water. Ensure it is swallowed whole.
- Be aware that sustained release form helps to prevent anginal attacks; it is not intended for immediate relief of angina.

Transdermal Ointment

- Using dose-determining applicator (paper application patch) supplied with package, squeeze prescribed dose onto this applicator. Using applicator, spread ointment in a thin, uniform layer to premarked 5.5 by 9 cm (2¼ by 3½ in.) square. Place patch with ointment side down onto nonhairy skin surface (areas commonly used: Chest, abdomen, anterior thigh, forearm). Cover with transparent wrap and secure with tape. Avoid getting ointment on fingers.
- Rotate application sites to prevent dermal inflammation and sensitization. Remove ointment from previously used sites before reapplication.

Transdermal Unit

- Apply transdermal unit (transdermal patch) at the same time each day, preferably to skin site free of hair and not subject to excessive movement. Avoid abraded, irritated, or scarred skin. Clip hair if necessary.
- Change application site each time to prevent skin irritation and sensitization.

Intravenous

- Check to see if patient has transdermal patch or ointment in place before starting IV infusion. The patch (or ointment) is usually removed to prevent overdosage.

PREPARE: **IV Infusion:** Nitroglycerin is available undiluted and premixed in D5W IV solutions of varying concentrations. ▪ *IV Infusion from Concentrate:* Use only non-PVC plastic or glass bottles and manufacturer-supplied IV tubing. ▪ Withdraw contents of one vial (25 or 50 mg) into syringe and inject immediately into 500 mL of IV solution to minimize contact with plastic; yields 50 mcg/mL or 100 mcg/mL. ▪ If less fluid is desired, add 5 mg to 100 mL to yield 50 mcg/mL. Other concentrations within the range of 25–400 mcg/mL may be used.

- Do not exceed 400 mcg/mL.

ADMINISTER: **IV Infusion:** Give by continuous infusion regulated exactly by an infusion pump. ▪ IV dosage titration requires careful and continuous hemodynamic monitoring.

INCOMPATIBILITIES: **Solution/additive: Caffeine, hydralazine, phenytoin. Y-site: Alteplase, levofloxacin.**

- Use only glass containers for storage of reconstituted IV solution. Polyvinyl chloride (PVC) plastic can absorb nitroglycerin and therefore should not be used.
- Non-polyvinyl-chloride (non-PVC) sets are recommended or provided by manufacturer.

ADVERSE EFFECTS CV: *Postural hypotension,* palpitations, tachycardia (sometimes with paradoxical bradycardia), increase in angina, syncope, and circulatory collapse. **CNS:** *Headache,* apprehension, blurred vision, weakness, vertigo, dizziness, faintness. **Skin:** Cutaneous vasodilation with flushing, rash, exfoliative dermatitis, contact dermatitis with transdermal patch; topical allergic reactions with ointment: Pruritic eczematous eruptions, anaphylactoid reaction characterized by oral mucosal and conjunctival edema. **GI:** Nausea, vomiting, involuntary passing of urine and feces, abdominal pain, dry mouth. **Hematologic:** Methemoglobinemia (high doses). **Other:** Muscle twitching, pallor, perspiration, cold sweat; local sensation in oral cavity at point of dissolution of sublingual forms.

DIAGNOSTIC TEST INTERFERENCE

Nitroglycerin may cause increases in determinations of ***urinary catecholamines*** and ***VMA;*** may interfere with the ***Zlatkis-Zak color reaction,*** causing a false report of decreased ***serum cholesterol.***

INTERACTIONS

Drug: Alcohol, ANTIHYPERTENSIVE AGENTS compound hypotensive effects; IV nitroglycerin may antagonize **heparin** anticoagulation. Vasodilating effects may be enhanced by **sildenafil, vardenafil,** or **tadalafil,** so this combination should be avoided.

PHARMACOKINETICS

Absorption: Significant loss to first pass metabolism after oral dosing. **Onset:** 2 min SL; 3 min PO; 30 min ointment. **Duration:** 30 min SL; 3–5 h PO; 3–6 h ointment. **Distribution:** Widely distributed; not known if distributes to breast milk. **Metabolism:** Extensively in liver. **Elimination:** Inactive metabolites in urine. **Half-Life:** 1–4 min.

NURSING IMPLICATIONS

Assessment & Drug Effects

- Administer IV nitroglycerin with extreme caution to patients with hypotension or hypovolemia since the IV drug may precipitate a severe hypotensive state.
- Monitor patient closely for change in levels of consciousness and for dysrhythmias.
- Be aware that moisture on sublingual tissue is required for dissolution of sublingual tablet. However, because chest pain typically leads to dry mouth, a patient may be unresponsive to sublingual nitroglycerin.
- Assess for headaches. Approximately 50% of all patients experience mild to severe headaches following nitroglycerin. Transient headache usually lasts about 5 min after sublingual administration and seldom longer than 20 min. Assess degree of severity and consult as needed with prescriber about analgesics and dosage adjustment.
- Supervise ambulation as needed, especially with older adult or debilitated patients. Postural hypotension may occur even with small doses of nitroglycerin. Patients may complain of dizziness or weakness due to postural hypotension.
- Take baseline BP and heart rate with patient in sitting position before initiation of treatment with transdermal preparations.
- One hour after transdermal (ointment or unit) medication has been applied, check BP and pulse again with patient in sitting position. Report measurements to prescriber.
- Assess for and report blurred vision or dry mouth.

- Assess for and report the following topical reactions: Contact dermatitis from the transdermal patch; pruritus and erythema from the ointment.

Patient & Family Education

- Store tablet form in its original container.
- Sit or lie down upon first indication of oncoming anginal pain.
- Relax for 15–20 min after taking tablet to prevent dizziness or faintness.
- Be aware that pain not relieved by 3 sublingual tablets over a 15-min period may indicate acute MI or severe coronary insufficiency. Contact prescriber immediately or go directly to emergency room.
- Note: Sublingual tablets may be taken prophylactically 5–10 min prior to exercise or other stimulus known to trigger angina (drug effect lasts 30–60 min).
- Keep record for prescriber of number of angina attacks, amount of medication required for relief of each attack, and possible precipitating factors.
- Remove transdermal unit or ointment immediately from skin and notify prescriber if faintness, dizziness, or flushing occurs following application.
- You can use a sublingual formulation while transdermal unit or ointment is in place.
- Report blurred vision or dry mouth. Both warrant withdrawal of drug.
- Change position slowly and avoid prolonged standing. Dizziness, light-headedness, and syncope (due to postural hypotension) occur most frequently in older adults.
- Report any increase in frequency, duration, or severity of anginal attack.

NITROPRUSSIDE SODIUM ⚠

(nye-troe-pruss'ide)

Nitropress

Classification: NONNITRATE VASODILATOR; ANTIHYPERTENSIVE

Therapeutic: ANTIHYPERTENSIVE; VASODILATOR

Prototype: Hydralazine

AVAILABILITY Solution for injection

ACTION & *THERAPEUTIC EFFECT* Potent, rapid-acting hypotensive agent that acts directly on vascular smooth muscle to produce peripheral vasodilation, with consequently marked lowering of arterial BP, mild decrease in cardiac output, and moderate lowering of peripheral vascular resistance. *Effective antihypertensive agent used for rapid reduction of high blood pressure.*

USES Short-term, rapid reduction of BP in hypertensive crises and for producing controlled hypotension during anesthesia to reduce bleeding.

UNLABELED USES Refractory CHF or acute MI.

CONTRAINDICATIONS Compensatory hypertension, as in atriovenous shunt or coarctation of aorta, acute heart failure, and for control of hypotension in patients with inadequate cerebral circulation, congenital optic atrophy, tobacco amblyopia; lactation (infant risk cannot be ruled out).

CAUTIOUS USE Hepatic insufficiency, hypothyroidism, severe renal impairment, hyponatremia, patients receiving anesthesia, older adult patients and patients who are poor surgical risks pregnancy (infant risk cannot be ruled out).

ROUTE & DOSAGE

Hypertensive Crisis

Adult: **IV** 0.3–0.5 mcg/kg/min (average 3 mcg/kg/min)
Child: **IV** 1 mcg/kg/min (average 3 mcg/kg/min) (max: 5 mcg/kg/min)

ADMINISTRATION

Intravenous

PREPARE: **Continuous:** Dissolve each 50 mg in 250–1000 mL of D5W. To yield 50–200 mcg/mL. ▪ Lower concentrations may be desirable depending on patient weight. ▪ Following reconstitution, solutions usually have faint brownish tint; if solution is highly colored, do not use it. ▪ Promptly wrap container with aluminum foil or other opaque material to protect drug from light.

ADMINISTER: **Continuous:** Administer by infusion pump or similar device that will allow precise measurement of flow rate required to lower BP. ▪ Give at the rate required to lower BP, usually between 0.3 and 10 mcg/kg/min.

▪ **Do not** exceed the maximum dose of 10 mcg/kg/min nor give this dose for longer than 10 min.

INCOMPATIBILITIES: **Solution/additive:** **Atracurium, dobutamine, nitroglycerin.** **Y-site:** **Acyclovir, amiodarone, amphotericin B conventional, ampicillin, ascorbic acid, atracurium, azathioprine, caspofungin, ceftazidime, chlorpromazine, cisatracurium, dantrolene, daunorubicin, diazepam, diazoxide, diphenhydramine, dobutamine, erythromycin, garenoxacin mesylate, haloperidol, hydralazine, hydroxyzine, imipenem/cilastatin, irinotecan, levofloxacin, mesna, mitomycin, mitoxantrone, moxifloxacin, mycophenolate, oritavancin, pantoprazole sodium, papaverine, pemetrexed, pentazocine, phenytoin, prochlorperazine, promethazine, propafenone hydrochloride, quinupristin/dalfopristin, sodium thiosulfate, sulfamethoxazole/trimethoprim, thiotepa, vinorelbine, voriconazole.**

▪ Store reconstituted solutions and IV solution at 20°–25° C (68°–77° F) protected from light; stable for 24 h.

ADVERSE EFFECTS **CV:** Bradycardia, ECG changes, flushing, palpitations, severe hypotension, substernal pain, tachycardia. **CNS:** Apprehension, dizziness, headache, increased intracranial pressure, restlessness. **Endocrine:** Hypothyroidism. **Skin:** Sweating, localized redness and streaking, rash. **GI:** Abdominal pain, intestinal obstruction, nausea, retching. **Musculoskeletal:** Muscle twitching. **Hematologic:** Decreased platelet count aggregation, methemoglobinemia.

PHARMACOKINETICS **Onset:** With-in 2 min. **Duration:** 1–10 min after infusion is terminated. **Metabolism:** Rapidly converted to cyanogen in erythrocytes and tissue, which is metabolized to thiocyanate in liver. **Elimination:** Excreted in urine primarily as thiocyanate. **Half-Life:** (Thiocyanate): 2.7–7 days.

NURSING IMPLICATIONS

Black Box Warning

Nitroprusside has been associated with precipitous drops in BP that can lead to irreversible ischemic injuries or death.

Assessment & Drug Effects

- Monitor constantly to titrate IV infusion rate to BP response.
- Relieve adverse effects by slowing IV rate or by stopping drug; minimize them by keeping patient supine.
- Notify prescriber immediately if BP begins to rise after drug infusion rate is decreased or infusion is discontinued.
- Monitor I&O.

NIVOLUMAB

(ni-vo′lu′mab)

Opdivo

Classification: IMMUNOMODULATOR; MONOCLONAL ANTIBODY; PROGRAMMED DEATH RECEPTOR-1 BLOCKER; ANTINEOPLASTIC

Therapeutic: IMMUNOMODULATOR; ANTINEOPLASTIC

Prototype: Basiliximab

AVAILABILITY Solution for injection

ACTION & *THERAPEUTIC EFFECT*

Is a monoclonal antibody that binds to the PD-1 (programmed cell death) receptor found on cytotoxic T-cells and prevents ligands produced by tumor cells from inhibiting the T-cell cytotoxic response, thus allowing tumor-specific cytotoxic T-cells to migrate into the tumor-inducing apoptosis. *Releases an immune pathway that restores the immune response to tumor cells causing tumor cell death.*

USES Treatment of patients with unresectable or metastatic melanoma; treatment of patients with metastatic squamous non-small-cell lung cancer (NSCLC) or small cell lung cancer (SCLC) with progression on or after platinum-based chemotherapy; advanced renal cell cancer; Hodgkin lymphoma; hepatocellular cancer; head/neck cancer, urothelial carconima, colorectal cancer.

CONTRAINDICATIONS Grade 3 or 4 immune-mediated pneumonitis from drug use; immune related encephalopathy due to drug use; severe or life-threatening infusion reactions; pregnancy—may cause fetal harm; lactation—infant risk cannot be ruled out.

CAUTIOUS USE Immune-mediated pneumonitis (Grade 1 or 2), colitis, hepatitis, hepatic impairment; endocrinopathies, nephritis, rash, renal dysfunction; thyroid disorders; hyperglycemia, women of childbearing age. Safety and efficacy in children younger than 12 y not established.

ROUTE & DOSAGE

Metastatic Melanoma, Metastatic Squamous Non-Small-Cell Lung Cancer, Advanced Renal Cell Cancer, Hepatocellular Cancer, Hodgkin Lymphoma

Adult: **IV** 240 mg over 60 min q2wk or 480 mg once q4w until disease progression or unacceptable toxicity

Toxicity Dosage Adjustment

Consult package insert for adjustment based on type and severity of toxicity experienced. See manufacturer's information for toxicities requiring drug discontinuation.

ADMINISTRATION

Intravenous

PREPARE: **IV Infusion:** Withdraw the required dose from the single-use vial and add to an IV bag of NS or D5W to produce a final concentration of 1 mg/mL to 10 mg/mL; for a final volume of 160 mL or less. Mix by gentle inversion but do not shake. IV infusion may be kept at room temperature for no more than 8 h including time of preparation and time for infusion.
ADMINISTER: **IV Infusion:** Give over 30 min through an IV line with a sterile, non-pyrogenic, low protein binding in-line filter (pore size of 0.2 micrometer to 1.2 micrometer). Flush at the end of infusion.
INCOMPATIBILITIES: **Y-site:** Do not coadminister other drugs through the same IV line.

- Store under refrigeration at 2°–8° C (36°–46° F) for no more than 24 h from the time of infusion preparation. Do not freeze. Protect from light.

ADVERSE EFFECTS (≥5%) **CV:** *Hypertension*. **Respiratory:** *Cough, dyspnea*, upper respiratory tract infection. **CNS:** *Headache*, peripheral neuropathy, sensory neuropathy. **Endocrine:** *Hyperglycemia*. **Skin:** Hand-foot syndrome, *rash*, pruritus. **GI:** *Abdominal pain, anorexia, constipation, nausea, vomiting, stomatitis*. **Musculoskeletal:** Arthralgia, *backache, musculoskeletal pain*. **Other:** *Fatigue*.

PHARMACOKINETICS **Half-Life:** 25 days.

NURSING IMPLICATIONS

Assessment & Drug Effects

- Monitor for and promptly report S&S of pneumonitis (e.g., fever, chills, coughing, shortness of breath, body aches, malaise).
- Monitor for and promptly report S&S of colitis (e.g., abdominal pain, blood or pus in stool, frequent diarrhea).
- Monitor for and promptly report S&S of pituitary, adrenal, and thyroid dysfunction.
- Monitor for and promptly report development of a rash.
- Monitor lab tests: Baseline and periodic LFT and renal function tests; pregnancy test prior to initiation of therapy in women of reproductive potential; periodic serum electrolytes, blood glucose levels, CBC with differential and platelet count, and thyroid function tests.

Patient & Family Education

- Report promptly to prescriber any of the following: New or worsening cough, chest pain, shortness of breath, severe diarrhea or vomiting, severe abdominal pain, easy bruising, jaundice, unusual fatigue or agitation, decreased urine output, blood in urine, or swollen ankles, changes in vision.
- Use effective contraception during treatment and for at least 5 mo after the last dose.
- Do not breast-feed while receiving this drug.

N

NIZATIDINE

(ni-za′ti-deen)

Classification: H_2-RECEPTOR ANTAGONIST; ANTISECRETORY
Therapeutic: ANTIULCER; ANTI-SECRETORY
Prototype: Cimetidine

AVAILABILITY Capsule; oral solution

ACTION & THERAPEUTIC EFFECT Inhibits secretion of gastric acid by reversible, competitive blockage of histamine at the H_2 receptor, particularly those in the gastric parietal cells. *Significantly reduces nocturnal gastric acid secretion for up to 12 h.*

USES Active duodenal ulcers; GERD, benign gastric ulcer.

UNLABELED USES Helicobacter pylori eradication, stress ulcer prophylaxis.

CONTRAINDICATIONS Hypersensitivity to nizatidine or other histamine H_2 antagonists; pregnancy—fetal risk cannot be ruled out; lactation—infant risk cannot be ruled out.

N

CAUTIOUS USE Hypersensitivity to other H_2-receptor antagonists; renal impairment or renal failure; older adults; children 12 y or older; children and elderly with CrCl of less than 50 mL/min.

ROUTE & DOSAGE

GERD

Adult/Adolescent: **PO** 150 mg bid × 12 wk

Duodenal Ulcer

Adult: **PO** 150 mg bid or 300 mg at bedtime for up to 8 weeks then 150 mg daily at bedtime

Benign Gastric Ulcer

Adult: **PO** 150 mg bid or 300 mg at bedtime for up to 8 weeks

Renal Impairment Dosage Adjustment

CrCl 20–50 mL/min: **PO** Decrease the dose to 150 mg once daily (active treatment)
CrCl less than 20 mL/min: **PO** Decrease the dose to 150 mg every other day (active treatment)

ADMINISTRATION

Oral

- Give drug usually once daily at bedtime. Dose may be divided and given twice daily.
- Administer oral liquid drug using a calibrated measuring device.
- Be aware that antacids consisting of aluminum and magnesium hydroxides with simethicone decrease nizatidine absorption by about 10%. Administer the antacid 2 h after nizatidine.

ADVERSE EFFECTS (>5%) **Respiratory:** Cough, nasal congestion, nasopharyngitis, *rhinitis*. **CNS:** Somnolence, fatigue Headache, dizziness. **Endocrine:** Hyperuricemia. **Skin**: Pruritus, sweating. **GI:** Abdominal pain, anorexia, constipation, Diarrhea, dry mouth, heart burn, nausea, and vomiting. **Other:** Irritability, fever.

DIAGNOSTIC TEST INTERFERENCE False-positive for urobilinogens using Multistix.

INTERACTIONS **Drug:** May decrease absorption of **delavirdine, didanosine, itraconazole, ketoconazole;** ANTACIDS may decrease absorption of nizatidine. Use caution with agents that may change acidity/solubility (e.g., **atazanavir, itraconazole, ketoconazole**).

May increase **alcohol** levels. Do not use with **dasatinib, delavirdine, pazopanib, risedronate**. **Food:** prolonged treatment may lead to malabsorption of **vitamin B12.**

PHARMACOKINETICS **Absorption:** Greater than 90% from GI tract. **Peak:** 0.5–3 h. **Metabolism:** In liver. **Elimination:** 60% in urine unchanged. **Half-Life:** 1–2 h.

NURSING IMPLICATIONS

Assessment & Drug Effects

- Monitor patient for alleviation of symptoms. Most ulcers should heal within 4 wk.
- Monitor for persistence of ulcer symptoms in patients who continue to smoke during therapy.
- Monitor lab tests: Periodic LFTs and renal function tests with long-term therapy, CBC, intragastric pH.

Patient & Family Education

- Take medications for the full course of therapy even though symptoms may be relieved.
- Do not take other prescription or OTC medications without consulting prescriber.
- Stop smoking; smoking adversely affects healing of ulcers and effectiveness of the drug.

NONOXYNOL-9

(noe-nox′ee-nole)

Conceptrol, Gynol II

Classification: SPERMICIDE CONTRACEPTIVE

Therapeutic: SPERMICIDE CONTRACEPTIVE

AVAILABILITY Gel; foam; sponge

ACTION & *THERAPEUTIC EFFECT* Nonionic surfactant spermicidal incorporated into foams, gels, jelly, or suppositories. Immobilizes sperm by cell membrane disruption. *Applied over the cervix, blocks entrance to uterus by sperm, traps and absorbs seminal fluid, then releases the immediately available spermicide.*

USES Prevention of pregnancy.

CONTRAINDICATIONS Cystocele, prolapsed uterus, sensitivity or allergy to polyurethane or to nonoxynol-9; vaginitis; history of TSS; immediately after delivery or abortion; lactation—infant risk cannot be ruled out.

CAUTIOUS USE HIV patients; menstruation; pregnancy.

ROUTE & DOSAGE

Contraceptive

Adult: **Topical** Apply or insert shortly before intercourse. Repeat before each intercourse. VCF film should be inserted at least 15 min but not more than 3 hours prior to intercourse.

ADMINISTRATION

Topical

- Apply foams, gels, jelly, cream: Fully load intravaginal applicator and insert about $^{2}/_{3}$ of its length [7.5–10 cm (3–4 in.)] into vagina.
- Use with diaphragm: Place 1–3 tsp spermicide formulation in dome prior to insertion. After diaphragm is in place, additional spermicide is recommended. Leave spermicide and diaphragm in place 6 h after intercourse.
- Store a room temperature and avoid exposure to heat or storage at temperatures exceeding 86° F.

ADVERSE EFFECTS **GU:** *Vaginal irritation and dryness; vaginal pain; irritation of penis.*

PHARMACOKINETICS Onset: Spermicidal action is prompt upon contact with sperm; minimal systemic absorption.

NURSING IMPLICATIONS

Patient & Family Education

- Stop using nonoxynol-9 if pregnancy is suspected.
- Report symptoms of vaginal infection to prescriber: Burning, inflammation, intense vaginal and vulvar itching, cheesy, curd-like discharge, painful intercourse, dysuria. Non-oxynol-9 antifungal properties are weaker than its antibacterial potency, thus vulvovaginal candidiasis frequently occurs.
- Use spermicide before the first and every subsequent act of intercourse.
- Remind patient to practice safe sex and the drug does not prevent disease transmission.

N

NOREPINEPHRINE BITARTRATE

(nor-ep-i-nef′rin)

Levophed, Noradrenaline

Classification: ADRENERGIC AGONIST; VASOPRESSOR

Therapeutic: VASOPRESSOR; CARDIAC INOTROPIC

Prototype: Epinephrine

AVAILABILITY Solution for injection

ACTION & *THERAPEUTIC EFFECT* Direct acting sympathomimetic amine identical to natural catecholamine norepinephrine. Acts directly and predominantly on alpha-adrenergic receptors; little action on beta receptors except in heart (beta$_1$ receptors). Causes vasoconstriction and cardiac stimulation; also produces powerful constrictor action on resistance and capacitance blood vessels. *Peripheral vasoconstriction and moderate inotropic stimulation of heart result in increased systolic and diastolic blood pressure, myocardial oxygenation, coronary artery blood flow, and workload of the heart.*

USES To restore BP in certain acute hypotensive states. Also as adjunct in treatment of cardiac arrest.

CONTRAINDICATIONS Use as sole therapy in hypovolemic states, except as temporary emergency measure; mesenteric or peripheral vascular thrombosis; profound hypoxia or hypercarbia; use during cyclopropane or halothane anesthesia; hypertension; hyperthyroidism; lactation.

CAUTIOUS USE Severe heart disease; older adult patients; within 14 days of MAOI therapy; patients receiving tricyclic antidepressants; pregnancy (category C). Safe use in children not established.

ROUTE & DOSAGE

Hypotension

Adult: **IV** Initial 8–12 mcg/min, titrate to response; maintenance dose usually 2–4 mcg/min

ADMINISTRATION

Intravenous

PREPARE: **IV Infusion:** Dilute a 4 mL ampule in 1000 mL of D5W or D5/NS. ▪ More concentrated solutions (e.g., 4 mg in 500 mL to yield 8 mcg/mL) may be used based on fluid requirements. ▪ Do not use solution if discoloration or precipitate is present. Protect from light.

ADMINISTER: **IV Infusion:** Initial rate of infusion is 2–3 mL/min (8–12 mcg/min), then titrated to maintain BP, usually

0.5–1 mL/min (2–4 mcg/min). ▪ An infusion pump is used. Usually give at the slowest rate possible required to maintain BP. Constantly monitor flow rate. ▪ Check infusion site frequently and immediately report any evidence of extravasation: Blanching along course of infused vein (may occur without obvious extravasation), cold, hard swelling around injection site. ▪ **Antidote for extravasation ischemia:** Phentolamine, 5–10 mg in 10–15 mL NS injection, is infiltrated throughout affected area (using syringe with fine hypodermic needle) as soon as possible. ▪ If therapy is to be prolonged, change infusion sites at intervals to allow effect of local vasoconstriction to subside. ▪ Avoid abrupt withdrawal; when therapy is discontinued, infusion rate is slowed gradually.

INCOMPATIBILITIES: **Solution/additive: Aminophylline, amobarbital, chlorothiazide, chlorpheniramine, nafcillin, pentobarbital, phenobarbital, phenytoin, sodium bicarbonate, sodium iodide, streptomycin, warfarin. Y-site: Aminophylline, amiodarone, amphotericin B (conventional and lipid), ampicillin, azathioprine, dantrolene, diazepam, diazoxide, folic acid, foscarnet, ganciclovir, gemtuzumab, haloperidol, hydralazine, indomethacin, insulin, mitomycin, nesiritide, pantoprazole, pentobarbital, phenobarbital, phenytoin, sodium bicarbonate, sulfamethoxazole.**

ADVERSE EFFECTS

CV: Palpitation, hypertension, reflex bradycardia, fatal arrhythmias (large doses), severe hypertension. **Respiratory:** Respiratory difficulty. **CNS:** Headache, violent headache, cerebral hemorrhage, convulsions. **HEENT:** Blurred vision, photophobia. **Endocrine:** Hyperglycemia. **Skin:** Tissue necrosis at injection site (with extravasation). **GI:** Vomiting. **Other:** Restlessness, anxiety, *tremors,* dizziness, weakness, insomnia, pallor, plasma volume depletion, edema, hemorrhage, intestinal, hepatic, or renal necrosis, retrosternal and pharyngeal pain, profuse sweating.

INTERACTIONS

Drug: ALPHA- and BETA-BLOCKERS antagonize pressor effects; ERGOT ALKALOIDS, **furazolidone, guanethidine, methyldopa,** TRICYCLIC ANTIDEPRESSANTS may potentiate pressor effects; **halothane, cyclopropane** increase risk of arrhythmias.

PHARMACOKINETICS

Onset: Very rapid. **Duration:** 1–2 min after infusion. **Distribution:** Localizes in sympathetic nerve endings; crosses placenta. **Metabolism:** In liver and other tissues by catecholamine O-methyltransferase and monoamine oxidase. **Elimination:** In urine.

NURSING IMPLICATIONS

Black Box Warning

Antidote for extravasation ischemia: To prevent sloughing and necrosis from extravasation, infiltrate the area as soon as possible with 10–15 mL of NS containing 5–10 mg of phentolamine. Use a syringe with a fine needle and infiltrated liberally throughout the area (identified by its cold, hard, and pallid appearance). Phentolamine causes immediate and conspicuous local hyperemic changes if the area is infiltrated within 12 h.

N

N

Assessment & Drug Effects

- Monitor constantly while patient is receiving norepinephrine. Take baseline BP and pulse before start of therapy, then q2min from initiation of drug until stabilization occurs at desired level, then every 5 min during drug administration.
- Adjust flow rate to maintain BP at low normal (usually 80–100 mm Hg systolic) in normotensive patients. In previously hypertensive patients, systolic is generally maintained no higher than 40 mm Hg below preexisting systolic level.
- Observe carefully and record mental status (index of cerebral circulation), skin temperature of extremities, and color (especially of earlobes, lips, nail beds) in addition to vital signs.
- Monitor I&O. Urinary retention and kidney shutdown are possibilities, especially in hypovolemic patients. Urinary output is a sensitive indicator of the degree of renal perfusion. Report decrease in urinary output or change in I&O ratio.
- Be alert to patient's complaints of headache, vomiting, palpitation, arrhythmias, chest pain, photophobia, and blurred vision as possible symptoms of overdosage. Reflex bradycardia may occur as a result of rise in BP.
- Continue to monitor vital signs and observe patient closely after cessation of therapy for clinical sign of circulatory inadequacy.

NORETHINDRONE

(nor-eth-in′drone)

Aygestin, Camila, Deblitane, Errin, Incassia, Jencycla, Lyleq, Norlyda, Tulana

NORETHINDRONE ACETATE

Aygestin ♣, Norlutate ♣

Classification: PROGESTIN

Therapeutic: PROGESTIN; CONTRACEPTIVE

AVAILABILITY Tablet

ACTION & *THERAPEUTIC EFFECT* Synthetic progestation hormone with androgenic, anabolic, and estrogenic properties. Progestin only contraceptives alter cervical mucus, exert progestational effect on endometrium, interfere with implantation, and, in some cases, suppress ovulation. *Contraceptive that suppresses the midcycle surge of luteinizing hormone (LH).*

USES Amenorrhea, abnormal uterine bleeding due to hormonal imbalance in absence of organic pathology; endometriosis. Also alone or in combination with an estrogen for birth control.

CONTRAINDICATIONS Thromboembolic disorders, cerebral vascular or coronary vascular disease; carcinoma of breast, endometrium, or liver; abnormal vaginal bleeding; known or suspected pregnancy - fetal risk cannot be ruled out; lactation—infant risk cannot be ruled out.

CAUTIOUS USE Cardiac disease; migraine; diabetes mellitus; CHF; history of thrombophlebitis or thromboembolic disease; children younger than 16 y.

ROUTE & DOSAGE

Amenorrhea

Adult: **PO Acetate** 2.5–10 mg on day 5 through day 10 of menstrual cycle

Endometriosis

Adult: **PO Acetate** 5 mg/day for 2 wk, increase by 2.5 mg/day q2wk up to 15 mg/day, dose may remain at this level for 6–9 mo or until breakthrough bleeding

Progestin-Only Contraception

Adult: **PO Norethindrone** starting on day 1 of menstrual flow, then continuing indefinitely

ADMINISTRATION

Oral

- Note: Dosing schedule is based on a 28-day menstrual cycle.
- NIOSH: use single gloves by anyone handling intact tablets or capsules or administering from a unit-dose package. Use double gloves and wear a protective gown when preparing tablets (cutting, crushing, handling). Wear single gloves and eye protection if the formulation is hard to swallow or if the patient may resist, vomit or spit up.
- Take exactly as directed and at the same time every day.
- Use or add a barrier contraceptive when starting the minipill regimen (progestin only contraception) for the first cycle or for 3 wk to ensure full protection.
- If dose is delayed by more than 3 hours, take the missed dose as soon as remembered; nonhormonal backup contraception is recommended for the next 48 hours of therapy.
- Protect drug from light and from freezing.
- Store tablet at controlled room temperature between 20 and 25° C (68 and 77° F). Excursions permitted between 15 and 30° C (59 and 86° F).

ADVERSE EFFECTS (common)

CNS: Headache. **GI:** Nausea. **GU:** *Breakthrough bleeding.* **Other:** *Breast tenderness.*

DIAGNOSTIC TEST INTERFERENCE

May changes results of some lab tests (coagulation factors, lipids, glucose tolerance, sex hormone binding globulin). Reduced response to ***metyrapone test***.

INTERACTIONS

Drug: CYP3A4 INDUCERS, BARBITURATES, **carbamazepine, fosphenytoin, modafinil, phenytoin, primidone, pioglitazone, rifampin rifabutin, rifapentine, topiramate, troglitazone** can decrease contraceptive effectiveness. Do not use with **ulipristal**.

PHARMACOKINETICS

Absorption: Readily absorbed from GI tract. **Metabolism:** In liver. **Elimination:** In urine and feces as metabolites.

NURSING IMPLICATIONS

Assessment & Drug Effects

- Monitor for S&S of thrombophlebitis (see Appendix F).
- Withhold drug and notify prescriber if any of the following occur: Sudden, complete, or partial loss of vision, proptosis, diplopia, or migraine headache.
- Monitor glucose tolerance and insulin requirements in prediabetic and diabetic women.

Patient & Family Education

- Wait at least 3 mo before becoming pregnant after stopping the

N

minipill to prevent birth defects. Use a barrier or nonhormonal method of contraception until pregnancy is desired.
- If you have not taken all your pills and you miss a period, consider the possibility of pregnancy after 45 days from the last menstrual period; stop using this drug until pregnancy is ruled out.
- If you have taken all your pills and you miss 2 consecutive periods, rule out pregnancy and use a barrier or nonhormonal method of contraception before continuing the regimen.
- Do not smoke during therapy; increase chance of heart attack and stroke.
- Promptly report prolonged vaginal bleeding or amenorrhea.
- Keep appointments for physical checkups (q6–12mo) while you are taking hormonal birth control.

N

NORMAL SERUM ALBUMIN, HUMAN

(al-byoo′min)

Albuminar, Albutein, Buminate, Plasbumin

Classification: PLASMA DERIVATIVE; PLASMA VOLUME EXPANDER

Therapeutic: PLASMA VOLUME EXPANDER

AVAILABILITY Solution for injection

ACTION & *THERAPEUTIC EFFECT* Plasma volume expander that increases the osmotic pressure of plasma. *Expands volume of circulating blood by osmotically shifting tissue fluid into general circulation.*

USES To restore plasma volume and maintain cardiac output in hypovolemic shock; for prevention and treatment of cerebral edema; as adjunct in exchange transfusion for hyperbilirubinemia and erythroblastosis fetalis; to increase plasma protein level in treatment of hypoproteinemia; and to promote diuresis in refractory edema. Also used for blood dilution prior to or during cardiopulmonary bypass procedures. Has been used as adjunct in treatment of adult respiratory distress syndrome (ARDS).

CONTRAINDICATIONS Hypersensitivity to albumin; severe anemia; cardiac failure; within 24 h of severe burns; heart failure; patients with normal or increased intravascular volume.

CAUTIOUS USE Low cardiac reserve, pulmonary disease, absence of albumin deficiency; liver or kidney failure, dehydration, hypertension, hypernatremia; restricted sodium intake; pregnancy (category C).

ROUTE & DOSAGE

Emergency Volume Replacement

Adult: **IV** 25 g, may repeat in 15–30 min if necessary (max: 250 g)

Colloidal Volume Replacement (Nonemergency)

Child: **IV** 12.5 g, may repeat in 15–30 min if necessary

Hypoproteinemia

Adult: **IV** 50–75 g (max: 2 mL/min)
Child: **IV** 25 g (max: 2 mL/min)

ADMINISTRATION

Intravenous

PREPARE: **IV Infusion:** Normal serum albumin, 5%, is infused without further dilution. ▪ Normal serum albumin, 20% and 25%, may be infused undiluted or diluted in NS or D5W (with sodium restriction).

ADMINISTER: **IV Infusion for Hypovolemic Shock:** Give initially as rapidly as necessary to restore blood volume. As blood volume approaches normal, rate should be reduced to avoid circulatory overload and pulmonary edema. ▪ Give 5% albumin at rate not exceeding 2–4 mL/min. Give 20% and 25% albumin at a rate not to exceed 1 mL/min. **IV Infusion with Normal Blood Volume:** Give 5% albumin human at a rate not to exceed 5–10 mL/min; give 20% and 25% albumin at a rate not to exceed 2 or 3 mL/min. **IV Infusion for Children:** Usual rate is 25%–50% of the adult rate.

INCOMPATIBILITIES: **Solution/additive: Amino acids, verapamil. Y-site: Fat emulsion, midazolam, vancomycin, verapamil.**

▪ Store at temperature not to exceed 37° C (98.6° F). ▪ Use solution within 4 h, once container is opened, because it contains no preservatives or antimicrobials. Discard unused portion.

ADVERSE EFFECTS

CV: Circulatory overload, pulmonary edema (with rapid infusion); hypotension, hypertension, dyspnea, tachycardia. **Skin:** Urticaria, rash. **GI:** Nausea, vomiting. **Other:** Fever, chills, flushing, increased salivation, headache, back pain.

DIAGNOSTIC TEST INTERFERENCE

False rise in ***alkaline phosphatase*** when albumin is obtained partially from pooled placental plasma (levels reportedly decline over period of weeks).

NURSING IMPLICATIONS

Assessment & Drug Effects

- Monitor BP, pulse and respiration, and IV albumin flow rate. Adjust flow rate as needed to avoid too rapid a rise in BP.
- Observe closely for S&S of circulatory overload and pulmonary edema (see Appendix F). If S&S appear, slow infusion rate just sufficiently to keep vein open, and report immediately to prescriber.
- Monitor I&O ratio and pattern. Report changes in urinary output. Increase in colloidal osmotic pressure usually causes diuresis, which may persist 3–20 h.
- Withhold fluids completely during succeeding 8 h, when albumin is given to patients with cerebral edema.

Patient & Family Education

- Report chills, nausea, headache, or back pain to prescriber immediately.

NORTRIPTYLINE HYDROCHLORIDE

(nor-trip'ti-leen)

Pamelor

Classification: TRICYCLIC ANTIDEPRESSANT (TCA)

Therapeutic: ANTIDEPRESSANT

Prototype: Imipramine

AVAILABILITY

Capsule; oral solution

ACTION & *THERAPEUTIC EFFECT*

Mechanism of mood elevation is unknown. Studies suggest that it may interfere with the transport, release, and storage of catecholamines. *Effective in improving depressive moods.*

USES Treatment of major depression.

UNLABELED USES Diabetic neuropathy, chronic lower back pain, irritable bowel syndrome, postherpetic neuralgia.

CONTRAINDICATIONS Hypersensitivity to tricyclic antidepressants; acute recovery period after MI; AV block; history of QT prolongation; suicidal ideation; during or within 14 days of MAO inhibitor therapy; pregnancy—fetal risk cannot be ruled out; lactation—infant risk cannot be ruled out.

CAUTIOUS USE Narrow-angle glaucoma, cardiac disease; history of suicidal tendencies; hyperthyroidism, concurrent use with electroshock therapy; history of urinary retention; poor CYP2D6 metabolizers history of suicides; Parkinson's disease; asthma; bipolar disorder; older adults; children.

N

ROUTE & DOSAGE

Antidepressant

Adult: **PO** 25 mg once daily, adjusted based on response to a typical dose of 25 mg 3–4 times/day (max 150 mg/day)
Geriatric: **PO** 30–50 mg/day given as single or divided doses, adjust based on patient response (max: 150 mg/day)
Adolescent: **PO** 30–50 mg/day in 3–4 divided doses or as single dose (max: 150 mg/day)

Pharmacogenetic Dosage Adjustment

Poor CYP2D6 metabolizers: monitor closely for response

ADMINISTRATION

Oral

- Give with food to decrease gastric distress.
- In older adults, total daily dose may be given once a day at bedtime (preferred).
- Be aware that nortriptyline is a 4% alcohol solution.
- Supervise drug ingestion to be sure patient swallows medication.
- Store at 20°–25° C (68°–77° F) in tightly closed container.

ADVERSE EFFECTS (common) GI: Constipation. **Other:** Hyperhidrosis.

INTERACTIONS Drug: May decrease response to ANTIHYPERTENSIVES; CNS DEPRESSANTS, **alcohol,** HYPNOTICS, BARBITURATES, SEDATIVES potentiate CNS depression; may increase hypoprothrombinemic effect of ORAL ANTICOAGULANTS; **levodopa,** SYMPATHOMIMETICS (e.g., **epinephrine, norepinephrine**) pose possibility of sympathetic hyperactivity with hypertension and hyperpyrexia; ANTICHOLINERGIC AGENTS may have increased adverse effects; MAO INHIBITORS pose possibility of severe reactions: Toxic psychosis, cardiovascular instability; **methylphenidate** increases plasma TCA levels; THYROID DRUGS may increase possibility of arrhythmias; **cimetidine** may increase plasma TCA levels. Agents impacting dopamine (ex ANTIPSHYCHOTICS, **bromopride**, or serotonergic ANTIDEPRESSANTS) may increase risk of movement related disorders. Do not use with other agents that prolong QT interval (e.g., **bepridil, dofetilide, pimozide, ziprasidone**) **Herbal: Ginkgo** may decrease seizure threshold. **St. John's wort** may cause serotonin syndrome. Kratom may enhance CNS depressant effect.

PHARMACOKINETICS **Absorption:** Rapidly from GI tract. **Peak:** 7–8.5 h. **Duration:** Crosses placenta; distributed in breast milk. **Metabolism:** In liver (CYP2D6, CYP3A4). **Elimination:** Primarily in urine. **Half-Life:** 16–90 h.

NURSING IMPLICATIONS

Black Box Warning

Nortriptyline hydrochloride has been associated with suicidal thinking and behavior in children, adolescents, and young adults.

Assessment & Drug Effects

- Monitor carefully for signs and symptoms of suicidality in children and adults.
- Monitor for S&S of serotonin syndrome (see Appendix F).
- Monitor BP and pulse rate during adjustment period of TCA therapy. If systolic BP falls more than 20 mm Hg or if there is a sudden increase in pulse rate, withhold medication and notify the prescriber.
- Monitor bowel elimination pattern and I&O ratio. Urinary retention and severe constipation are potential problems, especially in older adults.
- Observe patient with history of glaucoma. Symptoms that may signal acute attack (severe headache, eye pain, dilated pupils, halos of light, nausea, vomiting) should be reported promptly.
- Monitor labs: electrolytes.

Patient & Family Education

- Report immediately to prescriber signs of worsening mental status such as suicidal ideation, aggressiveness, agitation, anxiety, hostility, impulsivity, insomnia, irritability, panic attacks, and worsening of depression.
- Do not engage in hazardous activities until response to drug is known.
- Do not use OTC drugs unless prescriber approves.
- Consult prescriber about safe amount of alcohol, if any, that can be ingested.
- Report any change in heart rhythm.
- Avoid sudden discontinuation.
- Contact healthcare provider before an elective surgery.
- Nortriptyline enhances the effects of barbiturates and other CNS depressants are enhanced.

NYSTATIN

(nye-stat′in)

Bio-Statin, Nyamyc, Nyaderm ♦, Nystop

Classification: ANTIFUNGAL ANTIBIOTIC

Therapeutic: ANTIFUNGAL

Prototype: Amphotericin B

AVAILABILITY Tablet; capsule; oral suspension; cream; ointment; powder

ACTION & *THERAPEUTIC EFFECT* Nontoxic, nonsensitizing antifungal antibiotic that binds to sterols in fungal cell membrane, thereby changing membrane potential and allowing leakage of intracellular components that leads to fungi cell death. *Fungistatic and fungicidal activity against a variety of yeasts and fungi.*

USES Local infections of skin and mucous membranes caused by *Candida* sp. including *Candida albicans* (e.g., paronychia; cutaneous, oropharyngeal, vulvovaginal, and intestinal candidiasis).

CONTRAINDICATIONS Vaginal infections caused by *Gardnerella vaginalis* or *Trichomonas* sp. Hypersensitivity to nystatin; pregnancy—fetal risk cannot be ruled out; lactation—infant risk cannot be ruled out.

CAUTIOUS USE No precautions reported.

ROUTE & DOSAGE

Candida Infections

Adult: **PO** 500,000–1,000,000 units tid; **Topical** to affected areas twice daily until healing complete
Child: **Topical** to affected areas twice daily until healing

Oral Candidiasis Infections

Adult/Adolescent/Child: **Suspension:** 400,000–600,000 units qid swish and swallow.
Infant: **PO** 200,000–400,000 units qid

N

ADMINISTRATION

Oral

- Give reconstituted powder for oral suspension immediately after mixing. Shake well before use.
- Rinse mouth with 1–2 tsp oral suspension. Should be kept in mouth (swish) as long as possible (at least 2 min), then liquid should be spit out or swallowed (if "swish and swallow" is ordered).
- For children, infants: Apply drug with swab to each side of mouth. Avoid food or drink for 30 min after treatment.
- The troche dosage form should dissolve in mouth (about 30 min). Troches should not be chewed or swallowed. Food and drink should be avoided during period of dissolving and for 30 min after treatment.
- Store suspension and tablet at controlled room temperature between 20 and 25 degrees C (68 and 77 degrees F), with excursions permitted between 15 and 30 degrees C (59 and 86 degrees F). Protect suspension from light.

Topical

- Do not apply occlusive dressings over topical applications unless specifically directed to do so.
- Store cream and ointment at controlled room temperature between 15 and 30 degrees C (59 and 86 degrees F). Do not expose cream to excessive heat, above 40 degrees C (104 degrees F). Do not freeze ointment.

Intravaginal

- Store vaginal tablets at controlled room temperature between 15 and 30 degrees C (59 and 86 degrees F).

ADVERSE EFFECTS **Skin:** irritation. **Other:** Hypersensitivity reaction.

PHARMACOKINETICS **Absorption:** Poorly absorbed from GI tract. **Elimination:** In feces.

NURSING IMPLICATIONS

Assessment & Drug Effects

- Monitor oral cavity, especially the tongue, for signs of improvement.
- Monitor for local reactions.

Patient & Family Education

- This drug may cause contact dermatitis. Stop using the drug and report to prescriber if redness, swelling, or irritation develops.
- Take for oral candidiasis (thrush) treatment after meals and at bedtime.
- Care of dentures: Remove dentures before each rinse with oral suspension and before use of troche. Remove dentures at night (infection occurs more frequently in person who wears dentures 24 h a day).

slow-release potassium preparations in presence of delayed GI transit or Meckel's diverticulum; extensive tissue breakdown (such as severe burns); pregnancy (category C); lactation.

ROUTE & DOSAGE

Hypokalemia

Adult: **PO** 40–100 mEq/day in divided doses; **IV** Dose per package insert dependent on current serum potassium concentration

Child: **PO** 2–5 mEq/kg/day in divided doses; sustained release tablets not recommended; **IV** 0.25–0.5 mEq/kg/dose (max: 40 mEq/day)

Prevention of Hypokalemia

Adult: **PO** 20 mEq/day in 1–2 doses

Child: **PO** 1–2 mEq/kg/day in 1–2 doses

ADMINISTRATION

Oral

- Give while patient is sitting up or standing (never in recumbent position) to prevent drug-induced esophagitis. Some patients find it difficult to swallow the large sized KCl tablet.
- Do not crush or allow to chew any potassium salt tablets. Observe to make sure patient does not suck tablet (oral ulcerations have been reported if tablet is allowed to dissolve in mouth).
- Swallow whole tablet with a large glass of water or fruit juice (if allowed) to wash drug down and to start esophageal peristalsis.
- Follow exactly directions for diluting various liquid forms of KCl. In general, dilute each 20 mEq potassium in at least 90 mL water or juice and allow to dissolve completely before administration.
- Dilute liquid forms as directed before giving it through nasogastric tube.

Intravenous

PREPARE: **IV Infusion:** Add desired amount to 100–1000 mL IV solution (compatible with all standard solutions). ▪ Usual maximum is 80 mEq/1000 mL, however, 40 mEq/L is preferred to lessen irritation to veins. Note: **NEVER** add KCl to an IV bag/bottle which is hanging. ▪ After adding KCl invert bag/bottle several times to ensure even distribution.

ADMINISTER: **IV Infusion for Adult/Child:** KCl is **never** given direct IV or in concentrated amounts by any route. ▪ Too rapid infusion may cause fatal hyperkalemia. **IV Infusion for Adult:** Infuse at rate not to exceed 10 mEq/h; in emergency situations, may infuse very cautiously up to 40 mEq/h with continuous cardiac monitoring. **IV Infusion for Child:** Infuse at a rate not to exceed 0.5–1.0 mEq/kg/h.

INCOMPATIBILITIES: **Solution/additive:** **Amoxicillin/clavulanate furosemide, imipenem-cilastin pentobarbital, phenobarbital, succinylcholine.** **Y-site:** **Amphotericin B cholesteryl complex, azithromycin, dantrolene, diazepam, ergotamine, lansoprazole, methylprednisolone, phenytoin, sulfamethoxazole/trimethoprim.**

- Take extreme care to prevent extravasation and infiltration. At first sign, discontinue infusion and select another site.

P

ADVERSE EFFECTS **CV:** Asystole, bradycardia, chest pain, thrombosis, ventricular fibrillation. **Respiratory:** Dyspnea. **Endocrine:** Hyperkalemia. **Skin:** Skin rash, burning at injection site, erythema at injection site, injection site phlebitis. **GI:** Abdominal pain, diarrhea, flatulence, gastrointestinal hemorrhage, gastrointestinal irritation, nausea, vomiting.

INTERACTIONS **Drug:** POTASSIUM-SPARING DIURETICS, ANGIOTENSIN-CONVERTING ENZYME (ACE) INHIBITORS, ANTICHOLINERGIC AGENTS may cause hyperkalemia. Use with CALCIUM SALTS can cause metabolic acidosis. **Food:** Salty foods could increase the risk of hyperkalemia.

PHARMACOKINETICS **Absorption:** Readily from upper GI tract. **Elimination:** 90% in urine, 10% in feces.

NURSING IMPLICATIONS

Assessment & Drug Effects

P

- Monitor I&O ratio and pattern in patients receiving the parenteral drug. If oliguria occurs, stop infusion promptly and notify prescriber.
- Monitor for and report signs of GI ulceration (esophageal or epigastric pain or hematemesis).
- Monitor cardiac status of patients receiving parenteral potassium. Irregular heartbeat is usually the earliest clinical indication of hyperkalemia.
- Be alert for potassium intoxication (hyperkalemia, see S&S, Appendix E); may result from any therapeutic dosage, and the patient may be asymptomatic.
- The risk of hyperkalemia with potassium supplement increases (1) in older adults because of decremental changes in kidney function associated with aging, (2) when dietary intake of potassium suddenly increases, and (3) when kidney function is significantly compromised.
- Monitor lab tests: Baseline and periodic serum potassium.

Patient & Family Education

- Do not be alarmed when the tablet carcass appears in your stool. The sustained release tablet (e.g., Slow-K) utilizes a wax matrix as carrier for KCl crystals that passes through the digestive system.
- Learn about sources of potassium with special reference to foods and OTC drugs.
- Do not use any salt substitute unless it is specifically ordered by the prescriber. These contain a substantial amount of potassium and electrolytes other than sodium.
- Do not self-prescribe laxatives. Chronic laxative use has been associated with diarrhea-induced potassium loss.
- Notify prescriber of persistent vomiting because losses of potassium can occur.
- Report continuing signs of potassium deficit to prescriber: Weakness, fatigue, polyuria, polydipsia.
- Advise dentist or new prescriber that a potassium drug has been prescribed as long-term maintenance therapy.
- Do not open foil-wrapped powders and tablets before use.

POTASSIUM IODIDE

(poe-tass′ee-um)

SSKI

Classification: ANTITHYROID; EXPECTORANT

Therapeutic: ANTITHYROID; EXPECTORANT

AVAILABILITY oral solution; tablet

ACTION & THERAPEUTIC EFFECT Appears to increase secretion of respiratory fluids by direct action on bronchial tissue, thereby decreasing mucus viscosity. When the thyroid gland is hyperplastic, excess iodide ions temporarily inhibit secretion of thyroid hormone, foster accumulation in thyroid follicles, and decrease vascularity of gland. *Administration for hyperthyroidism is limited to short-term therapy. As an expectorant, the iodine ion increases mucous secretion formation in bronchi, and decreases viscosity of mucus.*

USES Block thyroidal update of radioactive isotopes; expectorant for the symptomatic treatment of chronic pulmonary disease complicated by mucous.

CONTRAINDICATIONS Hypersensitivity to iodine; dermatitis herpetiformis; hypocomplementemic vasculitis; nodular thyroid condition with heart disease; pregnancy (may cause hypothyroidism in fetus/newborn); lactation.

CAUTIOUS USE Renal impairment; cardiac disease; pulmonary tuberculosis; Addison's disease.

ROUTE & DOSAGE

Expectorant

Adult: **PO** 300–600 mg 3–4 times per day

Thyroid Blocking in Radiation Emergency

Adult/Adolescent (over 68 kg): **PO** 130 mg/day for 10–14 days
Adolescent (less than 68 kg)/ Child 3–12 years **PO** 65 mg/day
Child/Infant (younger than 3 y): **PO** 32.5 mg/day

ADMINISTRATION

Oral

- Give with meals in a full glass (240 mL) of water, milk, or fruit juice disguise salty taste and minimize gastric distress.
- Adhere strictly to schedule and accurate dose measurements when iodide is administered to prepare thyroid gland for surgery, particularly at end of treatment period when possibility of "escape" (from iodide) effect on thyroid gland increases.
- Store in airtight, light-resistant container.

ADVERSE EFFECTS **CV:** Cardiac arrhythmias, numbness, vasculitis. **Respiratory:** Dyspnea, rhinitis, wheezing. **CNS:** Confusion, fatigue, numbness, tingling sensation. **Endocrine:** Goiter, hypothyroidism, myxedema. **Skin:** Acne vulgaris, dermatitis, urticaria. **GI:** Diarrhea, nausea, vomiting, stomach pain, gastric distress, gastrointestinal haemorrhage, gingival pain, metallic taste, toothache. **Hematologic:** Eosinophilia, lymphedema, thyroid adenoma. **Musculoskeletal:** Arthralgia, weakness. **Other:** Hypersensitivity reaction. *Iodine poisoning (iodism):* Metallic taste, stomatitis, salivation, coryza, sneezing; swollen and tender salivary glands (sialadenitis), frontal headache, vomiting (blue vomitus if stomach contained starches, otherwise yellow vomitus), bloody diarrhea.

DIAGNOSTIC TEST INTERFERENCE Potassium iodide may alter ***thyroid function*** test results.

P

INTERACTIONS Drug: ANTITHYROID DRUGS, **lithium** may potentiate hypothyroid and goitrogenic actions; POTASSIUM-SPARING DIURETICS, POTASSIUM SUPPLEMENTS, ACE INHIBITORS increase risk of hyperkalemia.

PHARMACOKINETICS Absorption: Adequately absorbed from GI tract. **Distribution:** Crosses placenta. **Elimination:** Cleared from plasma by renal excretion or thyroid uptake.

NURSING IMPLICATIONS

Assessment & Drug Effects

- Keep prescriber informed about characteristics of sputum: Quantity, consistency, color.
- Monitor lab tests: Baseline and periodic serum thyroid function tests, potassium.

Patient & Family Education

- Report to prescriber promptly the occurrence of abdominal pain, distension, nausea, or vomiting.
- Report clinical S&S of iodism (see ADVERSE EFFECTS). Usually, symptoms will subside with dose reduction and lengthened intervals between doses.
- Avoid foods rich in iodine if iodism develops: Seafood, fish liver oils, and iodized salt.
- Be aware that sudden withdrawal following prolonged use may precipitate thyroid storm.
- Do not use OTC drugs without consulting prescriber. Many preparations contain iodides and could augment prescribed dose [e.g., cough syrups, gargles, asthma medication, salt substitutes, cod liver oil, multiple vitamins (often suspended in iodide solutions)].
- Be aware that optimum hydration is the best expectorant when taking KI as an expectorant. Increase daily fluid intake.

P

PRALATREXATE

(pra-la-trex′ate)

Folotyn

Classification: ANTINEOPLASTIC; ANTIMETABOLITE, ANTIFOLATE

Therapeutic: ANTINEOPLASTIC

Prototype: Methotrexate

AVAILABILITY Solution for injection

ACTION & *THERAPEUTIC EFFECT* Blocks folic acid participation in nucleic acid synthesis, thereby interfering with cell division (mitosis). Rapidly dividing cells, including cancer cells, are sensitive to this interference in the mitotic process. *Effective in treatment of relapsed or refractory peripheral T-cell lymphoma (PTCL).*

USES Treatment of relapsed or refractory peripheral T-cell lymphoma (PTCL) and non-Hodgkin's lymphoma.

CONTRAINDICATIONS Concomitant administration of hepatotoxity drugs; tumor lysis syndrome; pregnancy (category D); lactation.

CAUTIOUS USE Thrombocytopenia, neutropenia, anemia; moderate to severe renal function impairment; liver function impairment; pancreatic problems due to drug use; ulcerative colitis; poor nutritional status; older adults. Safety and efficacy in children not established.

ROUTE & DOSAGE

Peripheral T-Cell Lymphoma

Adult: **IV** 30 mg/m^2 over 3–5 min. Repeat weekly for 6 wk in 7-wk cycles.

Renal Impairment Dosage Adjustment

EGFR of 15–30 mL/min: Reduce dose to 15 mg/m^2

Toxicity and Organ Function Dosage Adjustments

See package insert

ADMINISTRATION

Intravenous

PREPARE: **Direct:** Withdraw from vial into syringe immediately before use. Do not dilute. Use gloves and other protective clothing during handling and preparation. ▪ Flush thoroughly if drug contacts skin or mucous membranes.

ADMINISTER: **Direct:** Give over 3–5 min via a side port of a free-flowing NS IV line. ▪ Withhold drug and notify prescriber for any of the following: Platelet count less than 100,000/mcL for first dose or less than 50,000/mcL for all subsequent doses, ANC less than 1000/mcL, or grade 2 or higher mucositis.

▪ Refrigerate at 2°–8° C (36°–46° F) until use and protect from light. ▪ Vials are stable at room temperature for up to 72 h if left in original carton.

ADVERSE EFFECTS **CV:** Tachycardia. **Respiratory:** *Cough, dyspnea, epistaxis,* pharyngolaryngeal pain, upper respiratory tract infection. **Endocrine:** Anorexia, elevated AST and ALT, hypokalemia. **Skin:** Pruritus, rash. **GI:** *Constipation, diarrhea, mucositis, nausea, vomiting,* stomatitis. **Musculoskeletal:** Back pain. **Hematologic:** *Anemia,* leukopenia, *neutropenia,* thrombocytopenia. **Other:** Abdominal pain, asthenia, *edema, fatigue,* night sweats, pain in extremity, *pyrexia,* sepsis.

INTERACTIONS **Drug: Probenecid** may increase pralatrexate levels. Drugs that are subject to substantial renal clearance (e.g., NSAIDS, **trimethoprim/sulfamethoxazole**) may delay the clearance of pralatrexate. Do not administer LIVE VACCINES.

PHARMACOKINETICS **Distribution:** 67% bound to plasma proteins. **Metabolism:** Not extensively metabolized. **Elimination:** Primarily excreted in the urine. **Half-Life:** 12–18 h.

NURSING IMPLICATIONS

Assessment & Drug Effects

- Monitor vital signs. Report immediately S&S of infection, especially fever of 100.5° F or greater.
- Monitor status of mucus membranes because mucositis is a dose-limiting toxicity.
- Monitor lab tests: Prior to each dose, CBC with differential and platelet count; baseline and periodic LFTs and renal function tests.

Patient & Family Education

- Practice meticulous oral hygiene.
- Monitor for S&S of an infection. Contact the prescriber immediately if an infection is suspected or if your temperature is elevated.
- Report promptly unexplained bleeding or symptoms of anemia (e.g., excessive weakness, fatigue, intolerance to activity, pale skin).
- Folic acid and vitamin B_{12} supplementation are recommended to reduce the risk of drug-related toxicities. Consult with prescriber.
- Use effective means of contraception to avoid pregnancy while taking this drug. If a pregnancy

P

does occur, notify prescriber immediately.

- Do not take aspirin or NSAIDS without consulting prescriber.

PRALIDOXIME CHLORIDE

(pra-li-dox′eem)

Protopam Chloride

Classification: CHOLINESTERASE RECEPTOR AGONIST; DETOXIFICATION AGENT

Therapeutic: ANTIDOTE; CHOLINESTERASE ENHANCER

AVAILABILITY Solution for injection

ACTION & *THERAPEUTIC EFFECT*

Reactivates cholinesterase by displacing the enzyme from its receptor sites; the free enzyme then can resume its function of degrading accumulated acetylcholine, thereby restoring normal neuromuscular transmission. *More active against effects of anticholinesterases at skeletal neuromuscular junction than at autonomic effector sites or in CNS respiratory center; therefore, atropine **must be** given concomitantly to block effects of acetylcholine and its accumulation in these sites.*

USES Antidote in treatment of poisoning by organophosphate insecticides and pesticides with anticholinesterase activity (e.g., parathion, TEPP, sarin) and to control overdosage by anticholinesterase drugs used in treatment of myasthenia gravis (cholinergic crisis).

CONTRAINDICATIONS Hypersensitivity to pralidoxime; use in poisoning by insecticide of the carbonate class (Sevin), inorganic phosphates, or organophosphates having no anticholinesterase activity.

CAUTIOUS USE Myasthenia gravis; renal insufficiency; asthma; peptic ulcer; severe cardiac disease; pregnancy (category C); lactation.

ROUTE & DOSAGE

Organophosphate Poisoning

Adult/Adolescent (17 y or older): **IV** 1–2 g in 100 mL NS infused over 15–30 min; or 1–2 g as 5% solution in sterile water over not less than 5 min, may repeat after 1 h if muscle weakness not relieved.; **IM** 600 mg, may repeat in 15 min to total dose of 1800 mg if IV route is not feasible.
Adolescent (younger than 17 y)/ Child/Infant: **IV** 20–50 mg/kg. May repeat in 1–2 h if needed (max dose: 2 g).

Anticholinesterase Overdose in Myasthenia Gravis

Adult: **IV** 1–2 g in 100 mL NS infused over 15–30 min, followed by increments of 250 mg q5min prn

ADMINISTRATION

Intramuscular

- Give only if unable to give IV; **not** preferred route.
- Reconstitute as for direct IV injection (see below).

Intravenous

PREPARE: **Direct:** Reconstitute 1-g vial by adding 20 mL sterile water for injection to yield 50 mg/mL (a 5% solution). ▪ If pulmonary edema is present, give without further dilution. **IV Infusion (preferred):** Further dilute reconstituted solution in 100 mL NS.
ADMINISTER: **Direct:** In pulmonary edema, 1 g or fraction thereof over 5 min; do not exceed 200 mg/

min. **IV Infusion (preferred):** Give over 15–30 min. ▪ Stop infusion or reduce rate if hypertension occurs.

ADVERSE EFFECTS **CV:** Tachycardia, hypertension (dose-related). **CNS:** Dizziness, headache, drowsiness. **HEENT:** Blurred vision, diplopia, impaired accommodation. **GI:** Nausea. **Other:** Hyperventilation, muscular weakness, laryngospasm, muscle rigidity.

INTERACTIONS **Drug:** May potentiate the effects of BARBITURATES.

PHARMACOKINETICS **Peak:** 5–15 min IV; 10–20 min IM. **Distribution:** Distributed throughout extracellular fluids; crosses blood–brain barrier slowly if at all. **Metabolism:** Probably in liver. **Elimination:** Rapidly in urine. **Half-Life:** 0.8–2.7 h.

NURSING IMPLICATIONS

Assessment & Drug Effects

- Monitor BP, vital signs, and I&O. Report oliguria or changes in I&O ratio.
- Monitor closely. It is difficult to differentiate toxic effects of organophosphates or atropine from toxic effects of pralidoxime.
- Be alert for and report immediately: Reduction in muscle strength, onset of muscle twitching, changes in respiratory pattern, altered level of consciousness, increases or changes in heart rate and rhythm.
- Observe necessary safety precautions with unconscious patient because excitement and manic behavior reportedly may occur following recovery of consciousness.
- Keep patient under close observation for 48–72 h, particularly when poison was ingested, because of likelihood of continued absorption of organophosphate from lower bowel.
- In patients with myasthenia gravis, overdosage with pralidoxime may convert cholinergic crisis into myasthenic crisis.

PRAMIPEXOLE DIHYDROCHLORIDE

(pra-mi-pex′ole)

Mirapex, Mirapex ER

Classification: NON-ERGOT DERIVATIVE DOPAMINE RECEPTOR AGONIST; ANTIPARKINSON

Therapeutic: ANTIPARKINSON

Prototype: Apomorphine

AVAILABILITY Tablet; extended release tablet

ACTION & *THERAPEUTIC EFFECT* A dopamine agonist with specificity for the D_2 subfamily dopamine receptor; shown to bind to D_3 and D_4 receptors stimulating dopamine activity on the nerves of the striatum and substantia nigra. *Effectiveness is indicated by improved control of neuromuscular functioning. Improves ADLs.*

USES Treatment of idiopathic Parkinson disease and moderate to severe primary restless legs syndrome (RLS).

CONTRAINDICATIONS Hypersensitivity to pramipexole or ropinirole; abrupt withdrawal; lactation.

CAUTIOUS USE Renal impairment; impulse control/compulsive behavior symptoms; history of

P

orthostatic hypotension; restless leg syndrome; older adults; pregnancy (insufficient information on the effect in pregnant women). Safety and efficacy in children not established.

ROUTE & DOSAGE

Parkinson Disease

Adult: **PO Immediate release** Start with 0.125 mg tid gradually increase every 5–7 days (max: 4.5 mg/day); **Extended release** 0.375 mg daily, may increase every 5–7 days (max: 4.5 mg/day)

Restless Legs Syndrome

Adult: **PO** 0.125 mg taken 2–3 h before bed; dose can be increased every 4–7 days (max: 0.75 mg/day)

Renal Impairment Dosage Adjustment

CrCl 35–59 mL/min: **PO Immediate release** Start with 0.125 mg bid; *CrCl 15–34 mL/min:* Start 0.125 mg once daily *CrCl 30–50 mL/min:* **PO Extended release** Start 0.375 mg every other day

P

ADMINISTRATION

Oral

- Ensure that extended release tablet is swallowed whole and not crushed, divided, or chewed.
- Administer with or without food to decrease nausea.
- For restless leg syndrome, administer 2 to 3 hours before bedtime.

ADVERSE EFFECTS **CV:** *Orthostatic hypotension,* peripheral edema. **Respiratory:** Dyspnea, nasal congestion. **CNS:** *Dizziness, insomnia, hallucinations, dyskinesia, extrapyramidal reaction,* drowsiness, headache, restless leg syndrome, confusion, fatigue, dystonia, abnormal gait, hypertonia, amnesia. **GI:** *Nausea, constipation,* anorexia, diarrhea, dry mouth, weight loss. **GU:** Urinary frequency. **Musculoskeletal:** Dyskinesia, asthenia, limb pain, muscle spasm. **Other:** Accidental injury, falls.

INTERACTIONS **Drug: Cimetidine** decreases clearance; BUTYROPHENONES, **metoclopramide**, PHENOTHIAZINES, ANTIPSYCHOTICS may antagonize effects. Closely monitor use with other CNS DEPRESSANTS; ANTIHYPERTENSIVES may have increased risk of hypotension.

PHARMACOKINETICS **Absorption:** Rapidly from GI tract, greater than 90% bioavailability. **Peak:** 2-6 h. **Distribution:** 15% protein bound. **Metabolism:** Minimally in the liver. **Elimination:** Primarily in urine. **Half-Life:** 8–12 h.

NURSING IMPLICATIONS

Assessment & Drug Effects

- Monitor Bp and Heart rate and for S&S of orthostatic hypotension, especially when the dosage is increased.
- Monitor cardiac status, especially in those with significant orthostatic hypotension.
- Monitor for and report signs of tardive dyskinesia (see Appendix E), CNS depression, and behavior changes
- Periodic skin examinations.
- Monitor for body weight changes.

Patient & Family Education

- Do not abruptly stop taking this drug. It should be discontinued over a period of 1 wk.
- Hallucinations are an adverse effect of this drug and occur more often in older adults.
- Make position changes slowly especially from a lying or sitting to standing.
- Use caution with potentially dangerous activities until response to drug is known; drowsiness is a common adverse effect.
- Avoid alcohol and use extra caution if taking other prescribed CNS depressants; both may exaggerate drowsiness, dizziness, and orthostatic hypotension.

PRAMLINTIDE

Symlin

Classification: ANTIDIABETIC; AMYLIN ANALOG

Therapeutic: ANTIHYPERGLYCEMIC

AVAILABILITY Solution for injection

ACTION & *THERAPEUTIC EFFECT* A synthetic analog of human amylin, a hormone secreted by pancreatic beta cells. Amylin reduces postmeal glucagon levels, thus lowering serum glucose level. *Pramlintide is an antihyperglycemic drug that controls postprandial blood glucose levels.*

USES Adjunct treatment of diabetes mellitus type 1 and type 2 in patients who use mealtime insulin therapy and who have failed to achieve desired glucose control despite optimal insulin therapy.

CONTRAINDICATIONS Hypersensitivity to pramlintide, metacresol; noncompliance with insulin regime or medical care; HbA1C greater than 9%; recurrent severe hypoglycemia; hypoglucemia unawareness; gastroparesis; dialysis.

CAUTIOUS USE Osteoporosis; alcohol; thyroid disease; older adults; pregnancy (category C); lactation. Safety and efficacy in children not established.

ROUTE & DOSAGE

Type 1 Diabetes Mellitus

Adult: **Subcutaneous** 15 mcg immediately before each major meal; may increase by 15 mcg increments if no clinically significant nausea for 3–7 days. If nausea or vomiting persists at 45 mcg or 60 mcg, reduce to 30 mcg.

Type 2 Diabetes Mellitus

Adult: **Subcutaneous** 60 mcg immediately before each major meal; may increase to 120 mcg if no clinically significant nausea for 3–7 days. If nausea or vomiting persists at 120 mcg, reduce to 60 mcg.

P

ADMINISTRATION

Subcutaneous

- Give subcutaneously into the abdomen or thigh (not the arm) immediately before each major meal. Rotate injection sites.
- Never mix pramlintide and insulin in the same syringe. Separate injection sites.
- Use a U100 insulin syringe to administer. One unit of pramlintide drawn from a 0.6 mg/mL vial contains 6 mcg of medication. Thus, a 30 mcg dose is equal to 5 units in a U100 syringe.

- Do not administer to patients with HbA1C greater than 9% or those taking drugs to stimulate GI motility.
- Note: When initiating pramlintide therapy, insulin dose reduction is required.
- Store at 2°–8° C (36°–46° F), and protect from light. Do not freeze. Discard vials that have been frozen or overheated. Discard open vials after 30 days.

ADVERSE EFFECTS **Respiratory:** *Coughing,* pharyngitis. **CNS:** Dizziness, fatigue, *headache.* **GI:** Abdominal pain, *anorexia, nausea, vomiting.* **Musculoskeletal:** Arthralgia. **Other:** *Allergic reaction, inflicted injury,* pancreatitis.

INTERACTIONS **Drugs:** Pramlintide can decrease rate and/or extent of GI absorption of other oral drugs. Significant slowing of gastric motility with ANTIMUSCARINICS.

PHARMACOKINETICS **Absorption:** 30–40% bioavailability. **Peak:** 20 min. **Distribution:** 60% protein bound. **Metabolism:** Extensive renal metabolism. **Half-Life:** 48 min.

P

NURSING IMPLICATIONS

Black Box Warning

Pramlintide use with insulin increases the risk of severe hypoglycemia, particularly in type 1 diabetics. When severe hypoglycemia occurs, it is seen within 3 h following a pramlintide injection. Serious injuries may occur.

Assessment & Drug Effects

- Monitor for severe hypoglycemia, which usually occurs within 3 h of injection. Hypoglycemia is worse in type 1 diabetics.
- Monitor diabetics for loss of glycemic control.
- Withhold drug and notify prescriber for clinically significant nausea or increased frequency or severity of hypoglycemia.
- Monitor for and report promptly S&S of pancreatitis (e.g., upper abdominal plain that radiates to back, nausea and vomiting).
- Monitor lab tests: Baseline and periodic HbA1C; frequent pre/postmeal plasma glucose levels.

Patient & Family Education

- Note: Patients should reduce a.c. rapid-acting or short-acting insulin dosages by 50% when pramlintide is initiated. Check with prescriber.
- Do not drive or engage in potentially hazardous activities until response to drug is known.
- Report any of the following to prescriber: Persistent, significant nausea; episodes of hypoglycemia (e.g., hunger, headache, sweating, tremor, irritability, or difficulty concentrating).

PRAMOXINE HYDROCHLORIDE

(pra-mox'een)

Pramox, ProctoFoam, Tronolane, Tronothane ✤

Classification: LOCAL ANESTHETIC (MUCOSAL); ANTIPRURITIC
Therapeutic: LOCAL ANESTHETIC; ANTIPRURITIC
Prototype: Procaine

AVAILABILITY Foam; gel; lotion; spray

ACTION & *THERAPEUTIC EFFECT* Produces anesthesia by blocking conduction and propagation of sensory nerve impulses in skin and mucous membranes.

Provides temporary relief from pain and itching on skin or mucous membrane.

USES Temporary relief of pain/itching associated with hemorrhoids or burns/cuts/scrapes.

CONTRAINDICATIONS Application to large areas of skin; prolonged use; preparation for laryngopharyngeal examination, bronchoscopy, or gastroscopy.

CAUTIOUS USE Extensive skin disorders; pregnancy (insufficient information related to use in pregnant women); lactation. Safety in children younger than 2 y not established.

ROUTE & DOSAGE

Relief of Minor Pain and Itching

Adult/Child (2 y or older):
Topical Apply tid or qid

ADMINISTRATION

Topical

- Clean thoroughly and dry rectal area before use for temporary relief of hemorrhoidal pain and itching.
- Administer rectal preparations in the morning and evening and after bowel movement or as directed by prescriber. Avoid insertion into rectum.
- Apply lotion or cream to affected surfaces with a gloved hand. Wash hands thoroughly before and after treatment. Apply sparingly, use minimal effective dose.
- Do not apply in or around eyes or nasal membranes.

ADVERSE EFFECTS **Skin:** Burning, stinging, sensitization.

PHARMACOKINETICS **Onset:** 3–5 min. **Duration:** Up to 5 h.

NURSING IMPLICATIONS

Assessment & Drug Effects

- Monitor for and report promptly significant tissue irritation or sloughing.

Patient & Family Education

- Drug is usually discontinued if condition being treated does not improve within 2–3 wk or if it worsens, or if rash or condition not present before treatment appears, or if treated area becomes inflamed or infected.
- Discontinue and consult prescriber if rectal bleeding and pain occur during hemorrhoid treatment.

PRASUGREL

(pra-soo′grel)

Effient

Classification: ANTIPLATELET; PLATELET INHIBITOR; ADP RECEPTOR ANTAGONIST

Therapeutic: PLATELET INHIBITOR

Prototype: Clopidogrel

AVAILABILITY Tablet

ACTION & THERAPEUTIC EFFECT An inhibitor of platelet activation and aggregation through irreversible binding to adenosine diphosphate (ADP) receptors on platelets. *Prasugrel prolongs bleeding time, thereby reducing atherosclerotic events in selected high risk patient managed with percutaneous coronary intervention (PCI).*

USES Prophylaxis of arterial thromboembolism in patients with acute coronary syndrome, including unstable angina, non–ST-elevation myocardial infarction (NSTEMI), or ST-elevation acute myocardial infarction (STEMI), who are being managed with percutaneous coronary intervention (PCI).

CONTRAINDICATIONS Active pathologic bleeding disorder; active bleeding; history of TIA or stroke; GI bleeding; within 7 days of CABG surgery or any surgery; adults over 75 y; concomitant use of NSAIDS or other drugs that increase risk of bleeding.

CAUTIOUS USE Severe hepatic impairment (Child-Pugh class C, total score greater than 10); end-stage renal disease; pts less than 60 kg; pregnancy (category B); lactation.

ROUTE & DOSAGE

Thromboembolism Prophylaxis

Adult (younger than 75 y, weight 60 kg or greater): **PO** 60 mg loading dose, then 10 mg once daily; *younger than 75 y, weight less than 60 kg:* 60 mg loading dose, then 5 mg once daily

P

ADMINISTRATION

Oral

- Give without regard to food.
- Daily aspirin is recommended with prasugrel.
- Do not administer to patient with active bleeding or who is likely to undergo urgent CABG.
- Store at 15°–30° C (59°–86° F).

ADVERSE EFFECTS **CV:** Hypertension. **Respiratory:** Epistaxis. **CNS:** Headache. **Endocrine:** Hypercholesterolemia, hyperlipidemia.

INTERACTIONS **Drug: Warfarin** or NSAIDS or ANTICOAGULANTS may increase the risk of bleeding. Do not use with PLATELET INHIBITOR or FIBRINOLYTICS.

PHARMACOKINETICS **Absorption:** 79% or higher. **Peak:** 30 min. **Metabolism:** Hydrolysis and oxidation to active metabolite. **Elimination:** Urine (68%) and feces (27%). **Half-Life:** 7 h.

NURSING IMPLICATIONS

Black Box Warning

Prasugrel has been associated with severe, sometimes fatal, bleeding (especially in patients with active pathological bleeding, history of TIA or stroke, or those age 75 and older).

Assessment & Drug Effects

- Monitor vital signs. Suspect bleeding if patient is hypotensive and has recently undergone an invasive or surgical procedure.
- Monitor for and report promptly any S&S of active bleeding.
- Monitor lab tests: Periodic Hct and Hgb.

Patient & Family Education

- Report promptly unexplained prolonged or excessive bleeding, or blood in urine or stool.
- Report immediately any of the following: Weakness, extremely pale skin, purple skin patches, jaundice, or fever.
- Inform all medical providers that you are taking prasugrel.
- Do not take OTC anti-inflammatory or pain medications without consulting prescriber.

PRAVASTATIN

(pra-vah-stat′in)

Pravachol

Classification: ANTIHYPERLIPEMIC; HMG-COA REDUCTASE INHIBITOR (STATIN)

 Common adverse effects in *italic;* life-threatening effects underlined; generic names in **bold;** classifications in SMALL CAPS; ♣ Canadian drug name; ⊙ Prototype drug; ⚠ Alert

Therapeutic: ANTILIPEMIC; STATIN
Prototype: Lovastatin

AVAILABILITY Tablet

ACTION & *THERAPEUTIC EFFECT* Competitively inhibits HMG-CoA reductase, the enzyme that catalyzes cholesterol biosynthesis. HMG-CoA reductase inhibitors (statins) increase serum HDL cholesterol, decrease serum LDL cholesterol, VLDL cholesterol, and plasma triglyceride levels. *It is effective in reducing total and LDL cholesterol in various forms of hypercholesterolemia.*

USES Hypercholesterolemia (alone or in combination with bile acid sequestrants) and familial hypercholesterolemia; atherosclerosis.

CONTRAINDICATIONS Hypersensitivity to pravastatin; active liver disease or unexplained elevated serum transaminases; hepatic encephalopathy, hepatitis, jaundice, rhabdomyolysis; pregnancy (category X); lactation.

CAUTIOUS USE Alcoholics, history of liver disease; renal impairment; renal disease; women of child-bearing age who use contraceptive measures. Safe use in children younger than 8 y not established.

ROUTE & DOSAGE

Hyperlipidemia /Stroke Prophylaxis

Adult: **PO** Initially 40 mg daily then may increase up to 80 mg/day
Adult (also taking cylcosporine): **PO** 10 mg daily may titrate up to 20 mg
Adolescent: **PO** 40 mg daily
Child (8–13 y): **PO** 20 mg daily

ADMINISTRATION

Oral

- Give without regard to meals.

ADVERSE EFFECTS **CV:** Chest pain. **CNS:** Headache. **Hepatic/GI:** Increased liver enzymes, nausea, vomiting.

INTERACTIONS **Drug:** May increase PT when administered with **warfarin.** IMMUNOSPRESSANTS may increase risk of myopathy. **Clarithromycin** may increase risk of toxicity. **Herbal:** Do not use with red yeast rice.

PHARMACOKINETICS **Absorption:** Poorly from GI tract; 17% reaches systemic circulation. **Onset:** 2 wk. **Peak:** 4 wk. **Distribution:** 43–55% protein bound; does not cross blood–brain barrier; crosses placenta; distributed into breast milk. **Metabolism:** Extensive first-pass metabolism in liver; has no active metabolites. **Elimination:** 20% of dose excreted in urine, 71% in feces. **Half-Life:** 1.8–2.6 h.

NURSING IMPLICATIONS

Assessment & Drug Effects

- Monitor diabetics and prediabetics for loss of glycemic control.
- Monitor coagulation studies with patients receiving concurrent warfarin therapy. PT may be prolonged.
- Monitor lab tests: Baseline LFTs, repeat at 4–12 wk, then annually. LFTs and CPK if symptoms warrant testing.

Patient & Family Education

- Report unexplained muscle pain, tenderness, or weakness, especially

if accompanied by malaise or fever, to prescriber promptly.
- Report signs of bleeding to prescriber promptly when taking concomitant warfarin therapy.
- Monitor blood glucose for loss of glycemic control if diabetic or prediabetic.

PRAZIQUANTEL

(pray-zi-kwon'tel)

Biltricide

Classification: ANTHELMINTIC

Therapeutic: ANTHELMINTIC

AVAILABILITY Tablet

ACTION & *THERAPEUTIC EFFECT* Increases permeability of parasite cell membrane to calcium. Leads to immobilization of their suckers and dislodgment from their residence in blood vessel walls. *Active against all developmental stages of schistosomes, including cercaria (free-swimming larvae). Also active against other trematodes (flukes) and cestodes (tapeworms).*

P

USES All stages of schistosomiasis (bilharziasis) caused by all *Schistosoma* species pathogenic to humans. Other trematode infections caused by Chinese liver fluke.

UNLABELED USES Lung, sheep liver, and intestinal flukes and tapeworm infections.

CONTRAINDICATIONS Hypersensitivity to praziquantel; ocular cysticercosis. Women should not breast-feed on day of praziquantel therapy or for 72 h after last dose of drug.

CAUTIOUS USE Hepatic disease; cardiac arrhythmias; pregnancy (category B); children younger than 4 y.

ROUTE & DOSAGE

Schistosomiasis

Adult/Child (4 y or older): **PO** 60 mg/kg in 3 equally divided doses at 4–6 h intervals on the same day, may repeat in 2–3 mo after exposure

Other Trematodes

Adult/Child (4 y or older): **PO** 75 mg/kg in 3 equally divided doses at 4–6 h intervals on the same day

Cestodiasis (Adult or Intestinal Stage)

Adult: **PO** 10–20 mg/kg as single dose

Cestodiasis (Larval or Tissue Stage)

Adult: **PO** 50 mg/kg in 3 divided doses/day for 14 days

ADMINISTRATION

Oral
- Give dose with food and fluids. Tablets can be broken into quarters but should **not** be chewed.
- Advise patient to take sufficient fluid to wash down the medication. Tablets are soluble in water; gagging or vomiting because of bitter taste may result if tablets are retained in the mouth.
- Store tablets in tight containers at less than 30° C (86° F).

ADVERSE EFFECTS CNS: *Dizziness, headache, malaise,* drowsiness, lassitude, CSF reaction syndrome (exacerbation of neurologic signs and symptoms such as seizures, increased CSF protein concentration, increased anticysticercal IgG levels, hyperthermia, intracranial hypertension) in patient treated for cerebral cysticercosis. **Skin:** Pruritus, urticaria. **Hepatic:** *Increased AST, ALT (slight).* **GI:** *Abdominal pain or discomfort with or without nausea;* vomiting, anorexia, diarrhea. **Other:** Fever, sweating, symptoms of host-mediated immunologic response to antigen release from worms (fever, eosinophilia).

DIAGNOSTIC TEST INTERFERENCE Be mindful that selected drugs may interfere with stool studies for ova and parasites: ***Iron, bismuth, oil (mineral*** or ***castor), Metamucil*** (if ingested within 1 wk of test), ***barium, antibiotics, antiamebic*** and ***antimalarial drugs,*** and ***gallbladder dye*** (if administered within 3 wk of test).

INTERACTIONS Drug: Phenytoin can lead to therapeutic failure. **Food: Grapefruit juice** (greater than 1 qt/day) may increase plasma concentrations and adverse effects.

PHARMACOKINETICS Absorption: Rapidly, 80% reaches systemic circulation. **Peak:** 1–3 h. **Distribution:** Enters cerebrospinal fluid. **Metabolism:** Extensively to inactive metabolites. **Elimination:** Primarily in urine. **Half-Life:** 0.8–1.5 h.

NURSING IMPLICATIONS

Assessment & Drug Effects

- Patient is reexamined in 2 or 3 mo to ensure complete eradication of the infections.

Patient & Family Education

- Do not drive or operate other hazardous machinery on day of treatment or the following day because of potential drug-induced dizziness and drowsiness.
- Usually, all schistosomal worms are dead 7 days following treatment.
- Contact prescriber if you develop a sustained headache or high fever.

PRAZOSIN HYDROCHLORIDE (Pr)

(pra'zoe-sin)

Minipress

Classification: ALPHA-ADRENERGIC RECEPTOR ANTAGONIST; ANTIHYPERTENSIVE

Therapeutic: ANTIHYPERTENSIVE

AVAILABILITY Capsule

ACTION & *THERAPEUTIC EFFECT* Causes selective inhibition of alpha-adrenergic receptors that produces vasodilation in both venous and arteriole vessels with the result that both peripheral vascular resistance and blood pressure are reduced. *Lowers blood pressure in supine and standing positions with most pronounced effect on diastolic pressure.*

USES Treatment of hypertension.

UNLABELED USES Benign prostatic hypertrophy; PTSD related nightmares and sleep disorders; Raynaud phenomenon.

CONTRAINDICATIONS Hypersensitivity to prazosin; hypotension.

CAUTIOUS USE Renal impairment; chronic kidney failure; hypertensive patient with cerebral thrombosis; angina; men with sickle cell trait; older adults; pregnancy (use during pregnancy may increase risk of birth defects); lactation; children.

ROUTE & DOSAGE

Hypertension

Adult: **PO** 1 mg bid or tid, may titrate to 20 mg/day in divided doses (max: 40 mg/day)

ADMINISTRATION

Oral

- Administer with or without food at the same time each day.
- Store at 20°C to 25°C (68°F to 77°F). Protect from moisture and light.

ADVERSE EFFECTS **CV:** Edema, syncope, postural hypotension, *palpitations*. **Respiratory:** Dyspnea, epistaxis, nasal congestion. **CNS:** *Dizziness, headache, drowsiness,* fatigue, nervousness, vertigo, depression. **HEENT:** Blurred vision. **Skin:** Rash. **GI:** Dry mouth, *nausea,* vomiting, diarrhea, constipation. **GU:** Urinary frequency. **Musculoskeletal:** Weakness.

DIAGNOSTIC TEST INTERFERENCE False positives may occur in screening for ***pheochromocytoma.***

INTERACTIONS **Drug:** DIURETICS, ANTIHYPERTENSIVE AGENTS and **alcohol** increase hypotensive effects. **Sildenafil, vardenafil,** and **tadalafil** may enhance hypotensive effects. Use with other ALPHA-BLOCKERS may increase adverse effects.

PHARMACOKINETICS **Absorption:** highly protein bound. **Onset:** 2 h. **Peak:** 2–4 h. **Duration:** 10–24 h. **Distribution:** Widely distributed, including into breast milk. **Metabolism:** Extensively in liver. **Elimination:** 6–10% in urine, rest in bile and feces. **Half-Life:** 2–3 h.

NURSING IMPLICATIONS

Assessment & Drug Effects

- Be alert for first-dose phenomenon (rare adverse effect: 0.15% of patients); characterized by a precipitous decline in BP, bradycardia, and consciousness disturbances (syncope) within 90–120 min after the initial dose of prazosin. Recovery is usually within several hours. Preexisting low plasma volume (from diuretic therapy or salt restriction), beta-adrenergic therapy, and recent stroke appear to increase the risk of this phenomenon.
- Monitor blood pressure, standing and sitting/supine. If it falls precipitously with first dose, notify prescriber promptly.
- Full therapeutic effect may not be achieved until 4–6 wk of therapy.

Patient & Family Education

- Avoid situations that would result in injury if you should faint, particularly during early phase of

P

treatment. In most cases, effect does not recur after initial period of therapy; however, it may occur during acute febrile episodes, when drug dose is increased, or when another antihypertensive drug is added to the medication regimen.

- Make position and direction changes slowly and in stages. Dangle legs and move ankles a minute or so before standing when arising in the morning or after a nap.
- Lie down immediately if you experience light-headedness, dizziness, a sense of impending loss of consciousness, or blurred vision. Attempting to stand or walk may result in a fall.
- Do not drive or engage in other potentially hazardous activities until response to drug is known.
- Take drug at same time(s) each day.
- Report priapism or impotence. A change in the drug regimen usually reverses these difficulties.
- Do not take OTC medications, especially remedies for coughs, colds, and allergy, without consulting prescriber.
- Be aware that adverse effects usually disappear with continuation of therapy, but dosage reduction may be necessary.

PREDNISOLONE

(pred-niss'oh-lone)

Rayos

PREDNISOLONE ACETATE

Pred Forte, Pred Mild

PREDNISOLONE SODIUM PHOSPHATE

Classification: ADRENAL CORTICOSTEROID

Therapeutic: ANTI-INFLAMMATORY; IMMUNOSUPPRESSANT

Prototype: Prednisone

AVAILABILITY **Prednisolone:** Tablet; delayed release tablet. **Acetate:** Ophthalmic suspension. **Sodium Phosphate:** Liquid; ophthalmic solution

ACTION & *THERAPEUTIC EFFECT* Has glucocorticoid activity similar to the naturally occurring hormone. It prevents or suppresses inflammation and immune responses. Its actions include inhibition of leukocyte infiltration at the site of inflammation, interference in the function of inflammatory mediators, and suppression of humoral immune responses. *Effective as an anti-inflammatory agent.*

USES Principally as an anti-inflammatory and immunosuppressant agent for a variety of diseases.

CONTRAINDICATIONS Hypersensitivity to prednisolone; systemic fungal infections; coadministration with live or attenuated virus vaccines; Kaposi sarcoma; pregnancy—fetal risk cannot be ruled out; lactation—infant risk cannot be ruled out.

CAUTIOUS USE Cataracts, herpes simplex, glaucoma; coagulopathy; hypertension; TB; adrenal insufficiency; hyperthyroidism; hypothyroidism, DM; psychotic tendencies; hepatic impairment; renal impairment; psychosis; emotional instability; GI disorders/bleeding; osteoporosis; older adults; children.

ROUTE & DOSAGE

Anti-Inflammatory

Adult: **PO** 10–60 mg/day in single or divided doses

Child: **PO** 0.1–2 mg/kg/day in divided doses

Ophthalmic See Appendix A-1

ADMINISTRATION

Oral

- Give with meals to reduce gastric irritation. If distress continues, consult prescriber about possible adjunctive antacid therapy.
- Ensure that delayed release tablets are swallowed whole and not crushed or chewed.
- Storage instructions vary between tablet, syrup, and suspension. See manufacturing directions for specific drug.

Alternate-Day Therapy (ADT) for Patient on Long-Term Therapy

- With ADT, the 48-h requirement for steroids is administered as a single dose every other morning.
- Be aware that ADT minimizes adverse effects associated with long-term treatment while maintaining the desired therapeutic effect.
- See PREDNISONE for numerous additional nursing implications.

ADVERSE EFFECTS (COMMON)

CV: Body fluid retention, hypertension. **CNS:** Headache. **HEENT:** Perforation of cornea (with topical drug), cataract, glaucoma. **Endocrine:** Decreased body growth, abnormal lipids. **Skin:** Ecchymotic skin lesions; acne, superinfection. Also see PREDNISONE. **GI:** Gastric irritation or ulceration. **Musculoskeletal:** Muscle weakness, osteoporosis. **Other:** Euphoria, psychotic disorder.

INTERACTIONS

Drug: BARBITURATES, **phenytoin, rifampin** increase steroid metabolism, therefore may need increased doses of prednisolone; **amphotericin B,** DIURETICS add to **potassium** loss; **neostigmine, pyridostigmine** may cause severe muscle weakness in patients with myasthenia gravis; VACCINES, TOXOIDS may inhibit antibody response. **Food: Licorice** may elevate plasma levels and adverse effects. **Herbal:** Echinacea may decrease therapeutic effect.

PHARMACOKINETICS

Absorption: Readily from GI tract. **Peak:** 1–2 h. **Duration:** 1–1.5 days. **Distribution:** Crosses placenta; distributed into breast milk. **Metabolism:** In liver. **Elimination:** HPA suppression: 24–36 h; in urine. **Half-Life:** 3.5 h.

NURSING IMPLICATIONS

Assessment & Drug Effects

- Be alert to subclinical signs of lack of improvement such as continued drainage, low-grade fever, and interrupted healing. In diseases caused by microorganisms, infection may be masked, activated, or enhanced by corticosteroids. Observe and report exacerbation of symptoms after short period of therapeutic response.
- Monitor vital signs.
- Monitor for changes in behavior, personality or emotional instability.
- Be aware that temporary local discomfort may follow injection of prednisolone into bursa or joint.

Patient & Family Education

- Adhere to established dosage regimen (i.e., do not increase, decrease, or omit doses or change dose intervals).
- Do not suddenly stop medication without first consulting healthcare provider.
- Report to provider any exposures to viral illnesses like chickenpox, measles, flu, or COVID-19.
- Report gastric distress or any sign of peptic ulcer.

P

PREDNISONE

(pred′ni-sone)

Apo-Prednisone ♣

Classification: ADRENAL CORTICOSTEROID

Therapeutic: IMMUNOSUPPRESSANT; ANTI-INFLAMMATORY

AVAILABILITY Tablet; solution; delayed release tablet

ACTION & *THERAPEUTIC EFFECT*

Immediate-acting synthetic analog of hydrocortisone with predominantly corticosteroid properties. *Has anti-inflammatory and immunosuppressant properties.*

USES Principally as an antiinflammatory and immunosuppressant agent.

UNLABELED USES Absence seizures. COPD exacerbation, Bells palsy.

CONTRAINDICATIONS Known hypersensitivity to prednisone; systemic fungal infections; history of optic neuritis; cerebral malaria; latent or active amebiasis; viral infections; live or attenuated vaccines; Kaposi sarcoma; pregnancy—fetal risk cannot be ruled out; lactation—infant risk cannot be ruled out.

CAUTIOUS USE Patients with infections; nonspecific ulcerative colitis; diverticulitis; active or latent peptic ulcer; renal insufficiency; cirrhosis; coagulopathy; psychosis; seizure disorders; adrenal insufficiency, thyroid disease; TB; thromboembolic disease; CHF; hypertension, recent MI; osteoporosis; glaucoma; MG; older adults; children.

ROUTE & DOSAGE

Anti-Inflammatory

Doses are highly individualized (ranges are provided)

Adult/Adolescent/Child: **PO** 10–60 mg/day in single or divided doses

Acute Asthma Exacerbation

Child (younger than 12 y): **PO** 1–2 mg/kg/day until peak expiratory flow is at 70% of personal best (max: 60 mg)

ADMINISTRATION

Oral

- Crush tablet and give with fluid of patient's choice if unable to swallow whole.
- Do not break, divide or chew delayed-release tablets.
- Give at mealtimes or with a snack to reduce gastric irritation.
- Dose adjustment may be required if patient is subjected to severe stress (serious infection, surgery, or injury) or if a remission or disease exacerbation occurs.
- Do not abruptly stop drug. Reduce dose gradually by scheduled decrements (various regimens) to prevent withdrawal symptoms and permit adrenals to recover from drug-induced partial atrophy.
- Store solution or tablet at controlled room temperature at 25° C (77° F), with excursions permitted between 15 and 30° C (59 and 86° F). Protect tablets from moisture.

Alternate-Day Therapy (ADT) for Patient on Long-Term Therapy

- With ADT, the 48-h requirement for steroids is administered as a single dose every other morning.
- Be aware that ADT minimizes adverse effects associated with

P

long-term treatment while maintaining the desired therapeutic effect.

ADVERSE EFFECTS (COMMON)

CV: Hypertension. **CNS:** Euphoria, disturbance in mood, psychosis. **Endocrine:** Body fluid retention, increased appetite, weight gain. **Musculoskeletal:** Osteoporosis, spontaneous fractures.

INTERACTIONS

Drug: BARBITURATES, **phenytoin, rifampin** increase steroid metabolism—increased doses of prednisone may be needed; **amphotericin B,** DIURETICS increase **potassium** loss; **neostigmine, pyridostigmine** may cause severe muscle weakness in patients with myasthenia gravis; may inhibit antibody response to VACCINES, TOXOIDS.

PHARMACOKINETICS

Absorption: Readily from GI tract. **Peak:** 1–2 h. **Duration:** 1–1.5 days. **Distribution:** Crosses placenta; distributed into breast milk. **Metabolism:** In liver. **Elimination:** Hypothalamus-pituitary axis suppression: 24–36 h; in urine. **Half-Life:** 2–3 h.

P

NURSING IMPLICATIONS

Assessment & Drug Effects

- Establish baseline and continuing data regarding BP, I&O ratio and pattern, weight, fasting blood glucose level, and sleep pattern. Start flow chart as reference for planning individualized pharmacotherapeutic patient care.
- Check and record BP during dose stabilization period at least 2 × daily. Report an ascending pattern.
- Monitor patient for evidence of HPA axis suppression during long-term therapy by determining plasma cortisol levels at weekly intervals.
- Be aware that older adult patients and patients with low serum albumin are especially susceptible to adverse effects because of excess circulating free glucocorticoids.
- Be alert to signs of hypocalcemia (see Appendix F). Patients with hypocalcemia have increased requirements for pyridoxine (vitamin B_6), vitamins C and D, and folates.
- Be alert to possibility of masked infection and delayed healing (anti-inflammatory and immunosuppressive actions). Prednisone suppresses early classic signs of inflammation. When patient is on an extended therapy regimen, incidence of oral *Candida* infection is high. Inspect mouth daily for symptoms: White patches, black furry tongue, painful membranes and tongue.
- Monitor bone density. Compression and spontaneous fractures of long bones and vertebrae present hazards, particularly in long-term corticosteroid treatment of rheumatoid arthritis or diabetes, in immobilized patients, and older adults.
- Be aware of previous history of psychotic tendencies. Watch for changes in mood and behavior, emotional stability, sleep pattern, or psychomotor activity, especially with long-term therapy, that may signal onset of recurrence. Report symptoms to prescriber.
- Monitor for withdrawal syndrome (e.g., myalgia, fever, arthralgia, malaise) and hypocorticism (e.g., anorexia, vomiting, nausea, fatigue, dizziness, hypotension, hypoglycemia, myalgia, arthralgia) with abrupt discontinuation of corticosteroids after long-term therapy.
- Ophthalmic exam recommended with prolonged use.

- Monitor lab tests: Periodic fasting blood glucose and serum electrolytes during long-term use.

Patient & Family Education

- Take drug as prescribed and do not alter dosing regimen or stop medication without consulting prescriber.
- Be aware that a slight weight gain with improved appetite is expected, but after dosage is stabilized, a sudden slow but steady weight increase [2 kg (5 lb)/wk] should be reported to prescriber.
- Avoid or minimize alcohol, which may contribute to steroid-ulcer development in long-term therapy.
- Avoid cigarette smoking.
- Report symptoms of GI distress to prescriber and do not self-medicate to find relief.
- Do not use aspirin or other OTC drugs unless they are prescribed specifically by the prescriber.
- Be fastidious about personal hygiene; give special attention to foot care, and be particularly cautious about bruising or abrading the skin.
- Report persistent backache or chest pain (possible symptoms of vertebral or rib fracture) that may occur with long-term therapy.
- Consult prescriber before taking any vaccines.
- Tell dentist or new prescriber about prednisone therapy.

PREGABALIN

Lyrica

Classification: ANTICONVULSANT; GABA-ANALOG; ANALGESIC/MISCELLANEOUS; ANXIOLYTIC

Therapeutic: ANTICONVULSANT; ANALGESIC; ANTI-ANXIETY

Prototype: Gabapentin

Controlled Substance: Schedule V

AVAILABILITY Capsule; oral solution

ACTION & *THERAPEUTIC EFFECT* An analog of gamma-aminobutyric acid (GABA) that increases neuronal GABA levels and reduces calcium currents in the calcium channels of neurons; this may account for its control of pain and anxiety. Its affinity for voltage-gated calcium channels may account for its antiseizure activity. *Has analgesic, anti-anxiety, and anticonvulsant properties.*

USES Management of neuropathic pain associated with diabetic peripheral neuropathy or spinal cord injury, adjunctive therapy for adult patients with partial-onset seizures, management of postherpetic neuralgia, fibromyalgia.

UNLABELED USES Treatment of generalized anxiety disorders, treatment of social anxiety disorder, treatment of moderate pain; myopathy related to drug use; restless leg syndrome, hot flashes.

CONTRAINDICATIONS Hypersensitivity to pregabalin or gabapentin; pregnancy—fetal risk cannot be ruled out; lactation—infant risk cannot be ruled out.

CAUTIOUS USE History of angioedema; renal impairment or failure, hemodialysis; respiratory impairment; history of suicidal tendencies or depression; history of drug abuse or alcohol; history of PR interval prolongation; CHF, NYHA (Class III or IV) cardiac status; older adults; Safe use in children younger than 1 month not established.

ROUTE & DOSAGE

Neuropathic Pain (Diabetic Peripheral Neuropathy)

Adult: **PO** 25–150 mg/day in 2–3 divided doses; may increase in increments of 25–150 mg/day at weekly intervals based on response

Partial-Onset Seizures

Adult: **PO** 150 mg/day divided into 2 or 3 doses; may increase based on response. *Child (over 4 y and over 30 kg):* 3.5 mg/kg/day in 2-3 divided doses (over 4 y and less than 30 kg): 2.5 mg/kg/day in 2–3 divided doses

Neuropathic Pain (Spinal Cord Injury)

Adult: **PO** 75 mg bid may increase to 150–600 mg/day

Fibromyalgia

Adult: **PO** 75 mg bid may increase up to 150 bid within first week, then up to 300–450 mg daily (divided)

Postherpetic Neuralgia

Adult: **PO** Initial dose 75 mg bid or 50 mg tid; may increase to 150–300 mg bid or 100–200 mg tid; Extended release 165 mg daily, may increase to 330 mg daily within 1 week based on response

Renal Impairment Dosage Adjustment (Immediate Release)

CrCl 30–60 mL/min: 75–300 mg/day given in 2 or 3 divided doses;
15–30 mL/min: 25–150 mg/day given in 1 or 2 divided doses; *less than 15 mL/min:* 25–75 mg once daily

Hemodialysis Dosage Adjustment

Dose based on renal function, give supplemental dose

ADMINISTRATION

Oral

- Dosage reduction is required with renal dysfunction.
- Drug should not be abruptly stopped; discontinue by tapering over a minimum of 1 wk.
- Give a supplemental dose immediately following dialysis.
- Do not split, crush or chew extended release tablet.
- Store at 15°–30° C (59°–86° F).

ADVERSE EFFECTS (≥5%) **CV:** Peripheral edema. **Respiratory:** Nasopharyngitis. **CNS:** *Ataxia, dizziness,* headache, incoordination, *somnolence,* tremor. **HEENT:** *Diplopia.* **Endocrine:** Increased appetite, *weight gain.* **GI:** Constipation, dry mouth. **Other:** Eupohria, disturbances in thinking, fatigue.

INTERACTIONS **Drug:** Concomitant use with THIAZOLIDINEDIONES may exacerbate weight gain and fluid retention. May enhance adverse effect of CNS DEPRESSANTS. **Herbal:** Do not use with kratom.

PHARMACOKINETICS **Absorption:** 90% bioavailability. **Peak:** 1.5 h. **Metabolism:** Negligible. **Elimination:** Primarily in the urine. **Half-Life:** 6 h.

NURSING IMPLICATIONS

Assessment & Drug Effects

- Monitor for and report promptly mental status or behavior changes

P

(e.g., anxiety, panic attacks, restlessness, irritability, depression, suicidal thoughts).

- Monitor for weight gain, peripheral edema, and S&S of heart failure, especially with concurrent thiazolidinedione (e.g., rosiglitazone) therapy.
- Monitor diabetics for increased incidences of hypoglycemia.
- Supervise ambulation especially when other CNS drugs are used concurrently.
- Consider more frequent ophthalmologicial assessments.
- Monitor lab tests: Baseline and periodic renal function tests; pregabalin levels, periodic platelet count.

Patient & Family Education

- Do not drive or engage in potentially hazardous activities until response to drug is known.
- Report any of the following to a healthcare provider: Changes in vision (i.e., blurred vision); dizziness and incoordination; weight gain and swelling of the extremities, muscle pain, weakness, behavior or mood changes, especially suicidal thoughts.
- Do not suddenly stop taking the drug without notifying the prescriber.
- Avoid alcohol consumption while taking this drug.
- Inform your prescriber if you plan to become pregnant or father a child.

PRIMAQUINE PHOSPHATE

(prim'a-kween)

Classification: ANTIMALARIAL
Therapeutic: ANTIMALARIAL
Prototype: Chloroquine

AVAILABILITY Tablet

ACTION & THERAPEUTIC EFFECT Acts on primary exoerythrocytic forms of *Plasmodium vivax* and *Plasmodium falciparum*. Destroys late tissue forms of *P. vivax* and thus effects radical cure (prevents relapse). *Gametocidal activity against all species of Plasmodia that infect humans; interrupts transmission of malaria.*

USES Malaria treatment

UNLABELED USES Treatment of *Pneumocystis carinii* pneumonia (PCP) in AIDS; malaria prophylaxis.

CONTRAINDICATIONS Hypersensitivity to primaquine or iodoquinol; rheumatoid arthritis; lupus erythematosus (SLE); hemolytic drugs, concomitant or recent use of agents capable of bone marrow depression (e.g., quinacrine; patients with G6PD deficiency), contraindicated in pregnancy; lactation—infant risk cannot be ruled out.

CAUTIOUS USE Bone marrow depression; hematologic disease; methemoglobin reductase deficiency; cardiac disease or hypertension, long QT syndrome, history of ventricular arrhythmia, bradycardia; hypokalemia, hypomagnesemia, children.

ROUTE & DOSAGE

Malaria Treatment

Screen for G6PD deficiency prior to initiating therapy
Adult: **PO** 30 mg daily for 14 days in combination with another appropriate agent

ADMINISTRATION

Oral

- Give drug at mealtime or with an antacid (prescribed); may prevent or relieve gastric irritation. Notify prescriber if GI symptoms persist.
- Do not administer to patients who have recently received quinacrine.
- Store at 25 degrees C (77 degrees F), with excursions permitted between 15 and 30 degrees C (59 and 86 degrees F).

ADVERSE EFFECTS **GI:** *Nausea, abdominal pain.* **Hematologic:** Hematologic reactions including granulocytopenia and acute hemolytic anemia in patients with G6PD deficiency, *leukopenia*, hemolytic anemia.

INTERACTIONS **Drug:** Avoid use with agents that prolong the QT interval (e.g., **dofetilide, dronedarone, pimozide, ziprasidone);** CYP2D6 INHIBITORS or CYP3A4 INDUCERS may decrease concentration of primaquine. **Food:** avoid grapefruit juice.

PHARMACOKINETICS **Absorption:** Readily from GI tract. **Peak:** 1–3 h. **Metabolism:** Rapidly in liver to active metabolites. **Elimination:** In urine. **Half-Life:** 3.7–9.6 h.

NURSING IMPLICATIONS

Assessment & Drug Effects

- Be aware drug may precipitate acute hemolytic anemia in patients with G6PD deficiency, an inherited error of metabolism carried on the X chromosome, present in about 10% of American Black males and certain White ethnic groups: Sardinians, Sephardic Jews, Greeks, and Iranians. Whites manifest more intense expression of hemolytic reaction than do blacks. Screen for prior to initiation of therapy.
- Monitor ECG in patients with cardiac disease, long QT syndrome, a history of a ventricular arrhythmia, uncorrected hypokalemia or hypomagnesemia, bradycardia or if the person is taking a drug to prolong the QT interval.
- Monitor lab tests: Periodic CBC with differential, and Hct and Hgb, pregnancy test prior to initiation of treatment for sexually active females of reproductive potential.

Patient & Family Education

- Examine urine after each voiding and to report to prescriber darkening of urine, red-tinged urine, and decrease in urine volume. Also report chills, fever, precordial pain, cyanosis (all suggest a hemolytic reaction). Sudden reductions in hemoglobin or erythrocyte count suggest an impending hemolytic reaction. Patient needs to stay hydrated through therapy.
- Review adverse effects with patient and/or caregiver.
- Tell patient to take the drug with food to minimize gastric irritation.

PRIMIDONE

(pri′mi-done)

Mysoline

Classification: ANTICONVULSANT; BARBITURATE

Therapeutic: ANTICONVULSANT

Prototype: Phenobarbital

AVAILABILITY Tablet

ACTION & *THERAPEUTIC EFFECT*

Antiepileptic properties result from raising the seizure threshold and changing seizure patterns. *Effective as an anticonvulsant in all types of seizure disorders except absence seizures.*

USES Alone or concomitantly with other anticonvulsant agents in the prophylactic management of complex partial (psychomotor) and generalized tonic-clonic (grand mal) seizures.

UNLABELED USES Essential tremor.

CONTRAINDICATIONS Hypersensitivity to barbiturates, porphyria; suicidal ideation; pregnancy (category D).

CAUTIOUS USE Chronic lung disease, sleep apnea; liver or kidney disease, dialysis; hyperactive children; mental status changes, major depression, suicidal tendencies; lactation; children.

ROUTE & DOSAGE

Seizures

Adult/Child (8 y or older): **PO** 125–250 mg/day, increased by 125–250 mg/wk (max: 2 g in 2–4 divided doses)
Child (younger than 8 y): **PO** 50–125 mg/day, increased by 50–125 mg/wk (max: 2 g/day in 2–4 divided doses)
Neonates: **PO** 12–20 mg/kg/day in 2–4 divided doses

ADMINISTRATION

Oral

- Give whole or crush with fluid of patient's choice.
- Give with food if drug causes GI distress.

ADVERSE EFFECTS CNS: *Drowsiness, sedation, vertigo, ataxia, headache,* excitement (children), confusion, unusual fatigue, hyperirritability, emotional disturbances, acute psychoses (usually patients with psychomotor epilepsy). **HEENT:** Diplopia, nystagmus, swelling of eyelids. **Skin:** Alopecia, maculopapular or morbilliform rash, edema, lupus erythematosus-like syndrome. **GI:** *Nausea, vomiting, anorexia.* **GU:** Impotence. **Hematologic:** *Leukopenia, thrombocytopenia,* eosinophilia, decreased serum folate levels, megaloblastic anemia (rare). **Other:** Lymphadenopathy, osteomalacia.

INTERACTIONS Drug: Alcohol, CNS DEPRESSANTS compound CNS depression; **phenobarbital** may decrease absorption and increase metabolism of ORAL ANTICOAGULANTS; increases metabolism of CORTICOSTEROIDS, ORAL CONTRACEPTIVES, ANTICONVULSANTS, **digitoxin,** possibly decreasing their effects; ANTIDEPRESSANTS potentiate adverse effects of primidone; **griseofulvin** decreases absorption of primidone. Do not use with **voriconazole. Herbal: Kava, valerian** may potentiate sedation.

PHARMACOKINETICS Absorption: Approximately 60–80% from GI tract. **Peak:** 4 h. **Distribution:** Distributed into breast milk. **Metabolism:** In liver to phenobarbital and PEMA. Affected cytochrome P450 isoenzymes and drug transporters: CYP2C9, CYP3A4, CYP1A2, CYP2C19, CYP2E1, UGT, and P-gp. **Elimination:** In urine. **Half-Life:** Primidone 3–24 h, PEMA 24–48 h; phenobarbital 72–144 h.

NURSING IMPLICATIONS

Assessment & Drug Effects

- Monitor primidone plasma levels (concentrations of primidone greater than 10 mcg/mL are usually associated with significant ataxia and lethargy). Therapeutic blood levels for primidone are 5–12 mcg/mL.

- Therapeutic response may not be evident for several weeks.
- Observe for S&S of folic acid deficiency: Mental dysfunction, psychiatric disorders, neuropathy, megaloblastic anemia. Determine serum folate levels if indicated.
- Monitor lab tests: Baseline CBC and complete metabolic panel, repeat q6mo; primidone blood level as needed.

Patient & Family Education

- Avoid driving and other potentially hazardous activities during beginning of treatment because drowsiness, dizziness, and ataxia may be severe. Symptoms tend to disappear with continued therapy; if they persist, dosage reduction or drug withdrawal may be necessary.
- Avoid alcohol and other CNS depressants unless otherwise directed by prescriber.
- Do not take OTC medications unless approved by prescriber.
- Pregnant women should receive prophylactic vitamin K therapy for 1 mo prior to and during delivery to prevent neonatal hemorrhage.
- Withdraw primidone gradually to avoid precipitating status epilepticus.

P

PROBENECID

(proe-ben′e-sid)

Benuryl ♣, Probalan

Classification: URICOSURIC; ANTIGOUT

Therapeutic: ANTIGOUT

AVAILABILITY Tablet

ACTION & *THERAPEUTIC EFFECT* Competitively inhibits renal tubular reabsorption of uric acid, thereby promoting its excretion and reducing serum urate levels. *Prevents formation of new tophaceous deposits and uric acid build-up in the serum and tissues. As an additive to penicillin, it increases serum concentration of penicillins and prolongs their serum concentration.*

USES Hyperuricemia in chronic gouty arthritis and tophaceous gout.

UNLABELED USES Adjuvant to therapy with penicillin G and penicillin analogs to elevate and prolong plasma concentrations of these antibiotics; to promote uric acid excretion in hyperuricemia secondary to administration of thiazides and related diuretics, furosemide, ethacrynic acid, pyrazinamide.

CONTRAINDICATIONS Blood dyscrasias; uric acid kidney stones; during or within 2–3 wk of acute gouty attack; over excretion of uric acid (greater than 1000 mg/day); patients with creatinine clearance less than 50 mg/min; use with penicillin in presence of known renal impairment; use for hyperuricemia secondary to cancer chemotherapy.

CAUTIOUS USE History of peptic ulcer; pregnancy (category B); lactation; children older than 2 y.

ROUTE & DOSAGE

Gout

Adult: **PO** 250 mg bid for 1 wk, then 500 mg bid (max: 3 g/day)

Adjunct for Penicillin or Cephalosporin Therapy

Adult: **PO** 500 mg qid or 1 g with single dose therapy (e.g., gonorrhea)

Child (2–14 y or weight less than 50 kg): **PO** 25–40 mg/kg/day in 4 divided doses

ADMINISTRATION

Oral

- Therapy is usually not initiated during an acute gouty attack. Consult prescriber.
- Minimize GI adverse effects by giving after meals, with food, milk, or antacid (prescribed). If symptoms persist, dosage reduction may be required.
- Give with a full glass of water if not contraindicated.
- Be aware that prescriber may prescribe concurrent prophylactic doses of colchicine for first 3–6 mo of therapy because frequency of acute gouty attacks may increase during first 6–12 mo of therapy.

ADVERSE EFFECTS

Respiratory: Respiratory depression. **CNS:** *Headache.* **Skin:** Dermatitis, pruritus. **GI:** *Nausea, vomiting, anorexia,* sore gums, hepatic necrosis (rare). **GU:** Urinary frequency. **Musculoskeletal:** Exacerbations of gout, uric acid kidney stones. **Hematologic:** Anemia, hemolytic anemia (possibly related to G6PD deficiency), aplastic anemia (rare). **Other:** Flushing, dizziness, fever, anaphylaxis.

DIAGNOSTIC TEST INTERFERENCE

False-positive ***urine glucose*** tests are possible with ***Benedict's solution*** or ***Clinitest*** [***glucose oxidase methods*** not affected (e.g., ***Clinistix, TesTape***)].

INTERACTIONS

Drug: SALICYLATES may decrease uricosuric activity; may decrease **methotrexate** elimination, causing increased toxicity; decreases **nitrofurantoin** efficacy and increases its toxicity. Decreases clearance of PENICILLINS, CEPHALOSPORINS, and NSAIDS.

PHARMACOKINETICS

Absorption: Readily from GI tract. **Onset:** 30 min. **Peak:** 2–4 h. **Duration:** 8 h. **Distribution:** Crosses placenta. **Metabolism:** In liver. **Elimination:** In urine. **Half-Life:** 4–17 h.

NURSING IMPLICATIONS

Assessment & Drug Effects

- Patients taking sulfonylureas may require dosage adjustment. Probenecid enhances hypoglycemic actions of these drugs (see DIAGNOSTIC TEST INTERFERENCES).
- Expect urate tophaceous deposits to decrease in size. Classic locations are in cartilage of ear pinna and big toe, but they can occur in bursae, tendons, skin, kidneys, and other tissues.
- Monitor lab tests: Periodic serum urate.

Patient & Family Education

- Drink fluid liberally (approximately 3000 mL/day) to maintain daily urinary output of at least 2000 mL or more. This is important because increased uric acid excretion promoted by drug predisposes to renal calculi.
- Prescriber may advise restriction of high-purine foods during early therapy until uric acid level stabilizes. Foods high in purine include organ meats (sweetbreads, liver, kidney), meat extracts, meat soups, gravy, anchovies, and sardines. Moderate amounts are present in other meats, fish, seafood, asparagus, spinach, peas, dried legumes, wild game.
- Avoid alcohol because it may increase serum urate levels.
- Do not stop taking drug without consulting prescriber. Irregular dosage schedule may sharply elevate serum urate level and precipitate acute gout.
- Report symptoms of hypersensitivity to prescriber. Discontinuation of drug is indicated.

- Do not take aspirin or other OTC medications without consulting prescriber. If a mild analgesic is required, acetaminophen is usually allowed.

PROCAINAMIDE HYDROCHLORIDE

(proe-kane-a′mide)

Classification: CLASS IA ANTIARRHYTHMIC

Therapeutic: CLASS IA ANTIARRHYTHMIC

AVAILABILITY Solution for injection

ACTION & *THERAPEUTIC EFFECT* Potent class IA antiarrhythmic that depresses excitability of myocardium to electrical stimulation, reduces conduction velocity in atria, ventricles, and His-Purkinje system. Produces peripheral vasodilation and hypotension, especially with IV use. *Effectively used for atrial arrhythmias; suppresses automaticity of His-Purkinje ventricular muscle.*

USES Prophylactically to maintain normal sinus rhythm following conversion of atrial flutter or fibrillation by other methods; to prevent recurrence of paroxysmal atrial fibrillation and tachycardia, paroxysmal AV junctional rhythm, ventricular tachycardia, ventricular and atrial premature contractions. Also cardiac arrhythmias associated with surgery and anesthesia.

UNLABELED USES Malignant hyperthermia; atrial fibrillation.

CONTRAINDICATIONS Hypersensitivity to procainamide or procaine, yellow dye 5 (tartrazine); blood dyscrasias; bundle branch block; complete AV block, second and third degree AV block unassisted by pacemaker; QT prolongation, torsades de pointes; non-life-threatening ventricular arrhythmias; leukopenia or agranulocytosis; SLE; concurrent use with other antiarrhythmic agents; myasthenia gravis.

CAUTIOUS USE Patient who has undergone electrical conversion to sinus rhythm; first-degree heart block; bone marrow suppression or cytopenia; hypotension, cardiac enlargement, CHF, MI, ischemic heart disease; coronary occlusion, ventricular dysrhythmia from digitalis intoxication, ventricular arrhythmias; hepatic or renal insufficiency; electrolyte imbalance; bronchial asthma; aspirin hypersensitivity; myasthenia gravis; cytopenia; pregnancy (category C); lactation.

ROUTE & DOSAGE

Arrhythmias

Adult: **IV** 100 mg q5min at a rate of 25–50 mg/min until arrhythmia is controlled or 1 g given, then 2–6 mg/min; **IV** ACLS recommendation is 20–50 mg/min until either the arrhythmia is suppressed, hypotension occurs, the QRS complex is widened by 50%, or the max dose of 17 mg/kg is given
Child: **IV** PALS recommendation is 15 mg/kg over 30–60 min

Renal Impairment Dosage Adjustment

CrCl 35–59 mL/min: Decrease initial maintenance dosage by approximately 30%.
CrCl 15–34 mL/min: Decrease initial maintenance dosage by 40–60%.
CrCl less than 15 mL/min: Individualize dosage

ADMINISTRATION

Intramuscular

- IM route should be used only when IV route is not feasible.

Intravenous

Use IV route for emergency situations.

PREPARE: **Direct:** Dilute each 100 mg with 5–10 mL of D5W or sterile water for injection. **IV Infusion:** Add 1 g of procainamide to 250–500 mL of D5W solution to yield 4 mg/mL in 250 mL or 2 mg/mL in 500 mL.

ADMINISTER: **Direct:** Usual rate is 20 mg/min. Faster rates (up to 50 mg/min) should be used with caution. **IV Infusion for Adult:** 2–6 mg/min. **IV Infusion for Child:** 20–80 mcg/kg/min. ▪ Control IV administration over several hours by assessment of procainamide plasma levels. ▪ Use an infusion pump with constant monitoring. ▪ Keep patient in supine position. ▪ Be alert to signs of too rapid administration of drug (speed shock: Irregular pulse, tight feeling in chest, flushed face, headache, loss of consciousness, shock, cardiac arrest).

INCOMPATIBILITIES: **Solution/additive:** **Bretylium, esmolol, ethacrynate, milrinone, phenytoin.** **Y-site:** **Acyclovir sodium, azathioprine sodium, carboplatin, carmustine, cefamandole, ceftizoxime, dantrolene sodium, diazepam, diazoxide, ganciclovir sodium, gemtuzumab ozogamicin, lansoprazole, metronidazole, milrinone acetate (amrinone), minocycline hydrochloride, phenytoin sodium, sulfamethoxazole-trimethoprim.**

- Store solution for up to 24 h at room temperature and for 7 days under refrigeration at 2°–8° C (36°–46° F). ▪ Slight yellowing does not alter drug potency, but discard solution if it is markedly discolored or precipitated.

ADVERSE EFFECTS

CV: Severe hypotension, pericarditis, <u>ventricular fibrillation</u>, AV block, tachycardia, flushing. **CNS:** Dizziness, psychosis. **Skin:** Maculopapular rash, pruritus, erythema, skin rash. **GI:** Diarrhea, nausea, taste disorder, vomiting. **Hematologic:** <u>Agranulocytosis with repeated use;</u> <u>*thrombocytopenia*</u>. **Other:** Fever, muscle and joint pain, angioneurotic edema, myalgia, *SLE-like syndrome (50% of patients on large doses for 1 y):* Polyarthralgias, pleuritic pain, pleural effusion.

INTERACTIONS

Drug: Other ANTIARRHYTHMICS add to therapeutic and toxic effects; ANTICHOLINERGIC AGENTS compound anticholinergic effects; ANTIHYPERTENSIVES add to hypotensive effects; **cimetidine** may increase levels with increase in toxicity; **fingolimod** increases antiarrhythmic effects.

PHARMACOKINETICS

Peak: 15–60 min IM; **Duration:** 3 h; 8 h with sustained release. **Distribution:** Distributed to CSF, liver, spleen, kidney, brain, and heart; crosses placenta; distributed into breast milk. **Metabolism:** In liver to *N*-acetylprocainamide (NAPA), an active metabolite (30–60% metabolized to NAPA). **Elimination:** In urine. **Half-Life:** 3 h procainamide, 6 h NAPA.

NURSING IMPLICATIONS

Black Box Warning

Procainamide has been associated with bone marrow depression.

Assessment & Drug Effects

- Check apical radial pulses before each dose during period of adjustment to the oral route.
- Patients with severe heart, liver, or kidney disease and hypotension are at particular risk for adverse effects.
- Monitor the patient's ECG and BP continuously during IV drug administration.
- Discontinue IV drug temporarily when (1) arrhythmia is interrupted, (2) severe toxic effects are present, (3) QRS complex is excessively widened (greater than 50%), (4) PR interval is prolonged, or (5) BP drops 15 mm Hg or more. Obtain rhythm strip and notify prescriber.
- Ventricular dysrhythmias are usually abolished within a few minutes after IV dose and within an hour after IM administration.
- Report promptly complaints of chest pain, dyspnea, and anxiety. Digitalization may have preceded procainamide in patients with atrial arrhythmias. Cardiotonic glycosides may induce sufficient increase in atrial contraction to dislodge atrial mural emboli, with subsequent pulmonary embolism.

Patient & Family Education

- Report to prescriber signs of reduced procainamide control: Weakness, irregular pulse, unexplained fatigability, anxiety.

P

PROCAINE HYDROCHLORIDE Pr

(proe'kane)

Novocain

Classification: LOCAL ANESTHETIC (ESTER-TYPE)

Therapeutic: LOCAL ANESTHETIC

AVAILABILITY Solution for injection

ACTION & *THERAPEUTIC EFFECT* Decreases sodium flux into nerve cell, thus depressing initial depolarization and preventing propagation and conduction of the nerve impulse. *Local anesthetic action produces loss of sensation and motor activity in circumscribed areas that are treated.*

USES Spinal anesthesia and epidural and peripheral nerve block by injection and infiltration methods.

CONTRAINDICATIONS Known hypersensitivity to procaine or to other drugs of similar chemical structure, to PABA, and to parabens; generalized septicemia, inflammation, or sepsis at proposed injection site; cerebrospinal diseases (e.g., meningitis, syphilis); heart block, hypotension, hypertension; bowel pathology, GI hemorrhage; coagulopathy, anticoagulants, *thrombocytopenia*.

CAUTIOUS USE Debilitated, acutely ill patients; obstetric delivery; increased intra-abdominal pressure; known drug allergies and sensitivities; impaired cardiac function, dysrhythmias; shock; older adults; pregnancy (category C); lactation; children.

ROUTE & DOSAGE

Spinal Anesthesia

Adult: **Intrathecal** 2 mL of 10% solution diluted with NS

Infiltration Anesthesia/Peripheral Nerve Block

Adult/Adolescent/Child:
Regional Up to 200 mL of a 0.5% solution, up to 100 mL of a 1% solution

ADMINISTRATION

- **0.5% Solution Preparation:** To prepare 60 mL of a 0.5% solution (5 mg/mL), dilute 30 mL of 1% solution with 30 mL of NS. Add 0.5–1 mL epinephrine 1:1000/100 mL anesthetic solution for vasoconstrictive effect (1:200,000–1:100,000).
- **0.25% Solution Preparation:** To prepare 60 mL of a 0.25% solution (2.5 mg/mL), dilute 45 mL of 1% solution with 45 mL of NS. Add 0.5–1 mL epinephrine 1:1000/100 mL anesthetic solution for vasoconstrictive effect (1:200,000–1:100,000).
- Do not use solutions that are cloudy, discolored, or that contain crystals. Discard unused portion of solutions not containing a preservative. Avoid use of solution with preservative for spinal, epidural, or caudal block.

INCOMPATIBILITIES: **Solution/additive: Aminophylline, amobarbital, chlorothiazide, magnesium sulfate, phenobarbital, phenytoin, secobarbital, sodium bicarbonate.**

ADVERSE EFFECTS

CV: Myocardial depression, arrhythmias including bradycardia (also fetal bradycardia); hypotension. **CNS:** Anxiety, nervousness, dizziness, circumoral paresthesia, tremors, drowsiness, sedation, convulsions, respiratory arrest. With spinal anesthesia: Postspinal headache, arachnoiditis, palsies, spinal nerve paralysis, meningism. **HEENT:** Tinnitus, blurred vision. **Skin:** Cutaneous lesions of delayed onset, urticaria, pruritus, angioneurotic edema, sweating, syncope, anaphylactoid reaction. **GI:** Nausea, vomiting. **GU:** Urinary retention, fecal or urinary incontinence, loss of perineal sensation and sexual function, slowing of labor and increased incidence of forceps delivery (all with caudal or epidural anesthesia).

INTERACTIONS

Drug: May antagonize effects of SULFONAMIDES; increased risk of hypotension with MAOIS, ANTIHYPERTENSIVES.

PHARMACOKINETICS

Absorption: Rapidly from injection site. **Onset:** 2–5 min. **Duration:** 1 h. **Metabolism:** Hydrolyzed by plasma pseudocholinesterases. **Elimination:** 80% of metabolites excreted in urine. **Half-Life:** 7.7 min.

P

NURSING IMPLICATIONS

Assessment & Drug Effects

- Be aware that reactions during dental procedure are usually mild, transient, and produced by epinephrine added to local anesthetic (e.g., headache, palpitation, tachycardia, hypertension, dizziness).
- Use procaine with epinephrine with caution in body areas with limited blood supply (e.g., fingers, toes, ears, nose). If used, inspect particular area for evidence of reduced perfusion (vasospasm): Pale, cold, sensitive skin.

- Hypotension is the most important complication of spinal anesthesia. Risk period is during first 30 min after induction and is intensified by changes in position that promote decreased venous return, or by preexisting hypertension, pregnancy, old age, or hypovolemia.

Patient & Family Education

- Understand that there will be temporary loss of sensation in the area of the injection.
- Do not consume hot liquids or foods until sensation returns when drug used for dental procedure.

PROCARBAZINE HYDROCHLORIDE

(proe-kar′ba-zeen)

Matulane

Classification: ANTINEOPLASTIC; ALKYLATING AGENT

Therapeutic: ANTINEOPLASTIC

Prototype: Cyclophosphamide

P

AVAILABILITY Capsule

ACTION & *THERAPEUTIC EFFECT* Hydrazine derivative with antimetabolite properties that is cell cycle–specific for the S phase of cell division. Suppresses mitosis at interphase and causes chromatin derangement. *Highly toxic to rapidly proliferating tissue.*

USES Treatment of stage III or IV Hodgkin lymphoma.

UNLABELED USES Solid CNS tumors.

CONTRAINDICATIONS Severe myelosuppression; pheochromocytoma; alcohol ingestion; foods high in tyramine content; diarrhea, sympathomimetic drugs. MAO inhibitors should be discontinued 14 days prior to therapy; tricyclic antidepressants discontinued 7 days before therapy; pregnancy—fetal risk cannot be ruled out; lactation—infant risk cannot be ruled out.

CAUTIOUS USE Hepatic or renal impairment; cardiac disease; bipolar disorder, mania, paranoid schizophrenia; G6PD deficiency; parkinsonism; following radiation or chemotherapy before at least 1 mo has elapsed; alcoholism; infection; children.

ROUTE & DOSAGE

Adjunct for Hodgkin Lymphoma

Adult: **PO** *as part of MOOP regimen* 100 mg/m^2 daily days 1–14; repeat cycle q28 days

ADMINISTRATION

Oral

- NIOSH recommends single gloves by anyone handling intact tablets or capsules or administering from a unit-dose package. Use double gloves and protective gown when cutting, crushing, or manipulating or handling of uncoated tablets. During administration uses single gloves and wear eye/face protection if the formulation is hard to swallow or if the patient may resist, vomit or spit up.
- Do not give if WBC count is less than 4000/mm^3 or platelet count is less than 100,000/mm^3. Consult prescriber.
- Avoid taking with high tyramine-containing foods.
- Store at 20 degrees C (68 degrees F). Protect from freezing, moisture, and light.

ADVERSE EFFECTS GI: *Severe nausea and vomiting.* **Hematologic:** Bone marrow suppression (*leukopenia*, anemia, *thrombocytopenia*).

INTERACTIONS Drug: Alcohol, PHENOTHIAZINES, and other CNS DEPRESSANTS add to CNS depression; TRICYCLIC ANTIDEPRESSANTS, MAO INHIBITORS, SYMPATHOMIMETICS, **ephedrine, phenylpropanolamine** may precipitate hypertensive crisis, hyperpyrexia; seizures or death. Procarbazine may enhance the effects of **CNS depressants.** Do not use with LIVE VACCINES; MYELOSUPPRESSIVE AGENTS AND IMMUNOSUPPRESSANTS increase risk of adverse effects. **Food: Tyramine**-containing foods may precipitate hypertensive crisis; alcohol may case disulfiram reaction. **Herbal:** Do not use with echinacea.

PHARMACOKINETICS Absorption: Readily from GI tract. **Peak:** 1 h. **Distribution:** Widely distributed with high concentrations in liver, kidneys, intestinal wall, and skin; crosses the blood–brain barrier. **Metabolism:** In liver. **Elimination:** In urine. **Half-Life:** 1 h.

NURSING IMPLICATIONS

Black Box Warning

Procarbazine should be given only under supervision of or by a physician experienced in the use of potent antineoplastic drugs. Adequate clinical and laboratory facilities should be available to patients for proper monitoring of treatment.

Assessment & Drug Effects

- Monitor baseline and periodic BP, weight, temperature, pulse, and I&O ratio and pattern.
- Protect patient from exposure to infection and trauma when nadir of leukopenia is approached. Note and report changes in voiding pattern, hematuria, and dysuria (possible signs of urinary tract infection). Monitor I&O ratio and temperature closely.
- Withhold drug and notify prescriber of any of the following: CNS S&S (e.g., paresthesias, neuropathies, confusion); leukopenia [WBC count less than 4000/mm^3; thrombocytopenia (platelet count less than 100,000/mm^3)]; hypersensitivity reaction, the first small ulceration or persistent spot of soreness in oral cavity, diarrhea, and bleeding.
- Monitor for and report any of the following: Chills, fever, weakness, shortness of breath, productive cough. Drug will be discontinued.
- Assess for signs of liver dysfunction: Jaundice (yellow skin, sclerae, and soft palate), frothy or dark urine, clay-colored stools.
- Tolerance to nausea and vomiting (most common adverse effects) usually develops by end of first week of treatment. Doses are kept at a minimum during this time. If vomiting persists, therapy will be interrupted.
- Monitor lab tests: Baseline and q3–4days Hgb, Hct, CBC with differential every 3–4 days during therapy and for a minimum of two weeks after administration, reticulocyte, and platelet count; baseline and weekly LFTs and renal function tests.

Patient & Family Education

- Avoid OTC nose drops, cough medicines, and antiobesity preparations containing ephedrine, amphetamine, epinephrine, and tricyclic antidepressants because they may cause hypertensive crises. Do not use OTC preparations without prescriber's approval.
- Report to prescriber any sign of impending infection.
- Avoid vaccines during therapy.
- Do not eat foods high in tyramine content (e.g., aged cheese, beer, wine).
- Avoid alcohol; ingestion of any form of alcohol may precipitate a disulfiram-type reaction (see Appendix F).
- Report to prescriber immediately signs of hemorrhagic tendencies: Bleeding into skin and mucosa, easy bruising, nose bleeds, or blood in stool or urine. Bone marrow depression often occurs 2–8 wk after start of therapy.
- Report stomatitis, or diarrhea.
- Avoid excessive exposure to the sun because of potential photosensitivity reaction: Cover as much skin area as possible with clothing, and use sunscreen lotion (SPF higher than 12) on all exposed skin surfaces.
- Avoid smoking during therapy.
- Use caution while driving or performing hazardous tasks until response to drug is known since drowsiness, dizziness, and blurred vision are possible adverse effects.
- Use contraceptive measures during procarbazine therapy. Drug may cause infertility in both men and women. Discuss family planning with healthcare provider before initiating therapy.

P

PROCHLORPERAZINE (Pr)

(proe-klor-per'a-zeen)

Compro

PROCHLORPERAZINE EDISYLATE

Classification: ANTIPSYCHOTIC; PHENOTHIAZINE; ANTIEMETIC

Therapeutic: ANTIPSYCHOTIC; ANTIEMETIC

AVAILABILITY Tablet; rectal suppositories. **Edisylate:** Solution for injection

ACTION & *THERAPEUTIC EFFECT* Strong antipsychotic effects thought to be due to blockade of postsynaptic dopamine receptors in the brain. Antiemetic effect is produced by suppression of the chemoreceptor trigger zone (CTZ). *Effective antipsychotic and antiemetic properties.*

USES To control severe nausea and vomiting.

UNLABLED USES Treatment of migraine; nausea/vomiting of pregnancy.

CONTRAINDICATIONS Hypersensitivity to prochlorperazine; blood dyscrasias, jaundice; comatose or severely depressed states; dementia-related psychosis in elderly; children weighing less than 9 kg (20 lb) or younger than 2 y of age; pediatric surgery; short-term vomiting in children or vomiting of unknown etiology; Reye's syndrome or other encephalopathies; pregnancy—fetal risk cannot be ruled out; lactation—infant risk cannot be ruled out.

CAUTIOUS USE Parkinson's disease; decreased GI motility; paralytic ileus; GI obstruction; CVD; cerebrovascular disease, history of cardiovascular impairment, hypovolemia; bone marrow depression, hepatic impairment; renal impairment; Alzheimer disease; narrow angle glaucoma; seizure disorders; urinary retention, BPH; children.

ROUTE & DOSAGE

Severe Nausea, Vomiting

Adult/Adolescent/Child (over 39 kg): **PO** 5–10 mg 3–4 × day (max: 40 mg/day); **IM** 5–10 mg 3–4 × day (max: 40 mg/day) **IV** 2.5–10 mg (max: 10 mg/dose or 40 mg/day); **PR** 25 mg bid
Child (2–12 y, weight 18–39 kg): **PO** 2.5 mg q8h or 5 mg q12h (max: 15 mg/day); *(weight 14–17 kg):* 2.5 mg q8–12h (max: 10 mg/day); *(weight 9–13 kg):* 2.5 mg q12–24h (max: 7.5 mg/day).

ADMINISTRATION

Oral

- Administer with food, milk, or a glass of water to decrease gastric irritation.
- Dosages for older adults, emaciated patients, and children should be increased slowly.
- Do not give oral concentrate to children.
- Avoid skin contact with oral concentrate or injection solution because of possibility of contact dermatitis.
- Store at 20 to 25 degrees C (68 to 77degrees F). Protect from light.

Rectal

- Ensure that suppository is inserted beyond the anal sphincter.
- Do not unwrap suppository until ready for use.
- Store at 20 to 25 degrees C (68 to 77degrees F).

Intramuscular

- Do not inject drug subcutaneously.
- Make injection deep into the upper outer quadrant of the buttock in adults. Follow agency policy regarding IM injection site for children.
- Keep patient in recumbent position for at least 30 min following injection to minimize hypotensive effects.
- Store at 20 to 25 degrees C (68 to 77degrees F). Protect from light. Clear or slightly yellow solutions may be used.

Intravenous

PREPARE: **Direct:** May be given undiluted or diluted in small amounts of NS. **IV Infusion:** Dilute in 50–100 mL of D5W, NS, D5/0.45% NaCl, LR, or other compatible solution.
ADMINISTER: **Direct: Do not** give a bolus dose. Give at a maximum rate of 5 mg/min. **IV Infusion:** Give over 15–30 min. Do not exceed direct IV rate.
INCOMPATIBILITIES: **Solution/additive: Aminophylline, chloramphenicol, chlorothiazide, furosemide, hydrocortisone, thiopental. Y-site: Acyclovir, aldesleukin, allopurinol, amifostine, aminocaproic acid, aminophylline, amphotericin B cholesteryl complex, amphotericin B lipid, ampicillin, azathioprine, aztreonam, bivalirudin, bretylium, calcium chloride, cangrelor, cefamanadole,**

cefazolin, cefepime, cefoperazone, cefotaxime, cefotetan, cefoxitin, ceftazidime, ceftizoxime, ceftriaxone, cefuroxime, chloramphenicol, clindamycin, dantrolene, dexamethasone, diazepam, diazoxide, epoetin alfa, ertapenem, etoposide, fenoldopam, filgrastim, fludarabine, fluorouracil, folic acid, foscarnet, fosphenytoin, furosemide, gallium, ganciclovir, gemcitabine, gemtuzumab, imipenem-cilastatin, indomethacin, insulin, ketorolac, lansoprazole, levofloxacin, midazolam, minocycline, mitomycin, nitroprusside, pantoprazole, pemetrexed, pentamidine, pentobarbital, phenytoin, piperacillin-tazobactam, sodium bicarbonate, streptokinase, SMZ/TMP, urokinase.

- Discard markedly discolored solutions; slight yellowing does not appear to alter potency.

ADVERSE EFFECTS

CV: Hypotension, prolonged QT interval. **CNS:** *Extrapyramidal reactions (akathisia, dystonia, or parkinsonism)*, persistent tardive dyskinesia.

DIAGNOSTIC TEST INTERFERENCE

Increased risk of false positives for phenylketouria and for pregnancy.

INTERACTIONS

Drug: Alcohol, CNS DEPRESSANTS increase CNS depression; **phenobarbital** increases metabolism of prochlorperazine; GENERAL ANESTHETICS increase excitation and hypotension; antagonizes antihypertensive action of **guanethidine; phenylpropanolamine** poses possibility of sudden death; do not use with **amisulpride** due to increased risk of neuroleptic malignant syndrome; TRICYCLIC ANTIDEPRESSANTS intensify hypotensive and anticholinergic effects; decreases seizure threshold—ANTICONVULSANT dosage may need to be increased; increased adverse effects when used with ANTICHOLINERGIC AGENTS. Risk of decreased efficacy when used with ANTIPARKINSON AGENTS. **Herbal: Kava** may increase risk and severity of dystonic reactions.

PHARMACOKINETICS

Absorption: Readily from GI tract. **Onset:** 30–40 min PO; 60 min PR; 10–20 min IM. **Duration:** 3–4 h PO/IM; PR 3–12 h. **Distribution:** Crosses placenta; distributed into breast milk. **Metabolism:** In liver. **Elimination:** In urine.

NURSING IMPLICATIONS

Black Box Warning

Prochlorperazine has been associated with increased mortality in older adults with dementia-related psychosis.

Assessment & Drug Effects

- Position carefully to prevent aspiration of vomitus; may have depressed cough reflex.
- Most older adult and emaciated patients and children, especially those with dehydration or acute illness, appear to be particularly susceptible to extrapyramidal effects. Be alert to onset of symptoms: Early in therapy watch for pseudoparkinson's and acute dyskinesia. After 1–2 mo, be alert to akathisia.
- Fall risk assessment.
- Monitor mental status and report significant changes in mood, behavior, or functional ability when used for long-term therapy.
- Be alert to signs of high core temperature: Red, dry, hot skin; full bounding pulse; dilated pupils; dyspnea; confusion; temperature

over 40.6° C (105° F); elevated BP. Exposure to high environmental temperature places this patient at risk for heat stroke. Inform prescriber and institute measures to reduce body temperature rapidly.

- Monitor lab tests: Periodic CBC with differential baseline and every 6 months thereafter, every 3 weeks for high risk patients, LFTs.

Patient & Family Education

- Take drug only as prescribed and do not alter dose or schedule. Consult prescriber before stopping the medication.
- Avoid hazardous activities such as driving a car until response to drug is known because drug may impair mental and physical abilities, especially during first few days of therapy.
- Be aware that drug may color urine reddish brown. It also may cause the sun-exposed skin to turn gray-blue.
- Protect skin from direct sun's rays and use a sunscreen lotion (SPF higher than 12) to prevent photosensitivity reaction.
- Withhold dose and report to the prescriber if the following symptoms persist more than a few hours: Tremor, involuntary twitching, exaggerated restlessness. Other reportable symptoms include light-colored stools, changes in vision, sore throat, fever, rash.

PROGESTERONE

(proe-jess'ter-one)

Crinone Gel, Prometrium

Classification: PROGESTIN

Therapeutic: PROGESTIN

AVAILABILITY Capsule; solution for injection; gel; vaginal insert; vaginal suppository

ACTION & THERAPEUTIC EFFECT Has estrogenic, anabolic, and androgenic activity. Transforms endometrium from proliferative to secretory state; suppresses pituitary gonadotropin secretion, thereby blocking follicular maturation and ovulation. *Relaxes estrogen-primed myometrium and prohibits spontaneous contraction of uterus. Sudden drop in blood levels of progestin (and estradiol) causes* "withdrawal bleeding" *from endometrium. Intrauterine placement of progesterone hypothetically inhibits sperm survival, and suppresses endometrial proliferation (antiestrogenic effect).*

USES Secondary amenorrhea, functional uterine bleeding, endometriosis, and premenstrual syndrome. Largely supplanted by new progestins, which have longer action and oral effectiveness. Treatment of infertile women with progesterone deficiency.

CONTRAINDICATIONS Hypersensitivity to progestins, known or suspected breast or genital malignancy; use as a pregnancy test; thrombophlebitis, thromboembolic disorders; ectopic pregnancy; cerebral apoplexy (or its history); severely impaired liver function or disease; undiagnosed vaginal bleeding, incomplete abortion; use during first 4 mo of pregnancy (category X); other than vaginal gel use for assisted reproductive technology (ART) in early pregnancy.

CAUTIOUS USE Anemia; diabetes mellitus; history of psychic depression; persons susceptible to acute intermittent porphyria or with conditions that may be aggravated by fluid retention (asthma, seizure disorders, cardiac or kidney function, migraine); impaired liver function; previous ectopic pregnancy; presence or history of salpingitis; venereal disease; unresolved abnormal Pap smear; genital bleeding of unknown etiology; previous pelvic surgery; lactation. **Vaginal gel:** In early first trimester (category B).

ROUTE & DOSAGE

Amenorrhea

Adult: **IM** 5–10 mg for 6–8 consecutive days; **PO** 400 mg at bedtime × 10 days; **Vaginal gel** 45 mg every other day (up to 6 doses)

Uterine Bleeding

Adult: **IM** 5–10 mg/day for 6 days

Premenstrual Syndrome

Adult: **PR** 200–400 mg/day

Assisted Reproductive Technology

Adult: **Vaginal** 90 mg gel daily or bid until placental autonomy OR 10–12 wk; 100 mg insert 2–3 × daily up to 10 wk

P

ADMINISTRATION

Oral

- Give at bedtime and advise caution with ambulation because drug may cause drowsiness or dizziness.
- Do not give oral capsules, which contain peanut oil, to patients allergic to peanuts.

Intramuscular

- Immerse vial in warm water momentarily to redissolve crystals (if present) and to facilitate aspiration of drug into syringe.
- Inject deeply IM. Injection site may be irritated. Inspect IM sites carefully and rotate areas systematically.

Rectal

- Ensure that suppository is inserted beyond the anal sphincter.

Vaginal

- A dosage increase from the 4% gel can only be accomplished by using the 8% gel. Increasing the volume of gel administered does not increase the amount of progesterone absorbed.
- Store drug at 15°–30° C (59°–86° F) unless otherwise specified by manufacturer. Protect from freezing and light.

ADVERSE EFFECTS

CV: Thromboembolic disorder, pulmonary embolism. **CNS:** Migraine headache, *dizziness,* lethargy, mental depression, somnolence, insomnia. **HEENT:** Change in vision, proptosis, diplopia, papilledema, retinal vascular lesions. **Endocrine:** Hyperglycemia, decreased libido, transient increase in sodium and chloride excretion, pyrexia. Gynecomastia, galactorrhea. **Skin:** *Acne,* pruritus, allergic rash, photosensitivity, urticaria, hirsutism, alopecia. **GI:** Hepatic disease, cholestatic jaundice; *nausea,* vomiting, *abdominal cramps.* **GU:** Vaginal candidiasis, chloasma, cervical erosion and changes in secretions, *breakthrough bleeding,* dysmenorrhea, amenorrhea, pruritus vulvae. **Other:** *Edema, weight changes;* pain at injection site; fatigue.

DIAGNOSTIC TEST INTERFERENCE

PROGESTINS may decrease levels of ***urinary pregnanediol*** and increase levels of ***serum alkaline phosphatase, plasma amino acids, urinary nitrogen,*** and

coagulation factors VII, VIII, IX, and ***X.*** They also decrease ***glucose tolerance*** (may cause false-positive ***urine glucose tests***) and lower ***HDL*** (high-density lipoprotein) levels.

INTERACTIONS

Drug: BARBITURATES, **carbamazepine, phenytoin, rifampin** may alter contraceptive effectiveness; **ketoconazole** may inhibit progesterone metabolism; may antagonize effects of **bromocriptine.**

PHARMACOKINETICS

Absorption: Rapid from IM site; PO peaks at 3 h. **Metabolism:** Extensively in liver. **Elimination:** Primarily in urine; excreted in breast milk. **Half-Life:** 5 min.

NURSING IMPLICATIONS

Black Box Warning

Progesterone in combination with estrogen has been associated with increased risk of invasive breast cancer.

Assessment & Drug Effects

- Record baseline data for comparative value about patient's weight, BP, and pulse at onset of progestin therapy. Report deviations promptly.
- Monitor lab tests: Periodic LFTs, blood glucose, and serum electrolytes.
- Monitor for and report immediately S&S of thrombophlebitis or thromboembolic disease.

Patient & Family Education

- If other intravaginal therapy is being used concurrently, allow at least 6 h before/after progesterone vaginal gel insertion.
- Small, white globules may appear as a vaginal discharge, possibly caused by progesterone vaginal gel accumulation, even several days after usage.
- Inform prescriber promptly if any of the following occur: Sudden severe headache or vomiting, dizziness or fainting, numbness in an arm or leg, pain in calves accompanied by swelling, warmth, and redness; acute chest pain or dyspnea.
- Report to prescriber promptly unexplained sudden or gradual, partial or complete loss of vision, ptosis, or diplopia.
- Monitor for loss of glycemic control if diabetic.
- Notify prescriber if you become or suspect pregnancy. Learn the potential risk to the fetus from exposure to progestin.

PROMETHAZINE HYDROCHLORIDE ⚠

(proe-meth'a-zeen)

Histantil ♣, Phenergan, Promethagen

Classification: ANTIHISTAMINE; ANTIEMETIC; ANTIVERTIGO

Therapeutic: ANTIHISTAMINE; ANTIEMETIC; ANTIVERTIGO

Prototype: Prochlorperazine

AVAILABILITY

Tablet; oral solution; rectal suppository; solution for injection

ACTION & *THERAPEUTIC EFFECT*

Exerts anti-serotonin, anticholinergic, and local anesthetic action. Antiemetic action thought to be due to depression of CTZ in medulla. *Long-acting derivative of phenothiazine with marked antihistamine activity and prominent sedative, amnesic, antiemetic, and anti-motion sickness actions.*

USES Motion sickness, nausea/vomiting, induction of sedation, treatment of allergic conditions.

UNLABELED USES hyperemesis gravidarum

CONTRAINDICATIONS Hypersensitivity to phenothiazines; acute MI; angina, atrial fibrillation, atrial flutter, cardiac arrhythmias, cardiomyopathy, uncontrolled hypertension; MAOI therapy; comatose or severely depressed states; lower respiratory tract symptoms, including history of asthma or sleep apnea; hepatic encephalopathy, hepatic diseases; acutely ill or dehydrated children; children with Reye's syndrome; pregnancy—fetal risk cannot be ruled out; lactation (infant risk cannot be ruled out); children younger than 2 y.

CAUTIOUS USE Impaired liver function; epilepsy; bone marrow depression; cardiovascular disease; peripheral vascular disease; acute or chronic respiratory impairment (particularly in children); narrow angle glaucoma; older adult or debilitated patients.

P

ROUTE & DOSAGE

Motion Sickness

Adult: **PO/PR** 25 mg 30–60 min before departure; repeat q8–12h prn

Child (2 y or older): **PO/PR** 0.5mg/kg 30–60 min before departure then q12h prn (max: 25 mg/dose)

Nausea

Adult: **PO/PR/IM/IV** 12.5–25 mg q4–6h prn

Child (2 y or older): **PO/PR/IM/IV** 1 mg/kg/dose q4–6h prn (max: 25 mg/dose)

Allergic Conditions

Adult: **PO/PR** 12.5 mg before meals and at bedtime or 25 mg at bedtime; **IM/IV** 25 mg, repeat in 2 h if necessary, switch to PO

Child (2 y or older): **PO** 0.125 mg/kg/dose (max 12.5 mg/dose) q6h prn and 0.5 mg at bedtime.

Sedation

Adult: **PO/IM/IV** 25–50 mg/dose

ADMINISTRATION

Oral

- Give with food, milk, or a full glass of water may minimize GI distress.
- Tablets may be crushed and mixed with water or food before swallowing.
- Oral doses for allergy are generally prescribed before meals and on retiring or as single dose at bedtime.
- Store at controlled room temperature between 20 and 25 degrees C (68 and 77 degrees F). Protect from light.

Rectal

- Ensure that suppository is inserted beyond the rectal sphincter.
- Refrigerate between 2 and 8 degrees C (36 and 46 degrees F).

Intramuscular

- Give IM injection deep into large muscle mass. Aspirate carefully before injecting drug. Intra-arterial injection can cause arterial or arteriolar spasm, with resultant gangrene.

Intravenous

PREPARE: **Direct:** The 25 mg/mL concentration may be given undiluted. ▪ Dilute the 50 mg/mL concentration in NS to yield no more than 25 mg/mL (e.g., diluting the

50 mg/mL concentration in 4 mL yields 10 mg/mL) and at a rate no greater than 25 mg/minute. ▪ Inspect parenteral drug before preparation. Discard if it is darkened or contains precipitate. Preferred administration through a central venous catheter

ADMINISTER: **Direct:** Give each 25 mg or fraction thereof over at least 1 min.

INCOMPATIBILITIES: **Solution/ additive:** **Aminophylline, cefotetan, chloramphenicol, chlorothiazide, floxacillin sodium, furosemide, heparin, hydrocortisone, methohexital, penicillin G sodium, phenobarbital, thiopental sodium.** **Y-site:** **Acyclovir, aldesleukin, allopurinol, aminophylline, amphotericin B, amphotericin B (lipid), ampicillin, asparaginase, azathioprine, bretylium, cangrelor, carmustine, cefamandole, cefepime, cefoperazone, cefotaxime, cefotetan, cefoxitin, ceftazidime, ceftobiprole, ceftriaxone, cefuroxime, chlorothiazide sodium, clindamycin, dantrolene, diazepam, diazoxide, dimenhydrinate, doxorubicin liposome, ertapenem, fluorescein, fluorouracil, folic acid, foscarnet, ganciclovir, gemtuzumab, inamrinone lactate, indomethacin, ketorolac, lansoprazole, methohexital sodium, methylprednisolone, minocycline, mitomycin, nafcillin, nitroprusside, oxacillin, pantoprazole, pentobarbital, phenobarbital, phenytoin, piperacillin/tazobactam, sodium bicarbonate, streptokinase, sulfamethoxazole-trimethoprim, ticarcillin disodium, urokinase.**

▪ Injection and oral: Store at 20°–25° C (68°–77° F) in tight, light-resistant container unless otherwise directed.

ADVERSE EFFECTS (≥5%)

CNS: Delerium *dizziness, drowsiness,* Parkinsonian-like syndrome. **GI:** *Nausea, vomiting, dry mouth.*

DIAGNOSTIC TEST INTERFERENCE

May produce false results with ***urinary pregnancy tests.*** Promethazine can cause significant alterations of ***flare response*** in ***intradermal allergen tests*** if performed within 4 days of patient receiving promethazine. May cause false positive with ***urine detection of amphetamine/methamphetamine;*** increased serum glucose may be seen with glucose tolerance tests.

INTERACTIONS

Drug: Alcohol and other CNS DEPRESSANTS add to CNS depression and anticholinergic effects. ANTICHOLINERGIC AGENTS increase the risk of adverse effects. Do not use with **metoclopramide, levosulpiride**.

PHARMACOKINETICS

Absorption: Readily from GI tract. **Onset:** 20 min PO/PR/IM; 5 min IV. **Duration:** 4–6 h. **Distribution:** Crosses placenta. **Metabolism:** In liver (CYP2D6, 2B6). **Elimination:** Slowly in urine and feces.

NURSING IMPLICATIONS

Black Box Warning

Promethazine has been associated with severe respiratory depression and death in pediatric patients younger than 2 y.

Assessment & Drug Effects

▪ Monitor respiratory function in patients with respiratory problems, particularly children. Drug may suppress cough reflex and cause thickening of bronchial secretions.

- Supervise ambulation. Promethazine sometimes produces marked sedation and dizziness.
- Monitor blood pressure and mental status.
- Monitor for and report promptly S&S of neuroleptic malignant syndrome.
- Monitor for seizures in those with a history of seizure disorders.
- Patients in pain may develop involuntary (athetoid) movements of upper extremities following parenteral administration. These symptoms usually disappear after pain is controlled.

Patient & Family Education

- For motion sickness: Take initial dose 30–60 min before anticipated travel and repeat at 8–12 h intervals if necessary. For duration of journey, repeat dose on arising and again at evening meal.
- Do not drive or engage in other potentially hazardous activities requiring mental alertness and normal reaction time until response to drug is known.
- Supervise children to avoid potential harm during play activities.
- Avoid sunlamps or prolonged exposure to sunlight.
- Avoid alcohol and other CNS depressants.
- Patients with a history of seizures should report any increased seizure activity.

P

PROPAFENONE

(pro-pa′fen-one)

Rythmol, Rythmol SR

Classification: CLASS IC ANTIARRHYTHMIC

Therapeutic: CLASS IC ANTIARRHYTHMIC

Prototype: Flecainide

AVAILABILITY Tablet; sustained release capsule

ACTION & *THERAPEUTIC EFFECT* Class IC antiarrhythmic drug with a direct stabilizing action on myocardial membranes. Reduces spontaneous automaticity. Exerts a negative inotropic effect on the myocardium. *Decreases rate of single and multiple PVCs and suppresses ventricular arrhythmias.*

USES Ventricular arrhythmias, atrial fibrillation, paroxysmal supraventricular tachycardia.

UNLABELED USES Wolff-Parkinson-White syndrome.

CONTRAINDICATIONS Hypersensitivity to propafenone; uncontrolled CHF, cardiogenic shock, sinoatrial, AV or intraventricular disorders (e.g., sick sinus node syndrome, AV block) without a pacemaker; cardiogenic shock; bradycardia, QT prolongation; marked hypotension; bronchospastic disorders; electrolyte imbalances; non-life-threatening arrhythmias.

CAUTIOUS USE CHF, COPD, chronic bronchitis; AV block; hepatic/renal impairment; older adult patients; pregnancy (category C); lactation. Safe use in children not established.

ROUTE & DOSAGE

Ventricular Arrhythmias

Adult: **PO Immediate release** Initiate with 150 mg q8h, may be increased at 3–4 days intervals (max: 300 mg q8h)

Atrial Fibrillation

Adult: **PO Extended release** 225 mg q12h increase to response (max: 425 mg q12h).

ADMINISTRATION

Oral

- Dosage increments are usually made gradually with older adults or those with previous extensive myocardial damage.
- Significant dose reduction is warranted with severe liver dysfunction. Consult prescriber.
- Store at 15°–30° C (59°–86° F).

ADVERSE EFFECTS **CV:** Arrhythmias, ventricular tachycardia, hypotension, bundle branch block, AV block, complete heart block, sinus arrest, CHF. **CNS:** *Blurred vision, dizziness,* paresthesias, fatigue, somnolence, vertigo, headache. **Skin:** Rash. **GI:** Nausea, abdominal discomfort, constipation, vomiting, dry mouth, *taste alterations,* cholestatic hepatitis. **Hematologic:** *Leukopenia*, granulocytopenia (both rare).

INTERACTIONS **Drug: Amiodarone, quinidine** increases the levels and toxicity of propafenone. May increase levels and toxicity of TRICYCLIC ANTIDEPRESSANTS, **cyclosporine, digoxin,** BETA-BLOCKERS, **theophylline,** and **warfarin** may increase levels of both **propafenone** and **diltiazem. Phenobarbital** decreases levels of **propafenone.** Use with caution in drugs that prolong the QT interval.

PHARMACOKINETICS **Absorption:** Readily from GI tract. **Peak:** 3.5 h. **Distribution:** 97% protein bound, concentrates in the lung. Crosses placenta, distributed into breast milk. **Metabolism:** Hepatic via CY2D6, CYPD3A4, CYP1A2. **Elimination:** 18.5–38% of dose excreted in urine as metabolites. **Half-Life:** 2–10 h in extensive metabolizers and 10–32 h in slow metabolizers.

NURSING IMPLICATIONS

Assessment & Drug Effects

- Monitor cardiovascular status frequently (e.g., ECG, Holter monitor) to determine effectiveness of drug and development of new or worsened arrhythmias.
- Monitor closely patients with preexisting CHF for worsening of this condition. Monitor for digoxin toxicity with concurrent use, because drug may increase serum digoxin levels.
- Report development of second- or third-degree AV block or significant widening of the QRS complex. Dosage adjustment may be warranted.

Patient & Family Education

- Report to prescriber any of following: Chest pain, palpitations, blurred or abnormal vision, dyspnea, or signs and symptoms of infection.
- Be aware when taking concurrent warfarin of possible increase in plasma levels that increase bleeding risk. Report unusual bleeding or bruising.
- Monitor radial pulse daily and report decreased heart rate or development of an abnormal heartbeat.
- Be aware of possibility of dizziness and need for caution with walking, especially in older adult or debilitated patients.

PROPANTHELINE BROMIDE
(proe-pan'the-leen)
Propanthel ♣
Classification: ANTICHOLINERGIC; ANTIMUSCARINIC; ANTISPASMODIC
Therapeutic: ANTICHOLINERGIC
Prototype: Atropine

AVAILABILITY Tablet

ACTION & *THERAPEUTIC EFFECT* Has potent postganglionic nicotinic receptor blocking action and diminishes gastric acid secretion. *Decreases motility (smooth muscle tone) resulting in antispasmodic action and decreases gastric acid secretion.*

USES Adjunct in treatment of peptic ulcer disease.

CONTRAINDICATIONS Narrow-angle glaucoma; tachycardia, MI; paralytic ileus, GI obstructive disease; hemorrhagic shock; myasthenia gravis.

CAUTIOUS USE CAD, CHF, cardiac arrhythmias; liver disease, ulcerative colitis, hiatus hernia, esophagitis; kidney disease; BPH; glaucoma; debilitated patients; hyperthyroidism; autonomic neuropathy; brain damage; Down's syndrome; spastic disorders; pregnancy (category C); lactation. Safe use in children not established.

ROUTE & DOSAGE

Peptic Ulcer Disease
Adult: **PO** 15 mg before each meal and 30 mg at bedtime

ADMINISTRATION
Oral
- Give 30–60 min before meals and at bedtime. Advise not to chew tablet; drug is bitter.
- Give at least 1 h before or 1 h after an antacid (or antidiarrheal agent).
- Store dry powder and tablets at 20°–25° C (68°–77° F); protect from freezing and moisture.

ADVERSE EFFECTS CNS: Drowsiness, confusion, headache, insomnia, nervousness. **HEENT:** Blurred vision, mydriasis, increased intraocular pressure. **GI:** *Constipation, dry mouth.* **GU:** Decreased sexual activity, difficult urination. Neuromuscular and skeletal muscle weakness.

INTERACTIONS Drug: Decreased absorption of **ketoconazole;** ORAL POTASSIUM may increase risk of GI ulcers. Use with other ANTIMUSCARINIC agents can increase side effects. **Food:** Food significantly decreases absorption.

PHARMACOKINETICS Absorption: Incompletely from GI tract. **Onset:** 30–45 min. **Duration:** 4–6 h. **Metabolism:** 50% in GI tract before absorption; 50% in liver. **Elimination:** Primarily in urine; some in bile. **Half-Life:** 9 h.

NURSING IMPLICATIONS
Assessment & Drug Effects
- Assess bowel sounds, especially in presence of ulcerative colitis, since paralytic ileus may develop, predisposing to toxic megacolon.
- Be aware that older adult or debilitated patients may respond to a

usual dose with agitation, excitement, confusion, drowsiness. Stop drug and report to prescriber if these symptoms are observed.
- Check BP, heart sounds and rhythm periodically in patients with cardiac disease.
- Monitor lab tests: Serum creatinine/BUN.

Patient & Family Education
- Avoid just prior to each dose to minimize risk of urinary hesitancy or retention. Record daily urinary volume and report problems to prescriber.
- Relieve dry mouth by rinsing with water frequently, chewing sugar-free gum, or sucking hard candy.
- Maintain adequate fluid and high-fiber food intake to prevent constipation.
- Make all position changes slowly and lie down immediately if faintness, weakness, or palpitations occur. Report symptoms to prescriber.
- Do not drive or engage in potentially hazardous activities until response to drug is known.

PROPOFOL
(pro′po-fol)

Diprivan, Fresenius Propoven, Propofol-Lipuro

Classification: GENERAL ANESTHESIA; SEDATIVE-HYPNOTIC

Therapeutic: SEDATIVE-HYPNOTIC; GENERAL ANESTHESIA

AVAILABILITY Solution for injection

ACTION & *THERAPEUTIC EFFECT* Sedative-hypnotic used in the induction and maintenance of anesthesia or sedation. Rapid onset (40 sec) and minimal excitation during induction of anesthesia. *Effectively used for conscious sedation and maintenance of anesthesia.*

USES Induction or maintenance of anesthesia as part of a balanced anesthesia technique; conscious sedation in mechanically ventilated patients.

CONTRAINDICATIONS Hypersensitivity to propofol or propofol emulsion, which contain soybean and soy products, and egg phosphatide; patients whom general anesthesia or sedation is contraindicated; obstetrical procedures; pregnancy—fetal risk cannot be ruled out; lactation—infant risk cannot be ruled out. Do not use for induction of anesthesia in children younger than 3 y and for maintenance of anesthesia in infants younger than 2 mo.

CAUTIOUS USE Patients with severe cardiac or respiratory disorders, hypotension, respiratory depression, hypoxemia, hypertension; history of epilepsy or seizures; hypovolemia; lipid metabolism disorders; zinc deficiencies; mitochondrial disease, patients with increased intercranial pressure or impaired cerebral circulation; renal impairment; older adults.

ROUTE & DOSAGE

Induction of Anesthesia

Healthy Adult: **IV** 1–2.5 mg/kg as total dose; administered as approximately 40 mg q10 sec until onset of anesthesia

P

Adolescent/Child (3 y or older): **IV** 2.5–3.5 mg/kg over 20–30 sec

Maintenance of Anesthesia

Adult: **IV** 50–200 mcg/kg/min titrate to clinical response

Child/Infant (2 mo or older): **IV** 125–300 mcg/kg/min

ADMINISTRATION

- Use strict aseptic technique to prepare propofol for injection; drug emulsion supports rapid growth of microorganisms.
- Inspect for particulate matter and discoloration. Discard if either is noted.
- Shake well before use. Inspect for separation of the emulsion. Do not use if there is evidence of separation of phases of the emulsion.

Intravenous

PREPARE: **IV Infusion:** Give undiluted or diluted in D5W to a concentration not less than 2 mg/mL. Begin drug administration immediately after preparation and complete within 12 h.

ADMINISTER: **IV Infusion:** Use syringe or volumetric pump to control rate. ▪ Rate is determined by patient weight in kg. Depending on the form of the drug, indication, and patient's health status and age, drug may be given by variable rate infusion or intermittent IV bolus (usually over 3–5 min). ▪ Avoid a rapid bolus in elderly, debilitated, or patient with increased risk of cardiorespiratory events. ▪ Administer immediately after spiking the vial. Complete infusion within 12 h.

INCOMPATIBILITIES: **Solution/additive: Remifentanil Y-site: Amikacin, amphotericin B, bretylium, calcium chloride, cefiderocol, ceftolozane-tazobactam, ciprofloxacin, cisatracurium, diazepam, digoxin, doripenem, doxorubicin, eravacycline, fosfomycin, gentamicin, hydrochloric acid, hydroxocobalamin, isavuconazonium sulfate, levofloxacin, methotrexate, methylprednisolone, metoclopramide, metronidazole, minocycline, mitoxantrone, netilmicin, nimodipine, phenytoin, plazomicin, temocillin sodium, tobramycin, verapamil.**

- Store unopened between 4° C (40° F) and 25° C (77° F). Do not freeze. Shake well before use. Protect from light.

ADVERSE EFFECTS (≥5%)

CV: Heart failure, hypertension. **GI:** Vomiting, nausea. **Musculoskeletal:** Involuntary movement. **Other:** Pain at injection site.

DIAGNOSTIC TEST INTERFERENCE

Propofol produces a temporary reduction in ***serum cortisol levels.*** However, propofol does not seem to inhibit adrenal responsiveness to ***ACTH.***

INTERACTIONS

Drug: Concurrent continuous infusions of propofol and **alfentanil** produce

P

higher plasma levels of **alfentanil** than expected. CNS DEPRESSANTS cause additive CNS depression. **Amiodarone** use (current or recent) can increase risk of hypotension. May enhance bradycardic effect of other agents.

PHARMACOKINETICS

Onset: 9–36 sec. **Duration:** 6–10 min. **Distribution:** Highly lipophilic, crosses placenta, excreted in breast milk. **Metabolism:** Extensively in the liver (CYP2B6, 2C9). **Elimination:** Approximately 88% of the dose is recovered in the urine as metabolites. **Half-Life:** 5–12 h.

NURSING IMPLICATIONS

Assessment & Drug Effects

- Monitor hemodynamic status and assess for dose-related hypotension.
- Monitor vital signs.
- Take seizure precautions. Tonic-clonic seizures have occurred following general anesthesia with propofol.
- Be alert to the potential for drug induced excitation (e.g., twitching, tremor, hyperclonus) and take appropriate safety measures.
- Provide comfort measures; pain at the injection site is quite common especially when small veins are used.
- Monitor lab tests: Urine zinc levels if administered for longer than 5 days or in patients experiencing burns, diarrhea, or major sepsis. Monitor urinalysis, triglycerides, CBC.

Patient & Family Education

- Avoid activities that require mental alertness and/or coordination until effects of the drug have cleared.

PROPRANOLOL HYDROCHLORIDE

(proe-pran'oh-lole)

Apo-Propranolol ♣, Inderal, Inderal LA, InnoPran XL, Novopranol ♣

Classification: BETA-ADRENERGIC RECEPTOR ANTAGONIST; ANTIHYPERTENSIVE; CLASS II ANTIARRHYTHMIC

Therapeutic: ANTIHYPERTENSIVE; CLASS II ANTIARRHYTHMIC; ANTIANGINAL

AVAILABILITY

Tablet; sustained release capsule; oral solution; solution for injection

ACTION & THERAPEUTIC EFFECT

Nonselective beta-blocker of both cardiac and bronchial adrenoreceptors that competes with epinephrine and norepinephrine for available beta receptor sites. In higher doses, it depresses cardiac function including contractility and arrhythmias. Lowers both supine and standing blood pressures in hypertensive patients. *Reduces heart rate, myocardial irritability (Class II antiarrhythmic), and force of contraction, depresses automaticity of sinus node and ectopic pacemaker, and decreases AV and intraventricular conduction velocity.*

Hypotensive effect is associated with decreased cardiac output. Has migraine prophylactic effects.

USES Management of cardiac arrhythmias, myocardial infarction, tachyarrhythmias associated with digitalis intoxication, anesthesia, and thyrotoxicosis, hypertrophic subaortic stenosis, angina pectoris due to coronary atherosclerosis, pheochromocytoma, hereditary essential tremor; also treatment of hypertension alone, but generally with a thiazide or other antihypertensives.

UNLABELED USES Anxiety states, migraine prophylaxis, essential tremors, schizophrenia, tardive dyskinesia, acute panic symptoms (e.g., stage fright), recurrent GI bleeding in cirrhotic patients, treatment of aggression and rage, drug-induced tremors.

CONTRAINDICATIONS Hypersensitivity to propranolol; greater than first-degree heart block; right ventricular failure secondary to pulmonary hypertension; ventricular dysfunction; sinus bradycardia, cardiogenic shock, significant aortic or mitral valvular disease; bronchial asthma or bronchospasm, severe COPD, pulmonary edema; major depression; PVD, Raynaud's disease; abrupt discontinuation.

CAUTIOUS USE History of anaphylactic reaction; peripheral arterial insufficiency; compensated heart failure; history of systemic insect sting reaction; history of psychiatric illness; patients prone to nonallergenic bronchospasm; major surgery; cerebrovascular disease, stroke; renal or hepatic impairment; pheochromocytoma, vasospastic angina; DM; patients prone to hypoglycemia; hyperthyroidism, cardiac arrhythmias; surgery; MG and other skeletal muscular diseases; Wolff-Parkinson-White syndrome; older adults; pregnancy (category C); lactation.

ROUTE & DOSAGE

Hypertension

Adult: **PO Immediate release** 40 mg bid, usually need 160–480 mg/day in divided doses; **InnoPran XL** dose 80 mg each night, may increase to 120 mg at bedtime; **Other extended release forms:** 80 mg daily increase up to 120–160 mg

Angina

Adult: **PO Immediate release** 10–20 mg/day in divided doses (increase up to 160–320 mg/day); **Extended release** 80 mg QD (increase to 160–320 mg/day)

Arrhythmias

Adult: **PO** 10–30 mg q6–8h **IV** 1–3 mg q4h

Post MI

Adult: **PO** 180–240 mg/day in divided doses

Acute MI

Adult: **IV** Total dose of 0.1 mg/kg given in 3 divided doses at 2–3 min intervals **PO Immediate release:** 180–320 mg/day in divided doses

Migraine Prophylaxis

Adult: **PO Immediate release** 80 mg/day in divided doses, may need 160–240 mg/day; **Extended release** 80 mg/day

Essential Tremor

Adult: **PO** 40 mg bid may increase to 120–320 mg/day in divided doses

ADMINISTRATION

- Take apical pulse and BP before administering drug. Withhold drug if heart rate less than 60 bpm or systolic BP less than 90 mm Hg. Consult prescriber for parameters.

Oral

- Do not give within 2 wk of an MAO inhibitor.
- Note that InnoPran XL should be given at bedtime.
- Be consistent with regard to giving with food or on an empty stomach to minimize variations in absorption.
- Ensure that sustained release form is not chewed or crushed. **Must be** swallowed whole.
- Reduce dosage gradually over a period of 1–2 wk and monitor patient closely when discontinued.

Intravenous

Note: Verify correct IV concentration and rate of infusion for neonates with prescriber.

- Take apical pulse and BP before administering drug. Withhold drug if heart rate less than 60 bpm or systolic BP less than 90 mm Hg. ▪ Consult prescriber for parameters.

PREPARE: **Direct:** May be given undiluted or dilute each 1 mg in 10 mL of D5W. **Intermittent:** Dilute a single dose in 50 mL of NS.

ADMINISTER: **Direct:** Give each 1 mg or fraction thereof over 1 min. **Intermittent:** Give each dose over 15–20 min.

INCOMPATIBILITIES: **Y-site: Amphotericin B (conventional and lipid), asparaginase, dantrolene, diazepam, diazoxide, indomethacin, insulin, lansoprazole, mitomycin, paclitaxel, pantoprazole, phenytoin, piperacillin/tazobactam, SMP/TMZ.**

- Store at 15°–30° C (59°–86° F) in tightly closed, light-resistant containers.

ADVERSE EFFECTS

CV: Palpitation, profound *bradycardia*, AV heart block, cardiac standstill, hypotension, angina pectoris, tachyarrhythmia, acute CHF, peripheral arterial insufficiency resembling Raynaud's disease, myotonia, paresthesia of *hands*. **Respiratory:** Dyspnea, <u>laryngospasm</u>, bronchospasm. **CNS:** Drug-induced psychosis, *sleep disturbances*, depression, *confusion*, agitation, giddiness, *lightheadedness*, *fatigue*, vertigo, *syncope*, weakness, *drowsiness*, insomnia, vivid dreams, visual hallucinations, delusions, reversible organic brain syndrome. **HEENT:** Dry eyes (gritty sensation), visual disturbances, conjunctivitis, tinnitus, hearing loss, nasal stuffiness. **Endocrine:** Hypoglycemia, hyperglycemia, hypocalcemia (patients with hyperthyroidism). **Skin:** Erythematous, psoriasis-like eruptions; pruritus, <u>Stevens–Johnson syndrome, toxic</u>

P

epidermal necrolysis, erythema multiforme, exfoliative dermatitis, urticaria. Reversible alopecia, hyperkeratoses of scalp, palms, feet; nail changes, dry skin. **GI:** Dry mouth, nausea, *vomiting*, heartburn, *diarrhea*, constipation, flatulence, abdominal cramps, mesenteric arterial thrombosis, ischemic colitis, pancreatitis. **GU:** Impotence or decreased libido. **Hematologic:** Transient eosinophilia, thrombocytopenic or nonthrombocytopenic purpura, agranulocytosis. **Other:** Fever; pharyngitis; respiratory distress, weight gain, LE-like reaction, cold extremities, *fatigue*, arthralgia, anaphylactic/anaphylactoid reactions.

DIAGNOSTIC TEST INTERFERENCE

BETA-ADRENERGIC BLOCKERS may produce false-negative test results in exercise tolerance ECG tests, and elevations in ***serum potassium, peripheral platelet count, serum uric acid, serum transaminase, alkaline phosphatase, lactate dehydrogenase, serum creatinine, BUN,*** and an increase or decrease in ***blood glucose*** levels in diabetic patients.

P

INTERACTIONS

Drug: PHENOTHIAZINES have additive hypotensive effects. BETA-ADRENERGIC AGONISTS (e.g., **albuterol**) antagonize effects. **Atropine** and TRICYCLIC ANTIDEPRESSANTS block bradycardia. DIURETICS and other HYPOTENSIVE AGENTS increase hypotension. High doses of **tubocurarine** may potentiate neuromuscular blockade. **Cimetidine** decreases clearance, increases effects. ANTACIDS, **ascorbic acid** may decrease absorption.

PHARMACOKINETICS

Absorption: Completely from GI tract; undergoes extensive first-pass metabolism. **Peak:** 60–90 min immediate release; 6 h sustained release; 5 min IV. **Distribution:** Widely distributed including CNS, placenta, and breast milk. **Metabolism:** Almost completely in liver (CYP1A2, 2D6). **Elimination:** 90–95% in urine as metabolites; 1–4% in feces. **Half-Life:** 2.3 h.

NURSING IMPLICATIONS

Black Box Warning

Propranolol has been associated with exacerbation of angina and MI following abrupt discontinuance.

Assessment & Drug Effects

- Obtain careful medical history to rule out allergies, asthma, and obstructive pulmonary disease. Propranolol can cause bronchiolar constriction even in normal subjects.
- Monitor apical pulse, respiration, BP for 2 h after initiation or dosage adjustment. Consult prescriber for acceptable parameters.
- Evaluate adequate control or dosage interval for patients being treated for hypertension by checking blood pressure near end of dosage interval or before administration of next dose.
- Monitor I&O ratio and daily weight as significant indexes for detecting fluid retention and developing heart failure.
- Monitor diabetics for loss of glycemic control.

Patient & Family Education

- Do not discontinue abruptly; can precipitate withdrawal syndrome (e.g., tremulousness, sweating, severe headache, malaise, palpitation, rebound hypertension, MI, and life-threatening arrhythmias in patients with angina pectoris).

- Learn usual pulse rate and take radial pulse before each dose. Report to prescriber if pulse is below the established parameter or becomes irregular.
- Be aware that propranolol suppresses clinical signs of hypoglycemia (e.g., BP changes, increased pulse rate) and may prolong hypoglycemia.
- Understand importance of compliance. Do not alter established regimen (i.e., do not omit, increase, or decrease dosage or change dosage interval).
- Be aware that drug may cause mild hypotension (experienced as dizziness or light-headedness) in normotensive patients on prolonged therapy. Make position changes slowly and avoid prolonged standing. Notify prescriber if symptoms persist.
- Do not drive or engage in potentially hazardous activities until response to drug is known.
- Inform dentist, surgeon, or ophthalmologist that you are taking propranolol (drug lowers normal and elevated intraocular pressure).

PROPYLTHIOURACIL (PTU) (Pr)

(proe-pill-thye-oh-yoor'a-sill)

Classification: ANTITHYROID

Therapeutic: ANTITHYROID

AVAILABILITY Tablet

ACTION & *THERAPEUTIC EFFECT* Interferes with use of iodine and blocks synthesis of thyroxine (T_4) and triiodothyronine (T_3); blocks conversion of T_4 to T_3 in peripheral tissues and T_3 stores in circulating blood and the thyroid. *Effective as an antithyroid agent in various hyperthyroid conditions.*

USES Hyperthyroidism in patients with Graves' disease or toxic multinodular goiter; amelioration of hyperthyroid symptoms prior to surgery.

CONTRAINDICATIONS Hypersensitivity to propylthiouracil; acute liver failure; exfoliative dermatitis; unexplained fever; pregnancy (nonteratogenic adverse effects, including fetal and neonatal hypothyroidism, goiter, and hyperthyroidism, have been reported following maternal).

CAUTIOUS USE Infection; bone marrow depression; impaired liver function; renal impairment; older adults; patients at risk for liver failure; lactation; children younger than 6 y.

ROUTE & DOSAGE

Hyperthyroidism

Adult: **PO** 300 mg/day divided q8h

ADMINISTRATION

Oral

- Give at the same time each day with relation to meals. Food may alter drug response by changing absorption rate.
- If drug is being used to improve thyroid state before radioactive iodine (RAI) treatment, discontinue 3 or 4 days before treatment to prevent uptake interference. PTU therapy may be resumed if necessary 3–5 days after the RAI administration.
- Store drug at 15°–30° C (59°–86° F) in light-resistant container.

ADVERSE EFFECTS **Cardiovascular:** Edema, periarteritis, vasculitis. **Respiratory:** Interstitial pneumonitis, pulmonary alveolar

P

hemorrhage. **CNS:** Paresthesias, headache, vertigo, drowsiness, neuritis. **Endocrine:** Hypothyroidism (goitrogenic), enlarged thyroid, periorbital edema, puffy hands and feet, bradycardia, cool and pale skin, worsening of ophthalmopathy, sleepiness, fatigue, mental depression, sensitivity to cold, nocturnal muscle cramps, changes in menstrual periods, unusual weight gain. **Skin:** Skin rash, urticaria, pruritus, skin pigmentation, exfoliative dermatitis, alopecia, Stevens-Johnson syndrome. **Hepatic/GI:** Nausea, vomiting, diarrhea, dyspepsia, loss of taste, stomach pain, hepatotoxicity, jaundice, hepatitis. **GU:** Acute renal failure, glomerulonephritis. **Hematologic:** Myelosuppression, lymphadenopathy, hypoprothrombinemia, *thrombocytopenia*, *leukopenia*, agranulocytosis, aplastic anemia, granulocytopenia, splenomegaly, hemorrhage. **Other:** Fever, lupus-like syndrome, arthralgia, myalgia.

INTERACTIONS

Drug: May increase myleosuppression with MYELOSUPRESSIVE AGENTS. Do not use with LIVE VACCINES.

PHARMACOKINETICS

Absorption: Rapidly from GI tract. **Peak:** 1–2 h. **Distribution:** Concentrates in thyroid gland; crosses placenta; some distribution into breast milk. **Metabolism:** Rapidly to inactive metabolites. **Elimination:** 35% in urine. **Half-Life:** 1–2 h.

NURSING IMPLICATIONS

Black Box Warning

Propylthiouracil has been associated with acute, sometimes fatal, liver injury.

Assessment & Drug Effects

- Be aware that about 10% of patients with hyperthyroidism have leukopenia less than 4000 cells/mm^3 and relative granulocytopenia.
- Observe for signs of clinical response to PTU (usually within 2 or 3 wk): Significant weight gain, reduced pulse rate, reduced serum T_4.
- Satisfactory euthyroid state may be delayed for several months when thyroid gland is greatly enlarged.
- Be alert to signs of hypoprothrombinemia: Ecchymoses, purpura, petechiae, unexplained bleeding. Warn ambulatory patients to report these signs promptly.
- Be alert for important diagnostic signs of excess dosage: Contraction of a muscle bundle when pricked, mental depression, hard and nonpitting edema, and need for high thermostat setting and extra blankets in winter (cold intolerance).
- Monitor for urticaria (occurs in 3–7% of patients during weeks 2–8 of treatment). Report severe rash.
- Monitor lab tests: Baseline and periodic T_3, T_4, and TSH; periodic LFTs and CBC with differential and platelet count.

Patient & Family Education

- Note that PTU treatment may be reinstituted if surgery fails to produce normal thyroid gland function.
- Report severe skin rash or swelling of cervical lymph nodes. Therapy may be discontinued.
- Report to prescriber sore throat, fever, and rash immediately (most apt to occur in first few months of treatment). Drug will be discontinued and hematologic studies initiated.

- Avoid use of OTC drugs for asthma, or cough treatment without checking with the prescriber. Iodides sometimes included in such preparations are contraindicated.
- Learn how to take pulse accurately and check daily. Report to prescriber continued tachycardia.
- Report diarrhea, fever, irritability, listlessness, vomiting, weakness; these are signs of inadequate therapy or thyrotoxicosis.
- Chart weight 2 or 3 × weekly; clinical response is monitored through changes in weight and pulse.
- Do not alter drug regimen (e.g., increase, decrease, omit doses, change dosage intervals).
- Check with prescriber about use of iodized salt and inclusion of seafood in the diet.

PROTAMINE SULFATE

(proe′ta-meen)

Classification: ANTIDOTE; HEPARIN ANTAGONIST
Therapeutic: ANTIHEMORRHAGIC

AVAILABILITY Solution for injection

ACTION & *THERAPEUTIC EFFECT* Combines with heparin to produce a stable complex; thus it neutralizes the anticoagulant effect of heparin. *Effective antidote to heparin overdose.*

USES Antidote for heparin overdosage (after heparin has been discontinued).

UNLABELED USES Antidote for heparin administration during extracorporeal circulation.

CONTRAINDICATIONS Hemorrhage not induced by heparin overdosage; lactation.

CAUTIOUS USE Cardiovascular disease; history of allergy to fish; vasectomized or infertile males; diabetes mellitus; patients who have received protamine-containing insulin; pregnancy (category C); children.

ROUTE & DOSAGE

Antidote for Heparin Overdose

Adult/Child: **IV** 1 mg for every 100 units of heparin to be neutralized (max: 100 mg in a 2 h period), give the first 25–50 mg by slow direct IV and the rest over 2–3 h

ADMINISTRATION

Note: Titrate dose carefully to prevent excess anticoagulation because protamine has a longer half-life than heparin and also has some anticoagulant effect of its own.

Intravenous

Note: Verify correct IV concentration and rate of infusion for infants or children with prescriber.

PREPARE: **Direct:** May be given as supplied direct IV. **Continuous:** Dilute in 50 mL or more of NS or D5W.

ADMINISTER: **Direct** Give each 50 mg or fraction thereof slowly over 10–15 min. ▪ NEVER give more than 50 mg in any 10 min period or 100 mg in any 2 h period.

Continuous: Do not exceed direct rate. Give over 2–3 h or longer as determined by coagulation studies.

INCOMPATIBILITIES: **Solution/additive:** RADIOCONTRAST MATERIALS, **furosemide.**

P

▪ Store protamine sulfate injection at 15°–30° C (59°–86° F).
▪ Solutions do not contain preservatives and should not be stored.

ADVERSE EFFECTS **CV:** *Abrupt drop in BP* (with rapid IV infusion), bradycardia. **GI:** Nausea, vomiting. **Hematologic:** Protamine overdose or "heparin rebound" (hyperheparinemia). **Other:** Urticaria, angioedema, pulmonary edema, anaphylaxis, dyspnea, lassitude; transient flushing and feeling of warmth.

PHARMACOKINETICS **Onset:** 5 min. **Duration:** 2 h.

NURSING IMPLICATIONS

Black Box Warning

Protamine can cause severe hypotension, cardiovascular collapse, noncardiogenic pulmonary edema, catastrophic pulmonary vasoconstriction, and pulmonary hypertension.

P

Assessment & Drug Effects

▪ Monitor closely for a hypersensitivity reaction. Risk factors include high doses or overdose, repeated doses, and previous protamine administration (including protamine-containing drugs).
▪ Monitor BP, HR, and respiratory status q15–30min, or more often if indicated. Continue for at least 2–3 h after each dose, or longer as dictated by patient's condition.
▪ Observe closely patients who have had cardiac surgery for bleeding (heparin rebound). Even with apparent adequate neutralization of heparin by protamine, bleeding may occur 30 min to 18 h after surgery.
▪ Monitor lab tests: Activated clotting time or aPTT 5–15 min after administration of protamine, and again in 2–8 h if desirable.

PROTEIN C CONCENTRATE (HUMAN)

(pro′teen)

Ceprotin

Classification: HEMATOLOGIC; THROMBOLYTIC; PROTEIN SYNTHESIS INHIBITOR

Therapeutic PROTEIN C REPLACEMENT THERAPY

AVAILABILITY Vial of lyophilized powder

ACTION & *THERAPEUTIC EFFECT* Protein C is a critical element in a pathway that provides a natural mechanism for control of the coagulation system. It prevents excess procoagulant responses to activating stimuli. *Protein C is necessary to decrease thrombin generation and intravascular clot formation.*

USES Treatment of patients with severe congenital protein C deficiency; protein C replacement therapy for the prevention and treatment of venous thrombosis and purpura fulminans in children and adults.

CONTRAINDICATIONS Hypersensitivity to human protein C; concurrent administration with tissue plasminogen activator (tPA); hypernatremia; lactation.

CAUTIOUS USE Concurrent administration of anticoagulants; heparin induced thrombocytopenia (HIT); renal impairment; hepatic impairment; older adults; pregnancy (category C); children.

ROUTE & DOSAGE

Acute Episodes of Venous Thrombosis and Purpura Fulminans and Short-Term Prophylaxis

Adult/Adolescent/Child/Infant: **IV** Initial dose 100–120 units/kg; then 60–80 units/kg q6h × 3; maintenance dose: 45–60 units/kg q6–12h.

ADMINISTRATION

Intravenous

PREPARE: **Direct/IV Infusion:** Bring powder and supplied diluent to room temperature. Insert supplied double-ended transfer needle into diluent vial, then invert and rapidly insert into protein C powder vial. (If vacuum does not draw diluent into vial, discard.) ▪ Remove transfer needle and gently swirl to dissolve. ▪ Resulting solution concentration is 100 units/mL and it should be colorless to slightly yellowish, clear to slightly opalescent and free from visible particles. ▪ Withdraw required dose with the supplied filter needle.

ADMINISTER: **Direct/IV Infusion:** Infuse at 2 mL/min. **Direct/IV Infusion for Child weighing greater than 10 kg:** Infuse at 0.2 mL/kg/min.

▪ Store at room temperature for no more than 3 h after reconstitution. ▪ Prior to reconstitution, protect from light.

ADVERSE EFFECTS **CV:** Hemothorax, hypotension. **CNS:** Lightheadedness. **Other:** Fever, hyperhidrosis, hypersensitivity reactions (rash, pruritus), restlessness.

INTERACTIONS **Drug:** Protein C concentrate can increase bleeding caused by **alteplase, reteplase,** or **tenecteplase.**

PHARMACOKINETICS **Peak:** 0.5–1 h. **Half-Life:** 9.9 h.

NURSING IMPLICATIONS

Assessment & Drug Effects

- Monitor for and promptly report S&S of bleeding or hypersensitivity reactions (see Appendix F).
- Monitor vital signs including BP and temperature.
- Monitor lab tests: Baseline and periodic protein C activity; periodic platelet count; frequent serum sodium with renal function impairment.

Patient & Family Education

- Report immediately early signs of hypersensitivity reactions including hives, generalized itching, tightness in chest, wheezing, difficulty breathing.
- Report immediately any signs of bleeding including black tarry stools, pink/red-tinged urine, unusual bruising.

P

PROTRIPTYLINE HYDROCHLORIDE

(proe-trip′te-leen)

Classification: TRICYCLIC ANTIDEPRESSANT

Therapeutic: ANTIDEPRESSANT

Prototype: Imipramine

AVAILABILITY Tablet

ACTION & *THERAPEUTIC EFFECT*

Believed to enhance actions of norepinephrine and serotonin by blocking their reuptake at the neuronal membrane. *Effective in the treatment of depressed individuals, particularly those who are withdrawn.*

USES Treatment of major depression.

CONTRAINDICATIONS Hypersensitivity to TCAs; concurrent use of MAOIs; concurrent use of cisapride; acute recovery phase following MI or within 14 days of use; QT prolongation, bundle branch block; cardiac conduction defects; suicidal ideation.

CAUTIOUS USE Hepatic, cardiovascular, or kidney dysfunction; DM; hyperthyroidism; history of alcoholism; patients with insomnia; asthma; bipolar disorder; suicidal tendencies; children and adolescents; pregnancy (adverse effects have not been observed in animal reproduction studies; tricyclic antidepressants may be associated with irritability, jitteriness, and convulsions in the neonate); lactation.

ROUTE & DOSAGE

Depression

Adult: **PO** 10–20 mg/day in 3–4 divided doses (max: 60 mg/day)

ADMINISTRATION

Oral

- Give whole or crush and mix with fluid or food.
- Give dosage increases in the morning dose to prevent sleep interference and because this TCA has psychic energizing action.
- Give last dose of day no later than mid-afternoon; insomnia rather than drowsiness is a frequent adverse effect.
- Store at 20°–25° C (68°–77° F) in tightly closed container.

ADVERSE EFFECTS **CV:** Cerebrovascular accident, flushing, *orthostatic hypotension, tachycardia,* arrhythmia. **CNS:** Insomnia, headache, confusion, anxiety, agitation, tingling of extremities. **HEENT:** Blurred vision, increased intraocular pressure, angle-closure glaucoma, tinnitus. **GI:** *Xerostomia, constipation,* paralytic ileus, dypepsia, nausea, abdominal cramps. **GU:** *Urinary retention,* breast hypertrophy, impotence, nocturia, testicular swelling, polyuria. **Other:** Suicidal ideation.

INTERACTIONS **Drug:** May decrease some response to ANTIHYPERTENSIVES; CNS DEPRESSANTS, **alcohol,** HYPNOTICS, BARBITURATES, SEDATIVES potentiate CNS depression; ORAL ANTICOAGULANTS may increase hypoprothrombinemic effects; **ethchlorvynol** causes transient delirium; **levodopa** SYMPATHOMIMETICS (e.g., **epinephrine, norepinephrine**) increases possibility of sympathetic hyperactivity with hypertension and hyperpyrexia; MAO INHIBITORS present possibility of severe reactions—toxic psychosis, cardiovascular instability; **methylphenidate** increases plasma TCA levels; THYROID DRUGS may increase possibility of arrhythmias; **cimetidine** may increase plasma TCA levels. There is an increased risk of ulcers with used with **potassium citrate**. Do not use with agents that prolong the QT interval (e.g., **dofetilide, dronedarone, ziprasidone**). **Herbal: Ginkgo** may decrease seizure threshold; **St. John's wort** may cause serotonin syndrome (headache, dizziness, sweating, agitation). Kratom can increase risk of CNS depression.

PHARMACOKINETICS **Absorption:** Rapidly from GI tract. **Peak levels:** 24–30 h. **Distribution:** Crosses placenta; distributed into breast milk. **Metabolism:** In liver. **Elimination:** Primarily in urine. **Half-Life:** 54–98 h.

NURSING IMPLICATIONS

Black Box Warning

Protriptyline has been associated with increased risk of suicidal thinking and behavior in children, adolescents, and young adults.

Assessment & Drug Effects

- Monitor therapeutic effectiveness. Onset of initial effect characterized by increased activity and energy is fairly rapid, usually within 1 wk after therapy is initiated. Maximum effect may not occur for 2 wk or more.
- Monitor adolescents as well as adults for changes in behavior that may indicate suicidality. Suicide is an inherent risk with any depressed patient and may remain until there is significant improvement.
- Monitor vital signs closely and CV system responses during early therapy, particularly in patients with cardiovascular disorders and older adults receiving daily doses in excess of 20 mg. Withhold drug and inform prescriber if BP falls more than 20 mm Hg or if there is a sudden increase in pulse rate.
- Monitor I&O ratio and bowel pattern during early therapy and when patient is on large doses.
- Assess and advise prescriber as indicated for prominent anticholinergic effects (xerostomia, blurred vision, constipation, paralytic ileus, urinary retention, delayed micturition).
- Assess condition of oral membranes frequently; institute symptomatic treatment if necessary. Xerostomia can interfere with appetite, fluid intake, and integrity of tooth surfaces.

Patient & Family Education

- Report promptly changes in mood or behavior indicative of suicidal thinking.
- Consult prescriber about safe amount of alcohol, if any, that can be taken. Actions of both alcohol and protriptyline are potentiated when used together for up to 2 wk after the TCA is discontinued.
- Consult prescriber before taking any OTC medications.
- Be aware that effects of barbiturates and other CNS depressants are enhanced by TCAs.
- Avoid potentially hazardous activities requiring alertness and skill until response to drug is known.
- Avoid exposure to the sun without protecting skin with sunscreen lotion (SPF higher than 12). Photosensitivity reactions may occur.

PRUCALOPRIDE

(proo-KAL-oh-pride)

Motegrity

Classifications: GI STIMULANT; PROKINETIC AGENT

Therapeutic: GI STIMULANT; ANTIEMETIC

Prototype: Metoclopramide

P

AVAILABILITY Oral tablet

ACTION & *THERAPEUTIC EFFECT* A selective, high affinity 5-HT_4 receptor agonist whose action at the receptor site promotes cholinergic and nonadrenergic, noncholinergic neurotransmission by enteric neurons. *Leads to stimulation of peristaltic reflex, intestinal secretions, and gastrointestinal motility.*

USES Treatment of Chronic Idiopathic Constipation (CIC).

CONTRAINDICATIONS Hypersensitivity to prucalopride or any component of the formulation; intestinal perforation or obstruction due to structural or functional disorder of the gut wall, obstructive ileus, or severe inflammatory conditions of the GI tract.

CAUTIOUS USE Renal impairment; elderly; pregnancy; lactation.

ROUTE & DOSAGE

Treatment of Chronic Idiopathic Constipation

Adult: **PO** 2 mg once daily

Renal Impairment Dosage Adjustment

CrCl less than 30 mL/min: 1 mg once daily
ESRD with dialysis: Avoid use

ADMINISTRATION

Oral

- Administer without regard to meals.
- Store at 20° to 25°C (68° to 77°F). Store in original container to protect from moisture.

P

ADVERSE EFFECTS **CNS:** Headache, dizziness. **GI:** Abdominal pain, nausea, diarrhea, abdominal distension.

INTERACTIONS No clinically relevant interactions reported.

PHARMACOKINETICS **Absorption:** 90% bioavailability. **Peak:** 2–3 h **Distribution:** 567 L (given IV); 30% protein bound. **Metabolism:** In the liver primarily by CYP3A4 (minor). **Elimination:** 84% in urine, 13% in feces. **Half-Life:** 24 h.

NURSING IMPLICATIONS

Assessment & Drug Effects

- Monitor frequency of bowel movements.
- Monitor for worsening of depression or emergence of suicidal thoughts or behavior.
- Assess for cardiovascular symptoms in patients with heart disease.
- Monitor lab tests: Baseline liver function tests, baseline renal function tests.

Patient & Family Education

- Notify health care provider if experiencing new or worse behavior or mood changes like depression or thoughts of suicide.
- Notify your doctor or get medical help right away if you have any of the following signs or symptoms of allergic reaction such as rash, hives, itching; red, swollen, blistered, or peeling skin with or without fever; wheezing; tightness in the chest or throat; trouble breathing, swallowing, or talking; unusual hoarseness; or swelling of the mouth, face, lips, tongue, or throat; or any dizziness or passing out.

PSEUDOEPHEDRINE HYDROCHLORIDE

(soo-doe-e-fed′rin)

Robidrine ♣, Sudafed

Classification: ALPHA- AND BETA-ADRENERGIC RECEPTOR AGONIST; DECONGESTANT

Therapeutic: NASAL DECONGESTANT

Prototype: Epinephrine

AVAILABILITY Tablet; sustained release tablet; liquid

ACTION & THERAPEUTIC EFFECT

Sympathomimetic amine that produces decongestion of respiratory tract mucosa by stimulating the sympathetic nerve endings including alpha-, $beta_1$-, and $beta_2$-receptors. *Effect is caused by vasoconstriction and thus increased nasal airway patency.*

USES Symptomatic relief of nasal congestion associated with rhinitis, coryza, and sinusitis.

CONTRAINDICATIONS Hypersensitivity to sympathomimetic amines; severe hypertension; severe coronary artery disease; use within 14 days of MAOIS; hyperthyroidism; prostatic hypertrophy.

CAUTIOUS USE Hypertension, heart disease, renal impairment; acute MI, angina; closed-angle glaucoma; severe narrowing of bowel; concurrent use of ACE INHIBITOR; thyroid disease, DM, elevated IOP; PVD; BPH; pregnancy (use of pseudoephedrine during the first trimester may be associated with a possible risk of gastroschisis, small intestinal atresia, and hemifacial microsomia; use during first trimester should be avoided); lactation. Safe use in children younger than 2 y **(PO)**, children younger than 12 y **(sustained release)** is not established.

ROUTE & DOSAGE

Nasal Congestion

Adult/Adolescent: **PO** 60 mg q4–6h or 120 mg sustained release q12h or 240 mg q24h (max: 240 mg/day)
Geriatric: **PO** 30–60 mg q6h prn
Child (2–6 y): **PO** 15 mg q4–6h (max: 60 mg/day); *6–11 y:* 30 mg q4–6h (max: 120 mg/day)

ADMINISTRATION

Oral

- Ensure that sustained release form is not chewed or crushed. **Must be** swallowed whole.

ADVERSE EFFECTS **CV:** Arrhythmias, palpitation, *tachycardia*. **Respiratory:** Dry nose, dyspnea, nasal congestion, pharyngeal edema, wheezing, thickening of bronchial secretions. **CNS:** *Nervousness,* dizziness, headache, insomnia, ataxia, neuritis, tremor, weakness. **HEENT:** Blurred vision, diplopia, tinnitus. **GI:** Anorexia, dry mouth, nausea, vomiting. **GU:** Difficult micturition, dysuria, urinary retention.

DIAGNOSTIC TEST INTERFERENCE May interfere with urine detection of amphetamine (false-positive).

INTERACTIONS **Drug:** Other SYMPATHOMIMETICS increase pressor effects and toxicity; MAO INHIBITORS may precipitate hypertensive crisis; BETA-BLOCKERS may increase pressor effects; do not use with ERGOT DERIVATIVES; may decrease antihypertensive effects and increase arrythomgenic effects of **guanethidine, methyldopa, reserpine.**

PHARMACOKINETICS **Absorption:** Readily from GI tract. **Onset:** 30 min. **Duration:** 4–6 h (8–12 h sustained release). **Distribution:** Crosses placenta; distributed into breast milk. **Metabolism:** Partially metabolized in liver. **Elimination:** In urine.

NURSING IMPLICATIONS

Assessment & Drug Effects

- Monitor HR and BP, especially in those with a history of cardiac disease. Report tachycardia or hypertension.
- Monitor for CNS changes.

P

Patient & Family Education

- Do not take drug within 2 h of bedtime because drug may act as a stimulant.
- Discontinue medication and consult prescriber if extreme restlessness or signs of sensitivity occur.
- Consult prescriber before concomitant use of OTC medications; many contain ephedrine or other sympathomimetic amines and might intensify action of pseudoephedrine.

PSYLLIUM HYDROPHILIC MUCILLOID

(sill'i-um)

Konsyl, Metamucil, Reguloid

Classification: BULK-PRODUCING LAXATIVE

Therapeutic: BULK LAXATIVE

AVAILABILITY Powder; granules

ACTION & *THERAPEUTIC EFFECT* Bulk-producing laxative that absorbs liquid in the GI tract, facilitating peristalsis and bowel motility. *Bulk-producing laxative that promotes peristalsis and natural elimination.*

USES Chronic atonic or spastic constipation and constipation associated with rectal disorders or anorectal surgery.

CONTRAINDICATIONS Esophageal and intestinal obstruction, dysphagia; nausea, vomiting, fecal impaction, acute abdomen; undiagnosed abdominal pain, appendicitis.

CAUTIOUS USE Diabetics; pregnancy (category C); children younger than 6 y.

ROUTE & DOSAGE

Constipation or Diarrhea

Adult: **PO** 2.5 to 30 g per day in divided doses

Child (6–12 y): **PO** 1.25 to 15 g/day in 1 to 3 divided doses

ADMINISTRATION

Oral

- Fill an 8-oz (240-mL) water glass with cool water, milk, fruit juice, or other liquid; sprinkle powder into liquid; stir briskly; and give immediately (if effervescent form is used, add liquid to powder). Granules should not be chewed.
- Follow each dose with an additional glass of liquid to obtain best results.
- Exercise caution with older adult patient who may aspirate the drug.

ADVERSE EFFECTS **GI:** Nausea and vomiting, diarrhea (with excessive use); GI tract strictures when drug used in dry form, abdominal cramps. **Hematologic:** Eosinophilia.

INTERACTIONS **Drug:** Psyllium may decrease absorption and clinical effects of ANTIBIOTICS, **warfarin, digoxin, nitrofurantoin,** SALICYLATES.

PHARMACOKINETICS **Absorption:** Not absorbed from GI tract. **Onset:** 12–24 h. **Peak:** 1–3 days.

NURSING IMPLICATIONS

Assessment & Drug Effects

- Report promptly to prescriber if patient complains of retrosternal pain after taking the drug. Drug may be lodged as a gelatinous mass (because of poor mixing) in the esophagus.

- Monitor therapeutic effectiveness. When psyllium is used as either a bulk laxative or to treat diarrhea, the expected effect is formed stools. Laxative effect usually occurs within 12–24 h. Administration for 2 or 3 days may be needed to establish regularity.
- Assess for complaints of abdominal fullness. Smaller, more frequent doses spaced throughout the day may be indicated to relieve discomfort of abdominal fullness.
- Monitor lab tests: Frequent warfarin and digoxin levels if either is given concurrently.

Patient & Family Education

- Note sugar and sodium content of preparation if on low-sodium or low-calorie diet. Some preparations contain natural sugars, whereas others contain artificial sweeteners.
- Understand that drug works to relieve both diarrhea and constipation by restoring a more normal moisture level to stool.
- Be aware that drug may reduce appetite if it is taken before meals.

PYRANTEL PAMOATE

(pi-ran'tel)

Pin-X

Classification: ANTHELMINTIC

Therapeutic: ANTHELMINTIC

Prototype: Praziquantel

AVAILABILITY Capsule; oral suspension

ACTION & *THERAPEUTIC EFFECT* Exerts selective depolarizing neuromuscular blocking action that results in spastic paralysis of worm. *Causes evacuation of worms from intestines.*

USES *Enterobius vermicularis* (pinworm) and *Ascaris lumbricoides* (roundworm) infestations.

UNLABELED USES Hookworm infestations; trichostrongylosis.

CONTRAINDICATIONS Hypersensitivity to pyrantel.

CAUTIOUS USE Liver dysfunction; malnutrition; dehydration; anemia; pregnancy (category C).

ROUTE & DOSAGE

Pinworm or Roundworm

Adult/Child: **PO** 11 mg/kg as a single dose (max: 1 g)

ADMINISTRATION

Oral

- Shake suspension well before pouring it to ensure accurate dosage.
- Give with milk or fruit juices and without regard to prior ingestion of food or time of day.
- Store below 30° C (86° F). Protect from light.

ADVERSE EFFECTS **CNS:** Dizziness, headache, drowsiness, insomnia. **Skin:** Skin rashes. **GI:** Anorexia, *nausea,* vomiting, abdominal distention, diarrhea, *tenesmus,* transient elevation of AST.

INTERACTIONS **Drug:** **Piperazine** and pyrantel may be mutually antagonistic.

PHARMACOKINETICS **Absorption:** Poorly from GI tract. **Peak:** 1–3 h. **Metabolism:** In liver. **Elimination:** Greater than 50% in feces, 7% in urine.

NURSING IMPLICATIONS

Assessment & Drug Effects

- Monitor stool for presence of eggs, worms, and occult blood.

Patient & Family Education

- Do not drive or engage in other potentially hazardous activities until response to drug is known.

CAUTIOUS USE History of gout or diabetes mellitus; impaired kidney function; alcoholism; history of peptic ulcer; acute intermittent porphyria; pregnancy (category C); lactation; children.

ROUTE & DOSAGE

Tuberculosis

Adult/Child: **PO** 15–30 mg/kg/day (max: 3 g/day)

Renal Impairment Dosage Adjustment

CrCl 10–50 mL/min: Extend interval to q48–72 hours; *CrCl less than 10 mL/min:* Extend interval to q72h

P

ADMINISTRATION

Oral

- Discontinue drug if hepatic reactions (jaundice, pruritus, icteric sclerae, yellow skin) or hyperuricemia with acute gout (severe pain in great toe and other joints) occurs.
- Store at 15°–30° C (59°–86° F) in tightly closed container.

ADVERSE EFFECTS **CNS:** Headache. **Endocrine:** *Rise in serum uric acid.* **Skin:** Urticaria. **GI:** Splenomegaly, fatal hemoptysis, aggravation of peptic ulcer, *hepatotoxicity, abnormal liver function tests.* **GU:** Difficulty in urination. **Hematologic:** Hemolytic anemia, decreased plasma prothrombin. **Other:** *Active gout,* arthralgia, lymphadenopathy.

DIAGNOSTIC TEST INTERFERENCE Pyrazinamide may produce a temporary decrease in ***17-ketosteroids*** and an increase in ***protein-bound iodine.***

INTERACTIONS **Drug:** Increase in liver toxicity (including fatal hepatoxicity in when treating latent TB) with **rifampin.**

PHARMACOKINETICS **Absorption:** Readily from GI tract. **Peak:** 2 h. **Distribution:** Crosses blood–brain barrier. **Metabolism:** In liver. **Elimination:** Slowly in urine. **Half-Life:** 9–10 h.

NURSING IMPLICATIONS

Assessment & Drug Effects

- Observe and supervise closely. Patients should receive at least one other effective antituberculosis agent concurrently.
- Examine patients at regular intervals and question about possible signs of toxicity: Liver enlargement or tenderness, jaundice, fever, anorexia, malaise, impaired vascular integrity (ecchymoses, petechiae, abnormal bleeding).
- Hepatic reactions appear to occur more frequently in patients receiving high doses.
- Monitor lab tests: Baseline and periodic LFTs and uric acid level.

Patient & Family Education

- Report to prescriber onset of difficulty in voiding. Keep fluid intake at 2000 mL/day if possible.
- Monitor blood glucose (diabetics) for possible loss of glycemic control.

PYRETHRINS

(peer′e-thrins)

A-200 Pyrinate, Barc, Blue, Pyrinate, Pyrinyl, R&C, RID, TISIT, Triple X

Classification: ANTIPARASITIC; PEDICULICIDE

Therapeutic: SCABICIDE

Prototype: Permethrin

AVAILABILITY Liquid; gel; shampoo

ACTION & *THERAPEUTIC EFFECT* Acts as a contact poison affecting the parasite's nervous system, causing paralysis and death. *Controls head lice, pubic (crab) lice, and body lice and their eggs (nits).*

USES External treatment of *Pediculus humanus* infestations.

CONTRAINDICATIONS Sensitivity to solution components; skin infections and abrasions.

CAUTIOUS USE Ragweed-sensitized patient; asthma; pregnancy (category C); lactation; infants; children.

ROUTE & DOSAGE

***Pediculus humanus* Infestations**

Adult: **Topical** See ADMINISTRATION for appropriate application

ADMINISTRATION

Topical

- Apply enough solution to completely wet infested area, including hair. Allow to remain on area for 10 min.
- Wash and rinse with large amounts of warm water.
- Use fine-toothed comb to remove lice and eggs from hair.
- Shampoo hair to restore body and luster.
- Repeat treatment once in 24 h if necessary.
- Repeat treatment in 7–10 days to kill newly hatched lice.
- Do not apply to eyebrows or eyelashes without consulting prescriber.
- Flush eyes with copious amounts of warm water if accidental contact occurs.

ADVERSE EFFECTS Other: Irritation with repeated use.

NURSING IMPLICATIONS

Patient & Family Education

- Do not swallow, inhale, or allow pyrethrins to contact mucosal surfaces or the eyes.
- Discontinue use and consult prescriber if treated area becomes irritated.
- Examine each family member carefully; if infested, treat immediately to prevent spread or reinfestation of previously treated patient.
- Dry clean, boil, or otherwise treat contaminated clothing. Sterilize (soak in pyrethrins) combs and brushes used by patient.
- Do not share combs, brushes, or other headgear with another person.

P

PYRIDOSTIGMINE BROMIDE

(peer-id-oh-stig′meen)

Mestinon, Regonol

Classification: CHOLINERGIC MUSCLE STIMULANT; ANTICHOLINESTERASE

Therapeutic: CHOLINESTERASE INHIBITOR; MUSCLE STIMULANT

Prototype: Neostigmine

AVAILABILITY Syrup; tablet; extended release tablet; solution for injection

ACTION & *THERAPEUTIC EFFECT*

Indirect-acting cholinergic agent that inhibits cholinesterase activity. Facilitates transmission of impulses across myoneural junctions by blocking destruction of acetylcholine. *Has direct stimulant action on voluntary muscle fibers and possibly on autonomic ganglia and CNS neurons. Produces increased tone in skeletal muscles.*

USES Myasthenia gravis and as an antagonist to nondepolarizing skeletal muscle relaxants (e.g., curariform drugs).

CONTRAINDICATIONS Hypersensitivity to anticholinesterase agents; mechanical obstruction of urinary or intestinal tract; hypotension; lactation.

CAUTIOUS USE Hypersensitivity to bromides; bronchial asthma; epilepsy; recent cardiac occlusion; renal impairment; vagotonia; hyperthyroidism; peptic ulcer; cardiac dysrhythmias; bradycardia; pregnancy (category C).

P

ROUTE & DOSAGE

Myasthenia Gravis

Adult: **PO** 60 mg–1.5 g/day spaced according to response of individual patient; **Sustained release** 180–540 mg 1–2 × day at intervals of at least 6 h; **IM/IV** Approximately $^1/_{30}$ of PO dose
Child: **PO** 7 mg/kg/day divided into 5–6 doses
Neonates: **PO** 5 mg q4–6h; **IM/IV** 0.05–0.15 mg/kg q4–6h

Reversal of Muscle Relaxants

Adult: **IV** 10–20 mg immediately preceded by IV atropine

ADMINISTRATION

Oral

- Give with food or fluid.
- Ensure that sustained release form is not chewed or crushed. **Must be** swallowed whole.
- Note: A syrup is available. Some patients may not like it because it is sweet; try to make it more palatable by giving it over ice chips. The syrup formulation contains 5% alcohol.

Intramuscular

- Note: Parenteral dose is about $^1/_{30}$ the oral adult dose.
- Give deep IM into a large muscle.

Intravenous

PREPARE: **Direct:** Give undiluted. **Do not** add to IV solutions.
ADMINISTER: **Direct:** Give at a rate of 0.5 mg over 1 min for myasthenia gravis; 5 mg over 1 min for reversal of muscle relaxants.

- Store at 15°–30° C (59°–86° F). Protect from light and moisture.

ADVERSE EFFECTS **CV:** Bradycardia, hypotension. **Respiratory:** Increased bronchial secretion, bronchoconstriction. **HEENT:** *Miosis.* **Skin:** Acneiform rash. **GI:** *Nausea, vomiting, diarrhea.* **Hematologic:** Thrombophlebitis (following IV administration). **Other:** *Excessive salivation and sweating,* weakness, fasciculation.

INTERACTIONS **Drug: Atropine** NONDEPOLARIZING MUSCLE RELAXANTS antagonize effects of pyridostigmine.

PHARMACOKINETICS **Absorption:** Poorly from GI tract. **Onset:** 30–45 min PO; 15 min IM; 2–5 min IV. **Duration:** 3–6 h. **Distribution:** Crosses placenta.

Metabolism: In liver and in serum and tissue by cholinesterases. **Elimination:** In urine.

NURSING IMPLICATIONS

Assessment & Drug Effects

- Report increasing muscular weakness, cramps, or fasciculations. Failure of patient to show improvement may reflect either underdosage or overdosage.
- Observe patient closely if atropine is used to abolish GI adverse effects or other muscarinic adverse effects because it may mask signs of overdosage (cholinergic crisis): Increasing muscle weakness, which through involvement of respiratory muscles can lead to death.
- Monitor vital signs frequently, especially respiratory rate.
- Observe for signs of cholinergic reactions (see Appendix F), particularly when drug is administered IV.
- Observe neonates of myasthenic mothers, who have received pyridostigmine, closely for difficulty in breathing, swallowing, or sucking.
- Observe patient continuously when used as muscle relaxant antagonist. Airway and respiratory assistance **must be** maintained until full recovery of voluntary respiration and neuromuscular transmission is assured. Complete recovery usually occurs within 30 min.

Patient & Family Education

- Be aware that duration of drug action may vary with physical and emotional stress, as well as with severity of disease.
- Report onset of rash to prescriber. Drug may be discontinued.
- Sustained release tablets may become mottled in appearance; this does not affect their potency.

PYRIDOXINE HYDROCHLORIDE (VITAMIN B_6)

(peer-i-dox'een)

Classification: VITAMIN
Therapeutic: VITAMIN B_6 REPLACEMENT

AVAILABILITY

Tablet; solution for injection

ACTION & *THERAPEUTIC EFFECT*

Water-soluble complex of three closely related compounds with B_6 activity. Converted in body to pyridoxal, a coenzyme that functions in protein, fat, and carbohydrate metabolism and in facilitating release of glycogen from liver and muscle. In protein metabolism, participates in enzymatic transformations of amino acids and conversion of tryptophan to niacin and serotonin. Aids in energy transformation in brain and nerve cells, and is thought to stimulate heme production. *Effectiveness is evaluated by improvement of B_6 deficiency manifestations: Nausea, vomiting, skin lesions resembling those of riboflavin and niacin deficiency, edema, CNS symptoms, hypochromic microcytic anemia.*

USES

Prophylaxis and treatment of pyridoxine deficiency, as seen with inadequate dietary intake, drug-induced deficiency (e.g., isoniazid, oral contraceptives), and inborn errors of metabolism (vitamin B_6–dependent convulsions or anemia).

UNLABELED USES

To treat acute toxicity caused by overdosage of cycloserine, hydralazine, isoniazid (INH); alcoholic polyneuritis. Has been used for management of many other conditions ranging from nausea and vomiting in radiation sickness and pregnancy.

P

CONTRAINDICATIONS IV: Cardiac disease.

CAUTIOUS USE Renal impairment; neonatal prematurity with renal impairment; cardiac disease; pregnancy (maternal pyridoxine plasma concentrations may decrease as pregnancy progresses and requirements may be increased in pregnant women).

ROUTE & DOSAGE

Dietary Deficiency

Adult: **IM/IV/PO** 10–20 mg/day × 3 wk followed by oral therapy
Child: **PO** 5–25 mg/day × 3 wk, then 2.5–5 mg/day in multivitamin

Pyridoxine Deficiency Syndrome

Adult: **PO/IM/IV** Initial dose up to 600 mg/day may be required; then up to 50 mg/day

Isoniazid-Induced Deficiency

Adult: **PO** 25–50 mg/day

P

ADMINISTRATION

Oral

- Ensure that sustained release and enteric forms are not chewed or crushed. **Must be** swallowed whole.

Intramuscular

- Give deep IM into a large muscle.

Intravenous

PREPARE: **Direct:** Give undiluted. **Continuous:** May be added to most standard IV solutions.
ADMINISTER: **Direct:** Give at a rate of 0.5 to 1 gram/minute.
INCOMPATIBILITIES: **Y-site: Amphotericin B, azathioprine, cefazolin, cefoperazone, ceftizoxime, chloramphenicol, dantrolene, diazepam, folic acid, furosemide, ganciclovir, hydrocortisone, imipenem, indomethacin, ketorolac, methylprednisolone, oxacillin, pentobarbital, phenobarbital. phenytoin, sulfamethoxazole/ trimethoprim.**

- Store at 20°–25° C (68°–77° F) in tight, light-resistant containers. Avoid freezing.

ADVERSE EFFECTS CNS: Seizures (particularly following large parenteral doses), ataxia, drowsiness, headache, neuropathy, paresthesia. **Endocrine:** Folate deficiency, acidosis. **GI/Hepatic:** Nausea, increased serum AST. **Other:** Hypersensitivity reaction.

INTERACTIONS Drug: Isoniazid and ORAL CONTRACEPTIVES may increase pyridoxine requirements; may reverse or antagonize therapeutic effects of **levodopa.**

PHARMACOKINETICS Absorption: Readily from GI tract. **Distribution:** Stored in liver; crosses placenta. **Metabolism:** In liver. **Elimination:** In urine.

NURSING IMPLICATIONS

Assessment & Drug Effects

- Monitor neurologic status to determine therapeutic effect in deficiency states.
- Record a complete dietary history so poor eating habits can be identified and corrected (a single vitamin deficiency is rare; patient can be expected to have multiple vitamin deficiencies).

Patient & Family Education

- Learn rich dietary sources of vitamin B_6: Yeast, wheat germ, whole grain cereals, muscle and glandular meats (especially liver), legumes, green vegetables, bananas.

- Do not self-medicate with vitamin combinations (OTC) without first consulting prescriber.

PYRIMETHAMINE

(peer-i-meth'a-meen)

Daraprim

Classification: FOLIC ACID ANTAGONIST

Therapeutic: ANTIMALARIAL

Prototype: Chloroquine

AVAILABILITY Tablet

ACTION & *THERAPEUTIC EFFECT* Selectively inhibits action of dehydrofolic reductase in parasites with resulting blockade of folic acid metabolism. *Prevents development of fertilized gametes in the mosquito and thus helps to prevent transmission of malaria.*

USES Treatment of toxoplasmosis (with a sulfonamide).

UNLABELED USES Cystoisosporiasis, pneumocystis pneumonia in patients with HIV.

CONTRAINDICATIONS Chloroguanide-resistant malaria; hypersensitivity to pyrimethamine or any component of the formulation; megaloblastic anemia caused by folate deficiency; lactation.

CAUTIOUS USE Convulsive disorders; asthma; bone marrow suppression; folate deficiency; hepatic disease; renal disease; seizure disorder; pregnancy (use with caution in patients with possible folate deficiency, including pregnant women); children.

ROUTE & DOSAGE

Toxoplasmosis

Adult: **PO** 50–75 mg/day for 1–3 wk, then decrease dose by half and continue for 4–5 weeks
Child: varies based on age, weight, concurrent medications and concurrent disease states, see package insert.

ADMINISTRATION

Oral

- Minimize GI distress by giving with meals.
- Give on same day each week for malaria prophylaxis. Begin when individual enters malarious area and continue for 10 wk after leaving the area.

ADVERSE EFFECTS **Cardiovascular:** Cardiac arrhythmia. **Respiratory:** Eosinophilic pneumonitis. **Skin:** Skin rashes, erythema multiforme, Stevens-Johnson Syndrome, toxic epidermal necrolysis. **GI:** Anorexia, vomiting, atrophic glossitis. **Hematologic:** *Folic acid deficiency (megaloblastic anemia, leukopenia, thrombocytopenia, pancytopenia).*

INTERACTIONS **Drug: Folic acid** may decrease effectiveness against toxoplasmosis. Do not use with **artemether, dapsone, lumefantrine** due to increased risk of adverse effects.

PHARMACOKINETICS **Absorption:** Readily from GI tract. **Peak:** 2 h. **Distribution:** Concentrates in kidneys, lungs, liver, and spleen; distributed into breast milk. **Elimination:** Slowly in urine. **Half-Life:** 80–95 h.

NURSING IMPLICATIONS

Assessment & Drug Effects

- Monitor patient response closely. Dosages required for treatment of toxoplasmosis approach toxic levels.
- Withhold drug and notify prescriber if hematologic abnormalities appear.
- Monitor lab tests: Twice weekly CBC, including platelets; LFTs and renal function tests.

Patient & Family Education

- Be aware that folic acid deficiency may occur with long-term use of pyrimethamine. Report to prescriber weakness, and pallor (from anemia), ulcerations of oral mucosa, superinfections, glossitis; GI disturbances such as diarrhea and poor fat absorption, fever. Folate (folinic acid) replacement may be prescribed. Increase food sources of folates (if allowed) in diet.

QUAZEPAM

(qua'ze-pam)

Doral

Classification: SEDATIVE-HYPNOTIC, NONBARBITUATE; BENZODIAZEPINE

Therapeutic: SEDATIVE

Prototype: Triazolam

Controlled Substance: Schedule IV

AVAILABILITY Tablet

ACTION & *THERAPEUTIC EFFECT* Believed to potentiate gamma-aminobutyric acid (GABA) neuronal inhibition in the limbic, neocortical, and mesencephalic reticular systems. *Significantly decreases total wake time and significantly increases sleep time. REM sleep is essentially unchanged.*

USES Insomnia characterized by difficulty in falling asleep, frequent nocturnal awakenings, or early morning awakenings.

CONTRAINDICATIONS Hypersensitivity to quazepam or benzodiazepines; sleep apnea; respiratory insufficiency; suicidal ideation; pregnancy (teratogenic effects have been observed with some benzodiazepines; hypoglycemia and respiratory problems in the neonate may occur); lactation.

CAUTIOUS USE Impaired liver and kidney function; history of seizures; depression; older adults; debilitated clients. Safety and efficacy in children younger than 18 y not established.

ROUTE & DOSAGE

Insomnia

Adult: **PO** 7.5 mg at bedtime; may increase to 15 mg if needed (intended for short-term use)

ADMINISTRATION

Oral

- Use lowest effective dose in older adults as soon as possible.
- Store at 20°–25° C (68°–77° F).

ADVERSE EFFECTS CNS: *Daytime sedation, headache*, fatigue, dizziness. **GI:** Dyspepsia, xerostomia. **Other:** Physiological or psychological dependence.

INTERACTIONS Drug: Alcohol, CNS DEPRESSANTS, ANTICONVULSANTS potentiate CNS depression; **cimetidine** increases quazepam plasma levels, increasing its toxicity; may decrease antiparkinsonism effects of **levodopa;** may increase **phenytoin** levels; **smoking** decreases sedative effects of quazepam. **Sodium oxybate** is contraindicated with quazepam. **Herbal: Kava, kratom, valerian** may potentiate sedation.

PHARMACOKINETICS **Absorption:** Readily from GI tract. **Onset:** 30 min. **Peak:** 2 h. **Distribution:** Crosses placenta; distributed into breast milk; highly protein bound. **Metabolism:** In liver to active metabolites. **Elimination:** In urine and feces. **Half-Life:** 73 h.

NURSING IMPLICATIONS

Black Box Warning

Concomitant use of benzodiazepines and opioids may result in profound sedation, respiratory depression, coma, and death. Reserve concomitant prescribing of these drugs for use in patients for whom alternative treatment options are inadequate. Limit dosages and durations to the minimum required. Follow patients for signs and symptoms of respiratory depression and sedation.

Assessment & Drug Effects

- Monitor for respiratory depression in patients with chronic respiratory insufficiency.
- Monitor for suicidal tendencies in previously depressed clients.
- Daytime drowsiness is more likely to occur in older adult clients.
- For inpatient use, institute safety measures to prevent falls.
- Monitor lab values: Baseline liver function.

Patient & Family Education

- Inform prescriber about any alcohol consumption and prescription or nonprescription medication that you take. Avoid alcohol use since it potentiates CNS depressant effects.
- Inform prescriber immediately if you become pregnant. This drug causes birth defects.
- Do not drive or engage in potentially hazardous activities until response to drug is known.
- Do not increase the dose of this drug; inform prescriber if the drug no longer works.
- This drug may cause daytime sedation, even for several days after drug is discontinued.

QUETIAPINE FUMARATE

(ke-ti-a′peen)

Seroquel, Seroquel XR

Classification: ATYPICAL ANTIPSYCHOTIC

Therapeutic: ANTIPSYCHOTIC

Prototype: Clozapine

AVAILABILITY Tablet; extended release tablet

ACTION & *THERAPEUTIC EFFECT* Antagonizes multiple neurotransmitter receptors in the brain including serotonin (5-HT_{1A} and 5-HT_2) as well as dopamine D_1 and D_2 receptors. *Effectiveness indicated by a reduction in psychotic behavior.*

USES Management of schizophrenia, maintenance of acute bipolar disorder, and add-on therapy for major depressive disorder.

UNLABELED USES Management of agitation with dementia; generalized anxiety disorder; PTSD, psychosis in Parkinson disease.

CONTRAINDICATIONS Hypersensitivity to quetiapine; alcohol use; suicidal ideation; dementia-related psychosis in older adults; NMS; lactation.

CAUTIOUS USE Liver function impairment; history of seizures or suicidal thoughts; or hepatic impairment; cardiovascular disease (history of MI or ischemic heart disease, heart failure, arrhythmias, congenital QT prolongation; CVA, hypotension, dehydration, treatment with antihypertensives); MDD; risk factors for diabetes; DM; abnormal lipid profile; breast cancer; Alzheimer disease, Parkinson disease; patient at risk for aspiration pneumonia; debilitated patients; BPH; decreased GI motility; cerebrovascular disease; hypothyroidism; older adults; pregnancy (antipsychotic use during the third trimester of pregnancy has a risk for abnormal muscle movements and/or withdrawal symptoms in newborns following delivery). Safe use in children younger than 10 y not established.

ROUTE & DOSAGE

Bipolar Disorder/Bipolar Depression

Adult/Adolescent: **PO Immediate release** 100–200 mg daily at bedtime on day 1; then increase by 100 mg/day in divided doses as tolerated to 400 mg/day on day 4 (max dose: 800 mg/day) or **Extended release** 300 mg daily at bedtime, increase to 600 mg on day 2 (max dose: 800 mg/day)
Child (older than 10 y): **PO Immediate release** 25 mg bid on day 1, 50 mg bid on day 2, 100 mg bid on day 3, 150 mg bid on day 4, and 200 mg bid beginning day 5, may increase as needed (max 600 mg/day) **Extended release** 50 mg daily on day 1, 100 mg daily on day 3, increase by 100 mg/day each day until target dose of 400 mg daily is reached.

Schizophrenia

Adult: **PO Immediate release** Start 25 mg bid, may increase by 25–50 mg bid to tid on the second or third day as tolerated to a target dose of 300–400 mg/day divided bid to tid, may adjust dose by 25–50 mg bid daily as needed (max: 800 mg/day); **Extended release** 300 mg daily at bedtime, titrate up to 400–800 mg daily (max: 800 mg/day)
Adolescent: **PO Immediate release** 25 mg bid then taper up by 50 mg each day to 200 mg bid **Extended release** 50 mg daily, then 100 mg daily on day 2 then increase in 100 mg/day increments to target dose of 400 mg daily.

Major Depressive Disorder (Adjunct)

Adult: **PO Extended release** 50 mg once daily × day 1 and day 2, then increase to 150 mg daily

Hepatic Impairment Dosage Adjustment

PO Immediate release Start with 25 mg dose and increase by 25–50 mg/day; **Extended release** Start with 50 mg on day 1, then increase by 50 mg/day to the lowest effective and tolerable dose

ADMINISTRATION

Oral

- Dose is usually retitrated over a period of several days when patient has been off the drug for longer than 1 wk.
- Follow recommended lower doses and slower titration for the older adults, the debilitated, and those with hepatic impairment or a predisposition to hypotension.
- May be administered with or without food. Swallow extended release tablets whole.
- Store at 25° C (77° F).

ADVERSE EFFECTS CV: *Increased diastolic Bp, increased systolic Bp, orthostatic hypotension, tachycardia.* **Respiratory:** Nasal congestion. **CNS:** *Dizziness, headache, somnolence*, agitation, extrapyramidal reaction, fatigue, withdrawal syndrome, irritability. **Endocrine:** Decreased HDL cholesterol, increased serum cholesterol, increased serum triglycerides, increased LDL cholesterol, weight gain. **Hepatic/GI:** *Dry mouth*, dyspepsia, nausea, constipation, *increased appetite*, increased liver enzymes. **Hematologic:** Leukopenia, decreased hemoglobin. **Other:** Increased risk of suicidal thinking.

DIAGNOSTIC TEST INTERFERENCE: May cause false positive TCA (serum) or methadone (urine) screen.

INTERACTIONS Drug: CYP3A4 inducers **carbamazepine, phenytoin, rifampin, thioridazine** may increase clearance of quetiapine. Quetiapine may potentiate the cognitive and motor effects of **alcohol,** enhance the effects of ANTIHYPERTENSIVE AGENTS. May decrease the effect of ANTIPARKINSON AGENTS. CYP3A4 inhibitors, **ketoconazole, itraconazole, fluconazole, erythromycin** may increase serum concentration of quetiapine and increase risk of adverse effects. There is potential for additive adverse effects with CNS DEPRESSANTS, OPIOIDS. Drugs that increase the QT interval (e.g., **amiodarone, clarithromycin,** ANTIARRHYTHMICS, **haloperidol, ziprasodone**) increase risk of cardiac effects. Other ANTIPSYCHOTICS increase the risk of adverse effects; increased risk of adverse effects with ANTICHOLINERGICS Do not use with **metoclopramide. Herbal: St. John's wort** may cause **serotonin** syndrome (see Appendix F).

PHARMACOKINETICS Absorption: Rapidly and completely absorbed from GI tract. **Peak:** 1.5 h. **Distribution:** 83% protein bound. **Metabolism:** In liver (CYP3A4). **Elimination:** 73% in urine, 20% in feces. **Half-Life:** 6 h.

NURSING IMPLICATIONS

Black Box Warning

Quetiapine has been associated with increased mortality in older adults with dementia-related psychosis, and with increased risk of suicidical thoughts and behavior in children, adolescents, and young adults.

Assessment & Drug Effects

- Monitor diabetics for loss of glycemic control.
- Monitor for changes in behavior that may indicate suicidality.
- Reassess need for continued treatment periodically.
- Withhold the drug and immediately report S&S of tardive dyskinesia or neuroleptic malignant syndrome (see Appendix F).

- Monitor Bp and ECG periodically, especially in those with known cardiovascular disease.
- Baseline cataract exam is recommended when therapy is started and at 6 mo intervals thereafter.
- Monitor patients with a history of seizures for lowering of the seizure threshold.
- Monitor lab tests: Periodic LFTs, lipid profile, thyroid function, HbA1C, CBC with differential.

Patient & Family Education

- Carefully monitor blood glucose levels if diabetic.
- Exercise caution with potentially dangerous activities requiring alertness, especially during the first week of drug therapy or during dose increments.
- Make position changes slowly, especially when changing from lying or sitting to standing to avoid dizziness, palpitations, and fainting.
- Avoid alcohol consumption and activities that may cause overheating and dehydration.

QUINAPRIL HYDROCHLORIDE

(quin′a-pril)

Accupril

Classification: ANGIOTENSIN-CONVERTING ENZYME (ACE) INHIBITOR; ANTIHYPERTENSIVE

Therapeutic: ANTIHYPERTENSIVE

Prototype: Enalapril

AVAILABILITY Tablet

ACTION & *THERAPEUTIC EFFECT* Potent, long-acting ACE inhibitor that lowers BP by interrupting the conversion sequences initiated by renin to form angiotensin II, a vasoconstrictor. Also decreases circulating aldosterone. Reduces PCWP, systemic vascular resistance, and mean arterial pressure, with concurrent increases in cardiac output, cardiac index, and stroke volume. *Lowers BP by producing vasodilation. Effective in the treatment of CHF since it improves cardiac indicators.*

USES Management of hypertension, heart failure.

UNLABELED USES: Non-ST elevation acute coronary syndrome, stable coronary artery disease, ST-elevation acute coronary syndrome.

CONTRAINDICATIONS Hypersensitivity to quinapril or other ACE inhibitors (angioedema specifically); cholestatic jaundice; concomitant use with aliskiren in diabetic patients; concomitant use with neprilysin inhibitor; pregnancy (exposure to an ACE inhibitor during the first trimester of pregnancy may be associated with an increased risk of fetal malformation).

CAUTIOUS USE History of angioedema; renal insufficiency; autoimmune disease, volume-depleted patients, aortic stenosis, hypertrophic cardiomyopathy; HF; renal artery stenosis, neutropenia; older adults; lactation. Safety and efficacy in children not established.

ROUTE & DOSAGE

Hypertension

Adult: **PO** 10–20 mg daily, may increase up to 80 mg/day in 1–2 divided doses
Geriatric: **PO** Start with 10 mg daily

Heart Failure

Adult: **PO** 5 mg bid may increase to 10–20 mg bid

 Common adverse effects in *italic;* life-threatening effects underlined; generic names in **bold;** classifications in SMALL CAPS; ♣ Canadian drug name; ⊙ Prototype drug; ⚠ Alert

Renal Impairment Dosage Adjustment

CrCl 30–60 mL/min: Start at 5 mg daily initially; *less than 10–30 mL/min:* 2.5 mg/day initially

ADMINISTRATION

Oral

- May be administered without regard to food.
- Store at 15°–30° C (59°–86° F) and protect from moisture.

ADVERSE EFFECTS **CV:** Hypotension, chest pain. **Respiratory:** *Cough*. **CNS:** *Dizziness*, fatigue, headache. **Endocrine:** *Hyperkalemia*. **GI:** Nausea, vomiting, diarrhea, intestinal angioedema. **Other:** Angioedema.

DIAGNOSTIC TEST INTERFERENCE May lead to false negative aldosterone/renin ratio.

INTERACTIONS **Drug:** POTASSIUM-SPARING DIURETICS, **aliskiren** may increase risk of hyperkalemia. May elevate serum **lithium** levels, resulting in **lithium** toxicity. May increase risk of hypotension with ANTIHYPERTENSIVES.

PHARMACOKINETICS **Absorption:** Rapidly from GI tract. **Onset:** 1 h. **Peak:** 2–4 h. **Duration:** Up to 24 h. **Distribution:** 97% bound to plasma proteins; crosses placenta; distributes into breast milk. **Metabolism:** Extensively metabolized in liver to its active metabolite, quinaprilat. **Elimination:** 50–60% in urine, primarily as quinaprilat; 30% in feces. **Half-Life:** 2 h.

NURSING IMPLICATIONS

Black Box Warning

Quinapril has been associated with fetal toxicity and death.

Assessment & Drug Effects

- Following initial dose, monitor for several hours for first-dose hypotension, especially in salt- or volume-depleted patients (e.g., those pretreated with a diuretic).
- Monitor BP at time of peak effectiveness, 2–4 h after dosing, and at end of dosing interval just before next dose.
- Report diminished antihypertensive effect toward end of dosing interval. Inadequate trough response may indicate need to divide daily dose.
- Observe for S&S of hyperkalemia (see Appendix F).
- Monitor lab tests: Baseline and periodic BUN, serum creatinine, and potassium; periodic CBC with differential.

Patient & Family Education

- Discontinue quinapril and report S&S of angioedema (e.g., swelling of face or extremities, difficulty breathing or swallowing) to prescriber.
- Notify prescriber immediately if you become or suspect you are pregnant.
- Maintain adequate fluid intake and avoid potassium supplements or salt substitutes unless specifically prescribed by prescriber.
- Light-headedness and dizziness may occur, especially during the initial days of therapy. If fainting occurs, stop taking quinapril until the prescriber has been consulted.

QUINIDINE SULFATE

(kwin′i-deen sul-fate)

Classification: CLASS IA ANTIARRHYTHMIC

Therapeutic: CLASS IA ANTIARRHYTHMIC

Prototype: Procainamide

AVAILABILITY Tablet.

ACTION & *THERAPEUTIC EFFECT* Depresses myocardial excitability, contractility, automaticity, and conduction velocity as well as prolongs refractory period. *Depresses myocardial excitability, conduction velocity, and irregularity of nerve impulse conduction.*

USES Premature atrial, AV junctional, and ventricular contraction; paroxysmal atrial tachycardia, chronic ventricular tachycardia (when not associated with complete heart block); maintenance therapy after electrical conversion of atrial fibrillation or flutter; life-threatening malaria; Wolff-Parkinson-White syndrome.

CONTRAINDICATIONS Hypersensitivity to quinine or quinidine; thrombocytopenic purpura resulting from prior use of quinidine or quinine; myasthenia gravis; intraventricular conduction defects, complete AV block, AV conduction disorders; bundle branch block; marked QRS widening; thyrotoxicosis; extensive myocardial damage, frank CHF, hypotensive states; history of drug-induced torsades de pointes.

Q

CAUTIOUS USE Incomplete heart block; impaired kidney or liver function; sick sinus syndrome; bronchial asthma or other respiratory disorders; potassium imbalance; pregnancy (crosses the placenta and can be detected in the amniotic fluid and neonatal serum); lactation. Safe use for children as an antiarrhythmic agent is not known.

ROUTE & DOSAGE

Conversion to and/or Maintenance of Sinus Rhythm
Sulfate Immediate Release

Adult: **PO** 200–300 mg q6–8h until sinus rhythm restored or toxicity occurs (max: 3–4 g)

Sulfate Extended Release

Adult: **PO** 300–600 mg q8–12h

ADMINISTRATION

Oral

- Give with a full glass of water on an empty stomach for optimum absorption (i.e., 1 h before or 2 h after meals). Administer drug with food if GI symptoms occur (nausea, vomiting, diarrhea are most common). Do not administer with grapefruit juice.
- Ensure that extended release tablets are swallowed whole. They should not be crushed or chewed.
- Store in tight, light-resistant containers away from excessive heat.

ADVERSE EFFECTS **CV:** Palpitations, angina pectoris, cardiac arrhythmia. **CNS:** Headache, fatigue, dizziness. **Skin:** Skin rash. **GI:** Diarrhea, upper gastrointestinal distress. **Other:** Weakness, fever.

INTERACTIONS **Drug:** Do not use with agents metabolized by CYP2D6. May increase **digoxin** levels by 50%; **amiodarone** may increase quinidine levels, increasing its risk of heart block; other ANTIARRHYTHMICS, PHENOTHIAZINES, **reserpine** add to cardiac depressant effects; ANTICHOLINERGIC AGENTS add to vagolytic effects; CHOLINERGIC AGENTS may antagonize cardiac effects; ANTICONVULSANTS, BARBITURATES, **rifampin** increase the metabolism of quinidine, thus decreasing its efficacy; CARBONIC ANHYDRASE INHIBITORS, **sodium bicarbonate,** CHRONIC ANTACIDS decrease renal elimination of quinidine, thus increasing its toxicity; **verapamil** causes significant hypotension; may increase hypoprothrombinemic effects of **warfarin.** Coadministration of other drug that prolongs the QT interval (e.g., **disopyramide, procainamide, amiodarone, bretylium, clarithromycin, levofloxacin**) may cause additive effects. **Diltiazem** may increase levels and decrease elimination of quinidine. **Food: Grapefruit juice** (greater than 1 qt/day) may decrease absorption.

PHARMACOKINETICS Absorption: Almost completely from GI tract. **Onset:** 1–3 h. **Peak:** 0.5–1 h. **Duration:** 6–8 h. **Distribution:** Widely distributed to most body tissues except the brain; crosses placenta; distributed into breast milk. **Metabolism:** In liver (CYP3A4, P-gp). **Elimination:** Greater than 95% in urine, less than 5% in feces. **Half-Life:** 6–8 h.

NURSING IMPLICATIONS

Black Box Warning

Quinidine has been associated with increased mortality (especially in those with structural heart disease) when used to treat non-life-threatening arrhythmias.

Assessment & Drug Effects

- Observe cardiac monitor and report immediately the following indications for stopping quinidine: (1) Sinus rhythm, (2) widening QRS complex in excess of 25% (i.e., longer than 0.12 sec), (3) changes in QT interval or refractory period, (4) disappearance of P waves, (5) sudden onset of or increase in ectopic ventricular beats (extrasystoles, PVCs), (6) decrease in heart rate to 120 bpm. Also report immediately any worsening of minor side effects.
- Monitor vital signs q1–2h or more often as needed during acute treatment. Count apical pulse for a full minute. Report any change in pulse rate, rhythm, or quality or any fall in BP.
- Severe hypotension is most likely to occur in patients receiving high oral doses.
- Monitor I&O. Diarrhea occurs commonly during early therapy; most patients become tolerant to this side effect. Evaluate serum electrolytes, acid-base, and fluid balance when symptoms become severe; dosage adjustment may be required.
- Monitor lab tests: Routine CBC and liver and renal function tests.

Patient & Family Education

- Report feeling of faintness to prescriber. "Quinidine syncope" is caused by quinidine-induced changes in ventricular rhythm resulting in decreased cardiac output and syncope.
- Do not self-medicate with OTC drugs without advice from prescriber.
- Do not increase, decrease, skip, or discontinue doses without consulting prescriber.
- Notify prescriber immediately of disturbances in vision, ringing in ears, sense of breathlessness, onset of palpitations, and unpleasant sensation in chest. Be sure to note the time of occurrence and duration of chest symptoms.

QUININE SULFATE

(kwye'nine)

Qualaquin, Novoquinine ♣

Classification: ANTIMALARIAL

Therapeutic: ANTIMALARIAL

Prototype: Chloroquine

AVAILABILITY Capsule

ACTION & *THERAPEUTIC EFFECT* Decreases oxygen uptake and carbohydrate metabolism; intercalates into DNA, disrupting the parasite's replication and transcription; cardiovascular effects similar to quinidine. Effective *against* Plasmodium vivax *and* Plasmodium malariae but not Plasmodium falciparum.

USES Treatment of malaria

UNLABELED USES Babesiosis.

CONTRAINDICATIONS Hypersensitivity to quinine or quinidine especially thrombocytopenia; prolonged QT interval; tinnitus, optic neuritis; myasthenia gravis; G6PD deficiency; severe hepatic impairment (Child-Pugh class C).

Q

CAUTIOUS USE Cardiac arrhythmias; restless leg syndrome. Same precautions as for quinidine sulfate when used in patients with cardiovascular conditions; chronic renal impairment; mild or moderate hepatic impairment; pregnancy (may cause significant maternal hypoglycemia and an increased risk of other adverse maternal events); lactation.

ROUTE & DOSAGE

Malaria Treatment

Adult: **PO** 648 mg q8h for 3–7 days

Child: **PO** 10 mg/kg/day q8h for 3–7 days

Renal Impairment Dosage Adjustment

GFR 10–50 mL/min administer q8–12h; GFR less than 10 mL/min administer q24h

ADMINISTRATION

Oral

- Give with or after meals or a snack to minimize gastric irritation. Swallow dose whole to avoid bitter taste.
- Avoid use of aluminum- or magnesium-containing antacids because of drug absorption problems.
- Store in tight, light-resistant containers.

ADVERSE EFFECTS **CV:** Angina, hypotension, tachycardia, <u>cardiovascular collapse</u>, appearance of u-wave on ECG. **Respiratory:** Asthma, dyspnea, pulmonary edema. **CNS:** Confusion, excitement, apprehension, syncope, delirium, convulsions, blackwater fever (extensive intravascular hemolysis with renal failure), <u>death</u>. **Hematologic:** <u>Leukopenia</u>, <u>thrombocytopenia</u>, <u>agranulocytosis</u>, hypoprothrombinemia, hemolytic anemia. **Other:** Cinchonism (tinnitus, decreased auditory acuity, dizziness, vertigo, headache, visual impairment, *nausea, vomiting, diarrhea*, fever); hypersensitivity (cutaneous flushing, visual impairment, pruritus, skin rash, gastric distress, dyspnea, tinnitus); <u>hypothermia, coma</u>.

DIAGNOSTIC TEST INTERFERENCE Quinine may interfere with quantitative urine dipstick protein assays and ***urinary steroids*** (via ***Zimmerman*** method); may cause false positive for OPIOIDS.

INTERACTIONS Drug: May increase **digoxin** levels; ANTICHOLINERGIC AGENTS add to vagolytic effects; CHOLINERGIC AGENTS may antagonize cardiac effects; ANTICONVULSANTS, BARBITURATES, CYP3A4 INDUCERS, **rifampin** increase the metabolism of quinine, thus decreasing its efficacy; CYP3A4 INHIBITORS decrease metabolism CARBONIC ANHYDRASE INHIBITORS, **sodium bicarbonate,** ANTACIDS decrease renal elimination of quinine, thus increasing its toxicity; **warfarin** may increase hypoprothrombinemic effects; may increase adverse effects of ANTIMALARIAL agents. **Amantadine, carbamazepine, phenobarbital** levels may be increased; use with QT Prolonging agents increase risk of cardiac adverse effects; ANTIHEPACIVIRAL COMBINATION PRODUCTS may increase serum concentrations; can increase adverse effects of drugs metabolized by P-glycoprotein (ex **betrixaban**). Avoid use with **ritonavir**. **Food: Grapefruit juice** (greater than 1 qt/day) may increase plasma concentrations and adverse effects.

PHARMACOKINETICS Absorption: Well from GI tract. **Peak:** 1–3 h. **Duration:** 6–8 h. **Distribution:** Widely distributed to most body tissues except the brain; crosses placenta; distributed into breast milk. **Metabolism:** In liver. **Elimination:** Greater than 95% in urine, less than 5% in feces. **Half-Life:** 8–21 h.

NURSING IMPLICATIONS

Black Box Warning

Quinine use for treatment or prevention of nocturnal leg cramps has been associated with serious and life-threatening hematologic reactions and renal impairment.

Assessment & Drug Effects

- Be alert for S&S of rising plasma concentration of quinine marked by tinnitus and hearing impairment, which usually do not occur until concentration is 10 mcg/mL or more.
- Follow the same precautions with quinine as are used with quinidine in patients with atrial fibrillation; quinine may produce cardiotoxicity in these patients.
- Baseline and periodic ECG.
- Baseline and periodic ophthalmologic examination.
- Monitor lab values: CBC with platelet count, LFTs, blood glucose.

Patient & Family Education

- Learn possible adverse reactions and report onset of any unusual symptom promptly to prescriber.

QUINUPRISTIN/ DALFOPRISTIN

(quin-u-pris'tin/dal'fo-pris-tin)

Synercid

Classification: STREPTOGRAMIN ANTIBIOTIC; CYCLIC MACROLIDE
Therapeutic: ANTIBIOTIC

AVAILABILITY Injection, powder for reconstitution

ACTION & *THERAPEUTIC EFFECT* Inhibits bacterial protein synthesis by binding to different sites on the 50S bacterial ribosomal subunit leading to cell death. *Effectiveness indicated by clinical improvement in S&S of life-threatening bacteremia. Active against gram-positive pathogens including vancomycin-resistant* Enterococcus faecium

Q

(VREF), as well as some gram-negative anaerobes.

USES complicated skin and skin structure infections caused by *Staphylococcus aureus* or *Streptococcus pyogenes.*

UNLABELED USES MRSA bacteremia, infective endocarditis (multidrug resistant), VREF meningitis.

CONTRAINDICATIONS Hypersensitivity to quinupristin/dalfopristin, pristinamycin, other streptogramins.

CAUTIOUS USE Renal or hepatic dysfunction; IBD; GI disease; pregnancy (adverse effects have not been observed in animal reproduction studies); lactation. Safe use in children younger than 16 y not established.

ROUTE & DOSAGE

Complicated Skin and Skin Structure Infections

Adult: **IV** 7.5 mg/kg infused over 60 min q12h × 7 days

Q

ADMINISTRATION

Intravenous

PREPARE: **Intermittent:** Reconstitute a single 500 mg vial by slowly adding 5 mL D5W or sterile water for injection to yield 100 mg/mL. ▪ Gently swirl to dissolve but **do not** shake. Allow solution to clear. ▪ Withdraw the required dose and further dilute by adding to 100 mL (central line) or 250–500 mL (peripheral site) of D5W.

ADMINISTER: **Intermittent:** Flush line before and after with D5W. **Do not** use saline. ▪ Administer over 1 h.

INCOMPATIBILITIES: **Solution/additive: Saline** (flush lines with **D5W** before infusing other drugs). **Y-site: Acyclovir, amifostine, aminocaproic acid, aminophylline, amphotericin B (conventional), amphotericin B (lipid), ampicillin, atenolol, azithromycin, bivalirudin, bumetanide, calcium chloride, calcium gluconate, cangrelor, cefazolin, cefepime, cefoperazone, cefotaxime, cefotetan, cefoxitin, ceftazidime, ceftizoxime, ceftriaxone, cefuroxime, clindamycin, dexamethasone, diazepam, digoxin, ertapenem, fludarabine, fluorouracil, foscarnet, fosphenytoin, furosemide, ganciclovir, gemtuzumab, heparin, hydrocortisone, imipenem/cilastatin, insulin, ketorolac, lepirudin, leucovorin, meropenem, mesna, methotrexate, methylprednisolone, metronidazole, nitroprusside, pantoprazole, pemetrexed, pentobarbital, phenobarbital, phenytoin, piperacillin, potassium salts, rituximab, sodium acetate, sodium bicarbonate, sulfamethoxazole/trimethoprim, thiopental, ticarcillin, tigecycline.**

▪ Refrigerate unopened vials. After reconstitution solution is stable for 5 h at room temperature and 54 h refrigerated.

ADVERSE EFFECTS **Skin:** Rash. **Hepatic/GI:** Hyperbilirubinemia, nausea, vomiting. **Other:** Myalgia, arthralgia. *Inflammation, pain, or edema at infusion site, other infusion site reactions.*

INTERACTIONS Drug: Inhibits CYP3A4 metabolism of **cyclosporine, midazolam, nifedipine,** PROTEASE INHIBITORS, **vincristine, vinblastine, docetaxel, paclitaxel, diazepam, tacrolimus, carbamazepine, quinidine, lidocaine, disopyramide.**

PHARMACOKINETICS Distribution: Moderately protein bound. **Metabolism:** Metabolized to several active metabolites. **Elimination:** Primarily in feces (75–77%). **Half-Life:** 3 h quinupristin, 1 h dalfopristin.

NURSING IMPLICATIONS

Assessment & Drug Effects

- Monitor for S&S of infusion site irritation; change infusion site if irritation is apparent.
- Monitor for cutaneous reaction (e.g., pruritus/erythema of neck, face, upper body).
- Monitor lab tests: Baseline C&S; conjugated bilirubin if indicated.

Patient & Family Education

- Report burning, itching, or pain at infusion site to prescriber.
- Report any sensation of swelling of face and tongue; difficulty swallowing.

RABEPRAZOLE SODIUM

(rab-e-pra′zole)

AcipHex

Classification: GASTRIC PROTON PUMP INHIBITOR

Therapeutic: ANTIULCER

Prototype: Omeprazole

AVAILABILITY Delayed release tablet; delayed release capsule

ACTION & *THERAPEUTIC EFFECT* Suppresses gastric acid secretion by inhibiting the parietal cell H+/K+ ATP pump in the parietal cells of the stomach. Produces an antisecretory effect on the hydrogen ion (H^+) in the parietal cells. *Effectiveness indicated by a negative for* H. pylori *with preexisting gastric ulcer; also by elimination of S&S of GERD or peptic ulcers.*

USES Healing and maintenance of healing of erosive or ulcerative gastroesophageal reflux disease (GERD); healing of duodenal ulcers; treatment of hypersecretory conditions; eradication of *H. pylori*.

CONTRAINDICATIONS Hypersensitivity to rabeprazole, or proton pump inhibitors (PPIs); concomitant use with rilpivirine-containing products; lactation.

CAUTIOUS USE Severe hepatic impairment; mild to moderate hepatic disease; Japanese heritage; older adults; pregnancy (category B); children.

ROUTE & DOSAGE

Healing of Erosive GERD

Adult: **PO** 20 mg daily × 4–8 wk, may continue up to 16 wk if needed

Symptomatic Therapy for GERD

Adult/Adolescent: **PO** 20 mg daily × 4–8 w
Child (weight greater than 15 kg): 10 mg daily × 12 wk; *weight less than 15 kg:* 5 mg daily × 12 wk

Healing Duodenal Ulcer

Adult: **PO** 20 mg daily × 4 wk

Hypersecretory Disease

Adult: **PO** 60 mg daily in 1–2 divided doses (max: 100 mg daily or 60 mg bid)

ADMINISTRATION

Oral

- Ensure that the tablet is swallowed whole. It should not be crushed or chewed. Capsule should be opened and sprinkled on a small amount of soft food 30 min before a meal. Do not chew or crush. May be administered with an antacid.
- Store at 15°–30° C (59°–86° F).

ADVERSE EFFECTS **CNS:** Headache. **GI:** Diarrhea, abdominal pain, vomiting, nausea.

INTERACTIONS **Drug:** Contraindicated with **atazanavir** or **rilpivirine.** May decrease concentration of **cefuroxime, ketoconazole, delaviridine, erlotinib, gefitinib, itraconazole, neratinib, pazopanib, rilpivirine, nelfinavir, velpatasvir;** may increase **digoxin** levels. May decrease effect of **risendronate. Herbal: Ginkgo** may decrease plasma levels.

DIAGNOSTIC TEST INTERFERENCE Falsely elevate serum chromogranin A (CgA) levels. Hyperresponse in gastrin secretion in adults in response to secretin stimulation test. False positive urine screening tests for tetrahydrocannabinol (THC) have been reported.

R

PHARMACOKINETICS **Absorption:** 52% bioavailability. **Distribution:** 96% protein bound. **Metabolism:** In liver by (CYP3A4, 2C19). **Elimination:** Primarily in urine. **Half-Life:** 1–2 h.

NURSING IMPLICATIONS

Assessment & Drug Effects

- Coadministered drugs: Monitor for changes in digoxin blood level.
- Monitor lab tests: Periodic magnesium level in patients on long-term treatment or those taking drugs that cause hypomagnesemia (e.g., digoxin, diuretics).

Patient & Family Education

- Report diarrhea, skin rash, other bothersome adverse effects to prescriber.

RALOXIFENE HYDROCHLORIDE

(ra-lox′i-feen)

Evista

Classification: SELECTIVE ESTROGEN RECEPTOR ANTAGONIST/ AGONIST

Therapeutic: OSTEOPOROSIS PROPHYLACTIC

Prototype: Tamoxifen

AVAILABILITY Tablet

ACTION & *THERAPEUTIC EFFECT* Exhibits selective estrogen receptor antagonist activity on uterus and breast tissue. Prevents tissue proliferation in both sites. Decreases bone resorption and increases bone density. *Effectiveness indicated by increased bone mineral density. Reduces the risk of invasive breast cancer in high risk postmenopausal women (e.g., breast cancer in situ, or atypical hyperplasia).*

USES Prevention and treatment of osteoporosis in postmenopausal women; breast cancer prophylaxis.

CONTRAINDICATIONS Active or past history of a thromboembolic event; drug induced venous thrombosis; hypersensitivity to raloxifene; severe hepatic impairment; pregnancy (category X); lactation.

CAUTIOUS USE Concurrent use of raloxifene and estrogen hormone replacement therapy and lipid-lowering agents; hyperlipidemia;

hepatic impairment; moderate or severe renal impairment.

ROUTE & DOSAGE

Prevention/Treatment of Osteoporosis

Adult: **PO** 60 mg daily

Breast Cancer Prophylaxis

Postmenopausal Adult: **PO** 60 mg daily

ADMINISTRATION

Oral

- Calcium and vitamin D supplementation are recommended with raloxifene: 1500 mg/day of elemental calcium and 400–800 units/day of vitamin D.
- Store at 15°–30° C (59°–86° F) in a tightly closed container and protect from light.

ADVERSE EFFECTS **CV:** *Hot flashes,* chest pain, peripheral edema, decreased serum cholesterol. **Respiratory:** Sinusitis, pharyngitis, cough, pneumonia, laryngitis. **CNS:** Migraine headache, depression, insomnia. **Skin:** Rash, sweating. **GI:** Nausea, dyspepsia, vomiting, flatulence, GI disorder, gastroenteritis, weight gain. **GU:** Vaginitis, UTI, cystitis, leukorrhea, endometrial disorder, breast pain, vaginal bleeding. **Other:** Infection, flu-like syndrome, leg cramps, fever, arthralgia, myalgia, arthritis.

INTERACTIONS **Drug:** Use of ESTROGENS not recommended; absorption reduced by **cholestyramine;** use with **warfarin** may result in changes in prothrombin time (PT). **Herbal: Soy isoflavones** should be used with caution.

PHARMACOKINETICS **Absorption:** 60% absorbed, absolute bioavailability 2%. **Metabolism:** Extensive first-pass metabolism in liver. **Elimination:** Primarily in feces. **Half-Life:** 27.7–32.5 h.

NURSING IMPLICATIONS

Black Box Warning

Raloxifene has been associated with increased risk of venous thromboembolism and death from stroke.

Assessment & Drug Effects

- Monitor carefully for and immediately report S&S of thromboembolic events.
- Do not give drug concurrently with cholestyramine; however, if unavoidable, space the two drugs as widely as possible.
- Monitor lab tests: Periodic LFTs.

Patient & Family Education

- Contact prescriber immediately if unexplained calf pain or tenderness occurs.
- Avoid prolonged restriction of movement during travel.
- Drug does not prevent and may induce hot flashes.
- Do not take drug with other estrogen-containing drugs.
- Raloxifene is normally discontinued 72 h prior to prolonged immobilization (e.g., postsurgical recovery, prolonged bed rest). Consult prescriber.

R

RALTEGRAVIR

(ral-te-gra′vir)

Isentress

Classification: ANTIRETROVIRAL; INTEGRASE INHIBITOR

Therapeutic: ANTIRETROVIRAL

AVAILABILITY Tablet; chewable tablet, oral suspension

ACTION & THERAPEUTIC EFFECT

Inhibits HIV-1 integrase, an enzyme required for integration of proviral DNA into the helper T-cell genome, thus preventing formation of the HIV-1 provirus. *Inhibiting integration prevents replication and proliferation of the HIV-1 virus.*

USES In combination with other antiretroviral agents for the treatment of HIV-1 infection.

CONTRAINDICATIONS Lactation.

CAUTIOUS USE Hepatitis; mild to moderate hepatic impairment; individuals at increased risk of myopathy or rhabdomyolysis; lactase deficiency; PKU; history of psychiatric disease or suicidal ideation; older adults; pregnancy (no increased risk of overall birth defects observed following first trimester exposure to raltegravir; use with caution during pregnancy); children younger than 2 y. Safety and efficacy in patients with severe hepatic impairment not established.

ROUTE & DOSAGE

HIV-1 Infection

Adult/Adolescent (over 25 kg): **PO (treatment naïve)** 400 mg bid or 1200 mg once daily **(treatment experienced)** 400 mg bid
Child (over 11 kg): **PO** 6 mg/kg bid (max: 300 mg/dose)
Child /infant (under 20 kg): **PO** 6 mg/kg bid (max: 100 mg/dose)

ADMINISTRATION

Oral

- May be given without regard to food.
- Film-coated tablets must be swallowed whole (400 mg). Chewable tablets (25 or 100 mg) may be chewed or swallowed whole.
- Give before dialysis.
- Store at 15–30° C (59–86° F).

ADVERSE EFFECTS **CNS:** Dizziness, headache, insomnia. **Hepatic/GI:** Increased serum ALT/AST/ALP, hyperbilirubinemia, abdominal pain, *diarrhea*, nausea, vomiting. **Hematologic:** Anemia, neutropenia.

INTERACTIONS **Drug: Aluminum**, **calcium carbonate, fosamprenavir, magnesium, rifampin** and **tipranavir/ritonavir** may decrease plasma levels of raltegravir.

PHARMACOKINETICS **Peak:** 3 h. **Distribution:** 83% protein bound. **Metabolism:** In the liver via UGT1A1. **Elimination:** Feces and urine. **Half-Life:** 9 h.

NURSING IMPLICATIONS

Assessment & Drug Effects

- Monitor for and report S&S of immune reconstitution syndrome (inflammatory response to residual opportunistic infections such as MAC, CMV, PCP, or reactivation of varicella zoster).
- Monitor diabetics for loss of glycemic control.
- Monitor for suicidal ideation.
- Monitor lab tests: Baseline and periodic CD4+ cell count and HIV RNA viral load; periodic CBC with differential, LFTs.

Patient & Family Education

- Inform prescriber immediately if you plan to become or become pregnant during therapy.
- Report promptly unexplained leg pain or muscle cramping.

RAMELTEON

(ra-mel'tee-on)

Rozerem

Classification: MELATONIN RECEPTOR AGONIST; SEDATIVE-HYPNOTIC

Therapeutic: SEDATIVE

AVAILABILITY Tablet

ACTION & *THERAPEUTIC EFFECT* A melatonin receptor agonist with high affinity for melatonin receptors in the brain. This activity is believed to promote sleep, as these receptors, in response to endogenous melatonin, are thought to be involved in maintaining the circadian rhythm underlying the normal sleep-wake cycle. *Effective in promoting onset of sleep.*

USES Treatment of insomnia characterized by difficulty with sleep onset.

CONTRAINDICATIONS Hypersensitivity to ramelteon; severe hepatic function impairment (Child-Pugh class C); severe sleep apnea or severe COPD; severe depression; suicidal ideation; lactation.

CAUTIOUS USE Moderate hepatic function impairment (Child-Pugh class B); depression with suicidal tendencies; older adults; pregnancy (adverse effects were observed in some animal reproduction studies). Safety and efficacy in children younger than 18 y not established.

ROUTE & DOSAGE

Insomnia

Adult: **PO** 8 mg within 30 min of bedtime (intended for short term use)

ADMINISTRATION

Oral

- Give within 30 min of bedtime. Avoid administering with or immediately after a high-fat meal.
- Do not administer to anyone on concurrent fluvoxamine therapy without alerting prescriber. This combination causes a dramatic increase in ramelteon blood level.
- Store at 15°–30° C (59°– 86° F).

ADVERSE EFFECTS Respiratory: Upper respiratory tract infection. **CNS:** Dizziness, fatigue, insomnia, somnolence. **GI:** Unpleasant taste, nausea.

INTERACTIONS Drug: Concurrent use with **ethanol** or CNS DEPRESSANTS produces additive CNS depressant effects; **ketoconazole, itraconazole,** and **fluvoxamine** increase ramelteon levels; other CYP1A2 INHIBITORS (e.g., **ciprofloxacin, enoxacin, mexiletine, norfloxacin**) may also increase ramelteon levels; **rifampin** decreases ramelteon levels. **Food:** High-fat meal, **grapefruit** or **grapefruit juice** increase ramelteon levels.

PHARMACOKINETICS Absorption: 84%. **Peak:** 45 min. **Distribution:** 82% protein bound. **Metabolism:** Rapid and extensive first pass hepatic metabolism; one metabolite, M-II, is active. **Elimination:** Primarily renal. **Half-Life:** 1–2.5 h.

NURSING IMPLICATIONS

Assessment & Drug Effects

- Monitor for and report worsening insomnia and cognitive or behavioral changes.

Patient & Family Education

- Do not take with or immediately after a high fat meal.

- Do not drive or engage in potentially hazardous activities until response to drug is known.
- Do not consume alcohol while taking this drug.
- Report any of the following to prescriber: Worsening insomnia, cognitive or behavioral changes, problem with reproductive function.

RAMIPRIL
(ram′i-pril)
Altace
Classification: ANGIOTENSIN-CONVERTING ENZYME (ACE) INHIBITOR; ANTIHYPERTENSIVE
Therapeutic: ANTIHYPERTENSIVE
Prototype: Enalapril

AVAILABILITY Capsule

ACTION & *THERAPEUTIC EFFECT* Reduces peripheral vascular resistance by inhibiting the formation of angiotensin II, a potent vasoconstrictor. This also decreases serum aldosterone levels and reduces peripheral arterial resistance (afterload) as well as improves cardiac output and exercise tolerance. *Lowers BP, and improves cardiac output as well as exercise tolerance.*

R

USES hypertension, heart failure post myocardial infarction, reduction in risk of MI, stroke, and death from CV causes.

UNLABELED USES Stable coronary artery disease, heart failure with reduced ejection fraction.

CONTRAINDICATIONS Hypersensitivity to ramipril or any other ACE inhibitor, history of angioneurotic edema; intestinal angioedema; jaundice; elevated hepatic enzymes; hyperkalemia; concurrent use of aliskiren in diabetic patients; concomitant use with neprilysin inhibitor; oliguria, or progressive azotemia; pregnancy (exposure to ACE inhibitor during first trimester of pregnancy may be associated with increased risk of fetal malformations); lactation.

CAUTIOUS USE Impaired kidney or liver function, surgery or anesthesia; CHF; SLE, scleroderma. Safety and efficacy in children not established.

ROUTE & DOSAGE

Hypertension

Adult: **PO** 2.5 mg daily, may titrate after 2–4 weeks up to 20 mg/day in 1–2 divided doses

Stroke/MI Risk Reduction

Adult: **PO** 2.5 mg daily × 1wk then 5 mg daily × 3wk, may increase up to 10 mg/day

Heart Failure Post Myocardial Infarction

Adult: **PO** 2.5 mg bid × 1 week then may titrate up every 3 weeks as needed (up to 5 mg bid)

Renal Impairment Dosage Adjustment

CrCl less than 40 mL/min: administer 25% of normal dose

ADMINISTRATION

Oral

- Swallow capsule whole; may open the capsule and mix contents with 120 mL of water, apple juice, or applesauce.
- Store at 15°–30° C (59°–86° F) and protect from moisture.

ADVERSE EFFECTS **CV:** *Hypotension.* **Respiratory:** *Cough.*

CNS: Dizziness, fatigue, headache. **Endocrine:** Hyperkalemia, hyponatremia. **Skin:** Stevens–Johnson syndrome. **Other:** Angioedema.

DIAGNOSTIC TEST INTERFERENCE

may cause false negative aldosterone/renin ratio; may cause false-positive results in urine acetone determination using **sodium nitroprusside** reagent; positive direct **Coombs test**.

INTERACTIONS

Drug: POTASSIUM-SPARING DIURETICS may increase risk of hyperkalemia. May elevate serum **lithium** levels, resulting in lithium toxicity. Use with **azathioprine** increases risk of hematologic side effects. **Pregabalin** use increases the risk of angioedema. Use with ANGIOTENSION II RECEPTOR ANTAGONISTS does not offer additional benefit. ANTIHYPERTENSIVES, **obinutuzumab** increase the risk of hypotension. May increase the risk of adverse effects with **iron**. Do not use with **lanthanum, telmisartan**.

PHARMACOKINETICS

Absorption: 60% from GI tract. **Onset:** 2 h. **Peak:** 6–8 h. **Duration:** Up to 24 h. **Distribution:** Crosses placenta; not known if distributed into breast milk. **Metabolism:** Rapidly metabolized in liver to active metabolite, ramiprilat. **Elimination:** 60% in urine, 40% in feces. **Half-Life:** 2–3 h.

NURSING IMPLICATIONS

Black Box Warning

Ramipril has been associated with fetal injury and death.

Assessment & Drug Effects

- Monitor BP at time of peak effectiveness, 3–6 h after dosing and at end of dosing interval just before next dose.
- Report diminished antihypertensive effect.
- Monitor for first-dose hypotension, especially in salt- or volume-depleted persons.
- Observe for S&S of hyperkalemia (see Appendix F).
- Monitor lab tests: Periodic BUN, serum creatinine, serum potassium, and CBC with differential

Patient & Family Education

- Notify prescriber immediately if you become or suspect you are pregnant.
- Discontinue drug and report S&S of angioedema to prescriber (e.g., swelling of face or extremities, difficulty breathing or swallowing).
- Maintain adequate fluid intake and avoid potassium supplements or salt substitutes unless specifically prescribed by the prescriber.
- Light-headedness and dizziness may occur, especially during the initial days of therapy. If fainting occurs, stop taking ramipril until the prescriber has been consulted.

RAMUCIRUMAB

(ram-u-cir'u-mab)

Cyramza

Classification: IMMUNOMODULATOR; MONOCLONAL ANTIBODY; VASCULAR ENDOTHELIAL GROWTH FACTOR RECEPTOR 2 (VEGFR2) ANTAGONIST

Therapeutic: IMMUNOMODULATOR

AVAILABILITY

Solution for injection

ACTION & *THERAPEUTIC EFFECT*

Inhibits vascular endothelial growth factor receptor 2 (VEGFR2) by binding to it and blocking its activation, thereby inhibiting proliferation and migration of endothelial cells.

VEGFR2 inhibition results in reduced tumor vascularity and growth.

USES Treatment of advanced gastric cancer or gastroesophageal junction adenocarcinoma, as a single-agent after prior fluoropyrimidine- or platinum-containing chemotherapy.

CONTRAINDICATIONS Uncontrolled severe hypertension; Grade 3–4 infusion-related reactions; urine protein greater than 3 mg/24 h; nephrotic syndrome; arterial thromboembolic events; GI perforation; Grade 3 or 4 bleeding; severe arterial thromboembolic event; Posterior Leukoencephalopathy Syndrome; lactation.

CAUTIOUS USE Hypertension; protein urea; infusion related reactions; concurrent NSAIDs or drug that increase bleeding risk; impaired wound healing; hepatic impairment; pregnancy (category C). Safety and efficacy in children younger than 18 y not established.

ROUTE & DOSAGE

Gastric Cancer

Adult: **IV** 8 mg/kg every 2 wk

Toxicity Dosage Adjustment

Infusion related reactions: Grade 1–2, decrease IV rate by 50%; Grade 3–4, permanently discontinue

Severe hypertension: Interrupt therapy until BP managed; permanently discontinue if BP cannot be controlled

Proteinuria: Urine protein levels 2g/24h or greater, interrupt therapy until levels are less than 2g/24h then reinitiate at 6 mg/kg q2wk (or 5 mg/kg q2wk in a recurrence); protein level is greater than 3mg/24h or nephrotic syndrome, permanently discontinue

Arterial Thromboembolic Events, GI Perforation, or Grade 3 or 4 Bleeding: Permanently discontinue

ADMINISTRATION

Intravenous

This drug is a cytotoxic agent and caution should be used to prevent any contact with the drug. Follow institutional or standard guidelines for preparation, handling, and disposal of cytotoxic agents.

PREPARE: **IV Infusion:** Dilute required dose in NS to a final volume of 250 mL. Invert gently to mix but do not shake. Discard unused portion of the vial.

ADMINISTER: **IV Infusion:** Give over 60 min through a 0.22 micron protein-sparing filter. **Do not** give IV push or bolus. Flush the line after infusion with NS. Reduce infusion rate (by 50%) for Grade 1 or 2 infusion reaction. Stop infusion for Grade 3 or 4 infusion reaction.

INCOMPATIBILITIES: Do not mix or infuse with any other drugs or solutions.

- Store diluted solutions at 2°–8° C (36°–46° F) for no longer than 24 h (do not freeze) or may store for 4 h at room temperature [below 25° C (77° F)].

ADVERSE EFFECTS **CV:** *Hypertension*. **CNS:** Headache. **Endocrine:** Hyponatremia, proteinuria. **Skin:** Rash. **GI:** *Diarrhea*, intestinal obstruction. **Hematological:** Arterial thromboembolic events, hemorrhage, neutropenia. **Other:** Infusion related reactions, epistaxis.

PHARMACOKINETICS

Half-Life: Dose related (200–300 h).

NURSING IMPLICATIONS

Black Box Warning

Ramucirumab has been associated with increased risk of hemorrhage, including severe and sometimes fatal hemorrhagic events. Permanently discontinue if severe bleeding occurs.

Assessment & Drug Effects

- Monitor closely for infusion related reactions.
- Monitor BP throughout therapy. Withhold drug and notify prescriber if severe hypertension occurs. Resume drug only after hypertension is medically controlled.
- If unexplained bleeding occurs, withhold drug and notify prescriber.
- Monitor for and report promptly S&S of liver dysfunction.
- Inspect wounds closely. If poor wound healing is suspected, withhold drug and notify prescriber.
- Monitor lab tests: Periodic LFTs, thyroid function, and urine protein.

Patient & Family Education

- Report promptly to prescriber if blood pressure is elevated or if symptoms of hypertension occur including severe headache, light-headedness, or neurologic symptoms.
- Contact prescriber for bleeding or symptoms of bleeding including light-headedness.
- Notify prescriber for severe diarrhea, vomiting, or severe abdominal pain.
- Monitor any wounds and report slow wound healing.
- Do not undergo surgery without first discussing the risk of poor wound healing with prescriber.

RANOLAZINE

(ra-no′la-zeen)

Ranexa

Classification: ANTIANGINAL; PARTIAL FATTY ACID OXIDATION (PFOX) INHIBITOR

Therapeutic: ANTIANGINAL

AVAILABILITY Extended release tablet

ACTION & *THERAPEUTIC EFFECT* A partial fatty-acid oxidation inhibitor that shifts myocardial metabolism away from fatty acids to glucose. This shift requires less oxygen for oxidation and results in decreased oxygen demand. *Improves exercise tolerance and angina symptoms.*

USES Treatment of chronic stable angina in combination with calcium channel blockers, beta-blockers, or nitrates.

CONTRAINDICATIONS Severe hepatic impairment; severe renal impairment, renal failure, hypokalemia, hypomagnesemia; history of acute MI; lactation.

CAUTIOUS USE History of QT prolongation or torsades de pointes; renal impairment; older adult; pregnancy (category C); children.

ROUTE & DOSAGE

Chronic Stable Angina

Adult: **PO** 500 mg bid (max: 1000 mg bid) (patients taking concurrent CYP3A4 inhibitors have a max dose of 500 mg bid)

R

ADMINISTRATION

Oral

- **Must be** swallowed whole. Should not be crushed, broken, or chewed.
- Store at 15°–30° C (59°–86° F).

ADVERSE EFFECTS **CV:** Palpitations. **Respiratory:** Dyspnea. **CNS:** *Dizziness,* headache. **HEENT:** Tinnitus, vertigo. **GI:** Abdominal pain, *constipation,* dry mouth, nausea, vomiting. **Other:** Peripheral edema.

DIAGNOSTIC TEST INTERFERENCE

Ranolazine is not known to interfere with any diagnostic laboratory test.

INTERACTIONS **Drug:** INHIBITORS OF P-GLYCOPROTEIN (e.g., **ritonavir, cyclosporine**) may increase ranolazine absorption. Ranolazine increases the plasma concentrations of **digoxin** and **simvastatin.** INHIBITORS OF CYP3A4 [e.g., **diltiazem, erythromycin, grapefruit juice,** HIV PROTEASE INHIBITORS, **ketoconazole,** MACROLIDE ANTIBIOTICS (especially **ketoconazole**), **verapamil**] can increase plasma levels and QT_c elevation. **Paroxetine,** a CYP2D6 INHIBITOR, increases the plasma levels of ranolazine. CLASS I OF III ANTIARRHYTHMICS (e.g., **quinidine, dofetilide, sotalol**), **thioridazine,** and **ziprasidone** can cause additive increases in QT_c elevation. **Food: Grapefruit juice.**

PHARMACOKINETICS **Absorption:** 73% of PO dose absorbed. **Peak:** 2–5 h. **Distribution:** 62% protein bound. **Metabolism:** Extensive hepatic metabolism. **Elimination:** 75% in urine; 25% in feces. **Half-Life:** 7 h.

NURSING IMPLICATIONS

Assessment & Drug Effects

- Monitor ECG at baseline and periodically for prolongation of the QT_c interval.
- Monitor blood levels of digoxin with concurrent therapy.
- When coadministered with simvastatin, monitor for and report unexplained muscle weakness or pain.
- Monitor lab tests: Baseline and periodic renal function tests with moderate-to-severe renal impairment.

Patient & Family Education

- Do not engage in hazardous activities until response to drug is known.
- Contact prescriber if you experience fainting while taking ranolazine.
- Do not drink grapefruit juice or eat grapefruit while taking this drug.

RASAGILINE

(ras-a-gi'leen)

Azilect

Classification: MONOAMINE OXIDASE-B (MAO-B) INHIBITOR; ANTIPARKINSON

Therapeutic: ANTIPARKINSON

AVAILABILITY Tablet

ACTION & *THERAPEUTIC EFFECT*

A potent monoamine oxidase B (MAO-B) inhibitor that prevents the enzyme monoamine oxidase B from breaking down dopamine in the brain. Rasagiline also interferes with dopamine reuptake at synapses in the brain. *Rasagiline helps to overcome dopaminergic motor dysfunction in Parkinson's disease.*

R

USES Treatment of Parkinson disease (monotherapy or adjunct).

CONTRAINDICATIONS Moderate to severe hepatic impairment; alcoholism; biliary cirrhosis; major psychotic disorders; uncontrolled hypertension; within 14 days of use of other MAOIs; concomitant use with cyclobenzaprine, dextromethorphan, or St. John's wort.

CAUTIOUS USE Mild hepatic dysfunction; cardiovascular disease; DM; asthma, bronchitis, hyperthyroidism; postural or orthostatic hypotension; migraine headaches; moderate to severe renal impairment, anuria; epilepsy or preexisting seizure disorders; pregnancy; (Adverse effects have been observed in animal reproduction studies.) lactation. Safety and efficacy in children not established.

ROUTE & DOSAGE

Parkinson Disease

Adult: **PO** 1 mg/day as monotherapy; 0.5–1 mg/day if used with levodopa as adjunctive therapy

Hepatic Impairment Dosage Adjustment

Mild Impairment: 0.5 mg/day

Concomitant Use of CYP1A2 Inhibitors Dosage Adjustment

Max dose: 0.5 mg once daily

ADMINISTRATION

Oral

- May be given without regard to food.
- Avoid foods containing high amounts of tyramine (> 150 mg) such as aged cheeses, cured meats, tap/draft beer, fava or broad bean pods, sauerkraut, soy sauce.
- Store at 25° C (77° F).

ADVERSE EFFECTS **Respiratory:** Flu-like symptoms. **CNS:** *Depression, fall, headache.* **HEENT:** Conjunctivitis. **GI:** Dyspepsia. **Musculoskeletal:** Arthralgia.

INTERACTIONS **Drug:** There are extensive drug interactions, consult a drug information database for a complete list, some significant interactions are highlighted below. INHIBITORS OF CYP1A2 (e.g., **atazanavir, ciprofloxacin, mexiletine**) may increase rasagiline plasma levels. Rasagiline increases the plasma levels of ANESTHETICS; thus it must be discontinued 14 days prior to elective surgery. Rasagiline can cause severe CNS toxicity, including hyperpyrexia and death, with ANTIDEPRESSANTS, SELECTIVE SEROTONIN REUPTAKE INHIBITORS (SSRI), SEROTONIN-NOREPINEPHRINE REUPTAKE INHIBITORS (SNRI), NONSELECTIVE MAO INHIBITORS, or SELECTIVE MAO-B INHIBITORS. Rasagiline can increase the plasma levels of **cyclobenzaprine** and SYMPATHOMIMETIC AMINES. Rasagiline and **dextromethorphan** can cause brief episodes of psychosis and bizarre behavior. Use with ALPHA OR BETA AGONISTS, AMPHETAMINES can cause hypertension. Rasagiline can potentiate the dopaminergic effects of **levodopa.** Rasagiline can increase the plasma levels of **meperidine, methadone, propoxyphene,** and **tramadol, acetaminophen,** resulting in coma, severe hypertension or hypotension, severe respiratory depression, convulsions, and death. **Food:** Caffeine or ethanol can cause significant side effects and caution should be used. Foods rich in tyramine can cause severe high blood pressure. **Herbal:** Rasagiline increases the plasma levels of **St. John's wort.**

PHARMACOKINETICS

Absorption: Rapidly absorbed with 36% bioavailability. **Peak:** 1 h. **Distribution:** 88–94% protein bound. **Metabolism:** Extensive hepatic metabolism (CYP1A2, CYP2C8/9). **Elimination:** Primarily renal (62%) with minor fecal elimination. **Half-Life:** 3 h.

NURSING IMPLICATIONS

Assessment & Drug Effects

- Monitor BP for new onset hypertension or hypertension not adequately controlled.
- Monitor for orthostatic hypotension especially in combination with levodopa.
- Monitor for and report to prescriber any of the following: Symptoms of parkinsonism; new or worsening mental status and behavioral changes; somnolence and falling asleep during activities of daily living.
- Perform baseline and periodic skin examination for presence of melanoma.
- Monitor lab values: Baseline and periodic liver and renal function tests.

R

Patient & Family Education

- Do not take any prescription or nonprescription drug without consulting prescriber.
- Periodic skin examinations should be scheduled with a dermatologist. If you notice changes in a skin mole or new skin lesion, contact the dermatologist.
- Avoid foods and beverages containing tyramine (e.g., aged cheeses and meats, tap beer, red wine, soybean products).
- Make position changes slowly, especially when standing from a lying or sitting position.
- Do not drive or engage in potentially hazardous activities until response to drug is known.
- Report immediately any of the following to a health care provider: Palpitations, severe headache, blurred vision, difficulty thinking, seizures, chest pain, unexplained nausea or vomiting, or any sudden weakness or paralysis.

RASBURICASE

(ras-bur'i-case)

Elitek, Fasturtec ✦

Classification: ANTIGOUT; ANTIMETABOLITE

Therapeutic: ANTIGOUT

AVAILABILITY

Powder for injection

ACTION & *THERAPEUTIC EFFECT*

A recombinant urate-oxidase enzyme produced by DNA technology. In humans, uric acid is the final step in the catabolic pathway of purines. Rasburicase catalyzes enzymatic oxidation of uric acid; thus it is only active at the end of the purine catabolic pathway. *Used to manage plasma uric acid levels in pediatric patients with leukemia, lymphoma, and solid tumor malignancies who are receiving anticancer therapy that results in tumor lysis, and therefore elevates plasma uric acid.*

USES

Initial management of increased uric acid levels secondary to tumor lysis.

CONTRAINDICATIONS

Severe hypersensitivity to rasburicase; deficiency in glucose-6-phosphate de-hydrogenase (G6PD); history of anaphylaxis; hemolytic reactions or methemoglobinemia reactions to rasburicase; lactation.

CAUTIOUS USE Patients at risk for G6PD deficiency (e.g., African or Mediterranean ancestry); asthma; bone marrow suppression, pregnancy (category C); children younger than 1 mo.

ROUTE & DOSAGE

Hyperuricemia

Adult/Child (1 mo or older): **IV** 0.2 mg/kg/day for up to 5 days

ADMINISTRATION

Intravenous

PREPARE: **IV Infusion:** Reconstitute each 1.5 mg vial or 7.5 mg vial with 1 or 5 mL, respectively, of the provided diluent and mix by swirling very gently. **Do not shake.** Discard if particulate matter is visible or if product is discolored after reconstitution. ▪ Remove the predetermined dose from the reconstituted vials and inject into enough NS in an infusion bag to achieve a final total volume of 50 mL.

ADMINISTER: **IV Infusion:** Give over 30 min. **Do not give bolus dose.** Infuse through an **unfiltered** line used for no other medications. ▪ If a separate line is not possible, flush the line with at least 15 mL of saline solution before/after infusion of rasburicase. ▪ Immediately discontinue IV infusion and institute emergency measures for S&S of anaphylaxis including chest pain, dyspnea, hypotension, and/or urticaria.

INCOMPATIBILITIES: Do not mix or infuse with other drugs.

ADVERSE EFFECTS **CNS:** *Headache,* anxiety. **Skin:** *Rash.* **GI:** *Mucositis, vomiting, nausea, diarrhea, abdominal pain.* **Hematologic:** Neutro-penia. **Other:** *Fever,* sepsis, severe hypersensitivity reactions including anaphylaxis at any time during treatment.

DIAGNOSTIC TEST INTERFERENCE May give false elevations for ***uric acid*** if blood sample is left at room temperature.

PHARMACOKINETICS **Half-Life:** 18 h.

NURSING IMPLICATIONS

Black Box Warning

Rasburicase has been associated with severe hypersensitivity reactions and with development of methemoglobinemia.

Assessment & Drug Effects

- Patients at higher risk for G6PD deficiency (e.g., patients of African or Mediterranean ancestry) should be screened prior to starting therapy as this deficiency is a contraindication for this drug.
- Monitor closely for S&S of hypersensitivity and be prepared to institute emergency measures for anaphylaxis.
- Monitor cardiovascular, respiratory, neurologic, and renal status throughout therapy.
- Monitor lab tests: Plasma uric acid levels (4 h after rasburicase administration and q6–8h until tumor lysis syndrome resolution); CBC as needed; baseline G6PD deficiency screening (in patients at high risk for deficiency).

Patient & Family Education

- Report immediately any distressing S&S to prescriber.

REGORAFENIB

(re-gor'a-fe-nib)

Stivarga

Classification: ANTINEOPLASTIC; KINASE INHIBITOR; MULTIKINASE INHIBITOR

Therapeutic: ANTINEOPLASTIC

Prototype: Erlotinib

AVAILABILITY Tablet

ACTION & *THERAPEUTIC EFFECT* Inhibits multiple kinase enzymes systems involved in normal cellular functions and in pathologic processes such as tumor development (oncogenesis), tumor angiogenesis, and maintenance of the tumor microenvironment. *Inhibits colorectal cancer tumor growth and metastasis.*

USES Metastatic colorectal cancer (CRC) in those previously treated with fluoropyrimidine-, oxaliplatin-, and irinotecan-based chemotherapy, an antivascular endothelial growth factor (VEGF) therapy, and, if cancer is a KRAS gene wild type, an anti-epidermal growth factor receptor (EGFR) therapy. Treatment of locally advanced, unresectable or metastatic gastrointestinal stromal tumors (GIST) in patients who have previously received imatinib and sunitinib; hepatocellular carcinoma.

CONTRAINDICATIONS Severe hepatic impairment (Child-Pugh class C); severe or life-threatening hemorrhage; severe or uncontrolled hypertension; posterior reversible encephalopathy syndrome; 2 wk before surgery; pregnancy (may cause fetal harm if administered during pregnancy); lactation.

CAUTIOUS USE Mild to moderate hepatic impairment; moderate-to-severe renal impairment; hypertension; history of myocardial ischemia. Safety and efficacy in children younger than 18 y not established.

ROUTE & DOSAGE

Colorectal Cancer, GIST, Hepatocellular Cancer

Adult: **PO** 160 mg once daily for the first 21 days of a 28 day cycle; repeat until disease progression or unacceptable toxicity

Dosing Modifications

Withhold drug and consult prescriber for any Grade 2 or higher reaction according to the National Cancer Institute (NCI) Common Terminology Criteria for Adverse Events (CTCAE). See package insert for more specific details.

Permanently discontinue if:

- Unable to tolerate 80 mg dose
- AST or ALT levels greater than 20 × ULN
- Reversible posterior leukoencephalopathy syndrome occurs
- AST or ALT levels greater than 3 × ULN with concurrent bilirubin greater than 2 × ULN
- Previously elevated AST or ALT levels return to greater than 5 × ULN despite dose reduction to 120 mg
- Any Grade 4 adverse reaction occurs (resume only if the potential benefit outweighs the risks)
- Severe hemorrhage

ADMINISTRATION

Oral

- Give at same time each day.
- Swallow tablet whole with water after a low-fat meal containing < 600 calories and < 30% fat.
- Avoid grapefruit juice.
- Store at 25° C (77° F). Keep tightly closed in original bottle and do not remove desiccant. Discard unused tablets 28 days after opening bottle.

ADVERSE EFFECTS **CV:** *Hypertension.* **Respiratory:** Nasopharyngitis. **CNS:** Headache, fatigue, pain. **HEENT:** Voice disorder. **Endocrine:** Hypocalcemia, hypokalemia, hyponatremia, hypophosphatemia, hypothyroidism, increased INR, increased lipase, *weight loss.* **Skin:** *Palmar-plantar erythrodysesthesia*, rash, alopecia. **Hepatic/GI:** *Diarrhea*, decreased appetite, *stomatitis*, nausea, vomiting, gastrointestinal pain, hepatotoxicity, increased liver enzymes, hyperbilirubinemia, increased serum amylase/lipase. **GU:** Proteinuria, urinary tract infection. **Musculoskeletal:** Asthenia, muscle spasms. **Hematological:** Anemia, lymphopenia, increased INR, hemorrhage, neutropenia, thrombocytopenia. **Other:** Fever, *infection.*

INTERACTIONS **Drug:** Coadministration of strong CYP3A4 inhibitors (e.g., **clarithromycin, itraconazole, ketoconazole, posaconazole, telithromycin, voriconazole**) increases the levels of regorafenib and decreases the levels of its active metabolites. Coadministration of strong CYP3A4 inducers (e.g., **carbamazepine, phenobarbital, phenytoin, rifampin**) decreases the levels of regorafenib and increases the levels of one of its active metabolites. May increase the concentration of drugs metabolized by CVRP/ABCG2 (ex **ozanimod, pazopanib, topotecan** etc.). **Food:** Grapefruit juice can increase the levels of regorafenib and decrease the levels of its active metabolites. **Herbal: St. John's wort** can decrease the levels of regorafenib and increase the levels of one of its active metabolites.

PHARMACOKINETICS **Absorption:** 69–83% bioavailable. **Peak:** 4 h. **Distribution:** Greater than 99% plasma protein bound. **Metabolism:** In liver to active metabolites. (CYP3A4 and UGT1A9). Also affects CYP2C9, CYP2B6, CYP2D6, UGT1A1, breast cancer resistance protein (BCRP). **Elimination:** Fecal (71%) and renal (19%). **Half-Life:** 28 h for parent drug, 25 h for one active metabolite, and 5 h for a second active metabolite.

NURSING IMPLICATIONS

Black Box Warning

Regorafenib has been associated with severe and sometimes fatal hepatotoxicity.

Assessment & Drug Effects

- Monitor BP weekly for first 6 wk then once every cycle or more often as needed. Notify prescriber for recurrent or persistently elevated BP (e.g., greater than 150/100).
- Monitor cardiac status and assess for S&S of myocardial ischemia.
- Monitor for and report promptly S&S dermatological toxicity (i.e., hand–foot skin reaction) or hepatotoxicity (see Appendix F).
- Add for 2 wk prior to surgery to allow for proper wound healing.
- Monitor lab tests: Baseline and biweekly LFTs first 2 mo and

R

monthly (or more frequently) thereafter; baseline and periodic CBC with differential, platelet count, and serum electrolytes, frequent INR with concurrent warfarin therapy.

Patient & Family Education

- Seek medical attention immediately if you experience any of the following: Chest pain, shortness of breath, dizziness, fainting, severe abdominal pain, persistent abdominal swelling, high fever, chills, nausea, vomiting, severe diarrhea, or dehydration.
- Report promptly any of the following: Redness, pain, blisters, bleeding, or swelling on the palms of hands or soles of feet; signs of bleeding; signs of high BP including severe headaches, lightheadedness, or changes in vision.
- Women and men should use effective means of birth control during therapy and for at least 2 mo following completion of therapy.
- Contact your prescriber immediately if you become pregnant during treatment.
- Do not breast-feed while receiving this drug.

REMDESIVIR

(rem-DE-si-vir)

Veklury

Classifications: ANTIVIRAL

Therapeutic: ANTIVIRAL

R

AVAILABILITY Solution for injection

ACTION & *THERAPEUTIC EFFECT*

An inhibitor of the SARS-CoV-2-2 RNA-dependent RNA polymerase which is essential for viral replication. It slows viral replication and can be used to improve patient outcomes in patient's diagnosed with COVID-19.

USES Treatment of coronavirus disease 2019 (COVID-19) requiring hospitalization.

CONTRAINDICATIONS Sensitivity to remdesivir or any component of the product; patients with impaired kidney function indicated by a GFR less than 30 mL/min; pregnancy—fetal risk cannot be ruled out; lactation—infant risk cannot be ruled out.

CAUTIOUS USE Concomitant use with chloroquine phosphate or hydroxychloroquine sulfate as it may result in a reduced antiviral activity; decreased liver function; impaired kidney function.

ROUTE & DOSAGE

COVID-19

Adult: **IV** 200 mg on day one, then 100 mg once daily for five days or hospital discharge, whichever is first. Duration can be extended for up to 10 days for certain patients.

ADMINISTRATION

Intravenous Only

- Dilute with normal saline prior to administration
- Lyophilized powder and solution available for intravenous administration. See package insert for specific instructions for mixing and administering times for infusion.
- Administer immediately after preparation.
- May store the final diluted solution in the infusion bags for up to 24 hours at room temperature (20 to 25° C or 68 to 77° F) or for 48 hours under refrigeration (2 to 8° C or 36 to 46° F).

- Do not administer simultaneously with other medication. IV compatibility with other solutions is unknown.
- Store vial of powder below 30° C (below 86° F) until required for use.
- Store vial of solution refrigerated between 2 and 8° C (36 and 46° F) until required for use. Prior to dilution, sealed vials may be stored up to 12 hours at room temperature between 20 and 25° C (68 and 77° F). Solution must be diluted the same day as administration. After dilution, solution may be stored at a room temperature between 20 and 25° C (68 and 77° F) for no more than 24 hours or refrigerated between 2 to 8° C (36 to 46° F) for no more than 48 hours. Discard any unused portion and do not reuse or save diluted solution for future use.

ADVERSE EFFECTS CV: Cardiac arrest, hypotension. **Skin:** Rash. **Hepatic**: ALT/SGPT elevation, increased aspartate aminotransferase serum levels, hepatotoxicity. **GI:** Nausea **Hematologic:** Prolonged prothrombin time.

INTERACTIONS Drug: Use alongside **chloroquine** or **hydroxychloroquine** may diminish therapeutic effect of remdesivir. Concomitant use should be avoided.

PHARMACOKINETICS Distribution: 88–94% protein bound. **Metabolism:** Hydrolysis through CES1. **Elimination:** 10% in urine. **Half-Life:** 1 h.

NURSING IMPLICATIONS

Assessment & Drug Effects

- Symptomatic improvement.
- Monitor blood pressure.
- Monitor for signs of anaphylactic reaction.
- Monitor labs: GFR, Prothrombin time, LFTs.

Patient & Family Education

- Review adverse effects with patient and caregivers.
- Report any light headedness or dizziness.

REMIFENTANIL HYDROCHLORIDE

(rem-i-fent′a-nil)

Ultiva

Classification: ANALGESIC, NARCOTIC (OPIATE AGONIST); GENERAL ANESTHESIA

Therapeutic: NARCOTIC ANALGESIC; GENERAL ANESTHESIA

Prototype: Morphine

Controlled Substance: Schedule II

AVAILABILITY Solution for injection

ACTION & *THERAPEUTIC EFFECT* Synthetic, potent narcotic agonist analgesic that is rapidly metabolized; therefore respiratory depression is of shorter duration when discontinued. *Used as the analgesic component of an anesthesia regime.*

USES Analgesic during induction and maintenance of general anesthesia, as the analgesic component of monitored anesthesia care.

CONTRAINDICATIONS Hypersensitivity to fentanyl analogs, epidural or intrathecal administration.

CAUTIOUS USE Head injuries, increased intracranial pressure; debilitated, morbid obesity, poor-risk patients; COPD, other respiratory problems, bradyarrhythmia; older adults; pregnancy (category C); lactation. Safety in labor and delivery not established.

R

ROUTE & DOSAGE

Adjunct to Anesthesia

Adult: **IV** 0.5–1 mcg/kg/min or 1 mcg/kg bolus
Child (birth–2 mo): **IV** 0.4–1 mcg/kg/min; *1–12 y:* 0.5–1 mcg/kg/min or 1 mcg/kg bolus

Obesity Dosage Adjustment

Dose based on IBW

ADMINISTRATION

- Clear IV tubing completely of the drug following discontinuation of remifentanil infusion to ensure that inadvertent administration of the drug will not occur at a later time.

Intravenous

IV administration to infants and children: Verify correct IV concentration and rate of infusion with prescriber.

PREPARE: **Direct/Continuous Infusion** Reconstitute by adding 1 mL of sterile water for injection, D5W, NS, D5NS, 1/2NS, or D5LR to each 1 mg of remifentanil to yield 1 mg/mL. Shake well to dissolve. ▪ Further dilute to a final concentration of 20, 25, 50, or 250 mcg/mL by adding the required dose to the appropriate amount of IV solution.

ADMINISTER: **Direct/Continuous Infusion** Give at the ordered rate according to patient's weight.

- Note that bolus doses should **not** be given during a continuous infusion of remifentanil.
- Flush IV tubing thoroughly following infusion.

INCOMPATIBILITIES: **Solution/additive:** Unknown. **Y-site: Amphotericin B, amphotericin B cholesteryl, chlorpromazine, diazepam.**

- Reconstituted solution is stable for 24 h at room temperature. Store vials of powder at 2°–25° C (36°–77° F).

ADVERSE EFFECTS **CV:** Hypotension, hypertension, bradycardia. **Respiratory:** Respiratory depression, apnea. **CNS:** Dizziness, headache. **Skin:** Pruritus. **GI:** *Nausea*, vomiting. **Other:** Muscle rigidity, shivering.

INTERACTIONS **Drug: Alcohol** and other CNS DEPRESSANTS potentiate effects; MAO INHIBITORS may precipitate hypertensive crisis.

PHARMACOKINETICS **Duration:** 12 min. **Distribution:** 70% protein bound. **Metabolism:** Hydrolyzed by nonspecific esterases in the blood and tissues. **Elimination:** In urine. **Half-Life:** 3–10 min.

NURSING IMPLICATIONS

Assessment & Drug Effects

- Monitor vital signs during postoperative period; observe for and immediately report any S&S of respiratory distress or respiratory depression, or skeletal and thoracic muscle rigidity and weakness.
- Monitor for adequate postoperative analgesia.

REPAGLINIDE

(rep-a-gli'nide)

Prandin, GlucoNorm ♣

Classification: ANTIDIABETIC; MEGLITINIDE

Therapeutic: ANTIHYPERGLYCEMIC

AVAILABILITY Tablet

ACTION & *THERAPEUTIC EFFECT* Hypoglycemic agent that lowers blood glucose levels by stimulating

 Common adverse effects in *italic;* life-threatening effects underlined; generic names in **bold;** classifications in SMALL CAPS; ♣ Canadian drug name; Prototype drug; Alert

release of insulin from the pancreatic islets. *Significantly reduces postprandial blood glucose in type 2 diabetes. Minimal effects on fasting blood glucose.*

USES Adjunct to diet and exercise in type 2 diabetes.

CONTRAINDICATIONS Hypersensitivity to repaglinide; insulin-dependent diabetes, diabetic ketoacidosis; lactation.

CAUTIOUS USE Hypoglycemia; loss of glycemic control due to secondary failure; hepatic impairment; severe renal impairment; older adults, surgery, fever, systemic infection, trauma; pregnancy (category C); Safety and efficacy in children not established.

ROUTE & DOSAGE

Type 2 Diabetes

Adult (initial dose): **PO** 0.5 mg 15–30 min a.c.; *initial dose for patients previously using glucose-lowering agents:* 1–2 mg 15–30 min a.c. (2–4 doses/day depending on meal pattern; max: 16 mg/day); *dosage range:* 0.5–4 mg 15–30 min a.c.

ADMINISTRATION

Oral

- Give within 30 min of beginning a meal.
- Store at 15°–30° C (59°–86° F) in a tightly closed container and protect from moisture.

ADVERSE EFFECTS **CV:** Chest pain, angina. **Respiratory:** URI, sinusitis, rhinitis, bronchitis. **CNS:** Headache. **Endocrine:** *Hypoglycemia*. **GI:** Nausea, diarrhea, constipation, vomiting, dyspepsia. **Other:** Arthralgia, back pain, paresthesia, allergy.

INTERACTIONS **Drug: Erythromycin, ketoconazole** may inhibit metabolism and potentiate hypoglycemia; BARBITURATES, **carbamazepine, rifabutin, rifampin, rifapentine, pioglitazone** may induce metabolism and cause hyperglycemia; **gemfibrozil** may increase risk of hypoglycemia and duration of action. Use with **deferasirox** requires a repaglinide dose reduction. **Herbal: Ginseng, garlic** may increase hypoglycemic effects. **Food: Grapefruit juice** (greater than 1 qt/day) may increase plasma concentrations and adverse effects.

PHARMACOKINETICS **Absorption:** Rapidly from GI tract, 56% bioavailability. **Peak:** 1 h. **Distribution:** 98% protein bound. **Metabolism:** In liver (CYP3A4). **Elimination:** 90% in feces. **Half-Life:** 1 h.

NURSING IMPLICATIONS

Assessment & Drug Effects

- Monitor carefully for S&S of hypoglycemia especially during the 1-wk period following transfer from a longer-acting sulfonylurea.
- Monitor lab tests: Frequent FBS, postprandial blood glucose, and HbA1C q3mo.

Patient & Family Education

- Take only with meals to lessen the chance of hypoglycemia. If a meal is skipped, skip a dose; if a meal is added, add a dose.
- Start repaglinide the morning after the other agent is stopped when changing from another oral hypoglycemia drug.
- Be alert for S&S of hyperglycemia or hypoglycemia (see Appendix F); report poor blood glucose control to prescriber.

R

RESLIZUMAB

(res-liz'ue-mab)

Cinqair

Classification: INTERLEUKIN-5 ANTAGONIST; ANTIINFLAMMATORY; MONOCLONAL ANTIBODY

Therapeutic: ANTIINFLAMMATORY; ANTIASTHMATIC

Prototype: Basiliximab

AVAILABILITY Solution for injection

ACTION & THERAPEUTIC EFFECT An antibody that acts as an interleukin-5 antagonist (IgG1 kappa). IL-5 is the major cytokine responsible for the growth and differentiation, recruitment, activation, and survival of eosinophils. Eosinophils are involved in the inflammation associated with the pathogenesis of asthma. *The inhibition of IL-5 signaling by reslizumab, reduces the production and survival of eosinophils.*

USES Treatment of patients with severe asthma 18 y and older with an eosinophilic phenotype; reslizumab should not be used for treatment of other eosinophilic conditions or for the relief of acute bronchospasm or status asthmaticus.

R

CONTRAINDICATIONS Hypersensitivity to reslizumab. Should not be used to treat acute asthma symptoms.

CAUTIOUS USE Use cautiously in patients with history of systemic neoplastic disease and in patients with a high risk of malignancy. Treat patients with preexisting helminth infections prior to initiating treatment with reslizumab. Do not discontinue systemic or corticosteroids abruptly upon initiation of reslizumab. Pregnancy and lactation data are insufficient to determine risk. Safety and efficacy in children and adolescents younger than 18 y not established.

ROUTE & DOSAGE

Severe Asthma

Adult: **IV** 3 mg/kg once every 4 wk

ADMINISTRATION

Intravenous

PREPARE: **IV Infusion:** Solution is clear to slightly hazy/opalescent, colorless to slightly yellow. Small particles may be translucent to white. Discard and do not use if discolored or other foreign particulate matter. ▪ Dilute in 50 mL of 0.9% sodium chloride. ▪ Reslizumab is compatible with polyvinylchloride (PVC) or polyolefin infusion bags. Gently invert the bag to mix. Do not shake.

ADMINISTER: **IV Infusion:** ▪ **Do not** administer IV push or bolus. Administer immediately after preparation. ▪ Use an infusion set with an in-line, low protein-binding filter (pore size of 0.2 micron). Compatible with polyethersulfone, polyvinylidene fluoride, nylon, cellulose acetate in-line filters. ▪ Infuse intravenously over 20–50 min. ▪ Do not infuse any other medication in the tubing. ▪ Stop infusion immediately if patient exhibits any signs of anaphylaxis and treat appropriately. ▪ Flush the intravenous administration set with 0.9% sodium chloride injection to ensure complete administration.

INCOMPATIBILITIES: **Solution/additive:** None listed (should be mixed with NS).

- Store intact vials in refrigerator at 2°–8° C (36°–46° F). Do not freeze or shake. Protect from light. If not used immediately, store in the refrigerator at 2°–8° C (36°–46° F) or at room temperature up to 25° C (77° F), protected from light for up to 16 h max. If refrigerated, warm to room temperature before administering. Single use vials; discard any unused portion.

ADVERSE EFFECTS **Respiratory:** Oropharyngeal pain. **Musculoskeletal:** Myalgia. **Other:** Elevated creatine phosphokinase, immunogenicity.

PHARMACOKINETICS **Metabolism:** Proteolytic degradation. **Half-Life:** 24 days.

NURSING IMPLICATIONS

Assessment & Drug Effects

- Assess for anaphylaxis has been noted to occur on the second dose, within 20 min after infusion is complete.
- Signs of anaphylaxis include dyspnea, decreased oxygen saturation, wheezing, and vomiting. If any symptoms occur, stop administration and notify prescriber.
- Assess respiratory status including pulse oximetry.
- Patients should be treated for parasitic helminth infections prior to administration of drug.

Patient & Family Education

- Women should use contraceptive measures.
- This is not a rescue drug and should not be used in an acute asthma attack.
- May experience sore throat and muscle pain.

RETAPAMULIN

(re-te-pam′ue-lin)

Altabax

Classification: ANTIBIOTIC; PLEUROMUTILIN

Therapeutic: TOPICAL ANTIBIOTIC

AVAILABILITY Topical ointment

ACTION & THERAPEUTIC EFFECT Selectively inhibits bacterial protein synthesis at a site on the 50S subunit of the bacterial ribosome. *Effective against* Staphylococcus *(MRSA) and* Streptococcus *organisms.*

USES Treatment of impetigo due to susceptible stains of *Staphylococcus aureus* (methicillin-sensitive strains only) or *Streptococcus pyogenes.*

CONTRAINDICATIONS Severe hypersensitivity to retapamulin.

CAUTIOUS USE Pregnancy (category B); lactation; children less than 9 mo.

ROUTE & DOSAGE

Impetigo Infection

Adult/Child/Infant (9 mo or older): Apply in thin layer bid × 5 days

ADMINISTRATION

Topical

- Apply a thin layer to infected region. May cover with gauze dressing.
- Store at 15°–30° C (59°–86° F).

ADVERSE EFFECTS **Respiratory:** Nasopharyngitis. **CNS:** Headache.

R

Endocrine: Creatinine phosphokinase increased. **Skin:** Eczema, pruritus. **GI:** Diarrhea, nausea. **Other:** Application-site irritation, pyrexia.

PHARMACOKINETICS

Absorption: Minimal systemic absorption. **Metabolism:** In liver.

NURSING IMPLICATIONS

Assessment & Drug Effects

- Monitor for excessive skin irritation. Report swelling, blistering, or oozing.

Patient & Family Education

- Report any of the following at application site: Redness, itching, burning, swelling, blistering, or oozing.

RETEPLASE RECOMBINANT

(re'te-plase)

Retavase

Classification: THROMBOLYTIC ENZYME, TISSUE PLASMINOGEN ACTIVATOR (T-PA)

Therapeutic: THROMBOLYTIC

Prototype: Alteplase

AVAILABILITY

10.4 international unit vials

ACTION & *THERAPEUTIC EFFECT*

DNA recombinant human tissue-type plasminogen activator (t-PA) that acts as a catalyst in the cleavage of plasminogen to plasmin. Responsible for degrading the fibrin matrix of a clot. *Has antithrombolytic properties.*

USES

Thrombolysis management of acute MI to reduce the incidence of CHF and mortality.

CONTRAINDICATIONS

Active internal bleeding, history of CVA, recent neurologic surgery or trauma, intracranial neoplasm, or aneurysm, bleeding disorders, severe uncontrolled hypertension.

CAUTIOUS USE

Any condition in which bleeding constitutes a significant hazard (i.e., severe hepatic or renal disease, CVA, hypertension, acute pancreatitis, septic thrombophlebitis); pregnancy (category C); lactation. Safety and efficacy in children not established.

ROUTE & DOSAGE

Thrombolysis during Acute MI

Adult: **IV** 10 units injected over 2 min. Repeat dose in 30 min (20 units total).

ADMINISTRATION

Intravenous

PREPARE: **Direct:** Reconstitute using only the diluent, syringe, needle, and dispensing pin provided with reteplase. ▪ Withdraw diluent with syringe provided. Remove needle from syringe, replace with dispensing pin and transfer diluent to vial of reteplase. Leave pin and syringe in place in vial and swirl to dissolve. **Do not** shake. ▪ When completely dissolved, remove 10 mL solution, replace dispensing pin with a 20-gauge needle.

ADMINISTER: **Direct:** Flush IV line before and after with 30 mL NS or D5W and **do not** give any other drug simultaneously through the same IV line. ▪ Give a single dose evenly over 2 min.

INCOMPATIBILITIES: **Solution/additive:** **Heparin.** **Y-site:** **Bivalirudin, heparin.**

- Store drug kit unopened at 2°–25° C (36°–77° F).

ADVERSE EFFECTS **CV:** Reperfusion arrhythmias. **Hematologic:** *Hemorrhage* (including *intracranial*, GI, genitourinary), anemia.

DIAGNOSTIC TEST INTERFERENCE Causes decreases in plasminogen and fibrinogen, making ***coagulation*** and ***fibrinolytic*** tests unreliable.

INTERACTIONS **Drug: Aspirin, dipyridamole, heparin** may increase risk of bleeding.

PHARMACOKINETICS **Elimination:** In urine. **Half-Life:** 13–16 min.

NURSING IMPLICATIONS

Assessment & Drug Effects

- Discontinue concomitant heparin immediately if serious bleeding not controllable by local pressure occurs and, if not already given, withhold the second reteplase bolus.
- Monitor carefully all potential bleeding sites; monitor for S&S of internal hemorrhage (e.g., GI, GU, intracranial, retroperitoneal, pulmonary).
- Monitor carefully cardiac status for arrhythmias associated with reperfusion.
- Avoid invasive procedures, arterial and venous punctures, IM injections, and nonessential handling of the patient during reteplase therapy.

Patient & Family Education

- Report changes in consciousness or signs of bleeding to prescriber immediately.

RHO(D) IMMUNE GLOBULIN

(row)

RhoGAM, Rhophylac, WinRho SDF

RHO(D) IMMUNE GLOBULIN MICRO-DOSE

BayRho-D Mini Dose, MICRho-GAM

Classification: BIOLOGICAL RESPONSE MODIFIER; IMMUNOGLOBULIN (IgG)

Therapeutic: IMMUNOGLOBULIN

Prototype: Immune globulin

AVAILABILITY **RhoGAM, MICRho-GAM:** Solution in prefilled syringe. **Rhophylac:** Prefilled syringe; **WinRho SDF:** Vial

ACTION & THERAPEUTIC EFFECT Provides passive immunity by suppressing active antibody response and formation of anti-Rho(D) in Rh-negative [Rho(D)-negative] individuals previously exposed to Rh-positive [Rho(D)-positive, D^u-positive] blood. *Effective against exposure to Rh-positive blood in Rh-negative individuals.*

USES To prevent isoimmunization in Rh-negative individuals exposed to Rh-positive RBC (see above). Rho(D) immune globulin microdose is for use only after spontaneous or induced abortion or termination of ectopic pregnancy up to and including 12 wk of gestation. Treatment of idiopathic thrombocytopenia purpura.

CONTRAINDICATIONS Rho(D)-positive patient; person previously immunized against Rho(D) factor, severe immune globulin hypersensitivity, bleeding disorders.

CAUTIOUS USE IgA deficiency; pregnancy (category C); neonates.

R

ROUTE & DOSAGE

Note: Only **WinRho SDF** and **Rhophylac** can be given IV. **BayRho-D** and **RhoGAM** are available in regular and mini-dose vials.

Antepartum Prophylaxis

Adult: **IM/IV** 300 mcg at approximately 28-wk gestation; followed by 1 vial of mini-dose or 120 mcg within 72 h of delivery if infant is Rh-positive

Postpartum Prophylaxis

Adult: **IM/IV** 300 mcg preferably within 72 h of delivery if infant is Rh-positive

Following Amniocentesis, Miscarriage, Abortion, Ectopic Pregnancy

Adult: **IM** If over 13-wk gestation, 300 mcg, preferably within 3 h but at least within 72 h; if less than 13 wk, give 50 mcg

Transfusion Accident

Adult: **IM/IV** 300 mcg for each volume of RBCs infused divided by 15, given within at least 72 h of accident

Child: **IV** Administer 600 mcg q8h until total dose given. Exposure to positive whole blood 9 mcg/mL, exposure to positive RBCs 18 mcg/mL. **IM** Administer 1200 mcg q12h until total dose given. Exposure to positive whole blood 12 mcg/mL, exposure to positive RBCs 24 mcg/mL.

Idiopathic Thrombocytopenia Purpura

Adult/Child: **IV** 50 mcg/kg, then 25–60 mcg/kg depending on response

R

ADMINISTRATION

- BayRho-D (HyperRHO S/D), MIC-RhoGam, and RhoGAM are administered by IM route only. NEVER give IV.
- WinRho SDF and Rhophylac may be given IM or IV depending on the indication.

Intramuscular

- Use the deltoid muscle. Give in divided doses at different sites, all at once or at intervals, as long as the entire dose is given within 72 h after delivery or termination of pregnancy.
- Observe patient closely for at least 20 min after administration. Keep epinephrine immediately available; systemic allergic reactions sometimes occur.

Intravenous

PREPARE: **Direct:** No dilution is required for products supplied in liquid form. ▪ **WinRho SDF:** Remove entire contents of vial to obtain the labeled dosage. If partial vial is needed for dosage calculation, withdraw the entire contents to ensure accurate calculation of dosage requirement. ▪ **Rhophylac:** Bring to room temperature before use.

ADMINISTER: **Direct: Rhophylac:** Give at a rate of 2 mL/15–60 sec for ITP. ▪ **WinRho SDF:** Give over 3–5 min.

▪ Refrigerate commercially prepared solutions, although it may remain stable up to 30 days at room temperature according to manufacturer. ▪ Discard solutions that have been frozen. ▪ Store powder at 2°–8° C (36°–46° F) unless otherwise directed; avoid freezing.

ADVERSE EFFECTS Other: Injection site irritation, slight fever, myalgia, lethargy.

INTERACTIONS Drug: May interfere with immune response to LIVE VIRUS VACCINE; should delay use of LIVE VIRUS VACCINES for 3 mo after administration of Rho(D) immune globulin.

PHARMACOKINETICS Peak: 2 h IV, 5–10 days IM. **Half-Life:** 25 days.

NURSING IMPLICATIONS

Black Box Warning

Rho(D) immune globulin has been associated with severe anemia, acute renal insufficiency, renal failure, DIC, and intravascular hemolysis leading to death.

Assessment & Drug Effects

- Obtain history of systemic allergic reactions to human immune globulin preparations prior to drug administration in patients with ITP.
- Monitor closely patients with ITP for at least 8 h after administration.
- Monitor for S&S of intravascular hemolysis, including back pain, shaking chills, fever, and discolored urine or hematuria.
- Monitor lab test: Dipstick urinalysis at baseline, 2 and 4 h after administration, and prior to the end of the monitoring period; periodic CBC, renal function tests, LFTs.

Patient & Family Education

- Report promptly early signs of allergic or hypersensitivity reactions to Rho(D) immune globulin, including anaphylaxis, chest tightness, generalized urticaria, hives, and wheezing.
- When treated for ITP, immediately report symptoms of intravascular hemolysis (i.e., back pain, decreased urine output, discolored urine, fluid retention/edema, fever, shaking chills, shortness of breath, and/or sudden weight gain).
- Be aware that administration of Rho(D) immune globulin (antibody) prevents hemolytic disease of the newborn in a subsequent pregnancy.

RIBAVIRIN

(rye-ba-vye′rin)

Rebetol, Virazole

Classification: ANTIHEPACIVIRIAL, NUCLEOSIDE

Therapeutic: ANTIVIRAL

Prototype: Acyclovir

AVAILABILITY Inhalation solution; tablet; capsule; oral solution

ACTION & *THERAPEUTIC EFFECT* Inhibits replication of DNA and RNA viruses; inhibits influenza virus RNA polymerase activity and inhibits the initiation and elongation of RNA fragments resulting in inhibition of viral protein synthesis. *Active against many RNA and DNA viruses.*

USES Aerosol product used for selected infants and young children with respiratory syncytial virus (RSV). Oral product used in combination with direct-acting antivirals to treat chronic hepatitis C infection.

UNLABELED USES viral hemorrhagic fever.

CONTRAINDICATIONS Mild RSV infections of lower respiratory tract; infants requiring simultaneous assisted ventilation; unstable cardiac disease; pancreatitis; autoimmune hepatitis; HCV infection;

renal failure; suicidal ideations; hemoglobinopathy; hepatic decompensation; hypersensitivity to ribavirin or any component of the formulation; concomitant use with didanosine; women who are of child bearing age; pregnancy (significant teratogenic and embryocidal effects; avoid pregnancy during therapy and for 6 months after completion of treatment in both female patients and female partners of male patients who are taking ribavirin therapy); lactation.

CAUTIOUS USE COPD, asthma; risk for severe anemia; history of MI, cardiac arrhythmias, cardiac disease; decreased renal, hepatic, or cardiac function; respiratory depression; severe anemia; history of depression or suicidal tendencies; older adults; children younger than 3 y.

ROUTE & DOSAGE

RSV

Child: **Inhalation** 6g continuous aerosolization administered over 12–18 h/day for 3–7 days **Inhalation** 2000 mg over 2 hours tid inn non mechanically ventilated patients for 3–7 days

Hepatitis C adjust per genotype

Adult/Adolescent/Child (weight greater than 80 kg): **PO** 1.2 g daily in 2 divided doses; *weight less than 75 kg:* 1 g daily in 2 divided doses
Child/Adolescent (weight 66–80 kg): **PO** 1000 mg/day in 2 divided doses; *weight 50–65 kg:* 800 mg/day in 2 divided doses; *weight 47–49 kg:* 600 mg/day in 2 divided doses; *3 y or older, weight less than 47 kg:* 15 mg/kg/day in divided doses

Renal Impairment Dosage Adjustment

CrCl less than 50 mL/min: varies per dosage form confirm with package insert.

ADMINISTRATION

Oral

- Give tablets/solution with food. Ensure that tablets and capsules are swallowed whole. Do not open, crush, or chew capsules.

Inhalation

- Administer only by SPAG-2 aerosol generator, following manufacturer's directions.
- Caution: Ribavirin has demonstrated teratogenicity in animals. Advise pregnant healthcare personnel of the potential teratogenic risks associated with exposure during ribavirin administration to patients.
- Do not give other aerosol medication concomitantly with ribavirin.
- Discard solution in the SPAG-2 reservoir at least q24h and whenever liquid level is low before fresh reconstituted solution is added.
- Store unopened vial in a dry place at 15°–25° C (59°–78° F) unless otherwise directed.
- Following reconstitution, store solution at 20°–30° C (68°–86° F) for 24 h.

ADVERSE EFFECTS **CV:** Chest pain. **Respiratory:** Cough, dyspnea, dyspnea on exertion, flu-like symptoms, pharyngitis, sinusitis, rhinitis, upper respiratory tract infection. **CNS:** Anxiety, depression, emotional lability, irritability, lack of concentration, nervousness, RUQ pain, rigors, malaise, memory impairment, mood changes, *dizziness, headache, insomnia, fatigue.* back pain. **HEENT:** Conjunctivitis, blurred vision. **Endocrine:** *Weight loss*, growth retardation, hyperuricemia, hypothyroidism, menstrual disease. **Hepatic/GI:** *Diarrhea, nausea, vomiting*, abdominal pain, anorexia, dyspepsia, xerostomia, decreased appetite, hyperbilirubinemia, constipation. **Skin:** Alopecia, dermatitis, diaphoresis, skin rash, xeroderma, eczema. **Hematologic:** *Neutropenia*, lymphocytopenia, hemolytic anemia (especially in combination with interferon alpha), leukopenia, thrombocytopenia. **Musculoskeletal:** Arthralgia, asthenia, musculoskeletal pain, myalgia, back pain. **Other:** Viral infection, bacterial infection, chills, fever, injection site reaction (erythema, inflammation).

INTERACTIONS **Drug:** Ribavirin may antagonize the antiviral effects of **zidovudine** against HIV; increased risk of fetal defects with **peginterferon.** Do not administer with LIVE VIRUS VACCINES. Increases risk of adverse effects with **azathioprine, cladribine, didanosine.**

PHARMACOKINETICS **Absorption:** Rapidly absorbed orally (44%) and systemically from lungs. **Peak:** Inhaled 60–90 min. PO 1.7–3 h. **Distribution:** Crosses placenta; distributed into breast milk. **Metabolism:** In cells to an active metabolite. **Elimination:** 85% in urine, 15% in feces. **Half-Life:** 24 h in plasma, 16–40 days in RBCs.

NURSING IMPLICATIONS

Black Box Warning

Ribavirin has been associated with hemolytic anemia which may worsen cardiac disease and cause MI, and with fetal toxicity.

Assessment & Drug Effects

- Monitor respiratory function and fluid status closely during therapy. Note baseline rate and character of respirations and pulse. Observe for signs of labored breathing: Dyspnea, apnea; rapid, shallow respirations, intercostal and substernal retraction, nasal flaring, limited excursion of lungs, cyanosis. Auscultate lungs for abnormal breath sounds.
- Monitor cardiac status, including ECG, especially in those with preexisiting cardiac dysfunction.
- Monitor lab tests: Baseline CBC with differential and platelet count, repeat at 2 and 4 wk, and periodically thereafter; baseline and periodic serum electrolytes, LFTs, renal function tests, CD4+ cell count, TSH and T4. Perform baseline pregnancy test.

Patient & Family Education

- Both male and female patients should take every precaution to prevent pregnancy during treatment and for 6 mo following the end of therapy.
- Inform prescriber immediately if a pregnancy occurs within 6 mo of completing therapy.
- Drink fluids liberally unless otherwise advised by prescriber.
- Use caution with hazardous activities until response to drug is known.

RIBOFLAVIN (VITAMIN B_2)

(rye′bo-flay-vin)

Classification: VITAMIN
Therapeutic: VITAMIN REPLACEMENT

AVAILABILITY Tablet; capsule

ACTION & *THERAPEUTIC EFFECT*

Component of flavoprotein enzymes that work together, which are necessary for normal tissue respiration; needed for activation of pyridoxine and conversion of tryptophan to niacin. *Evaluated by improvement of clinical manifestations of deficiency: Digestive disturbances, headache, burning sensation of skin (especially "burning" feet), cracking at corners of mouth (cheilosis), glossitis, seborrheic dermatitis (and other skin lesions), mental depression, corneal vascularization (with photophobia, burning and itchy eyes, lacrimation, roughness of eyelids), anemia, neuropathy.*

USES To prevent and treat riboflavin deficiency, also to treat microcytic anemia.

UNLABELED USE To prevent migraine headaches.

CAUTIOUS USE Pregnancy (riboflavin requirements may be increased in pregnant women); lactation.

ROUTE & DOSAGE

Dietary Supplement

Adult: **PO** 100 mg once or twice daily
Child: **PO** included in typical multivitamin

ADMINISTRATION

Oral

- Give with food to enhance absorption.
- Store in airtight containers protected from light.

ADVERSE EFFECTS GU: Urine discoloration (yellow-orange).

DIAGNOSTIC TEST INTERFERENCE

In large doses, riboflavin may produce yellow-green fluorescence in ***urine*** and thus cause false elevations in certain ***fluorometric determinations*** of ***urinary catecholamines.***

PHARMACOKINETICS Absorption: Readily absorbed from GI tract. **Distribution:** Little is stored; excess amounts are excreted in urine. **Elimination:** In urine. **Half-Life:** 66–84 min.

NURSING IMPLICATIONS

Assessment & Drug Effects

- Collaborate with prescriber, dietitian, patient, and responsible family member in planning for diet. A complete dietary history is an essential part of vitamin replacement so that poor eating habits can be identified and corrected. Deficiency in one vitamin is usually associated with other vitamin deficiencies.

Patient & Family Education

- Be aware that large doses may cause an intense yellow discoloration of urine.
- Note: Rich dietary sources of riboflavin are found in liver, kidney, beef, pork, heart, eggs, milk and milk products, yeast, whole-grain cereals, vitamin B–enriched breakfast cereals, green vegetables, and mushrooms.

RIFABUTIN
(rif-a-bu'tin)
Mycobutin
Classification: ANTIBIOTIC; ANTITUBERCULOSIS
Therapeutic: ANTITUBERCULOSIS
Prototype: Rifampin

AVAILABILITY Capsule

ACTION & *THERAPEUTIC EFFECT* Semisynthetic bacteriostatic antibiotic. Inhibits DNA-dependent RNA polymerase in susceptible bacterial cells but not in human cells. *Effective against* Mycobacterium avium *complex (MAC) (or* M. avium-intracellulare*) and many strains of* M. tuberculosis.

USES The prevention of disseminated *Mycobacterium avium* complex (MAC) disease in patients with advanced HIV infection.

CONTRAINDICATIONS Hypersensitivity to rifabutin or any other rifamycins; lactation.

CAUTIOUS USE Older adults, pregnancy (rifabutin crosses the placenta; use with caution); children.

ROUTE & DOSAGE

Prevention of MAC

Adult/Adolescent: **PO** 300 mg daily
Infant/Child: **PO** 10–20 mg/kg/dose daily (max 300 mg)

ADMINISTRATION

Oral

- Give the usual dose of 300 mg/day or in two divided doses of 150 mg with food if needed to reduce GI upset.
- Store at room temperature, 25° C (77° F).

ADVERSE EFFECTS **CNS:** *Headache.* **Skin:** Rash. **GI:** *Abdominal pain, nausea.* **Hematologic:** Thrombocytopenia, leukopenia, neutropenia. **Other:** *Turns urine, feces, saliva, sputum, perspiration, and tears orange. Soft contact lenses may be permanently discolored.*

INTERACTIONS **Drug:** Extensive drug interactions for complete list consult drug interaction database. May decrease levels of BENZODIAZEPINES, BETA-BLOCKERS, **clofibrate, dapsone, delavirdine, doravirine,** NARCOTICS, ANTICOAGULANTS, CORTICOSTEROIDS, HMG-COA REDUCTASE INHIBITORS, **cyclosporine, quinidine,** ORAL CONTRACEPTIVES, PROGESTINS, SULFONYLUREAS, **ketoconazole, fluconazole,** BARBITURATES, **theophylline,** ANTICONVULSANTS, and other medications metabolized by CYP3A4 or UGT1A4 resulting in therapeutic failure. ANTIFUNGALS, **atazanavir, darunavir**, **fosamprenavir,** may increase adverse effects. Do not use with LIVE VIRUS VACCINES. Efavirenz may decrease levels of rifabutin.

PHARMACOKINETICS **Absorption:** 12–20% of oral dose reaches the systemic circulation. **Peak:** 2–3 h. **Distribution:** 85% protein bound. Widely distributed, high concentrations in the lungs, liver, spleen, eyes, and kidney. Crosses placenta, distributed into breast milk. **Metabolism:** In the liver. Causes induction of hepatic enzymes. **Elimination:** Urine (53% as metabolites), 30% in feces. **Half-Life:** 16–96 h (average 45 h).

NURSING IMPLICATIONS

Assessment & Drug Effects

- Monitor patients for S&S of active TB. Report immediately.

- Evaluate patients on concurrent oral hypoglycemic therapy for loss of glycemic control.
- Review patient's complete drug regimen because dosage adjustment of a significant number of drugs may be needed when rifabutin is added to regimen.
- Monitor lab tests: Periodic LFTs, CBC with differential and platelet count.

Patient & Family Education

- Learn S&S of TB and MAC (e.g., persistent fever, progressive weight loss, anorexia, night sweats, diarrhea) and notify prescriber if any of these develop.
- Notify prescriber of following: Muscle or joint pain, eye pain or other discomfort, chest pain with dyspnea, rash, or a flu-like syndrome.
- Be aware that urine, feces, saliva, sputum, perspiration, tears, and skin may be colored brown-orange. Soft contact lens may be permanently discolored.
- Rifabutin may reduce the activity of a wide variety of drugs. Provide a complete and accurate list of concurrent drugs to the prescriber for evaluation.

R

RIFAMPIN Pr

(rif'am-pin)

Rifadin, Rofact ♣

Classification: ANTIBIOTIC; ANTITUBERCULOSIS

Therapeutic: ANTITUBERCULOSIS

AVAILABILITY Capsule; solution for injection

ACTION & *THERAPEUTIC EFFECT* Inhibits DNA-dependent RNA polymerase activity in susceptible bacterial cells, thereby suppressing RNA synthesis. *Active against* Mycobacterium tuberculosis, M. leprae, Neisseria meningitidis, *and a wide range of gram-negative and gram-positive organisms.*

USES Initial treatment and retreatment of tuberculosis; as short-term therapy to prevent meningococcal infection.

UNLABELED USES Chemoprophylaxis in contacts of patients with *Haemophilus influenzae* type B infection; leprosy (especially dapsone-resistant leprosy); endocarditis, pruritus.

CONTRAINDICATIONS Hypersensitivity to rifampin; obstructive biliary disease; meningococcal disease; intermittent rifampin therapy.

CAUTIOUS USE Hepatic disease; history of alcoholism; IBD. Concomitant use of other hepatotoxic agents; pregnancy (postnatal hemorrhages have been observed in the infant and mother with administration during the last weeks of pregnancy).

ROUTE & DOSAGE

Pulmonary Tuberculosis

Adults: **PO/IV** 10 mg/kg (max: 600 mg) daily for 2 mo with other agents
Child: **PO** 15–20 mg/kg/day (max: 600 mg/day) with other agents
Infant/Child (with HIV): **PO** 10–20 mg/kg once daily (max: 600 mg) daily for 2 mo with other agents

Meningococcal Prophylaxis

Adult: **PO** 600 mg q12h for 2 consecutive days

Adolescent/Child/Infant: **PO** 20 mg/kg/day in divided doses × 2 consecutive days (max: 600 mg/day)

ADMINISTRATION

Oral

- Give 1 h before or 2 h after a meal on an empty stomach with a glass of water. Peak serum levels are delayed and may be slightly lower when given with food; capsule contents may be emptied into fluid or mixed with food.
- Note: An oral suspension can be prepared from capsules for use with pediatric patients. Shake oral suspension well before using. May mix capsule contents with applesauce or jelly.
- Keep a desiccant in bottle containing capsules to prevent moisture causing instability.

Intravenous

PREPARE: **IV Infusion:** Reconstitute vial by adding 10 mL of sterile water for injection to each 600 mg to yield 60 mg/mL. Swirl to dissolve. ▪ Withdraw the ordered dose and further dilute in 500 mL of D5W (preferred) or NS. ▪ If absolutely necessary, 100 mL of D5W or NS may be used. ***ADMINISTER:*** **IV Infusion:** Infuse 500 mL solution over 3 h and 100 mL solution over 30 min. ▪ Note: A less concentrated solution infused over a longer period is preferred. Avoid extravasation. ***INCOMPATIBILITIES:*** **Solution/additive: ethambutol, isoniazid, minocycline. Y-site: diltiazem, tramadol.**

- Use NS solutions within 24 h and D5W solutions within 4 h of preparation.

ADVERSE EFFECTS **Cardiovascular:** Decreased Bp, flushing, shock, vasculitis. **Respiratory:** Dyspnea, flu-like symptoms, wheezing. **CNS:** Fatigue, drowsiness, headache, ataxia, confusion, dizziness, inability to concentrate, generalized numbness, peripheral pain, muscular weakness, behavioral changes. **HEENT:** Visual disturbances. **Endocrine:** Adrenocortical insufficiency, menstrual disease. **Skin:** Erythema multiforme, pemphigoid reaction, pruritis, skin rash, urticarial. **GI:** *Epigastric distress, nausea, vomiting, anorexia, flatulence, cramps, diarrhea,* staining of teeth, *elevated liver function tests* (bilirubin, BSP, alkaline phosphatase, ALT, AST), jaundice. **GU:** <u>Acute renal failure</u>, renal insufficiency, renal tubular necrosis, interstitial nephritis. **Hematologic:** <u>Thrombocytopenia</u>, transient <u>leukopenia</u>, anemia, including hemolytic anemia. **Musculoskeletal:** Myopathy. **Other:** Hypersensitivity (fever, pruritus, urticaria, skin eruptions, soreness of mouth and tongue, eosinophilia, hemolysis), flu-like syndrome. Increasing lethargy, liver enlargement and tenderness, jaundice, brownish-red or orange discoloration of skin, sweat, saliva, tears, and feces.

DIAGNOSTIC TEST INTERFERENCE

Rifampin interferes with contrast media used for ***gallbladder study;*** therefore, test should precede daily dose of rifampin. Inhibits standard assays for ***serum folate*** and ***vitamin*** $\boldsymbol{B_{12}}$, may cause false-positive opiate urine screen.

INTERACTIONS **Drug:** Extensive drug interactions, for complete list consult drug interaction database. Do not use with PROTEASE INHIBITORS and **nevirapine** as it may increase

R

treatment failure rate. **Alcohol, isoniazid, pyrazinamide**, **ritonavir,** saquinavir increase risk of drug-induced hepatotoxicity. decreases concentrations of **alfentanil, alosetron, alprazolam, amprenavir,** BARBITURATES, BENZODIAZEPINES, **carbamazepine, atovaquone, cevimeline, chloramphenicol, clofibrate,** CORTICOSTEROIDS, **cyclosporine, dapsone, delavirdine, diazepam, digoxin, diltiazem, disopyramide, estazolam, estramustine, fentanyl, fosphenytoin, fluconazole galantamine, indinavir, itraconazole, ketoconazole, lamotrigine, levobupivacaine, lopinavir, methadone, metoprolol, mexiletine, midazolam, nelfinavir,** ORAL SULFONYLUREAS, ORAL CONTRACEPTIVES, **phenytoin,** PROGESTINS, **propafenone, propranolol, quinidine, quinine, ritonavir, sirolimus, theophylline,** THYROID HORMONES, **tocainide, tramadol, verapamil, warfarin, zaleplon,** and **zonisamide,** drugs metabolized by CYP3A4 leading to potential therapeutic failure. Do not use with **simvastatin.**

R

PHARMACOKINETICS Absorption: Readily from GI tract. **Peak:** 2–4 h. **Distribution:** Widely distributed, including CSF; crosses placenta; distributed into breast milk; 80% protein bound. **Metabolism:** In liver to active and inactive metabolites; is enterohepatically cycled. **Elimination:** Up to 30% in urine, 60–65% in feces. **Half-Life:** 3 h.

NURSING IMPLICATIONS

Assessment & Drug Effects

- Monitor for extravasation during injection; local irritation and inflammation due to infiltration of the infusion may occur. If so, DC infusion and restart at another site.
- Check prothrombin time daily or as necessary to establish and maintain required anticoagulant activity when patient is also receiving an anticoagulant.
- Monitor lab tests: Periodic LFTs, serum creatinine, CBC, and platelet count.

Patient & Family Education

- Do not interrupt prescribed dosage regimen. Hepatorenal reaction with flu-like syndrome has occurred when therapy has been resumed following interruption.
- Be aware that drug may impart a harmless red-orange color to urine, feces, sputum, sweat, and tears. Soft contact lenses may be permanently stained.
- Report onset of jaundice, hypersensitivity reactions, and persistence of GI adverse effects to prescriber.
- Use or add barrier contraceptive if using hormonal contraception. Concomitant use of rifampin and oral contraceptives leads to decreased effectiveness of the contraceptive and to menstrual disturbances (spotting, breakthrough bleeding).
- Keep drug out of reach of children.

RIFAMYCIN

(rif-a-mye-sin)

Aemcolo

Classifications: ANTIDIARRHEAL; ANTIBIOTIC

Therapeutic: ANTIDIARRHEAL

Prototype: Rifampin

AVAILABILITY Oral tablet

ACTION & *THERAPEUTIC EFFECT* Inhibits bacterial synthesis by inhibiting the beta-subunit of the bacterial DNA-dependent RNA polymerase. *Used to treat travelers' diarrhea caused by noninvasive strains of Escherichia coli in adults.*

USES Treatment of traveler's diarrhea.

CONTRAINDICATIONS Hypersensitivity to rifamycin class antimicrobial agents or any component of the formulation.

CAUTIOUS USE Prolonged use may cause superinfection. Use with caution in the elderly, during pregnancy, and with lactation.

ROUTE & DOSAGE

Traveler's Diarrhea

Adult: **PO** 388 mg (two tablets) twice a day for three days

ADMINISTRATION

Oral

- Administer each dose with 6 to 8 ounces of nonalcoholic liquid, with or without food.
- Swallow tablets whole; do not crush, break, or chew.
- Store at 20° to 25° C (68° to 77° F).

ADVERSE EFFECTS **CNS:** Headache. **GI:** Constipation, abdominal pain.

INTERACTIONS Do not use with LIVE VACCINES.

PHARMACOKINETICS **Absorption:** <0.1% bioavailability. **Distribution:** 80% protein bound. **Elimination:** 86% excreted in the feces.

NURSING IMPLICATIONS

Assessment & Drug Effects

- Monitor for bloody stools as well as the frequency of diarrhea.

Patient & Family Education

- Notify your doctor or get medical help right away if you have any of the following signs or symptoms of allergic reaction such as rash, hives, itching; red, swollen, blistered, or peeling skin with or without fever; wheezing; tightness in the chest or throat; trouble breathing, swallowing, or talking; unusual hoarseness; or swelling of the mouth, face, lips, tongue, or throat; or any dizziness or passing out.

RIFAPENTINE

(rif'a-pen-teen)

Priftin

Classification: ANTIBIOTIC; ANTITUBERCULOSIS; MYCOBACTERIUM

Therapeutic: ANTITUBERCULOSIS

Prototype: Rifampin

AVAILABILITY Tablet

ACTION & *THERAPEUTIC EFFECT* Inhibits DNA-dependent RNA polymerase activity in susceptible bacterial cells, thereby suppressing RNA synthesis. *Effective against* Mycobacterium tuberculosis.

USES Active or latent pulmonary tuberculosis in conjunction with at least one other agent.

CONTRAINDICATIONS Hypersensitivity to any rifamycins (e.g., rifampin, rifabutin, rifapentine); porphyria; continuation phase of treatment in HIV-seropositive patients; soft contact lens; lactation.

CAUTIOUS USE Patients with abnormal liver function tests or hepatic disease; HIV disease; cavitary pulmonary lesions, bilateral pulmonary disease; older adults; pregnancy (limited information related to use in pregnant women); children.

R

ROUTE & DOSAGE

Active Tuberculosis

Adult/Adolescent: **PO** 600 mg twice weekly (at least 72 h apart) × 2 mo, then 600 mg once weekly × 4 mo

Latent Tuberculosis

Adult/Adolescent/Child (weight greater than 50 kg): **PO** 900 mg once weekly; *weight 32.1–50 kg:* 750 mg once weekly; *weight 25.1–32 kg:* 600 mg once weekly; *weight 14–25 kg:* 450 mg once weekly

ADMINISTRATION

Oral

- Give with an interval of NO LESS than 72 h between doses.
- Give with food to minimize GI upset. For patients who cannot swallow tablets, tablets may be crushed and added to small amount of semi-solid food and consumed immediately.
- Store at 25° C (77° F) in a tightly closed container and protect from excess moisture.

R

ADVERSE EFFECTS **CV:** Chest pain, edema. **Respiratory:** Hemoptysis, cough. **Skin:** Rash, diaphoresis. **GI/Hepatic:** Increased liver function tests (ALT, AST). **GU:** Uremia. **Hematologic:** Lymphocytopenia, anemia, leukopenia, thrombocytosis. **Musculoskeletal:** Back pain, arthralgia. **Other:** Hypersensitivity reaction.

DIAGNOSTIC TEST INTERFERENCE Inhibits standard assays for *serum folate* and *vitamin* B_{12}.

INTERACTIONS **Drug:** There are extensive drug interactions, consult a drug information database for a complete list. Decreased activity of ORAL CONTRACEPTIVES, **phenytoin, disopyramide, mexiletine, quinidine, tocainide, warfarin, fluconazole, itraconazole, ketoconazole, diazepam,** BETA-BLOCKERS, CALCIUM CHANNEL BLOCKERS, CORTICOSTEROIDS, **haloperidol,** SULFONYLUREAS, **cyclosporine, tacrolimus, levothyroxine,** NARCOTIC ANALGESICS, **quinine,** REVERSE TRANSCRIPTASE INHIBITORS, TRICYCLIC ANTIDEPRESSANTS, ANTIHEPACIVIRAL **sildenafil, theophylline,** drugs metabolized by CYP3A4. ANTFUNGAL AGENTS may increase the concentration of rifapentine.

PHARMACOKINETICS **Absorption:** 70% absorbed. **Peak:** 5–6 h. **Distribution:** 97.7% protein bound. **Metabolism:** Hydrolyzed by esterase enzyme to active metabolite in liver; inducer of cytochromes P450 3A4 and 2C8/9. **Elimination:** 70% in feces, 17% in urine. **Half-Life:** 13.3 h.

NURSING IMPLICATIONS

Assessment & Drug Effects

- Monitor carefully for S&S of toxicity with concurrent use of oral anticoagulants, digitalis preparations, or anticonvulsants.
- Monitor lab tests: Sputum smear and culture, baseline LFTs and repeat q4–6wk in those with preexisting hepatic impairment.

Patient & Family Education

- Follow strict adherence to the prescribed dosing schedule to prevent emergence of resistant strains of tuberculosis.
- Be aware that food may be useful in preventing GI upset.
- Report immediately any of the following to the prescriber: Fever, weakness, nausea or vomiting, loss of appetite, dark urine or yellowing of eyes or skin, pain or swelling of the joints, severe or persistent diarrhea.

- Use or add barrier contraceptive if using hormonal contraception.

RIFAXIMIN

(ri-fax′i-min)

Xifaxan

Classification: RIFAMYCIN ANTIBIOTIC; MYCOBACTERIUM

Therapeutic: MYCOBACTERIUM

Prototype: Rifampin

AVAILABILITY Tablet

ACTION & *THERAPEUTIC EFFECT* Inhibits bacterial RNA synthesis by binding to DNA-dependent RNA polymerase, thereby blocking RNA transcription. *Its spectrum of activity includes gram-positive and gram-negative aerobes and anaerobes.*

USES Treatment of traveler's diarrhea, prevention of hepatic encephalopathy, irritable bowel syndrome without constipation.

UNLABELED USES Crohn's disease, Clostridioides difficile infection, hepatic encephalopathy treatment, prophylaxis of traveler's diarrhea, diverticulitis.

CONTRAINDICATIONS Hypersensitivity to rifaximin, other rifamycin antimicrobial agents or to any of its components; dysentery; lactation.

CAUTIOUS USE Diarrhea with fever and/or blood in the stool, or diarrhea due to organisms other than *E. coli*; IBD, worsening diarrhea or diarrhea persisting for longer than 24–48 h; pregnancy (adverse events have been observed in some animal reproduction studies); children younger than 12 y.

ROUTE & DOSAGE

Traveler's Diarrhea Treatment

Adult/Adolescent: **PO** 200 mg tid for 3 days

Reduce Risk of Hepatic Encephalopathy Recurrence

Adult: **PO** 550 mg bid or 400 mg tid

Irritable Bowel Syndrome

Adult: **PO** 550 mg tid × 14 days

ADMINISTRATION

Oral

- May be given without regard to food.
- Store at 20°–25° C (68°–77° F).

ADVERSE EFFECTS **CV:** Peripheral edema. **Respiratory:** Dyspnea, nasopharyngitis. **CNS:** Headache, depression, dizziness, fatigue. **Skin:** Pruritis, skin rash. **GI/Hepatic:** Ascites, abdominal pain, C.diff colitis, nausea. **Musculoskeletal:** Arthralgia, increased CPK, muscle spasm, myalgia. **Hematologic:** Anemia. **Other:** Fever.

INTERACTIONS **Drug:** Do not administer cholera vaccine within 14 days of therapy. **Lasmiditan** may increase risk of adverse effects.

PHARMACOKINETICS **Absorption:** Less than 0.4% absorbed orally. **Peak:** 1.21 h. **Metabolized:** via CYP3A4 **Elimination:** In feces. **Half-Life:** 5.85 h.

NURSING IMPLICATIONS

Assessment & Drug Effects

- Withhold drug and notify prescriber if diarrhea worsens or lasts longer than 48 h after starting

R

drug; an alternative treatment should be considered.

- Report promptly the appearance of blood in the stool.
- Monitor lab values: Serum ammonia.

Patient & Family Education

- Report promptly any of the following: Fever; difficulty breathing; skin rash, itching, or hives; worsening diarrhea during or after treatment or blood in the stool.

RILPIVIRINE

(ril-pi′vi-reen)

Edurant

Classification: ANTIRETROVIRAL; NONNUCLEOSIDE REVERSE TRANSCRIPTASE INHIBITOR (NNRTI)

Therapeutic: ANTIRETROVIRAL; NNRTI

Prototype: Efavirenz

AVAILABILITY Tablet

ACTION & *THERAPEUTIC EFFECT* A nonnucleoside reverse transcriptase inhibitor (NNRTI) of human immunodeficiency virus type 1 (HIV-1). *Inhibits HIV-1 replication and slows/prevents disease progression.*

USES Treatment of HIV-1 infection in combination with other antiretroviral agents in adult patients who are treatment-naïve.

CONTRAINDICATIONS Concurrent drugs that significantly decrease rilpivirine plasma level such as anticonvulsants, antimycobacterials, proton pump inhibitors, systemic dexamethasone, St. John's wort; lactation.

CAUTIOUS USE Congenital prolonged QT interval or concurrent drugs that prolong the QT interval; depressive disorders or suicidal ideation; older adult; severe renal impairment; hepatic impairment; pregnancy (category B). Safety and efficacy in children not established.

ROUTE & DOSAGE

HIV-1 Infection (with Other Agents)

Adult: **PO** 25 mg once daily

ADMINISTRATION

Oral

- Give with a full meal.
- Swallow tablet whole with water.
- If antacids are prescribed, they must be given at least 2 h before or 4 h after rilpivirine.
- Store at 15–30° C (59–86° F) and protect from light.

ADVERSE EFFECTS **CNS:** Depression, headache, drowsiness, suicidal thoughts. **Endocrine:** Decreased plasma cortisol, increased serum cholesterol. **Hepatic:** Increased serum ALT, increased serum AST.

INTERACTIONS **Drug:** Strong CYP3A4 inhibitors (e.g., **atazanavir, clarithromycin, delaviridine, indinavir, itraconazole, ketoconazole, nefazodone, nelfinavir, ritonavir, saquinavir,** and **telithromycin**) **voriconazole,** can increase rilpivirine levels, while strong CYP3A4 inducers (e.g., **rifampin, dexamethasone, phenytoin, carbamazepine, efavirenz,** and **phenobarbital**) can decrease rilpivirine levels. Antacids, GLUCOCORTICOIDS, H_2 RECEPTOR ANTAGONISTS, **methadone** can decrease rilpivirine. Rilpivirine can decrease the levels of **methadone.** Rilpivirine has been associated with QT prolongation. Coadministration of other drug that prolongs the QT interval (e.g., **disopyramide, procainamide, amiodarone, bretylium, clarithromycin, levofloxacin**) may cause additive effects. **Food:** Administration with a meal enhances absorption. **Herbal: St. John's wort** may decrease the levels of rilpivirine.

PHARMACOKINETICS **Peak:** 4–5 h. **Distribution:** 99.7% plasma protein bound. **Metabolism:** In liver (CYP3A4). **Elimination:** Fecal (85%) and renal (6%). **Half-Life:** 50 h.

NURSING IMPLICATIONS

Assessment & Drug Effects

- Monitor closely for adverse effects in those with severe renal impairment.
- Monitor for and report promptly signs of depression or suicidal ideation.
- Monitor lab tests: Periodic plasma HIV RNA; baseline and periodic LFTs, cholesterol, and triglycerides.

Patient & Family Education

- Drug absorption is improved when taken with a full meal.
- Seek immediate medical assistance if you experience depression or thoughts of suicide.
- Do not self-treat depression with St. John's wort.
- Report to prescriber all prescription and nonprescription drugs and herbal products you use.
- Do not use over-the-counter stomach medications without consent of your health care provider.
- If you use an antacid, take it at least 2 h before or 4 h after taking rilpivirine.

RILUZOLE

(ri-lu'zole)

Exservan, Rilutek, Tiglutik

Classification: AMYOTROPHIC LATERAL SCLEROSIS (ALS) AGENT; GLUTAMATE ANTAGONIST

Therapeutic: ALS AGENT

AVAILABILITY Tablet; oral suspension; oral film

ACTION & THERAPEUTIC EFFECT Inhibits the presynaptic release of glutamic acid in the CNS, inactivates voltage-dependent sodium channels, and interferes with intracellular events that follow transmitter binding at excitatory amino acid receptors. *Believed to reduce the degeneration of neurons in ALS.*

USES Treatment of ALS.

CONTRAINDICATIONS Hypersensitivity to riluzole; ALT levels are 5 × ULN or if clinical jaundice develops; lactation.

CAUTIOUS USE Hepatic dysfunction, renal impairment; hypertension, history of other CNS disorders; older adults; pregnancy (adverse events have been observed in animal reproduction studies). Safe use in children younger than 12 y is not established.

ROUTE & DOSAGE

ALS

Adult: **PO** 50 mg q12h

ADMINISTRATION

Oral

- Give at same time daily and at least 1 h before or 2 h after a meal. Do not give before/after a high-fat meal. Place film on tongue and allow to dissolve. Do not administer with liquids. As film dissolves, swallow saliva in a normal manner but avoid chewing, spitting, or talking. Do not cut or split film.
- Store at room temperature; protect from bright light.

R

ADVERSE EFFECTS **CV:** Hypertension, tachycardia, peripheral edema. **Respiratory:** *Decreased lung function,* cough, apnea. **CNS:** Dizziness, insomnia. **Skin:** Pruritus, eczema. **GI/Hepatic:** Abdominal pain, *nausea,* vomiting, oral hypoesthesia, increased serum AST. **Other:** *Asthenia,* arthralgia.

INTERACTIONS **Drug:** Significant drug interactions exist, requiring dose/frequency adjustment or avoidance. Consult drug interactions database for more complete information. BARBITURATES, **allopurinol** may increase risk of hepatotoxicity.

PHARMACOKINETICS **Absorption:** Well absorbed from GI tract, 60% reaches systemic circulation. **Peak:** Steady-state levels by day 5. **Distribution:** 96% protein bound. **Metabolism:** In liver by CYP1A2. **Elimination:** 90% in urine. **Half-Life:** 12 h.

NURSING IMPLICATIONS

Assessment & Drug Effects

- Withhold drug and notify prescriber if liver enzymes are elevated.
- Monitor lab tests: Baseline ALT, then monthly for 3 mo, then periodically thereafter.

Patient & Family Education

- Report any febrile illness to prescriber.
- Do not engage in potentially hazardous activities until response to drug is known.
- Learn common adverse effects and possible adverse interaction with alcohol.

RIMANTADINE

(ri-man'ta-deen)

Classification: ANTIVIRAL; ADMANTANE

Therapeutic: ANTIVIRAL
Prototype: Amantadine

AVAILABILITY Tablet

ACTION & *THERAPEUTIC EFFECT* Exerts an inhibitory effect early in the viral replication cycle, probably by interfering with the viral uncoating procedure of the influenza A virus. Inhibits synthesis of both viral RNA and viral protein, thus causing viral destruction. *Prevents or interrupts influenza A infections.*

USES Prophylaxis and treatment of influenza A.

CONTRAINDICATIONS Hypersensitivity to rimantadine and amantadine; lactation; children younger than 1 y for prophylaxis treatment.

CAUTIOUS USE History of seizures; renal or hepatic impairment; older adults; pregnancy (adverse effects have been observed in animal reproduction studies). Safe use in children younger than 17 y for treatment of Influenza A is not known.

ROUTE & DOSAGE

Prophylaxis of Influenza A

Adult/Child (10 y or older): **PO** 100 mg bid × 7 days; *Child (1–9 y):* **PO** 5 mg/kg daily (max: 150 mg/day) in divided doses
Geriatric: **PO** 100 mg daily

Treatment of Influenza A

Adult/Adolescent (17 y or older): **PO** 100 mg bid started within 48 h of symptoms and continued for 5–7 days from initial symptoms; *Child (over 10 y):* **PO** 5 mg/kg daily in divided doses (max: 200 mg/day) *(1–9 y):* 6.6 mg/kg daily in divided doses (max: 150 mg/day)

Hepatic Impairment Dosage Adjustment

100 mg daily with severe liver disease

Renal Impairment Dosage Adjustment

CrCl 10–30 mL/min: 100 mg daily

ADMINISTRATION

Oral

- May administer with food.
- Store at 25° C (77° F).

ADVERSE EFFECTS CNS: Insomnia, lack of concentration. **GI:** Nausea, anorexia.

INTERACTIONS Drug: Intranasal influenza vaccine should not be used within 48 h.

PHARMACOKINETICS Absorption: Readily absorbed from GI tract. **Peak:** Serum levels 3.2–4.3 h. **Distribution:** Concentrates in respiratory secretions. **Metabolism:** Extensively in liver. **Elimination:** By kidneys. **Half-Life:** 20–36 h.

NURSING IMPLICATIONS

Assessment & Drug Effects

- Monitor carefully for seizure activity in patients with a history of seizures. Seizures are an indication to discontinue the drug.
- Monitor for adverse GI or CNS effects.

Patient & Family Education

- Report bothersome adverse effects to prescriber; especially hallucinations, palpitations, difficulty breathing, and swelling of legs.
- Use caution with hazardous activities until reaction to drug is known.

RIMEGEPANT

(ri-ME-je-pant)

Nurtec

Classifications: CGRP RECEPTOR ANTAGONIST;
Therapeutic: ANTIMIGRAINE

AVAILABILITY Orally disintegrating tablet

ACTION & *THERAPEUTIC EFFECT* Rimegepant is a calcitonin gene-related peptide receptor antagonist. The exact mechanism by which it exerts its clinical effects to relieve migraines is unknown.

USES Preventative treatment of migraines and acute treatment of migraine with or without aura.

CONTRAINDICATIONS History of hypersensitivity to rimegepant or to any of its components; pregnancy—fetal risk cannot be ruled out; lactation—infant risk cannot be ruled out; safety and efficacy in pediatric patients have not been established.

CAUTIOUS USE Hypersensitivity reactions, including delayed serious reactions, have occurred. Discontinue if suspected.

ROUTE & DOSAGE

Migraine treatment

Adult: **PO** 75 mg as needed; max dose of 75 mg a day

Migraine prevention

Adult: **PO** 75 mg every other day

Renal Impairment Dosage Adjustment

eGFR less than 15 mL/min: Avoid use

Hepatic Impairment Dosage Adjustment

Child-Pugh class C (Severe impairment): Avoid use

ADMINISTRATION

Oral

- Use dry hands when opening the blister pack.
- Peel back the foil and gently remove the disintegrating tablet.
- Gently place the tablet on or under the tongue. It will dissolve in saliva without additional liquid.
- Use immediately after opening; do not store outside of the blister pack for future use.
- Store blister pack at controlled room temperature between 20 and 25° C (68 and 77° F), with excursions permitted between 15 and 30° C (59 and 86° F).

ADVERSE EFFECTS **GI:** Abdominal pain, dyspepsia, nausea (not common less than 3%)

INTERACTIONS **Drug:** Avoid use with strong or moderate CYP3A4 inducers (**carbmazepine, phenytoin,** etc.) and CYP3A4 inhibitors (**clarithromycin**, **ketoconazole)**. Concomitant use with inhibitors of P-gp and BCRP efflux inhibitors can increase rimegepant exposure and should be avoided.

PHARMACOKINETICS **Absorption:** 64% bioavailability; absorption decreased following high fat meal. **Peak:** 1.5 h; delayed following high fat meal. **Distribution:** 96% protein-bound. **Metabolism:** Primarily by CYP3A4. **Excretion:** 51% excreted in urine; 42% in feces. **Half-Life:** 11 h.

NURSING IMPLICATIONS

Assessment & Drug Effects

- Monitor for improvement of migraine pain.

Patient & Family Education

- Review adverse effects.
- Remind patient to not open the blister pack until ready to use.
- Allow patient to self-administer medication if physically able to demonstrate proper technique of removing disintegrating tablet from the blister pack and proper placement on or under the tongue.

RIMEXOLONE

(rim-ex'o-lone)

Vexol

See Appendix A-1.

RISANKIZUMAB-RZA

(ris-an-kiz-ue-mab)

Skyrizi

Classifications: ANTIPSORIATIC AGENT; IL-23 INHIBITOR

Therapeutic: ANTIPSORIATIC

Prototype: Guselkumab

AVAILABILITY Subcutaneous Injection

ACTION & *THERAPEUTIC EFFECT*

A human IgG1 monoclonal antibody which selectively binds to the p19 subunit of interleukin (IL)-23 resulting in inhibition of the release of proinflammatory cytokines and chemokines. *Used to treat moderate-to-severe plaque psoriasis in adults who are candidates for systemic therapy or phototherapy.*

USES Treatment of moderate to severe plaque psoriasis in patients who are candidates for systemic therapy or phototherapy

CAUTIOUS USE Tuberculosis; infection; pregnancy; lactation.

ROUTE & DOSAGE

Plaque psoriasis

Adult: **Subcutaneous** Two injections of 75 mg (total 150 mg) at weeks 0, 4, and then every 12 weeks thereafter

ADMINISTRATION

Subcutaneous

- Administer the two consecutive injections subcutaneously at different sites such as thighs, abdomen, or back of upper arms. Do not inject into tissue that is tender, bruised, or hard, or affected by psoriasis. Self injection may occur after proper training.
- Store at 2° to 8° C (36° to 46° F) in the original carton; do not freeze. Protect from light. Do not shake.

ADVERSE EFFECTS **Respiratory:** Upper respiratory infection. **CNS:** Headache, fatigue. **Other:** Antibody development, infection.

INTERACTIONS **Drug:** Avoid the use of live vaccines in patients being treated with risankizumab. Do not use with IMMUNOSUPPRESANTS.

PHARMACOKINETICS **Absorption:** 89% bioavailability. **Peak:** 3–14 days. **Distribution:** 11.2 L. **Metabolism:** Similar to endogenous IgG; degraded into small peptides and amino acids through catabolic pathways. **Half-Life:** 28 days.

NURSING IMPLICATIONS

Assessment & Drug Effects

- Perform baseline and ongoing screening for tuberculosis or signs and symptoms of infection. Do not initiate therapy if active infection present.
- Monitor lab tests: Tuberculin skin testing.

Patient & Family Education

- Notify your health care provider if you currently have or experience any symptoms of infection including tuberculosis or if you have had a recent live vaccine.
- Talk with your provider before getting any vaccines or if you are pregnant, planning on getting pregnant, or are breastfeeding.
- Notify your doctor or get medical help right away if you have any of the following signs or symptoms of allergic reaction such as rash, hives, itching; red, swollen, blistered, or peeling skin with or without fever; wheezing; tightness in the chest or throat; trouble breathing, swallowing, or talking; unusual hoarseness; or swelling of the mouth, face, lips, tongue, or throat; or any dizziness or passing out.

RISEDRONATE SODIUM

(ri-se-dron′ate)

Actonel, Atelvia

Classification: BISPHOSPHONATE; BONE METABOLISM REGULATOR

Therapeutic: BONE RESORPTION INHIBITOR; OSTEOPOROSIS TREATMENT

Prototype: Etidronate disodium

AVAILABILITY Tablet; delayed release tablet

ACTION & *THERAPEUTIC EFFECT* Inhibits bone resorption via action on osteoclasts or

R

osteoclast precursors; decreases the rate of bone resorption leading to an indirect increase in bone mineral density. *Effectiveness indicated by decreased bone and joint pain and improved bone density.*

USES Paget's disease, prevention and treatment of osteoporosis.

UNLABELED USES Osteolytic metastases.

CONTRAINDICATIONS Hypersensitivity to risedronate or other bisphosphonates; hypocalcemia, vitamin D deficiency; severe renal impairment (CrCl less than 30 mL/min); esophageal stricture; lactation.

CAUTIOUS USE Renal impairment; CHF; hyperphosphatemia or vitamin D deficiency; hepatic disease; UGI disease; fever related to infection or other causes; pregnancy (category C). Safety and efficacy in children younger than 18 y not established.

ROUTE & DOSAGE

Paget's Disease

Adult: **PO** 30 mg daily for 2 mo, may repeat after 2 mo rest if necessary

Prevention and Treatment of Osteoporosis (post menopausal)

Adult (female): **PO** 5 mg daily OR 35 mg once weekly OR 150 mg once monthly; **Delayed release** 35 mg weekly
Adult (male): **PO** 35 mg weekly
Adult (with chronic systemic glucocorticoid): **PO** 5 mg daily

Osteoporosis (glucocorticoid-induced) Prevention

Adult: **PO** 5 mg daily

Renal Impairment Dosage Adjustment

CrCl less than 30 mL/min: Use not recommended

ADMINISTRATION

Oral

- Give on an empty stomach (at least 30 min before first food or drink of the day) with at least 6–8 oz plain water. Ensure that tablet is swallowed whole. It should not be crushed or chewed.
- Note: Patient should be upright. Maintain upright position and empty stomach for at least 30 min after administration.
- Space calcium supplements and antacids as far as possible from risedronate.
- Store at 15°–30° C (59°–86° F) in a tightly closed container and protect from light.

ADVERSE EFFECTS **CV:** Hypertension. **CNS:** Headache. **Skin:** Skin rash. **GI:** Gastrointestinal perforation, ulcers, or bleeding, diarrhea, nausea, abdominal pain. **GU:** Urinary tract infection.

DIAGNOSTIC TEST INTERFERENCE May interfere with the use of ***bone-imaging agents.***

INTERACTIONS **Drug: Calcium,** ANTACIDS significantly decrease absorption, use with NONSTEROIDAL ANTI-INFLAMMATORIES may increase risk of gastric ulcer. Do not use with ANTIHISTAMINES. Use caution with PPIs due to changes in bioavailability. **Food:** Any food will decrease bioavailability. Take at least 30 min before first food or drink of the day.

PHARMACOKINETICS **Absorption:** Minimally absorbed from GI tract, bioavailability 0.63%.

Peak: 1 h. **Distribution:** Approximately 60% of dose is distributed to bone. **Metabolism:** Not metabolized. **Elimination:** In urine; unabsorbed drug excreted in feces. **Half-Life:** 220 h.

NURSING IMPLICATIONS

Assessment & Drug Effects

- Monitor carefully for and immediately report S&S of GI bleeding and hypocalcemia.
- Monitor lab tests: Baseline and periodic electrolytes including serum calcium, phosphorus, and alkaline phosphatase.

Patient & Family Education

- Administration guidelines regarding upright position, empty stomach, and spacing relative to calcium supplements and antacids **must be** strictly followed.
- Report any of the following to prescriber: Eye irritation, significant GI upset, or flu-like symptoms.
- Preventive dental care important for at-risk populations.

RISPERIDONE

(ris-per'i-done)

Risperdal, Risperdal M-TAB, Risperdal Consta

Classification: ATYPICAL ANTIPSYCHOTIC

Therapeutic: ANTIPSYCHOTIC

Prototype: Clozapine

AVAILABILITY Tablet; oral disintegrating tablet; oral solution; solution for injection; suspension for injection

ACTION & *THERAPEUTIC EFFECT* Interferes with binding of dopamine to D_2-interlimbic region of the brain, serotonin (5-HT_2) receptors, and alpha-adrenergic receptors in the occipital cortex. It has low to moderate affinity for the other serotonin (5-HT) receptors. *Effective in controlling symptoms of schizophrenia as well as other psychotic symptoms.*

USES Treatment of schizophrenia; treatment of bipolar disorder; irritability associated with autism.

UNLABELED USES Insomnia in elderly patient, obsessive-compulsive disorder, stuttering, tardive dyskinesia, Tourette syndrome.

CONTRAINDICATIONS Hypersensitivity to risperidone; older adults with dementia-related psychosis; drug induced narcoleptic malignant syndrome (NMS); severe CNS depression, head trauma; lactation. **Risperdal Consta:** Lactation during use and for 12 wk after last injection.

CAUTIOUS USE Arrhythmias, hypotension, breast cancer, blood dyscrasia, cardiac disorders, cerebrovascular disease, hypotension, dehydration, DM; diabetic ketoacidosis, hyperglycemia, MI, obesity, orthostatic hypotension, mild or moderate CNS depression; GI obstruction, dysphagia; electrolyte imbalance, drug and alcohol abuse; heart failure, MI, ischemia; arrhythmias; renal or hepatic impairment; seizure disorder, suicidal tendencies; stroke, Parkinson's disease;

Alzheimer dementia; risks for aspiration pneumonia; PKU; older adults; pregnancy (may cause hyperprolactemia which may cause decrease in reproductive function in females). Safe use in children younger than 13 y for schizophrenia; children younger than 10 y for bipolar disease and children younger than 5 y for autism not established.

ROUTE & DOSAGE

Schizophrenia

Adult: **PO** 1–2 mg/day in 1 or 2 doses, may titrate in 24 hour increments (max: 16 mg/day); *Adult/Geriatric:* **IM** 25 mg once q2wk (max: 50 mg) **Subcutaneous:** 90–120 mg monthly
Geriatric: **PO** Start 0.5 mg bid and increase by 0.5 mg bid daily to an initial target of 1.5 mg bid (max: 4 mg/day)

Bipolar Disorder

Adult: **PO** 1–3 mg once daily in divided doses for up to 3 wk (max: 6 mg/day); **IM** Initiate Risperdal Consta with 25 mg every 2 wk; may increase to 37.5–50 mg every 2 wk
Geriatric: **PO** Start with 0.5 mg bid and increase by 0.5 mg bid daily to an initial target of 1.5 mg bid (max: 6 mg/day). May convert to once daily dosing after stabilized.
Adolescent (10 y or older): **PO** 0.5 mg once daily titrate to recommended target dose range of 1–2.5 mg/day

Irritability Associated with Autism

Adolescent/Child (5 y or older, weight 20 kg or greater): **PO** 0.5 mg daily; after 4 days, increase to 1 mg daily; can increase by 0.5 mg q2wk;
Child 5 y or older; weight 15–20 kg: 0.25 mg daily; after 4 days, increase to 0.5 mg daily; can increase by 0.25 mg q2wk

Renal Impairment Dosage Adjustment

CrCl less than 30 mL/min: Start with 0.5 mg bid, increase by 0.5 mg bid daily to an initial target of 1.5 mg bid, may increase by 0.5 mg bid at weekly intervals (max: 6 mg/day) **IM** Initial with oral dosing; then begin 25 mg IM q2weeks.

Hepatic Impairment Dosage Adjustment

Child Pugh Class C **PO** start with dose of 0.5 mg bid; **IM** Initial with oral dosing; then begin 25 mg IM q2weeks.

Enzyme Inducer or CYP2D6 Inhibitor Dosage Adjustment

See package insert

ADMINISTRATION

Oral

- The oral solution may be mixed with water, orange juice, low-fat milk, or coffee. It is not compatible with cola or tea.

- Orally disintegrating tablets should not be removed from the blister until immediately before administration. Tablets disintegrate immediately and may be swallowed with/without liquid.
- Store at 15°–30° C (59°–86° F).

Subcutaneous

- Administer SC into the abdomen only. Rotate injection sites. Do not rub injection site. Be aware of placement of any belts or clothing waistbands.

Intramuscular

- Reconstitute using only in the diluent supplied in the dose pack. Shake vigorously for at least 10 sec to produce a uniform, thick, milky suspension. If 2 min or more pass before injection, shake vial again.
- Give deep IM into the upper-outer quadrant of the gluteal muscle with the supplied needle; do not substitute. Follow the manufacturer's instructions for use of the SmartSite Needle-Free Vial Access Device and Needle-Pro device.
- Store unopened vials at 2°–8° C (36°–46° F). Protect from light.

ADVERSE EFFECTS **CV:** Prolonged QTc interval, tachycardia, orthostatic hypotension with initial doses. **Respiratory:** Rhinitis, *cough*, dyspnea, nasopharyngitis. **CNS:** *Sedation, drowsiness, headache,* transient blurred vision, *insomnia,* disinhibition, *agitation,* anxiety, increased dream activity, *dizziness,* catatonia, *extrapyramidal symptoms* (akathisia, dystonia, parkinsonism), especially with doses greater than 10 mg/day, neuroleptic malignant syndrome (rare), increased risk of stroke in elderly. **Endocrine:** Galactorrhea; Hyperglycemia, diabetes mellitus, *hyperprolactinemia, weight gain,* decrease in HDL cholesterol, increased serum cholesterol. **Skin:** Photosensitivity, sweating, skin rash. **GI:** *Dry mouth,* dyspepsia, nausea, *vomiting, diarrhea, constipation,* elevated liver function tests (AST, ALT). **GU:** Urinary retention, menorrhagia, incontinence, decreased sexual desire, erectile dysfunction, sexual dysfunction male and female. **Hematologic:** Anemia, neutropenia. **Musculoskeletal:** Tremor.

INTERACTIONS **Drug:** Risperidone may enhance the effects of certain ANTIHYPERTENSIVE AGENTS. May antagonize the antiparkinson effects of **bromocriptine, cabergoline, levodopa, pergolide, pramipexole, ropinirole, carbamazepine, phenytoin, phenobarbital, rifampin** may decrease risperidone levels. Monitor closely when used with CYP3A4 substrates. CYP2D6 inhibitors may increase the concentration of risperidone. **Clozapine** may increase risperidone levels. Do not use with nasal **azelastine, metoclopramide, orphenadrine, sulpiride, thalidomide, tiotropium.** Do not use with agents that prolong the QT interval (e.g., **dofetilide, dronedarone, procaine, ziprasidone**).

PHARMACOKINETICS **Absorption:** Rapidly; not affected by food. **Onset:** Therapeutic effect 1–2 wk. **Peak:** 1–2 h. **Distribution:** 0.7 L/kg; in animal studies, risperidone has been found in breast milk. **Metabolism:** Primarily in liver [CYP2D6, CYP3A4, P-glycoprotein (P-gp)]. **Elimination:** 70% in urine; 14% in feces. **Half-Life:** 20 h for slow metabolizers, 30 h for fast metabolizers.

R

NURSING IMPLICATIONS

Black Box Warning

Risperidone has been associated with increased mortality in older adults with dementia-related psychosis.

Assessment & Drug Effects

- Monitor diabetics for loss of glycemic control.
- Reassess patients periodically and maintain on the lowest effective drug dose.
- Monitor closely neurologic status of older adults.
- Monitor cardiovascular status closely; assess for orthostatic hypotension, especially during initial dosage titration.
- Monitor closely those at risk for seizures.
- Assess degree of cognitive and motor impairment and assess for environmental hazards.
- Monitor lab tests: Periodic CBC, electrolytes, renal function tests, LFTs, HbA1c, fasting lipid panel.

Patient & Family Education

- Carefully monitor blood glucose levels if diabetic.
- Do not engage in potentially hazardous activities until the response to drug is known.
- Be aware of the risk of orthostatic hypotension.
- Avoid alcohol while taking this drug.

R

RITONAVIR

(ri-ton'a-vir)

Norvir

Classification: PROTEASE INHIBITOR

Therapeutic: PROTEASE INHIBITOR

Prototype: Saquinavir

AVAILABILITY Tablet; capsule; oral solution; powder packets

ACTION & *THERAPEUTIC EFFECT* HIV protease inhibitor that renders the enzyme incapable of processing the polyprotein precursor necessary for the production of mature HIV-1 particles. *Protease inhibitor of both HIV-1 and HIV-2 resulting in the formation of noninfectious viral particles.*

USES Alone or in combination with other agents for treatment of HIV infection. Often used to increase the effect of other antiretrovirals.

CONTRAINDICATIONS Hypersensitivity to ritonavir; severe hepatic impairment; concurrent use of saquinavir and ritonavir in patients with conditions that affect cardiac electrical activity; coadministration with sedative hypnotics, alpha 1 adrenoreceptor antagonists, anitanginal, antiarrhythmics, anti fungals, anti gout medications, GI motility agents, St. John's wort, HMG-CoA reductase inhibitors, phosphodiesterase type-5 inhibitor; ergot alkaloids; antimicrobial resistance to protease inhibitors; pancreatitis; toxic epidermal necrolysis, lactation for HIV patients.

CAUTIOUS USE Mild to moderate hepatic diseases, liver enzyme abnormalities, or hepatitis, jaundice; cardiac myopathy, ischemic heart disease or structural heart disease; diabetes mellitus, diabetic ketoacidosis, hyperlipidemia, hypertriglyceridemia; pancreatitis; hemophilia A or B, renal insufficiency; Graves' disease; Guillain-Barre syndrome; pregnancy—fetal risk cannot be ruled out; lactation—infant risk cannot be ruled out.

Safe use in children younger than 1 mo not established.

ROUTE & DOSAGE

HIV

Adult: **PO** 600 mg bid

Child (1 mo or older): **PO** start with 250 mg/m^2 bid, increase by 50 mg/m^2 q2–3days up to 350–400 mg/m^2 bid (max: 600 mg bid)

ADMINISTRATION

Oral

- Give preferably with food; oral solution may be mixed with chocolate milk or nutritional therapy liquids within 1 h of dosing to improve taste.
- Capsules should be stored refrigerated at 2°–8° C (36°–46° F). Protect from light in tightly closed container. May be left at room temperature: Less than 25° C (77° F) if used within 30 days.
- Tablets should be stored at less than 30° C (86° F). May store at greater than 50° C (122° F) for up to 7 days.
- Store oral powder at less than 30° C (86° F).
- Store solution at 20°–25° C (68°–77° F).

ADVERSE EFFECTS **CV:** Edema, peripheral edema. **Respiratory:** Cough, throat pain. **CNS:** *Weakness*, *fatigue*, dizziness, *altered sensation like "pins and needles,"* peripheral neuropathy, headache. **HEENT:** Blurred vision. **Endocrine:** *Hypercholesterolemia*, increased triglycerides. **Skin:** Flushing, pruritus, *rash*. **Hepatic:** Increased gamma-glutamyl transferase, increased serum AST, increased serum ALT, hepatitis. **GI:** *Abdominal pain, diarrhea, nausea, vomiting*, altered taste, dyspepsia. **Musculoskeletal:** Joint pain, muscle pain, back pain. **Other:** Fever.

INTERACTIONS **Drug: Carbamazepine, dexamethasone, phenobarbital, phenytoin, rifabutin, rifampin,** smoking can decrease ritonavir levels. **Ritonavir** may increase serum levels and toxicity of **clarithromycin,** especially in patients with renal insufficiency (reduce **clarithromycin** dose in patients with CrCl less than 60 mL/min); **alfuzosin, amiodarone, bepridil, bupropion, clozapine, desipramine; dihydroergotamine, flecainide, fluticasone, meperidine, pimozide, piroxicam, propoxyphene, quinidine, rifabutin, saquinavir, trazodone.** Ritonavir decreases levels of ORAL CONTRACEPTIVES, **theophylline;** may increase **ergotamine** toxicity with **dihydroergotamine, ergotamine;** may increase systemic steroid exposure with **fluticasone.** Liquid formulation may cause disulfiram-like reaction with **alcohol** or **metronidazole.** Can not be used with **lovastatin.** Concurrent use of **dasatinib** requires dose reduction. Use with **darunavir** may increase risk of hepatoxicity. Use with lowest possible dose of **atorvastatin.** See the complete prescribing information for a comprehensive table of potential, but not studied, drug interactions. **Herbal: St. John's wort, garlic, red yeast rice,** may decrease antiretroviral activity.

PHARMACOKINETICS **Absorption:** Rapidly from GI tract. **Peak:** 2–4 h. **Distribution:** 98–99% protein bound. **Metabolism:** In liver (CYP3A4 and 2D6). **Elimination:** Primarily in feces (greater than 80%).

NURSING IMPLICATIONS

Black Box Warning

Coadministration of ritonavir with sedative hypnotics, antiarrhythmics, or ergot alkaloids has been associated with potentially serious and/or life-threatening adverse reactions.

Assessment & Drug Effects

- Withhold drug and notify prescriber in the presence of abnormal liver function.
- Assess for S&S of GI distress, peripheral neuropathy, and other potential adverse effects.
- Monitor lab tests: Periodic LFTs, uric acid, lipid profile, CPK, blood glucose, urinalysis, hepatitis C antibody levels, electrolytes, CBC with differential, and HbA1C.

Patient & Family Education

- Learn potential adverse reactions and drug interactions; report to prescriber use of any OTC or prescription drugs.
- Take this drug exactly as prescribed. Do not skip doses. Take at same time each day.
- Do not take ritonavir with any of the following drugs as fatal reactions may occur: **Amiodarone, astemizole, alfuzosin, bepridil, dihydroergotamine, ergotamine, flecainide, methylergonovine, midazolam, pimozide, propafenone, quinidine, triazolam, voriconazole.**

R

RITUXIMAB

(ri-tux'i-mab)

Rituxan

Classification: DISEASE-MODIFYING- ANTIRHEUMATIC DRUG (DMARD)

Therapeutic: ANTINEOPLASTIC; ANTIRHEUMATIC; DMARD

AVAILABILITY Solution for injection

ACTION & *THERAPEUTIC EFFECT* A monoclonal antibody against the protein CD20, which is primarily found on the surface of immune system B cells. It destroys B cells by attaching to CD20 and is therefore used to treat diseases which are characterized by excessive numbers of B cells, overactive B cells, or dysfunctional B cells. CD20 antigen is expressed in more than 90% of B-cell non-Hodgkin lymphomas. B cells are also believed to play a role in the pathogenesis of RA and associated chronic synovitis as they may be acting at multiple sites in the autoimmune/inflammatory process. *Rituximab effectiveness in both rheumatoid arthritis and non-Hodgkin's lymphoma is measured by induced depletion of peripheral B-lymphocytes.*

USES Rheumatoid arthritis, CLL, non-Hodgkin lymphoma, granulomatosis, microscopic polyangiitis.

UNLABELED USES Acute lymphocytic leukemia, idiopathic thrombocytopenic purpura, multiple sclerosis, hemolytic anemia, mantle cell lymphoma.

CONTRAINDICATIONS Hypersensitivity to murine proteins, rituximab; serious infection; life-threatening cardiac arrhythmias; severe infusion reactions to rituximab; drug-induced activation of hepatitis B virus (HBV); drug-induced progressive multifocal leukoencephalopathy (PML); tumor lysis syndrome; severe mucocutaneous reaction to rituximab; oliguria, rising serum creatinine; live vaccines; lactation (infant risk cannot be ruled out).

CAUTIOUS USE Prior exposure to murine-based monoclonal antibodies; history of allergies; asthma and other pulmonary disease (increased risk of bronchospasm); respiratory insufficiency; CAD; thrombocytopenia; history of cardiac arrhythmias; hypertension, renal impairment; older adults; pregnancy (fetal risk cannot be ruled out). Safety and efficacy in children not established.

ROUTE & DOSAGE

Non-Hodgkin Lymphoma

Adult: **IV** Varies based on disease-specific parameters, consult package insert

Rheumatoid Arthritis

Adult: **IV** 1000 mg on days 1 and 15 (with methotrexate); repeat every 24 wk

CLL

Adult: **IV** 375 mg/m^2 on day 1 of cycle 1 then 500 mg/m^2 (in combination with fludarabine/cyclophosphamide) on day 1 of cycles 2–6.

Granulomatosis/Microscopic Polyangiitis (Induction Therapy)

Adult: **IV** 375 mg/m^2 weekly × 4 wk

ADMINISTRATION

Intravenous ONLY

Premedicate before each infusion with acetaminophen and an antihistamine.

PREPARE: **IV Infusion:** Dilute ordered dose to 1–4 mg/mL by adding to an infusion bag of NS or D5W. ▪ Examples: 500 mg in 400 mL yields 1 mg/mL; 500 mg in 75 mL yields 4 mg/mL. ▪ Gently invert bag to mix. Discard unused portion left in vial.

ADMINISTER: **IV Infusion:** Infuse first dose at a rate of 50 mg/h; may increase rate at 50 mg/h increments q30min to maximum rate of 400 mg/h. ▪ For subsequent doses, infuse at a rate of 100 mg/h and increase by 100 mg/h increments q30min up to maximum rate of 400 mg/h. ▪ Slow or stop infusion if S&S of hypersensitivity appear (see Appendix F).

INCOMPATIBILITES: **Y-site: aldesleukin, amphotericin B colloidal, ciprofloxacin, cyclosporine, daunorubicin, doxorubicin, furosemide, levofloxacin, minocycline, ofloxacin, ondansetron, quinupristin/dalfopristin, sodium bicarbonate, topotecan, vancomycin.**

▪ Store unopened vials at 2°–8° C (36°–46° F) and protect from light. Solutions for infusion can be kept at room temperature for 24 h and an additional 24 h if refrigerated.

ADVERSE EFFECTS CV: Hypotension, hypertension, tachycardia, peripheral edema, *hypertension*. **Respiratory:** Bronchospasm, dyspnea, rhinitis, epistaxis, cough. **CNS:** Headache, dizziness, depression, insomnia. **Skin:** Pruritus, rash, urticaria. **GI:** *Nausea,* diarrhea, vomiting, throat irritation, anorexia, abdominal pain, hepatitis B reactivation with fulminant hepatitis, hepatic failure, and death. **Musculoskeletal:** Arthralgia, asthenia. **Hematologic:** Leukopenia, thrombocytopenia, anemia, neutropenia. **Infusion-related reactions:** *Fever, chills, rigors, pruritus, urticaria, pain, flushing,* chest pain, hypotension, hypertension, dyspnea; fatal infusion-related reactions have

R

been reported. **Other:** Angioedema, *fatigue,* night sweats, *fever, chills,* myalgia.

INTERACTIONS

Drug: Do not use with MONOCLONAL ANTIBODIES, DMARDS or TNF INHIBITORS. Avoid LIVE VACCINES. **Herbal:** Do not use with echinacea due to effect on immune system.

PHARMACOKINETICS

Duration: 6–12 mo. **Half-Life:** 60–174 h (increases with multiple infusions).

NURSING IMPLICATIONS

Black Box Warning

Rituximab has been associated with severe and sometimes fatal infusion reactions, severe mucocutaneous reactions, hepatitis B reactivation, and progressive multifocal leukoencephalopathy.

Assessment & Drug Effects

- Monitor carefully BP and ECG status during infusion and immediately report S&S of hypersensitivity (e.g., fever, chills, urticaria, pruritus, hypotension, bronchospasms; see Appendix F for others).
- Monitor for and report promptly S&S of progressive multifocal leukoencephalopathy (PML) (e.g., hemiparesis, visual field deficits, cognitive impairment, aphasia, ataxia, and/or cranial nerve deficits).
- Monitor lab tests: Baseline and periodic CBC with differential and platelet count, peripheral CD20+ B lymphocytes, LFTs, renal function tests, and serum uric acid.

Patient & Family Education

- Do not take antihypertensive medication within 12 h of rituximab infusions.
- Note: Use effective contraception during and for up to 12 mo following rituximab therapy.
- Report any of the following experienced during infusion: Itching, difficulty breathing, tightness in throat, dizziness, headache, or nausea.

RIVAROXABAN

(riv′a-rox′a-ban)

Xarelto

Classification: ANTICOAGULANT; ANTITHROMBOTIC; SELECTIVE FACTOR XA INHIBITOR

Therapeutic: ANTICOAGULANT; ANTITHROMBOTIC

AVAILABILITY

Tablet

ACTION & *THERAPEUTIC EFFECT*

A factor Xa inhibitor that selectively blocks the active site of factor Xa thus blocking activation of factor X to factor Xa (FXa) via the intrinsic and extrinsic pathways. *Inhibits the coagulation cascade thus preventing thrombosis formation.*

USES

Prevention or treatment of deep venous thrombosis (DVT); nonvalvular atrial fibrillation; treatment or prevention of venous thromboembolism; coronary artery disease (stable).

UNLABELED USE:

heparin-induced thrombocytopenia, superficial vein thrombosis.

CONTRAINDICATIONS

Hypersensitivity to rivaroxaban; major active bleeding; severe renal impairment (CrCl less than 30 mL/min); elderly with CrCl less than 50 mL/min. moderate-to-severe hepatic impairment (Child-Pugh class B or C); patients with

R

triple-positive antiphospholipid syndrome (APS); patients with prosthetic heart valves or who have had transcatheter aortic valve replacement; pregnancy—fetal risk cannot be ruled out; lactation—infant risk cannot be ruled out.

CAUTIOUS USE Spinal/epidural anesthesia or spinal puncture; concurrent platelet aggregation inhibitors, other antithrombotic agents, fibrinolytic therapy, thienopyridines and chronic use of NSAIDs; mild hepatic impairment (Child-Pugh class A); moderate renal impairment (CrCl 49–30 mL/min); elderly; surgical patients. Safety and efficacy in children younger than 18 y not established.

ROUTE & DOSAGE

Nonvalvular Atrial Fibrillation

Adult: **PO** 20 mg daily

Coronary Artery Disease

Adult: **PO** 2.5 mg daily with low dose aspirin and clopidogrel

Venous Thromboembolism Prophylaxis

Adult: **PO** 10 mg once daily × 31–39 days

Venous Thromboembolism Treatment

Adult: **PO** 15 mg bid × 21 days followed by 20 mg daily

Indefinite Anticoagulation

Adult: **PO** 10 mg qd

Hepatic Impairment Dosage Adjustment

Child-Pugh class B or C and hepatic disease with coagulopathy: Avoid use

Renal Impairment Dosage Adjustment

Varies based on indication; see package insert for details

ADMINISTRATION

Oral

- 2.5 mg and 10 mg tablets may be given without regard to food; 15 and 20 mg tablets should be taken with food at approximately the same time each day; food should immediately follow swallowing of medication.
- If unable to swallow whole tablets, may crush any strength table and mix with applesauce immediately prior to use; crushed tablets are stable in applesauce for up to 4 hours.
- *Following spinal/epidural anesthesia or spinal puncture:* Wait at least 18 h after the last dose of rivaroxaban to remove an epidural catheter. Do not give the next rivaroxaban dose earlier than 6 h after the removal of catheter. If traumatic puncture occurs, wait 24 h before giving rivaroxaban.
- Store at controlled room temperature at 25 degrees C (77 degrees F); with excursions permitted between 15°–30° C (59°–86° F).

R

ADVERSE EFFECTS (≥5%) **Hematologic:** *Bleeding complications, hemorrhage.*

DIAGNOSTIC TEST INTERFERENCE Use prolongs aPTT, **HepTest** and Russell viper venom time.

INTERACTIONS **Drug:** Concomitant use with drugs that are combined P-gp and CYP3A4 inhibitors (**ketoconazole, ritonavir, clarithromycin, erythromycin, itraconazole, lopinavir, indinavir, conivaptan, azithromycin,**

diltiazem, verapamil, quinidine, ranolazine, dronedarone, amiodarone, felodipine) may increase rivaroxaban exposure and increase bleeding risk. Concomitant use with drugs that are combined P-gp and CYP3A4 inducers (e.g., **rifampin, carbamazepine, phenytoin**) may decrease rivaroxaban levels. Concomitant use with ANTICOAGULANTS, ANTIPLATELTS, NSAIDS increase bleeding time and tendencies. Estrogens or PROGESTINS may decrease anticoagulant effects. **Herbal: St. John's wort** may decrease rivaroxaban levels.

PHARMACOKINETICS Absorption: 80–100% bioavailable. **Peak:** 2–4 h. **Distribution:** 92–95% plasma protein bound. **Metabolism:** Hepatic via CYP3A4/5 and CYP2J2. **Elimination:** Renal (66%) and fecal (28%). **Half-Life:** 5–9 h.

NURSING IMPLICATIONS

Black Box Warning

Rivaroxaban has been associated with epidural or spinal hematomas in those receiving neuraxial anesthesia or undergoing spinal puncture which may result in long-term or permanent paralysis.

R

Assessment & Drug Effects

- Monitor vital signs closely and report immediately S&S of bleeding and internal hemorrhage (e.g., intracranial and epidural hematoma, retinal hemorrhage, GI bleeding).
- Monitor frequently and report immediately S&S of neurologic impairment such as tingling, numbness (especially in the lower limbs), and muscular weakness.
- Report immediately neurologic impairment or an unexplained drop in BP or falling Hgb & Hct values.
- Monitor lab tests: Baseline renal and hepatic function tests; chromogenic anti-FXa assay; peak drug levels; CBC at initiation and at regular intervals; baseline and periodic Hgb & Hct.

Patient & Family Education

- Report promptly any of the following: Unusual bleeding or bruising; blood in urine or tarry stools; tingling or numbness (especially in the lower limbs); and muscular weakness.
- Notify prescriber immediately if you become pregnant or intend to become pregnant, or if you are breast-feeding or intend to breast-feed.
- Do not discontinue the drug without notifying the prescriber.
- Confer with prescriber before using a nonsteroidal anti-inflammatory drug (NSAID), aspirin, or herbal products as these may increase risk of bleeding.
- A missed dose should be taken as soon as possible on the same day. For the 15 mg twice daily schedule, 2 tablets can be taken together if necessary.

RIVASTIGMINE TARTRATE

(ri-vas′tig-meen)

Exelon

Classification: CHOLINESTERASE INHIBITOR; ANTIDEMENTIA
Therapeutic: ANTIALZHEIMER

AVAILABILITY Capsule; transdermal patch

ACTION & *THERAPEUTIC EFFECT*
Inhibits acetylcholinesterase G_1 form of this enzyme in the cerebral cortex and the hippocampus. The G_1 form of acetylcholinesterase is found in higher levels in the brains of patients with Alzheimer disease.

Inhibits acetylcholinesterase more specifically in the brain (hippocampus and cortex) than in the heart or skeletal muscle in Alzheimer disease.

USES Alzheimer dementia, Parkinson disease-related dementia.

CONTRAINDICATIONS Hypersensitivity to rivastigmine or carbamate derivatives; safety and efficacy has not been established in children; pregnancy—fetal risk cannot be ruled; lactation—infant risk cannot be ruled out.

CAUTIOUS USE History of toxicity to cholinesterase inhibitors; DM; sick sinus syndrome, bradycardia, or other supraventricular cardiac conduction conditions; asthma or obstructive pulmonary disease; GI disorders including intestinal obstruction; history of or at risk for PUD or GI bleeding; urogenital tract obstruction, BPH; history of seizures; smokers; hepatic or renal impairment; low body weight; elderly.

ROUTE & DOSAGE

Alzheimer/Parkinson Related Dementia

Adult/Geriatric: **PO** Start with 1.5 mg bid may increase by 1.5 mg/dose q2wk if tolerated, (max recommended: 6 mg bid)

Transdermal

Adult: Apply 4.6 mg patch daily, after 4 wk, can increase to 9.5 mg patch if tolerated, then 13.3 mg patch (max dose)

Hepatic Impairment Dosage Adjustment

Child-Pugh Class A and B: PO dose of 1.5 mg daily with slow titration up; Transdermal dose max 4.6 mg/24 hours

ADMINISTRATION

Oral

- Give capsules with food.
- For solution, use dosing syringe supplied. May swallow directly from the syringe or mix with water, cold fruit juice, or soda (do not mix with any other liquids). Stir well before drinking.
- Withhold drug and notify prescriber if significant anorexia, nausea, or vomiting occur.
- Store capsules below 25° C (77° F). Store solution in upright position and protect from freezing.

Transdermal

- Apply patch at same time each day to dry, hairless, healthy skin on the back, upper arm, or chest. Preferred site of application is the upper or lower back.
- Remove old patch before applying the new one.
- Rotate application sites and do not reapply to same site for at least 14 days.
- Do not tape or otherwise cover the patch.
- If a patch falls off, do not reapply. Replace with a new patch and remove it following the original schedule for replacement.
- Bathing and hot weather are acceptable when using the patch, but avoid long exposure to external heat sources.
- Store patch at controlled room temperature, 25 degrees C (77 degrees F); with excursions permitted to 15°–30° C (59°–86° F) in sealed pouch until ready to use.

ADVERSE EFFECTS (≥5%) CNS: *Dizziness, asthenia, headache, tremor.* **Endocrine:** *Weight loss.*

R

GI: *Nausea, vomiting, anorexia, dyspepsia, diarrhea, abdominal pain.*

INTERACTIONS **Drug:** May exaggerate muscle relations with **succinylcholine** and other NEUROMUSCULAR BLOCKING AGENTS, may attenuate effects of ANTICHOLINERGIC AGENTS. Do not use with BETA BLOCKING AGENTS due to increased bradycardia; use caution with other medications (**bromopride, ceritinib**) that cause bradycardia

PHARMACOKINETICS **Absorption:** Well absorbed. **Peak:** 1 h. **Duration:** 10 h. **Distribution:** Crosses blood–brain barrier with CSF peak concentrations in 1.4–2.6 h. **Metabolism:** By cholinesterase-mediated hydrolysis. **Elimination:** In urine. **Half-Life:** 1.5 h.

NURSING IMPLICATIONS

Assessment & Drug Effects

- Monitor cognitive function and ability to perform ADLs prior to driving and operating machinery.
- Monitor for and report S&S of GI distress or GI bleeding: Anorexia, weight loss, nausea, and vomiting.
- Monitor ambulation as dizziness is a common adverse effect.
- Monitor diabetics for loss of glycemic control.

Patient & Family Education

- Review instruction sheet provided with liquid form of the drug.
- Caution driving and operating machinery until effects of the drug are known.
- Monitor weight at least weekly.
- Report any of the following to the prescriber: Loss of appetite, weight loss, significant nausea and/or vomiting.
- Supervise activity since there is a high potential for dizziness.
- Contact healthcare professional if dose is missed for several days in a row; the drug may need to be restarted at a lower dose.

RIZATRIPTAN BENZOATE

(ri-za-trip'tan ben'zo-ate)

Maxalt, Maxalt-MLT

Classification: 5-HT_1 RECEPTOR AGONIST (TRIPTANS)

Therapeutic: ANTIMIGRAINE

Prototype: Sumatriptan

AVAILABILITY Tablet; disintegrating tablets

ACTION & *THERAPEUTIC EFFECT* Selective ($5\text{-HT}_{1B/1D}$) receptor agonist that reverses the vasodilation of cranial blood vessels associated with a migraine. *Activation of the $5\text{-HT}_{1B/1D}$ receptors reduces the pain pathways associated with the migraine headache as well as reversing vasodilation of cranial blood vessels.*

USES Acute migraine headaches with or without aura.

CONTRAINDICATIONS Hypersensitivity to rizatriptan; CAD; Prinzmetal's angina (potential for vasospasm); ischemic heart disease; risk factors for CAD such as hypertension, hypercholesterolemia, obesity, diabetes, smoking, and strong family history; hemiplegia; concurrent administration with ergotamine drugs or sumatriptan; concurrent administration with MAOIs; or within 14 days of use; stroke or TIA or history basilar or hemiplegic migraine.

R

CAUTIOUS USE Hypersensitivity to sumatriptan; renal or hepatic impairment; hypertension; asthmatic patients; pregnancy (category C); lactation (infant risk cannot be ruled out). Safety and efficacy in children younger than 18 y not established.

ROUTE & DOSAGE

Acute Migraine

Adult/Adolescent/Child (older than 6 y and weight greater than 40 kg): **PO** 5–10 mg, may repeat in 2 h if necessary (max: 30 mg/24 h); 5 mg with concurrent propranolol (max: 15 mg/24 h)

ADMINISTRATION

Oral

- Give any time after symptoms of migraine appear. If symptoms return, a second tablet may be given but no sooner than 2 h after the first.
- Do not exceed 30 mg (three doses) in any 24 h period.
- Do not give within 24 h of an ergot-containing drug or another 5-HT_1 agonist.
- Store at 15°–30° C (59°–86° F) and protect from light and moisture.

ADVERSE EFFECTS **CV:** Chest pain. **CNS:** Dizziness, weakness, sleepy. **GI:** Nausea. **Other:** Fatigue.

INTERACTIONS **Drug: Propranolol** may increase concentrations of rizatriptan, use smaller rizatriptan doses; **dihydroergotamine, methysergide,** MAOIs, other 5-HT_1 AGONISTS may cause prolonged vasospastic reactions; SSRIS have rarely caused weakness, hyperreflexia, and incoordination; MAOIS should not be used with 5-HT_1 AGONISTS or **dapoxetine. Herbal: St. John's wort** may increase triptan toxicity.

PHARMACOKINETICS **Absorption:** 45% of oral dose reaches systemic circulation. **Peak:** 1–1.5 h for oral tabs; 1.6–2.5 h for orally disintegrating tablets. **Metabolism:** Via oxidative deamination by monoamine oxidase A. **Elimination:** Primarily in urine (82%). **Half-Life:** 2–3 h.

NURSING IMPLICATIONS

Assessment & Drug Effects

- Monitor cardiovascular status carefully following first dose in patients at risk for CAD (e.g., postmenopausal women, men older than 40 y, persons with known CAD risk factors) or coronary artery vasospasms.
- ECG is recommended following first administration of rizatriptan to someone with known CAD risk factors.
- Report immediately to prescriber: Chest pain or tightness in chest or throat that is severe or does not quickly resolve.
- Monitor periodically cardiovascular status with continued rizatriptan use.

Patient & Family Education

- Do not exceed 30 mg (three doses) in 24 h.
- Allow orally disintegrating tablets to dissolve on tongue; no liquid is needed.
- Contact prescriber immediately if any of the following develop following rizatriptan use: Symptoms of angina (e.g., severe and/or persistent pain or tightness in chest or throat), hypersensitivity (e.g., wheezing, facial swelling, skin rash, or hives), abdominal pain.
- Report any other adverse effects (e.g., tingling, flushing, dizziness) at next prescriber visit.

R

ROFLUMILAST

(ro-flu'mi-last)

Daliresp

Classification: RESPIRATORY AGENT; ANTI-INFLAMMATORY; PHOSPHODIESTERASE 4 (PDE4) INHIBITOR

Therapeutic: ANTI-INFLAMMATORY; PDE4 INHIBITOR

AVAILABILITY Tablet

ACTION & *THERAPEUTIC EFFECT* Selectively inhibits phosphodiesterase 4 (PDE4), a major enzyme found in inflammatory and immune cells, thus indirectly suppressing the release of cytokines and other products of inflammation. *Has an anti-inflammatory effect in pulmonary diseases.*

USES Reduction of the prevalence of chronic obstructive pulmonary disease (COPD) exacerbations.

CONTRAINDICATIONS Moderate-to-severe liver impairment (Child-Pugh class B or C); suicidal ideation; lactation.

R

CAUTIOUS USE Mild hepatic impairment (Child-Pugh class A); history of psychiatric illness including anxiety, depression, or suicidal thoughts; clinically significant weight loss; pregnancy (category C). Safety and efficacy in children not established.

ROUTE & DOSAGE

Chronic Obstructive Pulmonary Disease

Adult: **PO** 500 mcg once daily

ADMINISTRATION

Oral

- May be given with or without food.
- Store at 15°–30° C (59°–86° F).

ADVERSE EFFECTS **Respiratory:** Rhinitis, sinusitis. **CNS:** Anxiety, depression, dizziness, headache, insomnia, tremor. **GI:** Abdominal pain, decreased appetite, *diarrhea*, dyspepsia, gastritis, nausea, vomiting, *weight loss*. **GU:** Urinary tract infection, acute renal failure. **Musculoskeletal:** Back pain, muscle spasms. **Other:** Influenza.

INTERACTIONS **Drug:** Coadministration with strong CYP3A4 or CYP3A4/CYP1A2 inhibitors (e.g., **cimetidine, ketoconazole, ritonavir, erythromycin, fluvoxamine**) may increase the levels of roflumilast. Coadministration with strong CYP3A4 inducers (i.e., **carbamazepine, phenobarbital, phenytoin,** RIFAMYCINS) may decrease the levels of roflumilast. Coadministration **gestodene** may increase the levels of roflumilast. **Food:** None listed. **Herbal: St. John's wort** may decrease the levels of roflumilast.

PHARMACOKINETICS **Absorption:** 80% Bioavailable. **Peak:** 1 h. **Distribution:** 99% plasma protein bound. **Metabolism:** In liver to active and inactive metabolites. **Elimination:** Primarily renal. **Half-Life:** 17 h (30 h for active metabolite).

NURSING IMPLICATIONS

Assessment & Drug Effects

- Monitor for and report promptly new onset or worsening insomnia, anxiety, depression, suicidal thoughts, or other significant mood changes.

- Monitor weight at regular intervals. Report significant weight loss to prescriber.

Patient & Family Education

- Roflumilast is not a bronchodilator and does not provide relief of acute bronchospasm.
- Report to prescriber any of the following: Disturbing mood changes such as anxiety or depression; difficulty sleeping; suicidal thoughts; persistent nausea and/or diarrhea.
- Monitor your weight and report unexplained weight loss.
- Do not self-treat depression with St. John's wort.

ROLAPITANT

(ro-la'pi-tant)

Varubi

Classification: CENTRALLY ACTING ANTIEMETIC; SUBSTANCE P/NEUROKININ 1 (NK1) ANTAGONIST

Therapeutic: ANTIEMETIC

Prototype Aprepitant

AVAILABILITY Tablets

ACTION & *THERAPEUTIC EFFECT* Acts at neurokinin-1 (NK-1) receptors in vomiting centers within the CNS to block their activation by substance P which is released as an unwanted consequence of chemotherapy. *Prevents both acute and delayed chemotherapy-induced nausea and vomiting.*

USES Prevention of chemotherapy-induced nausea and vomiting.

CONTRAINDICATIONS Hypersensitivity to rolapitant; concurrent use of thioridazine or CYP2D6 substrates with a narrow therapeutic window; severe hepatic impairment (Child-Pugh class C); children less than 2 y; safety and efficacy have not been established in pediatric patients; pregnancy—fetal risk cannot be ruled out; lactation—infant risk cannot be ruled out.

CAUTIOUS USE mild or moderate hepatic impairment (Child-Pugh class A or B); prolonged QT interval;

ROUTE & DOSAGE

Chemotherapy-Induced Nausea/Vomiting Prophylaxis

Adult: **PO** 180 mg single dose 1–2 h prior to chemotherapy;

Hepatic Impairment Dosage Adjustment

Severe impairment (Child-Pugh class C): Avoid use

ADMINISTRATION

Oral

- May give without regard to meals 1–2 h prior to chemotherapy.
- Capsule should be swallowed whole.
- Store at controlled room temperature between 20 and 25 degrees C (68 and 77 degrees F), with excursions permitted between 15°–30° C (59°–86° F).

ADVERSE EFFECTS (≥5%) **Respiratory:** *Hiccoughs.* **CNS:** *Dizziness.* **GI:** *Anorexia.* **Hematologic:** Neutropenia.

INTERACTIONS **Drug:** There are extensive drug interactions, consult a drug interaction database for a complete list. Rolapitant may increase the levels of coadministered drugs that require CYP2D6 for metabolism (e.g., **dextromethorphan, pimozide, thioridazine**),

are BCRP substrates (e.g., **irinotecan, methotrexate, topotecan**). Strong CYP3A4 inducers (e.g., **rifampin**) reduce the levels of rolapitant. Inhibits P-glycoprotein/ABCB1 so may increase concentration of drugs metabolized by that route.

PHARMACOKINETICS Peak: 4 h. **Distribution:** Highly plasma protein bound (>99.8%). **Metabolism:** In liver; primarily by CYP3A4. **Elimination:** Fecal (73%) and renal (14%). **Half-Life:** Approx. 7 d.

NURSING IMPLICATIONS

Assessment & Drug Effects

- Monitor for degree of emetic control.
- Monitor for sensitivity and anaphylaxis.

Patient & Family Education

- Report to prescriber if nausea and vomiting are not well controlled.
- Review adverse effects with patient and/or caregiver.
- Do not take rolapitant if taking thioridazine as the combination can cause serious or life-threatening heart rhythm changes.
- Do not take rolapitant more than once every 14 days.
- Inform prescriber when starting or stopping any concomitant medications.

R

ROMIDEPSIN

(rom-i-dep′sin)

Istodax

Classification: ANTINEOPLASTIC; HISTONE DEACETYLASE (HDAC) INHIBITOR

Therapeutic: ANTINEOPLASTIC

AVAILABILITY Powder for reconstitution for injection

ACTION & THERAPEUTIC EFFECT Inhibits histone deacetylase, an enzyme required for completion of the cell cycle in certain cancers, thus inducing cell cycle arrest and apoptosis in these cancer cells. The mechanism of antineoplastic effect has not been fully characterized. *Effective as a cytotoxic agent against cutaneous T-cell lymphoma.*

USES Treatment of cutaneous or peripheral T-cell lymphoma.

CONTRAINDICATIONS Severe bone marrow depression; pregnancy (category D); lactation.

CAUTIOUS USE Risk factors for potassium or magnesium imbalance, thrombocytopenia, or leukopenia; congenital long QT syndrome, history of significant CV disease; moderate-to-severe hepatic impairment; end-stage renal disease. Safe use in children not established.

ROUTE & DOSAGE

Cutaneous or Peripheral T-Cell Lymphoma (CTCL)

Adult: **IV** 14 mg/m^2 over 4 h on days 1, 8, and 15, repeat every 28 days. Repeat cycle until disease progression has been treated or unacceptable toxicity occurs.

Toxicity Dosage Adjustment (National Cancer Institute Common Toxicity Criteria, CTC)

For CTC grade 3 or 4 neutropenia or thrombocytopenia: Hold romidepsin until ANC is 1,500/mm^3 or higher and/or platelet count is 75,000/mm^3 or higher, or parameters return to baseline values. Then, resume romidepsin 14 mg/m^2.

For CTC grade 4 febrile neutropenia or thrombocytopenia requiring platelet transfusion: Hold romidepsin until cytopenia is no greater than grade 1 and permanently reduce dose to 10 mg/m^2.
For CTC grade 2 or 3 nonhematological toxicity: Hold romidepsin until toxicity is no greater than grade 1 or returns to baseline. Resume romidepsin 14 mg/m^2.
For recurrent CTC grade 3 nonhematological toxicity: Hold romidepsin until toxicity is no greater than grade 1 or returns to baseline and permanently reduce dose to 10 mg/m^2.
For CTC grade 4 nonhematological toxicity: Hold romidepsin until toxicity is no greater than grade 1 or returns to baseline and permanently reduce dose to 10 mg/m^2.
For recurrent CTC grade 3 or 4 nonhematological toxicity after dose reduction: Discontinue therapy.

ADMINISTRATION

Intravenous ONLY

This drug is a cytotoxic agent and caution should be used to prevent any contact with the drug. Follow institutional or standard guidelines for preparation, handling, and disposal of cytotoxic agents.

PREPARE: **IV Infusion:** Withdraw 2 mL of supplied diluent and inject slowly into the 10 mL powder vial to yield 5 mg/mL. Swirl to dissolve. ▪ Withdraw the required dose of reconstituted solution and add to 500 mL NS and invert container to dissolve. ▪ Should be administered as soon as possible after dilution.

ADMINISTER: **IV Infusion:** Give over 4 h. Note: Ensure that potassium and magnesium are within normal range before administration.

INCOMPATIBILITIES: **Solution/additive:** Do not mix with another drug. **Y-site:** Do not mix with another drug.

▪ Reconstituted vials are stable for 8 h and IV solutions are stable for 24 h at room temperature. Store unopened vials at 15°–30° C (59°–86° F).

ADVERSE EFFECTS **CV:** ECG ST-T wave changes, hypotension. **Endocrine:** Elevated ALT, elevated AST, hypermagnesemia, hyperuricemia, hypoalbuminemia, hypocalcemia, hypokalemia, hypomagnesemia, hyponatremia, hypophosphatemia. **Skin:** Pruritus, dermatitis, exfoliative dermatitis. **GI:** *Anorexia, constipation, diarrhea, dysgeusia, nausea, vomiting.* **Hematologic:** *Anemia, neutropenia,* leukopenia, lymphopenia, *thrombocytopenia*. **Other:** *Asthenia,* fatigue, hyperglycemia, *infections,* fever.

INTERACTIONS **Drug:** Coadministration of CYP3A4 inducers (e.g., **carbamazepine, phenobarbital, phenytoin, rifampin**) can decrease the levels of romidepsin. Coadministration of strong CYP3A4 inhibitors (e.g., **atazanavir, indinavir, itraconazole, ketoconazole, nefazodone, nelfinavir, ritonavir, saquinavir, telithromycin, voriconazole**) can increase the levels of romidepsin. Coadministration of drugs that prolong the QT interval (e.g., **amiodarone, bretylium, disopyramide, dofetilide, procainamide, quinidine, sotalol), arsenic trioxide, chlorpromazine, cisapride,**

R

dolasetron, droperidol, mefloquine, mesoridazine, moxifloxacin, pentamidine, pimozide, tacrolimus, thioridazine, and ziprasidone) may produce life-threatening arrhythmias. **Food:** Grapefruit juice can increase the levels of romidepsin. **Herbal:** **St. John's wort** can decrease the levels of romidepsin.

PHARMACOKINETICS

Distribution: 92–94% plasma protein bound. **Metabolism:** Extensive hepatic metabolism by CYP3A4. **Elimination:** Primarily biliary excretion. **Half-Life:** 3 h.

NURSING IMPLICATIONS

Assessment & Drug Effects

- Monitor ECG at baseline and periodically throughout treatment.
- Report immediately electrolyte imbalances or QT prolongation.
- Monitor lab tests: Baseline and prior to each dose: Serum electrolytes, CBC with differential including platelet count, LFTs and serum albumin.

Patient & Family Education

- Report promptly any of the following: Excessive nausea, chest pain, shortness of breath, or abnormal heart beat.
- Seek medical attention if unusual bleeding occurs.
- Women of childbearing age who use an estrogen-containing contraceptive should add a barrier contraceptive to prevent pregnancy.

R

ROPINIROLE HYDROCHLORIDE

(re-pin′i-role)

Requip XL

Classification: NON-ERGOT DERIVATIVE DOPAMINE AGONIST; ANTIPARKINSON

Therapeutic: ANTIPARKINSON
Prototype: Apomorphine

AVAILABILITY

Tablet; extended release tablet

ACTION & *THERAPEUTIC EFFECT*

Precise mechanism of action is unknown, but believed to be due to stimulation of postsynaptic dopamine D_2-type receptors within the caudate putamen in the brain. *Effectiveness indicated by improvement in idiopathic Parkinson disease.*

USES

Parkinson disease, restless legs syndrome.

CONTRAINDICATIONS

Hypersensitivity to ropinirole or any component of the product; major psychotic disorder; pregnancy—fetal risk cannot be ruled out; lactation—infant risk cannot be ruled out.

CAUTIOUS USE

Hepatic impairment; severe renal impairment; mental instability; concomitant use of CNS depressants; history of cardiovascular disease; elderly;. Safety and efficacy in children not established.

ROUTE & DOSAGE

Parkinson Disease

Adult: **PO Immediate release** Start with 0.25 mg tid, titrate daily based on response; usual dose 12–16 mg/day. (max: 24 mg/day); **Extended release** 2 mg daily for 1–2 wk then increase by 2 mg/day at one week intervals; usual dose 12–16 mg/day (max: 24 mg/day)

Restless Legs Syndrome

Adult: **PO** Take 0.25 mg 1–3 h before bed × 2 days, increase to 0.5 mg for the first wk, then increase by 0.5 mg qwk to a maximum of 4 mg

ADMINISTRATION

Oral

- Give with food to reduce occurrence of nausea.
- Do not crush extended release tablets. Ensure that they are swallowed whole.
- Drug should not be abruptly discontinued. Dose should be tapered over a period of days.
- Store tablet in a tightly closed container at a controlled room temperature between 20 and 25 degrees C (68 and 77 degrees F), with excursions permitted between at 15°–30° C (59°–86° F). Protect from light and moisture. Extended release tablets store at controlled room temperature of 25 degrees C (77 degrees F), with excursions permitted between 15 and 30 degrees C (59 and 86 degrees F).

ADVERSE EFFECTS (≥5%) **CV:** Hypertension, *orthostatic hypotension*. **CNS:** *Dizziness, somnolence, sudden sleep attacks*, hallucinations, *dyskinesia*. **GI:** *Nausea, vomiting, abdominal pain*. **Other:** *fatigue*.

INTERACTIONS **Drug:** Ropinirole levels may be increased by CYP 1A2 inhibitors; ESTROGENS, **diltiazem, erythromycin, fluvoxamine, mexiletine;** effects may be antagonized by PHENOTHIAZINES, BUTYROPHENONES, **metoclopramide** may increase ropinirole levels; may increase hypotensive effects of ANTIHYPERTENSIVES; may decrease the effect of ANTIPSYCHOTIC AGENTS.

PHARMACOKINETICS **Absorption:** Rapidly from GI tract; 55% bioavailability. **Peak:** 1–2 h. **Distribution:** 30–40% protein bound. **Metabolism:** In liver (CYP1A2). **Elimination:** Primarily in urine. **Half-Life:** 6 h.

NURSING IMPLICATIONS

Assessment & Drug Effects

- Monitor cardiac status. Report increases in BP and HR to prescriber.
- Monitor carefully for orthostatic hypotension, especially during dose escalation.
- Monitor level of alertness. Institute appropriate precautions to prevent injury due to dizziness or drowsiness.
- Monitor lab test: Periodic BUN and creatinine, and LFTs.

Patient & Family Education

- Be aware that hallucinations are a possible adverse effect and occur more often in older adults.
- Make position changes slowly, especially after long periods of lying or sitting. Postural hypotension is common, especially during early treatment.
- Reports of falling asleep during activities of daily living have been reported and if this occurs, contact healthcare provider. Effects are additive with alcohol or other CNS depressants.
- Avoid driving and other activities requiring mental alertness or coordination until the drug effects are realized.
- Avoid sudden discontinuation of the drug.
- Notify provider if patient starts or stops taking estrogen-containing drugs such as birth control pills during drug therapy.
- Report behavioral changes (e.g., impulsive behavior) to prescriber.

R

ROPIVACAINE HYDROCHLORIDE

(ro-piv′i-cane)

Naropin

Classification: LOCAL ANESTHETIC (ESTER-TYPE)

Therapeutic: LOCAL ANESTHETIC

Prototype: Procaine HCl

AVAILABILITY Solution for injection

ACTION & *THERAPEUTIC EFFECT* Blocks the generation and conduction of nerve impulses, probably by increasing the threshold for electrical excitability. *Local anesthetic action produces loss of sensation and motor activity in areas of the body close to the injection site.*

USES Local and regional anesthesia, postoperative pain management, anesthesia/pain management for obstetric procedures.

CONTRAINDICATIONS Hypersensitivity to ropivacaine or any local anesthetic of the amide type; generalized septicemia, inflammation or sepsis at the proposed injection site; cerebral spinal diseases (e.g., meningitis); heart block, hypotension, hypertension, GI hemorrhage.

R

CAUTIOUS USE Debilitated, older adult, or acutely ill patients; arrhythmias, shock; pregnancy (category B); lactation.

ROUTE & DOSAGE

Surgical Anesthesia

Adult: **Epidural** 25–200 mg (0.5–1% solution); **Nerve block** 5–250 mg (0.5%, 0.75% solution)

Labor Pain

Adult: **Epidural** 20–40 mg (0.2% solution) then 12–28 mg/h

Postoperative Pain Management

Adult: **Epidural** 12–28 mg/h (0.2% solution); **Infiltration** 2–200 mg (0.2–0.5% solution)

ADMINISTRATION

Intrathecal

- Avoid rapid injection of large volumes of ropivacaine. Incremental doses should always be used to achieve the smallest effective dose and concentration.
- Use an infusion concentration of 2 mg/mL (0.2%) for postoperative analgesia.
- Do not use disinfecting agents containing heavy metal ions (e.g., mercury, copper, zinc, etc.) on skin insertion site or to clean the ropivacaine container top.
- Discard continuous infusions solution after 24 h; it contains no preservatives.
- Store unopened at 20°–25° C (68°–77° F).

ADVERSE EFFECTS **CV:** *Hypotension,* bradycardia, hypertension, tachycardia, chest pain, fetal bradycardia. **CNS:** Paresthesia, headache, dizziness, anxiety. **Skin:** Pruritus. **GI:** Nausea. **GU:** Urinary retention, oliguria. **Hematologic:** Anemia. **Other:** Pain, fever, rigors, hypoesthesia.

INTERACTIONS **Drug:** Additive adverse effects with other LOCAL ANESTHETICS.

PHARMACOKINETICS **Onset:** 1–30 min (average 10–20 min) depending on dose/route of administration. **Duration:** 0.5–8 h depending on dose/route of administration. **Distribution:** 94% protein bound. **Metabolism:** In the liver by CYP1A. **Elimination:** In urine. **Half-Life:** 1.8–4.2 h.

NURSING IMPLICATIONS

Assessment & Drug Effects

- Monitor carefully cardiovascular and respiratory status throughout treatment period. Assess for hypotension and bradycardia.
- Report immediately S&S of CNS stimulation or CNS depression.

Patient & Family Education

- Report any of the following to prescriber immediately: Restlessness, anxiety, tinnitus, blurred vision, tremors.

ROSIGLITAZONE MALEATE

(ros-i-glit′a-zone)

Avandia

Classification: THIAZOLIDINEDIONE (GLITAZONE)

Therapeutic: ANTIHYPERGLYCEMIC

AVAILABILITY Tablet

ACTION & *THERAPEUTIC EFFECT* Lowers blood sugar levels by improving target cell response to insulin in Type 2 diabetics. It reduces cellular insulin resistance and decreases hepatic glucose output (gluconeogenesis). *Reduces hyperglycemia and hyperlipidemia, thus improving hyperinsulinemia without stimulating pancreatic insulin secretion. Effectiveness indicated by decreased HbA1C.*

USES Type 2 diabetes.

UNLABELED USES Polycystic ovary syndrome.

CONTRAINDICATIONS Hypersensitivity to rosiglitazone; patients with New York Heart Association Class III and IV cardiac status (e.g., CHF); symptomatic heart failure; initiation in patients with ischemic heart disease; active hepatic disease; ALT enzyme greater than 2.5 × ULN; high risk for bone fractures; Type I DM; lactation (infant risk cannot be ruled out).

CAUTIOUS USE CHF or risk for CHF; angina; patients with ongoing edema; anemia; hepatic impairment; older adults; pregnancy (category C). Safety and efficacy in children younger than 18 y not established.

ROUTE & DOSAGE

Type 2 Diabetes Mellitus

Adult: **PO** Start at 4 mg daily or 2 mg bid, may increase after 8–12 wk (max: 8 mg/day in 1–2 divided doses)

Hepatic Impairment Dosage Adjustment

If ALT is greater than 2.5 × ULN: Do not use

ADMINISTRATION

Oral

- May be given without regard to meals.
- Store at 15°–30° C (59°–86° F) in tight, light-resistant container.

ADVERSE EFFECTS CV: Edema. **Respiratory:** URI, nasopharyngitis. **CNS:** Headache. **Endocrine:** Weight gain, increased HDL cholesterol, increased LDL cholesterol. **Musculoskeletal:** Bone fracture.

INTERACTIONS Drug: Insulin may increase risk of heart failure or edema; enhance hypoglycemia with ORAL ANTIDIABETIC AGENTS,

ketoconazole, gemfibrozil may increase effect. **Bosentan, dabrafenib, rifampin** may reduce effect. **Cholestyramine** may decrease concentration of rosiglitazone. **Herbal: Garlic, ginseng, green tea** may potentiate hypoglycemic effects.

PHARMACOKINETICS **Absorption:** 99% from GI tract. **Peak:** 1 h, food delays time to peak by 1.75 h. **Duration:** Greater than 24 h. **Distribution:** Greater than 99% protein bound. **Metabolism:** In liver (CYP2C8) to inactive metabolites. **Elimination:** 64% urine, 23% feces. **Half-Life:** 3–4 h. Liver disease increases serum concentrations and increases half-life by 2 h.

NURSING IMPLICATIONS

Assessment & Drug Effects

- Monitor for S&S of hypoglycemia (possible when insulin/sulfonylureas are coadministered).
- Monitor for S&S of CHF or exacerbation of symptoms with preexisting CHF.
- Withhold drug and notify prescriber if ALT greater than 2.5 × normal or patient jaundiced.
- Monitor weight and notify prescriber of development of edema.
- Monitor lab tests: Baseline LFTs, and periodically thereafter or more often when elevated; periodic fasting serum glucose and HbA1C.

Patient & Family Education

- Report promptly any of the following: Rapid weight gain, edema, shortness of breath, or exercise intolerance.
- Be aware that resumed ovulation is possible in non ovulating premenopausal women.
- Use or add barrier contraceptive if using hormonal contraception.
- Report immediately to prescriber: S&S of liver dysfunction such as unexplained anorexia, nausea, vomiting, abdominal pain, fatigue, dark urine; or S&S of fluid retention such as weight gain, edema, or activity intolerance.
- Combination therapy: May need adjustment of other antidiabetic drugs to avoid hypoglycemia.

ROSUVASTATIN

(ro-su-va-sta′ten)

Crestor

Classification: STATIN

Therapeutic: ANTILIPEMIC; STATIN

Prototype: Lovastatin

AVAILABILITY Tablet

ACTION & *THERAPEUTIC EFFECT*

A potent inhibitor of HMG-CoA reductase, an enzyme that catalyzes the conversion of HMG-CoA to mevalonic acid, an early and rate-limiting step in cholesterol biosynthesis. This results in reducing the amount of mevalonic acid, a precursor of cholesterol. It increases the number of hepatic HDL receptors on the cell surface to enhance uptake and catabolism of LDL. It also inhibits hepatic synthesis of very low density lipoprotein (VLDL). *Reduces total cholesterol and LDL cholesterol; additionally, lowers plasma triglycerides and VLDL while increasing HDL.*

USES Adjunct to diet for the reduction of LDL cholesterol and triglycerides in patients with primary hypercholesterolemia, hypertriglyceridemia, and mixed dyslipidemia; prevention of cardiovascular disease.

CONTRAINDICATIONS Hypersensitivity to any component of

the product, active liver disease or unexplained persistent elevations of serum transaminases; rhabdomyolysis; pregnancy (fetal risk has been demonstrated), women of childbearing potential not using appropriate contraceptive measures; lactation—infant risk has been demonstrated.

CAUTIOUS USE Concomitant use of cyclosporine and gemfibrozil; Asian descent; DM; excessive alcohol use or history of liver disease; renal impairment; older adults; hypothyroidism. Safe use in children younger than 6 y not established.

ROUTE & DOSAGE

Hyperlipidemia/Slowing Atherosclerosis Progression

Adult/Adolescent/Child (10 y or older): **PO** 10–20 mg once daily (max: 40 mg/day)
Conservative Dosing: Initial dose of 5 mg/day

Homozygous Familial Hypercholesterolemia

Adult: **PO** 20 mg daily (max: 40 mg/day)

Prevention of Cardiovascular Disease

Adult: **PO** 5–40 mg daily

Renal Impairment Dosage Adjustment

CrCl less than 30 mL/min: 5 mg once daily (max: 10 mg/day)

Concurrent Medication Dosage Adjustment

If taking cyclosporine, gemfibrozil, lopinavir/ritonavir, start with 5 mg/day

ADMINISTRATION

Oral

- Persons of Asian descent may be slow metabolizers and may require half the normal dose.
- May give any time of day without regard to food.
- Do not give within 2 h of an antacid.
- Store between 20°–25° C (68°–77° F). Protect from light.

ADVERSE EFFECTS **CNS:** Headache. **GI:** Nausea, constipation. **Musculoskeletal:** Muscle pain, joint pain, weakness.

INTERACTIONS **Drug:** **Atazanavir, cyclosporine, gemfibrozil, niacin** may increase risk of rhabdomyolysis; ANTACIDS may decrease rosuvastatin absorption; may cause increase in INR with **warfarin.** **Herbal:** **Red yeast rice** increases rhabdomyolysis risk.

PHARMACOKINETICS **Absorption:** Well absorbed. **Peak:** 3–5 h. **Metabolism:** Limited metabolism in the liver (not CYP3A4). **Elimination:** Primarily in feces (90%). **Half-Life:** 20 h.

NURSING IMPLICATIONS

Assessment & Drug Effects

- Monitor for and report promptly S&S of myopathy (e.g., skeletal muscle pain, tenderness or weakness).
- Withhold drug and notify prescriber if CPK levels are markedly elevated (10 or more × ULN) or if myopathy is diagnosed or suspected.
- Monitor CV status, especially with a known history of hypertension or heart disease.
- Monitor diabetics for loss of glycemic control.

- Monitor lab tests: Baseline CPK and repeat with S&S of myopathy; periodic LFTs.

Patient & Family Education

- Do not take antacids within 2 h of taking this drug.
- Women should use reliable means of contraception to prevent pregnancy while taking this drug.

ROTIGOTINE

(roe-TIG-oh-teen)

Neupro

Classifications: ANTIPARKINSON AGENT; DOPAMINE AGONIST

Therapeutic: ANTIPARKINSON AGENT

Prototype: Apomorphine

AVAILABILITY Transdermal patch

ACTION & *THERAPEUTIC EFFECT*

A non-ergoline dopamine receptor agonist. The precise mechanism of action in treatment of Parkinson disease and restless legs syndrome is unknown, but thought to be related to the drug's ability to stimulate dopamine receptors. In Parkinson disease, it is thought to specifically stimulate dopamine receptors within the caudate-putamen in the brain. Used to improve symptoms of Parkinson disease (tremors, stiffness, slowed movements, and unsteadiness) and restless legs syndrome.

USES Parkinson disease; restless leg syndrome

CONTRAINDICATIONS Hypersensitivity to rotigotine or any component of the product; major psychotic disorder; pregnancy—fetal risk cannot be ruled out; lactation—milk effects are possible; safety and efficacy in children has not been established.

CAUTIOUS USE History of cardiac impairment, hypertension, CHF, renal insufficiency, patients with psychosis.

ROUTE & DOSAGE

Early stage Parkinson Disease

Adult: **Transdermal** 2 mg daily, increase by 2 mg/ 24 hours weekly (max dose: 6 mg/24hrs)

Advanced stage Parkinson Disease

Adult: **Transdermal** 4 mg daily, increase by 2 mg/ 24 hours weekly (max dose: 16 mg/24hrs)

ADMINISTRATION

Transdermal

- Apply the patch to clean, dry, intact, healthy, hairless skin (shaved at least 3 days prior) on front of the abdomen, thigh, hip, flank, shoulder, or upper arm that will not be rubbed by tight clothes. Avoid oily, irritated or damaged skin.
- Apply to a new site every day rotating from side to side and from upper to lower body; do not apply to the same site more than once every 14 days.
- After removing from protective liner, apply immediately by pressing in place for 30 seconds.
- Wear continually for 24 hours and apply a new patch at approximately the same time every day.
- If replacement patch is forgotten, or existing patch becomes dislodged, apply another patch for the remainder of the day then replace at the next regular time.
- Store unopened pouch between 20 and 25 degrees C (68 and

77 degrees F), with excursions permitted between 15 and 30 degrees C (59 and 86 degrees F). Use immediately after opening.

ADVERSE EFFECTS (≥5%) **CV:** *Orthostatic hypotension.* **CNS:** *Dizziness, dyskinesia, headache, sleep disorder, somnolence.* **Skin:** *Application site reaction*, diaphoresis. **GI:** Anorexia, *nausea, vomiting*, xerostomia **Other:** Compulsive behavior and hallucinations.

INTERACTIONS ANTIHYPERTENSIVES may have increased hypotensive effects. DOPAMINE AGONISTS, ANTIPSYCHOTICS may decrease effectiveness.

PHARMACOKINETICS **Distribution:** ·90% protein bound. **Metabolism:** Hepatic via CYP isoenzymes. **Elimination:** Urine **Half-Life:** 5-7 hours.

NURSING IMPLICATIONS

Assessment & Drug Effects

- Monitor for improved symptoms of tremor, stiffness, movement, and steadiness.
- Patient at risk for falls related to adverse effect of somnolence.
- Monitor blood pressure. Patient at risk for orthostatic hypotensive event.
- Monitor weight, and intake and output.
- Perform a thorough skin assessment.
- Monitor lab tests: renal function tests in patients with renal insufficiency

Patient & Family Education

- Avoid activities that require mental alertness or coordination until the effects of the drug are known. May cause somnolence up to 1 year after initiation.
- Advise patient that the patch contains aluminum and should be removed prior to a MRI or cardioversion.
- Avoid exposing the patch to direct heat as it may cause an increased drug absorption.
- Report signs of a site reaction: nausea, vomiting, dizziness, headache, insomnia, syncope, hallucinations, racing heart beat, swelling of extremities.
- Report any changes in moles and routinely inspect skin.
- Report any compulsive behavior: gambling, sexual urges, or binge eating.
- Review proper patch placement.
- Importance of not discontinuing the drug without consulting with the healthcare provider.
- Use extreme caution when taking alcohol, sedating medications or other CNS depressants when taking this drug.

SACUBITRIL AND VALSARTAN

(sac′u-bi-tril and val-sar-tan)

Entresto

Classification: CARDIOVASCULAR AGENT; NEPRILYSIN INHIBITOR; ANGIOTENSIN II RECEPTOR BLOCKER

Therapeutic: HEART FAILURE AGENT

AVAILABILITY Tablet

ACTIONS & *THERAPEUTIC EFFECT* Sacubitril is a prodrug that, when converted to an active metabolite (LBQ657), inhibits the enzyme, neprilysin, leading to increased levels of natriuretic peptides. Valsartan is an angiotensin receptor antagonist that selectively blocks the vasoconstriction and aldosterone-secreting effects of angiotensin II. *Decreases afterload thus facilitating increased cardiac output.*

S

USES Indicated for risk reduction of cardiovascular death and hospitalization from heart failure (HF) in patients with chronic HF (NYHA Class II-IV) and reduced ejection fraction; treatment of symptomatic HF with left ventricular systolic dysfunction in pediatric patients.

CONTRAINDICATIONS Hypersensitivity to any component; history of angioedema related to previous ACE inhibitor or ARB therapy; concomitant use with ACE inhibitors; concomitant use with aliskiren in patients with diabetes; severe hepatic impairment; pregnancy—fetal harm has been demonstrated; lactation—infant risk has been demonstrated.

CAUTIOUS USE Prior history of angioedema; African American ancestry; concomitant use of potassium-sparing diuretics, NSAIDs, or lithium; hypotension; renal impairment; mild to moderate hepatic impairment; potassium imbalance; risk factors for hyperkalemia including diabetes, hypoaldosteronism, or high potassium diet; older adults. Safety and efficacy established in children 1 y and older.

S

ROUTE & DOSAGE

Heart Failure with reduced ejection fraction

Adult: **PO** (Treatment naive or previous low dose ACE/ARB) Initial dose of sacubitril 24 mg/valsartan 26 mg bid or (previously taking moderate/high dose ACE or ARB) sacubitril 49 mg/valsartan 51 mg bid

Heart Failure with persevered ejection fraction

Adult: **PO** Sacubitril 49 mg/valsartan 51 mg bid; double dose as tolerated after ~2 weeks to target dose of sacubitril 97 mg/valsartan 103 mg bid

Heart Failure treatment

Adolescent/Child (over 1 yr): **PO** (Previously taking a moderate to high dose ACEI/ARB) *weight over 50 kg:* sacubitril 49 mg/valsartan 51 mg bid; *weight 40–50 kg:* sacubitril 24 mg/valsartan 26 mg bid

Hepatic Impairment Dosage Adjustment

Moderate impairment (Child-Pugh class B): Initial dose of sacubitril 24 mg/valsartan 26 mg bid

Severe impairment (Child-Pugh class C): Not recommended

Renal Impairment Dosage Adjustment

eGFR less than 30 mL/min: Initial dose of sacubitril 24 mg/valsartan 26 mg bid

ADMINISTRATION

Oral

- Correct volume or salt depletion prior to administration.
- May be given without regard to food.
- Store tablets at 20 to 25° C (68 to 77° F); excursions permitted between 15°–30° C (59°–86° F). Protect from moisture. Store suspension up to 15 days. Do not store above 25° C (77° F). Do not refrigerate and shake before each use.

ADVERSE EFFECTS (≥5%) CV: *Hypotension*, orthostatic hypotension. **CNS:** Dizziness. **Other:** Renal failure.

INTERACTIONS Drug: Concomitant use with an ANGIOTENSION CONVERTING ENZYME INHIBITOR increases the risk of angioedema and is contraindicated. Concomitant use of POTASSIUM SPARING DIURETICS (e.g., **amiloride, spironolactone, triamterene**) may lead to increased potassium levels. Concomitant use with NSAIDs in older adults, patients who are volume-depleted, or patients with compromised renal function may result in worsening of renal function. Sacubitril/valsartan may increase the levels of **lithium.** ANTIHEPACIVIRAL products may increase risk of adverse effects.

PHARMACOKINETICS Absorption: Sacubitril is greater than 60% bioavailable. **Peak:** Sacubitril 0.5 h.; LBQ657 2h.; valsartan 1.5 h. **Distribution:** Highly plasma protein bound (94–97%). **Metabolism:** Sacubitril is metabolized to an active metabolite, LBQ657; Valsartan minimal metabolism. **Elimination:** Sacubitril, 52–68% renal and 37–48% fecal; valsartan, 13% renal and 86% fecal. **Half-Life:** Sacubitril 1.4 h.; LBQ657 11.5 h.; valsartan 9.9 h.

NURSING IMPLICATIONS

Black Box Warning

The valsartan component of the drug has been associated with fetal toxicity. Discontinue use immediately if pregnancy is detected.

Assessment & Drug Effects

- Monitor cardiac status and BP frequently. Risk of hypotension increases with salt and/or volume depletion.
- Monitor activity tolerance and S&S of heart failure.
- Monitor for angioedema; if suspected, take measures necessary to ensure maintenance of a patent airway.
- Monitor for S&S of hyperkalemia (see Appendix F).
- Monitor for S&S of lithium toxicity with concurrent use.
- Monitor lab tests: Baseline and periodic LFTs and renal function tests; periodic serum potassium and Hct & Hgb.

Patient & Family Education

- Seek medical care immediately if experiencing swelling of face, lips, tongue, and throat (angioedema). Persons of African heritage are at greater risk for angioedema.
- Make position changes slowly, especially when standing from a lying or sitting position.
- Do not use potassium supplements, salt substitutes, or OTC nonsteroidal anti-inflammatory drugs (NSAIDs) without consulting prescriber.
- Women should use effective means of contraception while taking this drug. If pregnancy is suspected, stop taking this drug and report immediately to prescriber.
- Do not breast-feed while taking this drug.

SAFINAMIDE

(sa-fin′a-mide)

Xadago

Classification: MONOAMINE OXIDASE (MAO) B INHIBITOR

Therapeutic: ANTI-PARKINSON AGENT

S

AVAILABILITY Tablet

ACTION & *THERAPEUTIC EFFECT* Decreases dopamine catabolism via inhibition of type-B MAO which increases dopamine levels in the brain and subsequently increases dopaminergic activity. *Helpful adjunctive therapy in improving "off" episodes of Parkinson's disease.*

CONTRAINDICATIONS Hypersensitivity to safinamide or any component of the formulation; severe hepatic impairment (Child-Pugh class C); concomitant use of other monamine oxidase inhibitors (MAOIs) or other drugs that are potent inhibitors of monoamine oxidase, opioids, serotonin-norepinephrine reuptake inhibitors (SNRIs) tricyclic or triazolopyridine antidepressants, cyclobenzaprine, methylphenidate, amphetamines, and their derivatives, St. John's wort, dextromethorphan; lactation.

CAUTIOUS USE Hepatic impairment; ophthalmic disorders; psychotic disorders; pregnancy (category C).

ROUTE & DOSAGE

Parkinson's Disease

Adult: **Initial PO** 50 mg daily; after 2 wk titrate to 100 mg daily

Hepatic Impairment Dosage Adjustment

Moderate impairment (Child-Pugh class B): Max: 50 mg daily
Severe impairment (Child-Pugh class C): Do not use

ADMINISTRATION

Oral

- Administer without regard to meals at the same time every day. Always administer in association with levodopa/carbidopa.
- At doses 100 mg/day or less, interaction with tyramine-containing foods and beverages is unlikely, however, patients should avoid foods and beverages with very high (greater than 150 mg) tyramine concentrations. Food's freshness is also a consideration; improperly stored or spoiled food can create an environment where tyramine concentrations may increase.
- Store at 25° C (77° F); excursions permitted between 15°–30° C (59°–86° F).

ADVERSE EFFECTS **CV:** Hypertension. **CNS:** *Dyskinesia*, insomnia. **GI:** Nausea. **Other:** Falls, hallucinations, impulse control disorder, serotonin syndrome.

INTERACTIONS **Drug:** MAO-INHIBITORS or similar acting drugs (e.g., **linezolid**) may increase risk of nonselective MAO inhibition, which may lead to a hypertensive crisis; 14 days washout is appropriate between discontinuing safinamide and initiating another MAOI. SYMPATHOMIMETIC medications utilized with safinamide increases risk of hypertensive crisis (e.g., **methylphenidate, amphetamine,** and nasal or oral decongestants). Safinamide and **dextromethorphan** can cause brief episodes of psychosis and bizarre behavior. DOPAMINE ANTAGONISTS may decrease effectiveness of safinamide. Safinamide can increase the plasma levels of **cyclobenzaprine** and other serotonergic medications increasing the risk of serotonin syndrome; therefore the combination should be avoided [e.g., SELECTIVE SEROTONIN REUPTAKE INHIBITORS (SSRI), SEROTONIN-NOREPINEPHRINE REUPTAKE

INHIBITORS (SNRI)]. Selective OPIOIDS such as **tramadol** and **methadone** may also increase risk of serotonin syndrome when taken with safinamide, so the combination is contraindicated. Safinamide and its major metabolite may inhibit the breast cancer resistance protein, increasing concentrations of BCRP substrates; monitor use with substrates of BCRP (e.g., **methotrexate, irinotecan, topotecan**). **Food:** Tyramine containing foods (e.g., aged, fermented, cured, smoked, or pickled foods) may cause a release of norepinephrine resulting in a rise of blood pressure, and therefore should be avoided while on safinamide. **Herbal: St. John's wort** should be avoided.

PHARMACOKINETICS Absorption: 95% bioavailability. **Distribution:** 88% protein binding, volume of distribution 165 L. **Onset:** Time to peak 2–3 h. **Metabolism:** Primarily by cytosolic amidases and MAOA. **Elimination:** 76% in urine. **Half-Life:** 20–26 h.

NURSING IMPLICATIONS

Assessment & Drug Effects

- Monitor for an increase of daily "on" time without troublesome dyskinesia associated with Parkinson's disease may indicate efficacy.
- Monitor blood pressure.
- Monitor for new or increased impulse control or compulsive behaviors such as gambling, sexual, or spending urges, which may be unrecognizable by the patient.
- Monitor for visual changes in patients with a history of retinal or macular degeneration, uveitis, inherited retinal conditions, family history of hereditary retinal disease, albinism, retinitis pigmentosa, or any active retinopathy (diabetic retinopathy).

Patient & Family Education

- Notify all health care providers that this drug is being taken. This includes prescribers, doctors, nurses, pharmacists, and dentists.
- Avoid driving and doing other tasks or actions that require alertness until drug affects are known; some people have fallen asleep during activities.
- Monitor blood pressure at home as directed by prescriber; this drug may cause high blood pressure.
- Avoid foods high in tyramine (e.g., cheese, and red wine).
- Do not stop this drug without calling prescriber.
- Notify prescriber before drinking alcohol or using drugs and natural products that may slow actions.
- Notify prescriber if pregnant or have plans to get pregnant to discuss drug risks during pregnancy.
- Notify prescriber right away with S&S of an allergic reaction: Rash, hives, wheezing, chest tightness, trouble breathing, swelling in the mouth, face or lips
- Notify prescriber if experiencing symptoms of high blood pressure: Very bad headache, dizziness, passing out, or change in eyesight.
- Notify prescriber regarding the following: Movement control difficulty, hallucinations, confused or agitated feelings, strong urges that are hard to control, or experiencing falls.
- If this drug is taken along with drugs for depression, notify prescriber right away if experiencing the following: Agitation, change in balance, confusion, hallucinations, fast heart beat, muscle twitching or stiffness, seizure, shivering or shaking, profuse sweating, very bad diarrhea, upset stomach, vomiting, or very bad headache.

SALMETEROL XINAFOATE

(sal-me′ter-ol xin′a-fo-ate)

Serevent

Classification: BETA$_2$-ADRENERGIC RECEPTOR AGONIST

Therapeutic: BRONCHODILATOR

Prototype: Albuterol

AVAILABILITY Powder diskus for inhalation

ACTION & *THERAPEUTIC EFFECT* Long-acting beta$_2$-adrenoreceptor agonist that stimulates beta$_2$-adrenoreceptors, relaxes bronchospasm, and increases ciliary motility, thus facilitating expectoration. *Relaxes bronchospasm and increases ciliary motility, thus facilitating expectoration of pulmonary secretions.*

USES Maintenance therapy for asthma or bronchospasm associated with COPD. Prevention of exercise-induced bronchospasm.

CONTRAINDICATIONS Hypersensitivity to salmeterol or milk proteins; primary treatment of status asthmaticus; acute asthma; acute bronchospasm; acutely deteriorating COPD; MAOI therapy.

S

CAUTIOUS USE Cardiovascular disorders, cardiac arrhythmias, hypertension, QT prolongation, hypokalemia; history of seizures or thyrotoxicosis; hyperthyroidism; pheochromocytoma; liver and renal impairment; COPD; DM, sensitivity to other beta-adrenergic agonists; older adults; women in labor; pregnancy (category- C); lactation (infant risk cannot be ruled out). Safe use in children younger than 4 y not established.

ROUTE & DOSAGE

Asthma or Bronchospasm (COPD associated)

Adult/Child (4 y or older): **Inhalation** 1 powder diskus (50 mcg) bid approximately 12 h apart

Prevention of Exercise-Induced Bronchospasm

Adult/Child (4 y or older): **Inhalation** 1 powder diskus (50 mcg) 30–60 min before exercise

ADMINISTRATION

Inhalation

- Do not use to relieve symptoms of acute asthma.
- Activate diskus by moving lever until it clicks. Patient should exhale fully (not into diskus), place diskus in mouth, and inhale quickly and deeply through the diskus. Diskus should be removed and breath held for 10 sec.
- Store at room temperature, 15°–30° C (59°–86° F).

ADVERSE EFFECTS Respiratory: Congestion, bronchitis, throat irritation, cough, sinusitis, rhinitis. **CNS:** Headache, pain. **Musculoskeletal:** Muscle pain.

INTERACTIONS Drug: Effects antagonized by BETA-BLOCKERS, MAOIS. Avoid use of strong CYP3A4 inhibitors. Do not use with **cobicistat** or **telaprevir.** Do not use with other BETA 2-AGONISTS.

PHARMACOKINETICS Onset: 10–20 min. **Peak:** Effect 2 h. **Duration:** Up to 12 h. **Distribution:** 94–95% protein bound, excreted in breast milk. **Metabolism:** Salmeterol is extensively metabolized by hydroxylation. **Elimination:** Primarily in feces. **Half-Life:** 3–4 h.

NURSING IMPLICATIONS

Black Box Warning

Salmeterol has been associated with increased risk of asthma-related hospitalization and death.

Assessment & Drug Effects

- Withhold drug and notify prescriber immediately if bronchospasms occur following its use.
- Monitor cardiovascular status; report tachycardia.
- Monitor lab tests: Periodic serum glucose and serum potassium.

Patient & Family Education

- Never use a spacer device with the drug.
- Do not use this drug to treat an acute asthma attack.
- Notify prescriber immediately of worsening asthma or failure to respond to the usual dose of salmeterol.
- Do not use an additional dose prior to exercise if taking twice-daily doses of salmeterol.
- Take the preexercise dose 30–60 min before exercise and wait 12 h before an additional dose.

SALSALATE

(sal′sa-late)

Classification: NONSTEROIDAL ANTI-INFLAMMATORY DRUG (NSAID)

Therapeutic: NONNARCOTIC ANALGESIC, NSAID

Prototype: Aspirin

AVAILABILITY Tablet

ACTION & *THERAPEUTIC EFFECT* Anti-inflammatory and analgesic activity of salsalate may be mediated through inhibition of the prostaglandin synthetase enzyme complex. *Has analgesic, anti-inflammatory, and antirheumatic effects.*

USES Symptomatic treatment, rheumatoid arthritis, osteoarthritis, and related rheumatic disorders.

CONTRAINDICATIONS Hypersensitivity to salicylates or NSAIDs; chronic renal insufficiency; peptic ulcer; children younger than 12 y; hemophilia; chickenpox, influenza, tinnitus.

CAUTIOUS USE Liver function impairment; older adults; pregnancy (category C); lactation (infant risk cannot be ruled out). Safety and efficacy in children not established.

ROUTE & DOSAGE

Rheumatic Disorders

Adult: **PO** 3 g /day in 2 to 3 divided doses

ADMINISTRATION

Oral

- Give with a full glass of water or food or milk to reduce GI adverse effects.
- Store at controlled room temperature 15°–30° C (59°–86° F).

ADVERSE EFFECTS **CV:** Hypotension. **Respiratory:** Bronchospasm. **CNS:** Dizziness. **HEENT:** Auditory impairment, tinnitus. **Skin:** Rash, Stevens-Johnson syndrome, toxic epidermal necrolysis, urticaria. **Hepatic:** Increased liver function tests, hepatitis. **GI:** Abdominal pain, diarrhea, gastrointestinal hemorrhage, gastrointestinal perforation, gastrointestinal ulcer, nausea. **GU:** Decreased creatinine clearance, nephritis. **Hematologic:** Anemia.

S

DIAGNOSTIC TEST INTERFERENCE False-negative results for ***Clinistix;*** false-positives for ***Clinitest;*** false results for plasma T4.

INTERACTIONS **Drug: Aminosalicylic acid** increases risk of salicylate toxicity. ACIDIFYING AGENTS decrease renal elimination and increase risk of salicylate toxicity. ANTICOAGULANTS increase risk of bleeding. Do not use with NSAIDS. ORAL HYPOGLYCEMIC AGENTS increase hypoglycemic activity with salsalate doses greater than 2 g/day. CARBONIC ANHYDRASE INHIBITORS enhance salicylate toxicity. CORTICOSTEROIDS add to ulcerogenic effects. **Methotrexate** toxicity is increased. Low doses of salicylates may antagonize uricosuric effects of **probenecid** and **sulfinpyrazone. Herbal: Feverfew, garlic, ginger, ginkgo** may increase bleeding potential.

PHARMACOKINETICS **Absorption:** Readily absorbed from small intestine. **Peak:** 1.5–4 h. **Metabolism:** Hydrolyzed in liver, GI mucosa, plasma, whole blood, and other tissues. **Elimination:** In urine. **Half-Life:** 1 h.

NURSING IMPLICATIONS

Black Box Warning

NSAIDS may cause increased risk of serious cardiovascular thrombotic events, myocardial infarction, and stroke, which can be fatal.

Assessment & Drug Effects

- Symptom relief is gradual (may require 3–4 days to establish steady-state salicylate level).
- Monitor for adverse GI effects, especially in patient with a history of peptic ulcer disease.
- Monitor labs: CBC, fecal occult blood test, LFTs, BUN, creatinine, plasma salicylic acid.

Patient & Family Education

- Do not take another salicylate (e.g., aspirin) while on salsalate therapy.
- Monitor blood glucose for loss of glycemic control in diabetes; drug may induce hypoglycemia when used with sulfonylureas.
- Report tinnitus, hearing loss, vertigo, rash, or nausea.

SAQUINAVIR MESYLATE Pr

(sa-quin′a-vir mes′y-late)

Invirase

Classification: PROTEASE INHIBITOR

Therapeutic: PROTEASE INHIBITOR

AVAILABILITY Gelatin capsule; tablet

ACTION & *THERAPEUTIC EFFECT* Inhibits the activity of HIV protease and prevents the cleavage of viral polyproteins essential for the maturation of HIV. *Effectiveness indicated by reduced viral load (decreased number of RNA copies), and increased number of T helper CD4 cells.*

USES HIV infection (used with other antiretroviral agents).

CONTRAINDICATIONS Significant hypersensitivity to saquinavir; congenital long QT syndrome; severe hepatic impairment; AV block; hypokalemia, or hypomagnesia; antimicrobial resistance to other protease inhibitors; monotherapy; lactation (infant risk cannot be ruled out).

CAUTIOUS USE Hepatic insufficiency; severe renal impairment;

hepatitis B or C; DM, diabetic ketoacidosis; CHF, bradyarrhythmias, electrolyte imbalances; hemophilia A or B; older adults; pregnancy (category B). Safety and efficacy in HIV-infected children younger than 16 y not established.

ROUTE & DOSAGE

HIV

Adult/Adolescent: **PO** 1000 mg bid with ritonavir 100 mg bid

ADMINISTRATION

Oral

- Give with or up to 2 h after a full meal to ensure adequate absorption and bioavailability. Give with ritonavir.
- If patient is unable to swallow capsule, contents may be added to 3 tsps of jam or 15 mL of sugar syrup (sorbitol syrup for diabetic or glucose-intolerant patients); mix for 30–60 seconds.
- Do not administer to anyone taking rifampin or rifabutin because these drugs significantly decrease the plasma level of saquinavir.
- Store at 15°–30° C (59°–86° F) in a tightly closed bottle.

ADVERSE EFFECTS

CV: Atrioventricular block, prolonged QT interval, prolonged PR interval. **CNS:** Fatigue. **Endocrine:** Lipodystrophy. **GI:** Abdominal pain, diarrhea, nausea, vomiting.

INTERACTIONS

Drug: Do not use with **sildenafil, alfuzosin,** or **salmeterol.** Rifampin, **rifabutin** significantly decrease saquinavir levels. **Phenobarbital, phenytoin, dexamethasone, carbamazepine** may also reduce saquinavir levels. Saquinavir levels may be increased by **delavirdine, ketoconazole, ritonavir, clarithromycin, indinavir.** May increase serum levels of **triazolam, midazolam,** ERGOT DERIVATIVES, **nelfinavir, simvastatin.** PHENOTHIAZINES may increase arrhythmogenic effect of saquinavir. May increase risk of **ergotamine** toxicity of **dihydroergotamine, ergotamine.** Dosage adjustments are needed when used with **bosentan, tadalafil,** or **colchicine. Herbal: St. John's wort, garlic** may decrease antiretroviral activity. **Food: Grapefruit juice** (greater than 1 qt/day) may increase plasma concentrations and adverse effects.

PHARMACOKINETICS

Absorption: Rapidly from GI tract; food significantly increases bioavailability. **Distribution:** 98% protein bound. **Metabolism:** In liver (CYP3A4), first-pass metabolism. **Elimination:** Primarily in feces (greater than 80%). **Half-Life:** 13 h.

NURSING IMPLICATIONS

Assessment & Drug Effects

- Assess for buccal mucosa ulceration or other distressing GI S&S.
- Monitor weight periodically.
- Monitor for toxicity if any of the following drugs is used concomitantly: Calcium channel blockers, clindamycin, dapsone, quinidine, triazolam, or simvastatin.
- Monitor for and report S&S of peripheral neuropathy.
- Monitor lab tests: Baseline and periodic CD_4 count, serum electrolytes, hepatitis screening, LFTs, CBC with differential, fasting blood glucose, urinalysis, for women of child bearing potential base line pregnancy test, fasting blood glucose or HgbA1c at baseline and with modification, and lipid profile.

S

Patient & Family Education

- Take drug within 2 h of a full meal.
- Be aware of all drugs which should not be taken concurrently with saquinavir.
- Be aware that saquinavir is not a cure for HIV infection and that its long-term effects are unknown.
- Report any distressing adverse effects to prescriber.

SARECYCLINE

(sar-e-SYE-kleen)

Seysara

Classifications: TETRACYCLINE ANTIBIOTIC

Therapeutic: ANTIBIOTIC

Prototype: TETRACYCLINE

AVAILABILITY Oral tablet

ACTION & *THERAPEUTIC EFFECT* Bacteriostatic action that appears to be a result of reversible binding to ribosomal units of susceptible bacteria and inhibition of bacterial protein synthesis. *Effective against gram-positive and gram negative bacteria, but direct influence on acne vulgaris is unknown.*

USES Treatment of inflammatory acne vulgaris.

S

CONTRAINDICATIONS Known hypersensitivity to any of the tetraclines; pregnancy – fetal risk cannot be ruled out; lactation – infant risk cannot be ruled out.

CAUTIOUS USE Obese women of childbearing age, premature infants, approved for children 9 years or older.

ROUTE & DOSAGE

Acne vulgaris

Adult/Adolescent/Child (9 y or older, weight 33 to <55kg): **PO** 60 mg once daily
(weight 55 to <85kg): **PO** 100 mg once daily
(weight 85 to 136kg): **PO** 150 mg once daily

ADMINISTRATION

Oral

- Administer once daily with or without food; give with an adequate amount of fluid to prevent esophageal irritation and ulceration.
- Store at a controlled room temperature between 20 and 25 degrees of C (68 and 77 degrees F), with excursions permitted between 15 and 30 degrees C (59 and 86 degrees F). Protect from moisture and excessive heat.

ADVERSE EFFECTS CNS: Psuedotumor cerebri. **GI:** Nausea, Clostridium difficile diarrhea, staining of teeth. **Musculoskeletal:** delayed bone development and/or growth.

INTERACTIONS Drug: ANTACIDS, **calcium, magnesium**, and iron containing products bind sarecycline in gut and decrease absorption; may enhance effects of ANTICOAGULANTS (e.g., warfarin); increases **digoxin** absorption, thus increasing risk of **digoxin** toxicity. Do not use with **acitretin** or **isotretinoin.**

PHARMACOKINETICS Peak: 1.5–2h **Distribution:** 91.4–97 L,

62.5–74.7% protein bound. **Metabolism:** Minimal metabolism. **Elimination:** 42.6% and 44.1% excreted in feces and urine, respectively. **Half-Life:** 21–22h.

NURSING IMPLICATIONS

Assessment & Drug Effects

- Monitor for improvement in acne vulgaris lesion count.
- Assess for diarrhea. Risk for Clostridium difficile related diarrhea may occur 2 months after administration.
- Evaluate for visual disturbances, may indicate intracranial hypertension.

Patient & Family Education

- Report severe diarrhea.
- Review adverse effects.
- Avoid activities requiring mental alertness or coordination until drug effects are realized.
- Instruct patient to use sunscreen, wear protective clothing, and avoid tanning beds due to potential for photosensitivity.
- Report blurred vision or headaches, nausea, or vomiting as it may be indicative of intracranial hypertension.
- Make sure to take drug with adequate amounts of fluid to reduce the risk of esophageal irritation and ulceration.

SARGRAMOSTIM (GM-CSF)

(sar-gra′mos-tim)

Leukine

Classification: GRANULOCYTE-MACROPHAGE COLONY-STIMULATING FACTOR (GM-CSF)

Therapeutic: HEMAPOIETIC GROWTH FACTOR; GM-CSF

Prototype: Filgrastim

AVAILABILITY Solution for injection

ACTION & *THERAPEUTIC EFFECT* GM-CSF is a hematopoietic growth factor that stimulates proliferation and differentiation of progenitor cells in the granulocyte-macrophage pathways. *Effectiveness is measured by an increase in the number of mature white blood cells (i.e., neutrophil count).*

USES Febrile neutropenia, neutropenia caused by chemotherapy, peripheral blood stem cell (PBSC) mobilization.

UNLABELED USES Neutropenia secondary to other diseases; aplastic anemia, Crohn's disease, malignant melanoma.

CONTRAINDICATIONS Hypersensitivity to GM-CSF, yeast-derived products; excessive leukemic myeloid blasts in bone marrow or blood greater than or equal to 10%; within 24 h of chemotherapy or radiation treatment; if ANC exceeds 20,000 cells/mm^3 discontinue drug or use half the dose; increased growth of tumor size; pregnancy (fetal risk cannot be ruled out); lactation (infant risk cannot be ruled out).

CAUTIOUS USE Hypersensitivity to benzyl alcohol; history of cardiac arrhythmias, preexisting cardiac disease, renal or hepatic dysfunction, CHF, hypoxia, myelodysplastic syndromes; pulmonary infiltrates; fluid retention; kidney and liver dysfunction; use in AML for adults younger than 55 y. Safety and efficacy in children younger than 2 y not established.

S

ROUTE & DOSAGE

Neutropenia following Stem Cell Transplantation

Adult: **IV** 250 mcg/m²/day infused over 2 h for 21 days, begin 2–4 h after bone marrow transfusion and not less than 24 h after last dose of chemotherapy or 12 h after last radiation therapy

Following PBSC

Adult: **IV/Subcutaneous** 250 mg/m²/day

Neutropenia following Chemotherapy/Febrile Neutropenia

Adult: **IV/Subcutaneous** 250 mcg/m²/day starting ~day 11 or 4 days following induction chemotherapy

ADMINISTRATION

- Note: Do not give within 24 h preceding or following chemotherapy or within 12 h preceding or following radiotherapy.

Subcutaneous

- Reconstitute each 250 mcg powder vial with 1 mL of sterile water for injection (without preservative). Direct sterile water against side of vial and swirl gently. Avoid excessive or vigorous agitation. Do not shake. Use without further dilution for subcutaneous injection.

Intravenous

PREPARE: **IV Infusion:** Reconstitute powder vial as for subcutaneous, then further dilute reconstituted solution with NS. If the final concentration is less than 1 mcg/mL, add albumin (human) to NS before addition of sargramostim. ▪ Use 1 mg albumin/1 mL of NS to give a final concentration of 0.1% albumin. ▪ Administer as soon as possible and within 6 h of reconstitution or dilution for IV infusion. ▪ Discard after 6 h. ▪ Sargramostim vials are single-dose vials, do not re-enter or reuse. Discard unused portion.

ADMINISTER: **IV Infusion:** Give over 2, 4, or 24 h as ordered. ▪ Do not use an in-line membrane filter. ▪ Interrupt administration and reduce the dose by 50% if absolute neutrophil count exceeds 20,000/mm³ or if platelet count exceeds 500,000/mm³. Notify prescriber. ▪ Reduce the IV rate 50% if patient experiences dyspnea during administration. ▪ Discontinue infusion if respiratory symptoms worsen. Notify prescriber.

INCOMPATIBILITIES: **Y-site: Acyclovir, ampicillin, ampicillin/sulbactam, cefoperazone, chlorpromazine, ganciclovir, haloperidol, hydrocortisone, hydromorphone, hydroxyzine, imipenem/cilastatin, lorazepam, methylprednisolone, mitomycin, morphine, nalbuphine, ondansetron, piperacillin, sodium bicarbonate, tobramycin, vancomycin hydrochloride.**

- Refrigerate the sterile powder, the reconstituted solution, and store diluted solution at 2°–8° C (36°–46° F). ▪ Do not freeze or shake.

ADVERSE EFFECTS **CV:** *Hypertension, edema, pericardial effusion,* chest pain, peripheral edema, tachycardia. **Respiratory:** Pharyngitis, epistaxis, dyspnea. **CNS:** Weakness, joint pain, muscle pain, bone pain. **HEENT:** Retinal hemorrhage. **Endocrine:** *Weight loss,* *hyperglycemia,* hypercholesterolemia, hypomagnesemia. **Skin:** *Rash,* pruritis. **Hepatic:** *Hyperbilirubinemia.* **GI:** *Diarrhea, nausea, vomiting, abdominal pain,* anorexia, hematemesis, dysphagia, gastrointestinal hemorrhage. **GU:** UTI. **Musculoskeletal:** *Weakness,* bone pain, joint pain, muscle pain. **Other:** Fever.

INTERACTIONS

Drug: CORTICOSTEROIDS and **lithium** should be used with caution because it may potentiate the myeloproliferative effects.

PHARMACOKINETICS

Absorption: Readily from subcutaneous site. **Onset:** 3–6 h. **Peak:** 1–2 h. **Duration:** 5–10 days subcutaneous. **Elimination:** Probably in urine. **Half-Life:** 80–150 min.

NURSING IMPLICATIONS

Assessment & Drug Effects

- Discontinue treatment and notify prescriber if WBC 50,000/mm^3.
- Monitor cardiac status. Occasional transient supraventricular arrhythmias have occurred during administration, particularly in those with a history of cardiac arrhythmias. Arrhythmias are reversed with discontinuation of drug.
- Give special attention to respiratory symptoms (dyspnea) during and immediately following IV infusion, especially in patients with preexisting pulmonary disease.
- Use drug with caution in patients with preexisting fluid retention, pulmonary infiltrates, or CHF. Peripheral edema, pleural or pericardial effusion has occurred after administration. It is reversible with dose reduction.
- Notify prescriber of any severe adverse reaction immediately.
- Monitor lab tests: Baseline and biweekly CBC with differential and platelet count; biweekly LFTs and renal function tests in patients with established kidney or liver dysfunction.

Patient & Family Education

- Notify nurse or prescriber immediately of any adverse effect (e.g., dyspnea, palpitations, peripheral edema, bone or muscle pain) during or after drug administration.

SARILUMAB

(sar-il′ue-mab)

Kevzara

Classification: DISEASE MODIFYING ANTIRHEUMATIC (DMARD); INTERLEUKIN-6 RECEPTOR ANTAGONIST; MONOCLONAL ANTIBODY

Therapeutic: DISEASE-MODIFYING ANTIRHEUMATIC (DMARD)

AVAILABILITY

Subcutaneous injection

ACTION & *THERAPEUTIC EFFECT*

Inhibits interleukin-6 (IL-6)-mediated signaling by binding to IL-6 receptors that are both soluble and membrane-bound. *Inhibition of the IL-6 receptors by sarilumab leads to a reduction in CRP levels, which can improve inflammatory processes such as rheumatoid arthritis.*

USES

Treatment of rheumatoid arthritis that has failed or had insufficient response to other disease-modifying medications.

CONTRAINDICATIONS

Hypersensitivity to sarilumab or excipients, live vaccines. Limited available data to determine if sarilumab during pregnancy is associated with risk for major birth defects or miscarriage. Monoclonal antibodies,

S

like sarilumab, are transported across the placenta. There is no current data available on the presence of sarilumab in human milk or its effects on the breastfed infant or milk production.

CAUTIOUS USE History of diverticulitis or concomitant use of NSAIDS or corticosteroid use, active hepatic disease, or impairment.

ROUTE & DOSAGE

Rheumatoid Arthritis

Adult: **Subcutaneous** 200 mg every 2 wk

Hepatic Impairment Dosage Adjustment

ALT/AST greater than 3–5 × ULN: Hold therapy until ALT/ALT is less than 3 × ULN, then restart medication at 150 mg every 2 wk; increase to original dose as appropriate

ALT/AST greater than 5 × ULN: Discontinue therapy

ADMINISTRATION

Subcutaneous

- Allow to sit at room temperature for 30 min prior to administration; do not warm any other way.
- Solution should be clear and colorless to pale yellow.
- Do not shake.
- Not for IV administration.
- Rotate injection sites; do not inject where skin is tender, damaged, bruised, or scarred.
- Inject full amount of the prefilled syringe.
- If 3 days or less since missed dose, take as soon as possible; take next dose at regularly scheduled time.
- Store at 2°–8° C (36°–46° F) in the original carton to protect from light. Do not freeze or shake. May store at 25° C (77° F) or cooler for up to 14 days. After removal from the refrigerator, use within 14 days.

ADVERSE EFFECTS **Endocrine:** *Increased LFTs.* **Skin:** Injection site pruritis and erythema. **GU:** UTI. **Hematologic:** Neutropenia, leukopenia.

INTERACTIONS Do not give live virus vaccines to patients on sarilumab; not studied with the use of JAK inhibitors or other biological DMARD agents (such as TNF antagonists). Potential interaction with CYP450 substrates, specifically those with narrow therapeutic index or specific desired effectiveness (e.g., **warfarin, theophylline**, oral contraceptives).

PHARMACOKINETICS **Absorption:** 34% bioavailability. **Onset:** Peak effect in 2–4 days. **Metabolism:** Similar to endogenous IgG, undergoes catabolic metabolism to small peptides and amino acids. **Elimination:** Through proteolytic pathway. **Half-Life:** 8–10 days, dependent on dose.

NURSING IMPLICATIONS

Black Box Warning

Serious infections (e.g., bacterial, mycobacterial, invasive fungal, viral and opportunistic infections) which have led to hospitalization or death. Do not administer during active infections. Monitor patients for infection during use. Use caution in patients with TB exposure or history of serious opportunistic, chronic, or recurrent infection. Stop sarilumab if serious opportunistic infection develops.

Assessment & Drug Effects

- Monitor for improvement of signs or symptoms of rheumatoid arthritis.
- Monitor neutrophils and platelets: 4–8 wk after treatment initiation and approximately every 3 mo thereafter.
- Monitor for latent TB prior to initiation.
- Monitor for active TB in all patients, even if initial latent TB was negative.
- Monitor for S&S of infection during and after therapy.
- Monitor for gastrointestinal perforation.
- Monitor lab tests: ALT and AST levels 4–8 wk after treatment initiation and approximately every 3 mo thereafter. Other LFTs may be ordered if clinically indicated.

Patient & Family Education

- Do not take this drug if infection is present.
- TB has been seen in patients that take this drug.
- Notify health care provider right away of signs of infection such as fever, flu-like symptoms, chills, very bad sore throat, ear or sinus pain, cough, pain while urinating, mouth sores or sores that will not heal.
- Notify all health care providers that this drug is being taken. This includes prescribers, doctors, nurses, pharmacists, and dentists.
- Talk to prescriber before getting any vaccines.
- Birth control pills and other hormone-based birth control may not work to prevent pregnancy. Use another effective method for birth control while taking this drug.
- Notify prescriber if pregnant or plan to get pregnant.
- If pregnancy occurs while using this drug, notify your prescriber right away.
- Discuss possible breast-feeding risks with prescriber.
- Notify prescriber right away with S&S of an allergic reaction: Rash, hives, blistered skin, wheezing, chest tightness, unusual hoarseness, swelling of the mouth, face, lips, tongue or throat; very bad belly pain; vomiting dark brown coffee ground emesis, black tarry stools, shortness of breath, chest pain, dizziness, muscle pain or weakness, coughing up blood.

SAXAGLIPTIN

(sax-a-glip′tin)

Onglyza

Classification: DIPEPTIDYL PEPTIDASE-4 (DPP-4) INHIBITOR

Therapeutic: ANTIDIABETIC; HORMONE MODIFIER; DDP-4 INHIBITOR

Prototype: Sitagliptin

AVAILABILITY Tablet

ACTION & *THERAPEUTIC EFFECT* Slows inactivation of incretin hormones [e.g., glucagon-like peptide-1 (GLP-1) and glucose-dependent insulinotropic polypeptide (GIP)]. As plasma glucose rises, incretin hormones stimulate release of insulin from the pancreas and GLP-1 also lowers glucagon secretion, resulting in reduced hepatic glucose production. *In type 2 diabetics, saxagliptin elevates the level of incretin hormones, thus increasing insulin secretion and reducing glucagon secretion. It lowers both fasting and postprandial plasma glucose levels.*

USES Treatment of type 2 diabetes mellitus.

CONTRAINDICATIONS Hypersensitivity to saxagliptin; exfoliative skin condition; type 1 DM, concurrent administration with insulin.

CAUTIOUS USE Moderate to severe renal impairment; acute pancreatitis; history of angioedema with use of another DDP4 inhibitor; HF; lactose intolerance; older adults; pregnancy (category B) (fetal risk cannot be ruled out); lactation (infant risk cannot be ruled out). Safe use in children younger than 18 y not established.

ROUTE & DOSAGE

Type 2 Diabetes Mellitus

Adult: **PO** 2.5–5 mg daily. Limited to 2.5 mg daily when used with a strong CYP3A4/5 inhibitor.

Renal Impairment Dosage Adjustment

eGFR less than 45 mL/min/ 1.73 m²: 2.5 mg once daily

ADMINISTRATION

Oral

- May be taken without regard to meals.
- Ensure that tablets are taken whole; they must not be cut or split.
- Dosing in the older adults should be based on creatinine clearance.
- Store at 15°–30° C (59°–86° F).

ADVERSE EFFECTS **CV:** Peripheral edema. **Respiratory:** URI. **CNS:** Headache. **Endocrine:** Hypoglycemia. **GU:** UTI.

INTERACTIONS **Drug: Rifampin** and other inducers of CYP3A4/5 enzymes decrease saxagliptin levels. Moderate (e.g., **amprenavir, aprepitant, erythromycin, fluconazole, fosamprenavir, verapamil**) and strong (e.g., **atazanavir, clarithromycin, indinavir, itraconazole, ketoconazole, nefazodone, nelfinavir, ritonavir, saquinavir, telithromycin**) inhibitors of CYP3A4/5 increase saxagliptin levels. Decrease saxagliptin dose when used with INSULIN or ANTIDIABETIC drug to minimize risk of hypoglycemia. **Food: Grapefruit juice** increases saxagliptin levels.

PHARMACOKINETICS **Peak:** 2 h. **Distribution:** Negligible plasma protein binding. **Metabolism:** Hepatic metabolism to active and inactive compounds. **Elimination:** Renal (75%) and fecal (22%). **Half-Life:** 2.5–3.1 h.

NURSING IMPLICATIONS

Assessment & Drug Effects

- Monitor for and report S&S of significant GI distress including NV&D.
- Monitor for S&S of hypoglycemia when used in combination with a sulfonylurea or insulin.
- Monitor lab tests: Baseline and periodic creatinine clearance; periodic fasting and postprandial plasma glucose and HbA1C.

Patient & Family Education

- Carry out blood glucose monitoring as directed by prescriber.
- Consult prescriber during periods of stress and illness as dosage adjustments may be required.
- When taken alone to control diabetes, saxagliptin is unlikely to cause hypoglycemia because it only works when the blood sugar is rising after food intake.
- Stop taking drug immediately if you experience symptoms of a serious allergic reaction such as

S

swelling about the face or throat, or difficulty breathing or swallowing.

SCOPOLAMINE

(skoe-pol'a-meen)

Transderm Scop

SCOPOLAMINE HYDROBROMIDE

Classification: ANTICHOLINERGIC; ANTIMUSCARINIC; ANTISPASMODIC; ANTIVERTIGO

Therapeutic: ANTISPASMODIC; ANTI-EMETIC; ANTIVERTIGO

Prototype: Atropine

AVAILABILITY **Scopolamine:** Transdermal patch.

ACTION & THERAPEUTIC EFFECT Inhibits the action on acetylcholine (ACh) on postganglionic cholinergic nerves as well as on smooth muscles that lack cholinergic innervation. *Produces CNS depression with marked sedative and tranquilizing effects for use in anesthesia. Effective as a preanesthetic agent to control bronchial, nasal, pharyngeal, and salivary secretions. Additionally, it prevents nausea and vomiting associated with motion sickness.*

USES Prevention of nausea/vomiting associated with motion sickness and recovery from anesthesia.

CONTRAINDICATIONS Hypersensitivity to anticholinergic drugs; narrow angle glaucoma; severe ulcerative colitis, GI obstruction; urinary tract obstruction diseases; renal impairment; hepatic impairment; chronic lung disease; prostatic hypertrophy; infants under 6 months of age; toxemia of pregnancy; pregnancy—fetal risk cannot be ruled out; lactation—infant risk cannot be ruled out.

CAUTIOUS USE Remove patch before undergoing MRI to prevent burns at the patch site. Hypertension; patients older than 40 y, pyloric obstruction, autonomic neuropathy, myasthenia gravis; thyrotoxicosis, liver disease; CAD; CHF; tachycardia, or other tachyarrhythmias; paralytic ileus; hiatal hernia, mild or moderate ulcerative colitis, gastric ulcer, GERD; renal impairment; parkinsonism; COPD, asthma or allergies; hyperthyroidism; brain damage, psychosis; spastic paralysis; Down syndrome; older adults; children, infants.

ROUTE & DOSAGE

Motion Sickness

Adult: **Topical** 1 patch at least 4 h before anticipated travel and q3days as needed

ADMINISTRATION

Transdermal

- Apply transdermal disc system (Transderm Scōp, a controlled-release system) to dry hairless surface behind the ear. Wear gloves or wash hands thoroughly before and after application.
- Replace with another disc on another site behind the ear if disc system becomes dislodged.
- Upon removal, fold the used transdermal system in half with sticky sides together and discard in the household trash in a manner that prevents accidental contact or ingestion by children, pets, or others.
- Store patch in an upright position at a controlled room temperature

S

between 20 and 25 degrees C (68 and 77 degrees F). Do not bend or roll the pouch.

ADVERSE EFFECTS **CV:** Tachycardia. **CNS:** Amnesia (injection), somnolence (injection). **HEENT:** Dilated pupils. **Skin:** Local irritation from patch adhesive, rash, diminished sweating. **GI:** *Dry mouth and throat* (injection). **Other:** Local irritation.

INTERACTIONS **Drug: Amantadine,** ANTICHOLINERGIC AGENTS, ANTIHISTAMINES, TRICYCLIC ANTIDEPRESSANTS, **quinidine, disopyramide, procainamide** add to anticholinergic effects; decreases **levodopa** effects; **methotrimeprazine** may precipitate extrapyramidal effects; decreases antipsychotic effects (decreased absorption) of PHENOTHIAZINES; CNS DEPRESSANTS add to CNS related side effects; **clozapine** may have increased adverse effects. **Food: Grapefruit juice** (greater than 1 qt/day) may increase plasma concentrations and adverse effects.

DIAGNOSTIC TEST INTERFERENCE Interferes with ***gastric secretion test.***

PHARMACOKINETICS **Absorption:** Readily from GI tract and percutaneously. **Peak:** 24 hours. **Duration:** 72 hours. **Distribution:** Crosses placenta; distributed to CNS. **Metabolism:** In liver. **Elimination:** In urine.

NURSING IMPLICATIONS

Assessment & Drug Effects

- Observe patient closely; some patients manifest excitement, delirium, and disorientation shortly after drug is administered until sedative effect takes hold.
- Monitor I and Os and watch for improvement in nausea/vomiting.
- Use of side rails is advisable, particularly for older adults, because of amnesic effect of scopolamine.
- Monitor blood pressure.
- In the presence of pain, scopolamine may cause delirium, restlessness, and excitement unless given with an analgesic.
- Be aware that tolerance may develop with prolonged use.
- Terminate ophthalmic use if local irritation, edema, or conjunctivitis occur.

Patient & Family Education

- Vision may blur when used as mydriatic or cycloplegic; do not drive or engage in potentially hazardous activities until vision clears.
- Ophthalmic and injectable forms may cause photophobia. Wear sunglasses outside and avoid bright lights.
- Injectable form may impair heat regulation. Use caution with activities leading to an increased core temperature such as strenuous exercise, exposure to extreme heat, or dehydration.
- Review proper administration of ophthalmic drops.
- Place disc on skin site the night before an expected trip or anticipated motion for best therapeutic effect.
- Wash hands carefully after handling scopolamine. Anisocoria (unequal size of pupils, blurred vision can develop by rubbing eye with drug-contaminated finger).
- Avoid alcohol and any other drugs that affect the central nervous system.

SECNIDAZOLE
(sek-nik'a-zole)
Solosec
Classification: ANTIBACTERIAL; NITROIMIDAZOLE
Therapeutic: ANTIBACTERIAL; ANTIPROTOZOAL
Prototype: Metronidazole

AVAILABILITY Oral granules

ACTION & *THERAPEUTIC EFFECT* As a 5-nitroimidazole antimicrobial, produces radical anions within bacterial cells which interfere with bacterial DNA synthesis. *Secnidazole targets microorganisms often responsible for bacterial vaginosis in adult women.*

USES Bacterial vaginosis treatment; trichomoniasis.

CONTRAINDICATIONS Previous hypersensitivity to secnidazole or other nitroimidazole like medications.

CAUTIOUS USE May increase the incidence of vulvo-vaginal candidiasis, patients should be monitored for symptoms; the use of secnidazole in the absence of a suspected bacterial infection may increase the risk of drug-resistant microorganisms.

ROUTE & DOSAGE

Bacterial Vaginosis/ Trichomoniasis
Adult: **PO** 2 grams as a single dose

ADMINISTRATION

Oral
- Administer with or without food.
- Granules should not be crushed or chewed.
- Packet contents can be sprinkled onto food such as applesauce; granules are not intended to be dissolved in liquid.
- Granules should be consumed within 30 min of use.
- Avoid preparations containing ethanol or propylene glycol and consumption of alcohol during treatment and for at least 2 days after completing therapy.
- Store granule packet at 20°–25° C (68°–77° F), excursions permitted between 15 and 30° C (59 and 86° F) protected from moisture.

ADVERSE EFFECTS (≥5%) **GI:** Nausea. **GU:** Vulvo-vaginal candidiasis.

INTERACTIONS **Drug:** Alcohol increases adverse effects. Do not use with LIVE VACCINES.

PHARMACOKINETICS **Peak:** 4 h. **Distribution:** Less than 5% protein bound. **Metabolism:** Hepatic via CYP450. **Elimination:** Urine 15% (unchanged). **Half-Life:** 17 h.

NURSING IMPLICATIONS

Assessment & Drug Effects
- Monitor for vaginal discharge or allergic reaction.

Patient & Family Education
- Administer without regard to timing of meals. Sprinkle entire contents of one packet onto applesauce, yogurt, or pudding; granules will not dissolve; do not chew or crunch granules.

S

SECOBARBITAL SODIUM

(see-koe-bar′bi-tal)

Seconal

Classification: SEDATIVE-HYPNOTIC; BARBITURATE; ANXIOLYTIC

Therapeutic: SEDATIVE-HYPNOTIC

Controlled Substance: Schedule II

AVAILABILITY Capsule

ACTION & *THERAPEUTIC EFFECT* Short-acting barbiturate with CNS depressant effects as well as mood alteration from excitation to mild sedation, hypnosis, and deep coma. Depresses the sensory cortex, decreases motor activity, alters cerebellar function and produces drowsiness, sedation, and hypnosis. *Alters cerebellar function and produces drowsiness, sedation, and hypnosis.*

USES Preoperatively to provide basal hypnosis for general, spinal, or regional anesthesia; management of insomnia.

CONTRAINDICATIONS History of sensitivity to barbiturates; porphyria; hepatic coma; severe respiratory disease; parturition, fetal immaturity; uncontrolled pain; pregnancy (category D).

CAUTIOUS USE Pregnant women with toxemia or history of bleeding; labor and delivery; seizure disorders; aspirin hypersensitivity; liver function impairment; renal impairment; hyperthyroidism; diabetes mellitus; depression; history of suicidal tendencies or drug abuse; acute or chronic pain; severe anemia; older adults (short term use only), debilitated individuals; lactation; children younger than 6 y.

ROUTE & DOSAGE

Preoperative Sedative

Adult: **PO** 200–300 mg 1–2 h before surgery
Child: **PO** 2–6 mg/kg 1–2 h before surgery

Insomnia

Adult: **PO** 100 mg at bedtime

ADMINISTRATION

Oral

- Give hypnotic dose only after patient retires for the evening.
- Crush and mix with a fluid or with food if patient cannot swallow pill.

ADVERSE EFFECTS **Respiratory:** Respiratory depression, laryngospasm. **CNS:** Drowsiness, lethargy, hangover, paradoxical excitement in older adults.

INTERACTIONS **Drug: Phenmetrazine** antagonizes effects of secobarbital; CNS DEPRESSANTS, **alcohol,** SEDATIVES compound CNS depression; MAO INHIBITORS cause excessive CNS depression; **methoxyflurane** increases risk of nephrotoxicity. Do not use **nifedipine** concurrently. **Herbal: Kava, valerian** may potentiate sedation.

PHARMACOKINETICS **Absorption:** 90% from GI tract. **Onset:** 15–30 min. **Duration:** 1–4 h. **Distribution:** Crosses placenta; distributed into breast milk. **Metabolism:** In liver (CYP2C9, CYP2C19, CYP2E1, CYP3A, CYP1A2, UGT). **Elimination:** In urine. **Half-Life:** 30 h.

S

NURSING IMPLICATIONS

Assessment & Drug Effects

- Be alert to unexpected responses and report promptly. Older adults or debilitated patients and children sometimes have paradoxical response to barbiturate therapy (i.e., irritability, marked excitement as inappropriate tearfulness and aggression in children, depression, and confusion).
- Be aware that barbiturates do not have analgesic action, and may produce restlessness when given to patients in pain.
- Be alert for acute toxicity (intoxication) characterized by profound CNS depression, respiratory depression, hypoventilation, cyanosis, cold clammy skin, hypothermia, constricted pupils (but may be dilated in severe intoxication), shock, oliguria, tachycardia, hypotension, respiration arrest, circulatory collapse, and death.
- Monitor lab tests: Periodic LFTs, renal function tests and hematology tests during prolonged therapy.

Patient & Family Education

- Instances of sleep driving and sleep walking with no memory of the occurrence have been reported. Do not drive or engage in potentially hazardous activities until response to drug is established.
- Store barbiturates in a safe place; not on the bedside table or other readily accessible places. It is possible to forget having taken the drug, and in half-wakened conditions take more and accidentally overdose.
- Do not become pregnant. Use or add barrier contraception if using hormonal contraceptives.
- Report onset of fever, sore throat or mouth, malaise, easy bruising or bleeding, petechiae, or jaundice, rash to prescriber during prolonged therapy.
- Do not consume alcohol in any amount when taking a barbiturate. It may severely impair judgment and abilities.

SECUKINUMAB

(se-cu-kin′u-mab)

Cosentyx

Classification: MONOCLONAL ANTIBODY; INTERLEUKIN INHIBITOR; ANTIPSORIATIC

Therapeutic: ANTIPSORIATIC

Prototype: Basilixumab

AVAILABILITY Solution for injection

ACTION & *THERAPEUTIC EFFECT* Selectively binds to interleukin-17A (IL-17A) and inhibits its interaction with the IL-17 receptor. IL-17A is a naturally occurring cytokine involved in normal inflammatory and immune responses. *Inhibits the release of proinflammatory cytokines and chemokines, thus reducing psoriatic skin inflammation.*

USES Treatment of moderate to severe plaque psoriasis in adult patients who are candidates for systemic therapy or phototherapy; ankylosing spondylitis; psoriatic arthritis.

CONTRAINDICATIONS Serious hypersensitivity to secukinumab or any component of the formulation; active TB. Avoid live virus vaccines and understand that non-live vaccines may not elicit sufficient immune response. Pregnancy—fetal risk cannot be ruled out; lactation—infant risk cannot be ruled out.

CAUTIOUS USE Concurrent infectious disease; history of chronic or recurrent infection; Crohn's disease; latex allergy when using *Sensoready*® pen or prefilled syringe. Safety and efficacy in children younger than 6 y not established.

ROUTE & DOSAGE

Plaque Psoriasis

Adult: **Subcutaneous** 300 mg at wk 0, 1, 2, 3, and 4; then 300 mg q4wk
Adolescent/Child over 6 y (over 50 kg): **Subcutaneous** 150 mg weekly at wk 0, 1, 2, 3, and 4, then 150 mg q4w; (under 50 kg): 75 mg weekly at wk 0, 1, 2, 3, and 4, then 75 mg q4w

Ankylosing Spondylitis/Psoriatic arthritis

Adult: **Subcutaneous** 150 mg at wk 0, 1, 2, 3, and 4; then 150 mg q4wk

ADMINISTRATION

Subcutaneous ONLY

- Remove *Sensoready*® pen, prefilled syringe, or vial from refrigerator and allow to stand for 15–30 min to reach room temperature. Administer within 1 hour of removing from refrigerator.
- Vial reconstitution: Slowly inject 1 mL of SW onto the powder. Tilt vial 45° and gently rotate for about 1 min; do not shake or invert. Let vial stand at room temperature for approx. 10 min for powder to dissolve. Once again, tilt vial 45° and gently rotate for about 1 min; do not shake or invert. Allow vial to stand undisturbed at room temperature for about 5 min. Use immediately or store refrigerated for up to 24 h.
- Inject into outer thigh, lower abdomen (2 inches or greater away from the navel); rotate injection sites and avoid areas where the skin is tender, bruised, erythematous, indurated, or affected by psoriasis.
- Store intact vials, *Sensoready*® pens, and prefilled syringes refrigerated at 2°–8° C (36°–46° F). Store in original carton until administering and protect from light.

ADVERSE EFFECTS (≥5%) **Respiratory:** *Nasopharyngitis.* **Other:** Infectious disease.

INTERACTIONS **Drug:** Do not give LIVE VACCINES; IMMUNOSUPPRESSANTS may have additive effects. **Herbal:** Do not use with **echinacea.**

PHARMACOKINETICS **Absorption:** 55–77% bioavailable. **Peak:** 6 days. **Metabolism:** Peptide degradation. **Half-Life:** 22–31 days.

NURSING IMPLICATIONS

Assessment & Drug Effects

- Monitor for and report development of infection (e.g., nasopharyngitis, upper respiratory tract infection, and mucocutaneous candida infection).
- Monitor patients with Crohn's disease for exacerbations.
- Monitor improvement of plaque psoriasis.

Patient & Family Education

- Minimize exposure to persons with known, active infections as this drug may lower the ability of your immune system to fight infections.
- Immediately report to prescriber if you develop S&S of an infection.
- Do not breast-feed while taking this drug without consulting prescriber.
- Avoid live vaccinations during therapy.

SELEGILINE HYDROCHLORIDE (L-DEPRENYL)

(se-leg′i-leen)

Emsam, Zelapar

Classification: ANTIPARKINSON; ANTIDEPRESSANT (MAOI)

Therapeutic: ANTIPARKINSON; ANTI-DEPRESSANT

AVAILABILITY Tablet, capsule; orally disintegrating tablet; transdermal patch

ACTION & *THERAPEUTIC EFFECT* Effectiveness in parkinsonism is thought to be due to increased dopaminergic activity. It interferes with dopamine reuptake at the synapse of neurons as well as its inhibition of MAO type B dopaminergic activity in the brain. Interference with dopamine reuptake at the MAO type A dopaminergic receptors in the brain is thought to be the mechanism for antidepression. *Effectiveness is measured in decreased tremors, reduced akinesia, improved speech and motor abilities as well as improved walking. At slightly higher doses it is an effective antidepressant.*

USES Adjunctive therapy of Parkinson disease for patients being treated with levodopa and carbidopa who exhibit deterioration in the quality of their response to therapy, major depressive disorder.

UNLABELED USES Attention deficit/hyperactivity disorder.

CONTRAINDICATIONS Hypersensitivity to selegiline; uncontrolled hypertension; use with dextromethorphan, other MAO inhibitors (MAOIs), meperidine, methadone, propoxyphene, and tramadol; suicidal ideation; pregnancy—fetal risk cannot be ruled out; lactation infant risk cannot be ruled out.

CAUTIOUS USE Hypertension; hepatic or renal impairment; history of suicidal tendencies, bipolar disorder; restless leg disorder; impulse control disorder; psychosis; older adults. Safety and efficacy not established in pediatric patients.

ROUTE & DOSAGE

Parkinson Disease

Adult: **PO Tablet/Capsule** 5 mg bid with breakfast and lunch (max: 10 mg/day); **PO Orally disintegrating tablet** 1.25 mg daily × 6 wk (max: 2.5 mg daily)

Depression

Adult: **Transdermal** 6 mg/day, may increase by 3 mg/day q2wk up to 12 mg/day

Hepatic Impairment Dosage Adjustment

Child Pugh A and B: **Orally disintegrating tablet**: 1.25 mg once daily.

ADMINISTRATION

Oral

- Give orally disintegrating tablets before breakfast and lunch, without liquid. Do not push tablets through the foil backing; peel back the backing of blister with dry hands and gently remove tablet. Immediately place tablet on top of the tongue. Neither food nor liquids should be ingested for 5 min before/after administration.
- Store tablet and capsule at controlled room temperature between 20 and 25 degrees C

(68 to 77 degrees F). Store disintegrating tablet at controlled room temperature of 25 degrees C (77 degrees F), with excursions permitted between at 15°–30° C (59°–86° F).

Transdermal

- Do not cut or trim patch.
- Apply only one patch at approximately the same time every day.
- Before application wash the area with soap and warm water. Dry thoroughly.
- Apply to upper torso, upper thigh, or outer surface of upper arm. Do not apply to hairy, oily, irritated, broken, or calloused skin.
- Rotate sites.
- Avoid dermal contact with sticky side of the patch. Wash hands after application.
- Avoid exposure of application site to direct heat (e.g., heating pads, blankets, lamps, saunas, heated water beds, direct sunlight).

ADVERSE EFFECTS

Respiratory: *Rhinitis*. **CNS:** *Sleep disturbances* dyskinesia, dizziness, *headache*. **GI:** *nausea, indigestion xerostomia*. **Musculoskeletal:** Backache.

INTERACTIONS

Drug: There are extensive drug interactions, consult a drug interaction database for complete listing, some interactions of significance are listed here. TRICYCLIC ANTIDEPRESSANTS may cause hyperpyrexia, seizures; SSRIS may cause serotonin syndrome or hyperthermia, diaphoresis, tremors, seizures, delirium; SYMPATHOMIMETIC AGENTS, ALPHA AGONISTS, BETA-AGONISTS (e.g., **amphetamine, phenylephrine, phenylpropanolamine**), **guanethidine,** may cause hypertensive crisis; CNS DEPRESSANTS have additive CNS depressive effects; OPIATE ANALGESICS (especially **meperidine**) may cause hypertensive crisis and circulatory collapse; **buspirone,** hypertension; GENERAL ANESTHETICS: Prolonged hypotensive and CNS depressant effects; hypertension, headache, hyperexcitability reported with **dopamine, methyldopa, levodopa, tryptophan;** HYPOTENSIVE AGENTS and DIURETICS have additive hypotensive effects. **Food:** Aged meats or aged cheeses, protein extracts, sour cream, alcohol, anchovies, liver, sausages, overripe figs, bananas, avocados, chocolate, soy sauce, bean curd, natural yogurt, fava beans—**tyramine**-containing foods—may precipitate hypertensive crisis (less frequent with usual doses of **selegiline** than with other MAOIS). **Herbal: Ginseng, ephedra, ma huang, St. John's wort** may cause hypertensive crisis.

PHARMACOKINETICS

Absorption: Rapid; 73% reaches systemic circulation. **Onset:** 1–2 weeks (antidepressant). **Duration:** 1–3 days. **Distribution:** Crosses placenta; not known if distributed into breast milk. **Metabolism:** In liver to *N*-desmethyldeprenyl-amphetamine and methamphetamine. **Elimination:** In urine. **Half-Life:** 10 h.

NURSING IMPLICATIONS

Black Box Warning

Selegiline transdermal patch for depression has been associated with increased risk of suicidal thinking and behavior in children, adolescents, and young adults.

Assessment & Drug Effects

- Monitor vital signs, particularly during period of dosage

adjustment. Report alterations in BP or pulse. Indications for discontinuation of the drug include orthostatic hypotension, hypertension, and arrhythmias.

- Monitor for changes in behavior that may indicate increased suicidality, especially in adolescents or children being treated for depression.
- Monitor all patients closely for behavior changes (e.g., hallucinations, confusion, depression, delusions).

Patient & Family Education

- Do not exceed the prescribed drug dose.
- Report symptoms of MAO inhibitor-induced hypertension (e.g., severe headache, palpitations, neck stiffness, nausea, vomiting) immediately to prescriber.
- Do not drive or engage in potentially hazardous activities until response to drug is known.
- Make positional changes slowly and in stages. Orthostatic hypotension is possible as well as dizziness, light-headedness, and fainting.
- If the transdermal patch falls off, apply a new patch to a new area, and resume previous schedule.
- Only one should be worn at a given time. Remove the old transdermal patch.
- Routine screening by dermatologist for melanoma.

SELEXIPAG

(se-lex'i-pag)

Uptravi

Classification: PROSTAGLANDIN; PULMONARY ANTIHYPERTENSIVE

Therapeutic: PULMONARY ANTIHYPERTENSIVE

Prototype: Epoprostenol

AVAILABILITY Tablets, solution for injection

ACTION & THERAPEUTIC EFFECT Hydrolyzed in vivo to produce an active metabolite that acts as an agonist at the prostacyclin IP receptor. *Agonist action at the IP receptor produces inhibition of platelet function, a reduction in pulmonary vascular resistance, and relaxation of pulmonary vascular smooth muscle.*

USES Treatment of pulmonary arterial hypertension (PAH) in order to delay disease progression and reduce the risk of hospitalization.

CONTRAINDICATIONS Concomitant use with strong CYP2C8 inhibitors.

CAUTIOUS USE Avoid use in patients with severe hepatic impairment or pulmonary veno-occlusive disease (PVOD). Pregnancy—fetal risk cannot be ruled out; lactation—infant risk cannot be ruled out.

ROUTE & DOSAGE

Pulmonary Arterial Hypertension

Adult: **PO** 200 mcg bid; may increase weekly in 200 mcg increments (max dose: 1600 mcg)

Hepatic Impairment Dosage Adjustment

Moderate impairment (Child-Pugh class B): Reduce dosing interval to once daily

Severe impairment (Child-Pugh class C): Avoid use

ADMINISTRATION

Oral

- Administer without regard to food. Administering with food may improve tolerability.

S

- Do not split, crush, or chew tablets.
- Store at 15°–30° C (59°–86° F).

Intravenous

- Follow manufacturing instructions for detailed reconstitution and dilution instructions.
- Mix diluted infusion by gentle inversion of the glass container 5 times; do not shake.
- Diluted solutions should be clear and colorless. Discard if particulate matter is observed.
- Protect dilution from light at all times.
- Must be administered within 4 hours after the first puncture of the vial.
- Solution is for single administration. All remaining reconstituted product must be discarded.
- Administer infusion over 80 minutes using an infusion set made of DEHP-free polyvinyl chloride (PVC), natural latex rubber-free microbore tubing protected from light. Do not filter.
- Infusion solution should be kept at room temperature (20 to 25° C (68 to 77° F).

ADVERSE EFFECTS (≥5%) **CNS:** *Headache*. **GI:** *Diarrhea, nausea*. **Musculoskeletal:** *Jaw pain*.

INTERACTIONS **Drug:** Do not use with strong CYP2C8 inhibitors (e.g., **gemfibrozil**), may increase the levels of selexipag and its active metabolite. **Rifampin** may decrease serum concentrations.

PHARMACOKINETICS **Peak:** 3–4 h. **Distribution:** 99% plasma protein bound. **Metabolism:** Hydrolyzed to active metabolite; hepatic metabolism to inactive metabolites. Metabolized via CYP3A4, CYP2C8, UGT1A3. **Elimination:** Primarily fecal (93%). **Half-Life:** 6.2–13.5 h (active metabolite).

S

NURSING IMPLICATIONS

Assessment & Drug Effects

- Skin assessment for flushing and rash.
- Respiratory assessment, including pulse oximetry.
- Complaint of jaw, limb, muscle, or joint pain.

Patient & Family Education

- Women need to use appropriate contraceptive measures.
- Report any signs of significant reaction: Wheezing, chest tightness, fever, itching, swelling of face, lips, tongue, or throat.
- Patients may have decreased appetite.
- Report any shortness of breath, severe loss of strength or energy.
- Take a missed dose as soon as possible, but if the next dose is in less than 6 hours, skip the missed dose.
- Contact healthcare provider if drug is not take for 3 days or more for specific instructions.

SEMAGLUTIDE

(sem-a-gloo'tide)

Ozempic, Rybelsus, Wegovy

Classification: ANTIDIABETIC; GLUCAGON-LIKE PEPTIDE-1 RECEPTOR AGONIST; INCRETIN MIMETICS
Therapeutic: ANTIDIABETIC
Prototype: Exenatide

AVAILABILITY Solution for injection; pen injector; tablet

ACTION & *THERAPEUTIC EFFECT* Semaglutide is a glucagon-like peptide-1 (GLP-1) receptor agonist that causes increased insulin release and decreased glucagon release in the presence of elevated blood glucose, and delays the rate of gastric emptying. *Semaglutide lowers*

postprandial blood glucose levels and helps normalize HbA1C.

USES Treatment of type 2 diabetes mellitus in combination with diet and exercise; weight management (Wegovy only).

CONTRAINDICATIONS Family or personal history of medullary thyroid carcinoma (MTC); history of multiple endocrine neoplasia syndrome 2 (MEN 2); serious hypersensitivity reaction to semaglutide; Type 1 DM; pancreatitis; history of suicidal ideation or suicide attempt.

CAUTIOUS USE History of pancreatitis; alcohol abuse; history of cholethiasis; history of severe hypoglycemia; gastroparesis; history of angioedema; renal or hepatic impairment; concurrent use with insulin secretagogues (e.g., sulfonylureas); older adults; pregnancy—fetal risk canto be ruled out; lactation—infant risk cannot be ruled out. Safety and efficacy in children younger than 18 y not established.

ROUTE & DOSAGE

Type 2 Diabetes Mellitus

Adult: **Subcutaneous** Initial dose 0.25 mg once a wk for 4 wk, then increase to 0.5 mg weekly (max: 1mg once a wk) **PO** 3 mg daily × 30 days then 7 mg daily may increase to 14 mg daily after 30 days.

Weight management (Wegovy)

Adult: **Subcutaneous** 0.25 mg weekly weeks 1–4 then 0.5 mg weekly weeks 5–8 then 1 mg weekly weeks 9–12 then 1.7 mg weekly weeks 13–16 then 2.4 mg weekly

ADMINISTRATION

Oral

- Administer at least 30 minutes before the first food, beverage or other oral medications of the day and with no more than 4 ounces of plain water.
- Swallow tablets whole; do not split, chew or crush tablets.
- Taking two 7-mg tablets to achieve a 14-mg dose is not recommended.
- If a dose is missed, skip the missed dose and administer the next dose on the following day.
- Store tablet in original carton at a controlled room temperature between 20 to 25° C (68 and 77° F), excursions permitted between 15 and 30° C (59 and 86° F). Protect from moisture.

Subcutaneous

- Inject into abdomen, thigh, or upper arm without regard to meals.
- Rotate injection sites weekly. Administer on the same day each week.
- Administer separately from insulin (do not mix); may inject both medications in the same body region, but not adjacent to each other.
- Solution should be clear; do not use if particulate matter or color are seen.
- Do not mix with other injections in same syringe.
- Do not share pens with other patients, even if the needle is changed.
- Follow manufacturer instructions for missed doses.
- Store in refrigeration until first use, then either continue refrigeration or store at 15°–30 °C (59°–86° F) for up to 56 days.

ADVERSE EFFECTS (≥5%) **CNS:** *Headache.* **GI:** Nausea, vomiting, diarrhea, abdominal pain, constipation.

INTERACTIONS **Drug:** Avoid use with DPT4 INHIBITORS. Do not use with **liraglutide**. Due to its ability to slow gastric emptying, semaglutide can decrease absorption rate and plasma levels of oral medications; with other INSULIN SECRETAGOGUE (e.g., **sulfonylurea**) semaglutide may increase the risk of hypoglycemia.

PHARMACOKINETICS **Absorption:** 89% bioavailability. **Peak:** 1–3 days after single dose. **Distribution:** greater than 99% protein bound. **Metabolism:** Metabolized by endogenous proteolytic enzymes. **Elimination:** Urine, feces; 3% unchanged. **Half-Life:** 1 wk.

NURSING IMPLICATIONS

Black Box Warning

Semaglutide has been shown to cause thyroid C-cell tumors in animals. Clinical relevance in humans has not been established.

Assessment & Drug Effects

- Monitor for S&S of gall bladder disease.
- Monitor for worsening of depression, suicidal thoughts or behavior or any unusual mood changes.
- Monitor lab tests: Plasma glucose (HbA1C) at least twice yearly, renal function tests, triglycerides.

Patient & Family Education

- Wear medical alert ID bracelet.
- Check blood sugar as instructed by prescriber.
- Do not drive if blood sugar has been low.
- Report any changes in vision.
- Drink adequate fluids.
- Report any racing heart rate or palpitations.
- Have patient or care giver demonstrate proper technique of subcutaneous injection.
- Have bloodwork checked as ordered by prescriber.
- Talk with prescriber before drinking alcohol.

SENNA (SENNOSIDES)

(sen′na)

Black-Draught, Gentlax B, Senexon, Senokot, Senolax

Classification: STIMULANT LAXATIVE

Therapeutic: STIMULANT LAXATIVE

Prototype: Bisacodyl

AVAILABILITY Tablet; syrup

ACTION & *THERAPEUTIC EFFECT*

Senna glycosides are converted in colon to active aglycone, which stimulates peristalsis. Concentrate is purified and standardized for uniform action and is claimed to produce less colic than crude form. *Peristalsis stimulated by conversion of drug to active chemical resulting in a softening of the stool and relief from constipation.*

USES Acute constipation and preoperative and preradiographic bowel evacuation.

CONTRAINDICATIONS Hypersensitivity; appendicitis, fecal impaction; fluid and electrolyte imbalances; irritable colon, nausea, vomiting, undiagnosed abdominal pain, intestinal obstruction.

CAUTIOUS USE Diabetes mellitus; fluid and electrolyte imbalances; pregnancy; lactation (infant risk is minimal). Safe use in children younger than 2 y not established.

ROUTE & DOSAGE

Constipation

Adult: **PO** 1–2 tablets (max: 4 tablets); **Syrup, Liquid** 10–15 mL at bedtime

Child (6–11 y): **PO** 5–7.5mL at bedtime (max: 7.5 mL bid); *2–5 y:* 2.5–3.75mL at bedtime (max: 3.75 mL bid)

ADMINISTRATION

Oral

- Give at bedtime, generally.
- Avoid exposing drug to excessive heat; protect fluid extracts from light.
- Store between 15°–30° C (59°–86° F).

ADVERSE EFFECTS **Endocrine:** Electrolyte imbalance. **GI:** Abdominal pain, cramps, diarrhea, nausea, and vomiting. **GU:** Nephritis.

PHARMACOKINETICS **Onset:** 6–10 h; may take up to 24 h. **Metabolism:** In liver. **Elimination:** In feces.

NURSING IMPLICATIONS

Assessment & Drug Effects

- Reduce dose in patients who experience considerable abdominal cramping.

Patient & Family Education

- Be aware that drug may alter urine and feces color; yellowish brown (acid), reddish brown (alkaline).
- Continued use may lead to dependence. Consult prescriber if constipation persists beyond one week.
- See bisacodyl for additional nursing implications.

SERDEXMETHYLPHENIDATE AND DEXMETHYLPHENIDATE

(SER-dex-METH-il-FEN-I-date & dex-METH-il-FEN-I-date)

Azstarya

Classifications: CEREBRAL STIMULANT

Therapeutic: CEREBRAL STIMULANT

Controlled Substance: Schedule II

AVAILABILITY Oral capsule

ACTION & *THERAPEUTIC EFFECT*

A CNS stimulant and prodrug of dexmethylphenidate. The mode of therapeutic action in attention deficit disorder (ADHD) is not known.

USES Treatment of attention deficit hyperactivity disorder (ADHD) in patients 6 years of age and older.

CONTRAINDICATIONS Hypersensitivity to serdexmethylphenidate, methylphenidate, or other components of the product; concomitant use of MAOI currently or within 14 days from discontinuation of MAOI; patients with serious structural cardiac abnormalities, cardiomyopathy, serious heart rhythm abnormalities, or other serious cardiac conditions; pregnancy—fetal risk cannot be ruled out; lactation—infant risk cannot be ruled out. Not approved for children under the age of 6 y.

CAUTIOUS USE History of hypertension, tachycardic patients; pre-existing psychosis, depression, family history of suicide, bipolar disorder, history of priapism.

S

ROUTE & DOSAGE

Attention-Deficit/Hyperactivity Disorder

Child (6 yr or older): **PO** 39.2/7.8 mg every morning for one week; after one week dose increase can be considered for max daily dose of 52.3/10.4

ADMINISTRATION

Oral

- Administer in the morning with or without food.
- Capsules may be taken whole or opened and the entire contents sprinkled into 50 mL of water or over 2 tablespoons (30 mL) of applesauce. Consume all the drug/food immediately or within 10 minutes of mixing; do not store for future use.
- Store at controlled room temperature between 20 and 25° C (68 and 77° F), with excursions permitted between 15 and 30° C (59 and 86° C). Protect from light.

ADVERSE EFFECTS **CV:** Hypertension, tachycardia, sudden cardiac death, myocardial infarction, stroke. **CNS:** Dizziness, insomnia, anxiety. **Endocrine:** Weight loss. **GI:** Nausea, vomiting, dyspepsia, abdominal pain, decreased appetite. **GU:** Priapism. **Musculoskeletal:** Decreased linear skeletal growth; below expectation. **Other:** Psychotic disorder.

INTERACTIONS **Drug:** Additive stimulant effects with other STIMULANTS (including **amphetamine, caffeine**); concomitant use with MAO INHIBITORS and STIMULANTS may cause hypertensive crisis; May decrease effectiveness of medications used to treat high blood pressure. Concomitant use of halogenated anesthetics (halothane, etc.) should be avoided.

PHARMACOKINETICS **Absorption:** Serdexmethylphenidate: 3% bioavailability. **Peak:** Dexmethylphenidate: 2 h. **Distribution:** Serdexmethylphenidate: 56% protein-bound; Dexmethylphenidate: 47% protein-bound. **Metabolism:** Serdexmethylphenidate: Converted to dexmethylphenidate through gastrointestinal enzymes; Dexmethylphenidate: De-esterified in liver. **Elimination:** Serdexmethylphenidate: 62% excreted in urine (0.4% unchanged drug), 37% feces (11% unchanged drug). **Half-Life:** Serdexmethylphenidate: 5.7 h; Dexmethylphenidate: 11.7 h.

NURSING IMPLICATIONS

Black Box Warning

CNS simulants have a high potential for abuse and dependence. Assess the risk of abuse prior to prescribing, and monitor for signs of abuse and dependence while on therapy.

Assessment & Drug Effects

- Improvement in mental and behavioral symptoms of ADHD, including inappropriate inattention, impulsivity, hyperactivity, and cognitive performance, within 1 month is indicative of efficacy.
- Monitor for signs of toxicity: hypertension, tachycardia.
- Closely monitor growth (height and weight) in pediatric patients
- Observe for digital changes (e.g., peripheral vasculopathy, including Raynaud phenomenon).

Patient & Family Education

- Review administration directions with family.

- Report symptoms of serious heart effects (chest pain, racing heartbeat, unexplained dizziness).
- Inform family of pediatric patients that growth will be closely monitored.
- Review adverse effects with family.
- Report persistent and painful erection of the penis.
- Report any decrease of circulation to fingers causing a paleness or pain (Raynaud's phenomenon).

SERTACONAZOLE NITRATE

(ser-ta-con′a-zole)

Ertaczo

Classification: ANTIBIOTIC; AZOLE ANTIFUNGAL

Therapeutic: ANTIFUNGAL

Prototype: Fluconazole

AVAILABILITY Cream

ACTION & *THERAPEUTIC EFFECT* Believed to act primarily by inhibiting cytochrome P450-dependent synthesis of ergosterol, a key component of the cell membrane of fungi resulting in fungal cell injury. *Has a broad spectrum of activity against common fungal pathogens.*

USES Treatment of tinea pedis in immunocompetent patients.

CONTRAINDICATIONS Hypersensitivity to imidazoles.

CAUTIOUS USE History of hypersensitivity to azole antifungals; pregnancy (category C); lactation; children younger than 12 y.

ROUTE & DOSAGE

Tinea Pedis

Adult/Child (12 y or older):
Topical Apply thin layer to affected area twice daily for 4 wk

ADMINISTRATION

Topical

- Cleanse the affected area and dry thoroughly before application.
- Apply a thin layer of the cream to affected area between the toes and the immediately surrounding healthy skin. Gently rub into the skin.
- Store at 15°–30° C (57°–86° F).

ADVERSE EFFECTS **Skin:** Contact dermatitis, dry skin, burning, application site reaction, skin tenderness.

PHARMACOKINETICS **Absorption:** Negligible through intact skin.

NURSING IMPLICATIONS

Assessment & Drug Effects

- Monitor for clinical improvement, which should be seen about 2 wk after initiating treatment.

Patient & Family Education

- Report any of the following: Severe skin irritation, redness, burning, blistering, or itching.
- Do not stop using this medication prematurely. Athlete's foot takes about 4 wk to clear completely.
- Nursing mothers should ensure that this topical cream does not accidentally get on the breast.

SERTRALINE HYDROCHLORIDE

(ser′tra-leen)

Zoloft

Classification: ANTIDEPRESSANT; SELECTIVE SEROTONIN REUPTAKE INHIBITOR (SSRI)

Therapeutic: ANTIDEPRESSANT; SSRI

Prototype: Fluoxetine

AVAILABILITY Tablet; oral solution; capsule

ACTION & *THERAPEUTIC EFFECT*

Potent inhibitor of serotonin (5-HT) reuptake in the brain. Selective serotonin reuptake inhibitor (SSRI) Chronic administration results in downregulation of norepinephrine, a reaction found with other effective antidepressants. *Effective in controlling depression, obsessive-compulsive disorder, anxiety, and panic disorder.*

USES Major depression, obsessive-compulsive disorder, panic disorder, social anxiety disorder, premenstrual dysphoric disorder, post-traumatic stress disorder.

UNLABELED USES Eating disorders, generalized anxiety disorder, premature ejaculation, body dysmorphic disorder.

CONTRAINDICATIONS Patients taking MAO inhibitors or within 14 days of discontinuing MAO inhibitor; concurrent use of Antabuse or pimozide; suicidal ideation, hyponatremia; mania or hypomania; children with MDD; pregnancy—fetal risk cannot be ruled out.

CAUTIOUS USE Seizure disorders, major affective disorders, bipolar disorder, history of suicide; liver dysfunction, renal impairment; abrupt discontinuation; anorexia nervosa, recent history of MI or unstable cardiac disease, dehydration; DM; risk factor for QT prolongation; ECT therapy, older adults; pregnancy (category C); lactation—infant risk is minimal. Safe use for OCD in children younger than 6 y is not established.

ROUTE & DOSAGE

Depression

Adult: **PO** Begin with 50 mg/day, gradually increase every few weeks according to response (range: 50–200 mg) **PO** (Capsules) 150–200 mg daily after having been stabilized on tablet dose of at least 100 mg daily.
Geriatric: **PO** Start with 25 mg/day
Adolescent/Child (over 6y): **PO** 25 mg daily titrate in 12.5–25 mg increments weekly to usual effective dose of 50 mg daily.

Panic Disorder

Adult: **PO** 25 mg/day × 3–7 days then increase to 50 mg/day, may titrate dose up to 200 mg/day

PTSD

Adult: **PO** 25–50 mg daily, may increase in 25–50 mg increments weekly to max dose of 200 mg/day

Premenstrual Dysphoric Disorder

Adult: **PO** Begin with 25 mg/day for first cycle, then increase to 50 mg daily for next cycle; may titrate up to 200 mg/day

Obsessive-Compulsive Disorder

Adult /Adolescent: **PO** Begin with 50 mg/day, may titrate at weekly intervals up to 200 mg/day
Child (6–12 y): **PO** Begin with 25 mg/day, may increase by 50 mg/wk, as tolerated and needed, up to 200 mg/day

ADMINISTRATION

Oral

- Give in the morning or evening.
- Do not give concurrently with an MAO inhibitor or within 14 days of discontinuing an MAO inhibitor.
- Oral solution: Dilute concentrate before use with 4 oz of water, ginger ale, lemon/lime soda, lemonade, or orange juice ONLY. Give immediately after mixing. Caution with latex sensitivity, as the dropper contains dry natural rubber.

ADVERSE EFFECTS (≥5%) **CNS:** *Insomnia, headache, dizziness, somnolence,* tremor. **GI:** *Nausea, vomiting, diarrhea, constipation,* indigestion. **Other:** Fatigue, abnormal ejaculation, reduced libido.

DIAGNOSTIC TEST INTERFERENCE

May interfere with urine detection of benzodiazepines (false positive).

INTERACTIONS **Drug:** MAOIS (e.g., **selegiline, phenelzine**) should be stopped 14 days before sertraline is started because of serious problems with other SEROTONIN REUPTAKE INHIBITORS (shivering, nausea, diplopia, confusion, anxiety). **Sertraline** may increase levels and toxicity of **diazepam, pimozide, tolbutamide.** Use cautiously with other centrally acting CNS drugs; increase risk of **ergotamine** toxicity with **dihydroergotamine, ergotamine.** Avoid with agents that prolong the QT interval (e.g., **bepridil, dronedarone, ziprasidone**). May increase antiplatelet/anticoagulant effects of NSAIDS, **heparin**. Concentrate interacts with **disulfiram.** **Herbal:** **St. John's wort** may cause serotonin syndrome (headache, dizziness, sweating, agitation). **Food:** **Grapefruit juice** (greater than 1 qt/day) may increase plasma concentrations and adverse effects.

PHARMACOKINETICS **Absorption:** Slowly from GI tract. **Onset:** 2–4 wk. **Distribution:** 99% protein bound; distribution into breast milk unknown. **Metabolism:** Extensive first-pass metabolism in liver to inactive metabolites (substrate of CYP2B6, CYP2C9, CYP2D6, CYP3A4, and CYP2C19). **Elimination:** 40–45% in urine, 40–45% in feces. **Half-Life:** 24 h.

NURSING IMPLICATIONS

Black Box Warning

Sertraline has been associated with increased risk of suicidal thinking and behavior in children, adolescents, and young adults.

Assessment & Drug Effects

- Supervise patients at risk for suicide closely during initial therapy.
- Monitor for worsening of depression or emergence of suicidal ideation.
- Monitor for reductions in obsessive compulsive disorder, panic attacks or PTSD episodes depending on patient history and reason for medication.
- Monitor older adults for fluid and sodium imbalances.
- Monitor patients with a history of a seizure disorder closely.
- Monitor lab tests: Metabolic panel.

Patient & Family Education

- Report diarrhea, nausea, dyspepsia, insomnia, drowsiness, dizziness, or persistent headache to prescriber.
- Review dilution instructions and include permitted fluids (e.g., water, ginger ale, lemon/lime soda, lemonade or orange juice).
- Report emergence of agitation, irritability, hostility or aggression, mania.

S

- Avoid activities requiring mental alertness or coordination until drug effects are known.
- Report an changes in sexual function.
- Avoid sudden discontinuation of the drug, as this may precipitate discontinuation syndrome.
- Avoid alcohol.
- Report signs of bleeding promptly to prescriber when taking concomitant warfarin.

SEVELAMER HYDROCHLORIDE

(se-vel′a-mer)

Renagel, Renvela

Classification: ELECTROLYTE AND WATER BALANCE AGENT; PHOSPHATE BINDER

Therapeutic: PHOSPHATE BINDER

AVAILABILITY Tablet; oral powder for suspension

ACTION & *THERAPEUTIC EFFECT* Polymer that binds intestinal phosphate; interacts with phosphate by way of ion exchange and hydrogen binding. *Effectiveness indicated by a serum phosphate level 6.0 mg/dL or less.*

USES Hyperphosphatemia.

S

CONTRAINDICATIONS Hypersensitivity to sevelamer HCl; hypophosphatemia; fecal impaction; bowel obstruction; appendicitis; dysphagia, GI bleeding, major GI surgery; lactation.

CAUTIOUS USE GI motility disorders; vitamin deficiencies (especially vitamins D, E, and K and folic acid); pregnancy (category C); children younger than 18 y.

ROUTE & DOSAGE

Hyperphosphatemia

Adult: **PO** 800–1600 mg tid based on severity of hyperphosphatemia

ADMINISTRATION

Oral

- Give with meals.
- Give other oral medications 1 h before or 3 h after Renagel.
- Store at 15°–30° C (59°–86° F); protect from moisture.

ADVERSE EFFECTS CV: Hypertension, hypotension, thrombosis. **Respiratory:** Increased cough. **GI:** Diarrhea, dyspepsia, vomiting, nausea, constipation, flatulence. **Other:** Headache, infection, pain.

NURSING IMPLICATIONS

Assessment & Drug Effects

- Monitor lab tests: Periodic 24-hour urinary calcium and phosphorus, and serum magnesium; alkaline phosphatase q12mo or more often with elevated PTH; iPTH q3–12 mo depending on CKD severity.

Patient & Family Education

- Take daily multivitamin supplement approved by prescriber.

SILDENAFIL CITRATE

(sil-den′a-fil ci′trate)

Revatio, Viagra

Classification: PHOSPHODIESTERASE (PDE) INHIBITOR; IMPOTENCE; PULMONARY ANTIHYPERTENSIVE

Therapeutic: PULMONARY ANTIHYPERTENSIVE; IMPOTENCE

AVAILABILITY Tablet; solution for injection; powder for oral suspension

ACTION & THERAPEUTIC EFFECT Enhances vasodilation effect of nitric oxide in the corpus cavernosus of the penis, thus sustaining an erection. PDE-5 inhibitors increase pulmonary vasodilation by sustaining levels of cyclic guanosine monophosphate (cGMP). Additionally, sildenafil produces a reduction in the pulmonary to systemic vascular resistance ratio. *Effective for treatment of erectile dysfunction, whether organic or psychogenic in origin. Sildenafil produces a significant improvement in arterial oxygenation in pulmonary arterial hypertension (PAH).*

USES Erectile dysfunction, pulmonary arterial hypertension.

UNLABELED USES Altitude sickness, Raynaud's phenomenon, sexual dysfunction, anorgasmy.

CONTRAINDICATIONS Hypersensitivity to sildenafil. Patients with pulmonary veno-occlusive disease (PVOD) and patients taking nitrate/nitrite therapy.

CAUTIOUS USE CAD with unstable angina, heart failure, MI, cardiac arrhythmias, stroke within 6 mo of starting drug; hypotension and hypertension; risk factors for CVA; aortic stenosis; anatomic deformity of the penis; sickle cell anemia, polycythemia; multiple myeloma; leukemia; active bleeding or a peptic ulcer, GERD, hiatal hernia; coagulopathy; retinitis pigmentosa; visual disturbances, hepatic disease, hepatitis, cirrhosis; severe renal impairment; older adults; pregnancy (category B); lactation; children and infants.

ROUTE & DOSAGE

Erectile Dysfunction

Adult: **PO** 50 mg 0.5–4 h before sexual activity (dose range: 25 to 100 mg once/day)
Geriatric: **PO** 25 mg approximately 1 h before sexual activity

Pulmonary Arterial Hypertension

Adult: **PO** 5 mg or 20 mg tid (4–6 h apart); **IV** 2.5 mg or 10 mg tid

Hepatic Impairment Dosage Adjustment

Child-Pugh class A or B: Starting dose of 25 mg

Renal Impairment Dosage Adjustment

CrCl less than 30 mL/min: Starting dose of 25 mg

ADMINISTRATION

Oral

- For erectile dysfunction: Dose 1 h prior to sexual activity (effective range is 0.5–4 h).

Intravenous

PREPARE: **Direct:** Give undiluted.
ADMINISTER: **Direct:** Give as a bolus dose.

- Store at 15°–30° C (59°–86° F) in a tightly closed container; protect from light.

ADVERSE EFFECTS **CV:** Flushing, chest pain, MI, angina, AV block, tachycardia, palpitation, hypotension, postural hypotension, cardiac arrest, sudden cardiac death, heart failure, cardiomyopathy, abnormal ECG, edema. **Respiratory:** Nasal congestion, asthma, dyspnea, epistaxis, laryngitis, pharyngitis, sinusitis, bronchitis, cough. **CNS:** *Headache,* dizziness, migraine, syncope, cerebral thrombosis, ataxia, neuralgia, paresthesias, tremor, vertigo, depression, insomnia, somnolence, abnormal dreams. **HEENT:** Abnormal vision (color changes, photosensitivity, blurred vision, sudden vision loss). **Endocrine:** Gout, hyperglycemia, hyperuricemia, hypoglycemia, hypernatremia. **Skin:** Rash, urticaria, pruritus, sweating, exfoliative dermatitis. **GI:** Dyspepsia, diarrhea, abdominal pain, vomiting, colitis, dysphagia, gastritis, gastroenteritis, esophagitis, stomatitis, dry mouth, abnormal liver function tests, thirst. **GU:** UTI. **Hematologic:** Anemia, leukopenia. **Other:** Face edema, photosensitivity, shock, asthenia, pain, chills, fall, allergic reaction, arthritis, myalgia.

INTERACTIONS

Drug: NITRATES increase risk of serious hypotension; if used within 4 h of **doxazosin, prazosin, terazosin, tamsulosin; cimetidine, erythromycin, ketoconazole, itraconazole,** PROTEASE INHIBITORS increase sildenafil levels; **rifampin** can decrease sildenafil levels. Do not use with **telaprevir. Food: Grapefruit juice** (greater than 1 qt/day) may increase plasma concentrations and adverse effects.

PHARMACOKINETICS

Absorption: Rapidly from GI tract. **Peak:** 30–120 min. **Distribution:** 96% protein bound. **Metabolism:** In liver (CYP3A4 and 2C9). **Elimination:** 80% in feces, 12% in urine. **Half-Life:** 4 h.

NURSING IMPLICATIONS

Assessment & Drug Effects

- Monitor carefully for and immediately report S&S of cardiac distress.

Patient & Family Education

- Do not take sildenafil within 4 h of taking doxazosin, prazosin, terazosin, or tamsulosin.
- Consuming a high-fat meal before taking drug may cause delay in drug action.
- Report to prescriber: Headaches, flushing, chest pain, indigestion, blurred vision, sensitivity to light, changes in color vision.
- Seek medical attention if erection lasts for more than 4 h.

SILODOSIN

(sil′o-do-sin)

Rapaflo

Classification: ALPHA-1 ADRENERGIC RECEPTOR ANTAGONIST; GENITOURINARY SMOOTH MUSCLE RELAXANT

Therapeutic: GENITOURINARY SMOOTH MUSCLE RELAXANT

Prototype: Tamsulosin

AVAILABILITY

Capsule

ACTION & *THERAPEUTIC EFFECT*

Selective antagonist of post-synaptic alpha-1 adrenoreceptors located in the prostate, bladder base, bladder neck, prostatic capsule, and prostatic urethra. *Blockade of these alpha-1 adrenoreceptors causes the smooth muscle in these tissues to relax, resulting in improvement in urine flow and reduction in signs and symptoms of benign prostatic hyperplasia (BPH).*

USES

Treatment of the signs and symptoms of BPH.

CONTRAINDICATIONS

Severe renal impairment (CrCl less than 30 mL/min); severe hepatic impairment (Child-Pugh score greater than or equal to 10); hypersensitivity to silodosin or any other ingredients in the product; pregnancy—fetal risk cannot be ruled out; lactation—infant risk cannot be ruled out.

CAUTIOUS USE Moderate renal impairment; history of hypotension; cataract surgery; older adults. Safe use in children not established.

ROUTE & DOSAGE

Benign Prostatic Hyperplasia

Adult: **PO** 8 mg once daily with a meal

Renal Impairment Dosage Adjustment

CrCl 30–49 mL/min: 4 mg once daily; *less than 30 mL/min:* Contraindicated

ADMINISTRATION

Oral

- Give with meals.
- If unable to swallow whole, may sprinkle capsule contents on 1 Tablespoon of applesauce and swallow without chewing within 5 minutes; follow with 8 oz. of cool water.
- Store at controlled room temperature of 25 degrees C (77 degrees F), with excursions permitted between 15°–30° C (59°–86° F). Protect from light and moisture.

ADVERSE EFFECTS (≥ 5%) GU: *Retrograde ejaculation.*

DIAGNOSTIC TEST INTERFERENCE Increased ***prostate specific antigen (PSA).***

INTERACTIONS Drug: Strong CYP3A4 inhibitors (e.g., **idelalisib, itraconazole, ritonavir**) or strong P-GLYCOPROTEIN INHIBITORS (e.g., **ketoconazole**) greatly increases silodosin levels. Moderate CYP3A4 inhibitors (e.g., **clarithromycin, diltiazem, erythromycin, verapamil**) may increase silodosin levels. Other ALPHA-BLOCKERS can cause additive hypotensive effects. INHIBITORS OF UDP-GLUCURONOSYLTRANSFERASE 2B7 (e.g., **probenecid, valproic acid, fluconazole**) may increase silodosin levels.

PHARMACOKINETICS Absorption: 32% bioavailable. **Distribution:** Approximately 97% plasma protein bound. **Metabolism:** By CYP3A4 hepatic enzymes and is a P-glycoprotein (P-gp) substrate. **Elimination:** Feces and urine. **Half-Life:** 13.3 h.

NURSING IMPLICATIONS

Assessment & Drug Effects

- Monitor I&O and ease of voiding.
- Monitor orthostatic vital signs (lying and then standing) at the beginning of therapy. Report a systolic pressure drop of 15 mm Hg or greater and HR increase of 15 beats or greater upon standing.
- Monitor for orthostatic hypotension, especially at the beginning of therapy and in those taking concurrent antihypertensive drugs.

Patient & Family Education

- Make position changes slowly and in stages to minimize risk of dizziness and fainting.
- Take the drug once daily with a meal.
- Avoid hazardous activities until reaction to drug is known.
- Review adverse effects with patient and/or caregiver.
- Report unexplained skin eruptions or purple skin patches.
- If cataract surgery is planned, inform ophthalmologist that you are taking silodosin.
- Contact provider before taking any other medication or herbal supplement.

SILVER SULFADIAZINE

(sul-fa-dye'a-zeen)

Silvadene, SSD

Classification: SULFONAMIDE

Therapeutic: TOPICAL ANTI-INFECTIVE

AVAILABILITY Cream

ACTION & *THERAPEUTIC EFFECT* Silver salt is released slowly and exerts bactericidal effect only on bacterial cell membrane and wall. *Broad antimicrobial activity including many gram-negative and gram-positive bacteria and yeast.*

USES Prevention and treatment of sepsis in second- and third-degree burns.

CONTRAINDICATIONS Hypersensitivity to other sulfonamides; pregnant women at term.

CAUTIOUS USE Impaired kidney or liver function; porphyria; impaired respiratory function; G6PD deficiency; thrombocytopenia, leukopenia, hematological disease; pregnancy (category B); lactation; preterm infants; neonates younger than 2 mo.

ROUTE & DOSAGE

Burn Wound Treatment

Adult/Child: **Topical** Apply 1% cream 1–2 × day to thickness of approximately 1.5 mm ($^1/_{16}$ in.)

ADMINISTRATION

Topical

- Do not use if cream darkens; it is water soluble and white.
- Apply with sterile, gloved hands to cleansed, debrided burned areas. Reapply cream to areas where it has been removed by patient activity; cover burn wounds with medication at all times.
- Bathe patient daily (in whirlpool or shower or in bed) as aid to debridement. Reapply drug.
- Note: Dressings are not required but may be used if necessary. Drug does not stain clothing.
- Store at room temperature away from heat.

ADVERSE EFFECTS **Other:** Pain (occasionally), burning, itching, rash, reversible leukopenia. Potential for toxicity as for other SULFONAMIDES if applied to extensive areas of the body surface.

INTERACTIONS **Drug:** PROTEOLYTIC ENZYMES are inactivated by silver in cream.

PHARMACOKINETICS **Absorption:** Not absorbed through intact skin, however, approximately 10% could be absorbed when applied to second- or third-degree burns. **Distribution:** Distributed into most body tissues. **Metabolism:** In the liver. **Elimination:** In urine.

NURSING IMPLICATIONS

Assessment & Drug Effects

- Observe for and report hypersensitivity reaction: Rash, itching, or burning sensation in unburned areas.
- Observe patient for reactions attributed to sulfonamides.
- Note: Analgesic may be required. Occasionally, pain is experienced on application; intensity and duration depend on depth of burn.
- Continue treatment until satisfactory healing or burn site is ready for grafting, unless adverse reactions occur.

SIMEPREVIR

(sim-e-pre′vir)

Olysio

Classification: ANTIVIRAL; VIRAL PROTEIN INHIBITOR; DIRECT-ACTING ANTI-VIRUS; ANTIHEPATITIS

Therapeutic: ANTIHEPATITIS

AVAILABILITY Capsules

ACTION & *THERAPEUTIC EFFECT*

A direct-acting antiviral agent (DAA) that inhibits viral enzymes needed for critical steps in HCV replication; *prevents HCV replication.*

USES Treatment of chronic hepatitis C (CHC) infection in combination with other agents, in HCV genotype 1 infection.

CONTRAINDICATIONS Severe hepatic impairment (Child-Pugh class C); autoimmune hepatitis; decompensated liver disease; lactation.

CAUTIOUS USE Renal impairment; mild or moderate hepatic impairment; sulfa allergy; individuals of eastern Asian ancestry; older adults; pregnancy (category C). Safety and efficacy in children younger than 18 y not established.

ROUTE & DOSAGE

Hepatitis C Infection

Adult: **PO** 150 mg once a day for 12 wk in combination with other agents

Discontinuation Based on Inadequate Virologic Response

If HCV RNA 25 IU/mL or greater at wk 4: Discontinue all therapy

ADMINISTRATION

Oral

- Give with food and concurrently with peginterferon alfa and ribavirin.
- Capsules **must be** swallowed whole. They should not be cut or chewed.
- If peginterferon alfa or ribavirin is discontinued for any reason, simeprevir also **must be** discontinued.
- The dose of simeprevir **must not be** reduced or interrupted. If discontinued because of adverse reactions or inadequate response, treatment **must not be** reinitiated.
- Store at room temperature below 30° C (86° F). Protect from light.

ADVERSE EFFECTS **Respiratory:** *Dyspnea.* **CNS:** Dizziness, fatigue, headache, insomnia. **Skin:** Grade 3 photosensitivity, pruritus, *rash* (includes: cutaneous vasculitis, dermatitis exfoliative, eczema, erythema, maculopapular rash, photosensitivity reaction, toxic skin eruption, urticaria). **GI:** *Nausea.* **Musculoskeletal:** *Myalgia.* **Hematologic:** *Increased serum bilirubin,* increased serum alkaline phosphatase. **Other:** *Pruritus.*

INTERACTIONS **Drug:** Simeprevir may increase the levels of drugs that are substrates for OATP1B1/3 and P-gp transport (e.g., **digoxin,** HMG COA REDUCTASE INHIBITORS). Simeprevir may increase the levels of drugs requiring intestinal CYP3A4 for metabolism (e.g., CALCIUM CHANNEL BLOCKERS, **cisapride, midazolam, sildenafil, tadalafil, triazolam, vardenafil**). Co-administration of simeprevir with moderate or strong inhibitors of CYP3A4 (e.g., AZOLE ANTIFUNGALS, HIV PROTEASE INHIBITORS, MACROLIDES), may increase the levels of simeprevir. Co-administration with moderate or strong inducers of CYP3A4 (e.g., **carbamazepine, dexamethasone, efavirenz, phenobarbital, phenytoin**) may decrease the levels of simeprevir. **Food: Grapefruit** and **grapefruit juice** may increase the levels of simeprevir. **Herbal: Milk thistle** may increase the levels of simeprevir. **St. John's wort** may decrease the levels of simeprevir.

PHARMACOKINETICS **Absorption:** Orally bioavailable. **Peak:** 4–6 h. **Distribution:** 99.9% plasma protein bound, extensively distributed to gut and liver. **Metabolism:** In liver. **Elimination:** Primarily unchanged in feces. **Half-Life:** 10–13 h.

NURSING IMPLICATIONS

Assessment & Drug Effects

- Monitor for adverse dermatologic effects (e.g., including erythema, eczema, maculopapular rash, urticaria, toxic skin eruption, exfoliative dermatitis) and follow for progression and/or development of mucosal signs (e.g., oral lesions, conjunctivitis) or systemic symptoms. If rash becomes severe, report promptly to prescriber.
- Monitor lab tests: Baseline and periodic LFTs, uric acid; serum HCV-RNA at baseline and at wk 4, 12, 24, and end of treatment, and during treatment follow-up; pretreatment and monthly pregnancy tests and up to 6 mo after therapy is discontinued.

S

Patient & Family Education

- **Do not** reduce or interrupt the dose of simeprevir.
- Avoid excessive sunlight and tanning devices, and take precautions to limit exposure as drug (e.g., sunscreen) may cause moderate to severe phototoxicity reaction.
- Women of childbearing potential and male partners of pregnant women should use effective means of contraception while taking this drug and for at least 6 mo following discontinuation of therapy.

SIMVASTATIN

(sim-vah-sta′tin)

Zocor

Classification: HMG-COA REDUC-TASE INHIBITOR (STATIN)
Therapeutic: ANTILIPEMIC; STATIN
Prototype: Lovastatin

AVAILABILITY Tablet

ACTION & *THERAPEUTIC EFFECT* Inhibitor of HMG-CoA reductase. HMG-CoA reductase inhibitors increase HDL cholesterol, and decrease LDL cholesterol, and total cholesterol synthesis. *Effectiveness indicated by decreased serum triglycerides, decreased LDL, cholesterol, and modest increases in HDL cholesterol.*

USES Hypercholesterolemia (alone or in combination with other agents), familial hypercholesterolemia. Reduces risk of CHD death and nonfatal MI and stroke.

CONTRAINDICATIONS Hypersensitivity to simvastatin; active liver disease or unexplained elevation of serum transaminase, hepatic encephalopathy, hepatitis, jaundice, AST or ALT of 3 × ULN; rhabdomyolysis, acute renal failure; cholestasis; myopathy; MS; pregnancy (may cause fetal harm); lactation (harm to infant).

CAUTIOUS USE Homozygous familial hypercholesterolemia, history of liver disease, alcoholics;

renal disease, renal impairment; DM; ALS patients; seizure disorder; children younger than 10 y.

ROUTE & DOSAGE

Hypercholesterolemia, Hyperlipidemia, CV Prevention

Adult: **PO** 10–20 mg each evening; range 5–40 mg daily (max: 80 mg daily).
Adolescent/Child (10 y or older): **PO** 10 mg each night (may increase to 40 mg each day)

Homozygous Familial Hypercholesterolemia

Adult: **PO** 40 mg each evening

Renal Impairment Dosage Adjustment

CrCl less than 20 mL/min: Start with 5 mg each night

ADMINISTRATION

Oral

- Adjust dosage usually at 4-wk intervals.
- Shake suspension at least 20 sec prior to use and suspension should be taken on an empty stomach.
- Give in the evening.
- Store tablet at 5°–30° C (41°–86° F).
- Store suspension between 20°–25° C (68°–77° F). Do not freeze or refrigerate and protect from heat. Discard bottle 1 mo after first use.

ADVERSE EFFECTS **CV:** Atrial fibrillation. **Respiratory:** URI, bronchitis. **CNS:** Headache, vertigo. **Skin:** Eczema. **GI:** Abdominal pain, constipation, nausea. **Musculoskeletal:** Increased CPK levels.

INTERACTIONS **Drug:** Avoid use with **itraconazole, ketoconazole, erythromycin, clarithromycin, telithromycin,** PROTEASE INHIBITORS, **nefazodone.** Simvastatin dose will need to be decreased when given with **gemfibrozil, cyclosporine, danazole, amiodarone, verapamil, diltiazem.** May increase PT when administered with **warfarin. Cyclosporine, gemfibrozil, fenofibrate, clofibrate,** antilipemic doses of **niacin, fluconazole, miconazole, sildenafil, tacrolimus, amlodipine** may increase serum levels and increase risk of myopathy, rhabdomyolysis and acute kidney failure. Avoid use with **rifampin. Food: Grapefruit juice** (greater than 1 qt/day) may increase risk of myopathy, rhabdomyolysis. **Herbal: St. John's wort** may decrease efficacy.

PHARMACOKINETICS **Absorption:** Rapidly from GI tract. **Onset:** 2 wk. **Peak:** 4–6 wk. **Distribution:** 95% protein bound; achieves high liver concentrations; crosses placenta. **Metabolism:** Extensive first-pass metabolism to its active metabolite. **Elimination:** 60% in bile and feces.

NURSING IMPLICATIONS

Assessment & Drug Effects

- Assess for and report unexplained muscle pain. Determine CPK level at onset of muscle pain.
- Monitor coagulation studies with patients receiving concurrent warfarin therapy. PT may be prolonged.
- Monitor lab tests: Baseline and periodic lipid profile, LFTs, creatinine kinase.

Patient & Family Education

- Report unexplained muscle pain, tenderness, or weakness, especially if accompanied by malaise or fever, to prescriber.

S

- Report signs of bleeding to prescriber promptly when taking concurrent warfarin.
- Moderate intake of grapefruit juice while taking this medication.

SIPULEUCEL-T

(sip-u-lew'cel)

Provenge

Classification: BIOLOGIC RESPONSE MODIFIER; ACTIVE CELL IMMUNOTHERAPEUTIC; ANTINEOPLASTIC

Therapeutic: ANTINEOPLASTIC

AVAILABILITY Intravenous suspension

ACTION & *THERAPEUTIC EFFECT*

While the mechanism of action is unknown, sipuleucel-T is designed to induce an immune response against prostatic acid phosphatase (PAP), an antigen expressed on most prostate cancer cells. *Stimulation of humoral and T-cell mediated responses are thought to slow tumor progression and improve survival.*

USES Prostate cancer.

CONTRAINDICATIONS Pregnancy category undetermined; not for use in women.

CAUTIOUS USE Concomitant use of chemotherapy; history of infusion reactions.

ROUTE & DOSAGE

Prostate Cancer

Adult: IV 250 mL infusion q2wk for a total of 3 doses

ADMINISTRATION

Intravenous

▪ Use universal precautions when handling sipuleucel-T. ▪ Note: Premedication is recommended with oral acetaminophen and an antihistamine (e.g., diphenhydramine) approximately 30 min prior to administration.

PREPARE: **IV Infusion:** ▪ Product is intended only for autologous use (i.e., patient donates to self). ▪ Open the outer cardboard shipping box to verify the product and patient-specific labels located on the top of the insulated container. ▪ **Do not** remove the insulated container from the shipping box, or open the lid of the insulated container, until the patient is ready for infusion. Inspect for leakage. ▪ Contents of bag will be slightly cloudy, with a cream-to-pink color. Gently tilt bag to resuspend contents; inspect for clumps and clots that should disperse with gentle manual mixing. ▪ Do not administer if the bag leaks during handling or if clumps remain in the bag.

ADMINISTER: **IV Infusion:** ▪ Infusion must be started prior to the expiration date and time on *Cell Product Disposition Form* and label. Give over 60 min. ▪ Administer through a dedicated line and **do not** use a cell filter. Ensure that entire contents of bag are infused. ▪ Monitor closely during and for 1 h after infusion for an infusion reaction (e.g., dyspnea, hypertension, tachycardia, chills, fever, nausea). Infusion may be stopped or slowed depending on severity of reaction. ▪ Do not reinitiate infusion with a bag held at room temperature for more than 3 h.

S

INCOMPATIBILITIES: **Solution/additive:** Do not mix with another drug. **Y-site:** Do not mix with another drug.

ADVERSE EFFECTS **Respiratory:** Cough, dyspnea, upper respiratory infection. **CNS:** *Asthenia, dizziness, fatigue, headache*, insomnia, *paresthesia*, tremor. **Skin:** Rash, sweating. **GI:** Anorexia, *constipation*, diarrhea, *nausea, vomiting*, weight loss. **GU:** Hematuria, urinary tract infection. **Musculoskeletal:** *Back pain*, bone pain, *joint ache*, neck pain, *muscle ache*, muscle spasms, musculoskeletal chest pain, musculoskeletal pain, *pain in extremity*. **Hematologic:** *Anemia*. **Other:** *Chills, citrate toxicity, fever*, hot flush, influenza-like illness, *pain*, peripheral edema.

INTERACTIONS **Drug:** Due to the ability of sipuleucel-T to stimulate the immune system, concomitant use of immunosuppressive agents (e.g., **cortico-steroids**) may alter the efficacy and/or safety of sipuleucel-T.

NURSING IMPLICATIONS

Assessment & Drug Effects

- Observe closely during infusion and for at least 1 h following for an infusion reaction (see Administration). Monitor vital signs throughout observation period. Note that an acute infusion reaction is more likely after the second infusion.
- Report immediately to prescriber if an infusion reaction occurs.

Patient & Family Education

- Report immediately any of the following: Fever, chills, fatigue, breathing problems, dizziness, high blood pressure, palpitations, nausea, vomiting, headache, or muscle aches.

SIROLIMUS

(sir-o-li′mus)

Rapamune

Classification: IMMUNOMODULATOR; IMMUNOSUPPRESSANT

Therapeutic: IMMUNOSUPPRESSANT

Prototype: Cyclosporine

AVAILABILITY Tablet; oral solution

ACTION & *THERAPEUTIC EFFECT* Active in reducing a transplant rejection by inhibiting the response of helper T-lymphocytes and B-lymphocytes to cytokines [(interleukin) IL-2, IL-4, and IL-5]. *Inhibits antibody production and acute transplant rejection reaction in autoimmune disorders [e.g., systemic lupus erythematosus (SLE)]. Indicated by non rejection of transplanted organ.*

USES Prophylaxis of kidney transplant rejection; treatment of lymphangioleiomyomatosis.

CONTRAINDICATIONS Hypersensitivity to sirolimus; lung or liver transplant patients; soya lecithin (soy fatty acids) hypersensitivity; PML; lactation.

CAUTIOUS USE Hypersensitivity to tacrolimus; impaired renal function; renal transplant patients; dialysis patients; hepatic impairment; UV exposure, retransplant patients, multiorgan transplant recipients, African American transplant patients; interstitial lung disease; viral or bacterial infection; hyperlipidemia, DM, atrial fibrillation, CHF, hypervolemia, palpitations; hepatic disease; CAD; myelosuppression; older adults; pregnancy (category C); children younger than 13 y.

S

ROUTE & DOSAGE

Kidney Transplant

Adult/Adolescent (over 40 kg): **PO** 6 mg loading dose immediately after transplant, then 2 mg/day. Doses will need to be much higher if using cyclosporine or corticosteroids.

Adolescent (13 y or older, weight less than 40 kg): **PO** 3 mg/m^2 loading dose immediately after transplant, then 1 mg/m^2/day.

Lymphangioleiomyomatosis

Adult: **PO** 2 mg daily, then adjust to target concentration of 5–15 mg/mL

Hepatic Impairment Dosage Adjustment

Loading dose does not need to be modified.

Mild to moderate: Reduce maintenance does by 33% *Severe impairment:* Reduce maintenance by 50%

ADMINISTRATION

Oral

- Give 4 h after oral cyclosporine.
- Tablets should be swallowed whole. They should not be crushed or chewed.
- Add prescribed amount of sirolimus oral solution to a glass containing 2 oz (60 mL) or more of water or orange juice (do not use any other type of liquid). Stir vigorously and administer immediately. Refill glass with 4 oz (120 mL) or more of water or orange juice. Stir vigorously and administer immediately.
- Give consistently with respect to amount and type of food.
- Refrigerate; protect from light; use multidose bottles within 1 mo of opening.

ADVERSE EFFECTS

CV: *Hypertension,* atrial fibrillation, CHF, hypervolemia, hypotension, palpitation, peripheral vascular disorder, postural hypotension, syncope, tachycardia, thrombophlebitis, thrombosis, vasodilation. **Respiratory:** *Dyspnea, pharyngitis, upper respiratory tract infection,* asthma, atelectasis, bronchitis, cough, epistaxis, hypoxia, lung edema, pleural effusion, pneumonia, rhinitis, sinusitis. **CNS:** *Insomnia, tremor, headache,* anxiety, confusion, depression, dizziness, emotional lability, hypertonia, hyperesthesia, hypotonia, neuropathy, paresthesia, somnolence. **HEENT:** Abnormal vision, cataract, conjunctivitis, deafness, ear pain, otitis media, tinnitus. **Endocrine:** *Edema, hypercholesterolemia, hyperkalemia, hyperlipidemia, hypokalemia, hypophosphatemia, peripheral edema, weight gain,* Cushing's syndrome, diabetes, acidosis, hypercalcemia, hyperglycemia, hyperphosphatemia, hypomagnesemia, hypoglycemia, hypomagnesemia, hyponatremia; increased LDH, alkaline phosphatase, BUN, creatine phosphokinase, ALT, or AST; weight loss. **Skin:** *Acne, rash,* fungal dermatitis, hirsutism, pruritus, skin hypertrophy, skin ulcer, sweating. **GI:** *Constipation, diarrhea, dyspepsia, nausea, vomiting, abdominal pain,* anorexia, dysphagia, eructation, esophagitis, flatulence, gastritis, gastroenteritis, gingivitis, gum hyperplasia, ileus, mouth ulceration, oral moniliasis, stomatitis, abnormal liver function tests. **GU:** *UTI,* albuminuria, bladder pain, dysuria, hematuria, hydronephrosis, impotence, kidney pain, nocturia, renal tubular necrosis, oliguria, pyuria, scrotal edema, incontinence, urinary retention, glycosuria. **Hematologic:** *Anemia,* <u>thrombocytopenia,</u>

leukopenia, hemorrhage, ecchymosis, leukocytosis, lymphadenopathy, polycythemia, thrombotic, thrombocytopenic purpura. **Other:** *Asthenia, back pain, chest pain, fever, pain, arthralgia;* flu-like syndrome; generalized edema; infection; lymphocele; malaise; sepsis, arthrosis, bone necrosis, leg cramps, myalgia, osteoporosis, tetany, abscess, ascites, cellulitis, chills, face edema, hernia, pelvic pain, peritonitis.

INTERACTIONS **Drug:** Sirolimus concentrations increased by **clarithromycin, cyclosporine, diltiazem, erythromycin, ketoconazole, itraconazole, telithromycin;** sirolimus concentrations decreased by **rifabutin, rifampin;** VACCINES may be less effective with sirolimus; **tacrolimus** increases mortality, hepatic artery thrombosis, and graft loss. **Food: Grapefruit juice** significantly increases plasma levels. High fat meals increase levels. **Herbal: St. John's wort** decreases efficacy.

PHARMACOKINETICS **Absorption:** Rapidly with 14% bioavailability. **Peak:** 2 h. **Distribution:** 92% protein bound, distributes in high concentrations to heart, intestines, kidneys, liver, lungs, muscle, spleen, and testes. **Metabolism:** In liver (CYP3A4). **Elimination:** 91% in feces, 2.2% in urine. **Half-Life:** 62 h.

NURSING IMPLICATIONS

Black Box Warning

Sirolimus has been associated with increased susceptibility to infection and development of lymphoma.

Assessment & Drug Effects

- Monitor for S&S of graft rejection.
- Control hyperlipidemia prior to initiating drug.
- Monitor for and report promptly S&S of infection.
- Draw trough whole-blood sirolimus levels 1 h before a scheduled dose.
- Monitor lab tests: Periodic lipid profile, CBC with differential, LFTs, urinary protein, and creatinine, and serum sirolimus as indicated.

Patient & Family Education

- Avoid grapefruit juice within 2 h of taking sirolimus.
- Limit exposure to sunlight (UV exposure).
- Note: Decreased effectiveness possible for vaccines during therapy.
- Use or add barrier contraceptive before, during, and for 12 wk after discontinuing therapy.

SITAGLIPTIN (Prototype)

(sit-a-glip′tin)

Januvia

Classification: DIPEPTIDYL PEPTIDASE-4 (DPP-4) INHIBITOR

Therapeutic: ANTIDIABETIC; INCRETIN MODIFIER; DDP-4 INHIBITOR

AVAILABILITY Tablet

ACTION & *THERAPEUTIC EFFECT* Slows inactivation of incretin hormones [e.g., glucagon-like peptide-1 (GLP-1) and glucose-dependent insulinotropic polypeptide (GIP)] that are released by the intestine. As plasma glucose rises following food intake, incretin hormones stimulate release of insulin from the pancreas, and GLP-1 also lowers glucagon secretion, resulting in reduced hepatic glucose production. *Sitagliptin lowers both fasting and postprandial plasma glucose levels.*

USES Adjunct treatment of type 2 diabetes mellitus.

CONTRAINDICATIONS Serious hypersensitivity to sitagliptin; type I DM; diabetic ketoacidosis.

CAUTIOUS USE Moderate to severe renal impairment, renal failure, hemodialysis; heart failure, older adults; history of pancreatitis; pregnancy (fetal risk cannot be ruled out); lactation (infant risk cannot be ruled out). Safe use in children younger than 18 y not established.

ROUTE & DOSAGE

Type 2 Diabetes Mellitus

Adult: **PO** 100 mg/day

Renal Impairment Dosage Adjustment

CrCl between 30 mL/min and 50 mL/min: 50 mg/day; *less than 30 mL/min:* 25 mg/day

ADMINISTRATION

Oral

- May be given without regard to meals.
- Note that dosage adjustment is recommended for moderate to severe renal impairment.
- Store at 20°–25° C (68°–77° F).

S

ADVERSE EFFECTS **Respiratory:** Nasopharyngitis, URI. **CNS:** Headache. **Endocrine:** Hypoglycemia.

INTERACTIONS **Drug:** Sitagliptin may increase **digoxin** levels. QUINOLONES may increase blood glucose. Monitor closely with **insulin** or SULFONYLUREAS.

PHARMACOKINETICS **Absorption:** 87% absorbed. **Peak:** 1–4 h. **Distribution:** 38% protein bound. **Metabolism:** 20% metabolized in the liver. **Elimination:** Primarily renal (87%) with minor elimination in the kidneys. **Half-Life:** 12.4 h.

NURSING IMPLICATIONS

Assessment & Drug Effects

- Monitor for and report S&S of significant GI distress, including NV&D.
- Monitor for S&S of hypoglycemia when used in combination with a sulfonylurea drug or insulin.
- Monitor blood levels of digoxin with concurrent therapy.
- Monitor lab tests: Baseline and periodic CrCl; periodic fasting and postprandial plasma glucose and HbA1C.

Patient & Family Education

- Taking this drug with another drug that can lower your blood sugar, such as a sulfonylurea or insulin, increases your risk of hypoglycemia.
- Stop taking this drug and notify prescriber immediately if you have an allergic reaction (e.g., swelling of your face, lips, throat; difficulty swallowing or breathing); raised, red areas on your skin (hives); skin rash, itching, flaking or peeling.
- Contact prescriber if you experience unexplained symptoms of liver problems (e.g., nausea or vomiting, abdominal pain, unusual tiredness, loss of appetite, dark urine, yellowing of your skin or the whites of your eyes) or if swelling is noted in lower extremities.

SODIUM BICARBONATE NA(HCO_3)

(sod'i-um bi-car'bon-ate)

Sodium Bicarbonate

Classification: FLUID AND ELECTROLYTE BALANCE AGENT; ANTACID

Therapeutic: ANTACID

AVAILABILITY Tablet; solution for injection

ACTION & *THERAPEUTIC EFFECT*
Rapidly neutralizes gastric acid to form sodium chloride, carbon dioxide, and water. After absorption of sodium bicarbonate, plasma alkali reserve is increased and excess sodium and bicarbonate ions are excreted in urine, thus rendering urine less acid. *Short-acting, potent systemic antacid; rapidly neutralizes gastric acid or systemic acidosis.*

USES Systemic alkalinizer to correct metabolic acidosis (as occurs in diabetes mellitus, shock, cardiac arrest, or vascular collapse), to minimize uric acid crystallization associated with uricosuric agents, to increase the solubility of sulfonamides, and to enhance renal excretion of barbiturate and salicylate overdosage. Commonly used as home remedy for relief of occasional heartburn, indigestion, or sour stomach. Used topically as paste, bath, or soak to relieve itching and minor skin irritations such as sunburn, insect bites, prickly heat, poison ivy, sumac, or oak. Sterile solutions are used to buffer acidic parenteral solutions to prevent acidosis. Also as a buffering agent in many commercial products (e.g., mouthwashes, douches, enemas, ophthalmic solutions).

CONTRAINDICATIONS Prolonged therapy with sodium bicarbonate; patients losing chloride (as from vomiting, GI suction, diuresis); hypocalcemia; metabolic alkalosis; respiratory alkalosis; peptic ulcer.

CAUTIOUS USE Edema, sodium retaining disorders; heart disease, hypertension; preexisting respiratory acidosis; renal disease, renal insufficiency; hyperkalemia, hypokalemia; older adults; pregnancy (category C); children.

ROUTE & DOSAGE

Antacid

Adult: **PO** 0.3–2 g 1–4 × day or ½ tsp of powder in glass of water

Urinary Alkalinizer

Adult: **PO** 4 g initially, then 1–2 g q4h
Child: **PO** 84–840 mg/kg/day in divided doses

Cardiac Arrest

Adult: **IV** 1 mEq/kg initially, then 0.5 mEq/kg q10min depending on arterial blood gas determinations (8.4% solutions contain 50 mEq/50 mL), give over 1–2 min
Child: **IV** 0.5–1 mEq/kg q10min depending on arterial blood gas determinations, give over 1–2 min

Metabolic Acidosis

Adult/Child: **IV** Dose adjusted according to pH, base deficit, $Paco_2$, fluid limits, and patient response

ADMINISTRATION

Oral

- Do not add oral preparation to calcium-containing solutions.

Intravenous

PREPARE: **Direct/IV Infusion** May give 4.2% (0.5 mEq/mL) and 5% (0.595 mEq/mL) $NaHCO_3$ solutions undiluted. ▪ Dilute 7.5% (0.892 mEq/mL) and 8.4% (1 mEq/mL) solutions with compatible IV solutions to a maximum concentration of 0.5 mEq/mL.

▪ For infants and children, dilute to at least 4.2%.

ADMINISTER: **Direct:** Give a bolus dose over 1–2 min only in emergency situations. ▪ For neonates or infants younger than 2 y, use only 4.2% solution for direct IV injection. **IV Infusion:** Usual rate is 2–5 mEq/kg over 4–8 h; do not exceed 50 mEq/h. ▪ Flush line before/after with NS. ▪ Stop infusion immediately if extravasation occurs. Severe tissue damage has followed tissue infiltration.

INCOMPATIBILITIES: **Solution/additive:** **Alcohol 5%, lactated Ringer's, amoxicillin, ascorbic acid, bupivacaine, carboplatin, carmustine, ciprofloxacin, cisplatin, codeine, corticotropin, dobutamine, dopamine, epinephrine, glycopyrrolate, hydromorphone, imipenem/cilastatin, insulin, isoproterenol, labetalol, levorphanol, magnesium sulfate, meperidine, meropenem, methadone, metoclopramide, morphine, norepinephrine, oxytetracycline, penicillin G, pentazocine, pentobarbital, phenobarbital, procaine, promazine, streptomycin, succinylcholine, tetracycline, vancomycin, vitamin B complex with C.** **Y-site:** **Allopurinol, amiodarone, amphotericin B cholesteryl complex, calcium chloride, ciprofloxacin, cisatracurium, diltiazem, doxorubicin liposome, fenoldopam, hetastarch, idarubicin, imipenem/cilastatin, leucovorin, lidocaine, midazolam, milrinone acetate, nalbuphine, ondansetron, oxacillin, sargramostim, verapamil, vincristine, vindesine, vinorelbine.**

▪ Store in airtight containers. ▪ Note expiration date.

S

ADVERSE EFFECTS

Endocrine: Metabolic alkalosis; electrolyte imbalance: Sodium overload (pulmonary edema), hypocalcemia (tetany), hypokalemia, milk-alkali syndrome, dehydration. **Skin:** Severe tissue damage following extravasation of IV solution. **GI:** *Belching, gastric distention,* flatulence. **GU:** Renal calculi or crystals, impaired kidney function. **Other:** Rapid IV in neonates (hypernatremia, reduction in CSF pressure, <u>intracranial hemorrhage</u>).

DIAGNOSTIC TEST INTERFERENCE

Small increase in ***blood lactate*** levels (following IV infusion of sodium bicarbonate); false-positive ***urinary protein*** determinations (using ***Ames reagent, sulfacetic acid,*** heat and ***acetic acid*** or ***nitric acid ring method***); elevated ***urinary urobi-linogen*** levels (***urobilinogen*** excretion increases in alkaline urine).

INTERACTIONS

Drug: May decrease absorption of **ketoconazole;** may decrease elimination of **dextroamphetamine, ephedrine, pseudoephedrine, quinidine;** may increase elimination of **chlorpropamide, lithium,** SALICYLATES, TETRACYCLINES.

PHARMACOKINETICS

Absorption: Readily from GI tract. **Onset:** 15 min. **Duration:** 1–2 h. **Elimination:** In urine within 3–4 h.

NURSING IMPLICATIONS

Assessment & Drug Effects

▪ Be aware that long-term use of oral preparation with milk or calcium can cause milk-alkali syndrome: Anorexia, nausea, vomiting, headache, mental confusion, hypercalcemia,

hypophosphatemia, soft tissue calcification, renal and ureteral calculi, renal insufficiency, metabolic alkalosis.
- Observe for and report S&S of improvement or reversal of metabolic acidosis (see Appendix F).
- Monitor lab tests: Periodic measurements of acid–base status (blood pH, PO_2, PCO_2, HCO_3^-, and other electrolytes), usually several times daily during acute period.

Patient & Family Education

- Do not use sodium bicarbonate as antacid. A nonabsorbable OTC alternative for repeated use is safer.
- Do not take antacids longer than 2 wk except under advice and supervision of a prescriber. Self-medication with routine doses of sodium bicarbonate or soda mints may cause sodium retention and alkalosis, especially when kidney function is impaired.
- Be aware that commonly used OTC antacid products contain sodium bicarbonate (e.g., Alka Seltzer).

SODIUM FERRIC GLUCONATE

(so′di-um fer′ric glu′co-nate)

Ferrlecit

Classification: NUTRITIONAL SUPPLEMENT; IRON PREPARATION

Therapeutic: ANTIANEMIC; IRON REPLACEMENT

Prototype: Ferrous sulfate

AVAILABILITY Intravenous solution

ACTION & *THERAPEUTIC EFFECT* Stable iron complex used to restore iron loss in chronic kidney failure patients. The use of erythropoietin therapy and blood loss through hemodialysis require iron replacement. The ferric ion combines with transferrin and is transported to bone marrow where it is incorporated into hemoglobin. *Effectiveness indicated by improved Hgb and Hct, iron saturation, and serum ferritin levels.*

USES Treatment of iron deficiency anemia.

CONTRAINDICATIONS Any anemia not related to iron deficiency; hypersensitivity to sodium ferric gluconate complex; hemochromatosis, hemosiderosis; hemolytic anemia; thalassemia; neonates; pregnancy—fetal risk cannot be ruled out; lactation—infant risk cannot be ruled out.

CAUTIOUS USE Hypersensitivity to benzyl alcohol; active or suspected infection; cardiac disease; hepatic disease; dialysis patient; older adults. Safety and efficacy in children younger than 6 y not established.

ROUTE & DOSAGE

Iron Deficiency in Dialysis Patients

Adult: **IV** 125 mg infused over 1 h
Adolescent/Child (over 6 y): **IV** 1.5 mg/kg infused over 1 h (max:125 mg/dose); adjust based on iron status tests

ADMINISTRATION

Intravenous ONLY

PREPARE: **Direct for Adult:** May be given undiluted. **Direct for Child:** Dilute required doses in 25 mL NS. **IV Infusion for Adult/Child:** Dilute 125 mg in 100 mL of NS.

S

▪ Use immediately after dilution.
ADMINISTER: **Direct for Adult:** Give no faster than 12.5 mg/min. **IV Infusion for Adult/Child:** Give over **not** less than 60 min.
INCOMPATIBILITIES: **Solution/additive:** Do not administer with TPN.

▪ Store unopened ampules at 20°–25° C (68°–77° F), excursions permitted between 15 and 30° C (59 and 86° F). Do not freeze.

ADVERSE EFFECTS (≥5%) **CV:** Hypotension, hypertension, tachycardia. **Respiratory:** Dyspnea. **GI:** Vomiting, nausea, diarrhea. **CNS:** Dizziness, headache. **Skin:** Injection site reaction. **Musculoskeletal:** Muscle cramps. **Hematologic:** Red blood cell disorder. **Other:** Pain.

DIAGNOSTIC TEST INTERFERENCE May produce falsely elevated serum or transferring bound iron levels for up to 5 days after administration.

INTERACTIONS **Drug:** **Dimercaprol** may enhance nephrotoxic effects. **Amifostine** may increase hypotensive effects.

PHARMACOKINETICS **Half-life Elimination:** 1 h (bound iron).

S

NURSING IMPLICATIONS

Assessment & Drug Effects

- Monitor closely for S&S of severe hypersensitivity (see Appendix F) during IV administration.
- Monitor vital signs periodically during IV administration (transient hypotension possible especially during dialysis) and at least 30 minutes following the administration.
- Stop infusion immediately and notify prescriber if hypersensitivity is suspected.
- Monitor lab tests: Periodic Hgb, Hct, Fe saturation, and serum ferritin.

Patient & Family Education

- Report to prescriber immediately: Difficulty breathing, itching, flushing, rash, weakness, lightheadedness, pain, or any other discomfort during infusion.
- Advise patient that drug may decrease the absorption of any additional oral iron preparations.

SODIUM POLYSTYRENE SULFONATE

(pol-ee-stye′reen)

Kayexalate, SPS Suspension

Classification: ELECTROLYTE AND WATER BALANCE; CATION EXCHANGE
Therapeutic: CATION EXCHANGE

AVAILABILITY Suspension; powder

ACTION & *THERAPEUTIC EFFECT* Sulfonic cation-exchange resin that removes potassium by exchanging sodium ion for potassium, particularly in large intestine; potassium containing resin is then excreted through the bowel. *Removes potassium by exchanging sodium ion for potassium through the large intestine.*

USES Hyperkalemia.

CONTRAINDICATIONS Hypersensitivity to Kayexalate; GI obstruction; hypokalemia; lactation.

CAUTIOUS USE Acute or chronic kidney failure; low birth weight infants; neonates with reduced gut; patients receiving digitalis preparations; patients who cannot tolerate even a small increase in sodium load (e.g., CHF, severe hypertension, and marked edema); patients with constipation or bowel obstruction; renal insufficiency. older adults; pregnancy (category C); children.

ROUTE & DOSAGE

Hyperkalemia

Adult: **PO** 15 g 1–4 × per day **Rectal** 30–50 g q6h as warm emulsion high into sigmoid colon
Child: **PO** 1 g/kg q6h; **Rectal** 1 g/kg q2–6h

ADMINISTRATION

Oral

- Give as a suspension in a small quantity of water or in syrup. Usual amount of fluid ranges from 20–100 mL or approximately 3–4 mL/g of drug.

Rectal

- Use warm fluid (as prescribed) to prepare the emulsion for enema.
- Administer a cleansing enema (non-sodium-containing fluid) before and after rectal administration.
- Administer at body temperature and introduce by gravity, keeping suspension particles in solution by stirring. Flush suspension with 50–100 mL of fluid; then clamp tube and leave it in place.
- Urge patient to retain enema at least 30–60 min but as long as several hours if possible.
- Irrigate colon (after enema solution has been expelled) with 1 or 2 qt flushing solution (non-sodium containing). Drain returns constantly through a Y-tube connection.
- Store remainder of prepared solution for 24 h; then discard.

ADVERSE EFFECTS

Respiratory: Bronchitis, bronchopneumonia. **Endocrine:** Sodium retention, hypocalcemia, hypokalemia, hypomagnesemia, hypervolemia. **GI:** *Constipation, fecal impaction (in older adults);* anorexia, gastric irritation, nausea, vomiting, diarrhea (with sorbitol emulsions), gastrointestinal hemorrhage.

INTERACTIONS

Drug: ANTACIDS, LAXATIVES containing **calcium** or **magnesium** may decrease potassium exchange capability of the resin. Do not use with products containing sorbitol.

PHARMACOKINETICS

Absorption: Not absorbed systemically. **Onset:** Several hours to days. **Metabolism:** Not metabolized. **Elimination:** In feces.

NURSING IMPLICATIONS

Assessment & Drug Effects

- Serum potassium levels do not always reflect intracellular potassium deficiency. Observe patient closely for early clinical signs of severe hypokalemia (see Appendix F). ECGs are also recommended.
- Consult prescriber about restricting sodium content from dietary and other sources since drug contains approximately 100 mg (4.1 mEq) of sodium/g (1 tsp, 15 mEq sodium).
- Monitor lab tests: Daily serum potassium; periodic acid–base balance, and serum electrolytes.

Patient & Family Education

- Check bowel function daily. Usually, a mild laxative is prescribed to prevent constipation (common adverse effect). Older adult patients are particularly prone to fecal impaction.

SODIUM ZIRCONIUM CYCLOSILICATE

(sow′dee-um zir-koe′nee-um sye′kloe-sil′i-kate)

Lokelma
Classification: ELECTROLYTE AND WATER BALANCE; CATION EXCHANGE
Therapeutic: CATION EXCHANGE

AVAILABILITY Oral packet for suspension

ACTION & *THERAPEUTIC EFFECT* Sodium zirconium cyclosilicate is a nonabsorbed substance which has a high affinity for potassium ions, binding and increasing fecal elimination of free potassium. *Will lower potassium in nonemergent treatment of of hyperkalemia.*

USES Treatment of hyperkalemia.

CONTRAINDICATIONS Previous hypersensitivity to tildrakizumab or components of the formulation.

CAUTIOUS USE Avoid use in patients with gastroparesis, or motility disorders such as bowel obstruction or severe constipation. Contents may increase patient's risk of edema due to high sodium content. Should not be used for life-threatening hyperkalemia due to delayed onset of action. History of CHF or renal disease.

ROUTE & DOSAGE

Hyperkalemia

Adult: **Oral** 10 g 3 × day; titrated to serum potassium (max: 15 g/day)

ADMINISTRATION

Oral

- Empty entire contents of a packet into 3 or more tablespoons of water; stir contents and drink entire contents immediately.
- Administer other oral medications 2 h before or 2 h after this medication.
- Store packets at 15°–30° C (59°–86° F) in a dry place.

ADVERSE EFFECTS **CV:** Edema, peripheral edema. **Endocrine:** Hypokalemia.

INTERACTIONS Potential for sodium zirconium cyclosilicate to increase gastric pH, which may alter the absorption of medications with pH dependent solubility. Administering medications 2 h before or after may avoid this interaction.

PHARMACOKINETICS **Absorption:** Not systemically absorbed. **Metabolism:** Not subject to metabolism, due to lack of absorption. **Elimination:** Exclusively eliminated through feces.

NURSING IMPLICATIONS

Assessment & Drug Effects

- Assess for edema.
- Monitor lab tests: Serum potassium levels.

Patient & Family Education

- Review proper mixing instructions with patient and family.
- Any other oral medications should be taken 2 h before or 2 hs after sodium zirconium cyclosilicate.
- Follow low sodium diet since medication contains 400 mg of sodium in each 5-g dose.

SOFOSBUVIR

(so-fos′bu-vir)

Sovaldi
Classification: ANTIVIRAL; NUCLEOTIDE ANALOG; VIRAL POLYMERASE INHIBITOR
Therapeutic: ANTIHEPATITIS

AVAILABILITY Film-coated tablets

ACTION & THERAPEUTIC EFFECT A direct acting antiviral agent against HCV; is a prodrug converted to its active form via intracellular metabolism. *It inhibits HCV NS5B RNA-dependent RNA polymerase thus inhibiting viral replication.*

USES Treatment of chronic hepatitis C (CHC) infection as part of a combination treatment.

CONTRAINDICATIONS Inability to take concurrent peginterferon alfa/ribavirin or ribavirin alone; concomitant potent P-gp inducers (e.g., rifampin and St. John's wort); suicidal ideation; hepatic decompensation; pregnancy—fetal risk cannot be ruled out; lactation—infant risk cannot be ruled out.

CAUTIOUS USE Concomitant drugs that are P-gp inducers, anticonvulsants, antimycobacterials and amiodarone; post-liver transplant; chronic depression; history of suicide; severe renal impairment; ESRD; liver transplant. Safety and efficacy in children younger than 3 y not established.

ROUTE & DOSAGE

Hepatitis C Infection

Adult: **PO** (see manufacturer's guidelines for dosing by genotype)

ADMINISTRATION

Oral

- Give without regard to food.
- Do not chew pellets. If administered with food, sprinkle on one or more spoonful of non-acidic soft food or below room temperature pudding, chocolate syrup, mashed potatoes or ice cream. Take within 30 minutes of mixing.
- Do not use as monotherapy; use only in combination with ribavirin (with or without peginterferon alfa).
- If the other agents used in combination with sofosbuvir are permanently discontinued, sofosbuvir should also be discontinued.
- Store at room temperature below 30° C (86° F).

ADVERSE EFFECTS **CNS:** *Fatigue, headache, insomnia.* **Skin:** Pruritus. **GI:** Diarrhea. **Hematologic:** *Anemia.*

INTERACTIONS **Drug:** Co-administration with drugs that are potent P-gp inducers in the intestine (e.g., RIFAMYCINS) may decrease the levels of sofosbuvir. Co-administration with drugs that inhibit P-gp may increase the levels of sofosbuvir. Co-administration of sofosbuvir with **carbamazepine, phenytoin, phenobarbital,** or **oxcarbazepine** may decrease the levels of sofosbuvir. Do not use with **amiodarone,** may increase bradycardic effect. **Herbal: St. John's wort must not** be used with sofosbuvir because it is a potent P-gp inducer.

PHARMACOKINETICS **Peak:** 0.5–2 h. **Distribution:** 61–65% plasma protein bound. **Metabolism:** Converted to active metabolite. **Elimination:** Primarily renal. **Half-Life:** 27 h (active metabolite).

NURSING IMPLICATIONS

Assessment & Drug Effects

- Monitor for and report promptly changes in mental status such as depression or suicidal ideation.
- Monitor for S&S of infection or anemia.
- Monitor lab tests: Baseline and periodic LFTs, serum creatinine; serum

S

HCV-RNA at baseline during treatment, end of treatment, and during treatment follow-up; pretreatment and monthly pregnancy tests and up to 6 mo after therapy discontinued; periodic CBC with differential.

Patient & Family Education

- Report immediately to prescriber if patient experiences mental status changes such as depression, thoughts of suicide, anxiety, emotional instability, or illogical thinking.
- Review adverse effects with patient and/or caregiver.
- Women of childbearing potential and male partners of pregnant women should use effective means of contraception while taking this drug and for at least 6 mo following discontinuation of therapy when medication is combined with ribavirin and with peginterferon and ribavirin.
- Avoid taking St. John's Wort during therapy.

SOFOSBUVIR AND VELPATASVIR

(soe-fos'bue-vir and vel-pat'as-vir)

Epclusa

Classification: ANTIVIRAL; VIRAL POLYMERASE INHIBITOR; ANTIHEPATITIS

Therapeutic: ANTIHEPATITIS

S

AVAILABILITY Tablets; oral packet

ACTION & *THERAPEUTIC EFFECT*

Sofosbuvir is a prodrug that is metabolized to its active form (GS-461203) which then inhibits hepatitis C viral (HCV) NS5B RNA-dependent RNA polymerase, an enzyme required for viral replication. Velpatasavir inhibits HCV NS5A protein which is required for viral replication. *Inhibits replication of the HCV virus.*

USES Treatment of chronic hepatitis C virus (HCV) genotype 1, 2, 3, 4, 5, or 6 infection in adult patients without cirrhosis, with compensated cirrhosis, or in combination with ribavirin, with decompensated cirrhosis.

CONTRAINDICATIONS Combination with ribavirin is contraindicated in patients for whom ribavirin is contraindicated; Concomitant use with amiodarone; Concomitant use with P-glycoprotein inducers or moderate to potent CYP2B6, CYP2C8, CYP3A4; pregnancy—fetal risk cannot be ruled out; lactation—infant risk cannot be ruled out.

CAUTIOUS USE No data is available to establish safety and efficacy in patients with severe renal impairment or end stage renal disease. Use with caution with patients previously infected with hepatitis B virus (HBV) and hepatitis C (HCV).

ROUTE & DOSAGE

Hepatitis C Viral Infection

Adult/Adolescent/Child (over 3 y): **PO** Varies based on age, genotype and concurrent conditions, see package insert for specific dosing information.

ADMINISTRATION

Oral

- Take tablets without regard to food.
- If administered with ribavirin, take ribavirin with food.
- Oral pellets may be taken directly in the mouth or with food. In patients less than 6 years of age,

administer with food to increase tolerability.

- Sprinkle oral pellets on one or more spoonfuls of non-acidic soft food at or below room temperature (e.g., pudding, chocolate syrup, and ice cream). Take within 15 minutes of gently mixing food and swallow entire contents without chewing.
- Store below 30° C (86° F). Dispense only in original container.

ADVERSE EFFECTS **CNS:** *Headache*. **GI:** *Nausea*. **Other:** *Fatigue*.

INTERACTIONS **Drug:** Extensive drug interactions, consult a drug interaction database for a complete listing. Coadministration of inducers of P-gp and/or CYP2B6, CYP2C8, or CYP3A4 (e.g., **carbamazepine, phenobarbital, phenytoin, rifabutin, rifampin, rifapentine**) may decrease the levels of sofosbuvir and/or velpatasvir. ACID REDUCING AGENTS (e.g., ANTACIDS, **famotidine, omeprazole**) may decrease the levels of velpatasvir. Coadministration of **amiodarone** may result in serious symptomatic bradycardia. Sofosbuvir and/or velpatasvir may increase the levels of **digoxin, topotecan,** HMG-COA REDUCTASE INHIBITORS, and **tenofovir disoproxil fumarate. Efavirenz, ritonavir,** and **tipranavir** can decrease the levels of of sofosbuvir and/or velpatasvir. **Herbal: St. John's wort** may decrease the levels of sofosbuvir and/or velpatasvir.

PHARMACOKINETICS **Peak:** Sofosbuvir, 0.5–1 h; velpatasvir, 3 h. **Distribution:** Sofosbuvir, 61–65% plasma protein bound; velpatsavir, greater than 99.5% plasma protein bound. **Metabolism:** Hydrolytic and oxidative metabolism. **Elimination:** Sofosbuvir, renal (80%) and fecal (14%); velpatasvir, primarily fecal (95%). **Half-Life:** Sofosbuvir, 0.5 h; GS-r61203, 25 h; velpatasvir, 15 h.

NURSING IMPLICATIONS

Black Box Warning

Risk of Hepatitis B Virus Reactivation in Patients coinfected with HCV and HBV. Test all patients for evidence of current or prior hepatitis B virus (HBV) infection before initializing treatment. HBV reactivation has been reported in HCV/HBV coinfected patients who were undergoing or had completed treatment with HCV direct acting antivirals and were not receiving HBV therapy. Some cases have resulted in fulminant hepatitis, hepatic failure, and death.

Assessment & Drug Effects

- Monitor vital signs, as bradycardia and arrhythmias have been reported.
- Hepatitis C virus genotype checked prior to initiation of therapy.
- Monitor cognition: Irritability, insomnia, and depression have been reported.
- Monitor lab tests: LFTs, plasma hepatitis, pregnancy testing, serum creatinine/BUN.

Patient & Family Education

- Seek medical attention immediately if fainting or near fainting, fatigue, dizziness, shortness of breath, chest pain, and confusion or memory problems.
- Teach patient or caregiver how to take a pulse and contact healthcare provider if pulse falls below 60 bpm.
- Take antacid separately and allow 4 hours between antacid and drug administration.

S

- Make sure to keep a list of all medications that the patient is taking and share that information with all prescribers.
- Do not take any other over-the-counter medications, herbals, vitamins, or other prescription drugs without first checking with your health care provider.

SOLRIAMFETOL

(sol-ri-am-fe-tol)

Sunosi

Classifications: ANALEPTIC; DOPAMINE AND NOREPINEPHRINE REUPTAKE INHIBITOR (DNRI)

Therapeutic: ANTINARCOLEPTIC

Controlled Substance: Schedule IV

AVAILABILITY Oral tablet

ACTION & *THERAPEUTIC EFFECT*

Acts as a doapmine and norepinephrine reuptake inhibitor, although specific activity is unknown. *Solriamfetol causes wakefulness.*

USES Improve wakefulness in patients with narcolepsy or excessive sleepiness associated with obstructive sleep apnea.

CONTRAINDICATIONS Pregnancy—fetal risk cannot be ruled out; lactation—infant risk cannot be ruled out.

CAUTIOUS USE Patients with risk factors for major adverse cardiovascular events and those with moderate to severe renal impairment, history of psychosis or bipolar disorders, patient with ESRD and estimated glomerular filtration rate less than 15 mL/minute/1.73 m(2). Elderly; Safety and efficacy not established in children.

ROUTE & DOSAGE

Narcolepsy

Adult: **PO** 75 mg once daily

Obstructive Sleep Apnea

Adult: **PO** 37.5 mg once daily

Renal Impairment Dosage Adjustment

eGFR 30–59 mL/min: maximum dose 75 mg a day
eGFR 15–29 mL/min: maximum dose 37.5 mg a day
eGFR <15 mL/min: Avoid use

ADMINISTRATION

Oral

- Take upon awakening with or without food. Avoid taking within 9 hours of planned bedtime due to potential for interfering with sleep if taken too late in the day.
- Store at a controlled room temperature between 20 and 25 degrees C (68 and 77 degrees F), with excursions permitted between 15 and 30 degrees C (59 to 86 F).

ADVERSE EFFECTS **CNS:** *Headache, insomnia.* **GI:** *Decrease in appetite, nausea and vomiting.* **Other:** Psychiatric symptoms.

INTERACTIONS **Drug:** MAO INHIBITORS (e.g., **selegiline**) can precipitate hypertensive crisis (fatalities reported), do not administer solriamfetol during or within 14 days of these drugs; SYMPATHOMIMETIC medications utilized with solriametol increase risk of hypertensive crisis (e.g., **methylphenidate**, **amphetamine**, and nasal or oral decongestants). DOPAMINE AGONISTS (e.g., pramipexole, ropinirole) may have increase toxic effects; Solriamfetol may precipitate effects of medications which increase blood pressure of heart rate

PHARMACOKINETICS **Absorption:** 95% bioavailability. **Peak:** 2 h. **Distribution:** 199 L, 13.3–19.4% protein bound. **Elimination:** 95% excreted unchained in urine. **Half-Life:** 7.1 h

NURSING IMPLICATIONS

Assessment & Drug Effects

- Monitor for improved wakefulness and reduction in daytime sleepiness.
- Monitor pulse and blood pressure prior to initiating therapy and periodically throughout treatment, especially in patient with known cardiovascular and cerebrovascular disease, preexisting hypertension, and advanced age.
- Monitor for the development of psychiatric symptoms during treatment.
- Monitor elderly patients closely, particularly those with likelihood of decreased renal function
- Monitor for signs of misuse or abuse.
- Monitor lab tests: Renal function tests.

Patient & Family Education

- Teach patient and/or caregiver how to take blood pressure and have them report any elevations of blood pressure or pulse.
- Review side effects.
- Report psychiatric symptoms, symptoms of psychosis or bipolar disorder.

SOLIFENACIN SUCCINATE

(sol-i-fen′a-sin)

VESIcare

Classification: ANTICHOLINERGIC; ANTIMUSCARINIC; ANTISPASMODIC

Therapeutic: URINARY ANTISPASMODIC

Prototype: Oxybutynin

AVAILABILITY Tablet

ACTION & *THERAPEUTIC EFFECT* A selective muscarinic antagonist that depresses both voluntary and involuntary bladder contractions caused by detrusor overactivity. *Solifenacin improves the volume of urine/void and reduces the frequency of incontinent and urgency episodes.*

USES Treatment of overactive bladder (OAB); neurogenic detrusor overactivity.

CONTRAINDICATIONS Hypersensitivity to solifenacin; severe hepatic impairment (Child-Pugh class C); gastric retention; uncontrolled narrow-angle glaucoma; urinary retention; toxic megacolon; GI obstruction; ileus; pregnancy—fetal risk cannot be ruled out; lactation—infant risk cannot be ruled out.

CAUTIOUS USE Bladder outflow obstruction; concurrent use of ketoconazole or other potent CYP3A4 inhibitors; obstructive disorders; decreased GI motility; history of QT prolongation; controlled narrow-angle glaucoma; renal impairment; renal disease; mild to moderate hepatic impairment; older adults; myasthenia gravis. Safety and efficacy in children under the age of 2 y not established.

ROUTE & DOSAGE

Overactive Bladder

Adult: **PO** 5 mg once daily; may be increased to 10 mg once daily if tolerated (max: 5 mg/day if taking drugs that inhibit CYP3A4—see INTERACTIONS, Drug)

Hepatic Impairment Dosage Adjustment

Child-Pugh class B: Do not exceed 5 mg/day. *Child-Pugh class C:* Do not use

Renal Impairment Dosage Adjustment

CrCl less than 30 mL/min: Max dose 5 mg/day

ADMINISTRATION

Oral

- Tablets should be swallowed whole and followed by liquid (water). Without regard to food.
- Suspension: Any missed dose should be taken as soon as remembered, unless more than 12 hours have passed. If more than 12 hours have passed, the dose should be skipped and the next dose taken at the usual time.
- Store suspension at a controlled room temperature between 20 and 25 degrees C (68 and 77 degrees F), with excursions permitted between 15°–30° C (59°–86° F). Store in original bottle to protect from degradation. discard any unused product 28 days after opening the original bottle. Tablets should be stored at 25 degrees C (77 degrees C), with excursions permitted between 15°–30° C (59°–86° F).

S

ADVERSE EFFECTS (≥5%) **GI:** *Dry mouth, constipation.*

INTERACTIONS **Drug:** There are extensive drug interactions, consult a drug interaction database for complete listing, some interactions of significance are listed here. CYP3A4 inhibitors (e.g., **clarithromycin, delavirdine, diltiazem, efavirenz, erythromycin, fluconazole, fluvoxamine, itraconazole, nefazodone, norfloxacin, omeprazole,** PROTEASE INHIBITORS, **quinine, verapamil, voriconazole, zafirlukast**) may increase levels and toxicity (max: 5 mg/day); **amantadine, amoxapine, bupropion, clozapine, cyclobenzaprine, diphenhydramine, disopyramide, maprotiline, olanzapine, orphenadrine,** PHENOTHIAZINES, TRICYCLIC ANTIDEPRESSANTS have additive anticholinergic adverse effects. Do not use with agents that increase QT interval (e.g., **dofetilide, dronedarone, posaconazole, ziprasidone**). May increase ulcerogenic risk with **potassium. Food: Grapefruit juice** may increase solifenacin levels and toxicity.

PHARMACOKINETICS **Absorption:** 90% absorbed from GI tract.; 98% protein bound **Peak:** 3–8 h. **Metabolism:** Extensively metabolized in the liver by CYP3A4. **Elimination:** Primarily in urine, 22% in feces. **Half-Life:** 45–68 h.

NURSING IMPLICATIONS

Assessment & Drug Effects

- Monitor bladder function and report promptly urinary retention.
- Review adverse effects with patient and/or caregiver.
- Monitor ECG in patients with a known history of QT prolongation or patients taking medications that prolong the QT interval.

Patient & Family Education

- Stop taking this drug and report to prescriber if urinary retention occurs.
- Remind patient to take with water or milk, other liquids may cause a bitter taste.
- Report severe abdominal pain or constipation for more than 3 days.

- Avoid activities requiring mental alertness or coordination until drug effects are realized.
- Report promptly any of the following: Blurred vision or difficulty focusing vision, palpitations, confusion, or severe dizziness.
- Report to prescriber problems with bowel elimination, especially constipation lasting 3 days or longer.
- Exercise caution in hot environments, as the risk of heat prostration and impaired heat regulation increases with this drug.
- Review directions for missed dose with patient and/or caregiver described under administration.

SOMATROPIN

(soe-ma-troe′pin)

Genotropin, Genotropin MiniQuick, Humatrope, Norditropin, NuSpin, Omnitrope, Saizen, Serostim, Zomacton, Zorbtive

Classification: GROWTH HORMONE

Therapeutic: GROWTH HORMONE

AVAILABILITY Solution for injection

ACTION & *THERAPEUTIC EFFECT* Recombinant growth hormone with the natural sequence of 191 amino acids characteristic of endogenous growth hormone (GH), of pituitary origin. *Induces growth responses in children.*

USES Growth failure due to GH deficiency; replacement therapy prior to epiphyseal closure in patients with idiopathic GH deficiency; GH deficiency secondary to intracranial tumors or panhypopituitarism; inadequate GH secretion; short stature in girls with Turner's syndrome; AIDS wasting syndrome; short bowel syndrome; small for gestational age.

UNLABELED USES Growth deficiency in children with rheumatoid arthritis.

CONTRAINDICATIONS Hypersensitivity to somatropin or any ingredient; pediatric patient with closed epiphyses; underlying intracranial lesion or growing cranial tumor; acute critical illness caused by complications following open heart surgery or abdominal surgery, acute respiratory failure; acute diabetic retinopathy; during chemotherapy, radiation therapy, active neoplastic disease; selective cases of Prader-Willi syndrome who are severely obese or have severe respiratory impairment; children with an intracranial tumor; drug-induced acute pancreatitis.

CAUTIOUS USE Diabetes mellitus or family history of the disease, history of glucose intolerance; Prader-Willi syndrome with a diagnosis of growth hormone deficiency (GHD); skeletal abnormalities; Turner syndrome; HIV patients; history of upper airway obstruction, sleep apnea, or unidentified URI; concomitant or prior use of thyroid or androgens in prepubertal male; hypothyroidism; chronic renal failure; obesity; older adults; pregnancy (category B or category C depending on the brand); lactation; children.

ROUTE & DOSAGE

Note: Dosing will vary based on specific brand of product

Growth Hormone Deficiency (GHD)

Adult: **Subcutaneous Humatrope** Not more than 0.006 mg/kg once daily; dose may be increased (max: 0.0125 mg/kg/day); **Genotropin, Omnitrope** 0.04 mg/kg qwk divided into daily doses (max: 0.08 mg/kg/wk); **Norditropin** Initially 0.004 mg/kg/day (max: 0.016 mg/kg)

Child: **Subcutaneous Genotropin** 0.16–0.24 mg/kg/wk divided into 6–7 daily doses; **Humatrope** 0.18–0.3 mg/kg/wk (0.54 international unit/kg/wk) divided into equal doses given on either 3 alternate days or 6 × wk; **Norditropin** 0.024–0.034 mg/kg/day 6–7 × wk; **Omnitrope** 0.16–0.24 mg/kg/week divided into 6–7 injections

Small for Gestational Age

Child: **Subcutaneous Genotropin/Omnitrope** 0.48 mg/kg/week in divided doses; **Humatrope** 0.47 mg/kg divided into daily doses

AIDS Wasting or Cachexia

Adult (weight greater than 55 kg): **Subcutaneous Serostim** 6 mg each night; *weight 45–55 kg:* 5 mg each night; *weight 35–45 kg:* 4 mg each night; *weight less than 35 kg:* 0.1 mg/kg each night

Short Bowel Syndrome

Adult: **Subcutaneous Zorbtive** 0.1 mg/kg once daily for 4 wk (max: 8 mg/day)

ADMINISTRATION

Subcutaneous

- Reconstitute each brand following its manufacturer's instructions (vary from brand to brand).
- Read and carefully follow directions for use supplied with the Nutropin AQ Pen™ cartridge if this is the product being used.
- Rotate injection sites; abdomen and thighs are preferred sites. Do not use buttocks until the child has been walking for a year or more and the muscle is adequately developed.
- Store lyophilized powder at 2°–8° C (36°–46° F). After reconstitution, most preparations are stable for at least 14 days under refrigeration. **Do not freeze.**

ADVERSE EFFECTS **CV:** Chest pain, edema. **CNS:** Pain, headache, malaise, paresthesia, dizziness. **Endocrine:** *Hypercalciuria;* oversaturation of bile with cholesterol, hyperglycemia, ketosis; High circulating GH antibodies with resulting treatment failure, accelerated growth of intracranial tumor, pancreatitis. **GI:** Nausea, flatulence, abdominal pain, vomiting. **Musculoskeletal:** Arthralgia, limb pain, myalgia. **Other:** Pain, swelling at injection site; peripheral edema, myalgia. Fatalities reported in patients with Prader-Willi syndrome and one or more of the following: Severe obesity, history of respiratory impairment or sleep apnea, or unidentified respiratory infection, especially male patients.

INTERACTIONS **Drug:** ANABOLIC STEROIDS, **thyroid hormone,** ANDROGENS, ESTROGENS may accelerate epiphyseal closure; **ACTH,** CORTICOSTEROIDS may inhibit growth response to somatropin.

PHARMACOKINETICS **Metabolism:** In liver. **Elimination:** In urine. **Half-Life:** 15–50 min.

NURSING IMPLICATIONS

Assessment & Drug Effects

- Monitor growth at designated intervals.
- Hypercalciuria, a frequent adverse effect in the first 2–3 mo of therapy, may be symptomless; however, it may be accompanied by renal calculi, with these reportable symptoms: Flank pain and colic, GI symptoms, urinary frequency, chills, fever, and hematuria.
- Observe diabetics or those with family history of diabetes closely. Obtain regular fasting blood glucose and HbA1C.
- Examine patients with GH deficiency secondary to intracranial lesion frequently for progression or recurrence of underlying disease.
- Monitor lab test: Periodic serum and urine calcium and plasma glucose. Test for circulating GH antibodies (antisomatropin antibodies) in patients who respond initially but later fail to respond to therapy, thyroid function tests.

Patient & Family Education

- Be aware that during first 6 mo of successful treatment, linear growth rates may be increased 8–16 cm or more/year (average about 7 cm/y or approximately 3 in.). Additionally, subcutaneous fat diminishes but returns to pretreatment value later.
- Record accurate height measurements at regular intervals and report to prescriber if rate is less than expected.
- In general, growth response to somatropin is inversely proportional to duration of treatment.
- Bone age is typically assessed annually in all patients and especially those also receiving concurrent thyroid or androgen treatment, since these drugs may precipitate early epiphyseal closure. Take child for bone age assessment on appointed annual dates.

SONIDEGIB

(son-i-de′gib)

Odomzo

Classification: ANTINEOPLASTIC; BIOLOGICAL RESPONSE MODIFIER; SIGNAL TRANSDUCTION INHIBITOR; HEDGEHOG PATHWAY INHIBITOR

Therapeutic: ANTINEOPLASTIC

Prototype: Vismodegib

AVAILABILITY Capsules

ACTION & *THERAPEUTIC EFFECT* Hedgehog mutations associated with basal cell cancer can activate cell growth pathways resulting in unrestricted proliferation of skin basal cells. Sonidegib inhibits the Hedgehog pathway by binding to smoothened homologue (SMO), a transmembrane protein involved in Hedgehog signal transduction. Hedgehog regulates cell growth and differentiation in embryogenesis but is generally not active in adult tissue. Hedgehog regulates cell growth and differentiation in embryogenesis, but is generally not active in adult tissue. Hedgehog mutations associated with basal cell cancer can activate the pathway resulting in unrestricted proliferation of skin basal cells. *Inhibits the growth and differential of basal carcinoma cells.*

USES Treatment of adult patients with locally advanced basal cell carcinoma (BCC) that has recurred following surgery or radiation therapy, or those who are not candidates for surgery or radiation therapy.

CONTRAINDICATIONS Active TB infection; recurrent serum CK

S

greater than 5 × ULN; recurrent severe musculoskeletal reactions.

CAUTIOUS USE History of rhabdomyolysis with other drugs which inhibit the Hedgehog pathway; Crohn's disease. Concomitant use of CYP3A4 inhibitors; grapefruit consumption; pregnancy (category B); lactation. Safety and efficacy in children not established.

ROUTE & DOSAGE

Advanced BCC

Adult: **PO** 200 mg once daily

Toxicity Dosage Adjustment

Severe musculoskeletal reactions, first occurrence of serum CK 2.5–10 × ULN, or recurrent serum CK 2.5–5 × ULN: Temporarily discontinue, then resume at 200 mg upon resolution

Serum CK greater than 2.5 × ULN with worsening renal function: Permanently discontinue

Serum CK greater than 10 × ULN: Permanently discontinue

Recurrent serum CK greater than 5 × ULN: Permanently discontinue

Recurrent severe musculoskeletal reactions: Permanently discontinue

S

ADMINISTRATION

Oral

- Give on an empty stomach at least 1 h before or 2 h after a meal.
- Capsules should be swallowed whole.

ADVERSE EFFECTS **CNS:** *Dysgeusia, headache.* **Endocrine:** *Decreased appetite,* hyperglycemia, increased ALT/AST, increased amylase, increased lipase, increased serum creatinine, increased serum creatine kinase (CK), *weight loss.* **Skin:** *Alopecia, pruritus.* **GI:** *Abdominal pain, diarrhea, nausea, vomiting.* **Musculoskeletal:** *Muscle spasm, musculoskeletal pain, myalgia.* **Hematologic:** Anemia, lymphopenia. **Other:** *Fatigue, pain.*

INTERACTIONS **Drug:** Concomitant use with strong CYP3A4 inhibitors (e.g., **itraconazole, ketoconazole, nefazodone, posaconazole, saquinavir, telithromycin, voriconazole**) or moderate CYP3A4 inhibitors (e.g., **atanzavir, diltiazem, fluconazole**) increases the levels of sonidegib. Concomitant use with strong and moderate inhibitors (e.g., **carbamazepine, efavirenz, modafinil, phenobarbital, phenytoin, rifabutin, rifampin**) decreases the levels of sonidegib. **Food: Grapefruit** or **grapefruit juice** may increase the levels of sonidegib. **Herbal: St. John's wort** decreases the levels of sonidegib.

PHARMACOKINETICS **Absorption:** Less than 10% absorbed. **Peak:** 2–4 h. **Distribution:** Greater than 97% plasma protein binding. **Metabolism:** In liver by CYP450 enzymes. **Elimination:** Fecal (70%) and renal (30%). **Half-Life:** 28 days.

NURSING IMPLICATIONS

Black Box Warning

Sonidegib can cause embryo-fetal death or severe birth defects. Pregnancy status must be verified prior to initiating therapy. (See Patient & Family Education.)

Assessment & Drug Effects

- Monitor for and report to prescriber development of musculoskeletal pain, myalgia, dark urine, decreased urine output, or the inability to urinate.
- Monitor lab tests: Baseline pregnancy test; baseline and periodic serum creatine kinase (CK) and creatinine levels.

Patient & Family Education

- Women of childbearing age should discuss potential risks of this drug to fetal development.
- Women should use effective means of contraception while taking this drug and for at least 20 mo after the last dose.
- Women taking this drug or partners of males taking this drug should immediately report to prescriber if a pregnancy is suspected.
- Do not breast-feed while taking this drug.
- Males should use condoms (even after a vasectomy) during treatment and for at least 8 mo after the last dose to prevent exposure of females of childbearing age to this drug.
- Males should not donate semen during treatment and for at least 8 mo after the last dose.
- Report promptly any new unexplained muscle pain, tenderness or weakness occurring during treatment or that persists after discontinuing this drug.
- Report promptly dark urine, decreased urine output, or the inability to urinate.
- Avoid grapefruit products while taking this drug.

SORAFENIB

(sor-a-fe′nib)

Nexavar

Classification: ANTINEOPLASTIC; KINASE INHIBITOR; KINASE INHIBITOR

Therapeutic: ANTINEOPLASTIC

Prototype: Erlotinib

AVAILABILITY Tablet

ACTION & *THERAPEUTIC EFFECT* A multi-kinase inhibitor targeting enzyme systems in both tumor cells and tumor vasculature. It appears to be cytostatic, requiring continued drug exposure for tumor growth inhibition. *Sorafenib inhibits enzymes responsible for uncontrolled tumor cellular proliferation and angiogenesis.*

USES Treatment of advanced renal cell cancer; hepatocellular cancer; differentiated thyroid carcinoma.

UNLABELED USES Gastrointestinal stromal tumor.

CONTRAINDICATIONS Active infection; severe hypersensitivity to sorafenib or any other component of the product. severe renal impairment (less than 30 mL/min), or hemodialysis; concurrent use of gemcitabine and cisplatin in patients with squamous cell lung cancer; pregnancy – fetal risk cannot be ruled out. lactation – infant risk cannot be ruled out.

CAUTIOUS USE Previous myelosuppressive therapy, either radiation or chemotherapy; mild or moderate renal disease; hepatic disease; heart failure, ventricular dysfunction, cardiac disease, peripheral edema; females of childbearing age. Safe use in children younger than 18 y not established.

S

ROUTE & DOSAGE

Renal Cell Cancer/Hepatocellular Cancer/Differentiated Thyroid Carcinoma

Adult: **PO** 400 mg bid

Renal Impairment Dosage Adjustment

CrCl 20–39 mL/min: 200 mg bid; CrCl less than 20 mL/min dose not defined

Dosage Adjustments Toxicity

Varies by indication and specific level of toxicity; see package insert

ADMINISTRATION

Oral

- NIOSH: Use of single gloves by anyone handling intact tablets or capsules or administering from a unit-dose package is recommended. In preparation of tablets or capsules, including cutting, crushing or manipulating, or the handling of uncoated tablets, use double gloves and a protective gown. During administration, wear gloves, and wear single gloves and eye/face protection if the formulation is hard to swallow or if the patient may resist, vomit, or spit up.
- Tablets **must be** swallowed whole. They should not be crushed, broken, or chewed.
- Give on an empty stomach 1 h before or 2 h after eating.
- Store at 25 degrees C (77 degrees F), excursions permitted between 15°–30° C (59°–86° F). Protect from moisture.

ADVERSE EFFECTS (≥5%) **CV:** *Hypertension*. **Endocrine:** *Amylase elevation, hypoalbuminemia, hypocalcemia, elevated TSH, hypophosphatemia, lipase elevation, weight loss.* **Skin:** Acne, *alopecia, desquamation, dry skin,* erythema, exfoliative dermatitis, flushing, *hand-foot skin reaction, rash.* **Hepatic:** ALT/SGPT elevation, elevated aminotransferase serum level. **GI:** *Abdominal pain, anorexia, diarrhea, nausea,* *gastrointestinal hemorrhage*. **Hematologic:** *Hemorrhage, Lymphocytopenia,* thrombocytopenia. *fatigue* pain.

INTERACTIONS **Drug:** There are extensive drug interactions, consult a drug interaction database for complete listing, some interactions of significance are listed here. Sorafenib may increase levels of drugs requiring glucuronidation by the UGT1A1 and UGT1A9 pathways (e.g., **irinotecan**). Due to thrombocytopenic effects, sorafenib can contribute to increased bleeding from NONSTEROIDAL ANTI-INFLAMMATORY DRUGS, PLATELET INHIBITORS (e.g., **aspirin, clopidogrel**), THROMBOLYTIC AGENTS, and **warfarin.** Inducers of CYP3A4 (e.g., **carbamazepine, phenobarbital, phenytoin, rifampin**) may decrease the levels of sorafenib. Do not use with LIVE VACCINES. May increase adverse effects with MYELOSUPRESSIVE AGENTS **Food:** Food, especially high fat food, decreases the absorption of sorafenib. **Herbal: St. John's wort** may decrease the levels of sorafenib.

PHARMACOKINETICS **Absorption:** 38–49% absorbed. **Peak:** 3 h. **Distribution:** 99.5% protein bound. **Metabolism:** In the liver (CYP3A4 and UGT1A9). **Elimination:** Primarily fecal (77%) with minor elimination in the urine (19%). **Half-Life:** 25–48 h.

NURSING IMPLICATIONS

Assessment & Drug Effects

- Monitor for and report S&S of skin toxicity (e.g., rash, erythema, dermatitis, paresthesia, swelling, or pain in hands or feet). Severe reactions may require temporary suspension of therapy or dose reduction.
- Monitor for S&S of bleeding, especially in those on anticoagulation therapy.
- Monitor BP weekly for the first 6 wk of therapy and periodically thereafter. New-onset hypertension has been associated with sorafenib.
- Monitor blood levels of warfarin with concurrent therapy.
- ECG for QT interval prolongation in patients with CHF, bradyarrhythmia, or concurrent drug therapy known to prolong the QT interval.
- Monitor lab tests: Periodic CBC with differential and platelet count, serum electrolytes, TSH, LFTs, lipase, amylase, and alkaline phosphatase.

Patient & Family Education

- Report any of the following to a health care provider: Skin rash; redness, blisters, pain, or swelling of the palms or hands or soles of feet; signs of bleeding; unexplained chest, shoulder, neck and jaw, or back pain.
- Review adverse effects with patient and/or caregiver.
- Review administration guidelines discussed under administration.
- Do not take any prescription or nonprescription drugs without consulting the prescriber.
- Notify prescriber prior to any major surgical procedure as the drug may need to be temporarily discontinued.
- Female patients should use effective birth control during treatment and for at least 6 months following completion of treatment. Male patient with a female partner of reproductive potential to use effective contraception during therapy and for 3 months after the last dose.

SOTALOL

(so-ta'lol)

Betapace, Betapace AF, Sorine, Sotylize

Classification: BETA-ADRENERGIC ANTAGONIST; CLASS II AND III ANTIARRHYTHMIC

Therapeutic: CLASS II AND III ANTIARRHYTHMIC

Prototype: Amiodarone

AVAILABILITY Tablet; solution for injection

ACTION & *THERAPEUTIC EFFECT* Has both class II and class III antiar-rhythmic properties. Slows heart rate, decreases AV nodal conduction, and increases AV nodal refractoriness. Produces significant reduction in both systolic and diastolic blood pressure. *Antiarrhythmic properties are effective in controlling ventricular arrhythmias as well as atrial fibrillation/flutter.*

USES Treatment of life-threatening ventricular arrhythmias (sustained ventricular tachycardia) and maintenance of normal sinus rhythm in patients with atrial fibrillation/flutter.

CONTRAINDICATIONS Hypersensitivity to sotalol; bronchial asthma, acute bronchospasm; sinus bradycardia, second- and third-degree AV block without a functioning pacemaker, uncontrolled HF; cardiogenic shock; emphysema; major disease; congenital or acquired long QT prolongation; hypokalemia less than 4 mEq/L creatinine clearance of less than 40 mL/min; lactation.

CAUTIOUS USE CHF, electrolyte disturbances, within 14 days of MI, DM; sick sinus rhythm, PVD; untreated pheochromocytoma; MG; thyroid disease; history of psychiatric disease; hyperthroidism; renal impairment; excessive diarrhea, or profuse sweating; older adults; pregnancy (category B).

ROUTE & DOSAGE

Ventricular Arrhythmias (Betapace, Sorine, Sotylize)

Adult: **PO** Initial dose of 80 mg bid or 160 mg daily taken prior to meals, may increase every 3–4 days (most patients respond to 240–320 mg/day in 2 or 3 divided doses, doses greater than 640 mg/day have not been studied)

Renal Impairment Dosage Adjustment

CrCl greater than 60 mL/min: q12h; 30–60 mL/min: q24h; *10–30 mL/min:* q36–48h; *less than 10 mL/min:* Individualize carefully

Atrial Fibrillation/Flutter (Betapace AF, Sotylize)

Adult: **PO** Initial dose of 80 mg bid, may increase every 3–4 days (max: 240 mg/day in 1–2 divided doses); **IV** 75 mg bid may increase after 3 days depending on patient response

Renal Impairment Dosage Adjustment

CrCl 40–60 mL/min: Dose q24h; less than 40 mL/min contraindicated

ADMINISTRATION

Oral

- Sotalol and sotalol AF are **not** interchangeable because of significant differences in labeling (i.e., patient package insert, dosing administration, safety information).
- Give without regard to meals.
- Drug should be initiated and doses increased only under close supervision, preferably in a hospital with cardiac rhythm monitoring and frequent assessment.
- Use smallest effective dose for patients with nonallergic bronchospasms.
- Do not discontinue drug abruptly. Gradually reduce dose over 1–2 wk.
- Store at room temperature, 15°–30° C (59°–86° F).

Intravenous

PREPARE: **IV Infusion: Sotalol** infusion must be prepared to compensate for dead space in the infusion set. The directions that follow will yield 120 mL of prepared volume, but only 100 mL will be infused when using a volumetric infusion pump. Possible diluents include NS, D5W, and LR. For a target dose of 75 mg, use 6 mL sotalol injection and 114 mL diluent; for a target dose of 112.5 mg, use 9 mL sotalol injection and 111 mL diluent; for a target dose of 150 mg, use 12 mL sotalol injection and 108 mL diluent.
ADMINISTER: **IV Infusion:** Give at a constant rate over 5 h.

INCOMPATIBILITIES: Do not infuse with any other drugs or solutions.

ADVERSE EFFECTS **CV:** AV block, hypotension, aggravation of CHF, although the incidence of heart failure may be lower than for other beta-blockers, life-threatening ventricular arrhythmias, including polymorphous ventricular tachycardia or torsades de pointes, *bradycardia, dyspnea, chest pain, palpitation,* bleeding (less than 2%). **Respiratory:** Respiratory complaints. **CNS:** Headache, *fatigue, dizziness,* weakness, lethargy, depression, lassitude. **HEENT:** Visual disturbances. **Endocrine:** Hyperglycemia. **Skin:** Rash. Hyperglycemia. **GI:** Nausea, vomiting, diarrhea, dyspepsia, dry mouth. **GU:** Impotence, decreased libido.

INTERACTIONS **Drug:** Antagonizes the effects of BETA-AGONISTS. **Amiodarone** may lead to symptomatic bradycardia and sinus arrest. The hypoglycemic effects of ORAL HYPOGLYCEMIC AGENTS may be potentiated. May cause resistance to **epinephrine** in anaphylactic reactions. Should be used with caution with other ANTIARRHYTHMIC AGENTS, withhold Class I (e.g., **disopyramide, procainamide, quinidine**) or Class III ANTIARRHYTHMICS (e.g., **amiodarone, dofetilide**) for at least three half-lives prior to initiating sotalol. **Food:** Absorption may be reduced by food, especially **milk** and MILK PRODUCTS.

PHARMACOKINETICS **Absorption:** Slowly and completely from GI tract. Negligible first-pass metabolism. Reduced by food, especially milk and milk products. **Peak:** 2–3 h. **Duration:** 24 h. **Distribution:** Drug is hydrophilic and will enter the CSF slowly (about 10%). Crosses placental barrier. Distributed in breast milk. Not appreciably protein bound. **Metabolism:** Does not undergo significant hepatic enzyme metabolism and no active metabolites have been identified. **Elimination:** In urine with 75% of the drug excreted unchanged within 72 h. **Half-Life:** 7–18 h.

NURSING IMPLICATIONS

Black Box Warning

Sotalol initiation, reinitiation, and dosage adjustment have been associated with serious, life-threatening arrhythmias; thus patients should be in a facility that can provide continuous ECG monitoring, calculation of creatinine clearance, and cardiac resuscitation.

Assessment & Drug Effects

- Monitor ECG at baseline and periodically thereafter (especially when doses are increased) because proarrhythmic events most often occur within 7 days of initiating therapy or increasing dose.
- Monitor cardiac status throughout therapy. Exercise special caution when sotalol is used concurrently with other antiarrhythmics, digoxin, or calcium channel blockers.
- Monitor patients with bronchospastic disease (e.g., bronchitis, emphysema) carefully for inhibition of bronchodilation.
- Monitor diabetics for loss of glycemic control. Beta blockage reduces the release of endogenous insulin in response to hyperglycemia and may blunt symptoms of acute hypoglycemia (e.g., tachycardia, BP changes).
- Monitor lab test: Baseline and periodic creatinine clearance, and serum electrolytes. Correct

S

electrolyte imbalances of hypokalemia or hypomagnesemia prior to initiating therapy.

Patient & Family Education

- Be aware of risk for hypotension and syncope, especially with concurrent treatment with catecholamine-depleting drugs (e.g., guanethidine).
- Take radial pulse daily and report marked bradycardia (pulse below 60 or other established parameter) hold the dose and notify the prescriber.
- Type 2 diabetics are at increased risk for hyperglycemia. All diabetics are at risk of possible masking of symptoms of hypoglycemia.
- Do not abruptly discontinue drug because of the risk of exacerbation of angina, arrhythmias, and possible myocardial infarction.

SPINOSAD

(spin'oh-sad)

Natroba

Classification: SCABICIDE; PEDICULICIDE

Therapeutic: SCABICIDE; PEDICULICIDE

Prototype: Permethrin

AVAILABILITY Topical suspension

S

ACTION & *THERAPEUTIC EFFECT* Kills lice directly without measurable absorption into the human body. *Eliminates lice infestation in humans.*

USES Topical treatment of head lice infestations caused by *Pediculus capitis* in patients 4 y or older.

CONTRAINDICATIONS Contains benzyl alcohol and is not recommended for use in neonates and infants below the age of 6 months.

CAUTIOUS USE Inflammatory skin conditions (e.g., psoriasis, eczema); pregnancy (category B); lactation; children 4 y or older.

ROUTE & DOSAGE

Head Lice Infestation

Adult/Child (4 y or older): **Topical** May apply up to 120 mL to cover scalp/hair; may repeat in 7 d if necessary.

ADMINISTRATION

Topical

- Shake well immediately prior to use.
- Apply sufficient amount (up to one bottle) to cover dry scalp, then apply to dry hair; leave on 10 min, then rinse hair and scalp thoroughly with warm water.
- Store at 15°–30° C (59°–86° F).

ADVERSE EFFECTS **HEENT:** Ocular erythema. **Other:** Application-site erythema and irritation.

NURSING IMPLICATIONS

Assessment & Drug Effects

- Assess hair and scalp for presence of lice. If still present after 7 days of treatment, a second treatment should be applied.

Patient & Family Education

- Avoid contact with eyes. If spinosad gets in or near the eyes, rinse thoroughly with water.
- Wash hands after applying spinosad.
- Use on children only under direct supervision of an adult.

SPIRONOLACTONE

(speer-on-oh-lak'tone)

Aldactone, CaroSpir
Classification: POTASSIUM-SPARING DIURETIC
Therapeutic: POTASSIUM-SPARING DIURETIC; ANTIHYPERTENSIVE

AVAILABILITY Tablet; suspension

ACTION & THERAPEUTIC EFFECT Competes with aldosterone for cellular receptor sites in distal renal tubules. Promotes sodium and chloride excretion without loss of potassium. *A diuretic agent that promotes sodium and chloride excretion without concomitant loss of potassium. Lowers systolic and diastolic pressures in hypertensive patients. Effective in treatment of primary aldosteronism.*

USES Management of edema, heart failure, hypertension unresponsive to other therapies, primary hyperaldosteronism (tablet only).

UNLABELED USES Hirsutism in women with polycystic ovary syndrome or idiopathic hirsutism; hormone therapy for transgender females (male-to-female).

CONTRAINDICATIONS Anuria, acute renal insufficiency; renal failure; diabetic nephropathy; progressive impairment of kidney function, or worsening of liver disease; hyperkalemia; lactic acidosis; Addison disease; Concomitant eplerenone; pregnancy (fetal risk cannot be ruled out).

CAUTIOUS USE BUN of 40 mg/dL or greater, mild renal impairment; fluid and electrolyte imbalance; liver disease; severe heart failure; natremia; older adults; lactation (infant risk is minimal); children.

ROUTE & DOSAGE

Edema

Note: Tablet and suspension are not interchangeable

Adult: **PO Tablet** 100 mg daily in single or divided dose; titrate as needed (range 25–200 mg/day) **Suspension** 75 mg daily in single or divided dose

Hypertension

Adult: **PO Tablet** 25–50 mg/day in single or divided doses, may titrate at 2 wk intervals; **Suspension** 20–100 mg daily may titrate at 2 wk intervals

Primary Aldosteronism

Adult: **PO Tablet** 100–400 mg/day

Severe Heart Failure

Adult: **PO Tablet** 12.5–25 mg qd; may increase dose to 50 mg qd if needed

Renal Impairment Dosage Adjustment

eGFR 30–50 mL/min/1.73 m²: 25 mg/day (tablet); 10 mg/day (suspension)

ADMINISTRATION

Oral

- NIOSH recommends using single gloves when handling intact tablets or capsules or administering from unit package. If cutting or crushing or handling uncoated tablets, use double gloves and a protective gown. During administration, wear single gloves, and wear eye/face protection if the formulation is hard to swallow or if the patient may resist, vomit, or spit up.

S

- Give with food to enhance absorption. Avoid taking with potassium supplements and foods that are high in potassium (e.g., salt substitutes).
- Crush tablets and give with fluid of patient's choice if unable to swallow whole.
- Store in tight, light-resistant containers. Store suspension at 20°–25° C (68°–77° F). Store tablets below 25° C (77° F).

ADVERSE EFFECTS **CV:** Vasculitis. **CNS:** Ataxia, confusion, dizziness, drowsiness, headache, lethargy, nipple pain. **Endocrine:** Amenorrhea, decreased libido, electrolyte disturbance, hyperkalemia, hyponatremia, hypovolemia. **Skin:** Alopecia, chloasma, rash, Stevens–Johnson syndrome, toxic epidermal necrolysis, urticaria. **Hepatic:** Hepatotoxicity. **GI:** Abdominal cramps, diarrhea, gastritis, gastrointestinal hemorrhage, gastrointestinal ulcer, nausea, vomiting. **GU:** Erectile dysfunction, impotence, irregular menses, mastalgia, postmenopausal bleeding, Increased BUN, renal failure, renal insufficiency. **Musculoskeletal:** Leg cramps. **Hematologic:** Agranulocytosis, leukopenia, breast malignancy, thrombocytopenia. **Other:** Fever.

S

DIAGNOSTIC TEST INTERFERENCE May produce marked increases in ***plasma cortisol*** determinations by ***Mattingly fluorometric*** method; these may persist for several days after termination of drug (spironolactone metabolite produces fluorescence). There is the possibility of false elevations in measurements of ***digoxin serum levels*** by ***RIA*** procedures; may lead to false negative aldosterone/renin ratio.

INTERACTIONS **Drug:** Diuretic effect of spironolactone may be antagonized by **aspirin** and other SALICYLATES. **Digoxin** should be monitored for decreased effect of CARDIAC GLYCOSIDES. Hyperkalemia may result with **amiloride, cyclosporine, tacrolimus,** POTASSIUM SUPPLEMENTS, ACE INHIBITORS, ARBS, **heparin;** may decrease **lithium** clearance resulting in increased tenacity; may alter anticoagulant response in **warfarin.** Do not use with **eplerenone, darifenacin,** or **tranylcypromine.** **Food:** Salt substitutes may increase risk of hyperkalemia.

PHARMACOKINETICS **Absorption:** ~73% from GI tract. **Onset:** Gradual. **Peak:** 2–3 days; maximum effect may take up to 2 wk. **Duration:** 2–3 days or longer. **Distribution:** Crosses placenta, distributed into breast milk. **Metabolism:** In liver and kidneys to active metabolites; potent inhibitor of P-gp. **Elimination:** 40–57% in urine, 35–40% in bile. **Half-Life:** 1.4 hours (tablet) 1–2 hours (suspension).

NURSING IMPLICATIONS

Black Box Warning

Spironolactone has been associated with tumor development in laboratory animals. Unnecessary use of this drug should be avoided.

Assessment & Drug Effects

- Check blood pressure before initiation of therapy and at regular intervals throughout therapy.
- Assess for signs of fluid and electrolyte imbalance, and signs of digoxin toxicity.
- Monitor daily I&O and check for edema. Report lack of diuretic response or development of

edema; both may indicate tolerance to drug.

- Weigh patient under standard conditions before therapy begins and daily throughout therapy. Weight is a useful index of need for dosage adjustment. For patients with ascites, prescriber may want measurements of abdominal girth.
- Observe for and report immediately the onset of mental changes, lethargy, or stupor in patients with liver disease.
- Adverse reactions are generally reversible with discontinuation of drug. Gynecomastia appears to be related to dosage level and duration of therapy; it may persist in some after drug is stopped.
- Monitor lab tests: Periodic serum electrolytes especially during early therapy, blood glucose, BUN/creatinine, uric acid.

Patient & Family Education

- Be aware that the maximal diuretic effect may not occur until third day of therapy and that diuresis may continue for 2–3 days after drug is withdrawn.
- Report signs of hyponatremia or hyperkalemia (see Appendix F), most likely to occur in patients with severe cirrhosis.
- Avoid replacing fluid losses with large amounts of free water (can result in dilutional hyponatremia).
- Weigh 2–3 × each wk. Report gains/loss of 5 lb or more.
- Do not drive or engage in potentially hazardous activities until response to the drug is known.
- Avoid excessive intake of high potassium foods and salt substitutes.

STAVUDINE (D4T)

(sta′vu-deen)

Classification: ANTIRETROVIRAL; NUCLEOSIDE REVERSE TRANSCRIPTASE INHIBITOR (NRTI)
Therapeutic: ANTIRETROVIRAL; NRTI
Prototype: Lamivudine

AVAILABILITY Capsule

ACTION & *THERAPEUTIC EFFECT*

Appears to act by being incorporated into growing DNA chains by viral transcriptase, thus terminating viral replication. *Inhibits the replication of HIV in human cells and decreases viral load.*

USES HIV treatment. (not recommended in current treatment guidelines)

CONTRAINDICATIONS Hypersensitivity to stavudine; patient concurrently taking zidovudine or didanosine; lactic acidosis; pregnancy—fetal risk cannot be ruled out; lactation—infant risk cannot be ruled out.

CAUTIOUS USE Previous hypersensitivity to zidovudine, didanosine, or zalcitabine; folic acid or B_{12} deficiency; liver and renal insufficiency; alcoholism; peripheral neuropathy; history of pancreatitis or hepatitis C.

ROUTE & DOSAGE

HIV Infection

Adult/Adolescent (weight less than 60 kg): **PO** 30 mg q12h; *weight 60 kg or greater:* 40 mg q12h

S

Renal Impairment Dosage Adjustment

CrCl 25–50 mL/min: Reduce dose by 50%; *less than 25 mL/min:* Reduce dose by 50% and extend interval to q24h

ADMINISTRATION

Oral

- Adhere strictly to 12-h interval between doses.
- Take with or without food.
- Capsules may be stored at a controlled room temperature of 25° C (77° F), excursions permitted between 15 and 30 degrees C (59 to 86 degrees F). Protect powder from excessive moisture.

ADVERSE EFFECTS (≥5%) **CNS:** *Peripheral neuropathy, headache.* **Skin:** *Rash.* **Hepatic:** Abnormal liver function tests. **GI:** *Nausea, vomiting, diarrhea, increased pancreatic enzyme levels.* **Hematologic:** Macrocytosis.

INTERACTIONS **Drug:** **Didanosine, hydroxyurea** may increase risk of pancreatitis and hepatotoxicity; **zidovudine** may impact metabolism, avoid concurrent use. Use INTERFERONS, **ribavirin** cautiously. **Herbal:** Avoid use with echinacea.

PHARMACOKINETICS **Absorption:** Readily absorbed from GI tract; 82% reaches systemic circulation. **Peak:** 1 hour. **Distribution:** Distributes into CSF; excreted in breast milk of animals. **Metabolism:** intracellularly to active form. **Elimination:** In urine. **Half-Life:** 1–1.6 h.

NURSING IMPLICATIONS

Black Box Warning

Stavudine has been associated with lactic acidosis and severe, sometimes fatal, hepatomegaly with steatosis. Fatal lactic acidosis has been reported in pregnant females who received the combination of stavudine an didanosine with other antiretroviral agents. Fatal and nonfatal pancreatitis has occurred with patients when taking stavudine with didanosine.

Assessment & Drug Effects

- Monitor for peripheral neuropathy and report numbness, tingling, or pain, which may indicate a need to interrupt stavudine.
- Monitor for development of opportunistic infection.
- Monitor lab tests: Periodic measurement of acid–base balance, electrolytes, LFTs, renal function tests, urinalysis. CBC with differential and serum lipid profile at baseline and with modifications, fasting blood glucose and HbA1C at baseline and with modifications, viral loads, CD4 counts, at baseline and with modification of antiretroviral treatment.

Patient & Family Education

- Take drug exactly as prescribed.
- Educate patient on safe sex practice.
- Report to provider if pregnancy occurs.
- Report to prescriber any adverse drug effects that are bothersome.
- Report symptoms of peripheral neuropathy to prescriber immediately.
- The medication has several drug-drug interactions. Consult

S

healthcare provider before taking any new medications (including over-the-counter and herbal supplements).

STREPTOMYCIN SULFATE

(strep-toe-mye'sin)

Classification: AMINOGLYCOSIDE ANTIBIOTIC; ANTITUBERCULOSIS
Therapeutic: ANTIBIOTIC; ANTITUBERCULOSIS
Prototype: Gentamicin

AVAILABILITY Reconstituted solution for injection

ACTION & THERAPEUTIC EFFECT Inhibits bacterial protein synthesis through irreversible binding to the 30S ribosomal subunit of susceptible bacteria. *Active against a variety of gram-positive, gram-negative, and acid-fast organisms.*

USES Treatment of tuberculosis;. Used for tularemia, plague, and brucellosis, subacute bacterial endocarditis and in treatment of peritonitis, respiratory tract infections, granuloma inguinale, and chancroid when other drugs have failed.

UNLABELED USE: Mycobacterium avium complex infection.

CONTRAINDICATIONS History of toxic reaction or severe hypersensitivity to streptomycin; clinically significant reaction to other aminoglycosides; labyrinthine disease; concurrent or sequential use of neurotoxic and/or nephrotoxic drugs; myasthenia gravis; pregnancy—fetal risk cannot be ruled out.

CAUTIOUS USE Impaired renal function; prerenal azotemia; auditory dysfunction; older adults; lactation—infant risk is minimal; children.

ROUTE & DOSAGE

Endocarditis

Adult: **IM** 7.5 mg/kg q12h × 4 wk

Tuberculosis

Adult: **IM** 15 mg/kg daily or 25 mg/kg 3 times per week

Tularemia

Adult: **IM** 1 g bid for at least 10 days

Plague

Adult: **IM** 15 mg/kg (max 1 g) q12h × 10 days

Renal Impairment Dosage Adjustment

CrCl 10–50 mL/min: administer q24–72 h; *CrCl less than 10 mL/min:* administer q72–96 h

ADMINISTRATION

Intramuscular

- Give IM deep into large muscle mass to minimize possibility of irritation. Injections are painful. Preferred sites for the adult are upper outer quadrant of the buttock, or the midlateral thigh.
- Avoid direct contact with drug; sensitization can occur. Use gloves during preparation of drug.
- Use commercially prepared IM solution undiluted; intended only for IM injection (contains a preservative, and therefore is not suitable for other routes). Reconstituted solution may be stored for

S

1 week at room temperature and protected from light.

- Store dry powder at controlled room temperature between 20 and 25 degrees C (68 and 77 degrees F). Protect from light; exposure to light may slightly darken solution, with no apparent loss of potency.

ADVERSE EFFECTS

Respiratory: Respiratory depression. **CNS:** Paresthesias (peripheral, facial). **Skin:** Skin rashes, pruritus. **Hematologic:** Increased eosinophil count. *Fever.*

INTERACTIONS

Drug: May potentiate anticoagulant effects of **warfarin;** additive nephrotoxicity with **acyclovir, amphotericin B,** AMINOGLYCOSIDES, **carboplatin, cidofovir, cisplatin, cyclosporine, foscarnet, ganciclovir,** SALICYLATES, **tacrolimus, vancomycin.** Do not use with LIVE VACCINES.

PHARMACOKINETICS

Peak: 1–2 h. **Distribution:** Diffuses into most body tissues and extracellular fluids; crosses placenta; distributed into breast milk; 34% protein bound. **Elimination:** In urine. **Half-Life:** 2–3 h adults, 4–10 h newborns.

S

NURSING IMPLICATIONS

Black Box Warning

Streptomycin has been associated with increased risk of severe neurotoxic reactions, especially in those with impaired renal function.

Assessment & Drug Effects

- Be alert for and report immediately symptoms of ototoxicity (see Appendix F). Symptoms are most likely to occur in patients with impaired kidney function, patients receiving high doses (1.8–2 g/day) or other ototoxic or neurotoxic drugs, and older adults. Irreversible damage may occur if drug is not discontinued promptly.
- Early damage to vestibular portion of eighth cranial nerve (higher incidence than auditory toxicity) is initially manifested by moderately severe headache, nausea, vomiting, vertigo in upright position, difficulty in reading, unsteadiness, and positive Romberg sign.
- Be aware that auditory nerve damage is usually preceded by vestibular symptoms and high-pitched tinnitus, roaring noises, impaired hearing (especially to high-pitched sounds), sense of fullness in ears. Audiometric test should be done if these symptoms appear, and drug should be discontinued. Hearing loss can be permanent if damage is extensive. Tinnitus may persist several days to weeks after drug is stopped.
- Monitor I&O. Report oliguria or changes in I&O ratio (possible signs of diminishing kidney function). Sufficient fluids to maintain urinary output of 1500 mL/24 h are generally advised. Consult prescriber.
- Monitor lab tests: Baseline C&S; periodic BUN and creatinine; serum drug concentration as indicated.

Patient & Family Education

- Report any unusual symptoms. Review adverse reactions with prescriber periodically, especially with prolonged therapy.

- Report if the infection does not improve or worsens while taking the drug.
- Be aware of possibility of ototoxicity and its symptoms (see Appendix F).
- Report to prescriber immediately any of the following: Nausea, vomiting, vertigo, incoordination, tinnitus, fullness in ears, impaired hearing.
- Avoid taking any muscle relaxants while taking this drug.

STREPTOZOCIN

(strep-toe-zoe′sin)

Zanosar

Classification: ANTINEOPLASTIC, ALKYLATING; NITROSOUREA

Therapeutic: ANTINEOPLASTIC

Prototype: Cyclophosphamide

AVAILABILITY Solution for injection

ACTION & *THERAPEUTIC EFFECT* Inhibits DNA synthesis in cells and prevents progression of cells into mitosis, affecting all phases of the cell cycle (cell-cycle nonspecific). *Successful therapy with streptozocin (alone or in combination) produces a biochemical response evidenced by decreased secretion of hormones as well as measurable tumor regression. Thus, serial fasting insulin levels during treatment indicate response to this drug.*

USES Pancreatic cancer.

UNLABELED USES palliative treatment of metastatic carcinoid tumor.

CONTRAINDICATIONS Concurrent use with nephrotoxic drugs; pregnancy—fetal risk cannot be ruled out; lactation—infant risk cannot be ruled out; safety and efficacy in pediatrics are not approved by the FDA.

CAUTIOUS USE Renal impairment; hepatic disease, hepatic impairment; patients with history of hypoglycemia; DM.

ROUTE & DOSAGE

Islet Cell Carcinoma of Pancreas

Adult/Adolescent/Child: **IV** 500 mg/m^2/day on days 1–5 q6w or 1 g/m^2/wk for 2 wk, then increase to 1.5 g/m^2/wk × 4–6 wk

Renal Impairment Dosage Adjustment

CrCl 10–50 mL/min: Give 75% of dose; *CrCl less than 10 mL/min:* Give 50% of dose

ADMINISTRATION

Intravenous

This drug is a cytotoxic agent and caution should be used to prevent any contact with the drug. Follow institutional or standard guidelines for preparation, handling, and disposal of cytotoxic agents.

Use only under constant supervision by prescriber experienced in therapy with cytotoxic agents and only when the benefit to risk ratio is fully and thoroughly understood by patient and family.

PREPARE: **IV Infusion:** Reconstitute with 9.5 mL D5W or NS, to yield 100 mg/mL. Solution will be pale gold. ▪ May be further diluted with up to 250 mL of the original diluent. ▪ Protect reconstituted solution and vials of drug from light.

ADMINISTER: NIOSH recommends the use of gloves when handling the preparation of the powder and solution. Use double gloves and protective gown during administration. Eye/face protection may be needed. If there is a potential that the substance could splash or if the patient may resist, use eye/face protection. Use a closed system drug transfer device. **IV Infusion:** Give over 15–60 min. ▪ Inspect injection site frequently for signs of extravasation (patient complaints of stinging or burning at site, swelling around site, no blood return or questionable blood return). ▪ If extravasation occurs, area requires immediate attention to prevent necrosis. Remove needle, apply ice, and contact prescriber regarding further treatment to infiltrated tissue. Total storage time once the drug is in solution should not exceed 12 hours. Unopened vials should be refrigerated between 2 and 8 degrees C (35 to 46 degrees F) and protected from light.

INCOMPATIBILITIES: **Y-site:** **Acyclovir, allopurinol, amphotericin, aztreonam, cefepime, daptomycin, garenoxacin, levofloxacin, pantoprazole, piperacillin/tazobactam, trastuzumab.**

▪ Note: An antiemetic given routinely every 4 or 6 h and prophylactically 30 min before a treatment may provide sufficient control to maintain the treatment regimen (even if it reduces but does not completely eliminate nausea and vomiting).

▪ Discard reconstituted solutions after 12 h (contains no preservative and not intended for multidose use).

ADVERSE EFFECTS

CNS: *Confusion, lethargy.* **GI:** *Nausea.* **Other:** *Psychological depression.*

INTERACTIONS

Drug: MYELOSUPPRESSIVE AGENTS add to hematologic toxicity; nephrotoxic agents (e.g., AMINOGLYCOSIDES, **vancomycin, amphotericin B, cisplatin**) increase risk of nephrotoxicity; deferiprone may have increased risk of neutropenia. Do not administer LIVE VACCINES.

PHARMACOKINETICS

Absorption: Undetectable in plasma within 3 h. **Distribution:** Metabolite enters CSF. **Metabolism:** In liver and kidneys. **Elimination:** 70–80% of dose in urine. **Half-Life:** 35–40 min.

NURSING IMPLICATIONS

Black Box Warning

Streptozocin has been associated with severe, sometimes fatal, renal toxicity, and with severe GI, hepatic, and hematologic toxicities.

Assessment & Drug Effects

- Ensure that repeat courses of streptozocin treatment are not given until patient's liver, kidney,

S

 Common adverse effects in *italic;* life-threatening effects underlined; generic names in **bold;** classifications in SMALL CAPS; ♣ Canadian drug name; ⊙ Prototype drug; ⚠ Alert

and hematologic functions are within acceptable limits.

- Be alert to and report promptly early laboratory evidence of kidney dysfunction: Hypophosphatemia, mild proteinuria, and changes in I&O ratio and pattern.
- Mild adverse renal effects may be reversible following discontinuation of streptozocin, but nephrotoxicity may be irreversible, severe, or fatal.
- Be alert to symptoms of sepsis and superinfections or increased tendency to bleed (thrombocytopenia). Myelosuppression is severe in 10–20% of patients and may be cumulative and more severe if patient has had prior exposure to radiation or to other antineoplastics.
- Monitor and record temperature pattern to promptly recognize impending sepsis.
- Monitor lab tests: Weekly CBC; LFTs prior to each course of therapy; serial urinalyses, urine protein and kidney function tests; baseline and weekly serum electrolytes, then for 4 wk after termination of therapy.

Patient & Family Education

- Inspect site at weekly intervals and report changes in tissue appearance if extravasation occurred during IV infusion.
- Report symptoms of hypoglycemia (see Appendix F) even though this drug has minimal, if any, diabetogenic action.
- Drink fluids liberally (2000–3000 mL/day). Hydration may protect against drug toxicity effects.
- Report S&S of nephrotoxicity (see Appendix F).
- Do not take aspirin or NSAIDs without consulting prescriber.
- Avoid vaccines during therapy.
- Report to prescriber promptly any signs of bleeding: Hematuria, epistaxis, ecchymoses, petechiae.
- Report symptoms that suggest anemia: Shortness of breath, pale mucous membranes and nail beds, exhaustion, rapid pulse.
- Avoid alcohol, aspirin or ibuprofen during therapy.

SUCCINYLCHOLINE CHLORIDE

(suk-sin-ill-koe′leen)

Anectine, Quelicin

Classification: DEPOLARIZING SKELETAL MUSCLE RELAXANT

Therapeutic: SKELETAL MUSCLE RELAXANT

AVAILABILITY Solution for injection

ACTION & *THERAPEUTIC EFFECT*

Synthetic, ultra-short-acting depolarizing neuromuscular blocking agent with high affinity for acetylcholine (ACh) receptor sites. *Initial transient contractions and fasciculations are followed by sustained flaccid skeletal muscle paralysis produced by state of accommodation that develops in adjacent excitable muscle membranes.*

S

USES To produce skeletal muscle relaxation as adjunct to anesthesia; to facilitate intubation and endoscopy, to increase pulmonary compliance in assisted or controlled respiration, and to reduce intensity of muscle contractions in pharmacologically induced or electroshock convulsions.

CONTRAINDICATIONS Hypersensitivity to succinylcholine; family history of malignant hyperthermia; burns; trauma.

CAUTIOUS USE Kidney, liver, pulmonary, metabolic, or cardiovascular disorders; myasthenia gravis; dehydration, electrolyte imbalance, patients taking digitalis, severe burns or trauma, fractures, spinal cord injuries, degenerative or dystrophic neuromuscular diseases, low plasma pseudocholinesterase levels (recessive genetic trait, but often associated with severe liver disease, severe anemia, dehydration, marked changes in body temperature, exposure to neurotoxic insecticides, certain drugs); collagen diseases, porphyria, intraocular surgery, glaucoma; during delivery with cesarean section; pregnancy (category C); lactation; children.

ROUTE & DOSAGE

Surgical and Anesthetic Procedures

Adult: **IV** 0.3–1.1 mg/kg administered over 10–30 sec, may give additional doses prn; **IM** 2.5–4 mg/kg up to 150 mg
Child: **IV** 1–2 mg/kg administered over 10–30 sec, may give additional doses prn; **IM** 2.5–4 mg/kg up to 150 mg

Prolonged Muscle Relaxation

Adult: **IV** 0.5–10 mg/min by continuous infusion

Obesity Dosage Adjustment

Dose based on IBW

ADMINISTRATION

Intramuscular

- Give IM injections deeply, preferably high into deltoid muscle.

Intravenous

Use only freshly prepared solutions; succinylcholine hydrolyzes rapidly with consequent loss of potency.
- Give initial small test dose (0.1 mg/kg) to determine individual drug sensitivity and recovery time.

PREPARE: **Direct:** Give undiluted. **Intermittent/Continuous:** Dilute 1 g in 500–1000 mL of D5W or NS.
ADMINISTER: **Direct:** Give a bolus dose over 10–30 sec. **Intermittent/Continuous (Preferred):** Give at a rate of 0.5–10 mg/min. Do not exceed 10 mg/min.
INCOMPATIBILITIES: **Solution/additive:** **Pentobarbital, sodium bicarbonate.** **Y-site:** **Amphotericin B conventional, azathioprine, dantrolene, diazepam, diazoxide, ganciclovir, gemtuzumab, indomethacin, mitomycin, nafcillin, PENICILLINS, pentobarbital, phenobarbital, phenytoin, sodium bicarbonate.**

- Note: Expiration date and storage before and after reconstitution; varies with the manufacturer.

ADVERSE EFFECTS **CV:** *Bradycardia,* tachycardia, hypotension, hypertension, arrhythmias, sinus arrest. **Respiratory:** *Respiratory depression,* bronchospasm, hypoxia, apnea. **CNS:** *Muscle fasciculations,* profound and prolonged muscle relaxation, muscle pain. **Endocrine:** Myoglobinemia, hyperkalemia. **GI:** Decreased tone and motility of GI tract (large doses). **Other:** Malignant hyperthermia, increased IOP, excessive salivation, enlarged salivary glands.

INTERACTIONS **Drug: Aminoglycosides, colistin, cyclophosphamide, cyclopropane, echothiophate iodide, halothane, lidocaine,** MAGNESIUM SALTS, **methotrimeprazine,** NARCOTIC ANALGESICS, ORGANOPHOSPHAMIDE INSECTICIDES, MAO INHIBITORS, PHENOTHIAZINES, **procaine, procainamide, quinidine, quinine, propranolol** may prolong neuromuscular blockade; DIGITALIS GLYCOSIDES may increase risk of cardiac arrhythmias.

PHARMACOKINETICS **Onset:** 0.5–1 min IV; 2–3 min IM. **Duration:** 2–3 min IV; 10–30 min IM. **Distribution:** Crosses placenta in small amounts. **Metabolism:** In plasma by pseudocholinesterases. **Elimination:** In urine.

NURSING IMPLICATIONS

Black Box Warning

Succinylcholine has been associated with rare cases of acute rhabdomyolysis with hyperkalemia followed by ventricular arrhythmias, cardiac arrest, and death in children and adolescents.

Assessment & Drug Effects

- Be aware that transient apnea usually occurs at time of maximal drug effect (1–2 min); spontaneous respiration should return in a few seconds or, at most, 3 or 4 min.
- Have immediately available: Facilities for emergency endotracheal intubation, artificial respiration, and assisted or controlled respiration with oxygen.
- Monitor vital signs and keep airway clear of secretions.

Patient & Family Education

- Patient may experience postprocedural muscle stiffness and pain (caused by initial fasciculations following injection) for as long as 24–30 h.
- Be aware that hoarseness and sore throat are common even when pharyngeal airway has not been used.
- Report residual muscle weakness to prescriber.

SUCRALFATE

(soo-kral'fate)

Carafate, Sulcrate ♣

Classification: ANTIULCER; GASTROADHESIVE

Therapeutic: ANTIULCER; GASTRO-PROTECTANT

AVAILABILITY Tablet; suspension

ACTION & *THERAPEUTIC EFFECT* Sucralfate and gastric acid react to form a viscous, adhesive, paste-like substance that resists further reaction with gastric acid. This "paste" adheres to the GI mucosa with a major portion binding electrostatically to the positively charged protein molecules in the damaged mucosa of an ulcer crater or an acute gastric erosion. *Absorbs bile, inhibits the enzyme pepsin, and blocks back diffusion of H^+ ions. These actions plus adherence of the paste-like complex protect damaged mucosa against further destruction from ulcerogenic secretions and drugs.*

USES Duodenal ulcer.

UNLABELED USES Aspirin induced erosions, stress ulcer prophylaxis, suspension for chemotherapy-induced mucositis.

S

CONTRAINDICATIONS Hypersensitivity to sucralfate.

CAUTIOUS USE Chronic kidney failure or dialysis due to aluminum accumulation; pregnancy (category B); lactation. Safe use in children not established.

ROUTE & DOSAGE

Duodenal Ulcer (Active disease)

Adult: **PO** 1 g qid × 4–8 wk

Duodenal Ulcer (Maintenance)

Adult: **PO** 1g bid

ADMINISTRATION

Oral

- Use drug solubilized in an appropriate diluent by a pharmacist when given through nasogastric tube.
- Administer antacids prescribed for pain relief 30 min before or after sucralfate.
- Separate administration of quinolones, digoxin, phenytoin, tetracycline from that of sucralfate by 2 h to prevent sucralfate from binding to these compounds in the intestinal tract and reducing their bioavailability.
- Store in tight container at room temperature, 15°–30° C (59°–86° F). Stable for 2 y after manufacture.

ADVERSE EFFECTS **GI:** Nausea, gastric discomfort, *constipation*, diarrhea.

INTERACTIONS **Drug:** May decrease absorption of QUINOLONES (e.g., **ciprofloxacin, norfloxacin**), **digoxin, phenytoin, tetracycline.**

PHARMACOKINETICS **Absorption:** Minimally absorbed from GI tract (less than 5%). **Duration:** Up to 6 h (depends on contact time with ulcer crater). **Elimination:** 90% in feces.

NURSING IMPLICATIONS

Assessment & Drug Effects

- Be aware of drug interactions and schedule other medications accordingly.

Patient & Family Education

- Although healing has occurred within the first 2 wk of therapy, treatment is usually continued 4–8 wk.
- Be aware that constipation is a drug-related problem. Follow these measures unless contraindicated: Increase water intake to 8–10 glasses/day; increase physical exercise, increase dietary bulk. Consult prescriber: A suppository or bulk laxative (e.g., Metamucil) may be prescribed.

SULFACETAMIDE SODIUM

(sul-fa-see′ta-mide)

Bleph 10, Cetamide, Ophthacet, Ovace, Sebizon, Sodium Sulamyd, Sulf-10

SULFACETAMIDE SODIUM/SULFUR

Sulfacet, Rosula

Classification: SULFONAMIDE ANTIBIOTIC

Therapeutic: ANTIBIOTIC

Prototype: Silver sulfadiazine

AVAILABILITY **Sulfacetamide:** Lotion; solution; ointment; **Sulfacetamide/Sulfur:** Gel, lotion

S

ACTION & *THERAPEUTIC EFFECT*

Exerts bacteriostatic effect by interfering with bacterial utilization of PABA, thereby inhibiting folic acid biosynthesis required for bacterial growth. *Effective against a wide range of gram-positive and gram-negative microorganisms.*

USES Ophthalmic preparations are used for conjunctivitis, corneal ulcers, and other superficial ocular infections and as adjunct to systemic sulfonamide therapy for trachoma. The topical lotion is used for scaly dermatoses, seborrheic dermatitis, seborrhea sicca, and other bacterial skin infections.

CONTRAINDICATIONS Hypersensitivity to sulfonamides; neonates, pregnancy (category D near term).

CAUTIOUS USE Application of lotion to denuded or debrided skin; pregnancy (category C except near term); lactation. Safe use in children is not established.

ROUTE & DOSAGE

Conjunctivitis

Adult: **Ophthalmic** 1–3 drops of 10%, 15%, or 30% solution into lower conjunctival sac q2–3h, may increase interval as patient responds or use 1.5–2.5 cm (½–1 in.) of 10% ointment q6h and at bedtime

Seborrhea, Rosacea

Adult: **Topical** Apply thin film to affected area 1–3 × day

ADMINISTRATION

Instillation

- Be aware that ophthalmic preparations and skin lotion are not interchangeable.
- Check strength of medication prescribed.
- See patient instructions for instilling eye drops.
- Discard darkened solutions; results when left standing for a long time.
- Store at 8°–15° C (46°–59° F) in tightly closed containers unless otherwise directed.

ADVERSE EFFECTS **HEENT:** *Temporary stinging or burning sensation,* retardation of corneal healing associated with long-term use of ophthalmic ointment. **Other:** Hypersensitivity reactions (<u>Stevens–Johnson syndrome</u>, lupus-like syndrome), superinfections with nonsusceptible organisms.

INTERACTIONS **Drug: Tetracaine** and other LOCAL ANESTHETICS DERIVED FROM PABA may antagonize the antibacterial effects of SULFONAMIDES; SILVER PREPARATIONS may precipitate sulfacetamide from solution.

PHARMACOKINETICS **Absorption:** Minimal systemic absorption, but may be enough to cause sensitization. **Metabolism:** In liver to inactive metabolites. **Elimination:** In urine.

NURSING IMPLICATIONS

Assessment & Drug Effects

- Discontinue if symptoms of hypersensitivity appear (erythema, skin rash, pruritus, urticaria).

Patient & Family Education

- Wash hands thoroughly with soap and running water (before and after instillation).

S

- Examine eye medication; discard if cloudy or dark in color.
- Avoid contaminating any part of eye dropper that is inserted in bottle.
- Tilt head back, pull down lower lid. At the same time, look up while drop is being instilled into conjunctival sac. Immediately apply gentle pressure just below the eyelid and next to nose for 1 min. Close eyes gently, so as not to squeeze out medication.
- Report purulent eye discharge to prescriber. Sulfacetamide sodium is inactivated by purulent exudates.

SULFADIAZINE

(sul-fa-dye′a-zeen)

Classification: SULFONAMIDE ANTIBIOTIC

Therapeutic: ANTIBIOTIC

Prototype: Silver sulfadiazine

AVAILABILITY Tablet

ACTION & *THERAPEUTIC EFFECT* Exerts bacteriostatic effect by interfering with bacterial utilization of PABA, thereby inhibiting folic acid biosynthesis required for bacterial growth. *Effective against a wide range of gram-positive and gram-negative microorganisms.*

USES Used in combination with pyrimethamine for treatment of cerebral toxoplasmosis and chloroquine-resistant malaria.

CONTRAINDICATIONS Hypersensitivity to sulfonamides or to any ingredients in the formulation; porphyria; pregnancy (category D near term); lactation.

CAUTIOUS USE Application of lotion to denuded or debrided skin; dehydration; hepatic disease; impaired renal function; pregnancy (category C except near term).

ROUTE & DOSAGE

Mild to Moderate Infections

Adult: **PO Loading Dose** 2–4 g loading dose; **PO Maintenance Dose** 2–4 g/day in 4–6 divided doses

Child (2 mo or older): **PO Loading Dose** 75 mg/kg; **PO Maintenance Dose** 150 mg/kg/day in 4–6 divided doses (max: 6 g/day)

Rheumatic Fever Prophylaxis

Adult (weight less than 30 kg): **PO** 500 mg/day; *weight greater than 30 kg:* 1 g/day

Toxoplasmosis

Adult: **PO** 2–8 g/day divided q6h

Child (2 mo or older): **PO** 100–200 mg/kg/day divided q6h

Neonate: **PO** 50 mg/kg q12h × 12 mo

ADMINISTRATION

Oral

- Maintain sufficient fluid intake to produce urinary output of at least 1500 mL/24 h for children between 3000 and 4000 mL/24 h for adults. Concomitant administration of urinary alkalinizer may be prescribed to reduce possibility of crystalluria and stone formation.
- Store in tight, light-resistant containers.

ADVERSE EFFECTS CNS: Headache, peripheral neuritis, peripheral neuropathy, tinnitus, hearing loss, vertigo, insomnia, drowsiness, mental depression, acute psychosis, ataxia, convulsions, kernicterus (newborns). **HEENT:** Conjunctivitis, conjunctival or scleral infection, retardation of corneal healing (ophthalmic ointment). **Endocrine:** Goiter, hypoglycemia. **Skin:** Pruritus, urticaria, rash, erythema multiforme including Stevens–Johnson syndrome, exfoliative dermatitis, alopecia, photosensitivity, vascular lesions. **GI:** *Nausea, vomiting, diarrhea,* abdominal pains, hepatitis, jaundice, pancreatitis, stomatitis. **GU:** *Crystalluria,* hematuria, proteinuria, anuria, toxic nephrosis, reduction in sperm count. **Hematologic:** Acute hemolytic anemia (especially in patients with G6PD deficiency), aplastic anemia, methemoglobinemia, agranulocytosis, thrombocytopenia, leukopenia, eosinophilia, hypoprothrombinemia. **Other:** Headache, *fever,* chills, arthralgia, malaise, allergic myocarditis, serum sickness, anaphylactoid reactions, lymphadenopathy, local reaction following IM injection, fixed drug eruptions, diuresis, overgrowth of nonsusceptible organisms, LE phenomenon.

INTERACTIONS Drug: PABA-CONTAIN-ING LOCAL ANESTHETICS may antagonize sulfa's effects; ORAL ANTICOAGULANTS potentiate hypoprothrombinemia; may potentiate SULFONYLUREA-induced hypoglycemia. May decrease concentrations of **cyclosporine;** may increase levels of **phenytoin.**

PHARMACOKINETICS Absorption: Readily absorbed from GI tract. **Peak:** 3–6 h. **Distribution:** Distributed to most tissues, including CSF; crosses placenta. **Metabolism:** In liver. **Elimination:** In urine.

NURSING IMPLICATIONS

Assessment & Drug Effects

- Monitor hydration status.
- Monitor lab tests: Baseline and periodic urine C&S; frequent CBC and urinalysis; sulfadiazone blood levels with serious infections.

Patient & Family Education

- Take drug exactly as prescribed. Do not alter schedule or dose; take total amount prescribed unless prescriber changes the regimen.
- Drink fluids liberally unless otherwise directed.
- Report early signs of blood dyscrasias (sore throat, pallor, fever) promptly to the prescriber.

SULFAMETHOXAZOLE-TRIMETHOPRIM (SMZ-TMP)

(sul-fa-meth′ox-a-zole-tri-meth′o-prim)

Bactrim, Bactrim DS, Septra, Septra DS

Classification: URINARY TRACT ANTI-INFECTIVE; SULFONAMIDE
Therapeutic: URINARY TRACT ANTI-INFECTIVE
Prototype: Trimethoprim

AVAILABILITY Tablet; suspension; solution for injection

ACTION & *THERAPEUTIC EFFECT* Both components of the combination are synthetic folate antagonist anti-infectives. Principal action is by enzyme inhibition that prevents bacterial synthesis of essential nucleic acids and proteins. *Effective against Pneumocystis jiroveci pneumonitis (formerly PCP), Shigellosis enteritis, and severely complicated UTIs due to most strains of the Enterobacteriaceae.*

USES *Pneumocystis jiroveci* pneumonitis (formerly PCP), shigellosis enteritis, and severe complicated UTIs. Also children with acute otitis media due to susceptible strains of *Haemophilus influenzae,* and acute episodes of chronic bronchitis or traveler's diarrhea in adults.

UNLABELED USES Isosporiasis; cholera; genital ulcers caused by *Haemophilus ducreyi;* prophylaxis for *P. jiroveci* pneumonia (formerly PCP) in neutropenic patients.

CONTRAINDICATIONS Hypersensitivity to SMZ, TMP, sulfonamides, or bisulfites, carbonic anhydrase inhibitors; group A beta-hemolytic streptococcal pharyngitis; megaloblastic anemia due to folate deficiency; G6PD deficiency; hyperkalemia; porphyria; pregnancy (category D near term); lactation.

S

CAUTIOUS USE Impaired kidney or liver function; bone marrow depression; possible folate deficiency; severe allergy or bronchial asthma; hypersensitivity to sulfonamide derivative drugs (e.g., acetazolamide, thiazides, tolbutamide); pregnancy (category C except near term). Safe use in infants younger than 2 mo not established.

ROUTE & DOSAGE

(Weight-based doses are calculated on TMP component) Systemic Infections

Adult: **PO** 160 mg TMP/800 mg SMZ q12h; **IV** 8–10 mg/kg/day TMP divided q6–12h
Child (2 mo or older, weight less than 40 kg): **PO** 4 mg/kg/day TMP q12h; *weight greater than 40 kg:* 160 mg TMP/800 mg SMZ q12h
Child/Infant (2 mo or older): **IV** 6–10 mg/kg/day TMP divided q6–12h

***Pneumocystis jiroveci* Pneumonia (formerly PCP)**

Adult: **PO** 15–20 mg/kg/day TMP divided q6h
Adult/Adolescent/Child: **IV** 15–20 mg/kg/day TMP divided q6h

Prophylaxis for *Pneumocystis jiroveci* Pneumonia (formerly PCP)

Adult: **PO** 160 mg TMP/800 mg SMZ q24h
Child: **PO** 150 mg/m^2 TMP/750 mg/m^2 SMZ bid 3 consecutive days/wk (max: 320 mg TMP/day)

Renal Impairment Dosage Adjustment

CrCl 10–30 mL/min: Reduce dose by 50%; *less than 10 mL/min:* Reduce dose by 50–75%

ADMINISTRATION

Oral

- Give with a full glass of desired fluid.
- Maintain adequate fluid intake (at least 1500 mL/day) during therapy.
- Store at 15°–30° C (59°–86° F) in dry place protected from light. Avoid freezing.

Intravenous

PREPARE: **Intermittent:** Add contents of the 5 mL vial to 125 mL D5W. ▪ Use within 6 h. ▪ If less fluid is desired, dilute in 75 of 100 mL and use within 2 or 4 h, respectively.

ADMINISTER: **Intermittent:** Infuse over 60–90 min. ▪ Avoid rapid infusion.

INCOMPATIBILITIES: **Solution/additive:** Stability in **dextrose** and **normal saline** is concentration dependent, **fluconazole, linezolid, verapamil. Y-site: Alfentanil, amikacin, aminophylline, amphotericin B, ampicillin, ampicillin/sulbactam, atropine, azathioprine, benztropine, bumetanide, buprenorphine, butorphanol, calcium, caspofungin, cefamandole, cefazolin, cefmetazole, cefonicid, cefotaxime, cefotetan, cefoxitin, ceftazidime, ceftizoxime, ceftriaxone, cefuroxime, cephalothin, chloramphenicol, chlorpromazine, cimetidine, cisatracurium, clindamycin, codeine, cyanocobalamine, cyclosporine, dantrolene, dexamethasone, dexmedetomidine, diazepam, diazoxide, digoxin, diphenhydramine, dobutamine, dopamine, doxorubicin, doxycycline, ephedrine, epinephrine, epirubicin, epoetin alfa, erythromycin, famotidine, fentanyl, fluconazole, foscarnet, furosemide, ganciclovir, gentamicin, haloperidol, heparin, hydralazine, hydrocortisone, hydroxyzine, idarubicin, imipenem/cilastain, indomethacin, isoproterenol, ketorolac, lidocaine, mannitol, metaraminol, methicillin, methylprednisolone, metoclopramide, mezlocillin, miconazole, milrinone acetate, minocycline, midazolam, nafcillin, nalbuphine, naloxone, netilmicin, nitroglycerin, nitroprusside, norepinephrine, ondansetron, oxacillin, oxytocin, papaverine, penicillin, pentamidine, pentazocine, pentobarbital, phenobarbital, phentolamine, phenylephrine, phenytoin, phytonadione, piperacillin, potassium, prochlorperazine, promethazine, propranolol, protamine, pyridoxine, quinupristin/dalfopristin, ritodrine, succinylcholine, sufentanil, theophylline, ticarcillin, tobramycin, tolazoline, vancomycin, verapamil, vinorelbine.**

- Store unopened ampule at 15°–30° C (50°–86° F).

ADVERSE EFFECTS **Skin:** *Mild to moderate rashes (including fixed drug eruptions),* toxic epidermal necrolysis. **GI:** *Nausea, vomiting,* diarrhea, *anorexia,* hepatitis, pseudomembranous enterocolitis, stomatitis, glossitis, abdominal pain. **GU:** Kidney failure, oliguria, anuria, crystalluria.

Hematologic: Agranulocytosis (rare), aplastic anemia (rare), megaloblastic anemia, hypoprothrombinemia, thrombocy-topenia (rare). **Other:** Weakness, arthralgia, myalgia, photosensitivity, allergic myocarditis.

DIAGNOSTIC TEST INTERFERENCE

May elevate levels of ***serum creatinine, transaminase, bilirubin, alkaline phosphatase.***

INTERACTIONS

Drug: May enhance hypoprothrombinemic effects of ORAL ANTICOAGULANTS; may increase **methotrexate** toxicity. **Alcohol** may cause disulfiram reaction.

PHARMACOKINETICS

Absorption: Readily from GI tract. **Peak:** 1–4 h (oral). **Distribution:** Widely distributed, including CNS; crosses placenta; distributed into breast milk. **Metabolism:** In liver. **Elimination:** In urine. **Half-Life:** 8–10 h TMP, 10–13 h SMZ.

NURSING IMPLICATIONS

Assessment & Drug Effects

- Be aware that IV forms of the drug may contain sodium metabisulfite, which produces allergic type reactions in susceptible patients: Hives, itching, wheezing, anaphylaxis. Susceptibility (low in general population) is seen most frequently in asthmatics or atopic nonasthmatic persons.
- Monitor coagulation tests and prothrombin times in patient also receiving warfarin. Change in warfarin dosage may be indicated.
- Monitor I&O volume and pattern. Report significant changes to forestall renal calculi formation. Also report failure of treatment (i.e., continued UTI symptoms).
- Older adult patients are at risk for severe adverse reactions, especially if liver or kidney function is compromised or if certain other drugs are given. Most frequently observed: Thrombocytopenia (with concurrent thiazide diuretics); severe decrease in platelets (with or without purpura); bone marrow suppression; severe skin reactions.
- Be alert for overdose symptoms (no extensive experience has been reported): Nausea, vomiting, anorexia, headache, dizziness, mental depression, confusion, and bone marrow depression.
- Monitor lab tests: Baseline and periodic urinalysis; CBC with differential, platelet count, BUN and creatinine clearance with prolonged therapy.

Patient & Family Education

- Report immediately to prescriber if rash appears. Other reportable symptoms are sore throat, fever, purpura, jaundice; all are early signs of serious reactions.
- Monitor for and report fixed eruptions to prescriber. This drug can cause fixed eruptions at the same sites each time the drug is administered. Every contact with drug may not result in eruptions; therefore, patient may overlook the relationship.
- Drink 2.5–3 L (1 L is approximately equal to 1 qt) daily, unless otherwise directed.

SULFASALAZINE

(sul-fa-sal'a-zeen)

Azulfidine, PMS Sulfasalazine ♣, Salazopyrin ♣

Classification: ANTI-INFLAMMATORY; SULFONAMIDE

Therapeutic: GI ANTI-INFLAMMATORY; IMMUNOMODULATOR; DISEASE-MODIFYING ANTIRHEUMATIC DRUG (DMARD)
Prototype: Mesalamine

AVAILABILITY Tablet; sustained release tablet

ACTION & *THERAPEUTIC EFFECT* Exerts antibacterial and anti-inflammatory effects. Inhibits prostaglandins known to cause diarrhea and affect mucosal transport as well as interference with absorption of fluids and electrolytes from colon. Reduces *Clostridium* and *Escherichia coli* in the stools. *Anti-inflammatory and immunomodulatory properties are effective in controlling the S&S of ulcerative colitis and rheumatoid arthritis.*

USES Ulcerative colitis; juvenile rheumatoid arthritis; rheumatoid arthritis.

UNLABELED USES Granulomatous colitis, Crohn's disease, scleroderma, ankylosing spondylitis, psoriatic arthritis.

CONTRAINDICATIONS Sensitivity to sulfasalazine, other sulfonamides and salicylates, trimethoprim; folate deficiency; megaloblastic anemia; renal failure, renal impairment; agranulocytosis; intestinal and urinary tract obstruction; porphyria; pregnancy—fetal risk cannot be ruled out; lactation—milk effects are possible.

CAUTIOUS USE Severe allergy, or bronchial asthma; blood dyscrasias; hepatic or renal impairment; dehydration; men who plan biological fatherhood; G6PD deficiency; older adults. Safe use in children younger than 6 y not established.

ROUTE & DOSAGE

Ulcerative Colitis

Adult: **PO** 3–4 g/day in divided doses, then decrease to 2 g/day in divided doses.
Child: **PO** 30–70 mg/kg/day in 3–6 divided doses (max: 4000 mg/day)

Rheumatoid Arthritis

Adult: **PO** 500 mg daily, increase weekly to maintenance dose of 2g/day in divided doses. (max: 3 g/day)

Juvenile Rheumatoid Arthritis

Adolescent/Child (over 6 y): **PO** 30–50 mg/kg/day in 2 divided doses (max: 2 g/day)

ADMINISTRATION

Oral

- Give after eating to provide longer intestine transit time.
- Do not crush or chew sustained release tablets; **must be** swallowed whole.
- Use evenly divided doses over each 24-h period; do not exceed 8-h intervals between doses.
- Consult prescriber if GI intolerance occurs after first few doses. Symptoms are probably due to irritation of stomach mucosa and may be relieved by spacing total daily dose more evenly over 24 h or by administration of enteric-coated tablets.
- Store at 15°–30° C (59°–86° F) in tight, light-resistant containers, do not freeze.

ADVERSE EFFECTS (≥5%) CNS: Headache. **Skin:** Rash. **GI:** Abdominal pain, indigestion, *loss of appetite*, nausea, vomiting. **GU:** *low sperm count*.

INTERACTIONS **Drug: Iron,** ANTIBIOTICS may alter absorption of sulfasalazine. Do not use with **lasmiditan, voxilaprevir,** or **riluzole.**

PHARMACOKINETICS **Absorption:** 10–15% from GI tract unchanged; remaining drug is hydrolyzed in colon to sulfapyridine (most of which is absorbed) and 5-aminosalicylic acid (30% of which is absorbed). **Peak:** 1.5–6 h sulfasalazine; 6–24 h sulfapyridine. **Distribution:** Crosses placenta; distributed into breast milk; extensive protein binding. **Metabolism:** In intestines and liver. **Elimination:** All metabolites are excreted in urine. **Half-Life:** 5–10 h.

NURSING IMPLICATIONS

Assessment & Drug Effects

- Monitor for GI distress. GI symptoms that develop after a few days of therapy may indicate need for dosage adjustment. If symptoms persist, prescriber may withhold drug for 5–7 days and restart it at a lower dosage level.
- Be aware that adverse reactions generally occur within a few days to 12 wk after start of therapy; most likely to occur in patients receiving high doses (4 g or more).
- Monitor lab tests: Periodic RBC and folate in patients on high doses (more than 2 g/day), CBC with differential, LFTs, renal function tests, urinalysis, serum sulfapyridine levels.

Patient & Family Education

- Examine stools and report to prescriber if enteric-coated tablets have passed intact in feces. Some patients lack enzymes capable of dissolving coating; conventional tablet will be ordered.
- Take drug in evenly divided doses after meals. Swallow delayed-release tablets whole and do not chew or crush.
- Be aware that drug may color alkaline urine and skin orange-yellow.
- Contact healthcare provider immediately to report sore throat, fever, pallor, purpura, or jaundice.
- Maintain adequate hydration to prevent kidney stone formation.
- Remain under close medical supervision. Relapses occur in about 40% of patients after initial satisfactory response. Response to therapy and duration of treatment are governed by endoscopic examinations.

SULINDAC

(sul-in′dak)

Classification: NONSTEROIDAL ANTI-INFLAMMATORY DRUG (NSAID)
Therapeutic: NONNARCOTIC ANALGESIC; NSAID
Prototype: Ibuprofen

AVAILABILITY Tablet

ACTION & THERAPEUTIC EFFECT Anti-inflammatory action thought to result from inhibition of prostaglandin synthesis. *Exhibits anti-inflammatory, analgesic, and antipyretic properties.*

USES Acute and long-term symptomatic treatment of osteoarthritis, rheumatoid arthritis, ankylosing spondylitis; acute painful shoulder (acute subacromial bursitis or supraspinatus tendinitis); acute gouty arthritis.

CONTRAINDICATIONS Hypersensitivity to sulindac; hypersensitivity to aspirin (patients with "aspirin triad": Acute asthma, rhinitis, nasal polyps), other NSAIDs, or salicylates; significant kidney or liver dysfunction; CABG perioperative pain; GI bleeding; drug-induced CV event; pancreatitis; pregnancy (fetal risk of birth defects is known); lactation (infant risk cannot be ruled out).

CAUTIOUS USE History of upper GI tract disorders; anticoagulant therapy; CHF; moderate or mild renal impairment; hepatic impairment; infection; preexisting asthma; SLE; older adults, compromised cardiac function, hypertension. Safety and efficacy in children not established.

ROUTE & DOSAGE

Arthritis, Ankylosing Spondylitis, Acute Gouty Arthritis

Adult: **PO** 150–200 mg bid (max: 400 mg/day)

ADMINISTRATION

Oral

- Crush and give mixed with liquid or food if patient cannot swallow tablet.
- Administer with food, milk, or antacid (if prescribed) to reduce possibility of GI upset. Note: Food retards absorption and delays and lowers peak concentrations.

ADVERSE EFFECTS **CNS:** Dizziness, headache, feeling nervous. **Skin:** Rash. **GI:** Abdominal pain, constipation, diarrhea, indigestion, nausea.

DIAGNOSTIC TEST INTERFERENCE May lead to false-positive aldosterone/renin ratio.

INTERACTIONS **Drug:** Do not use with **ketorolac, acemetacin, aminolevulinic acid,** or **cidofovir. Heparin,** ORAL ANTICOAGULANTS may prolong bleeding time; may increase **lithium** or **methotrexate** toxicity; **aspirin,** other NSAIDS add to ulcerogenic effects; **dimethylsulfoxide (DMSO)** may decrease effects of sulindac; **altretamine** may cause hypoprothrombinemia. **Herbal: Feverfew, garlic, ginger, ginkgo** may increase bleeding potential.

PHARMACOKINETICS **Absorption:** 90% from GI tract. **Peak:** 3–4 h with food. **Duration:** 10–12 h. **Distribution:** Minimal passage across placenta; distributed into breast milk. **Metabolism:** In liver to active metabolite. **Elimination:** 75% in urine, 25% in feces. **Half-Life:** 7.8 h sulindac, 16.4 h sulfide metabolite.

NURSING IMPLICATIONS

Black Box Warning

Sulindac has been associated with increased risk of serious, potentially fatal, GI bleeding and cardiovascular events (e.g., MI and CVA); risk may increase with duration of use and may be greater in the older adult and those with risk factors for CV disease.

Assessment & Drug Effects

- Assess for and report promptly unexplained GI distress.
- Monitor for and report promptly S&S of CV thrombotic events (i.e., angina, MI, TIA, or stroke).
- Schedule auditory and ophthalmic examinations in patients receiving prolonged or high-dose therapy.
- Monitor lab tests: Baseline and periodic CBC and metabolic panel, fecal occult blood test, LFTs.

Patient & Family Education

- Do not drive or engage in potentially hazardous activities until response to drug is known.
- Report any incidence of unexplained bleeding or bruising immediately to prescriber (e.g., bleeding gums, black and tarry stools, coffee-colored emesis).
- Report onset of skin rash, itching, hives, jaundice, swelling of feet or hands, sore throat or mouth, shortness of breath, or night cough to prescriber.
- Be aware that adverse GI effects are relatively common. Report abdominal pain, nausea, dyspepsia, diarrhea, or constipation.
- Avoid alcohol and aspirin as they may increase risk of GI ulceration and bleeding tendencies.
- Monitor for and report promptly S&S of CV thrombotic events (i.e., angina, MI, TIA, or stroke).

SUMATRIPTAN

(sum-a-trip'tan)

Imitrex, Sumavel DosePro, Zembrace SymTouch

Classification: SEROTONIN 5-HT_1 RECEPTOR AGONIST

Therapeutic: ANTIMIGRAINE

AVAILABILITY Tablet; solution for injection; nasal spray.

ACTION & THERAPEUTIC EFFECT Selective agonist for a serotonin receptor (probably 5-HT_{1D}) that causes vasoconstriction of cranial blood vessels and reduces neurogenic inflammation. *Relieves migraine headache. Also relieves photophobia, phonophobia, nausea and vomiting associated with migraine attacks.*

USES Treatment of acute migraine attacks with or without aura, cluster headache.

CONTRAINDICATIONS Hypersensitivity to sumatriptan; ischemic CAD; acute MI, angina, arteriosclerosis; cerebrovascular disease; colitis; concurrent use with MAO inhibitors; uncontrolled hypertension; intracranial bleeding; PVD; Raynaud's disease; stroke; severe hepatic disease; Wolff-Parkinson-White syndrome; basilar or hemiplegic migraine.

CAUTIOUS USE Impaired liver or kidney function; MAO inhibitors; older adults; pregnancy (category C). Safety and efficacy in children not established.

ROUTE & DOSAGE

Migraine

Adult: **Subcutaneous** 6 mg any time after onset of migraine, if headache returns, may repeat with 6 mg subcutaneously at least 1 h after first injection (max: 12 mg/24 h); **PO** 50–100 mg once, if headache returns may repeat once after 2 h (max: 200 mg/24 hours); **Intranasal** 20 mg in one nostril, if headache returns, may repeat once after 2 h (max: 40 mg/24 h);

Cluster Headache

Adult: **Subcutaneous:** 6 mg once, pay repeat if headache recur after 1 hour. (max 12 mg in 24 hours).

ADMINISTRATION

Note: Do not give within 24 h of an ergot-containing drug.

Oral

- Give any time after symptoms of migraine appear.

- A second tablet may be given if symptoms return but no sooner than 2 h after the first tablet.
- Do not exceed 100 mg in a single oral dose or 300 mg/day.

Intranasal

- Note: A single dose is one spray into ONE nostril.

Subcutaneous

- A second injection may be given 1 h or longer following first injection if initial relief is not obtained or if migraine returns.
- Be aware that if adverse effects are dose limiting, a lower dose may be effective.
- Store all forms at room temperature, 15°–30° C (59°–86° F). Protect from light.

ADVERSE EFFECTS **CV:** Flushing. **CNS:** Tingling sensation, dizziness, vertigo, "hot" feeling. **Skin:** Injection site reaction, warm sensation at injection site.

INTERACTIONS **Drug: Dihydroergotamine**, ERGOT ALKALOIDS may cause vasospasm and a slight elevation in blood pressure. MAO INHIBITORS increase sumatriptan levels and toxicity (especially the oral form); do not use concurrently or within 2 wk of stopping MAO INHIBITORS; use with other serotonin altering drugs increases risk of serotonin syndrome (see Appendix F). **Herbal: St. John's wort** may increase triptan toxicity.

PHARMACOKINETICS **Onset:** 10–30 min after subcutaneous administration. **Duration:** 1–2 h. **Distribution:** Widely distributed, 10–20% protein bound. May be excreted in breast milk. **Metabolism:** Hepatically to inactive metabolite. **Elimination:** 57% in urine, 38% in feces. **Half-Life:** 2 h.

NURSING IMPLICATIONS

Black Box Warning

Sumatriptan has been associated with increased risk of serious, sometimes fatal, cardiovascular thrombotic reactions, MI, and CVA.

Assessment & Drug Effects

- Monitor cardiovascular status carefully following first dose in patients at relatively high risk for coronary artery disease (e.g., postmenopausal women, men over 40 years old, persons with known CAD risk factors) or who have coronary artery vasospasms.
- Report to prescriber immediately chest pain or tightness in chest or throat that is severe or does not quickly resolve following a dose of sumatriptan.
- Monitor therapeutic effectiveness. Pain relief usually begins within 10 min of injection, with complete relief in approximately 65% of all patients within 2 h.

Patient & Family Education

- Review patient information leaflet provided by the manufacturer carefully.
- Learn correct use of autoinjector for self-administration of subcutaneous dose.
- Pain or redness at injection site is common but usually disappears in less than 1 h.
- Notify prescriber immediately if symptoms of severe angina (e.g., severe or persistent pain or tightness in chest, back, neck, or throat) or hypersensitivity (e.g., wheezing, facial swelling, skin rash, or hives) occur.
- Do not take any other serotonin receptor agonist (Axert, Maxalt, Zomig, Amerge) within 24 h of taking sumatriptan.

S

- Check with prescriber before taking any new OTC or prescription drugs.
- Report any other adverse effects (e.g., tingling, flushing, dizziness) at next prescriber visit.

SUNITINIB

(sun-i-ti′nib)

Sutent

Classification: ANTINEOPLASTIC; KINASE INHIBITOR

Therapeutic: ANTINEOPLASTIC

Prototype: Erlotinib

AVAILABILITY Capsule

ACTION & *THERAPEUTIC EFFECT* An antineoplastic agent that is a selective inhibitor of receptors for tyrosine kinases (RTKs) in solid tumors. Carcinogenic activity within these tumors is a result of tumor angiogenesis and proliferation. *Sunitinib causes tumor regression and decreased tumor growth.*

USES Treatment of advanced renal cell cancer; treatment of gastrointestinal stromal tumors (GIST), pancreatic neuroendocrine tumor.

CONTRAINDICATIONS Hypersensitivity to sunitinib; acute MI; fever, hepatotoxicity; tumor lysis syndrome; pancreatitis; urine protein of at least 3 g per 24 h; RPLS; pregnancy (category D); lactation.

CAUTIOUS USE Cardiac dysfunction, CHF, poorly controlled hypertension, history of MI; history of QT_c prolongation; thyroid dysfunction; DM; CVA; hepatic impairment; renal insufficiency (CrCl of 60 mL/min or less); females of childbearing age; children.

ROUTE & DOSAGE

Advanced Renal Cell Cancer/GIST Tumor

Adult: **PO** 50 mg/day for 4 wk, followed by 2 wk off treatment.

Pancreatic Neuroendocrine Tumor

Adult: **PO** 37.5 mg daily

Dosage Adjustments with Concurrent Hepatic CYP3A4 Modifiers

CYP3A4 Inducers: Increase to maximum of 87.5 mg/day (GIST, RCC) or 62.5 mg/day (PNET)
CYP3A4 Inhibitors: Decrease to minimum of 37.5 mg/day (GIST, RCC) or 25 mg/day (PNET)

ADMINISTRATION

Oral

- Incremental dosage changes of 12.5 mg are recommended.
- May be administered with or without food.
- Store at 15°–30° C (59°–86° F).

ADVERSE EFFECTS CV: Hypertension, decreased left ventricular ejection fraction, peripheral edema, chest pain. **Respiratory:** Cough, dyspnea, epistaxis, nasopharyngitis, oropharyngeal pain, upper respiratory tract infection. **CNS:** Fatigue, glossalgia, headache, insomnia, chills, depression, dizziness. **Endocrine:** Increased uric acid, abnormal serum calcium, decreased serum albumin, decreased serum phosphate, increased serum glucose, abnormal serum potassium, abnormal serum sodium, decreased serum magnesium. **Skin:** Skin discoloration, hair discoloration, palmar-plantar erythrodysesthesia, xeroderma, skin rash, alopecia, erythema, pruritis. **Hepatic:**

Increased serum AST, increased serum ALT, increased serum ALP, increased serum bilirubin. **GI:** Diarrhea, nausea, increased serum lipase, anorexia, mucositis, dysgeusia, vomiting, abdominal pain, increased serum amylase, constipation, weight loss, flatulence, xerostomia, GERD. **GU:** Increased serum creatinine. **Musculoskeletal:** Increased creatine phosphokinase, limb pain, weakness, arthralgia, back pain, myalgia. **Hematologic:** Decreased hemoglobin, decreased neutrophils, abnormal absolute lymphocyte count, decreased platelet count, hemorrhage. **Other:** Fever.

INTERACTIONS **Drug:** Coadministration of CYP3A4 INDUCERS (e.g., **carbamazepine, dexamethasone, phenobarbital, phenytoin, rifabutin, rifampin, rifapentine**) may decrease plasma levels of sunitinib. Coadministration of CYP3A4 INHIBITORS (e.g., **atazanavir, clarithromycin, erythromycin, indinavir, itraconazole, ketoconazole, nefazodone, nelfinavir, ritonavir, saquinavir, telithromycin, voriconazole**) may increase plasma levels of sunitinib. Do not use with LIVE VACCINES, **bevacizumab, pimecrolimus, topical tacrolimus. Food: Grapefruit** and **grapefruit juice** may increase the plasma levels of sunitinib. **Herbal: St. John's wort** may decrease the plasma levels of sunitinib.

PHARMACOKINETICS **Peak:** 6–12 h. **Distribution:** 95–98% protein bound. **Metabolism:** Extensive hepatic metabolism (CYPE 3A4 substrate). **Elimination:** Primarily fecal (61%). **Half-Life:** 40–60 h.

NURSING IMPLICATIONS

Black Box Warning

Sunitinib has been associated with severe, sometimes fatal, hepatotoxicity.

Assessment & Drug Effects

- Monitor for and report S&S of bleeding (e.g., GI, GU, gingival).
- Monitor BP regularly and assess regularly for S&S of congestive heart failure. Withhold drug and notify prescriber if severe hypertension or signs of heart failure develop.
- Monitor for and report S&S of hepatotoxicity (see Appendix F).
- Monitor lab tests: At the beginning of each treatment cycle, urinalysis for proteinuria, CBC with differential and platelet count; periodic LFTs and serum electrolytes; thyroid function tests as indicated.

Patient & Family Education

- Do not use any prescription or nonprescription drugs without consulting a prescriber.
- Skin discoloration (yellow color) and/or loss of skin and hair pigmentation may occur with this drug.
- Report any of the following to a health care provider: Painful redness of palms and soles of feet; severe abdominal pain, vomiting, and diarrhea; signs of bleeding; chest pain or discomfort; shortness of breath; swelling of feet, legs, or hands; rapid weight gain.
- Women of childbearing age are advised not to become pregnant while taking sunitinib.

SUVOREXANT

(su-vor′ex-ant)

Belsomra
Classification:
SEDATIVE-HYPNOTIC; OXERIN RECEPTOR ANTAGONIST
Therapeutic: SEDATIVE-HYPNOTIC
Controlled substance:
Schedule IV

AVAILABILITY Tablet

ACTIONS & *THERAPEUTIC EFFECT* Promotes the natural transition from wakefulness to sleep by inhibiting the wakefulness-promoting orexin neurons of the arousal system. *Suvorexant improves sleep onset and sleep maintenance.*

USES Treatment of insomnia characterized by difficulties with sleep onset and/or sleep maintenance.

CONTRAINDICATIONS Narcolepsy; severe hepatic impairment; suicidal ideation.

CAUTIOUS USE Daytime somnolence; persistent insomnia after 7–10 days of treatment; complex nighttime behaviors while out of bed and not fully awake; concurrent CNS depressants or CYP3A4 inhibitors; alcohol use; history of drug abuse; depression; history of suicidal thoughts; behavioral changes; compromised respiratory function; obese individuals especially females; pregnancy (adverse effects have been observed in some animal reproduction studies); lactation. Safety and efficacy in children younger than 18 y not established.

S

ROUTE & DOSAGE

Insomnia

Adult: **PO** 10 mg no more than once per night and within 30 min of bedtime; dose can be increased to 20 mg if tolerated (intended for short term use only)

Concurrent Medication Dosage Adjustment

Significant interactions occur requiring modification of dosing/frequency. Consult a drug interaction database for more information.

Hepatic Impairment Dosage Adjustment

Severe impairment: Not recommended

ADMINISTRATION

Oral

- Give within 30 min of bedtime, with at least 7 h before the planned time of awakening.
- May be taken with or without food; effect may be delayed if taken with or soon after a meal.
- Store at 20°–25° C (66°–77° F).

ADVERSE EFFECTS **Respiratory:** Cough, upper respiratory tract infection. **CNS:** Drowsiness, dizziness, headache. **GI:** Diarrhea, dry mouth.

INTERACTIONS **Drug:** Extensive drug interactions, consult a drug interaction database for complete listing. Concomitant use with strong CYP3A4 inhibitors (e.g., **clarithromycin, conivaptan, indinavir, itraconazole, ketoconazole, nefazodone, nelfinavir, posaconazole, ritonavir, saquinavir, telaprevir, telithromycin**) or moderate CYP3A4 inhibitors (e.g., **amprenavir, aprepitant, atazanavir, ciprofloxacin, diltiazem, erythromycin, fluconazole, fosam-prenavir, imatinib, verapamil**) will increase the levels of suvorexant. Concomitant use with strong CYP3A4 inducers (e.g., **carbamazepine, phenytoin, rifampin**) will decrease the levels of suvorexant. Use with CNS DEPRESSANTS increases risk of adverse effects. **Food: Grapefruit juice** will increase the levels of suvorexant. **Herbal: St. John's wort** may decrease the levels of suvorexant.

PHARMACOKINETICS **Absorption:** 82% bioavailable. **Peak:** 2 h. **Distribution:** Greater than 99% plasma protein bound. **Metabolism:** In liver by CYP3A4 and CYP2C19. **Elimination:** Fecal (66%) and renal (23%). **Half-Life:** 12 h.

NURSING IMPLICATIONS

Assessment & Drug Effects

- Monitor for adverse effects. Note that dose reduction may be required in obese women due to adverse effects, and in those using other CNS depressant drugs due to potential additive effects.
- Monitor respiratory status and level of daytime alertness.
- Monitor for and report promptly signs of abnormal thinking, worsening of depression, suicidal thoughts, or other abnormal behaviors.

Patient & Family Education

- Do not take this drug if a full night of sleep is not anticipated.
- Report to prescriber if insomnia does not improve within 7–10 days.
- Avoid alcohol while taking this drug.
- Do not engage in potentially dangerous activities (e.g., driving) until response to drug is known.
- Report immediately to prescriber if experiencing any of the following: More outgoing or aggressive behavior than normal, confusion, agitation, memory loss, hallucinations, worsening depression or suicidal thoughts.
- Contact prescriber immediately if experiencing "sleep-walking" or doing other activities when asleep (e.g., eating, talking, driving a car).

TACROLIMUS

(tac-rol'i-mus)

Astagraf XL, Envarsus XR, Prograf, Protopic

Classification: BIOLOGIC RESPONSE MODIFIER; IMMUNOSUPPRESSANT

Therapeutic: IMMUNOSUPPRESSANT

Prototype: Cyclosporine

AVAILABILITY Capsule; injection; ointment; extended release capsule; extended release tablet

ACTION & *THERAPEUTIC EFFECT* Inhibits helper T-lymphocytes by selectively inhibiting secretion of interleukin-2, interleukin-3, and interleukin-gamma, thus reducing transplant rejection. *Inhibits antibody production (thus subduing immune response) by creating an imbalance in favor of suppressor T-lymphocytes.*

USES Prophylaxis for organ transplant rejection, moderate to severe atopic dermatitis (e.g., eczema).

UNLABELED USES Acute organ transplant rejection, severe plaque-type psoriasis, ulcerative colitis, myasthenia gravis, Crohn disease.

CONTRAINDICATIONS Hypersensitivity to tacrolimus or castor oil; postoperative oliguria or renal failure with CrCl greater than or

T

equal to 4 mg/dL; potassium sparing diuretics; lactation.

CAUTIOUS USE Renal or hepatic insufficiency, liver transplants; hyperkalemia, QT prolongation; CHF; serious infections; polyoma virus infections; CMV disease diabetes mellitus, gout, history of seizures, hypertension; cardiomyopathy, left ventricular dysfunction (e.g., heart failure); neoplastic disease, especially lymphoproliferative disorders; pregnancy (miscarriage, preterm delivery, birth defects, renal dysfunction, transient neonatal hyperkalemia, and fetal distress have been reported following in utero exposure to tacrolimus however pregnant patients were also taking a concomitant medication known to cause adverse pregnancy outcomes; tacrolimus monotherapy is the preferred immunosuppressant in patients who become pregnant following liver, kidney, heart, or uterine transplant). **Ointment:** Children younger than 2 y.

ROUTE & DOSAGE

Rejection Prophylaxis (Dose Varies Based on Concurrent Meds and type of transplant)

Adult: **PO** 0.075–0.2 mg/kg/day in divided doses q12h, start no sooner than 6 h after transplant; give first oral dose 8–12 h after discontinuing IV therapy; **IV** 0.01–0.05 mg/kg/day as continuous IV infusion, start no sooner than 6 h after transplant, continue until patient can take oral therapy
Child: **PO** 0.1–0.3 mg/kg/day **IV** 0.01–0.03 mg/kg/day

Atopic Dermatitis

Adult: **Topical** Apply thin layer of 0.1% ointment to affected area bid, continue until clearing of symptoms
Child (2–15 y): **Topical** Apply thin layer of 0.03% ointment to affected area bid, continue until clearing of symptoms

Renal Impairment Dosage Adjustment

Start with lower dose

Hepatic Impairment Dosage Adjustment

Start with lower dose and closely monitor serum concentrations.

ADMINISTRATION

Oral

- Patient should be converted from IV to oral therapy as soon as possible.
- Give first oral dose 8–12 h after discontinuing IV infusion.
- Administer with or without food.

Topical

- Ensure that skin is clean and completely dry before application.
- Apply a thin layer to the affected area and rub in gently and completely.
- Do not apply occlusive dressing over the site.

Intravenous

PREPARE: **IV Infusion:** Dilute 5 mg/mL ampules with NS or D5W to a concentration of 0.004–0.02 mg/mL (4–20 mcg/mL). ▪ Lower concentrations are preferred for children.
ADMINISTER: **IV Infusion:** Give as continuous IV, generally over 24 hours. ▪ PVC-free tubing is

T

recommended, especially at lower concentrations.

INCOMPATIBILITIES: Y-site: **Allopurinol, azathioprine, cefepime, dantrolene, diazepam, diazoxide, esomeprazole, gemtuzumab, iron sucrose, lansoprazole, levothyroxine, omeprazole, phenytoin, thiopental.**

- Store ampules at 5°–25° C (41°–77° F); store capsules at room temperature, 25° C (77° F). ▪ Store the diluted infusion in glass or polyethylene containers and discard after 24 h.

ADVERSE EFFECTS

CV: *Mild to moderate hypertension.* **Respiratory:** *Pleural effusion, atelectasis, dyspnea.* **CNS:** *Headache, tremors, insomnia, paresthesia, hyperesthesia* and/or sensations of warmth, circumoral numbness. **HEENT:** Blurred vision, photophobia. **Endocrine:** Hirsutism, *hyperglycemia, hyperkalemia, hypokalemia, hypomagnesemia,* hyperuricemia, decreased serum cholesterol. **Skin:** *Flushing, rash, pruritus, skin irritation,* alopecia, erythema, folliculitis, hyperesthesia, exfoliative dermatitis, hirsutism, photosensitivity, skin discoloration, skin ulcer, sweating. **GI:** *Nausea, abdominal pain, gas,* appetite changes, *vomiting, anorexia, constipation,* diarrhea, ascites. **GU:** UTI, oliguria, nephrotoxicity, nephropathy. **Hematologic:** *Anemia, leukocytosis,* thrombocytopenic *purpura.* **Other:** *Pain, fever, peripheral edema, increased risk of cancer.*

INTERACTIONS

Drug: Use with **cyclosporine** increases risk of nephrotoxicity. **Metoclopramide, lansoprazole,** CALCIUM CHANNEL BLOCKER, ANTIFUNGAL AGENTS, MACROLIDE ANTIBIOTICS, **bromocriptine, cimetidine, cyclosporine, methylprednisolone, omeprazole** may increase levels; **caspofungin, rifampin** may decrease levels. NSAIDS may lead to oliguria or anuria. Do not use with LIVE VACCINES OT IMMUNOSUPPRESANTS. **Herbal: St. John's wort** decreases efficacy. **Food: Grapefruit juice** (greater than 1 qt/day) may increase plasma concentrations and adverse effects.

PHARMACOKINETICS

Absorption: Erratic and incompletely from GI tract; absolute bioavailability approximately 14–25%; absorption reduced by food. **Peak:** PO 1–4 h. **Duration:** IV 12 h. **Distribution:** Within plasma, tacrolimus is found primarily in lipoprotein-deficient fraction; 75–97% protein bound; distributed into red blood cells; blood: plasma ratio reported greater than 4; animal studies have demonstrated high concentrations of tacrolimus in lung, kidney, heart, and spleen; distributed into breast milk. **Metabolism:** Extensively in liver (CYP3A4). **Elimination:** Metabolites primarily in bile. **Half-Life:** 8.7–11.3 h.

NURSING IMPLICATIONS

Black Box Warning

Tacrolimus has been associated with increased susceptibility to possible development of lymphoma and skin cancer.

Assessment & Drug Effects

- Monitor for and promptly report S&S of infection.
- Monitor kidney function closely; report elevated serum creatinine or decreased urinary output.
- Monitor for neurotoxicity, and report tremors, changes in mental status, or other signs of toxicity.
- Monitor cardiovascular status and report hypertension.

T

- Monitor for ECG for QT prolongation especially in those with renal or hepatic impairment.
- Monitor lab tests: Periodic serum tacrolimus, serum electrolytes, blood glucose, LFTs, and renal function tests.

Patient & Family Education

- Do not eat grapefruit or drink grapefruit juice while taking this drug.
- Report promptly unexplained hunger, thirst, and frequent urination.
- Be aware of potential adverse effects including increased risk for infection.
- Minimize exposure to natural or artificial sunlight while using the ointment.
- Notify prescriber of S&S of neurotoxicity.

TADALAFIL

(ta-dal′a-fil)

Adcirca, Cialis

Classification: IMPOTENCE; PHOSPHODIESTERASE (PDE) INHIBITOR; VASODILATOR
Therapeutic: IMPOTENCE; PULMONARY ANTIHYPERTENSIVE
Prototype: Sildenafil

AVAILABILITY Tablet

ACTION & *THERAPEUTIC EFFECT* PDE is responsible for degradation of cyclic GMP in the corpus cavernosum of the penis. Cyclic GMP causes smooth muscle relaxation in lung tissue and the corpus cavernosum, thereby allowing inflow of blood into the penis. PDE-5 inhibitors reduce pulmonary vasodilation by sustaining levels of cyclic guanosine monophosphate (cGMP). Additionally, tadalafil produces a reduction in the pulmonary-to-systemic vascular resistance ratio. *Tadalafil promotes sustained erection only in the presence of sexual stimulation. It also produces a significant improvement in arterial oxygenation in pulmonary hypertension.*

USES Treatment of erectile dysfunction, BPH, pulmonary hypertension.

CONTRAINDICATIONS Hypersensitivity to tadalafil, vardenafil, or sildenafil; MI within last 90 days; Class 2 or greater heart failure within last 6 mo; unstable angina or angina during intercourse; uncontrolled cardiac arrhythmias; nitrate/nitrite therapy; hypotension, uncontrolled hypertension; retinitis pigmentosa; CVA within last 6 mo; left ventricular outflow obstruction, aortic stenosis; severe (Child-Pugh class C) hepatic cirrhosis; women; lactation.

CAUTIOUS USE CAD, risk factors for CVA; renal insufficiency; mild to moderate (Child-Pugh class A or B) hepatic disease; anatomic deformity of the penis; sickle cell anemia; multiple myeloma; leukemia; active bleeding or a peptic ulcer; hiatal hernia, GERD; sickle cell disease; retinitis pigmentosa; severe renal impairment; concurrent use with other medicines for penile dysfunction; older adults; pregnancy (category B). Safety and efficacy for PAH in children younger than 18 y not established.

ROUTE & DOSAGE

Erectile Dysfunction

Adult: **PO** 2.5 mg daily OR 10 mg prior to anticipated sexual activity. May increase (max:

20 mg/day or reduce to 5 mg/day if needed)

Pulmonary Hypertension

Adult: **PO** 40 mg daily

BPH

Adult: **PO** 5 mg daily

Hepatic Impairment Dosage Adjustment

Mild to moderate impairment (Child-Pugh class A and B): Max 10 mg/day; not recommended with severe hepatic impairment *Severe hepatic impairment (Child-Pugh class C):* Not recommended

Renal Impairment Dosage Adjustment

CrCl 30–50 mL/min: Start at half normal dose; *less than 30 mL/min:* Max dose 5 mg and once daily dosing is not recommended

ADMINISTRATION

Oral

- If not on the daily dose regimen, tadalafil is taken approximately 30 min before expected intercourse, but preferably not after a heavy or high-fat meal.
- Store at 15°–30° C (59°–86° F).

ADVERSE EFFECTS **CV:** Angina, chest pain, hyper-tension, hypotension, MI, orthostatic hypotension, palpitations, syncope, sinus tachycardia. **Respiratory:** Nasal congestion, dyspnea, epistaxis, pharyngitis. **CNS:** *Head-ache,* dizziness, insomnia, somnolence, vertigo, hypesthesia, paresthesia. **HEENT:** Blurred vision, changes in color vision, conjunctivitis, eye pain, lacrimation, swelling of eyelids, sudden vision loss. **Endocrine:** Increased GGTP. **Skin:** Rash, pruritus, sweating. **GI:** Dyspepsia, nausea, vomiting, abdominal pain, abnormal liver function tests, diarrhea, loose stools, dysphagia, esophagitis, gastritis, GERD, xerostomia. **GU:** Spontaneous penile erection. **Musculoskeletal:** Arthralgia, myalgia, neck pain. **Other:** Flushing, back pain, asthenia, facial edema, fatigue, pain, transient global amnesia.

INTERACTIONS **Drug:** Do not use with any form of NITRATES or **riociguat** due to increased risk of hypotension. Do not use with **telaprevir.** May potentiate hypotensive effects of ETHANOL, **alfuzosin, doxazosin, prazosin, tamsulosin** (doses greater than 0.4 mg/day), **terazosin; erythromycin** (and other MACROLIDES), **indinavir,** PROTEASE INHIBITORS, **saquinavir,** may increase levels and toxicity of tadalafil; **barbiturates, bosentan, carbamazepine, dexamethasone, fosphenytoin, nevirapine, phenytoin, rifabutin, rifampin, troglitazone** may reduce level and effectiveness of tadalafil. If taking **ritonavir, itraconazole, ketoconazole,** or **voriconazole** (max dose: 10 mg q72h). **Food: Grapefruit juice** may increase levels and toxicity of tadalafil.

T

PHARMACOKINETICS **Absorption:** Rapidly absorbed, 15% reaches systemic circulation. **Onset:** 30–45 min. **Peak:** 2 h. **Duration:** Up to 36 h. **Metabolism:** In liver by CYP3A4. **Elimination:** In feces (61%) and urine (39%). **Half-Life:** 17.5 h.

NURSING IMPLICATIONS

Assessment & Drug Effects

- Monitor CV status and report angina or other S&S of cardiac dysfunction.
- Monitor for orthostatic hypotension.
- Monitor lab tests: Baseline and periodic PSA.

Patient & Family Education

- Do not take more than once/day.
- Note: With moderate renal insufficiency, the maximum recommended dose is 10 mg not more than once in every 48 h.
- Moderate use of alcohol when taking this drug.
- Do not take this drug without consulting prescriber if you are taking drugs called "alpha-blockers" or "nitrates" or any other drugs for high blood pressure, chest pain, or enlarged prostate.
- Report promptly any of the following: Palpitations, chest pain, back pain, difficulty breathing, or shortness of breath; dizziness or fainting; changes in vision; swollen eyelids; muscle aches; painful or prolonged erection (lasting longer than 4 h); skin rash, or itching.

TAMOXIFEN CITRATE Pr

(ta-mox′i-fen)

Soltamox

Classification: ANTINEOPLASTIC; SELECTIVE ESTROGEN RECEPTOR MODIFIER (SERM)

Therapeutic: ANTINEOPLASTIC; ANTIESTROGEN

AVAILABILITY Tablet

ACTION & *THERAPEUTIC EFFECT* Competes with estradiol at estrogen receptor (ER-positive) sites in target tissues such as breast, uterus, vagina, anterior pituitary. Estrogen is thought to increase breast cancer cell proliferation in ER-positive tumors. *Has effects on tumor with high concentration of estrogen receptors. Tamoxifen-receptor complexes move into the cell nucleus, decreasing DNA synthesis and estrogen responses.*

USES Palliative treatment of metastatic estrogen receptors (ER)-positive breast cancer in postmenopausal women, adjunctively with surgery in the treatment of breast carcinoma with positive lymph nodes; reduce incidence of breast cancer in high risk patient.

UNLABELED USES Gynecomastia, idiopathic male infertility.

CONTRAINDICATIONS Hypersensitivity to tamoxifen or any component of the formulation; concurrent warfarin therapy; history of DVT or pulmonary embolism; preexisting endometrial hyperplasia; intramuscular injections if platelets less than 50,000/mm^3; history of thromboembolic disease; pregnancy (in utero exposure to tamoxifen may cause fetal harm), especially during first trimester; lactation; children.

CAUTIOUS USE Vision disturbances; cataracts, visual disturbance; leukopenia, bone marrow suppression; thrombocytopenia; hypercalcemia; hypercholesterolemia, lipid protein abnormalities; women with ductal carcinoma in situ (DCIS).

ROUTE & DOSAGE

Breast Cancer Treatment

Adult: **PO** 20 mg daily for initial duration of 5 years; possibly up to 10 years

Breast Cancer Prophylaxis

Adult: **PO** 20 mg daily × 5 y

ADMINISTRATION

Oral

- Administer tablets or oral solution with or without food. Use supplied dosing cup for oral solution.
- Store at 20°–25° C (68°–77° F); protect from light. Oral solution should be used within 3 mo of opening.

ADVERSE EFFECTS **CV:** Flushing, hypertension, peripheral edema, vasodilation, chest pain. **Respiratory:** Pharyngitis, bronchitis, cough, dyspnea, flu-like symptoms, sinusitis, throat irritation (oral solution). **CNS:** Depression, fatigue, mood changes, pain, anxiety, dizziness, headache, insomnia, paresthesia. **HEENT:** Cataract. **Endocrine:** Amenorrhea, fluid retention, hot flash, weight loss, weight gain, infrequent uterine bleeding, menstrual disease. **Skin:** Skin rash, skin changes, alopecia, diaphoresis. **Hepatic/GI:** *Nausea, vomiting,* abdominal pain, constipation, diarrhea, dyspepsia, increased AST. **GU:** Irregular menses, vaginal discharge, vaginal hemorrhage, leukorrhea, mastalgia, urinary tract infection, vaginitis, vulvovaginitis. **Hematologic:** Lymphedema, anemia, neoplasm, thrombocytopenia. **Musculoskeletal:** Arthralgia, arthritis, asthenia, arthropathy, back pain, bone fracture, myalgia, ostealgia, osteoporosis. **Other:** Infection, sepsis, cyst.

DIAGNOSTIC TEST INTERFERENCE

Tamoxifen may produce elevation of T4.

INTERACTIONS **Drug:** May enhance hypoprothrombinemic effects of **warfarin;** may increase risk of thromboembolic events with CYTOTOXIC AGENTS; SSRI ANTIDEPRESSANTS may decrease effectiveness of tamoxifen; do not use with **anastrozole, ospermifene.** CYP 3A4 INHIBITORS may increase concentration of tamoxifen; CYP 3A4 INDUCERS may decrease concentration of tamoxifen; CYP 2D6 INHIBITORS may decrease concentration of tamoxifen.

PHARMACOKINETICS **Absorption:** Slowly from GI tract. **Distribution:** widely distributed; highly protein bound. **Peak:** 3–6 h. **Metabolism:** In liver (CYP2D6), enterohepatically cycled. **Elimination:** Primarily in feces. **Half-Life:** 7 days.

NURSING IMPLICATIONS

Black Box Warning

Tamoxifen has been associated with increased risk of uterine malignancies, stroke, and pulmonary embolism.

Assessment & Drug Effects

- Be aware that local swelling and marked erythema over preexisting lesions or the development of new lesions may signal soft-tissue disease response to tamoxifen. These symptoms rapidly subside.
- Monitor for signs and symptoms of DVT or PE.
- Baseline ophthalmic exam if vision problem.
- Monitor lab tests: Periodic CBC with platelet count, serum calcium, LFTs, lipid profile, INR, PT,

T

pregnancy test, and bone mineral density test (premenopausal women).

Patient & Family Education

- Do not change established dose schedule.
- Report to prescriber any of the following: Marked weakness or numbness in face or leg, especially on one side of the body; difficulty walking or loss of balance; unexplained sleepiness or mental confusion; edema; shortness of breath; or blurred vision.
- Report promptly any unexpected vaginal discharge or pain or pressure in your pelvis.
- Avoid OTC drugs unless specifically prescribed by the prescriber; particularly OTC pain medicines.
- Report onset of tenderness or redness in an extremity.

TAMSULOSIN HYDROCHLORIDE (Pr)

(tam′su-lo-sin)

Flomax

Classification: ALPHA-ADRENERGIC RECEPTOR ANTAGONIST

Therapeutic: SMOOTH MUSCLE RELAXANT OF BLADDER OUTLET & PROSTATE GLAND

AVAILABILITY Capsule

ACTION & *THERAPEUTIC EFFECT* Antagonist of the alpha$_{1A}$-adrenergic receptors located in the prostate. This blockage can cause smooth muscles in the bladder outlet and the prostate gland to relax, resulting in improvement in urinary flow and a reduction in symptoms of BPH. *Improves symptoms related to benign prostatic hypertrophy (BPH) related to bladder outlet obstruction.*

USES Benign prostatic hypertrophy.

CONTRAINDICATIONS Hypersensitivity to tamsulosin; women; lactation; children.

CAUTIOUS USE History of syncope, hypersensitivity to sulfonamides; hypotension; renal impairment, renal failure, renal disease; older adults; pregnancy (limited information related to use during pregnancy; use with caution).

ROUTE & DOSAGE

Benign Prostatic Hypertrophy

Adult: **PO** 0.4 mg daily 30 min after a meal, may increase up to 0.8 mg daily

ADMINISTRATION

Oral

- Give 30 min after the same meal each day.
- Instruct to swallow capsules whole; do not crush, chew, or open.
- If dose is interrupted for several days, reinitiate at the lowest dose, 0.4 mg.
- Store at 25° C (77° F).

ADVERSE EFFECTS CV: *Orthostatic hypotension (especially with first dose).* **Respiratory:** *Rhinitis,* dyspnea, epistaxis, increased cough, pharyngitis. **CNS:** *Headache, dizziness.* **HEENT:** Amblyopia. **GI:** Diarrhea, nausea. **GU:** *Abnormal ejaculation,* priapism. **Other:** Asthenia, back pain, infection.

INTERACTIONS Drug: Cimetidine may decrease clearance of tamsulosin. **Sildenafil, vardenafil,** and **tadalafil,** and alcohol may enhance hypotensive effects. CYP 3A4 INHIBITORS may increase concentration of tamsulosin; CYP 3A4 INDUCERS may decrease concentration of tamsulosin; may increase hypotensive effect with ANTIHYPERTENSIVES.

PHARMACOKINETICS Absorption: Rapidly from GI tract. Greater than 90% bioavailability. **Peak:** 4–5 h fasting, 6–7 h fed. **Distribution:** Widely distributed in body tissues, including kidney and prostate. **Metabolism:** In the liver via CYP3A4 and 2D6. **Elimination:** 76% in urine. **Half-Life:** 14–15 h.

NURSING IMPLICATIONS

Assessment & Drug Effects

- Monitor for signs of orthostatic hypotension; take BP lying down, then upon standing. Report a systolic pressure drop of 15 mm Hg or more or a HR 15 beats or more upon standing.
- Monitor patients on warfarin therapy closely.
- Monitor urinary symptoms.

Patient & Family Education

- Make position changes slowly to minimize orthostatic hypotension.
- Report dizziness, vertigo, or fainting to prescriber. Exercise caution with hazardous activities until response to drug is known.
- Be aware that concurrent use of cimetidine may increase the orthostatic hypotension adverse effect.

TAPENTADOL

(ta-pent'a-dol)

Nucynta, Nucynta ER

Classification: CENTRALLY ACTING NARCOTIC ANALGESIC; MU-OPIOID RECEPTOR AGONIST; INHIBITOR OF NOREPINEPHRINE REUPTAKE

Therapeutic: CENTRALLY ACTING NARCOTIC ANALGESIC

Controlled Substance: Schedule II

AVAILABILITY Tablet; extended release tablet

ACTION & *THERAPEUTIC EFFECT* Tapentadol is a centrally acting synthetic analgesic that is a mu-opioid agonist and also thought to inhibit norepinephrine reuptake. There is potential for opioid agonist abuse or addiction. *Effective in treatment of moderate to severe acute pain.*

USES Relief of acute moderate to severe pain, chronic pain (ER form only).

CONTRAINDICATIONS Hypersensitivity to tapentadol (e.g., anaphylaxis, angioedema); impaired pulmonary function (e.g., significant respiratory depression, acute or severe bronchial asthma, hypercapnia without monitoring or the absence of resuscitative equipment); known or suspected paralytic ileus; concomitant use of MAOI or use within 14 days; head injury, intracranial pressure (ICP); severe hepatic or renal impairment (CrCl less than 30 mL/min); alcohol consumption especially with tapentadol ER; labor and delivery; lactation.

CAUTIOUS USE Debilitated patients; upper airway obstruction; COPD; cor pulmonale; patients with decreased respiratory reserve; history of low blood pressure; cranial lesions without increased ICP; history of drug or alcohol abuse; history of seizures; mild or moderate renal or hepatic impairment; older adults; pregnancy (category C). Safe use in children younger than 18 y not established.

ROUTE & DOSAGE

Acute Moderate to Severe Pain

Adult: **PO** 50–100 mg q 4–6 h. On first day of dosing a second dose may be given 1 h later if initial dose ineffective (may titrate

T

to max total daily dose: 700 mg day 1 and 600 mg thereafter).

Chronic Pain (ER Form Only)

Adult: **PO** 100–250 mg bid

Hepatic Impairment Dosage Adjustment

Moderate impairment: Reduce initial dose to 50 mg q 8 h. *Severe impairment (Child-Pugh class C):* Not recommended for use.

ADMINISTRATION

Oral

- Extended release (ER) tablets must be swallowed whole. They must not be cut, chewed, dissolved, or crushed due to risk of rapid release of a potentially fatal dose.
- On day 1 of therapy, a second dose may be given as soon as 1 h after the initial dose if pain relief is inadequate. All subsequent doses should be at 4–6 h intervals.
- Do not exceed a total daily dose of 700 mg on day 1 or 600 mg on subsequent days.
- When extended-release (ER) tablets are discontinued, a gradual downward titration of the dose should be used to prevent S&S of drug withdrawal.
- Do not administer if a paralytic ileus is suspected.
- Do not give within 14 days of an MAOI.
- Store at 15°–30° C (59°–86° F).

T

ADVERSE EFFECTS CV: Hot flush. **Respiratory:** Nasopharyngitis, respiratory depression, upper respiratory tract infection. **CNS:** *Headache*, abnormal dreams, anxiety, confusional state, *dizziness*, insomnia, lethargy, *somnolence*, tremor. **Endocrine:** Decreased appetite. **Skin:** Hyperhidrosis, pruritus, rash. **GI:** *Constipation*, dry mouth, dyspepsia, *nausea, vomiting*. **GU:** Urinary tract infection. **Musculoskeletal:** Arthralgia. **Other:** Fatigue.

INTERACTIONS Drug: Other OPIOID AGONISTS, GENERAL ANESTHETICS, PHENOTHIAZINES, ANTIEMETICS, other TRANQUILIZERS, SEDATIVES, HYPNOTICS, or other CNS DEPRESSANTS may cause additive CNS depression. MAO INHIBITORS can raise **norepinephrine** levels resulting in adverse cardiovascular events.

PHARMACOKINETICS Absorption: 32% bioavailability. **Peak:** 1.25 h. **Metabolism:** In liver. **Elimination:** Primarily renal. **Half-Life:** 4 h.

NURSING IMPLICATIONS

Black Box Warning

Tapentadol ER has been associated with serious, sometimes fatal, respiratory depression and with neonatal withdrawal syndrome.

Assessment & Drug Effects

- Monitor degree of pain relief, mental status, and level of alertness.
- Monitor vital signs. Withhold drug and notify prescriber for a respiratory rate of 12/min or less.
- If an opioid antagonist is required to reverse the action of tapentadol, continue to monitor respiratory status since respiratory depression may outlast duration of action of the opioid antagonists.
- Monitor for signs of misuse, abuse, and addiction.
- Withhold drug and report promptly S&S of serotonin syndrome (see Appendix F).

- Monitor ambulation. Fall precautions may be warranted.

Patient & Family Education

- Avoid engaging in hazardous activities until reaction to drug is known.
- Avoid alcohol while taking the extended release (ER) form of this drug.
- Consult prescriber before taking OTC drugs.

TASIMELTEON

(tas-i-mel′tee-on)

Hetlioz

Classification:
SEDATIVE-HYPNOTIC; MELATONIN RECEPTOR AGONIST
Therapeutic: SEDATIVE
Prototype: Ramelteon

AVAILABILITY Capsule, oral suspension

ACTION & *THERAPEUTIC EFFECT* Agonist of melatonin receptors MT1 and MT2. Activation of MT1 is thought to induce sleepiness, and MT2 activation is thought to help regulate circadian rhythms. *Improves insomnia or excessive sleepiness related to abnormal synchronization between the 24-h light–dark cycle and endogenous circadian rhythms.*

USES Treatment of non-24 h sleep–wake disorder (non-24); nighttime sleep disturbances in Smith-Magenis syndrome.

CONTRAINDICATIONS Severe hepatic impairment.

CAUTIOUS USE Concomitant drugs (including alcohol) that cause CNS DEPRESSION; mild-to-moderate hepatic impairment; older adults; pregnancy (adverse effects were observed in some animal reproduction studies); lactation. Safety and efficacy in children younger than 16 y not established.

ROUTE & DOSAGE

Sleep-Wake Disorder (Non-24)

Adult: **PO** 20 mg once daily at the same time before bedtime

ADMINISTRATION

- Administer without food.
- Give with food at approximately same time every night before bedtime.
- Capsules **must be** swallowed whole. They should not be opened or chewed.
- Store at 15°–30° C (59°–86° F). Protect from light and moisture.

ADVERSE EFFECTS **Respiratory:** Upper respiratory tract infection. **CNS:** Headache, nightmare/abnormal dreams. **Endocrine:** Increased ALT. **GU:** Urinary tract infection.

INTERACTIONS **Drug:** Tasimelteon may enhance the effects of other CNS DEPRESSANTS. Coadministration with strong CYP1A2 inhibitors (e.g., **fluvoxamine**) or strong CYP3A4 inhibitors (e.g., **ketoconazole**) may increase the levels of tasimelteon. Coadministration with strong CYP3A4 inducers (e.g., **carbamazepine, phenytoin, rifampin**) may decrease the levels of tasimelteon. **Food: Grapefruit** and **grapefruit juice** may increase the levels of tasimelteon. **Herbal: St. John's wort** decreases the levels of tasimelteon. Kratom increases risk of CNS depression.

PHARMACOKINETICS **Peak:** 0.5–3 h. **Distribution:** 90% plasma

T

protein bound. **Metabolism:** Extensive metabolism in liver. **Elimination:** Primarily renal. **Half-Life:** 1.3 h.

NURSING IMPLICATIONS

Assessment & Drug Effects

- Monitor for and report worsening insomnia and cognitive or behavioral changes.
- Monitor urinary output and report immediately dysuria or difficulty urinating.
- Assess risk for falls in older adults and otherwise frail persons.
- Monitor lab test: Baseline LFTs.

Patient & Family Education

- If drug cannot be taken at approximately the same time on a given night, that dose should be skipped.
- Do not drive or engage in potentially hazardous activities until response to drug is known.
- Do not consume alcohol while taking this drug.
- Report any of the following to prescriber: Worsening insomnia, cognitive or behavioral changes, difficulty with urination.

TAZAROTENE

(ta-zar′o-teen)

Avage, Tazorac

Classification: RETINOID; ANTIACNE

Therapeutic: ANTIACNE

Prototype: Isotretinoin

AVAILABILITY Gel; cream

ACTION & *THERAPEUTIC EFFECT*

Retinoid prodrug that blocks epidermal cell proliferation and hyperplasia. Suppresses inflammation present in the epidermis of psoriasis. *Effectiveness indicated by improvement in acne or psoriasis.*

USES Topical treatment of plaque psoriasis on up to 20% of the body, mild to moderate acne, facial fine wrinkling, mottled hypo- and hyperpigmentation (blotchy skin discoloration), and benign facial lentigines.

CONTRAINDICATIONS Hypersensitivity to tazarotene; pregnancy (category X), women who are or may become pregnant; lactation.

CAUTIOUS USE Concurrent administration with drugs that are photosensitizers (e.g., thiazide diuretics, tetracyclines); retinoid hypersensitivity. Safety and efficacy in children younger than 12 y not established.

ROUTE & DOSAGE

Plaque Psoriasis

Adult: **Topical** Apply thin film to affected area once daily in evening

Acne

Adult: **Topical** After cleansing and drying face, apply thin film to acne lesions once daily in evening

Fine Wrinkles

Adult: **Topical** Apply thin film of cream to affected area once daily

ADMINISTRATION

Topical

- Dry skin completely before application of a thin film of medication.
- Apply medication to no more than 20% of body surface in those with psoriasis.
- Apply only to affected areas; avoid contact with eyes and mucous membranes.

ADVERSE EFFECTS Skin: *Pruritus, burning/stinging, erythema, worsening of psoriasis, irritation, skin pain,* rash, desquamation of skin, irritant contact dermatitis, inflammation, fissuring, bleeding, dry skin, sunburn.

INTERACTIONS Drug: Increased risk of photosensitivity reactions with QUINOLONES (especially **sparfloxacin**), PHENOTHIAZINES, SULFONAMIDES, SULFONYLUREAS, TETRACYCLINES, THIAZIDE DIURETICS.

PHARMACOKINETICS Absorption: Rapidly absorbed through skin. **Distribution:** Active metabolite greater than 99% protein bound; crosses placenta, distributed into breast milk. **Metabolism:** Undergoes esterase hydrolysis to active metabolite AGN 190299. **Elimination:** In both urine and feces. **Half-Life:** 18 h.

NURSING IMPLICATIONS

Assessment & Drug Effects

- Monitor for photosensitivity in those concurrently using any of the following: Thiazides, tetracyclines, fluoroquinolones, phenothiazines, sulfonamides.

Patient & Family Education

- Understand fully the risk of serious fetal harm. Use reliable forms of effective contraception. Discontinue treatment and notify prescriber if pregnancy occurs.
- Alert: Immediately rinse thoroughly with water if contact with eyes occurs.
- Avoid all unnecessary exposure to sunlight or artificial UV light. If brief exposure is necessary, cover as much skin surface as possible and use sunscreens (minimum SPF 15).
- Do not apply to sunburned skin.
- Discontinue medication and notify prescriber if any of the following occur: Pruritus, burning, skin redness, excessive peeling, worsening of psoriasis.
- Limit application of topicals with strong skin-drying effects to skin areas being treated with tazarotene.

TEDIZOLID PHOSPHATE

(ted-i-zo'lid)

Sivextro

Classification: OXAZOLIDINONE ANTIBIOTIC

Therapeutic: ANTIBIOTIC

Prototype: Linezolid

AVAILABILITY Tablets, lyophilized power for injection

ACTION & *THERAPEUTIC EFFECT* Prevents formation of a functional 70S essential for the bacterial translation process, thus inhibiting protein synthesis and cell proliferation. *Bacteriostatic against enterococci, staphylococci, and streptococci.*

USES Treatment of acute bacterial skin and skin structure infections (ABSSSI) caused by designated susceptible bacteria.

CONTRAINDICATIONS *Clostridium difficile*-associated diarrhea, except of treatment thereof; neutrophil counts less than 1,000 cells/mm^3.

CAUTIOUS USE Colitis; cardiac arrhythmia; history of anemia; pregnancy (adverse events were observed in animal reproduction studies); lactation. Safety and efficacy in children younger than 18 y not established.

T

ROUTE & DOSAGE

Skin and Skin Structure Infection

Adult: **PO or IV** 200 mg once daily for 6–14 days

ADMINISTRATION

Oral

- Give without regard to food.
- Store at 15°–30° C (59°–86° F).

Intravenous

PREPARE: **IV Infusion:** Reconstitute vial with 4 mL SW. **Do not** shake. Swirl gently and let stand until dissolved and foam disperses. If needed, invert vial to completely dissolve and swirl gently to prevent foaming. Place vial upright, tilt, and insert a syringe into bottom corner to remove 4 mL. **Do not** invert the vial during extraction. Further dilute in 250 mL of NS. Invert bag gently to mix but do not shake.
ADMINISTER: **IV Infusion:** Give over 1 h. **Do not** give IV push or bolus. Flush line before/after with NS if used for other drugs or solutions.
INCOMPATIBILITIES: **Solution/additive:** Solutions containing divalent cations (e.g., Ca^{+2}, Mg^{+2}), Lactated Ringer's, Hartmann's Solution. **Y-site:** **Albumin, calcium salts, caspofungin, cyclosporine, dobutamine, doxycycline, esmolol, gentamicin, isavuconazonium, magnesium sulfate, nicardipine, penicillin G, phenytoin, tobramycin.**

- Store reconstituted solution for up to 24 h at room temperature or under refrigeration at 2°–8° C (36°–46° F).

ADVERSE EFFECTS **CV:** Tachycardia. **CNS:** Headache. **HEENT:** Asthenopia, blurred vision, visual impairment, vitreous floaters. **Endocrine:** Decreased white blood cell count, increased ALT and AST, decreased platelet count. **Skin:** Dermatitis, pruritus, urticarial. **GI:** *Clostridium difficile* colitis, diarrhea, nausea, vomiting. **GU:** Vulvovaginal infection. **Hematological:** Anemia. **Other:** Infusion-related reaction, hypersensitivity reaction.

INTERACTIONS **Drug:** Tedizolid may increase the levels of other drugs (e.g., **aproclonidine, benzafibrate, bupropion, carbamazepine, levodopa,** SEROTONIN 5-HT1D RECEPTOR AGONISTS) that require MAO for metabolism. Do not use with LIVE VACCINES. May have increased risk of adverse effects with MYELOSUPPRESSIVE AGENTS.

PHARMACOKINETICS **Absorption:** 91% Bioavailable. **Peak:** 3 h. **Distribution:** 70–90% plasma protein bound; distributes into adipose and skeletal muscle tissue. **Elimination:** Fecal (82%) and renal (18%). **Half-Life:** 12 h.

NURSING IMPLICATIONS

Assessment & Drug Effects

- Monitor for S&S of superinfection, including *C. difficile*-associated diarrhea (CDAD) and pseudomembranous colitis that may develop months after treatment.
- Monitor lab tests: Baseline CBC with differential.

Patient & Family Education

- Report promptly to prescriber if you develop frequent watery or bloody diarrhea even 2 mo or more after last dose of antibiotic.
- Consult with prescriber if you are a female who is or plans to become pregnant.
- Do not breast-feed without consulting prescriber.

T

TELAVANCIN HYDROCHLORIDE

(tel-a-van'sin)

Vibativ

Classification: ANTIBIOTIC; GLYCOPROTEIN

Therapeutic: ANTIBIOTIC

Prototype: Vancomycin

AVAILABILITY Powder for reconstitution and injection

ACTION & *THERAPEUTIC EFFECT* Inhibits cell wall synthesis of bacteria. It binds to the bacterial membrane and disrupts the barrier function of the cell membrane of gram-positive bacteria. *Effective against a broad range of gram-positive bacteria.*

USES Treatment of complicated skin and skin structure infections hospital-acquired and ventilator-associated pneumonia.

CONTRAINDICATIONS Hypersensitivity to telavancin or any component of the formulation; concomitant use of IV unfractionated heparin; QT prolongation.

CAUTIOUS USE Moderate or severe renal impairment; renal disease; elderly; ulcerative colitis; severe hepatic impairment; women of childbearing potential; pregnancy (may cause fetal harm); lactation. Safe use in children younger than 18 y has not been established.

ROUTE & DOSAGE

Complicated Skin and Skin Structure Infections

Adult: **IV** 10 mg/kg q24h for 5–14 days

Hospital-Acquired and Ventilator-Associated Bacterial Pneumonia

Adult: **IV** 10 mg/kg q24h × 7–21 days

Renal Impairment Dosage Adjustment

CrCl 30–50 mL/min: Decrease to 7.5 mg/kg q 24 h; *10–29 mL/min:* Decrease to 10 mg/kg q 48 h

ADMINISTRATION

Intravenous

PREPARE: **Infusion:** Reconstitute each 250 mg with 15 mL or each 750 mg vial with 45 mL of D5W or NS to yield 15 mg/mL. Mix thoroughly to dissolve. For doses of 150–800 mg, must further dilute in 100–250 mL of IV solution. For doses less than 100 mg or greater than 800 mg, should be further diluted in D5W, NS, or LR to a final concentration in the range of 0.6–8 mg/mL.

ADMINISTER: **Infusion:** Infuse over 60 min to minimize infusion-related reactions. ▪ Do not infuse through the same line with any other drugs or additives.

▪ Storage: Reconstituted vials or infusion solution should be used within 4 h if at room temperature or 72 h if refrigerated. **Important note:** The total time holding time for reconstituted vials plus infusion solution cannot exceed 4 h at room temperature or 72 h refrigerated.

ADVERSE EFFECTS **CNS:** Dizziness, metallic taste. **Endocrine:** Decreased appetite, *increased serum creatinine.* **Skin:** Pruritus, rash. **GI:** Abdominal pain, diarrhea, diarrhea, *nausea, vomiting.*

GU: *Foamy urine*, increased serum creatinine, renal insufficiency, acute renal failure. **Other:** Rigors, infusion site erythema and pain.

DIAGNOSTIC TEST INTERFERENCE

Telavancin may cause increases in ***PT, INR, aPTT,*** and ***ACT.*** Telavancin interferes with ***urine qualitative dipstick protein assays,*** as well as quantitative ***dye methods*** (e.g., ***pyrogallol red-molybdate***).

INTERACTIONS

Drug: Do not administer LIVE VACCINES. May diminish effects of IV heparin.

PHARMACOKINETICS

Distribution: 93% bound to albumin. **Metabolism:** Metabolized to 3-hydroxylated metabolites. **Elimination:** Primarily via the urine. **Half-Life:** 8–9 h.

NURSING IMPLICATIONS

Black Box Warning

Telavancin has been associated with new-onset or worsening renal impairment and fetal harm.

Assessment & Drug Effects

- Monitor for flushing of upper body, urticaria, pruritus, or rash during infusion. If syndrome develops, slow infusion immediately. If reaction does not cease, stop infusion and notify prescriber.
- Withhold drug and notify prescriber for CrCl of 50 mL/min or less.
- Monitor for and report promptly the onset of watery diarrhea with or without fever, passage of tarry or bloody stools, pus, or mucus.
- Monitor ECG with concurrent use of drugs known to prolong the QT interval.
- Monitor lab tests: Baseline C&S. Baseline and frequent (q48–72h) renal function tests throughout therapy.

Patient & Family Education

- Report promptly appearance of rash or itching during drug infusion.
- Report promptly loose stools or diarrhea even after completion of drug.
- Women should use effective means of contraception while on this drug. Notify prescriber if pregnancy occurs during treatment.

TELBIVUDINE

(tel-bi'vu-deen)

Classification: ANTIRETROVIRAL; NUCLEOSIDE REVERSE TRANSCRIPTASE INHIBITOR (NRTI)

Therapeutic: ANTIRETROVIRAL; NRTI

Prototype: Lamivudine

AVAILABILITY

Tablet

ACTION & THERAPEUTIC EFFECT

Its metabolite inhibits HBV DNA polymerase (reverse transcriptase) by competing with the natural nucleoside substrate. Incorporation into HBV viral DNA causes DNA chain termination, resulting in inhibition of HBV replication. *Effectiveness is measured by reducing the viral load and preventing infection of new hepatocytes.*

USES

Chronic hepatitis B infection.

CONTRAINDICATIONS Hypersensitivity to telbivudine; concurrent use with peginterferon alfa-2a; lactic acidosis; severe hepatomegaly with steatosis; peripheral neuropathy; lactation.

CAUTIOUS USE Moderate to severe renal impairment, hemodialysis; alcoholism; obesity in females; risk of hepatic disease; individuals with organ transplants; older adults; pregnancy (in hepatitis B-infected women (not coinfected by HIV), treatment guidelines suggest antiviral therapy to reduce the risk of perinatal transmission of hepatitis B in HBsAg-positive pregnant women). Safe use in children younger than 16 y has not been established.

ROUTE & DOSAGE

Chronic Hepatitis B

Adults/Adolescents (16 y or older): **PO** 600 mg/day; duration is variable based on HBeAg status, duration of HBV suppression, presence of cirrhosis

Renal Impairment Dosage Adjustment

CrCl 30–49 mL/min: 600 mg q48h; *CrCl less than 30 mL/min (not requiring dialysis):* 600 mg q72h; *CrCl less than 5–10 mL/min (ESRD):* 600 mg q96h

ADMINISTRATION

Oral

- May be given without regard to food.
- Store at 25° C (77° F).

ADVERSE EFFECTS **Respiratory:** *Cough,* pharyngolaryngeal pain. **CNS:** Fatigue, headache, dizziness, insomnia. **Endocrine:** *Increased CPK levels,* increased serum ALT and AST. **Skin:** Rash. **GI:** *Abdominal pain, diarrhea.* **Musculoskeletal:** Arthralgia, back pain, myalgia. **Other:** Neutropenia.

INTERACTIONS **Drug:** Coadministration with drugs that alter renal function may alter plasma concentrations of telbivudine. Do not use with **pegylated interferon alfa-2a** or **interferon alfa-2b** because of increased risk of peripheral neuropathy.

PHARMACOKINETICS **Peak:** 1–4 h. **Distribution:** Minimal protein binding; widely distributed in tissues. **Elimination:** in urine. **Half-Life:** 40–49 h.

NURSING IMPLICATIONS

Black Box Warning

Telbivudine has been associated with lactic acidosis and severe hepatomegaly with steatosis.

Assessment & Drug Effects

- Monitor for and report S&S of lactic acidosis (e.g., anorexia, nausea, vomiting, bloating, abdominal pain, malaise, tachycardia or other arrhythmia, and difficulty in breathing).
- Monitor for signs and symptoms of peripheral neuropathy
- Monitor lab tests: Periodic LFTs during and for several months after discontinuation of telbivudine; periodic renal function tests, serum creatine kinase.

Patient & Family Education

- Notify your provider if you are pregnant or breastfeeding.

- Report any of the following to a health care provider: Loss of appetite, nausea and vomiting, abdominal pain, palpitations, or difficulty breathing.

TELITHROMYCIN

(tel-i-thro-my′sin)

Ketek

Classification: ANTIBIOTIC; KETOLIDE

Therapeutic: ANTIBIOTIC

Prototype: Erythromycin

AVAILABILITY Tablet

ACTION & *THERAPEUTIC EFFECT* Results in inhibition of RNA-dependent protein synthesis of bacteria, thus resulting in cell death. Telithromycin concentrates in phagocytes where it works against intracellular respiratory pathogens. *Its broad spectrum of activity is effective against respiratory pathogens, including erythromycin- and penicillin-resistant pneumococci.*

USES Treatment of community-acquired pneumonia.

UNLABELED USES Sinusitis.

CONTRAINDICATIONS Macrolide antibiotic hypersensitivity; QT prolongation; ongoing proarrhythmic conditions such as hypokalemia, hypomagnesemia, significant bradycardia, myasthenia gravis; severe renal impairment or renal failure; viral infections.

CAUTIOUS USE History of GI disease; hepatic disease; history of hepatitis or jaundice; pregnancy (category C); lactation. Safety and efficacy in children not established.

ROUTE & DOSAGE

Community-Acquired Pneumonia

Adult: **PO** 800 mg daily for 7–10 days

Renal Impairment Dosage Adjustment

CrCl less than 30 mL/min: 600 mg daily (400 mg daily with concomitant hepatic impairment)

ADMINISTRATION

Oral

- May be administered with or without food.
- Do not administer concurrently with simvastatin, lovastatin, atorvastatin, Class 1A (e.g., quinidine, procainamide) or Class III (e.g., dofetilide) antiarrhythmic agents.
- Store at 15°–30° C (59°–86° F). Keep container tightly closed. Protect from light.

ADVERSE EFFECTS **CV:** Potential to cause QT_c prolongation. **CNS:** Headache, dizziness. **HEENT:** Blurred vision, diplopia, difficulty focusing. **Endocrine:** Elevated LFTs, liver failure. **GI:** *Diarrhea,* nausea, vomiting, loose stools, dysgeusia. **Musculoskeletal:** May exacerbate myasthenia gravis.

INTERACTIONS **Drug: Pimozide** or CLASS IA or CLASS III ANTIARRHYTHMICS may cause life-threatening arrhythmias; may increase concentrations of **atorvastatin, lovastatin, sim-vastatin,** BENZODIAZEPINES; **rifampin** decreases telithromycin levels; ERGOT DERIVATIVES (**ergotamine, dihydroergotamine**) may cause severe peripheral vasospasm; **theophylline** may exacerbate adverse GI effects. **Food: Grapefruit juice** (greater than 1 qt/day) may increase plasma concentrations and adverse effects.

PHARMACOKINETICS **Absorption:** 57% bioavailable. **Peak:** 1 h. **Metabolism:** 50% in liver (CYP3A4), 50% by CYP-independent mechanisms. **Elimination:** In urine and feces. **Half-Life:** 10 h.

NURSING IMPLICATIONS

Black Box Warning

Telithromycin has been associated with fatal respiratory failure in patients with myasthenia gravis and is contraindicated in these patients.

Assessment & Drug Effects

- Monitor ECG in patients at risk for QT_C interval prolongation (i.e., bradycardia).
- Withhold drug and notify prescriber for S&S of QT_C interval prolongation such as dizziness or fainting.
- Monitor for and report promptly S&S of liver dysfunction: Fatigue, anorexia, nausea, clay-colored stools, etc.
- Monitor lab tests: Baseline and periodic LFTs.

Patient & Family Education

- Stop taking drug and notify prescriber for episodes of dizziness or fainting; report signs of jaundice (yellow color of the skin and/or eyes), unexplained fatigue, loss of appetite, nausea, dark urine, or clay-colored stool.
- Exercise caution when engaging in potentially hazardous activities; visual disturbances (e.g., blurred vision, difficulty focusing, double vision) are potential side effects of this drug. If visual problems occur, avoid quick changes in viewing between close and distant objects.

TELMISARTAN

(tel-mi-sar′tan)

Micardis

Classification: ANGIOTENSIN II RECEPTOR ANTAGONIST; ANTIHYPERTENSIVE

Therapeutic: ANTIHYPERTENSIVE

Prototype: Losartan potassium

AVAILABILITY Tablet

ACTION & *THERAPEUTIC EFFECT* Selectively blocks the binding of angiotensin II to the AT_1 receptors in many tissues (e.g., vascular smooth muscles, adrenal glands). Blocks the vasoconstricting and aldosterone-secreting effects of angiotensin II, thus resulting in an antihypertensive effect. *Effectiveness is indicated by a reduction in BP.*

USES Treatment of hypertension, cardiovascular risk reduction.

CONTRAINDICATIONS Hypersensitivity to telmisartan; development of angioedema due to use of telmisartan; women of child bearing age; concurrent use of aliskiren in diabetics; pregnancy (category D); lactation.

CAUTIOUS USE CAD; hypertropic cardiomyopathy; CHF; oliguria; hypotension in volume depleted patients; renal artery stenosis; advanced renal impairment; biliary obstruction; liver dysfunction; renal impairment; older adults; pregnancy (category C first trimester, discontinue use as soon as detected). Safety and efficacy in children younger than 18 y not established.

T

ROUTE & DOSAGE

Hypertension

Adult: **PO** 20–40 mg daily, may increase to 80 mg/day

CV Risk Reduction

Adult: **PO** 80 mg/day

ADMINISTRATION

Oral

- Do not remove tablets from blister pack until immediately before administration.
- May be administered without regard to meals.
- Store at 15°–30° C (59°–86° F).

ADVERSE EFFECTS **CV:** Intermittent claudication. **Respiratory:** Upper respiratory tract infection. **CNS:** Dizziness, fatigue.

DIAGNOSTIC TEST INTERFERENCE May lead to false-negative aldosterone/renin ratio

INTERACTIONS **Drug: Telmisartan** may increase **digoxin** or **lithium** levels. Increased risk of hyptension with ACE INHIBITORS or other ANTIHYPERTENSIVES.

PHARMACOKINETICS **Absorption:** Dose dependent, 42% of 40 mg dose is absorbed. **Peak:** 0.5–1 h. **Distribution:** Greater than 99% protein bound. **Metabolism:** Minimally metabolized. **Elimination:** Primarily in feces. **Half-Life:** 24 h.

NURSING IMPLICATIONS

Black Box Warning

Telmisartan has been associated with fetal toxicity and death.

Assessment & Drug Effects

- Monitor BP carefully after initial dose; and periodically thereafter. Monitor more frequently with preexisting biliary obstructive disorders or hepatic insufficiency.
- Monitor dialysis patients closely for orthostatic hypotension.
- Monitor concomitant digoxin levels throughout therapy.
- Monitor lab tests: Periodic serum electrolytes, creatinine clearance, and BUN.

Patient & Family Education

- Report pregnancy to prescriber immediately.
- Allow between 2 and 4 wk for maximum therapeutic response.

TEMAZEPAM

(te-maz′e-pam)

Restoril

Classification: BENZODIAZEPINE; SEDATIVE-HYPNOTIC

Therapeutic: SEDATIVE

Prototype: Triazolam

Controlled Substance: Schedule IV

AVAILABILITY Capsule

ACTION & THERAPEUTIC EFFECT Believed to potentiate gamma-aminobutyric acid (GABA) neuronal inhibition. The sedative and anticonvulsant actions involve GABA receptors located in the limbic, neocortical, and mesencephalic reticular systems. *Reduces night awakenings and early morning awakenings; increases total sleep times, absence of rebound effects.*

USES To relieve insomnia.

CONTRAINDICATIONS Hypersensitivity reaction including

T

angioedema; ethanol intoxication; drug abuse; narrow-angle glaucoma; psychoses; women of childbearing age; abrupt discontinuation of temazepam; pregnancy (teratogenic effects have been observed with some benzodiazepines; use during pregnancy is contraindicated); lactation.

CAUTIOUS USE Severely depressed patient or one with suicidal thinking; history of drug abuse or dependence, acute intoxication; alcoholism; chronic pulmonary insufficiency; COPD; liver or kidney dysfunction; sleep apnea; debilitated individuals; older adults. Safe use in children younger than 18 y not established.

ROUTE & DOSAGE

Insomnia

Adult: **PO** 7.5–15 mg at bedtime; may increase as needed to 30 mg.

Geriatric: **PO** 7.5 mg at bedtime

ADMINISTRATION

Oral

- Give 20–30 min before bedtime.
- Store at 15°–30° C (59°–86° F). Protect from light.

ADVERSE EFFECTS **CV:** Palpitations, *hypotension*. **CNS:** *Drowsiness,* dizziness, lethargy, hangover effect. **HEENT:** Blurred vision. **Endocrine:** Decreased libido. **Skin:** Diaphoresis, skin rash. **GI:** Diarrhea. **Musculoskeletal:** Weakness.

INTERACTIONS **Drug: Alcohol,** CNS DEPRESSANTS, ANTICONVULSANTS potentiate CNS depression; **cimetidine** increases temazepam plasma levels, thus increasing its toxicity; may decrease antiparkinsonism effects of **levodopa;** may increase **phenytoin** levels; smoking decreases sedative effects. Do not use with **sodium oxybate. Herbal: Kava, kratom, valerian** may potentiate sedation.

PHARMACOKINETICS **Absorption:** Readily from GI tract; 98% protein bound. **Onset:** 30–50 min. **Peak:** 2–3 h. **Duration:** 10–12 h. **Distribution:** Crosses placenta; distributed into breast milk. **Metabolism:** In liver to oxazepam. **Elimination:** In urine. **Half-Life:** 8–24 h.

NURSING IMPLICATIONS

Assessment & Drug Effects

- Be alert to signs of paradoxical reaction (excitement, hyperactivity, and disorientation) in older adults. Psychoactive drugs are the most frequent cause of acute confusion in this age group.
- CNS adverse effects are more apt to occur in the patient with hypoalbuminemia, liver disease, and in older adults. Report promptly incidence of bradycardia, drowsiness, dizziness, clumsiness, lack of coordination. Supervise ambulation, especially at night.
- Monitor respiratory and cardiovascular status.

Patient & Family Education

- Be aware that improvement in sleep will not occur until after 2–3 doses of drug.
- Notify prescriber if dreams or nightmares interfere with rest. An alternate drug or reduced dose may be prescribed.
- Be aware that difficulty getting to sleep may continue. Drug effect is evidenced by the increased amount of rest once asleep.

- Consult prescriber if insomnia continues in spite of medication.
- Do not smoke after medication is taken.
- Do not use OTC drugs (especially for insomnia) without advice of prescriber.
- Consult prescriber before discontinuing drug especially after long-term use. Gradual reduction of dose may be necessary to avoid withdrawal symptoms.
- Avoid use of alcohol and other CNS depressants.
- Do not drive or engage in other potentially hazardous activities until response to drug is known. This drug may depress psychomotor skills and cause sedation.

TEMOZOLOMIDE

(tem-o-zol′o-mide)

Temodar

Classification: ANTINEOPLASTIC; IMIDAZOTETRAZINE DERIVATIVE

Therapeutic: ANTINEOPLASTIC

AVAILABILITY Capsule; solution for injection

ACTION & *THERAPEUTIC EFFECT* Cytotoxic agent with alkylating properties that are cell cycle nonspecific. Interferes with purine (e.g., guanine) metabolism and thus protein synthesis in rapidly proliferating cells. *Effectiveness is indicated by objective evidence of tumor regression.*

USES Adult patients with refractory anaplastic astrocytoma, glioblastoma multiforme with radiotherapy.

UNLABELED USES Malignant melanoma.

CONTRAINDICATIONS Hypersensitivity to temozolomide, or dacarbazine; severe bone marrow suppression; pregnancy (category D); lactation.

CAUTIOUS USE Bacterial or viral infection; severe hepatic or renal impairment; myelosuppression; prior radiotherapy or chemotherapy; older adults; children younger than 3 y.

ROUTE & DOSAGE

Astrocytoma

Adult: **PO/IV** 150 mg/m^2 daily days 1–5/28-day treatment cycle (may increase to 200 mg/m^2/day); subsequent doses are based on absolute neutrophil count on day 21 or at least 48 h before next scheduled cycle (see prescribing information for dosage adjustments based on neutrophil count)

Glioblastoma Multiforme

Adult: **PO** 75 mg/m^2 daily for 42 days with focal radiotherapy; after 4 wk, maintenance phase of 150–200 mg/m^2 on days 1–5 of 28-day cycle

ADMINISTRATION

Oral

- Give consistently with regard to food.
- Do not administer unless absolute neutrophil count greater than 1500/microliter and platelet count greater than 100,000/microliter.
- Do not open capsules. Avoid inhalation or contact with skin or mucous membranes, if accidentally opened/damaged.
- Store at room temperature, 15°–30° C (59°–86° F).

Intravenous

PREPARE: **Infusion:** Bring the 100 mg vial to room temperature, then reconstitute with 41 mL sterile water to yield 2.5 mg/mL. Gently swirl to dissolve but do not shake, and do not further dilute. Must use within 14 h of reconstitution, including infusion time.
ADMINISTER: **Infusion:** Infuse over 90 min. Flush line before and after with NS. Note: May be administered in the same line with NS but not with any other IV solution.

ADVERSE EFFECTS **CV:** *Peripheral edema.* **Respiratory:** Upper respiratory tract infection, pharyngitis, sinusitis, cough. **CNS:** *Convulsions, hemiparesis, dizziness, abnormal coordination, amnesia, insomnia,* paresthesia, somnolence, paresis, ataxia, dysphasia, abnormal gait, confusion, anxiety, depression. **HEENT:** Diplopia, abnormal vision. **Endocrine:** Adrenal hypercorticism. **Skin:** Rash, pruritus. **GI:** *Nausea, vomiting, constipation, diarrhea,* abdominal pain, anorexia. **GU:** Urinary incontinence. **Hematologic:** Anemia, neutropenia, thrombocytopenia, leukopenia, lymphopenia. **Other:** *Headache, fatigue, asthenia, fever,* back pain, myalgia, weight gain; viral infection.

INTERACTIONS **Drug: Valproic acid** may decrease **temozolomide** levels.

PHARMACOKINETICS **Absorption:** Rapidly. **Peak:** 1 h. **Metabolism:** Spontaneously metabolized to active metabolite MTIC. **Elimination:** Primarily in urine. **Half-Life:** 1.8 h.

NURSING IMPLICATIONS

Assessment & Drug Effects

- Monitor for S&S of toxicity: Infection, bleeding episodes, jaundice, rash, CNS disturbances.
- Monitor lab tests: Periodic CBC with differential and platelet count; periodic LFTs and routine serum chemistry, including serum calcium.

Patient & Family Education

- Take consistently with respect to meals.
- Report to prescriber signs of infection, bleeding, discoloration of skin or skin rash, dizziness, lack of balance, or other bothersome side effects promptly.
- Exercise caution with hazardous activities until response to drug is known.
- Use effective methods of contraception; avoid pregnancy.

TEMSIROLIMUS

(tem-si-ro-li′mus)

Torisel

Classification: BIOLOGIC RESPONSE MODIFIER; ANTINEOPLASTIC; KINASE INHIBITOR; mTOR INHIBITOR
Therapeutic: ANTINEOPLASTIC
Prototype: Erlotinib

AVAILABILITY Injectable

ACTION & *THERAPEUTIC EFFECT* Inhibits an intracellular protein that controls cell division in renal carcinoma and other tumor cells. *Results in arrest of growth in tumor cells.*

USES Treatment of advanced renal cell carcinoma.

UNLABELED USES Astrocytoma, mantle cell lymphoma (MCL).

CONTRAINDICATIONS Hypersensitivity reaction including anaphylaxis; live vaccines; intracranial bleeding; bilirubin greater than 1.5 X ULN; interstitial lung disease; bowel perforation; acute renal failure; pregnancy (category D); lactation.

CAUTIOUS USE Hypersensitivity to temsirolimus, sirolimus, or polysorbate 80, renal impairment; DM; hyperlipemia; respiratory disorders; perioperative period due to potential for abnormal wound healing; CNS tumors (primary or by metastasis); hepatic impairment; older adults; children.

ROUTE & DOSAGE

Renal Cell Carcinoma

Adult: **IV** 25 mg qwk

Dosage Adjustment

Regimen with a strong CYP3A4 inhibitor: 12.5 mg/wk
Regimen with a strong CYP3A4 inducer: 50 mg based on tolerability

Hepatic Impairment Adjustment

Dose reduction req1uired

ADMINISTRATION

Intravenous

Patients should receive prophylactic IV diphenhydramine 25–50 mg (or similar antihistamine) 30 min before each dose.

PREPARE: **IV Infusion:** Inject 1.8 mL of supplied diluent into the 25 mg/mL vial to yield 10 mg/mL. ▪ Withdraw the required dose and inject rapidly into a 250 mL DEHP-free container of NS. Invert to mix.

ADMINISTER: **IV Infusion:** Use DEHP-free infusion line with a 5 micron or less in-line filter. ▪ Infuse over 30–60 min. ▪ Complete infusion within 6 h of preparation.

INCOMPATIBILITIES: **Solution/additive:** Do not add other drugs or agents to temsirolimus IV solutions.

▪ Store at 2°–8° C (36°–46° F). Protect from light. The 10 mg/mL drug solution is stable for up to 24 h at 15°–30° C (59°–86° F).

ADVERSE EFFECTS **CV:** Hypertension, thrombophlebitis, venous thromboembolism. **Respiratory:** Cough, dyspnea, epistaxis, interstitial lung disease, pharyngitis, pneumonia, rhinitis, upper respiratory tract infection. **CNS:** Depression, dysgeusia, headache, insomnia. **HEENT:** Conjunctivitis. **Endocrine:** *Elevated alkaline phosphatase, elevated AST, elevated serum creatinine,* hypokalemia, *hypophosphatemia,* hyperbilirubinemia, *hypercholesterolemia, hyperglycemia, hypertriglyceridemia,* weight loss. **Skin:** Acne, dry skin, nail disorder, pruritus, *rash*. **GI:** Abdominal pain, *anorexia,* constipation, diarrhea, fatal bowel perforation, *mucositis, nausea,* vomiting. **GU:** Urinary tract infection. **Musculoskeletal:** Arthralgia, back pain, myalgia. **Hematologic:** Decrease hemoglobin, *leukocytopenia, lymphopenia,* neutropenia, thrombocytopenia. **Other:** Allergic/hypersensitivity reactions, *asthenia,* chest pain, chills, *edema,* impaired wound healing, infections, pain, pyrexia.

INTERACTIONS Drug: AZOLE ANTIFUNGAL AGENTS (**fluconazole, itraconazole, ketoconazole, posaconazole, voriconazole), cyclosporine,** INHIBITORS OF CYP3A4 (HIV PROTEASE INHIBITORS, **clarithromycin, diltiazem**), **mycophenolate mofetil,** and **sunitinib** increase the plasma levels of **temsirolimus.** INDUCERS OF CYP3A4 (**dexamethasone, rifampin, rifabutin, phenytoin**) decrease the plasma level of temsirolimus. **Food: Grapefruit** and **grapefruit juice** increase the plasma level of temsirolimus. **Herbal: St. John's wort** decreases the plasma level of temsirolimus.

PHARMACOKINETICS Peak: 0.5–2 h. **Metabolism:** In liver. **Elimination:** Primarily in stool. **Half-Life:** 17.3 h.

NURSING IMPLICATIONS

Assessment & Drug Effects

- Withhold drug and notify prescriber for absolute neutrophil count less than 1000/mm³ or platelet count less than 75,000/mm³.
- Monitor for infusion-related reactions during and for at least 1 h after completion of infusion.
- Slow or stop infusion for infusion-related reactions. If infusion is restarted after 30–60 min of observation, slow rate to up to 60 min and continue observation.
- Monitor respiratory status and report promptly dyspnea, cough, S&S of hypoxia, fever.
- Monitor diabetics for loss of glycemic control.
- Monitor lab tests: Baseline and periodic CBC with differential and platelet count, lipid profile, LFTs, alkaline phosphatase, renal function tests, serum electrolytes, plasma glucose, and ABGs.

Patient & Family Education

- Avoid live vaccines and close contact with those who have received live vaccines.
- Use effective contraceptive measures to prevent pregnancy.
- Men with partners of childbearing age should use reliable contraception throughout treatment and for 3 mo after the last dose of temsirolimus.
- Report promptly any of the following: S&S of infection, difficulty breathing, abdominal pain, blood in stools, abnormal wound healing, S&S of hypersensitivity (see Appendix F).

TENAPANOR

(ten-A-pa-nor)

Ibsrela

Classifications: SODIUM/HYDROGEN EXCHANGER 3 (NHE3) INHIBITOR

Therapeutic: SODIUM/HYDROGEN EXCHANGER 3 (NHE3) INHIBITOR

AVAILABILITY Oral tablet

ACTION & *THERAPEUTIC EFFECT* A sodium/hydrogen exchange inhibitor which acts locally to reduce sodium absorption from the small intestine and colon. *Reduced sodium absorption results in increased intestinal lumen water secretion, accelerated intestinal transit time, and softening of stool consistency.*

USES Treatment of irritable bowel syndrome with constipation (IBS-C) in adults.

CONTRAINDICATIONS Patients < 6 years of age; known or suspected mechanical GI obstruction.

CAUTIOUS USE Use with caution if patient experiencing diarrhea or has existing renal impairment, is pregnant, or lactating.

ROUTE & DOSAGE

Irritable Bowel Syndrome with constipation (IBS-C)

Adult: **PO** 50 mg twice a day

ADMINISTRATION

Oral

- Administer immediately prior to breakfast or the first meal of the day and immediately before dinner.
- Store at 20° to 25° C (68° to 77° F). Store in original container to protect from moisture.

ADVERSE EFFECTS GI: Diarrhea, flatulence, abdominal distension.

INTERACTIONS No reported drug interactions

PHARMACOKINETICS Distribution: 99% protein bound. **Metabolism:** In the liver primarily by CYP3A4/5. **Elimination:** 65% in feces (unchanged drug).

NURSING IMPLICATIONS

Assessment & Drug Effects

- Monitor frequency of bowel movements and for signs and symptoms of dehydration in patients with diarrhea.
- Monitor lab tests: Serum potassium in patients with renal impairment.

Patient & Family Education

- Notify your doctor or get medical help right away if you have any of the following signs or symptoms of allergic reaction such as rash, hives, itching; red, swollen, blistered, or peeling skin with or without fever; wheezing; tightness in the chest or throat; trouble breathing, swallowing, or talking; unusual hoarseness; or swelling of the mouth, face, lips, tongue, or throat; or any dizziness or passing out.

TENECTEPLASE RECOMBINANT

(ten-ect′e-plase)

TNKase

Classification: THROMBOLYTIC ENZYME, TISSUE PLASMINOGEN ACTIVATOR (t-PA)

Therapeutic: THROMBOLYTIC ENZYME

Prototype: Alteplase

AVAILABILITY Vial

ACTION & *THERAPEUTIC EFFECT* Activates plasminogen, a substance created by endothelial cells in response to arterial wall injury that contributes to clot formation. Plasminogen is converted to plasmin which breaks down the fibrin mesh that binds the clot together, thus dissolving the clot. *Effective in producing thrombolysis of a clot involved in a myocardial infarction.*

USES Reduction of mortality associated with acute myocardial infarction (AMI).

CONTRAINDICATIONS Active internal bleeding; history of CVA; intracranial or intraspinal surgery with 2 mo; intracranial neoplasm; arteriovenous malformation, or aneurysm; known bleeding diathesis; brain tumor; increased intracranial pressure; coagulopathy; head trauma; stroke; surgery;

severe uncontrolled hypertension; lactation.

CAUTIOUS USE Recent major surgery, previous puncture of compressible vessels, CVA, recent GI or GU bleeding, recent trauma; hypertension, mitral valve stenosis, acute pericarditis, bacterial endocarditis; severe liver or kidney disease; hemorrhagic ophthalmic conditions; septic thrombophlebitis or occluded, infected AV cannula; advanced age; pregnancy (category C). Safety and efficacy in children not established.

ROUTE & DOSAGE

Acute Myocardial Infarction

Adult (weight less than 60 kg): **IV** Infuse dose over 5 sec 30 mg; *weight 60–70 kg:* 35 mg; *weight 70–80 kg:* 40 mg; *weight 80–90 kg:* 45 mg; *weight greater than 90 kg:* 50 mg

ADMINISTRATION

Intravenous

PREPARE: **Direct:** Read and follow instructions supplied with TwinPak™ Dual Cannula Device. ▪ Withdraw 10 mL of sterile water for injection from the supplied vial; inject entire contents into the TNKase vial directing the diluent stream into the powder. ▪ Gently swirl until dissolved but do not shake. The resulting solution contains 5 mg/mL. ▪ Withdraw the appropriate dose and discard any unused solution. ▪ Follow directions supplied with TwinPak™ for proper handling of syringe.

ADMINISTER: **Direct:** Dextrose-containing IV line **must be** flushed before and after bolus with NS. ▪ Give as a single bolus dose over 5 sec. ▪ The total dose given should not exceed 50 mg.

INCOMPATIBILITIES: **Solution/additive: Dextrose** solutions.

▪ Store unopened TwinPak™ at or below 30° C (86° F) or under refrigeration at 2°–8° C (36°–46° F).

ADVERSE EFFECTS **Hematologic:** Major bleeding, *hematoma,* GI bleed, bleeding at puncture site, hematuria, pharyngeal, epistaxis.

DIAGNOSTIC TEST INTERFERENCE Unreliable results for ***coagulation test I*** and measures of ***fibrinolytic activity.***

PHARMACOKINETICS **Metabolism:** In liver. **Half-Life:** 90–130 min.

NURSING IMPLICATIONS

Assessment & Drug Effects

- Avoid IM injections and unnecessary handling or invasive procedures for the first few hours after treatment.
- Monitor for S&S of bleeding. Should bleeding occur, withhold concomitant heparin and antiplatelet therapy; notify prescriber.
- Monitor cardiovascular and neurologic status closely. Persons at increased risk for life-threatening cardiac events include those with: A high potential for bleeding, recent surgery, severe hypertension, mitral stenosis and atrial fibrillation, anticoagulant therapy, and advanced age.
- Coagulation parameters may not predict bleeding episodes.

Patient & Family Education

- Notify prescriber of the following immediately: A sudden, severe headache; any sign of bleeding; signs or symptoms of hypersensitivity (see Appendix F).

T

- Stay as still as possible and do not attempt to get out of bed until directed to do so.

TENOFOVIR DISOPROXIL FUMARATE

(ten-o-fo′vir dy-so-prox′il fum′a-rate)

Viread

Classification: ANTIRETROVIRAL; NUCLEOTIDE REVERSE TRANSCRIPTASE INHIBITOR (NRTI)

Therapeutic: ANTIRETROVIRAL; NRTI

Prototype: Lamivudine

AVAILABILITY Tablet; oral powder

ACTION & *THERAPEUTIC EFFECT*

A potent inhibitor of retroviruses, including HIV-1. The active form of tenofovir persists in HIV-infected cells for prolonged periods, thus, it results in sustained inhibition of HIV replication. *It reduces the viral load (plasma HIV-RNA), and CD4 counts.*

USES In combination with other antiretrovirals for the treatment of HIV; chronic hepatitis B infection.

CONTRAINDICATIONS Hypersensitivity to tenofovir.

CAUTIOUS USE Hepatic dysfunction, alcoholism; renal impairment; obesity; low body weight; pathologic bone fractures; lactic acidosis, severe hepatomegaly, concurrent administration of nephrotoxic agents, acute renal failure; immune reconstitution syndrome; lactation; older adults; pregnancy (no increased risk of overall birth defects has been observed following first trimester exposure); children.

ROUTE & DOSAGE

HIV Infection

Adult: **PO** 300 mg once daily with meal
Adolescent/ Child: **PO** See package insert for weight based dose (approx. 8 mg/kg daily)

Chronic Hepatitis B

Adult/Child (12 y or older, weight 35 kg): **PO** 300 mg daily duration is variable based on HBeAg status, duration of HBV suppression, presence of cirrhosis
Child (2 y or older, weight at least 10 kg): **PO** 8 mg/kg once daily (max dose 300 mg/day)

Renal Impairment Dosage Adjustment

CrCl 30–49 mL/min: Dose q48h; *10–29 mL/min:* Dose q72–96 hours

Hemodialysis Dosage Adjustment

Dose weekly or after 12 h of dialysis

ADMINISTRATION

Oral

- Give at the same time each day with a meal.
- Measure powder form only with supplied dosing scoop. One level scoop contains 40 mg of tenofovir. Mix powder in 2–4 oz of soft food such as applesauce or yogurt (do not mix with liquid) and swallow immediately after mixing to avoid bitter taste.
- Store at room temperature; excursions to 25° C (77° F) are permitted.

ADVERSE EFFECTS **Respiratory:** Sinusitis, upper respiratory tract infection, nasopharyngitis, pneumonia. **CNS:** Headache, insomnia, pain, dizziness, depression, fatigue, anxiety, peripheral neuropathy. **Endocrine:** Increased *creatine kinase,* AST, ALT, serum amylase, cholesterol, triglycerides, serum glucose. **Skin:** Skin rash, pruritis. **GI:** *Nausea,* vomiting, diarrhea, flatulence, abdominal pain, anorexia. **GU:** Increased serum creatinine, renal failure. **Hematologic:** Neutropenia. **Musculoskeletal:** Decreased bone mineral density, increased CPK, weakness, back pain, arthralgia. **Other:** Fever.

INTERACTIONS **Drug:** May increase **didanosine** toxicity; **acyclovir, amphotericin B, cidofovir, foscarnet, ganciclovir, probenecid, valacyclovir, valganciclovir,** NSAIDs may increase tenofovir toxicity by decreasing its renal elimination. Do not use with **adefovir, diclofenac, ledipasvir.** **Food:** Food increases absorption.

PHARMACOKINETICS **Absorption:** Bioavailability 25% fasting, 40% with high fat meal. **Peak:** 1 h. **Distribution:** Less than 7% protein bound. **Metabolism:** Not metabolized by CYP450 enzyme system. **Elimination:** Renally eliminated. **Half-Life:** 11–14 h.

NURSING IMPLICATIONS

Black Box Warning

Tenofovir has been associated with lactic acidosis and severe, sometimes fatal, hepatomegaly with steatosis, and with posttreatment exacerbation of hepatitis.

Assessment & Drug Effects

- Withhold drug and notify prescriber if patient develops clinical or lab findings suggestive of lactic acidosis or pronounced hepatotoxicity (e.g., hepatomegaly and steatosis even in the absence of marked transaminase elevations).
- Monitor for S&S of bone abnormalities (e.g., bone pain, stress fractures).
- Monitor closely patients receiving other nephrotoxic agents for changes in serum creatinine and phosphorus. Withhold drug and notify prescriber for creatinine clearance less than 60 mL/min.
- Monitor lab tests: Baseline and periodic CBC with differential, reticulocyte count, creatine kinase, CD4 count, HIV RNA plasma levels, serum phosphorus, renal function tests, LFTs, urine protein, bone density, and HBV (prior to first treatment).

Patient & Family Education

- Take this drug exactly as prescribed. Do not miss any doses. If you miss a dose, take it as soon as possible and then take your next dose at its regular time. If it is almost time for your next dose, do not take the missed dose. Wait and take the next dose at the regular time. Do not double the next dose.
- Report any of the following to prescriber: Unexplained anorexia, nausea, vomiting, abdominal pain, fatigue, dark urine.

TERAZOSIN

(ter-ay′zoe-sin)

Classification: ALPHA-ADRENERGIC RECEPTOR ANTAGONIST; ANTIHYPERTENSIVE

T

Therapeutic: ANTIHYPERTENSIVE; BPH AGENT
Prototype: Prazosin

AVAILABILITY Capsule

ACTION & *THERAPEUTIC EFFECT* Selectively blocks alpha$_1$-adrenergic receptors in vascular smooth muscle in many tissues, including the bladder neck and the prostate. Promotes vasodilation, thus producing relaxation that leads to reduction of peripheral vascular resistance and lowered BP as well as increased urine flow. *Effectiveness is measured in lowering of blood pressure values and controlling the symptoms of benign prostate hypertrophy.*

USES Management of hypertension; to treat symptoms of benign prostatic hypertrophy (BPH).

CONTRAINDICATIONS Hypersensitivity to terazosin.

CAUTIOUS USE Prostate cancer; history of hypotensive episodes; angina; renal impairment, renal disease, renal failure; older adults; pregnancy (adverse effects have been noted in animal reproduction studies); lactation. Safe use in children is not established.

T

ROUTE & DOSAGE

Hypertension

Adult: **PO** Start with 1 mg daily, titrate based on response up to 20 mg daily (single or divided doses)

Benign Prostatic Hypertrophy

Adult: **PO** Start with 1 mg at bedtime, then titrate up as needed, most patients require 10 mg/day (max: 20 mg/day)

ADMINISTRATION

Oral

- Give initial dose at bedtime to reduce the potential for severe hypotensive effect. Administer at the same time each day.
- Store at 20°–25° C (68°–77° F) in tightly closed container away from heat and strong light. Do not freeze.

ADVERSE EFFECTS **CV:** Orthostatic hypotension, peripheral edema. **Respiratory:** *Nasal congestion.* **CNS:** Myasthenia, *dizziness,* drowsiness. **GI:** *Nausea.*

INTERACTIONS **Drug:** Antihypertensive effects may be attenuated by NSAIDS. **Sildenafil, vardenafil, tadalafil, obintuzumab,** and ANTIHYPERTENSIVES may enhance hypotensive effects. Avoid use of **alfuzosin** or **tranylcypromine** due to increased hypotension risk.

PHARMACOKINETICS **Absorption:** Readily from GI tract (90–94% protein bound). **Peak:** 1–2 h. **Metabolism:** In liver. **Elimination:** 60% in feces, 40% in urine. **Half-Life:** 9–12 h.

NURSING IMPLICATIONS

Assessment & Drug Effects

- Be alert for possible first-dose phenomenon (precipitous decline in BP with consciousness

disturbance). This is rare; occurs within 90–120 min of initial dose.
- Monitor BP at end of dosing interval (just before next dose) to determine level of antihypertensive control.
- Be aware that drug-induced decrease in BP appears to be more position dependent (i.e., greater in the erect position) during the first few hours after dosing than at end of 24 h.
- A greatly diminished hypotensive response at end of 24 h indicates need for change in dosage (increased dose or twice daily regimen). Report to prescriber.

Patient & Family Education

- Avoid situations that would result in injury should syncope (loss of consciousness) occur after first dose. If faintness develops, lie down promptly.
- Make position changes slowly (i.e., change in direction or from recumbent to upright posture). Dangle legs and move ankles a minute or so before standing when arising. Orthostatic hypotension (greatest shortly after dosing) can pose a problem with ambulation.
- Do not drive or engage in potentially hazardous activities for at least 12 h after first dose, after dosage increase, or when treatment is resumed after interruption of therapy.
- Do not alter established drug regimen. Consult prescriber if drug is omitted for several days. Drug will be started with the initial dosing regimen.
- Keep scheduled appointments for assessment of BP control and other clinically significant tests.

TERBINAFINE HYDROCHLORIDE

(ter-bin′a-feen)

Lamisil, Lamisil DermaGel

Classification: ANTIBIOTIC; ANTIFUNGAL

Therapeutic: ANTIFUNGAL

AVAILABILITY Tablet; cream; gel

ACTION & *THERAPEUTIC EFFECT*

Synthetic antifungal agent that inhibits sterol biosynthesis in fungi and ultimately causes fungal cell death. *Effective as an antifungal.*

USES Topical treatment of superficial mycoses such as interdigital tinea pedis, tinea cruris, and tinea corporis; oral treatment of onychomycosis due to tinea unguium.

CONTRAINDICATIONS Hypersensitivity to terbinafine; alcoholism; hepatic disease; hepatitis; jaundice; renal impairment; renal failure; lactation.

CAUTIOUS USE History of depression; pregnancy (category B). Safety and efficacy in children younger than 12 y not established.

ROUTE & DOSAGE

Tinea Pedis, Tinea Cruris, or Tinea Corporis

Adult: **Topical** Apply daily or bid to affected and immediately surrounding areas until clinical signs and symptoms are significantly improved (1–7 wk)

T

Onychomycosis

Adult: **PO** 250 mg daily × 6 wk for fingernails or × 12 wk for toenails

ADMINISTRATION

Oral

- Give tablets without regard to meals.
- Granules should be given with food. Sprinkle on a spoonful of soft, nonacidic food; do not mix granules with applesauce or other fruit-based foods. Entire spoonful should be swallowed without chewing.

Topical

- Apply externally. Avoid application to mucous membranes and avoid contact with eyes.
- Do not use occlusive dressings unless specifically directed to do so by prescriber.
- Store at 15°–30° C (59°–86° F).

ADVERSE EFFECTS **CNS:** *Headache.* **HEENT:** Taste disturbances, vision impairment. **Skin:** Pruritus, local burning, dryness, rash, vesiculation, redness, contact dermatitis at application site. **GI:** Diarrhea, dyspepsia, abdominal pain, liver test abnormalities, liver failure (rare). **Hematologic:** Neutropenia (rare).

T

INTERACTIONS **Drug:** May increase **theophylline** levels; may decrease **cyclosporine** levels; **rifampin** may decrease **terbinafine** levels.

PHARMACOKINETICS **Absorption:** 70% PO; approximately 3.5% of topical dose is absorbed systemically. **Elimination:** In urine. **Half-Life:** 36 h.

NURSING IMPLICATIONS

Assessment & Drug Effects

- Monitor for and report increased skin irritation.

Patient & Family Education

- Learn correct technique for application of cream.
- Notify prescriber if drug causes increased skin irritation or sensitivity.
- Be aware that medication **must be** used for full treatment time to be effective.

TERBUTALINE SULFATE

(ter-byoo′te-leen)

Classification: BETA-ADRENERGIC RECEPTOR AGONIST; BRONCHODILATOR

Therapeutic: RESPIRATORY SMOOTH MUSCLE RELAXANT; BRONCHODILATOR

Prototype: Albuterol

AVAILABILITY Tablet; solution for injection

ACTION & *THERAPEUTIC EFFECT* Synthetic adrenergic stimulant with selective $beta_2$-receptor activity in bronchial smooth muscles, inhibits histamine release from mast cells, and increases ciliary motility. *Relieves bronchospasm in chronic obstructive pulmonary disease (COPD) and significantly increases vital capacity. Increases uterine relaxation (thereby preventing or abolishing high intrauterine pressure).*

USES Asthma, prevention and reversal of bronchospasm.

UNLABELED USES To delay delivery in preterm labor.

CONTRAINDICATIONS Known hypersensitivity to sympathomimetic amines; severe hypertension and coronary artery disease; tachycardia with digitalis intoxication; within 14 days of MAO inhibitor therapy; angle-closure glaucoma; acute or maintenance tocolysis; prolonged use during preterm labor.

CAUTIOUS USE Angina, stroke, hypertension; DM; thyrotoxicosis; history of seizure disorders; MAOI therapy; cardiac arrhythmias; QT prolongation; thyroid disease; older adults; kidney and liver dysfunction; pregnancy (category C). Use caution in second and third trimester (may inhibit uterine contractions and labor). Children younger than 12 y.

ROUTE & DOSAGE

Bronchodilator

Adult/Adolescent (15 y or older): **PO** 5 mg tid at 6 h intervals (max: 15 mg/day); **Subcutaneous** 0.25 mg q20min for 3 doses
Adolescent (12–15 y): **PO** 2.5 mg tid at 6 h intervals (max: 7.5 mg/day); **Subcutaneous** 0.25 mg q15–30min up to 0.5 mg in 4 h

ADMINISTRATION

Oral

- Give with fluid of patient's choice; tablets may be crushed.
- Be certain about recommended doses: PO preparation, 2.5 mg; subcutaneous, 0.25 mg. A decimal point error can be fatal.
- Give with food if GI symptoms occur.
- Administer around-the-clock to promote less variation in peak and trough serum levels.

Subcutaneous

- Give subcutaneous injection into lateral deltoid area.
- Store all forms at 15°–30° C (59°–86° F); protect from light. Do not freeze.

ADVERSE EFFECTS **CNS:** Nervousness, restlessness. **Endocrine:** Decreased serum potassium, increased serum glucose. **Musculoskeletal:** Tremor.

DIAGNOSTIC TEST INTERFERENCE Terbutaline may increase ***blood glucose*** and free ***fatty acids.***

INTERACTIONS **Drug: Epinephrine,** other SYMPATHOMIMETIC BRONCHODILATORS may add to effects; MAO INHIBITORS, TRICYCLIC ANTIDEPRESSANTS potentiate action on vascular system; effects of both BETA-ADRENERGIC BLOCKERS and terbutaline antagonized.

PHARMACOKINETICS **Absorption:** 33–50% from GI tract. **Onset:** 30 min PO; less than 15 min subcutaneous; 5–30 min inhaled. **Peak:** 2–3 h PO; 30–60 min subcutaneous; 1–2 h inhaled. **Duration:** 4–8 h PO; 1.5–4 h subcutaneous; 3–4 h inhaled. **Distribution:** Into breast milk. **Metabolism:** In liver. **Elimination:** Primarily in urine, 3% in feces. **Half-Life:** 3–4 h.

NURSING IMPLICATIONS

Black Box Warning

Terbutaline has been associated with serious, sometimes fatal, adverse reactions in pregnant women including cardiac arrhythmias, myocardial ischemia, hypokalemia, and pulmonary edema.

T

Assessment & Drug Effects

- Assess vital signs: Baseline pulse and BP and before each dose. If significantly altered from baseline level, consult prescriber. Cardiovascular adverse effects are more apt to occur when drug is given by subcutaneous route or it is used by a patient with cardiac arrhythmia.
- Most adverse effects are transient, however, rapid heart rate may persist for a relatively long time.
- Aerosolized drug produces minimal cardiac stimulation or tremors.
- Be aware that muscle tremor is a fairly common adverse effect that appears to subside with continued use.
- Monitor patient being treated for premature labor for CV S&S for 12 h after drug is discontinued. Report tachycardia promptly.
- Monitor I&O ratio. Fluid restriction may be necessary. Consult prescriber.
- Monitor serum potassium, glucose.

Patient & Family Education

- Inhalator therapy: Review instructions for use of inhalator (included in the package).
- Learn how to take your own pulse and the limits of change that indicate need to notify the prescriber.
- Consult prescriber if breathing difficulty is not relieved or if it becomes worse within 30 min after an oral dose.
- Consult prescriber if symptomatic relief wanes; tolerance can develop with chronic use.
- Do not self-dose this drug, particularly during long-term therapy. In the face of waning response, increasing the dose will not improve the clinical condition and may cause overdosage. Understand that decreasing relief with continued treatment indicates need for another bronchodilator, not an increase in dose.
- Do not puncture container, use or store it near heat or open flame, or expose to temperatures above 49° C (120° F), which may cause bursting. Contents of the aerosol (inhalator) are under pressure.
- Do not use any other aerosol bronchodilator while being treated with aerosol terbutaline. Do not self-medicate with an OTC aerosol.
- Do not use OTC drugs without prescriber approval. Many cold and allergy remedies, for example, contain a sympathomimetic agent that when combined with terbutaline may cause harmful adverse effects.

TERCONAZOLE

(ter-con'a-zole)

Terazol 7, Terazol 3

Classification: AZOLE ANTIFUNGAL

Therapeutic: VAGINAL ANTIFUNGAL

Prototype: Fluconazole

AVAILABILITY Vaginal cream; vaginal suppository

ACTION & *THERAPEUTIC EFFECT* Thought to exert antifungal activity by disruption of normal fungal cell membrane permeability. *Exhibits fungicidal activity against* Candida albicans.

USES Local treatment of vulvovaginal candidiasis.

CONTRAINDICATIONS Hypersensitivity to terconazole or azole antifungals; use of tampons; lactation.

CAUTIOUS USE Pregnancy (category C). Safety and efficacy in children younger than 18 y not established.

ROUTE & DOSAGE

Candidiasis

Adult: **Intravaginal** One suppository (2.5 g) each night × 3 days; one applicator full of 0.4% cream each night × 7 days; one applicator full of 0.8% cream each night × 3 days

ADMINISTRATION

Intravaginal

- Insert applicator high into the vagina (except during pregnancy).
- Wash applicator before and after each use.
- Store away from direct heat and light.

ADVERSE EFFECTS **CNS:** *Headache*. **GU:** Vaginal itching, burning, irritation. **Other:** Rash, flu-like syndrome (fever, chills, headache, hypotension).

INTERACTIONS **Drug:** May inactivate **nonoxynol-9** spermicides.

PHARMACOKINETICS **Absorption:** Slow minimal absorption from vagina. **Onset:** Within 3 days. **Metabolism:** In liver. **Elimination:** Half in urine, half in feces. **Half-Life:** 4–11 h.

NURSING IMPLICATIONS

Assessment & Drug Effects

- Do not use if patient has a history of allergic reaction to other antifungal agents, such as miconazole.
- Monitor for sensitization and irritation; these may indicate need to discontinue drug.

Patient & Family Education

- Use correct application technique.
- Do not use tampons concurrently with terconazole.
- Learn potential adverse reactions, including sensitization and allergic response.
- Be aware that terconazole may interact with diaphragms and latex condoms; avoid concurrent use within 72 h.
- Refrain from sexual intercourse while using terconazole.
- Wear only cotton underwear; change daily.

TERIFLUNOMIDE

(ter-i-flu′no-mide)

Aubagio

Classification: IMMUNOMODULATOR; PYRIMIDINE SYNTHESIS INHIBITOR; ANTI-INFLAMMATORY

Therapeutic: IMMUNOMODULATOR; ANTI-INFLAMMATORY

AVAILABILITY Tablet

ACTION & *THERAPEUTIC EFFECT* An immunomodulatory agent with anti-inflammatory properties; exact mechanism of action unknown, but may involve a reduction in the number of activated lymphocytes in the CNS. *Reduces the number of MS relapses.*

USES Treatment of patients with relapsing forms of multiple sclerosis.

CONTRAINDICATIONS Severe liver impairment; coadministration with leflunomide; acute renal failure; pregnancy (category X); lactation.

CAUTIOUS USE Pre-existing liver disease; myelosuppression; serious infections; DM; history of

T

peripheral neuropathy; hypertension. Safety and efficacy in children younger than 18 y not established.

ROUTE & DOSAGE

Multiple Sclerosis

Adult: **PO** 7 or 14 mg once daily

ADMINISTRATION

Oral

- May give with or without food.
- Store at 15°–30° C (59°–86° F).

ADVERSE EFFECTS **CV:** Palpitations. **Respiratory:** Bronchitis, sinusitis, upper respiratory tract infection. **CNS:** Anxiety, burning sensation, carpal tunnel syndrome, headache, *paraesthesia*, sciatica. **HEENT:** Blurred vision, conjunctivitis. **Endocrine:** ALT and AST increased, gamma-glutamyl-transferase increased, hypophosphatemia, neutrophil count decreased, white blood cell count decreased hepatotoxicity. **Skin:** Acne, *alopecia*, pruritus. **GI:** Abdominal distension, *diarrhea, nausea*, toothache, upper abdominal pain, viral gastroenteritis. **GU:** Cystitis. **Musculoskeletal:** Musculoskeletal pain, myalgia. **Hematological:** Leukopenia, neutropenia. **Other:** *Influenza*, oral herpes, seasonal allergy.

T

INTERACTIONS **Drug:** Teriflunomide may increase the levels of other drugs requiring CYP2C8 for metabolism (e.g., **paclitaxel, pioglitazone, repaglinide, rosiglitazone**) and may decrease the levels of other drugs requiring CYP1A2 for metabolism (e.g., **alosetron, duloxetine, theophylline, tizanidine**). Teriflunomide may decrease the effectiveness of **warfarin.** Teriflunomide can increase the levels of **ethinylestradiol** and **levonorgestrel.**

PHARMACOKINETICS **Peak:** 1–4 h. **Distribution:** Greater than 99% plasma protein bound. **Metabolism:** Primarily unchanged in liver. **Elimination:** Fecal (61%) and renal (23%). **Half-Life:** 18–19 d.

NURSING IMPLICATIONS

Black Box Warning

Teriflunomide has been associated with severe liver injury, including fatal liver failure; it has also been associated with major birth defects.

Assessment & Drug Effects

- Monitor BP especially in those with a history of hypertension.
- Monitor for and report promptly S&S of hepatotoxicity (see Appendix F). Withhold drug until prescriber consulted if hepatotoxicity suspected.
- Assess for peripheral neuropathy (e.g., bilateral numbness or tingling of hands or feet) and S&S of hypokalemia (see Appendix F).
- Monitor lab tests: Baseline (within last 6 mo before beginning therapy) CBC with differential and LFTs; monthly LFTs for next 6 mo or more often when given with other potentially hepatotoxic drugs.

Patient & Family Education

- Report promptly any of the following: Numbness or tingling of hands or feet; unexplained nausea, vomiting, or abdominal pain; fatigue; anorexia; jaundice and/or dark urine; fever.
- Consult with prescriber before accepting a vaccination during

and for 6 mo following termination of therapy.

- Women should use effective contraception during treatment and until completion of an accelerated, drug-elimination procedure.
- Men should instruct their female partners to use reliable contraception. Those who wish to father a child should discontinue the drug and request an accelerated drug-elimination procedure.

TERIPARATIDE

(ter-i-par′a-tide)

Forteo

Classification: PARATHYROID HORMONE AGONIST

Therapeutic: PARATHYROID HORMONE AGONIST

AVAILABILITY Solution for injection

ACTION & *THERAPEUTIC EFFECT* Parathyroid hormone (PTH) is the primary regulator of calcium and phosphate metabolism in bone and kidney. Biological actions of PTH and teriparatide are similar in bone and kidneys. *Stimulates new bone formation by preferential stimulation of osteoblastic activity over osteoclastic activity; improves bone microarchitecture, and increases bone mass and strength by stimulating new bone formation.*

USES Treatment of osteoporosis.

CONTRAINDICATIONS Hypersensitivity to teriparatide; osteosarcoma; Paget's disease; unexplained elevations of alkaline phosphatase; bone metastases or a history of skeletal malignancies; metabolic bone diseases other than osteoporosis; preexisting hypercalcemia; prior history of radiation therapy involving the skeleton; pediatric patients or young adults with open epiphyses; lactation.

CAUTIOUS USE Active or recent urolithiasis, hypercalciuria; hypotension; concurrent use of digitalis; hepatic, renal, and cardiac disease; pregnancy (category C); children younger than 18 y.

ROUTE & DOSAGE

Osteoporosis

Adult: **Subcutaneous** 20 mcg daily

ADMINISTRATION

Subcutaneous

- Do not administer to anyone with hypercalcemia. Consult prescriber.
- Rotate subcutaneous injection sites.

ADVERSE EFFECTS **CV:** Hypertension, angina, syncope. **Respiratory:** Rhinitis, cough, pharyngitis, dyspnea, pneumonia. **CNS:** Headache, dizziness, depression, insomnia, vertigo. **Endocrine:** *Transient increase in calcium levels,* increase in serum uric acid, antibodies to teriparatide after 12 mo therapy. **Skin:** Rash, sweating. **GI:** Nausea, constipation, dyspepsia, vomiting. **Musculoskeletal:** *Arthralgia,* leg cramps. **Other:** *Pain,* asthenia, neck pain.

INTERACTIONS **Drug:** May increase risk of **digoxin** toxicity.

PHARMACOKINETICS **Absorption:** Extensively absorbed from subcutaneous site. **Onset:** 2 h for calcium concentration increase. **Peak:** Max calcium concentrations 4–6 h. **Duration:** 16–24 h. **Metabolism:** Parathyroid hormone is metabolized by nonspecific enzymes. **Elimination:** Primarily in urine. **Half-Life:** 1 h subcutaneous.

NURSING IMPLICATIONS

Black Box Warning

Teriparatide has been associated with development of osteosarcoma in laboratory animals, and it should not be prescribed for those at increased baseline risk for osteosarcoma.

Assessment & Drug Effects

- Monitor cardiovascular status including BP and subjective reports of angina.
- Concurrent drugs: Monitor closely for digoxin toxicity with concurrent use.
- Monitor lab tests: Periodic serum calcium, alkaline phosphatase, and uric acid.

Patient & Family Education

- Report unexplained leg cramps and bone pain.
- Learn correct technique for subcutaneous injection.

TESAMORELIN ACETATE

(tes′a-moe-rel′in as′e-tate)

Egrifta

Classification: GROWTH HORMONE RELEASING FACTOR ANALOG; GROWTH HORMONE MODIFIER

Therapeutic: GROWTH HORMONE MODIFIER

AVAILABILITY Powder for reconstitution and injection

ACTION & *THERAPEUTIC EFFECT* Binds to pituitary growth hormone-releasing factor receptors and stimulates the secretion of endogenous growth hormone which has anabolic and lipolytic properties. *Reduces fat deposition in those with HIV-associated lipodystrophy.*

USES Reduction of excess abdominal fat in HIV-infected patients with lipodystrophy.

CONTRAINDICATIONS Active malignancy; hypersensitivity to tesamorelin and/or mannitol; suppression of the hypothalamic-pituitary from hypophysectomy, hypopituitarism, pituitary tumor/surgery, head irradiation or trauma; pregnancy (category X); lactation.

CAUTIOUS USE Acute illness or trauma; injection site reactions; nonmalignant neoplasms; renal or hepatic impairment; conditions resulting in or associated with fluid retention (e.g., edema, carpal tunnel syndrome); glucose intolerance or diabetes; retinopathy; age 65 y and older. Safety and efficacy in children not established.

ROUTE & DOSAGE

Lipodystrophy in HIV Patients

Adult: **Subcutaneous** 2 mg once daily

ADMINISTRATION

Subcutaneous

- Use provided diluent only.
- Reconstitute 2 mg vial with 2.1 mL diluent; gently roll vial for 30 sec to mix; do not shake.
- When using 1 mg vials, to produce a 2 mg dose, reconstitute the first 1 mg vial with 2.2 mL diluent; gently roll vial (do not shake) for 30 sec to mix; reconstitute the second 1 mg vial with the entire solution from first vial; gently roll

vial (do not shake) for 30 sec to mix.

- Use immediately after preparation. Rotate injection sites.
- Store dry vials at 2°–8° C (36°–46° F). Protect from light. Reconstituted solution should be discarded if not used immediately.

ADVERSE EFFECTS **CV:** Hypertension, palpitations. **CNS:** Depression, hypesthesia, insomnia, paresthesia, peripheral neuropathy. **Endocrine:** Increased blood creatine phosphate. **Skin:** Hot flush, night sweats, pruritus, rash, urticarial. Erythema, hemorrhage, irritation, pain, pruritus, rash reaction, swelling, urticaria at injection site. **GI:** Dyspepsia, nausea, upper abdominal pain, vomiting. **Musculoskeletal:** *Arthralgia*, carpal tunnel syndrome, joint stiffness and swelling, muscle spasm, muscle pain, musculoskeletal pain, musculoskeletal stiffness, *myalgia, pain in extremity*. **Other:** Chest pain, pain, peripheral edema.

INTERACTIONS **Drug:** Tesamorelin may decrease the enzymatic activation of **cortisone** and **prednisone**. Tesamorelin may alter the metabolism of compounds requiring CYP450 enzymes; careful monitoring is suggested.

PHARMACOKINETICS **Peak:** 15 min. **Half-Life:** 26–38 min.

NURSING IMPLICATIONS

Assessment & Drug Effects

- Evaluate abdominal girth with periodic measurements at the level of the umbilicus.
- Assess for injections site reactions (i.e., erythema, pruritus, pain, irritation, and bruising).
- Monitor prediabetics and diabetics for loss of glycemic control.
- Monitor lab tests: Baseline and frequent IGF-1 level baseline and periodic FBG and HbA1C.

Patient & Family Education

- Seek immediate medical attention for any of the following: Rash or hives; swelling of face or throat; shortness of breath or trouble breathing; rapid heartbeat; feeling of faintness or fainting.
- Notify your prescriber if you experience swelling, an increase in joint pain, or pain or numbness in your hands or wrist (carpal tunnel syndrome).
- Women should discontinue tesamorelin and notify prescriber if pregnancy occurs.
- If diabetic, monitor fasting and postprandial blood glucose as directed.

TESTOSTERONE

(tess-toss′ter-one)

Androderm, AndroGel, Axiron, Foresta, Natesto, STRIANT, Testim, Testopel, Vogelxo

TESTOSTERONE CYPIONATE

Depo-Testosterone

TESTOSTERONE ENANTHATE

Delatestryl, Malogex ♣

Classification: ANDROGEN/ ANABOLIC STEROID; ANTINEOPLASTIC
Therapeutic: ANTINEOPLASTIC; ANABOLIC STEROID
Controlled Substance: Schedule III

T

AVAILABILITY **Testosterone:** Implantable pellet; transdermal patch; transdermal gel; intranasal gel; buccal tablet. **Testosterone Cypionate:** IM injection. **Testosterone Enanthate:** IM injection

ACTION & *THERAPEUTIC EFFECT* Synthetic steroid compound with both androgenic and anabolic activity. Controls development and maintenance of secondary sexual characteristics. **Androgenic activity:** Responsible for the growth spurt of the adolescent, onset of puberty, and for growth termination by epiphyseal closure. **Anabolic activity:** Increases protein metabolism and decreases its catabolism. Large doses suppress spermatogenesis, thereby causing testicular atrophy. *Antagonizes effects of estrogen excess on female breast and endometrium. Responsible for the growth spurt of the adolescent male and onset of puberty.*

USES Androgen replacement therapy, delayed puberty (male), hypogonadism, palliation of female mammary cancer (1–5 y postmenopausal), palliative treatment of breast cancer, and to treat postpartum breast engorgement. Available in fixed combination with estrogens in many preparations.

CONTRAINDICATIONS Hypersensitivity or toxic reactions to androgens; benzoic acid or benzyl alcohol hypersensitivity; serious cardiac, liver, or kidney disease; hypercalcemia; known or suspected prostatic or breast cancer in male; BPH with obstruction; asthenic males who may react adversely to androgenic overstimulation; conditions aggravated by fluid retention; hypertension; DVT; hepatic dysfunction as a result of use of testosterone; older adults; pregnancy (category X); possibility of virilization of external genitalia of female fetus; lactation.

CAUTIOUS USE Cardiac, liver, and kidney disease; prepubertal males; DM; history of MI; CAD; BPH; older adults; acute intermittent porphyria.

ROUTE & DOSAGE

Male Hypogonadism

Adult: **IM Cypionate, Enanthate** 50–400 mg q2–4wk; **IM Propionate** 10–25 mg 2–3/wk; **Topical** Start with 6 mg/day system applied daily, if scrotal area inadequate, use 4 mg/day system; **Androderm** Apply to torso; **AndroGel** Apply one packet to upper arms, shoulders, or abdomen once daily; **Striant** Apply one patch to the gum region just above the incisor tooth q12h

Delayed Puberty

Adult: **IM Cypionate, Enanthate** 50–200 mg q2–4wk; **Subcutaneous** 2–6 pellets inserted q3–6mo; **IM Propionate** up to 100 mg per mo

Metastatic Breast Cancer

Adult: **IM Cypionate, Enanthate** 200–400 mg q2–4wk; **IM Propionate** 50–100 mg 3 × wk

ADMINISTRATION

Buccal

- Apply buccal patch to gum just above the incisor tooth.

Nasal

- Instruct not to blow nose or sniff for 1 h after receiving Natesto.

Transdermal

- Apply transdermal system on clean, dry scrotal skin. Dry shave scrotal hair for optimal skin contact. Do not use chemical depilatories. Wear patch for 22–24 h.
- Topical gel preparations may be applied to shoulders and upper arms.
- Store at 15°–30° C (59°–86° F).

Intramuscular

- Give IM injections deep into gluteal musculature.
- Store IM formulations prepared in oil at room temperature. Warming and shaking vial will redisperse precipitated crystals.

ADVERSE EFFECTS **CV:** Skin flushing and vascularization. **CNS:** Excitation, insomnia. **Endocrine:** Hypercalcemia, hypercholesterolemia, *sodium and water retention (especially in older adults) with edema*. Renal calculi (especially in the immobilized patient); bladder irritability; female—suppression of ovulation, lactation, or menstruation; hoarseness or deepening of voice (often irreversible); hirsutism; oily skin; clitoral enlargement; regression of breasts; male-pattern baldness (in disseminated breast cancer); flushing, sweating; vaginitis with pruritus, drying, bleeding; menstrual irregularities. Male—prepubertal-premature epiphyseal closure, phallic enlargement, priapism. Postpubertal—testicular atrophy, decreased ejaculatory volume, azoospermia, oligospermia (after prolonged administration or excessive dosage), impotence, epididymitis, priapism, *gynecomastia*. **Skin:** *Acne*, injection site irritation and sloughing, pruritus. **GI:** Nausea, vomiting, anorexia, diarrhea, gastric pain, jaundice. **GU:** *Increased libido*. **Hematologic:** Leukopenia. Precipitation of acute intermittent porphyria. **Other:** Hypersensitivity to testosterone, anaphylactoid reactions (rare).

DIAGNOSTIC TEST INTERFERENCE Testosterone alters ***glucose tolerance*** tests; decreases ***thyroxine-binding globulin concentration*** (resulting in decreased ***total*** T_4 serum levels and increased ***resin of*** T_3 and T_4). Increases ***creatinine*** and ***creatinine*** excretion (lasting up to 2 wk after therapy is discontinued) and alters response to ***metyrapone test***. It suppresses ***clotting factors II, V, VII, X*** and decreases excretion of ***17-ketosteroids***. May increase or decrease ***serum cholesterol***.

INTERACTIONS **Drug:** ORAL ANTICOAGULANTS may potentiate hypoprothrombinemia. May decrease **insulin** requirements. May have increased concentration if used with **ceritinib, conivaptan, topotecan.**

PHARMACOKINETICS **Absorption:** **Cypionate** and **enanthate** are slowly absorbed from lipid tissue. **Duration:** 2–4 wk **cypionate** and **enanthate**. **Distribution:** 98% bound to sex hormone-binding globulin. **Metabolism:** Primarily in liver. **Elimination:** 90% in urine, 6% in feces. **Half-Life:** 10–100 min.

NURSING IMPLICATIONS

Assessment & Drug Effects

- Check I&O and weigh patient daily during dose adjustment period. Weight gain (due to sodium and water retention) suggests need for decreased dosage. When dosage is stabilized, urge patient to check weight at least twice weekly and to report increases, particularly if accompanied by edema in dependent areas. Dose adjustment and diuretic therapy may be started.
- Monitor serum calcium closely. Androgenic therapy is usually terminated if serum calcium rises above 14 mg/dL.
- Report S&S of hypercalcemia (see Appendix F) promptly. The immobilized patient is particularly prone to develop hypercalcemia,

T

which indicates progression of bone metastasis in patients with metastatic breast cancer. Treatment includes withdrawing testosterone and checking calcium, phosphate, and BUN levels daily.
- Instruct diabetic to report sweating, tremor, anxiety, vertigo. Testosterone-induced anabolic action enhances hypoglycemia (hyperinsulinism). Dosage adjustment of antidiabetic agent may be required.
- Observe patients on concomitant anticoagulant treatment for signs of overdosage (e.g., ecchymoses, petechiae). Report promptly to prescriber; anticoagulant dose may need to be reduced.
- Monitor prepubertal or adolescent males throughout therapy to avoid precocious sexual development and premature epiphyseal closure. Skeletal stimulation may continue 6 mo beyond termination of therapy.
- Monitor lab tests: Periodic serum cholesterol, serum electrolytes, and LFTs.

Patient & Family Education

- Review directions for application of transdermal patches.
- Report soreness at injection site, because a postinjection site boil may be an associated adverse reaction.
- Report priapism (sustained and often painful erections occurring especially in early replacement therapy), reduced ejaculatory volume, and gynecomastia to prescriber. Symptoms indicate necessity for temporary withdrawal or discontinuation of testosterone therapy.
- Notify prescriber promptly if pregnancy is suspected or planned. Masculinization of the fetus is most likely to occur if testosterone (androgen) therapy is provided during first trimester of pregnancy.
- Androgens may cause virilism in women at dosage required to treat carcinoma. Report increase in libido (early sign of toxicity), growth of facial hair, deepening of voice, male-pattern baldness. The onset of hoarseness can easily be overlooked unless its significance as an early and possibly irreversible sign of virilism is appreciated. Reevaluation of treatment plan is indicated.

TETRACAINE HYDROCHLORIDE

(tet′ra-kane)

Pontocaine

Classification: LOCAL ANESTHETIC (ESTER TYPE)

Therapeutic: LOCAL ANESTHETIC

Prototype: Procaine HCl

AVAILABILITY Solution for injection; powder; solution; cream; gel; ointment; ophthalmic solution

ACTION & *THERAPEUTIC EFFECT*

A potent and toxic local anesthetic that depresses initial depolarization phase of the action potential, thus preventing propagation and conduction of the nerve impulse. *Effectiveness indicated by loss of sensation and motor activity in circumscribed body areas close to injection or application site.*

USES Spinal anesthesia (high, low, saddle block) and topically to produce surface anesthesia. **Eye:** To anesthetize conjunctiva and cornea prior to superficial procedures (including tonometry, gonioscopy, removal of foreign bodies or sutures, corneal scraping). **Nose and Throat:** To abolish laryngeal and esophageal reflexes prior to bronchoscopy, esophagoscopy. **Skin:** To relieve pruritus, pain, burning.

T

CONTRAINDICATIONS Debilitated patients; prolonged use of ophthalmic preparations; known hypersensitivity to tetracaine or other local anesthetics of ester type (e.g., procaine, chloroprocaine, cocaine), sulfite, or to PABA or its derivatives; coagulopathy; anticoagulant therapy; thrombocytopenia; increased bleeding time; infection at application or injection site.

CAUTIOUS USE Shock; cachexia, cardiac decompensation; QT prolongation; older adults; pregnancy (category C); lactation; children younger than 16 y.

ROUTE & DOSAGE

Local Anesthesia

Adult: **Topical** Before procedure, 1–2 drops of 0.5% solution or 1.25–2.5 cm of ointment in lower conjunctival fornix or 0.5% solution or ointment to nose or throat; **Spinal** 1% solution diluted with equal volume of 10% dextrose injected in subarachnoid space

ADMINISTRATION

Topical

- Avoid use of solutions that are cloudy, discolored, or crystallized.
- When tetracaine is used on mucosa of larynx, trachea, or esophagus, the manufacturer recommends adding 0.06 mL of a 0.1% epinephrine solution to each mL tetracaine solution to slow absorption of the anesthetic.
- Store ophthalmic solution and ointment at 15°–30° C (59°–86° F); refrigerate topical. Avoid freezing. Use tight, light-resistant containers.

ADVERSE EFFECTS **CV:** Bradycardia, arrhythmias, hypotension. **CNS:** Postspinal headache, headache, spinal nerve paralysis, anxiety, nervousness, seizures. **HEENT:** Stinging; corneal erosion, retardation or prevention of healing of corneal abrasion, transient pitting and sloughing of corneal surface, dry corneal epithelium; dry mucous membranes, prolonged depression of cough reflex. **Other:** Anaphylactic reactions, convulsions, faintness, syncope.

INTERACTIONS **Drug:** May antagonize effects of SULFONAMIDES.

PHARMACOKINETICS **Onset:** 1 min eye; 3 min mucosal surface; 3 min spinal. **Duration:** Up to 15 min eye; 30–60 min mucosal surface; 1.5–3 h spinal. **Metabolism:** In liver and plasma. **Elimination:** In urine.

NURSING IMPLICATIONS

Assessment & Drug Effects

- Recovery from anesthesia to the pharyngeal area is complete when patient has feeling in the hard and soft palates and when muscles in the faucial (tonsillar) pillars contract with stimulation.
- Do not give food or liquids until these normal pharyngeal responses are present (usually about 1 h after anesthetic administration). The first small amount of liquid (water) should be given under supervision of care provider.
- Be aware that increased blood concentration of the drug may result from excess application of tetracaine to the skin (to relieve pruritus or burning), application to debrided or infected skin surfaces, or too rapid injection rate.
- High blood concentrations of tetracaine can lead to adverse systemic effects involving CNS and CV systems: Convulsions, respiratory arrest, dysrhythmias, cardiac arrest.

Patient & Family Education

- Do not use ophthalmic drug longer than prescribed period. Prolonged use to eye surface may cause corneal epithelial erosions and retard healing of corneal surface.
- Natural barriers to eye infection and injury are removed by the anesthesia. Do not rub eye after drug instillation until anesthetic effect has dissipated (evidenced by return of blink reflex). Patching for temporary protection of the corneal epithelium may be ordered.
- Wash or disinfect hands before and after self-administration of solutions or ointment.

TETRACYCLINE HYDROCHLORIDE

(tet-ra-sye′kleen)

Novotetra ✦, Sumycin

Classification: ANTIBIOTIC; TETRACYCLINE

Therapeutic: ANTIBIOTIC

AVAILABILITY Capsule; suspension

ACTION & *THERAPEUTIC EFFECT* Tetracyclines exert antiacne action by suppressing growth of *Propionibacterium acnes* within sebaceous follicles. *Effective against a variety of gram-positive and gram-negative bacteria and against most chlamydiae, mycoplasmas, rickettsiae, and certain protozoa (e.g., amebae). Exerts antiacne action against* Propionibacterium acnes.

USES Chlamydial infections (e.g., lymphogranuloma venereum, psittacosis, trachoma, inclusion conjunctivitis, nongonococcal urethritis); mycoplasmal infections (e.g., *Mycoplasma pneumoniae*); rickettsial infections (e.g., Q fever, Rocky Mountain spotted fever, typhus); spirochetal infections: Relapsing fever *(Borrelia)*, leptospirosis, syphilis (penicillin-hypersensitive patients); amebiasis; uncommon gram-negative bacterial infections [e.g., brucellosis, shigellosis, cholera, gonorrhea (penicillin-hypersensitive patients), granuloma inguinale, tularemia]; gram-positive infections (e.g., tetanus). Also used orally (solution) for inflammatory acne vulgaris.

UNLABELED USES Actinomycosis, acute exacerbations of chronic bronchitis; Lyme disease; pericardial effusion (metastatic); acute PID; sexually transmitted epididymo orchitis; with quinine for multi-drug-resistant strains of *Plasmodium falciparum* malaria; anti-infective prophylaxis for rape victims; recurrent cystic thyroid nodules; melioidosis; and as fluorescence test for malignancy.

CONTRAINDICATIONS Hypersensitivity to tetracyclines; severe renal or hepatic impairment, common bile duct obstruction; UV exposure; pregnancy (category D); lactation.

CAUTIOUS USE History of kidney or liver dysfunction; myasthenia gravis; history of allergy, asthma, hay fever, urticaria; undernourished patients; infants, children younger than 8 y.

ROUTE & DOSAGE

Systemic Infection

Adult: **PO** 250–500 mg bid–qid (1–2 g/day)

Child (8 y or older): **PO** 25–50 mg/kg/day in 2–4 divided doses

Acne

Adult/Child (8 y or older): **PO** 500–1000 mg/day in 4 divided doses

T

ADMINISTRATION

Oral

- Give with a full glass of water on an empty stomach at least 1 h before or 2 h after meals (food, milk, and milk products can reduce absorption by 50% or more).
- Do not give immediately before bed.
- Give with food if patient is having GI symptoms (e.g., nausea, vomiting, anorexia); do not give with foods high in calcium such as milk or milk products.
- Shake suspension well before pouring to ensure uniform distribution of drug. Use calibrated liquid measure to dispense.
- Check expiration date for all tetracyclines. Fanconi-like syndrome (renal tubular dysfunction) and also an LE-like syndrome have been attributed to outdated tetracycline preparations.
- Tetracycline decomposes with age, exposure to light, and when improperly stored under conditions of extreme humidity, heat, or cold. The resultant product may be toxic.
- Store at 15°–30° C (59°–86° F) in tightly covered container in dry place. Protect from light.

ADVERSE EFFECTS **CNS:** Headache, intracranial hypertension (rare). **HEENT:** Pigmentation of conjunctiva due to drug deposit. **Skin:** Dermatitis, *phototoxicity:* Discoloration of nails, onycholysis (loosening of nails); cheilosis; fixed drug eruptions particularly on genitalia; thrombocytopenic purpura; urticaria, rash, exfoliative dermatitis; with topical applications: Skin irritation, dry scaly skin, transient stinging or burning sensation, slight yellowing of skin at application site, acute contact dermatitis. **GI:** Reported mostly for oral administration, but also may occur with parenteral tetracycline (*nausea, vomiting,* epigastric distress, heartburn, *diarrhea,* bulky loose stools, steatorrhea, *abdominal discomfort, flatulence,* dry mouth); dysphagia, retrosternal pain, esophagitis, esophageal ulceration with oral administration, abnormally high liver function test values, decrease in serum cholesterol, fatty degeneration of liver [jaundice, increasing nitrogen retention (azotemia), hyperphosphatemia, acidosis, irreversible shock]; foul-smelling stools or vaginal discharge, stomatitis, glossitis; black hairy tongue (lingua nigra), diarrhea: Staphylococcal enterocolitis. **GU:** Particularly in patients with kidney disease; increase in BUN/serum creatinine, renal impairment even with therapeutic doses; Fanconi-like syndrome (outdated tetracycline) (characterized by polyuria, polydipsia, nausea, vomiting, glycosuria, proteinuria acidosis, aminoaciduria); vulvovaginitis, pruritus vulvae or ani (possibly hypersensitivity). **Other:** Drug fever, angioedema, serum sickness, anaphylaxis. Pancreatitis, local reactions: Pain and irritation (IM site), Jarisch-Herxheimer reaction.

DIAGNOSTIC TEST INTERFERENCE TETRACYCLINES may cause false increases in ***urinary catecholamines*** (by ***fluorometric methods***), and false decreases in ***urinary urobilinogen.*** Parenteral TETRACYCLINES containing ***ascorbic acid*** reportedly may produce false-positive ***urinary glucose*** determinations by ***copper reduction methods*** (e.g., ***Benedict's reagent, Clinitest***); TETRACYCLINES may cause false-negative results with ***glucose oxidase methods*** (e.g., ***Clinistix, TesTape***).

INTERACTIONS Drug: ANTACIDS, **calcium**, and **magnesium** bind tetracycline in gut and decrease absorption. ORAL ANTICOAGULANTS potentiate hypoprothrombinemia. ANTIDIARRHEAL AGENTS with **kaolin** and pectin may decrease absorption. Effectiveness of ORAL CONTRACEPTIVES decreased. **Methoxyflurane** may produce fatal nephrotoxicity. **Food:** Dairy products and **iron, zinc** supplements decrease tetracycline absorption.

PHARMACOKINETICS Absorption: 75–80% of dose absorbed. **Peak:** 2–4 h. **Distribution:** Widely distributed, preferentially binds to rapid growing tissues; crosses placenta; enters breast milk. **Metabolism:** Not metabolized; enterohepatic cycling. **Elimination:** 50–60% in urine within 72 h. **Half-Life:** 6–12 h.

NURSING IMPLICATIONS

Assessment & Drug Effects

- Report GI symptoms (e.g., nausea, vomiting, diarrhea) to prescriber. These are generally dose-dependent, occurring mostly in patients receiving 2 g/day or more and during prolonged therapy. Frequently, symptoms are controlled by reducing dosage or administering with compatible foods.
- Be alert to evidence of superinfections (see Appendix F). Regularly inspect tongue and mucous membrane of mouth for candidiasis (thrush). Suspect superinfection if patient complains of irritation or soreness of mouth, tongue, throat, vagina, or anus, or persistent itching of any area, diarrhea, or foul-smelling excreta or discharge.
- Withhold drug and notify prescriber if superinfection develops. Superinfections occur most frequently in patients receiving prolonged therapy, the debilitated, or those who have diabetes.
- Monitor I&O in patients receiving parenteral tetracycline. Report oliguria or any changes in appearance of urine or in I&O.
- Monitor lab tests: Periodic renal function tests, LFTs, and hematopoietic function tests, particularly during high-dose, long-term therapy.

Patient & Family Education

- Report onset of diarrhea to prescriber. It is important to determine whether diarrhea is due to irritating drug effect or superinfections or pseudomembranous colitis (caused by overgrowth of toxin-producing bacteria: *Clostridium difficile*) (see Appendix F). The latter two conditions can be life threatening and require immediate withdrawal of tetracycline and prompt initiation of symptomatic and supportive therapy.
- Reduce incidence of superinfection (see Appendix F) by meticulous care of mouth, skin, and perineal area. Rinse mouth of food debris after eating; floss daily and use a soft-bristled toothbrush.
- Avoid direct exposure to sunlight during and for several days after therapy is terminated to reduce possibility of photosensitivity reaction (appearing like an exaggerated sunburn).
- Exercise caution with potentially hazardous activities until reaction to drug is known.
- Report immediately sudden onset of painful or difficult swallowing (dysphagia) to prescriber. Esophagitis and esophageal ulceration have been associated with bedtime administration of tetracycline capsules or tablets with insufficient fluid, particularly to patients with hiatal hernia or esophageal problems.

- Response to acne therapy usually requires 2–8 wk, maximal results may not be apparent for up to 12 wk.

TETRAHYDROZOLINE HYDROCHLORIDE

(tet-ra-hye-drozz'a-leen)

Optigene, Visine

Classification: EYE AND NOSE PREPARATION; VASOCONSTRICTOR; DECONGESTANT

Therapeutic: NASAL DECONGESTANT; OCULAR VASOCONSTRICTOR

Prototype: Naphazoline

AVAILABILITY Ophthalmic solution; nasal solution

ACTION & *THERAPEUTIC EFFECT* Alpha-adrenergic agonist that causes intense vasoconstriction when applied topically to mucous membranes, and when applied as eyedrops. *Ophthalmic solution is effective for allergic reactions of the eye; nasal solution is anti-inflammatory and also decreases allergic congestion.*

USES Symptomatic relief of minor eye irritation and allergies and for nasopharyngeal congestion of allergic or inflammatory origin.

CONTRAINDICATIONS Hypersensitivity to tetrahydrozoline; use of ophthalmic preparation in glaucoma or other serious eye diseases; use within 14 days of MAO inhibitor therapy.

CAUTIOUS USE Hypertension; cardiovascular disease; hyperthyroidism; DM; pregnancy (animal reproduction studies have not been conducted); lactation. Use in children younger than 2 y; use of 0.1% or higher strengths in children younger than 6 y.

ROUTE & DOSAGE

Decongestant

Adult/Adolescent/Child (over 6y): **Ophthalmic** See Appendix A-1; **Nasal** 3–4 drops of 0.1% solution or spray in each nostril q3h prn

Child (2–6 y): **Nasal** 2–3 drops of 0.05% solution or spray in each nostril q4–6h prn

ADMINISTRATION

Instillation

- Make sure interval between doses is at least 4–6 h since drug action lasts 4–8 h.
- Place patient in upright position when using nasal spray. (If patient is reclining, a stream rather than a spray may be ejected, with consequent overdosage.)
- Use lateral, head-low position to administer nasal drops.
- Store at 30° C (86° F).

ADVERSE EFFECTS CV: Hypertension, palpitations, tachycardia. **HEENT:** *Transient stinging, sneezing,* **CNS:** Headache, tremors.

INTERACTIONS Drug: Do not use with MAO inhibitors.

PHARMACOKINETICS Absorption: May be absorbed from nasal mucosa. **Duration:** 4–8 h.

NURSING IMPLICATIONS

Patient & Family Education

- Discontinue medication and consult prescriber if relief is not obtained within 48 h or if symptoms persist or increase.

- Do not exceed recommended dosage. Rebound congestion and rhinitis may occur with frequent or prolonged use of nasal preparation.

THEOPHYLLINE

(thee-off′i-lin)

Elixophyllin, Pulmophylline ♣, Theo-24, Theochron, Uniphyl ♣

Classification: BRONCHODILATOR (RESPIRATORY SMOOTH MUSCLE RELAXANT); XANTHINE

Therapeutic: BRONCHODILATOR

AVAILABILITY Liquid; sustained release tablet; sustained release capsule; solution for injection

ACTION & THERAPEUTIC EFFECT Xanthine derivative that relaxes smooth muscle by direct action, particularly of bronchi and pulmonary vessels, and stimulates medullary respiratory center with resulting increase in vital capacity. *Effective for relief of bronchospasm in asthmatics, chronic bronchitis, and emphysema.*

USES Reversible airflow obstruction. Note: This is not a preferred agent for COPD nor is it recommended for use in asthma management in children 5 y or younger.

T

UNLABELED USES Treatment of apnea and bradycardia of premature infants and to reduce severe bronchospasm associated with cystic fibrosis and acute descending respiratory infection.

CONTRAINDICATIONS Hypersensitivity to theophylline; CAD or angina pectoris when myocardial stimulation might be harmful; severe renal or hepatic impairment.

CAUTIOUS USE Compromised cardiac or circulatory function, cardiac arrhythmias; hypertension; acute pulmonary edema; multiple organ failure; CHF; seizure disorders; hyperthyroidism; active peptic ulcer; prostatic hypertrophy; glaucoma; DM; older adults; pregnancy (category C); lactation; children; and neonates.

ROUTE & DOSAGE

Note: Dose individualized by steady state serum concentrations

Reversible Airflow Obstruction

Adult: **Immediate release** 300 mg/day in divided doses q6–8h; **Extended release** 12 h formulation 150 mg bid; **Extended release 24 h** formulation 300–400 mg daily

Obesity Dosage Adjustment

Dose based on IBW

ADMINISTRATION

Note: All doses based on ideal body weight.

Oral

- Wait 4–6 h after the last IV dose, when switching from IV to oral dosing.
- Give with a full glass of water and after meals to minimize gastric irritation.
- Give sustained release forms and enteric-coated tablets whole. Chewable tablets **must be** chewed thoroughly before swallowing. Sustained release granules from capsules can be taken on an empty stomach

or mixed with applesauce or water.

- Note: Timing of dose is critical. Be certain patient understands necessity to adhere to the correct intervals between doses.

Intravenous

PREPARE: Use as supplied with no further preparation.
ADMINISTER: **IV Infusion:** Infuse at a rate based on patient's weight.
INCOMPATIBILITIES: **Solution/additive: Ascorbic acid, ceftriaxone, cimetidine, hetastarch. Y-site: Hetastarch, phenytoin.**

ADVERSE EFFECTS **CV:** Cardiac flutter, tachycardia. **CNS:** Headache, insomnia, restlessness. **Endocrine:** Hypercalcemia. **GI:** GERD, gastrointestinal ulcer, nausea, vomiting. **GU:** Dysuria, diuresis. **Musculoskeletal:** Tremor.

DIAGNOSTIC TEST INTERFERENCE ***Plasma glucose, uric acid, free fatty acids, total cholesterol, HDL, HDL/LDL ratio,*** and ***urinary free cortisol excretion*** may be increased by **theophylline.** ***Probenecid*** may cause false high ***serum theophylline*** readings, and spectrophotometric methods of determining ***serum theophylline*** are affected by a furosemide, sulfathiazole, phenylbutazone, probenecid, theobromine.

INTERACTIONS **Drug:** Increases **lithium** excretion, lowering lithium levels; **cimetidine,** high-dose **allopurinol** (600 mg/day), QUINOLONES, MACROLIDE ANTIBIOTICS, and **zileuton** can significantly increase theophylline levels; **tobacco** use significantly decreases levels. **Herbal: St. John's wort** may decrease theophylline efficacy. **Daidzein** (in soy), **black pepper** increase serum concentrations and adverse effects.

PHARMACOKINETICS **Absorption:** Most products are 100% absorbed from GI tract. **Peak:** IV 30 min; uncoated tablet 1 h; sustained release 4–6 h. **Duration:** 4–8 h; varies with age, smoking, and liver function. **Distribution:** Crosses placenta. **Metabolism:** Extensively in liver. **Elimination:** Parent drug and metabolites excreted by kidneys; excreted in breast milk.

NURSING IMPLICATIONS

Assessment & Drug Effects

- Monitor vital signs. Improvement in respiratory status is the expected outcome.
- Observe and report early signs of possible toxicity: Anorexia, nausea, vomiting, dizziness, shakiness, restlessness, abdominal discomfort, irritability, palpitation, tachycardia, marked hypotension, cardiac arrhythmias, seizures.
- Monitor for tachycardia, which may be worse in patients with severe cardiac disease. Conversely, theophylline toxicity may be masked in patients with tachycardia.
- Monitor drug levels closely in heavy smokers. Cigarette smoking induces hepatic microsomal enzyme activity, decreasing serum half-life and increasing body clearance of theophylline. An increase of dosage from 50–100% is usual in heavy smokers.
- Monitor plasma drug level closely in patients with heart failure, kidney or liver dysfunction, alcoholism, high fever. Plasma clearance of xanthines may be reduced.
- Take necessary safety precautions and forewarn older adult patients

of possible dizziness during early therapy.

- Monitor patients on sustained release preparations for S&S of overdosage. Continued slow absorption leads to high plasma concentrations for a prolonged period.
- Note: Neonates of mothers using this drug have exhibited slight tachycardia, jitteriness, and apnea.
- Monitor **closely** for adverse effects in infants younger than 6 mo and prematures; theophylline metabolism is prolonged as is the half-life in this age group.
- Monitor lab tests: Theophylline plasma level when initiating therapy and with dosage increases.

Patient & Family Education

- Take medication at the same time every day.
- Avoid charcoal-broiled foods (high in polycyclic carbon content); may increase theophylline elimination and reduce the half-life as much as 50%.
- Limit caffeine intake because it may increase incidence of adverse effects.
- Cigarette smoking may significantly lower theophylline plasma concentration.
- Be aware that a low-carbohydrate, high-protein diet increases theophylline elimination, and a high-carbohydrate, low-protein diet decreases it.
- Drink fluids liberally (2000–3000 mL/day) if not contraindicated to decrease viscosity of airway secretions.
- Avoid self-dosing with OTC medications, especially cough suppressants, which may cause retention of secretions and CNS depression.

T

THIAMINE HYDROCHLORIDE (VITAMIN B_1)

(thye'a-min)

Classification: VITAMIN B_1

Therapeutic: VITAMIN B_1 REPLACEMENT THERAPY

AVAILABILITY Tablet; capsule; solution for injection

ACTION & *THERAPEUTIC EFFECT* Water-soluble B_1 vitamin and member of B-complex group used for thiamine replacement therapy. Functions as an essential coenzyme in carbohydrate metabolism and has a role in conversion of tryptophan to nicotinamide. *Effectiveness is evidenced by improvement of clinical manifestations of thiamine deficiency (e.g., anorexia, depression, loss of memory).*

USES Treatment and prophylaxis of thiamine deficiency.

CONTRAIDINDICATION Hypersensitivity to thiamine.

CAUTIOUS USE Pregnancy (thiamine requirements are increased during pregnancy).

ROUTE & DOSAGE

Thiamine Deficiency

Adult: **IV/IM** 10–30 mg daily
Child: **IV/IM** 10 mg daily × 2 wk then 3–5 mg **PO** × 6w

Wernicke's Encephalopathy

Adult: **IV** 200–500 mg tid × 2–7 days then 250 mg daily × 3–5 days or until on normal diet

ADMINISTRATION

Oral

- Do not crush or chew enteric-coated tablets. These **must be** swallowed whole.

Intramuscular

- Give deep IM into a large muscle; may be painful. Rotate sites and apply cold compresses to area if necessary for relief of discomfort.

Intravenous

Note: Intradermal test dose is recommended prior to administration in suspected thiamine sensitivity. Deaths have occurred following IV use.

PREPARE: **Direct:** Give undiluted. **IV Infusion:** Diluted in 1000 mL of most IV solutions.

ADMINISTER: **Direct:** Give IV push over 1 to 2 minutes. **IV Infusion:** Can be administered over a longer infusion time of 15 to 30 minutes.

INCOMPATIBILITIES: **Solution:** **amino acids.** **Y-site:** **aminophylline, amphotericin B, azathioprine, cefoperazone, ceftazidime, ceftizoxime, chloramphenicol, dantrolene, diazepam, diazoxide, folic acid, furosemide, ganciclovir, hydrocortisone, imipenem/cilastatin, iamrinone, indomethacin, methylprednisolone, pentobarbital, phenobarbital, phenytoin, sodium bicarbonate, SMZ/TMP.**

- Preserve in tight, light-resistant, nonmetallic containers. Thiamine is unstable in alkaline solutions (e.g., solutions of acetates, barbiturates, bicarbonates, carbonates, citrates) and neutral solutions.

ADVERSE EFFECTS

Respiratory: Cyanosis, pulmonary edema, pharyngeal edema. **Skin:** Urticaria, pruritus, diaphoresis. **GI:** GI hemorrhage, nausea. **Other:** Flushing sensation, restlessness, weakness, anaphylaxis.

INTERACTIONS

Drug: No clinically significant interactions established.

PHARMACOKINETICS

Absorption: Limited from GI tract. **Distribution:** Widely distributed, including into breast milk. **Elimination:** In urine.

NURSING IMPLICATIONS

Assessment & Drug Effects

- Record patient's dietary history carefully as an essential part of vitamin replacement therapy. Collaborate with prescriber, dietitian, patient, and responsible family member in developing a diet teaching plan that can be sustained by patient.

Patient & Family Education

- Food–drug relationships: Learn about rich dietary sources of thiamine (e.g., yeast, pork, beef, liver, wheat and other whole grains, nutrient-added breakfast cereals, fresh vegetables, especially peas and dried beans).
- Body requirement of thiamine is directly proportional to carbohydrate intake and metabolic rate; requirement increases when diet consists predominantly of carbohydrates.

T

THIOGUANINE (TG, 6-THIOGUANINE)

(thye-oh-gwah'neen)

Lanvis ♣, Tabloid

Classification: ANTINEOPLASTIC; ANTIMETABOLITE; PURINE ANTAGONIST

Therapeutic: ANTINEOPLASTIC

Prototype: Mercaptopurine

AVAILABILITY Tablet

ACTION & *THERAPEUTIC EFFECT* Tumor inhibitory properties may be caused by a sequential blockade of the synthesis and utilization of the purine nucleotides in DNA and DNA. *Interferes with nucleic acid biosynthesis, and has been found active against selected human neoplastic diseases.*

USES In combination with other antineoplastics for remission induction in acute myelogenous leukemia and as treatment of chronic myelogenous leukemia.

CONTRAINDICATIONS Patients with prior resistance to this drug; severe bone marrow depression; liver toxicity caused by drug; pregnancy (category D); lactation.

CAUTIOUS USE Resistance to mercaptopurine; hepatic disease; children.

ROUTE & DOSAGE

Leukemia

Adult: **PO** 2 mg/kg/day, may increase to 3 mg/kg/day if no response after 4 wk

ADMINISTRATION

Oral

- Withhold drug and notify prescriber if toxicity develops. There is no known antagonist; prompt discontinuation of the drug is essential to avoid irreversible myelosuppression from toxicity.
- Store at 15°–30° C (59°–86° F) in airtight container.

ADVERSE EFFECTS **CV:** Esophogeal varices, portal hypertension. **Endocrine:** Fluid retention, hyperuricemia, weight gain. **Hepatic:** Ascites, hepatomegaly, hepatotoxicity, hyperbilirubinemia, increased liver enzymes, jaundice, periportal fibrosis. **GI:** Anorexia, intestinal perforation, nausea, vomiting, stomatitis. **Musculoskeletal:** Bone hypoplasia. **Hematologic:** Anemia, bone marrow depression, granulocytopenia, hemorrhage, leukopenia, pancytopenia, splenomegaly, thrombocytopenia. **Other:** Infection.

INTERACTIONS **Drug:** Severe hepatotoxicity with **busulfan;** may decrease immune response to VACCINES; increase risk of bleeding with ANTICOAGULANTS; NSAIDS, SALICYLATES; PLATELET INHIBITORS, THROMBOLYTIC AGENTS; effects may be reversed by **filgrastim, sargramostim.** Do not use with **deferoprone, dipyrone, natalizumab, pimecrolimus, tacrolimus.**

PHARMACOKINETICS **Absorption:** Variable and incomplete absorption from GI tract. **Peak:** 8 h. **Distribution:** Crosses placenta. **Metabolism:** In liver. **Elimination:** In urine. **Half-Life:** 5–9 h.

NURSING IMPLICATIONS

Assessment & Drug Effects

- Determine hematologic parameters for withholding drug.
- Monitor I&O ratio and report oliguria.
- Observe patient's skin and sclera for jaundice. It should be reported promptly as a symptom of toxicity; drug will be discontinued promptly.
- Expect that the drop in leukocyte count may be slow over a period of 2–4 wk. Treatment is interrupted if there is a rapid fall within a few days.
- Monitor lab tests: Frequent CBC with differential and platelet count; weekly LFTs early in therapy and monthly thereafter.

Patient & Family Education

- Report promptly to prescriber any of the following: Fever, sore throat, jaundice, nausea, vomiting, signs of infection, bleeding from any site, or symptoms of anemia.
- Women should use effective means of contraception while taking this drug.

THIORIDAZINE HYDROCHLORIDE

(thye-o-rid'a-zeen)

Classification: ANTIPSYCHOTIC; PHENOTHIAZINE
Therapeutic: ANTIPSYCHOTIC
Prototype: Chlorpromazine

AVAILABILITY Tablet

ACTION & *THERAPEUTIC EFFECT* Blocks postsynaptic dopamine receptors in the mesolimbic system of the brain. The decrease in dopamine neurotransmission has been found to correlate to antipsychotic effects. *Effective in reducing excitement, hypermotility, abnormal initiative, affective tension, and agitation by inhibiting psychomotor functions. Also effective as an antipsychotic agent, and for behavioral disorders in children.*

USES Treatment of schizophrenia in patients who fail to respond adequately to treatment with other antipsychotics.

CONTRAINDICATIONS Hypersensitivity to phenothiazines; severe CNS depression; severe hyper-/hypotensive heart disease; family history of QT prolongation or cardiac arrhythmias; coadministration of drug that is known to prolong the QTc interval; suicidal ideation; older adults with dementia related psychosis; lactation.

CAUTIOUS USE Premature ventricular contractions; previously diagnosed breast cancer; patients exposed to extremes in heat or to organophosphorus insecticides; history of suicidal tendencies; Parkinson's disease; seizure disorders; closed-angle glaucoma; respiratory disorders; pregnancy (maternal antipsychotic use during the third trimester of pregnancy has a risk for abnormal muscle movements and withdrawal symptoms in newborns). Safe use in children younger than 2 y not established.

ROUTE & DOSAGE

Schizophrenia
Adult: **PO** 50–100 mg tid, may increase up to 800 mg/day as needed or tolerated
Child (2 y or older): **PO** 0.5 mg/kg/day in divided doses; (max: 3 mg/kg/day)

Pharmacogenetic Dosage Adjustment

Poor CYP2D6 metabolizers: reduce initial dose

ADMINISTRATION

Oral

- Administer with water, food, or milk to decrease GI upset.
- Schedule phenothiazine at least 1 h before or 1 h after an antacid or antidiarrheal medication.
- Add increases in dose to the first dose of the day to prevent sleep disturbance.
- Store at 20°–25° C (68°–77° F) in tightly covered, light-resistant containers unless otherwise indicated.

ADVERSE EFFECTS **CV:** ECG changes, hypotension, orthostatic hypotension, peripheral edema, prolonged QT_c interval. **CNS:** *Sedation,* dizziness, drowsiness, lethargy, extrapyramidal syndrome, nocturnal confusion, hyperactivity, headache, restlessness. **HEENT:** Nasal congestion, blurred vision, corneal opacity. **GI:** Xerostomia, *constipation,* weight gain. **GU:** Amenorrhea, breast engorgement, galactorrhea, sexual difficulty. **Hematologic:** Agranulocytosis, leukopenia.

DIAGNOSTIC TEST INTERFERENCE Possible false positive with urine detection of methadone and phencyclidine.

INTERACTIONS **Drug: Alcohol,** ANXIOLYTICS, SEDATIVE-HYPNOTICS, other CNS DEPRESSANTS add to CNS depression; additive adverse effects with other PHENOTHIAZINES. Use with other agents affecting QT interval can prolong QT_c interval resulting in arrhythmias. Use with ANTIPARKINSON AGENTS, ANTICHOLINERGIC AGENTS, ANTIPSYCHOTIC AGENTS results in increased adverse effects. Do not use with **aminolevulinic acid, amisulpride, asunaprevir, dapoxetine, eliglustat, glycopyrrolate**. **Herbal: Kava** may increase risk and severity of dystonic reactions.

PHARMACOKINETICS **Absorption:** Well absorbed from GI tract. **Onset:** Days to weeks. **Distribution:** Crosses placenta; distributed into breast milk. **Metabolism:** In liver (CYP2D6). **Elimination:** In urine. **Half-Life:** 5–27 h.

NURSING IMPLICATIONS

Black Box Warning

Thioridazine has been associated with prolongation of the QTc interval, development of torsades de pointes–type arrhythmias and sudden death; and with increased mortality in older adults with dementia-related psychosis.

Assessment & Drug Effects

- Monitor for changes in behavior that may indicate increased possibility of suicide ideation.
- Orthostatic hypotension may occur in early therapy. Monitor ambulation.
- Monitor ECG periodically throughout therapy, especially during a period of dose adjustment.
- Report promptly S&S of torsades de pointes (e.g., dizziness, palpitations, syncope).

- Monitor I&O ratio and bowel elimination pattern. Check for abdominal distention and pain. Encourage adequate fluid intake as prophylaxis for constipation and xerostomia. The depressed patient may not seek help for either symptom or for urinary retention.
- Obtain baseline and periodic ophthalmic exam.
- Monitor lab tests: Periodic CBC, serum electrolytes, lipid profile, fasting plasma glucose level, HbA1C, and LFTs.

Patient & Family Education

- Avoid alcohol during phenothiazine therapy. Concomitant use enhances CNS depression effects.
- Be aware that marked drowsiness generally subsides with continued therapy or reduction in dosage.
- Do not drive or engage in potentially hazardous activities until response to drug is known.
- Make position changes slowly, particularly from lying down to upright posture; dangle legs a few minutes before standing.
- Vasodilation produced by hot showers or baths or by long exposure to environmental heat may accentuate hypotensive effect.
- Do not use any OTC drugs unless approved by the prescriber.

THIOTEPA

(thye-oh-tep′a)

Tepadina

Classification: ANTINEOPLASTIC; ALKYLATING AGENT

Therapeutic: ANTINEOPLASTIC

Prototype: Cyclophosphamide

AVAILABILITY Solution for injection

ACTION & THERAPEUTIC EFFECT Cell-cycle nonspecific alkylating agent that selectively reacts with DNA phosphate groups to produce chromosome cross-linkage and consequent blocking of nucleoprotein synthesis. Highly toxic hematopoietic agent. *Myelosuppression is cumulative and unpredictable and may be delayed.*

USES To reduce the risk of graft rejection when with other agents as a preparative regimen for allogeneic hematopoietic progenitor (stem) cell transplantation in pediatric patients with class 3 beta-thalassemia.

UNLABELED USES Hematopoietic stem cell transplant, malignant meningeal neoplasms.

CONTRAINDICATIONS Hypersensitivity to thiotepa; acute leukemia; acute infection; concomitant use with live or attenuated vaccines; pregnancy (in utero exposure to thiotepa may cause fetal harm); lactation.

CAUTIOUS USE Chronic lymphocytic leukemia; myelosuppression produced by radiation; bone marrow invasion by tumor cells; impaired kidney or liver function; children.

ROUTE & DOSAGE

Hematopoietic stem cell transplant

Child/Adolescent: **IV** 300 mg/m^2 daily ×3 days beginning 8 days before transplant

T

ADMINISTRATION

Intravenous

Use only under constant supervision by prescribers experienced in therapy with cytotoxic agents. ▪ Avoid exposure of skin and respiratory tract to particles of thiotepa during solution preparation.
▪ Antiemetics may be recommended to prevent nausea and vomiting.
PREPARE: **Direct:** Reconstitute each 15 mg vial with 1.5 mL sterile water for infusion. Reconstituted concentration is 10 mg/mL. Solutions for IV infusion should be further diluted in NS. ▪ Filter solution through a 0.2 micron filter.
ADMINISTER: **Direct:** Administer over 3 hours via a central line. Infusion times may vary by protocol or dose for off-label uses; refer to specific protocols. Flush with 5 mL NS before and after infusion.
INCOMPATIBILITIES: **Solution/additive:** **Cisplatin. Y-site:** **Alemtuzumab, amiodarone, busulfan, cisplatin,** dantrolene, diazepam, **filgrastim,** gemtuzumab, **minocycline,** naloxone, nicardipine, nitroprusside, pantoprazole, phenytoin, **verapamil.**

▪ Store powder for injection and reconstituted solutions at 2°–8° C (35°–46° F); protect from light. ▪ Solutions reconstituted with sterile water only are stable for 8 h under refrigeration.

ADVERSE EFFECTS

CNS: Intracranial hemorrhage, seizure, dizziness, fatigue, headache. **Respiratory:** Pneumonia. **Skin:** Alopecia, contact dermatitis, skin depigmentation, rash, urticaria. **Hepatic/GI:** Anorexia, nausea, vomiting, stomatitis, abdominal pain, elevated liver enzymes, increased serum bilirubin. **GU:** Amenorrhea, interference with spermatogenesis. **Hematologic:** Neutropenia, thrombocytopenia, anemia, pancytopenia. **Other:** Cytomegalovirus disease, febrile reactions.

INTERACTIONS

Drug: May prolong muscle paralysis with **mivacurium;** ANTICOAGULANTS, NSAIDS, SALICYLATES, ANTIPLATELET AGENTS may increase risk of bleeding. Increased risk of adverse effects when used with IMMUNOSUPPRESSANT or MYELOSUPPRESSIVE AGENTS. Do not administer with LIVE VACCINES. CYP 3A4 INHIBITORS may decrease concentration of thiotepa. **Herbal:** Avoid use of echinacea.

PHARMACOKINETICS

Absorption: Rapidly cleared from plasma. **Onset:** Gradual response over several weeks. **Metabolism:** In liver. **Elimination:** 60% in urine within 24–72 h.

NURSING IMPLICATIONS

Assessment & Drug Effects

- Monitor closely for symptoms of dermatologic or CNS toxicity.
- Be aware that because of cumulative effects, maximum myelosuppression may be delayed 3–4 wk after termination of therapy.
- Withhold drug and notify prescriber if leukocyte count falls to 3000/mm^3 or below or if platelet count falls below 150,000/mm^3.
- Monitor lab tests: CBC with differential, LFTs, renal function tests, and platelet count at least weekly during therapy and for at least 3 wk after therapy is discontinued.

Patient & Family Education

- Be aware of possibility of amenorrhea (usually reversible in 6–8 mo).
- Report onset of fever, bleeding, a cold or illness, no matter how mild to prescriber; medical supervision may be necessary.

THIOTHIXENE HYDROCHLORIDE

(thye-oh-thix'een)

Navane ♣

Classification: ANTIPSYCHOTIC; PHENOTHIAZINE

Therapeutic: ANTIPSYCHOTIC

Prototype: Chlorpromazine

AVAILABILITY Capsule

ACTION & *THERAPEUTIC EFFECT* Mechanism of action is related to blockade of postsynaptic dopamine receptors in the mesolimbic region of the brain. Additionally, blockade of $alpha_1$-adrenergic receptors in the CNS produces sedation and muscle relaxation. *Possesses antipsychotic, sedative, adrenolytic, and antiemetic activity.*

USES Management of schizophrenia.

CONTRAINDICATIONS Hypersensitivity to thiothixene; CNS depression; coma; older adults with dementia related psychosis; circulatory collapse; blood dyscrasias; NMS; lactation.

CAUTIOUS USE History of convulsive disorders; alcohol withdrawal; glaucoma; prostatic hypertrophy; cardiovascular disease; older adults; patients who might be exposed to organophosphorus insecticides or to extreme heat; previously diagnosed breast cancer; pregnancy (adverse effects were observed in some animal reproduction studies). Safe use in children younger than 12 y not established.

ROUTE & DOSAGE

Schizophrenia

Adult/Adolescent: **PO** 2 mg tid, may increase up to 15 mg/day as needed or tolerated (max: 60 mg/day)

ADMINISTRATION

Oral

- Capsules may be opened and mixed with food or water for ease of administration.

ADVERSE EFFECTS **CV:** Tachycardia, *orthostatic hypotension,* cardiac arrest, ECG changes, peripheral edema, syncope. **Respiratory:** Asphyxia, nasal congestion. **CNS:** *Drowsiness,* insomnia, dizziness, cerebral edema, convulsions, *extrapyramidal symptoms (dose related),* paradoxical exaggeration of psychotic symptoms; sudden death, neuroleptic malignant syndrome, tardive dyskinesia, seizure, restlessness. **HEENT:** Blurred vision, pigmentary retinopathy. **Skin:** Rash, photosensitivity, contact dermatitis, diaphoresis, pruritis, skin discoloration (blue-gray). **Hepatic/GI:** Xerostomia, constipation, anorexia, nausea, stomach pain, elevated liver enzymes. **GU:** Impotence, gynecomastia, galactorrhea,

T

amenorrhea, breast hypertrophy, difficult micturition, ejaculatory disorder. **Hematologic:** Leukocytosis, leukopenia. **Other:** Fever.

DIAGNOSTIC TEST INTERFERENCE

may cause false positive pregnancy test

INTERACTIONS

Drug: Alcohol, ANXIOLYTICS, SEDATIVE-HYPNOTICS, other CNS DEPRESSANTS add to CNS depression; additive adverse effects with other PHENOTHIAZINES; Use with ANTIPARKINSON AGENTS, ANTICHOLINERGIC AGENTS, ANTIPSYCHOTIC AGENTS results in increased adverse effects. Do not use with **amisulpride, glycopyrrolate. Herbal: Kava** may increase risk and severity of dystonic reactions.

PHARMACOKINETICS

Absorption: Slowly absorbed from GI tract. **Duration:** Up to 12 h. **Distribution:** May remain in body for several weeks; crosses placenta. **Metabolism:** In liver, substrate of CYP1A2. **Elimination:** In bile and feces. **Half-Life:** 34 h.

NURSING IMPLICATIONS

Black Box Warning

Thiothixene has been associated with increased mortality in older adults with dementia-related psychosis.

T

Assessment & Drug Effects

- Monitor BP for excessive hypotensive response when thiothixene is added to drug regimen of patient on hypertensive treatment until therapy is stabilized.
- Report extrapyramidal effects (pseudoparkinsonism, akathisia, dystonia) to prescriber; dose adjustment or short-term therapy with an antiparkinsonism agent may provide relief.
- Be alert to first symptoms of tardive dyskinesia (see Appendix F). Withhold drug and notify prescriber.
- Monitor lab tests: Periodic electrolytes, lipid profile, LFTs, HbA1c, plasma fasting glucose.

Patient & Family Education

- Make position changes slowly, particularly from lying down to upright because of danger of light-headedness; sit a few minutes before walking.
- Do not drive or engage in potentially hazardous activities until response to drug is known.
- Avoid alcohol and other depressants during therapy.
- Take drug as prescribed; do not alter dosing regimen or stop medication without consulting prescriber. Abrupt discontinuation can cause delirium.
- Do not use any OTC drugs without approval of prescriber.
- Avoid excessive exposure to sunlight to prevent a photosensitivity reaction. If sun exposure is expected, protect skin with sunscreen lotion (SPF 12 or above).

- Schedule periodic eye exams and report blurred vision to prescriber.

THROMBIN

(throm'bin)

Recothrom, Thrombinar, Thrombostat

Classification: COAGULATOR; TOPICAL HEMOSTATIC

Therapeutic: COAGULATOR; HEMOSTATIC

AVAILABILITY Topical application

ACTION & *THERAPEUTIC EFFECT* Plasma protein prepared from prothrombin of bovine origin. Induces clotting of whole blood or fibrinogen solution without addition of other substances. *Facilitates conversion of fibrinogen to fibrin resulting in clotting of whole blood.*

USES Hemostasis aid.

CONTRAINDICATIONS Known hypersensitivity to any of thrombin components or to material of bovine origin; parenteral use; entry or infiltration into large blood vessels.

CAUTIOUS USE Older adults; pregnancy (category C). Safety and efficacy in children and infants not established.

ROUTE & DOSAGE

Hemostasis

Adult: **Topical** 100–2000 NIH units/mL, depending on extent of bleeding, may be used as solution, in dry form, by mixing thrombin with blood plasma to form a fibrin "glue," or in conjunction with absorbable gelatin sponge

ADMINISTRATION

Topical

- Ensure that sponge recipient area is free of blood before applying thrombin.
- Prepare solutions in sterile distilled water or isotonic saline.
- Use solutions within a few hours of preparation. If several hours are to elapse between time of preparation and use, solution should be refrigerated, or preferably frozen, and used within 48 h.
- Store lyophilized preparation at 2°–8° C (36°–46° F).

ADVERSE EFFECTS **Other:** Sensitivity, allergic and febrile reactions, <u>intravascular clotting and death when thrombin is allowed to enter large blood vessels</u>.

THYROID DESSICATED

(thye'roid)

Armour Thyroid, Nature-Thyroid, NP Thyroid, Westhroid, WP Thyroid

Classification: THYROID REPLACEMENT

Therapeutic: THYROID HORMONE REPLACEMENT

Prototype: Levothyroxine sodium

AVAILABILITY Tablet

ACTION & *THERAPEUTIC EFFECT* The mechanisms by which thyroid hormones exert their effects are not well understood. They enhance oxygen consumption, increase the basal metabolic rate and the metabolism of carbohydrates, lipids, and proteins. They exert a profound

T

influence on every organ system and are of particular importance in the development of the CNS. *Effectiveness indicated by diuresis, followed by sense of well-being, increased pulse rate, increased pulse pressure, increased appetite, increased psychomotor activity, loss of constipation, normalization of skin texture and hair, and increased T_3 and T_4 serum levels.*

USES Treatment of hypothyroidism of any etiology, and for the treatment or prevention of various types of euthyroid (non-toxic) goiter.

CONTRAINDICATIONS Thyrotoxicosis; acute MI not associated with hypothyroidism, cardiovascular disease; morphologic hypogonadism; nephrosis; uncorrected hypoadrenalism.

CAUTIOUS USE Angina pectoris, hypertension, older adults who may have occult cardiac disease; renal insufficiency; DM; history of hyperthyroidism; malabsorption states; pregnancy (category A); lactation (infant risk cannot be ruled out).

ROUTE & DOSAGE

Hypothyroidism

Adult/Adolescent: **PO** 30 mg/day, may increase by 15 mg q2–3 wk to 60–180mg/day
Infant/Child: See package insert for weight-based dosing.

ADMINISTRATION

Oral

- Give preferably on an empty stomach.
- Initiate dosage generally at low level and systematically increase in small increments to desired maintenance dose.
- Store in dark bottle to minimize spontaneous deiodination. Keep desiccated thyroid dry. Store at temperatures between 15°–30° C (59°–86° F).

ADVERSE EFFECTS **CV:** Palpitations and tachycardia (with excessive doses). **CNS:** Insomnia, tremor and restlessness (with excessive doses). **GI:** Diarrhea, nausea and vomiting (with excessive doses).

DIAGNOSTIC TEST INTERFERENCE Thyroid increases ***basal metabolic rate;*** may increase ***blood glucose levels, creatine phosphokinase, AST, LDH, PBI.*** It may decrease ***serum uric acid, cholesterol, thyroid-stimulating hormone (TSH), iodine 131*** uptake. Many medications may produce false results in ***thyroid function tests.***

INTERACTIONS **Drug:** ORAL ANTICOAGULANTS potentiate hypoprothrombinemia; may increase requirements for **insulin,** SULFONYLUREAS; **epinephrine** may precipitate coronary insufficiency; **cholestyramine,** aluminum, or calcium-containing products may decrease thyroid absorption. **Food:** Certain foods, beverages, and enteral feedings can inhibit the absorption of thyroid hormones.

PHARMACOKINETICS **Absorption:** Variably absorbed from GI tract. **Peak:** 1–3 wk. **Distribution:** Does not readily cross placenta; minimal amounts in breast milk. **Metabolism:** Deiodination in thyroid gland. **Elimination:** In urine and feces. **Half-Life:** T_3, 1–2 days; T_4, 6–7 days.

NURSING IMPLICATIONS

Assessment & Drug Effects

- Observe patient carefully during initial treatment for untoward reactions such as angina, palpitations, cardiac pain.
- Be alert for symptoms of overdosage (see ADVERSE EFFECTS) that may occur 1–3 wk after therapy is started.
- Monitor response until regimen is stabilized to prevent iatrogenic hyperthyroidism. In drug-induced hyperthyroidism, there may also be increased bone loss. Such a patient is vulnerable to pathologic fractures.
- Monitor vital signs: Assess pulse before each dose during period of dosage adjustment. Consult prescriber if rate is 100 or more or if there has been a marked change in rate or rhythm.
- TSH 4–8 wk after initiation or dose change, repeat at 6 mo, then q12 mo thereafter.

Patient & Family Education

- Be aware that replacement therapy for hypothyroidism is life-long; continued follow-up care is important.
- Monitor pulse rate and report increases greater than parameter set by prescriber.
- Report to prescriber onset of chest pain or other signs of aggravated CV disease (dyspnea, tachycardia).
- Report evidence of any unexplained bleeding to prescriber when taking concomitant anticoagulant.
- Use monthly height and weight measurement to monitor growth in juvenile undergoing treatment.

TIAGABINE HYDROCHLORIDE

(ti-a′ga-been)

Gabitril

Classification: ANTICONVULSANT; GABA INHIBITOR

Therapeutic: ANTICONVULSANT

Prototype: Valproic acid sodium (sodium valproate)

AVAILABILITY Tablet

ACTION & *THERAPEUTIC EFFECT*

Potent and selective inhibitor of GABA uptake into presynaptic neurons; allows more GABA to bind to the surfaces of postsynaptic neurons in the CNS. *Effectiveness indicated by reduction in seizure activity.*

USES Adjunctive therapy for focal (partial) seizures.

CONTRAINDICATIONS

Hypersensitivity to tiagabine; pregnancy—fetal risk cannot be ruled out; lactation—infant risk cannot be ruled out.

CAUTIOUS USE Liver function impairment; history of spike and wave discharge on EEG; taking other CNS depressants; status epilepticus. Safe use in children younger than 12 y not established.

ROUTE & DOSAGE

Seizures

Adult: **PO** Also on enzyme inducing medications. Start with 4 mg daily, may increase dose by 4–8 mg/day qwk (max: 56 mg/day in 2–4 divided doses) Not taking enzyme inducing medication will require a lower starting dose.
Adolescent (12–18 y): **PO** Start with 4 mg daily, after 2 wk may increase dose by 4–8 mg/day qwk (max: 32 mg/day in 2–4 divided doses)

ADMINISTRATION

Oral

- Give with food.
- Make dosage increases, when needed, at weekly intervals.
- Store at 20°–25° C (68°–77° F) in a tightly closed container and protect from light.

ADVERSE EFFECTS (≥5%) **Respiratory:** Pharyngitis. **CNS:** *Dizziness, asthenia, tremor, somnolence, nervousness,* difficulty concentrating, ataxia, insomnia, confusion. **GI:** Abdominal pain, nausea.

INTERACTIONS **Drug:** **Carbamazepine, mitotane, phenytoin, phenobarbital** decrease levels of tiagabine. Use with ANTIDEPRESSANTS, ANTIPSYCHOTICS, STIMULANTS, AMPHETAMINES, and NARCOTICS may increase seizure risk. Avoid use of **ceritinib, idelalisib, posaconazole,** as it may increase toxicity risk. CNS DEPRESSANTS have additive adverse effects. **Herbal:** **Ginkgo, kava** may decrease anticonvulsant effectiveness. **Evening primrose oil** may affect seizure threshold. Kratom has additive adverse effect. **Food:** Use of ethanol regularly may require lower tiagabine dose.

PHARMACOKINETICS **Absorption:** Rapidly absorbed; 90% bioavailability. **Peak:** 45 min. **Distribution:** 96% protein bound. **Metabolism:** In liver (CYP3A4). **Elimination:** 25% in urine, 63% in feces. **Half-Life:** 7–9 h (4–7 h with other enzyme-inducing drugs).

NURSING IMPLICATIONS

Assessment & Drug Effects

- Be aware that concurrent use of other anticonvulsants may decrease effectiveness of tiagabine or increase the potential for adverse effects.
- Monitor carefully for S&S of CNS depression and suicidal ideation.
- Monitor lab tests: Plasma tiagabine before and after changes are made in the drug regimen, LFTs.

Patient & Family Education

- Do not stop taking drug abruptly; may cause sudden onset of seizures.
- Take medication with food.
- Exercise caution while engaging in potentially hazardous activities because drug may cause dizziness.
- Use caution when taking other prescription or OTC drugs that can cause drowsiness.
- Report any of the following to the prescriber: Rash or hives; red, peeling skin; dizziness; drowsiness; depression; GI distress; nervousness or tremors; difficulty concentrating or talking.

TICAGRELOR

(tye′ka-gre-lor)

Brilinta

Classification: ANTIPLATELET INHIBITOR; ANTITHROMBOTIC

Therapeutic: PLATELET AGGREGATION INHIBITOR; ANTITHROMBOTIC

Prototype: Clopidogrel

AVAILABILITY Tablet

ACTION & *THERAPEUTIC EFFECT*

Ticagrelor and its major metabolite reversibly interact with the platelet ADP receptor to prevent signal transduction and platelet activation. *Prevents platelet activation and clot formation.*

USES Prophylaxis to prevent arterial thromboembolism in patients with acute coronary syndrome (ACS).

UNLABELED USES Unstable angina/non-ST elevation MI.

CONTRAINDICATIONS Hypersensitivity (e.g., angioedema) to ticagrelor; severe hepatic impairment; history of intracranial hemorrhage; active bleeding (e.g., peptic ulcer); use within 24 h.

CAUTIOUS USE Mild-to-moderate hepatic impairment; second or third AV block, sick sinus syndrome; history of bleeding disorders, percutaneous invasive procedures, and use of drugs that increase risk of bleeding (e.g., anticoagulant and fibrinolytic therapy, high dose aspirin, long-term NSAIDs); older adults; pregnancy (category C); lactation (infant risk cannot be ruled out). Safety and efficacy in children not established.

ROUTE & DOSAGE

Arterial Thromboembolism Prophylaxis

Adult: **PO** 180 mg loading dose (plus aspirin) followed by 90 mg bid (with 75–100 mg aspirin once daily) for 1 y; after 1 y 60 mg bid

ADMINISTRATION

Oral

- May be given without regard to food.
- Tablets may be crushed and mixed with water for oral or NG administration.
- Store at 15°–30° C (59°–86° F) and protect from moisture.

ADVERSE EFFECTS **CV:** Bradyarrhythmia. **Respiratory:** Dyspnea, pulmonary hemorrhage. **CNS:** Dizziness. **GU:** Increased serum creatinine.

INTERACTIONS **Drug:** Strong CYP3A4 inhibitors (e.g., **ketoconazole, itraconazole, voriconazole, clarithromycin, nefazodone, ritonavir, saquinavir, nelfinavir, indinavir, atazanavir,** and **telithromycin**) can increase ticagrelor levels, while potent CYP3A4 inducers (e.g., **rifampin, dexamethasone, phenytoin, carbamazepine,** and **phenobarbital**) can decrease ticagrelor levels. Ticagrelor can increase the levels of **simvastatin** and **lovastatin.** Avoid use with ANTIPLATELETS or ANTICOAGULANTS. Do not use with **avanafil, defibrotide.** **Herbal:** Do not use with **St. John's wort**.

PHARMACOKINETICS **Absorption:** 30–42% Bioavailable. **Onset:** 1.5–5 h. **Distribution:** Greater than 99% plasma protein bound. **Metabolism:** CYP3A4, CYP3A5, P-gp metabolism to active compound. **Elimination:** Fecal (58%) and renal (26%). **Half-Life:** 7 h (ticagrelor); 9 h (active metabolite).

NURSING IMPLICATIONS

Black Box Warning

Ticagrelor has been associated with serious, sometimes fatal, bleeding.

Assessment & Drug Effects

- Monitor cardiac status with ECG and frequent BP measurements. Report immediately development of hypotension in any one who has recently undergone coronary angiography, PCI, CABG, or other surgical procedures.
- Monitor for and report promptly S&S of bleeding or dyspnea. Monitor lab tests: CBC hemoglobin, hematocrit, renal functions, uric acid levels, and LFTs.

Patient & Family Education

- Report promptly to prescriber any of the following: Unexplained, prolonged, or excessive bleeding; blood in stool or urine; shortness of breath.
- Daily doses of aspirin **should not** exceed 100 mg. Do not take any other drugs that contain aspirin. Consult prescriber if taking a nonsteroidal anti-inflammatory drug (NSAID).
- Inform all healthcare providers that you are taking ticagrelor.

TICARCILLIN DISODIUM/ CLAVULANATE POTASSIUM

(tye-kar-sill′in/clav-yoo′la-nate)

Timentin

Classification: ANTIBIOTIC; EXTENDED-SPECTRUM PENICILLIN

Therapeutic: ANTIBIOTIC

Prototype: Piperacillin/ tazobactam

AVAILABILITY Solution for injection

ACTION & *THERAPEUTIC EFFECT* Used alone, clavulanic acid antibacterial activity is weak, but in combination with ticarcillin prevents degradation by beta-lactamase and extends ticarcillin spectrum of activity. *Combination drug extends ticarcillin spectrum of activity against many strains of beta-lactamase-producing bacteria (synergistic effect).*

T

USES Infections of lower respiratory tract and urinary tract and skin and skin structures, infections of bone and joint, and septicemia caused by susceptible organisms. Also mixed infections and as presumptive therapy before identification of causative organism.

CONTRAINDICATIONS Hypersensitivity to ticarcillin/clavulanate or penicillins or to cephalosporins, coagulopathy.

CAUTIOUS USE DM; GI disease; asthma; history of allergies; renal impairment; pregnancy (category B); lactation.

ROUTE & DOSAGE

Moderate to Severe Infections

Adult/Adolescent/Child (weight greater than 60 kg): **IV** 3.1 g q4–6h

Child/Infant (3 mo or older and weight less than 60 kg): **IV** 200–300 mg/kg/day divided q4–6h (based on ticarcillin)

Infant (younger than 3 mo and weight less than 60 kg): **IV** 200–300 mg/kg/day divided q6–8h (based on ticarcillin)

Renal Impairment Dosage Adjustment

CrCl 30–60 mL/min: Give 2 g q4h; *10–30 mL/min:* Give 2 g q8h; *less than 10 mL/min:* Give 2 g q12h

Hemodialysis Dosage Adjustment

2 g q12h, supplement with 3.1 g after dialysis

ADMINISTRATION

Intravenous

Note: Verify correct IV concentration and rate of infusion for administration to infants and children with prescriber.

PREPARE: **Intermittent:** Reconstitute by adding 13 mL sterile water for injection or NS injection to the 3.1 g vial to yield 200 mg/mL ticarcillin with 6.7 mg/mL clavulanic acid. Shake until dissolved. ▪ Further dilute the required does in NS, D5W, or LR to concentrations between 10–100 mg/mL. ▪ **Do not** use if discoloration or particulate matter is present.

ADMINISTER: **Intermittent:** Give over 30 min.

INCOMPATIBILITIES: **Solution/additive:** AMINOGLYCOSIDES, **sodium bicarbonate. Y-site: acyclovir, alatrofloxacin, amphotericin B cholesteryl complex, azathioprine, azithromycin, caspofungin, cefamandole, chlorpromazine, dantrolene, daunorubicin, diazepam, diazoxide, dobutamine, dolasetron, alfa, epirubicin, erythromycin, ganciclovir, gemtuzumab, haloperidol, hydroxyzine, idarubicin, inamrinone, lansoprazole, minocycline, mitomycin, mitoxantrone, mycophenolate, papaverine, pentamidine, pentazocine, phenytoin, promethazine, protamine, quinupristin/dalfopristin, SMZ/TMP, vancomycin.**

▪ Store vial with sterile powder at 21°–24° C (69°–75° F) or colder. ▪ If exposed to higher temperature, powder will darken, indicating degradation of clavulanate potassium and loss of potency. Discard vial. ▪ See package insert for information about storage and stability of reconstituted and diluted IV solutions of drug.

ADVERSE EFFECTS

CNS: Headache, blurred vision, mental deterioration, convulsions, hallucinations, seizures, giddiness, neuromuscular hyperirritability. **Endocrine:** Hypernatremia, transient increases in serum AST, ALT, BUN, and alkaline phosphatase; increases in serum LDH, bilirubin, and creatinine and decreased serum uric acid. **GI:** *Diarrhea, nausea,* vomiting, disturbances of taste or smell, stomatitis, flatulence. **Hematologic:** Eosinophilia, <u>thrombocytopenia</u>, <u>leukopenia</u>, neutropenia, hemolytic anemia. **Other:** Hypersensitivity reactions, pain, burning, swelling at injection site; phlebitis, thrombophlebitis; superinfections.

DIAGNOSTIC TEST INTERFERENCE

May interfere with test methods used to determine ***urinary proteins*** except for tests for urinary protein that use ***bromphenol blue. Positive direct antiglobulin (Coombs') test*** results, apparently caused by clavulanic acid, have been reported. This test may interfere with ***transfusion cross-matching procedures.***

INTERACTIONS

Drugs: May increase risk of bleeding with ANTICOAGULANTS; **probenecid** decreases elimination of ticarcillin.

PHARMACOKINETICS

Distribution: Widely distributed with highest concentrations in urine and bile; crosses placenta; distributed into breast milk. **Metabolism:** In liver. **Elimination:** In urine. **Half-Life:** 1.1–1.2 h ticarcillin, 1.1–1.5 h clavulanate.

NURSING IMPLICATIONS

Assessment & Drug Effects

- Be aware that serious and sometimes fatal anaphylactoid reactions have been reported in patients with penicillin hypersensitivity or history of sensitivity to multiple allergens. Reported incidence is low with this combination drug.
- Monitor cardiac status because of high sodium content of drug.

T

- Overdose symptoms: This drug may cause neuromuscular hyperirritability or seizures.
- Monitor lab tests: Baseline C&S; periodic LFTs and renal function tests, CBC, platelet count, and serum electrolytes.

Patient & Family Education

- Report urticaria, rashes, or pruritus to prescriber immediately.
- Report frequent loose stools, diarrhea, or other possible signs of pseudomembranous colitis (see Appendix F) to prescriber.

TICLOPIDINE HYDROCHLORIDE

(ti-clo′pi-deen)

Classification: ANTICOAGULANT; PLATELET AGGREGATION INHIBITOR; ADP RECEPTOR ANTAGONIST

Therapeutic: PLATELET AGGREGATION INHIBITOR

Prototype: Clopidogrel

AVAILABILITY Tablet

ACTION & *THERAPEUTIC EFFECT* Platelet aggregation inhibitor that interferes with platelet membrane functioning and therefore platelet interactions. Ticlopidine interferes with ADP-induced binding of fibrinogen to the platelet membrane at specific receptor sites. *Platelet adhesion and platelet aggregation are inhibited and prolong bleeding time.*

USES Reduction of the risk of thrombotic stroke; adjunctive therapy for stent thrombosis prophylaxis.

UNLABELED USES Prevention of venous thromboembolic disorders; maintenance of bypass graft patency and of vascular access sites in hemodialysis patients; improvement of exercise performance in patients with ischemic heart disease and intermittent claudication; prevention of postoperative deep venous thrombosis (DVT).

CONTRAINDICATIONS Hypersensitivity to ticlopidine; hematopoietic disease, coagulopathy; neutropenia thrombotic thrombocytopenic purpura (TTP) leukemia; pathologic bleeding; severe liver impairment; lactation.

CAUTIOUS USE Hepatic function impairment, renal impairment; patients at risk for bleeding from trauma, surgery, or a bleeding disorder; GI bleeding in patients with history of thienopyridine hypersensitivity; allergic cross-reactivity; pregnancy (category B). Safe use in children younger than 18 y not established.

ROUTE & DOSAGE

Prevention of Stroke/Stent Thrombosis

Adult: **PO** 250 mg bid with food

ADMINISTRATION

Oral

- Hold medication and notify provider if neutrophil count falls below 1200/mm^3.
- Give with food or just after eating to minimize GI irritation.
- Do not give within 2 h of an antacid.
- Store at 15°–30° C (59°–86° F).

ADVERSE EFFECTS **CNS:** Dizziness. **Endocrine:** Hypercholesterolemia. **Skin:** Urticaria, maculopapular rash, erythema nodosum (generally occur within the first 3 mo of therapy, with most

T

occurring within the first 3–6 wk). **GI:** Nausea, vomiting, diarrhea, abdominal cramps; dyspepsia, flatulence, anorexia; hypercholesterolemia, abnormal liver function tests (few cases of hepatotoxicity reported). **Hematologic:** Neutropenia (resolves in 1–3 wk), thrombocytopenia, leukopenia, agranulocytosis (usually within first 3 mo), and pancytopenia; hemorrhage (ecchymosis, epistaxis, menorrhagia, GI bleeding), thrombotic thrombocytopenic purpura (usually within first month).

DIAGNOSTIC TEST INTERFERENCE

Increases ***total serum cholesterol*** by 8–10% within 4 wk of beginning therapy. ***Lipoprotein ratios*** remain unchanged. Elevates ***alkaline phosphatase*** and ***serum transaminases.***

INTERACTIONS

Drug: ANTACIDS decrease bioavailability of ticlopidine. ANTICOAGULANTS increase risk of bleeding. **Cimetidine** decreases clearance of ticlopidine. CORTICOSTEROIDS counteract increased bleeding time associated with ticlopidine. May decrease **cyclosporine** levels. Increases **theophylline** serum levels. May increase levels of **citalopram, metoprolol, pimozide, phenytoin, tizanidine.** Can decrease levels of **clopidogrel.** Do not use with **defibrotide. Food:** Food may increase bioavailability of **ticlopidine. Herbal: Evening primrose oil** increases bleeding risk.

PHARMACOKINETICS

Absorption: 90% from GI tract; increased absorption when taken with food. **Onset:** Antiplatelet activity, 6 h; maximal effect at 3–5 days. **Peak:** Peak serum levels at 2h. **Duration:** Bleeding times return to baseline within 4–10 days. **Distribution:** 90% bound to plasma proteins. **Metabolism:** Rapidly and extensively metabolized in liver (CYP1A2, CYP2B6, CYP2C19). **Elimination:** 60% of metabolites excreted in urine, 23% in feces. **Half-Life:** 12.6 h; terminal half-life is 4–5 days with repeated dosing.

NURSING IMPLICATIONS

Black Box Warning

Ticlopidine has been associated with life-threatening neutropenia, agranulocytosis, thrombotic thrombocytopenic purpura (TTP), and aplastic anemia.

Assessment & Drug Effects

- Report promptly laboratory values indicative of neutropenia, thrombocytopenia, or agranulocytosis.
- Monitor for signs of bleeding (e.g., ecchymosis, epistaxis, hematuria, GI bleeding).
- Monitor lab tests: Baseline CBC with differentials and platelet count, repeat q2wk from second week to end of third month of therapy, repeat as indicated thereafter if S&S of infection develop, and LFTs.

Patient & Family Education

- Stop taking this drug and report promptly to prescriber any of the following: Nausea, diarrhea, rash, sore throat, or other signs of infection, signs of bleeding, or signs of liver damage (e.g., yellow skin or sclera, dark urine or clay-colored stools).
- Understand risk of GI bleeding; do not take aspirin along with ticlopidine.
- Do not take antacids within 2 h of ticlopidine.
- Keep appointments for regularly scheduled blood tests.

TIGECYCLINE

(ti-ge-cy'cline)

Tygacil

Classification: ANTIBIOTIC; GLYCYLCYCLINE

Therapeutic: ANTIBIOTIC

Prototype: Tetracycline

AVAILABILITY Solution for injection

ACTION & THERAPEUTIC EFFECT
Inhibits protein production in bacteria by binding to the 30S ribosomal subunit and blocking entry of transfer RNA molecules into ribosome of bacteria. This prevents formation of peptide chains within bacteria, thus interfering with their growth. *Tigecycline is active against a broad spectrum of bacterial pathogens and is bacteriostatic.*

USES Treatment of complicated skin and skin structure infections, community-acquired pneumonia, and complicated intra-abdominal infections.

CONTRAINDICATIONS Hypersensitivity to tigecycline; viral infections; pregnancy (category D); and during tooth development of the fetus.

T

CAUTIOUS USE Severe hepatic impairment (Child-Pugh class C); hypersensitivity to tetracycline, intestinal perforations, intra-abdominal infections; GI disorders; lactation. Safe use in children younger than 8 y not established.

ROUTE & DOSAGE

Community Acquired Pneumonia, Complicated Skin/ Intra-abdominal Infections

Adult: **IV** 100 mg initially, followed by 50 mg q12h over 30–60 min × 5–14 days

Hepatic Impairment Dosage Adjustment

Child-Pugh class C: Initial dose 100 mg, followed by 25 mg q12h

ADMINISTRATION

- Note that dosage adjustment is required with severe hepatic impairment.

Intravenous

PREPARE: **Intermittent:** Reconstitute each 50 mg with 5.3 mL of NS or D5W to yield 10 mg/mL. ▪ Swirl gently to dissolve; reconstituted solution should be yellow to orange in color. ▪ After reconstitution, immediately withdraw exactly 5 mL from each vial and add to 100 mL of NS or D5W for infusion. ▪ The maximum concentration in the IV bag should be 1 mg/mL (two 50 mg doses).
ADMINISTER: **Intermittent:** Give over 30–60 min through a dedicated line or Y-site; when using Y-site, flush IV line with NS or D5W before/after infusion.
INCOMPATIBILITIES: **Y-site: Amiodarone, amphotericin B, bleomycin, chloramphenicol, chlorpromazine, dantrolene, daunorubicin,**

diazepam, epirubicin, esomeprazole, idarubicin, methylprednisolone, nicardipine, omeprazole, phenytoin, quinuprustin/dalfopristin, verapamil, voriconazole.

- Store in the IV bag at room temperature for up to 6 h, or refrigerated at 2°–8° C (36°–46° F) for up to 24 h.

ADVERSE EFFECTS **CV:** Hypertension, hypotension, peripheral edema, phlebitis. **Respiratory:** Dyspnea, increased cough, pulmonary physical findings. **CNS:** Asthenia, dizziness, headache, insomnia. **Endocrine:** Alkaline phosphatase increased, ALT increased, amylase increased, AST increased, bilirubinemia, BUN increased, hyperglycemia, hypokalemia, hypoproteinemia, lactic dehydrogenase increased. **Skin:** Pruritus, rash, sweating. **GI:** Abdominal pain, constipation, diarrhea, dyspepsia, *nausea, vomiting*. **Musculoskeletal:** Back pain. **Hematologic:** Abnormal healing, anemia, infection, leukocytosis, thrombocythemia. **Other:** Abscess, fever, local reaction to injection, pain.

INTERACTIONS **Drug:** Increased concentrations of **warfarin** required close monitoring of INR. Efficacy of ORAL CONTRACEPTIVES may be decreased when used in combination with tigecycline.

PHARMACOKINETICS **Distribution:** 71–89% protein bound. **Metabolism:** Negligible. **Elimination:** Fecal (major) and renal. **Half-Life:** 27 h (single dose); 42 h (multiple doses).

NURSING IMPLICATIONS

Black Box Warning

Tigecycline has been associated with increased mortality, thus its use should be reserved for situations where alternative treatments are not suitable.

Assessment & Drug Effects

- Monitor for hypersensitivity reaction in those with reported tetracycline allergy.
- Monitor for and report S&S of superinfection (see Appendix F) or pseudomembranous enterocolitis (see Appendix F).
- Monitor diabetics for loss of glycemic control.
- Monitor lab tests: Baseline C&S, and periodic LFTs.

Patient & Family Education

- Avoid direct exposure to sunlight during and for several days after therapy is terminated to reduce risk of photosensitivity reaction.
- Report to prescriber loose stools or diarrhea either during or shortly after termination of therapy.
- Use a barrier contraceptive in addition to oral contraceptives if trying to avoid pregnancy.

TILDRAKIZUMAB

(til-dra-kiz′ue-mab)

Ilumya

Classification: ANTIPSORIATIC AGENT; IL-23 INHIBITOR; MONOCLONAL ANTIBODY

Therapeutic: ANTIPSORIATIC

AVAILABILITY Subcutaneous injection, prefilled syringe

T

ACTION & *THERAPEUTIC EFFECT*

Human monoclonal IgG1/k antibody that selectively binds with interleukin-23 receptor to inhibit the release of proinflammatory cytokines and chemokines. *Reduces inflammatory response in adults with moderate to severe plaque psoriasis.*

USES Treatment of moderate to severe plaque psoriasis in patients who are candidates for systemic therapy or phototherapy.

CONTRAINDICATIONS Previous hypersensitivity to tildrakizumab or components of the formulation; patients with active infection; pregnancy—fetal risk cannot be ruled out; lactation—infant risk cannot be ruled out.

CAUTIOUS USE Use of tildrakizumab increases the risk of serious infections. Patients should be evaluated for tuberculosis infection prior to use of tildrakizumab. Safety in children younger than 18 y not established.

ROUTE & DOSAGE

Psoriasis

Adult: **Subcutaneous** 100 mg at wk 0 and 4, and then every 12 wk thereafter

T

ADMINISTRATION

Subcutaneous

- To be administered by a health-care provider.
- Remove prefilled syringe from the refrigerator and allow to warm at room temperature for 30 min.
- Inspect solution for any particulate matter or discoloration; solution should be slightly opalescent, colorless, to lightly yellow.
- Injection should be given in abdomen, thighs, or upper arm. Avoid 2 inches around the belly button or any area that is tender, bruised, erythematous, indurated, or affected by psoriasis. Avoid scar tissue, stretch marks, or blood vessels.
- Store original carton at 2°–8° C (36°–46° F); do not freeze and protect from light. Solution may also be stored in original carton at room temperature not exceeding 25° C (77° F) for up to 30 days. Do not place back in refrigerator. Discard if not used within 30 days.

ADVERSE EFFECTS (≥5%) **Respiratory:** Upper respiratory infection.

INTERACTIONS **Drug:** Avoid the use of LIVE VACCINES in patients being treated with tildrakizumab. Avoid other IMMUNOSUPPRESSIVE agents.

PHARMACOKINETICS **Absorption:** 73–80% bioavailability. **Peak:** 6 days. **Metabolism:** Similar to endogenous IgG; degraded into small peptides and amino acids through catabolic pathways. **Half-Life:** 23 days.

NURSING IMPLICATIONS

Assessment & Drug Effects

- Assess skin for improvement of plaque psoriasis.
- Respiratory assessment for S&S of upper respiratory infection and TB (bad cough that lasts for at least 3 wk, coughing up blood or sputum, chest pain, weakness, fatigue, and weight loss).
- Monitor lab tests: TB screening prior to beginning treatment.

Patient & Family Education

- Report to prescriber any symptoms of itching, redness, soreness, difficulty breathing which may indicate an infection.

- Report to provider any signs of a respiratory infection (cough, fever, runny nose, congestion, coughing up blood, etc.). Local redness, swelling, soreness or itching at injection site or diarrhea.
- Avoid live vaccines during treatment.

TIMOLOL MALEATE

(tye'moe-lole)

Betimol, Istalol, Timoptic, Timoptic XE

Classification: BETA-ADRENERGIC ANTAGONIST; EYE PREPARATION; MIOTIC; ANTIHYPERTENSIVE; ANTIANGINAL

Therapeutic: ANTIGLAUCOMA; ANTIHYPERTENSIVE; ANTIANGINAL

Prototype: Propranolol

AVAILABILITY Tablet; ophthalmic solution; ophthalmic gel

ACTION & *THERAPEUTIC EFFECT* Exhibits antihypertensive, antiarrhythmic, and antianginal properties, and suppresses plasma renin activity. When applied topically, lowers elevated and normal intraocular pressure (IOP) by reducing formation of aqueous humor and possibly by increasing outflow. *Topically, lowers elevated and normal intraocular pressure (IOP). Orally, useful for mild hypertension, angina, and migraine headaches.*

USES Topically (ophthalmic solution) to reduce elevated IOP in chronic, open-angle glaucoma, aphakic glaucoma, secondary glaucoma, and ocular hypertension. Oral product is used as monotherapy or in combination with a thiazide diuretic to prevent reinfarction after MI and to treat mild hypertension; migraine prophylaxis.

UNLABELED USES Prophylactic management of stable, uncomplicated angina pectoris.

CONTRAINDICATIONS Bronchospasm; severe COPD; bronchial asthma or history there of; HF; abrupt discontinuation, acute bronchospasm, second- and third-degree AV block, sinus bradycardia, cardiogenic shock, acute pulmonary edema, Raynaud's disease.

CAUTIOUS USE Bronchitis, patients subject to bronchospasm, asthma; first-degree heart block, HF; renal impairment; hepatic disease; vasospastic angina; PVD; pheochromocytoma; thyrotoxicosis, hyperthyroidism; COPD; cerebrovascular insufficiency; stroke, CVD; depression; psoriasis; MG, DM, history of spontaneous hypoglycemia; older adults; pregnancy (category C). Safe use in children not established.

ROUTE & DOSAGE

Glaucoma

See Appendix A-1.

Hypertension

Adult: **PO** 10 mg bid (may increase to 20 mg bid)

Post-MI Reinfarction

Adult: **PO** 10 mg bid

Migraine Prophylaxis

Adult: **PO** 10 mg bid or up to 30 mg daily

ADMINISTRATION

Oral

- Give with fluid of patient's choice; tablet may be crushed.
- Dosage increases for hypertension should be made at weekly intervals.

ADVERSE EFFECTS **CV:** Palpitation, *bradycardia, hypotension*, syncope, AV conduction disturbances, CHF, aggravation of peripheral vascular insufficiency. **Respiratory:** Difficulty in breathing, bronchospasm. **CNS:** *Fatigue*, lethargy, weakness, somnolence, anxiety, *headache*, dizziness, *confusion*, psychic dissociation, *depression*. **HEENT:** *Eye irritation* including conjunctivitis, blepharitis, keratitis, superficial punctate keratopathy. **Endocrine:** Hypoglycemia, hypokalemia. **Skin:** Rash, urticaria. **GI:** Anorexia, *dyspepsia, nausea*. **Other:** Fever.

INTERACTIONS **Drug:** ANTIHYPERTENSIVE AGENTS, DIURETICS, SELECTIVE SEROTONIN REUPTAKE INHIBITORS potentiate hypotensive effects; NSAIDS may antagonize hypotensive effects.

PHARMACOKINETICS **Absorption:** 90% from GI tract; some systemic absorption from topical application. **Peak:** 1–2 h PO; 1–5 h topical. **Distribution:** Distributed into breast milk. **Metabolism:** 80% metabolized in liver to inactive metabolites. **Elimination:** In urine.

T

NURSING IMPLICATIONS

Black Box Warning

Timolol has been associated with exacerbation of angina and MI when abruptly discontinued following chronic administration.

Assessment & Drug Effects

- Check pulse before administering timolol, topical or oral. If there are extremes (rate or rhythm), withhold medication and notify prescriber.
- Assess pulse rate and BP at regular intervals and more often in patients with severe heart disease.
- Note: Some patients develop tolerance during long-term therapy.

Patient & Family Education

- Be aware that drug may cause slight reduction in resting heart rate. Learn how to assess pulse rate and report significant changes. Consult prescriber for parameters.
- Do not stop drug abruptly; angina may be exacerbated. Dosage is reduced over a period of 1–2 wk.
- Report promptly to prescriber difficulty breathing. Drug withdrawal may be indicated.

TINIDAZOLE

(tin'i-da-zole)

Classification: ANTIPROTOZOAL

Therapeutic: ANTIBIOTIC; ANTIPROTOZOAL; AMEBICIDE

Prototype: Metronidazole

AVAILABILITY Tablet

ACTION & *THERAPEUTIC EFFECT* Effective against dividing and nondividing cells of targeted bacteria and protozoa. It inhibits formation of their DNA helix and thus inhibits DNA synthesis of these organisms. This leads to bacterial and protozoal cell death. *Demonstrates activity against infections caused by protozoa and anaerobic bacteria.*

USES Treatment of trichomoniasis, giardiasis, amebiasis, bacterial vaginosis, and amebic liver abscess.

CONTRAINDICATIONS Hypersensitivity to tinidazole or other azole antibiotics; pregnancy (first trimester); lactation within 72 h of tinidazole use.

CAUTIOUS USE CNS diseases, liver dysfunction, alcoholism, ethanol intoxication; hematologic disease; neurologic disease; bone marrow depression; dialysis; candidiasis; pregnancy (second and third trimester); children younger than 3 y.

ROUTE & DOSAGE

Giardiasis

Adult: **PO** 2 g as single dose
Child (3 y or older): **PO** 50 mg/kg (up to 2 g) as single dose

Intestinal Amebiasis

Adult: **PO** 2 g once daily for 3 days
Child (3 y or older): **PO** 50 mg/kg/day (up to 2 g/day) once daily for 3 days

Amebic Liver Abscess

Adult: **PO** 2 g once daily for 3–5 days
Child (3 y or older): **PO** 50 mg/kg/day (up to 2 g/day) once daily for 3–5 days

Trichomoniasis

Adult/Adolescent: **PO** 2 g as single dose
Child (older than 3 y): **PO** 50 mg/kg as a single dose; (max: 2000 mg)

Bacterial Vaginosis

Adult/Adolescent: **PO** 2 g daily × 2 days OR 1 g daily × 5 days

Hemodialysis Dosage Adjustment
If dose given on dialysis day, give supplemental dose (½ regular dose) post-dialysis

ADMINISTRATION

Oral

- Give with food to minimize GI distress; may be crushed in artificial cherry syrup if tablets cannot be swallowed whole (suspension is stable for 7 days at room temperature).
- If given on a dialysis day, add a 50% dose of tinidazole at the end of hemodialysis.
- Separate the dosing of cholestyramine and tinidazole by 2–4 h when used concurrently.
- Do not give within 2 wk of the last dose of disulfiram.
- Store at 15°–30° C (59°–86° F). Protect from light.

ADVERSE EFFECTS GI: Altered taste, nausea. **GU:** Vulvovaginal candidiasis.

DIAGNOSTIC TEST INTERFERENCE May interfere with ***AST, ALT, triglycerides, glucose,*** and ***LDH*** testing.

INTERACTIONS Drug: May increase INR with **warfarin; alcohol** may cause **disulfiram**-like reaction; may increase the half-life of **fosphenytoin, phenytoin;** may increase levels and toxicity of **lithium, fluorouracil, cyclosporine, tacrolimus; cholestyramine** may decrease absorption of tinidazole; **cimetidine** or **ketoconazole** may increase levels.

PHARMACOKINETICS Peak: 2 h. **Distribution:** Crosses blood–brain barrier and placenta and is excreted in breast milk. **Metabolism:** In the liver by CYP3A4. **Elimination:** Primarily in urine. **Half-Life:** 12–14 h.

NURSING IMPLICATIONS

Black Box Warning

Carcinogenicity has been seen in animal studies with another agent

T

in the nitroimidazole class. Unnecessary use of tinidazole should be avoided.

Assessment & Drug Effects

- Withhold drug and notify prescriber for S&S of CNS dysfunction (e.g., seizures, numbness or paresthesia of extremities). Drug should be discontinued if abnormal neurologic signs appear.
- Monitor INR/PT frequently with concomitant oral anticoagulants. Continue monitoring for at least 8 days after discontinuation of tinidazole.
- Monitor serum lithium levels with concurrent use.
- Monitor for phenytoin toxicity with concurrent IV phenytoin.
- Monitor lab tests: CBC with differential if retreatment is required.

Patient & Family Education

- Stop taking the drug and report promptly: Convulsions, numbness, tingling, pain, or weakness in the hands or feet; dizziness or unsteadiness; fever.
- Harmless urine discoloration may occur while taking this drug.

TIOCONAZOLE

(ti-o-con′a-zole)

Vagistat-1

Classification: AZOLE ANTIFUNGAL

Therapeutic: ANTIFUNGAL

Prototype: Fluconazole

AVAILABILITY
Vaginal ointment

ACTION & THERAPEUTIC EFFECT
Broad-spectrum antifungal agent that inhibits growth of human pathogenic yeasts by disrupting normal fungal cell membrane permeability. *Effective against* Candida albicans, *other species of* Candida, *and* Torulopsis glabrata.

USES
Local treatment of vulvovaginal candidiasis.

CONTRAINDICATIONS
Hypersensitivity to tioconazole or other imidazole antifungal agents; lactation.

CAUTIOUS USE
Diabetes mellitus; HIV infections; immunosuppression; pregnancy (category C); children younger than 12 y.

ROUTE & DOSAGE

Candidiasis

Adult: **Intravaginal** One applicator full at bedtime × 1 day

ADMINISTRATION

Instillation

- Insert applicator high into the vagina (except during pregnancy).
- Wash applicator before and after each use.
- Store away from direct heat and light.

ADVERSE EFFECTS
GU: Mild erythema, burning, discomfort, rash, itching.

INTERACTIONS
Drug: May inactivate spermicidal effects of **nonoxynol-9.**

PHARMACOKINETICS
Absorption: Minimal absorption from vagina.

NURSING IMPLICATIONS

Assessment & Drug Effects

- Do not use for patient with a history of allergic reaction to other antifungal agents, such as miconazole.

- Monitor for sensitization and irritation; these may be an indication to discontinue drug.

Patient & Family Education

- Learn correct application technique.
- Understand potential adverse reactions, including sensitization and allergic response.
- Tioconazole may interact with diaphragms and latex condoms; avoid concurrent use within 72 h.
- Refrain from sexual intercourse while using tioconazole.
- Wear only cotton underwear; change daily.

TIOTROPIUM BROMIDE

(ti-o-tro′pi-um)

Spiriva HandiHaler, Spiriva Respimat

Classification: RESPIRATORY SMOOTH MUSCLE RELAXANT

Therapeutic: BRONCHODILATOR; ANTISPASMODIC

Prototype: Atropine

AVAILABILITY Capsule with powder for inhalation; respiratory spray

ACTION & *THERAPEUTIC EFFECT* A long-acting, antispasmodic agent. In the bronchial airways, it exhibits inhibition of muscarinic receptors of the smooth muscle resulting in bronchodilation. *Bronchodilation after inhalation of tiotropium is predominantly a site-specific effect.*

USES Maintenance treatment of bronchospasm associated with chronic obstructive pulmonary disease (COPD); reducing COPD exacerbations; long-term maintenance treatment of asthma.

CONTRAINDICATIONS Hypersensitivity to tiotropium, atropine, or ipratropium; acute bronchospasm.

CAUTIOUS USE Decreased renal function; BPH, urinary bladder neck obstruction; narrow-angle glaucoma; older adults; pregnancy (fetal risk cannot be ruled out); lactation (infant risk cannot be ruled out). Safe use in children younger than 6 y not established.

ROUTE & DOSAGE

COPD

Adult: **Inhaled Spiriva HandiHaler** 18 mcg OR **Spiriva Respimat** 2 inhalations once daily using inhaler device provided

Asthma

Adult: **Inhaled Spiriva Respimat** 2.5 mcg daily

ADMINISTRATION

Inhalation ONLY

- Place capsule in HandiHaler® and press button to puncture. Instruct patient to exhale deeply, then put the mouthpiece to the lips and breathe in the dose deeply and slowly; remove HandiHaler® and hold breath for at least 10 sec, and then exhale slowly; rinse mouth with water to minimize dry mouth.
- Ensure that drug does not contact the eyes.
- Store at 15°–30° C (59°–86° F). Do not expose to extreme temperature or moisture. Do not store in HandiHaler device.

ADVERSE EFFECTS **CV:** Chest pain, edema. **Respiratory:** Cough, pharyngitis, rhinitis, *URI*. **GI:** Dry mouth, abdominal pain, indigestion. **GU:** UTI.

T

INTERACTIONS Drug: May cause additive anticholinergic effects with other ANTICHOLINERGIC AGENTS. Do not use with inhaled form of **loxapine**.

PHARMACOKINETICS Absorption: 19.5% absorbed from the lungs. **Peak:** 5 min. **Metabolism:** Less than 25% of dose is metabolized in liver by CYP2D6 and 3A4. **Elimination:** 14% of dose excreted in urine; remaining is excreted in feces as nonabsorbed drug. **Half-Life:** 5–6 days.

NURSING IMPLICATIONS

Assessment & Drug Effects

- Withhold drug and notify prescriber if S&S of angioedema occurs.
- Monitor for anticholinergic effects (e.g., tachycardia, urinary retention).
- Monitor lab tests: Pulmonary function tests.

Patient & Family Education

- Do not allow powdered medication to contact the eyes, as this may cause blurring of vision and pupil dilation.
- Tiotropium bromide is intended as a once-daily maintenance treatment. It is not useful for treatment of acute episodes of bronchospasm (i.e., rescue therapy).
- Withhold drug and notify prescriber if swelling around the face, mouth, or neck occurs.
- Report any of the following: Constipation, increased heart rate, blurred vision, urinary difficulty.

T

TIPRANAVIR

(ti-pra′na-vir)

Aptivus

Classification: PROTEASE INHIBITOR

Therapeutic: ANTIRETROVIRAL

Prototype: Saquinavir

AVAILABILITY Capsule; oral solution

ACTION & THERAPEUTIC EFFECT Inhibits virus-specific processing of the viral polyproteins in HIV-1 infected cells, thus preventing the formation of mature viral particles. *Helps decrease viral load of HIV-1 strains resistant to other protease inhibitors.*

USES Treatment of HIV-1 infection in combination with other agents.

CONTRAINDICATIONS Known hypersensitivity to tipranavir; moderate to severe (Child-Pugh class B and C, respectively) hepatic impairment; drug induced hepatic decomposition or intracranial hemorrhage; pancreatitis; lactation (infant risk cannot be ruled out).

CAUTIOUS USE Hypersensitivity to sulfonamides; patients with chronic hepatitis B or hepatitis C coinfection; hepatic impairment, surgery and trauma patients; hemophilia; coagulopathy; elevated liver enzymes; diabetes mellitus or hyperglycemia; hyperlipidemia; autoimmune disorders, including Graves disease, polymyositis, & Guillain-Barr syndrome; pregnancy (fetal risk cannot be ruled out); children younger than 2 y.

ROUTE & DOSAGE

HIV-1 Infection

Adult: **PO** 500 mg (with 200 mg ritonavir) bid
Adolescent/Child (older than 2 y): **PO** 14 mg/kg bid OR 375 mg/m^2 bid (with ritonavir)

ADMINISTRATION

Oral

- Coadminister with ritonavir. Give with food.
- Store solution at 15°–30° C (59°–86° F). Once opened, use contents of bottle within 60 days.
- Store capsules prior to opening bottle at 2°–8° C (36°–46° F). After bottle is opened, may be stored at 25° C (77° F) for up to 60 days.

ADVERSE EFFECTS **CNS:** Headache, dizziness. **Endocrine:** *Hypertriglyceridemia*, hypercholesterolemia, increased amylase. **Skin:** Rash. **Hepatic:** Increased ALT/SGPT, increased AST/SGOT, *increased liver aminotransferase*. **GI:** Diarrhea, nausea, vomiting. **Other:** Fatigue, fever.

INTERACTIONS **Drug:** Do not use with **sildenafil, alfuzosin, salmeterol.** Do not use with ERGOT ALKALOIDS. Do not use with other PROTEASE INHIBITORS. Adjust **tipranavir** dosing when used with **bosentan, tadalafil, colchicine. Aluminum-** and **magnesium-**based ANTACIDS may decrease tipranavir absorption. AZOLE ANTIFUNGAL AGENTS, **clarithromycin, erythromycin,** and other inhibitors of CYP3A4 may increase tipranavir levels. **Efavirenz, loperamide,** NRTIS, and RIFAMYCINS (e.g., **rifampin**) may decrease tipranavir levels. Tipranavir increases **rifabutin** levels. Coadministration of tipranavir and **tenofovir** decreases the levels of both compounds. Tipranavir increases the concentration of BENZODIAZEPINES, **desipramine,** and numerous ANTIARRHYTHMIC AGENTS **(amiodarone, flecainide, propafenone, quinidine).** Combination use of tipranavir and HMG COA REDUCTASE INHIBITORS increases the risk of myopathy. Tipranavir capsules contain **alcohol** that can produce disulfiram-like reactions with **metronidazole** and **disulfiram.** Adjust **midazolam** dose. **Food:** Food enhances the bioavailability of tipranavir, avoid large doses of vitamin E. **Herbal: St. John's wort** decreases the levels of tipranavir.

PHARMACOKINETICS **Peak:** 3 h. **Distribution:** Greater than 99.9% protein bound. **Metabolism:** Extensive hepatic oxidation (CYP 3A4) to inactive metabolites (when given alone); minimal metabolism (when given with ritonavir). **Elimination:** Fecal (primary) and renal (minimal). **Half-Life:** 6 h.

NURSING IMPLICATIONS

Black Box Warning

Tipranavir has been associated with hepatitis, hepatic decompensation, and intracranial hemorrhage.

Assessment & Drug Effects

- Monitor for and report immediately S&S of liver toxicity (see Appendix F).
- Monitor for S&S of adverse drug reactions and toxicity from concurrently administered drugs. Many drugs interact with tipranavir.
- Monitor diabetics for loss of glycemic <u>control: Hyperglycemia</u>.
- Use barrier contraceptive if using hormonal contraceptive.
- Monitor blood levels of anticoagulants with concurrent therapy.
- Monitor lab tests: Baseline and frequent LFTs and lipid profile; CBC with differential, urinalysis, electrolytes, for women of childbearing potential (pregnancy test before starting therapy), viral

T

load, CD4 count, and fasting plasma glucose as indicated.

Patient & Family Education

- If a dose is missed, take it as soon as possible and then return to the normal schedule. Never double a dose.
- Inform prescriber of all medications and herbal products you are taking.
- Protect against sunlight exposure to minimize risk of photosensitivity.
- Report any of the following to prescriber: Fatigue, weakness, loss of appetite, nausea, jaundice, dark urine, or clay colored stools.

TIROFIBAN HYDROCHLORIDE

(tir-o-fi′ban)

Aggrastat

Classification: ANTICOAGULANT; ANTIPLATELET; GLYCOPROTEIN (GP) IIB/IIIA RECEPTOR INHIBITOR

Therapeutic: ANTIPLATELET

AVAILABILITY Solution for injection

ACTION & *THERAPEUTIC EFFECT* Binds to the glycoprotein IIb/IIIa receptor on platelets thus inhibiting platelet aggregation. *Effectiveness indicated by minimizing thrombotic events during treatment of acute coronary syndrome.*

T

USES Acute coronary syndromes (unstable angina, non ST elevation MI).

CONTRAINDICATIONS Hypersensitivity to tirofiban; active internal bleeding within 30 days; acute pericarditis; aortic dissection; intracranial aneurysm, intracranial mass, coagulopathy; history of aneurysm or AV malformation; history of intracranial hemorrhage or neoplasm; active abnormal bleeding; retinal bleeding; hemorrhagic retinopathy; major surgery or trauma within 3 days; stroke within 30 days; history of hemorrhagic stroke; thrombocytopenia following administration of tirofiban; history of thrombopenia due to prior exposure to tirofiban; severe rash during use of tirofiban; within 4 h of PCI; pregnancy—fetal risk cannot be ruled out; lactation infant risk cannot be ruled out.

CAUTIOUS USE Platelet count less than 150,000 mm^3; severe renal insufficiency. Safety and efficacy in children younger than 18 y not established.

ROUTE & DOSAGE

Unstable Angina, non ST-elevation MI

Adult: ***IV*** *25 mcg/kg over 5 min and then 0.15 mcg/kg/min for up to 18 h*

Renal Impairment Dosage Adjustment

CrCl less than or equal to 60 mL/min: Give 25 mcg/kg over less than 5 min and then 0.075 mcg/kg/min

ADMINISTRATION

Intravenous Only

PREPARE: **IV Infusion:** Use as supplied with no further preparation.

ADMINISTER: **IV Infusion:** Give an initial loading dose of 25 mcg/kg over 3 min and then 0.15 mcg/kg/min for up to 18 h.

INCOMPATIBILITIES: **Y-site: Amphotericin B, dantrolene, diazepam, lansoprazole, phenytoin.**

- Discard unused IV solution 24 h following start of infusion. ▪ Store unopened containers at 25 degrees C (77 degrees F), occasional excursions between 15°–30° C (59°–86° F) are permissible. ▪ Do not freeze and protect from light.

ADVERSE EFFECTS (≥5%) **CV:** Coronary artery dissection. **Hematologic:** *Bleeding (minor)*. **GU:** Pelvic pain.

INTERACTIONS **Drug:** Increased risk of bleeding with ANTICOAGULANTS, NSAIDS, SALICYLATES, ANTIPLATELET AGENTS. **Herbal: Feverfew, garlic, ginger, ginkgo, horse chestnut** may increase risk of bleeding.

PHARMACOKINETICS **Duration:** 4–8 h after stopping infusion. **Distribution:** 65% protein bound. **Metabolism:** Minimally metabolized. **Elimination:** 65% in urine, 25% in feces. **Half-Life:** 2 h.

NURSING IMPLICATIONS

Assessment & Drug Effects

- Withhold drug and notify prescriber if thrombocytopenia (platelets less than 100,000) is confirmed.
- Monitor carefully for and immediately report S&S of internal or external bleeding.
- Minimize unnecessary invasive procedures and devices to reduce the risk of bleeding.
- Monitor lab tests: Platelet count, Hgb and Hct before treatment, (within 6 h of infusing loading dose), and frequently throughout treatment; periodic APTT and ACT.

Patient & Family Education

- Report unexplained pelvic, leg or abdominal pain, dizziness, sweating, edema/swelling.
- Report episodes of bleeding or bruising. Review instructions that coffee ground emesis and black tarry stools are also a sign of bleeding as well as bright red blood.
- There are many drug-drug interactions. Consult healthcare provider before taking any new drug, over-the-counter, or herbal drugs.

TIZANIDINE HYDROCHLORIDE

(ti-zan'i-deen)

Zanaflex

Classification: CENTRAL ACTING SKELETAL MUSCLE RELAXANT; ALPHA 2 ADRENERGIC AGONIST

Therapeutic: SKELETAL MUSCLE RELAXANT; ANTISPASMODIC

Prototype: Cyclobenzaprine

AVAILABILITY Tablet; capsule

ACTION & *THERAPEUTIC EFFECT* Reduces spasticity by increasing presynaptic inhibition of motor neurons. Greatest effect on polysynaptic afferent reflex activity at the spinal cord level. *Site of action is the spinal cord; reduces skeletal muscle spasms. Effectiveness indicated by decreased muscle tone.*

USES Acute and intermittent management of spasticity.

CONTRAINDICATIONS Hypersensitivity to tizanidine; concomitant therapy with **ciprofloxacin** or **fluvoxamine** (potent CYP1A2 inhibitors); pregnancy—fetal risk cannot be ruled out; lactation infant risk cannot be ruled out. Effect of tizanidine on labor and delivery is unknown.

CAUTIOUS USE Patients with hepatic impairment, hepatic

T

disease; renal insufficiency (CrCl less than 25 mL/min), or renal failure; history of hypotension; psychosis; women taking oral contraceptives; history of QT prolongation; history of narcotic abuse; older adults because of renal impairment and orthostatic hypotension. Safety and efficacy in children not established.

ROUTE & DOSAGE

Spasticity

Adult: PO Start with 2 mg can be increased by 2–4 mg per day (max: 36 mg/day)

Renal Impairment Dosage Adjustment

CrCl less than 25 mL/min: If dose increases are needed increase dose not dosing frequency

ADMINISTRATION

Oral

- Can be given without regard to food, but patient should choose with food or without food and administer medication consistently.
- Dose increases are usually made gradually in 2- to 4-mg increments.
- Store at 25 degrees C (77 degrees F), excursions permitted from 15°–30° C (59°–86° F).

ADVERSE EFFECTS **CV:** *Hypotension.* **CNS:** *Somnolence, dizziness, asthenia.* **GI:** *Dry mouth.*

INTERACTIONS **Drug: Alcohol,** OPIOIDS and other CNS DEPRESSANTS increase CNS depression. Avoid concomitant therapy with **ciprofloxacin** or **fluvoxamine** (potent CYP1A2 inhibitors) due to increased risk of toxicity. Avoid use of agents that can prolong the QT interval (e.g., **dofetilide, dronedarone, pimozide, thioridazine, ziprasidone**); agents that cause bradycardia can have an additive adverse effect. CYP 1A2 INHIBITORS may increase concentration of tizanidine and increase adverse effects. **Herbal: Kava, valerian** may potentiate sedation.

PHARMACOKINETICS **Absorption:** Rapidly from GI tract; 40% bioavailability; tablets and capsules are bioequivalent in fasting conditions but not in nonfasting conditions. **Peak:** 1–2 h. **Duration:** 3–6 h. **Distribution:** Crosses placenta, distributed into breast milk. **Metabolism:** In the liver (CYP1A2). **Elimination:** 60% in urine, 20% in feces. **Half-Life:** 2.5 h.

NURSING IMPLICATIONS

Assessment & Drug Effects

- Monitor cardiovascular status and report orthostatic hypotension or bradycardia.
- Monitor closely older adults, those with renal impairment, and women taking oral contraceptives for adverse effects because drug clearance is reduced.
- Monitor lab tests: Baseline LFTs and 1 mo after max dose is achieved or if hepatic injury suspected, renal function tests.

Patient & Family Education

- Exercise caution with potentially hazardous activities requiring alertness since sedation is a common adverse effect. Effects are additive with alcohol or other CNS depressants.
- Make position changes slowly because of the risk of orthostatic hypotension.

- Report unusual sensory experiences; hallucinations and delusions have occurred with tizanidine use.
- Do not suddenly discontinue the drug.
- Drug has multiple drug-drug interactions. Consult healthcare provider prior to taking any new drug, over-the-counter drug or herbal supplement.

TOBRAMYCIN SULFATE

(toe-bra-mye′sin)

AKTob, Bethkis,TobraDex, Tobrex, Tobi Podhaler, Tobrasol

Classification: AMINOGLYCOSIDE ANTIBIOTIC

Therapeutic: ANTIBIOTIC

Prototype: Gentamicin sulfate

AVAILABILITY Solution for injection; nebulizer solution; capsule for inhalation; ophthalmic solution; ophthalmic ointment

ACTION & *THERAPEUTIC EFFECT*

Binds irreversibly to one of two aminoglycoside binding sites on the 30S ribosomal subunit of the bacteria, thus inhibiting protein synthesis, resulting in bacterial cell death. *Effective in treatment of gram-negative bacteria. Exhibits greater antibiotic activity against* Pseudomonas aeruginosa *than other aminoglycosides.*

USES Treatment of severe infections caused by susceptible organisms.

CONTRAINDICATIONS History of hypersensitivity to tobramycin and other aminoglycoside; pregnancy (category D).

CAUTIOUS USE Impaired kidney function; renal disease; dehydration; hearing impairment; myasthenia gravis; parkinsonism; older adults; lactation; premature, neonatal infants.

ROUTE & DOSAGE

Moderate to Severe Infections

Adult: **IV/IM** 3–6 mg/kg/day in 2–3 divided doses OR 4–7 mg/kg/day single dose
Adolescent/Child/Infant: **IM/IV** 2.5 mg/kg/dose q8h
Neonate: **IM/IV** 2.5 mg/kg q12–24h
Premature Neonate: **IV/IM** See package insert for dosage by weight and gestational age

Cystic Fibrosis

Adult: Child: **IM/IV** 10 mg/kg/dose q24h; **Nebulized** 300 mg inhaled bid × 28 days, may repeat after 28-day drug-free period
Podhaler: 112 mg (4 caps) q12h × 28 days may repeat after 28 drug-free days

Ocular Infection

Adults/Adolescents/Children/Infants 2 mo or older: **Topical** Apply a thin strip to the conjunctiva (about 1 cm) q8–12h; **Drops** 1–2 drops into the infected eye q4h

Renal Impairment Dosage Adjustment

Increase interval

Hemodialysis Dosage Adjustment

Administer dose after dialysis and monitor levels

Obesity Dosage Adjustment

Dose based on IBW; in morbid obesity, use dosing weight of IBW + 0.4 (Weight − IBW)

ADMINISTRATION

Note: Doses should be based on ideal body weight.

Inhalation

- Administer over 10–15 min using a handheld reusable nebulizer with a compressor (use only those supplied). Patient should sit upright and breathe normally through the nebulizer mouthpiece.

Intramuscular

- Give deep IM into a large muscle. Rotate injection sites.

Intravenous

Note: Verify correct IV concentration and rate of infusion to neonates, infants, or children with prescriber.

PREPARE: **Intermittent** ▪ Dilute each dose in 50–100 mL or more of D5W, NS or D5/NS. ▪ Final concentration should not exceed 5 mg/mL.

ADMINISTER: **Intermittent:** Infuse diluted solution over 20–60 min. ▪ Avoid rapid infusion.

INCOMPATIBILITIES: **Solution/additive:** **Alcohol 5% in dextrose, cefamandole, cefepime.** **Y-site:** **Allopurinol, amphotericin B cholesteryl complex, azathioprine sodium, azathioprine, azithromycin, cangrelor, cefazolin, cefoperazone, cefotetan, ceftobiprole, ceftriaxone, cloxacillin sodium, dacarbazine, dantrolene, defibrotide, dexamethasone, diazepam, diazoxide, folic acid, ganciclovir, garenoxacin mesylate, gemtuzumab, heparin, hetastarch, indomethacin, lansoprazole, oxacillin, pemetrexed, pentamidine, pentobarbital, phenytoin, piperacillin/tazobactam, propofol, sargramostim, SMZ/TMP.**

- Store at 15°–30° C (59°–86° F) prior to reconstitution. After reconstitution, solution may be refrigerated and used within 96 h. ▪ If kept at room temperature, use within 24 h.

ADVERSE EFFECTS

CNS: Neurotoxicity (including ototoxicity), *nephrotoxicity,* increased AST, ALT, LDH, serum bilirubin; anemia, fever, rash, pruritus, urticaria, nausea, vomiting, headache, lethargy, superinfections; hypersensitivity. **HEENT:** *Burning, stinging of eye after drug instillation;* eyelid itching and edema. **GU:** Oliguria, proteinuria.

INTERACTIONS

Drug: ANESTHETICS, SKELETAL MUSCLE RELAXANTS add to neuromuscular blocking effects; **acyclovir, amphotericin B, capreomycin,** CEPHALOSPORINS, **colistin, cisplatin, carboplatin, foscarnet, methoxyflurane, polymyxin B, vancomycin, furosemide, ethacrynic acid** increase risk of ototoxicity, nephrotoxicity. Do not use with **cidofovir** or **gallium.**

PHARMACOKINETICS

Peak: 30–90 min IM. **Duration:** Up to 8 h. **Distribution:** Crosses placenta; accumulates in renal cortex. **Elimination:** In urine. **Half-Life:** 2–3 h in adults.

NURSING IMPLICATIONS

Black Box Warning

Tobramycin has been associated with ototoxicity and nephrotoxicity.

Assessment & Drug Effects

- Weigh patient before treatment for calculation of dosage.

- Observe patient receiving tobramycin closely because of the high potential for toxicity, even in conventional doses.
- Monitor auditory, and vestibular functions closely, particularly in patients with known or suspected renal impairment and patients receiving high doses.
- Be aware that drug-induced auditory changes are irreversible (partial or total); usually bilateral. Partial or bilateral deafness may continue to develop even after therapy discontinued.
- Monitor I&O. Report oliguria, changes in I&O ratio, and cloudy or frothy urine (may indicate proteinuria). Keep patient well hydrated to prevent chemical irritation in renal tubules; older adults are especially susceptible to renal toxicity.
- Be aware that prolonged use of ophthalmic solution may encourage superinfection with nonsusceptible organisms including fungi.
- Report overdose symptoms for eye medication: Increased lacrimation, keratitis, edema and itching of eyelids.
- Monitor lab tests: Baseline C&S; baseline and periodic renal function tests; periodic peak and trough drug levels.

Patient & Family Education

- Report symptoms of superinfections (see Appendix F) to prescriber. Prompt treatment with an antibiotic or antifungal medication may be necessary.
- Report S&S of hearing loss, tinnitus, or vertigo to prescriber.

TOCILIZUMAB

(to-si-ly'zu-mab)

Actemra

Classification: DISEASE-MODIFYING ANTIRHEUMATIC DRUG (DMARD)

Therapeutic: DISEASE-MODIFYING ANTIRHEUMATIC DRUG (DMARD)

AVAILABILITY Solution for injection

ACTION & *THERAPEUTIC EFFECT* Binds to interleukin 6 (IL-6) receptors inhibiting IL-6 mediated signaling and suppressing systemic inflammatory responses; also reduces IL-6 production in joints affected by inflammatory processes such as rheumatoid arthritis. *Reduction of joint inflammation reduces joint pain and improves joint function and for improvement of cytokine release syndrome, Chimeric antigen T-cell induced, severe life threatening disease.*

USES Treatment of moderate to severe rheumatoid arthritis or juvenile idiopathic arthritis; cytokine release syndrome; COVID-19 in hospitalized patients.

CONTRAINDICATIONS History of anaphylaxis reaction with tocilizumab; severe neutropenia, severe thrombocytopenia; live vaccines; severe hepatic impairment; positive hepatitis B or hepatitis C virus serology; active hepatic disease; concomitant use of biological disease-modifying antirheumatic drugs such as tumor necrosis factor (TNF) antagonists, interleukin-1R antagonists, anti-CD20 monoclonal antibodies and selective co-stimulation modulators.

CAUTIOUS USE History of chronic or recurring infections; history of hypersensitivity; mild hepatic impairment; thrombocytopenia or neutropenia; risk for GI perforation; demyelinating disorders; preexisting or recent-onset demyelinating disorders; history of hyperlipidemia; older adults;

pregnancy (fetal risk cannot be ruled out); lactation (infant risk cannot be ruled out). Safety and efficacy in children younger than 2 y not established.

ROUTE & DOSAGE

Rheumatoid Arthritis

Adult: **IV** 4 mg/kg q4wk. May increase up to 8 mg/kg q4wk
Adult (weight greater than 100 kg): **Subcutaneous** 162 mg every wk
Adult (weight less than 100 kg): **Subcutaneous** 162 mg every other wk

Polyarticular Juvenile Idiopathic Arthritis

Child/Adolescent (older than 2 y and weight greater than 30 kg): **IV** 8 mg/kg q4wk; *older than 2 y and weight less than 30 kg:* **IV** 10 mg/kg q4wk

Systematic Juvenile Idiopathic Arthritis

Child/Adolescent (older than 2 y and weight greater than 30 kg): **IV** 8 mg/kg q2wk; **Subcutaneous** 162 mg/dose every 2 wk; *older than 2 y and weight less than 30 kg:* **IV** 12 mg/kg q2wks; **Subcutaneous** 162 mg/dose every 3 wk

Cytokine Release Syndrome

Adult (30 kg or more): **IV** 8 mg/kg (max: 800 mg/dose), may repeat for 3 additional doses (at least 8 h apart)
Adult/Adolescent/Child (weight less than 30 kg) **IV** 12 mg/kg (max: 800 mg/dose), may repeat for 3 additional doses (at least 8 h apart)

Giant Cell Arteritis

Adult: **Subcutaneous** 162 mg every other wk

COVID-19 in hospitalized patients

Adult (30 kg or more): **IV** 8 mg/kg as single dose (max: 800 mg/dose)
Adult (30 kg or less): **IV** 12 mg/kg as single dose (max: 800 mg/dose)

Absolute Neutrophil Count (ANC) Adjustment

ANC = 500–1000/mm³: Stop tocilizumab and restart at 4 mg/kg with an increase to 8 mg/kg as appropriate when ANC is greater than 1000 cells/mm³. *ANC less than 500/mm³:* Discontinue tocilizumab.

Platelet Count Dosage Adjustment

Platelet count 50,000–100,000/mm³: Stop tocilizumab and restart at 4 mg/kg with an increase to 8 mg/kg as appropriate when platelet count is greater than 100,000/mm³. *Platelet count less than 50,000/mm³:* Discontinue tocilizumab.

Hepatic Impairment Dosage Adjustment

Do not initiate tocilizumab if AST/ALT is greater than 1.5 × ULN. Mild impairment (AST and/or ALT 1–3 × ULN): Modify dose of concomitant DMARDs, if appropriate. For persistent increases in this range, reduce tocilizumab dose to 4 mg/kg or interrupt tocilizumab until AST/ALT have normalized. *Moderate impairment (AST and/or ALT greater than 3–5 × ULN confirmed by repeat testing):* Interrupt tocilizumab until AST/

ALT is less than 3 × ULN, then follow recommendations for 1–3 × ULN. *For persistent increases greater than 3 × ULN:* Discontinue tocilizumab. *Severe impairment (AST and/or ALT greater than 5 × ULN):* Discontinue tocilizumab.

ADMINISTRATION

Subcutaneous

- When transitioning from IV to subcutaneous route, give the first subcutaneous dose at the time of the next scheduled IV dose. Administer the full amount in the prefilled syringe. Allow to reach room temperature prior to use (30–45 min).
- Prefilled syringe or autoinjector for single use only.
- Prior to use remove prefilled syringe or autoinjector from the refrigerator and allow to sit at room temperature outside of the carton for 30 minutes (prefilled syringe) and 45 minutes for autoinjector. Do not warm in any other way.
- Solution should be clear and colorless to pale yellow.
- Inject full amount in syringe or autoinjector.
- Rotate injection sites; do not administer into areas of tenderness, bruising, reddened, hardened or scarred skin. Skin should be intact and avoid moles.
- Store prefilled syringes or autoinjectors in original package under refrigeration between 2 and 8° C (36 to 46° F). Do not freeze, protect from light and keep dry.

Intravenous

PREPARE: **IV Infusion:** For children weighing less than 30 kg, start with 50 mL of NS. For adults or children weighing 30 kg or more, start with 100 mL NS. From the bag of NS remove a volume of solution equal to the volume of tocilizumab necessary to deliver the required dose. Slowly add the required dose of tocilizumab to the IV bag, then gently invert to mix. Solution should reach room temperature prior to infusion. Discard unused drug remaining in vial.

ADMINISTER: **IV Infusion:** Give over 60 min. **Do not** give IV push or a bolus dose.

INCOMPATIBILITIES: **Solution/additive:** Do not mix with another drug. **Y-site:** Do not infuse tocilizumab concurrently with any drug in the same IV line.

- Store IV solution refrigerated for up to 24 h or at room temperature for up to 4 h. Protect from light. Store unopened vials refrigerated in original packaging to protect from light. Store in original package under refrigeration between 2 and 8° C (36 to 46° F). Do not freeze, protect from light and keep dry.

ADVERSE EFFECTS (≥5%) **CV:** Hypertension. **Respiratory:** Nasopharyngitis, upper respiratory infection. **CNS:** Headache, insomnia. **Skin:** Injection site reaction, *polyarticular juvenile idiopathic arthritis, systemic juvenile idiopathic arthritis.* **Hepatic:** *Increased ALT/SGPT, increased AST/SGOT.* **GI:** Diarrhea, constipation. **Hematologic:** Neutropenia. **Other:** Infusion-related reaction, anxiety.

INTERACTIONS **Drug:** Do not use with other biological DMARDs. Caution should be used when tocilizumab is combined with CYP3A4 substrate drugs (like **cyclosporine**) that have a narrow therapeutic index. Use with other

T

IMMUNE MODULATORS can increase risk of infection. Do not administer LIVE VACCINES.

PHARMACOKINETICS **Half-Life:** 14–16 days.

NURSING IMPLICATIONS

Black Box Warning

Tocilizumab has been associated with increased risk of serious infections that may lead to hospitalization or death.

Assessment & Drug Effects

- Monitor for signs of serious allergic reactions during and shortly following each infusion.
- Monitor for and promptly report S&S of infection, including TB or hepatitis B infection in carriers of HBV.
- Monitor for S&S of polyneuropathy.
- Monitor lab tests: Baseline latent TB screening; baseline and frequent (q4–8wk) WBC with differential and platelet count; baseline and periodic LFTs; periodic lipid profile.

Patient & Family Education

- Do not accept vaccinations with live vaccines while taking this drug.
- You should be tested for TB prior to taking this drug.
- Promptly report S&S of infection including: Chills, fever, cough, shortness of breath, diarrhea, stomach or abdominal pain, burning on urination, sores anywhere on your body, unexplained or excessive fatigue.
- Carriers of hepatitis B should report promptly signs of activation of the virus (e.g., clay-colored stools, dark urine, jaundice, unexplained fatigue).
- Teach patient or caregiver proper technique and placement for subq injections.
- Report promptly if you become pregnant.

TOFACITINIB (Pr)

(toe'fa-sye'ti-nib)

Xeljanz

Classification: BIOLOGICAL RESPONSE MODIFIER; JANUS KINASE (JAK) INHIBITOR; DISEASE-MODIFYING ANTIRHEUMATIC DRUG (DMARD)

Therapeutic: DISEASE-MODIFYING ANTIRHEUMATIC DRUG (DMARD)

AVAILABILITY

Tablet, extended release tablet, oral solution

ACTION & *THERAPEUTIC EFFECT*

Inhibits a specific tyrosine kinase enzyme and interferes with a signaling pathway that transmits extracellular information to the cell nucleus, influencing DNA transcription. *It improves rheumatoid arthritis by inhibiting the production of inflammatory mediators.*

USES

Treatment of moderately to severely active rheumatoid arthritis in patients who have had an inadequate response or intolerance to methotrexate. It may be used as monotherapy or in combination with methotrexate or other nonbiologic disease-modifying antirheumatic drugs (DMARDs). Treatment of active psoriatic arthritis. Treatment of moderately to severely active ulcerative colitis. Alternative to baricitinib in COVID-19 treatment.

CONTRAINDICATIONS

Serious uncontrolled infection, opportunistic infection or sepsis; live vaccines;

T

severe hepatic impairment; hepatitis B or C; pregnancy—infant risk cannot be ruled out; lactation—infant risk cannot be ruled out.

CAUTIOUS USE Renal transplant patients; active TB or history of latent or active TB; history of herpes virus infection or hepatitis B; history of chronic or recurrent infections; history of smoking; history or risk of GI perforation; DM; patients with history of hyperlipidemia; patients with history of melanoma, bradycardia, prolonged PR interval, conduction abnormalities; ischemic heart disease; patients at risk for interstitial lung disease; history of thrombosis; moderate or severe renal impairment; moderate hepatic impairment; Asian patients; malignancy; older adults; children.

ROUTE & DOSAGE

Rheumatoid Arthritis, Psoriatic Arthritis

Adult: **PO** Immediate release 5 mg bid; Extended release 11 mg daily

Ulcerative Colitis

Adult: **PO** Immediate release 10 mg bid × 8 wk then 5–10 mg bid; Extended release 22 mg daily × 8 w then 11 mg daily.

COVID-19 treatment

Adult: **PO** Immediate release 10 mg bid up to 14 days or hospital discharge, whichever is earlier.

Hepatic Impairment Dosage Adjustment

Moderate impairment (Child-Pugh class B): Reduce dose to 5 mg once daily (immediate release) or 11 mg daily (extended release)

Severe impairment (Child-Pugh class C): Not recommended

Renal Impairment Dosage Adjustment

Moderate to severe impairment: Reduce dose to 5 mg once daily (immediate release) or 11 mg daily (extended release)

Lymphopenia Dosage Adjustment

If less than 500 cells/m³: Discontinue

Neutropenia Dosage Adjustment

If ANC = 500–1000 cells/m³: Withhold until ANC is greater than 1000 cells/m³ then resume at normal dose

If ANC less than 500–1000 cells/m³: Discontinue

Anemia Dosage Adjustment

If hemoglobin is less than 8 g/dL or if decreased by greater than 2 g/dL: Withhold until hemoglobin levels normalize

ADMINISTRATION

Oral

- NIOSH recommends use of single gloves when handling intact tablets or capsules or administering from a unit-dosed package. Use double gloves if cutting or crushing the medication. During administration, use single gloves and wear eye/face protection if the formulation is hard to swallow or if the patient may resist, vomit, or spit up.
- May be given without regard to food.
- Swallow extended-release tablets whole, do not crush, split, or chew.

T

- Store tablets and solution at 20°–25° C (68°–77° F). Solution can have excursions permitted between 15 and 30° C (59 and 86° F). Protect solution from light. Use within 60 days of opening the bottle and discard any unused solution after 60 days.

ADVERSE EFFECTS **Respiratory:** Nasopharyngitis, URI. **CNS:** Headache. **Endocrine:** Increased HDL, increased LDL. **Other:** Infection.

INTERACTIONS **Drug:** Extensive drug interactions, consult drug interaction database for complete listing. Coadministration with potent inhibitors of CYP3A4 (e.g., **ketoconazole**) may increase the levels of tofacitinib. Coadministration with drugs that are moderate inhibitors of CYP3A4 and potent inhibitors of CYP2C19 (e.g., **fluconazole**) may increase the levels of tofacitinib. Coadministration with potent CYP3A4 inducers (e.g., **phenobarbital, phenytoin, rifampin**) may decrease the levels of tofacitinib. Coadministration with other potent immunosuppressive drugs (e.g., **azathioprine, tacrolimus, cyclosporine**) increases the risk of added immunosuppression. Do not use with LIVE VACCINES **Food: Grapefruit juice** may increase the levels of tofacitinib. **Herbal: St. John's wort** may decrease the levels of tofacitinib, use caution with **echinacea**.

T

PHARMACOKINETICS **Absorption:** 74% bioavailable. **Peak:** 0.5–1 h. **Distribution:** 40% plasma protein bound. **Metabolism:** Hepatic oxidation (substrate of CYP219 and CYP 3A4). **Elimination:** Hepatic (70%) and renal (30%). **Half-Life:** 3 h.

NURSING IMPLICATIONS

Black Box Warning

Tofacitinib has been associated with increased risk of developing serious infections that may lead to hospitalization or death.

Assessment & Drug Effects

- Evaluate for latent or active infection prior to administration of tofacitinib.
- Monitor closely for S&S of TB, including those who tested negative for latent TB prior to initiating therapy.
- Monitor for reactivation of viral infection (herpes zoster).
- Monitor closely for S&S of other infections during and after treatment. Withhold therapy and notify prescriber if an infection is suspected.
- Monitor for signs and symptoms of pulmonary embolism (e.g., shortness of breath, chest pain, anxiety, palpitations).
- Monitor lab tests: Baseline lymphocyte count and q3mo thereafter; baseline neutrophil count and Hgb, then q3mo after 4–8 wk of treatment; periodic LFTs; lipid profile 4–8 wk after initiation of therapy.

Patient & Family Education

- Report promptly to prescriber any new-onset abdominal symptoms, S&S of respiratory tract infection or any other type of infection.
- Female patients should avoid pregnancy during administration and for at least 4 weeks after discontinuation.
- Report any new or worsening skin lesions or moles.

TOLAZAMIDE

(tole-az′a-mide)

Classification: SULFONYLUREA
Therapeutic: ANTIDIABETIC
Prototype: Glyburide

AVAILABILITY Tablet

ACTION & *THERAPEUTIC EFFECT* Lowers blood glucose primarily by stimulating pancreatic beta cells to secrete insulin. Antidiabetic action is a result of stimulation of the pancreas to secrete more insulin in the presence of blood sugar; it requires functioning beta cells. *Effectiveness is measured in decreasing the serum blood level to within normal limits and decreasing HbA1C value to 6.5 or lower.*

USES Type 2 diabetes mellitus

CONTRAINDICATIONS Known sensitivity to sulfonylureas and to sulfonamides; type 1 diabetes complicated by ketoacidosis; infection; trauma; lactation (infant risk cannot be ruled out).

CAUTIOUS USE Renal disease; renal failure, renal impairment; adrenal or pituitary insufficiency; debilitated or malnourished patients; hemolytic anemia; hepatic insufficiency; stress from infection, fever, trauma or surgery; older adults; pregnancy (category C). Safety in children not established.

ROUTE & DOSAGE

Type 2 Diabetes Mellitus

Adult: **PO** 100 mg–250 mg daily, may adjust dose by 100–250 mg/day at weekly intervals (max: 1 g/day)

ADMINISTRATION

Oral

- Give in the morning with or before first main meal of the day.
- Divide dose of more than 500 mg and give bid
- Store at 20°–25° C (68°–77° F) in a tightly closed container unless otherwise directed. Protect from light. Keep drug out of the reach of children.

ADVERSE EFFECTS **CNS:** Dizziness, fatigue, headache, malaise, vertigo. **Endocrine:** Hypoglycemia, hyponatremia, SIADH. **Skin:** Rash, pruritis, photosensitivity, uritcaria. **Hepatic:** Jaundice. **GI:** Epigastric fullness, indigestion, nausea, anorexia, constipation, diarrhea, vomiting. **GU:** Diuretic effect. **Musculoskeletal:** Weakness. **Hematologic:** Agranulocytosis, aplastic anemia, hemolytic anemia, leukopenia, pancytopenia, thrombocytopenia.

INTERACTIONS **Drug: Alcohol** elicits disulfiram-type reaction in some patients; ORAL ANTICOAGULANTS, **chloramphenicol, clofibrate, phenylbutazone,** MAO INHIBITORS, SALICYLATES, **probenecid,** SULFONAMIDES may potentiate hypoglycemic actions; THIAZIDES may antagonize hypoglycemic effects; **cimetidine** may increase tolazamide levels, causing hypoglycemia; **aminolevulinic acid** may increase photosensitivity. **Herbal: Ginseng** may potentiate hypoglycemic effects.

PHARMACOKINETICS **Absorption:** Slowly from GI tract. **Onset:** 60 min. **Peak:** 4–6 h. **Duration:** 10–15 h (up to 20 h in some patients). **Distribution:** Distributed in highest concentrations in liver, kidneys, and intestines; crosses placenta; distributed into breast milk.

T

Metabolism: Extensively in liver. **Elimination:** 85% in urine, 15% in feces. **Half-Life:** 7 h.

NURSING IMPLICATIONS

Assessment & Drug Effects

- Monitor closely for daytime and nighttime hypoglycemia since tolazamide is long acting.
- Monitor for and report signs of an allergic reaction (e.g., rash, urticaria, pruritus).
- Monitor lab tests: Periodic HbA1C and frequent FBS; periodic CBC; renal function tests.

Patient & Family Education

- Check blood glucose daily or as ordered by prescriber. Important to continue close medical supervision for first 6 wk of treatment.
- Learn the S&S of hypoglycemia and hyperglycemia and check blood glucose level when either is suspected.
- Report to prescriber if you experience frequent and/or severe episodes of hypoglycemia.
- Do not take OTC preparations unless approved or prescribed by prescriber.
- Understand that alcohol can precipitate a disulfiram-type reaction.
- Many drugs interact with tolazamide. Monitor blood glucose more frequently whenever a new drug is added to your regimen.

T

TOLBUTAMIDE

(tole-byoo′ta-mide)

TOLBUTAMIDE SODIUM
Classification: SULFONYLUREA
Therapeutic: ANTIDIABETIC
Prototype: Glyburide

AVAILABILITY Tablet

ACTION & *THERAPEUTIC EFFECT*

Lowers blood glucose concentration by stimulating pancreatic beta cells to synthesize and release insulin. No action demonstrated if functional beta cells are absent. *Lowers blood glucose concentration by stimulating pancreatic beta cells to synthesize and release insulin.*

USES Management of mild to moderately severe, stable type 2 diabetes that is not controlled by diet and weight reduction alone.

CONTRAINDICATIONS Hypersensitivity to sulfonylureas or to sulfonamides; history of repeated episodes of diabetic ketoacidosis; type 1 diabetes as sole therapy; diabetic coma; severe stress, infection, trauma, or major surgery; severe renal insufficiency, liver or endocrine disease; lactation (infant risk cannot be ruled out).

CAUTIOUS USE Cardiac, thyroid, pituitary, or adrenal dysfunction; severe hepatic disease, renal disease, renal impairment, renal failure; history of peptic ulcer; alcoholism; infection; debilitated, malnourished, or uncooperative patient, older adults; stress caused by fever, infection, surgery, or trauma; pregnancy (category C). Safe use in children not established.

ROUTE & DOSAGE

Type 2 Diabetes

Adult: **PO** 1–2 g/day as a single dose in the morning or in divided doses

ADMINISTRATION

Oral

- Tablets may be crushed and given with full glass of water if patient desires.
- Do not give at bedtime because of danger of nocturnal hypoglycemia, unless specifically prescribed.
- Store at 20°–25° C (68°–77° F) in well-closed container. Protect from light.

ADVERSE EFFECTS CNS: Disulfiram-like reaction, headache. **Endocrine:** Hypoglycemia, hyponatremia, SIADH, build up of porphyrins. **Skin:** Rash, pruritis, photosensitivity, urticaria. **Hepatic:** Jaundice. **GI:** Altered sense of taste, epigastric fullness, heartburn, nausea. **Hematologic:** Agranulocytosis, aplastic anemia, hemolytic anemia, leukopenia, pancytopenia, thrombocytopenia.

DIAGNOSTIC TEST INTERFERENCE

The SULFONYLUREAS may produce abnormal ***thyroid function test*** results and reduced ***RAI uptake*** (after long-term administration).

INTERACTIONS Drug: Phenylbutazone increases hypoglycemic effects; THIAZIDE DIURETICS may attenuate hypoglycemic effects; **alcohol** may produce disulfiram reaction; BETA-BLOCKERS may mask symptoms of a hypoglycemic reaction. **Herbal: Ginseng,** may potentiate hypoglycemic effects.

PHARMACOKINETICS Absorption: Readily from GI tract. **Peak:** 3–5 h. **Distribution:** Into extracellular fluids. **Metabolism:** Principally in liver. **Elimination:** 75–85% in urine; some in feces. **Half-Life:** 7 h.

NURSING IMPLICATIONS

Assessment & Drug Effects

- Supervise closely during initial period of therapy until dosage is established. One or 2 wk of therapy may be required before full therapeutic effect is achieved.
- Monitor closely during adjustment period, watching for S&S of impending hypoglycemia (see Appendix F). Detection of a hypoglycemic reaction in a diabetic patient also receiving a beta-blocker, especially older adults, is difficult.
- Evaluate nondefinitive vague complaints; hypoglycemic symptoms may be especially vague in older adults. Observe patient carefully, especially 2–3 h after eating, check urine for sugar and ketone bodies and capillary blood glucose.
- Report repetitive complaints of headache and weakness a few hours after eating; may signal incipient hypoglycemia.
- Be aware that pruritus and rash, frequently reported adverse effects, may clear spontaneously; if these persist, drug will be discontinued.
- Monitor lab tests: Periodic HbA1C, fasting serum glucose and urine glucose.

Patient & Family Education

- Learn the S&S of hyperglycemia (see Appendix A) and check blood glucose level when hyperglycemia is suspected.
- Hypoglycemia is frequently caused by overdosage of hypoglycemic drug, inadequate or irregular food intake, nausea, vomiting, diarrhea, and added exercise without caloric supplement or dose adjustment. Learn the S&S of hypoglycemia (see

Appendix F) and check blood glucose level whenever hypoglycemia is suspected.

- Report any illness promptly. Prescriber may want to evaluate need for insulin.
- Do not self-medicate with OTC drugs unless approved or prescribed by prescriber.
- Be aware that alcohol, even in moderate amounts, can precipitate a disulfiram-type reaction (see Appendix F). A hypoglycemic response after ingesting alcohol requires emergency treatment.
- Protect exposed skin areas from the sun with a sunscreen lotion (SPF 12–15) because of potential photosensitivity (especially in the alcoholic).
- Monitor blood glucose daily or as directed by prescriber.
- Be alert to added danger of loss of control (hyperglycemia) when a drug that affects the hypoglycemic action of sulfonylureas (see DRUG INTERACTIONS) is withdrawn or added to the tolbutamide regimen. Monitor blood glucose carefully.
- Use or add barrier contraceptive if using hormonal contraceptives.

TOLCAPONE Pr

(tol′ca-pone)

Tasmar

Classification: ANTICHOLINERGIC; CATECHOLAMINE-O-METHYLTRANSFERASE (COMT) INHIBITOR

Therapeutic: ANTIPARKINSON

AVAILABILITY
Tablet

ACTION & *THERAPEUTIC EFFECT*
Selective and reversible inhibitor of catecholamine-O-methyltransferase (COMT). COMT is the enzyme responsible for metabolizing catecholamines and, therefore, levodopa. *Concurrent administration of tolcapone and levodopa increases the amount of levodopa available to control Parkinson's disease by increasing dopaminergic brain stimulation.*

USES
Idiopathic Parkinson disease as adjunct to levodopa/carbidopa.

CONTRAINDICATIONS
Hypersensitivity to tolcapone; liver disease; drug-induced signs of liver decompensation; history of nontraumatic rhabdomyolysis, history of hyperpyrexia and confusion related to a medication, MAOI therapy; history of major psychiatric disorder; pregnancy—fetal risk cannot be ruled out; lactation—infant risk cannot be ruled out.

CAUTIOUS USE
History of hypersensitivity to other COMT inhibitors (e.g., entacapone, nitecapone); anorexia nervosa; hematuria; hypotension; syncope; renal disease; renal impairment; history of liver insufficiency; history of dyskinesias, elderly. Safety and efficacy not established in pediatric patients.

ROUTE & DOSAGE

Parkinson Disease

Adult: **PO** 100 mg tid (max: 200 mg tid)

ADMINISTRATION

Oral

- Give with food if GI upset occurs.
- Give only in conjunction with levodopa/carbidopa therapy.
- Therapy with tolcapone **should not** be initiated if patient has ALT/AST greater than 2 × ULN or has known liver disease.
- Store at 20°–25° C (68°–77° F) in a tightly closed container.

ADVERSE EFFECTS (≥5%) **CV:** Orthostatic hypotension, syncope. **Respiratory:** URI. **CNS:** *Dyskinesia, dystonia, somnolence, confusion, dizziness*, headache. **Skin:** Sweating. **GI:** *Nausea, anorexia, diarrhea, vomiting*. **GU:** Hematuria. **Musculoskeletal:** Cramps. **Other:** Dream disorder, *sleep disorder*.

INTERACTIONS **Drug:** Will increase **levodopa** levels when taken simultaneously; CNS DEPRESSANTS may cause additive sedation; may have increased risk of hypotension when used with ANTIHYPERTENSIVES; do not give with nonselective MAOIS **(isocarboxazid, phenelzine, or tranylcypromine furazolidone, linezolid, procarbazine).** **Food:** Decreases levels. **Herbal:** Avoid use of **valerian, St. John's wort, kratom, kava.**

PHARMACOKINETICS **Absorption:** Rapidly from GI tract, bioavailability 65%. **Peak:** 2 h. **Distribution:** Over 99% protein bound. **Metabolism:** Extensively metabolized by COMT and glucuronidation. **Elimination:** 60% in urine, 40% in feces; clearance reduced by 50% in patients with liver disease. **Half-Life:** 2–3 h.

NURSING IMPLICATIONS

Black Box Warning

Tolcapone has been associated with risk of potentially fatal, acute fulminant liver failure.

Assessment & Drug Effects

- More frequent PT and INR when given concurrently with warfarin.
- Withhold drug and notify prescriber if liver dysfunction is suspected.
- Monitor carefully for and immediately report S&S of hepatic impairment (e.g., jaundice, dark urine).
- Monitor for new or increasing compulsive behaviors.
- Monitor level of consciousness.
- Monitor lab tests: Monthly LFTs for first 3 mo, every 6 wk for the next 3 mo, and periodically thereafter.

Patient & Family Education

- Notify prescriber promptly about any of following: Increased loss of muscle control, fainting, yellowing of skin or eyes, darkening of urine, severe diarrhea, hallucinations.
- Do not engage in hazardous activities until response to drug is known. Avoid use of alcohol or sedative drugs while on tolcapone.
- Rise slowly from a sitting or lying position to avoid a rapid drop in BP with possible weakness or fainting.
- Dermatological exams will be needed periodically to monitor for melanoma. Report any skin changes suggestive of melanoma.
- Report any intense urges or compulsive behavior such as gambling, sexual urges, or binge eating.
- Nausea is a common possible adverse effect especially at the beginning of therapy.
- Do not suddenly stop taking this drug. Doses **must be** gradually reduced over time.

T

TOLMETIN SODIUM

(tole′met-in)

Classification: NONSTEROIDAL ANTI-INFLAMMATORY (NSAID)

Therapeutic: NONNARCOTIC ANALGESIC, NSAID; DISEASE-MODIFYING ANTIRHEUMATIC DRUG (DMARD)

Prototype: Ibuprofen

AVAILABILITY Tablet; capsule

ACTION & THERAPEUTIC EFFECT Competitively inhibits both cyclooxygenase (COX) isoenzymes, COX-1 and COX-2, by blocking arachidonate binding to prostaglandin sites, and thus inhibits prostaglandin synthesis. *Possesses analgesic, antiinflammatory, antipyretic, and antirheumatic activity.*

USES In treatment of rheumatoid arthritis, juvenile rheumatoid arthritis, juvenile idiopathic arthritis.

CONTRAINDICATIONS History of intolerance or hypersensitivity to tolmetin, aspirin, and other NSAIDS; active peptic ulcer, CABG perioperative pain; in patients with active GI disease including peptic ulcer and ulcerative colitis; in patients with functional class IV rheumatoid arthritis (severely incapacitated, bedridden, or confined to a wheelchair). Safety during pregnancy (fetal risk cannot be ruled out); lactation (infant risk cannot be ruled out).

CAUTIOUS USE History of PUD or GI bleeding; impaired kidney function; SLE; hypertension; patients with fluid retention; CHF; compromised cardiac function; liver dysfunction; coagulation disorders; asthma; older adults. Safe use in children younger than 2 y not established.

ROUTE & DOSAGE

Arthritis

Adult: **PO** 400 mg tid (max: 2 g/day)

Juvenile Rheumatoid Arthritis

Child (2 y or older): **PO** 20 mg/kg/day in 3–4 divided doses (max: 30 mg/kg/day)

ADMINISTRATION

Oral

- Schedule to include a morning dose (on arising) and a bedtime dose.
- May be administered with magnesium or aluminum hydroxide containing antacids to minimize GI irritation. Administration with food or milk reduces bioavailability of the drug by 16%.
- Give with fluid of patient's choice; crush tablet or empty capsule to mix with water or food if patient cannot swallow tablet/capsule.
- Store at 20°–25° C (68°–77° F) in tightly capped and light-resistant container unless otherwise instructed.

ADVERSE EFFECTS **CV:** Hypertension, edema. **Respiratory:** Bronchospasm. **CNS:** Stroke, dizziness, headache. **Endocrine:** Weight changes. **Hepatic:** Hepatitis, increased LFTs, jaundice. **GI:** Nausea, abdominal pain, diarrhea, indigestion, flatulence, vomiting, constipation. **Musculoskeletal:** Weakness.

DIAGNOSTIC TEST INTERFERENCE Tolmetin prolongs ***bleeding time,*** inhibits ***platelet aggregation,*** elevates ***BUN, alkaline phosphatase,*** and ***AST*** levels. Metabolites may produce false-positive results for ***proteinuria*** [with tests that rely on acid precipitation (e.g., ***sulfosalicylic acid***)]. May interfere with urine detection of ***cannabinoids*** (false-positive); may lead to false-positive aldosterone/renin ratio.

INTERACTIONS Drug: ORAL ANTICOAGULANTS, **heparin** may prolong bleeding time; may increase **lithium** toxicity; **aspirin,** other NSAIDS add to ulcerogenic effects; may increase **methotrexate** toxicity. Do not use with **ketorolac** due to increased risk of toxicities. **Herbal: Feverfew,** cat's claw, **garlic, ginger, ginkgo** may increase bleeding potential.

PHARMACOKINETICS Absorption: Rapidly from GI tract. **Peak:** 30–60 min; therapeutic effect in 3–7 days. **Distribution:** Crosses blood–brain barrier and placenta; distributed into breast milk. **Metabolism:** In liver. **Elimination:** In urine. **Half-Life:** 60–90 min.

NURSING IMPLICATIONS

Black Box Warning

Tolmetin sodium has been associated with increased risk of serious, potentially fatal, GI bleeding and cardiovascular events (e.g., MI and CVA); risk may increase with duration of use and may be greater in the older adult and those with risk factors for CV disease.

Assessment & Drug Effects

- Monitor for and report promptly S&S of GI ulceration or bleeding. Significant GI bleeding may occur without prior warning.
- Monitor for and report promptly S&S of CV thrombotic events (i.e., angina, MI, TIA, or stroke).
- Monitor BP throughout the course of therapy.
- Monitor patients with kidney damage closely. Evaluate I&O ratio and encourage patient to increase fluid intake to at least 8 full glasses/day.
- Monitor lab tests: Periodic renal function tests with long-term therapy; CBC; Hct & Hgb if symptoms of anemia appear; C-reactive protein levels, erythrocyte sedimentation rate, LFTs, serum creatinine/BUN, and stool guaiac.

Patient & Family Education

- Stop taking drug and report promptly to prescriber if you experience S&S of GI ulceration: Stomach pain, frequent indigestion and nausea, bloody or tarry stools, vomit with blood or coffee-ground appearance.
- Monitor weight and report an increase greater than 2 kg (4 lb)/wk with impaired kidney or cardiac function; check for swelling in ankles, shins, hands, and feet.
- Report promptly signs of abnormal bleeding (ecchymosis, epistaxis, melena, petechiae bruising, bloody nose, black tarry stools, tiny, circular patches on skin), itching, skin rash, persistent headache, edema.
- Stop taking drug and report promptly to prescriber if you experience chest pain, shortness of breath, weakness, slurring of speech, or other signs of a cardiac or neurologic problem.
- Avoid potentially hazardous activities until response to drug is known because dizziness and drowsiness are common adverse effects.

T

TOLNAFTATE

(tole-naf'tate)

Pitrex ♣, Tinactin

Classification: ANTIFUNGAL ANTIBIOTIC

Therapeutic: ANTIFUNGAL

AVAILABILITY Cream; solution; gel; powder; spray

ACTION & THERAPEUTIC EFFECT

Distorts hyphae and stunts mycelial growth on susceptible fungi. *Fungistatic or fungicidal as well as anti-infective against bacteria, protozoa, and viruses.*

USES

Tinea pedis (athlete's foot), tinea cruris (jock itch), tinea corporis (body ringworm); prevention of tinea pedis.

CONTRAINDICATIONS

Skin irritations prior to therapy, previous hypersensitivity to tolnaftate, nail and scalp infections; immunosuppressed patients, diabetes mellitus, peripheral vascular disease; pregnancy—fetal risk cannot be ruled out; lactation—infant risk cannot be ruled out.

CAUTIOUS USE

Safe use in children younger than 2 y is not established.

ROUTE & DOSAGE

Tinea Infestations

Adult/Child: **Topical** Apply bid in morning and evening

ADMINISTRATION

Topical

- Cleanse site thoroughly with water and dry completely before applying. Massage thin layer gently into skin. Make sure area is not wet from excess drug after application.
- Shake aerosol powder or aerosol liquid container well before use. Apply powder or liquid aerosol liberally to affected areas from a distance of 6 to 10 inches.
- Apply powder to affected areas; can be applied to socks and shoes when treating foot infections.
- Note: Cream and powder are not recommended for nail or scalp infection.
- Use liquids (solutions) for scalp infection or to treat hairy areas.
- Store cream, gel, powder, and topical solution in light-resistant containers at 15°–30° C (59°–86° F); store aerosol container at 2°–30° C (38°–86° F). Avoid freezing.

ADVERSE EFFECTS

Skin: Local irritation, *pruritus.*

NURSING IMPLICATIONS

Assessment and Drug effects

- Monitor for symptomatic improvement and for local reactions (burning, itching, irritation).

Patient & Family Education

- Expect relief from pruritus, soreness, and burning within 24–72 h after start of treatment.
- Continue treatment for 2–3 wk after disappearance of all symptoms to prevent recurrence.
- Review application instructions with patient and/or caregiver.
- Instruct patient to not apply any other medicines or creams to affected skin area unless prescribed by a healthcare provider.
- Do not apply cosmetics or other skin products to affected areas.
- Return to prescriber in absence of improvement within 1 wk or if condition worsens.
- Note: If skin has thickened as a result of the infection, desired clinical response may be delayed for 4–6 wk.
- Avoid contact with eyes of all drug forms.
- Place container in warm water to liquify contents if solution solidifies. Potency is unaffected.

TOLTERODINE TARTRATE

(tol-ter′o-deen tar′trate)

Detrol, Detrol LA

Classification: ANTICHOLINERGIC; MUSCARINIC RECEPTOR ANTAGONIST

Therapeutic: ANTIMUSCARINIC; BLADDER ANTISPASMODIC

Prototype: Oxybutynin

AVAILABILITY Tablet; sustained release capsule

ACTION & *THERAPEUTIC EFFECT* Selective muscarinic urinary bladder receptor antagonist. Reduces urinary incontinence, urgency, and frequency. *Controls urinary bladder incontinence by controlling contractions.*

USES Overactive bladder.

CONTRAINDICATIONS Hypersensitivity to tolterodine or fesoterodine; uncontrolled narrow-angle glaucoma; gastric retention, obstruction, or pyloric stenosis; urinary retention; older patients with delirium or high risk for delirium; pregnancy—fetal risk cannot be ruled out; lactation—infant risk cannot be ruled out. **Extended release:** Severe hepatic impairment (Child-Pugh class C); if CrCl less than 10 mL/min.

CAUTIOUS USE Cardiovascular disease; liver disease; controlled narrow-angle glaucoma; significant urinary retention; severe hepatic impairment; obstructive GI disease; obstructive uropathy; myasthenia gravis; history of QT prolongation; paralytic ileus or intestinal atony; renal impairment; CrCl 10–30 mL/min; ulcerative colitis; older adults. Safety and efficacy in children not established.

ROUTE & DOSAGE

Overactive Bladder

Adult: **PO** 2 mg bid or **Sustained release:** 4 mg daily

Hepatic Impairment Dosage Adjustment

Reduce dose by 50%

Renal Impairment Dosage Adjustment

CrCl less than 30 mL/min: Reduce dose 50%

Medication Dosage Adjustment

Concurrent CYP3A4 inhibiting drugs: Reduce dose by 50%

ADMINISTRATION

Oral

- Do not crush or chew sustained release tablets. These **must be** swallowed whole.
- Doses greater than 1 mg bid are not recommended for those with significantly reduced liver function or kidney function or concurrently receiving macrolide antibiotics, azole antifungal agents, or other cytochrome P450 3A4 inhibitors.
- Store at 15°–30° C (59°–86° F) in a tightly closed container.

ADVERSE EFFECTS (≥5%) **CNS:** *Headache.* **GI:** *Dry mouth,* constipation, abdominal pain.

INTERACTIONS **Drug:** Additive anticholinergic effects with **amantadine, clozapine,** SEDATING H_1-BLOCKERS, PHENOTHIAZINES, TRICYCLIC ANTIDEPRESSANTS. Increased effects with CYP3A4 inhibitors (e.g., **clarithromycin, cyclosporine, erythromycin, itraconazole,** or **ketoconazole**). **Food: Grapefruit juice** may increase **tolterodine** levels in some patients.

PHARMACOKINETICS **Absorption:** 77% absorbed, decreased with food. **Peak:** 1–2 h. **Distribution:** 96% protein bound. **Metabolism:** In liver by CYP2D6 and CYP3A4. **Elimination:** 77% in urine, 17% in feces. **Half-Life:** 2–10 h (immediate release); 7–18 h (extended release)

NURSING IMPLICATIONS

Assessment & Drug Effects

- Monitor voiding pattern and report promptly urinary retention.
- Monitor vital signs carefully (HR and BP), especially in those with cardiovascular disease.
- Monitor lab tests: LFTs and renal function tests.

Patient & Family Education

- Notify prescriber promptly if you experience eye pain, rapid heartbeat, difficulty breathing, skin rash or hives, confusion, or incoordination.
- Avoid activities requiring mental alertness or coordination until drug effects are realized, as drug may cause blurred vision, dizziness, and drowsiness.
- Report blurred vision, sensitivity to light, and dry mouth (all common adverse effects) to prescriber if bothersome.
- Avoid the use of alcohol or OTC antihistamines.

T

TOLVAPTAN

(tol-vap'tan)

Samsca

Classification: ELECTROLYTE & WATER BALANCE AGENT; DIURETIC; VASOPRESSIN ANTAGONIST

Therapeutic: VASOPRESSIN ANTAGONIST; DIURETIC

Prototype: Conivaptan

AVAILABILITY Tablet

ACTION & *THERAPEUTIC EFFECT* Selective vasopressin V_2-receptor antagonist; antagonizes the effect of vasopressin and causes an increase in urine water excretion, decrease in urine osmolality, and increase in serum sodium concentrations. *Effectiveness is measured by increase in serum sodium level toward lower limit of normal, and/or decrease in sign and symptoms of hyponatremia.*

USES Treatment of hypervolemic and euvolemic hyponatremia.

CONTRAINDICATIONS Rapid correction of serum sodium (e.g., greater than 12 mEq/L/24 h); cognitively impaired; serious neurologic symptoms; hypovolemic hyponatremia; hypertonic saline; concurrent administration with strong CYP3A inhibitors; lactation.

CAUTIOUS USE Must be initiated or reinitiated in a hospital setting; cirrhosis; pregnancy (category C). Safe use in children younger than 18 y not established.

ROUTE & DOSAGE

Hyponatremia

Adult: **PO** Initially 15 mg once daily; may be adjusted up to 60 mg once daily

ADMINISTRATION

Oral

- Administer ONLY in setting where serum sodium can be closely monitored.
- Doses may be increased at 24 h intervals or greater.
- Do not administer if patient is unable to sense or respond to thirst.
- Store at 15°–30°C (59°–86°F).

ADVERSE EFFECTS Endocrine: Anorexia, *hyperglycemia*. **GI:** *Constipation, dry mouth, nausea.* **GU:** *Pollakiuria, polyuria*. **Other:** *Asthenia*, pyrexia, *thirst*.

INTERACTIONS Drug: Strong CYP3A4 INHIBITORS (e.g., **clarithromycin, ketoconazole, itraconazole, telithromycin, saquinavir, nelfinavir, ritonavir, nefazodone**) may increase tolvaptan levels. Moderate CYP3A INHIBITORS (e.g., **erythromycin, fluconazole, aprepitant, diltiazem, verapamil**) may increase tolvaptan levels. P-GLYCOPROTEIN INHIBITORS (e.g., **cyclosporine**) may require tolvaptan dosage reduction. CYP3A INDUCERS (e.g., **rifabutin, rifapentine, rifampin, barbiturates, phenytoin, carbamazepine**) decrease the levels of tolvaptan. Tolvaptan increases the levels of **digoxin.** BETA-BLOCKERS, ANGIOTENSIN RECEPTOR BLOCKERS, ANGIOTENSIN-CONVERTING ENZYME INHIBITORS and POTASSIUM-SPARING DIURETICS may cause hyperkalemia. **Food:** Administration with **grapefruit juice** may increase tolvaptan levels. **Herbal: St. John's wort** may decrease the levels of tolvaptan.

PHARMACOKINETICS Absorption: Approximately 40% absorbed. **Peak:** 2–4 h. **Distribution:** 99% plasma protein bound. **Metabolism:** In liver through CYP3A4. **Elimination:** Eliminated entirely by nonrenal routes. **Half-Life:** 12 h.

NURSING IMPLICATIONS

Black Box Warning

Tolvaptan has been associated with serious, sometime fatal, adverse events when hyponatremia is corrected too rapidly (e.g., more than 12 mEq/L per 24 h).

Assessment & Drug Effects

- Monitor vital signs frequently throughout therapy. Monitor ECG as warranted.
- Monitor weight and I&O closely as copious diuresis is expected.
- Fluid restriction should be avoided during the first 24 h of therapy.
- Monitor mental status throughout treatment. Report promptly changes in mental status (e.g., lethargy, confusion, disorientation, hallucinations, seizures).
- Report promptly symptoms of osmotic demyelination syndrome (ODS): Dysarthria, mutism, dysphagia, lethargy, affective changes, spasticity, seizures, or coma.
- Monitor digoxin levels closely with concurrent administration.
- Monitor lab tests: Baseline and frequent serum electrolytes; frequent serum sodium during initiation and titration.

Patient & Family Education

- Continue to drink fluid in response to thirst until otherwise directed. Fluid restrictions are usually required after the first 24 h of therapy.
- Report promptly any of the following: Trouble speaking or swallowing, drowsiness, mood changes, confusion, involuntary body movements, or muscle weakness in arms or legs.

TOPIRAMATE

(to-pir'a-mate)

Eprontia, Topamax, Qudexy XR, Trokendi XR

Classification: ANTICONVULSANT; GAMMA-AMINOBUTYRATE (GABA) ENHANCER

Therapeutic: ANTICONVULSANT; ANTIEPILEPTIC

AVAILABILITY Tablet; extended release capsule; sprinkle capsule

ACTION & *THERAPEUTIC EFFECT* Exhibits sodium channel-blocking action, as well as enhances the ability of GABA to induce a flux of chloride ions into the neurons, thus potentiating the activity of this inhibitory neurotransmitter (GABA). *Effectiveness indicated by a decrease in seizure activity or fewer migraines depending on indication.*

USES Adjunctive therapy for focal (partial) onset seizures; generalized tonic-clonic seizures primary; migraine prophylaxis.

UNLABELED USES Cluster headache, bulimia nervosa, neuropathic pain, infantile spasms, bipolar disorder, obesity.

CONTRAINDICATIONS Hypersensitivity to topiramate; suicidal ideation; visual field defects, or persistent or severe metabolic acidosis due to drug; abrupt withdrawal; pregnancy—fetal harm has been demonstrated; lactation—infant risk cannot be ruled out. Effect on labor and delivery is unknown. Recent alcohol use (i.e., within 6 h prior to and 6 h after administration).

T

CAUTIOUS USE Moderate and severe renal impairment, hepatic impairment; COPD; chronic acidosis; history of suicidal thoughts or psychiatric disturbances; concomitant use of CNS depressants; severe pulmonary disease; history of glaucoma; older adults. **Immediate release:** Children younger than 2 y.

ROUTE & DOSAGE

Seizures (Monotherapy)

Adult/Adolescent/Child (older than 10 y): **PO Immediate release** 50 mg/day; increase dose in 50 mg increments at weekly intervals based on response up to 200 mg/day; then may increase in 100 mg increments at weekly intervals up to 400 mg/day

Child (2–10 y): **PO** Weight-based dosing in package insert

Seizure (Adjunctive Therapy)

Adult: **PO Immediate release** 25–50 mg/day; increase in 25–50 mg increments at weekly intervals based on response up to 400 mg/day

Migraine Prophylaxis

Adult: **PO Immediate release** Initiate with 25 mg bid, increase by 25–50 mg/wk to 100 mg/day or max tolerated dose

Renal Impairment Dosage Adjustment

CrCl less than 70 mL/min: Decrease dose by 50%

ADMINISTRATION

Oral

- NIOSH guidelines: drug poses occupational hazard to men and women actively trying to conceive and women who are pregnant or may become pregnant and are breastfeeding. Use single gloves by anyone handling intact tablets or capsules and administering from a unit-dose package. Use double gloves and protective gown when cutting, crushing, manipulating, or handling uncoated tablets. For administration, wear single gloves, and eye/face protection if the formulations is hard to swallow or if the patient may resist, vomit, or spit up.

- May be taken without regard to meals.
- Capsule contents may be sprinkled on soft food and swallowed immediately. Do not chew.
- Make dosage increments of 50 mg at weekly intervals to the recommended dose, usually 400 mg/day.
- Do not break extended release tablets.
- See manufacturer guidelines for storage. Different guidelines exist for tablet, extended release and capsules.

ADVERSE EFFECTS (≥5%) **CNS:** *Somnolence, dizziness, ataxia, psychomotor slowing, confusion, paresthesia, memory difficulty, difficulty concentrating, nervousness,* mood disorder. **Endocrine:** *Abnormal bicarbonate level,* hyperammonemia (adolescents), metabolic acidosis. **GI:** *Anorexia,* weight loss. **Other:** *Fatigue, fever.*

INTERACTIONS **Drug:** Increased CNS depression with **alcohol** and other CNS DEPRESSANTS; may increase **phenytoin** concentrations; may decrease ORAL CONTRACEPTIVE, **valproate** concentrations; may increase risk of kidney stone formation with other CARBONIC ANHYDRASE INHIBITORS. **Carbamazepine, phenytoin, valproate** may decrease topiramate concentrations. Use cautiously with **metformin. Herbal: Ginkgo** may decrease anticonvulsant effectiveness.

PHARMACOKINETICS **Absorption:** Rapidly absorbed from GI tract; 80% bioavailability. **Peak:** 2 h. **Distribution:** 13–17% protein bound. **Metabolism:** Minimally metabolized in the liver. **Elimination:** Primarily in urine. **Half-Life:** 21 h.

NURSING IMPLICATIONS

Assessment & Drug Effects

- Monitor seizure activity, mental status and report significant cognitive impairment, depression, suicidal thoughts or behavior, unusual mood or behavior.
- Monitor lab tests: Monitor topiramate serum levels, periodic electrolytes and serum creatinine, ammonia levels (vomiting, lethargy or change in mental status), serum bicarbonate, serum pH.

Patient & Family Education

- Do not stop drug abruptly; discontinue gradually to minimize seizures.
- Report any change of behavior, depression, or suicidal ideation.
- Report immediately any skin rash.
- To minimize risk of kidney stones, drink at least 6–8 full glasses of water each day.
- Exercise caution with potentially hazardous activities. Sedation is common, especially with concurrent use of alcohol or other CNS depressants.
- Report any changes if vision.
- Use or add barrier contraceptive if using hormonal contraceptives.
- Be aware that psychomotor slowing and speech/language problems may develop while on topiramate therapy.
- Report adverse effects that interfere with activities of daily living.

T

TOPOTECAN HYDROCHLORIDE

(toe-po-tee′can)

Hycamtin

Classification: ANTINEOPLASTIC; CAMPTOTHECIN; DNA TOPOISOMERASE I INHIBITOR

Therapeutic: ANTINEOPLASTIC

AVAILABILITY Solution for injection; oral capsule

ACTION & THERAPEUTIC EFFECT Antitumor mechanism is related to inhibition of the activity of topoisomerase I, an enzyme required for DNA replication. Topoisomerase I is essential for the relaxation of supercoiled double-stranded DNA that enables replication and transcription to proceed. *Topotecan permits uncoiling of DNA strands but prevents recoiling of the two strands of DNA, resulting in a permanent break in the DNA strands.*

USES Metastatic ovarian cancer, cervical cancer, small cell lung cancer.

CONTRAINDICATIONS Previous hypersensitivity to topotecan, irinotecan, or other camptothecin analogs; acute infection; severe bone marrow depression; severe thrombocytopenia; neutropenic colitis; interstitial lung disease; pregnancy (category D); lactation.

CAUTIOUS USE Myelosuppression; mild to moderate renal impairment; history of bleeding disorders; previous cytotoxic or radiation therapy; older adults.

ROUTE & DOSAGE

Metastatic Ovarian Cancer and Small Cell Lung Cancer

Adult: **IV** 1.5 mg/m^2 daily for 5 days starting on day 1 of a 21-day course. Four courses of therapy recommended. Subsequent doses can be adjusted by 0.25 mg/m^2 depending on toxicity. **PO** 2.3 mg/m^2 × 5 days, repeat q21days

Cervical Cancer

Adult: 0.75 mg/m^2 days 1–3 every 3 weeks

Renal Impairment Dosage Adjustment

CrCl 20–39 mL/min: **IV** Use 0.75 mg/m^2 **PO** Reduce to 1.8 mg/m^2

Toxicity Dosage Adjustment

In severe neutropenia reduce dose by 0.4 mg/m^2 for subsequent courses

ADMINISTRATION

Oral

- Capsules must be swallowed whole. They must not be crushed, chewed, or opened.
- Avoid direct contact of the capsule contents with the skin or mucous membranes. If contact occurs, wash thoroughly with soap and water or wash eyes immediately with gently flowing water for at least 15 min.

Intravenous

▪ Initiate therapy only if baseline neutrophil count 1500/mm^3 or higher and platelet count 100,000/mm^3 or higher. ▪ Do not give subsequent doses until neutrophils 1000/mm^3 or higher, platelets 100,000/mm^3 or higher, and Hgb greater than 9.0 mg/dL.

This drug is a cytotoxic agent and caution should be used to prevent any contact with the drug. Follow institutional or standard guidelines for preparation, handling, and disposal of cytotoxic agents.

PREPARE: **IV Infusion:** Reconstitute each 4-mg vial with 4 mL sterile water for injection to yield 1 mg/mL. ▪ Withdraw the required dose and inject into 50–100 mL of NS or D5W.

ADMINISTER: **IV Infusion:** Give over 30 min immediately after preparation.

INCOMPATIBILITIES: Y-site: **Acyclovir, allopurinol, amifostine, aminophylline, amphotericin B, ampicillin/sulbactam, atenolol, bumetanide, calcium gluconate, cefepime, ceftazidime, clindamycin, dantrolene, dexamethasone, diazepam, digoxin, ertapenem, fluorouracil, foscarnet, fosphenytoin, ganciclovir, hydrocortisone, imipenem/cilastatin, ketorolac, meropenem, methohexital, mitomycin, nafcillin, pantoprazole, pemetrexed, pentobarbital, phenobarbital, phenytoin, piperacillin, piperacillin/tazobactam, potassium acetate, potassium phosphate, rituximab, sodium bicarbonate, sodium phosphate, SMZ/TMP, thiopental, ticarcillin, trastuzumab.**

- Store vials at 20°–25° C (68°–77° F); protect from light. Reconstituted vials are stable for 24 h.

ADVERSE EFFECTS **Respiratory:** *Dyspnea,* cough. **CNS:** *Headache, asthenia, pain.* **Skin:** *Alopecia, rash.* **GI:** *Nausea, vomiting, diarrhea, constipation, abdominal pain, stomatitis, anorexia,* transient elevations in liver function tests. **Hematologic:** Leukopenia, *neutropenia, anemia,* thrombocytopenia. **Other:** *Asthenia, fever, fatigue.*

INTERACTIONS **Drug:** Increased risk of bleeding with ANTICOAGULANTS, NSAIDS, SALICYLATES, ANTIPLATELET AGENTS. Avoid use with **clozapine, filgrastim, phenytoin, leflunomide, natalizumab, pimecrolimus, tacrolimus, tofacitinib,** and LIVE VACCINES.

PHARMACOKINETICS **Distribution:** 35% bound to plasma proteins. **Metabolism:** Undergoes pH-dependent hydrolysis. **Elimination:** ~30% in urine. **Half-Life:** 2–3 h.

NURSING IMPLICATIONS

Black Box Warning

Topotecan has been associated with severe bone marrow suppression.

Assessment & Drug Effects

- Assess for GI distress, respiratory distress, neurosensory symptoms, and S&S of infection throughout therapy.
- Monitor lab tests: Baseline and periodic CBC with differential; periodic renal function tests and LFTs.

Patient & Family Education

- Learn common adverse effects and measures to control or minimize when possible. Immediately report any distressing adverse effects to prescriber.
- Avoid pregnancy during therapy.

TORSEMIDE

(tor′se-mide)

Demadex

Classification: LOOP DIURETIC
Therapeutic: DIURETIC; ANTIHYPERTENSIVE
Prototype: Furosemide

AVAILABILITY Tablet

ACTION & *THERAPEUTIC EFFECT* Inhibits reabsorption of sodium and chloride primarily in the loop of Henle and renal tubules. Binds to the sodium/potassium/chloride carrier in the loop of Henle and in the renal tubules. *Long-acting potent "loop" diuretic and antihypertensive agent.*

USES Management of edema, hypertension.

CONTRAINDICATIONS Hypersensitivity to torsemide or sulfonamides; anuria; hepatic coma.

T

CAUTIOUS USE

Renal impairment; CVD; ventricular arrhythmias; gout or hyperuricemia; DM or history of pancreatitis; liver disease with cirrhosis and ascites; fluid and electrolyte depletion; hyperuricemia; hyperglycemia; hearing impairment; older adults; pregnancy (fetal risk cannot be ruled out); lactation (infant risk cannot be ruled out). Safety and efficacy in children not established.

ROUTE & DOSAGE

Edema of HF or Chronic Renal Failure

Adult: **PO** 10–20 mg once daily, may increase up to 200 mg/day as needed

Edema with Hepatic Cirrhosis

Adult: **PO** 5–10 mg once daily, may increase by doubling dose (max: dose 40 mg) administered with an aldosterone antagonist or potassium-sparing diuretic

Hypertension

Adult: **PO** 5 mg once daily, may increase to 10 mg/day if no response after 4–6 wk

ADMINISTRATION

- Note: With hepatic cirrhosis, use an aldosterone antagonist concomitantly to prevent hypokalemia and metabolic alkalosis.
- Store tablet at 15°–30° C (59°–86° F).

ADVERSE EFFECTS

GU: Polyuria.

DIAGNOSTIC TEST INTERFERENCE

May lead to false-negative aldosterone/renin ratio.

INTERACTIONS

Drug: NSAIDS may reduce diuretic effects. Also see furosemide for potential drug interactions such as increased risk of **digoxin** toxicity due to hypokalemia, prolonged neuromuscular blockade with NEUROMUSCULAR BLOCKING AGENTS, and decreased **lithium** elimination with increased toxicity. Do not use with **desmopressin, foscarnet, levosulpiride, promazine.** **Herbal: Ginseng** may decrease efficacy.

PHARMACOKINETICS

Absorption: Readily from GI tract. **Onset:** 60 min. **Peak:** 60–120 min. **Duration:** 6–8 h. **Metabolism:** In liver (CYP system). **Elimination:** 80% in bile; 20% in urine. **Half-Life:** 210 min.

NURSING IMPLICATIONS

Assessment & Drug Effects

- Monitor BP often and assess for orthostatic hypotension; assess respiratory status for S&S of pulmonary edema.
- Monitor ECG, as electrolyte imbalances predispose to cardiac arrhythmias.
- Monitor I&O with daily weights. Assess for improvement in edema.
- Monitor diabetics for loss of glycemic control.
- Monitor coagulation parameters and lithium levels in patients on concurrent anticoagulant and/or lithium therapy.
- Monitor lab tests: Periodic serum electrolytes, blood glucose.

Patient & Family Education

- Check weight at least weekly and report abrupt gains or losses to prescriber.
- Understand the risk of orthostatic hypotension.
- Report symptoms of hypokalemia (see Appendix F) or hearing loss immediately to prescriber.
- Monitor blood glucose for loss of glycemic control if diabetic.

TRAMADOL HYDROCHLORIDE

(tra′mad-ol)

ConZip, Rybix, Ryzolt, Ultram, Ultram ER, Zydol ♣

Classification: ANALGESIC; NARCOTIC (OPIATE AGONIST)

Therapeutic: NARCOTIC ANALGESIC

Prototype: Morphine sulfate

Controlled Substance: Schedule IV

AVAILABILITY Tablet; orally disintegrating tablet; extended release tablet; extended release capsule

ACTION & *THERAPEUTIC EFFECT* Centrally acting opiate receptor agonist that inhibits the uptake of norepinephrine and serotonin, suggesting both opioid and nonopioid mechanisms of pain relief. May produce opioid-like effects, but causes less respiratory depression than morphine. *Effective agent for control of moderate to moderately severe pain.*

USES Management of moderate or moderately severe pain.

CONTRAINDICATIONS Hypersensitivity to tramadol or other opioid analgesics including anaphylactoid reaction; severe respiratory depression; severe or acute asthmas; patients on MAO Inhibitors; substance abuse; suicidal; alcohol intoxication; lactation. **Extended release:** Do not administer to patients with severe hepatic impairment.

CAUTIOUS USE Debilitated patients; chronic respiratory disorders; respiratory depression; liver disease; renal impairment; myxedema, hypothyroidism, or hypoadrenalism; GI disease; acute abdominal conditions; increased ICP or head injury, increased intracranial pressure; history of seizures; older adults: pregnancy (category C); children younger than 16 y. **Extended release:** Do not use in children younger than 18 y.

ROUTE & DOSAGE

Pain

Adult: **PO Immediate release** 25 mg daily, titrated up to dose of 100 mg/day (max: 400 mg/day); **PO Extended release** 100 mg qd may titrate up q5d (max dose: 300 mg/day)
PO Disintegrating tablet 50 mg q4–6h may increase q3d to 200 mg/day

Renal Impairment Dosage Adjustment

CrCl less than 30 mL/min: Decrease to 50–100 mg q12h

Hepatic Impairment Dosage Adjustment

Cirrhosis: Decrease to 50–100 mg q12h

ADMINISTRATION

Oral

- Extended release tablets should be swallowed whole. They should not be crushed or chewed.
- Store at 15°–30° C (59°–86° F).

ADVERSE EFFECTS **CV:** Palpitations, vasodilation, orthostatic hypotension. **CNS:** Drowsiness, *dizziness, vertigo, fatigue, headache, somnolence,* restlessness, euphoria, confusion, anxiety, coordination disturbance, sleep disturbances, seizures. **HEENT:** Visual disturbances. **Skin:** Rash. **GI:** *Nausea, constipation,* vomiting, xerostomia, dyspepsia, diarrhea, abdominal pain, anorexia, flatulence. **GU:** Urinary retention/frequency, menopausal symptoms. **Other:** Sweating, <u>anaphylactic</u>

<u>reaction</u> (even with first dose), withdrawal syndrome (anxiety, sweating, nausea, tremors, diarrhea, piloerection, panic attacks, paresthesia, hallucinations) with abrupt discontinuation, flushing.

DIAGNOSTIC TEST INTERFERENCE Increased ***creatinine, liver enzymes;*** decreased ***hemoglobin; proteinuria.***

INTERACTIONS **Drug: Carbamazepine** significantly decreases tramadol levels (may need up to twice usual dose). Tramadol may increase adverse effects of MAO INHIBITORS, TRICYCLIC ANTIDEPRESSANTS, **cyclobenzaprine,** PHENOTHIAZINES, SELECTIVE SEROTONIN-REUPTAKE INHIBITORS (SSRIS), MAO INHIBITORS may enhance seizure risk with tramadol. May increase CNS adverse effects when used with other CNS DEPRESSANTS. **Herbal: St. John's wort** may increase sedation.

PHARMACOKINETICS **Absorption:** Rapidly absorbed from GI tract; 75% reaches systemic circulation. **Onset:** 30–60 min. **Peak:** 2 h. **Duration:** 3–7 h. **Distribution:** Approximately 20% bound to plasma proteins; probably crosses blood–brain barrier; crosses placenta; 0.1% excreted into breast milk. **Metabolism:** Extensively in liver by cytochrome P450 system. **Elimination:** Primarily in urine. **Half-Life:** 6–7 h.

T

NURSING IMPLICATIONS

Assessment & Drug Effects

- Assess for level of pain relief and administer PRN dose as needed but not to exceed the recommended total daily dose.
- Monitor vital signs and assess for orthostatic hypotension or signs of CNS depression.
- Withhold drug and notify prescriber if S&S of hypersensitivity occur.
- Assess bowel and bladder function; report urinary frequency or retention.
- Use seizure precautions for patients who have a history of seizures or who are concurrently using drugs that lower the seizure threshold.
- Monitor ambulation and take appropriate safety precautions.

Patient & Family Education

- Exercise caution with potentially hazardous activities until response to drug is known.
- Do not exceed the total number of mg prescribed for a 24 h period.
- Understand potential adverse effects and report problems with bowel and bladder function, CNS impairment, and any other bothersome adverse effects to prescriber.

TRAMETINIB

(tra-me′ti-nib)

Mekinist

Classification: ANTINEOPLASTIC; MITOGEN-ACTIVATED EXTRACELLULAR KINASE (MEK) INHIBITOR

Therapeutic: ANTINEOPLASTIC

Prototype: Erlotinib

AVAILABILITY Tablet

ACTION & *THERAPEUTIC EFFECT* A reversible inhibitor of certain kinases that transmit signals and promote cellular proliferation and cancer growth. *Trametinib inhibits BRAF V600 mutation-positive melanoma cell growth in vitro and in vivo.*

USES Treatment of unresectable or metastatic melanoma in patients with BRAF V600E or V600K mutations, as detected by an FDA-approved test.

 Common adverse effects in *italic*; life-threatening effects <u>underlined</u>; generic names in **bold;** classifications in SMALL CAPS; ♣ Canadian drug name; ⊙ Prototype drug; ⚠ Alert

CONTRAINDICATIONS Symptomatic cardiomyopathy or LVEF decreases by 10% below pre-treatment level and less than the LLN; drug-related loss of vision or other visual disturbances; drug-induced interstitial lung disease or pneumonitis; pregnancy (category D); lactation.

CAUTIOUS USE Severe renal impairment; moderate or severe hepatic impairment; cardiac disorders; CHF; respiratory disorders; ocular disorders; hypertension. Safety and efficacy in children not established.

ROUTE & DOSAGE

Malignant Melanoma

Adult: **PO** 2 mg once daily

Toxicity Dosage Adjustment

For specific toxicities see manufacturer guidelines.

ADMINISTRATION

Oral

- Give at least 1 h before or 2 h after a meal.
- Store at 2°–8° C (36°–46° F) and protect from moisture and light. Keep in original bottle and do not remove desiccant.

ADVERSE EFFECTS **CV:** Bradycardia, cardiomyopathy, hypertension. **CNS:** Dizziness, dysgeusia. **HEENT:** Dry eye, blurred vision. **Endocrine:** *Anemia, hypoalbuminemia, increased alkaline phosphatase, increased ALT/AST.* **Skin:** *Dermatitis acneiform,* cellulitis, dry skin, folliculitis, paronychia, pruritus, *rash.* **GI:** Abdominal pain and tenderness, aphthous stomatitis, *diarrhea,* mouth ulceration, mucosal inflammation, and stomatitis. **Musculoskeletal:** Rhabdomyolysis. **Hematologic:** Conjunctival hemorrhage, *edema,* epistaxis, gingival bleeding, hematochezia, hematuria, hemorrhoidal hemorrhage, *lymphedema,* melena, *peripheral edema,* rectal hemorrhage, and vaginal hemorrhage.

PHARMACOKINETICS **Absorption:** 72% bioavailable. **Peak:** 1.5 h. **Distribution:** 97.4% plasma protein bound. **Metabolism:** In liver. **Elimination:** Fecal (80%) and renal (20%). **Half-Life:** 3.9–4.8 d.

NURSING IMPLICATIONS

Assessment & Drug Effects

- Monitor cardiovascular status throughout therapy. Report promptly new-onset or worsening hypertension and S&S of heart failure.
- Monitor pulmonary status throughout therapy. Report promptly signs of interstitial lung disease including cough, dyspnea, and signs of hypoxia or pleural effusion.
- Monitor for and report promptly S&S of retinal detachment.
- Evaluate for signs of skin toxicity. Report to prescriber development of progressive rash or signs of skin infection.
- Monitor lab tests: Prior to therapy the presence of BRAF V600E or V600K mutation in tumor specimens must be confirmed.

Patient & Family Education

- Report to prescriber if you experience any of the following S&S of heart failure or lung problems: Rapid heart rate, shortness of breath, unproductive cough, swelling of ankles and feet, excessive fatigue.
- Report to prescriber if you experience blurred vision, see colored dots or halo around objects.
- Report promptly signs of skin toxicity such as skin rash, acne,

T

redness, swelling, peeling, or tenderness of hands or feet.

- Women should use highly effective contraception during treatment due to potential for serious fetal harm.
- Contact prescriber immediately if a pregnancy is suspected.

TRANDOLAPRIL

(tran-do'la-pril)

Classification: ANGIOTENSIN-CONVERTING ENZYME (ACE) INHIBITOR; ANTIHYPERTENSIVE

Therapeutic: ANTIHYPERTENSIVE; ACE INHIBITOR

Prototype: Enalapril

AVAILABILITY Tablet

ACTION & *THERAPEUTIC EFFECT* Inhibits ACE and interrupts conversion by renin which leads to the formation of angiotensin II from angiotensin I. Inhibition of ACE leads to vasodilation as well as to decreased aldosterone. Decreased aldosterone leads to diuresis and a slight increase in serum potassium. *Lowers blood pressure by specific inhibition of ACE. Unlike other ACE inhibitors, all racial groups respond to trandolapril, including low-renin hypertensives.*

USES Treatment of hypertension

T

UNLABELED USES: reduction of CV morbidity/mortality post MI in patients with heart failure; non ST elevation acute coronary syndrome.

CONTRAINDICATIONS Hypersensitivity to trandolapril or ACE inhibitors; history of angioedema related to previous treatment with an ACE inhibitor; history of idiopathic or hereditary angioedema; jaundice due to trandolapril; concomitant use of aliskiren in patients with diabetes, pregnancy—fetal risk cannot be ruled out and fetal injury and death have been reported; lactation—infant risk cannot be ruled out.

CAUTIOUS USE Renal impairment, hepatic insufficiency; patients prone to hypotension (e.g., CHF, ischemic heart disease, aortic stenosis, CVA, dehydration); systemic lupus erythematosus, scleroderma; patients being treated with hymenoptera venom. Safety and efficacy in children younger than 18 y not established.

ROUTE & DOSAGE

Hypertension

Adult: **PO** 1 mg once daily, may increase weekly to 2–4 mg once daily (max: 8 mg/day).

Renal Impairment Dosage Adjustment

CrCl less than 30 mL/min: Start with 0.5 mg once daily

Hepatic Impairment Dosage Adjustment

Hepatic cirrhosis: Start with 0.5 mg once daily

ADMINISTRATION

Oral

- Note: If concurrently ordered diuretic cannot be discontinued 2–3 days before beginning trandolapril therapy, initial dose is usually reduced to 0.5 mg.

- Dosage adjustments are typically made at intervals of at least 1 wk.
- Store at controlled room temperatures between 20 and 25 degrees C (59 to 77 degrees F). Capsules are stable for 2 years.

ADVERSE EFFECTS (≥5%)

CV: *Hypotension*, syncope. **Respiratory:** *Cough*. **CNS:** *Dizziness*. **Endocrine:** Hyperkalemia. **GI:** Dyspepsia. **GU:** elevated serum BUN.

DIAGNOSTIC TEST INTERFERENCE

may lead to false negative aldosterone/renin ratio.

INTERACTIONS

Drug: DIURETICS, ANTIHYPERTENSIVES, **rituximab** may enhance hypotensive effects. POTASSIUM-SPARING DIURETICS (**amiloride, spironolactone, triamterene**), POTASSIUM SUPPLEMENTS, POTASSIUM-CONTAINING SALT SUBSTITUTES, **aliskiren,** may increase risk of hyperkalemia. May increase serum levels and toxicity of **lithium.** NSAIDs may reduce the therapeutic response. Avoid use with **cyclosporine.** Increases adverse effects of **iron dextran, sodium phosphate.**

PHARMACOKINETICS

Absorption: Rapidly absorbed from GI tract and converted to active form, trandolaprilat, in liver; 70% of dose reaches systemic circulation as trandolaprilat. **Peak:** 4–10 h. **Distribution:** 80% protein bound; crosses placenta, secreted into breast milk of animals (human secretion unknown). **Metabolism:** In liver to trandolaprilat. **Elimination:** 33% in urine, 66% in feces. **Half-Life:** 6 h trandolapril, 22.5 h trandolaprilat.

NURSING IMPLICATIONS

Black Box Warning

Trandolapril has been associated with fetal toxicity.

Assessment & Drug Effects

- Monitor BP carefully for 1–3 h following initial dose, especially in patients using concurrent diuretics, on salt restriction, or volume depleted.
- Monitor serum lithium levels frequently with concurrent lithium therapy and assess for S&S of lithium toxicity; increase caution when diuretic therapy is also used.
- Monitor lab tests: Baseline LFTs and renal function tests; periodic serum potassium and sodium, fasting blood glucose, comprehensive metabolic panel, urinalysis, uric acid.

Patient & Family Education

- Discontinue drug and immediately report S&S of angioedema of face or extremities to prescriber. Seek emergency help for swelling of the tongue or any other sign of potential airway obstruction.
- Women with reproduction potential should be counseled on importance of birth control while taking this drug and if pregnancy occurs, notify provider right away. This medication is known to cause fetal harm.
- Review adverse effects with patient and/or caregiver.
- Be aware that lightheadedness can occur, especially during early therapy. Excess fluid loss of any kind will increase risk of hypotension and syncope.
- Patient should avoid activities requiring coordination until drug effects are realized as drug may cause dizziness.

- Report promptly if you are or suspect you are pregnant.

TRANYLCYPROMINE SULFATE

(tran-ill-sip′roe-meen)

Parnate

Classification: ANTIDEPRESSANT; MONOAMINE OXIDASE INHIBITOR (MAOI)

Therapeutic: ANTIDEPRESSANT; MAOI

Prototype: Phenelzine

AVAILABILITY Tablet

ACTION & *THERAPEUTIC EFFECT* Potent MAO with an antidepressant activity that arises from the increased availability of monoamines resulting from the inhibition of the enzyme MAO. This leads to increased concentration of neurotransmitters, such as epinephrine, norepinephrine, and dopamine in the CNS. *Drug of last choice for severe depression unresponsive to other MAO inhibitors.*

USES Major depression.

UNLABELED USES Orthostatic hypotension, panic disorder, social anxiety disorder.

CONTRAINDICATIONS Confirmed or suspected cerebrovascular defect, cardiovascular disease; hepatic disease or abnormal LFT; hypertension, pheochromocytoma history of severe or recurrent headaches; recent acute MI; angina; renal failure; suicidal ideation; anuria; lactation.

CAUTIOUS USE Bipolar disorder; Parkinson's disease; psychosis; schizophrenia, anxiety/agitation; CHF; DM; seizure disorders; hyperthyroidism; history of suicidal attempts; renal impairment; older adults; pregnancy (category C); children and adolescents with major depressive disorder or other psychiatric disorders.

ROUTE & DOSAGE

Major Depression

Adult: **PO** 30 mg/day in 2 divided doses, may increase by 10 mg/day at 2–3 wk intervals (max: 60 mg/day)

ADMINISTRATION

Oral

- Contraindicated drugs should be discontinued 1–2 wk before starting therapy.
- Crush tablet and give with fluid or mix with food if patient cannot swallow pill.
- Note: Doses given in the late evening may cause insomnia.

ADVERSE EFFECTS **CV:** *Orthostatic hypotension*, arrhythmias, hypertensive crisis. **CNS:** Vertigo, dizziness, tremors, muscle twitching, headache, blurred vision suicidality. **Skin:** Rash. **GI:** Dry mouth, anorexia, constipation, diarrhea, abdominal discomfort. **GU:** Impotence. **Other:** Peripheral edema, sweating.

INTERACTIONS **Drug:** TRICYCLIC ANTIDEPRESSANTS, SSRIS, AMPHETAMINES, **ephedrine, guanethidine, buspirone, methyldopa, dopamine, levodopa, tryptophan** may precipitate hypertensive crisis, and must be discontinued before **tranylcypromine** treatment. **Alcohol** and other CNS DEPRESSANTS add to CNS depressant effects; **meperidine** can cause fatal cardiovascular collapse; ANESTHETICS exaggerate hypotensive and CNS depressant effects;

metrizamide increases risk of seizures; DIURETICS and other ANTIHYPERTENSIVE AGENTS add to hypotensive effects. **Food: Tyramine**-containing foods may precipitate hypertensive crisis (e.g., aged or matured cheese, air-dried or cured meats including sausages and salamis; fava or broad bean pods, tap/draft beers, sauerkraut, soy sauce, and other soybean condiments). **Herbal: Ginseng, ephedra, ma huang, St. John's wort** may lead to hypertensive crisis; **ginseng** may lead to manic episodes.

PHARMACOKINETICS **Absorption:** Completely from GI tract. **Onset:** 10 days. **Metabolism:** Rapidly in liver to active metabolite. **Elimination:** Primarily in urine. **Half-Life:** 90–190 min.

NURSING IMPLICATIONS

Black Box Warning

Tranylcypromine sulfate has been associated with suicidal thinking and behavior in children, adolescents, and young adults.

Assessment & Drug Effects

- Monitor BP closely. Severe hypertensive reactions are known to occur with MAO inhibitors.
- Report immediately to prescriber signs of worsening mental status such as suicidal ideation, aggressiveness, agitation, anxiety, hostility, impulsivity, insomnia, irritability, panic attacks, and worsening of depression.
- Expect therapeutic response within 3 days, but full antidepressant effects may not be obtained until 2–3 wk of drug therapy.

Patient & Family Education

- Do not eat tyramine-containing foods (see FOOD–DRUG INTERACTIONS).
- Be aware that excessive use of caffeine-containing beverages (chocolate, coffee, tea, cola) can contribute to development of rapid heartbeat, arrhythmias, and hypertension.
- Report promptly emergence of anxiety, agitation, panic attacks, insomnia, irritability, hostility, aggressiveness, impulsivity, mania, worsening depression, suicidal ideation, or other unusual changes in behavior.
- Make position changes slowly, particularly from recumbent to upright posture.
- Avoid potentially hazardous activities until response to drug is known.
- Avoid alcohol or other CNS depressants because of their possible additive effects.

TRASTUZUMAB

(tra-stu'zu-mab)

Herceptin

Classification: IMMUNOMODULATOR; MONOCLONAL ANTIBODY; ANTINEOPLASTIC; ANTI-HUMAN EPIDERMAL GROWTH FACTOR (ANTI-HER)

Therapeutic: ANTINEOPLASTIC; IMMUNOMODULATOR; ANTI-HER

AVAILABILITY Solution for injection

ACTION & THERAPEUTIC EFFECT Recombinant DNA monoclonal antibody (IgG_1 kappa) that selectively binds to the human epidermal growth factor receptor-2 protein (HER_2). *Inhibits growth of human tumor cells that overexpress HER_2 proteins.*

USES Metastatic breast cancer in those whose tumors overexpress the HER_2 protein. HER_2-positive breast cancer after surgery.

CONTRAINDICATIONS Concurrent administration of anthracycline or radiation; anaphylaxis; angioedema; interstitial pneumonitis; acute respiratory distress syndrome; drug induced nephrotic syndrome; pregnancy (category D); lactation during and for 6 mo following administration of trastuzumab.

CAUTIOUS USE Preexisting cardiac dysfunction; pulmonary disease; previous administration of cardiotoxic therapy (e.g., anthracycline or radiation); hypersensitivity to benzyl alcohol; older adults.

ROUTE & DOSAGE

Metastatic Breast Cancer

Adult: **IV** 4 mg/kg, then 2 mg/kg qwk

ADMINISTRATION

Note: Trastuzumab and ado-trastuzumab emtansine are different products and are **not** interchangeable.

Intravenous

PREPARE: **IV Infusion:** Reconstitute each vial with 20 mL of supplied diluent (bacteriostatic water) to produce a multidose vial containing 21 mg/mL. ▪ Note: For patients with a hypersensitivity to benzyl alcohol, reconstitute with sterile water for injection; this solution **must be** used immediately with any unused portion discarded. ▪ Withdraw the ordered dose and add to a 250 mL of NS and invert bag to mix. ▪ Do not give or mix with dextrose solutions.

ADMINISTER: **IV Infusion:** Infuse loading dose (4 mg/kg) over 90 min; infuse subsequent doses (2 mg/kg) over 30 min. ▪ Do not give IV push or as a bolus dose.

INCOMPATIBILITIES: **Solution/additive: Dextrose** solution; do not mix or coadminister with other drugs. **Y-site: Aldesleukin, amikacin, amphotericin B, aztreonam, cefoperazone, cefotaxime, cefotetan, cefoxitin, chlorpromazine, clindamycin, cyclosporine, fludarabine, furosemide, idarubicin, irinotecan, levofloxacin, levorphanol, morphine, nalbuphine, netilmicin, ofloxacin, ondansetron, piperacillin, piperacillin/tazobactam, streptozocin, ticarcillin, topotecan.**

▪ Store unopened vials and reconstituted vials at 2°–8° C (36°–46° F). ▪ Discard reconstituted vials 28 days after reconstitution.

ADVERSE EFFECTS CV: CHF, cardiac dysfunction (dyspnea, cough, paroxysmal nocturnal dyspnea, peripheral edema, S3 gallop, reduced ejection fraction), tachycardia, *edema*, cardiotoxicity. **Respiratory:** *Cough, dyspnea*, rhinitis, pharyngitis, sinusitis. **CNS:** *Headache, insomnia, dizziness, paresthesias*, depression, peripheral neuritis, neuropathy myalgia. **Skin:** *Rash*, herpes simplex, acne. **GI:** *Diarrhea, abdominal pain, nausea, vomiting*, anorexia. **Hematologic:** *Anemia*, leukopenia, *thrombocytopenia, neutropenia*. **Other:** *Pain, asthenia, fever, chills*, flu syndrome, allergic reaction, *fatigue* bone pain, *arthralgia*, hypersensitivity (anaphylaxis, urticaria, bronchospasm, angioedema, or hypotension), *increased incidence of infections*, infusion reaction (*chills, fever*, nausea, vomiting, pain, rigors, headache, dizziness, dyspnea, hypotension, rash).

T

INTERACTIONS Drug: Paclitaxel may increase trastuzumab levels and toxicity.

PHARMACOKINETICS Half-Life: 5.8 days.

NURSING IMPLICATIONS

Black Box Warning

Trastuzumab has been associated with cardiomyopathy, infusion reactions, pulmonary toxicity, and embryo-fetal toxicity.

Assessment & Drug Effects

- Monitor for infusion reactions within 24 h of infusion. Stop infusion and notify prescriber if patients develop dyspnea, significant hypotension, or any other sign of infusion reaction. Monitor closely until symptoms resolve. chills and fever during the first IV infusion; these adverse events usually respond to prompt treatment without the need to discontinue the infusion. Notify prescriber immediately.
- Monitor carefully cardiovascular status at baseline and throughout course of therapy, assessing for S&S of heart failure (e.g., dyspnea, increased cough, PND, edema, S3 gallop). Those with preexisting cardiac dysfunction are at high risk for cardiotoxicity.
- Monitor lab tests: Periodic CBC with differential, platelet count, and Hgb and Hct.

Patient & Family Education

- Report promptly any unusual symptoms (e.g., chills, nausea, fever) during infusion.
- Report promptly any of the following: Shortness of breath, swelling of feet or legs, persistent cough, difficulty sleeping, loss of appetite, abdominal bloating.

TRAVOPROST

(tra'vo-prost)

Travatan

See Appendix A-1.

TRAZODONE HYDROCHLORIDE

(tray'zoe-done)

Oleptro

Classification: ANTIDEPRESSANT

Therapeutic: ANTIDEPRESSANT

Prototype: Imipramine

AVAILABILITY Tablet; extended release tablet

ACTION & *THERAPEUTIC EFFECT* Potentiates serotonin effects by selectively blocking its reuptake at presynaptic membranes in CNS. Produces varying degrees of sedation in normal and mentally depressed patients. *Increases total sleep time, decreases number and duration of awakenings in depressed patient, and decreases REM sleep. Has antianxiety effect in severely depressed patient.*

USES Major depressive disorder.

UNLABELED USES Adjunctive treatment of alcohol dependence, anxiety, panic disorder, insomnia.

CONTRAINDICATIONS Initial recovery phase of MI; ventricular ectopy; electroshock therapy; within 14 days of MAOIs use; initiation in patients treated with linezolid or methylene blue IV; suicidal ideation.

CAUTIOUS USE Bipolar disorder, MDD; older adults; history of suicidal tendencies; cardiac

T

arrhythmias or disease; patients at risk for QT prolongation; volume depleted individuals; hepatic disease, renal impairment; history of GI bleeding; older adults; pregnancy (category C); lactation. Safe use in children not established.

ROUTE & DOSAGE

Depression

Adult: **PO Immediate release** 150 mg/day in divided doses, may increase by 50 mg/day q3–4days (max: 400–600 mg/day); **PO Extended release** 150 mg daily may increase by 75 mg/day at 3 day intervals (max: 375 mg/day)

Pharmacogenetic Dosage Adjustment

Poor CYP2D6 metabolizer: Start with 80% of normal dose

ADMINISTRATION

Oral

- Ensure that extended release tablets are swallowed whole. They should not be crushed or chewed.
- Give drug with food; increases amount of absorption by 20% and appears to decrease incidence of dizziness or light-headedness. Maintain the same schedule for food-drug intake throughout treatment period to prevent variations in serum concentration.
- Store in tightly closed, light-resistant container at 15°–30° C (59°–86° F).

ADVERSE EFFECTS **CV:** Hypotension (including orthostatic hypotension), hypertension, syncope, shortness of breath, chest pain, tachycardia, palpitations, bradycardia, PVCs, ventricular tachycardia (short episodes of 3–4 beats). **CNS:** *Drowsiness*, light-headedness, tiredness, dizziness, insomnia, *nervousness*, headache, agitation, impaired memory and speech, disorientation. **HEENT:** Nasal and sinus congestion, blurred vision, eye irritation, sweating or clamminess, tinnitus. **Skin:** Skin eruptions, rash, pruritus, acne, photosensitivity. **GI:** *Dry mouth*, anorexia, constipation, abdominal distress, nausea, vomiting, dysgeusia, flatulence, diarrhea. **GU:** Hematuria, increased frequency, delayed urine flow, male priapism, ejaculation inhibition. **Musculoskeletal:** Skeletal aches and pains, muscle twitches. **Hematologic:** Anemia. **Other:** Weight change.

INTERACTIONS **Drug:** ANTIHYPERTENSIVE AGENTS may potentiate hypotensive effects; **alcohol** and other CNS DEPRESSANTS add to depressant effects; may increase **digoxin** or **phenytoin** levels; MAO INHIBITORS may precipitate hypertensive crisis; **ketoconazole, indinavir, ritonavir**, **saquinavir** may increase levels and toxicity. Use of other serotonergic agents may increase risk of serotonin syndrome. Do not use with **conivaptan, ivabradine, linezolid, mifepristone, saquinavir. Herbal: Ginkgo** may increase sedation.

PHARMACOKINETICS **Absorption:** Readily from GI tract. **Onset:** 1–2 wk. **Peak:** 1–2 h. **Distribution:** Distributed into breast milk. **Metabolism:** In liver (CYP2D6). **Elimination:** 75% in urine, 25% in feces. **Half-Life:** 5–9 h.

NURSING IMPLICATIONS

Black Box Warning

Trazodone hydrochloride has been associated with suicidal thinking and behavior in children, adolescents, and young adults.

T

Assessment & Drug Effects

- Monitor BP and heart rate and rhythm. Report to prescriber development of tachycardia, bradycardia, or palpitations.
- Monitor for orthostatic hypotension, especially in the elderly or those taking concurrent antihypertensive drugs.
- Monitor children and adolescents for changes in behavior that indicate increased suicidality.
- Observe patient's level of activity. If it appears to be increasing toward sleeplessness and agitation with changes in reality orientation, report to prescriber. Manic episodes have been reported.
- Be aware that overdose is characterized by an extension of common adverse effects: Vomiting, lethargy, drowsiness, and exaggerated anticholinergic effects.

Patient & Family Education

- Report immediately to prescriber signs of worsening mental status such as suicidal ideation, aggressiveness, agitation, anxiety, hostility, impulsivity, insomnia, irritability, panic attacks, and worsening of depression.
- Consult prescriber if drowsiness becomes a distressing adverse effect. Dose regimen may be changed so that largest dose is at bedtime.
- Limit or abstain from alcohol use. The depressant effects of CNS depressants and alcohol may be potentiated by this drug.
- Do not self-medicate with OTC drugs for colds, allergy, or insomnia treatment without advice of prescriber. Many of these drugs contain CNS depressants.
- Male patient should report inappropriate or prolonged penile erections. The drug may be discontinued.

TRETINOIN

(tret'i-noyn)

Atralin, Avita, Refissa, Renova, Retin-A, Retin-A Micro, Retinoic Acid, Tretin-X, Vesanoid

Classification: ANTINEOPLASTIC; ANTIACNE (RETINOID); ANTIPSORIATIC

Therapeutic: ANTINEOPLASTIC; ANTIACNE; ANTIPSORIATIC

Prototype: Isotretinoin

AVAILABILITY Cream; gel; capsule

ACTION & *THERAPEUTIC EFFECT*

Antiacne activity: Reverses retention hyperkeratosis and micro comedo formation in acne pathology. **Antineoplastic activity:** Induces cellular differentiation in malignant cells. Its exact mechanism of action is unknown. *Effective in early treatment and control of acne vulgaris grades I–III. Effective in treatment of (Acute Promyelocytic Leukemia) APL.*

USES Topical treatment of acne vulgaris grades I–III, especially during early stages when number of comedones is greatest; adjunctively in management of associated comedones and in treatment of flat warts; oral for remission induction treatment of acute promyelocytic leukemia; cream as adjunctive therapy for mitigation of fine wrinkles; palliation of fine wrinkles, mottled hyperpigmentation and facial skin roughness.

UNLABELED USES Psoriasis, senile keratosis, ichthyosis vulgaris, keratosis palmaris and plantaris, basal cell carcinoma, photodamaged skin (photoaging), and other skin conditions. **Orphan drug:** For squamous metaplasia of conjunctiva or cornea with mucous deficiency and keratinization.

T

CONTRAINDICATIONS Hypersensitivity to tretinoin or other retinoids; eczema; exposure to sunlight or ultraviolet rays, sunburn; pregnancy (high risk that a severely deformed infant will result if tretinoin capsules are administered during pregnancy).

CAUTIOUS USE Patient in an occupation necessitating considerable sun exposure or weather extremes; hepatic disease; lactation; children younger than 18 y.

ROUTE & DOSAGE

Acne

Adult: **Topical** Apply once/day at bedtime

Acute Promyelocytic Leukemia

Adult: **PO** 45 mg/m^2/day

Antiwrinkle Cream

Adult: **Topical** (0.05% cream) Apply to face once daily at bedtime

ADMINISTRATION

Oral

- Administer with a meal.
- Capsules must be swallowed whole; they cannot be opened, crushed, or chewed. Tretinoin has also been administered sublingually by squeezing the capsule contents beneath the tongue.

Topical

- Cleanse using a mild bland soap, and thoroughly dry areas being treated before applying drug. Avoid use of medicated, drying, or abrasive soaps and cleansers.
- Wash hands before and after treatment. Apply lightly over affected areas. Do not apply to nonaffected skin area.
- Avoid contact of drug with eyes, mouth, angles of nose, open wounds, mucous membranes.
- Store gel and liquid formulations below 30° C (86° F) and solution below 27° C (80° F).

ADVERSE EFFECTS **CV:** *Arrhythmias, flushing, hypotension, hypertension,* CHF, peripheral edema, chest discomfort, facial edema. **Respiratory:** *Dyspnea,* upper and/or lower respiratory complaint, pleural effusion, pulmonary infiltrates, pneumonia, rales, wheezing. **CNS:** *Dizziness, paresthesias, anxiety, insomnia, depression, headache,* cerebral hemorrhage, intracranial hypertension, hallucinations, malaise, shivering, pain, confusion, agitation. **HEENT:** Visual disturbances, eye disease, ear fullness, hearing loss. **Endocrine:** Hypercholesterolemia, hypertriglyceridemia, weight gain, weight loss. **Skin:** Cellulitis, pallor, diaphoresis, skin rash, xeroderma, pruritis, alopecia. **Hepatic/GI:** *Dry mucus membranes, nausea, vomiting, abdominal pain,* flank pain, *diarrhea, constipation, dyspepsia,* *GI hemorrhage,* mucositis, anorexia, dyspepsia, increased liver enzymes, hepatomegaly, splenomegaly. **GU:** Renal insufficiency, fluid imbalance, dysuria. **Musculoskeletal:** Ostealgia, myalgia. **Hematologic:** Hemorrhage, leucocytosis, DIC, lymphatic disease. **Other:** Infection, *fever.*

INTERACTIONS **Drug:** TOPICAL ACNE MEDICATIONS (including **sulfur, resorcinol, benzoyl peroxide,** and **salicylic acid**) may increase inflammation and peeling; topical products containing **alcohol** or **menthol** may cause stinging. PHOTOSENSITIZING AGENTS increase the risk of adverse effects. Do not use with **vitamin A** or multivitamins containing vitamin A due to risk of adverse effects. **Oral product:** PHOTOSENSITIZING AGENTS increase the risk of adverse effects. Do not use with **vitamin A** or multivitamins containing vitamin A due to risk of adverse effect

PHARMACOKINETICS Absorption: Minimally absorbed from intact skin, topical; 60% absorbed, PO. **Elimination:** About 0.1% of topical dose is excreted in urine within 24 h; 63% excreted in urine and 31% in feces, PO. **Half-Life:** 45 min, topical; 2–2.5 h, PO.

NURSING IMPLICATIONS

Assessment & Drug Effects

Topical

- Be aware that topical treatment to dark-skinned individuals may cause postinflammatory hyperpigmentation; reversible with termination of drug treatment.
- Clinical response to topical treatment should be evident in 2–3 wk; complete and satisfactory response (in 75% of the patients) may require 3–4 mo.
- Be aware that erythema and desquamation during the first 1–3 wk of topical treatment do not represent exacerbation of the skin problem but a probable response to the drug from deep previously unseen lesions.
- Monitor lab values: CBC with differential, coagulation profile, LFTs, triglyceride, and cholesterol.

Patient & Family Education

Topical

- As treatment is continued, lesions gradually disappear, leaving an inflammatory background; scaling and redness decrease after 8–10 wk of therapy.
- Wash face no more often than 2–3 × daily.
- Be aware that drug is not curative; relapses commonly occur within 3–6 wk after treatment has been discontinued.
- Avoid exposure to sun; when cannot be avoided, use a SPF 15 or higher sunscreen.
- Do not self-medicate with additional acne treatment because of danger of drug interactions.

TRIAMCINOLONE

(trye-am-sin′oh-lone)

TRIAMCINOLONE ACETONIDE

Kenalog, Nasacort Allergy 24h, Triderm, Triescence, Xipere, Zilretta

Classification: ADRENAL CORTICOSTEROID; GLUCOCORTICOID

Therapeutic: ANTI-INFLAMMATORY; IMMUNOSUPPRESSANT

Prototype: Prednisone

AVAILABILITY Triamcinolone: Tablet; syrup. **Triamcinolone acetonide:** Solution for injection; aerosol; inhaler; spray; nasal spray; cream, ointment, lotion; topical spray.

ACTION & *THERAPEUTIC EFFECT*

Long-acting corticosteroid with minimal sodium-retaining potential. Decreases inflammation by suppression of migration of polymorphonuclear leukocytes and reversal of increased capillary permeability; suppresses the immune system by reducing activity and volume of the lymphatic system; suppresses adrenal function at high doses. Possesses minimal sodium and water retention properties in therapeutic doses. *Anti-inflammatory and immunosuppressant drug*

T

that is effective in the treatment of bronchial asthma.

USES An anti-inflammatory or immunosuppressant agent. Orally inhaled: Bronchial asthma in patient who has not responded to conventional inhalation treatment. Therapeutic doses do not appear to suppress HPA (hypothalamic-pituitary-adrenal) axis.

CONTRAINDICATIONS Hypersensitivity to corticosteroids or benzyl alcohol; kidney dysfunction; glaucoma; acute bronchospasm; fungal infection.

CAUTIOUS USE Coagulopathy, hemophilia, diabetes mellitus, GI disease; CHF; herpes infection; infection; IBD; myasthenia gravis; MI; ocular exposure, ocular infection; osteoporosis; peptic ulcer disease; PVD; skin abrasion; pregnancy (adverse effects have been observed with corticosteroids in animal reproduction studies); lactation. Safe use in children younger than 6 y not established.

ROUTE & DOSAGE

Note: Doses depend on condition and response of patient. Lowest possible dose should be used to control condition.

Inflammation, Immunosuppression

Adult: **IM/Subcutaneous** 4–48 mg/day in divided doses; **Inhaled** 2–4 inhalations qid. **Topical** See Appendix A
Child: **IM/Subcutaneous** 0.11–0.16 mg/kg/day in 3–4 divided doses; **Intra-articular/Intradermal** 0.5–1 mg/kg/dose

ADMINISTRATION

Inhalation

- Follow manufacturer's directions for specific oral or nasal inhaler and instruct patient on proper administration technique.

Subcutaneous/Intramuscular

- Do not give triamcinolone injection IV.
- Shake well before use to ensure suspension is uniform.
- IM injections should only be given into a large, well developed muscle such as the gluteal muscle.
- Store at 15°–30° C (59°–86° F). Protect from light.

ADVERSE EFFECTS **CV:** Bradycardia, cardiac arrhythmia, edema. **CNS:** Euphoria, headache, insomnia, confusion, psychosis. **HEENT:** Cataracts. **Endocrine:** Cushingoid features, growth suppression in children, carbohydrate intolerance, hyperglycemia, hypokalemia. **Skin:** Burning, itching, folliculitis, hypertrichosis, hypopigmentation. **GI:** Nausea, vomiting, peptic ulcer. **Musculoskeletal:** Muscle weakness, delayed wound healing, muscle wasting, osteoporosis, aseptic necrosis of bone, spontaneous fractures, joint swelling. **Hematologic:** Nonthrombocytopenic purpura, petechia, purpuric rash.

INTERACTIONS **Drug:** BARBITURATES, **phenytoin, rifampin** increase steroid metabolism—may need increased doses of triamcinolone; **amphotericin B**, DIURETICS add to potassium loss; **neostigmine, pyridostigmine** may cause severe muscle weakness in patients with myasthenia gravis; may inhibit antibody response to VACCINES, TOXOIDS.

T

PHARMACOKINETICS **Absorption:** Readily absorbed from all routes. **Onset:** 24–48 h PO, IM. **Peak:** 1–2 h PO; 8–10 h IM. **Duration:** 2.25 days PO; 1–6 wk IM. **Metabolism:** In liver. **Elimination:** In urine. **Half-Life:** 2–5 h; HPA suppression, 18–36 h.

NURSING IMPLICATIONS

Assessment & Drug Effects

- Notify prescriber if wheezing occurs immediately following a dose of inhaled triamcinolone.
- Do not use occlusive dressing over topical application unless specifically ordered to do so.
- Monitor growth in children receiving prolonged, systemic triamcinolone therapy.
- Monitor for signs of negative nitrogen balance (e.g., muscle atrophy), especially in older or debilitated patients receiving prolonged therapy.
- Report to prescriber immediately if a local infection develops at site of topical application.
- Report symptoms of hypercortisolism or Cushing's syndrome (see Appendix F), hyperglycemia (see Appendix F), and glucosuria (e.g., polyuria). These may arise from systemic absorption after topical application, especially in children and if used over extensive areas for prolonged periods or if occlusive dressings are used.
- Monitor Bp, weight, intraocular pressure.
- Monitor lab values: Blood glucose, electrolytes.

Patient & Family Education

- Report promptly any of the following: Sore throat, fever, swelling of feet or ankles, or muscle weakness.
- Adhere to drug regimen; do not increase or decrease established regimen and do not discontinue abruptly.
- Asthmatics should report promptly worsening of asthma symptoms following oral inhalation.

TRIAMTERENE

(trye-am′ter-een)

Dyrenium

Classification: POTASSIUM-SPARING DIURETIC

Therapeutic: POTASSIUM-SPARING DIURETIC

Prototype: Spironolactone

AVAILABILITY Capsule

ACTION & *THERAPEUTIC EFFECT* Blocks epithelial sodium channels in the late distal convoluted tubule and collecting duct which inhibits sodium reabsorption from the lumen effectively reducing intracellular sodium; leads to potassium retention and decreased calcium, magnesium, and hydrogen excretion. *Has a diuretic action and a potassium-sparing effect.*

USES Treatment of edema.

CONTRAINDICATIONS Hypersensitivity to triamterene; anuria, severe or progressive kidney disease or dysfunction with possible exception of nephrosis; severe liver disease; diabetic neuropathy; elevated serum potassium; severe electrolyte or acid–base imbalance; coadministration of other potassium-sparing agents.

CAUTIOUS USE Impaired kidney or liver function; gout; history of gouty arthritis; CHF; arrhythmias; DM; history of kidney stones; older adults; pregnancy (category C). Safety and efficacy in children not established.

ROUTE & DOSAGE

Edema

Adult: **PO** 100 mg bid (max: 300 mg/day)

Renal Impairment Dosage Adjustment

CrCl less than 10 mL/min: Avoid use

ADMINISTRATION

Oral

- Empty capsule and give with fluid or mix with food, if patient cannot swallow capsule.
- Give drug with or after meals to prevent or minimize nausea.
- Schedule doses to prevent interruption of sleep from diuresis (e.g., with or after breakfast if a single dose is taken, or no later than 6 p.m. if more than one dose is prescribed). Consult prescriber.
- Withdraw drug gradually in patients on prolonged or high-dose therapy in order to prevent rebound increased urinary excretion of potassium.
- Store in tight, light-resistant containers at 15°–30° C (59°–86° F) unless otherwise directed.

ADVERSE EFFECTS **CNS:** Dizziness, fatigue, headache. **Endocrine:** Hyperkalemia, increased uric acid, metabolic acidosis. **Skin:** Photosensitivity, rash. **Hepatic/GI:** Jaundice, diarrhea, nausea, vomiting, xerostomia. **GU:** Azotemia, increased BUN, increased serum creatinine, nephrolithiasis. **Musculoskeletal:** Weakness. **Hematologic:** Anemia, thrombocytopenia. **Other:** Anaphylaxis.

DIAGNOSTIC TEST INTERFERENCE Pale blue fluorescence in urine interferes with ***fluorometric assay*** of ***quinidine*** and ***lactic dehydrogenase activity***. May lead to false-negative aldosterone/renin ratio.

INTERACTIONS **Drug:** May increase **lithium** levels, thus increasing its toxicity; **indomethacin** may decrease renal elimination of triamterene; ANGIOTENSIN-CONVERTING ENZYME (ACE) INHIBITORS, other POTASSIUM-SPARING DIURETICS may cause hyperkalemia. Do not use with **cyclosporine. Food: High potassium foods** may increase risk of hyperkalemia.

PHARMACOKINETICS **Absorption:** Rapidly but variably from GI tract. **Onset:** 2–4 h. **Duration:** 7–9 h. **Metabolism:** In liver to active and inactive metabolites. **Elimination:** In urine. **Half-Life:** 100–150 min.

NURSING IMPLICATIONS

Black Box Warning

Triamterene has been associated with increased risk of hyperkalemia.

Assessment & Drug Effects

- Monitor BP during periods of dosage adjustment. Hypotensive reactions, although rare, have been reported. Take care with ambulation, particularly for older adults.
- Weigh patient under standard conditions, prior to drug initiation and daily during therapy.
- Diuretic response usually occurs on first day of therapy; maximum effect may not occur for several days.
- Monitor and report oliguria and unusual changes in I&O ratio. Consult prescriber regarding allowable fluid intake.
- Be alert for S&S of kidney stone formation; reported in patients

taking high doses or who have low urine volume and increased urine acidity.

- Observe for S&S of hyperkalemia (see Appendix F), particularly in patients with renal insufficiency, on high-dose or prolonged therapy, older adults, and those with diabetes.
- Monitor diabetics closely for loss of glycemic control.
- Monitor lab tests: Baseline and periodic serum potassium; periodic renal function tests with known or suspected renal insufficiency.

Patient & Family Education

- Do not use salt substitutes; unlike most diuretics, triamterene promotes potassium retention.
- Do not restrict salt; there is a possibility of low-salt syndrome (hyponatremia). Consult prescriber.
- Report significant fatigue or weakness, malaise, fever, sore throat or mouth, and unusual bleeding or bruising to prescriber.
- Be aware that drug may cause photosensitivity; avoid exposure to sun and sunlamps.
- Drug may impart a harmless pale blue fluorescence to urine.

TRIAZOLAM (Pr)

(trye-ay'zoe-lam)

Halcion

Classification: SEDATIVE-HYPNOTIC; BENZODIAZEPINE

Therapeutic: SEDATIVE

Controlled Substance: Schedule IV

AVAILABILITY Tablet

ACTION & THERAPEUTIC EFFECT Blockade of cortical and limbic arousal results in hypnotic activity. *Decreases sleep latency and number of nocturnal awakenings, decreases total nocturnal wake time, and increases duration of sleep.*

USES Short-term management of insomnia.

CONTRAINDICATIONS Hypersensitivity to triazolam and benzodiazepines; ethanol intoxication; suicidal ideations; pregnancy (teratogenic effects have been observed with some benzodiazepines); lactation.

CAUTIOUS USE Depression; bipolar disorder; dementia; psychosis; myasthenia gravis; Parkinson's disease; debilitated patients; patients with suicidal tendency; impaired kidney or liver function; chronic pulmonary insufficiency; sleep apnea; older adults.

ROUTE & DOSAGE

Insomnia

Adult: **PO** 0.125–0.25 mg at bedtime (max: 0.5 mg/day) intended for short term use
Geriatric: **PO** 0.125 mg at bedtime

ADMINISTRATION

Oral

- Administer dose in bed; onset of drug action is rapid.
- Do not take with a meal or immediately after a meal. Tablet may be crushed or swallowed whole.
- Store at 20°–25° C (68°–77° F).

ADVERSE EFFECTS CNS: *Drowsiness,* headache, dizziness, ataxia, visual disturbances, confusion, *memory impairment, rebound insomnia.* **GI:** Nausea, vomiting. **Other:** Physiological dependence, psychological dependence, tolerance, withdrawal.

INTERACTIONS Drug: Alcohol, CNS DEPRESSANTS, ANTICONVULSANTS,

nefazodone, BENZODIAZEPINES potentiate CNS depression; Do not use with CYP3A4 inhibitors (e.g., **itraconazole, clarithromycin**) due to increases triazolam plasma levels, thus increasing its toxicity; may decrease antiparkinsonism effects of **levodopa**. Contraindicated with **cobicistat, delavirdine**, systemic AZOLE ANTIFUNGALS, PROTEASE INHIBITORS. **Herbal: Kava, kratom, valerian** may potentiate sedation. **St. John's wort** may decrease efficacy. **Food: Grapefruit juice** (greater than 1 qt/day) may increase plasma concentrations and adverse effects.

PHARMACOKINETICS **Absorption:** Readily from GI tract. **Onset:** 15–30 min. **Peak:** 1–2 h. **Duration:** 6–8 h. **Distribution:** Crosses placenta; distributed into breast milk. **Metabolism:** In liver via CYP3A4. **Elimination:** In urine. **Half-Life:** 2–3 h.

NURSING IMPLICATIONS

Assessment & Drug Effects

- Be aware that signs of developing tolerance or adaptation (with long-term use) include increased day-time anxiety, increased wakefulness during last one third of the night.
- Evaluate smoking habit. As with other benzodiazepines, smoking may decrease hypnotic effects.
- Monitor for symptoms of overdosage: Slurred speech, somnolence, confusion, impaired coordination, and coma. Monitor respiratory rate.

Patient & Family Education

- Do not drive or engage in potentially hazardous activities until response to drug is known.
- Avoid use of alcohol or other CNS depressants while on this drug; they may increase sedative effects.
- Do not stop taking drug suddenly, especially if you are subject to seizures. Withdrawal symptoms may occur and range from mild dysphoria to more serious symptoms (e.g., tremors, abdominal and muscle cramps, convulsions). Consult prescriber for schedule to discontinue therapy.
- Do not increase dose without prescriber's advice because of toxic potential of drug.

TRIFLUOPERAZINE HYDROCHLORIDE

(trye-floo-oh-per′a-zeen)

Classification: ANTIPSYCHOTIC; PHENOTHIAZIDE

Therapeutic: ANTIPSYCHOTIC

Prototype: Chlorpromazine

AVAILABILITY Tablet

ACTION & *THERAPEUTIC EFFECT* Phenothiazine with antipsychotic effects thought to be related to blockade of postsynaptic dopamine receptors in the brain. *Effectiveness indicated by increase in mental and physical activity.*

USES Management of schizophrenia.

CONTRAINDICATIONS Hypersensitivity to trifluoperazine, phenothiazines or any component of the formulation; comatose states; CNS depression; ethanol intoxication; blood dyscrasias; hematologic disease, bone marrow suppression; dementia related psychosis in older adults; hepatic disease; lactation.

CAUTIOUS USE Previously detected breast cancer; history of QT prolongation; significant cardiac disease or pulmonary disease; compromised respiratory function; seizure disorders; impaired liver function;

pregnancy (nonpharmacologic interventions should be considered first due to unknown maternal and fetal risk); children younger than 6 y.

ROUTE & DOSAGE

Schizophrenia

Adult: **PO** 2–5 mg once daily or bid, may increase up to 15–20 mg/day
Child (6–12 y): **PO** 1 mg 1–2 × day, may increase up to 15 mg/day

ADMINISTRATION

Oral

- May be taken with food to decrease GI upset; do not take within 2 hours of any antacids.
- Store in light-resistant container at 20°–25° C (68°–77° F) unless otherwise directed.

ADVERSE EFFECTS

CV: Orthostatic hypotension, *hypotension*. **Respiratory:** Nasal congestion. **CNS:** Dizziness, *extrapyramidal effects*, neuroleptic malignant syndrome, decreased seizure threshold, disruption of body temperature regulation, headache, tremor. **HEENT:** Corneal changes, lens disease, retinitis pigmentosa. **Endocrine:** Gynecomastia, galactorrhea, change in libido, change in menstrual flow, hyperglycemia, hypoglycemia, weight gain. **Skin:** Photosensitivity, skin rash, skin discoloration (blue-gray). **Hepatic/GI:** Constipation, nausea, stomach pain, vomiting, xerostomia, jaundice, hepatotoxicity. **GU:** Difficulty in micturition, ejaculatory disorder, lactation, mastalgia, priapism, urinary retention. **Hematologic:** Agranulocytosis, aplastic anemia, eosinophilia, haemolytic anemia, immune thrombocytopenia, leukopenia, pancytopenia.

DIAGNOSTIC TEST INTERFERENCE

May produce a false positive for phenylketonuria.

INTERACTIONS

Drug: Alcohol and other CNS DEPRESSANTS add to CNS depression. Do not use with agents that prolong QT interval (e.g., **bepridil, dofetilide, dronedarone, procaine, ziprasidone metoclopramide**, or **piribedil**). ANTICHOLINERGIC AGENTS and ANTIPARKINSON AGENTS may decrease effect. **Herbal: Kava** may increase risk and severity of dystonic reactions.

PHARMACOKINETICS

Absorption: Well absorbed from GI tract. **Onset:** Rapid onset. **Peak:** 2–3 h. **Duration:** Up to 12 h. **Metabolism:** In liver. **Elimination:** In bile and feces.

NURSING IMPLICATIONS

Black Box Warning

Trifluoperazine has been associated with increased risk of mortality in older adults with dementia-related psychosis.

Assessment & Drug Effects

- Monitor HR and BP. Hypotension is a common adverse effect.
- Hypotension and extrapyramidal effects (especially akathisia and dystonia) are most likely to occur in patients receiving high doses or in older adults. Withhold drug and notify prescriber if patient has dysphagia, neck muscle spasm, or if tongue protrusion occurs.
- Monitor I&O ratio and bowel elimination pattern. Check for abdominal distention and pain. Encourage adequate fluid intake

T

as prophylaxis for constipation and xerostomia.
- Expect maximum therapeutic response within 2–3 wk after initiation of therapy.
- Annual ocular examination.
- Monitor lab tests: Periodic CBC, serum electrolytes, LFTs, lipid profile, plasma glucose, and HbA1C.

Patient & Family Education
- Take drug as prescribed; do not alter dosing regimen or stop medication without consulting prescriber.
- Consult prescriber about use of any OTC drugs during therapy.
- Do not take alcohol and other depressants during therapy.
- Avoid potentially hazardous activities such as driving or operating machinery, until response to drug is known.
- Cover as much skin surface as possible with clothing when you **must be** in direct sunlight. Use an SPF higher than 12 sunscreen on exposed skin.

TRIFLURIDINE
(trye-flure′i-deen)
Classification: ANTIVIRAL
Therapeutic: ANTIVIRAL

AVAILABILITY Ophthalmic solution

ACTION & THERAPEUTIC EFFECT Interferes with viral replication. *Active against herpes simplex virus (HSV) types 1 and 2, vaccinia virus, and certain strains of adenovirus.*

USES Topically to eyes for treatment of primary keratoconjunctivitis and recurring epithelial keratitis caused by herpes simplex virus types 1 and 2.

CONTRAINDICATIONS Known sensitivity to trifluridine or any component of the formulation; lactation.

CAUTIOUS USE Dry eye syndrome; pregnancy (adverse effects have not been observed in animal reproduction studies); children younger than 6 y.

ROUTE & DOSAGE

Viral Infections of Eye

Adult: **Ophthalmic** 1 drop 1% ophthalmic solution into affected eye q2h during waking hours (max: 9 drops/day); when healing appears to be complete, dosage reduced to 1 drop q4h during waking hours for an additional 7 days (max: 5 drops/day); continuous administration beyond 21 days not recommended

ADMINISTRATION

Instillation
- Wash hands before and after instillation.
- Wait several minutes between applications when used concurrently with other eye drops. Remove contact lenses prior to use.
- Store refrigerated at 2°–8° C (36°–46° F) unless otherwise directed.

ADVERSE EFFECTS HEENT: Burning or stinging sensation in the eyes, epithelial keratopathy, eye irritation, hyperemia, increased ocular pressure, stromal edema, keratitis sicca, hyperemia, increased intraocular pressure.

PHARMACOKINETICS Absorption: penetrates cornea and aqueous humor (inflammation enhances penetration). Systemic absorption does not appear to be significant.

NURSING IMPLICATIONS

Assessment & Drug Effects

- Expect epithelial eye infections to respond to therapy within 2–7 days, with complete healing occurring in 1–2 wk; not for long-term use.

Patient & Family Education

- Inform prescriber of progress and keep follow-up appointments. Herpetic eye infections have a tendency to recur and can lead to corneal damage if not adequately treated.

TRIHEXYPHENIDYL HYDROCHLORIDE

(trye-hex-ee-fen′i-dill)

Classification: CENTRALLY ACTING CHOLINERGIC RECEPTOR ANTAGONIST; ANTIPARKINSON; ANTISPASMODIC
Therapeutic: ANTIPARKINSON; ANTISPASMODIC
Prototype: Benztropine

AVAILABILITY Tablet; oral solution

ACTION & THERAPEUTIC EFFECT Thought to act by blocking excess of acetylcholine at certain cerebral synaptic sites. Relaxes smooth muscle directly and has an indirect inhibitory effect on the parasympathetic nervous system. *Diminishes the characteristic tremor of Parkinson disease.*

USES Symptomatic treatment of all forms of parkinsonism (arteriosclerotic, idiopathic, postencephalitic). Also to treat drug-induced extrapyramidal disorders.

UNLABELED USES Huntington's chorea, spasmodic torticollis.

CONTRAINDICATIONS Hypersensitivity to trihexyphenidyl; narrow angle glaucoma.

CAUTIOUS USE Tardive dyskinesia; history of drug hypersensitivities; glaucoma; arteriosclerosis; hypertension; cardiac disease, kidney or liver disorders; MG; alcoholism; CNS diseases; obstructive diseases of GI or genitourinary tracts; BPH; older adults; pregnancy (animal reproduction studies have not been conducted); lactation. Safe use in children not established.

ROUTE & DOSAGE

Parkinsonism

Adult: **PO** 1 mg/day, increase by 2 mg increments at intervals of 3–5 days, up to 6–10 mg/day in divided doses.

Extrapyramidal Effects

Adult: **PO** 1 mg/day then increase as needed; usual dose 5–15 mg/day in 3–4 divided doses

ADMINISTRATION

Oral

- May be given before or after meals, depending on how patient reacts. Older adults and patients prone to excessive salivation (e.g., postencephalitic parkinsonism) may prefer to take drug after meals. If drug causes excessive mouth dryness, it may be better given before meals, unless it causes nausea.
- Store at 20°–25° C (68°–77°F) in tight container unless otherwise directed.

ADVERSE EFFECTS **CV:** Tachycardia. **CNS:** *Dizziness, nervousness,* insomnia, drowsiness, confusion,

T

agitation, delirium, delusions, hallucinations, headache, paranoia, psychotic manifestations, euphoria. **HEENT:** *Blurred vision*, mydriasis, increased ocular pressure, glaucoma. **Skin:** Skin rash. **GI:** *Dry mouth, nausea*, constipation, intestinal obstruction, parotitis, toxic megacolon. **GU:** Urinary retention. **Other:** Weakness.

INTERACTIONS **Drug:** Reduces therapeutic effects of **chlorpromazine, haloperidol**, PHENOTHIAZINES; increases bioavailability of **digoxin**; MAO INHIBITORS potentiate actions of trihexyphenidyl. ANTICHOLINERGIC AGENTS and ANTIPARKINSON AGENTS, PROKINETIC AGENTS may decrease effect. **Herbal: Betel nut** may increase risk of extrapyramidal symptoms.

PHARMACOKINETICS **Absorption:** Readily from GI tract. **Onset:** Within 1 h. **Peak:** 2–3 h. **Duration:** 6–12 h. **Elimination:** In urine and bile.

NURSING IMPLICATIONS

Assessment & Drug Effects

- Be aware that incidence and severity of adverse effects are usually dose related and may be minimized by dosage reduction. Older adults appear more sensitive to usual adult doses.
- Monitor vital signs. Pulse is a particularly sensitive indicator of response to drug. Report tachycardia, palpitations, paradoxical bradycardia, or fall in BP.
- Assess for and report severe CNS stimulation (see ADVERSE EFFECTS) that occurs with high doses, and in patients with arteriosclerosis, or those with history of hypersensitivity to other drugs.
- In patients with severe rigidity, tremors may appear to be accentuated during therapy as rigidity diminishes.
- Monitor daily I&O if patient develops urinary hesitancy or retention. Voiding before taking drug may relieve problem.
- Check for abdominal distention and bowel sounds if constipation is a problem.
- Baseline and periodic gonioscopic and intraocular pressure exams.

Patient & Family Education

- Learn measures to relieve drug-induced dry mouth; rinse mouth frequently with water and suck ice chips, sugarless gum, or hard candy. Maintain adequate total daily fluid intake.
- Do not to engage in potentially hazardous activities requiring alertness and skill. Drug causes dizziness, drowsiness, and blurred vision. Help walking may be indicated.

TRIMETHOBENZAMIDE HYDROCHLORIDE

(trye-meth-oh-ben′za-mide)

Tigan

Classification: ANTIEMETIC
Therapeutic: ANTIEMETIC
Prototype: Prochlorperazine

AVAILABILITY Solution for injection

ACTION & *THERAPEUTIC EFFECT* Acts centrally to inhibit the medullary chemoreceptor trigger zone by blocking emetic impulses to the vomiting center. *Less effective than phenothiazine antiemetics but produces fewer adverse effects.*

USES Control of nausea and vomiting.

CONTRAINDICATIONS Parenteral use in children or infants; rectal administration in prematures and newborns; hypersensitivity to trimethobenzamide or any component of the formulation.

CAUTIOUS USE Presence of high fever, dehydration, electrolyte imbalance; pregnancy (use of other agents during pregnancy is preferred); lactation; children.

ROUTE & DOSAGE

Nausea and Vomiting

Adult: **IM** 200 mg tid or qid prn

ADMINISTRATION

Intramuscular

- Give IM deep into upper outer quadrant of gluteal muscle.
- Minimize possibility of irritation and pain by avoiding escape of solution along needle track. Use Z-track technique. Rotate injection sites.
- Injection not for use in children or infants.

ADVERSE EFFECTS **CV:** Hypotension. **CNS:** Pseudoparkinsonism, coma, depression, disorientation, dizziness, drowsiness, extrapyramidal reaction, headache, opisthotonos, seizure. **HEENT:** Blurred vision. **Hepatic/GI:** Diarrhea, jaundice. **Musculoskeletal:** Muscle cramps. **Other:** Hypersensitivity reactions (including allergic skin reaction); pain, stinging, burning, redness, irritation at IM site.

INTERACTIONS **Drug:** Alcohol and other CNS DEPRESSANTS add to depressant activity; PHENOTHIAZINES, ANTICHOLINERGIC AGENTS may precipitate extrapyramidal syndrome. Do not use with **sodium oxybate.**

PHARMACOKINETICS **Onset:** 10–40 min PO; 15-35 min IM. **Duration:** 3–4 h PO; 2–3 h IM. **Elimination:** 30–50% of dose excreted unchanged in urine within 48–72 h.

NURSING IMPLICATIONS

Assessment & Drug Effects

- Monitor BP. Hypotension may occur particularly in surgical patients receiving drug parenterally.
- Report promptly and stop drug therapy if an acute febrile illness accompanies or begins during therapy.
- Antiemetic effect of drug may obscure diagnoses of GI or other pathologic conditions or signs of toxicity from other drugs. Avoid use in older adults.
- Monitor lab results: Renal function tests (in the elderly and patients with reduced renal function).

Patient & Family Education

- Report promptly to prescriber onset of rash or other signs of hypersensitivity (see Appendix F). Discontinue drug immediately.
- Do not drive or engage in potentially hazardous activities until response to drug is known.
- Do not drink alcohol or alcoholic beverages during therapy with this drug.

TRIMETHOPRIM (Pr)

(trye-meth'oh-prim)

Primsol

Classification: URINARY TRACT ANTI-INFECTIVE

Therapeutic: URINARY TRACT ANTI-INFECTIVE

AVAILABILITY Tablet; oral solution

ACTION & *THERAPEUTIC EFFECT*

Anti-infective and folic acid antagonist with slow bactericidal action.

Binds and interferes with bacterial cell growth. *Effective against most common UTI pathogens. Most pathogens causing UTI are in normal vaginal and fecal flora. Effective in treatment of acute otitis media.*

USES Initial episodes of acute uncomplicated UTIs, acute otitis media in children.

UNLABELED USES Treatment and prophylaxis of chronic and recurrent UTI in both men and women; treatment in conjunction with dapsone of initial episodes of *Pneumocystis carinii* pneumonia; treatment of travelers' diarrhea; acne; otitis media.

CONTRAINDICATIONS Hypersensitivity to trimethoprim; megaloblastic anemia secondary to folate deficiency; creatinine clearance less than 15 mL/min, impaired kidney or liver function; possible folate deficiency; children with fragile X chromosome associated with mental retardation.

CAUTIOUS USE Possible folate deficiency; risk factors for hyperkalemia; renal disease; mild or moderate renal impairment; hepatic impairment; older adults; pregnancy (category C); lactation; children younger than 12 y.

T

ROUTE & DOSAGE

Urinary Tract Infection

Adult/Adolescent: **PO** 100 mg bid or 200 mg once/day

ADMINISTRATION

Oral

- Give with 240 mL (8 oz) of fluid if not contraindicated.
- Store at 15°–30° C (59°–86° F) in dry, light-protected place.

ADVERSE EFFECTS **Endocrine:** Increased serum transaminases (ALT, AST), bilirubin, creatinine, BUN. **Skin:** *Rash, pruritus,* exfoliative dermatitis, photosensitivity. **GI:** Epigastric discomfort, nausea, vomiting, glossitis, abnormal taste sensation. **Hematologic:** Neutropenia, *megaloblastic anemia,* methemoglobinemia, leukopenia, thrombocytopenia (rare). **Other:** Fever.

DIAGNOSTIC TEST INTERFERENCE Interferes with serum ***methotrexate assays*** that use a competitive binding protein technique with a bacterial dihydrofolate reductase as the binding protein. May cause falsely elevated ***creatinine*** values when ***Jaffe reaction*** is used.

INTERACTIONS **Drug:** May inhibit **phenytoin** metabolism causing increased levels. Do not use with **dofetilide.**

PHARMACOKINETICS **Absorption:** Almost completely from GI tract. **Peak:** 1–4 h. **Distribution:** Widely distributed, including lung, saliva, middle ear fluid, bile, bone, CSF; crosses placenta; appears in breast milk. **Metabolism:** In liver. **Elimination:** 80% in urine unchanged. **Half-Life:** 8–11 h.

NURSING IMPLICATIONS

Assessment & Drug Effects

- Reinforce necessity to adhere to established drug regimen. Recurrent infection after terminating prophylactic treatment of UTI may occur even after 6 mo of therapy.

- Assess urinary pattern during treatment. Altered pattern (frequency, urgency, nocturia, retention, polyuria) may reflect emerging drug resistance, necessitating change of drug regimen. Periodically check for bladder distention.
- Be alert for toxic effects on bone marrow, particularly in older adults, malnourished, alcoholic, pregnant, or debilitated patients. Recognize and report signs of infection or anemia.
- Drug-induced rash, a common adverse effect, is usually maculopapular, pruritic, or morbilliform and appears 7–14 days after start of therapy with daily doses of 200 mg or less.
- Monitor lab tests: Baseline C&S.

Patient & Family Education

- Drink fluids liberally (2000–3000 mL/day, if not contraindicated) to help flush out urinary bacteria.
- Report pain and hematuria to prescriber immediately.
- Do not postpone voiding even though increases in fluid intake may cause more frequent urination.
- Do not use douches or sprays during treatment periods; practice careful perineal hygiene to prevent reinfection.
- Report to prescriber promptly any symptoms of a blood disorder (fever, sore throat, pallor, purpura, ecchymosis).
- Consult prescriber if severe traveler's diarrhea does not respond to 3–5 days therapy (i.e., persistence of symptoms of severe nausea, abdominal pain, diarrhea with mucus or blood, and dehydration).
- Drug-induced rash, a common adverse effect, may appear 7–14 days after start of therapy. Report rash to prescriber for evaluation.

TRIMIPRAMINE MALEATE

(tri-mip′ra-meen)

Classification: TRICYCLIC ANTIDEPRESSANT

Therapeutic: TRICYCLIC ANTIDEPRESSANT (TCA)

Prototype: Imipramine

AVAILABILITY Capsule

ACTION & *THERAPEUTIC EFFECT* Antidepressant effects are thought to result from postsynaptic sensitization to serotonin. *More effective in alleviation of endogenous depression than other depressive states.*

USES Treatment of depression.

CONTRAINDICATIONS Hypersensitivity to tricyclic antidepressants; prostatic hypertrophy; during recovery period after MI; AV block; QT prolongation; bundle-branch block; ileus; MAOI therapy; suicide ideation; concurrent use with linezolid or IV methylene blue.

CAUTIOUS USE Schizophrenia, electroshock therapy, psychosis, bipolar disease; Parkinson's disease; seizure disorders; increased intraocular pressure; history of urinary retention; history of narrow-angle glaucoma; hyperthyroidism, suicidal tendency; cardiovascular, liver, thyroid, kidney disease; pregnancy (tricyclic antidepressants may be associated with irritability, jitteriness, and convulsions in the neonate; pregnant women exposed to antidepressants during pregnancy are encouraged to enroll in the National Pregnancy Registry for Antidepressants); lactation. Safe use in children younger than 12 y not established.

T

ROUTE & DOSAGE

Depression

Adult: **PO** 25–50 mg daily in divided doses, may increase gradually up to 150 mg/day if needed (max dose: 300 mg/day)
Geriatric/Adolescent: **PO** 50 mg/day with gradual increases up to 100 mg/day

Pharmacogenetic Dosage Adjustment

Poor CYP2C19 metabolizer: Start with 50% of dose

ADMINISTRATION

Oral

- Give with food to decrease gastric distress. Administer maintenance doses as a single dose at bedtime.
- Store in tightly closed container at 20°–25° C (68°–77° F) unless otherwise specified.

ADVERSE EFFECTS **CV:** Tachycardia, *orthostatic hypotension*, hypertension, cardiac arrhythmia. **CNS:** Seizures, tremor, confusion, *agitation*, *anxiety*, suicidality, dizziness, drowsiness, headache. **HEENT:** Blurred vision. **Endocrine:** Change in libido, galactorrhea, gynecomastia. **Skin:** Photosensitivity, sweating, alopecia. **GI/Hepatic:** *Xerostomia, constipation*, paralytic ileus, dyspepsia, jaundice, increased liver enzymes. **GU:** *Urinary retention*, difficulty in micturition, impotence.

INTERACTIONS **Drug:** CNS DEPRESSANTS, **alcohol**, HYPNOTICS, BARBITURATES, SEDATIVES potentiate CNS depression; may increase hypoprothrombinemic effect of ORAL ANTICOAGULANTS; **levodopa**, SYMPATHOMIMETICS (e.g., **epinephrine, norepinephrine**) increase possibility of sympathetic hyperactivity with hypertension and hyperpyrexia; do not use with MAO INHIBITORS; **methylphenidate** increases plasma TCA levels; **cimetidine** may increase plasma TCA levels; potassium salts may increase risk of ulcer formation. **Herbal: Ginkgo** may decrease seizure threshold; **St. John's wort** may cause **serotonin** syndrome.

PHARMACOKINETICS **Absorption:** Rapidly absorbed from GI tract. **Peak:** 2 h. **Metabolism:** In liver (CYP2D6). **Elimination:** In urine and feces. **Half-Life:** 9.1 h.

NURSING IMPLICATIONS

Black Box Warning

Trimipramine maleate has been associated with increased risk of suicidal thinking and behavior in children, adolescents, and young adults.

Assessment & Drug Effects

- Monitor for changes in behavior that may indicate increased incidence of suicidality.
- Assess vital signs (BP and pulse rate) during adjustment period of tricyclic antidepressant (TCA) therapy. If BP falls more than 20 mm Hg or if there is a sudden increase in pulse rate, withhold medication and notify prescriber. Monitor for ECG changes.
- Orthostatic hypotension may be sufficiently severe to require protective assistance when patient is ambulating. Instruct patient to change position from recumbency to standing slowly and in stages.
- Report fine tremors, a distressing extrapyramidal adverse effect, to prescriber.
- Monitor bowel elimination pattern and I&O ratio. Severe

T

constipation and urinary retention are potential problems, especially in older adults. Advise increased fluid intake to at least 1500 mL/day (if allowed).

- Inspect oral membranes daily with high-dose therapy. Urge outpatient to report symptoms of stomatitis or xerostomia.
- Monitor lab values: Electrolytes, LFTs, blood glucose.

Patient & Family Education

- Report immediately to prescriber signs of worsening mental status such as suicidal ideation, aggressiveness, agitation, anxiety, hostility, impulsivity, insomnia, irritability, panic attacks, and worsening of depression.
- Be aware that your ability to perform tasks requiring alertness and skill may be impaired.
- Do not use OTC drugs unless approved by prescriber.
- Understand that the actions of both alcohol and trimipramine are increased when used together during therapy and for up to 2 wk after the TCA is discontinued. Consult prescriber about safe amounts of alcohol, if any, that can be taken.
- Be aware that the effects of barbiturates and other CNS depressants may also be enhanced by trimipramine.

TRIPTORELIN PAMOATE

(trip-tor′e-lyn)

Trelstar Depot, Trelstar LA, Triptodur

Classification: GONADOTROPIN RELEASING HORMONE (GNRH) AGONIST ANALOG

Therapeutic: GNRH AGONIST ANALOG

Prototype: Leuprolide acetate

AVAILABILITY Solution for injection

ACTION & *THERAPEUTIC EFFECT* An agonist analog of GnRH that causes suppression of ovarian and testicular hormone production due to decreased levels of LH and FSH with subsequent decrease in testosterone and estrogen levels. *In men, the level of serum testosterone is equivalent to a surgically castrated man.*

USES Palliative treatment of advanced prostate cancer; central percocious puberty.

UNLABELED USES Breast cancer hypersexuality, endometriosis, infertility, hirsutism.

CONTRAINDICATIONS Hypersensitivity to triptorelin, other LHRH agonists, or LHRH; dysfunctional uterine bleeding; pregnancy; lactation.

CAUTIOUS USE Prostatic carcinoma; hepatic or renal dysfunction; patients with impending spinal cord compression or severe urogenital disorder; premenstrual syndrome; renal insufficiency. Safety and efficacy in children not established.

ROUTE & DOSAGE

Prostate Cancer

Adult: IM 3.75 mg q4w OR 11.25 mg q12w or 22.5 mg q24w

Central Percocious Puberty (Triptodur)

Adolescent/Child (older than 2 y): IM 22.5 mg q24wk

ADMINISTRATION

Intramuscular

- Give deep into a large muscle.
- Alternate injection sites. Administer immediately after reconstitution.

ADVERSE EFFECTS **CV:** Hypertension, lower extremity edema. **CNS:** Headache, dizziness, insomnia, impotence, emotional lability. **Skin:** Pruritus, skin rash. **GI:** Diarrhea, vomiting, nausea, anorexia. **GU:** Urinary retention, UTI. **Musculoskeletal:** Musculoskeletal pain. **Hematologic:** Anemia. **Other:** *Hot flushes*, pain, leg pain, fatigue. Pain at injection site, hyperglycemia, increased serum testosterone, increased ALT/AST, increased BUN, decreased libido, gynecomastia.

DIAGNOSTIC TEST INTERFERENCE May interfere with tests for ***pituitary-gonadal function***.

INTERACTIONS **Drug:** Do not use with **corifollitropin alfa.** Use with QT prolonging agents (e.g., **amiodarone, citalopram, dofetilide**) should be avoided.

PHARMACOKINETICS **Peak:** 1–3 h. **Duration:** 1 mo. **Metabolism:** Unknown. **Elimination:** Eliminated by liver and kidneys. **Half-Life:** 3 h.

NURSING IMPLICATIONS

Assessment & Drug Effects

- Monitor for S&S of disease flare, especially during the first 1–2 wk of therapy: Increased bone pain, blood in urine, urinary obstruction, or symptoms of spinal compression.
- Monitor for S&S of emerging CV disease.
- Monitor lab tests: Periodic serum testosterone and HbA1C.

Patient & Family Education

- Disease flare (see ASSESSMENT & DRUG EFFECTS) is a common, temporary adverse effect of therapy; however, symptoms may become serious enough to report to the prescriber.
- Notify prescriber promptly of the following: S&S of an allergic reaction (itching, hives, swelling of face, arms, or legs; tingling in mouth or throat, tightness in chest or trouble breathing); weakness or loss of muscle control; rapid weight gain.

TROPICAMIDE

(troe-pik′a-mide)

See Appendix A-1.

TROSPIUM CHLORIDE

(tro-spi′um)

Classification: ANTICHOLINERGIC; ANTIMUSCARINIC; ANTISPASMODIC

Therapeutic: URINARY SMOOTH MUSCLE RELAXANT

Prototype: Oxybutynin

AVAILABILITY Tablet; extended release capsule

ACTION & *THERAPEUTIC EFFECT* Antagonizes the effect of acetylcholine on muscarinic receptors in smooth muscle. Its parasympatholytic action reduces smooth muscle tone of the bladder. *Decreases urinary frequency, urgency, and urge incontinence in patients with overactive bladders.*

USES Treatment of overactive (neurogenic) bladder, urinary incontinence.

CONTRAINDICATIONS Hypersensitivity to trospium; patients with or at risk for urinary retention; uncontrolled narrow-angle glaucoma; gastroparesis; GI obstruction, ileus, pyloric stenosis, toxic megacolon, severe ulcerative colitis.

CAUTIOUS USE Significant bladder obstruction, closed-angle glaucoma; BPH; ulcerative colitis, GERD, intestinal atony; myasthenia gravis, autonomic neuropathy; moderate or severe hepatic dysfunction; severe renal insufficiency, renal failure; older adults; pregnancy (category C); lactation. Safety in children not established.

ROUTE & DOSAGE

Overactive Bladder

Adult: **PO** 20 mg twice daily OR **Extended release** 60 mg daily
Geriatric (75 y or older): **PO Immediate release** 20 mg once daily

Renal Impairment Dosage Adjustment

CrCl less than 30 mL/min: **Immediate release** 20 mg once daily at bedtime

ADMINISTRATION

Oral

- Give at least 1 h before meals or on an empty stomach.
- Store at 20°–25° C (66°–77° F).

ADVERSE EFFECTS **CV:** Tachycardia. **Respiratory:** Nasopharyngitis, dry nose. **CNS:** Headache. **HEENT:** Dry eyes, blurred vision, skin rash. **GI:** *Dry mouth, constipation*, abdominal pain, dyspepsia, flatulence, vomiting. **GU:** Urinary retention, urinary tract infection. **Other:** Fatigue, dry skin.

INTERACTIONS **Drug:** Increased anticholinergic adverse effects with ANTICHOLINERGIC AGENTS. Do not use with **potassium citrate** due to increased ulerogenic effect.

PHARMACOKINETICS **Absorption:** Less than 10% absorbed orally. **Peak:** 5–6 h. **Metabolism:** In liver via CYP2D6. **Elimination:** Primarily in feces. **Half-Life:** 20 h.

NURSING IMPLICATIONS

Assessment & Drug Effects

- Monitor bowel and bladder function. Report urinary hesitancy or significant constipation.
- Withhold drug and notify prescriber if urinary retention develops.
- Monitor for and report worsening of GI symptoms in those with GERD.

Patient & Family Education

- Report promptly any of the following: Signs of an allergic reaction (e.g., itching or hives), blurred vision or difficulty focusing, confusion, dizziness, difficulty passing urine.
- Moderate intake of tea, coffee, caffeinated sodas, and alcohol to minimize side effects of this drug.
- Avoid situations in which overheating is likely, as drug may impair sweating, which is a normal cooling mechanism.
- Do not engage in hazardous activities until response to the drug is known.

ULIPRISTAL

(u-li-pris'tal)

Ella

Classification: PROGESTERONE AGONIST/ANTAGONIST; POSTCOITAL CONTRACEPTIVE
Therapeutic: POSTCOITAL CONTRACEPTIVE

AVAILABILITY Tablet

ACTION & *THERAPEUTIC EFFECT*

A selective progesterone receptor modulator with antagonistic and

U

partial agonistic effects. It binds to the progesterone receptor preventing the binding of progesterone. *If taken immediately before ovulation, it delays follicular rupture and inhibits ovulation. It may also alter the endometrium and interfere with implantation of a fertilized ovum.*

USES Postcoital contraception after unprotected intercourse or a known or suspected contraceptive failure.

CONTRAINDICATIONS Known or suspected pregnancy (use is contraindicated during a known or suspected pregnancy); lactation.

ROUTE & DOSAGE

Emergency Contraception

Adult: **PO** 30 mg as soon as possible but within 120 h of unprotected intercourse or known or suspected contraceptive failure; may repeat within 3 h if patient vomits initial dose

ADMINISTRATION

Oral

- Give within 120 h of unprotected intercourse.
- Administer with or without food at any time during menstrual cycle. If vomiting occurs within 3 hours of administration, consider repeating dose.
- Store at controlled room temperature 20°–25° C (68°–77° F).

U

ADVERSE EFFECTS **CNS:** *Headache.* **Endocrine:** Suppressed menstruation. **GI:** *Nausea,* abdominal pain. **GU:** Dysmenorrhea.

INTERACTIONS **Drug:** Coadministration of CYP3A4 inducers (e.g., **carbamazepine, phenobarbital, phenytoin, rifampin, topiramate**) can decrease the levels of ulipristal. Coadministration of strong CYP3A4 INHIBITORS (e.g., **itraconazole, ketoconazole**) can increase the levels of ulipristal. Will decrease effect of PROGESTINS. Do not use **topiramate** concurrently. **Food: Grapefruit juice** can increase the levels of ulipristal. **Herbal: St. John's wort** can decrease the levels of ulipristal.

PHARMACOKINETICS **Peak:** 1 h. **Distribution:** 94% plasma protein bound. **Metabolism:** Hepatic oxidation by CYP3A4 to active metabolite. **Half-Life:** 32.4 h.

NURSING IMPLICATIONS

Assessment & Drug Effects

- Monitor for vomiting. Drug may be re-administered if patient vomits within 3 h of initial dose.
- Evaluate for pregnancy or ectopic pregnancy if expected menses delayed for > or = 1 week following emergency contraception or if lower abdominal pain (3–5 weeks after administration) or persistent irregular bleeding develops.

Patient & Family Education

- Ulipristal is not intended for repeated use. It should not replace conventional means of contraception.
- Certain concurrently taken drugs may interfere with the contraceptive effects of ulipristal. Consult prescriber.
- Ulipristal may interfere with the length of the next menstrual cycle (i.e., cycle may occur sooner or later than expected).
- Ulipristal does not protect against sexually transmitted diseases.

UPADACITINIB

(ue-pad-a-sye-ti-nib)

Rinvoq

Classification: BIOLOGICAL RESPONSE MODIFIER; JANUS KINASE (JAK) INHIBITOR; DISEASE-MODIFYING ANTIRHEUMATIC DRUG (DMARD)

Therapeutic: DISEASE-MODIFYING ANTIRHEUMATIC DRUG (DMARD)

Prototype: Tofacitinib

AVAILABILITY Oral tablet

ACTION & *THERAPEUTIC EFFECT* Inhibits Janus kinase (JAK) enzymes which stimulate hematopoiesis and immune cell function through a signaling pathway. JAK enzymes activate signal transducers and activators of transcription (STATs) which regulate gene expression and intracellular activity. *Treats moderate to severe rheumatoid arthritis by inhibiting JAKs thereby preventing activation of STATs.*

USES Treatment of moderately to severely active rheumatoid arthritis in patients who have had an inadequate response or intolerance to methotrexate. It may be used as monotherapy or in combination with methotrexate or other nonbiologic disease-modifying antirheumatic drugs (DMARDs).

CAUTIOUS USE GI perforation; hematologic toxicity; impaired liver function; infection; malignancy; thrombosis; tuberculosis; pregnancy; lactation.

ROUTE & DOSAGE

Rheumatoid Arthritis

Adult: PO 15 mg once a day

Hepatic Impairment Dosage Adjustment

Severe impairment (Child-Pugh class C): Use not recommended

ADMINISTRATION

Oral

- Administer with or without food. Swallow tablet whole; do not crush, split, or chew.
- Store at 2° to 25° C (36° to 77° F). Store in the original bottle to protect from moisture.

ADVERSE EFFECTS **Respiratory:** Upper respiratory tract infection. **GI:** Nausea.

INTERACTIONS **Drug:** Coadministration with potent inhibitors of CYP3A4 (e.g., **ketoconazole**) may increase the levels of upadacitinib. Coadministration with potent CYP3A4 inducers (e.g., **phenobarbital, phenytoin, rifampin**) may decrease the levels of tofacitinib. Coadministration with other potent immunosuppressive drugs (e.g., azathioprine, tacrolimus, cyclosporine) increases the risk of added immunosuppression. **Food:** Grapefruit juice may increase the levels of upadacitinib. **Herbal:** St. John's wort may decrease the levels of upadacitinib.

PHARMACOKINETICS **Peak:** 2–4 h. **Distribution:** 52% protein bound. **Metabolism:** In the liver, through CYP3A4 (major) and CYP2D6 (minor). **Elimination:** 24% in urine, 38% in feces. **Half-Life:** 8–14 h.

NURSING IMPLICATIONS

Assessment & Drug Effects

- Monitor for signs and symptoms of infection, skin cancer, and thrombosis.

- Monitor lab tests: Baseline and periodic lymphocyte count, neutrophil count, hemoglobin, and LFTs; lipid levels 12 weeks after initiating therapy and periodically thereafter; baseline tuberculosis (TB) screen; baseline and periodic viral hepatitis screen.

Patient & Family Education

- Notify your healthcare provider if you experience swollen glands, night sweats, shortness of breath, stomach pain that is new or worse, change in bowel habits, or weight loss without trying.
- Notify your doctor or get medical help right away if you have any of the following signs or symptoms of allergic reaction such as rash, hives, itching; red, swollen, blistered, or peeling skin with or without fever; wheezing; tightness in the chest or throat; trouble breathing, swallowing, or talking; unusual hoarseness; or swelling of the mouth, face, lips, tongue, or throat; or any dizziness or passing out.

USTEKINUMAB

(us-te-kin′u-mab)

Stelara

Classification: IMMUNOMODULATOR; MONOCLONAL ANTIBODY; INTERLEUKIN-12 AND INTERLEUKIN-23 RECEPTOR ANTAGONIST

Therapeutic: IMMUNOSUPPRESSANT

Prototype: Basiliximab

U

AVAILABILITY Solution for injection

ACTION & *THERAPEUTIC EFFECT* A human monoclonal antibody that disrupts IL-12 and IL-23 mediated signaling and cytokine cascades. *Inhibits inflammatory and immune responses associated with plaque psoriasis thereby improving psoriasis.*

USES Treatment of moderate to severe plaque psoriasis; psoriatic arthritis, Crohn disease, ulcerative colitis.

CONTRAINDICATIONS Clinically significant hypersensitivity to ustekinumab; active infection (e.g., active TB); live vaccines; BCG vaccines within 1 y prior to, during, or 1 y following drug treatment; reversible posterior leukoencephalopathy syndrome (RPLS).

CAUTIOUS USE Chronic infection or history of recurrent infection (e.g., latent TB); prior malignancy; phototherapy; older adults; pregnancy (females and males with well-controlled psoriasis who are planning a pregnancy and wish to avoid fetal exposure can consider discontinuing ustekinumab 15 weeks prior to attempting pregnancy); lactation. Safety and efficacy in children younger than 6 y not established.

ROUTE & DOSAGE

Psoriasis

Adult 100 kg or less: **Subcutaneous** 45 mg initially and 4 wk later, followed by 45 mg q12wk
Adult over 100 kg: **Subcutaneous** 90 mg initially and 4 wk later, followed by 90 mg q12wk
Child (over 6 y and less than 60 kg): **Subcutaneous** 0.75 mg/kg at 0 and 4 week then 0.75 mg/kg q12w
Child (over 6 y and 60–100 kg): **Subcutaneous** 45 mg at 0 and 4 week then 45 mg/kg q12w

Child (over 6 y over 100 kg): **Subcutaneous** 90 kg at 0 and 4 week then 90 kg q12w

Psoriatic Arthritis

Adult: **Subcutaneous** 45 mg initially and 4 wk later then 45 mg q12w

Ulcerative colitis/Chron disease

Adult 55 kg or less: **Subcutaneous** 260 mg single dose then 90 mg q8w
Adult 55–85 kg: **Subcutaneous** 390 mg single dose then 90 mg q8w
Adult over 85 kg: **Subcutaneous** 530 mg single dose then 90 mg q8w

ADMINISTRATION

Subcutaneous

- Solution may contain a few small translucent or white particles. **Do not** shake.
- Note: Needle cover on prefilled syringe is natural rubber and should not be handled by latex sensitive persons.
- When using a single-use vial, withdraw dose using a 27 gauge syringe with a one-half inch needle.
- Rotate injection sites and do not inject into an area that is tender, bruised, red, or irritated.
- Store unopened vials upright in refrigerator. Discard unused portions in single-use vials.

Intravenous

- Infuse over at least 1 hour; use of IV set with an in-line, low-protein binding filter (0.2 micrometer) required. Do not infuse concomitantly in the same IV line with other agents.
- Store at 2°–7° C (36°–46° F). Do not freeze.

ADVERSE EFFECTS **Respiratory:** Nasopharyngitis, bronchitis. **CNS:** Headache. **Skin:** Injection-site erythema, pruritus. **GI:** Diarrhea, abdominal pain. **GU:** UTI, vulvovaginal candidiasis. **Other:** *Infection*, antibody development, fever, influenza.

INTERACTIONS **Drug:** LIVE VACCINES should not be administered concurrently with ustekinumab therapy. Do not use with IMMUNOSUPPRESANTS. Closely monitor use with narrow therapeutic index drugs (e.g., **warfarin**, **cyclosporine**).

PHARMACOKINETICS **Peak:** 7–13.5 days. **Metabolism:** Degraded to smaller proteins. **Half-Life:** 14.9–45.6 days.

NURSING IMPLICATIONS

Assessment & Drug Effects

- Monitor for and promptly report S&S of TB or other infection.
- Monitor neurologic status and report promptly: Seizures, problems with vision, headaches, or confusion.
- Note: BCG vaccines should not be given during treatment, for one year prior to initiating treatment, or one year following discontinuation of treatment.
- Monitor lab tests: CBC, complete metabolic panel, hepatitis C virus/hepatitis B virus (HBV) screening. Prior to initiation of therapy, test for latent TB.

Patient & Family Education

- Do not accept vaccinations with live vaccines while taking this drug. Note that nonlive vaccines may not be effective if given during a course of ustekinumab.

U

- You should be tested for TB prior to taking this drug.
- Report promptly S&S of infection including: Chills, fever, cough, shortness of breath, diarrhea, stomach or abdominal pain, burning on urination, sores anywhere on your body, unexplained or excessive fatigue.
- Report immediately seizures, problems with vision, headaches, or confusion.

VACCINIA IMMUNE GLOBULIN (VIG-IV)

(vac-cin'i-a)

Classification: BIOLOGIC RESPONSE MODIFIER; IMMUNOGLOBULIN

Therapeutic: IMMUNOGLOBULIN

Prototype: Immune globulin

AVAILABILITY Solution for injection

ACTION & *THERAPEUTIC EFFECT*

Vaccinia immune globulin, VIG (VIG-IV) is a purified human immunoglobulin G (IgG). VIG (VIG-IV) contains high titers of antivaccinia antibodies. *VIG is effective in the treatment of smallpox vaccine adverse reactions secondary to continued vaccinia virus replication after vaccination.*

USES Treatment of progressive vaccinia; severe generalized vaccinia; eczema vaccinatum; vaccinia infection in patients with skin conditions (e.g., burns, impetigo, varicella-zoster, poison ivy, or eczematous skin lesions); treatment or modification of aberrant infections induced by vaccinia virus.

V

CONTRAINDICATIONS Isolated vaccinia keratitis; history of anaphylaxis or prior severe systemic reaction associated with the parenteral administration of VIGIV or other human immune globulin preparations; IgA-deficient patients with antibodies against IgA and a history of IgA hypersensitivity, AIDS; chronic skin conditions; bone marrow suppression; chemotherapy; radiation therapy; corticosteroid therapy, eczema; hematologic disease, thrombosis; hypotension; herpes infection; postvaccinal encephalitis; aseptic meningitis syndrome (AMS); pulmonary edema; lactation.

CAUTIOUS USE Renal impairment; autoimmune disease; cardiomyopathy, impaired cardiac output, cardiac disease, history of hypercoagulation; elderly; pregnancy (no adequate and well-controlled studies in pregnant women have been conducted). Safe use in children not established.

ROUTE & DOSAGE

Vaccinia

Adults: IV 6,000 units/kg as soon as symptoms appear, may repeat based on symptom severity and response to treatment.

ADMINISTRATION

Intravenous

PREPARE: **IV Infusion:** No dilution required. Use solution as supplied. Do not shake. Avoid foaming.

ADMINISTER: **IV Infusion:** Begin infusion within 6 h of entering the vial. Complete infusion within 12 h of entering the vial. ▪ Use in-line filter (0.22 microns), infusion pump, and dedicated IV line [may infuse into a preexisting catheter if it contains NS, D2.5W, D5W, D10W, or D20W (or any combination of these)]. ▪ For patients < or = 50 kg, infuse at 0.04 mL/kg/minute. For patients > or = 50 kg, infuse at < or = 2 mL/minute. Maximum rate of administration is 4 mL/minute. Decrease rate of infusion in patients who develop minor adverse reactions and in patients with risk factors for thrombosis/thromboembolism and/or renal insufficiency.

ADVERSE EFFECTS **CV:** Peripheral edema. **CNS:** Dizziness, fatigue, feeling hot, pain, paresthesia, sensation of cold, *headache*. **Skin:** Erythema, diaphoresis, pallor. **GI:** Decreased appetite, nausea, vomiting. **Musculoskeletal:** Muscle spasm, tremor, weakness, back pain. **Other:** Injection site reaction.

INTERACTIONS **Drug:** May interfere with the immune response to LIVE VIRUS VACCINES. Vaccination with LIVE VIRUS VACCINES should be deferred until approximately 6 mo after administration of VIG-IV.

PHARMACOKINETICS **Half-Life:** 22 days.

NURSING IMPLICATIONS

Black Box Warning

Vaccinia immune globulin IV has been associated with serious renal dysfunction, acute renal failure, and death.

Assessment & Drug Effects

- Monitor vital signs continuously during infusion, especially after infusion rate changes.
- Slow infusion rate for any of the following: Flushing, chills, muscle cramps, back pain, fever, nausea, vomiting, arthralgia, and wheezing.
- Discontinue infusion, institute supportive measures, and notify prescriber for any of the following: Increase in heart rate, increase in respiratory rate, shortness of breath, rales, or other signs of anaphylaxis.
- Monitor lab values: Renal function.

Patient & Family Education

- Promptly report any discomfort that develops while drug is being infused.

VALACYCLOVIR HYDROCHLORIDE

(val-a-cy'clo-vir)

Valtrex

Classification: ANTIVIRAL; ANTIHERPES

Therapeutic ANTIVIRAL; ANTIHERPES

Prototype: Acyclovir

AVAILABILITY Tablet

ACTION & THERAPEUTIC EFFECT An antiviral agent hydrolyzed in the intestinal wall or liver to acyclovir, which interferes with viral DNA synthesis. *Active against herpes simplex virus types 1 (HSV-1) and 2 (HSV-2), varicella zoster virus, and cytomegalovirus. Inhibits viral replication.*

USES Herpes zoster (shingles) in immunocompetent adults. Treatment and suppression of recurrent genital herpes; suppression of recurrent herpes in HIV-positive patients; treatment of cold sores; treatment of varicella infection.

CONTRAINDICATIONS Hypersensitivity to valacyclovir, acyclovir, or any component of the formulation.

CAUTIOUS USE Renal impairment, patients receiving nephrotoxic drugs, advanced HIV disease, allogeneic bone marrow transplant and renal transplant recipients, treatment of disseminated herpes zoster, immunocompromised patients, pregnancy (studies show no increased rate of birth defects related to maternal exposure to valacyclovir); lactation; children younger than 2 y for chicken pox.

ROUTE & DOSAGE

Herpes Zoster

Adult/Adolescent: **PO** 1 g tid for 7 days, start within 48 h of onset of zoster rash

Renal Impairment Dosage Adjustment

CrCl 30–49 mL/min: 1 g q12h; *10–29 mL/min:* 1 g q24h; *less than 10 mL/min:* 500 mg q24h

Treatment of Recurrent Genital Herpes

Adult/Adolescent: **PO** 500 mg bid × 3 days

Renal Impairment Dosage Adjustment

CrCl 10 mL/min or less: 500 mg daily

Treatment of Cold Sores

Adult/Adolescent: **PO** 2 g 12 h × 1 day

Chickenpox Prophylaxis in immunocompromised patients

Adolescent/Child (2 y or older): **PO** 15–30 mg/kg tid (max: 1 g tid)

ADMINISTRATION

Oral

- If GI upset occurs, administer with meals.
- Give valacyclovir after hemodialysis.
- Store at 15°–25° C (59°–77° F).

ADVERSE EFFECTS

Respiratory: Nasopharyngitis. **CNS:** *Headache,* dizziness, fatigue, depression. **Skin:** Rash. **Hepatic/GI:** *Nausea, vomiting, diarrhea,* abdominal pain, elevated liver enzymes. **GU:** Dysmenorrhea. **Musculoskeletal:** Arthralgia.

INTERACTIONS

Drug: Zidovudine may cause increased drowsiness and lethargy. Do not use with **cladribine, foscarnet,** or LIVE VACCINES.

PHARMACOKINETICS

Absorption: Rapidly absorbed from GI tract; 54% reaches systemic circulation as acyclovir. **Peak:** 1.5 h. **Distribution:** 14–18% bound to plasma proteins; distributes into plasma, cerebrospinal fluid, saliva, and major body organs; crosses placenta; excreted in breast milk. **Metabolism:** Rapidly converted to acyclovir during first pass through intestine and liver. **Elimination:** 40–50% in urine. **Half-Life:** 2.5–3.3 h.

NURSING IMPLICATIONS

Assessment & Drug Effects

- Monitor kidney function in patients with kidney impairment or those receiving potentially nephrotoxic drugs.
- Monitor for S&S of hypersensitivity; if present, withhold drug and notify prescriber.
- Monitor lab tests: Urinalysis, BUN, serum creatinine, liver enzymes, and CBC.

Patient & Family Education

- Be aware of potential adverse effects; do not discontinue drug until full course is completed.
- Note: Post-herpes pain is likely to be present for several months after completion of therapy.

VALBENAZINE

(val-ben′a-zeen)

Ingrezza

Classification: CENTRAL MONOAMINE-DEPLETING AGENT; VMAT2-INHIBITOR

Therapeutic: CENTRAL NERVOUS SYSTEM AGENT

AVAILABILITY Capsule

ACTION & *THERAPEUTIC EFFECT* Thought to reversibly inhibit the vesicular monoamine transporter 2 (VMAT2) transporter, affecting the uptake of monoamines to the synaptic vesicle from the cytoplasm. *Improves stiff and jerky involuntary musculoskeletal movement.*

USES Treatment of tardive dyskinesia.

CONTRAINDICATIONS Avoid in patients with congenital long QT syndrome or cardiac arrhythmias associated with prolonged QT interval; patients with severe renal impairment or renal failure; patients taking monoamine oxidase inhibitor therapy (MAOI therapy). Data regarding valbenazine use in human pregnancy is insufficient to provide information on drug-associated risks; lactation.

CAUTIOUS USE History of hepatic disease. Safety in children not established.

ROUTE & DOSAGE

Tardive Dyskinesia

Adult: **PO** 40 mg daily; after 1 wk titrate to 80 mg daily

Renal Impairment Dosage Adjustment

CrCL less than 30 mL/min: Use is not recommended

Hepatic Impairment Dosage Adjustment

Moderate to Severe impairment (Child-Pugh class B or C): 40 mg daily

Concomitant CYP3A4 Inhibitor/Inducer

Strong CYP3A4 inducer: Do not use

Strong CYP3A4 inhibitor: Max dose: 40 mg daily

ADMINISTRATION

Oral

- May be administered with or without food.
- Store at 20°–25° C (68°–77° F); excursions permitted to 15°–30° C (59°–86° F).

ADVERSE EFFECTS **Respiratory:** Infection. **CNS:** Drowsiness, sedation, dizziness, falling, drooling, insomnia. **Endocrine:** Hyperglycemia, weight gain. **GI:** Vomiting. **Musculoskeletal:** Joint pain, involuntary movement.

INTERACTIONS CYP3A4 substrate; avoid use with strong CYP3A4 inducers (e.g., **carbamazepine**, **phenytoin**, **rifampin**); 40 mg daily max dose with CYP3A4 inhibitors (e.g., clarithyromycin, itraconazole, ketoconazole) **Herbal:** **St. John's wort** should not be combined with valbenazine.

PHARMACOKINETICS **Absorption:** 49% bioavailability, AUC and C_{max} decreased with high fat meals. **Distribution:** 99% protein bound. **Onset:** Peak effect in 0.5–1 h. **Metabolism:** Hepatic hydrolysis to an active metabolite, primarily by CYP3A4/5. **Elimination:** 30% in feces, 60% in urine. **Half-Life:** 15–22 h.

NURSING IMPLICATIONS

Assessment & Drug Effects

- Monitor for decrease in severity of tardive dyskinesia (abnormal involuntary movement) symptoms as indicative of efficacy.
- Monitor QT interval for patients at risk, prior to increasing the dose.
- EKG in patients at risk for QT prolongation.
- Monitor lab tests: Baseline LFTs.

Patient & Family Education

- Notify all health care providers that you this drug is being taken. This includes prescribers, doctors, nurses, pharmacists, and dentists.
- Avoid driving or other tasks that require alertness until drug affects are known.
- Notify prescriber if taking digoxin. Blood work will need to be monitored more closely.
- Notify prescriber of pregnancy or plan to get pregnant.
- Do not breast-feed while taking this drug or at least 5 days after final dose. Milk should be pumped and dumped during this time.
- Notify prescriber right away with S&S of an allergic reaction: Rash, hives, itching, blistered skin, fever, wheezing, chest or throat tightness, trouble breathing, unusual hoarseness, swelling of the mouth, face, lips, tongue, or throat.
- Notify prescriber right away with difficulties in focusing, blurred vision, difficulty urinating, a fast heartbeat that does not feel normal, or fainting.

V

VALGANCICLOVIR HYDROCHLORIDE

(val-gan-ci′clo-vir)

Valcyte

Classification: ANTIVIRAL

Therapeutic: ANTIVIRAL

Prototype: Acyclovir

AVAILABILITY Tablet; powder for oral solution

ACTION & *THERAPEUTIC EFFECT* Rapidly converted to ganciclovir by intestinal and hepatic enzymes. In cells infected with cytomegalovirus (CMV), ganciclovir is converted to ganciclovir triphosphate that inhibits viral DNA synthesis. *Effective antiviral that prevents replication of viral CMV DNA.*

USES Treatment or prevention of CMV retinitis; prevention of CMV disease in high-risk kidney, kidney-pancreas, and heart transplant patients (not effective in liver transplants).

UNLABELED USES CMV in solid organ transplant.

CONTRAINDICATIONS Hypersensitivity to valganciclovir, ganciclovir, or acyclovir; females of childbearing age; lactation.

CAUTIOUS USE Renal impairment; blood dyscrasias; older adults; pregnancy (based on animal reproduction studies, has the potential to cause birth defects in humans). Safe use in infants younger than 4 mo not established.

ROUTE & DOSAGE

Cytomegalovirus Prophylaxis

Adult/Adolescent: **PO** 900 mg once daily, duration depends on type of transplant, donor, and recipient CMV serostatus
Child/Infant (older than 4 mo): See package insert for dose calculation formula (max: 900 mg)

Cytomegalovirus Retinitis Treatment

Adult: **PO** 900 mg bid × 14–21 days then 900 mg daily

Renal Impairment Dosage Adjustment

CrCl 40–59 mL/min: 450 mg bid (induction) or daily (maintenance); *25–39 mL/min:* 450 mg daily (induction) or q2days (maintenance); *10–24 mL/min:* 450 mg q2days (induction) or twice weekly (maintenance)

ADMINISTRATION

Oral

- Exercise caution in handling tablets, powder for oral solution, and the oral solution. Do not crush or break tablets. Avoid direct contact of any form of the drug with skin or mucous membranes. Note that adults should receive tablets, not the oral solution.
- Give with food.
- Store tablets at 20°–25° C (68°–77° F). Store oral solution at 2°–8° C (36°–46° F) for no longer than 49 days.

ADVERSE EFFECTS **Cardiovascular:** Hypertension, hypotension, peripheral edema, cardiac arrhythmia. **Respiratory:** Cough, dyspnea, pharyngitis, URI. **CNS:** *Headache, insomnia*, peripheral neuropathy, paresthesia, seizure, psychosis, confusion, hallucinations, agitation, anxiety, chills, depression, dizziness, fatigue, malaise, pain, tremor. **HEENT:** *Retinal detachment*, eye pain, macular edema, deafness. **Endocrine:** Hyperkalemia, hypophosphatemia, weight loss. **Skin:** Dermatitis, increased wound secretion, night sweats, pruritis, cellulitis. **Hepatic/GI:** *Diarrhea, nausea, vomiting, abdominal pain*, abdominal distension, constipation, decreased appetite, dyspepsia, oral mucosa ulceration, dysgeusia, pancreatitis, increased serum ALT and AST. **GU:** Increased serum creatinine, hematuria, decreased creatinine clearance, renal impairment, renal failure. UTI. **Hematologic:** *Neutropenia, anemia*, <u>thrombocytopenia</u>, pancytopenia, <u>bone marrow suppression, aplastic anemia</u>, hemorrhage. **Musculoskeletal:** Arthralgia, back pain, muscle spasm, myalgia, weakness, limb pain. **Other:** *Fever*, graft rejection, organ transplant rejection, local and systemic infections, hypersensitivity reactions.

INTERACTIONS **Drug:** ANTINEOPLASTIC AGENTS, **amphotericin B, didanosine, dapsone, probenecid, zidovudine** may increase bone marrow suppression and other toxic effects of valganciclovir; may increase risk of nephrotoxicity from **cyclosporine**; ANTIRETROVIRAL AGENTS may decrease valganciclovir levels; valganciclovir may increase levels and toxicity of ANTIRETROVIRAL AGENTS; do not use with **cladribine**; may increase risk of seizures due to **imipenem-cilastatin**.

PHARMACOKINETICS **Absorption:** 60% reaches systemic circulation as ganciclovir. **Onset:** 3–8 days. **Peak:** 1–3 h. **Duration:** Clinical relapse can occur 14 days to 3.5 mo after stopping therapy; positive blood and urine cultures recur 12–60 days after therapy. **Distribution:** Distributes throughout body including CSF, eye, lungs, liver, and kidneys; crosses placenta in animals; not known if distributed into breast milk. **Metabolism:** Metabolized in intestinal wall to ganciclovir, ganciclovir is not metabolized. **Elimination:** 94–99% of dose is excreted unchanged in urine. **Half-Life:** 4 h (in adults).

NURSING IMPLICATIONS

Black Box Warning

Valganciclovir has been associated with granulocytopenia, anemia, and thrombocytopenia.

Assessment & Drug Effects

- Withhold drug and notify prescriber for any of the following: Absolute neutrophil count less than 500 cells/mm^3, platelet count less than 25,000/mm^3, hemoglobin less than 8 g/dL, declining creatinine clearance.
- Monitor for S&S of bronchospasm in asthma patients; notify prescriber immediately.
- Monitor lab tests: Baseline and frequent serum creatinine or creatinine clearance, CBC with differential, platelet count; pregnancy test prior to initiation in females of reproductive potential.

Patient & Family Education

- Schedule ophthalmologic follow-up examinations at least every 4–6 wk while being treated with valganciclovir.
- Keep all scheduled appointments for laboratory tests.
- Do not drive or engage in potentially hazardous activities until response to drug is known.
- Report any of the following immediately: Unexpected bleeding, infection.
- Use effective methods of contraception (barrier and other types) during and for at least 90 days following treatment.
- Discontinue drug and notify prescriber immediately in the event of pregnancy.

V

VALPROIC ACID (DIVALPROEX SODIUM, SODIUM VALPROATE) Pr

(val-proe′ic)

Depakote, Depakote ER, Depakote Sprinkle, Epival ✦

Classification: ANTICONVULSANT; GAMMA-AMINOBUTYRIC ACID (GABA) INHIBITOR

Therapeutic: ANTICONVULSANT

AVAILABILITY Capsule; sprinkle capsule; delayed release tablet; oral solution; solution for injection

ACTION & *THERAPEUTIC EFFECT*

Causes increased availability of gamma-aminobutyric acid (GABA), an inhibitory neurotransmitter, to brain neurons or may enhance the action of GABA or mimic its action at postsynaptic receptor sites. Blocks voltage-dependent sodium channels which results in suppression of high-frequency repetitive neuronal firing. *Depresses abnormal neuron discharges in the CNS, thus decreasing seizure activity.*

USES Alone or with other anticonvulsants in management of focal (partial) onset and generalized onset seizures; mania; migraine headache prophylaxis; bipolar disorder.

UNLABELED USES Status epilepticus refractory to IV diazepam, intractable migraine, bipolar major depression.

CONTRAINDICATIONS Hypersensitivity to valproic acid; hepatic function impairment; urea cycle disorders; hyperammonemia, encephalopathy; suicidal ideations; thrombocytopenia, patient with bleeding disorders or liver dysfunction or disease, drug induced pancreatitis; congenital metabolic disorders, mitochondrial disorders caused by mutations in mitochondrial DNA and children younger than 2 y who are suspected of having a mitochondial DNA polemerase related disorder; pancreatitis; pregnancy (risk of adverse fetal events including major congenital malformations, decreased IQ scores, and neurodevelopmental disorders; use during pregnancy is contraindicated); lactation.

CAUTIOUS USE History of suicidal tendencies; history of kidney disease, renal impairment or failure; history of mild or moderate liver impairment; congenital metabolic disorders, those with severe epilepsy; HIV; CMV-infected patients; hypoalbuminemia; organic brain syndrome or mental retardation; use as sore agent; older adults. Safe use in children with partial seizures younger than 10 y not established. Safe use for migraine use in children younger than 12 y not established.

ROUTE & DOSAGE

Note: May need to increase dose when converting from immediate release to extended release products

Management of Seizures

Adult/Child (10 y or older): **PO** 10–15 mg/kg/day in divided doses when total daily dose greater than 250 mg, increase by 5–10 mg/kg/day at weekly intervals until seizures are controlled or adverse effects develop (max: 60 mg/kg/day)
Conversion of PO to IV: Give normal dose in divided doses q6h

Migraine Headache Prophylaxis

Adult: **PO** 250 mg bid (max: 1000 mg/day) or **Depakote ER** 500 mg daily × 1 wk, may increase to 1000 mg daily
Child (over 5 y): **PO** 10–15 mg/kg/day in 2 divided doses (max: 250 mg/dose) titrate over 4–6w to 0–45 mg/kg/day.

Bipolar Disorder

Adult: **PO** 500–750 mg/day administered in divided doses may increase by 250–500 mg q1–3 days

Hepatic Impairment Dosage Adjustment

Dose reduction recommended

Renal Impairment Dosage Adjustment

Severe impairment may require close monitoring

ADMINISTRATION

Oral

- Give tablets and capsules whole; instruct patient to swallow whole and not to chew. Instruct to swallow sprinkle capsules whole or sprinkle entire contents on teaspoonful of soft food, and instruct to not chew food.

V

- Avoid using a carbonated drink as diluent for the syrup because it will release drug from delivery vehicle; free drug painfully irritates oral and pharyngeal membranes.
- Reduce gastric irritation by administering drug with food.

Intravenous

PREPARE: **IV Infusion:** Dilute each dose in 50 mL or more of D5W, NS, or LR.
ADMINISTER: **IV Infusion:** Give a single dose over at least 60 min (20 mg/min or less). ▪ Avoid rapid infusion.
INCOMPATIBILITIES: **Solution/additive:** Should avoid mixing with other drugs. **Y-site:** **Vancomycin**.

ADVERSE EFFECTS

CV: Edema, facial edema, orthostatic hypotension, tachycardia. **Respiratory:** Bronchitis, cough, dyspnea, pharyngitis, rhinitis, sinusitis. **CNS:** Breakthrough seizures, *sedation, drowsiness, headache*, dizziness, nervousness, insomnia, hallucinations, emotional lability, agitation, abnormal thinking. **HEENT:** Diplopia, visual disturbance, conjunctivitis, dry eyes, eye pain, deafness, otitis media, tinnitus. **Endocrine:** Amenorrhea, weight gain/loss. **Skin:** Skin rash, pruritis, ecchymoses, seborrhea, alopecia. **GI/Hepatic:** *Nausea, vomiting*, dyspepsia, abdominal pain, diarrhea, constipation, <u>increased liver enzymes, pancreatitis</u>. **Hematologic:** *Prolonged bleeding time*, thrombocytopenia, <u>bone marrow depression</u>, anemia. **Musculoskeletal:** Asthenia, tremor, arthralgia, back pain. **Other:** Infection, flu-like symptoms, fever, accidental injury.

DIAGNOSTIC TEST INTERFERENCE

Valproic acid produces false-positive results for ***urine ketones***, elevated ***AST***, ***ALT***, ***LDH***, and ***serum alkaline phosphatase***, prolonged ***bleeding time***, altered ***thyroid function tests***.

INTERACTIONS

Drug: Alcohol and other CNS DEPRESSANTS potentiate depressant effects; other ANTICONVULSANTS, BARBITURATES increase or decrease anticonvulsant and BARBITURATE levels; **haloperidol, loxapine, maprotiline**, MAOIS, PHENOTHIAZINES, THIOXANTHENES, TRICYCLIC ANTIDEPRESSANTS can increase CNS depression or lower seizure threshold; **aspirin, dipyridamole, warfarin** increase risk of spontaneous bleeding; **clonazepam** may precipitate absence seizures; SALICYLATES, **cimetidine, isoniazid** may increase valproic acid levels and toxicity. **Mefloquine** can decrease valproic acid levels; **meropenem** may decrease valproic acid levels; **cholestyramine** may decrease absorption. **Herbal: Ginkgo** may decrease anticonvulsant effectiveness.

PHARMACOKINETICS

Absorption: Readily from GI tract. **Peak:** 1–4 h valproic acid; 3–5 h divalproex. **Therapeutic Range:** 50–100 mcg/mL. **Distribution:** Crosses placenta; distributed into breast milk. **Metabolism:** In liver. **Elimination:** Primarily in urine; small amount in feces and expired air. **Half-Life:** 5–20 h.

NURSING IMPLICATIONS

Black Box Warning

Valproic acid, sodium valproate, and divalproex sodium have been associated with severe hepatotoxicity, life-threatening pancreatitis, and fetal harm.

Assessment & Drug Effects

- Monitor patient alertness especially with multiple drug therapy for seizure control.
- Monitor patient carefully during dose adjustments and promptly report presence of adverse effects. Increased dosage is associated with frequency of adverse effects.
- Monitor for and report promptly S&S of pancreatitis (e.g., abdominal pain, nausea, vomiting, and/or anorexia).
- Multiple drugs for seizure control increase the risk of hyperammonemia, marked by lethargy, anorexia, asterixis, increased seizure frequency, and vomiting. Report such symptoms promptly to prescriber. If they persist with decreased dosage, the drug will be discontinued.
- Monitor lab tests: Baseline LFTs, PT/PTT, CBC with platelet count, and serum ammonia; then repeat at least q2mo, especially during the first 6 mo of therapy. Serum valproate levels.

Patient & Family Education

- Women of childbearing age should be aware of the potential for birth defects should a pregnancy occur while taking this drug.
- Do not discontinue therapy abruptly; such action could result in loss of seizure control. Consult prescriber before you stop or alter dosage regimen.
- Notify prescriber promptly if spontaneous bleeding or bruising occurs (e.g., petechiae, ecchymotic areas, otorrhagia, epistaxis, melena).
- Withhold dose and notify prescriber for following symptoms: Visual disturbances, rash, jaundice, light-colored stools, protracted vomiting, diarrhea. Fatal liver failure has occurred in patients receiving this drug.
- Avoid alcohol and self-medication with other depressants during therapy.
- Consult prescriber before using any OTC drugs during anticonvulsant therapy, especially drugs containing aspirin or sedatives and medications for hay fever or other allergies.
- Do not drive or engage in potentially hazardous activities until response to drug is known.

VALRUBICIN

(val-roo′bi-sin)

Valstar

Classification: ANTINEOPLASTIC; (ANTIBIOTIC) ANTHRACYCLINE

Therapeutic: ANTINEOPLASTIC

Prototype: Doxorubicin hydrochloride

AVAILABILITY Solution

ACTION & *THERAPEUTIC EFFECT*

A cytotoxic agent that inhibits the incorporation of nucleosides in DNA and RNA, resulting in extensive chromosomal damage. It arrests the cell cycle of the HIV virus in the G2 phase by interfering with normal DNA action of topoisomerase II, which is responsible for separating DNA strands and resealing them. *Valrubicin has higher antitumor efficacy and lower toxicity than doxorubicin.*

USES Intravesical therapy of BCG-refractory carcinoma *in situ* of the urinary bladder.

CONTRAINDICATIONS Hypersensitivity to valrubicin, doxorubicin, anthracyclines, or castor oil; patients with a perforated bladder, concurrent UTI, active infection; severe irritable bladder symptoms; severe myelosuppression; lactation.

CAUTIOUS USE Within 2 wk of a transureteral resection; compromised bladder mucosa; mild to moderate myelosuppression; history of bleeding disorders; GI disorders, renal impairment; pregnancy (category C).

ROUTE & DOSAGE

BCG-Refractory Bladder Carcinoma *in situ*

Adult: **Intravesically** 800 mg once/wk × 6 wk

ADMINISTRATION

Instillation

Avoid skin reactions by using gloves during preparation/administration.
▪ Use only glass, polypropylene, or polyolefin containers and tubing.

Intravenous

PREPARE: Slowly warm 4 vials (5 mL each) to room temperature. ▪ When a precipitate is initially present, warm vials in hands until solution clears. ▪ Add contents of 4 vials to 55 mL of 0.9% NaCl injection to yield 75 mL of diluted solution.
ADMINISTER: Aseptically insert a urethral catheter and drain the bladder. ▪ Use gravity drainage to instill valrubicin slowly over several min. ▪ Withdraw catheter; instruct patient not to void for 2 h. ▪ Note: Do not leave a clamped catheter in place.

V

▪ Store vials in refrigerator. Do not freeze.

ADVERSE EFFECTS **CV:** Vasodilation. **Respiratory:** Pneumonia. **CNS:** Dizziness. **Skin:** Rash. **GI:** Diarrhea, flatulence, nausea, vomiting. **GU:** *Urinary frequency, urgency, dysuria, bladder spasm, hematuria, bladder pain, incontinence, cystitis, UTI,* nocturia, local burning, urethral pain, pelvic pain, gross hematuria, urinary retention. **Other:** Abdominal pain, asthenia, back pain, fever, headache, malaise, myalgia. Anemia, hyperglycemia, peripheral edema.

PHARMACOKINETICS **Absorption:** Not absorbed. **Distribution:** Penetrates bladder wall. **Metabolism:** Not metabolized. **Elimination:** Almost completely excreted by voiding the instillate.

NURSING IMPLICATIONS

Assessment & Drug Effects

- Therapeutic effectiveness: Indicated by regression of the bladder tumor.
- Notify prescriber if bladder spasms with spontaneous discharge of valrubicin occur during/shortly after instillation.

Patient & Family Education

- Expect red-tinged urine during the first 24 h after administration.
- Report prolonged passage of red-colored urine or prolonged bladder irritation.
- Drink plenty of fluids during 48 h period following administration.
- Use reliable contraception during therapy period (approximately 6 wk).

VALSARTAN

(val-sar'tan)

Diovan, Prexxartan

Classification: RENIN ANGIOTENSIN SYSTEM ANTAGONIST; ANTIHYPERTENSIVE

Therapeutic: ANTIHYPERTENSIVE; ANGIOTENSIN II RECEPTOR (AT_1) ANTAGONIST

Prototype: Losartan

AVAILABILITY Capsule; oral solution

ACTION & THERAPEUTIC EFFECT

An angiotensin II receptor antagonist that blocks the angiotensin converting enzyme (ACE). It inhibits the binding of angiotensin II to the AT_1 subtype receptors found in many tissues (e.g., vascular smooth muscle, adrenal glands). Angiotensin II is a potent vasoconstrictor and primary vasoactive hormone of the renin–angiotensin–aldosterone system (RAAS). *Blocking angiotensin II receptors results in vasodilation as well as decreasing the aldosterone-secreting effects of angiotensin II. These actions result in the antihypertensive effect of valsartan.*

USES Treatment of hypertension, heart failure; reduction of cardiovascular mortality in stable patients with left ventricular failure or left ventricular dysfunction (LVD) following acute myocardial infarction.

CONTRAINDICATIONS Hypersensitivity to valsartan or losartan; severe heart failure with compromised renal function; volume depletion; history of ACE inhibitor–induced angioedema concomitant use with aliskiren in patients with diabetes mellitus; children with CrCl of 30 mL/min/1.73 mm^3; pregnancy (category D); lactation.

CAUTIOUS USE Severe renal impairment; hyperuricemia; hyperglycemia; increases in cholesterol and triglycerides; acute angle-closure glaucoma; SLE; history of allergy or bronchial asthma; mild to moderate hepatic impairment; biliary stenosis; renal artery stenosis; hypovolemia; hyperkalemia; transient hypotension; use prior to surgery; history of angioedema; congestive heart failure; older adults; children younger than 6 y.

ROUTE & DOSAGE

Hypertension

Adult: **PO** 80 or 160 mg daily (max: 320 mg daily) **Oral solution** 40–80 mg bid
Adolescent/Child (6–16 y): **PO** 1.3 mg/kg (max: 40 mg/day); **Oral solution** 0.65 mg/kg/dose bid may titrate up (max dose: 160 mg/day)

Heart Failure

Adult: **PO** 20–40 mg bid and titrate up to 160 mg bid

Left Ventricular Dysfunction Post MI

Adult: **PO** 20 mg bid titrate to dose of 160 mg bid if tolerated

Hemodialysis Dosage Adjustment

Adjustment not needed

ADMINISTRATION

Oral

- May be given with or without food.
- Reduce dosage with severe hepatic or renal impairment.
- Note: Daily dose may be titrated up to 320 mg.
- Store at 15°–30° C (59°–86° F).

ADVERSE EFFECTS CV: Hypotension, orthostatic hypotension. **Respiratory:** Dry cough. **CNS:** Dizziness. Renal: Increased blood urea nitrogen.

DIAGNOSTIC TEST INTERFERENCE

May lead to false-negative aldosterone/renin ratio.

INTERACTIONS Do not use with **tranylcypromine**. Do not use within 12 h of **rituximab** administration. Use cautiously with **amifostine** due to increased risk of hypotension.

V

PHARMACOKINETICS **Absorption:** Rapidly from GI tract, 25% bioavailability. **Onset:** Blood pressure decreased in 2 wk. **Peak:** Plasma levels, 2–4 h; blood pressure effect 4 wk. **Distribution:** 99% protein bound. **Metabolism:** In the liver (CYP2C9). **Elimination:** Primarily in feces. **Half-Life:** 6 h.

NURSING IMPLICATIONS

Black Box Warning

Valsartan has been associated with fetal toxicity.

Assessment & Drug Effects

- Monitor BP periodically; take trough readings, just prior to the next scheduled dose, when possible.
- Monitor lab tests: Periodic electrolyte panel and renal function tests.

Patient & Family Education

- Inform prescriber immediately if you become pregnant.
- Note: Maximum pressure lowering effect is usually evident between 2 and 4 wk after initiation of therapy. Use precaution when changing positions.
- Notify prescriber of episodes of dizziness, especially those that occur when making position changes.
- Do not use potassium supplements or salt substitutes containing potassium without consulting the prescribing prescriber.

V

VANCOMYCIN HYDROCHLORIDE (Pr)

(van-koe-mye'sin)

Vancocin

Classification: ANTIBIOTIC; GLYCOPEPTIDE

Therapeutic: ANTIBIOTIC

AVAILABILITY Capsule; solution for injection

ACTION & THERAPEUTIC EFFECT Bactericidal action is due to inhibition of cell-wall biosynthesis and alteration of bacterial cell-membrane permeability and ribonucleic acid (RNA) synthesis. *Active against many gram-positive organisms.*

USES Parenterally for potentially life-threatening infections in patients allergic, nonsensitive, or resistant to other less toxic antimicrobial drugs. Used orally only in *Clostridium difficile* colitis and staphylococccal enterocolitis (not effective by oral route for treatment of systemic infections).

UNLABELED USES Rectal administration for complicated *C. difficile* infection.

CONTRAINDICATIONS Hypersensitivity to vancomycin.

CAUTIOUS USE Impaired kidney function, renal failure, renal impairment, hearing impairment; colitis, inflammatory disorders of the intestine; older adults; pregnancy (category B), children, neonates.

ROUTE & DOSAGE

Systemic Infections

Adult/Adolescent: **IV** 500 mg q6h or 1 g q12h or 15 mg/kg q12h
Child/Infant (1 mo or older): **IV** 30–40 mg/kg/day divided q6–8h
Neonate: **IV** 10–15 mg/kg q8–24h

***Clostridium difficile* Colitis**

Adult: **PO** 125 mg qid × 10 days
Child: **PO** 40 mg/kg/day divided q6h (max: 2 g/day)

Staphylococcal Enterocolitis

Adult: **PO** 500 mg–2g in 3–4 divided doses × 7–10 days
Child: **PO** 40 mg/kg/day divided q6h (max: 2 g/day)

Surgical Prophylaxis (in Patients Allergic to Beta-Lactams)

Adult/Adolescent/Child (weight at least 27 kg): **IV** 10–15 mg/kg starting 1 h before surgery
Child (weight less than 27 kg): **IV** 20 mg/kg starting 1 h before surgery

Endocarditis

Adult: **IV** 500 mg q6h or 1 g q12h *Infant older than 1 mo:* **IV** 10 mg/kg/dose q6h
Neonate: **IV** 15 mg/kg initial dose then 10 mg/kg q12h for first wk then q8h up to 1 mo old

Renal Impairment Dosage Adjustment

CrCl 40–60 mL/min: Dose q24h; *less than 40 mL/min:* Extend interval based on monitoring levels

Hemodialysis Dosage Adjustment

Not dialyzed

ADMINISTRATION

Oral

- May be given with or without food.
- Note: Some parenteral products may be administered orally; check manufacturer's package insert.

Intravenous

PREPARE: **Intermittent:** Reconstitute 500 mg vial, 750 mg vial, or 1 g vial with 10 mL, 15 mL, or 20 mL, respectively, of sterile water for injection to yield 50 mg/mL. ▪ Further dilute each 500 mg with at least 100 mL, each 750 mg with at least 150 mL, and each 1 g with at least 200 mL of D5W, NS, or LR.

ADMINISTER: **Intermittent:** Give a single dose at a rate of 10 mg/min or over **not less** than 60 min (whichever is longer). ▪ Avoid rapid infusion, which may cause sudden hypotension. ▪ Monitor IV site closely; necrosis and tissue sloughing will result from extravasation.

INCOMPATIBILITIES: **Solution/additive:** **Aminophylline**, BARBITURATES, **aztreonam** (high concentration), **calcium chloride, chloramphenicol, chlorothiazide, ciprofloxacin, dexamethasone, heparin, methicillin, pentobarbital, phenobarbital, sodium bicarbonate, sodium fusidate, warfarin.** **Y-site:** **Albumin, aminophylline, amphotericin B cholesteryl, azathioprine, aztreonam, bivalirudin, cefazolin, cefepime, cefoperazone, cefotaxime, cefotetan, cefoxitin, ceftazidime, ceftriaxone, cefuroxime, chloramphenicol, clorazepate, dantrolene, daptomycin, defibrotide, diazepam, diazoxide, dimenhydrinate, epoetin, fluorouracil, foscarnet, furosemide, ganciclovir, gemtuzumab, heparin, ibuprofen, idarubicin, indomethacin, ketorolac, lansoprazole, leucovorin, mitomycin, moxifloxacin, nafcillin, omeprazole,**

phenytoin, piperacillin/tazobactam, rituximab, sargramostim, streptokinase, SMZ/TMP, temocillin, ticarcillin, ticarcillin/clavulanate, valproate sodium, warfarin.

- Store oral and parenteral solutions in refrigerator for up to 14 days; after further dilution, parenteral solution is stable 24 h at room temperature.

ADVERSE EFFECTS **HEENT:** Ototoxicity (auditory portion of eighth cranial nerve). **GI:** Nausea, warmth. **GU:** Nephrotoxicity leading to uremia. **Hematologic:** Transient leukopenia, eosinophilia. **Other:** Hypersensitivity reactions (chills, fever, skin rash, urticaria, shock-like state), anaphylactoid reaction with vascular collapse, superinfections, severe pain, thrombophlebitis at injection site, generalized tingling following rapid IV infusion. Injection reaction that includes *hypotension accompanied by flushing and erythematous rash on face and upper body* ("red-neck syndrome") following rapid IV infusion.

INTERACTIONS **Drug:** Adds to toxicity of ototoxic and nephrotoxic drugs (AMINOGLYCOSIDES, **amphotericin B, colistin, capreomycin; cidofovir; cisplatin; cyclosporine; foscarnet; ganciclovir; IV pentamidine; polymyxin B; streptozocin; tacrolimus**). **Cholestyramine, colestipol** can decrease absorption of oral vancomycin; may increase risk of lactic acidosis with **metformin**.

PHARMACOKINETICS **Absorption:** Not absorbed. **Peak:** 30 min after end of infusion. **Distribution:** Diffuses into pleural, ascitic, pericardial, and synovial fluids; small amount penetrates CSF if meninges are inflamed; crosses placenta. **Elimination:** 80–90% of IV dose in urine within 24 h; PO dose excreted in feces. **Half-Life:** 4–8 h.

NURSING IMPLICATIONS

Assessment & Drug Effects

- Monitor BP and heart rate continuously through period of drug administration.
- Assess hearing. Drug may cause damage to auditory branch (not vestibular branch) of eighth cranial nerve, with consequent deafness, which may be permanent.
- Be aware that serum levels of 60–80 mcg/mL are associated with ototoxicity. Tinnitus and high-tone hearing loss may precede deafness, which may progress even after drug is withdrawn. Older adults and those on high doses are especially susceptible.
- Monitor I&O: Report changes in I&O ratio and pattern. Oliguria or cloudy or pink urine may be a sign of nephrotoxicity (also manifested by transient elevations in BUN, albumin, and hyaline and granular casts in urine).
- Monitor lab tests: Periodic renal function tests, urinalysis, and WBC count; serial vancomycin blood levels (peak and trough) in patients with borderline kidney function, in infants and neonates, and in patients older than 60 y.

Patient & Family Education

- Notify prescriber promptly of ringing in ears.
- Adhere to drug regimen (i.e., do not increase, decrease, or interrupt dosage. The full course of prescribed drug therapy **must be** completed).

VARDENAFIL HYDROCHLORIDE

(var-den′a-fil hy-dro-chlo′ride)

Levitra, Staxyn

Classification: IMPOTENCE AGENT; PHOSPHODIESTERASE (PDE) INHIBITOR; VASODILATOR

Therapeutic: IMPOTENCE; PDE TYPE 5 INHIBITOR

Prototype: Sildenafil

AVAILABILITY Tablet; orally disintegrating tablet

ACTION & *THERAPEUTIC EFFECT* Phosphodiesterases-5 (PDE5) is an enzyme that speeds up the degradation of cyclic guanosine monophosphate (cGMP), an enzyme needed to cause and maintain increased blood flow into the penis necessary for an erection. Vardenafil is a PDE5 inhibitor. *It enhances erectile function by increasing the amount of cGMP in the penis.*

USES Treatment of erectile dysfunction.

CONTRAINDICATIONS Hypersensitivity to vardenafil or sildenafil; coadministration of nitrates; QT prolongation, renal failure, severe renal impairment; retinitis pigmentosa. **Levitra:** Severe hepatic impairment (Child-Pugh class C); **Staxyn:** Moderate or severe hepatic impairment (Child-Pugh class B and C); lactation.

CAUTIOUS USE CAD, MI, or stroke within 6 mo; hypotension, or hypertension; risk factors for CVA; anatomic deformity of the penis; subaortic stenosis; sickle cell anemia, leukemia; multiple myeloma; leukemia; coagulopathy; active bleeding or a peptic ulcer; coagulopathy; GERD; hepatitis, cirrhosis; older adults; pregnancy (category B).

ROUTE & DOSAGE

Erectile Dysfunction

Adult: **PO** 10 mg approximately 60 min before sexual activity. May increase to max 20 mg/day (**Levitra** only) if needed.
Geriatric: **PO** Start with 5 mg 60 min before sexual activity (max: 20 mg/day)

Hepatic Impairment Dosage Adjustment

Moderate impairment: For **Levitra** reduce dose to 5 mg (max: 10 mg/day). For **Staxyn** dosing do not use in patients with moderate or severe (class B or C) hepatic impairment.

Drug Interaction Dosage Adjustment

If taking **Ritonavir**, max dose: 2.5 mg/72 h; if taking **erythromycin, indinavir, itraconazole, ketoconazole,** max dose: 2.5–5 mg/24 h

ADMINISTRATION

Oral

- Take approximately 1 h before expected intercourse, but preferably not after a heavy or high-fat meal.
- Store at 15°–30° C (59°–86° F).

ADVERSE EFFECTS **CV:** Angina, hypertension, hypotension, MI, orthostatic hypotension, palpitations, syncope, sinus tachycardia. **Respiratory:** Rhinitis, sinusitis, dyspnea, epistaxis, pharyngitis. **CNS:** *Headache*, dizziness, insomnia, somnolence, vertigo. **HEENT:** Tinnitus, sudden vision loss, blurred vision, changes in color vision. **Endocrine:** Increased creatine kinase. **Skin:** Photosensitivity, rash,

V

pruritus, sweating. **GI:** Dyspepsia, nausea, vomiting, abdominal pain, abnormal liver function tests, diarrhea, dysphagia, esophagitis, gastritis, GERD, xerostomia. **GU:** Ejaculation dysfunction. **Musculoskeletal:** Arthralgia, myalgia, hypertonia, hyperesthesia. **Other:** *Flushing*, flu-like syndrome, back pain, anaphylactoid reactions, asthenia, facial edema, pain, paresthesias.

INTERACTIONS **Drug:** May potentiate hypotensive effects of NITRATES, ALPHA-BLOCKERS, **alfuzosin, doxazosin, prazosin, tamsulosin, terazosin; amiodarone, dofetilide, procainamide, quinidine, sotalol** may increase QT_C interval leading to arrhythmias; dosage adjustment required with potent CYP3A4 inhibitors (**atazanavir, erythromycin, idinavir, itraconazole, ketaconazole**, etc.). If taking ritonavir, max dose is 2.5 mg/72 h. If taking erythromycin, indinavir, itraconazole, ketoconazole, max dose is 2.5–5 mg/24 h.

PHARMACOKINETICS **Absorption:** Rapidly absorbed, 15% reaches systemic circulation; 95% protein bound. **Onset:** Within 1 h. **Peak:** 0.5–2 h. **Metabolism:** In liver by CYP3A4, CYP3A5, and CYP2C. **Elimination:** Primarily in feces (90–95%). **Half-Life:** 4–5 h.

NURSING IMPLICATIONS

Assessment & Drug Effects

- Monitor CV status and report angina or other S&S of cardiac dysfunction.

Patient & Family Education

- Do not take more than once a day and never take more than the prescribed dose.
- Do not take this drug without consulting prescriber if you are taking drugs called "alpha-blockers" or "nitrates" or any other drugs for high blood pressure, chest pain, or enlarged prostate.
- Report promptly any of the following: Palpitations, chest pain, back pain, difficulty breathing, or shortness of breath; dizziness or fainting; changes in vision; dizziness; swollen eyelids; muscle aches; painful or prolonged erection (lasting longer than 4 h); skin rash, or itching.

VARENICLINE

(var-en'i-cline)

Chantix

Classification: SMOKING DETERRENT; NICOTINIC RECEPTOR AGONIST

Therapeutic: SMOKING CESSATION

Prototype: Nicotine

AVAILABILITY Tablet

ACTION & *THERAPEUTIC EFFECT*
Nicotine increases dopamine release in the brain and cravings for nicotine are stimulated by low levels of dopamine during periods of abstinence. Varenicline is a partial agonist at nicotinic acetylcholine receptors (nAChRs), the sites responsible for the dopamine effects of nicotine. It partially stimulates these receptors to produce a modest level of dopamine but blocks nicotine from binding to many of the nicotinic receptor sites. *By blocking nicotinic receptors, it reduces effects of nicotine in cases where patient relapses and uses tobacco.*

USES Adjunct for smoking cessation in patients experiencing nicotine withdrawal.

CONTRAINDICATIONS Suicidal ideation; chronic depression; serious psychiatric disease; lactation.

CAUTIOUS USE History of suicidal tendencies, depression; renal impairment, older adults; pregnancy (category C). Safe use in children younger than 18 y not known.

ROUTE & DOSAGE

Smoking Cessation

Adult: **PO** Begin with 0.5 mg/day for 3 days, increase to 0.5 mg bid for 4 days, then increase to 1 mg bid on day 8. Treat for 12 wk and may repeat an additional 12 wk.

Renal Impairment Dosage Adjustment

CrCl 50 mL/min or less: Titrate to 0.5 mg bid (max)

ADMINISTRATION

Oral

- Give after a meal with a full glass of water.
- Dose titration over 8 days (from 0.5 to 2 mg daily) is recommended to minimize adverse effects.
- Store at 15°–30° C (59°–86° F).

ADVERSE EFFECTS **CV:** Chest pain, hypertension. **Respiratory:** Dyspnea, epistaxis, respiratory disorder, rhinorrhea. **CNS:** *Abnormal dreams*, anorexia, anxiety, asthenia, disturbance in attention, depression, dizziness, drowsiness, emotional lability, *insomnia*, irritability, *nightmares*, restlessness, sensory disturbance, *sleep disorder*, <u>suicidality</u>. **HEENT:** Dysgeusia, xerostomia. **Endocrine:** Abnormal liver function test, appetite stimulation, weight gain. **Skin:** Hyperhidrosis, pruritus, rash. **GI:** Abdominal pain, *constipation*, diarrhea, dyspepsia, *flatulence*, gastroesophageal reflux, *nausea, vomiting*. **GU:** Menstrual irregularity, polyuria. **Musculoskeletal:** Arthralgia, back pain, muscle cramps, musculoskeletal pain, myalgia. **Other:** Fatigue, flushing, gingivitis, headache, influenza-like symptoms, lethargy, malaise, thirst.

INTERACTIONS **Drug: Cimetidine** increases systemic exposure to varenicline by 29%.

PHARMACOKINETICS **Absorption:** Complete absorption from GI tract. **Peak:** 3–4 h. **Distribution:** Less than 20% protein bound. **Metabolism:** Minimal. **Elimination:** Primarily eliminated unchanged in the urine. **Half-Life:** 24 h.

NURSING IMPLICATIONS

Black Box Warning

Varenicline has been associated with increased risk of depression, suicidal ideation, and suicide attempt.

Assessment & Drug Effects

- Monitor smoking cessation behavior and adverse effects.
- Monitor BP for new-onset hypertension.
- Monitor diabetics for loss of glycemic control.
- Monitor for increased suicidality, or increase in agitation or aggression.

Patient & Family Education

- Report persistent nausea, vomiting, or insomnia to a health care provider.
- Report new-onset of depressed mood, suicidal ideation, or changes in emotion and behavior resulting from the use of varenicline.

VARICELLA VACCINE

(var-i-cel'la)

Varivax

See Appendix J.

VASOPRESSIN INJECTION

(vay-soe-press'in)

Vasostrict

Classification: PITUITARY HORMONE; ANTIDIURETIC HORMONE (ADH)

Therapeutic: ADH REPLACEMENT

AVAILABILITY Solution for injection

ACTION & *THERAPEUTIC EFFECT* Produces concentrated urine by increasing tubular reabsorption of water (ADH activity), thus reabsorbing up to 90% of water in renal tubules. Causes contraction of smooth muscles of the GI tract as well as the vascular system, especially capillaries, arterioles, and venules. *Effective in reversing diuresis caused by diabetes insipidus. When given intravenously, it is effective as an adjunct in treating massive GI bleeding.*

USES Antidiuretic to treat diabetes insipidus, vasodilatory shock (Vasostrict only).

UNLABELED USES Test for differential diagnosis of nephrogenic, psychogenic, and neurohypophyseal diabetes insipidus; test to elevate ability of kidney to concentrate urine, and provocative test for pituitary release of corticotropin and growth hormone; emergency and adjunct pressor agent in the control of massive GI hemorrhage (e.g., esophageal varices).

CONTRAINDICATIONS Hypersensitivity to vasopression or any of the components in formulation; uncorrected nephritis accompanied by nitrogen retention; ischemic heart disease, PVCs, advanced arteriosclerosis; lactation.

CAUTIOUS USE Epilepsy; migraine; asthma; heart failure, angina pectoris; any state in which rapid addition to extracellular fluid may be hazardous; vascular disease; older adults; labor and delivery; pregnancy (category C); children.

ROUTE & DOSAGE

Diabetes Insipidus

Adult: **IM/Subcutaneous** 5–10 units aqueous solution 2–4 × day (5–60 units/day) or 1.25–2.5 units in oil q2–3days; **Intranasal** Apply to cotton pledget or intranasal spray

Child: **IM/Subcutaneous** 2.5–10 units aqueous solution 2–4 × day

Vasodilatory Shock

Adult: **IV** 0.03 units/min can titrate up by 0.005 units/min at 10–15 min intervals (max: 0.1 unit/min)

GI Hemorrhage

Adult: **IV** 20 units bolus then 0.2–0.4 units/min up to 0.9 units/min

Septic Shock

Adult: IV 0.01 units/min then can titrate up by 0.005 units/min (max: 0.07 units/min)

ADMINISTRATION

Intramuscular/Subcutaneous

- Give 1–2 glasses of water with vasopressin to reduce adverse

V

effects such as skin blanching, abdominal cramps and nausea.

- Give IM injection deeply into a large muscle.
- With subcutaneous injection, exercise caution not to inject intradermally.

Intravenous

PREPARE: **Direct/IV Infusion:** Dilute with NS or D5W to a concentration of 0.1–1 units/mL.

ADMINISTER: **Direct:** Give rapid bolus dose. **IV Infusion:** Titrate dose and rate to patient's response.

- Ensure patency prior to injection or infusion as extravasation may cause severe vasoconstriction with tissue necrosis and gangrene.

ADVERSE EFFECTS **CV:** Angina pectoris, atrial fibrillation, bradycardia, cardiac arrhythmia, peripheral vasoconstriction. **Respiratory:** Bronchoconstriction. **CNS:** Headache, vertigo. **Endocrine:** Hyponatremia, hypovolemic shock. **Skin:** Circumoral pallor, diaphoresis, urticaria. **Hepatic/GI:** Increased serum bilirubin, abdominal cramps, flatulence, nausea, vomiting. **GU:** Renal insufficiency. **Musculoskeletal:** Tremor. **Hematologic:** Decreased platelet count, hemorrhage. **Other:** Anaphylaxis.

DIAGNOSTIC TEST INTERFERENCE Vasopressin increases ***plasma cortisol*** levels.

INTERACTIONS **Drug: Alcohol, demeclocycline, epinephrine, heparin, lithium, phenytoin** may decrease antidiuretic effects of vasopressin; **guanethidine, neostigmine** increase vasopressor actions; **chlorpropamide, clofibrate, carbamazepine**, THIAZIDE DIURETICS may increase antidiuretic activity.

PHARMACOKINETICS **Duration:** 2–8 h in aqueous solution, 48–72 h in oil, 30–60 min IV infusion. **Distribution:** Extracellular fluid. **Metabolism:** In liver and kidneys. **Elimination:** In urine. **Half-Life:** 10–20 min.

NURSING IMPLICATIONS

Assessment & Drug Effects

- Monitor infants and children closely. They are more susceptible to volume disturbances (such as sudden reversal of polyuria) than adults.
- Establish baseline data of BP, weight, I&O pattern and ratio. Monitor BP and weight throughout therapy. (Dose used to stimulate diuresis has little effect on BP.) Report sudden changes in pattern to prescriber.
- Be alert to the fact that even small doses of vasopressin may precipitate MI or coronary insufficiency, especially in older adult patients. Keep emergency equipment and drugs (antiarrhythmics) readily available.
- Check patient's alertness and orientation frequently during therapy. Lethargy and confusion associated with headache may signal onset of water intoxication, which, although insidious in rate of development, can lead to convulsions and terminal coma.
- Monitor urine output, specific gravity, and serum osmolality while patient is hospitalized.
- Withhold vasopressin, restrict fluid intake, and notify prescriber if urine-specific gravity is less than 1.015.

Patient & Family Education

- Be prepared for possibility of anginal attack and have coronary vasodilator available (e.g., nitroglycerin) if there is a history of coronary artery disease. Report to prescriber.
- With diabetes insipidus, measure and record data related to

polydipsia and polyuria. Keep an accurate record of output. Understand that treatment should diminish intense thirst and restore undisturbed normal sleep.

- Avoid concentrated fluids (e.g., undiluted syrups), since these increase urine volume.

VECURONIUM BROMIDE

(vek-yoo-roe′nee-um)

Classification: NONDEPOLARIZING SKELETAL MUSCLE RELAXANT; ACETYLCHOLINE RECEPTOR ANTAGONIST

Therapeutic: SKELETAL MUSCLE RELAXANT

Prototype: Atracurium

AVAILABILITY Intravenous solution

ACTION & *THERAPEUTIC EFFECT* Intermediate-acting nondepolarizing skeletal muscle relaxant that inhibits neuromuscular transmission by competitively binding with acetylcholine at receptors located on motor endplate receptors. *Effective as a skeletal muscle relaxant.*

USES Adjunct for general anesthesia to produce skeletal muscle relaxation during surgery.

CONTRAINDICATIONS Hypersensitivity to vecuronium.

CAUTIOUS USE Severe liver disease; impaired acid–base, fluid and electrolyte balance; long-term use; severe obesity; adrenal or neuromuscular disease (myasthenia gravis, Eaton–Lambert syndrome); patients with slow circulation time (cardiovascular disease, old age, edematous states); obesity, pregnancy (category C); lactation; children younger than 1 y and older than 7 wk.

ROUTE & DOSAGE

Skeletal Muscle Relaxation

Adult/Child (10 y or older): **IV** 0.08–0.1 mg/kg initially, then after 25–40 min, 0.01–0.15 mg/kg q12–15min or 0.001 mg/kg/min by continuous infusion for prolonged procedures

Child (1–10 y)/Infant: **IV** Varies greatly; may require higher initial dose

Obesity Dosage Adjustment

Dose based on IBW

ADMINISTRATION

Note: Vecuronium is administered only by qualified clinicians.

Intravenous

PREPARE: **Direct:** Reconstitute the 10 or 20 mg vial with 10 or 20 mL, respectively, of sterile water for injection (supplied). **Continuous:** Further dilute the reconstituted solution in up to 100 mL D5W, NS, or LR to yield 0.1–0.2 mg/mL.

ADMINISTER: **Direct:** Give a bolus dose over 30 sec. **Continuous:** Give at the required rate.

INCOMPATIBILITIES: **Y-site: Amphotericin B cholesteryl complex, diazepam, etomidate, furosemide.**

- Refrigerate after reconstitution below 30° C (86° F), unless otherwise directed. Discard solution after 24 h.

ADVERSE EFFECTS **Respiratory:** Respiratory depression. **Other:** Skeletal muscle weakness, malignant hyperthermia.

INTERACTIONS **Drug:** GENERAL ANESTHETICS increase neuromuscular blockade and duration of action; AMINOGLYCOSIDES, **polymyxin B, clindamycin, lidocaine, parenteral magnesium, quinidine, quinine, trimethaphan, verapamil** increase neuromuscular blockade; DIURETICS may increase or decrease neuromuscular blockade; **lithium** prolongs duration of neuromuscular blockade; NARCOTIC ANALGESICS increase possibility of additive respiratory depression; **succinylcholine** increases onset and depth of neuromuscular blockade; **phenytoin** may cause resistance to or reversal of neuromuscular blockade.

PHARMACOKINETICS **Onset:** Less than 1 min. **Peak:** 3–5 min. **Duration:** 25–40 min. **Distribution:** Well distributed to tissues and extracellular fluids; crosses placenta; distribution into breast milk unknown. **Metabolism:** Rapid nonenzymatic degradation in bloodstream. **Elimination:** 30–35% in urine, 30–35% in bile. **Half-Life:** 30–80 min.

NURSING IMPLICATIONS

Assessment & Drug Effects

- Use peripheral nerve stimulator during and following drug administration to avoid risk of overdosage and to identify residual paralysis during recovery period. This is especially indicated when cautious use of drug is specified.
- Monitor vital signs at least q15min until stable, then q30min for the next 2 h. Also monitor airway patency until assured that patient has fully recovered from drug effects. Note rate, depth, and pattern of respirations. Obese patients and patients with myasthenia gravis or other neuromuscular disease may have ventilation problems.
- Evaluate patients for recovery from neuromuscular blocking (curare-like) effects as evidenced by ability to breathe naturally or take deep breaths and cough, to keep eyes open, and to lift head keeping mouth closed and by adequacy of hand grip strength. Notify prescriber if recovery is delayed.
- Note: Recovery time may be delayed in patients with cardiovascular disease, edematous states, and in older adults.
- Monitor lab tests: Baseline serum electrolytes, acid–base balance, LFTs, and renal function tests.

VEDOLIZUMAB

(ve-dol′i-zu-mab)

Entyvio

Classification: BIOLOGICAL RESPONSE MODIFIER; MONOCLONAL ANTIBODY; INTEGRIN INHIBITOR

Therapeutic: IMMUNOSUPPRESSANT

Prototype: Basiliximab

AVAILABILITY Lyophilized powder for reconstitution and injection

ACTION & *THERAPEUTIC EFFECT* Inhibits the migration of memory T-lymphocytes, which promote inflammation, across the endothelium into inflamed GI tissue. *Decreases inflammation and other responses.*

USES Treatment of moderate-to-severe ulcerative colitis (UC) and Crohn's disease (CD) in adults who have had inadequate response to a tumor necrosis factor (TNF) blocker or immunomodulator, or were unable to achieve corticosteroid-free remission.

CONTRAINDICATIONS Known serious or severe hypersensitivity to vedolizumab or any component

V

of the formulation; dyspnea, bronchospasm; progressive multifocal leukoencephalopathy (PML); active serious infection; jaundice or liver injury due to vedolizumab.

CAUTIOUS USE History of recurrent mild or moderate infection; liver impairment. Safety and efficacy in children younger than 18 y not established.

ROUTE & DOSAGE

Ulcerative Colitis or Crohn's Disease

Adult: **IV** 300 mg infusion, again at wk 2 and wk 6, then 300 mg every 8 wk; discontinue if no benefit after wk 14

ADMINISTRATION

Intravenous

PREPARE: **IV Infusion:** Reconstitute vial with 4.8 mL of SW. Swirl gently for at least 15 sec but do not vigorously shake or invert. Allow vial sit up to 20 min at room temperature to allow foam to settle; vial can be swirled during this time. If not fully dissolved after 20 min, allow another 10 min for dissolution. Do not use the vial if the drug is not dissolved in 30 min. Prior to withdrawing the reconstituted solution from the vial for dilution, gently invert vial 3 times. Withdraw 5 mL (300 mg) of reconstituted solution and add to 250 mL of NS and gently mix the infusion bag. Use as soon as possible.

ADMINISTER: **IV Infusion:** Give over 30 min. **Do not** give IV push or bolus. Flush line after infusion with 30 mL of NS. Observe closely during infusion (until complete) and monitor for hypersensitivity reactions; stop infusion if a reaction occurs.

INCOMPATIBILITIES: Do not add any other drugs or solutions to the IV line.

- Store up to 4 h at 2°–8° C (36°–46° F). Do not freeze.

ADVERSE EFFECTS **Respiratory:** Nasopharyngitis. **CNS:** Headache, fatigue. **Musculoskeletal:** Arthralgia. **Other:** Antibody development.

INTERACTIONS **Drug:** TUMOR NECROSIS FACTOR BLOCKERS may increase the risk of progressive multifocal leukoencephalopathy and other infections if given with vedolizumab. Concomitant use of vedolizumab with ANTINEOPLASTIC AGENTS, IMMUNOSUPPRESSIVES, IMMUNOMODULATING AGENTS, or **natalizumab** may enhance the risk of opportunistic infections.

PHARMACOKINETICS **Half-Life:** 25 d (300 mg dose).

NURSING IMPLICATIONS

Assessment & Drug Effects

- Monitor closely for S&S of a hypersensitivity reaction (see Appendix F). Interrupt infusion and notify prescriber if hypersensitivity is suspected.
- Monitor for and report promptly S&S of an infection, especially in the upper respiratory tract.
- Monitor for signs of hepatotoxicity (see Appendix F).
- Monitor lab test: Baseline TB screening; periodic LFTs.

Patient & Family Education

- Report immediately if you experience S&S of a hypersensitivity reaction (e.g., itching, rash, swelling about the mouth and face,

V

difficulty breathing, dizziness, feeling hot, or palpitations).

- Needed immunizations should be brought up to date before beginning therapy with vedolizumab.
- Report promptly to prescriber S&S of an infection (e.g., sinus infection, fever, cough, bronchitis, flu-like symptoms).
- Report to prescriber if you develop S&S of liver damage (e.g., tiredness, loss of appetite, pain on the right side of abdomen, dark urine, or yellowing of the skin and eyes).
- If you are pregnant or plan to become pregnant, immediately consult prescriber.
- Do not breast-feed while taking this drug without consulting prescriber.

VENLAFAXINE

(ven-la-fax′een)

Effexor, Effexor XR

DESVENLAFAXINE

Khedezla, Pristiq

Classification: ANTIDEPRESSANT; SEROTONIN NOREPINEPHRINE REUPTAKE INHIBITOR (SNRI)

Therapeutic: ANTIDEPRESSANT; SNRI

AVAILABILITY Tablet; sustained release capsule; extended release tablet. **Desvenlafaxine:** Extended release tablet

ACTION & *THERAPEUTIC EFFECT*
Potent inhibitor of neuronal serotonin and norepinephrine reuptake. *Antidepressant effect presumed to be due to potentiation of neurotransmitter activity in the CNS.*

USES Major depressive disorder, generalized anxiety disorder; premenstrual dysphoric disorder; social anxiety disorder.

UNLABELED USES Diabetic neuropathy, migraine prevention, obsessive-compulsive disorder, hot flashes, narcolepsy.

CONTRAINDICATIONS Hypersensitivity to venlafaxine or any component of the formulation; concurrent administration with MAO inhibitors or within 14 days of last dose; initiation in patients receiving linezolid or IV methylene blue; abrupt discontinuation; treatment for bipolar depression; serotonin syndrome symptoms; hyponatremia; suicidal ideation; lactation.

CAUTIOUS USE Renal and hepatic impairment, renal failure; anorexia nervosa, history of mania or other psychiatric disorders, history of suicidal tendencies or increase in suicidality especially in individuals younger than 24 y; elevated intraocular pressure, acute closed-angle glaucoma; cardiac disorders, recent MI, heart failure; hypertension; hyperthyroidism; CNS depression; history of seizures or seizure disorders; volume depleted individuals; hypertriglycerides; risk factors for interstitial lung disease; older adults; pregnancy (nonteratogenic adverse effects have been observed with venlafaxine and other SNRIs/SSRIs). Safety in children younger than 18 y not established.

ROUTE & DOSAGE

Depression

Adult: **PO Immediate release** 37.5–75 mg/day in 2–3 divided doses; **Extended release** 37.5–75 mg daily; **Desvenlafaxine:** 50 mg daily, may increase dose after 6 w to 100 mg/day (max: 400 mg/day)

V

Generalized Anxiety

Adult: **PO Sustained release** 37.5–75 mg daily and increase to 75 mg daily after 4–7 days then increase at 4 day intervals as tolerated (max: 225 mg/day)

Social Anxiety Disorder

Adult: **PO Extended release** 37.5 mg daily, increase to 75 mg/day after 1–2 weeks.

Renal Impairment Dosage Adjustment

Venlafaxine: *less than 30 mL/min:* Reduce total daily dose by 50%;
Desvenlafaxine: *CrCl 30–50 mL/min:* Max dose: 50 mg/day; *less than 30 mL/min:* Max dose: 50 mg every other day

Pharmacogenetic Dosage Adjustment

Poor CYP2D6 metabolizer: Start with 70% of dose

ADMINISTRATION

Oral

- Give with food. Extended-release *capsules* **must be** swallowed whole or carefully opened and sprinkled on a spoonful of applesauce. The applesauce mixture should be swallowed without chewing and followed with a glass of water. Extended release *tablets* should be swallowed whole and not divided, crushed, or chewed.
- Allow 14 days interval after discontinuing an MAO inhibitor before starting venlafaxine or desvenlafaxine.
- Do not abruptly withdraw drug after 1 wk or more of therapy.
- Store at room temperature, 15°–30° C (59°–86° F).

V

ADVERSE EFFECTS **CV:** Vasodilation. **CNS:** *Dizziness*, headache, *insomnia, drowsiness*, suicidality. **HEENT:** Visual disturbance. **Endocrine:** Decreased libido, hypercholesterolemia, abnormal orgasm, weight loss. **GI:** *Nausea, vomiting, dry mouth*, constipation, anorexia, diarrhea. **GU:** Impotence, abnormal ejaculation. **Other:** Diaphoresis, asthenia, tremor.

DIAGNOSTIC TEST INTERFERENCE False positive ***urine drug screen*** may occur for amphetamine or phencyclidine; use alternative tests to confirm results.

INTERACTIONS **Drug: Cimetidine**, MAO INHIBITORS, **desipramine, haloperidol** may increase levels and toxicity. Should not use in combination with MAO INHIBITORS: Do not start until greater than 14 days after stopping MAO INHIBITOR; do not start MAO INHIBITOR until 7 days after stopping venlafaxine/desvenlafaxine. **Trazodone** may lead to **serotonin** syndrome. May increase tachycardic effect of ALPHA- OR BETA- AGONISTS. May increase anticoagulant effect of heparin. **Herbal: St. John's wort, sour date nut** may cause **serotonin** syndrome.

PHARMACOKINETICS **Absorption:** Well absorbed from GI tract. **Onset:** 2 wk. **Peak:** Venlafaxine 1–2 h; metabolite 3–4 h. **Duration:** Extensively tissue bound. **Metabolism:** Undergoes substantial first-pass metabolism to its major active metabolite (CYP2D6). **Elimination:** ~60% in urine as parent compound and metabolites. **Half-Life:** Venlafaxine 3–4 h, desvenlafaxine ~11 h.

NURSING IMPLICATIONS

Black Box Warning

Venlafaxine has been associated with increased risk of suicidal thinking and behavior.

Assessment & Drug Effects

- Monitor for worsening of depression or emergence of suicidal ideation.
- Monitor cardiovascular status periodically with measurements of HR and BP.
- Monitor neurologic status and report excessive anxiety, nervousness, and insomnia.
- Monitor weight periodically and report excess weight loss.
- Assess safety, as dizziness and sedation are common.
- Monitor lab tests: Periodic lipid profile.

Patient & Family Education

- Be aware of potential adverse effects and notify prescriber of those that are bothersome.
- Report promptly worsening mental status, especially thoughts of suicide.
- Do not drive or engage in potentially hazardous activities until response to drug is known.
- Avoid using alcohol while on venlafaxine.
- Do not use herbal medications without consulting prescriber.

VERAPAMIL HYDROCHLORIDE

(ver-ap′a-mill)

Calan, Calan SR, Covera-HS, Isoptin SR, Verelan, Verelan PM

Classification: CALCIUM CHANNEL BLOCKER; ANTIHYPERTENSIVE; CLASS IV ANTIARRHYTHMIC

Therapeutic: CLASS IV ANTIARRHYTHMIC; ANTIHYPERTENSIVE; ANTIANGINAL

AVAILABILITY Tablet; sustained release tablet; sustained release capsule; solution for injection

ACTION & *THERAPEUTIC EFFECT* Inhibits calcium ion influx through slow channels into cells of myocardial and arterial smooth muscle. Dilates coronary arteries and arterioles and inhibits coronary artery spasm. Decreases and slows SA and AV node conduction without affecting normal arterial action potential or intraventricular conduction. Dilates peripheral arterioles, causing decreased total peripheral resistance, and this results in lowering the BP. *Decreases angina attacks by dilating coronary arteries and inhibiting coronary vasospasms. Decreases nodal conduction, resulting in an antiarrhythmic effect. Decreased total peripheral vascular resistance; and therefore, reduction in BP.*

USES Supraventricular tachyarrhythmias; Prinzmetal's (variant) angina, chronic stable angina; unstable, crescendo, or preinfarctive angina and essential hypertension.

UNLABELED USES Paroxysmal supraventricular tachycardia, atrial fibrillation; prophylaxis of migraine headache; and as alternate therapy in manic depression.

CONTRAINDICATIONS Severe hypotension (systolic less than 90 mm Hg), cardiogenic shock, cardiomegaly, digitalis toxicity, second- or third-degree AV block; Wolff–Parkinson–White syndrome including atrial flutter and fibrillation; accessory AV pathway, severe

V

left ventricular dysfunction, severe CHF, sinus node disease, sick sinus syndrome (except in patients with functioning ventricular pacemaker); lactation.

CAUTIOUS USE Duchenne's muscular dystrophy; hepatic and renal impairment; mild to moderate left ventricular heart failure; MI followed by coronary occlusion, aortic stenosis; MG; Duchenne muscular dystrophy; GI obstruction, GERD, hiatal hernia, ileus; older adults; pregnancy (category C). **Extended release:** Safe use in children younger than 18 y not established.

ROUTE & DOSAGE

Angina

Adult: **PO** 80 mg q6–8h, may increase up to 320–480 mg/day in divided doses (Note: **Covera-HS must be** given once daily at bedtime)

Hypertension

Adult: **PO Immediate release** 80 mg tid; **Sustained release tablet** 180 mg daily may increase to 240 mg daily (Note: Covera-HS **must be** given once daily at bedtime); **Sustained release capsule** 240 mg daily may adjust to response

Supraventricular Tachycardia, Atrial Fibrillation

Adult/Adolescent (15 y or older): **IV** 5–10 mg after 30 min may give 10 mg (max total dose: 20 mg)
Child/Adolescent (younger than 15 y): **IV** 0.1–0.3 mg/kg (do not exceed 5 mg)
Infant: **IV** 0.1–0.2 mg/kg may repeat after 30 min

Renal Impairment Dosage Adjustment

CrCl less than 10 mL/min: Give 50–75% of dose

Hemodialysis Dosage Adjustment

Supplemental dose not necessary

Hepatic Impairment Dosage Adjustment

Cirrhosis: Use 20–50% of normal dose

ADMINISTRATION

Oral

- Give with food to reduce gastric irritation.
- Capsules can be opened and contents sprinkled on food. **Do not** dissolve or chew capsule contents.
- Do not withdraw abruptly; may increase and extend duration of pain in the angina patient.

Intravenous

PREPARE: **IV Direct:** Given undiluted or diluted in 5 mL of sterile water for injection. ▪ Inspect parenteral drug preparation before administration. Make sure solution is clear and colorless.
ADMINISTER: **Direct:** Give a single dose over 2–3 min.
INCOMPATIBILITIES: **Solution/additive:** **Albumin, aminophylline, amphotericin B, hydralazine, trimethoprim/sulfamethoxazole.** **Y-site:** **Acyclovir, albumin, amphotericin B cholesteryl complex, ampicillin, azathioprine, cefperazone, ceftazidime, chloramphenicol, dantrolene, diazepam, diazoxide, ertapenem, fluorouracil, folic acid, foscarnet, ganciclovir, indomethacin, lansoprazole, nafcillin, oxacillin, pantoprazole,**

pentobarbital, phenobarbital, phenytoin, piperacillin/tazobactam, propofol, sodium bicarbonate, SMZ/TMP, thiotepa, tigecycline.

- Store at 15°–30° C (59°–86° F) and protect from light.

ADVERSE EFFECTS

CV: *Hypotension*, congestive heart failure, bradycardia, severe tachycardia, peripheral edema, AV block. **Respiratory:** Pharyngitis, sinusitus. **CNS:** Dizziness, vertigo, *headache*, fatigue, sleep disturbances, depression, syncope. **Skin:** Pruritus. **GI:** Nausea, abdominal discomfort, *constipation*, elevated liver enzymes. **Other:** Flushing, pulmonary edema, muscle fatigue, diaphoresis.

DIAGNOSTIC TEST INTERFERENCE

May cause false positive for ***urine screen*** detection of **methadone**.

INTERACTIONS

Drug: BETA-BLOCKERS increase risk of CHF, bradycardia, or heart block; significantly increased levels of **digoxin** and **carbamazepine** and toxicity; potentiates hypotensive effects of HYPOTENSIVE AGENTS; levels of **lithium** and **cyclosporine** may be increased, increasing their toxicity; **calcium salts** (IV) may antagonize verapamil effects. **Food: Grapefruit juice** may increase verapamil levels. **Herbal: Hawthorne** may have additive hypotensive effects. **St. John's wort** may decrease efficacy.

PHARMACOKINETICS

Absorption: 90% absorbed, but only 25–30% reaches systemic circulation (first pass metabolism). **Peak:** 1–2 h PO; 4–8 h sustained release; 5 min IV. **Distribution:** Widely distributed, including CNS; crosses placenta; present in breast milk. **Metabolism:** In liver (CYP3A4). **Elimination:** 70% in urine; 16% in feces. **Half-Life:** 2–8 h.

NURSING IMPLICATIONS

Assessment & Drug Effects

- Establish baseline data and periodically monitor BP and pulse with oral administration.
- Following IV infusion, instruct patient to remain in recumbent position for at least 1 h after dose is given to diminish subjective effects of transient asymptomatic hypotension that may accompany infusion.
- Monitor for AV block or excessive bradycardia when IV infusion is given concurrently with digitalis.
- Monitor I&O ratio during IV and early oral maintenance therapy. Renal impairment prolongs duration of action, increasing potential for toxicity and incidence of adverse effects. Advise patient to report gradual weight gain and evidence of edema.
- Monitor ECG continuously during IV administration. Essential because drug action may be prolonged and incidence of adverse reactions is highest during IV administration in older adults, patients with impaired kidney function, and patients of small stature.
- Check BP shortly before administration of next dose to evaluate degree of control during early treatment for hypertension.
- Monitor lab tests: Baseline and periodic LFTs and renal function tests.

Patient & Family Education

- Monitor radial pulse before each dose, notify prescriber of an irregular pulse or one slower than established guideline.

V

- Do not drive or engage in potentially hazardous activities until response to drug is known.
- Decrease intake of caffeinecontaining beverage (i.e., coffee, tea, chocolate).
- Change positions slowly from lying down to standing to prevent falls because of drug-related vertigo until tolerance to reduced BP is established.
- Notify prescriber of easy bruising, petechiae, unexplained bleeding.
- Do not use OTC drugs, especially aspirin, unless they are specifically prescribed by prescriber.

VIBEGRON

(vye-BEG-ron)

Gemtesa

Classifications: GENITOURINARY AGENT; BETA-3 ADRENERGIC AGONIST; ANTISPASMOTIC

Therapeutic: ANTISPASMOTIC

AVAILABILITY Oral tablet

ACTION & *THERAPEUTIC EFFECT* A selective beta-3 adrenergic receptor agonist that increases bladder capacity by relaxing the detrusor smooth muscle during bladder filling.

USES Treatment of overactive bladder.

CONTRAINDICATIONS Known hypersensitivity to vibegron or any components of the product; pregnancy—fetal risk cannot be ruled out; lactation—infant risk cannot be ruled out; safety and efficacy not established in pediatric patients.

CAUTIOUS USE Patients with a history of bladder outlet obstruction and those taking muscarinic antagonist medications for overactive bladder.

ROUTE & DOSAGE

Overactive Bladder

Adult: **PO** 75 mg once daily

Renal Impairment Dosage Adjustment

eGFR less than 15 mL/min: Not recommended

Hepatic Impairment Dosage Adjustment

Child-Pugh class C (Severe impairment): Not recommended

ADMINISTRATION

Oral

- Give with or without food.
- Swallow tablets whole with a glass of water.
- Tablets may be crushed, mixed with approximately 15 mL (one tablespoonful) of applesauce and taken immediately with a glass of water.
- Store at a controlled room temperature between 20 and 25° C (68 and 77° F), with excursions permitted between 15 and 30° C (59 and 86° F).

ADVERSE EFFECTS (not common) **Respiratory:** Nasopharyngitis. **CNS:** Headache. **GI:** Diarrhea, nausea. **GU:** Urinary tract infection, urinary retention.

INTERACTIONS **Drug:** Vibegron my increase concentrations of **digoxin**; carefully monitor serum digoxin levels during concomitant use.

PHARMACOKINETICS **Peak:** 1–3 h. **Distribution:** 50% protein-bound. **Metabolism:** Liver through CYP3A4. **Elimination:** 59% excreted in feces; 20% in urine. **Half-Life:** 31 h.

NURSING IMPLICATIONS

Assessment & Drug Effects

- Improvement in symptoms of an overactive bladder including urinary incontinence, urgency, and urinary frequency.
- Monitor for urinary retention

Patient & Family Education

- Report symptoms of urinary retention.
- Review adverse effects with patient and caregivers.
- Instruct a patient that has difficulty swallowing how to crush, mix with applesauce and follow with a glass of water immediately.

VILAZODONE

(vil-az'oh-done)

Vibryd

Classification: SELECTIVE SEROTONIN REUPTAKE INHIBITOR (SSRI); PSYCHOTHERAPEUTIC AGENT; ANTIDEPRESSANT

Therapeutic: ANTIDEPRESSANT; SSRI

Prototype: Fluoxetine

AVAILABILITY Tablet

ACTION & *THERAPEUTIC EFFECT* A selective serotonin reuptake inhibitor (SSRI). Antidepressant effect is presumed to be linked to inhibition of CNS neuronal uptake of the neurotransmitter, serotonin. *Improves mood in those with major depressive disorder.*

USES Treatment of major depressive disorder.

CONTRAINDICATIONS Concomitant use of MAOIs or MAOIs within the preceding 14 days; suicidal ideation.

CAUTIOUS USE History of suicidal thoughts; potential precursors to suicidal impulses (e.g., anxiety, agitation, panic attacks, insomnia, irritability, hostility, aggressiveness, impulsivity, psychomotor restlessness, hypomania, mania); history of seizure disorder; concurrent use of NSAIDs, aspirin, or other drugs that affect coagulation or bleeding; pregnancy (limited information related to use during pregnancy; patients exposed to antidepressants during pregnancy are encouraged to enroll in the National Pregnancy Registry for Antidepressants); lactation. Safety and efficacy in children younger than 18 y not established.

ROUTE & DOSAGE

Major Depressive Disorder

Adult: **PO** Initial dose of 10 mg once daily for 7 days, increase to 20 mg once daily for 7 days, then to 40 mg once daily

ADMINISTRATION

Oral

- Give with food to enhance absorption.
- Store at 25° C (77° F).

ADVERSE EFFECTS CNS: *Headache, dizziness,* fatigue, drowsiness, insomnia, suicidality. **Endocrine:** Decreased libido. **GI:** *Diarrhea,* dry mouth, dyspepsia, abdominal pain, *nausea*. **GU:** Erectile dysfunction.

INTERACTIONS Drug: Inducers of CYP3A4 (e.g., **phenytoin**) may reduce the levels of vilazodone. Coadministration or moderate (e.g., **erythromycin**) and strong (e.g., **ketoconazole**) increase the levels of vilazodone and require a dosage reduction to 20 mg once daily. MONOAMINE OXIDASE INHIBITORS

V

increase the levels of vilazodone and should not be used in combination with vilazodone. Coadministration of serotonergic agents (e.g, **busipirone, tramadol, thyptophan**, SELECTIVE SEROTONIN REUPTAKE INHIBITORS, SEROTONIN-NOREPINEPHRINE REUPTAKE INHIBITORS, TRIPTANS) increase the risk of serotonin syndrome. Vilazodone can increase the risk of bleeding if used in combination with **aspirin** or NSAIDs. **Food:** Ingestion of food enhances the absorption of vilazodone. Ethanol increases risk of adverse effects.

PHARMACOKINETICS **Absorption:** Bioavailability 72%. **Peak:** 4–5 h. **Distribution:** 96–99% plasma protein bound. **Metabolism:** Hepatic oxidative metabolism (CYP3A4). **Elimination:** Renal and fecal. **Half-Life:** 25 h.

NURSING IMPLICATIONS

Black Box Warning

Vilazodone has been associated with increased risk of suicidal thinking and behavior.

Assessment & Drug Effects

- Monitor closely and report promptly any of the following: Worsening of clinical symptoms; emergence of suicidal ideation; agitation, irritability, or unusual changes in behavior; signs of serotonin syndrome or neuroleptic malignant syndrome (see Appendix F).
- Supervise patients closely who are high suicide risks; be especially vigilant for changes in behavior and suicidal ideation in children and adolescents.
- Monitor those at risk for volume depletion (e.g., diuretics use) for S&S of hyponatremia.

Patient & Family Education

- Report promptly worsening of condition, suicidal thoughts or thoughts of self-harm.
- Do not abruptly stop taking this drug without consulting prescriber.
- Notify prescriber if you become pregnant or intend to breastfeed.
- Do not drive or engage in other hazardous activities until response to drug is known.
- Consult prescriber prior to using nonsteroidal anti-inflammatory drugs (NSAIDs), aspirin, or other drugs that affect coagulation.

VILOXAZINE

(vye-LOX-a-zeen)

Qelbree

Classifications: MISCELLANEOUS PSYCHOTHERAPEUTIC

Therapeutic: ADHD AGENT

AVAILABILITY Extended release oral capsule

ACTION & *THERAPEUTIC EFFECT*
It is believed that viloxazine inhibits norepinephrine uptake and can improve attention and focus.

USES Acute and maintenance treatment of attention-deficit/hyperactivity disorder (ADHD) in children ages 6 to 17.

CONTRAINDICATIONS Concomitant treatment with MAOI, or within 14 days following discontinuing an MAOI; concomitant administration of CYP1A2 substrates or CYP1A2 substrates with a narrow therapeutic range; pregnancy—fetal risk cannot be ruled out; lactation—infant risk cannot be ruled out. Not approved in pediatric patients under the age of 6 y.

CAUTIOUS USE History of hypertension and tachycardia; patients with bipolar disorder; patients with history of depression, anxiety, agitation, impulsive behavior, and suicidal ideation or behavior.

ROUTE & DOSAGE

Attention-deficit/hyperactivity disorder

Children 6 to 11 yr: **PO** 100 mg once a day; increase dose by 100 mg weekly to response. Max dose of 400 mg a day.
Children ≥12 yr: **PO** 200 mg once a day; may increase to 400 mg after one week based on response. Max dose of 400 mg a day.

Renal Impairment Dosage Adjustment

eGFR less than 30 mL/min: 100 mg once a day; increase dose by 50 to 100 mg weekly to response. Max dose of 200 mg a day.

ADMINISTRATION

Oral

- Give with or without food.
- Do not cut, crush, or chew the tablet
- Swallow capsule whole or may open the capsule and sprinkle the entire contents over a teaspoonful of applesauce; consume all sprinkles and applesauce without chewing within 2 hours of mixing; do not store for future use.
- Store between 20 and 25° C (68 and 77° F); excursions permitted between 15 and 30° C (59 and 86° F).

ADVERSE EFFECTS (>5%) CV: Increased diastolic blood pressure, tachycardia. **Respiratory:** Upper respiratory infection. **CNS:** Somnolence, headache, insomnia, fatigue. **GI:** Decreased appetite, abdominal pain, nausea, vomiting. **Other:** Irritability, suicidal behavior, suicidal thoughts.

INTERACTIONS Drug: CYP1A2 substrates (**duloxetine, ramelteon, tixanidine, clozapine**) should not be used with viloxazine. MAOIS may precipitate a hypertensive crisis; may attenuate effects of ANTIHYPERTENSIVE AGENTS.

PHARMACOKINETICS Absorption: 88% bioavailability; High fat meals may decrease overall availability. **Peak:** 5 h. **Distribution:** 76–82% protein bound. **Metabolism:** Metabolized by CYP2D6, UGT1A9, and UGT2B15. **Elimination:** Primarily renal; 90% in urine. **Half-Life:** ~7 h.

NURSING IMPLICATIONS

Black Box Warning

In clinical studies, higher rates of suicidal thoughts and behavior were reported in pediatric patients with ADHD. Close monitoring of all viloxazine-treated patients for clinical worsening and emergence of suicidal thoughts and behaviors is recommended.

Assessment & Drug Effects

- Improvement in hyperactivity and attention.
- Monitor pulse and blood pressure prior to initiating treatment, following increases in dosage, and periodically while on therapy.
- Monitor suicidal thoughts or behavior.
- Monitor weight.

V

Patient & Family Education

- Avoid activities requiring mental alertness or coordination, such as driving or operating heavy machinery, until drug effects are realized.
- Review adverse effects with patients and caregivers.
- Report new or worsening depression, suicidal ideation, or unusual changes in behavior including symptoms of mania or hypomania.
- Review instructions for mixing sprinkles with applesauce with caregiver if the patient is unable to swallow the capsule whole.

VINBLASTINE SULFATE

(vin-blast′een)

Classification: ANTINEOPLASTIC; MITOTIC INHIBITOR; VINCA ALKALOID

Therapeutic: ANTINEOPLASTIC

Prototype: Vincristine

AVAILABILITY Solution for injection

ACTION & *THERAPEUTIC EFFECT* Cell cycle–specific drug that binds to tubulin and inhibits microtubule formation by disrupting the mitotic spindle during metaphase. Has an effect on cell energy production needed for mitosis and interferes with nucleic acid synthesis. *Interrupts the cell cycle in metaphase, thus preventing cell replication and cancer cell proliferation.*

USES treatment of Hodgkin lymphoma. Kaposi sarcoma, Langerhans cell histiocytosis, testicular cancer and non-Hodgkin lymphomas. Used singly or in combination with other chemotherapeutic drugs.

UNLABELED USES treatment of bladder cancer, non small cell lung cancer.

CONTRAINDICATIONS Severe bone marrow suppression, significant granulocytopenia; bacterial infection; older adult patients with cachexia or skin ulcers; men and women of childbearing potential; pregnancy (females of reproductive potential should avoid becoming pregnant during vinblastine treatment); lactation.

CAUTIOUS USE Malignant cell infiltration of bone marrow; leukopenia; stomatitis; obstructive jaundice, hepatic impairment; history of gout; use of small amount of drug for long periods; use in eyes; children.

ROUTE & DOSAGE

Antineoplastic

Adult: **IV** dose varies based on protocol; usual range 5.5–7.4 mg/m^2 q7 days; (max dose: 18.5 mg/m^2)

Hodgkin Lymphoma

Child: **IV** 6 mg/m^2 on days 1 and 15 or days 1 and 8 (depends on protocol) of a 28 day cycle.

Hepatic Impairment Dosage Adjustment

bilirubin over 3 mg/dL: Administer 50% of dose

ADMINISTRATION

Intravenous

This drug is a cytotoxic agent and caution should be used to prevent any contact with the drug. Follow institutional or standard guidelines for preparation, handling, and disposal of cytotoxic agents.

PREPARE: **Direct:** Add 10 mL NS to 10 mg of drug to yield 1 mg/mL. Do not use other diluents. ▪ Avoid contact with eyes. Severe irritation and persisting corneal changes may occur. Flush immediately and thoroughly with copious amounts of water. Wash both eyes; do not assume one eye escaped contamination.

ADMINISTER: **Direct:** Drug is usually injected into tubing of running IV infusion of NS or D5W over period of 1 min. Prolonged administration over > 30–60 minutes may increase the risk of vein irritation and extravasation. ▪ Stop injection promptly if extravasation occurs. Use applications of moderate heat and local injection of hyaluronidase to help disperse extravasated drug. ▪ Observe injection site for sloughing. ▪ Restart infusion in another vein.

INCOMPATIBILITIES: **Y-site: Amphotericin B, cefepime, dantrolene, diazepam, furosemide, gemtuzumab, lansoprazole, pantoprazole, phenytoin.**

▪ Refrigerate reconstituted solution in tight, light-resistant containers up to 30 days without loss of potency.

ADVERSE EFFECTS **Cardiovascular:** Angina pectoris, ECG abnormality, hypertension, Raynaud's phenomenon, limb ischemia, myocardial infarction. **Respiratory:** Bronchospasm, dyspnea, pharyngitis. **CNS:** Mental depression, peripheral neuritis, numbness and paresthesias of tongue and extremities, loss of deep tendon reflexes, headache, convulsions. **HEENT:** Nystagmus, auditory disturbance, deafness, vestibular disturbance. **Endocrine:** SIADH. **Skin:** *Alopecia (reversible)*, dermatitis, photosensitivity, skin blister; phlebitis, cellulitis, and sloughing following extravasation (at injection site). **GI:** Vesiculation of mouth, stomatitis, pharyngitis, anorexia, *nausea, vomiting*, diarrhea, ileus, abdominal pain, constipation, rectal bleeding, hemorrhagic enterocolitis. **GU:** Urinary retention, *hyperuricemia*, azoospermia. **Hematologic:** Leukopenia, thrombocytopenia, *bone marrow depression*, *granulocytopenia*, thrombocytopenic purpura, anemia. **Musculoskeletal:** *Jaw pain*, myalgia, ostealgia, weakness.

INTERACTIONS **Drug: Mitomycin** may cause acute shortness of breath and severe bronchospasm; ALFA INTERFERONS, **erythromycin, itraconazole** may increase vinblastine toxicity. Increased risk of neutropenia when used with **deferiprone**. CYP 3A4 INHIBITORS (ex ketoconazole, clarithromycin, ritonavir) may increase concentration of vinblasine; CYP 3A4 INDUCERS may decrease concentration of vinblastine. Use with IMMUNOSUPPRESSANTS may have additive immunosuppressant effects. Do not administer LIVE VACCINES.

PHARMACOKINETICS **Distribution:** Concentrates in liver, platelets, and leukocytes; poor penetration of blood–brain barrier. **Metabolism:** Partially in liver (via CYP 3A4) **Elimination:** In feces and urine. **Half-Life:** 24 h.

NURSING IMPLICATIONS

Black Box Warning

Vinblastine extravasation has been associated with severe tissue irritation. Vinblastine is fatal if given intrathecally.

V

Assessment & Drug Effects

- Monitor for and report promptly unexplained bruising or bleeding.
- Adverse reactions seldom persist beyond 24 h with exception of leukopenia, and neurological adverse effects.
- Monitor GI adverse effects which may range from nausea and vomiting to severe constipation.
- Report promptly if oral mucosa tissue breakdown is noted.
- Monitor lab tests: Baseline and periodic CBC with differential, platelet count, serum uric acid, LFTs.

Patient & Family Education

- Be aware that temporary mental depression sometimes occurs on second or third day after treatment begins.
- Avoid exposure to infection, injury to skin or mucous membranes, and excessive physical stress.
- Report immediately to prescriber development of sore mouth, sore throat, fever, or chills.
- Notify prescriber promptly about onset of symptoms of agranulocytosis (see Appendix F). Do not delay seeking appropriate treatment.

VINCRISTINE SULFATE

(vin-kris′teen)

Classification: ANTINEOPLASTIC; MITOTIC INHIBITOR; VINCA ALKALOID

Therapeutic: ANTINEOPLASTIC

AVAILABILITY solution for injection

ACTION & *THERAPEUTIC EFFECT* Cell cycle–specific vinca alkaloid arrests mitosis at metaphase by inhibition of mitotic spindle function, thereby inhibiting cell division. *Induction of metaphase arrest in 50% of cells results in inhibition of cancer cell proliferation.*

USES Acute lymphoblastic leukemia, Hodgkin lymphoma, lymphosarcoma, neuroblastoma, Wilms tumor, rhabdomyosarcoma.

UNLABELED USES Central nervous system tumors, Ewing sarcoma, multiple myeloma.

CONTRAINDICATIONS Obstructive jaundice; active infection; adynamic ileus; radiation of the liver; patient with demyelinating form of Charcot–Marie–Tooth syndrome; men and women of childbearing potential; pregnancy (in utero exposure to vincristine may cause fetal harm); lactation.

CAUTIOUS USE Leukopenia; preexisting neuromuscular or neurologic disease; hypertension; hepatic or biliary tract disease; older adults; children.

ROUTE & DOSAGE

All

Adult: **IV** Varies based on concurrent medications usually 1.5 or 2 mg/m^2 *Child (weight greater than 10 kg):* **IV** Varies based on concurrent medications usually 1.5 mg/m^2 (max: 2 mg/m^2)

Hodgkin Lymphoma

Adult/Adolescent/Child: **IV** 1.4 mg/m^2 frequency varies based on concurrent medications

Non-Hodgkin Lymphoma

Adult/Adolescent/Child: **IV** usually 1.5 or 2 mg/m^2 frequency varies based on concurrent medications

Hepatic Impairment Dosage Adjustment

Bilirubin 1.5–3 mg/dL: Use 50% of dose

ADMINISTRATION

Intravenous

This drug is a cytotoxic agent and caution should be used to prevent any contact with the drug. Follow institutional or standard guidelines for preparation, handling, and disposal of cytotoxic agents.

PREPARE: **Direct:** No dilution is required. Administer as supplied. ▪ Avoid contact with eyes. Severe irritation and persisting corneal changes may occur. Flush immediately and thoroughly with copious amounts of water. Wash both eyes; do not assume one eye escaped contamination.

ADMINISTER: **Direct:** Administer minibag (25 to 50 mL bag) over 5 to 15 minutes. ▪ Stop injection promptly if extravasation occurs. Use applications of moderate heat and local injection of hyaluronidase to help disperse extravasated drug. ▪ Restart infusion in another vein. Observe injection site for sloughing.

INCOMPATIBILITIES: **Y-site: Amphotericin B colloidal, cefepime, diazepam, gemtuzumab, idarubicin, lansoprazole, nafcillin, pantoprazole, phenytoin.**

▪ Store solution in the refrigerator.

ADVERSE EFFECTS **CV:** Hypertension, hypotension, edema, ischemic heart disease, myocardial infarction, phlebitis. **Respiratory:** Bronchospasm, dyspnea. **CNS:** *Peripheral neuropathy*, neuritic pain, *paresthesias, especially of hands and feet*; foot and hand drop, sensory loss, athetosis, ataxia, loss of deep tendon reflexes, muscle atrophy, dysphagia, weakness in larynx and extrinsic eye muscles, ptosis, diplopia, mental depression, abnormal gait. **HEENT:** Optic atrophy with blindness; transient cortical blindness, ptosis, diplopia, photophobia, deafness. **Endocrine:** Hyperuricemia, hyperkalemia. **Skin:** Urticaria, rash, *alopecia*, cellulitis and phlebitis following extravasation (at injection site). **GI:** Stomatitis, pharyngitis, anorexia, nausea, vomiting, diarrhea, abdominal cramps, *severe constipation (upper-colon impaction), paralytic ileus (especially in children)*, rectal bleeding; <u>hepatotoxicity</u>. **GU:** Urinary retention, polyuria, dysuria, SIADH (high urinary sodium excretion, hyponatremia, dehydration, hypotension); uric acid nephropathy. **Other:** Convulsions with hypertension, malaise, fever, headache, pain in parotid gland area, weight loss.

INTERACTIONS **Drug: Mitomycin** may cause acute shortness of breath and severe bronchospasm; CYP 3A4 INHIBITORS (ex **ketoconazole, clarithromycin, ritonavir**) may increase concentration of vincristine; CYP 3A4 INDUCERS may decrease concentration of vincristine.

PHARMACOKINETICS **Distribution:** Concentrates in liver, platelets, and leukocytes; poor penetration of blood–brain barrier. **Metabolism:** Partially in liver (CYP3A4). **Elimination:** Primarily in feces. **Half-Life:** 10–155 h.

NURSING IMPLICATIONS

Black Box Warning

Vincristine extravasation has been associated with severe tissue irritation. Vincristine is fatal if given intrathecally.

Assessment & Drug Effects

▪ Monitor I&O ratio and pattern, BP, and temperature daily.

- Monitor respiratory status. Report promptly shortness of breath (bronchospasms) which may occur within minutes or hours of drug infusion.
- Be aware that neuromuscular adverse effects, most apt to appear in the patient with preexisting neuromuscular disease, usually disappear after 6 wk of treatment. Children are especially susceptible to neuromuscular adverse effects.
- Assess for hand muscular weakness, and check deep tendon reflexes (depression of Achilles reflex is the earliest sign of neuropathy). Also observe for and report promptly: Mental depression, ptosis, double vision, hoarseness, paresthesias, neuritic pain, and motor difficulties.
- Provide special protection against infection or injury during leukopenic days.
- Avoid use of rectal thermometer or intrusive tubing to prevent injury to rectal mucosa.
- Monitor ability to ambulate and supply support as needed.
- Start a prophylactic bowel regimen against constipation and paralytic ileus at beginning of treatment (paralytic ileus is most likely to occur in young children).
- Monitor for signs/symptoms of peripheral neuropathy.
- Monitor lab tests: Baseline and periodic CBC with differential; electrolytes; LFTs; and serum uric acid levels.

Patient & Family Education

- Notify prescriber promptly of stomach, bone, or joint pain, and swelling of lower legs and ankles.
- Report changes in bowel habit as soon as manifested.
- Report a steady gain or sudden weight change to prescriber.
- Women should use effective means of contraception during treatment.

V

VINORELBINE TARTRATE

(vin-o-rel′been)

Navelbine

Classification: ANTINEOPLASTIC; MITOTIC INHIBITOR; VINCA ALKALOID

Therapeutic: ANTINEOPLASTIC

Prototype: Vincristine

AVAILABILITY Solution for injection

ACTION & *THERAPEUTIC EFFECT* A semisynthetic vinca alkaloid with antineoplastic activity. Inhibits polymerization of tubules into microtubules, which disrupts mitotic spindle formation. *Arrests mitosis at metaphase, thereby inhibiting cell division in cancer cells.*

USES Non–small-cell lung cancer.

UNLABELED USES Breast cancer, ovarian cancer, Hodgkin lymphoma.

CONTRAINDICATIONS Hypersensitivity to vinorelbine, infection; severe bone marrow suppression; granylocyte counts greater than or equal to 1000 cells/mm^3; pulmonary toxicity to drug; constipation, ileus; pregnancy (may cause fetal harm if administered to a pregnant female); lactation.

CAUTIOUS USE Hypersensitivity to vincristine or vinblastine; leukopenia or other indicator(s) of bone marrow suppression; chickenpox or herpes zoster infection; hepatic insufficiency, severe liver disease; pulmonary disease; preexisting neurologic or neuromuscular disorders; older adults. Safety and efficacy in children not established.

ROUTE & DOSAGE

Non–Small-Cell Lung Cancer

Adult: **IV** 25–30 mg/m^2 weekly; may require toxicity adjustment

Hepatic Impairment Dosage Adjustment

Bilirubin 2.1–3 mg/dL: Use 50% of dose; *greater than 3 mg/dL:* Use 25% of dose

ADMINISTRATION

Intravenous

This drug is a cytotoxic agent and caution should be used to prevent any contact with the drug. Follow institutional or standard guidelines for preparation, handling, and disposal of cytotoxic agents.

PREPARE: **IV Infusion:** *Method One:* Dilute each 10 mg in a syringe with either 2 or 5 mL of D5W or NS to yield 3 mg/mL or 1.5 mg/L, respectively. *Method Two:* Dilute the required dose in an IV bag with D5W, NS, or LR to a final concentration of 0.5–2 mg/mL (e.g., 10 mg diluted in 19 mL yields 0.5 mg/mL).

ADMINISTER: **IV Infusion:** Give diluted solution over 6–10 min into the side port closest to an IV bag with free-flowing IV solution; follow by flushing with at least 75–125 mL of IV solution over 10 min. ▪ Take every precaution to avoid extravasation. If suspected, discontinue IV immediately and begin in a different site.

INCOMPATIBILITIES: Y-site: **Acyclovir, allopurinol, aminophylline, amphotericin B, amphotericin B cholesteryl complex, ampicillin, cefazolin, cefepime, cefoperazone, cefotetan, cefoxitin, ceftriaxone, cefuroxime, chloramphenicol, dantrolene, diazepam, fluorouracil, foscarnet, furosemide, ganciclovir, ketorolac, lansoprazole, methohexital, methylprednisolone, mitomycin, nafcillin, nitroprusside, pantoprazole, phenobarbital, phenytoin, piperacillin, sodium bicarbonate, SMZ/TMP, thiotepa.**

▪ Store at 2°–8° C (36°–46° F).

ADVERSE EFFECTS **Cardiac:** Chest pain. **CNS:** *Neurotoxicity, peripheral neuropathy.* **Skin:** Alopecia. **Hepatic/GI:** Paralytic ileus, *constipation, nausea, vomiting, diarrhea*, stomatitis, mucositis, hepatotoxicity *(elevated LFT)*, increased serum bilirubin. **GU:** Increased serum creatinine. **Hematologic:** *Anemia*, *febrile neutropenia, granulocytopenia*, thrombocytopenia, leukopenia. **Musculoskeletal:** Asthenia. **Other:** *Injection site reaction*, sepsis.

INTERACTIONS **Drug:** Increased severity of granulocytopenia in combination with **cisplatin**; increased risk of acute pulmonary reactions in combination with **mitomycin; paclitaxel** may increase neuropathy. CYP 3A4 INHIBITORS (ex **ketoconazole, clarithromycin, ritonavir**) may increase concentration of vinorelbine; CYP 3A4 INDUCERS may decrease concentration of vinorelbine; do not administer LIVE VACCINES. Use with IMMUNOSUPPRESSANTS may have additive adverse effects.

PHARMACOKINETICS **Distribution:** 60–80% bound to plasma proteins (including platelets and lymphocytes); sequestered in tissues, especially lung, spleen, liver, and kidney, and released slowly.

Metabolism: In liver (CYP3A4). **Elimination:** Primarily in bile and feces (50%), 10% in urine. **Half-Life:** 42–45 h.

NURSING IMPLICATIONS

Black Box Warning

Vinorelbine has been associated with severe granulocytopenia and increased risk of infection, and extravasation has been associated with severe local tissue necrosis.

Assessment & Drug Effects

- Withhold drug and notify prescriber if the granulocyte count is less than 1000 cells/mm^3.
- Monitor for neurologic dysfunction including paresthesia, decreased deep tendon reflexes, weakness, constipation, and paralytic ileus.
- Monitor for S&S of infection, especially during period of granulocyte nadir 7–10 days after dosing.
- Monitor lab results: CBC with differential (prior to each dose and after treatment); Periodic LFTs, kidney functions, and serum electrolytes. Verify pregnancy status prior to initiation of therapy.

Patient & Family Education

- Be aware of potential and inevitable adverse effects.
- Women should use reliable forms of contraception to prevent pregnancy.
- Notify prescriber of distressing adverse effects, especially symptoms of leukopenia (e.g., chills, fever, cough) and peripheral neuropathy (e.g., pain, numbness, tingling in extremities).
- Report changes in bowel habits as soon as manifested.

VISMODEGIB (Pr)

(vis-mo-de′gib)

Erivedge

Classification: ANTINEOPLASTIC; BIOLOGICAL RESPONSE MODIFIER; SIGNAL TRANSDUCTION INHIBITOR; HEDGEHOG PATHWAY INHIBITOR

Therapeutic: ANTINEOPLASTIC

AVAILABILITY Capsule

ACTION & *THERAPEUTIC EFFECT*

Inhibits the Hedgehog pathway which is needed to produce angiogenic factors and decrease activity of apoptotic genes that allow for tumor expansion. *Slow basal cell tumor growth and development.*

USES Treatment of adults with metastatic basal cell carcinoma, or locally advanced basal cell carcinoma.

CONTRAINDICATIONS Pregnancy (category D); lactation.

CAUTIOUS USE Renal and hepatic impairment; females of reproductive age. Safety and efficacy in children younger than 18 y not established.

ROUTE & DOSAGE

Basal Cell Carcinoma

Adult: **PO** 150 mg once daily

ADMINISTRATION

Oral

- May be given without regard to food.
- Ensure that capsules are swallowed whole. They should not be opened or crushed.
- Store at 15°–30° C (59°–86° F).

V

ADVERSE EFFECTS **Endocrine:** Azotemia, decreased appetite, hypokalemia, hyponatremia, *weight loss*. **GI:** Ageusia, constipation, diarrhea, *dysgeusia, nausea*, vomiting. **Musculoskeletal:** Arthralgias, *muscle spasms*. **Other:** *Alopecia*, fatigue.

INTERACTIONS **Drug:** Coadministration with drugs that inhibit P-glycoprotein (e.g., **clarithromycin, erythromycin, azithromycin**) may increase the levels of vismodegib. Drugs that alter the pH of the upper GI tract (e.g., PROTON PUMP INHIBITORS, H_2-RECEPTOR ANTAGONISTS, and ANTACIDS) may decrease the bioavailability of vismodegib.

PHARMACOKINETICS **Absorption:** 32% bioavailability. **Distribution:** Greater than 99% plasma protein bound. **Metabolism:** In the liver. **Elimination:** Primarily fecal (82%). **Half-Life:** 4 days.

NURSING IMPLICATIONS

Black Box Warning

Vismodegib has been associated with embryo-fetal death and severe birth defects.

Assessment & Drug Effects

- Ensure that women and men understand the risks associated with fetal exposure to this drug during a pregnancy. Advise males of the potential risk of vismodegib exposure through semen.
- Monitor lab tests: Baseline pregnancy test within 7 d before start of therapy; repeat pregnancy test anytime the possibility of a pregnancy arises.

Patient & Family Education

- If a dose is missed, skip the dose and wait for the next scheduled dose.
- Women should use a highly effective means of birth control during therapy and for at least 7 mo following completion of therapy. Contact your prescriber immediately if you become pregnant during treatment.
- Men (even those with a vasectomy) should always use a condom with a spermicide during sex with female partners during treatment and for 2 mo following completion of therapy. Report to prescriber immediately if your partner becomes pregnant or thinks she is pregnant while you are taking this drug.
- Do not breastfeed while receiving this drug.

VITAMIN A

(vye'ta-min A)

Aquasol A, Del-Vi-A

Classification: VITAMIN SUPPLEMENT

Therapeutic: VITAMIN A REPLACEMENT

AVAILABILITY Tablet; capsule; solution for injection

ACTION & *THERAPEUTIC EFFECT* Acts as a cofactor in mucopolysaccharide synthesis, cholesterol synthesis, and the metabolism of hydroxysteroids. *Essential for normal growth and development of bones and teeth, for integrity of epithelial and mucosal surfaces, and for synthesis of visual purple necessary for visual adaptation to the dark. Has antioxidant properties.*

USES Vitamin A deficiency and as dietary supplement during periods of increased requirements, such as pregnancy, lactation, infancy, and infections. Used during fat malabsorption diagnosis, ichthyosis, keratosis follicularis, measles.

CONTRAINDICATIONS History of sensitivity to vitamin A, hypervitaminosis A, oral administration to patients with malabsorption syndrome. Safe use in amounts exceeding 6000 international units during pregnancy (category X if greater than RDA) is not established.

CAUTIOUS USE Women on oral contraceptives, hepatic disease, hepatic dysfunction, hepatitis; renal disease; pregnancy (category A within RDA limit); lactation; children, low-birth weight infants.

ROUTE & DOSAGE

Severe Deficiency

Adult/Child (8 y or older): **PO** 500,000 international units/day for 3 days followed by 50,000 international units/day for 2 wk, then 10,000–20,000 international units/day for 2 mo; **IM** 100,000 international units/day for 3 days followed by 50,000 international units/day for 2 wk
Child (younger than 1 y): **PO/IM** 7500–15,000 international units/day for 10 days; *1–8 y:* 17,000–35,000 international units/day for 2 wk

Dietary Supplement

Child (younger than 4 y): **PO** 300 mcg/day; *4–8 y:* 400 mcg/day

V

ADMINISTRATION

Oral

- Give on an empty stomach or following food or milk if GI upset occurs.
- Store in tight, light-resistant containers.

Intramuscular

- Use IM route only if oral route not feasible.
- Inject deeply into a large muscle.

ADVERSE EFFECTS **CNS:** Irritability, headache, intracranial hypertension (pseudotumor cerebri), increased intracranial pressure, bulging fontanelles, papilledema, exophthalmos, miosis, nystagmus. **Endocrine:** Hypervitaminosis A syndrome (malaise, lethargy, abdominal discomfort, anorexia, vomiting), hypercalcemia. Polydipsia, polyurea. **Skin:** Gingivitis, lip fissures, excessive sweating, drying or cracking of skin, pruritus, increase in skin pigmentation, massive desquamation, brittle nails, alopecia. **GI:** Hepatosplenomegaly, jaundice. **GU:** Hypomenorrhea. **Musculoskeletal:** Slow growth; deep, tender, hard lumps (subperiosteal thickening) over radius, tibia, occiput; migratory arthralgia; retarded growth; premature closure of epiphyses. **Hematologic:** Leukopenia, hypoplastic anemias, vitamin A plasma levels greater than 1200 international units/dL, elevations of sedimentation rate and prothrombin time. **Other:** Anaphylaxis, death (after IV use).

DIAGNOSTIC TEST INTERFERENCE Vitamin A may falsely increase ***serum cholesterol*** determinations ***(Zlatkis-Zak reaction)***; may falsely elevate ***bilirubin*** determination (with ***Ehrlich's reagent***).

INTERACTIONS **Drug:** **Mineral oil, cholestyramine, orlistat** may decrease absorption of vitamin A.

PHARMACOKINETICS **Absorption:** Readily from GI tract in presence of bile salts, pancreatic lipase, and dietary fat. **Distribution:** Stored mainly in liver; small amounts also found in kidney and body fat; distributed into breast milk. **Metabolism:** In liver. **Elimination:** In feces and urine.

NURSING IMPLICATIONS

Assessment & Drug Effects

- Take dietary and drug history (e.g., intake of fortified foods, dietary supplements, self-administration or prescription drug sources). Women taking oral contraceptives tend to have significantly higher plasma vitamin A levels.
- Monitor therapeutic effectiveness. Vitamin A deficiency is often associated with protein malnutrition as well as other vitamin deficiencies. It may manifest as night blindness, restriction of growth and development, epithelial alterations, susceptibility to infection, abnormal dryness of skin, mouth, and eyes (xerophthalmia) progressing to keratomalacia (ulceration and necrosis of cornea and conjunctiva), and urinary tract calculi.

Patient & Family Education

- Avoid use of mineral oil while on vitamin A therapy.
- Notify prescriber of symptoms of overdosage (e.g., nausea, vomiting, anorexia, drying and cracking of skin or lips, headache, loss of hair).

VITAMIN B_1
See Thiamine HCl.

VITAMIN B_2
See Riboflavin.

VITAMIN B_3
See Niacin.

VITAMIN B_6
See Pyridoxine.

VITAMIN B_9
See Folic acid.

VITAMIN B_{12}
See Cyanocobalamin.

VITAMIN B_{12A}
See Hydroxocobalamin.

VITAMIN C
See Ascorbic acid.

VITAMIN D
See Calcitriol, Ergocalciferol.

VITAMIN E (TOCOPHEROL)
(vit'a-min E)

Aquasol E, Vita-Plus E, Vitec

Classification: VITAMIN SUPPLEMENT

Therapeutic: VITAMIN E SUPPLEMENT

AVAILABILITY Tablet; capsule; liquid

ACTION & *THERAPEUTIC EFFECT*

An antioxidant, it prevents peroxidation, a process that gives rise to free radicals (highly reactive chemical structures that damage cell membranes and alter nuclear proteins). *Prevents cell membrane and protein damage, protects against blood clot formation by decreasing platelet aggregation, enhances vitamin A utilization, and promotes normal growth, development, and tone of muscles.*

USES To treat and prevent hemolytic vitamin E deficiency; for the treatment of familial hypocholesterolemia. Also used topically for dry

V

or chapped skin and minor skin disorders.

UNLABELED USES Muscular dystrophy and a number of other conditions with no conclusive evidence of value. A component of many multivitamin formulations and of topical deodorant preparations as an antioxidant.

CONTRAINDICATIONS Bleeding disorders; thrombocytopenia.

CAUTIOUS USE Large doses may exacerbate iron deficiency anemia; pregnancy (category A within RDA); children.

ROUTE & DOSAGE

Vitamin E Deficiency

Adult: **PO** 60–75 international units/day
Child: **PO** 1 international unit/kg/day

Prophylaxis for Vitamin E Deficiency

Adult: **PO** 12–15 international units/day
Child: **PO** 7–10 international units/day
Neonate: **PO** 5 international units/day

Familial Hypocholesterolemia

Child/Infant: **PO** 50 international units/kg/day

ADMINISTRATION

Oral

- Give on an empty stomach or following food or milk if GI upset occurs.
- Ensure that capsules are swallowed whole. They should not be crushed or chewed.
- Store in tight containers protected from light.

ADVERSE EFFECTS **HEENT:** Blurred vision. **Endocrine:** Increased serum creatine kinase, cholesterol, triglycerides; decreased serum thyroxine and triiodothyronine; increased urinary estrogens, androgens; creatinuria. **Skin:** Sterile abscess, thrombophlebitis, contact dermatitis. **GI:** Nausea, diarrhea, intestinal cramps. **GU:** Gonadal dysfunction. **Other:** Skeletal muscle weakness, headache, fatigue (with excessive doses).

INTERACTIONS **Drug: Mineral oil, cholestyramine** may decrease absorption of vitamin E; may enhance anticoagulant activity of **warfarin**. Avoid use with **amprenavir, tipranavir** due to increased risk of bleeding.

PHARMACOKINETICS **Absorption:** 20–60% absorbed from GI tract if fat absorption is normal; enters blood via lymph. **Distribution:** Stored mainly in adipose tissue; crosses placenta. **Metabolism:** In liver. **Elimination:** Primarily in bile.

NURSING IMPLICATIONS

Patient & Family Education

- Natural sources of vitamin E are found in wheat germ (the richest source) as well as in vegetable oils (sunflower, corn, soybean, cottonseed), green leafy vegetables, nuts, dairy products, eggs, cereals, meat, and liver.

VORAPAXAR

(vor-a-pax′ar)

Zontivity

Classification: ANTIPLATELET; PROTEASE-ACTIVATED RECEPTOR-1 (PAR-1) ANTAGONIST

Therapeutic: PLATELET AGGREGATION INHIBITOR; ANTITHROMBOTIC

AVAILABILITY Tablet

ACTION & THERAPEUTIC EFFECT A reversible antagonist of the protease-activated receptor 1 (PAR-1) expressed on platelets; inhibits platelet aggregation induced by thrombin and thrombin receptor agonist peptide (TRAP). *Reduces the incidence of thrombus formation in those with preexisting risk factors.*

USES Reduction of thrombotic cardiovascular events in patients with a history of myocardial infarction (MI) or with peripheral arterial disease (PAD).

CONTRAINDICATIONS History of stroke, TIA, or intracranial hemorrhage (ICH); active pathological bleeding (e.g., hemorrhage, peptic ulcer bleeding); severe hepatic impairment; lactation.

CAUTIOUS USE Bleeding disorder; concomitant use of drugs that increase the risk for bleeding (e.g., anticoagulants, NSAIDs, SSRIs, SNRIs); depression; mild to moderate hepatic impairment; renal impairment; older adults; pregnancy (discontinue use if pregnancy detected due to potential for serious adverse effect of bleeding). Safety and efficacy in children younger than 18 y not established.

ROUTE & DOSAGE

Thromboembolism Prophylaxis

Adult: **PO** 2.08 mg once daily with aspirin and/or clopidogrel

ADMINISTRATION

Oral

- Give without regard to food.
- Store at 20°–25° C (68°–77° F) and protect from moisture.

ADVERSE EFFECTS **Hematologic:** Hemorrhage, bleeding. **GI:** GI hemorrhage. **Hematologic:** Anemia.

INTERACTIONS **Drug:** Strong inhibitors of CYP3A (e.g., **clarithromycin, conivaptan, indinavir, itraconazole, ketoconazole, nefazodone, nelfinavir, posaconazole, ritonavir, saquinavir, telaprevir, telithromycin**) can increase the levels of vorapaxar and can increase the risk of bleeding if used in combination. Strong inducers of CYP3A (e.g., **carbamazepine, phenytoin, rifampin**) can decrease the levels of vorapaxar. Use with ANTICOAGULANTS or ANTIPLATELETS may have additive adverse effects. **Herbal: St. John's wort** can decrease the levels of vorapaxar.

PHARMACOKINETICS **Absorption:** 100% bioavailable. **Peak:** 1 h. **Distribution:** Greater than 99% plasma protein bound. **Metabolism:** In liver to active and inactive metabolites. Substrate of CYP2J2 and CYP3A4. **Elimination:** Fecal (58%) and renal (25%). **Half-Life:** 8 days (range 5–13 days).

NURSING IMPLICATIONS

Black Box Warning

Vorapaxar has been associated with an increased risk of bleeding, including fatal bleeding events especially in those with a history of stroke, transient ischemic attack (TIA), or intracranial hemorrhage (ICH).

V

Assessment & Drug Effects

- Monitor for and report immediately S&S of bleeding. There is no antidote for vorapaxar-induced bleeding.
- Monitor closely those with risk factors for bleeding (e.g., older age, low body weight, reduced renal or hepatic function, history of bleeding disorders, and concomitant use of anticoagulants, NSAIDs, SSRIs, and SNRIs).
- Monitor lab test: Periodic Hct and Hgb.

Patient & Family Education

- Immediately report to prescriber if you experience any of the following: Bleeding that is severe or that you cannot control; pink, red, or brown urine; vomiting blood or your vomit looks like coffee grounds; red or black tarry stools; coughing up blood or blood clots.
- Consult prescriber before taking any new prescription or OTC drugs to determine possible interaction the vorapaxar.
- Be careful to avoid injury. Use a soft toothbrush and an electric razor.

VORICONAZOLE

(vor-i-con'a-zole)

Vfend

Classification: ANTIBIOTIC; AZOLE ANTIFUNGAL

Therapeutic: ANTIFUNGAL

Prototype: Fluconazole

AVAILABILITY Solution for injection; oral suspension

ACTION & *THERAPEUTIC EFFECT* Inhibits fungal cytochrome P450 enzymes used for an essential step in fungal ergosterol biosynthesis. The subsequent loss of ergosterol in the fungal cell wall is thought to be responsible for the antifungal activity. *Voriconazole is active against Aspergillus and* Candida.

USES Treatment of invasive aspergillosis, esophageal candidiasis, candidemia in nonneutropenic patients and disseminated skin infections, and abdomen, kidney, bladder wall, and wound infections due to *Candida*.

CONTRAINDICATIONS Known hypersensitivity to voriconazole; should be avoided in moderate or severe renal impairment (CrCl less than 50 mL/min) and severe Child-Pugh class C hepatic impairment; development of S&S of hepatic disease in response to voriconazole; history of galactose intolerance; Lapp lactase deficiency or glucose-galactose malabsorption; development of exfoliative cutaneous reaction; sunlight (UV) exposure; pregnancy (category D); lactation.

CAUTIOUS USE Mild to moderate hepatic cirrhosis, hepatitis, Child-Pugh class A and B hepatic disease; proarrhythmic conditions; renal disease; mild or moderate renal impairment; ocular disease; hypersensitivity to other azole antifungal agents such as fluconazole. Safety and efficacy in children younger than 12 y not established.

ROUTE & DOSAGE

Invasive Aspergillosis

Adult/Adolescent: **IV** 6 mg/kg q12h × 2 doses then 4 mg/kg q12h. Treatment continues until 7–14 days after symptom resolution; *weight greater than 40 kg:* **PO** 200 mg q12h; *weight less than 40 kg:* **PO** 100 mg q12h

Candidemia

Adult: **IV** 6 mg/kg q12h × 2 doses then 3–4 mg/kg q12h; *weight greater than 40 kg:* **PO** 200 mg q12h may titrate dose; *weight less than 40 kg:* 100 mg q12h, may titrate dose

Esophageal Candidiasis

Adult (weight greater than 40 kg): **PO** 200 mg q12h for a minimum of 14 days and for at least 7 days after resolution of symptoms (max: 600 mg daily); *weight less than 40 kg:* 100 mg q12h for a minimum of 14 days and for at least 7 days after resolution of symptoms (max: 300 mg daily)

Drug Interaction Dosage Adjustment

Needed for concomitant CYP 450 enzyme inducers/ substrates. See package insert for specific efavirenz and phenytoin adjustments.

Renal Impairment Dosage Adjustment

CrCl less than 50 mL/min: Switch to PO therapy after loading dose; hemodialysis does not require supplemental dose

Hepatic Impairment Dosage Adjustment

Child-Pugh class A or B: Reduce maintenance dose by 50%; *Child-Pugh class C:* Avoid drug use

ADMINISTRATION

Oral

- Give at least 1 h before or 1 h following a meal.
- Store tablets at 15°–30° C (59°–86° F).

Intravenous

PREPARE: **Intermittent:** Use a 20-mL syringe to reconstitute each 200 mg powder vial with exactly 19 mL of sterile water for injection to yield 10 mg/mL. Discard vial if a vacuum does not pull the diluent into vial. Shake until completely dissolved. ▪ Calculate the required dose of voriconazole based on patient's weight. ▪ From an IV infusion bag of NS, D5W, D5/NS, D5/.45NS, LR or other suitable solution, withdraw and discard a volume of IV solution equal to the required dose. ▪ Inject the required dose of voriconazole into the IV bag. The IV solution should have a final voriconazole concentration of 0.5–5 mg/ mL. ▪ Infuse immediately.

ADMINISTER: **Intermittent:** Infuse over 1–2 h at a maximum rate of 3 mg/kg/h. ▪ **Do not** give a bolus dose.

INCOMPATIBILITIES: **Solution/ additive:** Do not dilute with **sodium bicarbonate**; do not mix with any other drugs. **Y-site:** Do not infuse with other drugs.

- Store unreconstituted vials at 15°–30° C (59°–86° F).

ADVERSE EFFECTS

CV: Tachycardia, hypotension, hypertension, vasodilation. **CNS:** Headache, *hallucinations*, dizziness, chills. **HEENT:** *Abnormal vision (enhanced brightness, blurred vision, or color vision changes)*, photophobia. **Endocrine:** Increased alkaline phosphatase, AST, ALT, hypokalemia, hypomagnesemia, increased serum creatinine. **Skin:** *Rash*, pruritus. **GI:** *Nausea*, vomiting, abdominal pain, abnormal LFTs, diarrhea, cholestatic jaundice, dry mouth. **Other:** Peripheral edema, *fever*, chills.

V

INTERACTIONS **Drug:** Due to significant increased toxicity or decreased activity, the following drugs are contraindicated with voriconazole: BARBITURATES, **carbamazepine, efavirenz**, ERGOT ALKALOIDS, **pimozide, quinidine, rifabutin, sirolimus; fosphenytoin, phenytoin, rifampin**. Avoid use with CYP3A4 inhibitors (e.g., **atazanavir, itraconazole, ketoconazole, ritonavir**). PROTEASE INHIBITORS (except **indinavir**) may increase voriconazole toxicity; voriconazole may increase the toxicity of BENZODIAZEPINES, **cyclosporine**, NONNUCLEOSIDE REVERSE TRANSCRIPTASE INHIBITORS, **omeprazole, tacrolimus, vinblastine, vincristine, warfarin, fentanyl, oxycodone**, NSAIDS; **Food:** Absorption reduced with high-fat meals. **Herbal: St. John's wort** may decrease efficacy.

PHARMACOKINETICS **Absorption:** 96% absorbed. Has a nonlinear pharmacokinetic profile, a small change in dose may cause a large change in serum levels. Steady state not achieved until day 5–6 if no loading dose is given. **Peak:** 1–2 h. **Metabolism:** In liver by (and inhibits) CYP3A4, 2C9, and 2C19. **Elimination:** Primarily in urine. **Half-Life:** 6 h–6 days depending on dose.

NURSING IMPLICATIONS

Assessment & Drug Effects

- Visual acuity, visual field, and color perception should be monitored if treatment continues beyond 28 days.
- Withhold drug and notify prescriber if skin rash develops.
- Monitor cardiovascular status especially with preexisting CV disease.
- Concurrent drugs: Monitor PT/INR closely with warfarin as dose adjustments of warfarin may be needed. Monitor frequently blood glucose levels with sulfonylurea drugs as reduction in the sulfonylurea dosage may be needed. Monitor for and report any of the following: S&S of rhabdomyolysis in patient receiving a statin drug; prolonged sedation in patient receiving a benzodiazepine; S&S of heart block, bradycardia, or CHF in patient receiving a calcium channel blocker.
- Monitor lab tests: Baseline and periodic LFTs; frequent renal function tests; trough serum drug concentrations on day 5 and weekly thereafter for 4–6 wk; periodic CBC with platelet count, Hct and Hgb, serum electrolytes, blood glucose, and lipid profile.

Patient & Family Education

- Use reliable means of birth control to prevent pregnancy. If you suspect you are pregnant, contact prescriber immediately.
- Do not drive at night while taking voriconazole as the drug may cause blurred vision and photophobia.
- Do not drive or engage in other potentially hazardous activities until reaction to drug is known.
- Avoid strong, direct sunlight while taking voriconazole.

VORTIOXETINE

(vor-ti-ox′e-teen)

Trintellix

Classification: ANTIDEPRESSANT; SEROTONIN MODULATOR

Therapeutic: ANTIDEPRESSANT

AVAILABILITY Tablet

ACTION & *THERAPEUTIC EFFECT* Inhibits the reuptake of serotonin (5-HT), 5-HT3 receptor antagonism, and 5-HT1A receptor

V

agonism. *Enhanced serotonergic activity in the CNS is believed to produce an antidepressant effect.*

USES Treatment of major depressive disorder (MDD).

CONTRAINDICATIONS Hypersensitivity to vortioxetine; suicidal ideation; MAOIs within 14 days of starting vortioxetine or 21 days of stopping vortioxetine; serotonin syndrome; symptomatic hyponatremia; severe hepatic impairment; lactation.

CAUTIOUS USE History of suicidal thoughts; history of or family history of bipolar disorder, mania, or hypomania; history of bleeding disorders; history of GI bleeding; mild to moderate hepatic impairment; older adults; pregnancy (limited information related to use during pregnancy; patients exposed to antidepressants during pregnancy are encouraged to enroll in the National Pregnancy Registry for Antidepressants). Safety and efficacy in children not established.

ROUTE & DOSAGE

Major Depressive Disorder

Adult: **PO** 5–10 mg once daily; may increase to 20 mg or decrease to 5 mg as needed or tolerated

Metabolism Dosage Adjustment

Use with a strong CYP2D6 inhibitor: Decrease dose by 50%

Use with a strong CYP2D6 inducer: Increase dose; max increase is 3 times the normal dose

Use in patients who are poor CYP2D6 metabolizers: Maximum dose is 10 mg once daily

ADMINISTRATION

Oral

- May give without regard to food.
- To avoid adverse reactions, it is recommended that doses of 15–20 mg/day be decreased to 10 mg/day for 1 wk before discontinuation.
- Store at 25° C (77° F).

ADVERSE EFFECTS **CNS:** Abnormal dreams, *dizziness*. **Endocrine:** Hyponatremia. **Skin:** Pruritus. **GI:** Constipation, *diarrhea, dry mouth*, flatulence, *nausea*, vomiting. **GU:** Sexual dysfunction.

DIAGNOSTIC TEST INTERFERENCE May case false positive for methadone in urine assay.

INTERACTIONS **Drug:** Coadministration of other drugs that affect serotonin transmission (e.g., SSRIS, SNRIS, MAOIS, TRIPTANS, **buspirone, linezolid, tramadol**) may increase the risk of serotonin syndrome. Strong CYP2D6 inhibitors (e.g., **bupropion, fluoxetine, paroxetine, quinidine**) may increase the levels of vortioxetine. Strong CYP2D6 inducers (e.g., **carbamazepine, phenytoin, rifampin**) may decrease the levels of vortioxetine. May increase anticoagulant effect of heparin. **Food: Tryptophan** containing foods may increase the risk of serotonin syndrome.

PHARMACOKINETICS **Absorption:** 75% bioavailable. **Peak:** 7–11 h. **Distribution:** 98% plasma protein bound. **Metabolism:** Hepatic oxidation via CYP2D6, CYP3A4/5, CYP2C19, CYP2C9, CYP2A6, CYP2C8, and CYP2B6. **Elimination:** Renal (59%) and fecal (26%). **Half-Life:** 66 h.

V

NURSING IMPLICATIONS

Black Box Warning

Vortioxetine has been associated with suicidal thinking and behavior in children, adolescents, and young adults.

Assessment & Drug Effects

- Report immediately to prescriber signs of worsening mental status such as suicidal ideation, aggressiveness, agitation, anxiety, hostility, impulsivity, insomnia, irritability, panic attacks, and worsening of depression.
- Monitor for S&S of serotonin syndrome (see Appendix F). If serotonin syndrome is suspected withhold drug, notify prescriber and initiate supportive treatment.
- Monitor for and report promptly S&S of hyponatremia (see Appendix F) and any signs of abnormal bleeding.
- Monitor lab tests: Baseline and periodic LFTs.

Patient & Family Education

- Report promptly to prescribe suicidal ideation or behavior, aggressive or impulsive behavior, worsening depression or anxiety, mania or unusual changes in behavior or mood.
- Do not take OTC supplements such as tryptophan or St. John's wort without consulting prescriber.
- Inform prescriber if you are taking OTC nonsteroidal anti-inflammatory drugs (NSAIDs) or aspirin for pain relief.
- Report promptly any of the following: S&S of serotonin syndrome (see Appendix F); abnormal bleeding; S&S of low serum sodium (see hyponatremia Appendix F).
- Notify prescriber immediately if you are or suspect you are pregnant.
- Do not breast-feed while taking this drug.

VOXELOTOR

(vox-el-oh-tor)

Oxbryta

Classifications: HEMOGLOBIN S (HBS) POLYMERIZATION INHIBITOR

Therapeutic: HEMOGLOBINS (HbS) POLYMERIZATION INHIBITOR

AVAILABILITY Oral tablet

ACTION & *THERAPEUTIC EFFECT* An HbS polymerization inhibitor that reversibly binds to Hb and stabilizes the oxygenated Hb state. *Used to inhibit RBC sickling, improve RBC deformability, and reduce whole blood; may also extend RBC half-life and reduce anemia and hemolysis.*

USES Treatment of sickle cell disease in adults and pediatric patients older than 12 years old.

CONTRAINDICATIONS Hypersensitivity to voxelotor or any component of the formulation.

CAUTIOUS USE Hepatic impairment; pregnancy (no adverse effects observed in animal reproduction studies); lactation.

ROUTE & DOSAGE

Sickle Cell Disease

Adult: **PO** 1,500 mg once daily

Hepatic Impairment Dosage Adjustment

Severe impairment (Child-Pugh class C): **PO** 1,000 mg once daily

V

ADMINISTRATION

Oral

- Can be given with or without food.
- Swallow tablets whole; do not cut, crush, or chew tablets.
- Store at ≤30° C (86° F).

ADVERSE EFFECTS **CNS:** Headache, fatigue. **Skin:** Rash. **GI:** Diarrhea, abdominal pain, nausea. **Other:** Fever, hypersensitivity reaction.

INTERACTIONS **Drug:** Coadministration with potent inhibitors of CYP3A4 (e.g., **ketoconazole, fluconazole**) may increase the levels of voxelotor, increasing risk of toxicity; dose should be adjusted to 1,000 mg when interaction unavoidable. Coadministration with potent or moderate CYP3A4 inducers (e.g. **phenobarbital, phenytoin, rifampin**) may decrease the levels of voxelotor, dose should be adjusted to 2,500 mg when interaction unavoidable.

PHARMACOKINETICS **Absorption:** Plasma Cmax and AUC increased by 42% and 95% respectively, when administered with high-fat, high-calorie meal. **Peak:** 2 h. **Distribution:** 388 L, 99% protein-bound. **Metabolism:** In the liver, primarily through CYP3A4 oxidation (major). **Elimination:** 36% in urine, 63% in feces. **Half-Life:** 35.5 h

NURSING IMPLICATIONS

Assessment & Drug Effects

- Assess for signs/symptoms of hypersensitivity reaction.
- Monitor lab tests: Liver function tests.

Patient & Family Education

- Notify your doctor or get medical help right away if you have any of the following signs or symptoms of allergic reaction such as rash, hives, itching; red, swollen, blistered, or peeling skin with or without fever; wheezing; tightness in the chest or throat; trouble breathing, swallowing, or talking; unusual hoarseness; or swelling of the mouth, face, lips, tongue, or throat; or any dizziness or passing out.

WARFARIN SODIUM

(war'far-in)

Coumadin, Jantoven, Warfilone ♣

Classification: ANTICOAGULANT

Therapeutic: ANTICOAGULANT

AVAILABILITY Tablet

ACTION & THERAPEUTIC EFFECT Indirectly interferes with blood clotting by depressing hepatic synthesis of vitamin K-dependent coagulation factors: II, VII, IX, and X. *Deters further extension of existing thrombi and prevents new clots from forming.*

USES Prophylaxis and treatment of deep vein thrombosis and its extension, pulmonary embolism; treatment of atrial fibrillation with embolization. Also used as adjunct in treatment of coronary occlusion, cerebral transient ischemic attacks (TIAs), and as a prophylactic in patients with prosthetic cardiac valves; reduce the risk of death, recurrent MI, and thromboembolic events, post MI.

CONTRAINDICATIONS Hemorrhagic tendencies, hemophilia, coagulation factor deficiencies, dyscrasias; active bleeding; open wounds, active peptic ulcer, visceral carcinoma, esophageal varices, malabsorption syndrome; uncontrolled hypertension, cerebral vascular disease; heparin-induced thrombocytopenia (HIT); pericarditis; severe hepatic or renal disease; continuous tube drainage of any orifice; subacute bacterial endocarditis; recent surgery of brain, spinal cord, or eye; regional or lumbar block anesthesia; threatened abortion; unreliable patients; pregnancy (category X).

CAUTIOUS USE Alcoholism, allergic disorders, during menstruation, senility, psychosis; debilitated patients; CVD; renal impairment; hepatic impairment. Endogenous factors that may increase prothrombin time response (enhance anticoagulant effect): Carcinoma, CHF, collagen diseases, hepatic and renal insufficiency, diarrhea, fever, pancreatic disorders, malnutrition, vitamin K deficiency. Endogenous factors that may decrease prothrombin time response (decrease anticoagulant response): Edema, hypothyroidism, hyperlipidemia, hypercholesterolemia, chronic alcoholism, hereditary resistance to coumarin therapy; older adults; children.

ROUTE & DOSAGE

Anticoagulant

Adult: **PO** Usual dose 2–5 mg daily with dose adjusted to maintain a PT 1.2–2 × control or INR of 2–3 (target varies per disease state)

Pharmacogenetic Dosage Adjustment

Variations in CYP2C9 or VKORC1 may require dose adjustments (see package insert for tables)

W

ADMINISTRATION

Note: Antidote for bleeding—anticoagulant effect usually is reversed by omitting 1 or more doses of warfarin and by administration of specific antidote phytonadione (vitamin K_1) 2.5–10 mg orally. Prescriber may advise patient to carry vitamin K_1 at all times, but not to take it until after consultation. If bleeding persists or progresses to a severe level, vitamin K 10 mg IV is given, or a fresh whole blood transfusion may be necessary.

Oral

- Give tablet whole or crushed with fluid of patient's choice.

ADVERSE EFFECTS **GI:** Anorexia, nausea, vomiting, abdominal cramps, diarrhea, steatorrhea, stomatitis. **Other:** Major or minor hemorrhage from any tissue or organ; hypersensitivity (dermatitis, urticaria, pruritus, fever). Increased serum transaminase levels, hepatitis, jaundice, burning sensation of feet, transient hair loss, internal or external bleeding, paralytic ileus; skin necrosis of toes (purple toes syndrome), tip of nose, buttocks, thighs, calves, female breast, abdomen, and other fat-rich areas.

DIAGNOSTIC TEST INTERFERENCE Warfarin (coumarins) may cause alkaline urine to be red-orange; may enhance ***uric acid*** excretion, cause elevation of ***serum transaminases***, and may increase ***lactic dehydrogenase*** activity.

INTERACTIONS **Drug:** In addition to the drugs listed below, many other drugs have been reported to alter the expected response to warfarin; however, clinical importance of these reports has not been substantiated. The addition or withdrawal of any drug to an established drug regimen should be made cautiously, with more frequent ***INR*** determinations than usual and with careful observation of the patient and dose adjustment as indicated. The following may enhance the anticoagulant effects of warfarin: **Acetohexamide, acetaminophen**, ALKYLATING AGENTS, **allopurinol**, AMINOGLYCOSIDES, **aminosalicylic acid, amiodarone**, ANABOLIC STEROIDS, ANTIBIOTICS (ORAL), ANTIMETABOLITES, ANTIPLATELET DRUGS, **aspirin, asparaginase, capecitabine, celecoxib, chloramphenicol, chlorpropamide, chymotrypsin, cimetidine, clofibrate, cotrimoxazole, danazol, dextran, dextrothyroxine, diazoxide, disulfiram, erythromycin, ethacrynic acid, fluconazole, glucagons, guanethidine**, HEPATOTOXIC DRUGS, **influenza vaccine, isoniazid, itraconazole, ketoconazole**, MAO INHIBITORS, **meclofenamate, mefenamic acid, methyldopa, methylphenidate, metronidazole, miconazole, mineral oil, nalidixic acid, neomycin (oral)**, NONSTEROIDAL ANTI-INFLAMMATORY DRUGS, **oxandrolone, plicamycin**, POTASSIUM PRODUCTS, **propoxyphene, propylthiouracil, quinidine, quinine, rofecoxib, salicylates, streptokinase, sulindac**, SULFONAMIDES, SULFONYLUREAS, TETRACYCLINES, THIAZIDES, THYROID DRUGS, **tolbutamide**, TRICYCLIC ANTIDEPRESSANTS, **urokinase, vitamin E, zileuton**. The following may increase or decrease the anticoagulant effects of warfarin: **Alcohol** (acute intoxication may increase, chronic alcoholism may decrease effects), DIURETICS. The following may decrease the anticoagulant effects of warfarin: BARBITURATES, **carbamazepine, cholestyramine**, CORTICOSTEROIDS, **corticotropin, glutethimide, griseofulvin**, LAXATIVES, **mercaptopurine**, ORAL CONTRACEPTIVES, **rifampin, spironolactone, vitamin C, vitamin K.** **Herbal: Boldo, capsicum, celery, chamomile, chondroitin, clove, coenzyme Q10, danshen, devil's claw, dong quai, echinacea, evening primrose oil, fenugreek, feverfew, fish oil, garlic, ginger, ginkgo, glucosamine, horse chestnut, licorice root, passionflower herb, turmeric, willow bark** may increase risk of bleeding; **ginseng, green tea, seaweed, soy, St. John's wort** may decrease effectiveness of warfarin. **Food: Cranberry juice** may increase ***INR***. **Green leafy vegetables** may affect efficacy. **Avocado** may decrease effectiveness of warfarin.

PHARMACOKINETICS **Absorption:** Well absorbed from GI tract. **Onset:** 2–7 days. **Peak:** 0.5–3 days. **Distribution:** 97% protein bound; crosses placenta. **Metabolism:** In liver (CYP2C9). **Elimination:** In urine and bile. **Half-Life:** 0.5–3 days.

NURSING IMPLICATIONS

Black Box Warning

Warfarin has been associated with serious, sometimes fatal, bleeding events.

Assessment & Drug Effects

- Determine INP prior to initiation of therapy and then daily until maintenance dosage is established.
- Obtain a COMPLETE medication history prior to start of therapy and whenever altered responses to therapy require interpretation; extremely IMPORTANT since many drugs interfere with the activity of anticoagulant drugs (see INTERACTIONS).
- Dose is typically adjusted to maintain an INR of 2–4 depending on diagnosis.

- Note: Patients at greatest risk of hemorrhage include those whose INR is difficult to regulate, who have an aortic valve prosthesis, who are receiving long-term anticoagulant therapy, and older adult and debilitated patients.
- Monitor lab tests: INR prior to initiation of therapy and then daily until maintenance dosage is established. For maintenance dosage, INR determinations at 1–4-wk intervals depending on patient's response; periodic urinalyses, stool guaiac, and LFTs.

Patient & Family Education

- Understand that bleeding can occur even though INR are within therapeutic range. Stop drug and notify prescriber immediately if bleeding or signs of bleeding appear: Blood in urine, bright red or black tarry stools, vomiting of blood, bleeding with tooth brushing, blue or purple spots on skin or mucous membrane, round pinpoint purplish red spots (often occur in ankle areas), nosebleed, bloody sputum; chest pain; abdominal or lumbar pain or swelling, profuse menstrual bleeding, pelvic pain; severe or continuous headache, faintness or dizziness; prolonged oozing from any minor injury (e.g., nicks from shaving).
- Stop drug and report immediately any symptoms of hepatitis (dark urine, itchy skin, jaundice, abdominal pain, light stools) or hypersensitivity reaction (see Appendix F).
- Take drug at same time each day, and **do not** alter dose.
- Risk of bleeding is increased for up to 1 mo after receiving the influenza vaccine.
- Fever, prolonged hot weather, malnutrition, and diarrhea lengthen INR (enhanced anticoagulant effect).
- A high-fat diet, sudden increase in vitamin K–rich foods (cabbage, cauliflower, broccoli, asparagus, lettuce, turnip greens, onions, spinach, kale, fish, liver), coffee or green tea (caffeine), or by tube feedings with high vitamin K content shorten INR.
- Avoid excess intake of alcohol.
- Use a soft toothbrush and floss teeth gently with waxed floss.
- Use barrier contraceptive measures; if you become pregnant while on anticoagulant therapy the fetus is at great potential risk of congenital malformations.
- Do not take any other prescription or OTC drug unless specifically approved by prescriber or pharmacist.

ZAFIRLUKAST

(za-fir-lu'kast)

Accolate

Classification: RESPIRATORY SMOOTH MUSCLE RELAXANT; LEUKOTRIENE RECEPTOR ANTAGONIST (LTRA); BRONCHODILATOR

Therapeutic: BRONCHODILATOR; LTRA

AVAILABILITY Tablet

ACTION & *THERAPEUTIC EFFECT*

Selective leukotriene receptor antagonist (LTRA) that inhibits binding of leukotriene D_4 and E_4, thus inhibiting inflammation and bronchoconstriction. Leukotriene production and receptor affinity have been correlated with the pathogenesis of asthma. *Zafirlukast helps to prevent the signs and symptoms of asthma, including airway edema, smooth muscle constriction, and altered cellular activity due to inflammation.*

 Common adverse effects in *italic;* life-threatening effects underlined; generic names in **bold;** classifications in SMALL CAPS; ♣ Canadian drug name; Prototype drug; Alert

USES Prophylaxis and chronic treatment of asthma in adults and children older than 5 y (not for acute bronchospasm).

UNLABELED USES Chronic urticaria.

CONTRAINDICATIONS Hypersensitivity to zafirlukast; acute asthma attacks, including status asthmaticus, acute bronchospasm; hepatic impairment including cirrhosis; lactation.

CAUTIOUS USE Patients 65 y or older, pregnancy (category B); children younger than 5 y.

ROUTE & DOSAGE

Asthma

Adult/Child (12 y or older): **PO** 20 mg bid
Child (5 y or older): **PO** 10 mg bid

ADMINISTRATION

Oral

- Give 1 h before or 2 h after meals.
- Store at 20°–25° C (68°–77° F); protect from light and moisture.

ADVERSE EFFECTS **CNS:** Headache, dizziness.

INTERACTIONS **Drug:** May increase ***prothrombin time (PT)*** in patients on **warfarin. Erythromycin** decreases bioavailability of zafirlukast. Avoid use with CYP2C8 inhibitors and strong CYP2C9 inhibitors/inducers. Do not use with **loxapine**.

PHARMACOKINETICS **Absorption:** Rapidly from GI tract, bioavailability significantly reduced by food. **Onset:** 1 wk. **Peak:** 3 h. **Distribution:** Greater than 99% protein bound; secreted into breast milk. **Metabolism:** In liver (CYP2C9). **Elimination:** 90% in feces, 10% in urine. **Half-Life:** 10 h.

NURSING IMPLICATIONS

Assessment & Drug Effects

- Assess respiratory status and airway function regularly.
- Monitor closely phenytoin level with concurrent phenytoin therapy.
- Monitor lab tests: Periodic LFTs, and INR with concurrent warfarin therapy.

Patient & Family Education

- Taking medication regularly, even during symptom-free periods.
- Note: Drug is not intended to treat acute episodes of asthma.
- Report S&S of hepatic toxicity (see Appendix F) or flu-like symptoms to prescriber. Follow-up lab work is very important.
- Notify prescriber immediately if condition worsens while using prescribed doses of all antiasthmatic medications.

ZALEPLON

(zal′ep-lon)

Classification: SEDATIVE-HYPNOTIC; NONBARBITUATE
Therapeutic: SEDATIVE-HYPNOTIC
Prototype: Zolpidem
Controlled Substance: Schedule IV

AVAILABILITY Capsule

ACTION & THERAPEUTIC EFFECT Short-acting nonbenzodiazepine with sedative-hypnotic, muscle relaxant. *Reduces difficulty in initially falling asleep. Preserves deep sleep (stages 3 through 4) at hypnotic dose with minimal-to-absent rebound insomnia when discontinued.*

USES Short-term treatment of insomnia.

CONTRAINDICATIONS Hypersensitivity to zaleplon or any component of the formulation; severe hepatic impairment; suicidal ideation.

CAUTIOUS USE Hypersensitivity to salicylates; chronic depression; history of suicidal thoughts; history of drug abuse; COPD; respiratory insufficiency; hepatic impairment; pulmonary disease; older adults; pregnancy (adverse effects observed in some animal reproduction studies; use during pregnancy not recommended by manufacturer); lactation. Safe use in children not established.

ROUTE & DOSAGE

Insomnia

Adult: **PO** 5–10 mg at bedtime (max: 20 mg at bedtime)
Geriatric: **PO** 5 mg at bedtime (max: 10 mg at bedtime)

Hepatic Impairment Dosage Adjustment

Mild-Moderate impairment: 5 mg at bedtime.

ADMINISTRATION

Oral

- Give immediately before bedtime; not while patient is still ambulating.
- Avoid taking with or after a heavy, high-fat meal as it reduces absorption.
- Ensure that extended release tablets are swallowed whole and are not crushed or chewed.
- Sublingual tablets should not be given with water and should not be swallowed.
- Oral spray container must be primed before first use. Ensure that a full dose (5 mg) is sprayed directly into the mouth over the tongue. For a 10 mg dose, administer a second spray.
- Store at 20°–25° C (68°–77° F).

ADVERSE EFFECTS **CNS:** Headache, amnesia, dizziness, drowsiness. **HEENT:** Eye pain. **GI:** Abdominal pain, nausea. **GU:** Dysmenorrhea. **Other:** Asthenia.

INTERACTIONS **Drug: Alcohol, imipramine, thioridazine, topiramate**, BARBITURATES, CNS DEPRESSANTS may cause additive CNS impairment; **rifampin** increases metabolism of **zaleplon; cimetidine** increases serum levels of **zaleplon**. Do not use with **sodium oxybate. Herbal: Valerian, kratom, melatonin** may produce additive sedative effects. **Food: High-fat meals** may delay absorption.

PHARMACOKINETICS **Absorption:** Rapidly and completely absorbed, 30% reaches systemic circulation. **Onset:** 15–20 min. **Peak:** 1 h. **Duration:** 3–4 h. **Distribution:** 60% protein bound. **Metabolism:** Extensively in liver (CYP3A4) to inactive metabolites. **Elimination:** 70% in urine, 17% in feces. **Half-Life:** 1 h.

NURSING IMPLICATIONS

Assessment & Drug Effects

- Monitor behavior and notify prescriber for significant changes. Use extra caution with preexisting clinical depression.
- Provide safe environment and monitor ambulation after drug is ingested.
- Monitor respiratory status with preexisting compromised pulmonary function.

Patient & Family Education

- Exercise caution when walking; avoid all hazardous activities after taking zaleplon.
- Do not take in combination with alcohol or any other sleep medication.

- Note: Exhibits altered effectiveness if taken with/immediately after high-fat meal.
- Do not use longer than 2–3 wk.
- Expect possible mild/brief rebound insomnia after discontinuing regimen.
- Report use of OTC medications to prescriber (e.g., cimetidine).
- Report pregnancy to prescriber immediately.

ZANAMIVIR

(zan'a-mi-vir)

Relenza

Classification: ANTIVIRAL; NEURAMINIDASE INHIBITOR

Therapeutic: ANTIINFLUENZA

Prototype: Oseltamivir

AVAILABILITY Powder for inhalation

ACTION & *THERAPEUTIC EFFECT* Inhibitor of influenza A and B viral enzyme; does not permit the release of newly formed viruses from the surface of the infected cells. *Prevents viral spread across the mucus lining of the respiratory tract, and inhibits the replication of influenza A and B virus. Relieves flu-like symptoms.*

USES Treatment of uncomplicated acute influenza in patients symptomatic less than 2 days; prophylaxis for influenza.

CONTRAINDICATIONS Hypersensitivity to zanamivir or milk protein; severe renal impairment, renal failure; COPD; severe asthma.

CAUTIOUS USE Renal impairment; cardiac disease; severe metabolic disease; older adults; pregnancy (an increased risk of adverse neonatal or maternal outcomes has not been observed following use of zanamivir during pregnancy); lactation. **Acute influenza:** Safety and efficacy in children younger than 7 y not established. **Influenza prophylaxis:** Safe use in children younger than 5 y not established.

ROUTE & DOSAGE

Influenza Treatment

Adult/Child (7 y or older): **Inhaled** 2 inhalations (one 5 mg blister/inhalation) bid × 5 days

Influenza Prophylaxis

Adult/Child (5 y or older): **Inhaled** 2 inhalations daily for 10 days (household prophylaxis) or for 28 days (community outbreak)

ADMINISTRATION

Inhalation

- Most effective if initiated within 48 h of onset of flu-like symptoms. Administer at approximately the same time each day (with the exception of the first dose).
- Give any scheduled inhaled bronchodilator before zanamivir.
- Store at 25° C (77° F).

ADVERSE EFFECTS **Respiratory:** Nasal symptoms, bronchitis, cough, sinusitis. **CNS:** Dizziness. **Skin:** Urticaria. **GI:** Abdominal pain.

INTERACTIONS **Drug:** Do not use with LIVE VACCINES.

PHARMACOKINETICS **Absorption:** 4–17% of inhaled dose is systemically absorbed. **Peak:** 1–2 h. **Distribution:** Less than 10% protein bound. **Metabolism:** Not metabolized. **Elimination:** In urine. **Half-Life:** 2.5–5.1 h.

NURSING IMPLICATIONS

Patient & Family Education

- Start within 48 h of onset of flu-like symptoms for most effective response.
- Use any scheduled inhaled bronchodilator first; then use zanamivir.
- Monitor for any change in behavior.

ZICONOTIDE

(zi-con'o-tide)

Prialt

Classification: MISCELLANEOUS ANALGESIC; N-TYPE CALCIUM CHANNEL ANTAGONIST

Therapeutic: MISCELLANEOUS ANALGESIC

AVAILABILITY Solution for injection

ACTION & *THERAPEUTIC EFFECT*

Ziconotide binds to N-type calcium channels located on the afferent nerves in the dorsal horn in the spinal cord. It is thought that these binding blocks of N-type calcium channels lead to a blockade of excitatory neurotransmitter release in the afferent nerve endings. *Ziconotide is effective in controlling severe chronic pain that is intractable to other analgesics.*

USES Management of severe chronic pain in patients for whom intrathecal (IT) therapy is warranted.

CONTRAINDICATIONS Hypersensitivity to ziconotide; preexisting history of psychosis; epidural or intravenous administration; sepsis; depression with suicidal ideation; cognitive impairment; bipolar disorder; schizophrenia; dementia; presence of infection at the injection site, uncontrolled bleeding, or spinal canal obstruction that impairs circulation of CSF; coagulopathy; seizures; lactation.

CAUTIOUS USE Renal, hepatic, and cardiac impairment; older adults; pregnancy (adverse events and maternal toxicity were observed in animal reproduction studies). Safe use in children and infants not established.

ROUTE & DOSAGE

Severe Chronic Pain

Adult: **Intrathecal** Initial dose up to 0.1 mcg/h; may titrate up 0.1 mcg/h q2–3days to 0.8 mcg/h (19.2 mcg/day)

ADMINISTRATION

Intrathecal

- May be administered undiluted (25 mcg/mL in 20 mL vial) or diluted using the 100 mcg/mL vials. Diluted ziconotide is prepared with NS without preservatives.
- Administer using an implanted variable-rate microinfusion device or an external microinfusion device and catheter.
- Note: Due to serious adverse events, 19.2 mcg/day (0.8 mcg/h) is the maximum recommended dose.
- Doses should normally be titrated upward by no more than 2.4 mcg/day (0.1 mcg/h) at intervals of 2–3 × wk.
- Refrigerate all ziconotide solutions after preparation and begin infusion within 24 h. Discard any unused portion left in a vial.

ADVERSE EFFECTS **CV:** Hypotension, orthostatic hypotension, peripheral edema. **Respiratory:** Sinusitis. **CNS:** *Dizziness*, confusion, memory impairment, drowsiness abnormal gait, ataxia, speech disorder, headache, aphasia, hallucination, abnormal thinking, amnesia, anxiety, dysarthria, paresthesia, rigors, vertigo, insomnia. **HEENT:** Blurred vision, nystagmus. **Skin:** Pruritis, diaphoresis. **GI:** *Nausea*, vomiting, diarrhea, anorexia, dysgeusia. **GU:**. Urinary retention. **Musculoskeletal:** *Increased CPK*, weakness, tremor, muscle spasm, limb pain. **Hematologic:** Anemia, ecchymosis. **Other:** Fever.

INTERACTIONS Drug: Ethanol and other CNS DEPRESSANTS may increase drowsiness, dizziness, and confusion.

PHARMACOKINETICS Distribution: 50% protein bound. **Metabolism:** Hydrolyzed by peptidases. **Half-Life:** 4.6 h.

NURSING IMPLICATIONS

Black Box Warning

Ziconotide has been associated with severe psychiatric symptoms and neurologic impairment.

Assessment & Drug Effects

- Monitor for and report S&S of meningitis, cognitive impairment, hallucinations, changes in mood or consciousness, or other psychiatric symptoms.
- Monitor lab values: Serum CPK (every other week for first month then monthly).

Patient & Family Education

- Report any of the following to prescriber: Muscle pain, soreness, or weakness, confusion, unusual behavior, symptoms of depression or suicidal thoughts, fever, headache, stiff neck, nausea or vomiting, seizures.
- Note: Taking this drug with other depressants (e.g., alcohol, sedatives, tranquilizers) will increase the risk of side effects.

ZIDOVUDINE (ZDV) (FORMERLY AZIDOTHYMIDINE, AZT)

(zye-doe′vyoo-deen)

Retrovir

Classification: ANTIVIRAL; NUCLEOSIDE REVERSE TRANSCRIPTASE INHIBITOR

Therapeutic: ANTIVIRAL; NRTI

Prototype: Lamivudine

AVAILABILITY Tablet; capsule; syrup; solution for injection

ACTION & *THERAPEUTIC EFFECT* A thymidine analog which interferes with the HIV viral RNA-dependent DNA polymerase resulting in inhibition of viral replication. *Zidovudine has antiviral action against HIV, LAV (lymphadenopathy-associated virus), and ARV (AIDS-associated retrovirus).*

USES Treatment of HIV (along with other antiretroviral agents), prevention of perinatal transfer of HIV during pregnancy.

UNLABELED USES Postexposure chemoprophylaxis, thrombocytopenia.

CONTRAINDICATIONS Life-threatening allergic reactions to any of the components of the drug; drug induced lactic acidosis; pronounced hepatotoxicity; lactation.

CAUTIOUS USE Severe renal impairment; or impaired hepatic function, alcoholism; anemia; chemotherapy; radiation therapy; bone marrow depression; older adults; pregnancy (high level of transfer across the placenta; in general,

ART is recommended for pregnant females living with HIV); children.

ROUTE & DOSAGE

HIV Infection

Adult/Adolescent/Child (weight 30 kg or greater): **PO** 300 mg bid; **IV** 1 mg/kg given q4h around the clock *Adolescent/Child/Infant (older than 4 wk, weight 9–30 kg):* 9 mg/kg/dose bid; *weight less than 9 kg:* 12 mg/kg/dose bid

Prevention of Maternal-Fetal Transmission

Maternal: **IV** (preferred route) During labor, 2 mg/kg loading dose, then 1 mg/kg/h until clamping umbilical cord

Toxicity Dosage Adjustment

Hemoglobin falls below 7.5 g/dL or falls 25% from baseline: Interrupt therapy. *ANC falls below 750 cells/mm^3 or decreases 50% from baseline:* Interrupt therapy.

Renal Impairment Adjustment (Adult)

CrCl less than 15 mL/min: 100 mg tid (oral) or 1 mg/kg q6–8h (IV)

ADMINISTRATION

Oral

- May be given with or without food.

Intravenous

PREPARE: **Intermittent:** Withdraw required dose from vial and dilute with D5W to a concentration not to exceed 4 mg/mL. ***ADMINISTER:*** **Intermittent for HIV infection:** Give calculated dose at a constant rate over 60 min; avoid rapid infusion or bolus injection. **IV Infusions for Prevention of Maternal-Fetal Transmission:** Give maternal loading dose over 1 h, then continuous infusion at 1 mg/kg/h. **Intermittent Infusion for Prevention of Maternal Transmission of HIV to Neonate:** Give calculated dose at a constant rate over 30 min. ***INCOMPATIBILITIES:*** **Y-site: Dexrazoxane, gemtuzumab, lansoprazole.**

- Store at 15°–25° C (59°–77° F) and protect from light. Store diluted IV solutions refrigerated for 24 h.

ADVERSE EFFECTS

Cardiac: Cardiac failure, ECG abnormality, edema, left ventricular dilation. **Respiratory:** *Cough, wheezing,* nasal congestion, rhinorrhea, abnormal breath sounds. **CNS:** *Headache,* insomnia, anxiety, restlessness, agitation, hyporeflexia, irritability, nervousness, chills, fatigue, neuropathy. **Endocrine:** <u>Lactic acidosis</u>, weight loss, increased amylase. **Skin:** *Rash,* itching, diaphoresis. **Hepatic/GI:** *Nausea,* diarrhea, *vomiting, anorexia,* GI pain, constipation, stomatitis, abdominal pain/cramps, dyspepsia, hepatomegaly, elevated liver enzymes. **GU:** Hematuria. **Hematologic:** <u>*Bone marrow depression, granulocytopenia, anemia, macrocytosis*</u>, lymphadenopathy, neutropenia, splenomegaly, thrombocytopenia. **Musculoskeletal:** Asthenia, arthralgia, musculoskeletal, myalgia. **Other:** *Fever,* injection site reaction.

INTERACTIONS

Drug: Acetaminophen, ganciclovir, interferon alfa may enhance bone marrow suppression; **aspirin, dapsone, doxorubicin, fluconazole, flucytosine, methadone, pentamidine, vincristine, valproic acid**

may increase risk of **AZT** toxicity; **probenecid** will decrease **AZT** elimination, resulting in increased serum levels and thus toxicity. **Nelfinavir, rifampin, ritonavir** may decrease zidovudine (**AZT**) concentrations; other ANTIRETROVIRAL AGENTS may cause lactic acidosis and severe hepatomegaly with steatosis; **stavudine, doxorubicin** may antagonize **AZT** effects. Do not administer LIVE VACCINES; use with MYELOSUPPRESSIVE AGENTS may have additive adverse effects.

PHARMACOKINETICS **Absorption:** Readily from GI tract; 60–70% reaches systemic circulation (first-pass metabolism). **Peak:** 0.5–1.5 h. **Distribution:** Crosses blood–brain barrier and placenta. **Metabolism:** In liver. **Elimination:** 63–95% in urine. **Half-Life:** 1 h.

NURSING IMPLICATIONS

Black Box Warning

Zidovudine has been associated with hematologic toxicity (including neutropenia and severe anemia), myopathy, lactic acidosis, and severe hepatomegaly with steatosis.

Assessment & Drug Effects

- Evaluate patient at least weekly during the first month of therapy.
- Myelosuppression results in anemia, which commonly occurs after 4–6 wk of therapy, and granulocytopenia in 6–8 wk.
- Monitor for common adverse effects, especially severe headache, nausea, insomnia, and myalgia.
- Monitor lab tests: Baseline and periodic CBC with differential; LFTs; serum creatinine; HIV viral load and CD4 count.

Patient & Family Education

- Contact prescriber promptly if health status worsens or any unusual symptoms develop.
- Report to prescriber any of the following: Muscle weakness, shortness of breath, symptoms of hepatitis or pancreatitis, or any other unexpected adverse reaction.
- Understand that this drug is not a cure for HIV infection; you will continue to be at risk for opportunistic infections.
- Do not share drug with others; take drug exactly as prescribed.
- Drug does **not** reduce the risk of transmission of HIV infection through body fluids.

ZILEUTON

(zi-leu′ton)

Zyflo, Zyflo CR

Classification: RESPIRATORY SMOOTH MUSCLE RELAXANT; BRONCHODILATOR; LEUKOTRIENE RECEPTOR ANTAGONIST (LTRA)

Therapeutic: BRONCHODILATOR; LTRA

Prototype: Zafirlukast

AVAILABILITY Immediate release tablet; controlled release tablet

ACTION & *THERAPEUTIC EFFECT* Inhibits 5-lipoxygenase, the enzyme needed to start the conversion of arachidonic acid to leukotrienes, which are important inflammatory agents that induce bronchoconstriction and mucus production. *Zileuton helps to prevent the signs and symptoms of asthma including airway edema, smooth muscle constriction, and altered cellular activity due to inflammation.*

USES Prophylaxis and chronic treatment of asthma in adults and children older than 12 y.

CONTRAINDICATIONS Hypersensitivity to zileuton or zafirlukast, active liver disease, status asthmaticus; QT prolongation; lactation.

CAUTIOUS USE Hepatic insufficiency; alcoholism; fever; infection; history of QT prolongation; older females; older adults; pregnancy (category C). Safety and efficacy in children younger than 12 y not established.

ROUTE & DOSAGE

Asthma

Adult/Child (12 y or older): **PO Controlled release** 1200 mg bid OR **Immediate release** 600 mg qid

ADMINISTRATION

Oral

- Ensure that controlled release tablets are swallowed whole. Do not crush or chew.
- Give without regard to meals.
- Store at room temperature, 15°–30° C (59°–86° F); protect from light.

ADVERSE EFFECTS **CV:** Chest pain. **Respiratory:** Upper respiratory tract infection, sinusitis. **CNS:** Headache, pain.

INTERACTIONS **Drug:** May double **theophylline** levels and increase toxicity. Increases hypoprothrombinemic effects of **warfarin**. May increase levels of BETA-BLOCKERS (especially **propranolol**), leading to hypotension and bradycardia. Do not use with **loxapine, pimozide**.

PHARMACOKINETICS **Absorption:** Rapidly from GI tract. **Peak:** 1.7 h. **Duration:** 5–8 h. **Distribution:** 93% protein bound; secreted in the breast milk of rats. **Metabolism:** In liver primarily via glucuronide conjugation. Substrate of CYP1A2, CYPD2C9, CYP3A4. **Elimination:** Primarily in urine (94%). **Half-Life:** 2.5 h.

NURSING IMPLICATIONS

Assessment & Drug Effects

- Assess respiratory status and airway function regularly.
- Monitor closely each of the following with concurrent drug therapy: With theophylline, theophylline levels; with warfarin, PT and INR; with phenytoin, phenytoin level; with propranolol, HR and BP for excessive beta blockade.
- Monitor lab tests: Baseline and periodic LFTs.

Patient & Family Education

- Take medication regularly even during symptom-free periods.
- Drug is not intended to treat acute episodes of asthma.
- Report to prescriber promptly S&S of hepatic toxicity (see Appendix F) or flu-like symptoms. Follow-up lab work is very important.
- Notify prescriber if condition worsens while using prescribed doses of all antiasthmatic medications.

ZIPRASIDONE HYDROCHLORIDE

(zip-ra-si′done)

Geodon

Classification: ATYPICAL ANTIPSYCHOTIC

Therapeutic: ANTIPSYCHOTIC

Prototype: Clozapine

AVAILABILITY Capsule; solution for injection

ACTION & *THERAPEUTIC EFFECT* Exerts antischizophrenic effects through dopamine (D_2) and serotonin ($5\text{-}HT_{2A}$) receptor antagonism. Exerts antidepressant effects through $5\text{-}HT_{1A}$ agonism, $5\text{-}HT_{1D}$ antagonism, and serotonin/norepinephrine reuptake inhibition. *Improves signs and symptoms of schizophrenia, schizoaffective disorder, and psychotic depression.*

USES Treatment of schizophrenia, bipolar disorder, agitation associated with psychiatric disorder.

UNLABELED USES Psychosis associated with dementia, major depressive disorder.

CONTRAINDICATIONS Hypersensitivity to ziprasidone; history of QT prolongation including congenital long QT syndrome or with other drugs known to prolong the QT interval; recent MI or uncompensated heart failure; NMS; older adults with dementia-related psychosis; lactation.

CAUTIOUS USE History of seizures, CVA, dementia, Parkinson's disease, or Alzheimer disease; known cardiovascular disease, conduction abnormalities, cerebrovascular disease; hepatic impairment; seizure disorder, seizures; breast cancer; risk factors for elevated core body temperature; esophageal motility disorders and risk of aspiration pneumonia; schizophrenia; suicide potential; DM; pregnancy (antipsychotic use during third trimester of pregnancy may cause increased risk for abnormal muscle movements and/or withdrawal symptoms in newborns); children older than 7 y for use in Tourette's syndrome only. Safety and efficacy in children or adolescents (except for treatment of Tourette's syndrome) not established.

ROUTE & DOSAGE

Schizophrenia

Adult: **PO** Start with 20 mg bid with food, may increase slowly as needed (normal dose 40–80 mg bid)

Acute Episodes of Agitation/ Acute Psychosis

Adult: **IM** 10 mg q2h or 20 mg q4h up to max of 40 mg/day

Acute Mania/Bipolar Disorder

Adult: **PO** Start with 40 mg bid with food; may increase q2days up to 80 mg bid if needed

ADMINISTRATION

Oral

- Administer with a meal containing at least 500 calories.
- Store at 25° C (77° F).

Intramuscular

- Give deep IM into a large muscle.
- Store at 25° C (77° F).

ADVERSE EFFECTS **CV:** Orthostatic hypotension, prolonged QT_c interval. **Respiratory:** Rhinitis, respiratory tract infection. **CNS:** *Drowsiness*, dizziness, extrapyramidal effects, headache, anxiety, akathisia. **HEENT:** Visual disturbances. **Endocrine:** Weight gain. **Skin:** Rash. **GI:** *Nausea*, constipation, dyspepsia, diarrhea, dry mouth, vomiting. **Musculoskeletal:** Weakness, myalgia. **Other:** Pain at injection site.

INTERACTIONS **Drug: Carbamazepine** may decrease **ziprasidone** levels; **ketoconazole** may increase **ziprasidone** levels; increased risk of arrhythmias and heart block due to prolonged QT_c interval with agents that affect QT interval (ex ANTIARRHYTHMIC AGENTS, **amoxapine, arsenic trioxide, chlorpromazine, clarithromycin, citalopram, daunorubicin, diltiazem, dolasetron, doxorubicin, droperidol, erythromycin, halofantrine, indapamide, levomethadyl**, LOCAL ANESTHETICS, **maprotiline, mefloquine, mesoridazine, octreotide, pentamidine, pimozide, levofloxacin, moxifloxacin, sparfloxacin**, TRICYCLIC ANTIDEPRESSANTS, **tacrolimus, thioridazine, troleandomycin)**; additive CNS depression with SEDATIVE-HYPNOTICS, ANXIOLYTICS, **ethanol**, OPIATE AGONISTS.

PHARMACOKINETICS Absorption: Well absorbed with 60% reaching systemic circulation. **Peak:** 6–8 h. **Metabolism:** In liver (CYP3A4). **Elimination:** Feces and urine. **Half-Life:** 7 h.

NURSING IMPLICATIONS

Black Box Warning

Ziprasidone has been associated with increased mortality in older adults with dementia-related psychosis.

Assessment & Drug Effects

- Monitor diabetics for loss of glycemic control.
- Monitor for S&S of torsade de pointes (e.g., dizziness, palpitations, syncope), tardive dyskinesia (see Appendix F) especially in older adult women and with prolonged therapy, and the appearance of an unexplained rash. Withhold drug and report to prescriber immediately if any of these develop.
- Monitor for signs and symptoms of suicidality.
- Monitor I&O ratio and pattern: Notify prescriber if diarrhea, vomiting or any other conditions develops which may cause electrolyte imbalance.
- Monitor BP lying, sitting, and standing. Report orthostatic hypotension to prescriber.
- Monitor cognitive status and take appropriate precautions.
- Monitor for loss of seizure control, especially with a history of seizures or dementia.
- Baseline and annual ocular examination.
- Monitor lab tests: Baseline and periodic CBC with differential; electrolytes; fasting blood glucose; lipid panel; LFTs.

Patient & Family Education

- Carefully monitor blood glucose levels if diabetic.
- Be aware that therapeutic effect may not be evident for several weeks.
- Report any of the following to a health care provider immediately: Palpitations, faintness or loss of consciousness, rash, abnormal muscle movements, vomiting, or diarrhea.
- Do not drive or engage in potentially hazardous activities until response to drug is known.
- Make position changes slowly and in stages to prevent dizziness upon arising.
- Avoid strenuous exercise, exposure to extreme heat, or other activities that may cause dehydration.

ZIV-AFLIBERCEPT

(ziv-a-fli'ber-cept)

Zaltrap

Classification: BIOLOGICAL RESPONSE MODIFIER; GROWTH FACTOR INHIBITOR; SIGNAL TRANSDUCTION INHIBITOR; RECOMBINANT FUSION PROTEIN; ANTINEOPLASTIC

Therapeutic: ANTINEOPLASTIC

AVAILABILITY Solution

ACTION & *THERAPEUTIC EFFECT* Binds to certain vascular growth factors thus inhibiting their binding to and activation of receptors that stimulate neovascularization (new blood vessel growth) and increased vascular permeability. *Decreased neovascularization in tumors slows growth of metastatic colorectal tumors.*

USES Treatment of metastatic colorectal cancer in combination chemotherapy with 5-flurouracil, leucovorin, and irinotecan in patients whose condition has progressed or is resistant to an oxaliplatin-containing combination

CONTRAINDICATIONS Severe hemorrhage; GI perforation; compromised wound healing; fistula development; 4 wk before or after elective surgery; hypertensive crisis or hypertensive encephalopathy; drug induced arterial thromboembolic event or nephrotic syndrome; reversible posterior leukoencephalopathy syndrome (RPLS); lactation.

CAUTIOUS USE Hypersensitivity to ziv-aflibercept; hemorrhage; history of GI perforation; poor wound healing; severe hypertension or hypertension; thromboembolic events; proteinuria; infection; diarrhea and dehydration; older adults; pregnancy (category C). Safety and efficacy in children younger than 18 y not established.

ROUTE & DOSAGE

Colorectal Cancer

Adult: **IV** 4 mg/kg q2wk; administer prior to 5-flurouracil, leucovorin, and irinotecan

Toxicity Dosage Adjustments

Recurrent of severe hypertension: Hold therapy until hypertension is controlled; permanently reduce dose to 2 mg/kg for subsequent cycles

Proteinuria: Hold therapy until proteinuria is less than 2 g/24 h; permanently reduce dose to 2 mg/kg for subsequent cycles

ADMINISTRATION

Intravenous

PREPARE: **IV Infusion:** Withdraw required dose of ziv-aflibercept and dilute to a final concentration of 0.6–8 mg/mL in NS or D5W (enter vial only once to withdraw dose). Dilute in PVC infusion bags containing bis (2-ethylhexyl) phthalate (DEHP) or polyolefin.

ADMINISTER: **IV Infusion:** Infuse over 1 h through a 0.2 micron polyethersulfone filter. Do not use filters made of polyvinylidene fluoride or nylon. **Do not** give IV push or as bolus dose. Use an infusion set made of PVC containing DEHP or one of the other materials approved by manufacturer.

INCOMPATIBILITIES: **Solution/additive:** Do not combine ziv-aflibercept with other drugs in the same IV solution. **Y-site:** Do not administer ziv-aflibercept in the same IV line with other drugs

- Store diluted solution at 2°–8° C (36°–46° F) for up to 4 h.

ADVERSE EFFECTS **CV:** Deep venous thrombosis, pulmonary embolism, *hypertension.* **Respiratory:** Dysphonia, dyspnea, epistaxis, nasopharyngitis, oropharyngeal pain, pulmonary embolism, rhinorrhea, upper respiratory tract infection. **CNS:** Headache. **HEENT:** Blurred vision, cataract, *conjunctival hemorrhage*, conjunctival hyperemia, corneal edema, corneal erosion, detachment of the retinal pigment epithelium, *eye pain*, eyelid edema, foreign body sensation in the eyes, increased intraocular pressure, increased lacrimation, retinal pigment epithelium tear, tooth infection, vitreous detachment, vitreous floaters. **Endocrine:** *Decreased appetite*, dehydration, *increased ALT and AST*, *weight decreased*. **Skin:** Palmar-plantar erythrodysesthesia syndrome, skin hyperpigmentation. **GI:** *Abdominal pain*, *diarrhea*, hemorrhoids, proctalgia, rectal hemorrhage, *stomatitis*, GI perforation. **GU:** *Proteinuria*, *serum creatinine increased*, urinary tract infections. **Hematologic:** *Leukopenia*, *neutropenia*, *thrombocytopenia*, hemorrhage. **Other:** Asthenia, *fatigue*, catheter site infection, hypersensitivity, injection site hemorrhage, injection site pain, pneumonia.

PHARMACOKINETICS Peak: 1–3 d. **Metabolism:** Via proteolysis. **Half-Life:** 5–6 d.

NURSING IMPLICATIONS

Black Box Warning

Ziv-aflibercept has been associated with severe, sometimes fatal hemorrhage, GI perforation, and seriously compromised wound healing.

Assessment & Drug Effects

- Monitor vital signs, especially BP for exacerbation of hypertension.
- Monitor for and report immediately S&S of bleeding and GI perforation.
- Monitor for diarrhea and dehydration, especially in the older adult.
- Monitor lab tests: Baseline and prior to each cycle, CBC with differential; periodic LFTs, renal function tests, and urinalysis for proteinuria; 24 h urine when urinary protein creatinine ratio is greater than 1.

Patient & Family Education

- Report promptly any of the following: S&S of bleeding including light-headedness; S&S of hypertension including severe headache, or dizziness; severe diarrhea, vomiting, or abdominal pain.
- Frequent monitoring of BP is advised. Contact prescriber if BP is elevated beyond usual parameters.
- Men and women should use effective means of birth control during therapy and for at least 3 mo following completion of therapy.
- Contact your prescriber immediately if you or your partner becomes pregnant during treatment with ziv-aflibercept.
- Do not breast-feed while receiving this drug without consultation with prescriber.

ZOLEDRONIC ACID

(zo-le-dron′ic)

Aclasta ♣, Reclast

Classification: BISPHOSPHONATE; BONE METABOLISM REGULATOR

Therapeutic: BONE METABOLISM REGULATOR

Prototype: Etidronate disodium

AVAILABILITY Solution for injection

ACTION & THERAPEUTIC EFFECT Zoledronic acid inhibits various stimulatory factors of osteoclastic activity produced by bone tumors.

Common adverse effects in *italic*; life-threatening effects underlined; generic names in **bold**; classifications in SMALL CAPS; ♣ Canadian drug name; Prototype drug; Alert

It also induces osteoclast apoptosis. *Zoledronic acid blocks osteoclastic resorption of bone, thus reducing the amount of calcium released from bone.*

USES Treatment of hypercalcemia of malignancy, multiple myeloma, and bony metastases from solid tumors, Paget's disease (Reclast), postmenopausal or glucocorticoid-induced osteoporosis (Reclast).

CONTRAINDICATIONS Hypersensitivity to zoledronic acid preexisting hypocalcemia (**Reclast** only); serum creatinine less than 35 mL/min; pregnancy (category D); lactation.

CAUTIOUS USE Aspirin-sensitive asthma; cancer chemotherapy; renal and/or hepatic impairment; dental work; multiple myeloma; Paget disease; hypoparathyroidism, malabsorption syndrome; QT prolongation, cardiac arrhythmias; neurologic events; older adults. Safety and efficacy in children not established.

ROUTE & DOSAGE

Hypercalcemia of Malignancy

Adult: **IV** 4 mg over a minimum of 15 min. May consider retreatment if serum calcium has not returned to normal, may repeat after 7 days

Multiple Myeloma and Bone Metastases from Solid Tumors

Adult: **IV** 4 mg q3–4wk

Osteoporosis (Reclast)

Adult: **IV** 5 mg infusion once/year

Osteoporosis Prophylaxis in Postmenopausal Women (Reclast)

Adult: **IV** 5 mg every other year

Paget's Disease (Reclast)

Adult: **IV** 5 mg dose, retreatment may be necessary

Renal Impairment Dosage Adjustment (for Oncology Uses)

CrCl 50–60 mL/min: 3.5 mg; *40–49 mL/min:* 3.3 mg; *30–39 mL/min:* 3 mg; *less than 30 mL/min:* Do not use

Renal Impairment Dosage Adjustment (Reclast)

CrCl less than 35 mL/min: Do not use

ADMINISTRATION

Intravenous

Do not administer to anyone who is dehydrated or suspected of being dehydrated. Consult prescriber.
▪ Do not administer until serum creatinine values have been evaluated by the prescriber.

PREPARE: **IV Infusion:** *Reclast:* No further preparation is necessary. *Zometa concentrate:* Further dilute in 100 mL NS or D5W. *Powder for injection:* Reconstitute with 5 mL of sterile water for injection (provided) to yield 0.8 mg/mL. Further dilute in 100 mL NS or D5W prior to administration. ▪ If not used immediately, refrigerate. The total time between reconstitution and end of infusion must not exceed 24 h.

ADMINISTER: **IV Infusion:** Infuse a single dose over NO LESS than 15 min. Flush line with 10 mL NS following infusion.

INCOMPATIBILITIES: **Solution/additive and Y-site:** Do not mix or infuse with **calcium**-containing solutions (e.g.,

lactated Ringer's). Alemtuzumab, dantrolene, dauorubicin, diazepam, gemtuzumab, pheytoin.

- Store at 2°–8° C (36°–46° F) following dilution. ▪ **Must be** completely infused within 24 h of reconstitution.

ADVERSE EFFECTS **CV:** Lower extremity edema, hypotension. **Respiratory:** Dyspnea, cough. **CNS:** *Fatigue*, headache, dizziness, insomnia, depression, anxiety, agitation, confusion, hypoesthesia, rigors. **Endocrine:** Dehydration, hypophosphotemia, hypokalemia, hypomagnesemia. **Skin:** Alopecia, dermatitis. **GI:** *Nausea*, vomiting, *constipation*, diarrhea, anorexia, weight loss, abdominal pain, dyspepsia, decreased appetite. **GU:** Urinary tract infection, renal insufficiency. **Musculoskeletal:** *Ostealgia*, weakness, myalgia, arthralgia, back pain, paresthesia, limb pain. **Hematologic:** Anemia, progression of cancer, neutropenia. **Other:** *Fever*, candidiasis.

INTERACTIONS **Drug:** NSAIDS may increase the risk of GI toxicity. **Thalidomide** and other NEPHROTOXIC DRUGS may increase risk of renal toxicity.

PHARMACOKINETICS **Onset:** 4–10 days. **Duration:** 3–4 wk. **Metabolism:** Not metabolized. **Elimination:** In urine. **Half-Life:** 146 h.

NURSING IMPLICATIONS

Assessment & Drug Effects

- Notify prescriber immediately of deteriorating renal function as indicated by rising serum creatinine levels over baseline value.
- Withhold zoledronic acid and notify prescriber if serum creatinine is not within 10% of the baseline value.
- Monitor closely patient's hydration status. Note that loop diuretics should be used with caution due to the risk of hypocalcemia.
- Monitor for S&S of *bronchospasm* in aspirin-sensitive asthma patients; notify prescriber immediately.
- Baseline dental exam prior to initiation of therapy for patients at risk for osteonecrosis including all cancer patients.
- Monitor lab tests: Baseline renal function tests prior to each dose and periodically thereafter; periodic ionized calcium or corrected serum calcium levels, serum phosphate and magnesium, electrolytes, CBC with differential, Hct and Hgb.

Patient & Family Education

- Maintain adequate daily fluid intake. Consult with prescriber for guidelines.
- Report unexplained weakness, tiredness, irritation, muscle pain, insomnia, or flu-like symptoms.
- Use reliable means of birth control to prevent pregnancy. If you suspect you are pregnant, contact prescriber immediately.

ZOLMITRIPTAN

(zol-mi-trip′tan)

Zomig, Zomig ZMT

Classification: SEROTONIN 5-HT_1 RECEPTOR AGONIST

Therapeutic: ANTIMIGRAINE

Prototype: Sumatriptan

AVAILABILITY Tablet; orally disintegrating tablet; nasal spray

ACTION & THERAPEUTIC EFFECT

Selective serotonin ($5\text{-}HT_{1B/1D}$) receptor agonist. The agonist effects at $5\text{-}HT_{1B/1D}$ reverse the vasodilation of cranial blood vessels and inhibit release of proinflammatory neuropeptides. *Vasoconstricts dilated cranial blood vessels and decreased neuropeptide release relieve the pain of a migraine headache.*

USES Acute migraine headaches with or without aura.

CONTRAINDICATIONS Hypersensitivity to zolmitriptan; history of stroke or TIA; ischemic heart disease (angina, arteriosclerosis, ECG changes, history of MI or Prinzmetal's angina); cardiac arrhythmias associated with cardiac accessory conduction pathway disorders; symptomatic Wolff–Parkinson–White syndrome, uncontrolled hypertension; patients with other cardiac risk factors, such as diabetes, obesity, cigarette smoking, high cholesterol levels; hemiplegia or basilar migraine; concurrent administration of ergotamine or sumatriptan; concurrent use of MAOIs or within 14 days of use; vasospasm-related events; lactation.

CAUTIOUS USE Men older than 40 y; postmenopausal women; strong family history of CAD; GI disease, PVD, ischemic colitis, Raynaud's disease, hepatic impairment; adults older than 65 y; pregnancy (category C); children younger than 12 y.

ROUTE & DOSAGE

Acute Migraine

Adult: **PO** 1.25–2.5 mg, may repeat in 2 h if necessary (max: 10 mg/24 h); **Orally disintegrating tablet** 2.5 mg

Adult/Adolescent: **Nasal Spray** One spray into one nostril

Hepatic Impairment Dosage Adjustment

Moderate to severe: 1.25 mg tablet (max: 5 mg)

ADMINISTRATION

Oral

- Give any time after symptoms of migraine appear. Give 2.5 mg or less by breaking a 5 mg tablet in half. If headache returns, may repeat q2h up to 10 mg in 24 h.
- **Do not** give zolmitriptan within 24 h of an ergot-containing drug or other $5\text{-}HT_1$ agonist.
- Discard unused tablets that have been removed from the packaging.

Intranasal

- Unit-dose spray device delivers a 5 mg dose. Do not exceed the maximum dose of 10 mg in 24 h.
- Store at 2°–25° C (36°–77° F) and protect from light.

ADVERSE EFFECTS **CNS:** Dizziness, paresthesia, drowsiness. **GI:** Unpleasant taste, nausea.

INTERACTIONS **Drug: Dihydroergotamine, methysergide**, ERGOT ALKALOIDS, other $5\text{-}HT_1$ AGONISTS may cause prolonged vasospastic reactions; SSRIS have rarely caused weakness, hyperreflexia, and incoordination; MAOIS should not be used with 5-HT_1 AGONISTS; **cimetidine** increases half-life of zolmitriptan. **Herbal: St. John's wort** may increase TRIPTAN toxicity.

PHARMACOKINETICS

Absorption: Rapidly absorbed, 40% bioavailability. **Peak:** 2–3 h. **Distribution:** 25% protein bound. **Metabolism:** In liver to active metabolite. **Elimination:** Primarily in urine (65%), 30% in feces. **Half-Life:** 3 h.

NURSING IMPLICATIONS

Assessment & Drug Effects

- Monitor for therapeutic effectiveness: Relief or reduction of migraine pain within 1–4 h.
- Monitor cardiovascular status carefully following first dose in patients at risk for CAD (e.g., postmenopausal women, men older than 40 y, persons with known CAD risk factors) or coronary artery vasospasms.
- Periodic cardiovascular evaluation is recommended with long-term use.
- Report to prescriber immediately chest pain, nausea, or tightness in chest or throat that is severe or does not quickly resolve.

Patient & Family Education

- Carefully review patient information insert and guidelines for taking drug.
- **Do not** take zolmitriptan during the aura phase, but as early as possible after onset of migraine.
- Do not remove orally disintegrating tablet from blister until just prior to dosing.
- Concurrent oral contraceptive use may increase incidence of adverse effects.
- Contact prescriber immediately if any of the following occur after zolmitriptan use: Symptoms of angina (e.g., severe or persistent pain or tightness in chest or throat, sudden nausea), hypersensitivity (e.g., wheezing, facial swelling, skin rash, hives), fainting, or abdominal pain.
- Report any other adverse effects (e.g., tingling, flushing, dizziness) at next prescriber visit.

ZOLPIDEM (Pr)

(zol'pi-dem)

Ambien, Ambien CR, Edluar, Zolpimist

Classification: SEDATIVE-HYPNOTIC, NONBARBITUATE

Therapeutic: SEDATIVE-HYPNOTIC

Controlled Substance: Schedule IV

AVAILABILITY

Tablet; extended release tablet; sublingual tablet; oral solution

ACTION & *THERAPEUTIC EFFECT*

An agonist that binds the gamma-aminobutyric acid (GABA)-A receptor chloride channel, thus inhibiting its action potential in the cortical region of the brain. *Effective as a sedative.*

USES

Short-term treatment of insomnia.

CONTRAINDICATIONS

Hypersensitivity of zolpidem or any component of the formulation; suicidal ideation; patients who have experienced complex sleep behaviors after taking zolpidem.

CAUTIOUS USE Depressed patients, psychiatric disorders; history of suicidal tendencies; hepatic/renal impairment, alcohol or drug abuse; patients with compromised respiratory status, COPD, sleep apnea; chronic depression; older adults; pregnancy (severe neonatal respiratory depression and sedation have been reported when zolpidem was used at the end of pregnancy). Safe use in children younger than 18 y not established.

ROUTE & DOSAGE

Short-Term Treatment of Insomnia

Adult: **PO Immediate release** 5 mg (female) or 10 mg (male) immediately before bedtime OR **Extended release** 6.25 mg (female) or 12.5 mg (male) immediately before bedtime **PO** Sublingual tablet form 1.75 mg (women) or 3.5 mg (men) once/night if needed
Geriatric: Avoid use

Hepatic Impairment Dosage Adjustment

Immediate release 5 mg OR **Extended release** 6.25 mg at bedtime Sublingual tablet 1.75 mg once per night

ADMINISTRATION

Oral

- Give immediately before bedtime; for more rapid sleep onset, **do not** give with or immediately after a meal.
- Ensure that sublingual tablets are not swallowed.
- Extended release tablets should be swallowed whole. Ensure that they are not crushed or chewed.
- Store at room temperature, 15°–30° C (59°–86° F).

ADVERSE EFFECTS CNS: *Headache on awakening, drowsiness, fatigue*, dizziness. Doses greater than 10 mg may be associated with anterograde amnesia or memory impairment.

DIAGNOSTIC TEST INTERFERENCE Increases aminotransferase (ALT/AST), bilirubin; decreases RAI uptake.

INTERACTIONS Drug: CNS DEPRESSANTS, **alcohol**, PHENOTHIAZINES by augmenting CNS depression. **Food:** Extent and rate of absorption of zolpidem are significantly decreased.

PHARMACOKINETICS Absorption: Readily from GI tract. 70% reaches systemic circulation. **Onset:** 7–27 min. **Peak:** 0.5–2.3 h. **Duration:** 6–8 h. **Distribution:** Highly protein bound. Lowest concentrations in CNS, highest concentrations in glandular tissue and fat. Crosses placenta. **Metabolism:** In the liver to 3 inactive metabolites. **Elimination:** 79–96% in the bile, urine, and feces. **Half-Life:** 1.7–2.5 h.

NURSING IMPLICATIONS

Assessment & Drug Effects

- Assess respiratory function in patients with compromised respiratory status. Report immediately to prescriber significantly depressed respiratory rate (less than 12/min).
- Monitor patients for S&S of depression (see Appendix F); zolpidem may increase level of depression.

- Monitor closely older adult or debilitated patients for impaired cognitive or motor function and unusual sensitivity to the drug's effects. Institute fall risk precautions.

Patient & Family Education

- Avoid taking alcohol or other CNS depressants while on zolpidem.
- Do not drive or engage in other potentially hazardous activities until response to drug is known.
- Report vision changes to prescriber.
- Note: Onset of drug is more rapid when taken on an empty stomach.

ZONISAMIDE

(zon-i′sa-mide)

Zonegran

Classification: ANTICONVULSANT; SULFONAMIDE

Therapeutic: ANTICONVULSANT

AVAILABILITY Capsule

ACTION & *THERAPEUTIC EFFECT* A broad-spectrum anticonvulsant that facilitates dopaminergic and serotonergic neurotransmission but does not potentiate the activity of gamma-aminobutyric acid (GABA) in the synapses of the CNS neurons. *Suppresses focal spike discharges and electroshock seizures. Effective against a variety of seizure types.*

USES Adjunctive therapy for focal partial onset seizures.

UNLABELED USES Binge eating disorder.

CONTRAINDICATIONS Hypersensitivity to sulfonamides or zonisamide; suicidal ideation; worsening of depression; severe metabolic acidosis; abrupt discontinuation; lactation.

CAUTIOUS USE Depressive individuals; CNS effects; history of suicidal tendencies; renal or hepatic insufficiency, dehydration, hypovolemia; renal impairment; older adults; pregnancy (limited information related to use during pregnancy; patients exposed to zonisamide during pregnancy are encouraged to enroll in the NAAED Pregnancy Registry). Safety and efficacy in children younger than 16 y not established.

ROUTE & DOSAGE

Partial Seizures

Adult/Adolescent/Child (16 y or older): **PO** Start at 100 mg daily, may increase after 2 wk to 200 mg/day, may then increase q2wk, if necessary (max: 400 mg/day in 1–2 divided doses)

ADMINISTRATION

Oral

- Do not crush or break capsules; ensure capsules are swallowed whole with adequate fluid.
- Withdraw drug gradually when discontinued to minimize seizure potential.
- Store at 25° C (77° F); room temperature permitted. Protect from light and moisture.

ADVERSE EFFECTS **CNS:** Agitation, irritability, ataxia, confusion, depression, difficulty concentrating, difficulty with memory, *dizziness*, fatigue, *headache*, insomnia, mental slowing, nervousness, paresthesia, *somnolence*, abnormal gait, incoordination. **HEENT:** Nystagmus, diplopia, speech abnormalities, taste perversion, amblyopia, tinnitus. **Endocrine:** Metabolic acidosis. **GI:** Abdominal pain, *anorexia*, diarrhea, nausea. **GU:** Nephrolithiasis. **Hematologic:** Agranulocytosis, aplastic anemia. **Other:** Flu-like syndrome.

INTERACTIONS **Drug:** **Phenytoin, carbamazepine, phenobarbital, valproic acid** may decrease half-life of zonisamide. CNS DEPRESSANTS have additive sedative effect. May enhance the arrhythmogenic effect of **lamotrigine**.

PHARMACOKINETICS **Peak:** 2–6 h. **Distribution:** 40% protein bound, extensively binds to erythrocytes. **Metabolism:** Acetylated in liver by CYP3A4. **Elimination:** Primarily in urine. **Half-Life:** 63–105 h.

NURSING IMPLICATIONS

Assessment & Drug Effects

- Withhold drug and notify prescriber if an unexplained rash or S&S of hypersensitivity appear (see Appendix F).
- Monitor for and report S&S of CNS impairment (somnolence, excessive fatigue, cognitive deficits, speech or language problems, incoordination, gait disturbances); oligohidrosis (lack of sweating) and hyperthermia in pediatric patients.
- Monitor lab tests: Periodic BUN, metabolic profile, serum creatinine, serum bicarbonate, ammonia level.

Patient & Family Education

- Do not abruptly stop taking this medication.
- Increase daily fluid intake to minimize risk of renal stones. Notify prescriber immediately of S&S of renal stones: Sudden back or abdominal pain, and blood in urine.
- Report any of the following: Dizziness, excess drowsiness, frequent headaches, malaise, double vision, lack of coordination, persistent nausea, sore throat, fever, mouth ulcers, or easy bruising.
- Exercise special caution with concurrent use of alcohol or CNS depressants.
- Do not drive or engage in other potentially hazardous activities until response to drug is known.

ZOSTER VACCINE

(zos'ter)

Zostavax

See Appendix J.

APPENDICES

◆ APPENDIX A

(Generic names are in **bold**)

APPENDIX A-1

OCULAR MEDICATIONS

BETA-ADRENERGIC BLOCKERS Prototype for classification: Betaxolol Use: Intraocular hypertension and chronic open-angle glaucoma.

Betaxolol HCl Betoptic S, 0.25% suspension, 0.5% solution	*Adult:* Topical 1 drop in affected eye bid for 0.25% suspension; 1–2 drops in affected eye for 0.5% solution.
Carteolol HCl Ocupress, 1% solution	*Adult:* Topical 1 drop bid
Levobunolol Betagan, 0.25%, 0.5% solution	*Adult:* Topical 1–2 drops of 0.25% solution bid or 1–2 drops of 0.5% solution daily.
Metipranolol HCl 0.3% solution	*Adult:* Topical 1 drop bid
Timolol maleate Betimol, Istalol, Timoptic, Timoptic XE, 0.25%, 0.5% solution	*Adult:* Topical 1 drop of 0.25–0.5% solution bid; may decrease to daily. Apply gel daily. Apply Istalol solution once daily.

ADVERSE EFFECTS/CLINICAL IMPLICATIONS May cause *mild ocular stinging* and discomfort; tearing; may also have the adverse effects of systemic beta-blockers. May precipitate thyroid storm in patients with hyperthyroidism. Patients with impaired cardiac function and the elderly should report to prescriber signs and symptoms of heart failure. Monitor BP for hypotension and heart rate for bradycardia.

MIOTICS Prototype for classification: Pilocarpine HCl Use: Open-angle and angle-closure glaucomas; to reduce IOP and to protect the lens during surgery and laser iridotomy; to counteract effects of mydriatics and cycloplegics following surgery or ophthalmoscopic examination.

Apraclonidine HCl Iopidine, 0.5%, 1% solution	**Intraoperative and Postsurgical Increase in IOP:** *Adult:* **Topical** 1 drop of 1% solution in affected eye 1 h before surgery and 1 drop in same eye immediately after surgery. **Open-Angle Glaucoma:** *Adult:* **Topical** 1 drop of 0.5% solution in affected eye tid
Brimonidine tartrate Alphagan P,0.1%, 0.15%, 0.2% solution	**Glaucoma:** *Adult:* **Topical** 1 drop in affected eye(s) tid approximately 8 h apart. *Child (2 y or older):* **Topical** 1 drop in affected eye tid approximately 8 h apart.

Brinzolamide Azopt, 1% suspension	**Ocular Hypertension or Open-Angle Glaucoma:** *Adult:* **Topical** 1 drop in affected eye(s) tid
Carbachol Miostat 1.5%, 3% solution	**Glaucoma:** *Adult:* **Topical** 2 drops in affected eye(s) up to 3 × daily.
Dorzolamide Trusopt, 2% solution	**Ocular Hypertension or Open-Angle Glaucoma:** *Adult, Child:* **Topical** 1 drop in affected eye(s) tid
Echothiophate 0.125% solution	**Ocular Hypertension:** *Adult:* **Topical** 1 drop in affected eye(s) bid
Pilocarpine HCl Isopto Carpine, 1%, 2%, 4% solution	**Acute Glaucoma:** *Adult:* **Topical** 1 drop of 1–2% solution in affected eye q5–10min for 3–6 doses, then 1 drop q1–3h until IOP is reduced. **Chronic Glaucoma:** *Adult:* **Topical** 1 drop of 0.5–4% solution in affected eye q4–12h or 1 ocular system (Ocusert) q7days. **Miotic:** *Adult:* **Topical** 1 drop of 1% solution in affected eye.

ADVERSE EFFECTS/CLINICAL IMPLICATIONS **Ocular:** Ciliary spasm with brow ache, twitching of eyelids, eye pain with change in eye focus, miosis, *diminished vision in poorly illuminated areas,* blurred vision, reduced visual acuity, sensitivity, contact allergy, lacrimation, follicular conjunctivitis, conjunctival irritation, cataract, retinal detachment. **CNS:** *Headache, drowsiness,* depression, syncope. **GI:** Abnormal taste, dry mouth. **Clinical Implications:** Wait 15 min after instillation before inserting soft contact lenses to avoid staining lenses. Use with MAO inhibitors may increase risk of hypertensive emergency. May increase the effects of beta-blockers and other antihypertensives on blood pressure and heart rate. TCAs may reduce the effects of **brimonidine. Brinzolamide** is a carbonic anhydrase inhibitor (prototype: Acetazolamide) and is a sulfonamide. It should not be used by patients with sulfa allergies. Reconstituted solutions of **echothiophate** remain stable for 1 mo at room temperature. Expiration date should appear on label. The length of time solutions remain stable under refrigeration varies with manufacturer. **Echothiophate** therapy is generally discontinued 2–6 wk before surgery. If necessary, alternate therapy is substituted. Medication should be given in the evening. Give at least 5 min apart from other topical ophthalmic drugs.

PROSTAGLANDINS **Prototype for classification: Latanoprost**

Use: Open-angle glaucoma and intraocular hypertension.

Bimatoprost Lumigan, 0.01%, 0.03% solution	*Adult:* **Topical** 1 drop in affected eye(s) once daily in the evening.
Latanoprost Xalatan, 0.005% solution	*Adult:* **Topical** 1 drop (1.5 mcg) in affected eye(s) once daily in the evening.

Trafluprost Zioptan 0.015 mg/Ml	*Adult:* **Topical** 1 drop in the conjunctival sac of the affected eye(s) once daily in the evening.
Travoprost Travatan, 0.004% solution	*Adult:* **Topical** 1 drop in affected eye(s) once daily in the evening.

ADVERSE EFFECTS **Ocular:** *Conjunctival hyperemia, growth of eyelashes, ocular pruritus,* ocular dryness, visual disturbance, ocular burning, foreign body sensation, eye pain, pigmentation of the periocular skin, blepharitis, cataract, superficial punctate keratitis, eyelid erythema, ocular irritation, eyelash darkening, eye discharge, tearing, photophobia, allergic conjunctivitis, increases in iris pigmentation (brown pigment), conjunctival edema. **Body as a Whole:** Headaches, abnormal liver function tests, asthenia, and hirsutism. **Clinical Implications:** Should instill in the evening. Wait 15 min after instillation before inserting soft contact lenses to avoid staining the lenses. Give at least 5 min apart from other topical ophthalmic drugs.

MYDRIATIC **Prototype for classification: Homatropine HBr**
Use: Mydriatic for ocular examination and as cycloplegic to measure errors of refraction. Also inflammatory conditions of uveal tract, ciliary spasm, as a cycloplegic and mydriatic in preoperative and postoperative conditions, and as an optical aid in select patients with axial lens opacities.

Cyclopentolate HCl Cyclogyl, 0.5%, 1%, 2% solution	**Cycloplegic Refraction:** *Adult:* **Topical** 1 drop of 1% solution in eye 40–50 min before procedure, followed by 1 drop in 5 min; may need 2% solution in patients with darkly pigmented eyes. *Child:* **Topical** 1 drop of 0.5–1% solution in eye 40–50 min before procedure, followed by 1 drop in 5 min; may need 2% solution in patients with darkly pigmented eyes.
Homatropine HBr Homatropaire, Isopto Homatropine, 2%, 5% solution	**Cycloplegic Refraction:** *Adult:* **Topical** 1–2 drops of 2% or 5% solution in eye repeated in 5–10 min if necessary. **Ocular Inflammation:** *Adult:* **Topical** 1–2 drops of 2% or 5% solution in eye up to q3–4h.
Phenylephrine HCl AK-Dilate Ophthalmic, Mydfrin, 0.12%, 2.5%, 10% solution	**Ophthalmoscopy:** *Adult:* **Topical** 1 drop of 2.5% or 10% solution before examination. *Child:* **Topical** 1 drop of 2.5% solution before examination. **Vasoconstrictor:** *Adult:* **Topical** 2 drops of 0.12% solution q3–4h as necessary.
Tropicamide Mydriacyl, Tropicacyl, 0.5%, 1% solution	**Refraction:** *Adult:* **Topical** 1–2 drops of 1% solution in each eye, repeat in 5 min; if patient is not seen within 20–30 min, an additional drop may be instilled. **Examination of Fundus:** *Adult:* **Topical** 1–2 drops of 0.5% solution in each eye 15–20 min prior to examination; may repeat q30min if necessary.

CONTRAINDICATED IN Primary (narrow-angle) glaucoma or predisposition to glaucoma; children younger than 6 y. **Cautious Use in:** Increased IOP, infants, children, pregnancy (category C), the elderly or debilitated; hypertension; hyperthyroidism; diabetes; cardiac disease. **Adverse Effects:** Increased IOP, *blurred vision, photophobia*. **Prolonged Use:** Local irritation, congestion, edema, eczema, follicular conjunctivitis. **Excessive Dosage/Systemic Absorption:** Symptoms of atropine poisoning (flushing, dry skin, mouth, nose; decreased sweating; fever, rash, rapid/irregular pulse; abdominal and bladder distention; hallucinations, confusion). **CNS:** Psychotic reaction, behavior disturbances, ataxia, incoherent speech, restlessness, hallucinations, somnolence, disorientation, failure to recognize people, grand mal seizures. **Clinical Implications:** Carefully monitor **cyclopentolate** patients with seizure disorders, since systemic absorption may precipitate a seizure. Photophobia associated with mydriasis may require patient to wear dark glasses. Since drug causes blurred vision, supervision of activity may be indicated.

VASOCONSTRICTOR; DECONGESTANT Prototype for classification: Naphazoline HCl Use: Ocular vasoconstrictor.

Naphazoline HCl 0.012%, 0.02%, 0.1% solution	*Adult:* **Topical** 1–3 drops of 0.1% solution q3–4h prn or 1–2 drops of a 0.012–0.03% solution q4h prn.
Tetrahydrozoline HCl Opti-Clear, Visine Original, 0.05% solution	*Adult:* **Topical** 1–2 drops of 0.05% solution in eye bid or tid

CONTRAINDICATED IN Narrow-angle glaucoma; concomitant use with MAO INHIBITORS or TRICYCLIC ANTIDEPRESSANTS **Cautious Use in:** Hypertension, cardiac irregularities, advanced arteriosclerosis; diabetes; hyperthyroidism; elderly patients. **Adverse Effects:** Pupillary dilation, increased intraocular pressure, rebound redness of the eye, headache, hypertension, nausea, weakness, sweating. **Overdosage:** Drowsiness, hypothermia, bradycardia, shocklike hypotension, coma.

CORTICOSTEROID, ANTI-INFLAMMATORY Prototype for classification: Hydrocortisone Use: Inflammation. **Unlabeled Use:** Anterior uveitis.

Difluprednate Durezol, 0.05% suspension	*Adult:* **Topical** 1 drop in conjunctival sac qid for the first 24 h; qid for 2 wk; then bid for 2 wk.
Fluorometholone Flarex, FML Forte, FML Liquifilm, 0.1%, 0.25% suspension; 0.1% ointment	*Adult/Child (2 y or older):* **Topical** 1–2 drops of suspension in conjunctival sac q.h. for the first 24–48 h; then bid to qid; or a thin strip of ointment q4h for the first 24–48 h; then 1–3 × day.

Loteprednol etabonate Alrex, Lotemax, 0.2%, 0.5% suspension	*Adult:* **Topical** 1–2 drops in conjunctival sac qid during initial treatment, may increase to q1h if necessary.
Prednisolone sodium phosphate Inflamase Mild, Pred Mild, Prednisol, Inflamase Forte, 0.11%, 0.12%, 0.9% suspension	*Adult:* **Topical** 1–2 drops in conjunctival sac q.h. during the day; then q2h at night; may decrease to 1 drop tid or qid
Rimexolone Vexol, 1% solution	**Postoperative Ocular Inflammation:** *Adult:* **Topical** 1–2 drops qid beginning 24 h after surgery, continue through first 2 wk postoperatively. **Anterior Uveitis:** *Adult:* **Topical** 1–2 drops in affected eye every hour while awake for first wk, then q2h for second wk, then taper frequency until uveitis resolves.

CONTRAINDICATED IN Ocular fungal diseases, *herpes simplex* keratitis, ocular infections, ocular mycobacterial infections, viral disease of cornea or conjunctiva such as vaccinia, varicella. **Adverse Effects: Ocular:** Blurred vision, photophobia, conjunctival edema, corneal edema, erosion, eye discharge, dryness, irritation, pain. **Prolonged Use:** Glaucoma, ocular hypertension, damage to optic nerve, defects in visual acuity and visual fields, posterior subcapsular cataract formation, secondary ocular infections. **Other:** Headache, taste perversion. **Clinical Implications:** Shake all products well before use.

OCULAR ANTIHISTAMINES **Prototype for classification: Emedastine Use:** Relief of signs and symptoms of allergic conjunctivitis.

Azelastine HCl OPTIVAR, 0.05% solution	*Adult/Child (3 y or older):* **Topical** 1 drop in affected eye(s) bid
Bepotastine Bepreve, 1.5% solution	*Adult:* **Topical** 1 drop in affected eye(s) bid
Cetirizine Zerviate, 0.24% solution	*Adult:* **Topical** 1 drop in each eye bid
Cromolyn sodium Crolom, Opticrom, 4% solution	*Adult:* **Topical** 1–2 drops in each eye 4–6 × day.
Emedastine difumarate 0.05% solution	*Adult/Child (3 y or older):* **Topical** 1 drop in affected eye(s) up to qid
Epinastine hydrochloride Elestat, 0.05% solution	*Adult/Child (3 y or older):* **Topical** 1 drop in affected eye(s) up to bid

Ketotifen fumarate Zaditor, 0.025% solution	*Adult:* **Topical** 1 drop in affected eye(s) q8–12h.
Lodoxamide Alomide, 0.1% solution	*Adult/Child (2 mo or older):* **Topical** 1–2 drop in affected eye(s) qid for up to 3 mo.
Nedocromil sodium Alocril, 2% solution	*Adult/Child (3 y or older):* **Topical** 1–2 drops in affected eye(s) bid
Olopatadine HCl Patanol, 0.1% solution; Pataday, 0.2% solution; Pazeo, 0.7% solution	*Adult/Child (3 y or older):* **Topical** 1–2 drops in affected eye(s) bid at least 6–8 h apart.

ADVERSE EFFECTS **Ocular:** Allergic reactions, *burning, stinging,* discharge, dry eyes, eye pain, eyelid disorder, itching, keratitis, lacrimation disorder, mydriasis, photophobia, rash. **CNS:** Drowsiness, fatigue, headache. **Other:** Dry mouth, cold syndrome, pharyngitis, rhinitis, sinusitis, taste perversion. **Clinical Implications:** Wait 10 min after instilling drops before inserting soft contact lenses.

OCULAR NONSTEROIDAL ANTI-INFLAMMATORY DRUGS **Prototype for classification: Ibuprofen Use:** Treatment of ocular pain and inflammation associated with cataract surgery.

Bromfenac Xibrom, 0.09% solution	*Adult:* **Topical** 1 drop into affected eye(s) bid beginning 24 h after cataract surgery and continuing for 14 days.
Diclofenac 0.1% solution	*Adult:* **Topical** 1–2 drops in affected eye(s) within 1 h prior to surgery then 1–2 drops 15 min after surgery, then daily beginning 4–6 h after surgery, continue up to 3 days.
Flurbiprofen Ocufen, 0.03% solution	*Adult:* **Topical** 1 drop q30min beginning 2 h prior to surgery for total of 4 drops.
Ketorolac Acular, Acular LS, Acuvail, 0.4% 0.45%, 0.5% solution	*Adult:* **Topical** 1 drop to affected eye(s) 4 × day beginning 24 h after surgery and continuing for 14 days.
Nepafenac Nevanac, 0.1% suspension	*Adult/Child (10 y or older):* **Topical** 1 drop into affected eye(s) tid beginning 24 h after cataract surgery and continuing for 14 days.

ADVERSE EFFECTS **Ocular:** Conjunctival hyperemia, ocular hypertension, foreign body sensation, decreased visual acuity, headache, iritis, ocular inflammation (e.g., edema, erythema), ocular irritation (burning/stinging), ocular pruritus, ocular pain, photophobia, lacrimation, abnormal sensation in the eye, delayed wound healing, keratitis, lid margin crusting, corneal erosion, corneal perforation, corneal thinning, and epithelial breakdown. Continued use can lead to ulceration or perforation. **Clinical Implications: Nepafenac** suspension **must be** shaken well prior to use.

OCULAR ANTIBIOTIC, QUINOLONE Prototype for classification: Ciprofloxacin Use: Treatment of ocular infection.

Besifloxacin Besivance, 0.6% suspension	*Adult/Adolescent/Child (1 y or older):* **Topical** 1 drop in affected eye(s) tid × 7 days
Ciprofloxacin Ciloxin, 0.3% solution	*Adult/Adolescent/Child (1 y or older):* **Topical** 1–2 drops in affected eye(s) q2h × 2 days then q4h × 5 days.
Levofloxacin 0.5% solution	*Adult/Adolescent/Child (6 y or older):* **Topical** 1–2 drops in affected eye(s) q2h (up to 8 × day) on days 1 and 2 then q4h (up to 4 × day)
Moxifloxacin Vigamox, 0.5% solution Moxeza, 0.5% solution	*Adult/Child (1 y or older):* **Topical** (Vigamox) 1 drop in affected eye(s) tid × 7 days. (Moxeza) 1 drop in affected eye(s) bid × 7 days
Ofloxacin Ocuflox 0.3% solution	*Adult/Adolescent/Child:* **Ophthalmic** Instill 1–2 drops q2–4h for first 2 days, then qid × 5 additional days

ADVERSE EFFECTS Ocular: Conjunctival redness, blurred vision, irritation, pain, pruritus. **CNS:** Headache.

APPENDIX A-2

LOW MOLECULAR WEIGHT HEPARINS

ANTICOAGULANT, LOW MOLECULAR WEIGHT HEPARIN Prototype for classification: Enoxaparin Use: Prevention and treatment of DVT following hip or knee replacement or abdominal surgery, unstable angina, acute coronary syndromes.

Dalteparin sodium Fragmin, 10,000 international units/mL, 25,000 international units/mL	**DVT Prophylaxis, Abdominal Surgery:** *Adult:* **Subcutaneous** 2500 international units daily starting 1–2 h prior to surgery and continuing for 5–10 days postoperatively. DVT Prophylaxis, Total Hip Arthroplasty: *Adult:* **Subcutaneous** 2500–5000 international units daily starting 1–2 h prior to surgery and continuing for 5–14 days postoperatively. Acute Thromboembolism:

	Adult: **Subcutaneous** 120 international units/kg bid for at least 5 days. Recurrent Thromboembolism: *Adult:* **Subcutaneous** 5000 international units bid for 3–6 mo. Unstable Angina/Non–Q-Wave MI: *Adult:* **Subcutaneous** 120 international units/kg (max: 10,000 international units) q12h. **DVT Prophylaxis with risk of PE:** *Adult:* **Subcutaneous** 5000 international units once daily for 12–14 days. **Extended Treatment of VTE or Proximal DVT:** *Adult:* **Subcutaneous** 200 international units/kg daily for 1 mo, then 150 international units/kg daily for 2–6 mo.
Enoxaparin Lovenox, 100 mg/mL	**Prevention of DVT after Hip or Knee Surgery:** *Adult:* **Subcutaneous** 30 mg subcutaneously bid for 10–14 days starting 12–24 h post-surgery. **Prevention of DVT after Abdominal Surgery:** *Adult:* **Subcutaneous** 40 mg daily starting 2 h before surgery and continuing for 7–10 days (max: 12 days). **Treatment of DVT and Pulmonary Embolus:** *Adult:* **Subcutaneous** 1 mg/kg bid; monitor anti-Xa activity to determine appropriate dose. **Acute Coronary Syndrome:** *Adult:* **Subcutaneous** 1 mg/kg q12h × 2–8 days. Give concurrently with aspirin 100–325 mg/day.

CONTRAINDICATED IN Hypersensitivity to ardeparin, other low molecular weight heparins, pork products, or parabens; active major bleeding, thrombocytopenia that is positive for antiplatelet antibodies with ardeparin; uncontrolled hypertension; nursing mothers. **Tizaparin** contraindicated in patients over 90 years old with CrCl less than 60 mL/min. **Cautious Use in:** Hypersensitivity to heparin; history of heparin-induced thrombocytopenia; bacterial endocarditis; severe and uncontrolled hypertension, cerebral aneurysm or hemorrhagic stroke, bleeding disorders, recent GI bleeding or associated GI disorders (e.g., ulcerative colitis), thrombocytopenia, or platelet disorders; severe liver or renal disease, diabetic retinopathy, hypertensive retinopathy, invasive procedures; pregnancy (category C). **Adverse Effects: Body as a Whole:** Allergic reactions (rash, urticaria), arthralgia, pain and inflammation at injection site, peripheral edema, fever. **CNS:** *CVA,* dizziness, headache, insomnia. **CV:** Chest pain. **GI:** Nausea, vomiting. **Hematologic:** *Hemorrhage,* thrombocytopenia, ecchymoses, anemia. **Respiratory:** Dyspnea. **Skin:** Rash, pruritus. **Drug Interactions: Aspirin,** NSAIDS, **warfarin** can increase risk of hemorrhage **Clinical Implications:** Alternate injection sites using the abdomen, anterior thigh, or outer aspect of upper arms. **Lab Tests:** CBC with platelet count, urinalysis, and stool for occult blood should be tested throughout therapy. Routine coagulation tests are not required. Carefully monitor for and immediately report S&S of excessive anticoagulation (e.g., bleeding at venipuncture sites or surgical site) or hemorrhage (e.g., drop in BP or Hct). Patients on oral anticoagulants, platelet inhibitors, or with impaired renal function **must be** very carefully monitored for hemorrhage. Patient should be sitting or lying supine for injection. Inject deep subcutaneously with entire length of needle inserted into skin fold. Hold skin fold gently throughout injection and do not rub site after injection.

APPENDIX A-3

INHALED CORTICOSTEROIDS (ORAL AND NASAL INHALATIONS)

CORTICOSTEROID, ANTIINFLAMMATORY Prototype for classification: Hydrocortisone Use: Oral inhalation to treat steroid-dependent asthma, nasal inhalation for the management of the symptoms of seasonal or perennial rhinitis.

Beclomethasone dipropionate Beconase AQ, Qnasl	**Asthma:** *Adult:* **Oral Inhaler** 40–80 mcg bid may try to reduce systemic steroids after 1 wk of concomitant therapy; (max: 320 mcg/day). *Child (4–11 y):* **Oral Inhaler QVAR Redihaler** 40 mcg bid (max: 160 mcg/day). **Allergic Rhinitis:** *Adult:* **Nasal Inhaler** 1–2 spray/nostril bid. *Child (older than 6 y):* 1 spray daily.
Budesonide Pulmicort Flexhaler	**Asthma, Maintenance Therapy:** *Adult:* **Oral Inhalation** 360 mcg bid (max: 720 mcg bid). *Child (6 y or older):* **Oral Inhalation** 180 mcg bid (max: 400 mcg bid). *Child (6 mo–8 y):* **Nebulization** 0.5 mg/day in 1–2 divided doses. **Rhinitis:** *Adult/Child (6 y or older):* **Intranasal** 1–2 sprays each/nostril each day.
Ciclesonide Alvesco, Omnaris, Zetonna	**Rhinitis:** *Adult/Child (2 y or older):* **Intranasal** 1–2 sprays/nostril once daily (depends on product used). **Asthma:** *Adult/Child (12 y and older):* **Inhaled** 80 mcg bid; may increase to 320 mcg bid depending on previous therapies
Flunisolide 0.025% nasal solution	**Allergic Rhinitis:** *Adult/Adolescent:* **Intranasal** 2 sprays intranasally/nostril, bid; may increase to tid, if needed. *Child:* **Intranasal** 6–14 y, 1 spray intranasally/nostril tid or 2 sprays bid
Fluticasone ArmonAir RespiClick, Flonase, Flovent, Flovent HFA, 44 mcg, 110 mcg, 220 mcg aerosol, **Veramyst,** 27.5 mcg/actuation	**Seasonal Allergic Rhinitis:** *Adult:* **Intranasal** 100 mcg (1 inhalation)/nostril 1–2 × daily (max: 4 × daily). **Inhalation** 1–2 inhalations daily. *Child (4 y or older):* **Intranasal** 1 spray/nostril once daily. May increase to 2 sprays/nostril once daily if inadequate response, then decrease to 1 spray/nostril once daily. when control is achieved. *Adult/Adolescent/Child (12 y or older):* **Intranasal (Veramyst)** 2 sprays/nostril daily then reduce to 1 spray daily. *Child (2–11 y):* **Intranasal (Veramyst)** 1 spray/nostril daily, may increase to 2 sprays/nostril daily if necessary. *Adult/Adolescent:* **Inhaled (Advair)** 1–2 inhalations q12h.

Fluticasone/ Vilanterol Breo Ellipta, 100 mcg/25 mcg powder for inhalation	*Adult:* **Inhalation** 1 inhalation every 24 h.
Mometasone furoate Asmanex, Sinuva 220 mcg/ inhalation, 50 mcg/inhalation	**Allergic Rhinitis:** *Adult/Child (12 y or older):* **Intranasal** 2 sprays (50 mcg each) in each nostril once daily. *Child (2 y–11 y):* **Intranasal** 1 spray in each nostril once daily. *Adult/Child (12 y or older):* **Powder for Inhalation** 1 inhalation (220 mcg) once or twice daily (max: 400 mcg bid). *Child (4–11 y):* **Powder for Inhalation** 110 mcg/inhalation (may increase to 440 mcg) bid
Triamcinolone acetonide Nasacort, 100 mcg/ inhalation	*Adult:* **Inhalation** 2 puffs 3–4 × day (max: 16 puffs/ day) or 4 puffs bid **Nasal Spray** 2 sprays/nostril once daily (max: 8 sprays/day). *Child (6–12 y):* **Inhalation** 1–2 sprays tid or qid (max: 12 sprays/ day) or 2–4 sprays bid **Intranasal** 1 spray in each nostril daily.

CONTRAINDICATED IN Hypersensitivity to any component of the formulation; severe hypersensitivity to milk proteins; primary treatment of status asthmaticus, acute attack of asthma, acute episode of COPD. **Cautious Use in:** Patients receiving systemic corticosteroids; use with extreme caution if at all in respiratory tuberculosis, untreated fungal, bacterial, or viral infections, and ocular herpes simplex; nasal inhalation therapy for nasal septal ulcers, nasal trauma, or surgery. **Adverse Effects: Oral Inhalation:** *Candidal infection of oropharynx* and occasionally larynx, hoarseness, dry mouth, sore throat, sore mouth, otitis media, respiratory infection, rhinitis, headache, nasopharyngitis, fatigue, malaise, headache. **Nasal (Inhaler):** *Transient nasal irritation, burning, sneezing,* epistaxis, bloody mucus, nasopharyngeal itching, dryness, crusting, and ulceration; headache, nausea, vomiting. **Other:** With excessive doses, symptoms of hypercorticism. Increased risk of adverse effects if Advair is used with other long-acting beta-agonists. **Clinical Implications:** Note that oral inhalation and nasal inhalation products are not to be used interchangeably. **Oral Inhaler:** Emphasize the following: (1) Shake inhaler well before using. (2) After exhaling fully, place mouthpiece well into mouth with lips closed firmly around it. (3) Inhale slowly through mouth while activating the inhaler. (4) Hold breath 5–10 sec, if possible, then exhale slowly. (5) Wait 1 min between puffs. Clean inhaler daily. Separate parts as directed in package insert, rinse them with warm water, and dry them thoroughly. Rinsing mouth and gargling with warm water after each oral inhalation removes residual medication from oropharyngeal area. Mouth care may also delay or prevent onset of oral dryness, hoarseness, and candidiasis. **Nasal Inhaler:** Directions for use of nasal inhaler provided by manufacturer should be carefully reviewed with patient. Emphasize the following points: (1) Gently blow nose to clear nostrils. (2) Shake inhaler well before using. (3) If 2 sprays in each nostril are prescribed, direct one spray toward upper, and the other toward lower part of nostril. (4) Wash cap and plastic nosepiece daily with warm water; dry thoroughly. Inhaled steroids do not provide immediate symptomatic relief and are not prescribed for this purpose.

APPENDIX A-4

TOPICAL CORTICOSTEROIDS

CORTICOSTEROID, ANTI-INFLAMMATORY Prototype for classification: Hydrocortisone Use: As a topical corticosteroid, the drug is used for the relief of the inflammatory and pruritic manifestations of corticosteroid-responsive dermatoses.

Drug	Dosage
Hydrocortisone Aeroseb-HC, Alphaderm, Cetacort, Cortaid, Cortenema, Dermolate, Hytone, Rectacort, Synacort, Caldecort, 0.5%, 1%, 2.5% cream, lotion, ointment, spray	*Adult:* **Topical** Apply a small amount to the affected area 1–4 × day. **PR** Insert 1% cream, 10% foam, 10–25 mg suppository, or 100 mg enema nightly.
Hydrocortisone acetate Anusol HC, Carmol HC, Colifoam, Cortaid, Cort-Dome, Corticaine, Cortifoam, Epifoam, 0.5%, 1% ointment, cream	
Alclometasone dipropionate 0.05% cream, ointment	*Adult:* **Topical** Apply sparingly bid or tid; may use occlusive dressing for resistant dermatoses.
Amcinonide 0.1% cream, lotion, ointment	*Adult:* **Topical** Apply thin film bid or tid
Betamethasone dipropionate Diprolene, Diprolene AF, Diprosone, Maxivate, 0.05% cream, gel, lotion, ointment	*Adult:* **Topical** Apply thin film bid
Betamethasone valerate Luxiq, Valisone, Psorion, Beta-Val, 0.1% cream, ointment, lotion; 0.12% aerosol foam	*Adult:* **Topical** Apply sparingly bid
Clobetasol propionate Clobex, Cormax, Embeline, Olux, Tovate, 0.05% cream, gel, ointment, lotion, aerosol foam	*Adult:* **Topical** Apply sparingly bid (max: 50 g/wk) for up to 2 weeks.

Drug	Dosage
Clocortolone pivalate Cloderm, 0.1% cream	*Adult:* **Topical** Apply thin layer tid
Desonide Desonate, DesOwen, Tridesilon, Verdeso, 0.05% cream, ointment, lotion, gel, foam	*Adult:* **Topical** Apply thin layer bid to tid (lotion) or bid to qid (cream, ointment) or bid (foam, gel)
Desoximetasone Topicort, 0.05%, 0.25% cream, gel, ointment; 0.25% topical spray	*Adult:* **Topical** Apply thin layer bid if no improvement in 4 weeks reassess diagnosis
Diclofenac Flector, Pennsaid, 1.3% topical patch; 1% topical gel	*Adult:* **Topical** Up to 4 g 4 × day on affected joint (max: 16 g).
Diflorasone diacetate ApexiCon E, Psorcon E, Psorcon, 0.05% cream, ointment	*Adult:* **Topical** Apply thin layer 1–3 × day.
Fluocinolone acetonide Capex, Synalar, 0.025% ointment, cream; 0.2% cream; 0.01% cream, solution, shampoo	*Adult:* **Topical** Apply thin layer bid to qid
Fluocinonide Vanos, 0.05% cream, ointment, solution, gel; 0.1% cream	*Adult:* **Topical** Apply thin layer bid to qid
Flurandrenolide Cordran, Nolix, 0.025% cream; 0.05% cream, lotion; 4 mcg/cm^2 tape	*Adult/Child:* **Topical** Apply thin layer bid or tid; apply tape 1–2 × day
Fluticasone Beser, Cutivate, 0.05% cream, lotion; 0.005% ointment	*Adult/Child (3 mo or older):* **Topical** Apply a thin layer to affected area once or twice daily if no improvement within 2 weeks reassess diagnosis.
Halcinonide Halog, 0.1% cream, ointment, solution	*Adult:* **Topical** Apply thin layer bid or tid *Child:* **Topical** Apply thin layer once/day.
Halobetasol Ultravate, 0.05% cream, ointment	*Adult:* **Topical** Apply sparingly bid
Mometasone furoate Elocon, 0.1% cream, lotion, ointment	*Adult:* **Topical** Apply a thin film of cream or ointment or a few drops of lotion to affected area once/day.

Triamcinolone Kenalog, Triderm, 0.025%, 0.5%, 0.1% cream, ointment; 0.025%, 0.1% lotion	*Adult:* **Topical** Apply sparingly bid or tid

CONTRAINDICATED IN Topical steroids contraindicated in presence of hypersensitivity, varicella, vaccinia, on surfaces with compromised circulation, lesions exuding serum or in intertriginous areas (tape), and in children younger than 1 y. **Cautious Use in:** Children; diabetes mellitus; stromal *herpes simplex;* glaucoma, tuberculosis of eye; osteoporosis; untreated fungal, bacterial, or viral infections **Adverse Effects: Skin:** Skin thinning and atrophy, *acne, impaired wound healing,* secondary infection (oral candidiasis, sinus infection); skin rash, pruritis; hypopigmentation or hyperpigmentation, hyperglycemia, hypothalamic-pituitary-adrenal axis dysfunction, pseudotumor cerebri, glycosuria hirsutism, acneiform eruptions, subcutaneous fat atrophy; allergic dermatitis, urticaria, intracranial hypertension, localized burning, local irritation, fatigue, malaise, headache, arthralgia. **Clinical Implications:** Administer retention enema preferably after a bowel movement. The enema should be retained at least 1 h or all night if possible. If an occlusive dressing is to be used, apply medication sparingly, rub until it disappears, and then reapply, leaving a thin coat over lesion. Completely cover area with transparent plastic or other occlusive device or vehicle. Avoid covering a weeping or exudative lesion. Usually, occlusive dressings are not applied to face, scalp, scrotum, axilla, and groin. Inspect skin carefully between applications for ecchymotic, petechial, and purpuric signs, maceration, secondary infection, skin atrophy, striae or miliaria; if present, stop medication and notify prescriber. Warn patient not to self-dose with OTC topical preparations of a corticosteroid more than 7 days. They should not be used for children younger than 2 y. If symptoms do not abate, consult prescriber. Usually, topical preparations are applied after a shower or bath when skin is damp or wet. Cleansing and application of prescribed preparation should be done with extreme gentleness because of fragility, easy bruisability, and poor-healing skin. Hazard of systemic toxicity is higher in small children because of the greater ratio of skin surface area to body weight. Apply sparingly. Urge patient on long-term therapy with topical corticosterone to check expiration date.

APPENDIX A-5

TOPICAL ANTIFUNGAL AGENTS

USES Treatment of fungal infections managed by topical agents. This could include: Tinea (pityriasis) versicolor due to *M. furfur* (formerly *P. orbiculare*), interdigital tinea pedis (athlete's foot), tinea corporis (ringworm) and tinea cruris (jock itch) due to *E. floccosum, T. mentagrophytes, T. rubrum,* and *T. tonsurans*. Shampoo for treatment of seborrheic dermatitis.

Butenafine Lotrimin Ultra, Mentax, 1% cream	*Adult:* **Topical** Apply 1–2 × daily for 2–4 wk.

Drug	Dosage
Ciclopirox Ciclodan, Loprox, Penlac, 8% solution, 1% shampoo, 0.77% gel	*Adult:* **Topical** Apply twice daily (morning and evening). Nail lacquer solution should be applied once daily.
Econazole Ecoza, 1% cream, 1% foam	*Adult:* **Topical** Apply once daily × 2–4 wk (depending on area).
Efinaconazole Jublia, 10% solution	*Adult:* **Topical** Apply daily to affected toenail × 48 wk.
Ketoconazole 2% cream	*Adult:* **Topical** Apply to affected area daily × 2 wk.
Luliconazole Luzu, 1% cream	*Adult:* **Topical** Apply to affected area daily × 1–2 wk.
Miconazole 2% cream	*Adult:* **Topical** Apply to affected area bid × 2–4 weeks
Naftifine Naftin, 1%, 2% cream; 1%, 2% gel	*Adult:* **Topical** Apply cream once daily or gel twice daily to affected areas × 2–4 wk.
Oxiconazole Oxistat, 1% cream	*Adult:* **Topical** Apply to affected area 1–2 times daily × 2–4 wk.
Sertaconazole Eratczo, 2% cream	*Adult:* **Topical** Apply to affected area bid × 4 wk.
Sulconazole Exelderm, 1% cream; 1% solution	*Adult:* **Topical** Apply to affected area 1–2 times daily × 3–4 wk.
Tavaborole Kerydin 5% solution	*Adult:* **Topical** Apply to affected toenails daily × 48 wk.
Terbinafine Lamisil, 1% cream	*Adult:* **Topical** Apply to affected area 1–2 times daily for at least 1 week
Tolnaftate Fungi-Guard, Fongoid-D, Lamisil AF Defense, Mycocide Clinical NS, Tinactin, Tinaspore, 1% solution, 1% powder, 1% cream, 1% aerosol, 1% aerosol powder	*Adult/Adolescent/Child (2 y or older):* **Topical** Apply to affected area 1–2 times daily × 4 wk.

CONTRAINDICATED IN Patients with known or suspected sensitivity to agent.

CAUTIOUS USE Pregnancy or lactation, cautious use in children (except tolnaftate), avoid use with occlusive dressing.

ADVERSE EFFECTS **Skin:** Stinging/burning at application site, contact dermatitis, erythema, irritation, itching. **Dermatologic:** Ingrown toenail.

CLINICAL IMPLICATIONS If symptoms not resolving within recommended therapy duration patient needs to be re-evaluated. Patients using a nail product should avoid pedicures, or use of nail polish during treatment.

◆ APPENDIX B U.S. SCHEDULES OF CONTROLLED SUBSTANCES

Schedule I

High potential for abuse and of no currently accepted medical use. Examples: heroin, LSD, ecstasy peyote. Not obtainable by prescription but may be legally procured for research, study, or instructional use.

Schedule II

High abuse potential and high liability for severe psychological or physical dependence. Prescription required and cannot be renewed.[a] Includes opium derivatives, other opioids, and short-acting barbiturates. Examples: Amphetamine, cocaine, meperidine, morphine, fentanyl.

Schedule III

Potential for abuse is less than that for drugs in Schedules I and II. Moderate to low physical dependence and high psychological dependence. Includes certain stimulants and depressants not included in the above schedules and preparations containing limited quantities of certain opioids. Examples: Ketamine, anabolic steroids, testosterone. Prescription required.[a,b]

Schedule IV

Lower potential for abuse than Schedule III drugs. Examples: Certain psychotropics (tranquilizers), chlordiazepoxide, diazepam, meprobamate, phenobarbital. Prescription required.[a,b]

Schedule V

Abuse potential less than that for Schedule IV drugs. Preparations contain limited quantities of certain narcotic drugs; generally intended for antitussive and antidiarrheal purposes and may be distributed without a prescription provided that:

1. Such distribution is made only by a pharmacist.
2. Not more than 240 mL or not more than 48 solid dosage units of any substance containing opium, nor more than 120 mL or not more than 24 solid dosage units of any other controlled substance may be distributed at retail to the same purchaser in any given 48-hour period without a valid prescription order.
3. The purchaser is at least 18 years old.

4. The pharmacist knows the purchaser or requests suitable identification.
5. The pharmacist keeps an official written record of: name and address of purchaser, name and quantity of controlled substance purchased, date of sale, initials of dispensing pharmacist. This record is to be made available for inspection and copying by U.S. officers authorized by the Attorney General.
6. Other federal, state, or local law does not require a prescription order.

Under jurisdiction of the Federal Controlled Substances Act:
[a]Except when dispensed directly by a practitioner, other than a pharmacist, to an ultimate user, no controlled substance in Schedule II may be dispensed without a *written* prescription, except that in emergency situations such drug may be dispensed upon oral prescription and a written prescription must be obtained within the time frame prescribed by law. No prescription for a controlled substance in Schedule II may be refilled.
[b]Refillable up to 5 × within 6 mo, but only if so indicated by prescriber.

◆ APPENDIX C FDA PREGNANCY INFORMATION

In December 2014 the FDA released a final rule replacing the historic *letter categories* (listed below) with new detailed subsections describing the risk of medication exposure in the real-world context of caring for pregnant patients. The final rule requires the use of three subsections in the labeling titled, *Pregnancy, Lactation,* and *Females and Males of Reproductive Potential* that provide details about use of the drug or biological product. The historic categories described by the FDA are as follows:

Category A

Controlled studies in women fail to demonstrate a risk to the fetus in the first trimester (and there is no evidence of risk in later trimesters), and the possibility of fetal harm appears remote.

Category B

Either animal-reproduction studies have not demonstrated a fetal risk but there are no controlled studies in pregnant women, or animal-reproduction studies have shown an adverse effect (other than a decrease in fertility) that was not confirmed in controlled studies in women in the first trimester (and there is no evidence of a risk in later trimesters).

Category C

Either studies in animals have revealed adverse effects on the fetus (teratogenic or embryocidal effects or other) and there are no controlled studies in women, or studies in women and animals are not available. Drugs should be given only if the potential benefit justifies the potential risk to the fetus.

Category D

There is positive evidence of human fetal risk, but the benefits from use in pregnant women may be acceptable despite the risk (e.g., if the drug is needed in a life-threatening situation or for a serious disease for which safer drugs cannot be used or are ineffective). There will be an appropriate statement in the "warnings" section of the labeling.

Category X

Studies in animals or human beings have demonstrated fetal abnormalities or there is evidence of fetal risk based on human experience, or both, and the risk of the use of the drug in pregnant women clearly outweighs any possible benefit. The drug is contraindicated in women who are or may become pregnant. There will be an appropriate statement in the "contraindications" section of the labeling.

Drugs approved after June 2015 will not have a *pregnancy category* but will instead include the categories of *Pregnancy, Lactation, and Females and Males of Reproductive Potential.*

◆ APPENDIX D PRESCRIPTION COMBINATION DRUGS*

Acanya (ANTIACNE) *gel:* benzoyl peroxide 2.5%/clindamycin (see p. 380) 1.2%.

Accuretic (ANTIHYPERTENSIVE) *tablet:* quinapril (see p. 1442) 10 mg/hydrochlorothiazide (see p. 809) 12.5 mg; 20 mg quinapril (see p. 1442)/12.5 mg hydrochlorothiazide; 20 mg quinapril/25 mg hydrochlorothiazide.

Activella (HORMONE REPLACEMENT THERAPY) *tablet:* estradiol (see p. 650) 1 mg/norethindrone acetate (see p. 1194) 0.5 mg.

Actonel with Calcium (BISPHOSPHONATE) *tablet:* risedronate (see p. 1448) 35 mg/1250 calcium carbonate (see p. 249).

ACTOplus Met (ANTIDIABETIC) *tablet:* pioglitazone (see p. 1351) 15 mg/metformin (see p. 1051) 500 mg; pioglitazone 15 mg/metformin 850 mg.

Advair Diskus (BRONCHODILATOR) *Inhalation powder:* fluticasone propionate (see p. 737) 100 mcg/salmeterol (see p. 1517) 50 mcg; fluticasone propionate 250 mcg/salmeterol 50 mcg; fluticasone propionate 115 mcg/salmeterol 21 mcg; fluticasone propionate 230 mcg/salmeterol 21 mcg; fluticasone propionate 45 mcg/salmeterol 21 mcg.

Advicor (ANTILIPEMIC) *tablets, sustained release:* niacin (see p. 1164) 500 mg/lovastatin (see p. 1001) 20 mg; niacin 1000 mg/lovastatin 20 mg.

Aggrenox (ANTIPLATELET) *extended release capsule:* dipyridamole (see p. 529) 200 mg/aspirin (see p. 126) 25 mg.

AirDuo RespiClick (BRONCHODILATOR) *inhalation powder:* fluticasone (see p. 737) 113 mcg/salmeterol (see p. 1517) 14 mcg; fluticasone 232 mcg/salmeterol 14 mcg; fluticasone 55 mcg/salmeterol 14 mcg.

Akynzeo (ANTIEMETIC) *solution:* reconsitituted fosnetupitant 235 mg/plonosetron 0.25 mg.

Aldactazide 25/25 (DIURETIC) *tablet:* spironolactone (see p. 1577) 25 mg/hydrochlorothiazide (see p. 809) 25 mg.

Aldactazide 50/50 (DIURETIC) *tablet:* spironolactone (see p. 1577) 50 mg/hydrochlorothiazide (see p. 809) 50 mg.

Allegra D 12 hour (ANTIHISTAMINE, DECONGESTANT) *tablet, extended release:* fexofenadine (see p. 708) 60 mg/pseudoephedrine (see p. 1429) 120 mg.

Allegra D 24 hour (ANTIHISTAMINE, DECONGESTANT) *tablet, extended release:* fexofenadine (see p. 708) 180 mg/pseudoephedrine (see p. 1429) 240 mg.

Anexsia 5/325 (NARCOTIC ANALGESIC [schedule III]) *tablet:* hydrocodone (see p. 811) 5 mg/acetaminophen (see p. 13) 325 mg.

Anexsia 7.5/325 (NARCOTIC ANALGESIC [schedule III]) *tablet:* hydrocodone (see p. 811) 7.5 mg/acetaminophen (see p. 13) 325 mg.

Angeliq (HORMONE) *tablet:* drospirenone 0.5 mg/estradiol (see p. 650) 1 mg.

Apresazide 25/25 (ANTIHYPERTENSIVE) *capsule:* hydralazine hydrochloride (see p. 807) 25 mg/hydrochlorothiazide (see p. 809) 25 mg.

*For a complete list that includes nonprescription drugs, please see our companion website at www.prenhall.com

Apresazide 50/50 (ANTIHYPERTENSIVE) *capsule:* hydralazine hydrochloride (see p. 807) 50 mg/hydrochlorothiazide (see p. 809) 50 mg.

Apresodex (ANTIHYPERTENSIVE) *tablet:* hydralazine hydrochloride (see p. 807) 25 mg/hydrochlorothiazide (see p. 809) 15 mg.

Aralen Phosphate with Primaquine Phosphate (ANTIMALARIAL) *tablet:* chloroquine phosphate (see p. 340) 500 mg (300 mg base)/primaquine phosphate (see p. 1395) 79 mg (45 mg base).

Arthrotec 50 (NSAID) *tablet:* diclofenac sodium (see p. 499) 50 mg/misoprostol (see p. 1108) 200 mcg.

Arthrotec 75 (NSAID) tablet: diclofenac sodium (see p. 499) 75 mg/misoprostol (see p. 1108) 200 mcg.

Atacand HCT (ANTIHYPERTENSIVE) *tablet:* candesartan (see p. 258) 32 mg/hydrochlorothiazide (see p. 809) 12.5 mg; candesartan 16 mg/hydrochlorothiazide 12.5 mg.

Atripla (ANTIRETROVIRAL) *tablet:* 600 mg efavirenz (see p. 581)/200 mg emtricitabine (see p. 594)/300 mg tenofovir (see p. 1628).

Augmentin (ANTIBIOTIC) *tablet:* amoxicillin (see p. 86) 250 mg/clavulanic acid 125 mg; amoxicillin 500 mg/clavulanic acid 125 mg; amoxicillin 875 mg/clavulanic acid 125 mg; amoxicillin 1000 mg/clavulanic acid 125 mg; *chewable tablet:* amoxicillin 125 mg/clavulanic acid 31.25 mg; amoxicillin 200 mg/clavulanic acid 28.5 mg; amoxicillin 250 mg/clavulanic acid 62.5 mg; amoxicillin 400 mg/clavulanic acid 57 mg; *suspension (per 5 mL):* amoxicillin 125 mg/clavulanic acid 31.25 mg; amoxicillin 200 mg/clavulanic acid 28.5 mg; amoxicillin 250 mg/clavulanic acid 62.5 mg; amoxicillin 400 mg/clavulanic acid 57 mg; amoxicillin 600 mg/clavulanic acid 42.9 mg.

Avalide (ANTIHYPERTENSIVE) *tablet:* irbesartan (see p. 886) 150 mg/hydrochlorothiazide (see p. 809) 12.5 mg; irbesartan 300 mg/hydrochlorothiazide 12.5 mg; irbesartan 300 mg/hydrochlorothiazide 25 mg.

Avandamet (HYPOGLYCEMIC AGENT) *tablet:* 1 mg rosiglitazone maleate (see p. 1509)/500 mg metformin HCl (see p. 1051); 2 mg rosiglitazone/500 mg metformin; 4 mg rosiglitazone/500 mg metformin; 2 mg rosiglitazone/1000 mg metformin; 4 mg rosiglitazone/1000 mg metformin.

Avandaryl (HYPOGLYCEMIC AGENT) *tablet:* rosiglitazone (see p. 1509) 4 mg/glimepiride (see p. 776) 1 mg; rosiglitazone 4 mg/glimepiride 2 mg; rosiglitazone 4 mg/glimepiride 4 mg.

Azo Gantanol (URINARY ANTI-INFECTIVE, ANALGESIC) *tablet:* sulfamethoxazole (see p. 1591) 500 mg, phenazopyridine hydrochloride (see p. 1325) 100 mg.

Azo Gantrisin (URINARY ANTI-INFECTIVE, ANALGESIC) *tablet:* sulfisoxazole (see p. 1008) 500 mg/phenazopyridine hydrochloride (see p. 1325) 50 mg.

Azor (ANTIHYPERTENSIVE) *tablet:* amlodipine (see p. 84) 5 mg/olmesartan (see p. 1210) 20 mg; amlodipine 5 mg/olmesartan 40 mg; amlodipine 10 mg/olmesartan 20 mg; amlodipine 10 mg/olmesartan 40 mg.

B-A-C (ANALGESIC) acetaminophen (see p. 13) 650 mg/caffeine (see p. 243) 40 mg/butalbital 50 mg.

Bacticort Ophthalmic (ANTI-INFLAMMATORY) suspension: hydrocortisone (see p. 812) 1%/neomycin sulfate (see p. 1157) 0.35%/polymyxin B (see p. 1365) 10,000 units.

Bactrim (URINARY TRACT AGENT) *tablet:* sulfamethoxazole (see p. 1591) 400 mg/trimethoprim (see p. 1591) 80 mg.

Bactrim DS (URINARY TRACT AGENT) *tablet:* sulfamethoxazole (see p. 1591) 800 mg/trimethoprim (see p. 1726) 160 mg.

Benicar HCT (ANTIHYPERTENSIVE) *tablet:* 20 mg olmesartan medoxomil (see p. 1210)/12.5 mg hydrochlorothiazide (see p. 809); 40 mg olmesartan medoxomil/12.5 mg hydrochlorothiazide; 40 mg olmesartan medoxomil/25 mg hydrochlorothiazide.

Betoptic Pilo Suspension (ANTIGLAUCOMA) *suspension:* betaxolol (see p. 188) 0.25%/pilocarpine (see p. 1343) 1.75%.

Bevespi Aerosphere (ANTICHOLINERGIC/BETA AGONIST) inhaler: glycopyrrolate 9 mcg/formoterol fum 4.8 mcg.

Beyaz (ORAL CONTRACEPTIVE) *tablet:* drosperinone 3 mg/ethinyl estradiol 0.02 mg/levomefolate calcium 0.451 mg.

BiDil (ANTIHYPERTENSIVE) *tablet:* isosorbide dinitrate (see p. 901) 20 mg/hydralazine (see p. 807) 37.5 mg.

Breo Ellipta (BRONCHODIALATOR) *powder for inhalation:* fluticasone (see p. 737) 100 mcg/vilanterol 25 mcg.

Blephamide (OPHTHALMIC STEROID, SULFONAMIDE) *suspension:* prednisolone acetate (see p. 1389) 0.2%/sulfacetamide sodium (see p. 1588) 10%.

Blephamide S.O.P. (OPHTHALMIC STEROID, SULFONAMIDE) *ointment:* prednisolone acetate (see p. 1389) 0.2%/sulfacetamide sodium (see p. 1588) 10%.

Brevicon (MONOPHASIC ORAL CONTRACEPTIVE [ESTROGEN, PROGESTIN]) *tablet:* ethinyl estradiol 35 mcg/norethindrone (see p. 1194) 0.5 mg.

Bromfed (DECONGESTANT, ANTIHISTAMINE) *sustained release capsule:* pseudoephedrine hydrochloride (see p. 1194) 120 mg/brompheniramine maleate (see p. 220) 12 mg.

Bromfed-PD (DECONGESTANT, ANTIHISTAMINE) *sustained release capsule:* pseudoephedrine hydrochloride (see p. 1429) 60 mg/brompheniramine maleate (see p. 220) 6 mg.

Bronchial Capsules (ANTIASTHMATIC) *capsule:* theophylline (see p. 1648) 150 mg/guaifenesin (see p. 793) 90 mg.

Byvalson (ANTIHYPERTENSIVE) tablet: nebivolol 5 mg/valsartan 80 mg.

Caduet (ANTIHYPERTENSIVE/ANTILIPEMIC) *tablet:* 2.5 mg amlodipine (see p. 84)/10 mg atorvastatin (see p. 135); 2.5 mg amlodipine/20 mg atorvastatin; 2.5 mg amlodipine/40 mg atorvastatin; 5 mg amlodipine/10 mg atorvastatin; 10 mg amlodipine/10 mg atorvastatin; 5 mg amlodipine/20 mg atorvastatin; 10 mg amlodipine/20 mg atorvastatin; 5 mg amlodipine/40 mg atorvastatin; 10 mg amlodipine/40 mg atorvastatin; 5 mg amlodipine/80 mg atorvastatin; 10 mg amlodipine/80 mg atorvastatin.

Cafergot Suppositories (ANTIMIGRAINE) *suppository:* ergotamine tartrate (see p. 627) 2 mg/caffeine (see p. 243) 100 mg.

Cam-Ap-Es (ANTIHYPERTENSIVE) suspension, *tablet:* hydrochlorothiazide (see p. 809) 15 mg/hydralazine hydrochloride (see p. 807) 25 mg.

Carisoprodol Compound (SKELETAL MUSCLE RELAXANT, ANALGESIC) *tablet:* carisoprodol (see p. 281) 200 mg/aspirin (see p. 126) 325 mg.

Celestone-Soluspan (GLUCOCORTICOID) *injection (suspension) (per mL):* betamethasone acetate (see p. 185) 3 mg/betamethasone sodium phosphate (see p. 185) 3 mg.

Cetacaine (TOPICAL ANESTHETIC) *gel, liquid, ointment, aerosol:* benzocaine (see p. 180) 14%/tetracaine hydrochloride (see p. 1642) 2%/ butamben 2%/benzalkonium chloride (see p. 179) 0.5%.

Cheracol Syrup (NARCOTIC ANTITUSSIVE, EXPECTORANT [schedule V]) *syrup (per 5 mL):* codeine phosphate (see p. 400) 10 mg/ guaifenesin (see p. 793) 100 mg/ alcohol 4.75%.

Cipro HC Otic (ANTI-INFECTIVE/ANTI-INFLAMMATORY) *topical:* ciprofloxacin (see p. 365) 2 mg/ dexamethasone (see p. 481) 10 mg otic suspension.

Ciprodex Otic (ANTI-INFECTIVE/ANTI-INFLAMMATORY) *topical:* ciprofloxacin (see p. 365) 0.3%/dexamethasone (see p. 481) 0.1% otic suspension.

Claritin D (ANTIHISTAMINE, DECONGESTANT) loratadine (see p. 995), 5 mg/pseudoephedrine (see p. 1429) 120 mg; loratadine 10 mg/ pseudoephedrine 240 mg.

Clarinex D 24 hr (ANTIHISTAMINE, DECONGESTANT) *tablet:* desloratadine (see p. 477) 5 mg/pseudoephedrine (see p. 1429) 240 mg.

Climara Pro (HORMONE REPLACEMENT THERAPY) *transdermal patch:* estradiol (see p. 650) 0.045 mg/ levonorgestrel acetate 0.015 mg.

Coly-Mycin S Otic (OTIC: STEROID, ANTIBIOTIC) *suspension (per mL):* hydrocortisone acetate (see p. 812) 1%/neomycin sulfate (see p. 1157) 3.3 mg/colistin sulfate 3 mg/thonzonium bromide 0.05%.

Combigan (GLAUCOMA) *ophthalmic solution:* brimonidine (see p. 215) 0.2%/timolol (see p. 1671) 0.5%.

CombiPatch (HORMONE REPLACEMENT THERAPY) *transdermal patch:* estradiol (see p. 650) 0.05 mg/norethindrone acetate (see p. 1194) 0.14 mg; estradiol 0.05 mg/ norethindrone acetate 0.25 mg.

Combivent Respimat (BETA-AGONIST/ANTICHOLINERGIC BRONCHODILATOR) *inhalation solution:* 100 mcg albuterol sulfate/20 mcg ipratropium

Combivir (ANTIVIRAL) *tablet:* zidovudine (see p. 1791) 300 mg/ lamivudine (see p. 931) 150 mg.

Complera (ANTIRETROVIRAL) *tablet:* rilpivirine 25 mg/emtricitabine 200 mg/tenofovir 300 mg.

Cortisporin (OPHTHALMIC STEROID, ANTIBIOTIC) *suspension (per mL):* hydrocortisone (see p. 812) 1%/ neomycin sulfate (see p. 1157) (equivalent to 0.35% neomycin base)/polymyxin B sulfate (see p. 1324) 10,000 units.

Cortisporin Ointment (OPHTHALMIC STEROID, ANTIBIOTIC) *ointment:* hydrocortisone (see p. 812) 1%/ neomycin sulfate (see p. 1157) (equivalent to 0.35% neomycin base)/bacitracin zinc (see p. 160) 400 units, polymyxin B sulfate (see p. 1365) 10,000 units/g.

Corzide (ANTIHYPERTENSIVE) *tablet:* nadolol (see p. 1128) 40 mg/bendroflumethiazide 5 mg; nadolol 80 mg/bendoflumethiazide 5 mg.

Cosopt (OPHTHALMIC, GLAUCOMA) *ophthalmic solution:* dorzolamide (see p. 550) 2%/timolol (see p. 1671) 0.5%.

Cyclomydril (OPHTHALMIC DECONGESTANT) *ophthalmic solution:* atropine hydrochloride 0.2%/ phenylephrine hydrochloride (see p. 1334) 1%.

Decadron with Xylocaine (GLUCOCORTICOID) *injection (per mL):* dexamethasone sodium phosphate (see p. 481) 4 mg/lidocaine hydrochloride (see p. 966) 10 mg.

Deconamine (DECONGESTANT, ANTIHISTAMINE) *syrup (per 5 mL):* pseudoephedrine hydrochloride (see p. 1429) 30 mg/chlorpheniramine maleate (see p. 344) 2 mg; *tablet:* pseudoephedrine hydrochloride 60 mg/chlorpheniramine maleate 4 mg.

Deconamine SR (DECONGESTANT, ANTIHISTAMINE) *sustained release capsule:* pseudoephedrine hydrochloride (see p. 1429) 120 mg/chlorpheniramine maleate (see p. 344) 8 mg.

Depo-Testadiol (ESTROGEN, ANDROGEN) *injection (per mL):* estradiol cypionate (see p. 650) 2 mg/testosterone cypionate (see p. 1639) 50 mg.

Descovy (REVERSE TRANSCRIPTASE INHIBITOR) *tablet:* emtricitabine (see p. 595) 200 mg/tenofovir alafenamide (see p. 1648) 25 mg.

Diclegis (ANTIEMETIC) *tablet:* doxylamine 10 mg/pyridoxine (see p. 1436) 10 mg.

Diovan HCT (ANTIHYPERTENSIVE) *tablet:* hydrochlorothiazide (see p. 809) 12.5 mg/valsartan (see p. 1513) 80 mg; hydrochlorothiazide 12.5 mg/valsartan 160 mg; hydrochlorothiazide 25 mg/valsartan 160 mg; hydrochlorothiazide 12.5 mg/valsartan 320 mg; hydrochlorothiazide 25 mg/valsartan 320 mg.

Donnatal (GASTROINTESTINAL ANTICHOLINERGIC, SEDATIVE) *tablet, elixir:* atropine sulfate (see p. 141) 0.0194 mg/scopolamine hydrobromide (see p. 1528) 0.0065 mg/hyoscyamine hydrobromide or sulfate (see p. 826) 0.1037 mg/phenobarbital (see p. 1329) 16.2 mg. The elixir contains alcohol 23%/5 mL.

Donnatal Extentab (GASTROINTESTINAL ANTICHOLINERGIC, SEDATIVE) *tablet:* atropine sulfate (see p. 141) 0.0582 mg/scopolamine hydrobromide (see p. 1528) 0.0195 mg/hyoscyamine sulfate (see p. 826) 0.3111 mg/phenobarbital (see p. 1329) 48.6 mg.

Duac (ANTIACNE) *gel:* clindamycin (see p. 380) 1%/benzoyl peroxide 5%.

Duavee (HORMONE REPLACEMENT) tablet conjugated estrogen 0.45 mg/bazedoxifene 20 mg.

Duetact (ANTIDIABETIC) *tablet:* pioglitazone (see p. 1351) 30 mg/glimepiride (see p. 776) 2 mg; pioglitazone 30 mg/glimepiride 4 mg.

Duexis (ANTIULCERATIVE) *tablet:* ibuprofen 800 mg/famotidine 26.6 mg.

Dulera (CORTICOSTEROID/BETA-AGONIST) *inhaler:* mometasone 100 mcg/fomoterol 5 mcg; mometasone 200 mcg/fomoterol 5 mcg.

DuoNeb (BETA-AGONIST/ANTICHOLINERGIC BRONCHODILATOR) *inhalation solution:* 2.5 mg albuterol sulfate (see p. 39)/0.5 mg ipratropium bromide (see p. 885) per 3 mL.

Duzallo (ANTIGOUT) *tablet:* lesinurad (see p. 946) 200 mg/allopurinol (see p. 48) 200 mg; lesinurad 200 mg/allopurinol 300 mg.

Dyazide (DIURETIC) *capsule:* triamterene (see p. 809) 37.5 mg/hydrochlorothiazide (see p. 809) 25 mg.

Dymista (ANTIHISTAMINE) *Nasal spray:* azelastine 137 mcg/fluticasone 50 mcg.

Edarbyclor (ANTIHYPERTENSIVE) *tablet:* azilsartan 40 mg/chlorthalidone 12.5 mg; azilsartan 40 mg/chlorthalidone 25 mg.

EluRyng (CONTRACEPTIVE) *vaginal ring:* ethinyl estradiol 0.015 mg/etonogestrel 0.12 mg.

Embeda (ANALGESIC [schedule II]) *tablet:* morphine (see p. 1119) 20 mg/naltrexone (see p. 1139) 0.8 mg; morphine 30 mg/naltrexone 1.2 mg; morphine 50 mg/naltrexone 2 mg; morphine 60 mg/naltrexone 2.4 mg; morphine 80 mg/naltrexone 3.2 mg; morphine 100 mg/naltrexone 4 mg.

Endocet (NARCOTIC ANALGESIC [schedule II]) *tablet:* oxycodone (see p. 1249) 7.5 mg/acetaminophen (see p. 13) 325 mg; oxycodone 7.5 mg/acetaminophen 500 mg; oxycodone 10 mg/acetaminophen 325 mg; oxycodone 10 mg/acetaminophen 650 mg.

Enlon Plus (ANTICHOLINESTERASE) *solution:* edrophonium 10 mg/atropine 0.14 mg.

Entresto (NAPRILYSIN INHIBITOR/ANGIOTENSION II BLOCKER) *tablet:* sacubitril 24 mg/valsartan 26 mg; sacubitril 49 mg/valsartan 51 mg; sacubitril 97 mg/valsartan 103 mg.

Epiduo (ANTIACNE) *gel:* adapalene (see p. 28) 0.1%/benzoyl peroxide 2.5%.

Epclusa (ANTIVIRAL) *tablet:* sofosbuvir 400 mg/velpatasvir 100 mg.

Epzicom (ANTIRETROVIRAL AGENT) *tablet:* abacavir (see p. 1) 600 mg/lamivudine (see p. 931) 300 mg.

Estratest (ESTROGEN, ANDROGEN) *tablet:* esterified estrogens (see p. 658) 1.25 mg/methyltestosterone (see p. 1078) 2.5 mg.

Estratest H.S. (ESTROGEN, ANDROGEN) *tablet:* esterified estrogens (see p. 658) 0.625 mg/methyltestosterone (see p. 1078) 1.25 mg.

Evotaz (ANTIVIRAL/PROTEASE INHIBITOR) *tablet:* atazanavir (see p. 129) 300/cobicistat 150.

Exforge (ANTIHYPERTENSIVE) *tablet:* amlodipine (see p. 84) 5 mg/valsartan (see p. 1513) 160 mg; amlodipine 10 mg/valsartan 160 mg; amlodipine 5 mg/valsartan 320 mg; amlodipine 10 mg/valsartan 320 mg.

Exforge HCT (ANTIHYPERTENSIVE) *tablet:* amlodipine (see p. 84) 5 mg/valsartan (see p. 1513) 160 mg/hydrochlorothiazide (see p. 809) 12.5 mg; amlodipine 5 mg/valsartan 160 mg/hydrochlorothiazide 25 mg; amlodipine 10 mg/valsartan 160 mg/hydrochlorothiazide 12.5 mg; amlodipine 10 mg/valsartan 160 mg/hydrochlorothiazide 25 mg.

Fioricet with Codeine (NONNARCOTIC AGONIST ANALGESIC) *capsule:* acetaminophen (see p. 13) 300 mg/ butalbital 50 mg/caffeine (see p. 243) 40 mg/codeine (30 mg).

Fiorinal (NONNARCOTIC AGONIST ANALGESIC [schedule III]) *capsule,* aspirin (see p. 126) 325 mg/butalbital 50 mg/caffeine (see p. 243) 40 mg.

Fiorinal with Codeine (NARCOTIC AGONIST ANALGESIC [schedule III]) *capsule:* codeine phosphate (see p. 395) 30 mg/aspirin (see p. 126) 325 mg/caffeine (see p. 243) 40 mg/butalbital 50 mg.

Fosamax Plus D (BISPHOSPHONATE) *tablet:* alendronate (see p. 41) 70 mg/vitamin D (see p. 1775) 2800 international units.

Glucovance (ANTIDIABETIC) *tablet:* glyburide (see p. 780) 1.25 mg/metformin (see p. 1051) 250 mg; glyburide 2.5 mg/metformin 500 mg; glyburide 5 mg/metformin 500 mg.

Harvoni (ANTIVIRAL) *tablet:* ledipasvir (see p. 942) 90 mg/sofosbuvir (see p. 942) 400 mg.

Helidac (ANTIULCER, ANTIBIOTIC) *tablet:* bismuth subsalicylate (see p. 198) 262.4 mg/metronidazole (see p. 1086) 250 mg/tetracycline (see p. 1644) 500 mg.

Herceptin Hylecta (ANTINEOPLASTIC) *solution for injection:* trastuzumab 600 mg/hyaluronidase 10,000 units/5 mL

Hycodan (ANTITUSSIVE [schedule III]) *tablet, syrup:* hydrocodone bitartrate (see p. 811) 5 mg/homatropine methylbromide 1.5 mg.

Hycotuss Expectorant (ANTITUSSIVE [schedule III]) guaifenesin (see p. 793) 100 mg/hydrocodone (see p. 811) 5 mg.

Hyzaar (ANTIHYPERTENSIVE) *tablet:* losartan (see p. 1000) 50 mg/hydrochlorothiazide (see p. 809) 12.5 mg/losartan 100 mg/hydrochlorothiazide 12.5 mg/losartan 100 mg/hydrochlorothiazide 25 mg.

Inderide 40/25 (ANTIHYPERTENSIVE) *tablet:* propranolol hydrochloride (see p. 1418) 40 mg/hydrochlorothiazide (see p. 809) 25 mg.

Invokamet (ANTIDIABETIC) *tablet:* canagliflozin (see p. 257) 150/metformin (see p. 1051) 1000 mg; canagliflozin 50/metformin 500 mg.

Jalyn (BPH AGENT) *capsule:* dutasteride (see p. 577) 0.5 mg/tamsulosin (see p. 1628) 0.4 mg.

Janumet (ANTIDIABETIC) *tablet:* sitagliptin (see p. 1554) 50 mg/metformin (see p. 1051) 500 mg; sitagliptin 50 mg/metformin 1000 mg.

Janumet XR (ANTIDIABETIC) *extended release tablet:* sitagliptin 100 mg/metformin 1000 mg; sitagliptin 50 mg/metformin 1000 mg; sitagliptin 50 mg/metformin 500 mg.

Jentadueto (ANTIDIABETIC) *tablet:* linagliptan 2.5 mg/metformin 1000 mg; linagliptan 2.5 mg/metformin 500; mglinagliptan 2.5 mg/metformin 850 mg.

Jusvisync (ANTIDIABETIC) *tablet:* sitagliptin 100 mg/simvastatin 10 mg; sitagliptin 100 mg/simvastatin 20 mg; sitagliptin 100 mg/simvastatin 40 mg.

Kazano (ANTIDIABETIC) *tablet:* alogliptin (see p. 52) 12.5 mg/metformin (see p. 1051) 500 mg alogliptin 12.5 mg/metformin 1000 mg.

Kisqali Femara (ANTINEOPLASTIC) *tablet*: letrozole (see p. 949) 2.5 mg/ribociclib 200 mg; letrozole 2.5 mg/ribociclib 400 mg; letrozole 2.5 mg/ribociclib 600 mg.

Kombiglyze XR (ANTIDIABETIC) *extended release tablet:* saxagliptin 5 mg/metformin 500 mg; saxagliptin 2.5 mg/metformin 1000 mg; saxagliptin 5 mg/metformin 1000 mg.

LidoSite (LOCAL ANESTHETIC) *transdermal patch:* lidocaine (see p. 966) 100 mg/epinephrine (see p. 609) 1.05 mg.

Limbitrol (PSYCHOTHERAPEUTIC [schedule IV]) *tablet:* chlordiazepoxide (see p. 338) 5 mg/amitriptyline (see p. 80) 12.5 mg; chlordiazepoxide 10 mg/amitriptyline 25 mg.

Limbitrol DS (PSYCHOTHERAPEUTIC [schedule IV]) *tablet:* chlordiazepoxide (see p. 338) 10 mg/amitriptyline (see p. 82) 25 mg.

Liptruzet (LIPID-LOWERING AGENT) *tablet:* atorvastatin (see p. 135) 10 mg/ezetimibe (see p. 686) 10 mg atorvastatin 20 mg/ezetimibe 10 mg atorvastatin 40 mg/ezetimibe 10 mg atorvastatin 80mg/ezetimibe 10 mg.

Loestrin 1/20 (ORAL CONTRACEPTIVE) *tablet:* ethinyl estradiol 20 mcg/norethindrone acetate (see p. 1194) 1 mg.

Loestrin 1/20 Fe (ORAL CONTRACEPTIVE) *tablet:* ethinyl estradiol 20 mcg/norethindrone acetate (see p. 1194) 1 mg/ferrous fumarate 75 mg in last 7 tablets.

Loestrin 1.5/30 (ORAL CONTRACEPTIVE) *tablet:* ethinyl estradiol 30 mcg/norethindrone acetate (see p. 1161) 1.5 mg.

Loestrin 1.5/30 Fe (ORAL CONTRACEPTIVE) *tablet:* ethinyl estradiol 30 mcg/norethindrone acetate (see p. 1194) 1.5 mg/ferrous fumarate 75 mg in last 7 tablets.

Lomotil (ANTIDIARRHEAL) *tablet:* diphenoxylate (see p. 527) 2.5 mg/atropine (see p. 141) 0.025 mg.

Lo/Ovral 28 (ORAL CONTRACEPTIVE) tablet: ethinyl estradiol 30 mcg/norgestrel 0.3 mg.

Lopressor HCT (ANTIHYPERTENSIVE) *tablet:* metoprolol tartrate (see

p. 1083) 50 mg/hydrochlorothiazide (see p. 809) 25 mg; meto-prolol tartrate 100 mg/hydrochlorothiazide 25 mg; metoprolol tartrate 100 mg/hydrochlorothiazide 50 mg.

LoSeasonique (ORAL CONTRACEPTIVE) *tablet:* ethinyl estradiol 0.01 mg/ethinyl estradiol 0.02 mg/levonorgestrel (see p. 962) 0.1 mg.

Lotensin HCT (ANTIHYPERTENSIVE) *tablet:* hydrochlorothiazide (see p. 809) 25 mg/benazepril (see p. 176) 20 mg; hydrochlorothiazide 12.5/benazepril 20 mg; hydrochlorothiazide 12.5 mg/benazepril 10 mg.

Lotrel (ANTIHYPERTENSIVE) *tablet:* amlodipine (see p. 84) 2.5 mg/benazepril (see p. 176) 10 mg; amlodipine 5 mg/benazepril 10 mg; amlodipine 5 mg/benazepril 20 mg; amlodipine 10 mg/benazepril 20 mg; amlodipine 10 mg/benazepril 40 mg.

Lotrisone (CORTICOSTEROID, ANTIFUNGAL) *cream:* betamethasone (see p. 185) (as dipropionate) 0.05%/clotrimazole (see p. 397) 1%.

Malarone (ANTIMALARIAL) *tablet:* atovaquone (see p. 136) 250 mg/proguanil HCl 100 mg; atovaquone 62.5 mg/proguanil HCl 25 mg.

Maxitrol (OPHTHALMIC STEROID, ANTIBIOTIC) *ophthalmic ointment, ophthalmic suspension:* dexamethasone (see p. 481) 0.1%/neomycin sulfate (see p. 1157) (equivalent to 0.35% neomycin base)/polymyxin B sulfate (see p. 1365) 10,000 units.

Maxzide (DIURETIC) *tablet:* triamterene (see p. 1718) 75 mg/hydrochlorothiazide (see p. 809) 50 mg.

Maxzide 25 (DIURETIC) *tablet:* triamterene (see p. 1718) 37.5 mg/hydrochlorothiazide (see p. 809) 25 mg.

Metaglip (HYPOGLYCEMIC AGENT) *tablet:* glipizide (see p. 777) 2.5 mg/metformin HCl (see p. 1051) 250 mg; glipizide 2.5 mg/metformin 500 mg; glipizide 5 mg/metformin 500 mg.

Micardis HCT (ANTIHYPERTENSIVE) *tablet:* telmisartan (see p. 1619) 40 mg/hydrochlorothiazide (see p. 809) 12.5 mg; telmisartan 80 mg/hydrochlorothiazide 12.5 mg; telmisartan 80 mg/hydrochlorothiazide 25 mg.

Minizide (ANTIHYPERTENSIVE) *capsule:* polythiazide 0.5 mg/prazosin hydrochloride (see p. 1387) 1 mg; polythiazide 0.5 mg/prazosin hydrochloride 2 mg; polythiazide 0.5 mg/prazosin hydrochloride 5 mg.

Modicon 28 (ORAL CONTRACEPTIVE) *tablet:* ethinyl estradiol 35 mcg/norethindrone (see p. 1194) 0.5 mg.

Moduretic (DIURETIC) *tablet:* amiloride hydrochloride (see p. 70) 5 mg/hydrochlorothiazide (see p. 809) 50 mg.

Mycitracin (OPHTHALMIC ANTIBIOTIC) *ophthalmic ointment:* polymyxin B sulfate (see p. 1365) 10,000 units/neomycin sulfate (see p. 1157) 3.5 mg/bacitracin (see p. 160) 500 units/g.

Mycolog II (CORTICOSTEROID, ANTIFUNGAL) *cream, ointment:* triamcinolone acetonide (see p. 1716) 0.1%/nystatin (see p. 1198) 100,000 units/g.

Mydayis (ATTENTION DEFICIT DISORDER AGENT [schedule II]) *extended release capsule:* amphetamine aspartate 3.125 mg, amphetamine sulfate (see p. 89) 3.125 mg, dextroamphetamine saccharate 3.125 mg, dextroamphetamine sulfate (see p. 491) 3.125 mg.

Neo-Cortef (CORTICOSTEROID ANTIBIOTIC) *water-soluble cream, topical ointment:* hydrocortisone acetate (see p. 812) 1%/neomycin sulfate (see p. 1157) 0.5%.

Neosporin (OPHTHALMIC ANTIBIOTIC) *ophthalmic drops:* polymyxin B sulfate (see p. 1365) 10,000 units/neomycin sulfate (see p. 1157) 1.75 mg/gramicidin 0.025 mg/mL; *ophthalmic ointment:* polymyxin B sulfate 10,000 units/neomycin sulfate 3.5 mg/bacitracin zinc (see p. 160) 400 units/g.

Neosporin G.U. Irrigant (ANTIBIOTIC) *solution:* neomycin sulfate (see p. 1157) 40 mg/polymyxin B sulfate (see p. 1365) 200,000 units/mL.

Neutra-Phos (PHOSPHORUS REPLACEMENT) *capsule, powder:* phosphorus 250 mg/potassium (see p. 1372) 231 mg/sodium (see p. 1555) 167 mg/combination of monobasic, dibasic, sodium, and potassium phosphate.

Nexlizet (ANTILIPEMIC AGENT) *tablet:* bempedoic acid 180 mg/ezetimibe 10 mg

Norco (NARCOTIC AGONIST ANALGESIC [schedule III]) *tablet:* hydrocodone bitartrate (see p. 811) 10 mg/acetaminophen (see p. 13) 325 mg; hydrocodone bitartrate 7.5 mg/acetaminophen 325 mg.

Nordette 28 (ORAL CONTRACEPTIVE) *tablet:* ethinyl estradiol 30 mcg/levonorgestrel (see p. 962) 0.15 mg.

Norgesic (SKELETAL MUSCLE RELAXANT) *tablet:* orphenadrine citrate (see p. 1230) 25 mg/aspirin (see p. 126) 385 mg/caffeine (see p. 243) 30 mg.

Norgesic Forte (SKELETAL MUSCLE RELAXANT, ANALGESIC) *tablet:* orphenadrine citrate (see p. 1230) 50 mg/aspirin (see p. 126) 770 mg/caffeine (see p. 243) 60 mg.

Norinyl 1+35 (ORAL CONTRACEPTIVE) *tablet:* ethinyl estradiol 35 mcg/norethindrone (see p. 1194) 1 mg.

Norinyl 1+50 (ORAL CONTRACEPTIVE) *tablet:* mestranol 50 mcg/norethindrone (see p. 1194) 1 mg.

NuvaRing (CONTRACEPTIVE) *vaginal ring:* ethinyl estradiol (see p. 650) 0.015 mg/etonogestrel 0.12 mg.

Odefsey (NUCLEOSIDE REVERSE TRANSCRIPTASE INHIBITOR/NONNUCELOSIDE REVERSE TRANSCRIPTASE INHIBITOR) *tablet:* emtricitabine (see p. 594) 200 mg/rilpivirine (see p. 1483) 25 mg/tenofovir alafenamide (see p. 1628) 25 mg.

Oriahnn (ESTROGEN/PROGESTIN) *capsule:* elagolix 300 mg/ estradiol 1 mg/norethindrone 0.5 mg

Ortho Evra (CONTRACEPTIVE) *transdermal patch:* norelgestromin 0.15 mg/ethinyl estradiol 0.02 mg.

Osensi (ANTIDIABETIC) *tablet:* alogliptin 25 mg/pioglitazone (see p. 1351) 15 mg; alogliptin 25 mg/pioglitazone 30 mg; alogliptin 25 mg/pioglitazone 45 mg; alogliptin 12.5 mg/pioglitazone 15 mg; alogliptin 12.5 mg/pioglitazone 30 mg; alogliptin 12.5 mg/pioglitazone 45 mg

Oxycet (NARCOTIC ANALGESIC [schedule II]) *tablet:* acetaminophen (see p. 13) 325 mg/ oxycodone (see p. 1249) 5 mg.

Paremyd (MYDRIATIC) ophthalmic *solution:* 1% hydroxyamphetamine hydrobromide, 0.25% tropicamide (see p. 1731).

Percocet (NARCOTIC ANALGESIC [schedule II]) *tablet:* oxycodone (see p. 1249) 2.5 mg/acetaminophen (see p. 13) 325 mg; oxycodone 7.5 mg/acetaminophen 325 mg; oxycodone 10 mg/acetaminophen 325 mg; oxycodone 10 mg/acetaminophen 650 mg.

Percodan (NARCOTIC ANALGESIC [schedule II]) *tablet:* oxycodone hydrochloride (see p. 1249) 4.5 mg/oxycodone terephthalate 0.38 mg/aspirin (see p. 126) 325 mg.

Phesgo (ANTINEOPLASTIC) *solution for injection:* pertuzumab 60 mg/trastuzumab 60 mg/hyaluronidase 2000units/mL; pertuzumab 80 mg/trastuzumab 40 mg/hyaluronidase 2000units/mL.

Polysporin Ointment (ANTI-INFECTIVE [OPHTHALMIC]) *ophthalmic ointment:* polymyxin B sulfate (see p. 1365) 10,000 units/bacitracin zinc (see p. 160) 500 units/g.

Prandimet (HYPOGLYCEMIC AGENT) *tablet:* repaglinide (see p. 1466) 1 mg/metformin (see p. 1051) 500 mg; repaglinide 2 mg/metformin 500 mg.

Premphase (ESTROGEN, PROGESTERONE) *tablet:* conjugated estrogens (see p. 658) 0.625 mg/medroxyprogesterone acetate (see p. 1026) 5 mg.

Prempro (ESTROGEN, PROGESTIN) *tablet:* conjugated estrogens (see p. 658) 0.3 mg/medroxyprogesterone (see p. 1026) 1.5 mg; conjugated estrogen 0.45 mg/ medroxyprogesterone 1.5 mg; conjugated estrogen 0.625 mg/ medroxyprogesterone 2.5 mg; conjugated estrogen 0.625 mg/ medroxyprogesterone 5 mg.

Prestalia (ACE INHIBITOR/CALCIUM CHANNEL BLOCKER) *tablets:* perindopril 14 mg/amlodipine besylate 10 mg; perindopril 3.5 mg/amlodipine besylate 2.5 mg; perindopril 7 mg/amlodipine besylate 5 mg.

Prevacid NapraPAC (PROTON PUMP INHIBITOR/ANTI-INFLAMMATORY) capsules and *tablets:* lansoprazole (see p. 935) 15 mg capsule/naproxen sodium (see p. 1142) 375 mg table; lansoprazole 15 mg capsule/naproxen sodium 500 mg tablet.

Prevpac (ANTIBIOTIC/ANTISECRETORY) capsules and *tablets:* amoxicillin (see p. 86) 500 mg capsules, clarithromycin (see p. 375) 500 mg tablets, lansoprazole (see p. 935) 30 mg capsules.

Prinzide (ANTIHYPERTENSIVE) *tablet:* hydrochlorothiazide (see p. 809) 12.5 mg/lisinopril (see p. 983) 10 mg; hydrochlorothiazide 12.5 mg/lisinopril 20 mg; hydrochlorothiazide 25 mg/lisinopril 20 mg.

Probenecid and Colchicine (ANTIGOUT) *tablet:* probenecid (see p. 1398) 500 mg/colchicine (see p. 402) 0.5 mg.

Pyridium Plus (ANALGESIC) *tablet:* phenazopyridine hydrochloride (see p. 1325) 150 mg/hyoscyamine hydrobromide (see p. 826) 0.3 mg/butalbital 15 mg.

Qsymia (ANTIOBESITY) *extended release capsule:* phentermine 3.75/topiramate 23 mg; phentermine 7.5 mg/topiramate 46 mg; phentermine 11.25 mg/topiramate 69 mg phentermine 15 mg/ topiramate 92 mg.

Qtren (ANTIDIABETIC) *tablet:* dapagliflozin (see p. 448) 10 mg/saxagliptin (see p. 1527) 5 mg.

Quartette (ORAL CONTRACEPTIVE) *tablet:* various combinations of levonorgestrel and ethinyl estradiol.

Rebetron (INTERFERON, ANTIVIRAL) ribavirin (see p. 1473) tablet polythiazide 2 mg.

Recarbrio (ANTIBIOTIC) *solution for injection:* imipenem (see p. 845) 500 mg/cilastatin 500 mg/relebactam 250 mg.

Rifamate (ANTITUBERCULOSIS) *capsule:* isoniazid (see p. 898) 150 mg/ rifampin (see p. 1477) 300 mg.

Rifater (ANTITUBERCULOSIS) *tablet:* rifampin (see p. 1477) 120 mg/isoniazid (see p. 898) 50 mg/pyrazinamide 300 mg.

Rimactane/INH Dual Pack (ANTITUBERCULOSIS) *pack:* 30 isoniazid (see p. 898) 300 mg tablets, sixty rifampin (see p. 1477) 300 mg capsules.

Rondec (DECONGESTANT, ANTIHISTAMINE) *tablet:* pseudoephedrine hydrochloride (see p. 1429) 60 mg/ carbinoxamine maleate 4 mg; *drops (per mL):* pseudoephedrine hydrochloride 25 mg/

carbinoxamine maleate 2 mg; *syrup (per mL):* pseudoephedrine hydrochloride 60 mg/carbinoxamine maleate 4 mg.

Roxicet (NARCOTIC ANALGESIC [schedule II]) *tablet:* oxycodone (see p. 1249) 5 mg/acetaminophen (see p. 13) 325 mg.

Ryzodeg 70/30 (INSULIN); *injection:* insulin degludec 70/insulin aspart 30.

Seglentis (ANALGESIC) *tablet:* celecoxib 56 mg/tramadol 44 mg

Simcor (ANTILIPIDEMIC) extended release *tablet:* niacin (see p. 1164) 1000 mg/simvastatin (see p. 1549) 20 mg; niacin 1000 mg/simvastatin 40 mg, niacin 500 mg/simvastatin 20 mg; niacin 500 mg/simvastatin 40 mg, niacin 750 mg/simvastatin 20 mg.

Soliqua (ANTIDIATBETIC) *injection:* insulin glargine (see p. 869) 100 units/lixisenatide (see p. 987) 33 mg.

Soma Compound (SKELETAL MUSCLE RELAXANT) *tablet:* carisoprodol (see p. 281) 200 mg/aspirin (see p. 126) 325 mg.

Soma Compound with Codeine (SKELETAL MUSCLE RELAXANT [schedule III]) *tablet:* carisoprodol (see p. 281) 200 mg, aspirin (see p. 126) 325 mg/codeine phosphate 16 mg.

Stalevo (ANTIPARKINSON AGENT) *tablet:* carbidopa (see p. 270) 12.5 mg/levodopa (see p. 957) 50 mg/entacapone (see p. 603) 200 mg; carbidopa 18.75 mg/levodopa 75 mg/entacapone 200 mg; carbidopa 25 mg/levodopa 100 mg/entacapone 200 mg; carbidopa 31.25 mg/levodopa 125 mg/entacapone 200 mg; carbidopa 37.5 mg/levodopa 150 mg/entacapone 200 mg.

Stiolto (BRONCHODIALATOR) *powder for inhalation:* tiotropium 2.5 mcg/ olodaterol 2.5 mcg.

Suboxone (ANALGESIC) sublingual *tablet:* buprenorphine (see p. 225) 2 mg/naloxone (see p. 1138) 0.5 mg; buprenorphine 8 mg/naloxone 2 mg.

Symbicort (MINERALOCORTICOID/BRONCHODILATOR) *inhaler:* budesonide (see p. 221) 0.08 mg/formoterol (see p. 743) 0.045 mg; budesonide 0.16 mg/formoterol 0.045 mg.

Symbyax (ATYPICAL ANTIPSYCHOTIC/SSRI) *capsule:* olanzapine (see p. 1208) 6 mg/fluoxetine (see p. 729) 25 mg; olanzapine 6 mg/fluoxetine 50 mg; olanzapine 12 mg/fluoxetine 25 mg; olanzapine 12 mg/fluoxetine 50 mg.

Synera (LOCAL ANESTHETIC) *transdermal patch:* lidocaine (see p. 966) 70 mg/tetracycline (see p. 1644) 70 mg.

Syntest D.S. (ESTROGEN, ANDROGEN) *tablet:* esterified estrogens (see p. 658) 1.25 mg/methyltestosterone (see p. 1078) 2.5 mg.

Syntest H.S. (ESTROGEN, ANDROGEN) *tablet:* esterified estrogens (see p. 658) 0.625 mg/methyltestosterone (see p. 1078) 1.25 mg.

Taclonex Scalp (NSAID) *topical suspension:* betamethasone (see p. 185) 0.064%/calcipotriene (see p. 245) 0.005%.

Tanafed DP (DECONGESTANT, ANTIHISTAMINE) *suspension:* pseudoephedrine (see p. 1429) 75 mg/chlorpheniramine tannate 4.5 mg.

Tarka (ANTIHYPERTENSIVE) *tablet:* trandolapril (see p. 1707) 2 mg/verapamil HCl (see p. 1761) 180 mg; trandolapril 4 mg/verapamil HCl 240 mg; trandolapril 1 mg/verapamil HCl 240 mg, trandolapril 2 mg/verapamil HCl 240 mg.

Technivie (ANTIVIRAL) *tablet:* ombitasvir 12.5 mg/paritaprevir 75 mg/ritonavir 50 mg.

Tekamlo (ANTIHYPERTENSIVE) *tablet:* aliskiren 150 mg/amlodipine 10 mg; aliskiren 150 mg/amlodipine 5 mg; aliskiren 300 mg/amlodipine 10 mg; aliskiren 300 mg/amlodipine 5 mg.

Tekurna HCT (ANTIHYPERTENSIVE) *tablet:* aliskiren (see p. 46) 150 mg/hydrochlorothiazide (see p. 809) 12.5 mg.

Tenoretic 50 (ANTIHYPERTENSIVE) *tablet:* chlorthalidone (see p. 351) 25 mg/atenolol (see p. 131) 50 mg.

Tenoretic 100 (ANTIHYPERTENSIVE) *tablet:* chlorthalidone (see p. 351) 25 mg/atenolol (see p. 131) 100 mg.

Terra-Cortril Suspension (OCULAR STEROID AND ANTIBIOTIC) *suspension:* hydrocortisone acetate (see p. 812) 1.5%/oxytetracycline 0.5%.

Teveten HCT (ANTIHYPERTENSIVE) *tablet:* eprosartan mesylate (see p. 620) 600 mg/hydrochlorothiazide (see p. 809) 12.5 mg; eprosartan 600 mg/hydrochlorothiazide 25 mg.

Timolide (ANTIHYPERTENSIVE) *tablet:* hydrochlorothiazide (see p. 809) 25 mg/timolol maleate (see p. 1671) 10 mg.

Tobradex (ANTI-INFECTIVE) *ophthalmic suspension:* dexamethasone (see p. 481) 0.1%/tobramycin (see p. 1681) 0.3%; ophthalmic ointment: dexamethasone 0.1%/tobramycin 0.3%.

Treximet (ANALGESIC) *tablet:* naproxen (see p. 1142) 500 mg/sumatriptan (see p. 1597) 85 mg.

Triacin-C Cough Syrup (ANTITUSSIVE [schedule V]) *syrup:* pseudoephedrine (see p. 1429) 30 mg/triprolidine 1.25 mg/codeine (see p. 400) 10 mg.

Tribenzor (ANTIHYPERTENSIVE) *tablet:* olmesartan 20 mg/amlodipine 5 mg/hydrochlorothiazide 12.5 mg; olmesartan 40 mg/amlodipine 10 mg/hydrochlorothiazide 12.5 mg; olmesartan40 mg/amlodipine 10 mg/hydrochlorothiazide 25 mg; olmesartan 40 mg/amlodipine 5 mg/hydrochlorothiazide 12.5 mg; olmesartan 40 mg/amlodipine 5 mg/hydrochlorothiazide 25 mg.

Trijardy XR (ANTIDIABETIC) *tablet:* empagliflozin (see p. 592) 10 mg/linagliptin (see p. 970) 5 mg/metformin (see p. 1051) 1000 mg; empagliflozin 25 mg/linagliptin 5 mg/ metformin (see p. 1051) 1000 mg; empagliflozin 5 mg/linagliptin 2.5 mg/ metformin 1000 mg; empagliflozin 12.5 mg/linagliptin 2.5 mg/ metformin 1000 mg

Tri-Hydroserpine (ANTIHYPERTENSIVE) *tablet:* hydrochlorothiazide (see p. 809) 15 mg/hydralazine hydrochloride (see p. 807) 25 mg.

Tri-Luma Cream (STEROID) *cream:* 4% hydroquinone (see p. 818)/0.05% tretinoin (see p. 1043)/0.01% fluocinolone acetonide (see p. 726).

Tri-Norinyl 28 (ORAL CONTRACEPTIVE) *tablet:* ethinyl estradiol (see p. 650) 35 mcg/norethindrone (see p. 1194) 0.5 mg × 7 d, ethinyl estradiol 35 mcg/norethindrone 1 mg × 9 d, ethinyl estradiol 35 mcg/norethindrone 0.5 mg × 5 d.

Triple Antibiotic (OPHTHALMIC ANTIBIOTIC) *ophthalmic ointment:* hydrocortisone (see p. 812) 1%/neomycin sulfate (see p. 1157) 0.5%/bacitracin zinc (see p. 160) 400 units/polymyxin B sulfate (see p. 1365) 10,000 units/g.

Triumeq (ANTIRETROVIRAL) *tablet:* abacavir (see p. 1) 600 mg/dolutegravir (see p. 542) 50 mg/lamivudine (see p. 931) 300 mg.

Trizivir (REVERSE TRANSCRIPTASE INHIBITOR) *tablet:* abacavir (see p. 1) 300 mg/lamivudine (see p. 931) 150 mg/zidovudine (see p. 1791) 300 mg.

Truvada (NUCLEOSIDE REVERSE TRANSCRIPTASE INHIBITOR) *tablet:* emtricitabine (see p. 588) 200 mg/tenofovir disoproxil fumarate (see p. 1628) 300 mg.

Tussicap (ANTITUSSIVE [schedule III]) *extended release capsule:* chlorpheniramine (see p. 344) 8 mg/hydrocodone (see p. 811) 10 mg.

Twinrix (VACCINE) *injection:* hepatitis A vaccine (see p. 804) 720 ELU/hepatitis B recombinant vaccine (see p. 804) 20 mcg per single dose vial.

Twyneo Cream (STEROID) *cream:* benzoyl peroxide 1%/tretinoin 3%

Twynsta (ANTIHYPERTENSIVE) *tablet:* telmisartan 40 mg/amlodipine 5 mg; telmisartan 40 mg/amlodipine 10 mg; telmisartan 80 mg/amlodipine 5 mg; telmisartan 80 mg/amlodipine 10 mg.

Tylenol with Codeine No. 3 (NARCOTIC AGONIST ANALGESIC [schedule III]) *tablet:* acetaminophen (see p. 13) 300 mg/codeine phosphate 30 mg.

Tylenol with Codeine No. 4 (NARCOTIC AGONIST ANALGESIC [schedule III]) *tablet:* acetaminophen (see p. 13) 300 mg/codeine phosphate 60 mg.

Ultracet (ANALGESIC/ANTIPYRETIC) *tablet:* tramadol (see p. 1704) 37.5 mg/acetaminophen (see p. 13) 325 mg.

Uniretic (ANTIHYPERTENSIVE) *tablet:* moexipril (see p. 1116) 7.5 mg/hydrochlorothiazide (see p. 809) 12.5 mg; moexipril 15 mg/hydrochlorothiazide 12.5 mg, moexipril 15 mg/hydrochlorothiazide 25 mg.

Urised (URINARY ANTI-INFECTIVE) *tablet:* methenamine (see p. 1058) 40.8 mg/phenyl salicylate 18.1 mg/atropine sulfate (see p. 141) 0.03 mg/hyoscyamine (see p. 826) 0.03 mg/benzoic acid 4.5 mg/methylene blue 5.4 mg.

Vabomere (ANTI-INFECTIVE) *solution for injection:* meropenem (see p. 1045) 1 g/vaborbactam 1 g.

Valturna (ANTIHYPERTENSIVE) *tablet:* aliskiren (see p. 46) 150 mg/valsartan (see p. 1513) 160 mg; aliskiren 300 mg/valsartan 320 mg.

Vaseretic (ANTIHYPERTENSIVE) *tablet:* enalapril maleate (see p. 595) 10 mg/hydrochlorothiazide (see p. 809) 25 mg.

Vasocidin (OPHTHALMIC CORTICOSTEROID, ANTI-INFECTIVE) *ophthalmic solution:* prednisolone sodium phosphate (see p. 1389) 0.23%/sulfacetamide sodium (see p. 1588) 10%.

Veltin (ANTIACNE) *gel:* clindamycin 1/2%/tretinoin 0.025%.

Viekira XR (ANTIVIRAL) *tablet:* ombitasvir 8.33 mg/paritaprevir 50 mg/ritonavir 33.33 mg/dasabuvir 200 mg.

Vimovo (ANALGESIC) *tablet:* naproxen 375 mg/esomeprazole 20 mg; naproxen 500 mg/esomperazole 20 mg.

Vosevi (ANTIVIRAL) *tablet:* sofosbuvir (see p. 1561) 400 mg/velpatasvir 100 mg/voxilaprevir 100 mg.

Vytorin (ANTILIPEMIC AGENT) *tablet:* ezetimibe (see p. 686) 10 mg/simvastatin (see p. 1549) 10 mg; ezetimibe 10 mg/simvastatin 20 mg; ezetimibe 10 mg/simvastatin 40 mg; ezetimibe 10 mg/simvastatin 80 mg.

Vyxeos (ANTINEOPLASTIC) *powder for injection:* daunorubicin (see p. 461) 44 mg/cytarabine (see p. 429) 100 mg.

Xerese (TOPICAL ANTIINFECTIVE) *cream:* acyclovir 5%/hydrocortisone 1%.

Yasmin (ORAL CONTRACEPTIVE) *tablet:* ethinyl estradiol 30 mcg/drospirenone 3 mg.

Yosprala (ANTIPLATELET/ANTIULCERATIVE) *tablet:* aspirin 81 mg/omeprazole 40 mg; aspirin 325 mg/omeprazole 40 mg.

Zepatier (ANTIVIRAL/PROTEASE INHIBITOR) *tablet:* elbasvir 50 mg/grazoprevir 100 mg.

Zestoretic (ANTIHYPERTENSIVE) *tablet:* hydrochlorothiazide (see p. 809) 12.5 mg/lisinopril (see p. 983) 10 mg; hydrochlorothiazide 12.5 mg/lisinopril 20 mg; hydrochlorothiazide 25 mg/lisinopril 20 mg.

Ziac (ANTIHYPERTENSIVE) *tablet:* bisoprolol (see p. 199) 2.5 mg/hydrochlorothiazide (see p. 809) 6.25 mg; bisoprolol 5 mg/hydrochlorothiazide 6.25 mg; bisoprolol 10 mg/hydrochlorothiazide 6.25 mg.

Ziana (ANTIACNE) *gel:* clindamycin 0.5%/tretinoin 0.025%.

Zubsolv (ANALGESIC) *sublingual tablet:* buprenorphine 1.4 mg/naloxone 0.36 mg; buprenorphine 2.9 mg/naloxone 0.71 mg; buprenorphine 5.7 mg/naloxone 1.4 mg; buprenorphine 8.6 mg naloxone 2.1 mg; buprenorphine 11.4 mg/naloxone 2.9 mg.

Zylet (OPHTHALMIC ANTIBIOTIC) *solution:* loteprednol etabonate (see p. 1001) 0.5%/tobramycin (see p. 1681) 0.3%.

Zyrtec-D (ANTIHISTAMINE/DECONGESTANT) *sustained release tablet:* cetirizine (see p. 328) 5 mg/pseudoephedrine (see p. 1429) 120 mg.

◆ APPENDIX E GLOSSARY OF KEY TERMS, CLINICAL CONDITIONS, AND ASSOCIATED SIGNS AND SYMPTOMS

acute coronary syndrome an acute ischemic event with or without marked ST segment elevation.

acute dystonia extrapyramidal symptom manifested by abnormal posturing, grimacing, spastic torticollis (neck torsion), and oculogyric (eyeball movement) crisis.

adverse effect unintended, unpredictable, and nontherapeutic response to drug action. Adverse effects occur at doses used therapeutically or for prophylaxis or diagnosis. They generally result from drug toxicity, idiosyncrasies, or hypersensitivity reactions caused by the drug itself or by ingredients added during manufacture (e.g., preservatives, dyes, or vehicles).

afterload resistance that ventricles must work against to eject blood into the aorta during systole.

agranulocytosis sudden drop in leukocyte count; often followed by a severe infection manifested by high fever, chills, prostration, and ulcerations of mucous membrane such as in the mouth, rectum, or vagina.

akathisia extrapyramidal symptom manifested by a compelling need to move or pace, without specific pattern, and an inability to be still.

analeptic restorative medication that enhances excitation of the CNS without affecting inhibitory impulses.

anaphylactoid reaction excessive allergic response manifested by wheezing, chills, generalized pruritic urticaria, diaphoresis, sense of uneasiness, agitation, flushing, palpitations, coughing, difficulty breathing, and cardiovascular collapse.

anticholinergic actions inhibition of parasympathetic response manifested by dry mouth, decreased peristalsis, constipation, blurred vision, and urinary retention.

bioavailability fraction of active drug that reaches its action sites after administration by any route. Following an IV dose, bioavailability is 100%; however, such factors as first-pass effect, enterohepatic cycling, and biotransformation reduce bioavailability of an orally administered drug.

blood dyscrasia pathological condition manifested by fever, sore mouth or throat, unexplained fatigue, easy bruising, or bleeding.

cardiotoxicity impairment of cardiac function manifested by one or more of the following: hypotension, arrhythmias, precordial pain, dyspnea, electrocardiogram (ECG) abnormalities, cardiac dilation, congestive failure.

cholinergic response stimulation of the parasympathetic response manifested by lacrimation, diaphoresis, salivation, abdominal cramps, diarrhea, nausea, and vomiting.

circulatory overload excessive vascular volume manifested by increased central venous pressure (CVP), elevated blood pressure, tachycardia, distended neckveins, peripheral edema, dyspnea, cough, and pulmonary rales.

CNS stimulation excitement of the CNS manifested by hyperactivity, excitement, nervousness, insomnia, and tachycardia.

CNS toxicity impairment of CNS function manifested by ataxia, tremor, incoordination, paresthesias, numbness, impairment of pain or touch sensation, drowsiness, confusion, headache, anxiety, tremors, and behavior changes.

congestive heart failure (CHF) impaired pumping ability of the heart manifested by paroxysmal nocturnal dyspnea, cough, fatigue or dyspnea on exertion, tachycardia, peripheral or pulmonary edema, and weight gain.

Cushing's syndrome fatty swellings in the interscapular area (buffalo hump) and in the facial area (moon face), distention of the abdomen, ecchymoses following even minor trauma, impotence, amenorrhea, high blood pressure, general weakness, loss of muscle mass, osteoporosis, and psychosis.

dehydration decreased intracellular or extracellular fluid manifested by elevated temperature, dry skin and mucous membranes, decreased tissue turgor, sunken eyes, furrowed tongue, low blood pressure, diminished or irregular pulse, muscle or abdominal cramps, thick secretions, hard feces and impaction, scant urinary output, urine specific gravity above 1.030, an elevated hemoglobin.

disulfiram-type reaction Antabuse-type reaction manifested by facial flushing, pounding headache, sweating, slurred speech, abdominal cramps, nausea, vomiting, tachycardia, fever, palpitations, drop in blood pressure, dyspnea, and sense of chest constriction. Symptoms may last up to 24 hours.

enzyme induction stimulation of microsomal enzymes by a drug resulting in its accelerated metabolism and decreased activity. If reactive intermediates are formed, drug-mediated toxicity may be exacerbated.

extravasation escape of fluids or drugs into the subcutaneous tissue; a complication of intravenous infusion.

first-pass effect reduced bioavailability of an orally administered drug due to metabolism in GI epithelial cells and liver or to biliary excretion. Effect may be avoided by use of sublingual tablets or rectal suppositories.

fixed drug eruption drug-induced circumscribed skin lesion that persists or recurs in the same site. Residual pigmentation may remain following drug withdrawal.

gamma-glutamyl transpeptidase screening test for possible liver damage and/or suspected alcohol abuse.

half-life ($t_{1/2}$) time required for concentration of a drug in the body to decrease by 50%. Half-life also represents the time necessary to reach steady state or to decline from steady state after a change (i.e., starting or stopping) in the dosing regimen. Half-life may be affected by a disease state and age of the drug user.

heart failure left- and/or right-sided failure associated with systolic and/or diastolic dysfunction.

heat stroke a life-threatening condition manifested by absence of sweating; red, dry, hot skin; dilated pupils; dyspnea; full bounding pulse; temperature above 40° C (105° F); and mental confusion.

hepatotoxicity impairment of liver function manifested by jaundice, dark urine, pruritus, light-colored stools, eosinophilia, itchy skin or rash, and persistently high elevations of alanine aminotransferase (ALT) and aspartate aminotransferase (AST).

hyperammonemia elevated level of ammonia or ammonium in the blood manifested by lethargy, decreased appetite, vomiting, asterixis (flapping tremor), weak pulse, irritability, decreased responsiveness, and seizures.

hypercalcemia elevated serum calcium manifested by deep bone and flank pain, renal calculi, anorexia, nausea, vomiting, thirst, constipation, muscle hypotonicity, pathologic fracture, bradycardia, lethargy, and psychosis.

hyperglycemia elevated blood glucose manifested by flushed, dry skin, low blood pressure and elevated pulse, tachypnea, Kussmaul's respirations, polyuria, polydipsia; polyphagia, lethargy, and drowsiness.

hyperkalemia excessive potassium in blood, which may produce life-threatening cardiac arrhythmias, including bradycardia and heart block, unusual fatigue, weakness or heaviness of limbs, general muscle weakness, muscle cramps, paresthesias, flaccid paralysis of extremities, shortness of breath, nervousness, confusion, diarrhea, and GI distress.

hypermagnesemia excessive magnesium in blood, which may produce cathartic effect, profound thirst, flushing, sedation, confusion, depressed deep tendon reflexes (DTRs), muscle weakness, hypotension, and depressed respirations.

hypernatremia excessive sodium in blood, which may produce confusion, neuromuscular excitability, muscle weakness, seizures, thirst, dry and flushed skin, dry mucous membranes, pyrexia, agitation, and oliguria or anuria.

hypersensitivity reactions excessive and abnormal sensitivity to given agent manifested by urticaria, pruritus, wheezing, edema, redness, and anaphylaxis.

hyperthyroidism excessive secretion by the thyroid glands, which increases basal metabolic rate, resulting in warm, flushed, moist skin; tachycardia, exophthalmos; infrequent lid blinking; lid edema; weight loss despite increased appetite; frequent urination; menstrual irregularity; breathlessness; hypoventilation; congestive heart failure; excessive sweating.

hyperuricemia excessive uric acid in blood, resulting in pain in flank; stomach, or joints, and changes in intake and output ratio and pattern.

hypocalcemia abnormally low calcium level in blood, which may result in depression; psychosis; hyperreflexia; diarrhea; cardiac arrhythmias; hypotension; muscle spasms; paresthesias of feet, fingers, tongue; positive Chvostek's sign. Severe deficiency (tetany) may result in carpopedal spasms, spasms of face muscle, laryngospasm, and generalized convulsions.

hypoglycemia abnormally low glucose level in the blood, which may result in acute fatigue, restlessness, malaise, marked irritability and weakness, cold sweats, excessive hunger, headache, dizziness, confusion, slurred speech, loss of consciousness, and death.

hypokalemia abnormally low level of potassium in blood, which may result in malaise, fatigue, paresthesias, depressed reflexes, muscle weakness and cramps, rapid, irregular pulse, arrhythmias, hypotension, vomiting, paralytic ileus, mental confusion, depression, delayed thought process, abdominal distention, polyuria, shallow breathing, and shortness of breath.

hypomagnesemia abnormally low level of magnesium in blood, resulting in nausea, vomiting, cardiac arrhythmias, and neuromuscular symptoms (tetany, positive Chvostek's and Trousseau's signs, seizures, tremors, ataxia, vertigo, nystagmus, muscular fasciculations).

hyponatremia a decreased serum concentration (less than 125 mEq) of sodium that results in intracellular swelling. The resulting signs and symptoms include nausea, malaise, headache, lethargy, obtundation, seizures, and coma. There is significant variability in the symptomatology of hyponatremia manifested in patients.

hypophosphatemia abnormally low level of phosphates in blood, resulting in muscle weakness, anorexia, malaise, absent deep tendon reflexes, bone pain, paresthesias, tremors, negative calcium balance, osteomalacia, osteoporosis.

hypothyroidism condition caused by thyroid hormone deficiency that lowers basal metabolic rate and may result in periorbital edema, lethargy, puffy hands and feet, cool, pale skin, vertigo, nocturnal cramps, decreased GI motility, constipation, hypotension, slow pulse, depressed muscular activity, and enlarged thyroid gland.

hypoxia insufficient oxygenationin the blood manifested by dyspnea, tachypnea, headache, restlessness, cyanosis, tachycardia, dysrhythmias, confusion, decreased level of consciousness, and euphoria or delirium.

immune reconstitution inflammatory syndrome (IRIS) describes a collection of inflammatory disorders associated with worsening of preexisting infectious processes following initiation of highly active antiretroviral therapy in HIV-infected individuals. Usually the inflammatory reaction is self-limiting but long-term sequelae and fatal outcomes may occur, particularly when neurologic structures are involved.

international normalizing ratio measurement that normalizes for the differences obtained from various laboratory readings in the value for thromboplastin blood level.

ischemic colitis blood flow to part of the colon is reduced due to narrowing or blocked arteries resulting in insufficient oxygen to those cells. Signs and symptoms can include pain, tenderness, or cramping in the abdomen which can occur suddenly or gradually, bright red or maroon-colored blood in stool, or passage of blood alone from the rectum, a feeling of urgency to defecate, and diarrhea.

lactic acidosis is characterized by low pH (pH less than 7.35) in body tissues and blood (acidosis) accompanied by buildup of lactate. Lactate buildup results from metabolizing glucose anaerobically (low oxygen). Signs and symptoms include nausea, vomiting, hyperventilation, abdominal pain, lethargy, anxiety, hypotension, irregular heart rate, tachycardia, and severe anemia.

leukopenia abnormal decrease in number of white blood cells, usually below 5000 per cubic millimeter, resulting in fever, chills, sore mouth or throat, and unexplained fatigue.

liver toxicity manifested by anorexia, nausea, fatigue, lethargy, itching, jaundice, abdominal pain, dark-colored urine, and flu-like symptoms.

metabolic acidosis decrease in pH value of the extracellular fluid caused by either an increase in hydrogen ions or a decrease in bicarbonate ions. It may result in one or more of the following: lethargy, headache, weakness, abdominal pain, nausea, vomiting, dyspnea, hyperpnea progressing to Kussmaul breathing, dehydration, thirst, weakness, flushed face, full bounding pulse, progressive drowsiness, mental confusion, combativeness.

metabolic alkalosis increase in pH value of the extracellular fluid caused by either a loss of acid from the body (e.g., through vomiting) or an increased level of bicarbonate ions (e.g., through ingestion of sodium bicarbonate). It may result in muscle weakness, irritability, confusion, muscle twitching, slow and shallow respirations, and convulsive seizures.

microsomal enzymes drug-metabolizing enzymes located in the endoplasmic reticulum of the liver and other tissues chiefly responsible for oxidative drug metabolism (e.g., cytochrome P450).

myopathy any disease or abnormal condition of striated muscles manifested by muscle weakness, myalgia, diaphoresis, fever, and reddish-brown urine (myoglobinuria) or oliguria.

nephrotoxicity impairment of the nephrons of the kidney manifested by one or more of the following: oliguria, urinary frequency, hematuria, cloudy urine, rising BUN and serum creatinine, fever, graft tenderness or enlargement.

neuroleptic malignant syndrome (NMS) potentially fatal complication associated with antipsychotic drugs manifested by hyperpyrexia, altered mental status, muscle rigidity, irregular pulse, fluctuating BP, diaphoresis, and tachycardia.

orphan drug (as defined by the Orphan Drug Act, an amendment of the Federal Food, Drug, and Cosmetic Act which took effect in January 1983): drug or biological product used in the treatment, diagnosis, or prevention of a rare disease. A rare disease or condition is one that affects fewer than 200,000 persons in the United States, or affects more than 200,000 persons but for which there is no reasonable expectation that drug research and development costs can be recovered from sales within the United States.

ototoxicity impairment of the ear manifested by one or more of the following: headache, dizziness or vertigo, nausea and vomiting with motion, ataxia, nystagmus.

pharmacogenetic genetic variation affecting response to different drugs.

post-transplant lymphoproliferative disorder (PTLD) of B-cell proliferation that is a life-threatening complication after hematopoietic stem cell or organ transplant due to therapeutic immunosuppression after transplant. The majority of cases are associated with Epstein-Barr virus (EBV), while other causes are endogenous anti-T cell cytokine and anti-T cell antibodies, or production of interleukin-10. Some of the B cell mutations can result in lymphoma.

prodrug inactive drug form that becomes pharmacologically active through biotransformation.

protein binding reversible interaction between protein and drug resulting in a drug-protein complex (bound drug) which is in equilibrium with free (active) drug in plasma and tissues. Since only free drug can diffuse to action sites, factors that influence drug-binding (e.g., displacement of bound drug by another drug, or decreased albumin concentration) may potentiate pharmacologic effect.

pseudomembranous enterocolitis life-threatening superinfection characterized by severe diarrhea and fever.

pseudoparkinsonism extrapyramidal symptom manifested by slowing of volitional movement (akinesia), mask facies, rigidity and tremor at rest (especially of upper extremities); and pill rolling motion.

pulmonary edema excessive fluid in the lung tissue manifested by one or more of the following: shortness of breath, cyanosis, persistent productive cough (frothy sputum may be blood tinged), expiratory rales, restlessness, anxiety, increased heart rate, sense of chest pressure.

QT prolongation longer than normal time interval from the Q wave (QRS complex) to the end of the T wave; may be congenital or drug-induced.

renal insufficiency reduced capacity of the kidney to perform its functions as manifested by one or more of the following: dysuria, oliguria, hematuria, swelling of lower legs and feet.

serotonin syndrome may include several of the following: Confusion, agitation or restlessness, dilated pupils, headache, status changes, nausea and/or vomiting, diarrhea, rapid heart rate, tremor, loss of muscle coordination, twitching muscles, shivering, or diaphoresis.

somogyi effect rebound phenomenon clinically manifested by fasting hyperglycemia and worsening of diabetic control due to unnecessarily large p.m. insulin doses. Hormonal response to unrecognized hypoglycemia (i.e., release of epinephrine, glucagon, growth hormone, cortisol) causes insensitivity to insulin. Increasing the amount of insulin required to treat the hyperglycemia intensifies the hypoglycemia.

superinfection new infection by an organism different from the initial infection being treated by antimicrobial therapy manifested by one or more of the following: black, hairy tongue; glossitis, stomatitis; anal itching; loose, foul-smelling stools; vaginal itching or discharge; sudden fever; cough.

tachyphylaxis rapid decrease in response to a drug after administration of a few doses. Initial drug response cannot be restored by an increase in dose.

tardive dyskinesia extrapyramidal symptom manifested by involuntary rhythmic, bizarre movements of face, jaw, mouth, tongue, and sometimes extremities.

torsade de pointes a form of ventricular tachycardia nearly always due to drugs; characterized by a long QT interval.

vasovagal symptoms transient vascular and neurogenic reaction marked by pallor, nausea, vomiting, bradycardia, and rapid fall in arterial blood pressure.

water intoxication (dilutional hyponatremia) less than normal concentration of sodium in the blood resulting from excess extracellular and intracellular fluid and producing one or more of the following: lethargy, confusion, headache, decreased skin turgor, tremors, convulsions, coma, anorexia, nausea, vomiting, diarrhea, sternal fingerprinting, weight gain, edema, full bounding pulse, jugular vein distention, rales, signs and symptoms of pulmonary edema.

◆ APPENDIX F ABBREVIATIONS

ABGs	arterial blood gases
ABW	adjusted body weight
a.c.	before meals (*ante cibum*)
ACD	acid-citrate-dextrose
ACE	angiotensin-converting enzyme
ACh	acetylcholine
ACIP	Advisory Committee on Immunization Practices
ACLS	advanced cardiac life support
ACS	acute coronary syndrome
ACT	activated clotting time
ACTH	adrenocorticotropic hormone
AD	Alzheimer's disease
ADCC	antibody-dependent cell-mediated cytotoxicity
ADD	attention deficit disorder
ADH	antidiuretic hormone
ADLs	activities of daily living
ad lib	as desired (*ad libitum*)
ADP	adenosine diphosphate
ADT	alternate-day drug (administration)
AED	antiepileptic drug
AF	atrial fibrillation
AFL	atrial flutter
AIDS	acquired immunodeficiency syndrome
AIP	acute intermittent porphyria
alpha1-PI	alpha1-proteinase inhibitor
ALS	amyotrophic lateral sclerosis
ALT	alanine aminotransferase (formerly SGPT)
AMI	acute myocardial infarction
AML	acute myelogenous leukemia
AMP	adenosine monophosphate
ANA	antinuclear antibody(ies)
ANC	absolute neutrophil count
ANG I	angiotensin I
ANG II	angiotensin II
ANH	atrial natriuretic hormone
ANLL	acute nonlymphocytic leukemia
AntiXa	antifactor Xa
APL	acute promyelotic leukemia
aPTT	activated partial thromboplastin time
ARC	AIDS-related complex
ARDS	adult respiratory distress syndrome
ASHD	arteriosclerotic heart disease
AST	aspartate aminotransferase (formerly SGOT)
ATIII	antithrombin III
AT_1	angiotensin II receptor subtype I
AT_2	angiotensin II receptor subtype II

ATP	adenosine triphosphate
AUV	area under the curve
AV	atrioventricular
b.i.d.	two times a day
BMD	bone mineral density
BMI	body mass index
BMR	basal metabolic rate
BP	blood pressure
BPH	benign prostatic hypertrophy
bpm	beats per minute
BSA	body surface area
BSE	breast self-exam
BSP	bromsulphalein
BT	bleeding time
BUN	blood urea nitrogen
C	centigrade, Celsius
CAD	coronary artery disease
cAMP	cyclic adenosine monophosphate
CBC	complete blood count
CCR5	cellular chemokine coreceptor-5
CD	Crohn's disease
CDAD	clostridium difficile-associated diarrhea
CDC	Centers for Disease Control and Prevention
CDC	complement-dependent cytotoxicity
CF	cystic fibrosis
cGMP	cyclic guanosine monophosphate
CHC	chronic hepatitis C
CHF	congestive heart failure
CKD	chronic kidney disease
CLL	chronic lymphocytic leukemia
cm	centimeter
CML	chronic myeloid leukemia
CMV	cytomegalovirus-I
CNS	central nervous system
Coll	collyrium (eye wash)
COMT	catecholamine-O-methyl transferase
COPD	chronic obstructive pulmonary disease
COX-1	cyclooxygenase-1
COX-2	cyclooxygenase-2
COVID 19	Coronovirus Disease
CPK	creatinine phosphokinase
CPR	cardiopulmonary resuscitation
CRC	colorectal cancer
CrCl	creatinine clearance
CRF	chronic renal failure
CRFD	chronic renal failure disease
C&S	culture and sensitivity
CSF	cerebrospinal fluid

CSP	cellulose sodium phosphate
CSSSI	complicated skin and skin structure infections
CT	clotting time
CTZ	chemoreceptor trigger zone
CV	cardiovascular
CVA	cerebrovascular accident
CVP	central venous pressure
CYP	cytochrome P450 system of enzymes
CYP3A4	cytochrome 3A4
D5W	5% dextrose in water
D&C	dilation and curettage
DIC	disseminated intravascular coagulation
DKA	diabetic ketoacidosis
dL	deciliter (100 mL or 0.1 liter)
DM	diabetes mellitus
DMARD	disease-modifying antirheumatic drug
DNA	deoxyribonucleic acid
DPD	dihydropyrimidine dehydrogenase
DTC	differentiated thyroid cancer
DTRs	deep tendon reflexes
DVT	deep venous thrombosis
ECG, EKG	electrocardiogram
ECT	electroconvulsive therapy
EEG	electroencephalogram
EENT	eye, ear, nose, throat
e.g.	for example (*exempli gratia*)
EGFR	epidermal growth factor receptor
eGFR	estimated glomerular filtration rate
EIB	exercise-induced bronchoconstriction
ENT	ear, nose, throat
EPS	extrapyramidal symptoms (or syndrome)
ER	estrogen receptor
ESRF	end-stage renal failure
F	Fahrenheit
FBS	fasting blood sugar
FDA	Food and Drug Administration
FSH	follicle-stimulating hormone
FTI	free thyroxine index
5-FU	5-fluorouracil
FUO	fever of unknown origin
g	gram
G6PD	glucose-6-phosphate dehydrogenase
GABA	gamma-aminobutyric acid
GERD	gastroesophageal reflux disease
GFR	glomerular filtration rate
GGT	gamma-glutamyl transferase
GGTP	gamma-glutamyl transpeptidase
GH	growth hormone

GI	gastrointestinal
GIST	gastrointestinal stomal tumor
GLP-1	glucagon-like peptide-1
GM-CSF	granulocyte-macrophage colony-stimulating factor
GnRH	gonadotropic releasing hormone
GPIIb/IIIa	glycoprotein IIb/IIIa
GTT	glucose tolerance test
GU	genitourinary
GVHD	graft-versus-host disease
h	hour
HACA	human antichimeric antibody
HbA1C	glycosylated hemoglobin
hBNP	human B-type natriuretic peptide
HBV	viral hepatitis B
HCG	human chorionic gonadotropin
Hct	hematocrit
HCV	hepatitis C virus
HDD-CKD	hemodialysis-dependent chronic kidney disease
HDL-C	high-density-lipoprotein cholesterol
HER	human epidermal growth factor
HF	heart failure
Hgb	hemoglobin
5-HIAA	5-hydroxyindoleacetic acid
HIT	heparin-induced thrombocytopenia
HIV	human immunodeficiency virus
HMG-CoA	3-hydroxy-3-methyl-glutaryl coenzyme A
HPA	hypothalamic–pituitary–adrenocortical (axis)
HPV	human papillomavirus
HR	heart rate
HSV-1	herpes simplex virus type 1
HSV-2	herpes simplex virus type 2
5-HT	5-hydroxytryptamine (serotonin receptor)
IBD	inflammatory bowel disease
IBW	ideal body weight
IC	intracoronary
ICH	intracranial hemorrhage
ICP	intracranial pressure
ICU	intensive care unit
ID	intradermal
IFN	interferon
Ig	immunoglobulin
IGF-1	insulin-like growth factor 1
IL	interleukin
IM	intramuscular
INR	international normalized ratio
IOP	intraocular pressure
IPPB	intermittent positive pressure breathing
iPTH	idiopathic parathyroid hormone

IT	intrathecal
ITP	idiopathic thrombocytopenic purpura
IV	intravenous
JRA	juvenile rheumatoid arthritis
kg	kilogram
KGF	keratinocyte growth factor
17-KGS	17-ketogenic steroids
17-KS	17-ketosteroids
KVO	keep vein open
L	liter
LABA	long-acting beta-2 agonist
LDH	lactic dehydrogenase
LDL	low density lipoprotein
LDL-C	low-density-lipoprotein cholesterol
LE	lupus erythematosus
LFT	liver function test
LH	luteinizing hormone
LLN	lower limit of normal
LR	lactated Ringer's
LSD	lysergic acid diethylamide
LTRA	leukotriene receptor antagonist
LVEDP	left ventricular end diastolic pressure
LVEF	left ventricular ejection fraction
M	molar (strength of a solution)
m^2	square meter (of body surface area)
MAC	mycobacterium avium complex
MAO	monoamine oxidase
MAOI	monoamine oxidase inhibitor
MBD	minimal brain dysfunction
MCH	mean corpuscular hemoglobin
MCHC	mean corpuscular hemoglobin concentration
mCi	millicurie
MCL	mantle cell lymphoma
mcg	microgram (1/1000 of a milligram)
MDD	major depressive disorder
MDI	metered dose inhaler
MDR	minimum daily requirements
MDS	muscular dystrophy syndrome
mEq	milliequivalent
mg	milligram
MI	myocardial infarction
MIC	minimum inhibitory concentration
min	minute
mL	milliliter (0.001 liter)
mm	millimeter
mo	month
MPS I	mucopolysaccharidosis I
MRSA	methicillin-resistant *Staphylococcus aureus*
MS	multiple sclerosis

MTC	medullary thyroid cancer
mTOR	mammalian target or rapamycin
mu-m	micrometer
N	normal (strength of a solution)
NADH	reduced form of nicotine adenine dinucleotide
NAPA	*N*-acetyl procainamide
nb	note well (*nota bene*)
NDD	non-hemodialysis dependent
NDD-CKD	non-hemodialysis-dependent chronic kidney disease
ng	nanogram (1/1000 of a microgram)
NMDA	N-methyl-D-aspartic acid
NMS	neuroleptic malignant syndrome
NNRTI	nonnucleoside reverse transcriptase inhibitor
NON-PVC	nonpolyvinyl chloride IV bag or tubing
NPN	nonprotein nitrogen
NPO	nothing by mouth
NRTI	nucleoside reverse transcriptase inhibitor
NS	normal saline
NS 3/4A	nonstructural protein (NS) 3/4A protease inhibitor
NSAID	nonsteroidal anti-inflammatory drug
NSCLC	non-small-cell lung cancer
NSR	normal sinus rhythm
NVAF	non-valvular atrial fibrillation
NYHA Class I, II, III, IV	New York Heart Association classes of heart failure
OA	osteoarthritis
OAB	overactive bladder
OATP	organic anion transporting polypeptide
OC	oral contraceptive
OCD	obsessive compulsive disorder
ODT	oral disintegrating tablet
17-OHCS	17-hydroxycorticosteroids
OTC	over the counter (nonprescription)
P450	cytochrome P450 system of enzymes
PABA	*para*-aminobenzoic acid
PAR-1	protease-activated receptor-1
PAS	*para*-aminosalicylic acid
PAWP	pulmonary artery wedge pressure
PBI	protein-bound iodine
PBP	penicillin-binding protein
p.c.	after meals (*post cibum*)
PCI	percutaneous coronary intervention
PCP	*Pneumocystis carinii* pneumonia
PCWP	pulmonary capillary wedge pressure
PD-1	programmed cell death receptors
PDD	peritoneal dialysis dependent
PDD-CKD	peritoneal dialysis-dependent chronic kidney disease

PDE	phosphodiesterase
PDE5	phosphodiesterase type-5
PE	pulmonary embolism
PERRLA	pupils equal, round, react to light and accommodation
P-gp	P-glycoprotein transporter
PG	prostaglandin
PGE_2	prostaglandin E_2
pH	hydrogen ion concentration
Ph	Philadelphia (chromosome)
PI	protease inhibitor
PID	pelvic inflammatory disease
PJP	*Pneumocystis jirovecii* pneumonia
PKU	phenylketonuria
PMDD	premenstrual dysphoric disorder
PML	progressive multifocal leukoencephalopathy
PND	paroxysmal nocturnal dyspnea
PNE	primary nocturnal enuresis
PO	by mouth or orally (*per os*)
PPES	Plantar Palmar Erythrodysesthesia
PPI	proton pump inhibitor
PPM	parts per million
PR	rectally (*per rectum*)
PRES	posterior reversible encephalopathy syndrome
prn	when required (*pro re nata*)
PSA	prostate-specific antigen
PSP	phenolsulfonphthalein
PSVT	paroxysmal supraventricular tachycardia
PT	prothrombin time
PTCL	peripheral T-cell lymphocyte
PTH	parathyroid hormone
PTLD	post-transplant lymphoproliferative disorder
PTSD	post-traumatic stress disorder
PTT	partial thromboplastin time
PUD	peptic ulcer disease
PVC	polyvinyl chloride IV bag or tubing
PVC	premature ventricular contraction
PVD	peripheral vascular disease
PZI	protamine zinc insulin
q.i.d.	four times daily
RA	rheumatoid arthritis
RAAS	renin angiotensin aldosterone system
RAI	radioactive iodine
RAR	retinoic acid receptor
RAST	radioallergosorbent test
RBC	red blood (cell) count
RDA	recommended (daily) dietary allowance
RDS	respiratory distress syndrome
REM	rapid eye movement

rem	radiation equivalent man
RES	reticuloendothelial system
RIA	radioimmunoassay
RNA	ribonucleic acid
ROM	range of motion
RSV	respiratory syncytial virus
RT	reverse transcriptase
RTK	receptor tyrosine kinase
RT_3U	total serum thyroxine concentration
S&S	signs and symptoms
SA	sinoatrial
SARA	selective aldosterone receptor antagonist
SBE	subacute bacterial endocarditis
SC	subcutaneous
S_{cr}	serum creatinine
SE	systemic embolism
sec	second
SERMs	selective estrogen receptor modulators
SGGT	serum gamma-glutamyl transferase
SGLT2	sodium-glucose cotransporter 2 in proximal tubule of kidney
SGOT	serum glutamic–oxaloacetic transaminase (*see* AST)
SGPT	serum glutamic–pyruvic transaminase (*see* ALT)
SIADH	syndrome of inappropriate antidiuretic hormone
SI Units	International System of Units
SK	streptokinase
SL	sublingual
SLE	systemic lupus erythematosus
SLL	small lymphocytic lymphoma
SMA	sequential multiple analysis
SMZ/TMP	sulfamethoxazole/trimethoprim
SNRI	serotonin norepinephrine reuptake inhibitor
SOS	if necessary (*si opus cit*)
sp	species
SPF	sun protection factor
sq	square
SR	sedimentation rate
SRS-A	slow-reactive substance of anaphylaxis
SSRI	selective serotonin reuptake inhibitor
stat	immediately
STD	sexually transmitted disease
STEMI	ST elevated MI
SVT	supraventricular tachyarrhythmias
SW	sterile water
$t_{1/2}$	half-life
T_3	triiodothyronine
T_4	thyroxine
TCA	tricyclic antidepressant

TG total triglycerides
TIA transient ischemic attack
t.i.d. three times a day (*ter in die*)
TKI tyrosine kinase inhibitor
TNF tumor necrosis factor
tPA tissue plasminogen activator
TPN total parenteral nutrition
TPR temperature, pulse, respirations
TSH thyroid-stimulating hormone
TSS toxic shock syndrome
TT thrombin time
TTP thrombotic cyclopenic purpura
UA urinary analysis
UC ulcerative colitis
ULN upper limit of normal
URI upper respiratory infection
USP United States Pharmacopeia
USPHS United States Public Health Service
UTI urinary tract infection
UV-A, UVA ultraviolet A wave
VDRL Venereal Disease Research Laboratory
VEGF vascular endothelial growth factor
VEGFR2 vascular endothelial growth factor receptor 2
VLDL very low density lipoprotein
VMA vanillylmandelic acid
VREF vancomycin-resistant *Enterococcus faecium*
VRSA vancomycin-resistant *Staphylococcus aureus*
VS vital signs
wk week
WBC white blood (cell) count
WBCT whole blood clotting time
y year

◆ APPENDIX G HERBAL AND DIETARY SUPPLEMENT TABLE

As patient interest in dietary supplements and other natural products increases, there is an increased need for information on this topic. These products are not standardized or stringently regulated by FDA guidelines; therefore, caution should be used when discussing these products. Consumers should note that since rigid quality control standards are not required for these products, substantial variability can occur in both potency and purity of a given product, especially between different commercial companies.

Many of these products have limited research on safety; thus, side effects and potential drug interactions are not well understood. Dietary supplements may either increase or decrease the level of a drug in the patient's body.

This table provides basic information on some of the most commonly sold dietary supplements. For additional information, a specialty resource on herbal and/or dietary supplements should be consulted.

Name	Common Use	Significant Safety Concerns
Bilberry	Eye health	Long-term, high-dose use can cause liver problems
Black cohosh	Menopausal symptoms	Should be avoided in pregnant patients
Cranberry	Urinary tract infections	Considered safe at usual doses; high dose may increase bleeding risk
Echinacea	Infections	May cause allergic reactions; should be used only short-term
Eleuthera (Siberian ginseng)	Energy	Avoid use with digoxin
Evening primrose	Menopausal symptoms	May affect seizure threshold
Garcinia cambogia	Weight loss	Mild GI side effects
Flax	Cholesterol	Minor GI side effects
Garlic	Cholesterol	Significant drug interactions with drugs metabolized by CYP system
Ginger	Nausea	Overdoses may cause cardiac arrhythmias

Name	Common Use	Significant Safety Concerns
Ginkgo	Memory enhancement	Potential increased bleeding risk
Ginseng (American ginseng)	Energy	Should not be used with MAO inhibitors; may affect anticoagulants
Glucosamine	Osteoarthritis	Considered safe at usual doses; at higher doses, possible interaction with warfarin and other coumarin anticoagulants
Green tea	Energy, weight loss	High doses may cause cardiovascular side effects
Horny goat weed	Sexual function	Should be avoided in pregnant/lactating women
Horse chestnut	Congestive heart failure	Potential hepatotoxicity
Kratom	Reduce fatigue	Risk of addiction/abuse/dependence, reports of fatal drug interactions with CNS Depressants
Milk thistle	Liver function	May affect CYP metabolism and interact with drugs metabolized by this system
Saw palmetto	Benign prostatic hyperplasia	Adverse effects appear mild
Soy	Menopausal symptoms	GI-related side effects may be significant for some patients
St. John's wort	Depression	Significant drug interactions with several drugs metabolized by CYP system
Turmeric	Arthritis, inflammatory conditions	May reduce blood glucose levels and have additive effect with other ANTIDIABETEIC AGENTS
Valerian	Sleep disorder	Potentially hepatotoxic
Yohimbe	Sexual function	Do not use with drugs affecting serotonin system

◆ APPENDIX H VACCINES

The Centers for Disease Control and Prevention (CDC) contains detailed listings of what vaccinations are recommended for various age groups as well as patients with multiple concurrent disease states. The full recommendations are available at: www.cdc.gov/vaccines/.

COVID-19 Vaccination: The Advisory Committee on Immunization Practices (ACIP) currently recommends COVID-19 vaccines for everyone ages 5 yr and older within the scope of the Emergency Use Authorization or Biologics License Application for the particular vaccine. COVID-19 vaccines can be administered on the same day as other vaccines. The CDC has expanded recommendations for booster shots to now include all adults 18 yr and older who received a Pfizer-BioNTech, Moderna, or Johnson and Johnson (mRNA) COVID-19 vaccine as part of the series. Please review the most up to date information regarding COVID-19 vaccines at **www.cdc.gov/vaccines/covid-19/info-by-product/index.html**

Dosing information is provided for some common vaccines. There are many other vaccines and vaccine formulations. Please consult the package insert for specific details regarding each of the following:

BCG (BACILLUS CALMETTE-GUERIN) VACCINE

Tice, TheraCys

USES To protect groups with excessive rates of TB infection.

Adult/Adolescent/Child (1 mo or older): **Percutaneous** 0.2–0.3 mL of a 50 mg/mL vaccine **Intradermal** 0.1 mL. If tuberculin test is negative post-vaccination and indications for immunization remain, administer full vaccine dose after 2 to 3 months.
Child (younger than 1 mo): **Percutaneous** 0.2 to 0.3 mL of 25 mg/mL solution for 1 dose. If tuberculin test is negative post-vaccination and indications for immunization remain, administer full vaccine dose when older than 1 year.
Children (1 month to 1 year): 0.2 to 0.3 mL of a 50 mg/mL solution for 1 dose. If tuberculin test is negative post-vaccination and indications for immunization remain, administer full vaccine dose when older than 1 year.

CONTRAINDICATIONS Hypersensitivity to any vaccine component; active or past mycobacterial infection; congenital or acquired immunosuppression whether due to disease or cancer therapy or immunosuppressive therapy. Concurrent febrile illness, UTI or gross hematuria, immunosuppressed patients, biopsy, transurethral resection or traumatic catheterization, active tuberculosis.

DIPHTHERIA TOXOID/TETANUS TOXOID/ACELLULAR PERTUSSIS VACCINE, ADSORBED (DTaP/Tdap)

Adacel, Boostrix, Daptacel, Infanrix

USES Prevention of tetanus, diphtheria, and pertussis.

Adult/Adolescent/Child (2 months old or older): **IM** 0.5 mL

CONTRAINDICATIONS Severe allergic reaction to any component of the formulation; encephalopathy within 7 days of a previous dose of pertussis antigen; progressive neurologic disorder.

HAEMOPHILUS B CONJUGATE VACCINE (HIB)

ActHIB, Hiberix, Liquid PedvaxHIB

USES To provide active immunity to H. influenzae type b (Hib) infection.

Infant: **IM** 0.5 mL at 2, 4, and 6 mo and a booster at 15 through 18 months. (ActHIB)
Infant/Child: **IM** 0.5 mL at 2 and 4 mo and again at 11 to 14 mo (Liquid PedvaxHIB)

Child (15–71 mo previously unvaccinated): **IM** 0.5 mL as booster (PedvaxHIB(R))

CONTRAINDICATIONS Hypersensitivity to any vaccine components; fever of unknown etiology; infants younger than 6 weeks.

HEPATITIS A VACCINE

Havrix, Vaqta

USES To provide active immunity to hepatitis A.

Adult: **IM** 1 mL dose then 1 mL 6–18 mo later
Child (1–18 y): **IM** 1 mL then 1 mL booster dose 6–12 mo later

CONTRAINDICATIONS Hypersensitivity to any vaccine component; neomycin hypersensitivity.

HEPATITIS B IMMUNE GLOBULIN

HepaGam B, HyperHep, Nabi-HB

USES To provide passive immunity to hepatitis B infections in individuals exposed to HBV or Hbs Ag-positive materials; to prevent hepatitis B recurrence in post-liver transplant (HepaGam B).

Adult/Child: **IM** 0.06 mL/kg as soon as possible (preferably within 7 days) post-exposure, then repeat 28–30 day post-exposure
Neonate: **IM** 0.5 mL within 12 h of birth, follow up with hepatitis B vaccine.
Adult: **HepaGam B IV** 20,000 U/dose daily every 2 wk (2–12 wk) then monthly (liver transplant)

CONTRAINDICATIONS Hypersensitivity to parenteral human globulin, IgA deficiency.

HEPATITIS B VACCINE (RECOMBINANT)

Engerix-B, Recombivax HB, Heplisav-B

USES To provide active immunity to individuals at high risk for exposure.

Adult (older than 20 yr): Engerix-B: 20 mcg/1 mL IM as a 3-dose series: 0, 1, and 6 months. *Recombivax HB*: 10 mcg/mL 1 dose (1 mL) IM as a 3-dose series given on a 0, 1, and 6-month schedule. *Heplisav-B (only for 18 yr or older):* 0.5 mL IM at 0 and 1 month.
Adult (younger than 20 yr)/Adolescent/Child/Infant: Engerix-B: **IM** 10 mcg/0.5mL within 24 hours of birth and at 1 month, and 6 months; for older children that

did not start the series at birth: 0, 1, 6 months. *Recombivax HB:* 5mcg/0.5 mL 1 dose (0.5 1 mL) **IM** as 3-dose series given within 24 hours of birth, 1 month, 6 months. For older children that did not start the series at birth: 0, 1, and 6 months. For teens age 11–15 years, 1.0 mL at 0 and 4–6 months.

CONTRAINDICATIONS Hypersensitivity to any vaccine component; yeast hypersensitivity.

HUMAN PAPILLOMAVIRUS BIVALENT (RECOMBINANT)

Cervarix for females only

USES To prevent disease associated with HPV exposure.

Adult/Adolescent/Child (9 y or older): **IM** 0.5 mL dose at 0 (before the 15 yr birthday), 1–2.5, and 5–12 months. If an adolescent receives two doses less than 5 months apart, a third dose of HPV vaccine will be required. For teens and adults ages 15 through 26 years old, 3-dose schedule at 0, 2, and 6 months is recommended. For immunocompromised individuals (including those with HIV), the 3-dose schedule is recommended for ages 9 through 26 years of age.

CONTRAINDICATIONS Hypersensitivity to any vaccine component; yeast hypersensitivity, pregnancy, moderate or severe acute illness.

HUMAN PAPILLOMAVIRUS QUADRIVALENT VACCINE (RECOMBINANT)

Gardasil females, transgender persons and males

USES To prevent HPV-related disease; to prevent genital warts; to prevent anal cancer.

Adult/Child (11 y or older): **IM** 0.5 mL followed by doses at 2 and 6 months.

CONTRAINDICATIONS Hypersensitivity to any vaccine component; yeast hypersensitivity; monitor for 15 minutes after vaccine because episodes of syncope have been reported that could result in fall and injury.

HUMAN PAPILLOMAVIRUS 9-VALENT VACCINE

Gardasil 9 females and males

USES To prevent HPV-related disease; to prevent genital warts; to prevent anal cancer.

Adult/Child (9–26 y): **IM** 0.5 mL for first dose and followed by doses at 2 and 6 months: make sure there is at least 4 weeks between the first and second interval, a 12-week interval between the second and third interval, and a 5-month minimum interval between the first and third dose.

CONTRAINDICATIONS Hypersensitivity to any vaccine component; yeast hypersensitivity; previous use of other brand of HPV vaccine, monitor for 15 minutes after vaccine because episodes of syncope have been reported that could result in fall and injury.

INFLUENZA VACCINE

Afluria Quadrivalent, FLUAD, Fluarix, Flublok, FluLaval, Fluzone, Flumist, FluMist Quadrivalent

USES To prevent influenza.

Adult & child (2–49 y): **Intranasal** *Flumist* 0.2 mL dose (0.1 per nostril); Afluria, *Fluarix Quadravalent, FluLaval Quadravalent* **IM** 0.5 mL; *Geriatric: FLUAD* formulation **IM** 0.5mL
Child (> 3 y): Afluria **IM** 0.5 mL
Infant/Child (6–35 mo): Fluzone Quadrivalent **IM** 0.25 mL dose.

CONTRAINDICATIONS Hypersensitivity to egg, kanamycin, neomycin, or polymyxin concomitant aspirin or salicylate-containing therapy in children and adolescents: children age 2y–4y with diagnosis of asthma; children and adults who are immunocompromised; close contact with those who are severely immunocompromised; pregnancy-live vaccine, receipt of influenza antiviral medication within the past 48 hours.

MENINGOCOCCAL DIPHTHERIA TOXOID CONJUGATE

Menveo, Menactra

USES To provide prophylaxis against meningococcal infection.

Adult (younger than 55 y)/Adolescent/Child (2 y or older): **IM** 0.5 mL injection
Infant/Child (9 mo to 2 years): Menactra only: 0.5 mL injection (2 dose series); *Menveo (2 months to less than 3 months) IM 0.5 mL/dose given as a 4-dose series at 2,4,6, and 12 months of age.*

CONTRAINDICATIONS Hypersensitivity to any vaccine component; history of Guillain-Barré syndrome, latex hypersensitivity, moderate to severe illness.

MEASLES, MUMPS AND RUBELLA VIRUS VACCINE

M-M-R II

USES Vaccination against measles, mumps, and rubella.

Child (over 12 mo): **Subcutaneous** 0.5 mL at ages 12–15 mo; second dose at ages 4–6 y

CONTRAINDICATIONS Hypersensitivity to any component of the vaccine, including gelatin. Do not administer to patients who are pregnant, receiving immunosuppressive therapy, currently ill with febrile illness.

MENINGOCOCCAL GROUP B VACCINE

Bexsero, Trumenba

USES To provide prophylaxis against meningococcal infection.

Adult/Adolescent/Child (ages 10–25 y): **IM** 0.5 mL/dose as part of a 2 or 3 dose series

CONTRAINDICATIONS Hypersensitivity to the meningococcal group B vaccine or any component of the formulation.

PNEUMOCOCCAL 13-VALENT VACCINE, DIPHTHERIA

Prevnar 13

USES To provide routine prophylaxis for infants and children as part of the primary childhood immunization schedule.

Adult (19 to 64 y): **IM** 0.5 mL as a single dose

Geriatric (≥65 y): Only in special circumstances; not routine. **IM** 0.5 mL as a single dose.

Child/Adolescent (6–17 y): **IM** 0.5 mL as single dose
Infant and children (6 wk–15 mo): **IM** 0.5 mL dose initiated between 6 and 8 wk, then repeated at 4 mo, 6 mo, 12 mo, 15 mo (total of 4 doses); see CDC guidelines for catch-up schedule if infant did not receive this recommended schedule.

CONTRAINDICATIONS Hypersensitivity to any vaccine component.

PNEUMOCOCCAL POLYSACCHARIDE VACCINE, 23-VALENT
Pneumovax 23

USES Pneumococcal disease prevention

Adult/Adolescent/Child (2 y or older): **Subcutaneous/IM** 0.5 mL; revaccination may be necessary in some patients with concurrent immunocompromised disease states.

CONTRAINDICATIONS Severe allergic reaction to pneumococcal vaccine or any component of the formulation.

RABIES VACCINE
RabAvert, Imovax

USES Pre-exposure rabies prophylaxis

Adult/Adolescent/Children/Infant: **IM** Series of 3 injections 1 mL on days 0, 7, 21, or 28

CONTRAINDICATIONS Anaphylaxis to vaccine or vaccine component.

ROTAVIRUS VACCINE
Rotarix, RotaTeq

USES To prevent gastroenteritis caused by rotavirus infection.

Infant (6–32 wk) (RotaTeq only): **PO** 2 mL at 6–12 wk, followed by 2 other doses given at 4–10 wk intervals and to be completed by 32 wk.

Infant (6–24 wk) (Rotarix only): **PO** 1 mL at 6 wk; then second dose to follow at least 4 wk later and completed by 24 wk.

CONTRAINDICATIONS Hypersensitivity to any vaccine component, history of intussusception, or severe combined immunodeficiency; history of uncorrected congenital malformation of the GI tract that would predispose to risk of intussusception.

VARICELLA VACCINE
Varivax

USES To provide vaccination against varicella.

Adult/Adolescent: **Subcutaneous** 0.5 mL followed by a second dose 4–8 wk later
Child (1–12 y): **Subcutaneous** 0.5 mL and allow at least 3 months to elapse before a second 0.5 mL dose is given.

CONTRAINDICATIONS Hypersensitivity to any vaccine component; febrile illness; untreated tuberculosis; AIDS; bone marrow suppression; concurrent chemotherapy or corticosteroid therapy; gelatin hypersensitivity; hypogammaglobulinemia; current leukemia or lymphoma; neomycin hypersensitivity; pregnancy (avoid pregnancy for 3 months following vaccination); tuberculosis; concurrent radiation therapy.

ZOSTER VACCINE INACTIVATED
Shingrix

USES To prevent herpes zoster in people over 18 y old.

Adult (50 y or older): **IM** Administer 0.5 mL as a 2-dose series administered at 0 and 1–2 months 4 weeks later.

Adult (18 y to 49 y): **IM** 0.5 mL administered as a 2-dose series at 0 and 1–2 months.

CONTRAINDICATIONS Hypersensitivity to any vaccine component; person known to be seronegative for varicella; person experiencing an acute episode of herpes zoster, pregnant and lactating women; adults with moderate to severe acute illness.

BIBLIOGRAPHY

American Hospital Formulary Service (AHFS) Drug Information. 2021. Bethesda, MD: American Society of Health-System Pharmacists.

Food and Drug Administration. http://www.fda.gov. 2021.

Lexi-Drugs. Lexicomp [Online database]. Hudson, OH: Wolters Kluwer Health, Inc.; 2021. http://online.lexi.com/.

Micromedex [Online database]. Greenwood Village, CO: Truven Health Analytics; 2021. http://www.micromedexsolutions.com/

National Institute of Health. *Daily Med*. http://daily med.nlm.gov. 2021.

Trissel's 2 Clinical Pharmaceutics [Online database]. Hudson, OH: Wolters Kluwer 2021. https://online.lexi.com/lco/action/ivcompatibility/trissels

INDEX

Drug categories are in SMALL CAPS. Prototypes are in **bold.**
Generic drug names are given in parentheses.

Drug categories are in SMALL CAPS. Prototypes are in **bold.**
Generic drug names are given in parentheses.

Drug categories are in SMALL CAPS. Prototypes are in **bold.**
Generic drug names are given in parentheses.

Drug categories are in SMALL CAPS. Prototypes are in **bold.**
Generic drug names are given in parentheses.

Drug categories are in SMALL CAPS. Prototypes are in **bold.**
Generic drug names are given in parentheses.

Drug categories are in SMALL CAPS. Prototypes are in **bold.**
Generic drug names are given in parentheses.

B

Drug categories are in SMALL CAPS. Prototypes are in **bold.**
Generic drug names are given in parentheses.

Drug categories are in SMALL CAPS. Prototypes are in **bold.**
Generic drug names are given in parentheses.

C

Drug categories are in SMALL CAPS. Prototypes are in **bold.**
Generic drug names are given in parentheses.

Drug categories are in SMALL CAPS. Prototypes are in **bold.**
Generic drug names are given in parentheses.

D

Drug categories are in SMALL CAPS. Prototypes are in **bold.**
Generic drug names are given in parentheses.

Drug categories are in SMALL CAPS. Prototypes are in **bold.**
Generic drug names are given in parentheses.

Drug categories are in SMALL CAPS. Prototypes are in **bold.**
Generic drug names are given in parentheses.

G

Drug categories are in SMALL CAPS. Prototypes are in **bold.**
Generic drug names are given in parentheses.

I

Drug categories are in SMALL CAPS. Prototypes are in **bold.**
Generic drug names are given in parentheses.

L

Drug categories are in SMALL CAPS. Prototypes are in **bold.**
Generic drug names are given in parentheses.

Drug categories are in SMALL CAPS. Prototypes are in **bold.**
Generic drug names are given in parentheses.

N

Drug categories are in SMALL CAPS. Prototypes are in **bold.**
Generic drug names are given in parentheses.

O

Drug categories are in SMALL CAPS. Prototypes are in **bold.**
Generic drug names are given in parentheses.

P

Drug categories are in SMALL CAPS. Prototypes are in **bold.**
Generic drug names are given in parentheses.

Drug categories are in SMALL CAPS. Prototypes are in **bold.**
Generic drug names are given in parentheses.

Drug categories are in SMALL CAPS. Prototypes are in **bold.**
Generic drug names are given in parentheses.

Drug categories are in SMALL CAPS. Prototypes are in **bold.**
Generic drug names are given in parentheses.

Drug categories are in SMALL CAPS. Prototypes are in **bold.**
Generic drug names are given in parentheses.

Drug categories are in SMALL CAPS. Prototypes are in **bold.**
Generic drug names are given in parentheses.

U

Drug categories are in SMALL CAPS. Prototypes are in **bold.**
Generic drug names are given in parentheses.

W

Drug categories are in SMALL CAPS. Prototypes are in **bold.**
Generic drug names are given in parentheses.

	AMINOPHYLLINE	DOBUTAMINE	DOPAMINE	HEPARIN	MEPERIDINE	MORPHINE	NITROGLYCERIN	ONDANSETRON	POTASSIUM CL
acyclovir	C	I	I	C	I/C	I/C	C	I	C
alteplase		I	I	I			I		
amikacin	C	C	C	I/C	C	C	C	C	C
amino acids (TPN)	I/C	C	I/C	I/C	C	C	C	I/C	C
aminophylline	C	I	C	C	C	C	C	I	C
amiodarone	I	I/C	C	I	C	C	C	C	I/C
ampicillin	I	I	I/C	I/C	I/C	I/C	I/C	I	I/C
ampicillin/sulbactam	I/C	I	I/C	I/C	I/C	I/C	I/C	I	I/C
aztreonam	C	C	C	C	C	C	C	C	C
bretylium	C	C	C	C	C	C	C	C	C
bumetanide	C	C	C	C	C	C	C	C	C
calcium chloride	C	C	C	C	C	C	C	C	C
cefazolin	C	I	I	C	C	C	C	C	C
cefotaxime	C	I	C	C	C	C	C	C	C
cefotetan	C	I	C	C	I/C	C	C	I/C	C
cefoxitin	C	I	C	C	C	C	C	C	C
ceftazidime	C	I/C	C	C	C	C	C	I/C	C
ceftizoxime	C	C	C	C	C	C	C	C	C
ceftriaxone	C	I	C	C	C	C	C	I/C	C
cefuroxime	C	I	C	C	C	C	C	C	C
chloramphenicol	C	I	I	C	I/C	C	C	I	C
cimetidine	C	C	C	C	C	C	C	C	C
ciprofloxacin	I	C	C	I	C	C		C	C
clindamycin	C	C	C	C	C	C	C	C	C
dexamethasone	C	I	C	C	I/C	C	C	C	C
diazepam	I	I/C	I	I	I	I/C	I	I/C	I
digoxin	C	C	C	C	C	C	C	C	C

COMMON DRUG IV-SITE COMPATIBILITY CHART

	AMINOPHYLLINE	DOBUTAMINE	DOPAMINE	HEPARIN	MEPERIDINE	MORPHINE	NITROGLYCERIN	ONDANSETRON	POTASSIUM CL
diltiazem	I/C	C	C	I/C	C	C	C	C	C
diphenhydramine	I	C	C	I/C	C	C	C	C	C
dobutamine	I	C	C	I/C	C	C	C	C	C
dopamine	C	C	C	C	C	C	C	C	C
doxycycline	C	C	C	I	C	C	C	C	C
enalaprilat	C	C	C	C	C	C	C	C	C
epinephrine	I/C	C	C	C	C	C	C	C	C
eptifibatide	C	C	C	C	C	C	C	C	C
erythromycin	C	C	C	I/C	C	C	C	C	C
esmolol	C	C	C	C	C	C	C	C	C
famotidine	C	C	C	C	C	C	C	C	C
filgrastim	C			I	C	C		C	C
fluconazole	C	C	C	C	C	C	C	C	C
foscarnet	C	I	C	C	C	C	C	I	C
furosemide	C	I/C	I/C	I/C	I/C	I/C	I/C	I	C
ganciclovir	I	I	I	C	I	I	C	I	C
gentamicin	C	C	C	I/C	C	C	C	C	C
heparin	C	I/C	C	C	I/C	C	C	C	C
hydrocortisone	C	I	C	C	I/C	C	C	C	I/C
hydromorphone	C	C	C	C		C	C	C	C
imipenem/cilastatin	I/C	I/C	C	C	I/C	C	C	C	C
inamrinone	I/C	I/C	I/C	I	I/C	I	I/C	I	C
insulin (regular)	C	I/C	I/C	I/C	C	I/C	C	I/C	C
isoproterenol	I/C	C	C	C	C	C	C	C	C
labetolol	C	C	C	I/C	C	C	C	C	C
lansoprazole	I	I	I	C	I	I	I	I	I
lidocaine	C	C	C	C	C	C	C	C	C
lorazepam	C	C	C	C	I	C	C	I	C

methylprednisolone	C	C	C	I/C	I/C	C	C	I/C	C
metoclopramide	C	C	C	C	C	C	C	C	C
metoprolol	C	C	C	C	C	C	I/C	C	C
metronidazole	C	C	C	C	C	C	C	C	C
micofungin	C	I	C	C	I	I	C	I	C
midazolam	I	I/C	C	C	C	C	C	C	I
milrinone	C	C	C	C	C	C	C	I	C
morphine	C	C	C	C	C	C	C	C	C
nafcillin	C	C	C	C	I	C	C	C	I/C
nitroglycerin	C	C	C	C	C	C	C	C	C
nitroprusside	C	I/C	C	C	C	C	C	C	C
norepinephrine	I/C	C	C	C	C	C	C	C	C
ondansetron	I	C	C	C	C	C	C	C	C
pantoprazole	C	I	I/C	I/C	I	I/C	I/C	I	I/C
penicillin G	I/C	I	C	C	C	C	C	C	C
phenylephrine	C	C	C	C	C	C	C	C	C
phenytoin	I	I	I	I	I	I	I	I	I
piperacillin	C	I	C	C	C	C	C	I/C	I/C
piperacillin/tazobactam	C	I	C	C	C	C	C	C	I/C
potassium Cl	C	C	C	C	C	C	C	C	C
procainamide	C	C	C	C	C	C	C	C	C
propofol	C	I/C	I/C	C	C	I/C	I/C		I/C
ranitidine	C	C	C	C	C	C	C	C	C
sargramostim	C		C	C	C	I		I	I/C
sodium bicarbonate	C	I	I	C	I	C	C	I	C
sulfamethoxazole-trimethoprim	I	I	I	I/C	I/C	I/C	I	I	C
ticarcillin/clavulanate	C	I	C	C	C	C	C	C	I/C
tobramycin	C	C	C	I/C	C	C	C	C	C
vancomycin	I	C	C	I/C	C	C	C	C	C

C = compatible; I = incompatible; I/C = conflicting data.